PATHOPHYSIOLOGY
CLINICAL CONCEPTS OF DISEASE PROCESSES

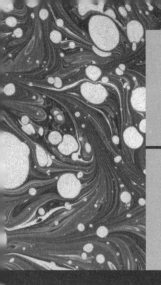
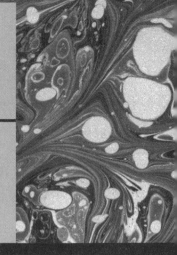

PATHOPHYSIOLOGY

CLINICAL CONCEPTS OF DISEASE PROCESSES

SYLVIA ANDERSON PRICE, RN, PhD

Professor, College of Nursing
University of Tennessee at Memphis
Memphis, Tennessee

LORRAINE McCARTY WILSON, RN, PhD

Professor and MSN Program Director
Pathophysiology Instructor
Eastern Michigan University
Ypsilanti, Michigan

FIFTH EDITION

Illustrations by

Margaret Croup Brudon

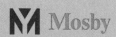 Mosby

St. Louis Baltimore Boston Carlsbad Chicago Naples New York Philadelphia Portland
London Madrid Mexico City Singapore Sydney Tokyo Toronto Wiesbaden

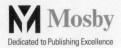

A Times Mirror
Company

Vice President and Publisher: Nancy L. Coon
Senior Editor: Sally Schrefer
Developmental Editor: Gail Brower
Associate Developmental Editor: Rae Robertson
Project Manager: Patricia Tannian
Project Specialist: Betty Hazelwood
Book Design Manager: Gail Morey Hudson
Manufacturing Supervisor: Karen Lewis
Cover Designer: Teresa Breckwoldt
Cover Art: Marbling by Gail Morey Hudson

FIFTH EDITION

Printed in the United States of America
Composition by Graphic World, Inc.
Lithography/color film by Color Dot Graphics, Inc.
Printing/binding by Von Hoffmann Press, Inc.

Mosby–Year Book, Inc.
11830 Westline Industrial Drive
St. Louis, Missouri 63146

Library of Congress Cataloging in Publication Data

Pathophysiology: clinical concepts of disease processes / [edited by]
   Sylvia Anderson Price, Lorraine McCarty Wilson; illustrations by
   Margaret Croup Brudon.—5th ed.
        p.   cm.
   Includes bibliographical references and index.
   ISBN 0-8151-6621-4
   1. Physiology, Pathological.   I. Price, Sylvia Anderson.
II. Wilson, Lorraine McCarty.
   [DNLM: 1. Pathology—nurses' instruction.   QZ 4 P302 1996]
RB113.P363   1996
616.07—dc20
DNLM/DLC
for Library of Congress   96-15023
                                                              CIP

96 97 98 99 00 / 9 8 7 6 5 4 3 2 1

This book is affectionately dedicated to our husbands
JOE and **HAROLD**
without whose help, understanding, and support
this book would not have been possible

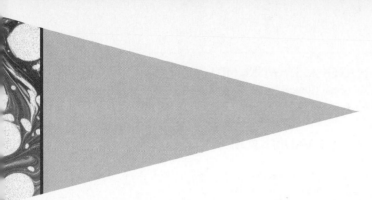

Contributors

GERALD D. ABRAMS, MD

Professor of Pathology
University of Michigan
Medical Center
Ann Arbor, Michigan

CATHERINE M. BALDY, RN, MS, OCN

Clinical Nurse Specialist in Hematology
Henry Ford Hospital
Detroit, Michigan

BETTY J. BEARD, RN, PhD

Professor, Department of Nursing
Eastern Michigan University
Ypsilanti, Michigan

MARJORIE A. BOLDT, RN, MS, JD

Former Head Nurse
Coronary Care Unit
Beth Israel Hospital
Boston, Massachusetts

MARGARET CROUP BRUDON, BS

Former President, Association of Medical Illustrators;
Staff Medical Illustrator and Assistant Professor of Medical
and Biological Illustrations
University of Michigan
Ann Arbor, Michigan

PENNY FORD CARLETON, RN, MS, MPA

Cardiovascular Clinical Nurse Specialist
Anesthesia Bioengineering Unit
Massachusetts General Hospital;
Research Associate
Harvard Medical Center
Boston, Massachusetts

MICHAEL A. CARTER, RN, DNSc

Professor and Dean
College of Nursing
University of Tennessee
Memphis, Tennessee

PATRICIA HENRY FOLCARELLI, RN, PhC, MA

Vascular Unit
Beth Israel Hospital;
Instructor in Surgery
Harvard Medical School
Boston, Massachusetts

MARY S. HARTWIG, RN, PhD

Professor and Chair
Department of Nursing
Arkansas State University
State University, Arkansas

GLENDA N. LINDSETH, RN, PhD

Associate Professor
College of Nursing
University of North Dakota
Grand Forks, North Dakota

MARY CARTER LOMBARDO, RN, MSN, CEN

Clinical Nurse Specialist, Neurology
Howard County General Hospital
Columbia, Maryland

MADELINE M. O'DONNELL, RN, MS

Cardiac Clinical Specialist
Intensive Care Nursing Service
Massachusetts General Hospital
Boston, Massachusetts

EVELYN J. PIEHL, MSN, CRNP

Clinical Nurse Specialist, Obstetrics
University of Michigan
Medical Center
Ann Arbor, Michigan

DAVID E. SCHTEINGART, MD

Professor of Internal Medicine
University of Michigan
Medical Center
Ann Arbor, Michigan

CYNTHIA C. SENERCHIA, RN, MS

Cardiovascular Clinical Nurse Specialist
Project Director
Cardiovascular Data Analysis Center
Beth Israel Hospital
Boston, Massachusetts

WILLIAM R. SOLOMON, MD

Professor of Internal Medicine
University of Michigan
Medical Center
Ann Arbor, Michigan

MARILYN SAWYER SOMMERS, RN, PhD

Associate Professor
College of Nursing
University of Cincinnati
Cincinnati, Ohio

MAREK A. STAWISKI, MD

Associate Clinical Professor of Internal Medicine
Michigan State University
East Lansing, Michigan

JAMES L. VANDENBOSCH, PhD

Associate Professor
Department of Biology
Eastern Michigan University
Ypsilanti, Michigan

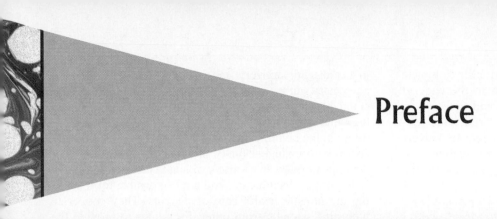

Preface

Pathophysiology deals with the *dynamic* aspects of disease processes. It is the study of disordered or altered functions—the physiologic mechanisms altered by disease in the living organism. Pathophysiology provides the basic link between the scientific realm of anatomy, physiology, and biochemistry and its application to clinical practice. The study of pathophysiology is essential to understand the rationale for diagnosis and therapeutic intervention in disease conditions.

The fifth edition of *Pathophysiology: Clinical Concepts of Disease Processes* retains the same philosophy and organizational framework as the four previous editions. Our focus is on alterations in biologic processes that affect the body's dynamic equilibrium or homeostasis, a conceptual approach designed to integrate knowledge from the basic and clinical sciences.

The conceptual framework is designed to present the general concepts of disease processes. The various dysfunctions of an organ or organ system are then examined. Emphasis is on understanding the etiology and pathogenesis of a given disorder, which is an essential factor in the development of insight.

This new edition has been thoroughly updated and revised and incorporates many significant changes suggested by faculty, students, and practitioners. One of the most significant additions is the new chapter on the neurophysiology of pain. The pain chapter incorporates material on two major pain problems—headache and back pain. The chapters on genetics, basic immunologic principles, and acquired immunodeficiency syndrome (AIDS) have been completely rewritten for the fifth edition to reflect the growing knowledge base resulting from scientific study in these rapidly developing fields. A major new section on calcium, phosphate, and magnesium metabolism and imbalances has been added to Part Four on Fluid and Electrolyte Disorders. New content on the hyperfiltration theory clearly explains the mechanisms of progressive renal failure, especially in persons with diabetes mellitus. The role of angiotensin-converting enzyme inhibitors and protein restriction in slowing this progression is then related to this theory.

Throughout this edition, the authors and many expert contributors have incorporated recent research findings, new diagnostic procedures and preventive measures, and current treatment measures. Through the past four editions, students and faculty alike have experienced tremendous user satisfaction with this textbook. Several of the features that have contributed to this are highlighted below. These features have been retained in the fifth edition, and many have been enhanced even more.

- One of the hallmarks of this textbook has been the short chapters. Students usually find pathophysiology to be a very complex and intimidating subject, so the short chapters are offered to make the content easier to read and synthesize. The textbook is divided into 13 parts according to the traditional body systems approach. It is further divided into 82 short chapters, presenting the challenging concepts of pathophysiology to students in manageable increments.

- A comprehensive illustration program has been a mainstay of this textbook since its first edition. More than 680 photographs and drawings throughout the textbook help clarify the more difficult concepts and demonstrate the normal as well as the disease processes. One hundred new illustrations have been added to this edition, and more than 75 have been updated.

- The Color Plate section of this new edition has been expanded to include a total of 54 color photographs. The color plates clearly depict certain disease manifestations and enhance the content for students. Twenty-four of the plates are new to this edition. The new plates illustrate the topics of hematology and conditions related to AIDS and HIV infection. All of the color plates have been grouped together and moved to the front of the text for easy access. Students can quickly turn to the plates for reference as they read the related content in the textbook.

- The end-of-chapter study questions have always been a popular feature with students and instructors. No other text offers a "built-in study guide" like this one. The questions include a combination of matching, short answer, true/false, and multiple choice—a total of nearly 3300 questions in all! Complete answers to the questions are given in the back of the book so students can self-test and assess their level of comprehension of the material. This self-instructional method enables the student to actively participate in the learning process by reading, reasoning, and demonstrating in writing his or her mastery of the concepts.

An *Instructor's Manual and Test Bank to Accompany Pathophysiology: Clinical Concepts of Disease Processes* provides additional teaching and learning devices to help instructors teach and to help students comprehend the study of pathophysiology. Divided by chapters to correspond with the textbook, each chapter of the *Instructor's Manual and Test Bank* includes a complete chapter outline, key terms with page numbers for easy reference to the text discussion of those terms, and a list of the learning objectives for the particular chapter. The Test Bank is extremely comprehensive and complete, offering instructors a wide array of test questions to include in their examinations. The Test Bank includes more than 2000 questions! All of the questions are multiple choice, and all are keyed to the chapter objectives. A new section of case studies has been added to the *Instructor's Manual and Test Bank* to help instructors teach clinical application of the content. These case studies cover each of the body systems and include answers to the questions posed.

This textbook provides the reader with a comprehensive presentation of pathophysiologic mechanisms in disease processes. The authors have emphasized relevant concepts that will enable the practitioner to function effectively in the health care delivery system. Our intent is to offer a textbook that not only is informative, but also will challenge and broaden the horizons of the health care professional.

This textbook of pathophysiology is designed to meet the more sophisticated needs of health care consumers and health professionals alike. Changes in the pattern of health care delivery have made it ever more important for consumers of the health care system to better understand the reasoning behind the care they are given. Rapid advances in biomedical sciences, coupled with the changes in health care delivery and its effect on consumerism, have made nurses and other health care professionals accountable for creating an environment that promotes high-quality, patient-centered care. The role of the practitioner in the health care system and that of the consumer continue to change. Nurses are functioning as independent practitioners in a variety of health care settings, such as in primary health care, and are responsible for managing the holistic health care of patients. They cooperate with professionals from other disciplines to provide the best possible care to meet the patients' needs. It is essential that these professionals synthesize pathophysiologic concepts to understand the rationale for preventive measures and therapeutic interventions. And it is becoming more incumbent on those who receive the health care to take an active role in maintaining or improving their health.

ACKNOWLEDGMENTS

Our sincere appreciation to Sally Schrefer, senior editor, nursing editorial department, for her valuable contributions during the planning and execution of this revision; to Gail Brower and Rae Robertson, developmental editors at Mosby–Year Book, for the excellent quality of their editorial assistance; to Betty Hazelwood, project specialist, for her meticulous attention to detail; to Therese Savia, research assistant to Marjorie Boldt, for her assistance in the cardiovascular section; to Anne Stawiski, for her assistance with word processing in preparing the manuscript; and to Margaret Croup Brudon, for the creative illustrations that she prepared for this and all previous editions of the book. We also appreciate the comprehensive review of and suggestions for changes in the manuscript offered by Mary Morgan, Jacqueline Newsome, and Mary Standridge.

Sylvia Anderson Price
Lorraine McCarty Wilson

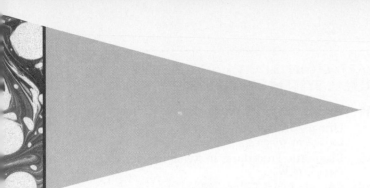

Contents

COLOR PLATES

COLOR PLATE CREDITS

Plates 1, 2, 3, 4, 5, 6, 7, and 8 from Grimes DE, Grimes RM: *AIDS and HIV infection,* St Louis, 1994, Mosby; courtesy The Centers for Disease Control and Prevention.

Plates 9, 10, 11, 14, 15, 16 17, 18, 19, 20, 21, 23, and 26 courtesy Herminia Bigornia, MT, and Muhammad S. Shurafa, MD, Division of Hematology/Oncology, Henry Ford Hospital, Detroit, Mich.

Plates 12, 22, and 24 courtesy Kolichi Maeda, MD, Division of Hematology/Oncology, Henry Ford Hospital, Detroit, Mich.

Plates 13 and 25 courtesy Sheikh Saeed, MD, Division Head of Hematopathology, Henry Ford Hospital, Detroit, Mich.

Plate 27 from Doughty D: *Gastrointestinal disorders,* St Louis, 1993, Mosby.

Plates 28 and 29 from Hill M: *Skin disorders,* St Louis, 1994, Mosby.

Plates 30, 39, 41, 42, 43, 44, 45, 46, 47, 50, 52, and 54 from Fitzpatrick TB et al, editors: *Dermatology in general medicine,* ed 2, New York, 1979, McGraw-Hill.

Plates 31, 32, 33, 34, 35, 36, 37, 38, 40, 48, 49, 51, and 53 courtesy Marek A. Stawiski, MD, Associate Clinical Professor of Internal Medicine, Michigan State University, East Lansing, Mich.

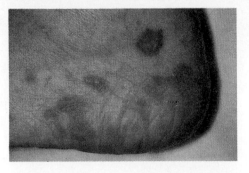

1 Kaposi's sarcoma of heel and lateral foot.

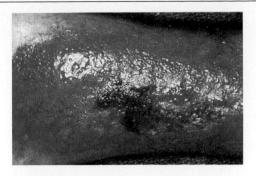

2 Kaposi's sarcoma of distal leg and ankle.

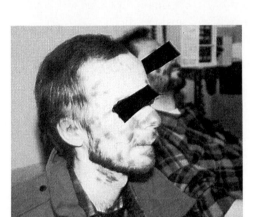

3 Kaposi's sarcoma of face.

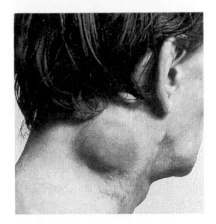

4 Lymphoma on neck.

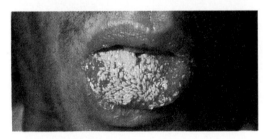

5 Severe pseudomembranous candidiasis of tongue in patient with acquired immunodeficiency syndrome (AIDS).

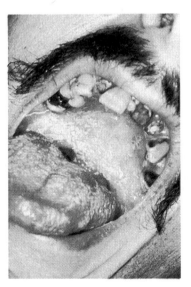

7 Candidiasis of tongue in AIDS patient resistant to fluconazole.

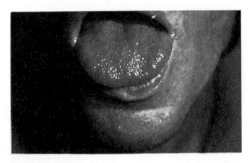

6 Candidiasis of tongue in patient shown in Plate 5 after 48 hours of treatment with fluconazole.

For color plate credits see p. xvi.

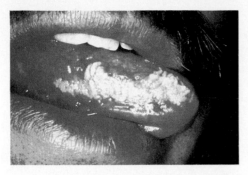

8 **Oral hairy leukoplakia** often presents as white plaques on lateral tongue and is associated with Epstein-Barr virus infection.

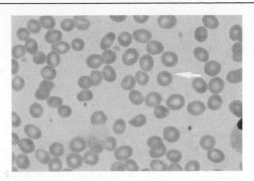

9 **Normal red blood cells** (RBCs) are round, possess an area of central pallor, appear slightly smaller than nucleus of mature lymphocyte *(lower right)*, and vary little in size or shape.

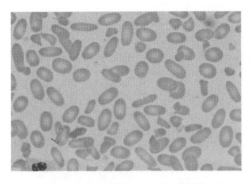

10 **Anisocytosis and poikilocytosis:** RBCs that vary in size and shape, respectively.

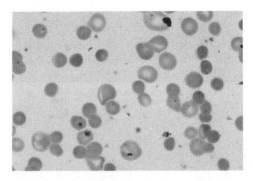

11 **Spherocytes** are smaller than normal RBCs and do not have central pallor, stain deeper, and tend to hemolyze readily.

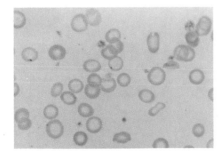

12 Hypochromic, microcytic RBCs characteristic of **iron deficiency anemia.** Poikilocytosis is seen.

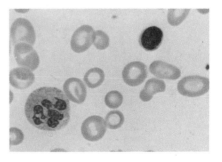

13 Peripheral blood findings seen in **megaloblastic (macrocytic) anemia.** Hypersegmented neutrophil and ovalocytes (large, oval-shaped RBCs) are evident.

For color plate credits see p. xvi.

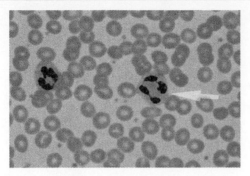

14 Normal mature **neutrophil** (PMN). PMN has segmented nucleus (two to five lobes) with heavy, clumped chromatin; fine neutrophilic (lilac-colored) granules are dispersed throughout its cytoplasm.

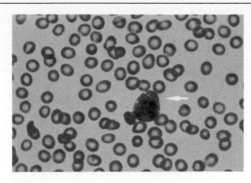

15 Normal **eosinophil.** Nucleus is bilobed, and cytoplasm contains purplish red granules.

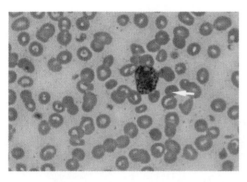

16 Normal **basophil** contains large, dark-blue granules that fill cell and obscure nucleus.

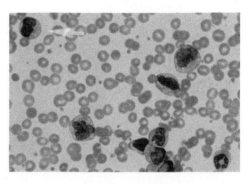

17 Normal **monocyte** is large cell with indented or folded nucleus containing loose, strandlike chromatin; cytoplasm has blue-gray color and usually contains fine, azurophilic granules.

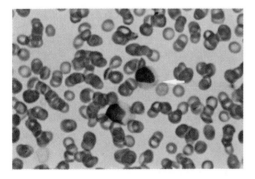

18 Normal **lymphocytes** have small, round or slightly indented nucleus with abundant, dark-staining condensed chromatin. Only thin external rim of slightly basophilic cytoplasm is visible.

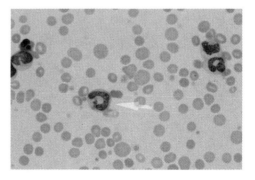

19 **Band neutrophil** is a slightly immature neutrophil with bandlike nucleus, usually shaped like a horseshoe. Numbers rise in acute bacterial infections.

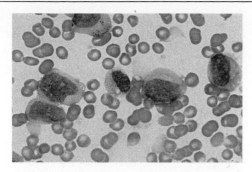

20 **Myeloblasts in acute myelogenous leukemia.** Cells have large nucleus with fine nuclear chromatin, very little cytoplasm, and usually two to five nucleoli.

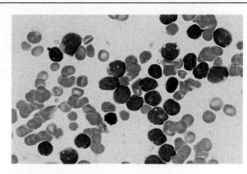

21 **Lymphoblast in acute lymphocytic leukemia.** Cells have fine chromatin nuclei with minimal cytoplasm and usually one or two nucleoli.

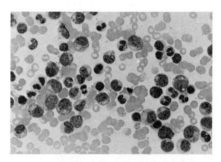

22 Bone marrow characteristic of **chronic granulocytic leukemia.** Marrow is hypercellular with an increase in granulocytic line.

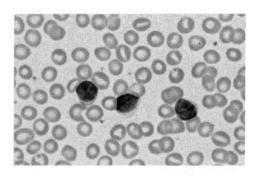

23 **Chronic lymphocytic leukemia.** Mature lympho-cytes with coarse nuclear chromatin and thin cytoplasm.

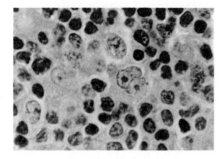

24 **Reed-Sternberg cell:** giant binucleated cell *(center)* typically seen in **Hodgkin's disease.** Small, mature lymphocytes are seen in background. To left of Reed-Sternberg cell is eosinophil containing red-orange cytoplasmic granules.

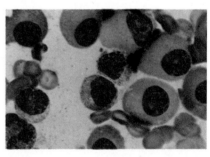

25 Bone marrow aspirate depicting cells seen in **multiple myeloma.**

26 **Platelets** (or **thrombocytes**) lack a nucleus because they are derived from cytoplasmic fragments of megakaryocytes. Platelets show central granular region with prominent purple-staining granules and nongranular periphery that stains pale transparent blue.

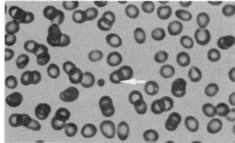

For color plate credits see p. xvi.

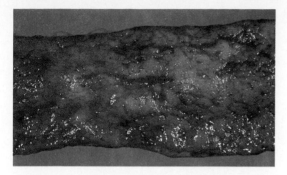

27 **Ulcerative colitis** showing severe mucosal edema and inflammation with ulcerations and bleeding.

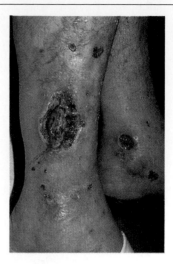

28 **Pyoderma gangrenosum** of legs in patient with ulcerative colitis.

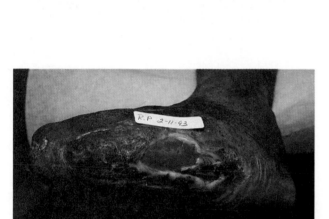

29 **Diabetic foot ulcer** caused by abnormal pressure distribution secondary to diabetic neuropathy. Vascular disease with diminished blood supply also contributes to development of the lesion, and infection is common.

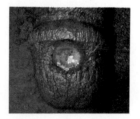

30 **Primary syphilis.** Painless papule.

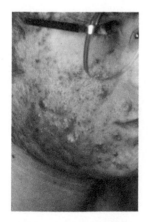

31 **Acne grade IV.** Conglobate, cysts, and scars.

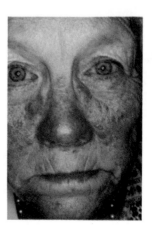

32 **Acne rosacea.** Central facial erythema and pustules.

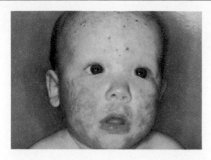

33 **Infantile eczema.** Weeping, erythematous patches.

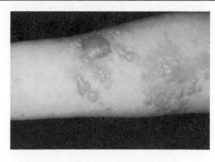

34 **Poison ivy.** Vesticles in linear and grouped configuration.

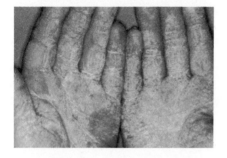

35 **Hand eczema.** Scaliness, fissures.

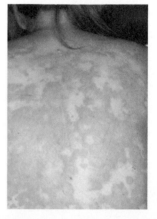

36 **Urticaria (hives).** Annular and arciform wheals.

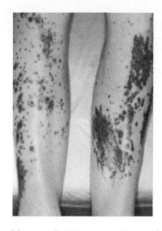

37 **Vasculitis.** Hemorrhagic, necrotic patches and papules.

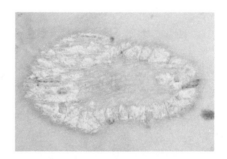

38 **Psoriasis.** Sharply marginated plaque with thick white scale.

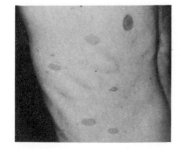

39 **Pityriasis rosea.** Oval-shaped patches on trunk.

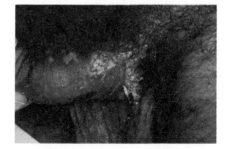

40 **Chronic herpes simplex** in AIDS patient. Chronic ulceration 3 months in duration with positive herpetic culture.

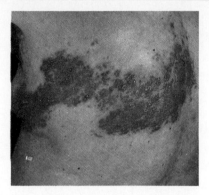

41 Herpes zoster. Linear vesicles on erythematous base along one dermatome.

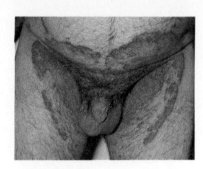

42 Tinea cruris. Peripheral extension of sharply marginated plaques.

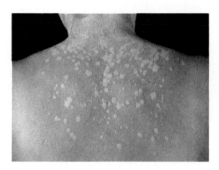

43 Tinea versicolor. Whitish, scaly confluent macules.

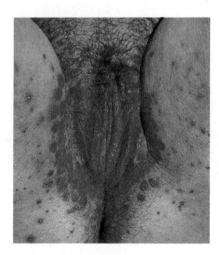

44 Intertriginous candidiasis. Sharply marginated, scaly plaque and satellite pustules.

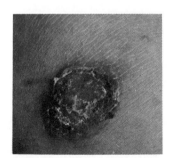

45 Impetigo. Crusts, erosion, and moist patch.

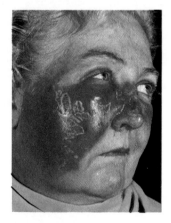

46 Facial erysipelas. Bright-red, sharply marginated, painful hot lesion.

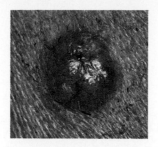

47 **Basal cell carcinoma.** Early nodule with pearly appearance and peripheral telangiectatic vessels.

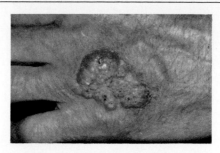

48 **Early squamous cell carcinoma.** Erythematous, infiltrating, ulcerated tumor on sun-exposed area.

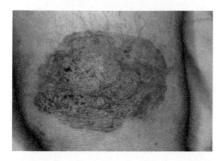

49 **Bowen's disease.** Erythematous, scaly patch with irregular configuration on sun-exposed area.

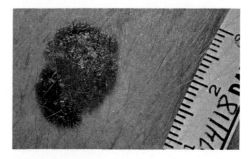

50 **Superficial spreading melanoma.** Variegated colors and infiltration of surrounding skin with diffusion of pigment.

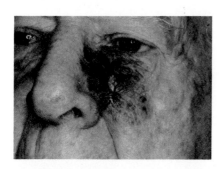

51 **Lentigo maligna melanoma.** Brown-black patch with central black nodule of melanoma arising.

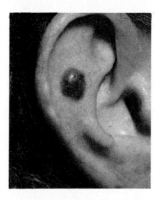

52 **Blue nevus.** Blue, uniform color of a benign nevus.

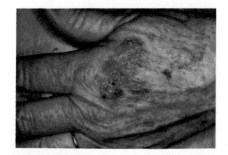

53 **Actinic keratosis.** Erythematous, scaly, firm papulation on plaque.

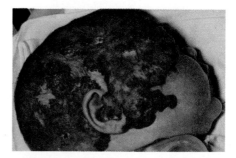

54 Extensive **capillary** ("strawberry") **hemangioma.**

For color plate credits see p. xvi.

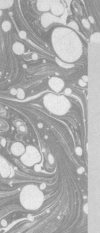

PART ONE

INTRODUCTION TO GENERAL PATHOLOGY

MECHANISMS OF DISEASE

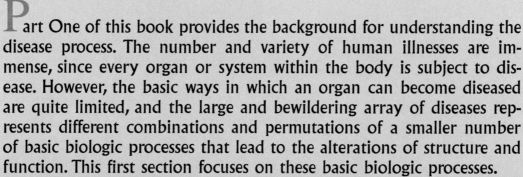

Part One of this book provides the background for understanding the disease process. The number and variety of human illnesses are immense, since every organ or system within the body is subject to disease. However, the basic ways in which an organ can become diseased are quite limited, and the large and bewildering array of diseases represents different combinations and permutations of a smaller number of basic biologic processes that lead to the alterations of structure and function. This first section focuses on these basic biologic processes.

Pathology is the science or study of disease. In its broadest sense, pathology is literally abnormal biology, the study of biologic processes gone awry, or the study of individuals who are ill or disordered. As a basic biologic science, pathology includes fields such as plant pathology, insect pathology, and veterinary and comparative pathology, as well as human pathology.

Pathology, in the context of human medicine, is not only a basic or theoretic science but also a clinical medical specialty. Pathologists are physicians who specialize in laboratory medicine; they consult with other physicians, thereby assisting in the diagnosis and treatment of disease. The scope of laboratory medicine includes all the studies performed on patient samples, including samples of tissue, blood, and other body fluids. Laboratory studies involving *anatomic pathology* examine and assess morphologic alterations in cells and tissues. Surgical pathology, cytopathology, and autopsy pathology are included in this category. Many studies are performed using other means. These areas of *clinical pathology* include clinical chemistry, microbiology, hematology, immunology, and immunohematology. *Pathophysiology* deals with the dynamic aspects of the disease process. It is the study of disordered or altered functions, for example, the physiologic changes caused by disease in a living organism.

Fundamental disease processes, such as inflammation, neoplasia, and immunologic injury, are described in this part of the textbook. The details of specific illnesses are addressed in later parts of the text. ▼

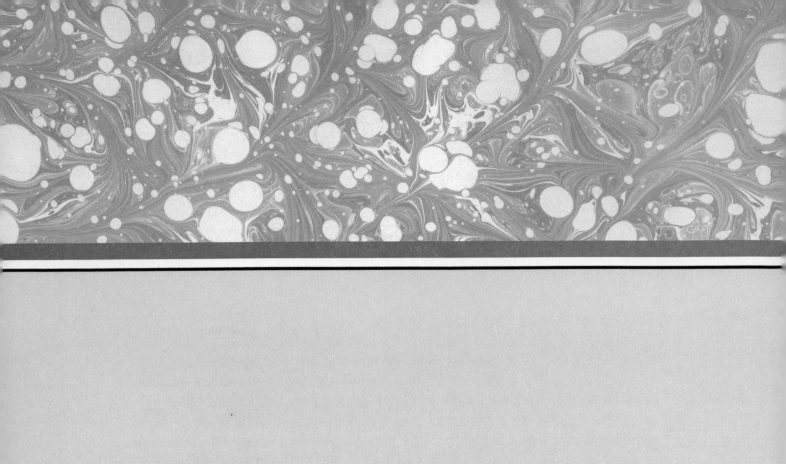

CHAPTER 1

General Concepts of Disease

HEALTH VERSUS DISEASE

GERALD D. ABRAMS

CONCEPT OF NORMALCY

Most people have some notion of *normal* and would define disease or illness as a deviation from or an absence of that normal state. However, on closer scrutiny, the concept of normalcy turns out to be complex and cannot be defined succinctly; correspondingly, the concept of disease is far from simple.

Any parameter of measurement applied to an individual or group of individuals has some sort of average value that is considered normal. Average values for height, weight, and blood pressure are derived from observation of many individuals and include a certain amount of variation.

Variations in normal values occur for several reasons. First, individuals differ from one another in their genetic makeup. Thus no two individuals in the world, except those derived from the same fertilized ovum, have exactly the same genes. Second, individuals differ in their life experiences and in their interaction with the environment. Third, in every individual there are variations in physiologic parameters because of the way in which the control mechanisms of the body function. For instance, blood glucose concentrations in a healthy person vary significantly at different times during the day, depending on food intake, activities of the individual, and so forth. These variations generally occur within a certain range.

The situation is somewhat analogous to a thermostatically controlled room. The temperature may dip slightly below the desired level before such a drop is sensed by the thermostat. The corrective action triggered by the thermostat may, in turn, overshoot the ideal slightly before the heat input is halted. Indeed, such variations in body temperature, even in the normal state, occur in all individuals. Finally, for physiologic parameters measured by fairly intricate means, a significant amount of variation in observed values may result from error or imprecision inherent in the measurement process itself.

Because of these considerations, determining a normal range of variation from an average value is a complex matter. This complexity includes knowing the degree of physiologic oscillation of a particular measurement, accounting for the degree of variation among normal individuals even under baseline conditions, and evaluating the precision of the measurement method. Finally, the biologic significance of the measurement must be estimated. Single measurements, observations, or laboratory results that seem to indicate abnormality must always be judged in the context of the entire situation of the individual. A single reading of elevated blood pressure does not make an individual hypertensive; a single slightly elevated blood glucose level does not mean that the individual is diabetic; and a single hemoglobin value lower than average does not necessarily indicate anemia.

To place such considerations in perspective, concepts of normalcy and even of disease are, to an extent, arbitrary and influenced by cultural values as well as by biologic realities. For example, in our culture a defect of a central nervous system function may produce a significant reading disability and would be an abnormality, whereas the same defect might never be noted in a culture in which reading is not an important aspect of everyday life. Furthermore, a trait that might be average and thus normal in one population might be considered distinctly abnormal in another. Consider, for instance, how a "normal" person from our population would be viewed by a group of central African pygmies; or conversely, how an infant from a less developed area, in which chronic diarrhea and relatively low weight gain are "normal" for that population, might be viewed in one of our well-baby clinics.

CONCEPT OF DISEASE

Disease can be defined as changes in individuals that cause their health parameters to fall outside the range of normal. The most useful biologic yardstick for normalcy relates to the individual's ability to meet the demands placed on the body and to adapt to these demands or changes in the external environment so as to maintain reasonable constancy of the internal environment. All cells in the body need a certain amount of oxygen and nutrients for their continuing survival and function, and they also require an environment that provides narrow ranges of temperature, water content, acidity, and salt concentration. Thus the maintenance of internal conditions within fairly narrow limits is an essential feature of the normal body. When some of the structures and functions of the body deviate from the norm to the point where the ability to maintain homeostasis is destroyed or threatened or where the individual can no longer meet environmental challenges, disease is said to exist. A person's subjective perception of disease is related to impairment of the ability to carry on daily activities comfortably.

Disease does not involve the development of a completely new form of life but rather is an extension or distortion of the normal life processes present in the individual. Even in the case of an obviously infectious disease, where the body is literally invaded, the infectious agent itself does not constitute the disease but only evokes the changes that ultimately are manifested as disease. Thus disease is actually the sum of the physiologic processes that have been distorted. To understand and adequately treat the disease, the identity of the normal processes interfered with, the character of the disturbances, and the secondary effects of such disturbances on other vital processes must be taken into account.

Historically, it was believed that disease is actually a new form of life, a sort of possession of the body by an outside agent. From this notion it would follow that some form of "exorcism" to drive out the disease agent is proper therapy. However, even in the instance of an invasive infectious agent, attempted treatment with antibiotics alone may not cure the patient if proper attention is not directed toward the intrinsic body processes that have become deranged.

A theme that recurs, with variations, throughout this volume is that above all, disease is "part and parcel" of the patient. *Normal and abnormal processes represent different points on the same continuous spectrum.* In fact, the seeds of disease often lie within the adaptive mechanisms of the body itself, mechanisms that constitute a po-

tential two-edged sword. For example, the leukocytes, which are essential in responding to microbial invaders, may themselves become agents of tissue injury. The mechanisms that allow persons to become immune to certain infections also form the basis for allergic reactions such as hay fever and asthma. Similarly, the mechanism of cellular proliferation that allows persons to repair wounds and constantly renew cell populations in various tissues may run amok, giving rise to cancer.

DEVELOPMENT OF DISEASE

Etiology

Etiology, in its most general definition, is the assignment of causes or reasons for phenomena. A decription of the cause of a disease includes the identification of those factors that provoke the particular disease. Thus the tubercle bacillus is designated as the etiologic agent of tuberculosis. Other etiologic factors in the development of tuberculosis include the age, nutritional status, and even the occupation of the individual. Even in the case of an infectious disease, such as tuberculosis, the agent itself does not constitute the disease. Rather, all the resulting responses to that agent, all the perversions of biologic processes taken together, constitute the disease. In the etiology of a particular disease, therefore, a range of extrinsic or exogenous factors in the environment must be considered along with a variety of intrinsic or endogenous characteristics of the individual.

Pathogenesis

Pathogenesis of a disease refers to the development or evolution of the disease. To continue with the previous example, the pathogenesis of tuberculosis would include the mechanisms whereby the invasion of the body by the tubercle bacillus ultimately leads to the observed abnormalities.

Such an analysis would relate the proliferation and spread of tubercle bacilli to the evolving inflammatory responses, to the immunologic defenses of the body, and to the destruction of cells and tissues. The pattern and extent of the tissue damage would ultimately be related to the overt manifestations of clinical disease. Pathogenesis also takes into account the sequential occurrence of certain phenomena and the temporal aspects of the evolving disease. A given disease is not static; it is a dynamic phenomenon with a rhythm and pattern of its own. Thus each disease has a characteristic *natural history*—a typical pattern of evolution, impact, and duration that is seen unless the disease is successfully modified by some intervention. In the diagnostic evaluation of patients and the assessment of therapy, it is essential to keep in mind this concept of natural history and the range of variation among different diseases with regard to their natural history. Some diseases characteristically have a rapid response, whereas others have a long prodrome. Some diseases are self-limited; that is, they resolve spontaneously in a brief time. Others become chronic, and still others are subject to frequent remissions and exacerbations.

Manifestations

Early in the development of a disease, the etiologic agent or agents may provoke a number of changes in biologic processes that can be detected by laboratory analysis even though the patient has no subjective symptoms. Thus many diseases have a *subclinical stage,* during which the patient functions normally even though the disease processes are well established. The structure and function of many organs provide a large reserve or safety margin, and functional impairment may become evident only when the disease has become quite advanced. For example, chronic renal disease could completely destroy one kidney and partly destroy the other before any symptoms related to decreased renal function would be perceived. However, some diseases seem to begin as functional derangements and actually become clinically evident although no anatomic abnormalities can be detected at the time. Such functional illnesses may lead to secondary structural abnormalities.

As certain biologic processes are encroached on, the patient begins to feel subjectively that something is wrong. These subjective feelings are called symptoms of disease. By definition, *symptoms* are subjective and can be reported only by the patient to an observer. However, when manifestations of the disease can be objectively identified by an observer, these are termed *signs* of the disease. Nausea, malaise, and pain are symptoms, whereas fever, reddening of the skin, and a palpable mass are signs of disease. A demonstrable structural change produced in the course of a disease is referred to as a *lesion.* Lesions may be evident at a gross and/or a microscopic level. The outcome of a disease is sometimes referred to as a *sequela* (plural, *sequelae*). For example, the sequela to an inflammatory process in a given tissue might be a scar in that tissue. The sequela to acute rheumatic inflammation of the heart might be scarred, deformed cardiac valves. A *complication* of a disease is a new or separate process that may arise secondarily because of some change produced by the original entity. For example, bacterial pneumonia may be a complication of viral infection of the respiratory tract. Fortunately, many diseases can also undergo what is termed *resolution,* and the host returns to a completely normal state, without sequelae or complications. Resolution can occur spontaneously, that is, resulting from body defenses, or it can result from successful therapy.

Finally, it is essential to reemphasize that disease is dynamic rather than static. The manifestations of disease in a given patient may change from day to day as biologic equilibria shift and as compensatory mechanisms are brought into play. Environmental influences brought to bear on the patient also affect the disease. Therefore every disease has a range of manifestations and a spectrum of expressions that may vary from patient to patient.

QUESTIONS

▼ *Answer the following on a separate sheet of paper.*

1. Formulate definitions for pathology and pathophysiology.
2. Explain the difference between anatomic and clinical pathology. List at least three examples of types of studies included under each of these categories.
3. What is meant by pathogenesis of a disease?
4. Describe the complex factors associated with the concept of normalcy.
5. Explain why a given disease is not a static phenomenon.

▼ *Circle the letter preceding each item below that correctly answers the question or completes the statement. More than one answer may be correct.*

6. The study and evaluation of morphologic alterations in cells and tissues are referred to as:
   a. Pathophysiology
   b. Anatomic pathology
   c. Clinical pathology
   d. Comparative pathology
7. Etiology refers to the:
   a. Study of the cause of a disease
   b. Degree of injury sustained
   c. Development of a new form of life
   d. Mechanism of the disease process
8. The outcome of disease is termed a:
   a. Sequela
   b. Complication
   c. Manifestation
   d. Lesion
9. Resolution of a disease refers to which of the following?

a. When the host returns to a normal state without sequelae or complication
   b. New or separate process that arises
   c. Both a and b
   d. Neither a nor b
10. In the course of an illness, a demonstrable structural change produced by a disease process is termed a:
   a. Symptom
   b. Sign
   c. Lesion
   d. Complication
11. Which of the following would be considered a sign of a disease?
   a. Nausea
   b. Fever
   c. Malaise
   d. Headache

CHAPTER 2

Heredity, Environment, and Disease

INTERACTION OF HEREDITY AND ENVIRONMENT

JAMES L. VANDENBOSCH

This chapter opens with a brief review of molecular genetics followed by an introduction to human molecular genetics and patterns of inheritance. The chapter also describes genetic disorders and their diagnosis and therapies. The focus of this chapter is on human genetics and its applications to pathology. It describes neither the mechanisms by which mutations occur nor how these changes are prevented from occurring; both of these topics are better covered in a course on genetics. An understanding of bacterial and viral genetics would be very helpful in understanding diseases caused by these organisms, but it is outside the scope of this chapter; these subjects should be handled in a microbiology course. This chapter demonstrates that many diseases are caused directly or exclusively at the genetic level. It also provides insight into the patterns of inheritance and the genetic tests performed in the diagnosis of these diseases. Finally, it helps the health care worker in understanding the principles of genetic therapies that are and will be available in the treatment of these disorders. All these insights are important in the diagnosis, treatment, and counseling of afflicted individuals and their families.

EXTRINSIC AND INTRINSIC FACTORS IN DISEASE

Extrinsic Factors

Some important causes of human disease include infectious agents, mechanical trauma, toxic chemicals, radiation, extremes of temperature, nutritional problems, and psychologic stress. Although these *extrinsic factors* are important causes of human misery, a view of disease that takes into account only these factors is incomplete. Because disease is actually "part and parcel" of the life of the afflicted individual, the intrinsic response mechanisms of that individual and all the biologic processes affected by a particular extrinsic agent must also be considered.

Intrinsic Factors

Many characteristics of the individual are *intrinsic factors* in disease, since they have a significant impact on the evolution of various conditions. Age, gender, and even abnormalities acquired in the course of previous illnesses are factors to be considered in the pathogenesis of a disease. Above all, the genetic constitution, or genome, of the individual is an essential part of the "equation." This is because the anatomic characteristics of the host, the myriad of physiologic mechanisms of everyday life, and the modes of responding to injury are all determined by the genetic information assembled at the moment of conception. In studying the biology of disease, heredity and environment must always be taken into account.

Interaction Between Extrinsic and Intrinsic Factors

One often hears the question, "Is this disease hereditary?" In a sense, that question is improper. Intrinsic factors are almost always involved in disease. Therefore the question should be phrased, "To what extent is heredity important in this disease?" Exceptions to this principle are relatively few and quite extreme. Admittedly, heredity is not significant when the patient is involved in an explosion or struck by a speeding truck; however, such instances aside, it is always a factor. Even in a clearly exogenous infection, genetic factors can and do influence susceptibility to the infectious agent and the pattern of disease produced.

A broad spectrum exists in the balance of heredity and environment in the causation of disease. At one end of the spectrum are those diseases largely determined by some environmental agent regardless of the individual's hereditary background. At the other end are diseases that result from faulty genetic programming. These diseases are expressed in almost any bearer of the faulty genetic information, regardless of extrinsic influences. These latter diseases are usually identified as hereditary diseases. Most human diseases lie between these two ends of the spectrum and involve a significant interplay between genetic and extrinsic factors.

MOLECULAR ARCHITECTURE AND PROCESSING OF GENETIC INFORMATION

Molecular Structures

The understanding of genetics requires a basic knowledge of the chemistry of at least three different classes of molecules: deoxyribonucleic acid (DNA), ribonucleic acid (RNA), and proteins.

Deoxyribonucleic acid

DNA is a polymer of deoxyribonucleotides, each of which is composed of a phosphorylated sugar (deoxyribose) and a nitrogenous base (either a purine or a pyrimidine). All the nucleotides have the same sugar but have only one of four different bases (adenine, thymine, cytosine, or guanine). Because chemists assign numbers to the carbons in the sugar ribose, one can say that the phosphate is on the $5'$-carbon, the oxygen has been removed from the $2'$-carbon, and a hydroxyl group is on the $3'$-carbon (Fig. 2-1, *A*).

The nucleotides are held together in the polymer by phosphodiester bonds, in which the phosphate joins the $5'$-carbon of one nucleotide to the $3'$-carbon of another. As a consequence, for a long polymer of nucleotides, all but one of its $5'$-carbons is attached to the $3'$-carbon of another nucleotide. Similarly, all but one of its $3'$-carbons are joined to the $5'$-carbon of another nucleotide. These unattached carbons are considered the $5'$ and $3'$ ends of the polymer, respectively.

The DNA polymers almost never exist in humans as the single strands shown in Fig. 2-1, *C*. Instead, DNA is usually found in the double-stranded form, in which two sugar "backbones" are parallel but are aligned in the opposite $5'$ to $3'$ orientation (Fig. 2-1, *D*). The two strands are held together by specific hydrogen bonding between complementary pairs of bases: adenine pairing with thymine and guanine with cytosine. Because the base pairing is specific, the same information is present in both strands, but one strand has the information in the "antisense" form, similar to a negative of a photograph. Each of these long, linear, double-stranded DNA polymers is the nucleic acid portion of a *chromosome.*

Ribonucleic acid

RNA is very similar to DNA. It is a polymer of ribonucleotides, each of which differs from deoxynucleotides in having a hydroxyl group on the $2'$-carbon (Fig. 2-1, *B*). RNA also differs from DNA in having the base uracil rather than thymine. As with DNA, RNA nucleotides are held together by phosphodiester bonds between the $5'$-carbon of one nucleotide and the $3'$-carbon of another. Therefore RNA also has $5'$ and $3'$ ends. Unlike DNA, RNA is rarely found as a double-stranded molecule. It is usually single stranded, but these single strands may fold back on themselves to allow for elaborate structures that are stabilized by complementary base pairings between bases on the same linear strand of RNA. These structures are essential to the proper functioning of transfer RNA (tRNA) and ribosomal RNA (rRNA).

Proteins

Proteins are polymers of amino acids joined by peptide bonds between the amino group of one amino acid and the carboxyl group of the preceding amino acid. As with DNA and RNA, proteins have distinct ends: the amino- (or *N*-) terminus and the carboxy- (or *C*-) terminus. As

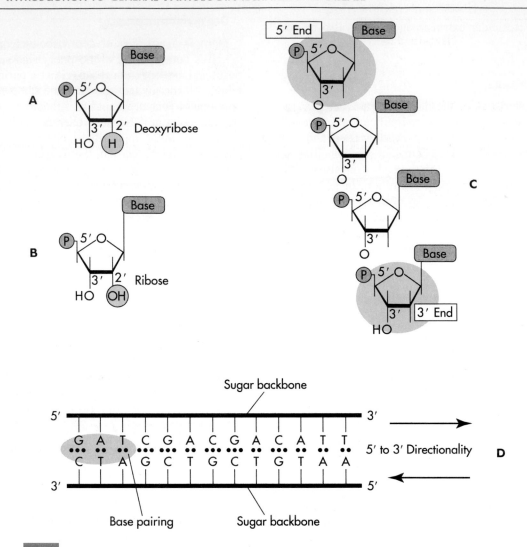

FIG. 2-1   Nucleic acids. **A**, Deoxyribonucleotide. **B**, Ribonucleotide. **C**, Polymer of deoxyribonucleotides joined by phosphodiester bonds. **D**, Double-stranded deoxyribonucleic acid (DNA) held together by complementary base pairs.

with RNA, they are usually highly folded to form specific structures essential for the molecule's function and for it to associate with other proteins to form larger, functional complexes. Proteins can be structural components for the cell, enzymes that catalyze chemical reactions, or regulatory molecules that alter the sites of DNA or RNA polymerization.

Processes

To function as the repository of inheritable information, the DNA must be manipulated in at least two ways. First, the DNA must be copied with very high fidelity for the genetic information to be transmitted reliably from a dividing cell to its two daughter cells and, on a larger scale, from parents to their children. Second, the information in the DNA must be expressed. If the information were retained only as DNA, it would be of little use. To be functional, the information must be used to form the RNA and

proteins that carry out the various activities for cell functioning and viability.

Replication

Copies of the DNA polymer are made in the nucleus by the process of replication. In *replication,* a group of proteins separates the two strands of DNA and forms two new strands using the original strands as templates. The enzyme that actually forms the new DNA strand is termed a *DNA polymerase.* As it moves from 3' to 5' on an existing DNA strand, it forms a new strand in the 5' to 3' order. That is, the last nucleotide added always constitutes the 3' end of the polymer (Fig. 2-2). Although the replication process is fairly fast (about 100 bases are added per second by each enzyme), the large size of the human genome requires that each chromosome have a thousand or more sites at which replication is initiated simultaneously. The mechanism by which this is coordinated is not clear. In addition to being fast, replication is

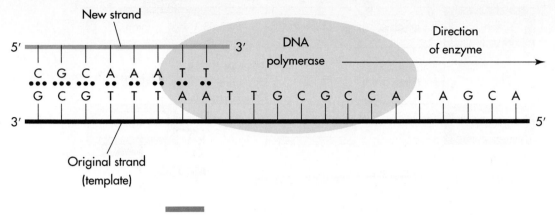

FIG. 2-2   DNA polymerase replicating DNA.

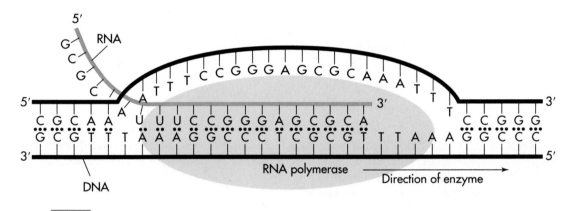

FIG. 2-3   Ribonucleic acid (RNA) polymerase forming RNA by transcribing a DNA template.

highly accurate (errors are made at less than once in a million bases added). Because the human genome has more than 1000 million bases, however, this low rate of replication errors is sufficient to introduce changes (mutations) continually into DNA. These spontaneous mutations that arise during replication are one source of defective genes that can lead to genetic diseases.

Transcription

RNA polymers containing the information from DNA are formed in the nucleus by the process of transcription. In *transcription,* an enzyme complex separates the two strands of DNA and forms a strand of RNA using one of the DNA strands as a template. The enzyme complexes that carry out transcription are termed *RNA polymerases,* of which there are three different types in humans. As with the DNA polymerases, the RNA polymerases move from 3' to 5' on an existing DNA strand, forming a new RNA strand in the 5' to 3' order (Fig. 2-3). The process of transcription is initiated from a site called the *promoter,* where the RNA polymerase binds to the DNA. Transcription stops at a site called the *terminator.*

The RNA made by the RNA polymerase (i.e., the transcript) is usually not the final form of the RNA. Indeed, it is called hnRNA (*h*eterogenous *n*uclear RNA) because it is found only in the nucleus and is processed before it is transported to the cytoplasm. An important component of this processing is *splicing* (Fig. 2-4). In most structural genes, this involves the removal of RNA stretches termed *introns* (*int*ervening sequences) and the joining of the flanking RNA regions termed *exons* (*ex*pressed sequences). mRNA is the product of splicing and several other processing events. The splicing process is regulated so that different exons may remain in the final mRNA. Therefore the same transcript of a particular gene may yield different mRNAs, depending on the developmental stage of the organism or the tissue in which the cell is located.

Translation

After RNA is transcribed, processed, and exported from the nucleus to the cytoplasm, it may be translated. In *translation,* ribosomes (complexes of rRNA and proteins) polymerize amino acids to form proteins. The order

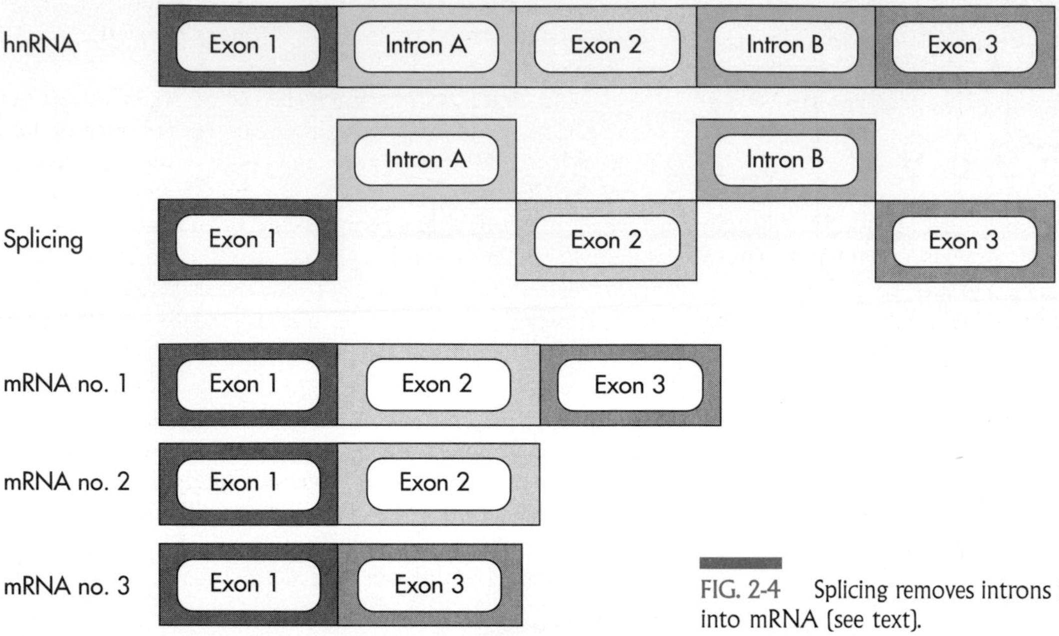

FIG. 2-4   Splicing removes introns in the conversion of hnRNA into mRNA (see text).

of the amino acids is determined by the order of bases in the mRNA template. The ribosomes "read" these bases in groups of three bases. Each of these triplets constitutes a *codon*. All codons either encode for one specific amino acid or do not encode for any amino acid. Therefore the UUA codon encodes leucine and UCA encodes serine. Those that do not encode an amino acid (e.g., UAA) cause translation to stop and, hence, are called *stop codons*.

Genes

The human genome is believed to contain nearly 100,000 genes. Each gene is a transcriptional unit. That is, a gene can be defined as a region of DNA that will be transcribed to form RNA. Some transcripts (e.g., rRNA and tRNA) will remain as RNA. Most of the RNA transcripts, however, will subsequently be translated to form proteins. Those genes that encode proteins are termed *structural genes*.

Because genes are discrete physical entities, they can be designated as having a particular *locus* (plural, *loci*), or location, on a chromosome. For all individuals, a given gene is normally found at the same locus of a given chromosome. Although they have the same location, copies of a gene from different individuals are likely to have a slightly different sequence of bases. If this difference results in differences in the RNA or protein formed, they are considered to be different *alleles* of the same gene. Loci can also be assigned or named for regions of the DNA that are not genes. These regions may not encode

for any product but may be involved in other functions such as the binding of regulatory proteins.

Regulation

It is essential for an organism to regulate which genes are expressed in each cell at any given time. Regulation may affect the initiation of transcription or may control gene expression posttranscriptionally by affecting translation, hnRNA processing, or the half-life of the mRNA. Transcription is not initiated spontaneously through the interaction of the RNA polymerase with the DNA. Instead, the binding of the RNA polymerase to the DNA is controlled by regulatory proteins termed *transcription factors*. These factors may increase the expression of a gene by binding to an *enhancer* site and thereby encourage the binding of the RNA polymerase to the promoter by either changing the shape (conformation) of the DNA or interacting directly with the polymerase. A transcription factor may act alone to control expression or may require the direct interaction of a second factor. In this latter case, the two dissimilar transcription factors usually bind to the DNA as a mixed pair *(heterodimer)*. In this way the cell can require two signals to turn on a gene, with each signal eliciting the formation or binding of a different transcription factor that combines as a dimer to control transcription. In addition to enhancers, there are also regulatory sites, or *silencers,* that decrease transcription. The combined effects of enhancers and silencers control the timing and cell specificity of most gene expression. The abnormal regulation of a normal gene can affect an organism as profoundly as an abnormal gene.

CELLULAR ARCHITECTURE AND PROCESSING OF GENETIC INFORMATION

Cytogenetic Structures

Chromosomes

The picture of a chromosome becomes more complex when the three-dimensional view is considered. These long, double-stranded DNA polymers do not lie flat but normally twist to form a *double helix*. Furthermore, in the cell these double helixes are wrapped around groups of proteins called *histones* to form *nucleosomes*. The combination of chromosome, histones, and other associated proteins is termed *chromatin*. Usually the chromatin is relatively dispersed within the nucleus, so that, if the nucleus is broken open and the DNA is stained, no particular structures can be seen with the light microscope. When a cell is ready to divide, however, the chromatin becomes tightly condensed to form the structures commonly thought of as chromosomes. These *metaphase chromosomes* are used to identify chromosome number and type for the genetic analysis of individuals.

Each of the metaphase chromosomes consists of two *chromatids* (identical pieces of chromosomal DNA and associated proteins) joined at a region called the *centromere* (Fig. 2-5). The centromeres are essential for the proper segregation of the chromatids into the daughter cells during mitosis. If the centromere fails to function properly, nondisjunction will occur, giving rise to daughter cells with an improper contingent of chromosomes. With the exception of the gametes (spermatozoa and ova), all normal human cells have 46 chromosomes, 44 *somatic chromosomes,* or *autosomes,* and two *sex chromosomes.* The autosomes consist of 22 homologous pairs, each member of a pair having the same genes. The two sex chromosomes, in the case of normal females,

have the same genes (i.e., two X chromosomes) or, in the case of the normal male, have different genes (i.e., an X chromosome and a Y chromosome).

DNA, therefore, has many levels of organization. At the simplest level, it is a single, linear polymer of nucleotides. Most single-gene defects (e.g., cystic fibrosis, sickle cell anemia) are now understood to result from discrete changes in the specific order of these bases. At the next level, DNA is a linear, double-stranded molecule of complementary bases aligned in an antiparallel orientation spatially organized as a double helix. At a higher level, the chromosomal DNA is complexed with proteins, including histones and other proteins. These protein-DNA complexes constitute the chromatin, which can condense during metaphase to form the two chromatid chromosomes often used in genetic analysis. Chromosomal disorders (e.g., Down's syndrome, Klinefelter's syndrome) are frequently diagnosed by changes in gross chromosomal number or type.

Karyotype

The complete set of chromosomes in a somatic cell is the *karyotype.* Therefore the karyotype is 46,XY for a normal male and 46,XX for a normal female. The somatic chromosome pairs are each numbered in descending order of size. Thus chromosome 1 is the largest and chromosome 22 the smallest. Each chromosome is distinguishable by its size, the placement of the centromere, and distinct banding patterns that appear with certain stains. These characteristics allow geneticists to microscopically examine chromosomes from cells at metaphase and determine the karyotype (Fig. 2-6). Karyotype analysis can determine if any chromosomes are absent or present in excess numbers to confirm gender or diagnose disorders such as Down's syndrome (trisomy 21; Fig. 2-6, *B*). The analysis can also detect gross malformations of the chromosomes, such as breakage and loss of a chromatid, or the exchange of one chromatid fragment for another.

Meiosis and Mitosis

Cells undergo two different types of division. All cells undergo mitotic division. In *mitosis* the two sister chromatids separate and are distributed equally into the daughter cells. The result of this process is that each daughter cell will receive one chromatid from each chromosome and, hence, a full complement of chromosomes. None of the genetic information of the mother cell is lost for either daughter cell. Germline cells undergo an additional type of division termed *meiosis* (Fig. 2-7, *A*). Meiosis involves two divisions. In the first division, pairs of chromatids are separated into the daughter cells in such a manner that each cell receives only one chromosome of each type (e.g., each cell will receive one chromatid pair for chromosome 21). The second division is similar to mitotic division in that the sister chromatids are

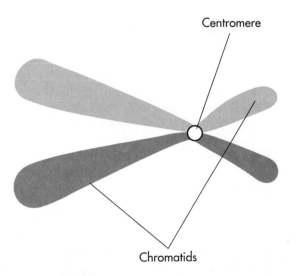

Centromere

Chromatids

FIG. 2-5   Chromosome structure.

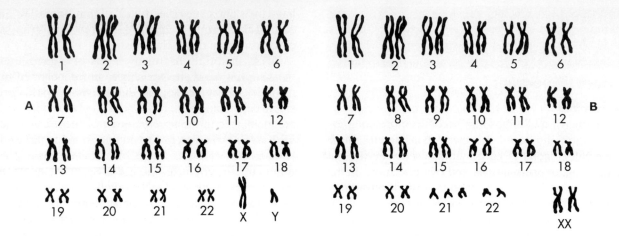

FIG. 2-6 **A,** Example of a karyotype of a normal male displayed in the standard format. **B,** Karyotype of a female with Down's syndrome. In the position conventionally designated as 21, three chromosomes exist instead of two (trisomy 21).

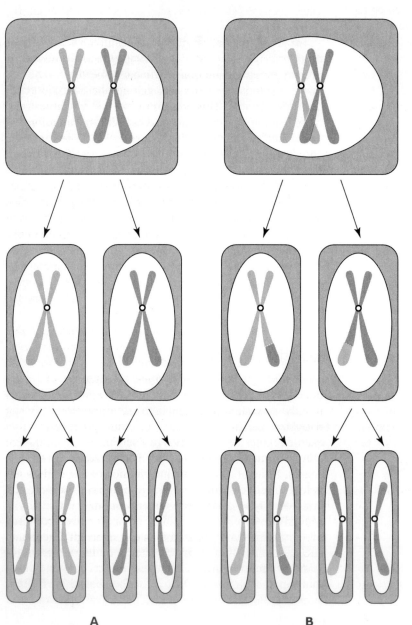

FIG. 2-7 Chromosomal and chromatid segregation during meiosis. **A,** Simple segregation of chromosomes into daughter cells. **B,** Segregation and meiotic recombination.

separated and, unless meiotic recombination has occurred (see following discussion), each of the two daugther cells from this division obtains the same genetic information. The consequence of the first division is that each daughter cell receives only half the genetic information present in the cell before division. Furthermore, the segregation of the chromosomes into the daughter cells is random, providing for a very large number (2^{23}) of possible genetic combinations in the daughter cells. Therefore each germline cell is likely to have a unique set of genetic information. When spermatozoa and ova combine, the resultant zygote will have a complete set of chromosomes consisting of 22 pairs of somatic chromosomes and two sex chromosomes. Both meiotic and mitotic divisions require the proper centromere functioning in the separation of chromosomes or chromatids to the opposite poles of the cell. This process is termed *disjunction.* If disjunction fails, the nondisjunction results in daughter cells with an inappropriate contingent of chromosomes or chromatids. This situation is termed *aneuploidy,* and the related disorders are described later as chromosomal disorders.

Genetic diversity is also increased by a second process during meiosis. This process, termed *meiotic recombination,* results in the exchange of equivalent portions of chromatids between different chromosome pairs (Fig. 2-7, *B*). Meiotic recombination is believed to occur many times during each meiotic division. As a consequence, a given chromosome may have exchanged chromatid segments more than once during the formation of any spermatozoon or ovum. The genetic diversity is thereby increased enormously. With the exception of identical twins, each individual is truly unique.

Human Genome Project

Knowledge of human genetics is expanding at an unparalleled rate. The rate of this explosion in information is largely attributable to the Human Genome Project, which was first proposed in 1988 and begun in 1990. Its principal aim is to construct a physical map of the entire 3.2 billion base pairs present in the human genome. The project will eventually isolate and identify all 50,000 to 100,000 genes in the human genome. Although the project started in the United States, it has spread internationally, involving Britain, France, Japan, and other countries in investigations coordinated by an international group, the Human Genome Organization. An important side benefit of the project has been the changes in genetic research infrastructure. Since its proposal in 1988, the project has supported the development of major new techniques, including the polymerase chain reaction (PCR), yeast artificial chromosomes (YACs), and fluorescence in situ hybridization (FISH). These techniques have made possible, respectively, the amplification, cloning, and visualization of large segments of human DNA. Combined, these techniques are leading to the almost daily mapping of new genetic elements of human disease.

PATTERNS OF INHERITANCE

Genetic Variation

Some genes have a reasonably high frequency of different alleles at a given locus. Good examples of this genetic polymorphism are the ABO blood group locus and the HLA antigens (human leukocyte antigens). Individuals with two alleles that can be distinguished as different for a given locus are considered to be *heterozygous* for that locus. If the two alleles are not distinguishable, the individual is *homozygous* for that allele.

The molecular basis for allelic variation is *mutation,* a change in the order or arrangement of DNA bases. Mutations are generated at an average rate of one per cell per cell division. As a result, almost every cell in the human body has some genetically unique feature. Usually these mutations affect genes in somatic cells, and therefore only a limited set of cells will receive the mutation. Because most mutations are likely to occur in regions between genes and because any cell will express only a small proportion of its genes, it is unlikely that a given mutation will have any detectable effect. Furthermore, even a somatic mutation that causes the loss of a gene important to a particular cell may not be detected at the organismal level. This is because the individual will exhibit *mosaicism,* having some cells with the mutation and other somatic cells lacking the mutation. These normal cells are still available to carry out the same function for the organism. Sometimes somatic mutations arise in genes critical to controlling cell growth. Such mutations are a frequent cause of cancer. Unlike somatic mutations, mutations that arise in germline cells can be passed on to the progeny. These mutations are present in all the cells of the organism, and almost all its genes are required at some point in the development of any organism. If a germline cell mutation significantly affects the expression of any gene, it is highly likely that it will be detected at the organismal level.

Mutations may arise by a number of mechanisms. Despite the high fidelity of the polymerization process, normal replication and the accompanying error correction mechanisms generate mutations. Mutations also arise during the repair of DNA damage from *mutagens*, exogenous agents such as chemicals, and ultraviolet (UV) or ionizing radiation. These replication and repair errors usually result in substitutions of one base for another or the deletion or insertion of one or a few bases of DNA. A second source of mutation is the movement of mobile genetic elements called *transposons* and insertion sequences. These normal constituents of our genome do not have fixed loci but move within it. In moving from one locus to another, these elements can interrupt a gene and cause deletions and rearrangements of large regions of DNA. A third source of mutation is the introduction of new genes or modified alleles from outside the body. This occurs naturally with some viral infections when the vi-

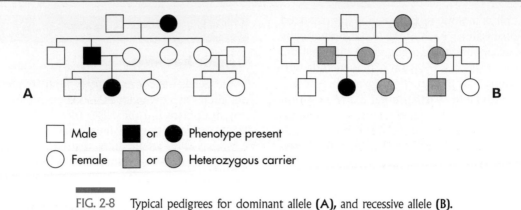

- □ Male   ■ or ● Phenotype present
- ○ Female ▦ or ⬤ Heterozygous carrier

FIG. 2-8   Typical pedigrees for dominant allele **(A)**, and recessive allele **(B)**.

ral genome is integrated into DNA or when a virus accidentally brings in genes of a previous host cell. In some cases, these new additions to the genome can give rise to genetic disorders. Conversely, the emerging field of gene therapy is using viruses and other means to introduce into the body genes that can correct or mollify existing genetic disorders.

Dominance

The particular genetic makeup of an individual is the *genotype*. An observable trait arising from expression of the genotype is the *phenotype*. Phenotypes have long been used by geneticists and animal breeders to construct *pedigrees* to demonstrate patterns of inheritance (Fig. 2-8). If an individual is heterozygous for a given gene, the two alleles may not contribute equally to the resultant phenotype. A phenotype is *dominant* if it is observable in the heterozygote. For dominant alleles, therefore, the associated phenotype will be expressed by all individuals with that allele. Dominant alleles generally encode for some positive attribute (i.e., the product of the allele does something that can be detected). An example would be an allele that encodes for an out-of-control enzyme. In a cell with an allele for a normal enzyme and a second allele for an unregulated enzyme, the phenotype of the cell would be that conferred by the unregulated enzyme in spite of the presence of the normal enzyme. Two or more alleles may be *codominant* if both phenotypes are detected in the heterozygote. The A and B alleles of the ABO blood type are codominant because the heterozygotes are AB. An allele is *recessive* if it is observable only in the homozygote. An individual heterozygous for that allele, therefore, would be a *carrier* of the allele. Although they would not display the phenotype, they would be able to pass it on to their progeny. Recessive alleles generally fail to encode for some positive attribute (i.e., the product of the allele fails to do something that can be detected). An example would be an allele that encodes for an inactive enzyme. In the heterozygote the cells would have both a functional enzyme and a nonfunctional enzyme. Although some effect may be associated with the decreased level of the enzyme activity, the overall phenotype would most likely be of an individual with only the normal functional enzyme.

Punnet Squares

The random segregation of chromosomes into daughter cells during meiosis and the subsequent merging of genomes in gamete fusion result in a reasonably simple and predictable set of gene distributions in the progeny. Since the basic rules for these inheritance patterns were established in the 19th century by Gregor Mendel, the study of patterns of inheritance is often referred to as *mendelian genetics*. The predictions of mendelian genetics are usually expressed as probabilities, and the underlying rationale is made apparent by the use of Punnet squares (Fig. 2-9). Assume that a given gene has two different alleles, *A* and *a*. If an individual is homozygous for the allele (e.g., *AA*), all that individual's gametes will share that allele *(A)*. If that person mates with an individual homozygous for the other allele *(aa)*, all the progeny will be heterozygous for that gene (Fig. 2-9, *A*). If a heterozygote mates with either a homozygote (Fig. 2-9, *B*) or another heterozygote (Fig. 2-9, *C*), approximately half the offspring will be heterozygous and half homozygous. In the former case, however, all of the homozygous progeny will be homozygous for the same allele *(aa)*. In the latter case, approximately a quarter of the progeny will be homozygous for one allele *(aa)* and a quarter for the other allele *(AA)*. If one of these homozygous conditions *(aa)* results in a disease, an offspring from the mating of two heterozygotes would have a one in four chance of having that disease.

Linkage

Because chromosomes segregate as units, two genes with loci on the same chromosome are much more likely to segregate into the same gamete than two genes on different chromosomes. This process is not absolute, however, because meiotic recombination can move a particular allele to a different chromosome. The closer any two loci

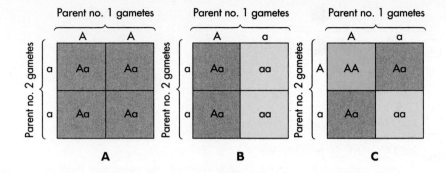

FIG. 2-9   Examples of Punnet squares. **A,** Parents homozygous with different alleles (*AA* and *aa*) will produce only heterozygous progeny (*Aa*). **B,** Heterozygous parent (*Aa*) and homozygous parent (*aa*) will produce homozygous progeny (*aa*) half the time and heterozygous progeny (*Aa*) half the time. **C,** Heterozygous (*Aa*) parents will produce homozygous progeny (*AA* or *aa*) half the time and heterozygous progeny (*Aa*) half the time.

are on a given chromosome, the less likely that meiotic recombination will occur at a site between them and thereby distribute them to different chromosomes. Conceptually, the two loci can be considered to be more or less tightly linked to each other. This *linkage* can be measured as a probability and quantified in centimorgans (cM) as the genetic length resulting in meiotic recombination 1% of the time. Linkage is important in the diagnosis of genetic disorders. Sometimes the actual gene causing a disorder is unknown or its presence cannot be readily assayed. Within a family or larger population, however, the disfunctional gene may be tightly linked to some other locus that can be readily measured (e.g., see later discussion on RFLPs). In these cases the diagnosis is based on the presence of this second, linked locus, and the probability that the diagnosis is correct depends on how tightly the two loci are linked.

GENETIC DISORDERS

Single-gene Disorders

Currently, more than 3000 different genetic disorders involve mutant alleles. These single-gene disorders involve different tissues and organs and are present in approximately 1% of all live births. As a consequence, health care providers in every specialty will encounter these disorders. The enormous number of these disorders precludes any attempt to describe even a small percentage of them. It is important, however, to understand the general principles by which these disorders arise and the patterns of inheritance that might reveal a particular disease to have a hereditary basis. The box on the right lists a few examples of single-gene disorders.

Autosomal dominant disorders

Autosomal dominant disorders are manifested by both homozygous and heterozygous individuals. Individuals

EXAMPLES OF SINGLE-GENE DISORDERS

AUTOSOMAL DOMINANT

Achondroplasia
Familial hypercholesterolemia
Hereditary spherocytosis
Huntington's disease
Marfan's syndrome
Neurofibromatosis type 1
Osteogenesis imperfecta
Polycystic kidney disease
von Willebrand's disease

AUTOSOMAL RECESSIVE

Albinism
Color blindness
Cystic fibrosis
Galactosemia
Glycogen storage disease
Mucopolysaccharidosis
Phenylketonuria (PKU)
Sickle cell anemia
Tay-Sachs' disease

X LINKED

Duchenne's muscular dystrophy
Hemophilia
Ornithine transcarbamylase deficiency

Y LINKED

Gonadal dysgenesis, XY type

MITOCHONDRIAL

Leber's hereditary optic neuropathy
Myoclonic epilepsy and ragged red fiber disease

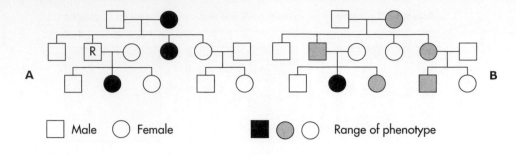

□ Male   ○ Female   ■ ◉ ○   Range of phenotype

FIG. 2-10   Typical pedigrees for a dominant allele with reduced penetrance (male *R*) **(A)** and a dominant allele with variable expressivity **(B).**

homozygous for the mutant allele usually have a much more extreme phenotype. Because the underlying mutations usually arise only infrequently, most cases reflect the inheritance of the disorder from a parent with the disease-associated allele. The pattern of inheritance is, therefore, almost always apparent, and the pedigree readily reveals the lineage of the defect through each succeeding generation (Fig. 2-10, *A*). For autosomal disorders, the gene is on a chromosome other than the X or Y chromosomes, and therefore the trait is usually displayed equally by males and females. Either parent may donate the mutated allele, and all progeny have an equal chance of inheriting the disorder. Despite these odds, the actual distribution may deviate significantly from what would be predicted based strictly on probabilities. The small size of any given family often results in large deviations from the probabilities of inheritance derived for populations. Similarly, phenotypes that are apparent early in life (e.g., achondroplastic dwarfism) may be reperesented by new mutations more frequently than predicted because affected individuals have fewer offspring. Conversely, those phenotypes that develop only late in life (e.g., Huntington's chorea) have traditionally had little effect on reproductive decisions because they could not be diagnosed until after most people had their families.

An autosomal dominant disorder may exhibit a broad range of phenotypes in different individuals. The phenomenon is termed *variable expressivity* and reflects the differences in context (both genotypic and environmental) that a gene experiences in different individuals (Fig. 2-10, *B*). As a result of variable expressivity, some individuals with neurofibromatosis may have many prominent fibromas, whereas other, related individuals may have only a few discolored spots. In some cases, individuals may have the mutated allele but not show the corresponding phenotype at all. The percentage of individuals with a given genotype who display the corresponding phenotype is the *penetrance* of that allele. When an allele has reduced penetrance, a disorder may appear to be arising from a new mutation when it is, in fact, inherited from the previous generation (Fig. 2-10, *A*). Reduced penetrance can make genetic counseling more difficult, since it may not be clear whether an individual has the

mutated allele until the phenotype is seen in the progeny (see male *R* in Fig. 2-10, *A*). Diagnosis is now being made more reliable by direct tests of the DNA either for the mutated allele itself or for a closely linked sequence of DNA.

Neurofibromatosis type 1 is the most frequent autosomal dominant single-gene disorder affecting humans (1:3000). The disorder is highly penetrant, has extremely variable expressivity, and may affect a wide range of organs. Symptoms range from café au lait spots to learning disabilities, mental retardation, and a wide range of malignancies. Of interest, the variability within a family is as great as the variability among families. The gene responsible for the disorder, NF-1, was isolated from human chromosome 17 in 1990. The mutant allele usually arises by mutations in the paternal germline but, unlike disorders such as achondroplasia, is not influenced by paternal age. The high mutation rate has been ascribed in part to the rather large size of the gene (about tenfold larger than most genes) and also to possible local conditions in the DNA. It is thought that the NF-1 product regulates the activity of a protein, p21, in stimulating cell proliferation of many human cells. The loss of NF-1 function would permit p21 to continue to stimulate cell proliferation, resulting in many of the symptoms associated with type 1 neurofibromatosis.

Autosomal recessive disorders

Autosomal recessive disorders are usually apparent in individuals homozygous for the mutated allele, whereas individuals heterozygous for the mutant allele rarely display the disorder-associated phenotype. Because carriers do not display the phenotype, the pedigree usually reveals little of the lineage for the mutated allele through the succeeding generations, but a cluster of affected individuals will appear in a set of siblings (Fig. 2-11). Because the allele is autosomal, the phenotype will be displayed equally by the male and female siblings. When the disorder appears, it reflects the inheritance of the disorder from both parents, each contributing one copy of the disorder-associated allele. The parents both must be heterozygous carriers, and any subsequent children would have a 25% probability of having the disorder and a 50% probability

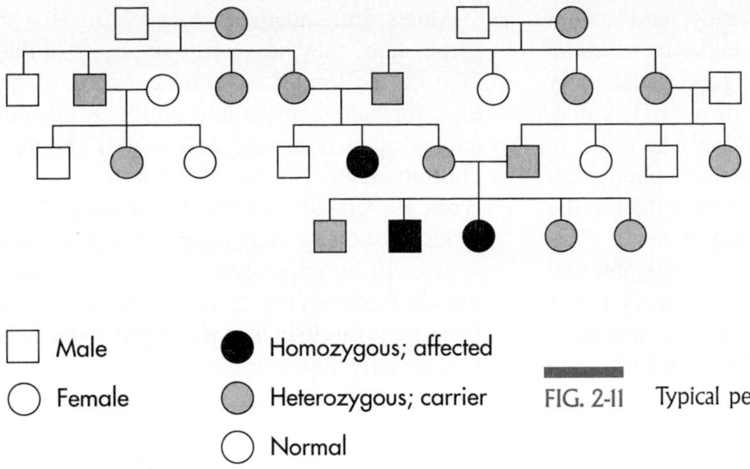

□ Male   ● Homozygous; affected

○ Female   ◐ Heterozygous; carrier

                ○ Normal

FIG. 2-11   Typical pedigree for a recessive allele.

of being a carrier (see Fig. 2-9, *C*). All the offspring of the homozygous recessive individual will obtain at least one copy of the mutated allele. Some autosomal recessive genes are reasonably common (e.g., sickle cell anemia occurs in 1:400 African Americans; cystic fibrosis occurs in 1:2000 Caucasians), and the probability of unrelated heterozygotes marrying and having children with the disorder is significant. Many other autosomal recessive alleles are reasonably uncommon, and the probability of two unrelated heterozygotes having children is very low. When such a rare disorder appears, therefore, family histories may reveal a common ancestor.

Sickle cell anemia is an extremely common autosomal recessive disease in African Americans, with a 1 in 12 frequency of heterozygous carriers of the mutant allele and a 1 in 400 incidence of sickle cell disease in that population. The disease results from a single base-pair change in the coding portion of the β-globin gene on chromosome 11. The substitution of a thymine for an adenine results in the replacement of a glutamic acid with a valine. The resultant change in charge on the protein causes it to deform under low oxygen tensions. This protein deformation decreases the red blood cell (RBC) flexibility and alters the shape to an elongate "sickle," causing them to occlude the vasculature. The lysis and removal of deformed cells lead to anemia, while the vascular occlusions cause organ damage and pain in the bones and joints. Treatment is currently limited to supportive care, including pain management and increased fluid intake. The high frequency of the sickle cell allele has been explained by its ability to confer to the heterozygote increased resistance to malaria. *Malaria* is a major cause of death and debility in those regions where the allele is most common. The heterozygote carrier, therefore, benefits from the increased resistance without undergoing the more profound negative effects associated with the homozygote.

Cystic fibrosis is the most common inherited disease in the Caucasian population, in whom it has a mutant allele frequency of 1 in 20 and a disease incidence of 1 in 2000.

All the known mutations associated with the disease are in the CFTR gene, which was isolated in 1989. CFTR encodes a chloride transporter responsible for the transport of chloride ions across epithelial cells, particularly those lining the pulmonary tree, intestine, pancreas, and apocrine sweat glands. When chloride transport is impeded, the secretions are less hydrated and become extremely viscous. The altered viscosity interferes with organ function. As a consequence, the pulmonary tree retains mucus, which not only directly interferes with gas exchange, but also results in a significant increase in respiratory infections, most often by the bacterium *Pseudomonas aeruginosa.* The median age of death for those afflicted with cystic fibrosis is 26. Death is usually associated with complications of pulmonary infection or right-sided heart failure resulting from pulmonary hypertension. Other organ systems are also affected. In the apocrine sweat glands, chloride reabsorption is affected, leading to an elevated chloride ion concentration in sweat. This provides the basis for the *chloride sweat test,* a convenient, noninvasive test indicating cystic fibrosis. Similarly, the intestinal tract is affected, leading to a range of malabsorptive pathologies, including the neonatal ileum meconium highly associated with the disorder. Treatment is limited primarily to mucolytic agents, vitamins, antibiotics, and other agents providing supportive care designed to alleviate many of the symptoms. In rare cases, heart-lung transplants have sustained the patient. Because cystic fibrosis is an autosomal recessive disorder, it is a good prospect for gene therapy, and efforts are now being directed toward improved delivery and expression in the target tissues (see Chapter 38).

The autosomal recessive disorder *phenylketonuria* (PKU) is caused by a lack of the enzyme phenylalanine hydroxylase (PAH), the gene for which was cloned in 1985. PAH normally converts phenylalanine to the essential amino acid tyrosine. When a functional PAH is lacking, phenylalanine levels increase in the blood to toxic levels and some of the breakdown products are excreted in the urine. If untreated in the neonate, the disorder causes rashes, seizures, growth deficiency, and severe mental retardation. If diagnosed very early in neonatal life, the disorder can be treated with good success by strictly constraining the dietary intake of phenylalanine. As a result, tests for the disorder are routinely included in neonatal screening programs. Unfortunately, phenylalanine is maintained at higher levels in the fetus than in the maternal blood, and fetuses of any genotype in PKU mothers often develop a related syndrome (maternal PKU) despite dietary control of the mother. Nearly 1% of individuals of Northern European descent are heterozygous for 1 of 40 known PKU alleles. The high incidence and multiple types of the PKU alleles have led to the suggestion that a selective advantage may be associated with PKU heterozygosity. In support of this idea, it has been shown that the heterozygous fetus is more resistant to certain fungal toxins that contaminate foods in cool, wet climates.

Sex-linked disorders

Unlike the autosomal chromosomes, the sex chromosomes (X and Y) are not present in two copies for every normal individual. As a consequence, the disorders encoded on these chromosomes are termed *X-linked* if they are encoded on the X chromosome and *Y-linked* if they are encoded on the Y chromosome. As expected, their patterns are distinct from those of autosomal disorders. All normal females have two X chromosomes and no Y chromosomes, whereas all normal males have a single X and a single Y chromosome. Several concepts follow from this. The Y chromosome must encode for functions unique to the male and cannot encode any functions essential for viability. Females must have received an X chromosome from each parent and are equally likely to donate either X chromosome to their children, regardless of gender. Males must have received their X chromosome from their mothers and can only donate it to their daughters.

Males are said to be *hemizygous* for the X chromosome, since they have only one copy of the chromosome. One of the important consequences of hemizygosity is that, for males, any allele on the X chromosome will be expressed as if it were dominant. Females, having two X chromosomes, can have dominant and recessive phenotypes associated with the X chromosome. Therefore disorders associated with recessive alleles on the X chromosome will be expressed in males at a much higher rate than in females (Fig. 2-12, *A*). Males will inherit the trait from their mothers and pass it on to their daughters, who will usually be asymptomatic carriers (see female *C* in Fig. 2-12, *A*). Because only the males will display the phenotype, the trait will appear to skip generations. For some alleles, the associated disorder may be so severe as to be lethal for the male fetus.

If the allele is dominant, a similar pattern will emerge, except females will also display the disorder. When the disorder is lethal for male fetuses, only females will display the phenotype. As with autosomal alleles, the X-linked disorders can display variable expressivity. This phenotypic variability will be most pronounced for females, since their heterozygosity will allow for the normal allele to influence the phenotype (Fig. 2-12, *B*). The range of variability for the female is often greater for the X-linked gene than for autosomal genes because of the phenomenon of X chromosome inactivation.

X chromosome inactivation arises when the developing female fetus reduces the gene dosage associated with having two X chromosomes. Early in fetal development, one X chromosome in each somatic cell is inactivated. When the inactivation occurs, it is random and each X chromosome has a 50% chance of being inactivated. The progeny of these cells, however, always keep the same X chromosome inactive or active as the parent cell. As a consequence, the female will have some cells that express the genes on one X chromosome and others that express the genes on the other X chromosome. This results

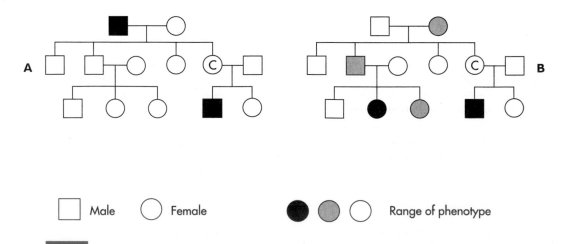

☐ Male   ◯ Female   ● ◐ ◯ Range of phenotype

FIG. 2-12   Typical X-linked pedigrees for a recessive allele **(A)** and a dominant allele with variable expressivity **(B)**. Female *C* is an asymptomatic carrier.

in *mosaics,* in which some cells express only the disorder-associated allele and are affected as profoundly as cells of the hemizygous male. Other cells will express the genes on the other X chromosomes, which will include the normal allele, and these cells, therefore, will be totally unaffected. The clinical symptoms for the heterozygous carrier depend on the percentage of cells inactivating the normal allele for each tissue. This ratio varies depending on the randomness of the initial inactivation process and with any preferences for subsequent cell growth and survival.

One of the most common X-linked disorders is *Duchenne's muscular dystrophy,* with an incidence of 1 in 3500 males. The disorder results in a progressive deterioration of skeletal, cardiac, and in some cases smooth muscle. It is usually diagnosed in the second year of life and progresses with a loss of ambulation by age 11. Death normally ensues by age 20. In all cases the protein dystrophin is missing or reduced. This protein is related to α-actinin and is normally found in all muscle cells and some cells of the central nervous system (CNS). In the neurologic tissues, dystrophin has a different first exon from that in the muscle. The dystrophin gene was cloned in 1987 from the short arm of the X chromosome. The high frequency of mutations is largely attributable to the enormous size of the gene, which, at two megabases, represents 0.1% of the human genome. This is approximately 100 times larger than the average human gene. The large size of the gene reflects both the size of the protein and the amount of the gene allocated to introns. A similar but less severe syndrome, *Becker's muscular dystrophy,* is also associated with the dystrophin gene. Most mutations associated with the two syndromes are deletions or duplications of parts of the gene. As might be predicted, the mutations associated with Becker's muscular dystrophy have a less profound effect on the protein.

Mitochondrial disorders

A different pattern of inheritance arises with disorders associated with nonnuclear genes. In addition to the genes found in the nucleus, the human cell also has genes within the mitochondria in the form of mitochondrial DNA (mtDNA). The mtDNA includes 13 genes required for oxidative phosphorylation and other genes associated with the maintenance and expression of the mtDNA. A somatic cell may have hundreds of mitochondria in it. It has been believed that all these mitochondria are derived from the mitochondria in the ova and none from the spermatozoa. Therefore all the mitochondrial genes would be inherited from the mother and their lineage strictly matriarchal. The resulting disorders would, therefore, also be strictly of matriarchal lineage: all the children of an affected female but none of the children of an affected male would have the disorder. It has now been shown that mice have a low level of paternal mitochondrial transfer. For humans, therefore, mitochondria may also be rarely inherited from the father. As with other types of genetic disorders, mitochondrial disorders may display variable expressivity. The multiplicity of mitochondria in a cell contributes to this variability, since the degree of affliction often represents the percentage of the mitochondria carrying the mutant allele in a particular cell or tissue.

One of the best-studied mitochondrial genetic disorders is *Leber's hereditary optic neuropathy* (LHON), which is usually associated with a single base change in a NADH dehydrogenase gene (ND4). LHON is a maternally inherited adult-onset disease in which blindness results from death of the optic nerve. Characteristically, the peripheral vision is retained, whereas the central vision is lost. The most common mutation can be confirmed by restriction fragment length polymorphism (RFLP) analysis (see later discussion) by the resultant loss of a *Sfa*Ni restriction endonuclease site and the creation of an *Mae*I site.

Another mitochondrial disease is *myoclonic epilepsy and ragged red fiber disease* (MERRF), which results from a mutation in a mitochondrial tRNA gene. The consequent decrease in protein production and the associated decrease in oxidative phosphorylation may cause a progressive disease as patients age and their mitochondrial oxidative phosphorylation capacity declines. The disease is evidenced by an uncontrolled myoclonic epilepsy (periodic jerking) and myochondrial myopathy. Deafness, dementia, and respiratory failure may also occur. The degree of debility and the age of onset are affected in part by the percentage of mitochondria with the defective allele.

Genomic imprinting

In mendelian genetics, it is usually assumed that the expression of any allele is independent of the source of that allele. That is, it should not matter whether a given chromosome came from the mother or the father. It is now becoming apparent, however, that some alleles are altered, presumably during the formation of the sperm or ova, in such a way that the origin of the allele affects the level of expression of that allele throughout the life of the individual. This effect is termed parental or *genomic imprinting.* Some geneticists believe that genomic imprinting is responsible for the lack of parthenogenesis in mammals. *Parthenogenesis* is a reproductive strategy seen in numerous animals such as insects. It allows an animal to reproduce from an unfertilized egg. With imprinted genes, there must be both paternal and maternal chromosomes, or some genes will be expressed at too high a level and others at too low a level.

The *Beckwith-Wiedemann syndrome* is an inherited disorder with an incidence of 1 in 13,770 that appears to be an example of genomic imprinting in humans. In this syndrome, neonates have a variety of craniofacial abnormalities (including a large tongue), umbilical defects, and a high frequency of tumors. Within families the syndrome appears to be associated with a single autosomal dominant gene encoded on chromosome 11. It also occurs sporadically as a partial duplication of a small region of chromosome 11. The pattern of inheritance, however, is odd. It has been suggested that the disorder arises from the overexpression of some or all of the genes in a small region of chromosome 11. Included in this region is IGF-2, an insulin-like growth factor, which stimulates cell metabolism and proliferation. IGF-2 has been shown in mice to be imprinted during ovum formation and is expressed only when it is from the father. Unlike X chromosome inactivation, which affects the entire chromosome, imprinting seems to be gene specific because the nearby gene H19 is imprinted during spermatozoa formation and is expressed only from the maternal chromosome. H19 appears to balance or counteract the action of IGF-2. In humans with Wilms' tumor, the imprinting of the maternal chromosome is changed to that resembling the paternal chromosome. It appears as if the Beckwith-Wiedemann syndrome occurs when one or more paternal genes of the IGF-2 region are overexpressed. A recent investigation of eight sporadic cases of Beckwith-Wiedemann syndrome demonstrated that both copies of chromosome 11 were of paternal origin. In those cases where extra copies of this region are found, the extra copy is usually of paternal origin.

Multifactorial Disorders

Most genetic disorders do not appear to follow any of the patterns of inheritance previously described. Diseases such as coronary heart disease and breast cancer often tend to run in families without any clear pattern. The obscurity of the pattern results from both the strong influence of extrinsic factors (e.g., diet, exposure to mutagens) and frequently the polygenic requirements underlying the disorder. For these multifactorial disorders, multiple genes may be required to contribute in an additive or synergistic manner to create the final phenotype. Because these genes may be on different chromosomes, their conjunction in any one individual is much less predictable. Furthermore, the diseases may also require a particular environmental influence so that they are expressed only after some form of chemical or physical injury. Because the confluence of any particular set of genes is so difficult to predict and because the experiences for any given individual may be so variable, the occurrence of a disorder is difficult to predict and the determination of the underlying genetic contributions is similarly complicated.

Despite these obstacles, the search to understand multifactorial disorders is extraordinarily important. These disorders are extremely common, probably representing more afflictions than all the single-gene disorders and chromosomal abnormalities combined. As a consequence, advances made in the diagnosis and treatment of these disorders will have a correspondingly great impact on the health of the entire population. The role of extrinsic factors is also important, since changes in behavior may profoundly influence the likelihood of the individual

subsequently developing the disorder. Identification of the contributing intrinsic genetic factors, therefore, will provide the diagnostic tools that can alert the individual before the onset of any symptoms to initiate behavioral interventions to avoid or delay the development of the more serious complications of the disorder.

Chromosomal Disorders

Chromosomal disorders include abnormalities in both chromosome number and chromosome structure. An abnormal number of chromosomes, *aneuploidy,* involve the gain or loss of one or more chromosomes, usually arising from nondisjunction during cell division. Defects in chromosome structure reflect major changes in the content of a chromosome and can be generated by a number of mechanisms. One of the most common structural changes, translocation, typically arises from meiotic recombination (see previous discussion) or during the recombinational events required for the maturation of the immune system. The pathologies resulting from chromosomal disorders may reflect changes in gene dosage (gene number), changes in gene regulation, or the formation of mutant genes.

Aneuploidy usually results in a somatic cell having either only a single copy of a chromosome *(monosomy)* or three copies of a chromosome *(trisomy).* Aneuploidy is quite common, occurring in 3% to 4% of all recognized pregnancies, including first-term spontaneous abortions. The most common trisomy is *Down's syndrome (trisomy 21),* which usually arises from nondisjunction during meiosis of the maternal germline. The frequency of this trisomy increases dramatically with maternal age, rising from approximately 0.1% in mothers 30 years of age to 1% by age 40 and to nearly 4% by age 45. Now that the chromosomes derived from each parent can be identified, it has also become apparent that *advanced paternal age* carries an increased risk of abnormal chromosomal segregation. Abnormal chromosomal segregation (meiotic nondisjunction) may be paternal in origin in 33% of trisomic individuals. The syndrome is apparent at birth and results in morphologic changes, mental retardation, and personality alterations. Aneuploidies of sex chromosomes are also frequent (approximately 0.2% of live births), but the consequences may not be apparent until puberty or later in life. Common examples are 47,XXY males *(Klinefelter's syndrome)*, 45,X females *(Turner's syndrome),* 47,XXX females, and 47,XYY males.

Structural disorders include large deletions, duplications, inversions, and translocations. These abnormalities can usually be seen in a karyotype analysis of chromosome structure and banding patterns of the affected cells. Partial deletion of the short arm of chromosome 5 produces a unique syndrome called *cri-du-chat* (cry of the cat). Hypoplasia of the larnyx produces a weak, shrill cry during infancy that sounds like the mewing of a cat. Infants with cri-du-chat commonly exhibit low birth

TUMORS RESULTING FROM CHROMOSOMAL STRUCTURAL CHANGES

NONFUSIONS (INTACT GENES MOVED NEAR A PROMOTER)

Acute lymphocytic leukemia
B cell lymphoma
Burkitt's lymphoma
Chronic lymphocytic leukemia
Diffuse large-cell lymphoma
Follicular lymphoma
Non-Hodgkin's lymphoma
Prolymphocytic leukemia

GENE FUSIONS (TWO GENES FUSED TOGETHER)

Acute lymphocytic leukemia
Acute mylogenous leukemia
Acute promyelocytic leukemia
Acute undifferentiated leukemia
B cell lymphoma
Chronic myelomonocytic leukemia
Chronic mylogenous leukemia
Ewing's sarcoma
Liposarcoma
Melanoma
Myelodysplasia
Myeloid
Non-Hodgkin's lymphoma
Papillary thyroid carcinoma
Rhabdomyosarcoma
Synovial sarcoma
T cell lymphoma

c-MYC protein and turns on other genes in the cell, leading to cancer. Similarly, many T cell acute leukemias arise from the translocation of other transcription factor genes to a locus adjacent to other genes active in immune cells. Many leukemias and lymphomas arise by translocations (see box on left). This is because many genes specifically expressed by cells of the immune system normally require structural changes (deletions or other rearrangements) to become functional. The pathologic translocations, therefore, represent errors in a normal process.

Translocations, deletions, and inversions may also cause the formation of a new gene. In these cases the breaks in the chromosome occur within genes, and when the ends are rejoined, a new gene is encoded by the fusion of these two DNA fragments. These gene fusions encode for *chimeric proteins,* which combine parts of the functions of the two contributing genes. In many of these cases, one of the contributing genes is a transcription factor. The chimeric protein may now retain its ability to increase the expression of other genes, but the protein responds differently to regulatory signals within the cell. The fusion of a particular gene with another gene may result in different tumors, depending on the identity of the two genes. For example, in *Ewing's sarcoma*, a gene termed *EWS* may fuse with the transcription factor genes ERG or FL11. However, when the EWS gene fuses with the transcription factor gene ATF-1, a malignant melanoma results. Conversely, when the transcription factor gene ERG fuses with the FUS gene, acute mylogenous leukemia may result.

DIAGNOSIS AND PREVENTION

Diagnosis

Progress in the understanding of human molecular genetics is initiating a shift in health care from postsymptomatic treatment to disease prediction and prevention. With the evolution of these new diagnostic tools, potential problems can be detected by prenatal screening, before the onset of symptoms in the neonate, or at very early stages of disease in the older individual. The prenatal diagnosis of a potentially lethal condition gives the parents the opportunity to choose termination of the pregnancy. The prenatal diagnosis of correctable abnormalities allows the family to plan neonatal management strategies, including surgery and referral to special care centers. For diagnoses made after birth, counseling can lead to life-style changes early in the course of diseases that can delay or avoid the onset of symptoms. It can be anticipated that the continued evolution of these diagnostic tools for genetic disorders will also raise new ethical questions that will need to be confronted by patients, their health care providers, and society in general. Among these are likely to be changes in health, life, and disabil-

weight, microcephaly with severe mental retardation, and failure to thrive. In some cases, translocations may involve the exchange of chromatid fragments between two different chromosomes (e.g., chromosome 21 and chromosome 22). Because genetic information is rearranged and not lost, the rearrangement is considered balanced for that individual. Although such individuals usually appear normal, a high proportion of their gametes have an unbalanced set of chromosomes. As a consequence, these individuals may experience a high rate of spontaneous abortions or have children with physical abnormalities resulting from the unbalanced rearrangement.

Structural disorders, particularly translocations, in somatic cells can also lead to cancer by two basic mechanisms. In one case, a gene encoding a transcription factor may be moved adjacent to the promoter for another gene. A good example of this is *Burkitt's lymphoma,* which usually arises from a translocation event in which a gene encoding the transcription factor c-MYC is brought near the promoter for the antibody genes. When such a cell expresses this gene to make antibody, it produces the

ity insurance. It is, therefore, helpful to understand some of the methods already in use and those emerging in the diagnosis of these diseases.

Phenotypic screening

Many genetic disorders can be diagnosed by a phenotype that they generate. This allows for the more or less direct measure of the consequences of metabolic and physiologic disorders. Therefore cystic fibrosis currently is diagnosed by the chloride sweat test (see earlier discussion on autosomal recessive disorders) and PKU by determining phenylalanine concentrations in the neonate's blood.

Some developmental disorders can be diagnosed prenatally by changes in phenotype. Neural tube defects and ventral wall defects often lead to an elevation of the α-fetoprotein concentrations in the maternal serum. The basis for this is somewhat less direct than the chemical tests mentioned earlier. α-Fetoprotein is a glycoprotein normally produced only in fetal tissues. Because any α-fetoprotein found in the maternal serum originates in the fetus, the concentration in the maternal serum can be suggestive of the state of the fetus. Neural tube and ventral wall defects allow the fetal internal organs either to come in direct contact with the amniotic fluid or to be separated from it by only a thin membrane. Thus the level of α-fetoprotein in the amniotic fluids is elevated in these disorders, and this elevation is reflected with abnormally high concentrations in the maternal serum. Although it is important to keep in mind that the α-fetoprotein levels can also be elevated for other causes (e.g., multiple fetus pregnancies), the concentrations in maternal serum can be an important first indicator of a disorder. Some of these neural tube defects are strongly associated with chromosomal aberrations, such as trisomy 13, trisomy 18, and triploidy. It is interesting to note that the α-fetoprotein levels in maternal serum may be low in patients with Down's syndrome. One of the advantages of screening for α-fetoprotein in the maternal serum is that it is noninvasive of the fetus. Furthermore, coupled with an indicated fetal karyotype analysis, more than 80% of significant neural tube defects can be detected within the first two trimesters.

In addition to sampling maternal serum, the phenotypes of developmental abnormalities can also be detected by ultrasonography. Various structural disorders become detectable at different stages. A few can be detected in the first trimester, but most structural disorders (e.g., spina bifida, hydrocephaly) are first detectable in the second trimester. Some disorders (e.g., heterozygous achondroplasia) are not clearly detectable until the third trimester.

Fetal cell sampling

Although much can be inferred from samples of the maternal serum and visualizations of the fetus by ultrasound, the actual genetic analysis of an individual, whether fetus or adult, requires the acquisition of the DNA. This almost always requires sampling methods that yield intact cells. In prenatal diagnosis, this is usually accomplished by either amniocentesis or chorionic villus sampling.

Amniocentesis, as practiced for more than 40 years, involves using a needle to remove amniocentesis fluid, usually early in the second trimester. The fluid consists largely of fetal urine but also has sloughed off cells from the skin and developing mucosal membranes. Historically, these cells have been collected aseptically and grown for 2 to 3 weeks in the laboratory before genetic testing. This period of growth has been required to obtain sufficient DNA for testing and also allows the cells to be arrested in metaphase for karyotyping.

Chorionic villus sampling (CVS) involves the direct acquisition of cells, not from the fluid, but from the villi of chorion frondosum of the placental bed. This sampling technique, which has been widely used only for the past 10 years, has the advantage of being able to be performed late in the first trimester. Cells are removed from the villi either transcervically with a catheter or transabdominally with a needle. CVS yields more cells than amniotic fluid, a greater percentage of the cells are viable, and these cells are more rapidly dividing. In some cases, karyotype analysis can be accomplished in 24 to 48 hours without growth of the cells. In other cases, the growth period is considerably less (1 to 2 weeks) than that required for samples obtained by amniocentesis. Because the actual site of the sampling is the placenta and not the fetus, nonrepresentative samples (e.g., mosaicism) can be obtained in the sample that are not present in the fetus.

When a rapid determination of karyotype is important (e.g., after findings of CVS mosaicism) or the diagnosis of the disorder rests on hemotologic findings (e.g., some genetically undefined forms of β-thalassemia), fetal blood can be obtained. This is usually done by sampling the umbilical cord (*cordocentesis*) in a manner analogous to amniocentesis. Similarly, other fetal tissues (skin, liver, muscle) have been obtained for enzyme analysis when the genetic defect has not been defined.

A still largely experimental technique is *preimplantation embryo analysis.* In this technique, an embryo arising by in vitro fertilization is allowed to develop to the four- or eight-cell stage, and then a few cells are removed by micromanipulation. These cells are grown in parallel with the embryo until they can be analyzed for a genetic defect. If found free of the defect (this has been done for several cases of suspected cystic fibrosis), the embryo is implanted and a normal fetus develops. The technique has exciting possibilities in reducing both physical and psychologic trauma and in offering reproductive options to couples at risk for genetic diseases but for whom premature termination of a pregnancy is not an acceptable choice.

Molecular genetic analysis

Although the chemical analysis of fluid and tissue samples has allowed for important gains in prenatal analysis, the diagnostic strategies that are evolving most

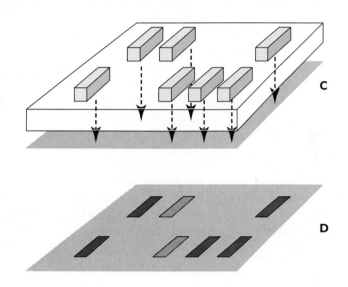

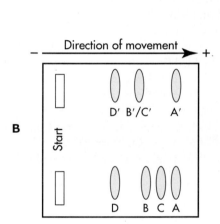

FIG. 2-13   Restriction fragment length polymorphism (RFLP) analysis. **A,** DNA from two individuals is digested with a restriction endonuclease (in this case *Eco*RI), producing DNA fragments with lengths of 1000, 1500, 2000, and 6000 base pairs for one set of DNA and lengths of 1000, 3500, and 6000 base pairs for the other. The difference is attributable to the substitution of a G for an A, which destroys the restriction site between fragments B and C for the second individual. **B,** DNA fragments are separated electrophoretically according to their rate of migration through the gel. **C,** DNA fragments are transferred (blotted) from the gel onto a membrane. **D,** Fragment B is detected by using a DNA probe complementary to the fragment B DNA. If a particular mutation is designated by the open box (⬜), it would be closely linked to the presence of the 3500-base-pair fragment. Any member of a related population having the 3500-base-pair fragment would therefore be likely to also have the mutation.

rapidly and hold the greatest future promise are based on molecular genetics. The direct detection of mutations is difficult, however, since in most cases the responsible gene(s) is not known. In those cases for which the gene responsible for a disease is known, the corresponding allele could, theoretically, be obtained from the patient's cells and sequenced. Although this process would reveal all mutations in a gene, it is too slow and expensive for diagnostic purposes. As a consequence, a variety of techniques have emerged to screen for particular mutations.

The most common of these techniques is *restriction fragment length polymorpism* (RFLP) analysis (Fig. 2-13). RFLP analysis is normally carried out directly on that DNA extracted from cells. As such, it requires the DNA from many cells and, hence, the need to grow cells obtained by amniocentesis. The procedure is based on the ability of a class of enzymes, termed *restriction endonucleases,* to cut DNA at specific sites. Each enzyme has its own specific set of sites, all of which have the same sequence of bases. As an example, the restriction enzyme *Bam*HI cuts DNA within the sequence GGATCC, whereas the restriction enzyme *Eco*RI cuts DNA within the sequence GAATTC. In each of these examples, the

base sequence recognized by the enzyme is six bases long. These sites, therefore, occur at an average of once in every 4096 base pairs (4^6), and a single digestion of a cell genome with one of these enzymes would yield approximately a million unique fragments. These fragments can be sorted according to their length by forcing them through a gel matrix with an electric current. This process, known as *gel electrophoresis,* allows the smaller DNA fragments to move through the gel faster and, therefore, progress further. The two strands of the DNA fragments can then be separated by adjusting the pH and the salt concentration and blotted onto a nitrocellulose or nylon membrane. A particular band can be located on the membrane by using *Southern hybridization,* in which a labeled DNA probe is allowed to bind to the DNA fragments stuck onto the membrane. Because the probe DNA will bind to the appropriate affixed DNA by hydrogen bonding between complementary base pairs, the binding will be specific.

RFLP analysis is rarely used as a direct measure of a particular genetic mutation. Usually a particular mutant allele will be associated with a closely linked RFLP within a given pedigree. The RFLP analysis demonstrates whether a given individual has inherited a particular RFLP. This subsequently is interpreted to determine the probability that the individual has also received the linked, mutant allele. Sometimes, however, the RFLP is a direct detection of the mutation. A good example of this is in the diagnosis of sickle cell disease by using the enzyme *Mst*II, which recognizes the sequence CCTNAGG (where N is any nucleotide). In the disease the *A* is the base most frequently substituted. Therefore the gain and loss of a restriction site can be used to determine if an individual is heterozygous or homozygous for the mutant allele.

The development of the *polymerase chain reaction* (PCR) has radically altered the potential for molecular genetic analyses. PCR provides for the enzymatic amplification of DNA so that a single strand of DNA can be accurately copied into millions of identical strands within hours. The theory of PCR is quite simple (Fig. 2-14). Briefly, the DNA to be amplified is placed in a tube with a special DNA polymerase (often the enzyme Taq polymerase), the nucleotides needed to make more DNA, and a high concentration of a specific set of short, single-stranded pieces of DNA called *primers.* The sequence of the primers is complementary to specific sites flanking the region to be amplified. The tube is heated to separate (melt) the two strands of the DNA to be amplified and then cooled enough to allow specific complementary base pairing *(annealing)* to occur. Because the primers are the most plentiful, they bind to their complementary sites on the DNA before the other strand can bind. The DNA polymerase can now extend the 3′ end of the primer, copying the original DNA. Each time the tube is heated and cooled, the process is repeated, the number of copies is doubled, and each copy can serve as a template for the next round. Since repeating the cycle 20 times yields more than 1 million copies, a much smaller sample size is needed than described for RFLP analysis. PCR, however, does require specific primers and can usually only amplify a short section of DNA.

PCR can yield samples for RFLP analysis and, more

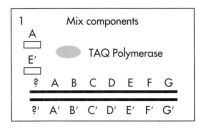

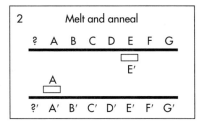

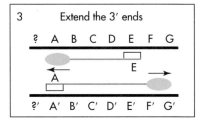

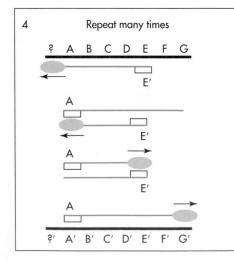

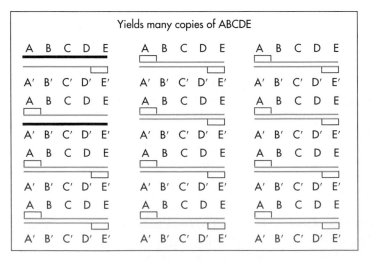

FIG. 2-14   Amplification of DNA by the polymerase chain reaction (PCR).

important, has led to the development of a wide variety of new tests. These tests include single-strand conformation polymorphism (SSCP), ligation chain reaction (LCR), allele-specific oligonucleotides (ASOs), heteroduplex analysis (HET), cleavage fragment length polymorphisms (CFLP), and ribonuclease (RNase) mismatch cleavage. Although a description of these procedures is beyond the scope of this chapter, the reader should appreciate that these and others will become a part of their vocabulary in the near future. The availability of these tests will lead to the rapid and inexpensive diagnosis of many genetic disorders. An important adjunct of this information is that the precise identification of the lesions as provided by these procedures will also allow for the effective application of gene therapy.

Gene Therapy

In the past the diagnosis of genetic disorders has provided few options for patients, their families, or their health care providers. Counseling could help couples decide whether to have children, whether to terminate pregnancies, and what changes to their life-style could prolong or improve the quality of life of the afflicted individual. The era is now beginning in which the underlying causes of these disorders can be corrected. The goals of gene therapy are to replace or correct for genetic defects. These changes may be transient or permanent.

Patients with recessive disorders are the most likely candidates for *replacement therapy*. These individuals generally produce a nonfunctional protein, too little of a protein, or no protein at all. In theory, therapy merely involves placing additional, functional copies of the gene in the cell to replace the function of the defective gene. In practice, targeting the gene to the correct cells is often problematic and, even more important, ensuring the appropriate regulation of the new gene is even more difficult. In some cases the cells targeted for gene therapy are removed from the patient and the new gene is put into the cell ex vivo. Although entry of the gene into the cells may be accomplished mechanically or chemically, the delivery of the new genes to the target cells is most often accomplished by packaging the genes into viruses in place of some viral genes. The virus brings the gene into the cell and inserts the gene into the recipient cell chromosome. Because the virus has lost key genes, it cannot replicate in the new host cell and, therefore, cannot cause disease. When a viral delivery system is used, the target cell specificity of the virus can ensure that the appropriate cells receive the new gene, allowing the infection to be carried out in vivo.

The first human gene therapy approved by the National Institutes of Health (NIH) was conducted in 1990 on a young girl with severe combined immunodeficiency that resulted from the lack of a functional adenosine deaminase, encoded by the gene ADA. The failure to deaminate adenosine leads to toxic levels of adenosine in T cells.

One of the advantages of this disorder is that the normal range of ADA gene expression is very broad, varying 500-fold among individuals. As a consequence, obtaining acceptable levels of expression was less problematic. To carry out the therapy, the normal genes of a retrovirus were removed and replaced with a functional ADA gene. Peripheral T cells were obtained from the girl by venipuncture, and the cells were infected with this modified virus. The virus inserted the new ADA gene into the recipient T cell chromosome. After four rounds of this therapy, the girl developed acceptable levels of T cells in her blood and could begin a normal life after years of isolation. Studies since 1993 have used stem cells from the umbilicus of neonates known to be afflicted with the disorder. These cells appear able to populate the bone marrow and provide an even more stable source of T cells. Gene replacement therapy is also being tested for cystic fibrosis and other genetic diseases.

Dominant disorders may be treated with replacement therapy or may require some form of correction therapy. Familial hypercholesterolemia, which results from the lack of the low-density lipoprotein (LDL) receptor, is being treated by a replacement therapy protocol in which hepatocytes are infected ex vivo with a retroviral vector carrying the functional LDL gene. The need for correction therapy is associated with either the overproduction of a protein or the production of an abnormal protein, the dysfunction of which leads to the disorder. In these patients either the defective gene can be replaced by exchanging it with a corrected gene, or the overproduction of a gene can be down-regulated. A broadly applicable strategy for controlling the overproduction of a protein is the use of antisense genes. When an antisense gene is expressed, the mRNA made is the complement (i.e., antisense) of the mRNA for a defective gene it is designed to control. The antisense mRNA forms complementary base pairs with the mRNA encoded by the defective gene. As a result, the ribosome will not be able to bind to the mRNA, and no protein will be made. Antisense genes limit the expression of the defective gene by controlling its translation.

In addition to congenital defects, gene therapy is also being applied to various somatic cell mutations that result in cancer. In some cancer therapies the tumor cells are returned to near-normal patterns of regulation by the gene replacement of a tumor suppressor gene (e.g., p53) that is defective in these cells. Control of regulation in the cell can also be accomplished by inserting an antisense gene. In other strategies the tumor cells become labeled by receiving a completely new gene that causes them to present a new molecule on their surface. This allows the immune system to recognize these cells more readily and respond more robustly against them. A strategy being employed against some brain tumors is to make the tumor cells susceptible to an antiviral drug. The genes are delivered to the tumor by injecting into the tumor fibroblasts engineered to produce a retrovirus continually, which in turn will bring the thymidine kinase gene into the tumor cells. The thymidine kinase gene renders these cells sensitive to the drug gancyclovir. An interesting aspect of this therapy is that a strong "bystander" effect occurs. Because these cells form gap junctions, the tumors regress in 50% of the cases even when only 10% of the tumor cells express the thymidine kinase gene. In still other procedures the cells targeted for gene therapy are not the defective cells but are cells of the immune system that normally control and prevent these tumors. In this strategy, T cells directed against the tumor are isolated from the patient and genetically modified to produce high levels of tumor necrosis factor (TNF). When these cells are returned to the patient, they infiltrate the tumor and deliver concentrations of TNF locally to the tumor, which would be toxic to the patient if administered systemically.

Gene therapy also has its associated problems. Whenever a gene is inserted, there is the risk of generating new mutations from the insertion. This can be limited by the use of adeno-associated viruses that always cause the insertion into a known site in chromosome 19 or by adenoviruses that do not insert. There is concern that the viral vectors may interact with normal viruses the patient encounters during or after therapy and that a recombinant virus could result. In part, this has been limited by stringent quality controls in the production of the viruses and by a prudent choice of vectors (e.g., no herpesvirus protocols have been considered). A different problem arises in cases of correcting for gene deletions. In this situation, the expression of a new gene in a cell may cause that cell to be recognized as foreign by the recipient. If this occurs, cells producing the protein may be attacked by the recipient's immune system in a manner identical to organ transplant rejection.

Philosophically and ethically, gene therapy can be divided into two broad categories. In somatic cell gene *insertion* the genes of the recipient's somatic cells are modified by either replacement or addition. Because the changes are confined to the recipient, such therapy can be thought of in terms analogous to organ transplants. In contrast, the *modification* of the genes of germline cells necessarily involves changes in the genomes of future generations. Each of these categories presents a unique set of ethical problems that are currently being intensely debated. As a consequence, the Recombinant DNA Advisory Committee of the NIH at this time is not considering any proposals that would modify human germline cells.

QUESTIONS

▼ *Answer the following on a separate sheet of paper.*

1. Describe the flow of genetic information from mother cell to daughter cells at the molecular (replication) and cellular (meiosis and mitosis) levels.
2. Describe the flow of genetic information from DNA to RNA (transcription) and protein (translation), including key enzymes, specific sites, and regulators.
3. What determines whether an allele is dominant or recessive?
4. Construct a Punnet square for the mating of two heterozygotes (*Bb* with *Bb*), where *B* is the normal allele and *b* is a recessive mutant allele. What is the probability that a progeny would have the mutant phenotype?
5. How does X chromosome inactivation contribute to variable expressivity for females?
6. Why are translocations often associated with hematologic cancers?
7. What are the advantages and disadvantages of chorionic villus sampling compared with amniocentesis?
8. How can antisense genes be used in correcting dominant disorders?

▼ *Circle the letter preceding each item below that correctly completes the statement. More than one answer may be correct.*

9. Extrinsic factors in disease include:
   a. Infectious agents
   b. Age
   c. Race
   d. Toxins
10. Karyotype analysis can determine:
   a. The number of each type of chromosome
   b. Large structural changes to chromosomes
   c. Gender
   d. The presence of single base-pair mutations
11. When the same mutation causes different degrees of disease among individuals in a given population, it is said to exhibit:
   a. Mosaicism
   b. Penetrance
   c. Variable expressivity
   d. Dominance

12. An individual with only a single copy of a given gene is _____ for that gene.
   a. Autosomal
   b. Homozygous
   c. Heterozygous
   d. Hemizygous
13. The high frequency of muscular dystrophy has been attributed to:
   a. The large size of the gene
   b. X chromosome inactivation
   c. Genomic imprinting
   d. Trisomy 18
14. To prevent their expression in the progeny, genes may be modified during the formation of ova and spermatozoa by the process of:
   a. X chromosome inactivation
   b. Genomic imprinting
   c. Parthenogenesis
   d. Translocations
15. Patterns of inheritance are most difficult to recognize in:
   a. Mitochondrial disorders
   b. X-linked disorders
   c. Autosomal recessive disorders
   d. Multifactorial disorders

QUESTIONS—cont'd

16. The disorder most frequently associated with aneuploidy is:
    a. Down's syndrome
    b. Muscular dystrophy
    c. Sickle cell anemia
    d. Cystic fibrosis

17. Diagnosis of developmental disorders by α-fetoprotein concentrations:
    a. Requires a direct sampling of the fetal serum
    b. Uses samples acquired by amniocentesis
    c. Is not affected by the presence of a multiple-fetus pregnancy
    d. Is an indirect measure of phenotype

18. Preimplantation embryo analysis has the advantage of:
    a. Permitting genetic analysis before pregnancy
    b. Sampling the genotype, not the phenotype
    c. Being invasive of only the mother
    d. Not posing any risk to the embryo

19. Among the potential risks associated with gene therapy are:
    a. The formation of new mutations when a gene is inserted
    b. The formation of new viruses
    c. Immune rejection of cells carrying new genes

▼ Circle T if the answer is true and F if it is false. Correct any false statements.

20. T F Unlike RNA, DNA is usually a short-lived, single-stranded molecule.

21. T F The chromosome consists of DNA and proteins.

22. T F Splicing of hnRNA is part of the process of forming mRNA.

23. T F Enhancers are binding sites for transcription factors that will increase the expression levels of a gene.

24. T F Autosomal chromosomes are those chromosomes found in nongermline cells.

25. T F Meiotic recombination contributes to genetic diversity.

26. T F Mutations in germline cells are more likely than similar mutations in somatic cells to generate profound phenotypes.

27. T F Autosomal recessive disorders often appear to skip generations.

28. T F X-linked disorders are more common in females.

29. T F Female progeny are more likely than male progeny to display mitochondrial disorders.

30. T F The frequency of trisomy 21 increases greatly with maternal age.

31. T F RFLP analysis is usually a direct measure of mutation.

32. T F Persons with recessive disorders are less likely than those with dominant disorders to be good candidates for replacement therapy.

33. T F PCR has strongly influenced molecular diagnosis of genetic disorders by eliminating the need to obtain the patient's DNA.

▼ Match the genetic disorder in column A with the type of defect in column B.

Column A	Column B
34. _____ Leber's hereditary optic neuropathy	a. Translocations
35. _____ Klinefelter's syndrome	b. Mitochondrial
36. _____ Leukemia	c. Genomic imprinting
37. _____ Down's syndrome	d. Aneuploidy
38. _____ Myoclonic epilepsy and ragged red fiber disease	
39. _____ Beckwith-Wiedemann syndrome	

▼ Match the genetic condition in column A with the type of inheritance in column B.

Column A	Column B
40. _____ Phenylketonuria	a. X-linked
41. _____ ABO blood group	b. Autosomal dominant
42. _____ Sickle cell anemia	c. Autosomal recessive
43. _____ Cystic fibrosis	d. Codominant
44. _____ Neurofibromatosis type 1	
45. _____ Muscular dystrophy	

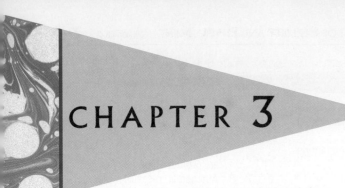

CHAPTER 3

Cellular Injury and Death

GERALD D. ABRAMS

CELLULAR ORGANIZATION

Although the body contains many different types of cells with highly specialized functions, all cells, to a large extent, have similar life-styles and similar structural elements. They have parallel requirements for oxygen and nutrient supplies, for a constant temperature, for water supply, and for a means of waste disposal. The cell is literally the unit of life, the smallest entity that manifests the various phenomena associated with living. Therefore the cell is also the basic unit of disease.

The organization of a hypothetic "typical" cell is diagramed in Fig. 3-1. The cell is bounded by a cell membrane, which gives the cell its shape and attaches it to other cells. The cell membrane is the gateway to and from the cell, allowing only certain things to pass in either direction and even actively transporting some things in a selective fashion. The cell membrane also receives many of the control signals from around the body and transmits these signals to the interior of the cell.

Within the cell is the *nucleus*, which serves as the control center because the deoxyribonucleic acid (DNA) is concentrated within it. The instructions coded within the nuclear DNA are actually executed within the *cytoplasm*, the portion of the cell outside the nucleus. The cytoplasm is a watery medium containing many structures so small that they can be seen only with an electron microscope. These ultramicroscopic organs are called *organelles*, and they are highly specialized as to function even within the confines of a single cell.

The *mitochondria* are organelles devoted to energy production within the cell. They are the power plant of the cell. Within them, various foodstuffs are oxidized to produce the driving force for other cellular activities. The *endoplasmic reticulum* and *Golgi apparatus* constitute a sort of manufacturing, processing, and plumbing system within the cytoplasm. The endoplasmic reticulum is a network of interconnecting tubules and cisterns, and the Golgi complex is a closely related array of flattened cisterns and associated vesicles. Protein synthesis is carried out along the endoplasmic reticulum under control of ribonucleic acid (RNA) in the *ribosomes*. The cytoplasmic RNA is produced and directed by nuclear DNA to act as a kind of assembly team in relation to the executive role of the DNA. The ribosomes carry out protein synthesis by assembling amino acids into complex molecules according to the directions supplied by the DNA. The Golgi apparatus is a packaging device that wraps the cell products for export (secretion) or for storage within the cell. Certain glycoprotein complexes are also elaborated within the Golgi apparatus. The *lysosomes* are membrane-bound packages of digestive enzymes prepared by the cell and held inactive until needed. Still other organelles not shown in Fig. 3-1 account for additional special functions within the cell, such as providing rigidity and movement in the manner of a musculoskeletal system. The various organelles represent a total organism in microcosm, and their activity must be closely coordinated and controlled to preserve cellular integrity.

Individual cells relate to one another in a variety of ways as they assemble into tissues and organs. Some tis-

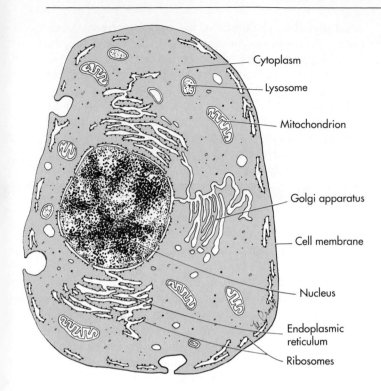

FIG. 3-1 Diagram of a hypothetic typical cell. The structural basis for division of labor within the cell is shown. It should be noted that in the living body, the cell membrane not only bounds the cell and controls access to the interior, but also joins the cell with others to form tissues.

Cytoplasm
Lysosome
Mitochondrion
Golgi apparatus
Cell membrane
Nucleus
Endoplasmic reticulum
Ribosomes

sues, such as lining or covering epithelia, consist of densely packed cells directly and tightly adherent to one another with little intervening space. Groups of cells of this type are soft and pliable and could not maintain the form of various organs or the strength of the entire body. It is actually connective tissue that holds the body together because of its *intercellular substance*—literally, material between the cells. This substance includes *collagen,* which is a protein produced in the form of extremely tough fibers (similar to those in tendons and ligaments), and *elastin,* which is also a protein assembled into fibers, but which also has elastic properties. Between these fibers is a gelatinous matrix, or *ground substance.* The combination of tough and elastic fibers and the matrix gives the body its strength, form, and resiliency. In the skeleton the intercellular substance is impregnated with calcium salts, producing the rigid bony support of the body.

MODALITIES OF CELLULAR INJURY

Cells can be injured or killed in many ways, but important types of injury tend to fall into just a few categories.

One of the most common factors in cellular injury is a *deficiency of oxygen or other critical nutrient material.* Cells depend on a continuous supply of oxygen, because it is the energy of oxidative chemical reactions that drives the machinery of the cell and maintains the integrity of the various components of the cell. Therefore without oxygen the various maintenance and synthesizing activities of cells quickly come to a halt.

A second type of injury is *physical,* which involves actual disruption of cells or at least disturbance of the usual spatial relationships among the various organelles or of the structural integrity of one or more types of organelles. Thus mechanical and thermal means of injury are significant causes of human disease.

Living *infectious agents* constitute a third means of cellular injury, and particular organisms injure cells in a variety of ways.

Finally, *chemical agents* are a common means of cellular injury. Not only do toxic substances find their way into cells from the environment, but accumulation of endogenous substances (as with genetically determined metabolic "errors") also may injure cells.

THE CELL UNDER ATTACK

When an injurious stimulus is applied to a cell, the first important effect is a *biochemical lesion.* This involves a change in the chemistry of one or more metabolic reactions within the cell. Few types of injury are actually understood at this initial level. Although biochemical changes can be noted in injured cells, often the abnormalities noted are second- or third-order effects rather than evidence of the primary biochemical lesion. When a biochemical lesion is established, the cell may or may not manifest a functional abnormality. In the case of many injuries, the cell possesses sufficient reserve to perform without significant functional impairment; in other instances, there can be a failure of contraction, secretion, or other activities of the cell. Particularly important determinants in this regard are the extent of impairment of energy production (with adenosine triphosphate [ATP] depletion) and the extent of impairment of cell membrane functions.

A cell with biochemical and functional abnormalities may or may not display a detectable morphologic change. The limitation here is one of technique. Changes that are evident on routine microscopic examination are generally late changes, since many biochemical and functional abnormalities may have occurred before the anatomic abnormality became evident. With the advent of electron microscopy, increasingly earlier detection of microscopic lesions of the various organelles is becoming possible. However, with presently available techniques, many functionally impaired cells may not yield evidence of their impairment in morphologic terms.

The result of an attack on a cell is not always impairment of function. In fact, there are cellular mechanisms of adaptation to various kinds of adversity. For example, a common reaction of a muscle cell placed under abnormal stress is to increase strength by enlargement, a process called *hypertrophy*. Thus the heart muscle cells of an individual with high blood pressure will enlarge to cope with the strain of pumping against increased resistance. A similar type of adaptation occurs in regard to certain chemical challenges. Barbiturates and certain other substances are usually metabolized in liver cells, under the influence of enzyme systems found within these cells in association with the endoplasmic reticulum. An individual taking barbiturates often has a striking increase in the amount of endoplasmic reticulum within liver cells, and this is associated with an increased enzyme content in these cells and an increased ability to metabolize the drug.

MORPHOLOGIC CHANGES IN SUBLETHALLY INJURED CELLS

When cells are injured but not killed, they often manifest easily identifiable morphologic changes. These sublethal changes are at least potentially reversible. That is, if the injurious stimulus can be withdrawn, the cells return to their previous state of health. On the other hand, these changes may be a step toward cell death if the noxious influence cannot be corrected. Sublethal changes in cells are traditionally called *degenerations* or *degenerative changes*. Although any cells of the body may manifest such changes, metabolically active cells such as those in liver, kidney, and heart are typically involved. Degenerative changes tend to involve the cytoplasm of cells, whereas nuclei maintain their integrity as long as the cell is not lethally injured. Although an extremely large number of injurious agents or specific ways of attacking cells exist, the repertory of morphologic expression of injury is actually quite limited.

The most common form of cellular degenerative change involves the *accumulation of water* within the affected cells. The injury in effect causes loss of volume control on the part of the cells. To maintain constancy of its internal environment, a cell must expend metabolic energy to pump sodium ions out of the cell. This occurs at the level of the cell membrane. Anything that disturbs energy metabolism in the cell or slightly injures the cell membrane may render the cell unable to pump out a sufficient amount of sodium ions. The natural osmotic result of increased intracellular concentration of sodium is an influx of water into the cell. The result is a morphologic change termed *cellular swelling*. A previous name for this change was cloudy swelling, because an organ whose cells suffered this change acquired a peculiar parboiled appearance grossly, and the affected cells acquired an unusual granular appearance of the cytoplasm microscopically. When water accumulates within the cytoplasm, the cytoplasmic organelles also absorb it, causing mitochondrial swelling, dilation of the endoplasmic reticulum, and so forth.

Microscopically, the changes of cellular swelling are quite subtle and involve simply an enlargement of the cell and slight change in its texture. The gross counterpart of this is the enlargement of the affected tissue or organ, which is usually detectable by a moderate increase in weight. If the noxious influence producing cellular swelling can be removed, after a time the cells usually begin to extrude sodium, and along with it water, and the volume returns to normal. This change is only a slight perturbation in the normal state of affairs.

If a severe influx of water occurs, some of the cytoplasmic organelles, such as the endoplasmic reticulum, may be converted into water-filled sacs. When examined under a microscope, the cytoplasm of the cell is seen to be vacuolated (Fig. 3-2). This is termed *hydropic change* or sometimes vacuolar change. The gross appearance of affected organs and the significance of the change are identical to those of cellular swelling.

A more significant change than simple cellular swelling involves the intracellular accumulation of lipid within affected cells. This type of change usually involves the kidneys, heart muscle, and liver, particularly the latter. Microscopically, the cytoplasm of the affected cells appears vacuolated in a manner similar to that seen in hydropic change, but the content of the vacuoles is lipid instead of water. In the case of the liver, the amount

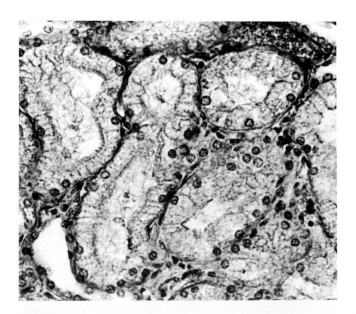

FIG. 3-2   Hydropic change in renal tubular epithelium. The epithelial cells lining these convoluted tubules are enlarged and have vacuolated, lacy-appearing cytoplasm because of intracellular accumulation of water. (Photomicrograph, ×500.)

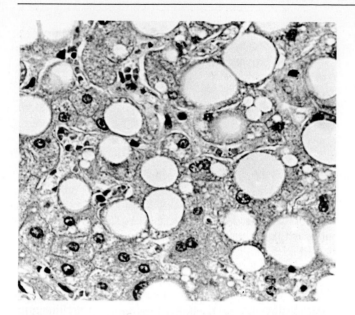

FIG. 3-3   Fatty change in liver. Many liver cells have several small "holes" in their cytoplasm or a single huge vacuole that distorts the entire cell. These apparently empty spaces once contained abundant lipid, which was dissolved during histologic preparation. The liver cells at the lower left are virtually normal. (Photomicrograph, ×500.)

of lipid accumulating within a cell is often relatively large, so that the nucleus of the cell is pushed to one side and the cytoplasm of the cell is occupied by one lipid-containing vacuole (Fig. 3-3). The counterpart of such changes with respect to the gross appearance of affected tissues involves swelling of the tissues, increase in weight of the affected organ, and often a distinct yellowish cast to the tissue caused by the contained lipid. Severely affected livers are often bright yellow and greasy to touch. This type of change is called *fatty change* or *steatosis* (or sometimes fatty degeneration or fatty infiltration).

Steatosis occurs often because it can be produced by so many different mechanisms, particularly in the liver. Hepatocytes (and other types of cells) normally are involved in an active metabolic exchange of lipids. These substances are constantly mobilized from adipose tissue into the bloodstream, from which they are extracted by the liver cells. Some of the lipid absorbed by the cell is oxidized, whereas some of it is combined with protein synthesized by the cell and then exported from the cell (i.e., into the bloodstream) in the form of lipoprotein.

Accumulation of fat within the cell can be produced by interfering with the usual exchange processes at any of several points. For example, if an excess of lipid is presented to the liver cell, the metabolic and synthetic capabilities of the cell may be exceeded, and then the lipid will accumulate intracellularly. If, on the other hand, normal amounts of lipid reach the cell but oxidation is im-

paired by some cellular injury, lipid will accumulate. Finally, if the process of lipoprotein synthesis and export is interfered with at any of several points, lipid will also accumulate. For these reasons, a fatty liver may be encountered in diverse situations, ranging from malnutrition, which impairs protein synthesis, to overfeeding, which swamps the liver with lipids. Hypoxia sufficiently impairs cellular metabolism to produce fatty accumulation, and numerous toxic substances from the environment affect the cells in such a manner as to promote lipid accumulation. One of the most potent and widespread toxins in our environment that produces fatty livers is alcohol. This substance is directly toxic to liver cells, as well as being indirectly injurious to individuals whose alcohol intake is extreme, since this often leads to malnutrition. Fatty change is potentially reversible, but it frequently reflects a severe injury to the cell and, thus, is a step on the way to cell death.

Another response of cells under attack is to undergo a reduction in mass, literally a shrinkage. Such an acquired reduction in the size of a cell, a tissue, or an organ is referred to as *atrophy*. The atrophic cell or tissue seems to be able to achieve an equilibrium under the adverse conditions imposed on it by reducing the total demand it must meet. Grossly, atrophic tissues or organs are smaller than normal.

In the course of becoming atrophic, the cell must absorb some of its constituent parts. This involves *autophagocytosis* or *autophagy*, literally a self-eating process, in which enzymes digest portions of the cell contained within cytoplasmic vacuoles. This same process occurs not only in the cell undergoing atrophy, but also in the "wear and tear" of everyday cellular existence. When cytoplasmic organelles become damaged, they are sequestered within cytoplasmic vacuoles and digested enzymatically. The digestion process tends to leave traces of residual indigestible material, which gradually accumulate within the cells. This material is derived for the most part from membranous structures within the cells and generally has a dark-brown color. As cells age, they accumulate more and more of this intracytoplasmic pigment, referred to as *lipofuscin, aging pigment,* or *wear-and-tear pigment*. As cells become atrophic, lipofuscin may become even more concentrated because of increased autophagocytic activity. Sometimes the atrophic tissue is pigmented even grossly; the process responsible is called *brown atrophy*. Insoluble residual material may also accumulate as the result of *heterophagocytosis* or *heterophagy*, which is the cellular uptake of materials from outside the cell.

A discussion of degenerative changes must inevitably focus on the topic of aging. Clearly, the process of aging or senescence is exceedingly complex and involves many genetic, endocrine, immunologic, and environmental factors. The process is poorly understood at all levels, that is, from the level of the whole individual down to the level of single cells. It has been postulated that aging may result from an actual genetic limitation on the replicative ability of cells, coupled with the progressive accumulation of small injuries in cells that no longer proliferate. However, it has not yet been possible to identify any cellular features specific to the process of aging, and the true functional implications of even the nonspecific changes are not known.

CELLULAR DEATH

If a noxious influence on a cell is severe enough or continued long enough, the cell will reach a point at which it can no longer compensate and cannot carry on metabolically. At some hypothetic point of no return, the processes become irreversible and the cell is in effect dead. At this hypothetic instant of death, when the cell just reaches the point of no return, it may not be possible to recognize morphologically that the cell is irreversibly dead. However, if a group of cells that has reached this state remains in the living host for even a few hours, additional events occur that permit the recognition of the cells or the tissue as being dead. All cells have within them a variety of enzymes, many of them lytic. While the cell is alive, these enzymes do no damage to the cell, but they are released when the cell dies and begin to dissolve various cellular constituents. In addition, as the dead cells change chemically, the living tissues immediately adjacent respond to the changes and mount an acute inflammatory reaction (see Chapter 4). Part of this latter reaction is the delivery of many leukocytes or white blood cells to the area, and these assist in the digestion of the dead cells. Thus from their own digestive enzymes or as a result of the inflammatory process, the cells that have reached the point of no return begin to undergo discernible morphologic changes.

When a cell, a group of cells, or tissue in a living host is recognizably dead, it is referred to as *necrotic*. Necrosis, therefore, represents local cell death.

Morphologic Changes of Necrosis

In general, although the lytic changes in necrotic tissue may involve the cytoplasm of cells, the nuclei manifest the changes most clearly indicative of cell death. Typically, the nucleus of the dead cell shrinks, develops an irregular outline, and stains densely with the usual dyes used by pathologists. This process is referred to as *pyknosis,* and the nuclei are said to be *pyknotic.* Alternatively, nuclei may crumble, leaving scattered fragments of chromatin material within the cell. This process is referred to as *karyorrhexis.* Finally, in some instances, the nuclei of dead cells lose their staining ability and simply disappear, the process being referred to as *karyolysis* (Fig. 3-4).

The morphologic appearance of necrotic tissue varies, depending on the results of lytic activities within the dead

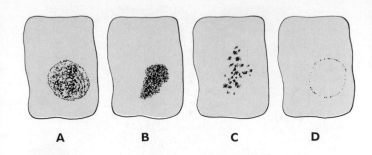

FIG. 3-4   Nuclear changes in cell death. The morphologic changes most clearly indicative of cell death involve the nucleus. **A,** Normal nucleus; **B,** pyknotic nucleus; **C,** karyorrhectic nucleus; and **D,** nucleus that has undergone karyolysis.

tissue. If the activity of lytic enzymes is inhibited somewhat by local conditions, the necrotic cells will maintain their outline and the tissue will maintain its architectural features for some time. This type of necrosis is called *coagulative necrosis* and is particularly common when necrosis has been caused by deprivation of blood supply (Fig. 3-5). In general, coagulative necrosis is the most frequently encountered type of necrosis. In some instances, the necrotic tissue gradually liquefies by enzymatic action; the process is called *liquefactive necrosis.* This is likely to occur in an area of necrotic brain, and the result is literally a hole in the brain filled with fluid (Fig. 3-6). In other situations, the necrotic cells disintegrate but the finely divided cellular fragments remain in the area for months or even years, virtually undigested. This type of necrosis is referred to as *caseous necrosis* because the affected area has the appearance of crumbly cheese when viewed grossly (Fig. 3-7). A standard situation giving rise to caseous necrosis is tuberculosis, although this type of necrosis can arise in many other situations.

Certain special local conditions produce other variants of necrosis. *Gangrene* is defined as coagulative necrosis, usually caused by deprivation of blood supply, with superimposed growth of saprophytic bacteria. Gangrene occurs in necrotic tissues that are exposed to living bacteria. This is common in the extremities (Fig. 3-8) or in a segment of bowel that becomes necrotic (Fig. 3-9). Sometimes the shriveled, blackened tissue of a gangrenous area on an extremity is described as being the seat of *dry gangrene,* whereas on an internal area that cannot become desiccated, it is designated as *moist gangrene.* In either situation the process involves the growth of saprophytic bacteria superimposed on necrotic tissue.

Necrotic adipose tissue constitutes another special case. If the duct system of the pancreas is ruptured, either by trauma or in the course of spontaneous disease of the pancreas, the pancreatic enzymes ordinarily carried within the duct may be spilled into the surrounding tissues. The secretions of the pancreas contain many powerful hydrolytic enzymes, including lipases that cleave the lipids of adipose tissue. When this cleavage occurs,

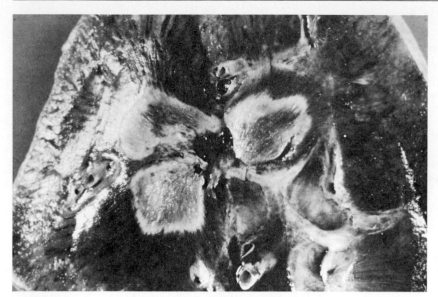

FIG. 3-5   Coagulative necrosis. In this close-up of the cut surface of a kidney, three pale areas of necrosis can be seen approximately in the center of the field. The architectural outlines are obviously maintained in the dead tissue, hence the designation of coagulative necrosis. (Because the renal papillae are involved, this condition is specifically termed *renal papillary necrosis.*)

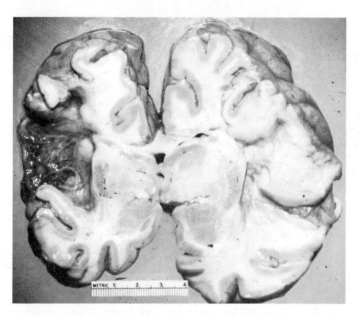

FIG. 3-6   Liquefactive necrosis. A large defect is seen at the left in this section of the brain. The brain substance in this area became necrotic because of deprivation in the blood supply. As is generally true in this organ, the necrotic tissue gradually softened, then liquefied, leaving a permanent defect.

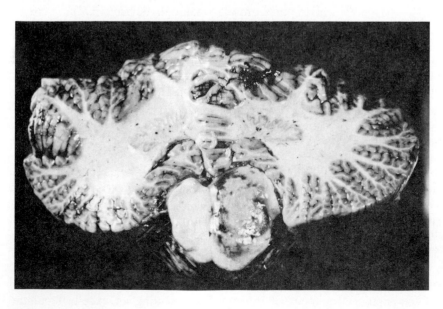

FIG. 3-7   Caseous necrosis. A large necrotic area is evident in the brain stem at the right of center. In this instance the dead tissue crumbled but did not liquefy. Because of an apparent gross resemblance to cheese, this type of necrosis is termed *caseous.* (This particular lesion was the result of tuberculosis, one of many causes of caseation.)

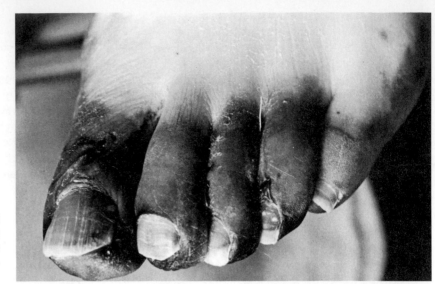

FIG. 3-8   Gangrene. The toes of this foot have become necrotic because of poor blood supply. Saprophytic microorganisms are growing in the blackened dead tissue. On the extremities, gangrene of this type is frequently termed *dry*.

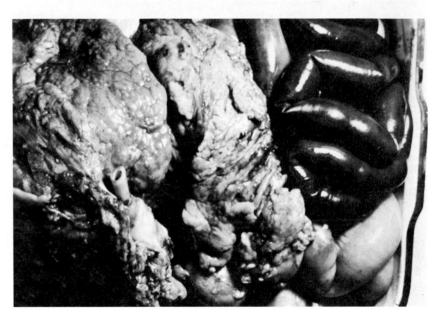

FIG. 3-9   Gangrene. In this instance a major portion of small intestine has been deprived of its blood supply. The gangrenous loops of intestine at the upper right contrast with the viable ones at the lower right. Saprophytes flourish in the necrotic tissue. Internal gangrene of this type is inevitably *moist* as contrasted to that on the extremities.

free fatty acids are formed by enzymatic action and these are rapidly combined with cations (e.g., calcium ions) in the area, producing deposits of soaps. This enzymatic (or pancreatic) fat necrosis is largely restricted to the abdominal cavity, since this is the area exposed to leaking pancreatic enzymes. If adipose tissue elsewhere becomes necrotic, spillage of lipid from the dead cells may evoke an inflammatory response but there is no formation of the yellow, chalky deposits characteristic of enzymatic fat necrosis.

In recent years, another pattern of cell death referred to as *apoptosis* has been recognized. This form of cell death is actually programmed by genetic information already within the cell; that is, the events leading to cell death are triggered by gene activation or by release of some process from normal inhibition. Apoptosis can be triggered by a variety of extrinsic injurious stimuli, but it can also be part of the physiologic relationship of cell populations. The process usually involves single cells or groups of a few cells, and as the cells die, they fragment into membrane-bound pieces that are rapidly phagocytosed by adjacent cells or macrophages. The process is morphologically subtle, with little or none of the obvious inflammatory response seen in conjunction with various patterns of necrosis.

Effects of Necrosis

The most obvious effect of necrosis is loss of function in the dead area. If the necrotic tissue represents a small fraction of an organ with a large reserve (e.g., the kidney), there may be no functional impact on the body, whereas if the area of necrosis is in a portion of brain, a severe neurologic deficit or even death might result. In addition, the necrotic area in some instances can become a focus of infection, representing an excellent culture medium for the growth of certain organisms that might then spread elsewhere in the body. Even without becoming infected, the presence of necrotic tissue within the body may evoke certain systemic changes (e.g., fever), increased numbers of leukocytes within the circulating blood, and a variety of subjective symptoms. Finally, the necrotic tissue often leaks its constituent enzymes into the bloodstream as the cells die and the permeability of cell membranes increases. It is possible to analyze a specimen of blood and determine the level of various enzymes, such as creatine phosphokinase (CPK), lactic dehydrogenase (LDH), or aspartate aminotransferase (AST). Then an increased level of one or another enzyme may indicate that the patient has an area of necrosis hidden deep in some tissue. This principle has given rise to an important diagnostic field, *clinical enzymology*.

FATE OF NECROTIC TISSUE

When an area of tissue becomes necrotic, the event usually evokes an *inflammatory response* from the adjacent tissues (see Chapter 4). As a result of this inflammatory response, the dead tissue is ultimately demolished and removed, making way for the reparative process that replaces the necrotic area with regenerating cells of the sort lost or, in many instances, with scar tissue. If the necrotic tissue is located on a body surface (e.g., along the lining of the gastrointestinal tract), it may slough off, leaving a gap in the continuity of the surface, which is referred to as an *ulcer*. Finally, if the necrotic area is neither demolished nor cast off, it often is encapsulated by fibrous connective tissue and ultimately is impregnated with calcium salts precipitated from the circulating blood in the area of necrosis. This process of calcification may lead to the necrotic area becoming stony hard and remaining so for the life of the individual.

PATHOLOGIC CALCIFICATION

The deposition of insoluble calcium salts from the bloodstream, which renders tissues rigid and hard, is perfectly normal in the formation of bones and teeth. When such a phenomenon occurs elsewhere, it is abnormal and is referred to as *pathologic calcification* or *heterotopic calcification*. This may occur in several situations.

Dystrophic Calcification

Often, as described earlier, injured tissue or necrotic tissue that is not quickly demolished may become a site of calcification. This particular form of calcification is referred to as *dystrophic*. Because an area of caseous necrosis by its very nature remains undigested for long periods, it typically becomes calcified. Thus because tiny foci of

tuberculosis or other infections occur in the lung and in the lymph nodes draining the lung, small foci of dystrophic calcification often appear in these areas. They are not particularly important biologically, but they often appear on radiographs because of the opacity of the dense deposits of calcium salts. Another common site of dystrophic calcification is in the wall of arteries that have become atherosclerotic (see Chapter 7). In fact, the texture of this "hardening of the arteries" is caused by the calcium deposition. Calcium salts also tend to deposit, with advancing age, in previously cartilaginous areas such as the rib cartilages. Ultimately, dystrophic calcific deposits in any location may undergo actual conversion to bone; the process is called *heterotopic ossification*.

Metastatic Calcification

Calcium salts may also be deposited in the soft tissues of the body in the absence of prior tissue damage or necrosis. This type of calcification is referred to as *metastatic calcification*. This process occurs not because of an abnormality of tissues, but because an abnormal concentration of calcium and phosphorus salts exists within the circulating blood. Specifically, if the concentration of these substances rises beyond a certain critical level, their solubility product is exceeded and precipitation occurs in a variety of tissues, especially lung, kidney, stomach, and the walls of blood vessels. The concentrations of calcium and phosphates in the blood are affected by activity of the parathyroid glands, renal function, intake of calcium and vitamin D in the diet, and the integrity of the skeleton. Thus metastatic calcification may be seen with hyperparathyroidism, decreased renal function, abnormal diet, and destructive lesions of the skeletal system that liberate large quantities of calcium salts from the bones.

Stone Formation

Calcium salts may also be deposited in the form of stones, or *calculi,* within the duct systems of a variety of organs. Calculi may be formed from calcium or from a variety of other locally available substances within the secretions of the particular organ. Thus although they frequently contain calcium as one constituent, many calculi are not primarily calcific. Some calculi form as a result of encrustation of necrotic debris within a duct, whereas others form because of an imbalance in the constituents of a particular secretion so that there is precipitation from what is ordinarily a dissolved state. For a variety of reasons, therefore, calculi are often encountered in the biliary tract (Fig. 3-10), the pancreas, the salivary glands, the prostate, and the urinary system.

Although calculi are often silent and discovered incidentally if at all, many move along the duct system of the particular organ and cause pain and bleeding. Calculi may lodge in the narrow part of the duct system and produce obstruction of the outflow of the particular secretion. When this occurs, there is often infection

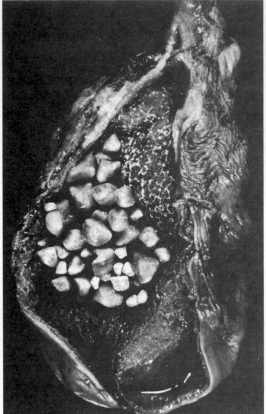

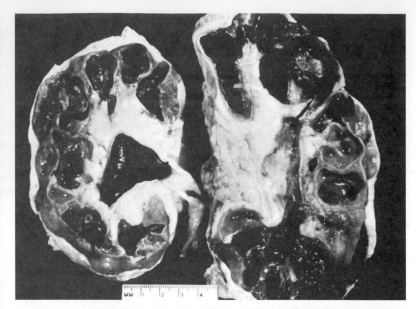

FIG. 3-11 Renal calculi. Numerous large stones are present within the calyces and pelvis of these hemisected kidneys. The associated obstruction of urine flow and infection have led to marked loss of renal parenchyma.

FIG. 3-10 Gallstones within the gallbladder. Calculi of this type are composed largely of bile pigments and cholesterol. It is apparent that stones of this size may be propelled into the common bile duct, where they can obstruct the flow of bile.

of the obstructed organ and atrophy of the parenchyma (Fig. 3-11).

SOMATIC DEATH

Death of the entire individual, as contrasted to localized death or necrosis, is referred to as *somatic death*. In the past the definition of somatic death was a relatively simple matter. An individual was declared dead when "vital functions" such as heart action and respiration ceased beyond any chance of reversal. Thus if an individual stopped breathing and could not be resuscitated, the heart rather quickly stopped beating as a result of anoxia and the individual was indisputably dead. Today, with technologic advances, a patient can be attached to a mechanical ventilator if breathing stops. If the patient's heart begins to falter, an electronic pacemaker may be put in place. With such "life-sustaining" machinery available, the definition of death becomes a different matter. In fact, not all cells of the body die at once. Living tissue cultures have been established from tissues removed from corpses. In hospitals today, a common definition of so-

matic death concerns the activity of the central nervous system, specifically the brain. Clearly, if the brain is actually dead, there is no chance for the subject to regain a conscious existence. Such "brain death" involves irreversible loss of responsivity, including certain key reflexes, and irreversible loss of electrical activity, as indicated by an isoelectric or "flat" electroencephalogram (EEG). When the absence of electrical activity has been demonstrated for a predetermined period under rigidly defined circumstances, medical authorities consider the patient dead despite the fact that the heart and lungs could be kept going artificially for some time.

Postmortem Changes

After death, certain so-called postmortem changes ensue. Because of a chemical reaction in the muscles of the dead subject, a stiffness called *rigor mortis* develops. The phrase *algor mortis* refers to the inevitable cooling of a dead subject as the body temperature approaches environmental temperature. Another set of changes is referred to as *livor mortis* or postmortem lividity. Generally, such lividity results because when the circulation stops, the blood within the vessels settles according to the pull of gravity, and the tissues lowermost in the body develop a purple discoloration because of their increased content of blood. At a microscopic level, as the individual tissues within the corpse die, their enzymes are released locally and lytic reactions begin. These reactions, termed *postmortem autolysis* (literally self-dissolution), are very similar to the changes seen in necrotic tissue but, of course, are not accompanied by an inflammatory reaction. Finally, unless prevented by special measures (e.g., embalming), massive bacterial overgrowth and putrefaction will occur. The speed of onset of various postmortem changes is extremely variable, depending on individual and associated environmental characteristics. Thus the amazingly accurate pinpointing of the time of death by medical authorities in detective fiction is largely just that—fiction.

QUESTIONS

▼ *Circle the letter preceding each item below that correctly completes the statement. More than one answer may be correct.*

1. The part of the cell that serves as the control center because DNA is concentrated within it is the:
   a. Cell membrane   c. Mitochondria
   b. Cytoplasm   d. Nucleus

2. Within the cytoplasm of the cell, protein synthesis is carried out in association with:
   a. Lysosomes
   b. Endoplasmic reticulum
   c. Mitochondria
   d. Lipofuscin granules

3. The first significant effect of an injurious stimulus applied to a cell is referred to as:
   a. Degeneration
   b. Functional abnormality
   c. Biochemical lesion
   d. Hypertrophy

4. Structural alterations in cells that are reversible include all the following except:
   a. Cloudy swelling or cellular swelling
   b. Hydropic change
   c. Fatty infiltration
   d. Karyolysis

5. Accumulation of lipid within liver cells may be related to:
   a. Starvation of the patient
   b. Excessive alcohol intake by the patient
   c. Obesity
   d. Toxic injury to liver cells
   e. All the above

6. An increase in the size of a tissue or an organ because of an increase in the size of the individual cells without an increase in the number of component cells would be termed:
   a. Atrophy   c. Autophagocytosis
   b. Hypertrophy   d. Karyolysis

7. The process by which dystrophic calcification undergoes conversion to bone is:
   a. Heterotopic ossification
   b. Heterophagy
   c. Metastatic calcification
   d. None of the above

8. The death of cells or tissue within a living host is:
   a. Somatic death   c. Necrosis
   b. Putrefaction   d. Inflammation

9. Necrosis that results in a cheeselike appearance of affected tissue because of disintegration of the dead cells and that is frequently caused by tuberculosis is termed:
   a. Liquefactive necrosis
   b. Caseous necrosis
   c. Coagulative necrosis
   d. Enzymatic fat necrosis

10. A common type of necrosis caused by deprivation of blood supply is termed:
    a. Coagulative necrosis
    b. Caseous necrosis
    c. Enzymatic fat necrosis
    d. Liquefactive necrosis

11. Gangrene is most likely to develop in a large area of ischemic necrosis in the:
    a. Heart   c. Brain
    b. Pancreas   d. Intestine

12. A type of calcification that occurs when damaged or dead cells cannot be eliminated from the body is:
    a. Dystrophic   c. Calcinosis
    b. Metastatic   d. Hypertrophic

13. Enzymatic fat necrosis is usually found in the:
    a. Lungs
    b. Abdominal cavity
    c. Kidney
    d. Wall of the arteries

14. Cellular uptake of materials from outside the cell is:
    a. Metastatic calcification
    b. Calculi
    c. Heterophagy
    d. Autophagy

15. Dystrophic calcification occurs in the:
    a. Soft tissues of the body in the absence of prior tissue damage
    b. Atherosclerotic arteries
    c. Duct systems of several organs
    d. Lung in an area of caseous necrosis

▼ *Fill in the blanks with the correct words.*

16. The sequence of events involved in cellular degeneration includes _____, _____, and finally _____ alterations.

17. Somatic death concerns the activity of the _____ system, especially the _____.

18. Two major categories of pathologic calcification are _____ and _____.

19. After death, a chemical reaction in the muscles causing them to stiffen produces _____.

▼ *Match the type of necrosis in column A with its characteristic manifestation or description in column B.*

Column A	Column B
20. _____ Coagulative necrosis	a. Massive necrosis with superimposed bacterial growth
21. _____ Liquefactive necrosis	b. Characteristic of tuberculosis or fungal infections
22. _____ Caseation	c. Events leading to cell death triggered by gene activation
23. _____ Enzymatic fat necrosis	d. Characteristic necrosis of heart and kidney resulting from ischemia
24. _____ Gangrene	e. Related to rupture of the pancreatic duct system
25. _____ Apoptosis	f. Characteristic of brain

CHAPTER 4

Response of the Body to Injury

INFLAMMATION AND REPAIR

GERALD D. ABRAMS

INFLAMMATORY REACTION

Whenever cells or tissues of the body are injured or killed, as long as the host survives, the surviving adjacent tissues make a striking response called *inflammation.* More specifically, inflammation is a vascular reaction whose net result is the delivery of fluid, dissolved substances, and cells from the circulating blood into the interstitial tissues in an area of injury or necrosis.

There is a natural tendency to view inflammation as something undesirable, since an inflamed throat, skin, soft tissue, or the like can cause considerable discomfort. However, inflammation is actually a beneficial and defensive phenomenon. The net result is the neutralization and elimination of an offending agent, the demolition of necrotic tissue, and the establishment of conditions necessary for repair and restitution. The beneficial character of the inflammatory reaction is dramatically demonstrated by what happens when the body cannot produce a needed inflammatory reaction, for example, when it becomes necessary to administer high dosages of drugs that also suppress such reactions. Under these conditions, a high incidence of extremely severe, rapidly spreading, or even lethal infections is caused by ordinarily harmless microorganisms.

The inflammatory reaction is actually a dynamic and continuous succession of well-coordinated events. To manifest an inflammatory reaction, a tissue must be alive and in particular must possess a functional microcirculation. If an area of tissue necrosis is extensive, the inflammatory reaction will be found not in its midst but rather at its edges, that is, at the interface between the dead tissue and living tissue with an intact circulation. Also, if a particular injury kills the host instantly, no evidence exists of an associated inflammatory reaction, because this would take time to develop.

The causes of inflammation are numerous and varied, and it is essential to understand that *inflammation and infection are not synonymous.* Thus *infection* (the presence of living microorganisms within the tissue) is just one cause of inflammation. Inflammation can easily occur under conditions of perfect sterility, such as when a portion of tissue dies because of deprivation of blood supply. Because of the broad range of situations that result in inflammation, an understanding of the process is basic to much of biology and health care. Without an understanding of the process, it is impossible to comprehend the principles of infectious disease; the principles of surgery, wound healing, and the response to a variety of trauma; or the principles of how the body copes with catastrophes of tissue death such as cerebrovascular accidents (CVAs, strokes), "heart attacks," and the like.

Despite the large number of causes of inflammation and the variety of situations in which it appears, the events set in motion generally tend to be the same, with various types of inflammation differing in their quantitative detail. Therefore the inflammatory reaction can be studied as a general phenomenon, and the quantitative variations can be dealt with secondarily.

GROSS FEATURES OF ACUTE INFLAMMATION

Acute inflammation is the immediate response of the body to injury or cell death. The gross features were described some 2000 years ago and are still known as *cardinal signs of inflammation;* they include redness, warmth, pain, and swelling, or in the classic Latin, *rubor,*

calor, dolor, and *tumor.* A fifth cardinal sign, altered function, or *functio laesa,* was added in the past century.

Rubor (Redness)

Rubor, or redness, is usually the first thing to be noted in an area becoming inflamed. As the inflammatory reaction begins, the arterioles supplying the area dilate, thus allowing more blood into the local microcirculation. Capillaries previously empty or perhaps only partly distended quickly become packed with blood (Fig. 4-1). This condition, termed *hyperemia* or *congestion,* accounts for the local blush of acute inflammation. The production of hyperemia at the start of an inflammatory reaction is controlled by the body both neurogenically and chemically, via the release of substances such as histamine.

Calor (Heat)

Calor, or heat, parallels the redness of an acute inflammatory reaction. Actually, heat is a characteristic only of inflammatory reactions at the body surface, which is normally cooler than the 37° C core temperature. An area of cutaneous inflammation becomes warmer than its surroundings because there is more blood (at 37° C) being conducted from the inside of the body to the surface in the affected area than there is in a normal area. This phenomenon of local warmth is not observed in inflamed areas deep within the body, since such tissues are already at

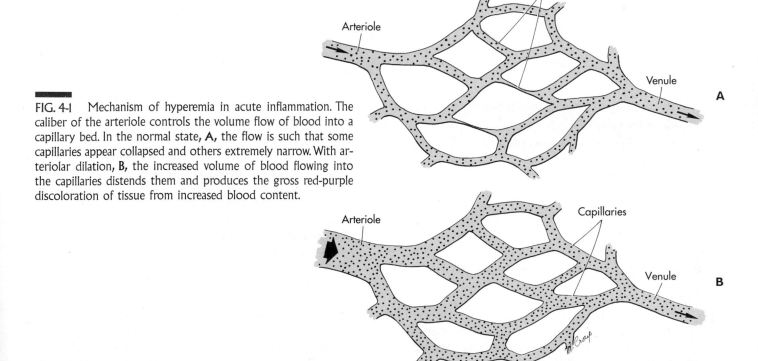

FIG. 4-1   Mechanism of hyperemia in acute inflammation. The caliber of the arteriole controls the volume flow of blood into a capillary bed. In the normal state, **A,** the flow is such that some capillaries appear collapsed and others extremely narrow. With arteriolar dilation, **B,** the increased volume of blood flowing into the capillaries distends them and produces the gross red-purple discoloration of tissue from increased blood content.

the core temperature of 37° C and local hyperemia would make no difference.

Dolor (Pain)

The dolor, or pain, of an inflammatory reaction is probably produced in a variety of ways. Change in local pH or in the local concentration of certain ions can stimulate nerve endings. Similarly, the release of certain chemicals, such as histamine or other bioactive chemicals, can stimulate the nerves. In addition, swelling of inflamed tissues leading to increased local pressure can undoubtedly produce pain.

Tumor (Swelling)

Perhaps the most striking aspect of acute inflammation is the tumor, or local swelling produced by fluid and cells transferred from the bloodstream to the interstitial tissues. This mixture of fluid and cells that accumulates in an area of inflammation is called an *exudate*. Early in the course of inflammatory reactions, most of the exudate is fluid, such as that which appears quickly within a blister after a minor burn of the skin. Somewhat later, white blood cells, or leukocytes, leave the bloodstream and accumulate as part of the exudate.

Functio Laesa (Altered Function)

Functio laesa, or altered function, is a familiar part of the inflammatory reaction. In a superficial way, it is easy to understand why a swollen, painful part with an abnormal circulation and abnormal local chemical environment should function abnormally. However, we do not understand in detail the means whereby function of an inflamed tissue is impaired.

FLUID ASPECTS OF INFLAMMATION

Exudation

To understand the rapid flux of fluid across vessel walls into inflamed tissue, it is necessary to recall the principles governing normal fluid transport. Ordinarily, the walls of the smallest vascular channels (e.g., capillaries, venules) allow small molecules to pass but retain large molecules, such as plasma proteins, within the vascular lumen. The semipermeable character of the vessels produces an osmotic force that tends to keep fluid within the vasculature. This is counterbalanced by the outward thrust of hydrostatic pressure within the vessels. A simplified diagram of the balance of forces is shown in Fig. 4-2. The lymphatics siphon off fluid that reaches the interstices of

the tissue, and an equilibrium is thus normally maintained.

Shifts of fluid in the evolving inflammatory reaction are exceedingly rapid, as illustrated by the previously cited example of a blister following thermal injury. Such inflammatory exudates contain significant amounts of plasma protein. Thus a key event in acute inflammation is the alteration of permeability of the tiny vessels in the area, which leads to protein leakage. This is followed by a shift in osmotic balance, and water follows the protein, producing swelling of the tissues. The arteriolar dilation that produces local hyperemia and redness also results in an increase in intravascular pressure locally as vessels become engorged. This, too, augments the fluid shift (Fig. 4-2). The major factor, however, is the increase in vascular permeability to protein.

The endothelial cells that line the small vessels are responsible for the usual semipermeable character of the vessels, and it is these cells that change their relationship to one another in acute inflammation, producing the leakage of protein and fluid. Fig. 4-3 diagrams this situation. In the normal small vessel in *A,* the endothelial lining cells are joined tightly to one another. The dots in the lumen represent large molecules, such as those of serum proteins or of large marker particles injected experimentally to simulate protein molecules. Ordinarily, these large molecules or particles cannot penetrate the intercellular junctions. However, if an inflammatory reaction occurs locally, an actual separation between contiguous endothelial cells develops in the area and the marker particles (and presumably the protein molecules) exit from the lumen, as shown in Fig. 4-3, *B.* If a pigmented marker particle is used for such an experiment, entire vessels become discolored and it becomes possible to see which part of the microcirculation is actually leaking in the course of inflammation. In most instances studied in this fashion, the leak seems to occur chiefly at the venular end of the microcirculation rather than within the true capillaries (Fig. 4-3, *C*).

Lymphatics and Flow of Lymph

Events in the lymphatic system parallel those in the blood vascular system in the acute inflammatory reaction. Ordinarily, interstitial fluid slowly percolates into lymphatic channels and the lymph is carried centrally in the body, ultimately to rejoin venous blood. As an area becomes inflamed, there is usually a striking increase in the flow of lymph draining from the area. In the course of acute inflammation, the contiguous lining cells of the smallest lymphatics separate somewhat, just as they do within the venules, allowing more ready access to material from the interstices of tissues into the lymphatics. Lymphatic channels probably are maintained in an open position as a tissue swells by a system of connective tissue fibers anchored to the walls of the lymphatics. In any event, not

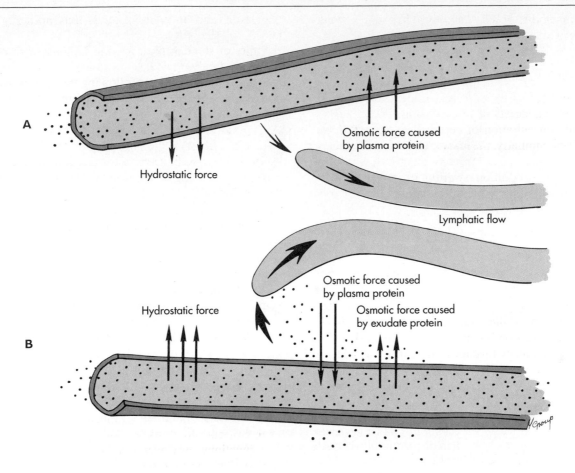

Hydrostatic force

Osmotic force caused
by plasma protein

Lymphatic flow

Hydrostatic force

Osmotic force caused
by plasma protein

Osmotic force caused
by exudate protein

FIG. 4-2   Factors involved in fluid exchange between blood vessels and tissues. In the normal or resting state, **A,** hydrostatic forces tend to push fluid into the interstitial spaces. This is largely balanced by the osmotic force exerted by plasma proteins *(dots)* that ordinarily do not pass through vessel walls. The fluid that does pass into the interstices drains via the lymphatics. In acute inflammation, **B,** protein escapes from the vessels as permeability increases. This, along with a smaller contribution from the increased hydrostatic pressure related to hyperemia, accounts for a significant fluid flux. Lymphatic flow is correspondingly increased.

only does the flow of lymph increase, but the protein and cell content of the lymph likewise increases during acute inflammation.

On the one hand, this increased flow of material through lymphatics is beneficial, since it tends to minimize the swelling of the inflamed tissue by draining off a portion of the exudate. However, potentially injurious agents can be carried by the lymphatics from a primary site of inflammation to distant points in the body. By such means, infectious agents may spread. The spread is often limited by the filtering action of regional lymph nodes through which the lymph flows, but agents or materials carried within the lymph may pass through the nodes and eventually reach the bloodstream.

For these reasons, the possible involvement of the lymphatic system must always be considered in inflammation of any cause. *Lymphangitis* is the inflammation of a lymphatic vessel; *lymphadenitis* is the inflammation of a lymph node. Regional lymphadenitis often accompanies inflammation. One familiar example is the enlarged, tender cervical lymph nodes seen with tonsillitis. The more general term *lymphadenopathy* is used to describe virtually any abnormality of lymph nodes. In practice, the term refers not only to lymphadenitis, but to any enlargement of lymph nodes, since most nodal reactions are accompanied by enlargement.

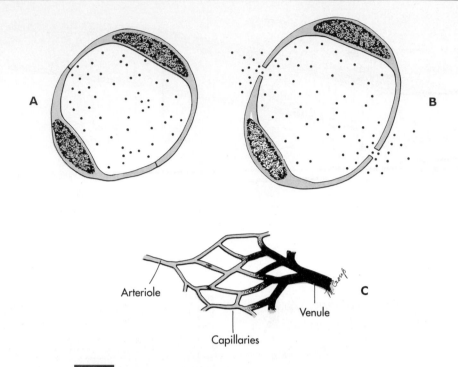

FIG. 4-3   Mechanism of increased vascular permeability in acute inflammation. In normal vessels, **A,** the junctions between endothelial lining cells are sufficiently tight to keep large molecules *(dots)* within the lumen. In acute inflammation, **B,** contraction of endothelial cells creates gaps that allow leakage of macromolecules. As shown in **C,** the permeability change is at the venular side of the microcirculatory bed.

CELLULAR ASPECTS OF INFLAMMATION

Margination and Emigration

As arterioles dilate early in acute inflammation, the flow of blood into the inflamed area increases. However, the character of the blood flow soon changes. As fluid leaks out of the microcirculation with its increased permeability, large numbers of formed elements (red blood cells, platelets, white blood cells) are left behind and the viscosity of the blood increases. The circulation within the affected area then slows, leading to some important consequences. Normally, the flow of blood is more or less streamlined (Fig. 4-4, *A*) and the formed elements do not bump against the sides of the vessel appreciably. As the viscosity of the blood increases and the flow slows, the leukocytes begin to *marginate;* that is, they move to the periphery of the stream, along the lining of the vessel (Fig. 4-4, *B*). As the phenomenon progresses, the marginated leukocytes begin to adhere to the endothelium, producing an appearance reminiscent of a cobblestone street, which is why this is known as *pavementing.* Margination and pavementing are preludes to the emigration of leukocytes from the blood vessels to the surrounding tissue.

Fig. 4-4, *C,* illustrates leukocytic emigration. Leukocytes move in an ameboid fashion. They seem able to extend a pseudopod into the potential space between two endothelial cells and then gradually push through to appear on the other side, a process requiring a matter of minutes. The net result, since this event is repeated in innumerable venules and since more and more leukocytes are delivered into the area via the circulating blood, is that tremendous numbers of cells are delivered into the area of inflammation in a relatively short time. Literally millions of cells emigrate into even a small area of inflammation within several hours.

Chemotaxis

The movement of the leukocytes in the interstices of inflamed tissues once they emigrate is apparently not random but is directionally oriented by a variety of chemical "signals." This phenomenon is referred to as *chemotaxis.* Various agents may provide a chemotactic signal to attract leukocytes, including infectious agents, damaged tissues, and substances activated within the protein fraction of plasma leaking from the bloodstream. Thus a smooth combination of increased delivery of leukocytes to the area (as a result of hyperemia), changes in blood flow resulting in margination and pavementing, and

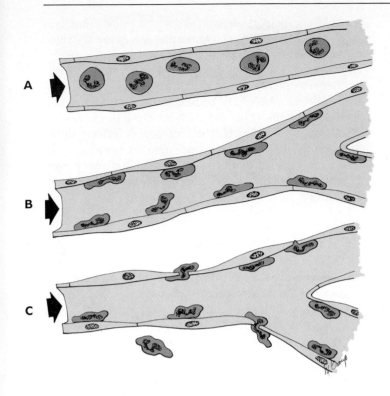

FIG. 4-4   Blood flow and cellular phenomena in acute inflammation. Normally, **A,** formed elements of the blood, especially the leukocytes shown, are carried in the main stream. As the circulation slows, **B,** margination of leukocytes occurs. This is a prelude to emigration of leukocytes between endothelial cells, **C.**

chemotactic orientation of leukocyte motion results in the rapid accumulation of a significant leukocytic component in the exudate.

MEDIATION OF INFLAMMATION

The dramatic vascular, fluid, and cellular phenomena of inflammation are obviously under meticulous control. Although some injuries directly damage vascular endothelium and by themselves lead to leakage of protein and fluid in the zone of injury, in most cases injury triggers the formation and/or release of chemical substances within the body and these mediators elicit the phenomena of inflammation. Many types of injuries can activate the same endogenous mediators, which would explain the stereotyped character of the inflammatory response to diverse stimuli. The period of latency between the injurious stimulus and the development of inflammatory response also points to the role of mediators; the ability to circumvent certain aspects of the reaction with pharmacologic blocking agents emphasizes the importance of mediators.

Many endogenously released substances have been identified as mediators of the inflammatory response. This sort of knowledge has, on the one hand, led to a better understanding of deficiencies and perturbations of the inflammatory response and, on the other hand, suggested the means of suppressing unwanted inflammation when dictated by the clinical setting. Although the list of proposed mediators is long and complex, the better recognized mediators fall into the following classes:

1. Vasoactive amines
2. Substances produced by plasma enzyme systems
3. Arachidonic acid metabolites
4. Miscellaneous cell products

Histamine

The most important vasoactive amine is histamine, which is capable of producing vasodilation and increased vascular permeability. Large amounts of histamine are stored within the granules of connective tissue cells known as *mast cells,* which are widely distributed in the body (histamine is also present in blood basophils and platelets). The stored histamine is inactive and exerts its vascular effects only when released. Many physical injuries cause mast cell degranulation and histamine release. Some injuries first trigger activation of the serum complement system (described later and in Chapter 5), certain components of which then lead to histamine release. Some immunologic reactions (detailed in Chapter 5) also trigger release of this mediator from mast cells. Histamine seems particularly important early in inflammation and is a prime mediator in some common allergic reactions. Antihistamines are drugs designed to block the mediator effects of histamine.

Plasma Factors

Blood plasma is a rich source of a number of important mediators. These are formed through the action of certain proteolytic enzymes that make up a sort of interconnected defensive system. The key agent coordinating these systems is the *Hageman factor (factor XII),* which is present in the plasma in an inactive form and which can be activated by a variety of injuries. Activated Hageman factor triggers the clotting cascade, leading to the formation of fibrin (see Chapter 19). Clotting, per se, is an important defensive reaction to injury, but certain products derived from fibrin also act as vasoactive mediators in inflammation. Hageman factor also activates the plasminogen system, liberating plasmin or fibrinolysin. This protease not only splits fibrin, but also activates the complement system. Several components of the complement system function as important inflammatory mediators. For example, derivatives of the third and fifth components, the *anaphylatoxins,* release histamine and affect vascular permeability. A derivative of the fifth component and a complex of the fifth, sixth, and seventh components are potent chemotactic agents when activated in tissues. These effects are important in many examples of inflammation, not just in immunologically provoked reactions (although, as described in Chapter 5, union of antigen and certain antibodies is a potent activator of the complement system). Activated Hageman factor also converts *prekallikrein* (an inactive substance in plasma) to *kallikrein* (a proteolytic enzyme). This, in turn, acts on plasma kininogen to liberate *bradykinin,* a peptide that dilates blood vessels and increases permeability.

Arachidonic Acid Metabolites

In recent years, attention has been directed to arachidonic acid metabolites as important inflammatory mediators.

Arachidonic acid is derived from the phospholipid of many cell membranes when phospholipases are activated by injury (or by other mediators). Subsequently, arachidonic acid can be metabolized by two different pathways, the *cyclooxygenase pathway* and the *lipoxygenase pathway,* yielding a variety of prostaglandins, thromboxanes, and leukotrienes (Fig. 4-5). These substances show a broad range of vascular and chemotactic effects in inflammation, and some are important in hemostasis as well. It is now recognized that aspirin and many nonsteroidal antiinflammatory drugs inhibit the cyclooxygenase pathway.

Miscellaneous Cell Products

In addition to the mediators just mentioned, a variety of cell-derived substances have properties that may also be important in inflammation. A partial list would include oxygen metabolites produced by neutrophils and macrophages, lysosomal contents of these cells (following discussion), and cytokines released by a variety of cells, particularly activated lymphocytes and macrophages. Cytokines that have an important role in mediating inflammation include *interleukins 1 and 8* (IL-1, IL-8) and *tumor necrosis factor* (TNF). *Nitric oxide* (NO) is another cell-derived mediator discovered within recent years. This substance, produced by macrophages, endothelial cells, and other cells, can have important vasomotor effects and can affect platelet function and can even act as a cytotoxic free radical. Finally, the mediation of leukocyte adhesion and transmigration has been shown to involve the binding of complementary adhesion molecules on the surfaces of endothelial cells and leukocytes. These molecules include *selectins, endothelial adhesion molecules,* and *integrins.* Certain mediators such as histamine and certain cytokines can stimulate the expression of

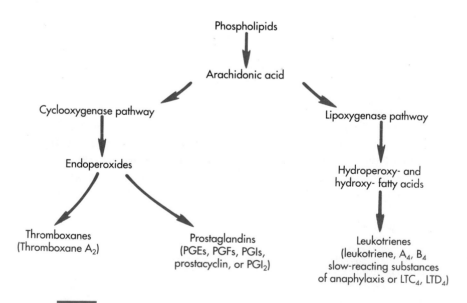

FIG. 4-5   Arachidonic acid metabolism and inflammatory mediators.

selectins and other adhesion molecules (e.g., intercellular adhesion molecule 1 [ICAM-1], vascular cell adhesion molecule 1 [VCAM-1]) on endothelial surfaces. Then, as leukocytes are activated, integrins on their surfaces interact with the endothelial adhesion molecules and the ultimate result is leukocyte extravasation.

Thus the total list of proposed mediators of inflammation is extensive, and knowledge of which substances are significantly involved in a given reaction is still quite limited. Considerable overlap and redundancy appear to be involved in effectively blocking inflammatory reactions.

TYPES OF LEUKOCYTES AND THEIR FUNCTIONS

The leukocytes that circulate in the bloodstream and emigrate into inflammatory exudates originate in the bone marrow, where red blood cells and platelets are also continuously produced (see Chapter 17). Normally within the bone marrow, large numbers of immature leukocytes of various types may be found, and a "pool" of mature leukocytes are held in reserve for release into the circulating blood. The numbers of each type of leukocyte circulating in the peripheral blood are closely limited (see Chapter 18) but are altered "on demand" when an inflammatory process arises. That is, with the instigation of an inflammatory response, feedback signals to the bone marrow alter the rate of production and release of one or more kinds of leukocytes into the bloodstream.

Granulocytes

Granulocytes, a class of leukocytes including neutrophils, eosinophils, and basophils, are so named because of the granules within the cytoplasm visible after the application of certain dyes. Two other types of leukocytes, monocytes and lymphocytes, do not contain the numerous cytoplasmic granules that characterize the previously listed cells. Although each of the types of cells listed is available in the circulating blood, leukocytes do not randomly appear within exudates, but probably as a result of specific chemotactic signals arising in the evolution of the inflammatory process.

The first cells to appear in large numbers within exudates in the early hours of inflammation are neutrophils. The nuclei of these cells are irregularly lobed or polymorphous (Fig. 4-6). These cells are, therefore, called *polymorphonuclear neutrophils, PMNs,* or *"polys."* These cells have a developmental sequence within the bone marrow that requires approximately 2 weeks for completion. When they are released into the circulating blood, their circulatory half-life is 6 hours or so. Approximately 5000 neutrophils per cubic millimeter of blood are in circulation at any given time, with approximately 100 times this number being held in reserve as mature cells within the bone marrow ready to be released on sig-

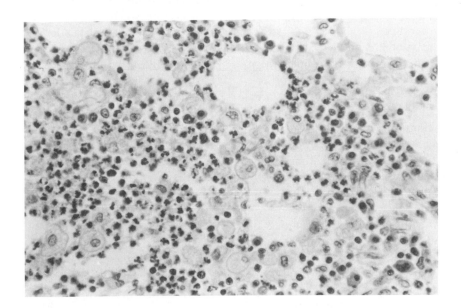

FIG. 4-6   Macrophages and neutrophils in connective tissue. These cells are part of a voluminous exudate that is formed, in this instance in response to bacterial infection. Most of the cells shown are neutrophils. Their cytoplasmic granules cannot be seen at this magnification, but their irregularly lobed (polymorphous) nuclei are evident. The macrophages are several-fold larger and, in this particular exudate, have a bubbly appearing cytoplasm. They are scattered but are prominent in the lower center and lower left of the field. (Photomicrograph, ×500.)

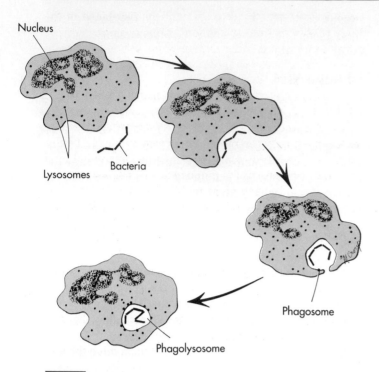

Nucleus

Lysosomes

Bacteria

Phagosome

Phagolysosome

FIG. 4-7   Diagram of phagocytosis. Neutrophils and monocytes ingest particles by flowing their cytoplasm around the objects and internalizing them in an envelope of cell membrane, the phagosome. The digestive enzymes of the lysosomes are then released into the phagolysosomes.

nal. Although literally billions of neutrophils per day are replaced by the bone marrow, their production and release are quite rigidly controlled.

When released into the bloodstream, PMNs are usually incapable of further cell division or significant synthesis of cellular enzymes. The numerous granules visible within the cytoplasm of the neutrophils, however, actually represent membrane-bound packets of enzymes *(lysosomes)* produced during maturation of the cells. These enzymes include a variety of hydrolases, including proteases, lipases, and phosphatases. In addition, associated with the granules are a variety of antimicrobial substances. Thus, in effect, the mature PMN is a suitcase of enzyme-loaded and antimicrobial particles.

PMNs are capable of active ameboid motion and are able to engulf a variety of materials by a process called *phagocytosis.* As illustrated in Fig. 4-7, the neutrophil approaches the particle (e.g., a bacterium) to be phagocytosed, flows its cytoplasm around the particle, and eventually takes the particle into the cytoplasm enveloped in a membrane-bound vesicle that pinches off from the cell membrane of the neutrophil. This phagocytic process is aided by certain substances that coat the object to be ingested and render it more easily internalized by the leukocyte. These kinds of leukocytosis-promoting substances, called *opsonins,* include immunoglobulins (antibodies) and components of the complement system (see

Chapter 5). Having ingested a particle and incorporated it into the cytoplasm in a *phagocytic vacuole* or *phagosome,* the leukocyte's next task is to kill the particle, if it is a living microbial agent, and to digest it. Living agents may be killed in a variety of ways, including altering the intracellular pH after phagocytosis, releasing antibacterial substances into the phagocytic vacuole, and producing antibacterial substances such as hydrogen peroxide (and other highly reactive oxygen metabolites) as a result of cellular metabolic processes initiated after the phagocytic event. The phagocytosed particles are generally digested within the vacuoles formed by fusion of lysosomes with phagosomes. The previously inactive digestive enzymes are now activated within these *phagolysosomes,* resulting in the enzymatic digestion of the objects.

Under certain circumstances, digestive enzymes and oxygen metabolites of the neutrophils may be released into the host tissues rather than into intracellular phagolysosomes. When this occurs, the neutrophils become potent agents of tissue injury. This extracellular release occurs with death and disintegration of neutrophils; it occurs after phagocytosis of certain crystals, such as urates, by neutrophils (because phagocytosis of these crystals is followed by rupture of phagolysosomes); it also occurs when neutrophils attempt to ingest immune complexes under certain circumstances. These types of situations are described more fully later.

The *eosinophil* is another type of granulocyte that may appear in inflammatory exudates, although usually in relatively small numbers. Eosinophils have irregular nuclei much like neutrophils, but the cytoplasmic granules stain a bright red when dyed with eosin and are much more prominent than the lavender-colored granules of neutrophils. The granules of eosinophils are packets of enzymes quite similar to those of neutrophils. In fact, eosinophils have many of the same functions: they respond to chemotactic stimuli; they phagocytose various kinds of particles; and they even kill certain microorganisms. What appears to be distinctive about eosinophils, however, is that they respond to certain unique chemotactic stimuli generated in the course of allergic reactions and they contain substances toxic to certain parasites and substances that may mediate inflammatory reactions. Also, eosinophils tend to accumulate in significant concentrations at the site of parasitic infestation and allergic reactions.

The third type of granulocyte is the *basophil,* whose cytoplasm is crowded with large granules that stain a deep blue with basic dyes. Although these cells come from the bone marrow as do other granulocytes, they have many features in common with certain cells of the connective tissues called *mast cells* or *tissue basophils.* The granules of both of these types of cells contain a variety of enzymes, heparin, and histamine. *Blood basophils* seem to respond to chemotactic signals released in the course of certain immunologic reactions. Ordinarily, they are present in small numbers in exudates. Blood basophils and tissue mast cells are stimulated to release the contents of their granules into the surroundings in a variety of injurious circumstances, including both immunologic and nonspecific reactions. The mast cells are a major source of histamine early in any acute inflammatory reaction. The immunologic means of stimulating granule release by mast cells or basophils is discussed in Chapter 5.

Monocytes and Macrophages

The *monocyte* is a form of leukocyte that differs from the granulocyte because of its nuclear morphology and its relatively agranular cytoplasm (see Fig. 4-6). The monocyte also originates within the bone marrow, but its circulatory life is three to four times longer than that of granulocytes. In the course of acute inflammatory reactions, monocytes begin to emigrate at approximately the same time as neutrophils but they do so in much smaller numbers and at a slower rate. Consequently, in the early hours of inflammation, there are relatively few such cells within exudate. However, as exudates age, the percentage of these cells usually increases. The same cell that is called a monocyte in the circulating blood is called a *macrophage* when it appears within exudates. In fact, the same type of cell is found wandering in small numbers through the connective tissues of the body even in the absence of overt inflammation. These wandering macrophages in the connective tissues are known as *histiocytes*.

Macrophages have functions similar to those of PMNs, in that macrophages are actively motile cells that respond to chemotactic stimuli, are actively phagocytic, and are able to kill and digest a variety of agents. Several important differences between macrophages and PMNs exist. First, macrophages may survive weeks or even months within the tissues, in contrast to the short-lived PMNs. Second, when the monocyte leaves the bone marrow, enters the bloodstream, and then passes into the tissues, it is not a fully mature cell in the same sense as the neutrophil. Third, PMNs are incapable of further division and are also incapable of active synthesis of digestive enzymes. Monocytes, on the other hand, can be stimulated under some circumstances to divide within the tissues, and they are capable of responding to local conditions by synthesizing a variety of intracellular enzymes. This ability to undergo "on-the-job training" is a vital property of macrophages, particularly in certain immunologic reactions where they are trained by lymphocytes. In such circumstances, macrophages increase their metabolic activities, become more effective in phagocytosis, and become more efficient in killing and digesting certain microbes. Macrophages may also alter their form as they undergo such changes, giving rise to cells known as epithelioid cells. Macrophages are also able to fuse together to form multinucleated giant cells. These forms are illustrated in Figs. 4-13 and 4-14.

Although macrophages are significant components of various exudates, they are also widely distributed in the body under normal conditions. This was recognized many years ago, and the term *reticuloendothelial system* (RES) was coined to denote mononuclear cells sharing the same property, namely, phagocytosis. *Monocyte-macrophage system* is the current name applied to the RES because it is actually more descriptive. As typically conceived, the RES, or monocyte-macrophage system, includes not only the blood monocytes and tissue histiocytes, or wandering macrophages, but a large population of more or less fixed mononuclear phagocytic cells closely related to the more mobile members of the system. This population of less mobile cells includes lining cells along blood channels within the spleen, the liver (where the cells are known as *Kupffer's cells*), and the bone marrow. Similar fixed macrophages are present along many of the lymphatic channels within the lymph nodes of the body. In addition, many macrophages are present within the serosal cavities of the body, within the lungs (alveolar macrophages), and even within the central nervous system (microglial cells).

The important functions of this system involve the vigorous phagocytic activities of the component cells. These cells clean the blood, the lymph, and the interstitial spaces of foreign material, thus performing a vital defensive function. Even if millions of microorganisms are injected into the circulating blood, they would be removed within a matter of a few hours by the many millions of macrophages located strategically around the body. This is exceedingly important, since at least a few microorganisms may be released into the circulating fluids of the body with vigorous brushing of the teeth, with defecation, or with certain medical or dental manipulations. Because of the phagocytic activities of the macrophage system, such episodes of bacteremia are transient and trivial. The macrophages in the body cavities and connective tissues perform a similar police function. In addition, the uptake of foreign material by macrophages is an essential first step in the chain of events that leads to the induction of an immune response (see Chapter 5).

An important everyday function of the monocyte-macrophage system involves the processing of the hemoglobin of red blood cells that have reached the end of their life span. Macrophages trap and recycle the components of this essential substance by splitting hemoglobin into an iron-containing portion and a non-iron-containing portion. The iron is recycled for the building of other red blood cells in the bone marrow; the non-iron-containing portion is further processed, liberating a substance known as *bilirubin,* which is carried in the bloodstream to the liver, where the hepatocytes extract it and secrete it as part of the bile.

Lymphocytes

One type of leukocyte, the lymphocyte, has not yet been mentioned. *Lymphocytes* generally are present in exudates only in small numbers until the exudates are quite old; that is, until the inflammatory reactions have become chronic. Because the known functions of lymphocytes are all within the immunologic realm, these cells are more fully described in Chapter 5.

• • •

Each component of the inflammatory response has a unique importance. Vasodilation early in acute inflammation brings to the area the "raw materials" for the reaction. If the arteriolar dilation and increased blood flow are circumvented by local conditions or by the administration of certain drugs, later aspects of the inflammatory reaction are significantly frustrated. The increased vascular permeability not only accomplishes the outpouring of fluid, which may dilute noxious agents, but also transfers important protein substances such as opsonins or other antibodies to the "battleground." Furthermore, one of the proteins that leaks into the area of inflammation is *fibrinogen,* which is quickly converted to form *fibrin,* which may act as kind of a sealer or "glue" in wounds. Because of its fibrillar character, fibrin may act as a scaffold for migration of phagocytic leukocytes and ultimately for the cells that form scar tissue in the reparative phase. Mobilized leukocytes not only apprehend invading microbes, but also demolish tissue debris so that repair processes can begin.

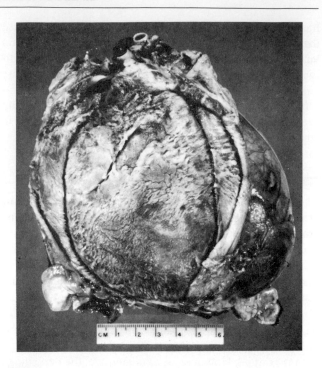

FIG. 4-8   Fibrinous exudate on the surface of the heart. The pericardium has been opened, and instead of the normally smooth epicardial surface, a shaggy layer of fibrin is evident. This has formed from fibrinogen exuded from underlying vessels. Classically, this condition has been termed "bread-and-butter heart."

PATTERNS OF INFLAMMATION

Although the inflammatory reaction tends to follow the mechanisms described earlier, various patterns of inflammation can emerge, based on the type of exudate that is formed, the particular organ or tissue involved, and the duration of the inflammatory process. The nomenclature of inflammatory processes takes into account each of these variables. Different types of exudates are given descriptive names. The duration of the inflammatory response is designated as *acute* during the phase of active exudation, as *chronic* when there is evidence of advanced repair along with the exudation, and as *subacute* when there is only early evidence of repair along with the exudation. The location of the inflammatory reaction is designated by the organ or tissue name, to which is appended the suffix *-itis* (e.g., appendicitis, tonsillitis, arthritis).

Noncellular Exudates
Serous exudate

In some instances of inflammation, the exudate consists almost entirely of fluid and dissolved substances with few leukocytes. The simplest type of noncellular exudate is a *serous exudate,* which consists basically of the protein that leaks from permeable blood vessls in an area

of inflammation along with the accompanying fluid. The most familiar example of serous exudate is blister fluid. Similar accumulations of serous exudate are common within body cavities, such as the pleural cavity or the peritoneal cavity, and although not as striking, serous exudates often spread through connective tissues.

Sometimes collections of fluid occur in body cavities for reasons other than inflammation, usually increased hydrostatic pressure or depletion of plasma protein. Such noninflammatory collections are termed *transudates* and are protein poor and cell poor compared with exudates.

Fibrinous exudate

A second type of noncellular exudate is *fibrinous exudate,* which forms when the protein extravasated in an area of inflammation contains abundant fibrinogen. This fibrinogen is converted to fibrin, a sticky, elastic meshwork (perhaps more familiar as the backbone of a blood clot). Fibrinous exudates are often encountered on inflamed serosal surfaces such as the pleura and the pericardium, where the precipitated fibrin compacts to a shaggy layer on the involved membrane (Fig. 4-8). When such a shaggy layer of fibrin accumulates on serosal surfaces, it is frequently accompanied by pain when one surface rubs on another. Thus, for instance, the patient with pleuritis feels pain on respiration when the roughened surfaces rub together during inspiration. This rubbing of shaggy surfaces also produces a sign called *friction rub,* which is audible through the stethoscope over the affected area, whether it is the pleura, pericardium, or similar structure.

Mucinous exudate

Another noncellular exudate is the *mucinous* or *catarrhal* exudate. This type of exudate forms only on the surface of a mucous membrane, where there are cells capable of secreting mucin. This type of exudate differs from others in that it represents a cellular secretion rather than something that escapes from the bloodstream. Mucin secretion is a normal property of mucous membranes, and mucinous exudate represents nothing more than an acceleration of a basic physiologic process. The most familiar example of a mucinous exudate is the runny nose that accompanies many upper respiratory infections.

Cellular Exudates

Neutrophilic exudate

The most common exudates consist predominantly of PMNs, in such numbers as to overshadow the fluid and proteinaceous parts of exudate. Such neutrophilic exudates are referred to as *purulent.* Purulent exudates (Fig. 4-9) are usually formed in response to bacterial infection. They are also seen in response to many aseptic injuries and are prominent almost anywhere in the body where tissues have become necrotic.

Bacterial infection often causes extremely high concentrations of PMNs to accumulate in a tissue, and many of these cells die and liberate their powerful hydrolytic enzymes into the surroundings. Under such circumstances, the enzymes of the PMNs literally digest the underlying tissue and liquefy it. This combination of neutrophil aggregation and liquefaction of underlying tissues is referred to as *suppuration,* and the exudate thus formed is called *suppurative exudate,* or more commonly, *pus.* Thus pus consists of living, dying, and disintegrated PMNs; liquefied, digested underlying tissue; fluid exudate of the inflammatory process; and often the inciting bacteria. The significant difference between suppurative and purulent inflammation is that with suppuration, there is liquefactive necrosis of underlying tissue. Fig. 4-10 illustrates this liquefactive necrosis of suppuration. (Although a significant difference exists between purulent and suppurative inflammation, many unfortunately use the terms interchangeably.)

When localized suppuration occurs within a solid tissue, the resulting lesion is termed an *abscess.* As seen in Fig. 4-10, an abscess is quite literally a hole filled with pus in the involved tissue. Abscesses are difficult lesions for the body to handle because of their tendency to expand with the liquefaction of more tissue, their tendency to burrow, and their resistance to healing. When an abscess forms, it is difficult to deliver therapeutic agents

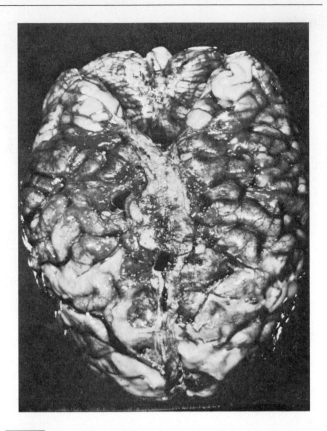

FIG. 4-9   Purulent exudate within the cerebral meninges. The membranes covering the brain contain literally millions of neutrophils forming a purulent exudate. The creamy patches of exudate are especially prominent at the bottom. The gyri in the center of the photograph are dark because of intense vascular congestion, part of the inflammatory response. (This is pneumococcal meningitis.)

such as antibiotics into the abscess via the bloodstream. In general, the handling of abscesses by the body is greatly aided by draining them surgically, thus allowing the closed space previously filled with pus to collapse and heal. If abscesses are not surgically drained by pathways chosen by the surgeon, they tend to expand, destroying additional structures in their path. An abscess in a lung might burrow until it communicates with the pleural cavity, and if the contents are discharged into the pleural cavity and infection spreads, the result might be *empyema,* which is a purulent inflammatory process involving the entire pleural cavity. Occasionally an abscess ruptures onto a surface and produces a draining tract that ends blindly in the space of the abscess. Any such blind tract communicating with a surface is referred to as a *sinus.* If, on the other hand, an abscess extends to two separate surfaces, it might result in an abnormal tract connecting two organs or connecting the lumen of a hollow organ and the body surface. Such an abnormal connection is referred to as a *fistula.* (Fistulas are named according to their communications, e.g., gastrocolic, bronchopleural, colocutaneous.)

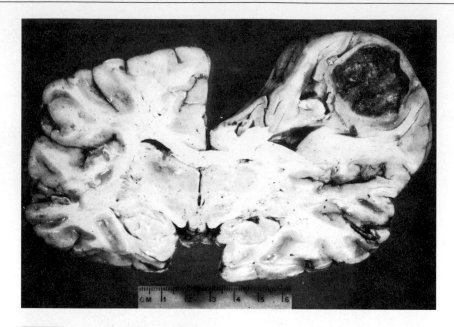

FIG. 4-10 Brain abscess. As a result of bacterial infection in the cerebral hemisphere on the right, large numbers of neutrophils emigrated into the region. Liquefaction of the regional tissue by lysosomal enzymes of the neutrophils produced the defect illustrated.

Another common example of suppurative inflammation is the *furuncle,* or boil, which is a cutaneous abscess forming in a hair follicle as a result of bacterial infection. A *carbuncle* is a more deep-seated area of suppuration involving the subcutaneous tissue, with multiple areas of discharge onto the skin surface.

When purulent inflammation extends diffusely through a tissue, the process is referred to as phlegmonous, or more often, the term *cellulitis* is used clinically to describe an area of phlegmonous inflammation. Such a spreading purulent process is seen usually as a result of bacterial infection when the particular agent is capable of spreading rapidly through the loose connective tissue of the body.

Mixed exudates

As one would expect, there are frequently mixtures of noncellular and cellular exudates, and these are named accordingly. Thus there are *fibrinopurulent* exudates, which consist of fibrin and PMNs; *mucopurulent* exudates consisting of mucin and PMNs; *serofibrinous* exudates; and so forth. Certain exudates, such as mucinous and mucopurulent, are unique to mucous membranes.

Occasionally, in association with damage to mucous membranes, a necrotic area may actually slough off, leaving a gap in the continuity of the mucosal surface. Such a defect is termed an *ulcer.* Most often, fibrinopurulent exudate emanating from the underlying blood vessels forms the surface of an ulcer bed (Fig. 4-11). Sometimes, broad areas of mucous membrane will become necrotic and the dead cells may become enmeshed in a web of

fibrinopurulent exudate, which coats the mucosal surface. Such an area grossly resembles a ragged mucous membrane, and hence this type of process is referred to as *pseudomembranous inflammation* (Fig. 4-12). The classic example of pseudomembranous inflammation in the past was the pseudomembrane of diphtheria within the respiratory tract. Thus such membranes are occasionally referred to as *diphtheritic.* Pseudomembranous inflammation may be observed within the gastrointestinal tract, particularly the colon, as the result of an upset in the microbial ecology of the tract, usually brought about by the administration of antibiotics.

Granulomatous Inflammation

A unique and distinctive pattern of inflammation that can occur virtually anywhere is granulomatous inflammation. This type of inflammation is characterized by the massing of large numbers of macrophages and their aggregation into nodular clumps referred to as *granulomas.* Although many inflammatory exudates contain appreciable numbers of macrophages, in granulomatous inflammation the field is dominated by sheets of these cells or their derivatives, such as epithelioid cells or multinucleated giant cells. Granulomas take time to evolve and generally pass through rather nondescript acute stages where there is exudation of fluid, neutrophils, and protein. The continued emigration of monocytes and the local proliferation of these cells lead to their massing as a granuloma. Granulomas usually form because of the persistence within the tissues of some offensive agent resistant to the

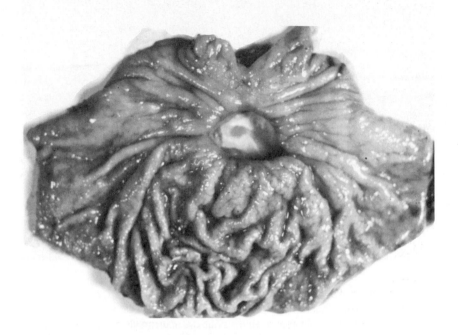

FIG. 4-11   Gastric ulcer. This type of gap in the continuity of a surface is termed an *ulcer*. An inflammatory reaction is invariably present in the base. Blood vessels may be eroded, giving rise to hemorrhage, or the full thickness of the wall may be perforated.

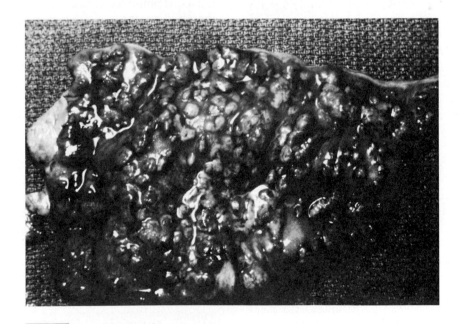

FIG. 4-12   Pseudomembranous colitis. The many plaquelike lesions on the colonic mucosal surface are patches of *pseudomembrane* consisting of fibrinopurulent exudate and necrotic epithelial debris.

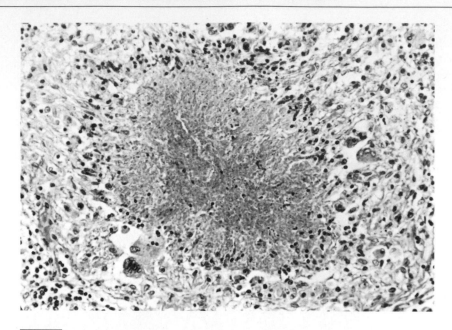

FIG. 4-13   Epithelioid tubercle. A tubercle is a mass of macrophages that have acquired an epithelioid appearance. The zone of poorly defined, light-staining cells at the periphery of the field (outer third) consists of epithelioid macrophages and multinucleated giant cells (3 o'clock and 7 o'clock). The center of the tubercle has undergone caseous necrosis. The small, dark cells are lymphocytes. (Photomicrograph, ×315.)

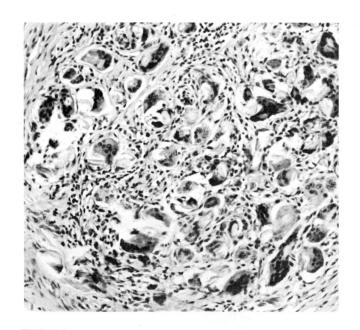

FIG. 4-14   Foreign body granuloma. In this instance the granuloma is a mass of macrophages that have fused to form many giant cells. Many of these have engulfed fibrils, which represent fragments of suture material. (Photomicrograph, ×200.)

efforts of the body to dispose of it. Such agents can include insoluble but sterile materials or particularly resistant microorganisms. The prototypical microorganism that evokes the formation of granulomas is the *Mycobacterium tuberculosis,* or tubercle bacillus. The response to this organism is characteristically granulomatous, and usually the macrophages mass in nodular aggregates of epithelioid cells and giant cells. This type of a nodular mass of epithelioid cells is referred to as a *tubercle* (Fig. 4-13). Granulomas also form in response to foreign bodies such as suture materials (Fig. 4-14). In general, the presence of a granuloma is the hallmark of "tissue indigestion." As the granuloma evolves in some instances, the macrophages acquire increasing ability to handle the offensive agent, in which case it is eliminated. In other instances the agent remains refractory, and the net effect of the granuloma formation is to wall off that agent from the remainder of the body.

FATE OF THE INFLAMMATORY REACTION

Given the presence of an inflammatory reaction, the best result that can be obtained occurs when little or no destruction of underlying tissue has occurred. In such instances, when the offending agent has been neutralized and removed, the stimulus for continuing exudation of fluid and cells gradually disappears. The small blood vessels in the area regain their usual semipermeability, fluid flux ceases, and emigration of leukocytes likewise stops. The fluid that has been previously exuded is gradually absorbed by the lymphatics, and the cells of the exudate disintegrate, wander off via the lymphatics, or are actually eliminated from the body (e.g., lung exudates being coughed up). The net result of this process is that the previously inflamed tissue is left precisely as it was before the reaction started. This phenomenon is called *resolution.*

In contrast, when significant amounts of tissue have been destroyed, resolution cannot occur. The destroyed tissue must be repaired by proliferation of adjacent surviving host cells. Repair actually involves two separate but coordinated components. The first, *regeneration,* actually involves proliferation of parenchymal elements identical to those lost, the net result being replacement of those lost elements by the same type of cells. The second component of repair involves the proliferation of connective tissue elements, leading to the formation of *scar tissue.* In most tissues there is a combination of these two activities.

Various cells and tissues differ widely in their ability to regenerate. Most epithelial tissues, such as the covering of the skin and the lining of the mouth, pharynx, and gas-

trointestinal tract, regenerate easily after a portion of the tissue has been lost. Other epithelial cells, such as those of the liver parenchyma, renal tubules, or the secretory elements of certain glands, regenerate well, provided the outlines of the tissue are maintained without extensive collapse during the inflammatory process. Complex specialized structures such as renal glomeruli do not regenerate if destroyed. Some types of cells regenerate very poorly or not at all. Useful regneration is extremely limited in involuntary and voluntary muscle if it is present at all, and no regeneration occurs in heart muscle, which is unfortunate given the frequency of necrosis of portions of myocardium. Finally, it should be stressed that no regeneration of neurons or nerve cells occurs within the central nervous system. When such cells are lost, the loss is permanent.

Repair by formation of scar tissue is an efficient process in virtually any tissue of the body. Formation of scar tissue involves proliferating connective tissue from areas adjoining the necrotic tissue extending into the area as the tissue is demolished by the inflammatory reaction. Such ingrowth of a proliferating young connective tissue into an area of inflammation is referred to as *organization,* and the connective tissue itself is referred to as *granulation tissue.* The components of granulation tissue actually include proliferating fibroblasts, proliferating capillary sprouts (the endothelial cells are sometimes re-

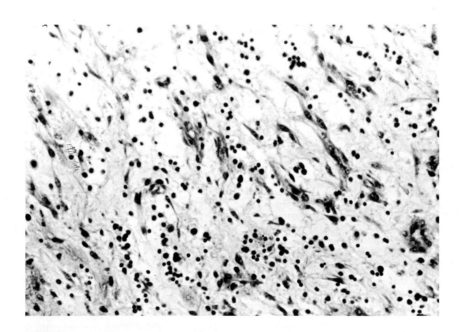

FIG. 4-15   Early organization. The field depicts granulation tissue growing into an area of repair. The elongated, spindle-shaped cells are fibroblasts. Capillary sprouts are recognized as tubular structures, round in cross section (as at the lower right). The small, dark cells are leukocytes, and the interstitial spaces contain exudate fluid and connective tissue ground substance. Compare with Fig. 4-16. (Photomicrograph, ×315.)

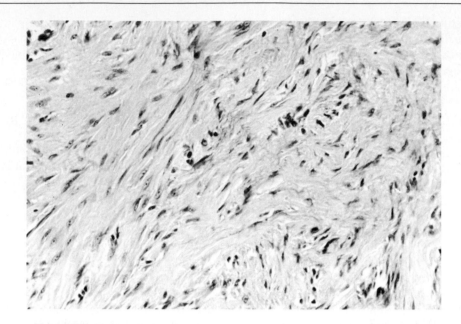

FIG. 4-16   Maturing scar. As granulation tissue matures, the fibroblasts synthesize collagen, which forms the tough scar. In this field the interstitial material has a "stringy" appearance because of abundant collagen in fibrillar form. As the scar ages, it becomes less cellular and more densely collagenous. (Photomicrograph, ×315.)

ferred to as *angioblasts*), various leukocytes of the inflammatory process, fluid portions of the exudate, and a loose semifluid connective tissue ground substance. Organization occurs when abundant tissue has become necrotic, when inflammatory exudates persist and do not resolve, and when masses of blood (hematomas) or blood clots do not resolve quickly. The fibroblasts and angioblasts of granulation tissue originate from preexisting fibroblasts and capillaries in the surroundings, and their migration is somehow oriented so that this tissue gradually extends into the appropriate area (Fig. 4-15).

The earliest evidence of organization usually occurs several days after the start of the inflammatory reaction. By the end of a week or so, the granulation tissue is still very loose and cellular. At this point the fibroblasts of the granulation tissue gradually begin to secrete the soluble precursors of the protein collagen, which gradually precipitates as fibrils in the interstices of the granulation tissue. Over time, more and more collagen is deposited in the granulation tissue, which is now gradually maturing to a rather dense collagenous connective tissue or scar (Fig. 4-16). Although the scar achieves much of its strength by the end of 2 weeks or so, a continuing remodeling process and increase in the density and strength of the scar occur over the ensuing weeks. The granulation tissue, which at first was quite cellular and vascular, gradually becomes less cellular and less vascular and more densely collagenous. The gross counterpart of this evolu-

tion is familiar in the appearance of healing incisions, where the resulting scar is at first somewhat loose and quite pink because of the vascularity, and ultimately becoming denser and paler as the blood vessels regress.

Wound Healing

The coordination of scar formation and regeneration is perhaps most easily illustrated through the healing of cutaneous wounds. The simplest type of healing is that seen in the body's handling of wounds such as surgical incisions, where the wound edges can be brought together for the healing process to begin. Such healing is referred to as *primary healing* or *healing by first intention.* As seen in Fig. 4-17, *A,* immediately after wounding the wound edges are bound together by part of a blood clot, the fibrin of which acts somewhat like a glue. Immediately thereafter, an acute inflammatory reaction develops at the edges of the wound, and the inflammatory cells, particularly macrophages, enter the blood clot and begin to demolish it. After this exudative inflammatory reaction, the ingrowth of granulation tissue into the area formerly occupied by the clot begins. Thus over several days the wound is bridged by granulation tissue destined to mature to a scar. While this is occurring (Fig. 4-17, *B),* the surface epithelium at the edges begins to regenerate, and within a few days a thin layer of epithelium migrates across the wound surface. As the scar be-

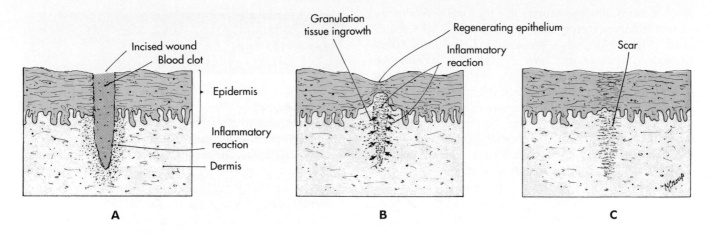

FIG. 4-17   Healing of an incised, primarily closed wound. The wound edges are initially held together by a blood clot, **A,** and perhaps also by sutures. An acute inflammatory response is mounted in the adjacent tissue, which leads to ingrowth of granulation tissue after several days, **B.** At this stage, epidermal regeneration is under way. The usual result is complete epidermal regeneration and a compact dermal scar, which forms as the granulation tissue matures, **C.**

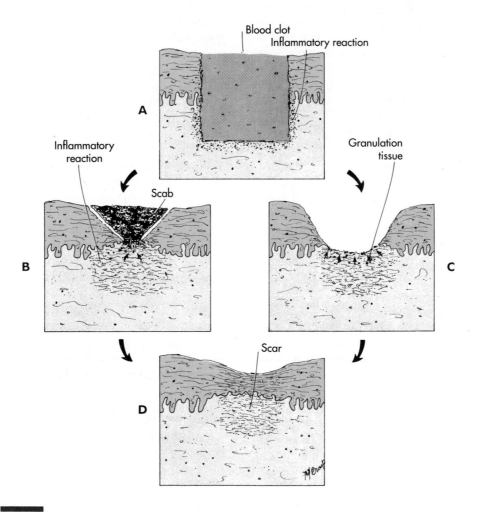

FIG. 4-18   Healing of an open wound by second intention. The process is qualitatively similar to that shown in Fig. 4-17 but involves more extensive epithelial regeneration and formation of more abundant scar. **A,** The situation shortly after wounding; **B,** healing under a scab; **C,** an open wound with visible granulation tissue. **D,** The end result involves a large scar and often a thin area of "new" epidermis devoid of hair and other appendages.

neath matures, this epithelium also thickens and matures so that it comes to resemble the adjacent skin. The net result (Fig. 4-17, *C*) is a reconstituted skin surface and an underlying scar that may be virtually invisible or barely visible as a thickened line. Many skin wounds heal in this manner with no medical attention. In others, sutures are placed to hold the wound edges in apposition until healing occurs. Sutures can be removed when organization and epithelial regeneration have progressed to the point where the edges will not gape when the sutures are removed. Thus, in an area of skin where there is relatively little tension, sutures can be removed in several days, long before maximal strength of the scar has been achieved and before appreciable amounts of collagen have been laid down. In areas under stress, sutures must be left in place longer to hold the tissue together until a tough scar can form.

A second pattern of healing occurs when the wounding of skin is such that the edges cannot be brought together during the healing process. This is referred to as *healing by second intention* or sometimes *healing by granulation* (Fig. 4-18). This type of healing is qualitatively identical to that previously described. The difference lies only in that much more granulation tissue is formed, much more epithelial regeneration is necessary, and usually a larger scar is formed. The entire process, of course, takes longer than healing by primary intention. Often in such large open wounds, granulation tissue can be observed covering the floor of the wound as a delicate nappy carpet that bleeds easily on touch. In other situations, the granulation tissue actually grows beneath a scab and epithelial regeneration likewise occurs beneath the scab. Ultimately in such circumstances, the scab is cast off when healing is complete. Most of us can recall having impatiently removed a scab approximately in the stage shown in Fig. 4-18, *B,* to reveal a central pinpoint of bleeding granulation tissue where epithelial regeneration was not yet total. Although identical in many ways to healing by primary intention, secondary healing is less desirable (not that there is often a choice!) because of the time involved and the termination in a much larger and potentially disfiguring scar.

Healing in virtually any tissue of the body occurs by a process paralleling that described for the skin, with local variations depending on the ability of the tissues to regenerate, and so forth.

The designation of an inflammatory process as acute, subacute, or chronic reflects the duration in terms of the extent of repair. *Acute* inflammation, by definition, has no reparative aspects; it consists only of the exudative phenomena of inflammation. In *subacute* inflammation, there is beginning granulation tissue ingrowth and perhaps beginning regeneration. In *chronic* inflammation, there is evidence of advanced repair side by side with continuing exudation. Evidence of advanced repair includes extensive regenerative proliferation and extensive formation of scar with abundant collagen.

FACTORS AFFECTING INFLAMMATION AND HEALING

In some situations the inflammatory process may be impaired from the beginning, that is, in its exudative stages. The entire inflammatory process depends on an intact circulation to the affected area. Thus, when blood supply to an area is deficient, the result may be sluggish inflammatory processes, persistent infections, and poor healing. Another requisite for efficient exudative inflammation is a liberal supply of leukocytes in the circulating blood. Patients whose marrow is destroyed or depressed (e.g., from malignant disease or adverse reaction to drugs) are unable to produce cellular exudates with normal function and as a result are susceptible to severe infections. More rarely, the functions of leukocytes, even when they are present in normal numbers, may be impaired (e.g., abnormal chemotaxis, abnormal phagocytosis, abnormal intracellular killing and digestion), and the patient is rendered similarly susceptible to aggressive infections. Because leukocyte function is assisted by certain antibodies (see Chapter 5), the inflammatory reaction is also less than normally effective in immunodeficient patients. Finally, certain drugs, in sufficiently high doses, are capable of inhibiting essential aspects of the inflammatory response. For example, if a patient were receiving high doses of corticosteroids or other antiinflammatory drugs, inflammation and healing might be impaired.

Many factors can affect the healing of wounds or other areas of tissue injury and inflammation. The healing process, because of its dependence on cellular proliferation and synthetic activity, is particularly sensitive to local deficiencies of blood supply (with attendant impairment of raw material delivery) and is also sensitive to the patient's nutritional state. Patients who are extremely malnourished do not heal wounds optimally. The healing of wounds is also adversely affected by the presence of foreign material or necrotic tissue in the wound, by the presence of wound infection, and by incomplete immobilization and apposition of wound edges. In extreme cases, with failure of healing, a surgical wound might even undergo *dehiscence,* breaking open.

Complications of Healing

Even if healing proceeds adequately on a cellular level, complications occasionally occur as an end result. It is in the nature of scar tissue to shorten and to become more dense and compact over time. The result is sometimes *contracture,* which may disfigure an area or limit motion at a joint. If the scar tissue encircles a tubular structure (e.g., the urethra), the result may be a *stricture,* which narrows the structure in question and may produce serious difficulty. When serosal surfaces are inflamed and the exudate does not resolve, granulation tissue and eventually scar tissue may eventually bind serosal surfaces together, forming *adhesions.* In many areas, such as the pleura or the pericardium, adhesions generally have a negligible effect on organ function. Within the peritoneal cavity, however, adhesions, whether between loops of bowel or between abdominal viscera and the body wall, may produce webs that can constrict portions of the GI tract or can actually entrap them, forming *internal hernias* that may strangulate and become gangrenous. Another complication seen occasionally in healing wounds of the body wall is the *incisional hernia.* In this situation, the granulation tissue and scar that bridge the surgical defect in the body wall gradually yield to intraperitoneal pressure and a bulging sac in the incision is formed. Another minor local complication of healing is the protrusion of a piece of granulation tissue above the surface of the healing wound, forming what is sometimes called "proud flesh." Healing generally proceeds well when such excrescences are cauterized or nipped off. A complication of healing occasionally encountered is the *amputation,* or *traumatic, neuroma,* which simply represents regenerative proliferation of nerve fibers into the area of healing, where they become entrapped in dense scar. Such a neuroma may constitute an unsightly or even painful lump within a scar. Finally, some individuals, apparently on a genetic basis, handle the production and/or remodeling of collagen in a healing wound abnormally such that excess collagen is formed, leading to a protrusion called a *keloid.* These are somewhat more common in blacks and Asians and in younger patients. Keloids are biologically trivial but cosmetically may assume great importance.

SYSTEMIC ASPECTS OF INFLAMMATION

The emphasis of the previous discussion was on the local aspects of the response to injury. It should be noted, however, that important and prominent systemic effects accompany local inflammatory reactions. These *acute-phase reactions* are apparently mediated by cytokines produced by leukocytes participating in the inflammatory reactions. One familiar reaction is *fever,* which is produced by cytokine action on hypothalamic temperature-regulating centers. *Leukocytosis,* an increase in the number of circulating leukocytes, results from cytokine-medicated stimulation of leukocyte maturation and release from the bone marrow. Other acute-phase reactions include increased hepatic synthesis of "acute-phase proteins" such as C-reactive protein and serum amyloid-associated (SAA) protein, and components of the coagulation and complement system. The increase in some proteins is associated with an increased erythrocyte sedimentation rate (ESR), giving rise to a blood test for the presence of inflammation that is sometimes useful clinically. Severe injuries can cause striking metabolic and endocrine changes. Local inflammatory reactions are accompanied by a variety of poorly defined "constitutional symptoms," including malaise, anorexia or loss of appetite, and varying degrees of disability or even prostration. These symptoms are presumably also mediated by substances released from the areas of inflammation.

QUESTIONS

▼ *Circle the letter preceding each item below that correctly answers the question or completes the statement. More than one answer may be correct.*

1. The best definition of inflammation is:
   a. Accumulation of water in the cells because of failure of the sodium pump
   b. Invasion of tissue by living pathogenic organisms
   c. Margination of leukocytes along the vascular lining
   d. Local reaction of the tissues to an injury
2. The ultimate purpose of the inflammatory response is to:
   a. Increase fatty infiltration in the affected tissue in preparation for the process of healing
   b. Release lysosomes, which promote the synthesis of cellular proteins to promote healing

   c. Localize, destroy, neutralize, and remove injurious agents in preparation for the process of healing
   d. Restore function by promoting hydropic changes in cells
3. An acute inflammatory reaction in the host can be expected:
   a. After cell injury by pathogenic bacteria
   b. After introduction of a sterile but irritating foreign material
   c. Around an area of necrosis in a sterile area
   d. In the center of a necrotic area
   e. Shortly after death
4. Which of the following are cardinal signs of acute inflammation?
   a. Calor
   b. Rigor
   c. Functio laesa
   d. Algor
   e. Rubor

5. Which of the cardinal signs of inflammation result from increased blood flow in the affected area?
   a. Swelling
   b. Heat
   c. Pain
   d. Redness
6. Manifestations of inflammation resulting from increased vascular permeability include:
   a. Swelling
   b. Heat
   c. Pain
   d. Redness
7. Which of the following are believed to be causes of pain in an inflamed area?
   a. Pressure of the exudate
   b. Changes in the pH caused by acidic breakdown products
   c. Release of chemical mediators that stimulate nerve endings

Continued.

d. Increased flow of lymph

8. The two major forces that normally govern the transport of fluid between the intravascular and interstitial spaces are:
   a. The hydrostatic pressure of the blood
   b. The contractility of endothelial cells
   c. The osmotic pressure of the plasma proteins
   d. The permeability of connective tissue

9. Which one of the following reactions occurs in an acute inflammatory response?
   a. Lymph flow decreases, producing edema.
   b. Arterioles in the area dilate to produce active congestion.
   c. Protein follows water into the interstitial spaces.
   d. The permeability of the venules decreases because of the release of local chemical mediators.

10. An exudate differs from a transudate in that:
    a. Exudates contain more cells derived from the blood.
    b. Transudates are much smaller in quantity.
    c. A transudate is a result of a noninflammatory situation.
    d. Exudates have a higher protein content than transudates.

11. In an acute inflammatory reaction, the initial cause of fluid moving into the injured area is:
    a. Decreased intravascular hydrostatic pressure
    b. Separation of intercellular endothelial junctions
    c. Decreased colloid osmotic pressure
    d. Decreased lymphatic flow

12. Which of the following best describes histamine?
    a. It produces vasoconstriction.
    b. It increases vascular permeability.
    c. It is released from mast cells early in inflammation.
    d. It has an important role in chronic inflammation.

13. Hageman factor is known to:
    a. Increase vascular permeability
    b. Be present in plasma in an active form
    c. Trigger the clotting cascade system
    d. Be an important inflammatory mediator

14. The cyclooxygenase pathway is responsible for generating which of the following mediators of inflammation?
    a. Histamine
    b. Hageman factor
    c. Prostaglandins
    d. Leukotrienes

15. In an acute inflammatory reaction, the first cells to appear at the site of injury are generally the:
    a. Monocytes
    b. Lymphocytes
    c. Plasma cells
    d. Polymorphonuclear neutrophils (PMNs)

16. The cells least likely to be found in large numbers (dominant in the exudate) in chronic inflammation are:
    a. Lymphocytes
    b. Plasma cells
    c. Macrophages
    d. Fibroblasts
    e. PMNs

17. A process by which bacteria are rendered more susceptible to phagocytosis is:
    a. Pavementing
    b. Margination
    c. Opsonization
    d. Chemotaxis

18. Phagocytosis of bacteria in acute inflammation is associated with:
    a. PMNs
    b. Lymphocytes
    c. Erythrocytes
    d. Monocytes

19. Basophils:
    a. Have many features in common with mast cells in connective tissue
    b. Have cytoplasmic granules that stain deep blue with basic dyes
    c. Are generally present in large numbers in exudates
    d. Are granulocytes that contain histamine and heparin in their cytoplasmic granules

20. The mechanisms of leukocytosis in the course of an inflammatory reaction include:
    a. Increased production of leukocytes by the bone marrow
    b. Increased life span of leukocytes during inflammation
    c. Increased release of leukocytes from the bone marrow reserves into the blood
    d. Stimulation of the vascular endothelium by pyrogens

21. The monocyte-macrophage system:
    a. Was originally called the reticuloendothelial system
    b. Provides a major defense against the spread of infection in the body
    c. Removes foreign material from circulating blood, lymph, and tissue spaces
    d. Includes as components blood monocytes, wandering macrophages, and fixed mononuclear phagocytic cells
    e. Is present in the bone marrow, spleen, lymph nodes, and liver

22. Epithelioid cells:
    a. Are altered epithelial cells
    b. Are common components of granulomatous inflammation
    c. Serve to wall off an agent that cannot be destroyed or eliminated from the body
    d. Are altered macrophages

23. The distinct feature(s) of eosinophils is (are):
    a. They are associated with allergic reactions.
    b. They release digestive enzymes and oxygen metabolites into host tissues.
    c. They form a significant concentration at site of parasitic infestation.
    d. They respond to chemotactic signals in immunologic reactions.

24. Pus contains:
    a. Dead and dying neutrophils
    b. Microorganisms
    c. Tissue debris
    d. Water and solutes

25. Which of the following cells are capable of regeneration after necrosis?
    a. Myocardial cells
    b. Epithelial cells of the gastrointestinal tract
    c. Neurons
    d. Hepatocytes
    e. Lymphoid cells

26. What two cell types play the primary role in organization?
    a. Fibroblasts producing collagen
    b. Osteoblasts producing mature scar tissue
    c. Endothelial cells producing new blood vessels
    d. Parenchymal cells producing new connective tissue

27. Which of the following may organize?
    a. Unresolved exudate
    b. Necrotic tissue

QUESTIONS—cont'd

c. Persistent blood clots
d. Collagen fibers

28. In comparison with healing by first intention, healing by second intention involves:
a. Good apposition of wound edges
b. A longer time for the process to be completed
c. Less scarring
d. Formation of more granulation tissue
e. A greater amount of exudate

29. The outcome of inflammation is affected by:
a. Vascularity of the tissue
b. Patient's nutritional status
c. Presence of debris
d. Immunologic capability

30. Systemic manifestations associated with inflammation include:
a. Leukocytosis
b. Malaise (vague feeling of discomfort)
c. Fever
d. Agranulocytosis

31. Cytokines are released primarily by activated:
a. Macrophages
b. Fibroblasts
c. Eosinophils
d. Lymphocytes

32. Leukocyte adhesion and transmigration involve the binding of which of the following complementary adhesion molecules?
a. Endothelial adhesion molecules
b. Selectins
c. Integrins
d. None of the above

33. The primary function(s) of nitric oxide include(s) which of the following?
a. Causes vasomotor effects that can affect platelet function
b. Acts as tumor necrosis factor
c. Acts as cytotoxic free radical
d. Stimulates the expression of selections

▼ *Circle T if the statement is true and F it if is false. Correct any false statements.*

34. T F Nitric oxide (NO) is a cell-derivated mediator produced by cells such as macrophages and endothelial cells.

35. T F Three cytokines that are important in mediating inflammation are IL-1, IL-8, and TNF.

36. T F When a specific area of the body is infected, the regional lymph nodes may act as filters, preventing further spread of the bacteria in the body.

37. T F A chemotactic effect can be exerted only by the injurious agent.

38. T F Monocytes and neutrophils both respond to chemotactic signals.

39. T F Mast cells are the primary source of histamine.

40. T F Lysosomes are packets of digestive enzymes within the cytoplasm of neutrophils and other cells.

41. T F Monocytes differ from neutrophils in that they are capable of synthesizing intracellular enzymes and dividing after migration to the tissues, whereas neutrophils are not.

42. T F When a circulating monocyte appears in an exudate, it is called a mast cell.

43. T F Granulation tissue consists primarily of proliferating young connective tissue.

44. T F Healing by second intention requires a longer time and leaves a larger scar than healing by primary intention.

45. T F Granulomas may result from a foreign material such as a nonabsorbable suture left in the body or from certain bacteria, such as the tubercle bacillus, which are resistant to phagocytosis or enzymatic digestion.

46. T F Granuloma formation indicates that the body cannot easily overcome or eliminate the agent responsible.

47. T F Giant cells are formed by the fusion of neutrophils in chronic granulomatous inflammation.

48. T F Subacute inflammation shows evidence of advanced repair along with exudation.

49. T F A keloid represents disordered wound healing and is caused by the proliferation of nerve fibers and their entrapment in dense scar tissue.

50. T F Arachidonic acid is derived from cell membrane phospholipids when phospholipases are activated by injury.

51. T F Prostaglandins are important vascular and chemotactic mediators of inflammation.

▼ *Match the following types of exudates in column A with the statements in column B.*

Column A	Column B
52. _____ Catarrhal	a. Poorly limited spreading or diffuse inflammation
53. _____ Suppurative	b. Occurs only on mucous membranes and contains mucin
54. _____ Phlegmonous (cellulitis)	c. Includes a web of fibrinopurulent exudate coating the necrotic mucosal surface
55. _____ Serous	d. Contains very few cells (e.g., blister fluid)
56. _____ Pseudomembranous	e. Contains many living and dead neutrophils and debris liquefied by enzymes released from the dead neutrophils

---

▼ *Fill in the blanks with the correct words.*

57. A(n) _____ is a lesion within solid tissue and contains dead cells, liquefied tissue, neutrophils, and often bacteria.

58. A(n) _____ is a local gap in the continuity of the mucosal surface.

59. The accumulation of pus in the pleural cavity is called _____.

Continued.

? QUESTIONS—cont'd

60. An abnormal communication tract between two organs or the lumen of a hollow organ and the body surface is called a(n) _____.
61. The suffix for inflammation is _____.
62. _____ is the term describing the movement of leukocytes from the axial stream to the periphery of the blood vessel lumen.
63. _____ is the term used to describe leukocytes inserting pseudopodia in intercellular junctions and sliding and wriggling through to the extravascular spaces.
64. The resorption of exudate with return of the area to normal is called _____.
65. _____ is the replacement of dead or injured tissues by new cells of parenchymal or stromal origin.
66. Inflammation of the lymph nodes is termed _____.
67. The correct sequence of the following events as they occur in an inflammatory reaction is _____.
    a. Tissue injury
    b. Increased local blood flow, leading to heat and redness
    c. Emigration of leukocytes
    d. Slowing of blood flow; margination of leukocytes
    e. Increased vascular permeability

CHAPTER 5

Response of the Body to Immunologic Challenge

MARILYN SAWYER SOMMERS

The function of the immune system in the human body is to differentiate "self" from "nonself." All organisms are a delicate integration of cells, tissues, and organs, with each necessary for the sustenance of life. To support life, an organism must be able to protect itself against threats to its individuality. These threats can exist externally (e.g., a splinter stuck beneath the skin, a virus or bacterium ingested or inhaled) or internally (e.g., a neoplasm or tumor derived from the body's own cells).

IMMUNITY: OVERVIEW AND DEFINITIONS

To protect itself against threats to individuality, the human body has developed cellular defense reactions that are labeled the *immune response*. The terms *immunology* and *immunity* are derived from the Latin word *immunitas*, which was used in Roman times to describe the protection from civic duties and legal prosecution that Roman senators received during their terms of office. Historically the terms have come to describe protection from infectious disease. In order for the human body to protect itself, it requires mechanisms to differentiate its own cells (self) from invading agents (nonself).

These mechanisms can be described as the body's *immunity*, a state of protection (primarily against infectious agents) that is characterized by memory and specificity. *Memory* is the heightened ability of an organism to respond to an *antigen* (cell or molecule that promotes an immune response; also known as an *immunogen*) because of previous exposure to the antigen. *Specificity* is the property that immune system cells demonstrate when they have the ability to react with one and only one antigenic determinant. Immunity has three primary functions: (1) its role in *defense* is to provide resistance to invaders such as microorganisms; (2) its role in *surveillance* is to identify and destroy the body's own cells that mutate and have the potential to form neoplasms (tumors); and (3) its role in *homeostasis* is to remove cellular debris and waste so that cell types remain uniform and unchanged.

Self Versus Nonself

An important key to the body's ability to distinguish self from nonself is the *major histocompatibility complex* (MHC), a single gene cluster on the short arm of the sixth chromosome. The MHC gene cluster controls the production of one particular set of molecules that serve as cellular antigens, "self-markers," to indicate that all cells belong to one particular organism. These surface antigens are inherited and unique to each person. They serve as cellular labels; recognition of the MHC antigen by the body's own immune system causes the development of *self-tolerance* (the body's ability to restrain from attacking native cells). In humans, MHC antigens are often called the *human leukocyte antigens* (HLAs) because they were first detected on white blood cells (WBCs).

Role of Antigens (Immunogens)

Although the terms *antigen* and *immunogen* are often used interchangeably, they have subtle differences. An antigen is a molecule or cell that reacts with *antibodies* (also known as *immunoglobulins,* which are plasma glycoproteins secreted by activated B lymphocytes). Immunoglobulins are capable of binding with the specific antigen that stimulated their production. An immunogen is a molecule or cell that induces an immune response. For the most part, either term (antigen or immunogen) is appropriate unless the molecule involved is a *hapten* (an antigen that is not an immunogen unless it is bound to a larger carrier molecule). A hapten, therefore, cannot initiate an immunogenic response by itself; it is an antigen but not an immunogen. Penicillin G is an example of a medication that serves as a hapten and results in a severe allergic reaction in some people. Other haptens include toxins and certain hormones. Although most haptens are small molecules, some high-molecular-weight nucleic acids are also haptens.

Several features of molecules determine their potential ability to evoke an immune response. Molecules that are nonself are distinctly different from body cells. The *foreignness* of molecules, therefore, is an essential characteristic of molecules that elicit an immune response. The *size* of molecules is also important. The strongest immunogens are proteins with a molecular weight greater than 100,000 daltons. Molecules with a low molecular weight of less than 10,000 daltons are weakly immunogenic, and very small molecules such as haptens need a carrier protein to become immunogenic. The *chemical complexity* is also an important consideration. Complex molecules such as polymers (matter formed by a combination of two or more molecules of the same substance) are more immunogenic than a single amino acid. In addi-

tion, the *concentration* of an immunogen has to be of sufficient quantity to elicit an immune response.

A final important feature of immunogens is the presence of *epitopes* (some authors refer to an epitope as an *antigenic determinant*). An epitope is a small chemical group on the immunogen that can elicit an immune response and can react with an immunoglobulin (Fig. 5-1). Most immunogens have more than one type of epitope and are considered "multivalent." Other immunogens have repeated epitopes. Usually an epitope is about five amino acids or sugars in size. The specificity of the immune response depends on the response to epitopes. Immunoglobulins are produced that are specific for the epitope rather than the whole immunogen cell or molecule. The immunoglobulin, therefore, does not bind to an entire cell or molecule but rather to the epitopes on the immunogen's surface.

Common foreign immunogens include microorganisms such as bacteria, viruses, and fungi and organic substances such as pollen or house dust. When organs, tissues, cells, or molecules from other humans or even other species are introduced into a person through transplant surgery, blood transfusion, or vaccination, they also serve as immunogens. Native immunogens can also evoke an immune response, particularly when body cells mutate and become cancer cells.

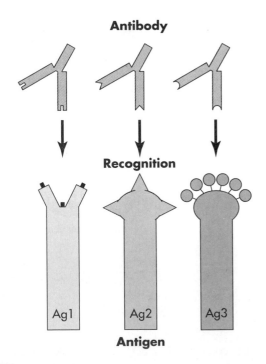

FIG. 5-1 Antigens, molecules that generate an immune response, each have a set of epitopes (antigenic determinants). The epitopes on one antigen (*Ag1, Ag2*) are usually different from those on another, although antigens such as Ag3 may have repeated epitopes. Epitopes are molecular shapes recognized by the antibodies and T cell receptors of the adaptive immune system.

OVERVIEW OF THE IMMUNE SYSTEM

The human body's lymphoid system works together with the monocyte-macrophage system (defense-related phagocytosis; see Chapter 4) to discriminate self from nonself. The lymphoid system defends the body against invaders through the use of two immune responses: cell-mediated immunity and humoral immunity. *Cell-mediated immunity,* or cellular immune response, is the immune response carried out by T lymphocytes. When the body is exposed to an immunogen, the T cells proliferate and direct a host of cellular and subcellular interactions to react to the specific epitope. *Humoral immunity,* or antibody-mediated immunity, is specific immunity mediated by the production of immunoglobulins (antibodies) by B lymphocytes in response to an epitope. Humoral immunity is also assisted by the *complement system,* an amplification system that completes the action of immunoglobulins to kill nonself immunogens.

The Lymphoid (Immune) System

The *lymphoid (immune) system* is composed of cells, tissues, and organs in which lymphocyte precursors and derivatives originate, differentiate, mature, and lodge. All blood cells originate from the common precursor, the stem cell. *Stem cells* are self-replicating cells found in the bone marrow and other hematopoietic tissues that give rise to all the blood components (e.g., erythrocytes, platelets, granulocytes, macrophages, lymphocytes). Stem cells differentiate and mature into specific blood cells (Fig. 5-2) under the direction of a variety of *colony-stimulating factors* (group of substances that increase the production of various types of hematologic cells) and additional cell-derived growth factors. Three types of lymphocytes are derived from stem cells: *T lymphocytes* (known as T cells), *B lymphocytes* (known as B cells), and *natural killer cells* (NK cells) (Table 5-1). NK cells are sometimes classified as a type of T cell because they share some characteristics with T cells and have other individual characteristics. These three cell types are differ-

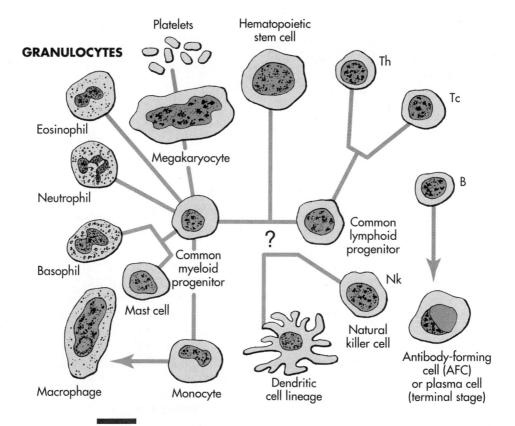

FIG. 5-2   All the cells involved in the immune system response are derived from pluripotential stem cells in the bone marrow. The stem cells give rise to two main lineages: lymphoid cells and myeloid cells. The common lymphoid progenitor differentiates into either a T cell or a B cell; the myeloid progenitor differentiates into the committed cells shown on the left. The term *granulocyte* is sometimes used for neutrophils, eosinophils, and basophils.

▶ TABLE 5-1   Types of Lymphocytes

Characteristics	T Cells	B Cells	Natural Killer (NK) cells
Origin	Stem cell	Stem cell	Stem Cell
Maturation	Thymus	? Bone marrow	? Bloodstream
Peripheral sites	Lymph nodes (paracortical area)	Lymph nodes (cortex)	Bloodstream
	Spleen (white pulp)	Spleen (white and red pulp)	
	Gut-associated lymphoid tissue (GALT, or Peyer's patches)	GALT, BALT	
	Bronchus-associated lymphoid tissue (BALT)		
Percentage of total lymphocytes	65-80	20-30	5-15
Type of immunity	Cell mediated	Humoral	Nonspecific
Subpopulations	CD4 (helper)	Plasma cells	None
	CD8 (cytotoxic)	Memory B cells	
	CD8 (suppressor)		
	Memory T cells		
Products	Lymphokines	Immunoglobulins	Perforins
	Interleukins: IL-2, IL-3, IL-4, IL-5, IL-6, IL-9, IL-10	Lymphokines: IL-6	
	Gamma interferon		
	Colony-stimulating factors		
	Tumor necrosis factor (TNF)		
	Perforins		
Protection against	Viruses (intracellular)	Bacteria	Viruses (extracellular)
	Fungi	Viruses	Tumor cells
	Parasites		Allografts
	Tumor cells		
	Allografts (transplanted tissue)		
Other characteristics			
Surface immunogen receptors	Yes	Yes	No
Memory	Yes	Yes	No
CD proteins on surface	Yes: CD3 and others	No	Yes: CD2 and CD16
Immunoglobulins on surface	No	Yes	No

entiated from each other by protein markers on their cell surfaces called *clusters of differentiation* (CD). CD proteins are used to differentiate T cells, NK cells, and B cells from each other and are also useful markers to identify subsets of T cells.

Primary Lymphoid Organs

Although lymphocytes exist in all parts of the body, they tend to be highly concentrated in several lymphoid organs, including the bone marrow, the thymus, the spleen, the lymph nodes, and in the organ-associated lymphoid tissues (Fig. 5-3). The bone marrow and thymus are considered the *primary lymphoid organs*. In the initial stages of lymphocyte development from stem cells in the bone marrow, lymphocytes do not produce receptors for reaction with immunogens. As they mature under the control of colony-stimulating factors, they begin to express (present on their cell surface) immunogen receptors and become responsive to immunogenic stimulation. They also develop into the three different subclasses. T cells mi-

grate from the bone marrow to the thymus gland for further maturation and are considered "thymus-dependent" lymphocytes. B cells probably remain in the bone marrow and are considered "thymus-independent" lymphocytes. NK cells are lymphocytes with some T cell markers. A primary difference between NK cells and T cells, however, is that NK cells are "prethymic"; that is, they do not pass through the thymus to mature.

The *thymus* is a two-lobed organ that is located in the mediastinum anterior to and above the heart. At birth the thymus weighs 10 to 15 g and increases in size to its maximum at puberty, when it weighs as much as 40 g. During adulthood and older age, it undergoes involution until it weighs less than 15% of its size at puberty. The thymus is a highly vascular organ with many lymphatic vessels that drain into the mediastinal lymph nodes. The thymus has both an outer cortex and an inner medulla (Fig. 5-4). The cortex contains a heavy concentration of *thymocytes* (T lymphocytes found in the thymus), whereas the medulla is more sparsely populated. *Hassall's corpuscles,* groups of tightly packed epithelial cells

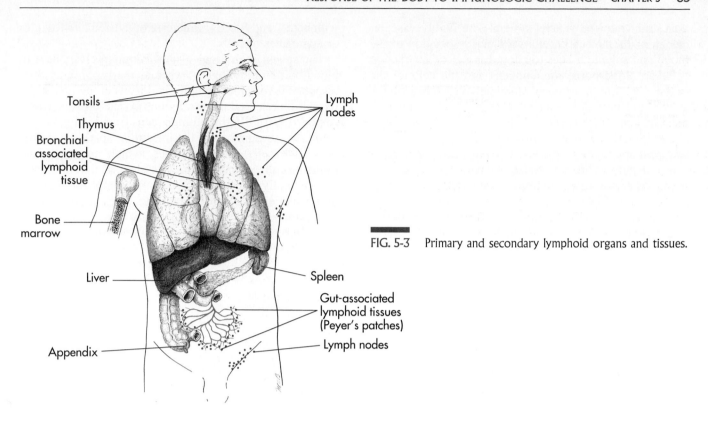

FIG. 5-3   Primary and secondary lymphoid organs and tissues.

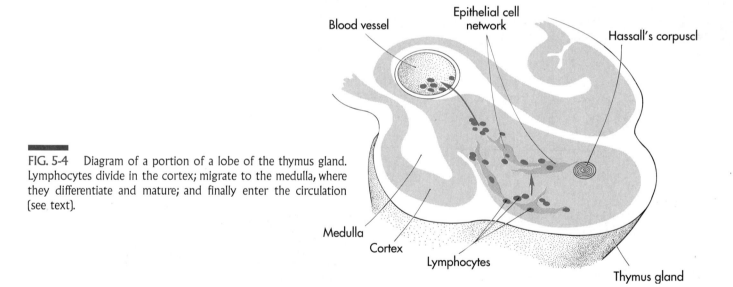

FIG. 5-4   Diagram of a portion of a lobe of the thymus gland. Lymphocytes divide in the cortex; migrate to the medulla, where they differentiate and mature; and finally enter the circulation (see text).

that may be areas of cell degeneration, are found in the medulla. The thymocytes are T lymphocytes that have arrived from the bone marrow via the bloodstream and are at various stages of maturation.

Secondary Lymphoid Organs

The *secondary lymphoid organs* include the spleen, the lymph nodes, and nonencapsulated (without a capsule) tissue. Examples of nonencapsulated tissue are the ton-

sils, adenoids, and patches of lymphoid tissue in the lamina propria (fibrous connective tissue that lies directly beneath surface epithelium of a mucous membrane) and in the submucosa of the gastrointestinal (GI), respiratory, and genitourinary (GU) tracts. The *spleen* weighs approximately 150 g in adults and is located in the left upper quadrant of the abdomen behind the stomach. Blood supply arrives via the splenic artery, which divides into progressively smaller branches. When the branches divide into arterioles, they drain into vascular sinusoids that then drain into the venous system. The highly vascular design of the spleen provides a close association of the blood and splenic tissues to allow for a close interaction between blood-borne immunogens and the cells of the immune system. In essence, blood percolates through the spleen and comes in contact with a larger number of macrophages (phagocytic WBCs) and lymphocytes, which initiate the immune response. The spleen contains two primary types of tissues: *red pulp* and *white pulp*. The red pulp is mainly concerned with destruction of worn-out erythrocytes (red blood cells [RBCs]) but also contains macrophages, platelets, and lymphocytes (B cells in particular). The white pulp of the spleen is dense, lymphoid tissue arranged around a central arteriole. This arrangement is often called the *periarteriolar lymphoid sheath* (PALS) (Fig. 5-5). The PALS contains cell areas

with both T and B cells, which are organized into follicles or aggregates of cells.

The spleen is the major site of immune responses to blood-borne immunogens, whereas the *lymph nodes* are responsible for processing immunogens in the lymph derived from regional tissues. Lymph nodes form a network responsible for filtering immunogens from the lymph and from fluid draining from the interstitial space (space between the cells). Lymph nodes, which are small and round or kidney-shaped structures 1 to 20 mm in diameter, generally occur at branches of lymphatic vessels. Lymph node clusters are found in the neck, axillae, groin, mediastinum, and abdominal cavity (Fig. 5-6). Lymph flows into the lymph nodes through afferent (inflowing) lymphatics into the subcapsular sinuses (Fig. 5-7). The lymph then flows toward the hilus (a central terminus for

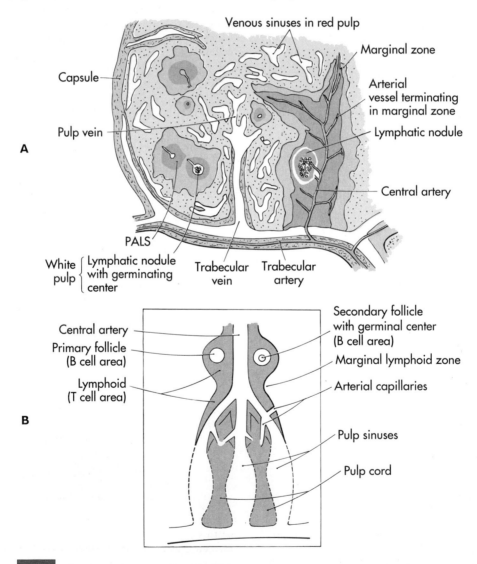

FIG. 5-5   Structure of the spleen. **A,** The white pulp is composed of periarteriolar lymphoid sheaths *(PALS),* which contain germinal centers with mantle zones. The red pulp contains venous sinuses separated by splenic cords. **B,** In white pulp, B cell areas are primary and secondary follicles and the marginal lymphoid zone, whereas T cell areas are lymphoid cells around the follicles and arterial capillaries. (**B** redrawn from Videback A et al: *The spleen in health and disease,* Chicago, 1982, Mosby.)

blood and lymph) and then exits through the efferent (outflowing) lymphatics.

Lymph nodes are surrounded by a connective tissue capsule and are organized into three main areas: the cortex, the paracortex, and the medulla. The *cortex* contains clusters of B cells called *lymphoid follicles* (primary follicles). When the body is exposed to an immunogen, B cells in this area form *germinal centers* (secondary follicles). Within these active centers, B cells divide, proliferate, and mature rapidly into immunoglobulin-producing cells. The *paracortex*, or inner cortex, is populated primarily by T cells and macrophages. Macrophages,

other phagocytic cells, and B cells are also known as *antigen-presenting cells* (APCs) because they engulf and degrade immunogens and present epitopes on the cell surface to activate T lymphocytes. The paracortex is an important area where immunogens are presented on the macrophage, and T cells become activated as a result. The *medulla,* the smallest portion of lymph nodes, contains both T cells and B cells. Medullary sinuses drain into terminal sinuses to provide a mechanism for the lymph to drain out of the lymph node into the general lymphatic circulation.

Several areas of nonencapsulated lymphoid tissue exist in body systems. This tissue, often described as *mucosa-associated lymphoid tissue* (MALT), is organized into diffuse clumps of cells or nodules containing germinal centers (secondary follicles) similar to those in the spleen. MALT acts as a guard to protect the body at several submucosal entry sites in the GI, respiratory, and GU tracts and the skin. MALT is further divided into subclassifications organized by their location. *Gut-*

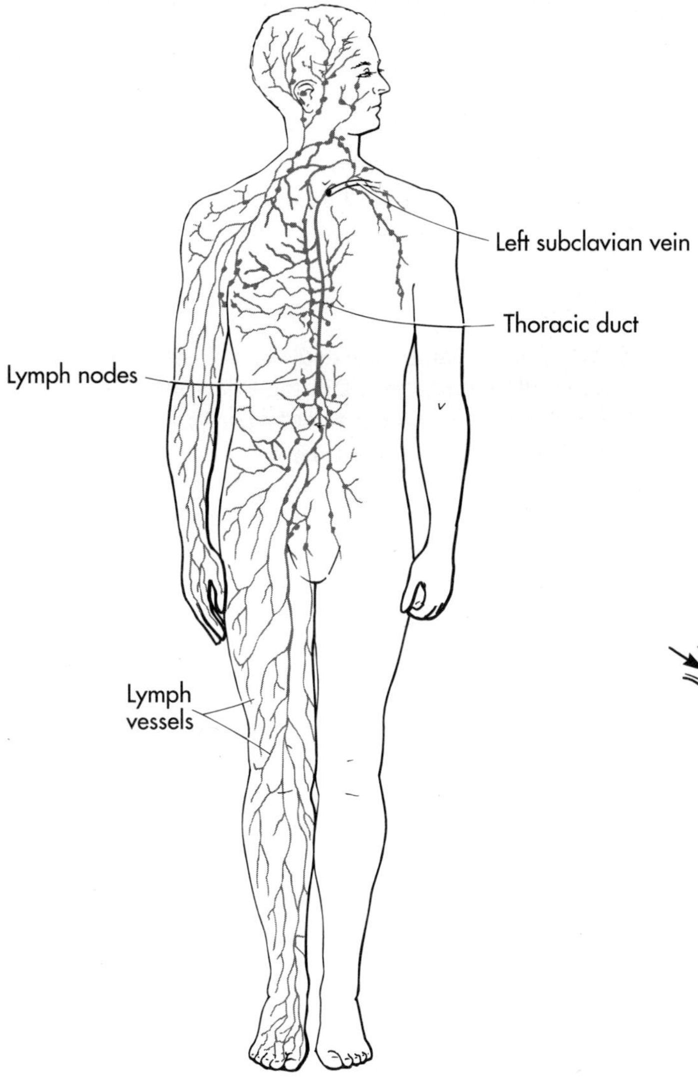

FIG. 5-6   The lymphatic system. Lymph nodes are found at junctures of lymphatic vessels and·form a complete network, draining and filtering lymph derived from the tissue spaces. They are either superficial or visceral, draining the skin or deep tissues and internal organs of the body. The lymph eventually reaches the thoracic duct, which drains into the left subclavian vein and thus back into the circulation.

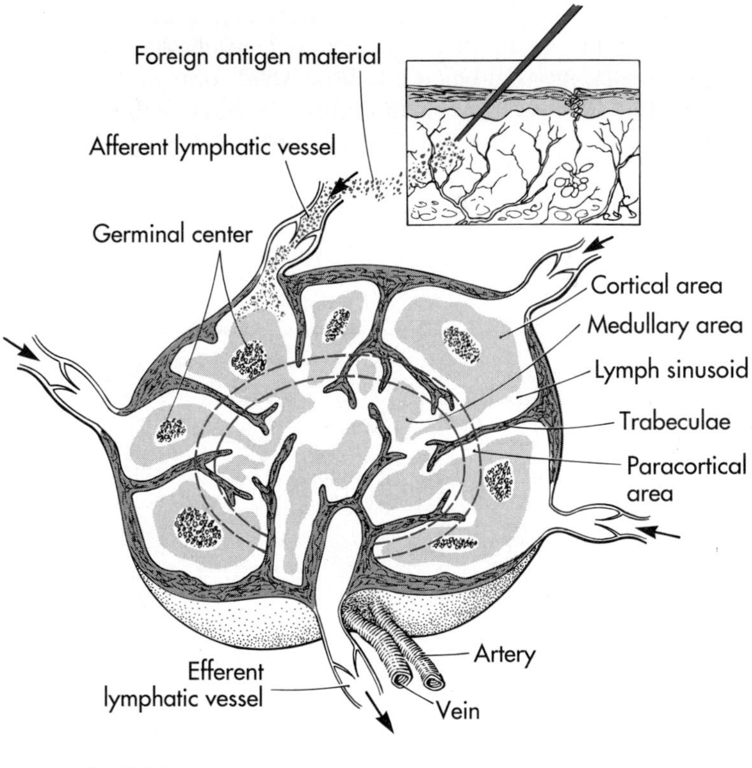

FIG. 5-7   Structure of a lymph node. Lymph nodes are organized into three main areas: the outer cortex, where B cells proliferate and mature; the deeper paracortex, populated mainly by macrophages and T cells; and the inner medulla, containing both B cells and T cells. Macrophages, B cells, and T cells interact with each other, often in the presence of antigen percolating through the node, resulting in the inductive phase of the immune response.

associated lymphoid tissue (GALT) includes the tonsils, which are strategically positioned to intercept airborne and ingested immunogens. Peyer's patches (nodules of lymphoid tissue on the outer wall of the intestine) and the appendix have T and B cell areas and can also respond to alimentary immunogens. Immunoglobulins produced in GALT migrate to the GI tract, tear ducts, and salivary glands to defend against nonself penetration of epithelial surfaces. *Bronchus-associated lymphoid tissue* (BALT) resembles GALT and is found at the bifurcations of larger branches of the respiratory tree. *Skin-associated lymphoid tissue* (SALT) is found in the epidermis of the skin, where lymphocytes identify foreign invaders in the epidermis and transport the epitopes to a regional lymph node for processing.

Lymphocytic Traffic Within the Body

The various components of the lymphoid system are joined together by a sort of "double-plumbing" system—the blood vascular system and the lymphatic system (Fig. 5-8). At any given time, millions of lymphocytes are moving within the blood and the lymph. The various lymphatic channels in the body drain fluid from the interstices of organs and tissues. The lymph is conducted into large central channels that join together and enter the bloodstream via the thoracic duct. A constant flow of lymph back into the blood and a constant formation of lymph by the movement of fluid from the blood into the tissues therefore occur. Similarly, lymphocytes are constantly recirculated. The lymph within the thoracic duct contains many lymphocytes. Sufficient numbers of lymphocytes flow through the thoracic duct to replace the total number in circulation in the bloodstream several times per day.

Most lymphocytes flowing in the thoracic duct are being "recycled." Lymphocytes leave the bloodstream by specialized venules within lymphoid tissues, spend variable lengths of time within the lymphoid tissues, and then circulate via the lymph to rejoin the lymphocytes in the circulating blood. Lymphocytes differ from one another with respect to their movements around the body. Some lymphocytes are remarkably long-lived (many months or even years) and travel and recycle extensively. Other lymphocytes are relatively short-lived and do not move around quite as freely. It also appears that certain groups of lymphocytes have preferential "homing" patterns with respect to various parts of the lymphoid system. The key point is that a provision exists within the lymphoid system for moving lymphocytes from one area to another. The biologic importance of this fact is that members of a particular clone of lymphocytes that initially proliferate in one given location may circulate around the body and be available for interaction with immunogens at many locations.

Cell-mediated Immunity

The role of T cells can be divided into two major functions: the regulator functions and the effector functions. The *regulator functions* are primarily performed by one subset of T cells, the *helper T cells* (also known as CD4 cells because the cluster of differentiation marker on the cell surface has been assigned the number 4). The CD4

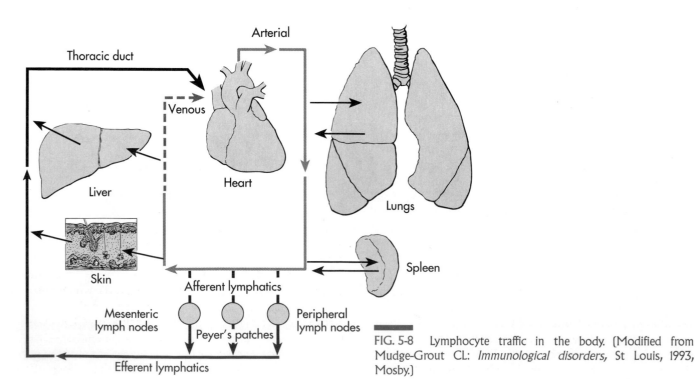

FIG. 5-8   Lymphocyte traffic in the body. (Modified from Mudge-Grout CL: *Immunological disorders,* St Louis, 1993, Mosby.)

cells perform their regulator function by releasing molecules known as *lymphokines* (small-molecular-weight proteins secreted by lymphocytes). Many other cell types release the same or related molecules; in aggregate, these proteins are termed *cytokines*. Lymphokines from CD4 cells regulate immune processes such as the production of immunoglobulins by B cells, the activation of other T cells, and the activation of macrophages. The *effector functions* are performed by *cytotoxic T cells* (formerly known as killer T cells but not to be confused with NK cells; currently known also as CD8 cells because the cluster of differentiation has been assigned the number 8). CD8 cells are able to kill virus-infected cells, tumor cells, and transplanted tissues by injecting chemicals called *perforins* into the "foreign" target.

Thymic education

Both CD4 and CD8 cells undergo "thymic education" in the thymus gland so that they learn their functions. The *theory of clonal deletion* provides one explanation of how the T cells learn their functions. When immature T cells reach the thymus, they have no epitope-binding receptor and no CD4 or CD8 protein. The role of an epitope receptor in a mature T cell is to bind an antigenic epitope. The role of the CD4 or CD8 proteins in a mature T cell is to stabilize the interaction between a T cell and other cells (Fig. 5-9). A mature T cell leaving the thymus, therefore, has a receptor to bind with an epitope and either a CD4 protein (making the cell a *CD4 T cell,* also known as a *helper T cell*) or a CD8 protein (making the cell a *CD8 T cell,* also known as a *cytotoxic* or *suppressor T cell*).

If the T cell is to be ready to perform its functions when it leaves the thymus, therefore, it needs first to recognize nonself epitopes and second to have functioning CD4 or CD8 protein. Successful thymic education thus produces either CD4 or CD8 T cells with the following functions: (1) cells that recognize other self cells from the MHC antigen and do not bind with them (i.e., the T cell protein receptor will not have a good "fit" with other self cells); (2) cells that recognize nonself cells as invaders; and (3) cells that can bind with nonself cells with a functioning CD4 or CD8 protein to stabilize the interaction between the two cells (see Fig. 5-9). Cells potentially reactive with self antigens *and* MHC components are probably also produced but are deleted within the thymus. They may be either killed by other cells or made to undergo *apoptosis* (programmed death).

Regulator functions of CD4 cells

The CD4 cells are found primarily in the medulla of the thymus, tonsils, and blood. They make up approximately 65% of the total circulating T lymphocytes. One essential regulatory function of CD4 cells is their role in linking the *monocyte-macrophage system* (system containing defense-related phagocytic WBCs such as monocytes and macrophages) to the lymphoid system. When a

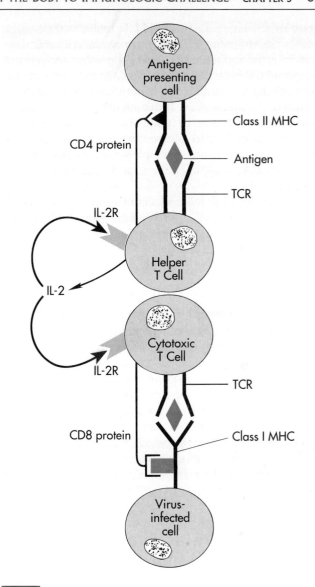

FIG. 5-9   Activation of T cells. The antigen-presenting cell (APC) presents the antigen by means of class II MHC to the helper T cell. The reaction is stabilized by the CD4 protein. The helper T cell is activated to produce interleukin-2 *(IL-2),* which binds to the receptors and further activates the cells. The virally infected cell presents the antigen by means of class I MHC to the cytotoxic T cell, and in conjunction with IL-2 produced by the helper T cell, the cytotoxic T cell is activated to destroy the virally infected cell. The reaction is stabilized by the CD8 protein.

macrophage ingests an immunogen such as a bacterium, it degrades the immunogen by the processes described in Chapter 4. The bacteria's epitopes are one of the products of bacterial destruction. An epitope binds with the macrophage's MHC antigen (MHC class II), which raises the MHC-epitope complex "like a flag" on the macrophage's cell surface. This "flag" activates CD4 cells, whose antigen receptor also binds with the epitope-MHC complex. This interaction between phagocytic cells and the lymphoid cells is an essential link that allows the body to defend against invaders. It unites two powerful body systems, the monocyte-macrophage system and the lymphoid system, into a defense system that protects self from nonself throughout the person's life. The interaction between the APC and the CD4 cells leads to an additional regulator function. CD4 cells in this reaction release gamma- (γ-)interferon (a lymphokine) once the APC and the CD4 cell are bound. The release of γ-interferon by the CD4 cell attracts other macrophages into the area, activates them, and amplifies the tissue reaction to the foreign antigen.

The CD4 cell has other important regulatory functions, particularly those involved with immunoglobulin production. When an APC presents an epitope, the APC interacts with a CD4 cell and activates it. The activated CD4 cell produces chemicals or lymphokines such as interleukins 2, 4, and 5 (IL-2, IL-4, IL-5). These lymphokines and other interactions stimulate B cells to divide and differentiate into *plasma cells,* the mature B cells that are capable of producing immunoglobulins. CD4 cells are essential, therefore, to stimulate B cells to produce immunoglobulins. Furthermore, the pattern of cytokines to which B cells are exposed affects gene rearrangements that determine the type of antibody to be secreted.

CD4 cells have other regulator functions. For example, when they interact with an APC, IL-2 production is also important for the growth of other CD4 and CD8 cells; this role promotes cell-mediated immunity. In addition, some T cells will develop into *memory T cells,* which are capable of rapid activation on exposure to the epitope at a later time.

Controversy exists as to whether a distinct subset exists of CD8 cells that have a regulatory function in the body. Some immunologists suggest that certain CD8 cells have a suppressor function that modulates or "turns off" the action of helper (CD4) and cytotoxic (CD8) T cells so that they do not cause harmful responses. At present, however, immunologists are not able to identify a specific subset of suppressor CD8 cells that have this "moderating" role. Although CD8 cells do have suppressor function, current thinking is that suppressor CD8 cells and cytotoxic CD8 cells are not distinguishable.

Effector functions of CD8 cells

CD8 lymphocytes, which are found primarily in human bone marrow and GALT, make up about 35% of all circulating T lymphocytes. The CD8 cells perform two primary effector functions: delayed hypersensitivity and cytotoxicity. *Delayed hypersensitivity* occurs when immunogens of intracellular organisms such as fungi or mycobacteria cause an allergic response.

Cytotoxicity is concerned primarily with destruction of virus-infected cells, graft rejection, and destruction of tumor cells. All cells of the body contain one type of MHC antigens (MHC Class I) that can display a viral epitope on the cell surface. CD8 cells recognize that MHC-epitope complex and, with the help of CD4 cells, develop

a clone of CD8 cells specific to the viral epitope. The CD8 cells then release *perforins,* toxic chemicals that damage the infected cell's outer membrane. Perforins form a channel through the cell membrane, allowing extracellular fluid to enter and the cell to lyse. When the virus-infected cell dies, the CD8 cell is unharmed and continues to kill other cells infected with the same virus.

When a foreign organ or tissue is transplanted, the recipient's CD8 cells recognize that the MHC antigens on the transplanted cells' surface are not self. With the help of CD4 cells, the CD8 cells develop a clone of cells that are specific to the destruction of the nonself epitopes on the transplanted cells' surface. The CD8 cells kill the cells in the foreign tissue by the release of perforins. A similar process occurs with tumor cells. As tumors grow, they often develop new immunogens (different from the self components on normal body cells) on their surface. Relevant epitopes are recognized by CD8 cells, which form a clone to serve as tumor surveillance, ideally to kill neoplasms as they develop.

Major functions of cell-mediated immunity

In summary, cell-mediated immunity has four frequently cited functions:

1. CD8 T cells have a *cytotoxic* function. CD8 cells cause direct cell death of target cells such as virally infected cells or tumor cells. The CD8 cells perform this function by binding with the virally infected cell and releasing perforins to cause cell death.
2. T cells also cause *delayed hypersensitivity reactions* when they produce lymphokines that lead to inflammation. The lymphokines not only directly affect tissues, but also activate other cells such as APCs.
3. T cells have the capability to provide *memory.* Memory T cells allow for an accelerated immune response the second time the body is exposed to an immunogen and often long after the initial immunizing exposure.
4. T cells also have an important role in *regulation* or control. CD4 and CD8 cells facilitate and/or suppress cell-mediated and humoral immune responses.

Natural killer cells

Although NK cells are not truly T cells, they also perform important effector functions. NK cells specialize in destroying virus-infected cells and neoplasms by secreting perforins similar to those produced by CD8 cells. They are named "natural killer" cells because they are active without prior exposure to a "sensitizing" epitope. They recognize nonself cells by nonimmunologic means such as unusual electrical charges on the cell surface. The primary differences between CD8 cells and NK cells are that they are not specific for the epitope and are not enhanced by the earlier exposure. The NK cells, however, perform an important function. They are always available to attack cells displaying "foreign" markers without prior sensitization and probably kill these nonself cells before cell-mediated immunity is fully activated.

Approximately 5% to 15% of all circulating lymphocytes are NK cells. Although they have some T cell markers, they do not pass through the thymus to mature, they have no immunologic memory, and they have no T cell receptor.

Humoral Immunity

B cells have two essential functions: (1) they differentiate into plasma cells that produce immunoglobulins, and (2) they are one group of APCs. In fetal life, B cell precursors are first found in the liver and then migrate into the bone marrow. B cells mature in two stages but, unlike T cells, do not mature in the thymus. The first phase of B cell maturation is *antigen-independent*. In this phase, which probably takes place in the bone marrow, stem cells mature first to pre–B cells and then to B cells that express immunoglobulin M (IgM) on their surface. Surface IgM production is independent of an immunogen (i.e., it is not a result of a reaction with an epitope). Both IgM and immunoglobulin D (IgD) can be epitope receptors on the surface of B cells.

In the second, *antigen-dependent*, phase, B cells interact with an immunogen, become activated, and form plasma cells capable of secreting immunoglobulins. *Clonal selection* is a theory that explains how immunoglobulins are produced. Each person has a pool of approximately 10^7 B cells, each of which has IgM or IgD on its surface that can react to one immunogen (or a closely related group of immunogens). An immunogen interacts with the B cell that shows the best "fit" with the immunoglobulin on its surface. When the B cell is activated by this reaction, it is stimulated to proliferate and form a clone of cells. The clone cells mature into plasma cells, which secrete an immunoglobulin specific for the immunogen that initiated this sequence.

The B cell surface immunoglobulin-immunogen complex can also undergo *endocytosis* (ingestion of a foreign substance by a cell). The B cell then presents the epitope on its surface in the binding cleft of an MHC antigen. The epitope-MHC complex is recognized by a CD4 T cell (helper T), which produces interleukins that stimulate growth and differentiation of the B cell. A clone of B cells forms and produces immunoglobulins specific to the epitope. In addition, some activated B cells become memory B cells, which stay inactive for months or years until re-exposure to the immunogen a second time. Most B cell responses require T cell help.

Immunoglobulins

Immunoglobulins (antibodies), which make up approximately 20% of the protein in blood plasma, are the primary product of plasma cells. In addition to blood plasma, immunoglobulins are found in tears; saliva; mucosal secretions of the respiratory, GI, and GU tracts; and colostrum. Immunoglobulins react with specific immunogens that stimulate their production. Although immuno-

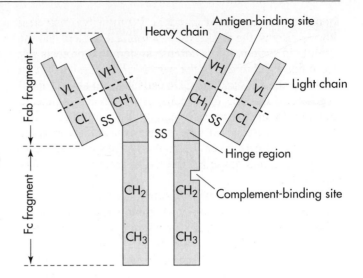

FIG. 5-10   Molecular structure of an antibody showing two light *(L)* and two heavy *(H)* polypeptide chains held together by disulfide bonds *(SS).* The molecules have a variable *(V)* portion, constant *(C)* portion, and flexible hinge region, which can be cleaved at this site by the enzyme papain in experimental studies. The variable portion or antibody-binding *(Fab)* region of the molecule binds with the antigen epitope. It is also called the N-terminal end of the immunoglobulin. The constant region or C-terminal end of the immunoglobulin is called the Fc fragment and functions as the site for various nonspecific interactions, such as complement fixation and cell receptor binding.

globulins of all classes do not have the exact same structure, many have a basic structure similar to Fig. 5-10, with a characteristic Y shape. Immunoglobulins are composed of light-molecular-weight (L) and heavy-molecular-weight (H) polypeptide chains. Although some differences exist, immunoglobulins have two H chains and two L chains variably linked by disulfide bonds. The L chains usually have one variable portion and one constant portion; the H chains usually have one variable portion and three constant portions. Table 5-2 summarizes the characteristics and functions of the five classes of immunoglobulins, and Fig. 5-11 depicts their structure.

The variable portion of the structure (at the "top" of the Y structure) is composed of distinctive amino acid sequences that form the epitope-binding site. This portion has molecular variability because of the immune system's specificity. A host of epitope-specific immunoglobulins are needed by the body to combine with a host of different epitopes; therefore different immunoglobulins with many different variable portions have to be produced to bind with millions of different epitopes. The variable portion of immunoglobulins provides one aspect of the immune system's specificity through the large variation in amino acid sequence. The constant portion has an amino acid sequence that remains consistent among antibodies of different binding specificity. The variable and constant portions that make up each arm of the Y shape

▶ TABLE 5-2   Classification of Immunoglobulins

Class	Percentage in Serum; Serum Concentration	Location	Description	Functions
IgM	5%-10%; 80-170 mg/dl	Serum Surface of B cells	Most primitive and largest Ig with short half-life Circulates as pentamer (group of five) First to form in response to bacterial/viral infection First Ig formed by fetus	Responsible for primary response Most efficient Ig in agglutination and complement fixation Binds with immunogen on B cell surface Forms Ig against immunogens on foreign red blood cell (transfusion reactions)
IgG	75%-80%; 700-1700 mg/dl	Serum Interstitial fluid	Most abundant Ig in blood Only Ig that crosses placenta Has four subclasses	Responsible for secondary response Provides passive immunity for newborn Important in opsonization, precipitation, and agglutination Fixes complement
IgA	10%-15%; 170-280 mg/dl	Main Ig in secretions; colostrum, saliva, tears, and secretions of respiratory, GI, and GU tracts Serum	Monomer in serum (single Y) but dimer (double) or trimer (triple) forms present in secretions Complexed with secretory piece from epithelial cells to pass between epithelial cells into serosal fluids Synthesized by lymphoid tissues near mucous membranes	Neutralizes toxins in blood Primary defense against invasion of mucous membranes; prevents attachment of bacteria and virus to mucous membranes Coupled with a polypeptide for passage to mucosal surfaces
IgD	<1% <1 mg/dl	Serum Surface of B cells	Found in very low concentrations in blood	Function uncertain; may function as an immunogen receptor or in B cell differentiation
IgE	<1% <1 mg/dl	Serum Interstitial fluid Exocrine secretions	Able to fix to receptors on mast cells and basophils	Acts as receptor for allergen when body triggers allergic response; triggers release of histamine and other mediators during allergic response Involved in type I hypersensitivity reactions Defense of parasitic infections

are called the *Fab fragment,* whose function is epitope binding.

The lower portion of the immunoglobulin is important for various biologic functions such as cell receptor binding and complement fixation. The base of the Y is called the *Fc fragment* and is made up of four constant portions. A *flexible hinge region* (Hi region) lies at the intersection of the Fab and Fc fragments and gives the immunoglobulin great physical flexibility. The arms of the immunoglobulin can reach out as much as 180 degrees to bind an immunogen.

Functions of immunoglobulins

Immunoglobulins have several specific functions. One is *agglutination,* the process that causes immunoglobulins and immunogens to clump together. Immunoglobulins can directly attack immunogens by agglutination, a process that may lead to *neutralization* (in-

activation) and lysis of the immunogen (Fig. 5-12). Immunoglobulins can also cause neutralization of toxins (poisons) released from bacteria by binding with them. The toxin and the immunoglobulins bind, a process that does not allow the toxins to bind to tissue cells and exert harmful effects. When the complexes are formed, they undergo *precipitation* (process that causes the complexes to fall out of solution). The products of all these processes are destroyed by phagocytic cells, and this degradation is promoted by immunoglobulin binding.

Immunoglobulins can activate *anaphylaxis* (systemic allergic reaction in a previously sensitized individual) by releasing histamine and other proinflammatory mediators into surrounding tissue fluid and the blood after exposure to an immunogen. The reintroduction of a sensitizer also may induce more limited forms of *hypersensitivity reaction.* This reaction causes the release of mediators from mast cells and basophils when the person is exposed to an

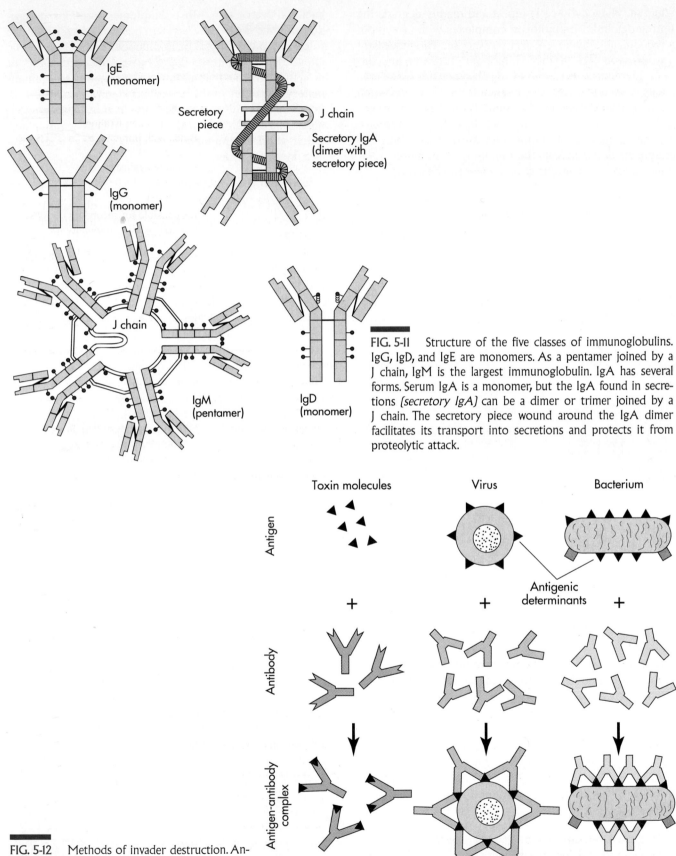

FIG. 5-11   Structure of the five classes of immunoglobulins. IgG, IgD, and IgE are monomers. As a pentamer joined by a J chain, IgM is the largest immunoglobulin. IgA has several forms. Serum IgA is a monomer, but the IgA found in secretions *(secretory IgA)* can be a dimer or trimer joined by a J chain. The secretory piece wound around the IgA dimer facilitates its transport into secretions and protects it from proteolytic attack.

FIG. 5-12   Methods of invader destruction. Antibodies can neutralize bacterial exotoxins, neutralize viruses, and lead to opsonization of bacteria.

allergen. Phagocytic cells ingest and readily degrade the immunoglobulin-immunogen complexes with or without a recognizable hypersensitivity response. The process of *opsonization* is another important function of immunoglobulins. An *opsonin* is a substance that makes the bacteria more "tasty" to phagocytic cells, which often have surface receptors that bind IgG. When immunoglobulins (IgG in particular) coat the exterior surface of an immunogen by binding with surface epitopes, the phagocyte easily ingests the immunogen. Immunoglobulins can also activate the *complement (C) cascade.*

Structure and Function of Complement

The *complement (C) system* consists of approximately 20 proteins that are found in human serum and tissue fluids. The term *complement* was initially coined by Paul Ehrlich to describe the ability of these proteins to complete or augment the actions of immunoglobulins during

bacterial destruction. Most complement proteins are produced in the liver. The C system has three major biologic roles: (1) to cause lysis of immunogens such as bacteria, allografts, and tumor cells; (2) to produce mediators or protein fragments that modulate the immune and inflammatory responses of the body; and (3) to cause opsonization, which is additive to that produced by immunoglobulins. The overall role of the C system is to act as an amplifier of all the immune reactions occurring in response to a nonself invader.

Complement functions

A major function of the C system is cell *lysis*. Its role in bacterial lysis occurs because of the activation of the C cascade. As C components are sequentially activated (Fig. 5-13), they interact with each other to build a *membrane attack complex* (MAC) on the surface of a target cell. The MAC inserts pore-forming molecules into the cell membrane of the immunogen. The cell membrane becomes disrupted, water and electrolytes enter the cell, and the target cell ruptures and dies.

A second function of complement, the *production of immune mediators,* contributes importantly to immune inflammation. The proteins of the C system lead to vasodilation at the site of inflammation. When tissues vasodilate, more blood and immune cells can circulate to the area. In addition, C fragments (particularly C5a and the complex C567) attract neutrophils and macrophages to the area to contribute to phagocytosis. This process of attracting phagocytic cells to areas of inflammation is termed *chemotaxis.* Several fragments (C3a, C4a, C5a) cause *degranulation* (emptying out of vesicles containing histamine) of mast cells and basophils. The histamine that is released causes increased vascular permeability and smooth muscle contraction. Because these changes resemble the tissue effects following IgE-dependent reactions such as anaphylaxis, responsible C fragments are often called *anaphylatoxins.*

A third function of the C system is *opsonization.* Phagocytic cells are often able to ingest materials more easily if these immunogens are coated with complement (particularly C3b). Many phagocytic cells have C3b receptors on their surface. When the immunogen is coated with complement, the phagocytic cell receptors for complement are bound and phagocytosis proceeds rapidly.

Complement activation

The C system becomes activated in one of two ways. Activation can occur because of the formation of immunogen-immunoglobulin complexes of IgG or IgM *(classic pathway)* or by a variety of molecules *(alternative pathway),* such as endotoxins (gram-negative bacterial lipopolysaccharides), fungal cell walls, and viral outer envelopes. Of the two pathways, the alternative pathway is more important to host defense the first time a person is infected because the immunoglobulin necessary to trigger the classic pathway is not present. Both the

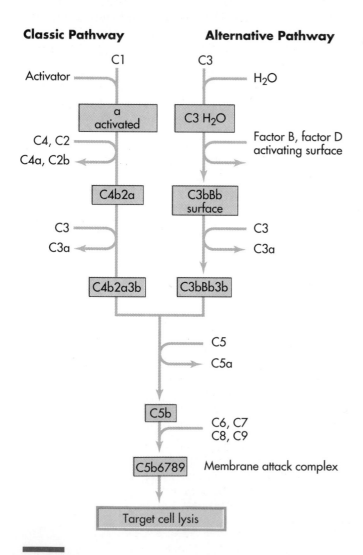

Classic Pathway   **Alternative Pathway**

FIG. 5-13   The classic and alternative pathways of the complement cascade.

classic and the alternative pathways lead to the formation of the central C molecule, C3b, which has two important functions: opsonization and in the formation of the MAC.

MAJOR HISTOCOMPATIBILITY COMPLEX

The MHC, also known as HLA complex, depends on a region on the short arm of human chromosome 6 (Fig. 5-14). Each person has two sets of these genes (haplotypes): one from the mother's chromosomes and one from the father's. This group of genes is responsible for producing *alloantigens* (antigens that differ among individual organisms of the same species), some of which are found on the surface of all nucleated cells. These alloantigens identify every nucleated cell in an individual as self cells.

Classes of MHC Antigens

The proteins encoded by the MHC are generally divided into three classes: class I, class II, and class III MHC antigens. *Class I MHC antigens* are found on the surface of all nucleated cells and platelets except spermatozoa.

When any cell becomes infected with a virus, the viral epitope is presented on the surface of the cell by class I MHC molecules. In this complex the epitope is recognized by a CD8 T cell (cytotoxic T cell) bearing an appropriate T cell receptor (TCR) (Fig. 5-15). The CD8 protein on the CD8 cell stabilizes the interaction, and the CD8 cell becomes activated to continue the immune response.

Class II MHC molecules are involved in types of cellular reactions different from those of class I MHC components. When an APC such as a macrophage presents a processed epitope onto its surface, it is bound to the class II MHC antigen. A CD4 T cell (helper T cell) recognizes the epitope and binds to the immunogen-MHC complex with its TCR complex. The CD4 protein from the CD4 T cell stabilizes the interaction, and the CD4 cell becomes activated to continue the immune response. Therefore all nucleated cells have class I MHC antigens. When cells are infected with viruses, therefore, the class I MHC antigen presents the viral immunogen on its surface to activate CD8 cells. The class II MHC antigens, however, are associated with APCs presenting cells such as macrophages, monocytes, and B cells. When an antigen is presented on the APC by a class II MHC antigen, CD4 cells are activated.

Class III MHC antigens are actually part of the C cas-

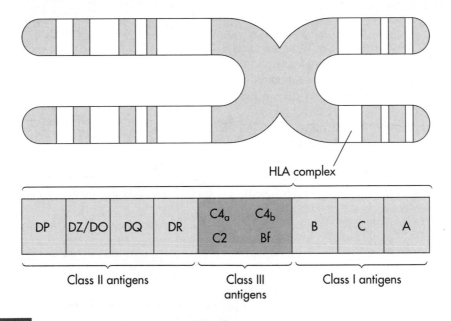

HLA complex

| DP | DZ/DO | DQ | DR | C4ₐ   C4ᵦ | B | C | A |
| | | | | C2   Bf | | | |

Class II antigens   Class III   Class I antigens
                            antigens

FIG. 5-14   The major histocompatibility complex (MHC), or human leukocyte antigen *(HLA)* complex, is located on the short arm of chromosome 6. It is the site of genes that encode HLA antigens. This gene complex is important for immune recognition, cell-cell interaction, and the coding of cell surface histocompatibility antigens that are essential for evoking an immune response. HLA complex antigens are divided into three groups. Class I antigens (loci: *HLA A, B,* and *C)* are found on the surface of most cells in the body and are important in immune recognition, tissue graph rejection, and elimination of virally infected cells. Class II antigens are found on immunocompetent cells (B cells, T cells, macrophages, monocytes) and are important in providing regulatory communication between these cells. Class III antigens are involved in both classic and alternative pathways of the complement system.

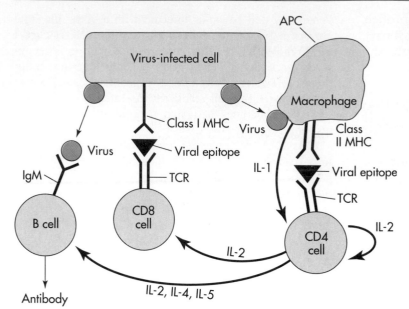

FIG. 5-15   Sequence of cell-mediated immunity and action of antibody against a viral infection. Virus released by the infected cell is ingested and processed by an antigen-presenting cell *(APC),* (e.g., a *macrophage).* The viral epitope is presented in association with a class II MHC protein to the virus-specific T cell receptor *(TCR)* on the CD4 cell. The macrophage makes IL-l, which helps to activate the CD4 cell. The activated CD4 cell makes interleukins (e.g., *IL-2,* which activates the CD8 cell to attack the virus-infected cell, and *IL-4* and *IL-5,* which activate the B cell to produce antibody). The specificity of the cytotoxic response mounted by the CD8 cell is provided by its TCR, which recognizes the viral epitope presented by the virus-infected cell in association with the class I MHC protein.

cade (C2 and C4) and are involved in both the alternative and the classic pathways of the C system. Two mediators, *tumor necrosis factor* (TNF) and *lymphotoxin,* as well as some apparently unrelated substances, are also coded in the class III MHC region.

Role of MHC Antigens in Transplants and Autoimmunity

Each person has two MHC *haplotypes* (the combination of several alleles in a gene cluster; *alleles* are one of two or more different genes containing the specific inheritable characteristics that occupy corresponding positions on a pair of chromosomes). Each parent passes his or her own haplotype to the offspring, who shares one haplotype with each parent. The more similar two persons are in their MHC makeup, the more likely that an organ or tissue transplant between them will be successful. *Tissue typing,* a process used in paternity testing and selection of donors for tissue transplantation, is the mechanism used to identify individual cellular specificities on the MHC.

Autoimmunity is defined as a condition in which structural or functional cellular damage may be caused by the reaction of lymphocytes or immunoglobulins with apparently normal components of the body. Many autoimmune diseases occur with increased frequency in people who carry certain MHC genes. The cause of these often strong associations is not completely clear. However, it appears that certain MHC gene products and not others can present immunogens (including self antigens) for a possible immunologic response.

Usually a person is tolerant to tissue immunogens that are recognized as self. In certain situations, however, tolerance to self may be lost and immune reactions may develop to self immunogens. Bacteria, viruses, and medications have all been implicated as the source of tissue

changes that trigger activation of T cells and B cells to attack self cells.

The term *molecular mimicry* is used to explain this situation. The trigger bacteria or virus resembles a component of the body with sufficient similarity that an immune attack is directed against the body components rather than the trigger. Many autoimmune diseases have a marked family incidence *(genetic predisposition)* that can be linked to the MHC antigen. Autoimmune diseases that may be caused by molecular mimicry include rheumatic heart disease, systemic lupus erythematosus, rheumatoid arthritis, type I diabetes mellitus, myasthenia gravis, multiple sclerosis, and Graves' disease. Chapter 12 discusses additional mechanisms possibly initiating autoimmunity.

PUTTING IT ALL TOGETHER: THE IMMUNE RESPONSE

The immune response is a complex interaction (Fig. 5-16) between APCs, the cells of the immune system, and other proteins such as the C system and a host of cytokines (small-molecular-weight proteins that are secreted by cells participating in the immune response). The body has several mechanisms to encourage phagocytosis of nonself immunogens. Although APCs can ingest bacteria and viruses without opsonization, when an immunogen is coated with complement or immunoglobulins, the process of phagocytosis is amplified. When either an APC or a virally infected cell presents an epitope on the cell surface, T cells bind with the epitope and T cell activation occurs. The class I and class II MHC antigens are essential to present the immunogenic epitope and stabilize the cell-to-cell interaction, which leads to a clone of either CD8 or CD4 T cells. The class I MHC

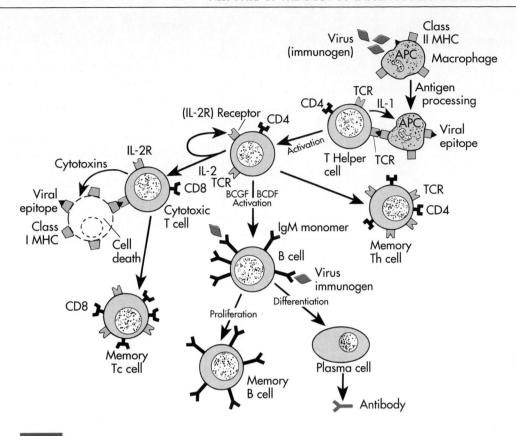

FIG. 5-16   Overview of the process by which the cell-mediated immune response and the humoral immune response are induced (see text).

antigens stabilize reactions with virus-infected cells and CD8 (cytotoxic) T cells, whereas the class II MHC antigens stabilize reactions with APCs and CD4 (helper) T cells. The APC produces IL-1 to help the T cells activate, and the T cells in turn produce other interleukins to cause T cell differentiation and proliferation. Interleukins also stimulate B cells to produce immunoglobulins and affect the type of immunoglobulin produced.

Complement amplifies the response to aid in immunogen lysis and destruction. The "invading" immunogen is destroyed because of direct cytotoxic action by the CD8 T cells. Destruction and neutralization may also reflect immunoglobulin-mediated reactions that result in agglutination, precipitation, neutralization, opsonization, and activation of C enzymes and cell lysis. Memory T cells and B cells are developed to provide a more rapid response to the immunogen when it is next encountered.

Afferent and Efferent Limbs of the Immune Response

The immune response can be described in two phases: the afferent limb and the efferent limb. The *afferent limb,* also known as the *induction phase,* is the part of the immune response that leads to immunogen recognition and generation of responsive elements. The cells responsible for this aspect of the immune response are the lymphocytes (both T and B cells) and APCs, which proliferate during the afferent limb. The *efferent limb,* also known as the *effector phase,* occurs when immunocompetent lymphocytes and reactive antibodies are widely spread throughout the body. The role of these fixed and circulating components in the immune response is to react with the immunogen and render it inactive. The effector cells or immunoglobulin molecules participate in the efferent limb virtually anywhere in the body.

Primary and Secondary Immune Responses

A final important distinction in the immune response is the number of times the body has "seen" the immunogen. When a immunogen is first encountered by the body, immunologic events termed the *primary response* occur. Appearance of a specific antibody usually occurs within 7 to 10 days, reflecting production by a clone of B cells and plasma cells for the particular immunogen. Specific serum immunoglobulin level continues to increase for approximately 4 weeks and then decreases gradually. The first immunoglobulins to appear are IgM, followed by IgG and IgA (Fig. 5-17).

Months or even years after the person is exposed to the immunogen, when a second exposure occurs, the person

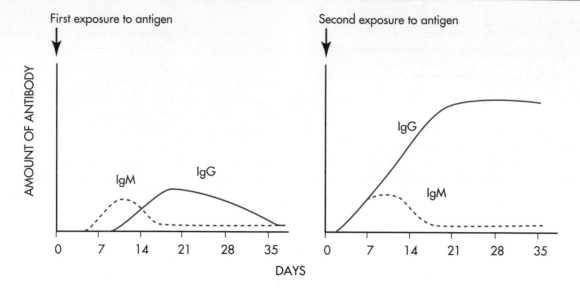

FIG. 5-17   Primary and secondary immune responses. The introduction of antigen induces a response dominated by two classes of antibodies, IgM and IgG. IgM predominates and is the first to appear in the primary response, with some IgG appearing later. After the host's immune system is primed, exposure to the same antigen induces the secondary response, in which some IgM and large amounts of IgG are produced.

has a *secondary response.* The secondary response is more rapid because of the presence of the memory cells from the first contact with the immunogen. The memory cells proliferate to form a large clone of cells capable of producing IgM as during the primary response. The production of IgG is much larger, however, than during the primary response, and levels tend to persist much longer than during the first contact with the immunogen. In addition, the immunoglobulins tend to bind with the immunogen more tightly and inactivate or clear it from the body more effectively.

TYPES OF IMMUNITY

Several types of immunity occur in individuals during the life span depending on age and disease management. *Natural immunity* (native immunity, innate resistance) is the potential for resistance to a foreign "agent" without prior contact. Natural immunity is considered "nonspecific" because it is maintained by NK cells, the C cascade, the interferons, and the skin and mucous membranes without depending on specific immune mechanisms. Body processes such as phagocytosis and inflammation also contribute to natural immunity. Species-dependent immunity is one aspect of natural immunity. Humans do not contract diseases specific to other species, such as cows, pigs, and horses.

Acquired immunity occurs after an exposure to an immunogen after birth. Acquired immunity can be either ac-

tive or passive. *Active immunity* is resistance to an immunogen that occurs as a result of contact with the foreign immunogen. Contact may consist of an infection, immunization with live or killed immunogen, exposure to bacterial products such as endotoxin or toxoids, or transplantation of foreign cells or organs. In active immunity the individual actively produces immunoglobulins and/or sensitized lymphocytes in response to the specific immunogen. The main advantage to active immunity is that resistance is long-term. Its main disadvantage is that active immunity has a relatively slow onset. Active immunity occurs when a person comes in contact with a virus such as the one that causes chickenpox; the virus stimulates a response that makes the person resistant or immune during reexposure. Whole or parts of killed or weakened viruses, their toxic products, or genetically engineered antigens such as the hepatitis B surface antigen can also confer active immunity.

Passive immunity is relative resistance that depends on the production of immunoglobulins by another person or host. Passive immunity can occur naturally as maternal IgG is passed to the fetus or the newborn receives IgA in colostrum. It can also be induced artificially as treatment with an immune serum to prevent infections (e.g., smallpox, rabies, measles) or to neutralize toxins (e.g., diphtheria, tetanus, botulism, snake venoms). The primary advantage of passive immunity is that it is promptly available with large amounts of immunoglobulin. The major disadvantages are that passive immunization has a short life span and may produce an allergic reaction, especially if derived from "nonhuman" sources.

PHYSIOLOGY OF HYPERSENSITIVITY REACTIONS

Humoral and cell-mediated immunity clearly have an adaptive value to the body. The term *immunity* generally refers to such beneficial phenomena mediated by the immune system. However, the price humans pay for having adaptive immune machinery is that occasionally the interaction of immunoglobulins or T cells with immunogens may result in injury to the body. These injurious reactions are referred to as *hypersensitivity reactions*. The term *allergy* is also used to describe certain frequently observed hypersensitivity reactions in humans.

In the past, hypersensitivity reactions mediated by immunoglobulins were called *immediate-type* (or *humoral*) hypersensitivity reactions, whereas those mediated by cellular immune mechanisms were called *delayed* (or *cell-mediated*) hypersensitivity reactions. Although this terminology is still used today, considerable overlapping in the appearance rates of the various reactions deprives these terms of precision. A more useful classification of immunologic injuries developed by Gel and Coombs is used to classify them as types I, II, III, and IV reactions (Table 5-3).

Type I (Anaphylactic) Reactions

In *type I reactions* (anaphylactic-type reactions, immediate hypersensitivity reactions), the individual is sensitized to a particular immunogen by a previous exposure. During the initial contact, IgE is made, circulates throughout the body, and becomes fixed to the surface of mast cells and basophils. When the immunogen is reintroduced, its interaction with mast cell–fixed antibody results in the explosive release of proinflammatory substances such as histamine contained within these cells. If the amount of immunogen introduced to the person is small and in a well-defined, local area, the mediator release is local as well. In this situation the result is a small area of vasodilation with increased permeability and some local swelling. This reaction is also the basis for skin testing by the allergist. However, if a larger amount of immunogen is introduced intravenously into the sensitized person, the release of mediators may be massive and widespread, producing an anaphylactic reaction. Common causes of type I reactivity are insect venoms, pollens, animal allergens, fungi, and foods.

A classic example of this type of generalized anaphylactic reaction occurs when a previously sensitized person receives an intravenous infusion of an allergen such as penicillin. Signs of distress appear within a few minutes or less, and the person may die quickly after a period of agitation, seizures, bronchospasm, and/or circulatory collapse. An anaphylactic reaction such as this occurs because of bronchial obstruction, which leads to trapping of inspired air within the lungs, ventilatory failure, and oxygen deficit or to factors such as severe hypotension, laryngeal swelling, or cardiac rhythm disturbances. The chain of events is the result of the release of mediator substances from mast cells that target airway and vascular smooth muscle. Less severe reactions include allergic rhinitis (hay fever), angioedema, and urticaria (hives).

Type II (Cytotoxic) Reactions

Type II reactions are cytotoxic in nature. Circulating IgG or IgM unites with epitopes on the immunogen's surface or MHC antigens presented on the cell surface. The net result of the interaction might be accelerated phagocytosis of the target cell or actual lysis of the target cell af-

TABLE 5-3   Summary of Hypersensitivity Reactions

Type	Mechanisms	Examples
Type I: anaphylactic	Antigen reacts with IgE antibody bound to surface of mast cells; results in mediator release and mediator effects.	Positive allergy scratch test Anaphylaxis Respiratory allergies Insect venom
Type II: cytotoxic	Antibody unites with antigen that is part of body's cell or tissue; leads to complement activation, lysis, or phagocytosis of target cell and possibly antibody-dependent, cell-mediated cytotoxicity.	Immune hemolytic anemias Goodpasture's syndrome
Type III: immune complex	Union of antigen and antibody forms a complex that activates complement, attracting leukocytes and leading to tissue damage from leukocyte products.	Serum sickness Some forms of glomerulonephritis Lesions of systemic lupus erythematosus
Type IV: cell mediated	Reaction of T lymphocytes with antigen leads to lymphokine release, direct cytotoxicity, and recruitment of reactive cells.	Allergic contact dermatitis Allograft rejection Tuberculosis lesions/skin test

ter activation of the C system. If the target cell is a foreign invader, such as a bacterium, the outcome of this reaction is beneficial. If the target cell is one of the body's own cells, such as an erythrocyte, the result may be a form of hemolytic anemia. Another kind of type II reaction is called *antigen-dependent, cell-mediated cytotoxicity* (ADCC). In this type of reaction, immunoglobulin directed against surface antigens of a cell binds to that cell. Leukocytes such as neutrophils and macrophages having receptors for a particular portion (the Fc portion) of the immunoglobulin molecules then bind to the cell and destroy it. Common examples of type II reactions include erythrocyte destruction during ABO-incompatible blood transfusions, myasthenia gravis, and Goodpasture's syndrome (attack on renal and lung basement membranes).

Type III (Immune Complex) Reactions

Type III reactions take a number of forms but are mediated ultimately by immune complexes (complexes of immunogen with immunoglobulin, usually IgG) that are deposited in tissues, arteries, and veins. A well-studied example of this type of reaction is the *Arthus reaction.* Classically, this reaction is elicited by first sensitizing a person to a foreign protein. Then the person is challenged by an intradermal injection of the same immunogen. The reaction evolves over several hours, when the area initially becomes swollen and red and eventually becomes necrotic and hemorrhagic in severe situations.

The basic mechanisms for these changes involve the formation of immunogen-immunoglobulin complexes in vessel walls. A key element in the reaction is activation of the C cascade by the immune complexes deposited within the vascular walls, although the vascular cells are not the source of the immunogen; rather, the immunogen diffuses into the walls from the blood. C activation results in the formation of chemotactic factors that attract neutrophils from the circulation. Vessel damage continues as neutrophils degranulate (release lytic enzymes) into surrounding areas. Damage to surrounding tissue include microthrombi, increased vascular permeability, and enzyme release leading to inflammation, tissue damage, and even tissue death. Type III reactions differ from type II reactions. Cell destruction during type II reactions is localized to a certain type of cell that is a specific "target," whereas type III reactions destroy tissue or organs anywhere the immune complexes are deposited. For example, glomerulonephritis can result if immune complexes are deposited in the kidneys, and systemic lupus erythematosus and arthritis can result if immune complexes are deposited in the skin and joints. Another example of a type III reaction is serum sickness, which develops 1 to 2 weeks after a person is injected with a foreign serum. Immune complexes are deposited on vessel walls, leading to complement activation and the resulting edema, fever, and inflammation.

Type IV (Cell-mediated) Reactions

Type IV reactions (cell-mediated reactions, delayed hypersensitivity reactions) are mediated by the contact of sensitized T cells with the corresponding immunogen. These reactions tend to occur 12 to 24 hours after the initial exposure to the immunogen. CD4 cells (helper T cells) release lymphokines that attract and stimulate macrophages to release inflammatory mediators. If the immunogen persists, tissue damage caused by this process may develop into a chronic granulomatous reaction such as a collection of mononuclear cells in an area of damaged tissue.

A variety of immunogens, such as viruses, bacteria, fungi, haptens, and medications, can initiate a type IV reaction. The tubercle bacillus appears to cause a cell-mediated response leading to lymphotoxicity. Poison ivy, detergents, and perfumes can also cause a cell-mediated allergic dermatitis. Type IV reactions are also a principal source of rejection that occurs with some transplanted organs. When living tissue from one individual is grafted into another, whether it is a patch of skin or an entire organ, unless the donor and recipient are genetically identical, the graft tissue is sensed by the recipient's immune system as being foreign and nonself. After a brief induction phase, lymphocytes specifically sensitized to the MHC antigens from the donor invade the graft. These lymphocytes lead to graft destruction or rejection by a number of mechanisms involving either direct lymphocytotoxicity or involvement of macrophages. Although T cells play a major role in graft rejection, under some circumstances, immunoglobulins play a significant parallel role. It is these types of rejection reactions that limit the ability to replace defective organs in one individual with organs taken from another.

IMMUNODEFICIENCY

The existence of a competent immune system is essential to defend the individual from foreign antigens. Therefore an individual may develop disease because of a deficiency in any of the components of the immune system. These diseases are manifested clinically as an unusual susceptibility to infections, which may be so severe as to be lethal. The pattern of infection depends on the precise type of deficiency.

Immunologic deficiencies may be primary or secondary. *Primary immunologic deficiencies* have a genetic basis, and various parts of the immune system may be involved. An example of a defect in humoral immunity is *X-linked agammaglobulinemia* resulting from a deficiency of B cells. This condition results in almost total absence of immunoglobulin production, with consequent recurrent or chronic infections most often caused by pyrogenic bacteria such as *Haemophilus influenzae, Streptococcus pneumoniae,* and staphylococci. Humoral immunodeficiency can be of one particular immunoglobulin, such as *isolated IgA deficiency;* individuals with this condition have an increased number of respiratory and GI infections and may have severe anaphylactic reactions when transfused with normal blood (since they may develop significant levels of antibodies to IgA). There are also primary deficiencies of the T cell system (e.g., *DiGeorge syndrome*) or even *severe combined immunodeficiency disease* (SCID). SCID involves functional impairment of both humoral and cell-mediated immunity. Infants with this condition are susceptible to devastating bacterial, fungal, and viral infections and often die within the first year of life. Complement abnormalities are another category of immunodeficiency (some of the primary immunodeficiency disorders are discussed in Chapter 14).

LIFE SPAN CONSIDERATIONS

The ability to maintain a functioning immune system is impaired at both the beginning and the end of the life span. Although questions exist about the relatively poor immune response in newborns, T cell function appears to be inadequate. The newborn relies primarily on passive immunity to remain healthy. Antibodies are primarily supplied by the transfer of maternal IgG across the placenta before birth. Another protective mechanism for newborns is the high quantity of IgA in colostrum, which protects the newborn from respiratory and GI infections. By 3 to 6 months, however, little maternal IgG remains and the risk of infection rises. Fetuses and newborns do have the capability for immunoglobulin production. The fetus can produce IgM in response to certain immunogens, such as the organisms that cause congenital syphilis. Shortly after birth, the newborn also begins to produce his or her own IgG and IgA, and levels of these immunoglobulins rise progressively after 4 to 6 months.

In elderly persons the ability to mount an immune response generally diminishes from uncertain causes. Elderly individuals have a decreased ability to produce IgG in response to immunogens. In addition, they have fewer T cells and a delayed and diminished hypersensitivity response. To complicate matters, they have an increased level of circulating immunoglobulins against self (autoantibodies).

Elderly persons also have a decrease in the surveillance function of the immune system. When T cells and NK cells are less able to identify and destroy mutating cells, tumor cells may proliferate and the risk of cancer increases. For these reasons, infections in both newborns and elderly persons have increased in both frequency and severity. Elderly persons are also at higher risk for the emergence of malignancies and neoplasms than in other periods during the life span.

QUESTIONS

▼ *Circle the letter preceding each item below that correctly answers each question or completes the statement. Only one answer is correct.*

1. Which of the following is the best definition of immunity?
   a. Immunity is a hypersensitivity reaction to certain antigens.
   b. Immunity constitutes all the physiologic mechanisms that allow the body to recognize materials as foreign to itself and neutralize or eliminate them.
   c. Immunity refers to the resistance of the body to microbes (viruses, bacteria) and other unicellular and multicellular organisms.
   d. Immunity refers to the production of immunoglobulins by B cells to eliminate bacteria and other foreign material from the body.
2. The fundamental basis of immunity depends on immune cells' ability to:
   a. Destroy harmful microorganisms
   b. Distinguish self from nonself
   c. Maintain homeostasis
   d. Destroy mutant cells, thus preventing malignancy
3. Features of molecules that determine their potential ability to evoke an immune response include all the following *except:*
   a. Must be recognized as foreign to the body
   b. Usually a protein with a molecular weight greater than 10,000 daltons
   c. Chemically complex
   d. Very low concentration in body
4. An important feature of immunogens (antigens) is the presence of epitopes because:
   a. The molecule is not an immunogen unless it is bound to a larger carrier molecule.
   b. They are the smallest portion of the immunogen that can elicit an immune response and can interact with immunoglobulins.
   c. They build the membrane attack complex (MAC).
   d. They coat bacteria and make them more appetizing to antigen-presenting cells (APCs).
5. Haptens are small molecules that join with larger carrier molecules to function as:
   a. Immunoglobulins
   b. Cell mediators
   c. Effectors
   d. Immunogens
6. Which of the following is considered a primary lymphoid organ?
   a. Spleen
   b. Lymph nodes
   c. Thymus
   d. Gut-associated lymphoid tissue (GALT)
7. Lymphocytes that are independent of the thymus in their development are called:
   a. B cells
   b. T cells
   c. Lymphokines
   d. Antibodies

Continued.

? QUESTIONS—cont'd

8. A primary lymphoid organ that is important in the maturation and "education" of T lymphocytes is the:
   a. Bone marrow
   b. Thymus
   c. Spleen
   d. Lymph nodes

9. The cell marker that distinguishes a T cell as a helper T cell is:
   a. CD2   c. CD7
   b. CD4   d. CD8

10. Cytokines are:
    a. A portion of the CD4 T cell membrane
    b. Mature T cells that are "educated" by the thymus
    c. Small proteins secreted by immune cells
    d. Small fragments of the complement system

11. An essential regulator function of CD4 cells is to:
    a. Link the mononuclear phagocytic system to the lymphoid system by binding with the epitope presented on the APC's surface
    b. Initiate the delayed hypersensitivity reaction when an immunogen such as fungi causes an allergic response
    c. Cause cytotoxicity, with destruction of virus-infected cells and tumor cells
    d. Identify "nonself" cells in transplanted organs

12. An important site in the lymph node where immunogens are presented on the macrophage cell surface and T cells become activated is the:
    a. Paracortex
    b. Lymphoid follicles in the cortex
    c. Germinal centers in the cortex
    d. Lymphoid centers in the medulla

13. The role of natural killer (NK) cells is to:
    a. Perform the regulator function of T cells
    b. Act as APCs
    c. Secrete cytokines that activate CD4 and CD8 cells
    d. Recognize "nonself" cells by their unusual surface charges.

14. Class I MHC antigens:
    a. Are involved with APCs by raising the processes' epitope of the cell's surface
    b. Are involved with presenting a viral epitope on a virally infected cell to activate other parts of the immune system

c. Are part of the complement cascade
d. Act as an opsonin to enhance phagocytosis of APCs

15. CD8 cells (cytotoxic or killer T cells) directly attack virally infected cells, causing their death by the release of a cytokine called:
    a. Perforin
    b. Interleukin-1 (IL-1)
    c. Interleukin-2 (IL-2)
    d. Colony-stimulating factor

16. B cell maturation:
    a. Occurs in the thymus gland, where the B cell learns to differentiate self from nonself
    b. Occurs in two stages, in the bone marrow and during reactions with immunogens
    c. Is independent of immunogens
    d. Can occur only when B cells interact with plasma cells

17. Induction of antibody production (afferent limb of the immune response) in response to an immunogen requires interaction with and cooperation of all the following *except:*
    a. Macrophage (APC)
    b. B cell
    c. CD4 T cell
    d. Transfer factor

18. Plasma cells are:
    a. Macrophages that devour bacteria
    b. Activated B lymphocytes that produce immunoglobulins
    c. Antigens that produce a diffuse response
    d. Monocytes that are found in an exudate

19. The importance of the variable portion of the immunoglobulin is that it is composed of:
    a. Varying amino acid sequences that form the epitope binding sites and provide binding sites for a host of antigens
    b. A constant amino acid sequence to provide stability to the molecule
    c. Varying amino acid sequences that allow for cell receptor binding and complement fixation
    d. A constant amino acid sequence that provides a flexible hinge to allow for the immunoglobulin to reach out as much as 180 degrees to bind

20. An immunoglobulin that guards mucosal surfaces and is present in many body secretions is:
    a. IgG

b. IgM
c. IgA
d. IgD
e. IgE

21. An important function of IgG is:
    a. Protection of the mucosal surfaces
    b. Defense against infections with pyogenic bacteria
    c. Mediation of the tuberculin skin test
    d. Participation in anaphylactic reactions

22. Complement functions include:
    a. Maturation of T cells in the thymus and B cells in the bone marrow
    b. Production of immunoglobulins
    c. Maturation of stem cells and storage of B cells in the spleen
    d. Lysis of the target cell through the MAC and production of immune mediators

23. One of the functional mechanisms of the complement system, specifically the MAC (C5 to C9), is to:
    a. Damage the cell membrane of the antigen and cause cell lysis
    b. Increase the density of the cell membrane
    c. Induce the antigen to produce a specific antibody
    d. Cause the release of histamine from mast cells

24. Complement activation via the classic pathway would be anticipated with:
    a. Reactions of antigens with IgE bound to mast cells
    b. Reactions of antigens with IgG
    c. Reactions of antigens with activated T lymphocytes
    d. Addition of antigens alone to complement-rich serum

25. A major group of genes that control the immune response and allow an individual to recognize that a substance is foreign (nonself) is called the _____ and is located on the short arm of chromosome _____.
    a. Homozygous complex; 1
    b. Major histocompatibility complex (MHC); 6
    c. Haplotype complex; X
    d. Philadelphia complex; 21

26. Characteristics of the secondary immune response include all the following *except:*
    a. The secondary immune response is more rapid than the primary immune response.
    b. Memory B lymphocytes develop

❓ QUESTIONS—cont'd

after the first contact with the immunogen.

c. The production of IgM is greater than that of IgG during the secondary response.

d. Immunoglobulins have a stronger destructive effect on the immunogen during the secondary response.

27. The nurse administers tetanus toxoid to a client in the emergency room as a prophylaxis against the development of tetanus. The type of immunity that has been conferred on the client is classified as:
    a. Natural immunity
    b. Passive immunity
    c. Actively acquired immunity
    d. Borrowed immunity

28. A type II hypersensitivity reaction:
    a. Is cytotoxic in nature by increasing phagocytosis of the target cell or increasing target cell lysis

b. Is an anaphylactic reaction that occurs immediately in a sensitized person

c. Occurs when immune complexes are deposited in tissues, arteries, and veins

d. Occurs up to 24 hours after the initial exposure and is caused by viruses, bacteria, fungi, and medications

29. Rejection of an organ transplantation (e.g., kidney) would be an example of a hypersensitivity immune reaction that is:
    a. Type I (anaphylactic)
    b. Type II (cytotoxic)
    c. Type III (immune complex)
    d. Type IV (cell mediated)

30. Which of the following statements related to autoimmunity is false?
    a. Autoimmunity is a condition in which the body's immune mechanisms attack the body's own tissues.

b. One explanation for autoimmune disease is molecular mimicry of a component of the body by a bacterium or virus.

c. Many autoimmune diseases can be linked to a particular MHC genetic makeup in afflicted individuals.

d. Autoantibodies occur less frequently in elderly persons.

31. When an antibody reacts with its corresponding antigen:
    a. A precipitate may be produced from a previously soluble antigen.
    b. A biologically "toxic" complex may be formed.
    c. The elimination of the antigen (in the intact host) may be accelerated.
    d. A particular antigen may be caused to agglutinate.
    e. All the above are correct.

▼ *Match the term in column A related to the basic structures of an immunoglobulin and the complement system with its description in column B.*

Column A	Column B
32. _____ Fab region	a. Only activated by immune complexes with IgG and IgM
33. _____ Fc region of IgE	
34. _____ Classic pathway of complement activation	b. Does not require an antigen-antibody reaction for activation (e.g., may be activated by a bacterial endotoxin)
35. _____ Alternate pathway of complement activation	c. Antigen binding site in antigen-antibody interactions
	d. Cell membrane receptors are on the mast cell or blood basophil

---

▼ *Match the immunoglobulin (Ig) in column A with its description in column B.*

Column A	Column B
36. _____ IgA	a. Most primitive and largest Ig; responsible for the primary immune response
37. _____ IgD	b. Mediates anaphylaxis
38. _____ IgE	c. Function uncertain
39. _____ IgG	d. Most abundant Ig in blood; responsible for secondary immune response
40. _____ IgM	e. Main Ig in secretions such as tears, saliva, and GI and GU secretions

CHAPTER 6

Response of the Body to Infectious Agents

GERALD D. ABRAMS

Infection is a universal aspect of life. Plants and animals of all sizes and descriptions are infested with a variety of living microbes, and humans are no exception. The purpose of the following discussion is not to catalog the many specific infections to which human beings fall victim, but rather to discuss in a more general way the biologic principles that govern the interaction between host and infectious agents. In particular, a goal of this chapter is to provide a proper perspective of the universe of infection, that is, to establish firmly the view that infectious disease is only an occasional outcome of the interaction between the host and the microbe.

HOST DETERMINANTS OF INFECTION

A requirement for the production of any infection is that the infectious organism must be able to *adhere to, colonize,* or *invade* the host and proliferate at least to some extent. Not surprisingly, therefore, animal species, including humans, have evolved certain elaborate defense mechanisms at the various interfaces with the environment.

Skin and Oropharyngeal Mucosa

A major interface between the environment and the human body is the skin. Fig. 6-1 shows the structure of a typical area of human skin. Clearly the intact skin, with its keratinized or horny layer at the outer surface and multilayered epithelium beneath, constitutes an excellent mechanical barrier to infection. Ordinarily it is exceedingly difficult for any microorganism to breach this mechanical barrier. However, cuts, abrasions, or areas of maceration (e.g., those folds of the body that are kept constantly moist) may allow infectious agents to enter. In addition to being a simple mechanical barrier, the skin also has a certain ability to decontaminate itself. Thus organisms that adhere to the outer layers of skin (assuming they do not simply die as they dry out) are shed as the outer flakes of skin fall off. In addition to this physical type of decontamination, a chemical decontamination is attributable to the properties of sweat and sebaceous secretions that bathe the surface of the skin. Finally, associated with the skin is the normal flora (described more fully later in this chapter), which may exert a type of biologic decontaminative effect by inhibiting the multiplication of organisms that land on the cutaneous surface.

The lining of the mouth and much of the pharynx is similar to the skin in that it has a surface with a multilayered epithelium that constitutes a formidable mechanical barrier to microbial invasion. This mechanical barrier, however, may be breached along gingival margins and in the region of the tonsils. The oropharyngeal mucosa is

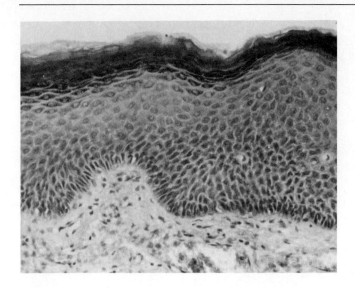

FIG. 6-1   Skin. The epidermis *(upper two thirds of field)* consists of multiple layers of cells, the most superficial of which are flattened, keratinized, and without nuclei. These layers constitute a formidable mechanical barrier. (Photomicrograph, ×300.)

also decontaminated by the flow of saliva, which simply washes many particles away. In addition, substances in the saliva inhibit certain microorganisms. Finally, a rich microbial flora within the mouth and pharynx may also impair the growth of some potential invaders.

Gastrointestinal Tract

The gastric mucosa is of a glandular type and is not a particularly impressive mechanical barrier. Typically, there are small defects or erosions of the gastric lining, but these are of no consequence in relation to infection, since the gastric environment is extremely hostile to many mi-

croorganisms. This is largely because of the pronounced acidity of gastric secretions. Also, the stomach tends to empty its contents relatively rapidly into the small intestine. The lining of the small intestine (Fig. 6-2) is likewise not particularly tough mechanically, and it may be easily penetrated by many bacteria. However, peristaltic propulsion of the intestinal contents is extremely rapid in the small intestine, and bacterial populations are kept quite sparse within the lumen. When intestinal motility is impaired, microbial counts are sharply elevated within the small intestine and invasion of the mucosa may then occur. Several other features of the small intestine assist in the rapid propulsion of organisms through the tract. Abundant mucus is constantly secreted by intestinal lining cells, forming a viscous blanket over the intestinal surface, trapping bacteria, and propelling them distally by peristalsis. In addition, adhesion of bacteria to the mucosal surface is inhibited by the presence of antibodies within the intestinal secretions. In the large intestine (Fig. 6-3) the lining is likewise not particularly tough mechanically. In this location, propulsion is not especially rapid, and intestinal contents are relatively stagnant. Here the major defense against establishment of invading microbes is the presence of astronomic numbers of "normal" microbial inhabitants that coexist peacefully with the host. This mass of normal bacteria has many ecologic ways of discouraging invaders either by competing for foodstuffs or by actually secreting antibacterial (antibiotic) substances.

Respiratory Tract

Fig. 6-4 presents a microscopic view of the mucosal surface typical of conducting portions of the respiratory tract, for example, the lining of the nose, the nasopharynx, the trachea, and the bronchi. The epithelium consists of tall cells, some of which are mucus-secreting, but most of which are equipped with cilia at their luminal surfaces.

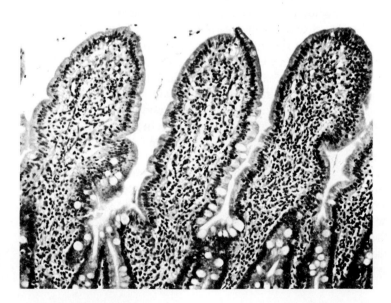

FIG. 6-2   Small intestine. The epithelium separating bowel contents from underlying tissue is actually quite delicate and is not a particularly good mechanical barrier. The surface is protected by mucus secreted by the light-staining "goblet cells," by antibody produced by the underlying lymphoid tissues, and by peristaltic emptying. (Photomicrograph, ×200.)

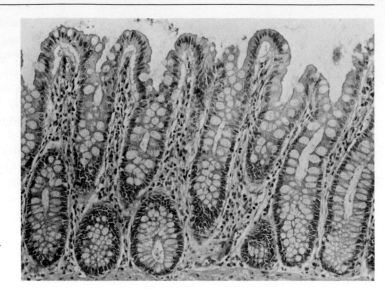

FIG. 6-3   Colon. This epithelium contains many mucus-secreting cells. During life the surface is bathed in a layer of mucus, but after tissue processing, only wisps remain *(upper right)*. The rich microbial flora that "defends" the colon is not visible in this preparation. (Photomicrograph, ×315.)

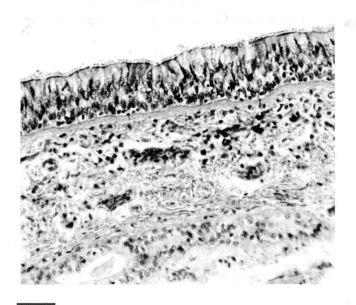

FIG 6-4   Trachea. This type of epithelium is equipped with cilia, visible as a fringe along the upper surface. These are responsible for propelling a protective mucous blanket over the exposed surface of the air passages. (Photomicrograph, ×315.)

These tiny projections beat like whips, with the action stroke directed upward toward the mouth, nose, and exterior of the body. The mucus-secreting cells produce a sticky blanket that rides on top of the cilia and glides continuously upward. If microbes are inhaled, they tend to impinge on the mucous blanket, to be moved outward and either expectorated or swallowed. This protective action is enhanced by the presence of antibodies within the secretions. If some agents elude these defenses and reach the air spaces in the lung itself, the macrophages always present there provide another line of defense.

Other Defensive Barriers

Other surfaces in the body are similarly equipped with defensive mechanisms. Within the urinary tract the lining is a multilayered epithelium that provides a mechanical barrier, but one of the main antimicrobial defenses is the flushing action of urine flow. Anything that interferes with the normal flow of urine, whether obstruction of a ureter or simply bad habits of long-delayed micturition, will promote infection. The ocular conjunctiva is likewise defended in part mechanically and in part by the flow of tears. The vaginal mucosa is a tough, multilayered epithelium whose mechanical properties are augmented by a rich resident flora and by mucous secretions.

Inflammation as a Defense

If an infectious agent manages to penetrate one or another of the barriers of the body and enter the tissues, the next line of defense is the *acute inflammatory reaction*. From the discussion in Chapter 4, the value of the inflammatory reaction should be evident. The inflammatory reaction is an arena in which humoral (antibody) and cellular aspects of body defense converge. The antimicrobial activities of the phagocytes, for instance, are augmented by the opsonizing effects of antibodies and complement components. The defensive properties of macrophages, as another example, may be enhanced by cellular immune mechanisms (see Chapter 5).

If the acute inflammatory reaction is not sufficient to handle the invader, the infection may spread elsewhere in the body. The usual means of spread is largely passive in regard to microbial action and usually involves currents of body fluid carrying the organisms. Locally, even the outpouring of exudate fluid may move the organisms about, and a phagocyte may actually be an agent of spread if it does not kill the ingested organism but wanders to another location. Spread tends to occur across natural spaces. For example, if something perforates part of the gastrointestinal (GI) tract and the contained microorganisms enter the peritoneal cavity, they may spread along the entire peritoneal surface. If some agent reaches a connective tissue plane, such as that along a muscle, it may spread rapidly along that plane. When infectious organisms gain access to the meninges (the coverings around the central nervous system), they may rapidly spread along the entire cerebrospinal axis.

Lymphatics in Infection

For reasons outlined in Chapter 4, the flow of lymph is accelerated in acute inflammation. This means, unfortunately, that infectious agents occasionally may also spread quite rapidly along the course of lymphatics with the flowing lymph. Sometimes, lymphangitis is the result, but more often the infectious agents are carried directly to the lymph nodes, where they are rapidly phagocytosed by macrophages. In such instances the effluent lymph moving centrally beyond a lymph node may be free of living organisms.

The Final Defenses

If spreading infectious agents are not arrested within lymph nodes or if such agents directly invade venous

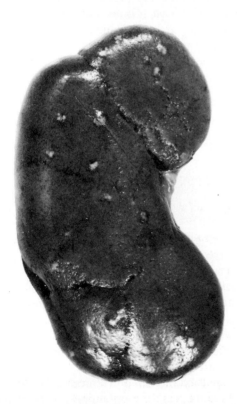

FIG 6-5   Kidney in septicopyemia. The light-colored lesions scattered over the cortical surface are actually small abscesses formed as a result of lodgement of blood-borne bacteria.

channels at the primary site, the bloodstream itself may be infected. Bursts of bacteria in the bloodstream do occur, and these episodes of bacteremia are usually handled quickly and effectively by the macrophages of the monocyte-macrophage system. If large numbers of organisms are fed into the bloodstream and if these organisms are sufficiently resistant, the macrophage system may be overwhelmed. This will result in persistence of organisms in circulation, with associated symptoms of malaise, prostration, and signs of fever, chills, and so forth. This condition is called *septicemia* or *sepsis,* often referred to by lay persons as "blood poisoning." Finally, in some instances, organisms reach such high numbers that they are circulating in clumps, lodging in many organs, and producing myriads of microabscesses (Fig. 6-5). This overwhelming situation is called *septicopyemia,* or simply *pyemia.*

MICROBIAL DETERMINANTS OF INFECTION

Transmissibility

An obviously essential feature in the production of infection is the transport of the living infectious agent to the body. Perhaps the most obvious means of transmission of infection is directly from person to person, for example, by coughing, sneezing, and kissing.

Organisms are transmitted indirectly in a variety of ways. Infected individuals shed organisms into the environment, and these are deposited on various surfaces and can be resuspended in air at a later time, thus spreading indirectly to others. Similarly, organisms can get into the soil, the water, the food, or other chains of indirect transmission. In hospitals, infection can also be spread via exudates and excreta. Blood transfusions may also be a means of spreading infection, as in the case of viral hepatitis. More complex types of indirect transmission involve vectors such as insects. These may act in a strictly mechanical fashion, carrying the microbial agents from one place to another, or may act in a biologic fashion, that is, by serving as intermediate hosts in some essential part of a life cycle of the infectious agent.

Certain intrinsic characteristics of microorganisms sharply influence their transmissibility or communicability. Organisms that are very resistant to drying, such as spore-forming organisms, are readily transmissible through the environment. On the other hand, some organisms, such as the spirochetes of syphilis, are extremely sensitive to drying and temperature change, factors that sharply limit the mode of this transmission. Another natural selective factor that influences the communicability of microbial agents is their resistance to antibiotics. It is distressingly common to find antibiotic-resistant strains of microorganisms emerging and then being communicated relatively freely in the hospital environment. A concern exists that antibiotic-resistant strains may also arise and spread in the community setting, especially with the use of suboptimal treatment regimens that permit such emergence.

Invasiveness

Once communicated to a new host, the microbial agent must establish itself on or in the body to produce infection. Great variability exists in the means adopted by various infectious agents for becoming established on or in the individual. Cholera, for instance, is caused by an organism that never invades the tissues but only colonizes the lining of the intestine, apparently by being able to adhere to some component of the surface and thus avoid being washed away. Some other organisms, such as those that produce bacillary dysentery, invade only the superficial lining of the bowel but never go any farther into the body. Still other organisms, such as the causative agent of typhoid, not only invade the superficial lining of the bowel, but eventually reach the bloodstream and disseminate throughout the body. Another efficient spreader is the spirochete of syphilis, which penetrates mucous membrane or skin at the portal of entry and is disseminated via the bloodstream with great rapidity.

Some organisms, after gaining access to the tissues and becoming established, never spread to any extent. The organisms that produce tetanus, for instance, do not actually spread throughout the body. When they grow locally, they secrete a toxin that is carried via the bloodstream to produce the widespread effects that characterize the disease. The reasons for these differences in invasiveness of various organisms are not clearly understood, but they undoubtedly are related to specific chemical requirements of the organism and the extent to which these requirements can be met in various locales.

Microorganisms have evolved certain ways of breaching host barriers or eluding defense mechanisms. For example, some organisms develop a slimy capsule so that the phagocytic cells of the host cannot ingest them efficiently. Other organisms have developed the enzymatic means of spreading through the ground substance of connective tissue by a chemical digestive process. Yet, other organisms secrete toxins that kill leukocytes, thus eluding capture. Some organisms have even evolved a resistance to the intracellular environment within phagocytes, and these organisms (e.g., the tubercle bacillus) tend to persist as intracellular parasites.

Ability to Produce Disease

Our knowledge of the chemical or molecular way an infectious agent produces disease has been relatively meager and is only now growing. Best understood are those situations in which the infectious agent actually secretes a soluble exotoxin, which then circulates and produces well-defined physiologic changes by acting on specific cells. Thus the chemical mechanisms of disease production in tetanus and in diphtheria are relatively well understood.

Many other microorganisms, such as the gram-negative bacteria, contain as part of their structure a complex endotoxin that is released with lysis of the microorganism. Although the biologic role of such endotoxins is far from completely understood, it is known that the release of endotoxin can be associated with the production of fever and, under more extreme circumstances, such as gram-negative septicemias, with the production of a shock syndrome.

Some organisms actually injure the host, largely by immunologic means. The tubercle bacillus, for instance, appears to have no direct toxin of its own. Rather, the patient becomes allergic to the tubercle bacillus (cell-mediated immune mechanism) and the caseous necrosis typical of the disease is produced on an immunologic basis. In a similar vein, some organisms affect the body by contributing to the formation of antigen-antibody complexes that may subsequently be injurious, such as via the development of immune complex glomerulonephritis.

At the far end of the spectrum are viruses that are obligate intracellular parasites. In effect, viruses are simply chunks of genetic material (deoxyribonucleic [DNA] and ribonucleic [RNA] acids) equipped to insert themselves into host cells. The cells are subsequently injured (if at all) by the new genetic information being expressed in altered cell function. One expression of such added genetic information is the replication of additional infectious virus, which may be accompanied by lysis of the affected cell. The cell may also be altered without actually becoming necrotic. In fact, the cell may even be stimulated to proliferate, as in the case of virally induced tumors. Viruses may also injure the host by evoking a variety of immunologic reactions in which part of the virus or the virus-infected cell behaves as an antigen.

INTERACTION OF HOST AND MICROBE

The interaction between a host and an infectious agent is usually viewed in terms of all-out war or a "fight to the death." There is a great tendency to view infectious agents as intrinsically "bad" things, designed to produce disease. However, the real "business," biologically speaking, of any living agent is not to produce disease, but to produce more of the same kind of agent. In effect, a given microbial agent "could not care less" about producing disease in the host individual. In fact, an ideal infectious agent would simply reproduce within a given host (who constitutes a food supply) and not harm the host or otherwise "rock the boat."

Thinking in evolutionary terms, if a particular infectious agent were to be so effective in producing disease that it would be lethal to each host it entered, the organism would rapidly run out of a food supply and quickly become extinct. The other side of the coin is that if a particular host species is to survive in the course of evolution, one of the things that it must face successfully is infectious agents within the environment. Natural selection obviously would favor the hardier hosts. Therefore in the course of evolution, more resistant hosts and less lethal infectious agents tend to be developed. Thus the dictates of evolution are such that most interactions between host and infectious agent should turn out eventually to be rather "happy" ones, producing significant harm to neither party. When a relationship between host and infectious agent is inoffensive to either species, that type of interaction is referred to as *commensalism.* When the interaction affords both parties some benefit, the interaction is referred to as *mutualism.* Commensalism and mutualism are the most frequent outcomes of infectious interactions in nature, and the production of infectious disease is in an evolutionary sense (and numerically) an aberrant circumstance.

By this line of reasoning, it would be predicted that most infectious diseases should be mild or even that most infections should be unaccompanied by disease. For most microbial "pathogens," the presence of the organism on or in the host is most usually trivial or inapparent and only as the exception is significant disease produced. Thus for every individual with an infectious disease of a particular type, several individuals in the population probably are infected with the same organism and are not sick. Pneumococci, staphylococci, meningococci, and many other pathogens can be recovered easily from perfectly healthy individuals in the population.

There are certainly exceptions to the principle that infection is most often mild or even inapparent. These exceptions can usually be explained on evolutionary grounds. Rabies, for instance, is almost 100% fatal to humans. Our species has not evolved with the virus but is only accidentally inserted into the chain of infection, which usually involves other mammalian species better adapted to the infection. The same is true of many other animal diseases in which humans "get in the way"; they become much more ill than the particular animal species adapted to that infection. Another sort of evolutionary exception is seen when "new" organisms are introduced into previously isolated human populations. Thus when isolated populations are suddenly invaded by individuals from the outside world or when island populations are exposed to agents that are commonplace in human experience (e.g., measles), the attack and fatality rates may be striking. This same evolutionary principle is involved in the spread of certain strains of influenza virus around the world. In this latter instance the virus behaves as if it were "new" because of the development of antigenic traits that are unknown to the population at risk.

Simply knowing the line of transmission of an infectious agent from host to host does not explain fully the incidence of an infectious disease. To understand the epidemiology of such a disease completely, one must understand those aspects of the interaction between host and microbe that convert an ordinarily innocuous or inapparent infection into a clinically significant infectious disease.

OPPORTUNISTIC INFECTION

The concept of opportunistic infection reflects the fact that many organisms are not regarded as doing much to a healthy individual but, given the right circumstances, will take over and produce an infectious disease. Such organisms are referred to as *opportunists* because they seemingly take advantage of the special circumstances of the host. Many opportunists are organisms that reside constantly within the body, and these are sometimes referred to as *endogenous infectious agents.* Some exogenous agents are likewise opportunistic in their behavior.

Opportunistic infections emerge when some factor or set of factors has compromised intrinsic defense mechanisms of the body or in some way has altered the ecology of the normal resident microbes (see later discussion). Many opportunistic infections are seen in hospital patients who have been significantly debilitated by diseases that impair their nutrition, their immunologic reactions, or their ability to produce effectively functioning leukocytes. Leukemias and other forms of cancer are high on the list of such diseases associated with opportunistic infections. Similarly, pharmacologic agents used to treat certain diseases may have as an undesirable side effect the suppression of immunologic or inflammatory reactions, thus paving the way for opportunistic infections. Adrenal corticosteroids, which behave in many ways as antiinflammatory agents, are high on this list, as are cytotoxic agents given in the course of cancer chemotherapy or immunosuppressive therapy. Antimicrobial therapy sometimes leads to opportunistic infection, apparently via suppression of part of the normal microbial flora. It may alter the critical ecologic balance so that another member of the flora may emerge and grow out of all proportion, thus producing disease. Antimicrobial therapy may also render the body more susceptible to some agent that ordinarily could not get a foothold because of the normal microbial flora.

Many other things happen to hospitalized patients that tend to favor an infectious organism. These include certain phenomena associated with anesthesia, shock, and burns. Many diseases predispose individuals to the occurrence of infectious diseases. For example, certain cancers that involve the lymphoid tissues of the body result in defective cellular immune reactions. Individuals with these deficiencies develop infectious diseases caused by agents ordinarily controlled by the lymphocyte-macrophage system. Finally, one infectious disease may predispose to another. For example, an individual may develop a viral "cold" and thereby become likely to develop bacterial pneumonia as a complication.

Numerous environmental factors in the community at large favor a particular organism rather than the host. An example of such an environmental factor involving a single individual would be occupational exposure, such as exposure to silica dust predisposing to tuberculosis. Entire populations of individuals may be involved at one time, as in famine conditions, where depression of host response results in virtual epidemics of diseases such as tuberculosis. Finally, meteorologic changes may also influence the incidence of infectious disease as compared with infection. A variety of studies have indicated that certain infectious agents can be found within human populations the year round, but symptomatic infections with those agents have a seasonal incidence, perhaps related to the weather.

None of the previous discussion is intended to belittle the importance of germs in disease or to discourage attempts at interrupting the cycle of transmission of infectious agents among individuals. It should be emphasized, however, that a given organism may be a necessary condition for the production of a particular disease without being a sufficient condition. It is the complex interaction of many host and environmental factors that ultimately determines the precise outcome in a given instance of infection. For these reasons, considering the "virulence" or the "pathogenicity" of a particular microorganism must be done in relation to the status of the given host at that time.

NORMAL MICROBIAL FLORA

The previous discussion mentioned the normal or indigenous microbial flora. It should be emphasized that the host together with this microbial flora constitute a sort of ecosystem whose equilibria are an essential part of what is considered to be health.

Quantitatively, the normal microbial flora of animal hosts (including humans) represents a staggering load. For example, a significant fraction of the dry weight of feces actually consists of bacterial carcasses. Humans excrete trillions of organisms each day from the GI tract. The skin also has a large resident flora, estimated to be in concentration of greater than 10,000 organisms per square centimeter of skin. These are not simply organisms adhering to dirty skin, but organisms that live deep within the various epithelial structures of the skin (and in fact are shed in larger numbers with scrubbing). Astronomic numbers of organisms also live within the mouth. Scrapings taken from the surfaces of teeth or gums may contain millions of organisms per milligram of material, and saliva may contain as many as 100 million organisms per milliliter.

This impressive microbial flora is not a random population. Of the many species of microbes encountered within the environment as humans move about each day, only relatively few have become adapted in the course of their own evolution to the particular environments that humans afford in various tissues. Therefore, within certain limits the flora of a given animal species is predictable and within a given species, such as humans, the flora of particular tissues is quite predictable. In most tissues that have been studied carefully, the anaerobic bacteria seem to outnumber the aerobic bacteria. This is especially true in the bowel, where the ratio is as high as 1000:1.

Biologists have known of the existence of the normal microbial flora for many decades, but opinions concerning the significance of the flora have varied tremendously through the years. In the early years of the 20th century, some authorities had a very dim view of the flora, judging it at best to be a neutral mass and at worst to be a cause of the degenerative diseases of aging. Gradually this view has been replaced with the increasing recognition that no animal species would evolve with a particular flora in a disadvantageous relationship. To the contrary, it would be predicted that a mutually advantageous relationship should evolve.

Clearly, indigenous microbes perform many good actions for humans. Many chemical reactions within the lumen of the bowel, for instance, are actually carried out by the resident microbes. The ecologic functions of such microbes in repelling potential invaders has already been discussed. Many traits of humans have evolved as they did partly as a result of the presence of the microbial associates. This means that a number of anatomic and physiologic traits considered normal and innate actually developed as a response to the presence of the flora. In other words, to a significant extent the body depends for normalcy on the microbial flora. For example, the structure and function of the lining of the GI tract are influenced by the presence of the flora, the motility of the tract is influenced by the flora, and many of the reactions of the tract to challenge are similarly conditioned by the flora.

Although such considerations are perhaps more obvious within the GI tract, the direct and indirect effects of the indigenous flora are not limited to that area. There is reason to believe that even immunologic function and leukocyte function are influenced by the flora.

The actual means by which the microbial flora acts on the body are not well understood. In fact, even the identity of some components of the flora in humans is far from clear. We are only now beginning to learn what controls the usual ecologic balance of the flora itself: a combination of factors involving microbe-to-microbe and host-to-microbe interactions. What is evident at this point, however, is that when one disrupts the normal ecology of the microbial flora, it is done at significant risk to the host.

QUESTIONS

▼ *Answer the following on a separate sheet of paper.*

1. What are the criteria used to determine whether a body is infected? Does an infected individual necessarily have an infectious disease?

2. Name at least five portals of entry of infectious agents into the body. Describe the characteristics of the defenses at each of these portals.

3. Briefly describe what can occur if an acute inflammatory reaction is unable to contain an invading microorganism locally.

4. What is the final line of defense against widespread dissemination of an infectious agent throughout the body?

5. What is meant by an opportunistic infection?

6. What are some situations that can change an inapparent infection into an infectious disease?

7. Briefly discuss the interaction of the human host and the bacteria forming the normal flora on body surfaces. What value does this relationship provide for the host?

8. List several known mechanisms causing tissue injury by infectious agents.

▼ *Circle the letter preceding each item below that correctly answers each question or completes the statement. More than one answer may be correct.*

9. All the following may directly deter or prevent the invasion and spread of infectious agents *except:*
   a. Inflammatory response
   b. Intact skin
   c. Alveolar macrophages
   d. Fibroblasts
   e. Monocyte-macrophage system

10. When microorganisms reach such a high number in the circulation that they lodge in tissues and form abscesses, the condition is termed:
    a. Septicemia
    b. Bacteremia
    c. Septicopyemia
    d. Polycythemia

11. In relationships between hosts and infectious agents, evolution has favored:
    a. Weak, nonresistant hosts
    b. Hardier, resistant hosts
    c. Very lethal infectious agents
    d. Less lethal infectious agents

12. A relationship between the host and infectious agent that is inoffensive to either species is referred to as:
    a. An opportunistic infection
    b. Mutualism
    c. Commensalism
    d. Immune reaction

13. Septicemia is also called:
    a. Pyemia
    b. Blood poisoning
    c. Bacteremia
    d. None of the above

▼ *Match the organisms listed in column A with their specific invasive characteristic in column B.*

Column A	Column B
14. _____ *Vibrio cholerae*	a. Penetrates the mucous membrane or skin and enters the bloodstream; disseminated widely in body
15. _____ Typhoid bacillus	b. Invades the lining of the bowel and enters the bloodstream
16. _____ Syphilis spirochete	c. Colonizes bowel lumen; never invades
17. _____ Tetanus bacillus	d. Remains local but secretes a toxin that is carried in the bloodstream

▼ *Match the terms in column A, which indicate the type of relationship between two dissimilar organisms living in close association (e.g., human and microorganism), with their correct interpretation in column B.*

Column A	Column B
18. _____ Commensalism	a. The association is beneficial to one but detrimental to the other.
19. _____ Parasitism	b. The association is without injury to either organism.
20. _____ Mutualism	c. The association is beneficial to both.

CHAPTER 7

Disturbances in Circulation

GERALD D. ABRAMS

CONGESTION (HYPEREMIA)

Congestion is an overabundance of blood within the vessels in a given region. Another word for congestion is *hyperemia*. When observed grossly, an area of tissue or an organ that is congested has a deeper red (or purplish) color than usual because of the increase in blood within the tissue. Microscopically the capillaries in a hyperemic tissue are dilated and engorged with blood. Basically, congestion may be produced by two mechanisms: (1) an increase in the amount of blood flowing into an area and (2) a decrease in the amount of blood draining from an area.

Active Congestion

When the flow of blood into an area is increased and produces congestion, the phenomenon is called *active congestion*, in that more blood than usual is actively flowing into the area. This increase in local blood flow is caused by dilation of arterioles, which behave as valves governing the flow into the local microcirculation. One common example of active congestion is the hyperemia accompanying acute inflammation; this accounts for the redness described in Chapter 4 (see Fig. 4-1). Another example of active congestion is a blush, which is basically a matter of vasodilation produced in response to a neurogenic stimulus. A physiologic example of active congestion is the delivery of more blood on "demand" of a working tissue, such as an actively contracting muscle. This is also called *functional hyperemia*. By its very nature, active congestion is often short-lived. As the stimulus to arteriolar dilation is withdrawn, the flow of blood to the affected area is decreased and the situation returns to normal.

Passive Congestion

As the name suggests, *passive congestion* does not involve an increase in the amount of blood flowing into an area, but an impairment in drainage of blood from the area. Anything that compresses the venules and veins draining a tissue may produce passive congestion. When an elastic tourniquet is placed about the arm before drawing blood from a vein, an artificial form of passive congestion is induced. A similar and more significant change could be produced, for instance, by a tumor compressing the local venous drainage from an area. In addition to such local causes of passive congestion, central or systemic reasons exist for impaired venous drainage. Sometimes the heart fails in its pumping action (see Part Six), and this leads to impaired venous drainage. For instance, if the left side of the heart fails in its pumping action, the flow of blood returning to the heart from the lung is somewhat impaired. Under such circumstances, blood is dammed back into the lung, producing passive congestion of the pulmonary vasculature. Similarly, if the right side of the heart fails, the damming of blood affects systemic venous return and many tissues throughout the body become passively congested. Patients typically have simultaneous right-sided and left-sided cardiac failure.

Passive congestion may be relatively short-lived, in which case it is called *acute passive congestion,* or it may be longstanding, in which case it is called *chronic passive congestion.* If the passive congestion is short-lived, there are no effects on the involved tissue. Chronic passive congestion, however, may cause permanent changes in the tissues. These changes generally take place in a passively congested area, and if the change in blood flow is severe enough, tissue hypoxia may lead to shrinkage or even loss of cells of the involved tissue. In certain organs this also leads to an increase in the amount of fibrous connective tissue. In many areas there is also evidence of local breakdown of red blood cells (RBCs), which results in the deposition of hemoglobin-derived pigments within the tissues.

The effects of chronic passive congestion are particularly notable in the lungs and the liver. In the lungs (Fig. 7-1) the walls of air spaces tend to become thickened and numerous macrophages are found to contain hemosiderin pigment, a product of the breakdown of hemoglobin from RBCs that escape the congested vessels into the air spaces. Such hemosiderin-containing macrophages are called *heart failure cells* and can be found in the sputum of patients with chronic left-sided cardiac failure. In the liver, chronic passive congestion leads to marked dilation of the blood channels in the center of each hepatic lobule, with shrinkage of liver cells in this area. The result of this is a striking gross appearance of the liver (Fig. 7-2) produced by the hyperemic centrilobular zone alternating with the less affected peripheral areas of each lobule. This gross appearance is sometimes referred to as "nutmeg liver" because of the fancied resemblance of the cut surface of such a liver to the cut surface of a nutmeg.

Another effect of chronic passive congestion is dilation of the veins in the affected area. As the walls of affected veins are chronically stretched, they become somewhat fibrotic, and the veins also tend to lengthen. Because veins are fixed at various points along their length, they necessarily become tortuous as they lengthen; that is, they twist back and forth between points of fixation. Dilated, somewhat tortuous, thick-walled veins are referred to as *varicose veins* or *varices.* Varicose veins in the legs are a familiar sight. Also common are *hemorrhoids,* which are actually varicose veins of the anus (in the hemorrhoidal plexus of veins). More important, venous varices sometimes form in the lower esophagus in cases of chronic liver disease (see Chapter 23), and rupture of such congested varices may lead to fatal hemorrhage.

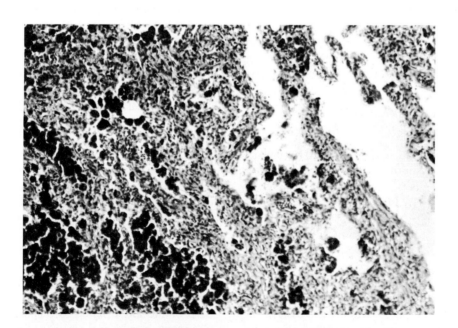

FIG. 7-1   Chronic passive congestion of lung. Alveolar septa are thickened *(evident at the right),* and many air spaces contain deeply pigmented macrophages containing hemosiderin. [Photomicrograph, ×200.]

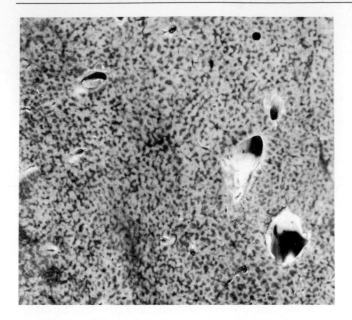

FIG. 7-2   Chronic passive congestion of liver. Dark areas on this cut surface are hyperemic centrilobular zones, and light areas are less affected peripheral zones. The result is this typical "nutmeg" pattern.

EDEMA

Edema is an accumulation of excess fluid between the cells of the body or within the various body cavities. (Some authors also include in the definition the accumulation of excess fluids intracellularly.) When fluid accumulates in the cavity, it is usually called an *effusion,* such as pericardial effusion and pleural effusion. An accumulation of fluid in the peritoneal cavity is usually called *ascites.* Massive generalized edema is typically referred to as *anasarca.* Hydrops and dropsy are older terms also referring to edema.

Etiology and Pathogenesis

The development of edema can be explained by considering the various forces normally controlling fluid exchange across vessel walls (see Fig. 4-2 and Chapter 4). Local factors include the hydrostatic pressure within the microcirculation and the permeability of vessel walls. Increases in hydrostatic pressure tend to force fluid into the interstitial spaces of the body. For this simple reason, congestion and edema tend to develop together. As explained in the discussion of inflammation, a local increase in the permeability of vessel walls to protein allows these large molecules to escape the vessels, and fluid follows osmotically. Therefore edema is a prominent part of the acute inflammatory reaction. Another local cause of edema formation is obstruction of lymphatic channels, which normally drain the interstitial fluid.

When these channels become obstructed for any reason, an important drainage pathway of fluid is lost, leading to accumulation of fluid, which is called *lymphedema.* Lymphedema is seen in a variety of inflammatory conditions affecting the lymphatics but is perhaps most frequently encountered after either excision or irradiation of local lymphatics as part of cancer therapy. A specific example of this type of edema is the swelling of the upper extremity sometimes seen after radical mastectomy with dissection of axillary lymph nodes.

Systemic factors may also favor edema formation. Because fluid balance depends on osmotic properties of serum protein, conditions accompanied by a lower concentration of this protein may lead to edema. In nephrotic syndrome, massive amounts of protein are lost in the urine and the patient becomes hypoproteinemic and edematous. The hypoproteinemia of advanced liver disease may also favor the formation of edema. In famine situations, massive edema may likewise accompany the nutritional hypoproteinemia.

Transudates Versus Exudates

When fluid accumulates in a tissue or space because of increased vascular permeability to protein, this accumulation is called an *exudate.* Thus inflammatory edema is an exudate. When fluid accumulates in the tissues or spaces for reasons other than changes in vascular permeability, the accumulation is called a *transudate.* Cardiac failure is a leading cause of transudate formation. Sometimes it becomes important clinically to determine whether a particular fluid accumulation represents a transudate or an exudate. Exudates, by their very nature, tend to contain more protein that transudates and therefore tend to have higher specific gravities. In addition, the protein of exudates often includes fibrinogen, which precipitates as fibrin, causing clotting of the exudate fluid. Transudates generally do not clot. Finally, exudates usually contain leukocytes as part of the inflammatory process, whereas transudates tend to be cell-poor.

Morphology

The morphology of edema involves simply a swelling of the affected part because of too much fluid contained within the interstices. The swelling is generally soft, and unless it is largely intracellular, the fluid can be moved about. This latter feature is used clinically in diagnosing subtle degrees of edema. Although a massively swollen ankle is easily diagnosed on sight, a slight degree of edema may be present without being particularly visible. In this instance, gentle pressure of a thumb against the side of the ankle tends to displace some of the edema fluid temporarily, and when the thumb is removed after a few moments, a depression is left in the tissues. This is referred to as *pitting edema.* This same mobility of edema fluid within the interstices of tissues accounts for certain postural effects. Sometimes, when first admitted to the hospital, a patient has demonstrably edematous ankles, because in the ambulatory situation the edema moves with gravity toward the lower extremities. However, when the patient has been in bed for a time with the lower extremities not in a dependent position, the ankles may become slimmer and edema may become demonstrable over the sacrum instead.

Effects

Edema is an important indicator of something being amiss. In other words, the swollen ankles per se do not harm the patient other than perhaps in a cosmetic sense, but they do serve as an indicator of protein loss or congestive heart failure. In certain locations, edema itself is extremely important. Edema of the lungs, as in left-sided heart failure, is an acute medical emergency if extensive. If a sufficient number of air spaces in the lungs fill with edema fluid, the patient may literally drown. Massive pulmonary edema can be lethal within minutes. Lesser degrees of pulmonary edema that can be tolerated in a ventilatory sense may be dangerous to bedridden patients. In such instances the fluid may collect posteriorly at the lung bases and serve as a focus for the development of bacterial pneumonia, sometimes called *hypostatic pneumonia*. Edema is also life-threatening when it affects the brain, because the skull is a closed space with no room to spare. As the brain becomes edematous, it swells and is compressed against the bony confines of the skull. At some point, in severe cases, increased intracranial pressure will compromise blood flow within the brain, leading to death.

HEMORRHAGE

Hemorrhage is the escape of blood from the cardiovascular system, with accumulation in tissues or spaces of the body or with actual escape from the body. Special terms are used to designate various types of hemorrhage. An accumulation of blood within tissues is called a *hematoma*. When the blood escapes into various spaces in the body, it is named according to the space, for example, hemopericardium, hemothorax (hemorrhage into the pleural space), hemoperitoneum, and hematosalpinx (hemorrhage into the fallopian tube). Pinpoint hemorrhages visible on cutaneous or mucosal surfaces or on cut surfaces of organs are called *petechiae*. Larger, blotchy areas of hemorrhage are referred to as *ecchymoses,* and a condition characterized by widespread blotchy hemorrhages is referred to as *purpura.*

Etiology

The most common cause of hemorrhage is the loss of integrity of vascular walls, which permits the escape of blood. This is usually the result of external trauma, such as the injuries everyone occasionally experiences accompanied by bruising. The discoloration of a bruise is caused by the blood accumulated in the interstices of the traumatized tissue. Vascular walls may be disrupted as a result of disease as well as of trauma.

A number of mechanisms exist within the body to counteract hemorrhage (see Part Three). One mechanism of hemostasis involves the blood platelets, which are made in the bone marrow and circulate in the blood in large numbers. Platelets act directly to plug small leaks in vessels by aggregating in the area and blocking the flow. Platelets also lead to hemostasis by triggering the clotting mechanism of the blood. The "backbone" of a blood clot is fibrin, which is precipitated from its circulating precursor, fibrinogen. The precipitation of fibrin is controlled by a number of clotting factors that are activated under certain circumstances (see Chapter 19).

Hemorrhage may be caused by an abnormality of these hemostatic mechanisms. For instance, hemorrhage accompanies a state of *thrombocytopenia,* a deficiency in the number of circulating platelets. Thrombocytopenia may arise because of destruction or suppression of the bone marrow (e.g., by malignancy or some drug), with consequent failure of platelet production. Thrombocytopenia may also occur if circulating platelets are rapidly destroyed, as occurs in certain diseases. When the platelet count in the peripheral blood drops below a certain point, the patient begins to bleed "spontaneously," meaning that the trauma of normal motion leads to widespread hemorrhages. A deficiency of any of the various clotting factors may likewise lead to hemorrhage. Such deficiency may be hereditary (e.g., hemophilia) but may also be acquired. Some of the blood-clotting factors are synthesized in the liver, and with advanced hepatic disease the level of such factors available in the blood may drop precipitously. Paradoxically, in certain situations, excessive clotting of the blood may lead to an acquired deficiency of platelets and/or clotting factors. Usually this involves the formation of myriads of tiny clots around the body, *disseminated intravascular coagulation* (DIC), and the acquired deficiency state is sometimes referred to under the general heading of *consumptive coagulopathy* (see Chapter 19).

Effects

The *local* effects of hemorrhage are related to the presence of extravasated blood in the tissues and can range from trivial to lethal. Perhaps the most trivial local effect is a bruise, which may be of only cosmetic importance. The initial bluish discoloration of the bruise is related directly to the presence of spilled RBCs accumulated in the tissue. These extravasated erythrocytes break down fairly rapidly and are phagocytized by macrophages arriving as part of the associated inflammatory response. These macrophages process the hemoglobin in the same manner as used in the normal recycling of old RBCs but in a much more accelerated, concentrated fashion. As the hemoglobin is metabolized within these cells, an iron-containing complex called *hemosiderin* is formed, along with a non-iron-containing moiety, which in tissues is termed *hematoidin* (although it is chemically identical with bilirubin). Hemosiderin has a rusty-brown color, and hematoidin is light yellow. The interaction of these pigments in a resolving bruise produces the familiar range of colors as the "black-and-blue mark" fades through varying shades of brown and yellow, ultimately to disappear as the macrophages wander off, and restitution of the tissue is complete. Sometimes, when a hematoma is of considerable volume, it may actually organize rather than resolve completely, leaving some degree of local scarring.

At the other extreme, a strictly local hemorrhage may be fatal, even if of small volume, if it is in the wrong place. Thus, as seen in Fig. 7-3, a relatively small volume of hemorrhage in a vital area of the brain can produce death. Similarly, if a few hundred milliliters of blood are aspirated into the tracheobronchial tree, the patient may suffocate. Another area wherein a relatively small volume of hemorrhage may produce death is the pericardial sac. If hemopericardium develops quickly and the tough, fibrous pericardial sac does not have the opportunity to stretch, pressure within the sac builds up rapidly as blood accumulates. Sometimes, with accumulation of only a few hundred milliliters, the pressure is sufficient to impair diastolic filling of the heart, leading to death by *cardiac tamponade.*

The *systemic* effects of blood loss are related directly to the volume of blood extravasated. If a major portion of the circulatory volume is lost, as with massive trauma, the patient may quickly die of exsanguination. A patient may exsanguinate with absolutely no external evidence of hemorrhage. This occurs when the extravasated blood accumulates within a large body cavity such as the pleural cavity or peritoneal cavity. This type of lethal internal hemorrhage is seen all too often in crushing injuries associated with motor vehicle accidents, when broken ribs lacerate a lung or abdominal trauma results in rupture of the spleen or liver. (In emergency room practice, such internal hemorrhage is identified by needle aspiration of the cavity in question.) The effects of a given volume of hemorrhage are also related to the rate at which the loss occurs, a larger volume loss being better tolerated if it occurs gradually rather than instantaneously.

Short of death, the rapid loss of a sufficient volume of blood may lead to a condition of *shock.* A detailed consideration of the various shock syndromes is beyond the scope of this discussion, but it should be pointed out that shock can be produced not only by the loss of blood volume, but also by neurogenic causes, cardiac causes, or even accompanying systemic sepsis. Although the various shock syndromes differ in detail, they are all basically accompanied by a decrease in blood pressure and by an element of loss of control over the regulation of blood flow, leading ultimately to inadequate perfusion and oxygenation of the vital tissues of the body.

If a patient survives the acute loss of a given volume of blood, the circulatory volume is quickly regained by an influx of fluid into the cardiovascular system. This leads to a relative dilution of the RBC mass remaining, and the patient at that point would be somewhat anemic. Under such conditions, the marrow is stimulated to produce RBCs at an accelerated rate and the anemia is gradually corrected. Under conditions of chronic loss of even relatively small volumes of blood, the compensatory abilities of the marrow may be exceeded and the patient may become progressively more anemic. Patients with chronic loss of blood may have signs and symptoms of the ane-

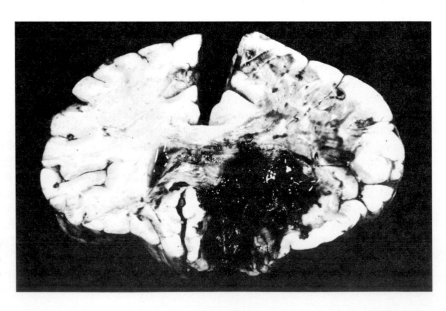

FIG. 7-3   Cerebral hemorrhage. In an instance such as this, a relatively small volume of hemorrhage may lead to death because of local destructive effects.

mia rather than of the blood loss itself. Thus many patients with cancer of the colon, which oozes blood for many months unnoticed into the feces, may ultimately seek medical attention because of fatigue, pallor, or lack of energy. Therefore occult blood loss is a consideration in the investigation of many anemias.

THROMBOSIS

The process of formation of a blood clot or coagulum within the vascular system (i.e., blood vessels or heart) during life is referred to as *thrombosis*. The coagulum of blood is called a *thrombus*. The accumulation of blood that clots outside of the vascular system (e.g., a hematoma) is not referred to as a thrombus. Furthermore, the clots that form after death within the cardiovascular system are not called thrombi. They are called postmortem clots.

Thrombosis is of great adaptive value in case of hemorrhage; a thrombus acts as an effective hemostatic plug. However, thrombosis may also occur inappropriately when the normal control mechanisms are defective and, under these circumstances, prove to be harmful.

Etiology and Pathogenesis

Three sets of factors ordinarily guard against inappropriate thrombus formation. First, the normal vascular system has a smooth, slick lining of endothelial cells to which platelets and fibrin do not readily adhere. Second, the normal flow of blood within the vascular system is fairly streamlined so that platelets are not hurled against lining surfaces. Finally, the clotting mechanism (see Chapter 19) has built into it a number of chemical checks and balances to control clot formation. Correspondingly, there are three basic situations in which clots form inappropriately: (1) an abnormality exists in the vessel wall and lining; (2) blood flow is abnormal; and (3) the coagulability of the blood itself is increased.

The flow of blood on the arterial side of the circulation is a high-pressure flow of rapid velocity, and the arteries themselves are rather thick-walled and not easily deformed. For these reasons, the usual cause of arterial thrombosis is disease in the lining and wall of the artery, particularly atherosclerosis (see later discussion). On the venous side of the circulation, the blood flow has a low pressure and relatively lower velocity, and the veins are sufficiently thin-walled that they can be deformed readily by external pressures. For these reasons, the usual causes of thrombosis on the venous side of the circulation relate to diminished flow of blood. Finally, chemical changes occur in the blood of patients with a variety of diseases, leading to a hypercoagulable state that may further complicate any of the situations just mentioned.

Morphology and Fate of Thrombi

Thrombi consist of varying combinations of aggregated platelets, precipitated fibrin, and enmeshed RBCs and white blood cells (WBCs, leukocytes). The precise configuration of a thrombus depends on the conditions under which it was formed. If the thrombus begins to form in flowing blood, often the first element is a clump of platelets adhering to the endothelium. This may occur because of abnormal flow allowing platelets to settle against or to be hurled against the endothelium; it also may occur because of a roughening of the endothelial lining, which would produce a nidus for platelet aggregation. As platelets aggregate, they release substances that encourage the precipitation of fibrin so that soon the platelet aggregates become surrounded by fibrin and trapped blood cells. Successive waves of events of this type can lead to a complex, ribbed structure of a thrombus. On the other hand, if a thrombus forms in a vessel in which the flow has virtually stopped, the clot may simply consist of a diffuse meshwork of fibrin trapping the formed elements in the blood more or less homogeneously. However, in contrast to the processes just described, postmortem clotting occurs quite slowly so that the formed elements of the blood layer out before the clot solidifies, giving rise to a stratified structure in which RBCs, WBCs, and fibrin may be quite separate. Such postmortem clots tend to be more elastic than true thrombi and are much less likely to adhere to vascular walls. These distinctions may become important at autopsy.

Thrombi may occur in any part of the cardiovascular system and for a variety of causes. Fig. 7-4 illustrates a thrombus from a large, deep vein of the leg. Such thrombi are common in hospitalized, bedridden patients. Their occurrence is generally related to the decreased rate of flow through these veins, in turn secondary to the loss of pumping action of muscular activity. The situation is aggravated in many instances by sluggish peripheral circulation related to chronic cardiac failure. *Phlebothrombosis*, the formation of thrombi in veins, is an ever-present danger for bedridden or immobilized patients. Such thrombi may develop relatively silently or may be accompanied by signs and symptoms of inflammation of the vein wall, which are presumably secondary to the presence of the thrombus. When inflammatory signs dominate, the condition is called *thrombophlebitis*. The most feared consequence of such venous thrombi is the breaking off of a portion, which is then transported in the bloodstream to lodge at a distant site.

Fig. 7-5 illustrates a thrombus within the left atrium of the heart. In this case the thrombus formed because of an abnormal flow and a pattern of circulation through the atrium related to stenosis of the mitral valve. Occasionally, such an atrial thrombus may behave as a "ball valve," suddenly occluding the atrioventricular orifice and producing instant death. More often such thrombi act

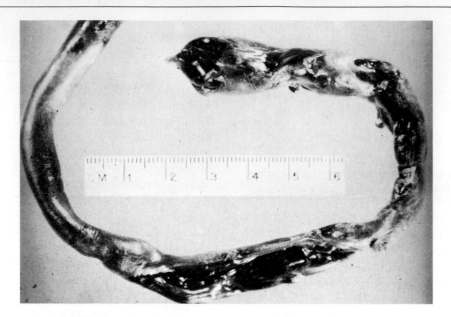

FIG. 7-4   Venous thrombus. This thrombus was extracted from a leg vein at autopsy. Such a finding is unfortunately quite common and is associated with many dire consequences. Reference to the scale emphasizes the magnitude of the clot.

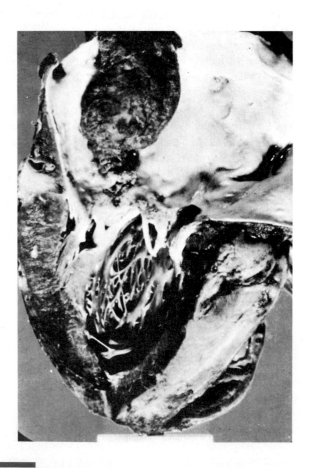

FIG. 7-5   Atrial thrombus. A huge thrombus formed in the left atrium because of malfunction of the scarred mitral valve. The position of this clot renders it a great potential danger.

as the source of fragments that are propelled distally in the bloodstream.

Fig. 7-6 illustrates a thrombus on a cardiac valve. In this instance, the cause is bacterial infection of the valve and the thrombus is called a *vegetation.* Vegetations of infective endocarditis are exceedingly dangerous because of local damage to the valve and because fragments may be propelled to other sites in the body, where additional vessels may become occluded and infected.

Fig. 7-7 illustrates a thrombus within the left ventricle of the heart. When a thrombus such as this adheres to the wall of the cardiovascular system but does not totally occlude the area, it is referred to as a *mural thrombus.* The usual reason for the formation of a ventricular mural thrombus is hypokinesis of the heart wall caused by disease or death of the underlying myocardium.

Fig. 7-8 illustrates a thrombus within an artery. Clearly evident are the thickening and roughening of the artery wall that have given rise to the thrombus. The roughening in this instance is caused by a disease (atherosclerosis) and is a precipitating cause of thrombosis.

Often, when the subject survives the formation of a thrombus, the thrombus may undergo resolution. The body possesses fibrinolytic mechanisms that, along with the action of leukocytes, may lead to the dissolution of clots. Everyone probably forms tiny thrombi now and then, and these are resolved without ever reaching the clinical horizon. On the other hand, some large thrombi undergo organization, with granulation tissue growing from an adjacent vascular lining. In such instances the involved vessel may become permanently plugged by scar

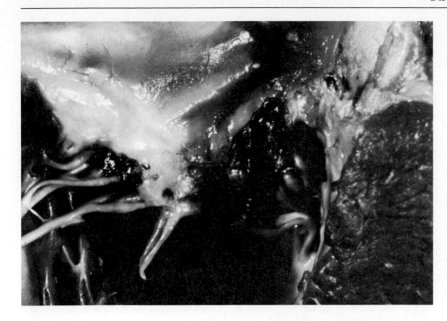

FIG 7-6   Infective endocarditis. The dark vegetations on this mitral valve are actually thrombotic masses formed around foci of bacterial infection of the valve. The valve was previously scarred (note thickening of leaflets and chordae) and therefore was susceptible to infection during a burst of bacteremia.

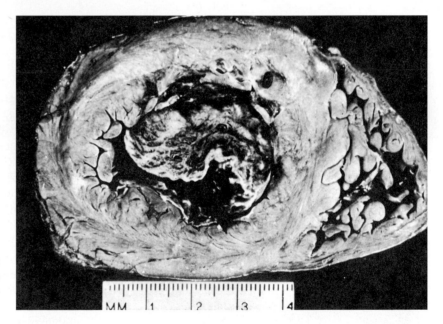

FIG. 7-7   Mural thrombus in heart. In this transverse section a large mural thrombus overlies an area of previous myocardial necrosis in the wall of the left ventricle.

tissue. Sometimes the vascular channels within the young granulation tissue organizing a thrombus may anastomose and provide new channels through the area occupied by a thrombus. This phenomenon is referred to as *recanalization.* Unfortunately, before the thrombus either organizes or resolves, portions of it often break off and are propelled in the bloodstream, ultimately lodging elsewhere and occluding additional vessels.

Effects

The consequences of thrombosis are perhaps most obvious with arterial thrombi. If an artery is occluded by a thrombus, the tissues served by that artery lose their blood supply. The results of this may range from functional abnormality of tissue to death of the tissue or death of the subject. The consequences of venous thrombi are somewhat different. If one vein is plugged, the blood is likely to find its way back to the heart via some anastomosing channel. Only when a large vein is occluded by a thrombus do local problems with passive congestion become evident. The most ominous problem associated with venous thrombi is their fragmentation and transport to distant points in the body. Similarly, the effects of cardiac thrombi are largely related to their moving elsewhere within the cardiovascular system.

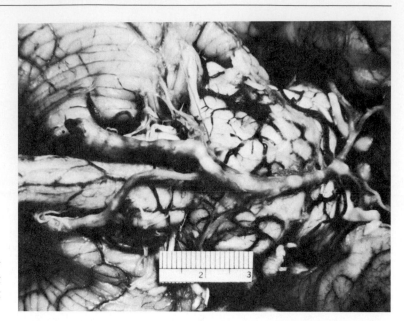

FIG. 7-8   Thrombus in a sclerotic artery. The artery above the brain stem *(left of center)* is atherosclerotic and gnarled. The lumen is occluded by a thrombus that protrudes from the cut end at the left.

EMBOLISM

Definition and Types

The transportation of a physical mass in the bloodstream from one place to another with lodgement in the new location is called *embolism*. The physical mass itself is called an *embolus*. The most common emboli in humans are derived from thrombi and are called *thromboemboli*. Many other things, however, can become embolic. Bits of tissue can embolize if they enter the vascular system, usually with trauma. Cancer cells may embolize, constituting a devastating means of spread of the disease (see Chapter 8). Foreign materials injected into the cardiovascular system also may embolize. Droplets of liquid that form in the circulation under a variety of circumstances or are injected into the circulation may embolize, and even gas bubbles may become embolic.

Pathogenesis, Routes, and Effects

The most common sources of emboli within the body are venous thrombi, most often in the deep veins of the legs or the pelvis. When fragments of such venous thrombi break off and float with the flow of blood, they enter the vena cava and then the right side of the heart. Such fragments do not lodge along this path because of the large size of the vessels and cardiac chambers involved. The blood leaving the right ventricle, however, flows into the main pulmonary artery, which branches into right and left pulmonary arteries, which in turn branch to smaller vessels. For these anatomic reasons, emboli originating in venous thrombi usually terminate as pulmonary arterial emboli. When a large fragment of a thrombus becomes an embolus, a major portion of the pulmonary arterial sup-

ply may suddenly be occluded (Fig. 7-9). This can cause virtually instantaneous death of the subject. On the other hand, smaller pulmonary arterial emboli may be silent, may lead to pulmonary hemorrhage secondary to the vascular damage, or may actually result in necrosis of a portion of lung. Pulmonary emboli of various sizes can be found in a significant number of patients dying after being bedridden; sometimes the pulmonary emboli contribute to the death of the subject, and sometimes they are only of incidental importance. Showers of tiny pulmonary emboli over a long period may produce sufficient occlusion of the pulmonary vascular bed to cause the right side of the heart to become overloaded and to fail.

Emboli that lodge on the arterial side of the circulation originate from the "left side" of the circulatory system, either in the left cardiac chambers or in the large arteries. The only way that an embolus originating on the venous side of the circulation could lodge on the arterial side is to bypass the lungs via a defect in the interatrial or interventricular septum of the heart. This situation, called *paradoxical embolism*, is exceedingly rare. Most often an arterial embolus is found to have originated from an intracardiac thrombus or, more rarely, from a mural thrombus in the aorta or one of its large branches.

Gas bubbles may become embolic in a variety of circumstances. One such circumstance, called *caisson disease,* is popularly known as "the bends." This situation arises when a subject has been living under markedly increased atmospheric pressure, such as that within a pressurized caisson or in underwater diving gear. In such circumstances, increased amounts of atmospheric gases are dissolved within the bloodstream. If decompression is sufficiently abrupt, the result is analogous to what is seen when a warm bottle of a carbonated beverage is suddenly opened. The myriads of tiny gas bubbles appearing

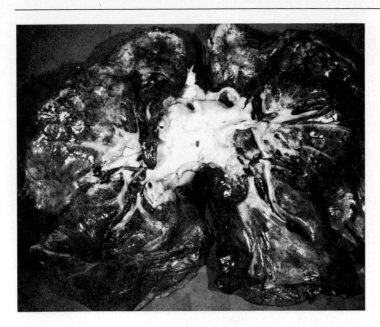

FIG. 7-9   Massive pulmonary emboli. The opened pulmonary arteries supplying these lungs are seen in the center of the photograph. The several dark cylindric masses are emboli that originated from venous thrombus in a leg, similar to that shown in Fig. 7-4. The patient died within moments of lodgement of the emboli.

within the circulation are carried to a variety of places in the body, where they lodge in the microcirculation and occlude the blood flow to those tissues. An analogous circumstance sometimes arises when atmospheric air enters venous channels as a result of faulty handling of an intravenous infusion or indwelling vascular catheter, or sometimes in the course of a surgical procedure when large vascular channels must be traversed. With massive air embolism, a large *bolus* of air may enter the right side of the heart and at autopsy a large, foamy mass of air and blood is seen distending the heart and pulmonary vessels.

An example of embolism of liquid droplets is *traumatic fat embolism*. As the name suggests, these emboli, composed of fat globules, tend to form within the circulation after trauma. The usual point of lodgement is the microcirculation of the lung. Minor degrees of fat embolism probably follow most surgical procedures when fatty tissue is incised and lipidic material is allowed to enter vascular channels. In such circumstances the few scattered emboli that lodge in the lung are completely silent and trivial. A similar circumstance arises when bones are fractured, apparently with liberation of lipid into the sinusoids of the bone marrow. Again, such scattered pulmonary fat emboli are trivial and clinically inapparent. Occasionally, however, after traumatic injury, fat embolism may be massive. It is not clear whether all the fat droplets in such a circumstance originate from trauma to adipose cells. Some evidence suggests that in this type of circumstance the lipid normally carried within the bloodstream coalesces. In any event, with sufficiently massive fat embolism, symptoms of respiratory distress may appear, usually in the first day or two after trauma. In severe instances, the emboli lodge in a variety of places in the body beyond the lungs, including the skin and, more important, the central nervous system. In both

these latter areas, each microscopic fat embolus is associated with a petechial hemorrhage. In the brain a tiny focus of necrosis surrounds each occluded vessel. In these rare instances, fat embolism can be fatal, usually because of cerebral damage.

ATHEROSCLEROSIS

Arteriosclerosis, or "hardening of the arteries," is an exceedingly important disease phenomenon in most developed countries. The term *arteriosclerosis* actually encompasses any condition of arterial vessels that results in a thickening and/or hardening of the walls. Three conditions are generally included under this heading: Mönckeberg's sclerosis, arteriolosclerosis, and atherosclerosis. *Mönckeberg's sclerosis* involves the deposition of calcium salts in the muscular wall of medium-sized arteries. Although this can be detected grossly and even seen on radiographs, this form of arteriosclerosis is not clinically significant, since the lining of the involved vessel is not roughened and the lumen is not narrowed. *Arteriolosclerosis* refers to a thickening of arterioles and is typically seen in patients with elevated blood pressure and to some extent in association with aging. The most important type of arteriosclerosis is atherosclerosis, and generally when the term arteriosclerosis is used, it is used synonymously with atherosclerosis.

Atherosclerosis involves the aorta, its large branches, and medium-sized arteries, such as those supplying portions of the extremities, brain, heart, and major internal viscera. Atherosclerosis does not involve arterioles and or the venous side of the circulation. The disease is multifocal, and the unit lesion, or *atheroma* (also termed *athero-*

sclerotic plaque), consists of an elevated mass of fatty material associated with fibrous connective tissue, very often with secondary deposits of calcium salts and blood products. The plaques of atherosclerosis begin in the intima or inner layer of the vessel wall and project into the lumen, but with growth they may extend to encroach on the media or musculoelastic portion of the vessel wall.

Morphology

The typical gross appearance of moderately severe atherosclerosis is shown in Fig. 7-10. A smooth endothelial lining of vessels is an important protection against throm-bus formation, so it is not difficult to realize why atherosclerosis should involve considerable liability to arterial thrombosis. The microscopic appearance of an atheroma is illustrated in Fig. 7-11. The dominance of both fibrous and fatty material in the lesion is evident (*athero* refers to the mushy and *sclerosis* to the hard character of the lesions). In large vessels, such as the aorta, even numerous and severe atheromas generally do not lead to occlusion of the lumen but only to roughening of the lining surface. In smaller vessels, the atheromas may actually become circumferential, leading to marked narrowing of the lumen (Fig. 7-12).

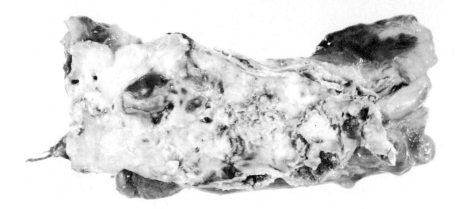

FIG. 7-10   Atherosclerosis of aorta. This photograph depicts the intimal (lining) surface of the opened abdominal aorta. Instead of being pearly and smooth, the surface is a roughened mass of atherosclerotic plaques.

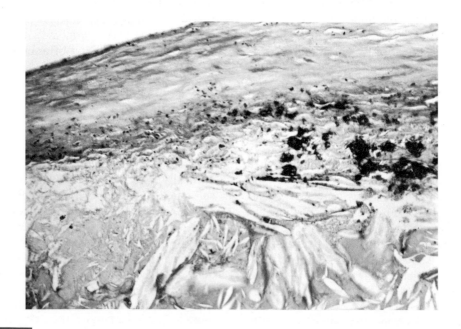

FIG. 7-11   Atherosclerotic plaque. The cleft in the depths of the plaque represents large deposits of cholesterol. The dark material at the right is a dystrophic calcific deposit, and the horizontal band across the top is a fibrous "cap" of the lesion. The elevated rough lesions in Fig. 7-10 have this microscopic appearance.

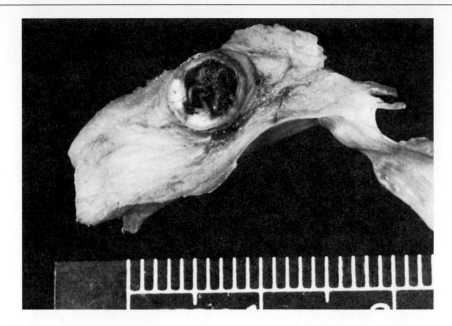

FIG. 7-12   Atherosclerotic coronary artery. The circumferential atheroma has left only a tiny lumen (at 8 o'clock) in this cross section of coronary artery. Consequences in terms of blood flow are obvious.

Etiology and Incidence

Many factors contribute to the development of atherosclerosis, and it is therefore not possible to cite a single or dominant cause. The various factors are so widespread in the populations of the more affluent countries that only the youngest individuals are spared by the disease. In fact, autopsies performed on otherwise healthy young adults who died as a result of trauma often reveal lesions of atherosclerosis, sometimes surprisingly severe. The earliest fatty deposits may be seen in young children, and these generally tend to increase with age. The rate at which atheromas increase in size and number is influenced by a variety of factors. Genetic factors are important, and atherosclerosis and its complications often tend to run in families. Subjects with elevated levels of serum cholesterol are often susceptible to accelerated atherosclerosis, as are individuals with diabetes mellitus. Blood pressure is an important factor in the incidence and severity of atherosclerosis. Patients with hypertension are much more likely to have earlier and more severe atherosclerosis; the severity of the disease is correlated with the blood pressure even in the normal range. Atherosclerosis is not seen within the pulmonary arteries (usually a low-pressure circuit) unless the pressure is abnormally elevated, a state called *pulmonary hypertension.* Another risk factor in the development of atherosclerosis is cigarette smoking, which is a major environmental factor leading to increased severity of atherosclerosis. The precise way in which these various factors contribute to the pathogenesis of the lesions of atherosclerosis has not been completely elucidated.

Consequences

The consequences of atherosclerosis depend in part on the size of the artery involved. If the artery is a medium-sized one, such as a major branch of the coronary artery, with a lumen perhaps a few milliliters in diameter, atherosclerosis may lead gradually to narrowing or even total obstruction of the lumen.

In contrast to this slowly developing occlusion, complications of atherosclerosis may lead to an abruptly developing occlusion. One such circumstance is thrombus formation superimposed on the intimal roughening produced by atherosclerotic plaques. Thrombosis tends to be occlusive in a small or medium-sized artery, but it may be in the form of a relatively thin mural deposit in a large vessel such as the aorta. Another complication of atherosclerosis is hemorrhage in the soft center of the plaque. In a vessel the size of the coronary artery, this may result in swelling of the plaque with sudden occlusion of the lumen. Another complication that may lead to acute arterial occlusion is a rupture of the plaque with welling up of the soft lipidic contents into the lumen and lodgement in a narrower "downstream" segment of the vessel. Finally, if extensive and severe enough, lesions of atherosclerosis may encroach on the muscular and elastic wall (the media) of an artery, thus weakening it. In the abdominal aorta, a common site of severe atherosclerosis, the result of such medial damage may be the formation of an atherosclerotic *aneurysm,* which is a ballooning of the weakened arterial wall (Fig. 7-13). Although a thrombus may form within such an aneurysm because of the abnormal swirling of the blood and because of the roughened

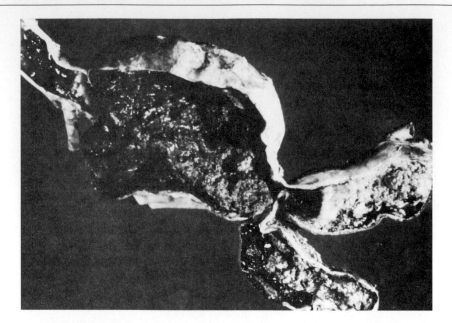

FIG. 7-13   Atherosclerotic aneurysms. A large aneurysm distorts the distal aorta and each iliac artery. The walls of such aneurysms are prone to rupture.

intima, the most dangerous complication of an aneurysm is rupture with exsanguination.

ISCHEMIA AND INFARCTION

Ischemia is simply an inadequate blood supply in an area. When tissues are rendered ischemic, they are deprived of necessary oxygen and nutrients. The accumulation of metabolic wastes within the poorly perfused tissue may also contribute to tissue damage. Anything that affects the flow of blood may produce tissue ischemia. The most obvious cause is local arterial obstruction related to atherosclerosis, thrombosis, or embolism. Less often, venous obstruction may lead to ischemia when the flow of blood through the tissue virtually reaches a standstill. There are even systemic causes of tissue ischemia. For instance, if heart failure is sufficiently severe, a tissue might become ischemic simply because of the low level of perfusion. Similarly, prolonged shock may lead to significant tissue ischemia.

The effects of ischemia vary, depending on the intensity of the ischemia, the rate of onset, and the metabolic demands of the particular tissue. In some instances of ischemia, usually involving muscular tissues, pain may be a symptom of diminished blood supply. For example, an elderly person with atherosclerosis of the leg arteries and consequent decrease in blood flow may have sufficient blood supply when at rest but not during activity. When such an individual walks briskly, increasing the meta-bolic demand of the leg muscles, the onset of relative ischemia may cause pain and limping. The same event occurs in the heart muscle with narrowing of the coronary arterial circulation. In this case, with activity a patient may develop a feeling of oppression or squeezing pain within the chest, a phenomenon referred to as *angina pectoris.* By definition, anginal pain recedes with rest, when the metabolic demand of the heart muscle diminishes to the point where the narrowed coronary arterial circulation is adequate.

Another effect of ischemia if it is of gradual onset and prolonged duration is that the involved tissue may atrophy, or shrink. A common example of this is observed in a patient who has atherosclerosis that diminishes the circulation to the lower extremities. Often the legs exhibit loss of muscle mass, and the skin becomes smooth, thin, and hairless, all the results of chronic ischemia.

The most extreme effect of ischemia is the death of the ischemic tissue. An area of ischemic necrosis is termed an *infarct,* and the process of forming an infarct is termed *infarction.* Whether an ischemic area actually undergoes infarction depends on a variety of local and systemic factors. For example, a degree of arterial occlusion is better tolerated if it occurs slowly, if the metabolic demand of the tissue is low, and if there is development of collateral circulation (i.e., auxiliary supply of the involved area by branches of neighboring arteries). In addition, the effects of a given degree of ischemia are worsened if the oxygen transport within the blood is diminished for any reason.

The morphologic features of infarcts vary from organ

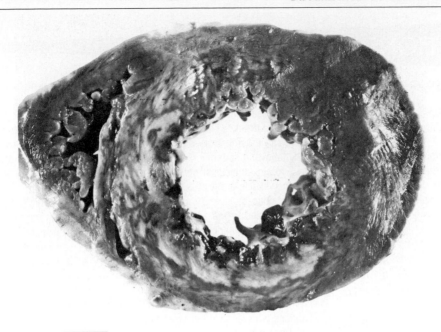

FIG. 7-14   Myocardial infarct. Myocardial ischemia has resulted in coagulative necrosis *(light area)* of much of the septum and ventricular wall.

to organ, but in general the tissue necrosis produced by ischemia is accompanied by an element of hemorrhage from damaged vessels at the edges of the infarcted area. In loose tissues, such as the lung, this hemorrhage is extensive and the infarcted area literally becomes stuffed with blood, producing a hemorrhagic or red infarct. In other organs (e.g., kidney, heart), the hemorrhage accompanying infarction is minimal and the infarct tends to be pale. In hemorrhagic as well as in pale infarcts, the basic cause of the damage is ischemia of the tissues. In most infarcts, the necrosis produced by ischemia is coagulative and the outlines of the tissue are maintained (Fig. 7-14). In the lung, hemorrhage dominates the picture, whereas in the brain, an area of infarction gradually softens and undergoes liquefactive change so that the result is a hole in the tissue (see Fig. 3-6).

The presence of infarcted tissue excites an inflammatory reaction at the margins interfacing with viable tissue. Neutrophils and macrophages rapidly invade the dead area to begin the job of demolition. Subsequently, the area is gradually organized as demolition proceeds and the usual outcome is scarring of the infarcted area. In many organs an infarct itself is not particularly important, given the amount of reserve of that organ. Thus even a moderately large renal infarct will not endanger the person's life because of the ability of one kidney or even part of one kidney to maintain homeostasis. The presence of a pulmonary infarct likewise is not particularly threatening in terms of ventilatory function. In this latter instance, however, the occurrence of pulmonary infarction is somewhat ominous, since it is usually the result of pulmonary embolism. Therefore there is always concern that larger and more threatening emboli may originate from the source of the first embolus. In the brain and myocardium the results of infarction are much more significant because there is less reserve in these organs, with each area being important, and in particular because in these two areas no possibility exists of regeneration of infarcted elements. Finally, in some areas exposed to bacterial populations, the infarcted tissue will serve as a focus of growth of saprophytic microorganisms. Thus infarcts of the bowel quickly become gangrenous, and infarcts of portions of an extremity are initially recognized as areas of gangrene.

QUESTIONS

▼ *Answer the following on a separate sheet of paper.*

1. Describe how the mechanisms involved in active congestion differ from those in passive congestion.
2. Explain how congestion could be produced by a cardiac problem.
3. What effects do acute passive congestion and chronic passive congestion have on the involved tissue?
4. Define edema.

▼ *Circle the letter preceding each term below that correctly answers the question or completes the statement. More than one answer may be correct.*

5. Which of the following are examples of active congestion?
   a. The lung in acute left ventricular failure
   b. The tissues of the leg in femoral vein thrombosis
   c. The red "halo" around an area of cutaneous inflammation
   d. A blush
6. The individual with chronic right-sided heart failure who develops persistent hyperemia of the liver has which type of congestion?
   a. Active
   b. Chronic active
   c. Chronic passive
   d. Acute passive
7. Chronic passive congestion may lead to which of the following changes in the liver?
   a. Dilation of the blood channels in the centrilobular zone of each hepatic lobule
   b. Enlargement of liver cells of each hepatic lobule
   c. Constriction of blood channels in the peripheral zone of each hepatic lobule
   d. Shrinkage of liver cells in the centrilobular zone of each hepatic lobule
8. The accumulation of fluid in the peritoneal cavity is called:
   a. Pericardial effusion
   b. Peritonitis
   c. Ascites
   d. Anasarca
9. Which of the following would be likely to contribute to the formation of edema?
   a. Elevation of venous pressure in a tissue
   b. Dehydration

c. Marked decrease in serum protein
d. Arterial obstruction in a tissue
e. Increased phagocytosis in the lymph nodes draining the area

10. In acute inflammatory states, which of the following statements apply?
    a. Protein molecules move from inside the vessels of the area to the interstitial spaces.
    b. Arterioles in the area dilate to produce active congestion.
    c. Water "follows" protein into the interstitial spaces.
    d. Edema develops because of diminution of lymphatic drainage.
11. Which of the following edematous conditions is potentially the *most* serious?
    a. Pleural effusion
    b. Ascites
    c. Cerebral edema
    d. Lymphedema
12. Exudates differ from transudates in that:
    a. Exudates tend to contain more leukocytes.
    b. Transudates have a higher specific gravity than exudates.
    c. Exudates have a higher protein content than transudates.
    d. Exudates usually do not clot.
13. Pinpoint hemorrhages visible on cutaneous or mucosal surfaces are referred to as:
    a. Ecchymoses
    b. Petechiae
    c. Hematomas
    d. Purpura
14. Dilation of the blood channels in the center of each hepatic lobule with shrinkage of liver cells in this area is seen in:
    a. Active congestion
    b. Acute passive congestion
    c. Chronic passive congestion
    d. None of the above

▼ *Answer the following on a separate sheet of paper.*

15. What is the most common cause of a hemorrhage?
16. What are two basic mechanisms for stopping hemorrhage?
17. Describe the local and systemic effects of hemorrhage.
18. Describe two clinical implications of thrombosis.

19. List some local causes of ischemia.
20. Describe possible effects of ischemia.

▼ *Circle the letter preceding the item below that correctly answers each question or completes the statement. More than one answer may be correct.*

21. Thrombi consist of which of the following?
    a. Aggregated platelets
    b. Precipitated fibrin
    c. Enmeshed leukocytes
    d. Enmeshed erythrocytes
22. In the formation of a thrombus, which event usually occurs first?
    a. Platelet aggregation
    b. Precipitation of fibrin
    c. Vascular dilation
    d. Hemolysis
23. Thrombosis is favored by all the following *except:*
    a. Decreased viscosity of the blood
    b. Venous stasis
    c. Increase in blood platelets
    d. Rough vessel lining
24. The transport of a physical mass in the bloodstream from one place to another with lodgement in the new location is:
    a. Ischemia
    b. Infarction
    c. Embolism
    d. Thrombosis
25. Emboli that lodge on the arterial side of the circulation generally originate from a(n):
    a. Mural thrombus in the aorta
    b. Right atrium
    c. Intracardiac thrombus
    d. Femoral vein
26. If decompression is sufficiently abrupt or when atmospheric air enters venous channels, gas bubbles may appear within the circulation, where they lodge in the microcirculation and occlude the blood flow to the area. Examples of this condition would include:
    a. A diver who has been living under increased atmospheric pressure
    b. A surgical procedure in which large vascular channels were traversed
    c. A patient with a fractured femur
    d. Generalized traumatic injury involving adipose tissue
27. All the following conditions contribute to atherosclerosis *except:*
    a. Certain genetic factors
    b. Increased serum cholesterol levels

QUESTIONS—cont'd

c. Diabetes mellitus
d. Hypotension
e. Cigarette smoking

28. The atherosclerotic plaque usually initially involves the:
    a. Arterioles
    b. Intima of an artery
    c. Media of an artery
    d. Intima of a vein

29. A ventricular mural thrombus usually forms because of:
    a. Hypokinesis of the wall of a diseased heart
    b. Stenosis of the mitral valve
    c. Infarction of the underlying myocardium
    d. All the above

30. All the following generally cause ischemia *except:*
    a. Diminished clotting factors
    b. Local arterial obstruction

c. Thrombosis
d. Atherosclerosis

31. Which of the following describes an infarcted area located in the lung?
    a. The hemorrhage accompanying infarction is minimal, and the infarction tends to be pale.
    b. The hemorrhage is extensive, and the infarcted area tends to be red.
    c. The infarction gradually softens and undergoes liquefactive change.

▼ *Circle T if the statement is true and F if it is false. Correct any false statements.*

32. T   F   Mönckeberg's sclerosis is a clinically significant form of arteriosclerosis, since the lining of the involved vessel is roughened and the lumen is narrowed.

33. T   F   Atherosclerosis is the most important form of arteriosclerosis.

34. T   F   An atheroma is an elevated mass of fatty material and associated fibrous connective tissue.

35. T   F   Atherosclerosis can usually be ascribed to a single or dominant cause.

36. T   F   Complications of atherosclerosis may lead to an abruptly developing occlusion.

37. T   F   The results of infarction in the brain and myocardium are very significant, particularly because there is no possibility of regeneration of infarcted elements.

38. T   F   Infarct is a term used to denote a type of circulatory abnormality.

CHAPTER 8

Disturbances in Growth, Cellular Proliferation, and Differentiation

GERALD D. ABRAMS

This chapter focuses on a number of extremely diverse conditions having different causes and consequences. The unifying concept is that each of the conditions discussed is characterized by an abnormality in (1) the size and/or number of cells in a tissue, (2) the mode of cellular proliferation, or (3) the character of cellular differentiation. These abnormalities may lead to tissues that are smaller or larger than normal and to tissues that have abnormal functional specialization. At the extreme the abnormal cells may form masses, the behavior of which is generally beyond the influence of normal homeostatic controls.

ORGANS AND TISSUES SMALLER THAN NORMAL

Occasionally a tissue, organ, or part of the body that is smaller than normal is encountered. This situation can arise in two ways: the organ or tissue may never have grown to normal size, or it may have reached normal size and then shrunk.

Agenesis and Aplasia

In the course of development, the embryonic rudiment of an organ may never form. This phenomenon is called *agenesis,* and the result is the absence of the particular organ; for example, some individuals are born with only a single kidney. A related situation is *aplasia,* when the embryonic rudiment of an organ fails to grow at all once it has formed. (Some use the terms agenesis and aplasia interchangeably, and little practical difference exists.)

Hypoplasia

Sometimes the embryonic rudiment forms and grows but never quite reaches definitive or adult size, yielding a dwarfed organ. This phenomenon is called *hypoplasia.* Hypoplasia, as with agenesis and aplasia, may involve any portion of the body, one of a pair of organs, or even both organs of a pair. Minor degrees of hypoplasia of some organ might be well tolerated for long periods, the net effect being some encroachment on the usual degree of reserve of that organ.

Atrophy

Organs that reach definitive size in the course of development and then shrink are referred to as *atrophic*. Atrophy has a variety of causes, and in some instances it is actually normal or physiologic, such as when certain parts of the embryo or fetus atrophy in the course of development. Some forms of atrophy are inevitable with advancing age, such as the endocrine atrophy that occurs when hormonal support is withdrawn from a tissue such as the mammary gland. An extremely common cause of atrophy is chronic ischemia. Another common type of atrophy, primarily involving skeletal muscle, is *disuse atrophy*. When a broken leg is placed in an immobilizing cast for weeks or months, the mass of the extremity is significantly reduced because of atrophy of the unused muscle. In this situation the individual muscle cells are of reduced size, but the state is a reversible one. In other instances of atrophy, actual loss of cellular elements occurs.

ORGANS AND TISSUES LARGER THAN NORMAL

Hypertrophy

Hypertrophy is defined as an enlargement of a tissue or organ because of enlargement of individual cells. Hypertrophy can be seen in a variety of tissues, but it is prominent in various types of muscle. An increased workload on a muscle is a strong stimulus to hypertrophy. The bulging muscles of the weight lifter are an obvious example of muscular hypertrophy. The same type of event occurs as an important adaptive response in the myocardium. If a subject has an abnormal cardiac valve that imposes an unusual mechanical load on the left ventricle or if the ventricle is pumping against an elevated systemic blood pressure, the result is hypertrophy of the myocardium with thickening of the ventricular wall. A similar phenomenon can occur in smooth muscle that is forced to work against an increased load. Thus the wall of the urinary bladder may become hypertrophic when there is obstruction to the free outflow of urine. In each of these instances, hypertrophic enlargement of cells is actually accompanied by an increase in the contractile elements of the tissue, and thus the response is adaptive. Hypertrophy is stimulus-related, so it tends to regress, at least to some extent, if the abnormal workload is withdrawn.

Hyperplasia

Hyperplasia is an increase in the absolute number of cells within a tissue, leading to an increase in the size of that tissue or organ. This obviously occurs only in a tissue capable of cell division; in such tissues, hyperplasia may also be accompanied by hypertrophy of individual cells. Hyperplasia occurs in a variety of tissues under many different circumstances, some of them completely physiologic. For example, with the hormonal stimulus of pregnancy and lactation, extensive proliferation of epithelial elements occurs within the breast, with an increase in the size of breast tissue caused by this hyperplasia. An example of nonphysiologic hyperplasia is the enlargement of the prostate gland, often seen in aging men. Another example of hyperplasia that is nonphysiologic but still adaptive is a callus, or thickening of skin, developing in response to a mechanical stimulus. Microscopic examination of a callus reveals a marked increase in the number of epidermal cells and layers of cells in the epidermis, clearly an adaptive response.

Many examples of hyperplasia represent "rational" responses of the body to some imposed demand. As with hypertrophy, if the abnormal circumstance is reversed, the signal to cellular proliferation is withdrawn, and the hyperplasia regresses and more normal conditions return. In the previous examples, the enlarged breast shrinks to a more normal size after lactation and the callus gradually disappears when the mechanical stimulus to the skin is no longer applied. Unfortunately, the stimulus leading to prostatic hyperplasia is not understood and the excess tissue often must be resected surgically.

ABNORMAL DIFFERENTIATION: DEFINITIONS

Metaplasia

The character of cellular differentiation in a given tissue may also change under abnormal circumstances. *Differ-*

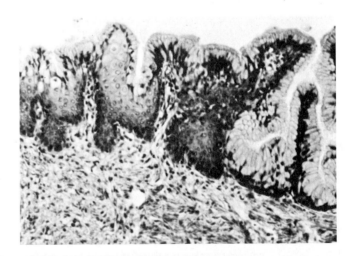

FIG. 8-1   Squamous metaplasia. In this lining epithelium of uterine cervix, the usual cell type is columnar, as at the right. Most of the epithelium has altered its differentiation to form an epidermis-like squamous epithelium. (Photomicrograph, ×200.)

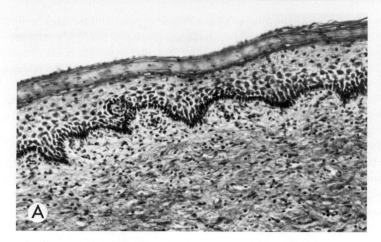 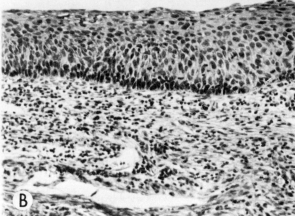

FIG. 8-2   Dysplasia versus normal cells. **A,** In the normal epithelium the cells are very regular in a given zone and layering is orderly. **B,** In dysplasia there is marked morphologic variation in the cells and layering is disordered. (Photomicrograph, ×200.)

entiation is the process by which the progeny of dividing stem cells become specialized to perform a particular task. For instance, dividing cells in the deepest layer of the epidermis gradually migrate upward and as they do so, they acquire the specialized protective characteristics of outer epidermal cells and produce a proteinaceous substance known as *keratin.* Similarly, within the lining of the respiratory tract, some of the dividing cells in the epithelium develop into tall, columnar cells with cilia on their luminal surfaces.

When differentiating cell systems of this type are placed under adverse circumstances, the pattern of differentiation may change so that the dividing cells begin to differentiate into types of cells not usually found in the area but that would be normal elsewhere in the body. This phenomenon is referred to as *metaplasia.* For example, when the lining of the uterine cervix is chronically irritated, portions of the columnar epithelium are replaced by an epidermis-like squamous epithelium (Fig. 8-1). Presumably, this "squamous metaplasia" is adaptive; that is, the squamous epithelium is more resistant to irritation than the original epithelium. The process of metaplasia seems to be under tight control; that is, the "new" type of differentiation is regular as well as adaptive. Metaplasia is potentially reversible, so if the cause of the original change can be eliminated, the stem cells once again will differentiate to form the specialized types of cells usually found in that locale.

Dysplasia

Dysplasia is an abnormality in the differentiation of proliferating cells, resulting in an abnormal degree of variation in the size, shape, and appearance of the cells and a disturbance in the usual arrangement of those cells (Fig. 8-2). In dysplasia there is a loss of control over the af-

fected cell population. Minor degrees of dysplasia are potentially reversible if the irritant stimulus can be reversed. However, in most instances the stimulus leading to dysplasia cannot be identified and the changes may become progressively more severe, terminating eventually in the development of malignant disease. In the uterine cervix, dysplasia is common and its natural history has been extensively studied. In this location, dysplasia is termed *cervical intraepithelial neoplasia* (CIN). Dysplasia may progress from mild to moderate to severe grades (CIN I to CIN II or III), with severe dysplasia actually representing preinvasive cancer. Destruction of foci of CIN can prevent the development of frankly invasive cancer.

NEOPLASIA

A *neoplasm,* literally a "new growth," is an abnormal mass of proliferating cells. The cells of a neoplasm are derived from previously normal cells, but in undergoing neoplastic change, they acquire a certain degree of autonomy. Neoplastic cells grow at a rate that is uncoordinated with the needs of the host and function quite independently of the usual homeostatic controls. The growth of neoplastic cells is usually progressive; that is, it does not reach equilibrium but results in an ever-increasing mass of cells having the same properties. A neoplasm serves no beneficial adaptive purpose and is often harmful. Finally, because of the autonomous character of neoplastic cells, even if the stimulus that caused the neoplasm is withdrawn, the neoplasm will continue to grow progressively.

The term *tumor* is more or less synonymous with the term *neoplasm.* Originally, tumor meant simply swelling or lump, and occasionally the phrase "true tumor" is used to differentiate a neoplasm from some other sort of lump. Neoplasms are distinguished by their behavior; some are benign, whereas others are malignant. *Cancer* is a general term referring to any malignant neoplasm, and many tumors or neoplasms are noncancerous.

CHARACTERISTICS OF NEOPLASMS

Benign Neoplasms

A *benign* (i.e., noncancerous) neoplasm is a strictly local affair. The proliferating cells that constitute the neoplasm tend to be quite cohesive, so that as the mass of neoplastic cells grows, there is centrifugal expansion of the mass with a fairly well-defined border. Because the proliferating cells do not fall away from each other, the edges of the neoplasm tend to move outward more or less smoothly, pushing adjacent tissue away in the process. In so doing, benign neoplasms may acquire a capsule of compressed connective tissue that separates them from their surroundings. Above all, as indicated in Fig. 8-3, *A,* the benign neoplasm does not spread to a distant site. The rate of growth of benign neoplasms is often rather leisurely, and some seem to plateau and remain at a more or less stable size for many months or years.

Malignant Neoplasms

Many characteristics of malignant neoplasms contrast sharply with those of their benign counterparts. *Malig-*

nant neoplasms generally grow more rapidly than benign ones and almost always grow in a relentlessly progressive manner if not removed. The cells of a malignant neoplasm are not very cohesive, and consequently the pattern of expansion of a malignant neoplasm is often quite irregular (Fig. 8-3, *B*). Malignant neoplasms tend to be unencapsulated, and unlike benign neoplasms, they usually are not easily separable from their surroundings. Malignant neoplasms characteristically invade their surroundings rather than simply push them aside. Malignant cells, whether in clusters, cords, or singly, seem to cut their way through adjacent tissue in a destructive fashion. The gross features of benign and malignant neoplasms are contrasted in Figs. 8-4 and 8-5.

The proliferating cells of malignant neoplasms have the ability to break away from the parent *(primary)* tumor and enter the circulation to float elsewhere. When such embolic cancer cells lodge, they are able to extravasate, continue their proliferation, and form a *secondary* tumor. A single primary focus of cancer can give rise to numerous embolic fragments that, in turn, may form dozens or even hundreds of secondary nodules at considerable distance from the primary. This process of discontinuous spread of malignant neoplasms is referred to as *metastasis,* and the daughter foci or areas of secondary growth are called *metastases* (singular, *metastasis*). Thus cancers or malignant neoplasms are distinguished from noncancerous or benign neoplasms by their ability to invade normal tissue and form metastases. A benign neoplasm has neither of these abilities.

Metastasis can occur by a variety of routes. Invasion of vascular channels gives rise to hematogenous metastasis

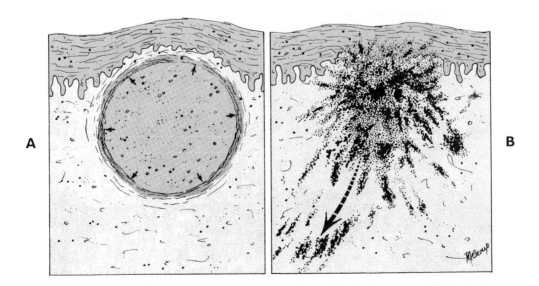

FIG. 8-3 Diagrams of benign versus malignant growth. **A,** "Typical" benign neoplasm is cohesive, centrifugally expanding, smooth bordered, and often encapsulated. Adjacent tissue is compressed. **B,** Malignant neoplasm is less cohesive, has an irregular border, and invades adjacent tissue. Malignant cells are also capable of metastasis *[dotted arrow].*

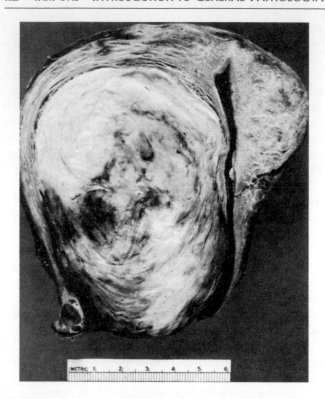

FIG. 8-4   Benign neoplasm. In this section of uterus the right half is normal. On the left is a large, benign neoplasm (leiomyoma).

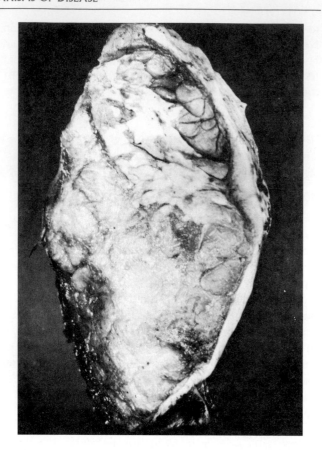

FIG. 8-5   Malignant neoplasm. In this section of breast a whitish tissue infiltrates the breast to the left of center. This is a malignant neoplasm, specifically, a carcinoma. Contrast the gross features of this with the benign neoplasm in Fig. 8-4.

in a pattern that at first may be quite predictable. If cancer cells originating from a primary location in the wall of the gastrointestinal tract enter the venous drainage of the tract, they are likely to lodge in the liver, since portal venous blood must flow through that organ before returning to the heart. On the other hand, hematogenously borne cells originating from a malignant neoplasm in the leg will flow via the vena cava to the right side of the heart and then to the lungs, where the secondary foci may grow. In an analogous manner, malignant cells may invade lymphatic channels and float with the streaming of lymph. In such instances, metastases would be expected to appear in the regional lymph node group filtering the lymph emanating from a particular organ. Thus lymphogenous metastases from a primary cancer of the breast may be anticipated in the axillary lymph nodes, and lymphogenous metastases from a primary cancer in the oral cavity would be sought in cervical lymph node groups. As cancers progress, floating malignant cells may pass through capillary beds and regional lymph nodes and circulate widely. Then the precise location of metastases depends on the "fit" between the metabolic needs of the embolic cancer cells and the environment provided by a particular tissue. Metastases can become established in virtually any organ of the body. In addition to metastasizing via blood vessels and lymphatics, cancer cells may

metastasize directly by being transported across a body cavity (e.g., peritoneal cavity) and implanting on a distant surface of that cavity. In this way a malignant neoplasm that invades through the entire thickness of the wall of an abdominal organ may "seed" the entire peritoneal cavity, producing literally hundreds of metastases by the direct route. Similarly, if malignant cells are picked up on surgical instruments in the course of a procedure, they may be implanted elsewhere in the incision, ultimately to grow into metastatic foci. Figs. 8-6 to 8-8 illustrate metastases encountered at autopsy.

In all likelihood, most cancer cells that enter the blood or lymphatic circulation or various body cavities fail to form progressively growing metastases. This is partly because the growth of such cells is inhibited by various body defenses (e.g., immunologic defenses) and also because growth conditions in an organ of secondary lodgement may not be adequate for the particular cells. Presumably on this basis, many cancers have characteristic patterns of metastases that become important in diagnosis and treatment.

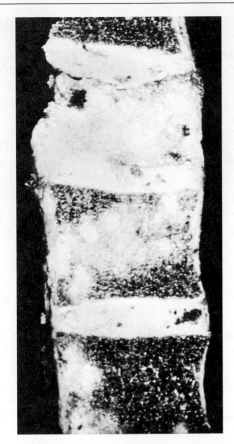

FIG. 8-6   Vertebral metastases. The whitish nodules of metastatic carcinoma within the bone grew from cells originating in the lung and spreading hematogenously.

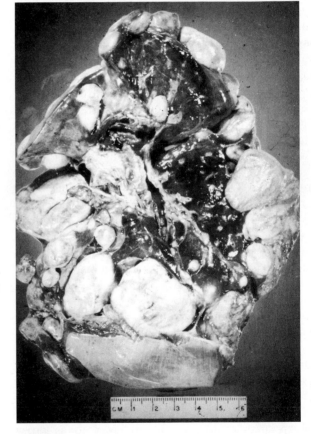

FIG. 8-7   Pulmonary metastases. This lung is extensively replaced (as was the contralateral lung) by a malignant neoplasm that originated in the kidney.

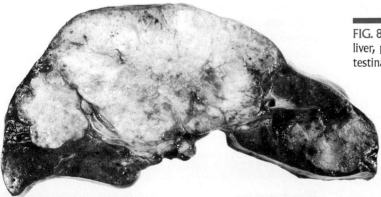

FIG. 8-8   Hepatic metastases. Many neoplasms spread to the liver, particularly, as in this case, those arising in the gastrointestinal tract. The whitish tissue is metastatic carcinoma.

NEOPLASM-HOST INTERACTION

Effects of Neoplasms on the Host

Neoplasms affect the host in a variety of ways. Because benign neoplasms do not invade or metastasize, the problems they cause are generally local. These can range from trivial to lethal. For example, a small, strictly benign tumor in the loose subcutaneous tissue of the arm might constitute a cosmetic problem but little else. At the opposite end of the spectrum, a perfectly benign tumor growing in a vital area, such as the cranial cavity, might actually kill the patient by exerting pressure on some vital part of the brain as the neoplasm expands locally. For such reasons, "benign" does not necessarily mean inconsequential.

Local problems caused by benign neoplasms might involve plugging of various body passages. A vein or a part of the gastrointestinal (GI) tract might become obstructed by a perfectly benign neoplasm impinging on it. Benign neoplasms can become ulcerated and infected, and they may give rise to significant hemorrhage. Finally, benign tumors can produce striking effects that are not mechanical but are related to the metabolic properties of the tumor cells. For example, the cells of the islets of Langerhans of the pancreas may give rise to a benign neoplasm only a few millimeters in diameter that would never produce mechanical problems. Sometimes, however, such neoplastic cells retain the function of the parent cells and produce insulin. Because neoplasms do not respond appropriately to homeostatic signals, such a neoplasm of islet cells might produce insulin inappropriately and in great excess, causing abnormally low blood sugar levels. Patients with such neoplasms might have a variety of systemic signs and symptoms of hypoglycemia.

Malignant neoplasms do everything that benign tumors do, but usually in a much more aggressive, destructive manner because of the generally faster growth rate of malignant neoplasms and their ability to invade, destroy local tissues, and spread to form distant metastases. Patients with advanced cancers often have the appearance of severe malnutrition, a state referred to as *tumor cachexia*. This condition has a complex origin, probably related to the effects of cytokines generated within the tumor or as part of the response to the tumor. Such debilitated patients with advanced cancer usually succumb to an episode of pneumonia or systemic sepsis.

Host Impact on Neoplasms

Although a key event in the life history of any neoplasm is the development of a "runaway" clone of proliferating cells that are unresponsive to homeostatic signals within the body, even highly malignant neoplasms are not completely autonomous. Neoplasms need a supply of oxygen and nutrients for the proliferating neoplastic cells, and these must be supplied by the body. Neoplastic cells are

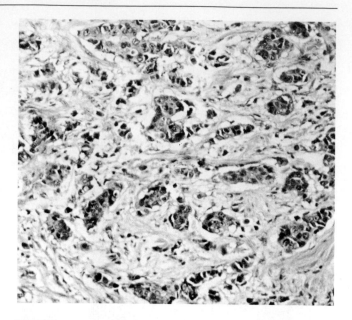

FIG. 8-9   Microscopic structure of a neoplasm. The dark clumps of cells are the actual carcinoma cells (i.e., cells of the malignant clone), while the remaining tissue is a fibrovascular stroma supplied by the host tissue.

able to evoke from the neighboring nonneoplastic tissues the formation of a vascular supply to nourish the tumor cells. Thus the supporting framework or *stroma* of neoplasms includes not only a fibrous connective tissue, but also numerous finely branching, thin-walled blood vessels (Fig. 8-9). The connective tissue cells and blood vessels are actually not part of the neoplastic clone of cells, but they represent nonneoplastic host cells whose proliferation has been stimulated by substances released from the tumor cells.

Various body processes may modulate the growth of neoplastic cells and in effect constitute antineoplastic defenses. Many neoplastic cells are sufficiently different antigenically from the corresponding normal cells that the body may mount an immunologic reaction against the neoplasm. Although such immunologic defenses exist, the current state of knowledge about them does not yet permit the routine widespread use of immunotherapeutic measures. There have been promising beneficial immunologic treatments of certain neoplasms, and the immunologic status of the host is considered in planning and conducting various modes of antineoplastic therapy and even in manipulating the immune system to suppress neoplastic growth.

STRUCTURE OF NEOPLASMS

Neoplasms are made up of proliferating neoplastic cells associated with a support system called a stroma. The organization of tumor cells and stroma varies widely among neoplasms, and the relative balance of stromal elements may lend the neoplasm distinctive characteristics. A tumor that contains an extremely dense fibrous stroma is hard grossly and is sometimes referred to as *scirrhous.* A tumor that consists predominantly of neoplastic cells with little stroma is much softer and is sometimes referred to as *medullary.*

Because neoplastic cells are derived from previously normal cell populations, they may have many characteristics of normal cell populations metabolically and microscopically. However, tumors vary in their degree of resemblance to normal tissues. If the microscopic resemblance of tumor cells to their normal ancestors is close, the neoplasm is said to be *well-differentiated* (Fig. 8-10). If the resemblance of neoplastic cells to their forebears is very slight, so that the tumor consists largely of unspecialized proliferating elements, the neoplasm is often termed *poorly differentiated, undifferentiated,* or *anaplastic.* The neoplasm in Fig. 8-9 is rather poorly differentiated. The level of differentiation may be expressed in terms of the structure of individual cells, in terms of the production of some cell products, such as mucin or keratin, or in the arrangement of neoplastic cells in relation to one another. Thus a well-differentiated neoplasm arising from a mucin-producing glandular epithelium may be composed of tumor cells that individually resemble the nonneoplastic glandular tissue, are arranged in a pattern of tubules or glands resembling the parent tissue, and may manifest mucin secretion. An anaplastic tumor arising from such as tissue might lack individual cellular resemblance or glandular arrangement and might manifest

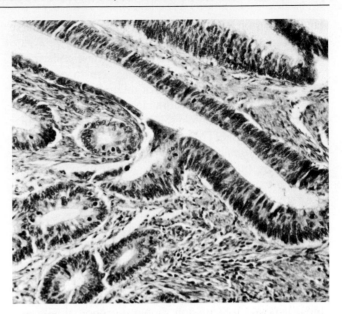

FIG. 8-10   Well-differentiated adenocarcinoma. This carcinoma of the colon resembles the parent tissue to the extent of forming glands that are easily recognizable (see Fig. 6-3); thus it is "well-differentiated." (Photomicrograph, ×200.)

no evidence of mucin secretion. In general, benign neoplasms are well differentiated; they resemble parent tissues very closely. Malignant neoplasms occupy a rather broad spectrum with regard to differentiation. Many highly aggressive destructive cancers are poorly differentiated or anaplastic microscopically, but in some in-

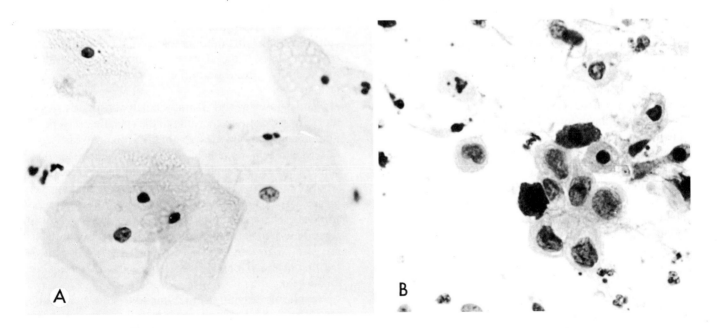

FIG. 8-11   Benign and malignant cells in vaginal cytologic smears. In **A** the cells are benign. The ratio of nucleus to cytoplasm is small, and nuclei are regular. In **B,** taken from a patient with carcinoma of the uterine cervix, the ratio of the nucleus to cytoplasm is increased, and the nuclei are irregular. These features allow the diagnosis of malignancy. (Photomicrograph, ×800.)

stances even well-differentiated neoplasms may behave in a malignant fashion.

In many malignant neoplasms, individual cells manifest morphologic abnormalities that seem to mirror the malignant behavioral potential of the cells. Many cancer cells have an altered ratio of nuclear volume to cytoplasmic volume, irregular contour of nuclei, and irregular chromatin patterns. These individual cytologic manifestations of malignancy form the basis of cytopathologic examination, that is, the examination of individual cells that have exfoliated or dropped from the surface of tissues into the secretion bathing those tissues or that have been brushed from the surface of a tumor or aspirated from a mass through a fine needle. The familiar Pap smear, named after George Papanicolaou, is a smear made from a sample of cervicovaginal mucus. Specimens for cytologic examination can often be obtained with minimal inconvenience to the patient and provide valuable diagnostic information should morphologically malignant cells be found on the smear. Fig. 8-11 illustrates benign and malignant cells seen in a cytologic smear. Even dysplastic cells (CIN) can be identified in Pap smears.

CLASSIFICATION AND NOMENCLATURE OF NEOPLASMS

A classification of neoplasms helps predict the possible or probable course of disease in a particular patient and aids in planning rational modes of therapy. The usual contemporary scheme of classification of neoplasms uses several sets of criteria. The most important is the distinction between benign and malignant biologic behavior. If a particular neoplasm has already invaded neighboring nonneoplastic tissue or has produced metastases, it is obviously malignant. However, even in the absence of such established invasion or metastasis, the pathologist can classify a neoplasm as malignant if its potential for malignant behavior can be predicted; that is, a particular neoplasm will be designated as malignant on the basis of its microscopic appearance alone if experience has shown that neoplasms of that type will invade and metastasize if not treated. Other parts of the classification scheme take into account the cell type of origin of the neoplasm and the organ of origin of the neoplasm. Years of accumulated experience have shown that a tumor with a particular appearance of cells, of a certain level of differentiation, arranged in a certain way, and originating in a certain organ will behave with a degree of predictability. This allows the health care team to plan therapy based on the knowledge of what has happened to many patients with similar neoplasms in the past.

This kind of classification of neoplasms uses a system of naming that serves as a sort of shorthand, condensing abundant information into a relatively few terms. The entire system of tumor nomenclature will not be covered at this point, but a few generalizations are provided here as a basis for further discussion. Abundant specific information is given in subsequent chapters.

Many neoplasms arise from epithelium, which includes cells covering surfaces, lining organs, and forming glands of various kinds. The root *adeno-* denotes something of glandular origin. The suffix *-oma* refers to a neoplasm (with some exceptions). Thus in the usual system of nomenclature, an adenoma is a benign neoplasm of glandular epithelial origin. Examples of such neoplasms would include adenomas of the thyroid gland, the adrenal gland, or the lining glandular epithelium within the GI tract. In the instance of neoplasms arising and projecting from lining epithelia, less specific topographic terms are sometimes used. Thus an adenoma of the colonic lining epithelium, which projects into the lumen either as a broad-based mass or hangs into the lumen on a "stem," is often called a *polyp*. Such a growth projecting into the lumen of an organ in fingerlike projections is often referred to as a *papilloma*. These topographic terms are not restricted in their use, however, so that the usual nasal polyp, for instance, is not a neoplasm at all but a polypoid fold of swollen nasal mucosa. A malignant neoplasm arising from epithelium is referred to as *carcinoma*. Various qualifying prefixes and adjectives can then be added to the name. A malignancy of glandular epithelium would be referred to as an *adenocarcinoma*, whereas a malignant neoplasm arising from a squamous epithelium would be called a *squamous cell carcinoma*. The designation of a neoplasm might also include some comment about the level of differentiation, for example, "well-differentiated, mucin-forming adenocarcinoma" or "well-differentiated, keratinizing squamous cell carcinoma." In addition, topographic descriptors may be used, such as "papillary adenocarcinoma" or "fungating (literally, mushrooming) carcinoma" for a projecting lesion.

Neoplasms derived from the supporting tissues of the body are named according to the specific tissue of origin. Thus a benign neoplasm of fibrous tissue would be termed a *fibroma,* a benign neoplasm of bone would be called an *osteoma,* and a benign neoplasm of cartilage would be referred to as a *chondroma.* A malignant neoplasm derived from supporting tissue is referred to as a *sarcoma.* The specific tissue of origin is prefixed to this term. Thus a malignant neoplasm arising from fibrous tissue is a *fibrosarcoma,* one arising from bone is an *osteosarcoma,* and one arising from cartilage is a *chondrosarcoma.*

Neoplasms arising from lymphoid tissue are called *lymphomas.* Such neoplasms generally behave in a malignant manner, so that the term lymphoma generally is synonymous with malignant lymphoma. Lymphomas may arise from lymphoid tissue anywhere in the body, that is, not only from lymph nodes and spleen, but also

▶ TABLE 8-1   Classification of Neoplasms

Cell or Tissue of Origin	Benign	Malignant
Epithelium		
Stratified, squamous	Squamous papilloma	Squamous cell carcinoma (epidermoid carcinoma)
Glandular (lining fluid-filled spaces)	Adenoma (cystadenoma)	Adenocarcinoma (cystadenocarcinoma)
Melanocytes	Nevus	Melanoma
Connective tissue		
Fibrous	Fibroma	Fibrosarcoma
Adipose	Lipoma	Liposarcoma
Cartilage	Chondroma	Chondrosarcoma
Bone	Osteoma	Osteosarcoma
Muscle		
Smooth	Leiomyoma	Leiomyosarcoma
Striated	Rhabdomyoma	Rhabdomyosarcoma
Endothelium		
Blood vessel	Hemangioma	Hemangiosarcoma
Lymphatic	Lymphangioma	Lymphangiosarcoma
Nervous tissue		
Nerve sheath	Neurofibroma	Neurofibrosarcoma
Glial cells	—	Glioma, glioblastoma
Meninges	Meningioma	
Lymphoid tissue/bone marrow	—	
Hematopoietic lymphoid tissue	—	
Lymphoid tissue	—	Lymphoma, Hodgkin's disease
	Lymphocytic leukemia	
		Plasmacytoma (multiple myeloma)
Bone marrow	—	Granulocytic (myelogenous, monocytic, erythroleukemia, polycythemia rubra vera)
Germinal tissue	Teratoma	Malignant teratoma, teratocarcinoma, seminoma, embryonal carcinoma

from lymphoid cells in virtually any organ. Lymphomas may involve the bone marrow extensively, and in many patients the lymphoma cells circulate in the blood in large numbers, giving rise to leukemia. *Leukemia* literally means "white blood" and pertains not only to lymphoid malignancy, but also to malignancy of bone marrow cells with circulating malignant elements. The nomenclature of leukemias and lymphomas is discussed more fully in Part Three.

Many special names are used for neoplasms arising in specific sites and from particular specialized tissues. Thus gliomas arise from glial supportive cells in the central nervous system (CNS), mesotheliomas arise from the lining cells of body cavities, retinoblastomas arise within the eye, and so forth. Table 8-1 provides a simplified summary of the classification of neoplasms.

CARCINOGENESIS

As indicated earlier, cancer cells are derived from previously normal cells, with the transformation accomplished through a series of events that ultimately confers new behavioral properties on the cells of the affected population. This newly acquired behavior could be described as "antisocial" with regard to other cells of the body. Cancer cells disobey the usual territorial rules and grow in inappropriate locations. They do not respond to the usual restraints on the size of the cell populations or their rate of growth. Many of these important abnormalities of cancer cells seem to be related to cell membrane functions. The membrane of the cell is responsible for receiving regulatory signals from other nearby cells and from distant points in the body. It appears that genes and proteins that are involved in *signal transduction* (conversion of an extracellular signal into a series of intracellular events) are also involved in the transformation of normal into malignant cells.

Carcinogenesis appears to involve genetic changes in the affected cells, especially those involving regulatory genes normally associated with growth promotion and growth inhibition. Genes that promote normal growth of cells, referred to as *proto-oncogenes,* may be converted to cancer-causing genes, or *oncogenes.* This can occur by actual mutation in one or more genes or by altered expression of these genes. Similarly, some genes that normally regulate growth and potentially act as *tumor suppressors*. Mutations in such genes, in effect, allow unbridled cell proliferation. Current evidence suggests that most cancers involve at least several gene alterations, with activation of multiple oncogenes and loss of a number of suppressor genes. Once a single cell has acquired the genetic changes, proliferation of that cell and its progeny produces an expanding clone of similarly endowed cells, which then constitute the tumor.

Many different types of agents can produce the genetic changes necessary for malignant transformation. Ultraviolet radiation (as in sunlight) can produce errors in deoxyribonucleic acid (DNA) replication and lead to skin cancer (see Chapter 81). Ionizing radiation (gamma rays, x-rays, atomic particles) is associated with a variety of types of cancer. Many chemicals, most of which are mutagenic, can initiate or promote the chain of events leading to the formation of cancer. Aromatic hydrocarbons and amines, nitrosamines, and azo dyes are recognized carcinogens, as are a number of naturally occurring substances (e.g., aflatoxin, which is derived from a common fungus). Certain viruses have been recognized as carcinogenic in animals, and there is no longer any doubt that the same is true for humans.

Although the changes necessary for carcinogenesis may occur in somatic cells, it is becoming evident that some genetic abnormalities may actually be inherited, yielding a predisposition for the development of a tumor in a given family. Thus cancers of the breast "run" or are evident in some families and cancer of the colon runs in others. With the advent of molecular methods of analysis, the specific genes and gene products involved in these familial cancer syndromes are being identified in increasing numbers. Therefore persons at higher-than-normal risk of developing various tumors can be identified and appropriate preventive or intervention strategies can be designed and implemented.

Although it is important to emphasize the role of genetic alteration in carcinogenesis, it is evident that the wide variations in the incidence of different tumors reflect the powerful influence of environmental factors. The list of known environmental carcinogens is very diverse, ranging from sunlight, to alcohol, to tobacco smoke, and to sexually transmitted human papillomaviruses. One cannot hope to lead a life completely free of risk, but the previous examples point the way to meaningful risk reduction through relatively straightforward behavioral modifications.

CLINICAL ASPECTS OF NEOPLASIA

The variety of signs and symptoms that can be produced by neoplasms is virtually endless. Therefore the possibility of neoplasm could be considered with many different modes of patient presentation. Fig. 8-12 provides information about the incidence of various kinds of cancers in different organs in the two genders. A clue of particular value is the *persistence* (if not progression) of a given manifestation, for example, a *sore that does not heal* or *chronic hoarseness*. The age of the patient must also be

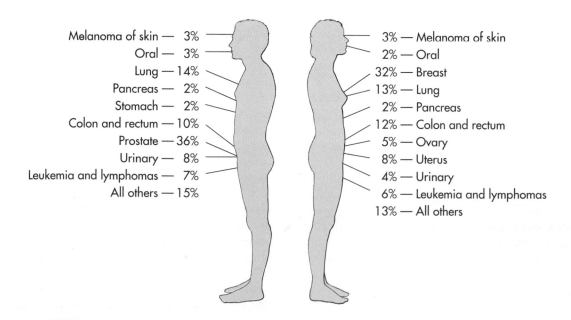

Melanoma of skin — 3%
Oral — 3%
Lung — 14%
Pancreas — 2%
Stomach — 2%
Colon and rectum — 10%
Prostate — 36%
Urinary — 8%
Leukemia and lymphomas — 7%
All others — 15%

3% — Melanoma of skin
2% — Oral
32% — Breast
13% — Lung
2% — Pancreas
12% — Colon and rectum
5% — Ovary
8% — Uterus
4% — Urinary
6% — Leukemia and lymphomas
13% — All others

FIG. 8-12   Estimated new cancer cases, United States, percent distribution of sites by gender for 1995. Statistics do not include basal and squamous cell skin cancers and in situ carcinomas except for the bladder. [From Wingo P, Tong T, Bolden S: *Ca J Clin* 45[8]:11, 1995. Reproduced with permission from the American Cancer Society, Michigan Division.]

considered. For example, hoarseness in a young child suggests a different list of possibilities (and approaches) than the same sign would in a 60-year-old smoker. An iron deficiency anemia in an elderly patient might be associated with a chronically bleeding colonic cancer, whereas the same finding in a teenage girl may be explained by a nutritionally inadequate diet combined with the onset of menstrual blood loss.

Whether the index of suspicion is based on circumstances or on physical findings, the presence of the neoplasm must be definitively confirmed, because nonneoplastic conditions can also produce identical manifestations. In a few instances, certain blood tests may provide additional circumstantial evidence of a particular neoplasm. Ultimately, a space-occupying mass must be identified and delineated, whether by simple palpation during physical examination or by radiography, ultrasonography, radionuclide scanning, or any of several endoscopic procedures for direct visualization of internal structures. A final diagnostic step involves morphologic confirmation by the pathologist based on microscopic examination of the tissue in question. The diagnostic biopsy may be curative, such as when the questionable lump is totally excised and found to be benign. In other cases a wedge biopsy might be performed, a tiny core of tissue might be removed from the mass with a special biopsy needle, or a small amount of fluid containing neoplastic cells might be aspirated by needle from the mass.

A cytologic smear made from some fluid or secretion bathing the area in question may also yield valuable diagnostic information. A cytologic examination indicating the presence of cancer cells is usually confirmed by biopsy before treatment is undertaken. The Pap smear may contain cancer cells from an area not visible by ordinary examinations (e.g., the upper endocervical canal) and thereby may direct attention to that precise area. Pap smears also provide samples from large numbers of individuals on a routine basis even when signs and symptoms of abnormality may not have been noted. Obviously, routine biopsy of asymptomatic people is not feasible; however, sampling cervicovaginal mucus is an innocuous procedure that may yield some "positives," leading to the diagnosis of dysplasia or possibly of cancer in an early stage.

Microscopic examination of the tissue is essential in distinguishing neoplastic from nonneoplastic and malignant from benign conditions, and it has additional value in planning therapy. Precise identification of a cancer allows some important general predictions of its likely behavior, for instance, whether a particular neoplasm might have an extremely high probability of metastases in regional lymph nodes, lungs, or other sites, even in the absence of clinical evidence. In this situation, simple excision of the primary lesion with no additional therapy generally would not be successful. Predictions about certain malignant neoplasms may be more accurate if they take into account the *histologic grade* of the neoplasm, which

is based on the microscopic appearance, arrangement, and degree of differentiation of the cancer cells (i.e., the extent to which they resemble normal cells), features that may correlate with the behavioral aggressiveness of the tumor.

These predictions are general and provide correspondingly broad guidelines for therapy. However, decisions regarding treatment can be refined by determining the clinical stage of the cancer in the patient. *Staging* is based on an estimate of the progression of the neoplasm within the patient's body. A patient with a small, limited primary tumor would be at an earlier clinical stage and less likely to have metastases in local lymph nodes than in a patient with a larger, more deeply invasive tumor of the same type. A patient with established lymph nodal metastases would be at a more advanced stage than one without and would be more likely to have occult distant metastases. A patient with overtly evident distant metastases would, of course, be in an extremely advanced stage of the disease. These considerations have led to extensive use of the *TNM system* of staging. In this system, *T* refers to the primary tumor, and a T1 lesion would be smaller than a T4 lesion. *N* is the status of regional lymph nodes, with N0 designating absence of nodal metastases and N1, N2, or N3 indicating increasing metastatic involvement. *M* refers to distant metastasis, with appropriate adscripts. The precise definition of T, N, and M varies for different cancers, but the system provides a widely applicable shorthand for tumor staging.

Clinical staging not only helps determine the prognosis but also helps to plan rational therapy, preferably a step ahead of the neoplasm. The patient in a late stage of disease requires an entirely different treatment regimen than a patient in an early stage, and the regimen may have risks and morbidity that render it undesirable unless it is clearly indicated. Because different types of neoplasms have strikingly different natural histories, the staging schemes and methods vary accordingly. For example, a patient with cervical carcinoma will be staged differently than a patient with lymphoma in the neck. Staging may involve physical examination, various radiologic techniques, or even surgical biopsy of certain tissues distant from the primary.

Several different modalities of cancer treatment may be employed simultaneously or serially. Each modality attempts to eradicate the cancerous tissue with an acceptable degree of loss or damage to normal tissues.

The oldest and best known treatment is *surgical removal* of the cancerous tissue. This is extremely effective if excision of the primary tumor, along with a margin of normal tissues and perhaps the regional lymph nodes, eliminates all cancer cells from the body (or, some would claim, reduces the total body load of cancer cells to the point where host defenses can eliminate the remainder). However, many tumors are "inoperable." Sometimes this is because the primary cannot be totally excised without sacrificing essential local structures. In other cases, distant metastases may be evident; therefore removal of the primary tumor would not eradicate all the neoplasm. Also, the natural history of some diseases (e.g., leukemia) renders surgery inappropriate at any stage.

Another mode of treatment is *radiotherapy,* which is the application of ionizing radiation to the neoplasm. Because the lethal effect of radiation is greater on proliferating, poorly differentiated cancer cells than on adjacent normal cells, the normal tissues may be injured to a tolerable, reparable degree, whereas the cancer cells are eliminated. In a favorable situation a cure can be effected without sacrificing some vital structure. This mode of therapy also has limitations. Some tumors are radioresistant, being no more sensitive to the effects of irradiation than the surrounding normal cells. Widespread tumors cannot be treated by radiotherapy, since irradiation of broad areas of the body would risk unacceptable morbidity or could be lethal.

A rapidly evolving treatment modality is *chemotherapy,* which exposes proliferating cancer cells and normal cells to a variety of cytotoxic agents. Widely disseminated cancer cells beyond the confines of surgical or radiation therapy might be eliminated by a systemically administered drug whose toxic effects on normal cells are low enough to be acceptable. However, various cancers are sensitive to different drugs or combinations of drugs, and no one regimen is applicable to all tumors. Unfortunately, chemotherapy is often limited by the toxicity of the agents for rapidly proliferating normal cells, such as the hematopoietic cells or the lining epithelial cells of the bone marrow or the GI tract. However, reports are continually emerging of previously uncontrollable neoplasms proving to be sensitive to new chemotherapeutic approaches.

Immunotherapy is also being tried in the treatment of cancers. Cancer cells often differ antigenically from normal cells to a degree that immunologic reactions may be mounted against them. Such reactions are demonstrable in laboratory situations but are not yet controllable at a practical clinical level. However, therapeutic measures aimed at immunologic stimulation of the cancer patient have shown promise in some instances.

The approach to the cancer patient is not limited to the use of a single treatment modality, but it involves a team approach tailored to the unique needs of the individual with a particular neoplasm at a given clinical stage. Even if a neoplasm is deemed "incurable," several modes of therapy may provide dramatic palliation, significantly prolonging the span of comfortable, useful life for the cancer patient.

? QUESTIONS

▼ *Match the term in column A with its proper description in column B.*

Column A	Column B
1. _____ Aplasia	a. Abnormal degree of variation in size, shape, and appearance of the cells with an abnormal arrangement of cells
2. _____ Hyperplasia	b. Lack of differentiation or specialization in a group of neoplastic cells; representation as a mass of pleomorphic primitive cells
3. _____ Hypertrophy	c. Failure of structure to grow in the course of organogenesis
4. _____ Metaplasia	d. Increase in the absolute number of cells, leading to an increase in the size of that tissue or organ
5. _____ Dysplasia	e. Differentiation of dividing cells into types of cells not ordinarily found in the area, but types of cells that would be perfectly reasonable elsewhere
6. _____ Neoplasia	f. Increase in size of existing cells without an increase in their number
7. _____ Anaplasia	g. Formation of an abnormal mass of proliferating cells, possessing a significant degree of autonomy

▼ *Circle the letter preceding each item below that correctly answers the question or completes the statement. More than one answer may be correct.*

8. Which of the following are types of abnormal development?
   a. Hyperplasia   c. Aplasia
   b. Agenesis   d. Atrophy

9. Failure to reach definitive or adult size is:
   a. Atrophy
   b. Hypoplasia
   c. Both a and b
   d. Neither a nor b

10. The pressure of an enlarged prostate causes urethral obstruction. The resultant thickening of the bladder wall muscle is referred to as:
    a. Hypertrophy
    b. Hypoplasia
    c. Atrophy
    d. Neoplasia

11. A callus formed on the hand of a gardener from handling a hoe is an example of:
    a. Dysplasia   c. Metaplasia
    b. Hyperplasia   d. Neoplasia

12. Neoplasia differs from all other pathologic processes in that it:
    a. Involves proliferation of the cells of affected tissues
    b. Is relatively autonomous of the body's controls
    c. Is detrimental to the host
    d. May affect the host's nutritional state adversely

13. Malignant neoplasms differ from benign neoplasms in that malignant neoplasms:
    a. Have an infiltrative pattern of growth
    b. Are encapsulated
    c. Give rise to metastases
    d. Compress adjacent tissue

14. A carcinoma of the stomach would be most likely to produce its earliest metastases in:
    a. Bone

QUESTIONS—cont'd

b. Lung
c. Liver
d. Kidney

15. An osteosarcoma of the femur would be most likely to produce its earliest metastases in the:
   a. Kidney
   b. Liver
   c. Brain
   d. Lung

16. A malignant neoplasm of glandular epithelial origin would be termed a(n):
   a. Adenoma
   b. Myoma
   c. Adenocarcinoma
   d. Chondroma

17. A malignant neoplasm arising in fibrous tissue (mesenchymal origin) would be termed a:
   a. Fibroma
   b. Carcinoma
   c. Fibrocarcinoma
   d. Fibrosarcoma

18. A malignant neoplasm arising from the glial supportive cells in the central nervous system would be called a:
   a. Neurofibrosarcoma
   b. Neuroma
   c. Neurofibroma
   d. Glioblastoma

19. A benign neoplasm of fibrous tissue would be called a(n):
   a. Fibroma
   b. Osteoma
   c. Chrondroma
   d. Fibrosarcoma

20. Genes that promote normal growth of cells are:
   a. Oncogenes

b. Proto-oncogenes
c. Lymphokines
d. Interferon

▼ *Circle T if the statement is true and F if it is false. Correct any false statements.*

21. T F Genes and proteins involved in signal transduction are also responsible for the transformation of normal into malignant cells.

22. T F Neoplastic cells are sufficiently different antigenically from the normal host cells that the body may mount an immunologic reaction against the neoplasm.

23. T F A tumor that contains dense fibrous stroma and hard growth is referred to as a medullary tumor.

24. T F Benign neoplasms tend to be well differentiated; that is, they closely resemble parent tissues.

25. T F Evidence indicates that most cancers involve several gene mutations, with activation of multiple oncogenes and loss of suppressor genes.

26. T F A malignant neoplasm of the smooth muscles is classified as a rhadomyosarcoma.

27. T F A Papanicolau smear is a cytologic diagnostic preparation made from a sample of cervicovaginal mucus.

▼ *Fill in the blanks with the correct words.*

28. Some causes of atrophy are _____, _____, and _____ .

29. Two dangerous properties of malignant neoplasms that distinguish them from benign neoplasms are _____ and _____ .

▼ *Answer the following on a separate sheet of paper.*

30. List at least three pathways by which malignant neoplasms disseminate through the body.

31. How do neoplasms (benign and malignant) affect the host?

32. What are the criteria used in the classification of neoplasms?

33. Explain the importance of cervical intraepithelial neoplasia (CIN) with regard to severe grades of dysplasia (CIN II or III).

34. What is the significance of the condition referred to as tumor cachexia?

35. What is happening at a cellular level during the "transformation" or carcinogenesis?

36. List at least four types of agents that can produce genetic changes that are necessary for malignant transformation.

37. In terms of cellular control mechanism, explain the "phenotypic" expression of malignancy in cells.

38. What is the TNM system for tumor staging?

39. Why is it important to identify the genetic abnormalities that may be inherited in relation to the development of neoplasia in families?

40. What are the means and criteria used to establish the diagnosis and to determine the therapeutic modalities for treatment of neoplasia?

BIBLIOGRAPHY ▼ PART 1

Abbas AK, Lichtman AH, Pober JS: *Cellular and molecular immunology,* Philadelphia, 1994, Saunders.

Bellanti JA: *Immunology and medicine,* Philadelphia, 1985, Saunders.

Berg P, Singer M: *Dealing with genes, the language of heredity,* Mill Valley, Calif, 1992, University Science Books.

Catin RS, Kumer V, Robbins SL: *Robbins pathologic basis of disease,* ed 5, Philadelphia, 1994, Saunders.

Cotton GH: Current methods of mutation detection, *Mutation Res* 285:125-144, 1993.

DeVita VT Jr, Hellman S, Rosenberg SA: *Cancer: principles and practice of oncology,* ed 4, Philadelphia, 1993, Lippincott.

Eisenbarth GS, Bellgrau D: Autoimmunity, *Sci Am Sci Med* 1(2):38-47, 1994.

Frohlich EE, editors: *Pathophysiology: altered regulatory mechanisms in disease,* Philadelphia, 1983, Lippincott.

Griffiths AJF et al: *An introduction to genetic analysis,* ed 5, New York, 1993, Freeman.

Hartl DL: *Genetics,* ed 3, Boston, 1994, Jones & Bartlett.

Healy DP, Robertson WL: *Immune system function and immune-based therapy: a primer for the practicing pharmacist,* Module A and B, No 679-105-92-023/024, Columbus, Ohio, 1992, Council of Ohio Colleges of Pharmacy.

Henry JD: *Clinical diagnosis and management by laboratory methods,* ed 18, Philadelphia, 1989, Saunders.

Human genetic disorders, *J NIH Res* 6:115-134, 1994.

Janeway CA: How the immune system recognizes invaders, *Sci Am* 269(3):22-29, 1993.

Johnson HM, Russell JK, Pontzer C: Superantigens in human disease, *Sci Am* 266(4):92-101, 1992.

Klug WS, Cummings MR: *Concepts of genetics,* ed 4, New York, 1994, Macmillan.

Leder P, Clayton DA, Rubenstein E: *Introduction to molecular medicine,* New York, 1992, Scientific American.

Levinson W, Jawetz E: *Medical microbiology and immunology,* ed 3, East Norwalk, Conn, 1993, Appleton & Lange.

Levinson WWE, Jawetz D: *Medical microbiology and immunology,* East Norwalk, Conn, 1994, Appleton & Lange.

Luciano D, Vander A, Sherman J: *Human anatomy and physiology: structure and function,* ed 2, New York, 1983, McGraw-Hill.

Marrack P, Kappler JW: How the immune system recognizes the body, *Sci Am* 269(3):80-89, 1993.

Mudge-Grout CL: *Immunologic disorders,* St Louis, 1993, Mosby.

Munro JM, Cotran RS: The pathogenesis of atherosclerosis: pathogenesis and inflammation, *Lab Invest* 58:249-261, 1988.

Peacock EE: *Wound repair,* ed 3, Philadelphia, 1984, Saunders.

Rabbitts H: Chromosomal translocations in human cancer, *Nature* 372:143-149, 1994.

Roitt IM, Brostoff J, Male DK: *Immunology,* ed 3, St Louis, 1993, Mosby.

Rubin E, Farber JL, editors: *Pathology,* ed 3, Philadelphia, 1993, Lippincott.

Ruddon RW: *Cancer biology,* ed 3, New York, 1988, Oxford University Press.

Russell PJ: *Fundamentals of genetics,* New York, 1994, Harper Collins.

von Boehmer H, Kisielow P: How the immune system learns about self, *Sci Am* 265(4):74-81, 1991.

Wallace DC: Diseases of the mitochondrial DNA, *Annu Rev Biochem* 61:1175-1212, 1992.

Weissman IL, Cooper MD: How the immune system develops, *Sci Am* 269(3):64-71, 1993.

Wingo P, Tong T, Bolden S: Cancer statistics, 1995, *Ca J Clin* 45(8):8-11, 1995.

Wyngaarden JB, Smith LH: *Cecil textbook of medicine,* ed 19, Philadelphia, 1991, Saunders.

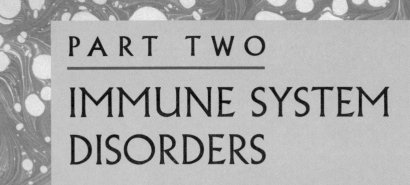

PART TWO
IMMUNE SYSTEM DISORDERS

Unfavorable effects of immune processes underlie much human disease and may impair the function of any major organ system. In addition, characteristic changes in immune reactants that provide essential diagnostic clues *accompany* many conditions as effects or parallel events. Normal antibody and cell-mediated responses involve a series of steps, each modulated by groups of specific cells. Defects in these control processes may cause excessive or inappropriate immune reactions. Less often, disease results when normally protective immediate and delayed hypersensitivity mechanisms become impaired or fail to develop properly. Various immunologic states may be viewed as a *balance* between the pathogenic effects of two groups of factors: potentially harmful foreign agents of disease (e.g., microorganisms) and the body's defensive responses, which may cause incidental tissue damage or disordered function.

Protective immunity and allergic diseases share common processes of tissue response to substances recognized as "foreign." Immune mechanisms provide essential defense against invasion by injurious organisms and the emergence of malignant tumors, functions that have ensured their retention throughout vertebrate evolution. However, these same processes may be activated by relatively innocuous extrinsic agents and occasionally may focus the reaction on host tissue components. In these circumstances the *net* effects of exposure and host response are unfavorable; patterns of overt illness that result are recognized as immunologic diseases. These conditions are diverse and range from trivial, chronic disorders of the skin or mucous membranes to catastrophic events that may be fatal within seconds. The tissue processes responsible and their relationship to a practical classification of human immunologic disorders are described in Chapter 5. Because these diseases are determined by host reactivity as well as by the type and strength of antigenic exposure, regional differences in their prevalence are prominent. Overall, however, these disorders are remarkably common and their impact on human comfort and productivity is evident universally. ▼

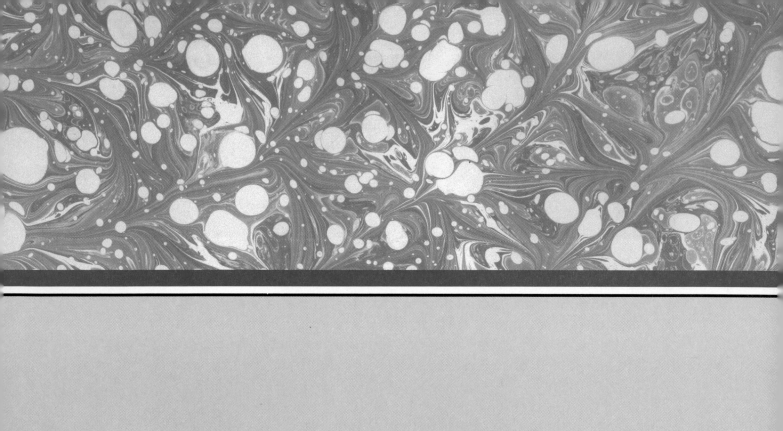

CHAPTER 9

Familiar Allergic Disorders

ANAPHYLAXIS AND THE ATOPIC DISEASES

WILLIAM R. SOLOMON

Clinical reactions of immediate or delayed hypersensitivity can result when prior contact with a specific, chemically characterizable entity ("antigen") has sensitized the individual to that particular agent. Reexposure to the agent may cause sensitized cells, as well as one or more types of immunoglobulins, to react in a specific "defensive" response. Clinical hypersensitivity reactions in humans often show more than one immunologic process, each with its specific amplification system(s). Such complexity seems sensible when the "invader" is antigenically complex (e.g., a microorganism), but the reaction also can be elicited by single, defined proteins (see Chapter 5).

After exposure to a *single* antigen, humoral (antibody-dependent) and cell-mediated immune responses may develop together or separately. The size and form of the antigen and the route of exposure, as well as the respondent's age, health, and prior experience with that sensitizer, will affect the responding immunoglobulin (Ig) class(es). For example, first exposure to an injected agent (e.g., a vaccine) usually elicits an IgM response that, in days, changes to IgG synthesis. Reexposure typically elicits only IgG production. Very low antigen does often favor IgE synthesis, whereas mucosal exposure promotes an IgA response, often localized to the challenged organ. A single antigen-antibody interaction can also provoke different effects, depending on the circumstances in which it is observed. Human IgG molecules specific for an antigen may separate the antigen from solution, agglutinate insoluble particles coated with the antigen, or activate complement proteins after interacting with the antigen in either form. The effects depend largely on antigen-antibody concentrations, the relative proportions of these reactants, and the presence of additional components, which often serve as "indicators" in laboratory tests. When such interactions occur in vivo, their effects reflect similar factors as well as local tissue responses to the primary antigen-antibody reaction and to activation of secondary amplification mechanisms (see also Chapter 5).

Antigen-binding specificity is directed by paired combining sites on the antibody fragment (Fab) portions of immunoglobulin molecules. Events that follow binding are directed by the crystallizable fragment (Fc fragment) portion of antibodies, which is shared by immunoglobulins of a defined class (isotype). Receptors on phagocytic cells may recognize this region, facilitating adhesion and removal of antigen-antibody complexes and other particles bearing surface-bound immunoglobulins. Activation of the "classic" complement pathway (see Fig. 5-13) also involves the Fc region; as a result, target cell lysis, leukocyte attraction, and release of permeability-enhancing factors may be generated. In addition, the class-specific properties of immunoglobulins that determine their tissue localization and specificity as antigens (to "antiimmunoglobulin" antibodies) are expressed on the Fc region.

Although levels of IgE normally are the lowest of the five antibody classes, these molecules play a disproportionately major role in human allergic* responses. IgE molecules readily bind to surface receptors of tissue mast

---

*The term *allergy* was proposed by von Pirquet in 1906 to denote all instances of acquired altered reactivity that promote "supersensitivity." Current usage equates allergy with common, clinically evident responses of immediate or delayed hypersensitivity.

TABLE 9-1 Some Mediators of Inflammation Released by Human Mast Cells and Basophils

Mediator*	Chemical Characteristics	Biologic Activity
Histamine	Simple amine; mol wt 111	Contracts visceral smooth muscle; increases permeability of capillaries; increases respiratory mucous gland activity; produces sensation of itching
Prostaglandin D	mol wt 352	Contracts smooth muscle; increases mediator release by basophils
Platelet-activating factor (PAF)	Phospholipid(s?), mol wt 500-550	Aggregates and degranulates platelets; contracts some smooth muscle; produces wheal and flare skin responses; variably attracts neutrophils
Leukotrienes (C, D, and E)†	Acid lipids	Causes prolonged visceral smooth muscle spasm; dilates and increases permeability of venules
Prostaglandin-generating factor of anaphylaxis	Simple peptide; mol wt 1450	Stimulates production of prostaglandins, leukotrienes, and related products of arachidonic acid
Neutral proteases (including tryptase, chymase, and carboxypeptidase)	Small protein enzymes; mol wt <50,000	Cleaves tissue components, such as collagen and complement factors; may generate kinins
Acid hydrolases (including beta-glucuronidase and arylsulfatase)	Fairly large proteins	Cleaves sugars from complex carbohydrates and glycoproteins
Superoxide dismutase	Enzymatic protein	Converts superoxide (O_2^-) to H_2O_2
Heparin	Peptide chain bearing long-chain sulfated amino sugars	Anticoagulant; modulates activities of other mediators
Eosinophil chemotactic factor of anaphylaxis (ECF-A)	Pair of acidic tetrapeptides	Attracts eosinophils selectively
Neutrophil chemotactic factor (NCF-A)	Large protein; mol wt >500,000	Causes directed migration of neutrophils
Basophil kallikrein‡	Not defined	Causes formation of bradykinin

*Serotonin is present in human platelets and in the mast cells of other species.

†Formerly called SRS-A; many additional arachidonic acid products of activated mast cells (including thromboxanes and prostacycline) may contribute to tissue inflammation.

‡Released from basophils, but not as yet described from mast cells.

cells and blood basophils. As a result, bound IgE is concentrated primarily in the respiratory and gastrointestinal (GI) tracts as well as in the circulating blood and skin. When adjacent IgE molecules combine with groupings of a multiply reactive antigen, a series of events (Fig. 9-1) can occur with the cell liberating tissue-reactive "mediator" substances, including histamine, leukotrienes (formerly termed SRS-A), and eosinophil chemotactic factor(s) of anaphylaxis (ECF-A); substances that attract neutrophils and lead to the formation of kinins also have been described. Additional products may include an anticoagulant (heparin), proteolytic enzymes (tryptase and chymase), and a highly reactive oxygen radical (superoxide) as well as prostaglandins and related arachidonic acid products. Individual characteristics of some of these agents are summarized in Table 9-1; their combined effects promote dilation and hyperpermeability of small blood vessels (principally venules), spasm of the walls of hollow viscera, and increased secretion by mucous membranes. Heightened venule permeability should lower the circulating blood volume and the arterial pressure as well

as promote collections of fluid outside of vessels. In fact, these effects are all easily observed in clinically significant human responses involving IgE.

As Fig. 9-1 suggests, the release of mediator substances from mast cell granules is modulated by cellular levels of agents, especially cyclic nucleotides, with cyclic adenosine monophosphate (AMP) depressing and guanosine monophosphate (GMP) facilitating secretion. Both cholinergic and alpha-adrenergic stimuli seem to increase GMP, whereas beta-adrenergic agents promote adenylate cyclase activity and augment AMP. Cell activation triggered by IgE begins within seconds, releasing mediators such as histamine that are preformed and stored. Minutes later, newly synthesized agents such as leukotrienes appear. Clinically, the resulting "immediate" reactions reach peak intensity in 10 to 20 minutes and then subside. In addition, "late" IgE-dependent reactions may follow, 4 to 8 hours after the eliciting antigen was introduced. Reappearance of several mediators characterizes late responses, which probably reflect secretion by cells newly attracted to the reaction site.

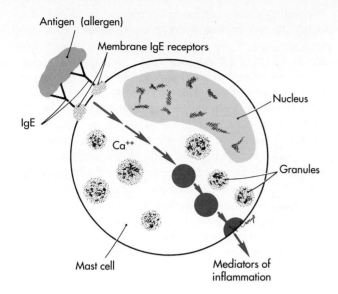

FIG. 9-1 Mast cell secretion provoked by bridging of adjacent IgE molecules by multivalent antigen or allergen. The process is calcium dependent and proceeds after membrane IgE receptors are brought together. The secretion process is affected by levels of cyclic nucleotides (cyclic AMP and GMP) within the mast cell (see Fig. 10-7). Many drugs can affect mast cell activity by their effects on cyclic nucleotides, although separate membrane receptors also occur for these and other substances.

TYPE I DISORDERS

Anaphylaxis

Acute systemic reactions, often fatal, were first recognized in several species during immunization experiments with foreign toxins. In many animals, sensitization did not confer protection; rather, when the toxin was readministered, there was prompt development of shock, airway obstruction, and/or visceral congestion in species-specific patterns. The term anaphylaxis (*ana,* against; *phylaxis,* protection) reflected this paradoxical outcome. Similar human reactions were noted early in the 20th century and remain the most rapidly developing and dangerous form of allergic response. Acute systemic reactions generally follow the *injection* of a potent antigen (allergen) into a highly sensitive subject, although, rarely, reaction may follow ingestion of an offending agent. In the past, antiserums derived from other species (especially horses) were most often responsible for these reactions; more recently, injected antibiotics have become principal offenders, with serums, insulin, and other drugs less often implicated. Murine (mouse) monoclonal antibodies, used increasingly in organ transplantation, provoke similar problems. Comparable reactions also may follow insect stings and bites in previously sensitized subjects.

Acute systemic reactions generally begin within minutes after exposure to an allergen; a delay longer than 1 hour is distinctly rare. In extreme sensitivity, injection of an allergen may cause death or a sublethal reaction almost instantly, and, generally, the most severe reactions begin most rapidly. Affected persons report a sense of uneasiness, rapidly followed by lightheadedness, which may lead to syncope (loss of consciousness). Itching of the palms and scalp may herald hives (urticaria) that cover much of the skin surface. Localized tissue swellings (angioedema) may appear within minutes and distort especially the eyelids, lips, tongue, hands, feet, and genitalia. *Angioedema* is a discrete swelling, involving deeper tissues of skin or mucous membranes, produced by a localized increase in vascular permeability without injury to the small veins and capillaries involved. Angioedema is often reversible within a short time and differs from other forms of swelling (edema) in which abnormal pressure or blood vessel damage promotes passage of fluid into tissues. Edema of the uvula and larynx are less evident to casual inspection but are especially prominent in human anaphylaxis and may cause death by respiratory obstruction. Laryngeal edema induces prominent air hunger, impaired speech, noisy breathing, and a "barking" cough. Respiratory difficulty also may arise because of bronchial narrowing, with audible wheezes mimicking spontaneous asthma (see Chapter 10). Less often, spasm of the gut, bladder, or uterus is prominent, with cramping pain, loss of visceral contents, or vaginal spotting. Fig. 9-2 summarizes the principal manifestations of human anaphylaxis.

Clinical anaphylaxis involves a sudden multifocal reaction of allergen with mast cell–bound, specific IgE, followed by widespread tissue response to the released mediator substances such as histamine and leukotrienes. Many features of these responses, including urticaria, can be induced by injection of agents that *directly* release mediators from mast cells in vivo, although not by injection of histamine alone. Systemic reactions to certain injected agents (e.g., radiologic contrast media) may exemplify such nonimmunologic mast cell secretion, since rises in plasma levels of mediators and activated complement components have been shown to occur. In addition, narcotic analgesics, dextrans, certain antibiotics, and other drugs directly stimulate mediator secretion by mast cells. The resulting nonimmunologic responses, which may closely resemble anaphylaxis, are termed *anaphylactoid.*

The first and most important step in managing an anaphylactic reaction is to ensure a patent airway and maintain arterial oxygen levels. Careful and continuous observation is essential, since it may become necessary to perform oropharyngeal intubation or tracheostomy to prevent asphyxia from laryngeal edema. Hypotension principally reflects vessels leaking intravascular fluid; if it is severe or prolonged, it may lead to brain, kidney, or heart damage. Hypotension may be corrected most directly by restoring plasma volume with normal saline solution, half-normal saline solution, or plasma. Several liters of fluid are often required to normalize blood pressure. Vasoconstrictor drugs such as norepinephrine may be of help, but without adequate volume replacement, they have limited benefit. Epinephrine is the preferred drug to limit or reverse the anaphylactic process. A dose of 0.3 ml of 1:1000 epinephrine may be injected subcutaneously (see Chapter 10) and repeated several times, if needed, at intervals of 15 minutes; small children may receive 0.022 ml/kg to a maximum of 0.3 ml per dose. The absorption of epineprine from subcutaneous depots is slow with severe hypotension; when shock is present, the drug may be diluted to 1:10,000 and slowly infused intravenously to provide comparable total doses. Injected antihistaminics, such as diphenhydramine or chlorpheniramine, may speed the resolution of urticaria and relieve cramps originating in hollow viscera. Adrenocortical steroids are often given for their favorable effects on inflammation and abnormal vascular permeability; however, they are not immediately beneficial. Although the steroids rarely may be lifesaving in prolonged shock, they should be given only after the airway is secure, volume repletion has been initiated, and epinephrine administered.

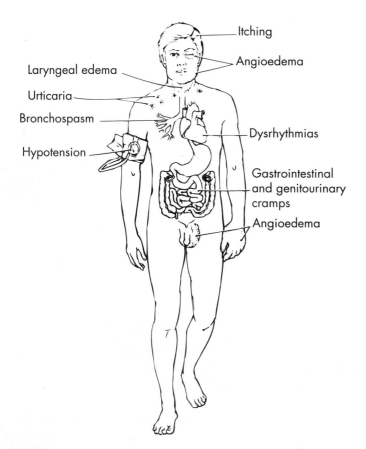

FIG. 9-2   Prominent manifestations of anaphylaxis. Laryngeal edema and profound hypotension usually pose the greatest dangers; cardiac effects may be primary or secondary to profound lowering of blood pressure.

Avoiding known offenders (allergens) is critical in reducing the risk of anaphylaxis; see Chapter 13 for drug considerations. Typical systemic reactions may follow specific foods (e.g., nuts, shellfish) and stings of insects such as bee, wasp, hornet, and yellow jacket and, rarely, insect bites (e.g., by deerflies). These responses appear to be IgE-mediated and can be fatal without treatment. Besides avoiding situations favored by stinging insects, susceptible persons are urged to carry commercially prepared, preloaded syringes of epinephrine whenever feasible. Such persons must be prepared to self-administer the drug in 0.3 ml subcutaneous doses and to apply a proximal tourniquet if an extremity has been attacked. Immunotherapy or hyposensitization with incremental injected doses of purified, diluted venoms is extremely effective in reducing risks of sting anaphylaxis when adequate doses are administered over many months. However, scrupulous avoidance is the only proven approach for food-sensitive subjects.

Atopic Diseases

Anaphylactic sensitization generally requires the injection of potent allergens, and certain GI and respiratory parasites also can elicit prominent IgE responses. In addition, a substantial minority of persons demonstrate specific IgE responses to mucosal contact (i.e., by inhalation or ingestion) with quite innocuous materials, including foods, pollens, and animal emanations (danders). Allergen-specific IgE, fixed to tissue, may be demonstrated by performing skin tests and observing the development 5 to 15 minutes of local redness (erythema), often with a central hive (wheal). Some persons, easily sensitized for such type I (IgE-mediated) responses by mucosal exposure, also manifest one or more related illnesses, such as allergic rhinitis, allergic (extrinsic) asthma, and *atopic* dermatitis. In addition, GI allergy, allergic conjunctivitis, and instances of acute urticaria and angioedema may coexist. Those with GI allergy may show (in response to specific foods) perioral pruritus (itching), tongue and mucous membrane swelling, difficulty in swallowing (dysphagia), nausea, vomiting, abdominal cramps, diarrhea, and perianal itching—singly or in combination. Food allergy also may affect distant organs, including the skin and bronchi, and rarely may underlie generalized reactions. These common conditions often are grouped as *atopic* diseases, and the predisposition that favors their occurrence is termed *atopy.**

The pathophysiologic basis of atopy still is not entirely clear; however, prominent IgE production from mucosal exposure to (benign) allergens appears to be a principal marker and one fundamental characteristic. In addition, health histories of affected subjects typically include

---

*Atopy is derived from the Greek ατοπια, which means strange or out of place. The term probably was chosen to express the inappropriateness of an immune response to entirely innocuous environment agents.

more than one of the atopic conditions, for example, eczema in infancy, then allergic rhinitis and/or asthma. Furthermore, familial clustering of these conditions is very prominent, although it seems to be the atopic tendency, rather than any specific form of illness, that is hereditable. In most North American reports, more than one half of overtly affected subjects have close relatives with atopic conditions, whereas in subjects free of atopic disease, a positive family history is definable in only about 10%.

Allergic rhinitis

Nasal allergy is the most frequently encountered atopic condition, affecting as many as 20% of pediatric and young-adult populations in North America and Western Europe. Elsewhere, rates of this and other atopic illnesses appear to be lower, especially in less developed countries. Persons with allergic rhinitis experience prominent nasal stuffiness and may report excessive nasal secretion *(rhinorrhea)* and sneezes occurring in rapid succession. *Pruritus* (Fig. 9-3) of the nasal mucosa, throat, and ears often is distressing and is accompanied by conjunctival redness, ocular pruritus, and lacrimation. The involved mucous membranes show dilation of blood vessels (especially venules) and extensive edema with prominent accumulation of eosinophils in both tissue and secretions. Some of these features, including the pruritus, can be duplicated by applying histamine alone to the normal mucosa, and allergic rhinitis may reflect the straightforward tissue effects of recognized mast cell–derived mediator substances (see earlier discussion). A release of hista-

mine, leukotrienes, prostaglandin D, and so on from the mucosa has been shown after direct nasal challenge of sensitive subjects with pollen allergens.

Although no absolute distinction is implied, allergic rhinitis is often divided into "seasonal" and "perennial" forms. Seasonal allergic rhinitis, or "hay fever," usually involves a specific period of symptoms in successive years, reflecting sensitivity principally to airborne pollens and fungus spores (Fig. 9-4) with defined schedules of prevalence. Seasonal rhinitis is mild in many persons who do not seek medical care, but it can be an exhausting illness for some because of continual sneezing, copious rhinorrhea, and unremitting pruritus. Intense pallor and swelling of mucous membranes usually accompany these dramatic symptoms, and eosinophils abound in nasal secretions (Fig. 9-5). In contrast, perennial rhinitis seldom shows major annual variations in severity, and symptoms often are dominated by unremitting nasal obstruction; prominent offenders include house dust mites and animal emanations to which daily exposure is commonplace. Not surprisingly, persons with multiple clinical sensitivities often experience perennial rhinitis as well as one or more predictable seasonal flares.

Perennial allergic rhinitis rarely is a source of dramatic symptoms. However, persistent partial nasal obstruction can promote distressing complications, such as mouth breathing, with resulting complaints of snoring and oropharyngeal dryness. Dark circles and redundant tissue often develop beneath the eyes. Although popularly termed "allergic shiners," these changes may reflect longstanding nasal obstruction of any cause. The swollen mucosa

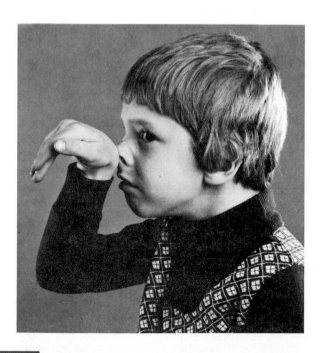

FIG. 9-3 Upward deflection of the nasal tip is a common mannerism among children with allergic rhinitis. This "allergic salute" briefly reduces pruritus and opens the nasal airway.

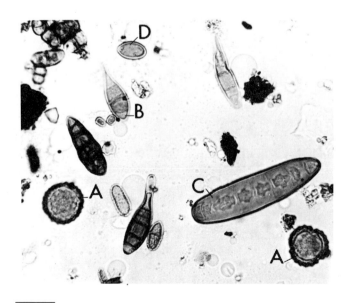

FIG. 9-4 Particles recovered during atmospheric sampling in late summer. Prominent sources of hay fever including ragweed pollen grain *(A)*, and fungus spores of *Alternaria (B)* and *Helminthosporium (C)* species are evident. Many spores, such as those of mushrooms *(D)*, remain to be evaluated as allergens.

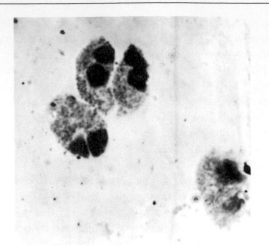

FIG. 9-5 Eosinophils from nasal secretions of a child with florid ragweed hay fever. Bilobed nuclei and discrete, round granules are familiar features of these cells, when suitably stained.

readily sustains bacterial infection, and obstruction of paranasal sinus openings is common; these lead to recurrent or chronic sinusitis. Drainage from foci of nasal infection promotes sore throat and leads to bronchial soiling and bronchitis. Especially with recurrent infection, the swollen nasal mucosa is prone to form local projections, or *polyps,* that further obstruct the airway. In addition, especially in children, the pharyngeal openings of the eustachian tubes are readily blocked by swollen mucosa, enlarged lymphoid tissue, or exudate. Without normal access to air, the middle ears develop negative pressure and fill with fluid, creating a chronic serous otitis with at least transient hearing loss and, often, recurrent middle ear infection.

Although allergic rhinitis sufferers tend to develop bronchial asthma with above-normal frequency, the extent of this increased risk remains unclear. In one population of rhinitic persons, unselected for symptom severity, less than 10% were observed to develop asthma as a new manifestation. However, this sequence has been recorded much more often in persons who eventually were evaluated by an allergist. In general, the risk of subsequent asthma appears to rise with increasing severity of rhinitis, with prominent sinobronchial infection, and when asthma was present in the past.

Although the pruritus, repetitive sneezing, and watery, profuse rhinorrhea of hay fever are characteristic, they are not unique to this disorder, and the symptoms of perennial rhinitis readily mimic those of other conditions. The distinctive feature of allergic rhinitis is that compatible symptoms appear or worsen predictably in response to specific allergen exposures. Therefore, in diagnosis, careful analysis of factors precipitating rhinitis is of overriding importance. Many persons with nonallergic "vasomotor" rhinitis have similar nasal stuffiness and marked rhinorrhea, some also showing intense nasal

eosinophilia. However, this group is without response to identifiable allergens. Instead, their complaints relate largely to airborne irritants, extremes of temperature and humidity, pregnancy, stages of the menstrual cycle, and emotional factors. Longstanding nasal complaints caused by recurrent or chronic infection, nasal polyps, marked deviation of the nasal septum, hypothyroidism, and anti-hypertensive or ovulatory suppressant drugs also must be distinguished from perennial allergic and nonallergic forms of rhinitis.

A clinical history of symptoms on exposure provides the clearest indication of offenders in respiratory allergy. Symptom variations during and after travel deserve special attention, and the effects of overt exposure to house dust mites, animals and fur products, feathers, seed derivatives, silk, and so forth may be sought directly. When casual observations are insufficient, history may be "created" by markedly increasing and/or reducing specific exposures, such as to foods or house pets, for brief periods to observe the results. In addition, the time or place of symptom occurrence may furnish etiologic clues not readily evident to the patient. Specific pollen sensitivities, for example, may be deduced if the resulting symptoms can be dated precisely and "seasons" of prevalence for local airborne pollens are known (Fig. 9-6). Similarly, recognition of the heavy fungus exposures associated with leaf collection, lawn care, and gardening as well as with hiking in tall vegetation helps to explain associated symptoms.

Skin tests eliciting a wheal-and-flare reaction provide useful correlates for a detailed clinical evaluation and are widely performed. However, even strongly positive reactions indicate only the immunologic "apparatus" for response and provide no *assurance* that symptoms arise from exposure to the allergens in question. The ultimate value of skin tests is to support or oppose impressions formed during clinical fact-finding. For tests of immediate reactivity, aqueous extracts are used, and testing is performed by pricking the skin through applied drops of these materials to produce epidermal or "prick" tests or by injecting small quantities (usually 0.02 ml) intracutaneously (Figs. 9-7 and 9-8, respectively). Because even this volume of highly diluted extract may be hazardous in exquisitely sensitive persons, prick tests are usually done first and persons with negative reactions are considered for intracutaneous (IC) testing. Because occasional persons manifest whealing with any skin trauma *(dermographism),* all reactions must be compared with those at negative control sites tested with sterile diluent alone. Wheal and erythema reactions may be reduced factitiously by antihistamine drugs (see later in this section); some recently developed agents (e.g., astemizole) cause suppression lasting many weeks. Cortisone-like drugs, by contrast, have little effect on immediate skin reactivity, whereas suppression by theophylline and sympathomimetic amines is trivial, at best.

Few additional test procedures help evaluate respira-

SEASONAL
AEROALLERGENS

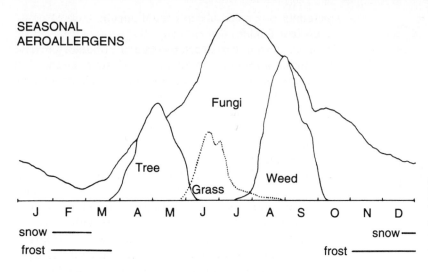

FIG. 9-6   Patterns of airborne allergen prevalence typical of central North America. The relationship of the patient's symptoms to tree, grass, and weed pollen sensitivity can often be deduced from their periods of occurrence.

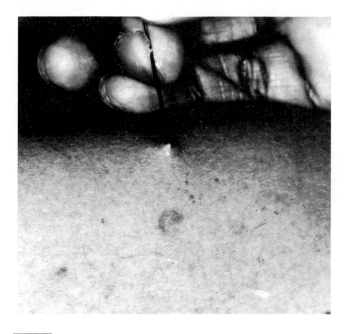

FIG. 9-7   Technique of epidermal (prick) testing using a sterile, straight needle. Because only the epidermis is penetrated, bleeding should not occur.

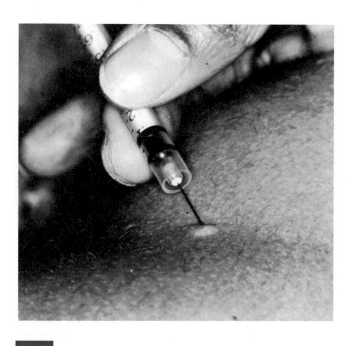

FIG. 9-8   Technique of intradermal (intracutaneous) skin testing.

tory allergy. Initial hopes that levels of *total* serum IgE could distinguish clearly between symptomatic atopic patients and others have not been sustained. Recently, in vitro measurement of allergen-specific IgE has become possible using venous blood. One approach, the radioallergosorbent test (RAST), diagrammed in Fig. 9-9, offers certain logistic advantages over direct testing and eliminates rare adverse reactions that accompany that procedure. Alternative in vitro procedures, such as ELISA (enzyme-linked immunosorbent assay) and FAST (fluorescent antibody staining technique), also are available. However, neither the sensitivity nor the specificity of these approaches now exceeds that of conventional skin tests.

The demonstration of eosinophils as the predominant cell in nasal or lacrimal secretions suggests an associated type I allergic inflammatory process but may occur also in nonallergic conditions. In suitably stained material the bilobed nuclei and abundant, discrete, red, refractile granules of eosinophils are evident by oil-immersion microscopy (see Fig. 9-5).

Three principal considerations dominate the management of allergic rhinitis: (1) efforts to reduce allergen (and irritant) exposure, (2) suppressive medications to mitigate symptom severity nonspecifically, and (3) specific hyposensitization* to reduce responsiveness to un-

---

*Generally now termed *immunotherapy*.

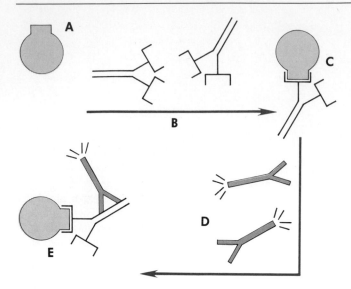

FIG. 9-9   The radioallergosorbent test (RAST), a technique for quantitating *allergen-specific* immunoglobulin E. In this procedure, allergens are linked chemically to carrier particles **(A)**, and the resulting conjugate is reacted with serum presumably containing specific IgE **(B)**. If IgE is bound **(C)**, it will react with and bind radiolabeled antihuman IgE **(D)** to form a radioactive complex **(E)**. By counting radioactivity, the amount of specific IgE originally present may be estimated.

avoidable allergens. Avoidance measures are most feasible for allergens associated with home and work situations, such as house dust mites, animal emanations, and agricultural products. However, even pollen exposure can be reduced significantly by the patient remaining indoors with windows closed—a strategy that usually requires air conditioning for success. Avoidance of dust mites is fostered by smooth, simple surfaces that facilitate cleaning (e.g., bare floors, uncluttered table and dresser tops) as well as by elimination or plastic encasing of bedding and upholstered furnishings (Fig. 9-10). High-efficiency filters are helpful where central forced-air heating is used, but they do not replace a careful antidust program at room level. Avoidance of indoor dampness also effectively limits dust mite populations.

Where symptoms result from sensitivity to animal emanations (dander), total avoidance of the source usually is justified. Although danders are popularly equated with hair, far more potent allergen sources include epidermal scales, saliva, lacrimal secretions, and even urine. House pets are the most persistently troublesome animal allergen sources. However, occupational exposures also may plague laboratory workers, veterinarians, and livestock handlers. In addition, products from animal sources may retain sensitizing properties for long periods; these include feather- and down-filled materials, fur-trimmed clothing and toys, furniture and rug pads (cattle and horse hair), and raw silk. Mohair and camel hair fabrics are occasionally implicated as allergen sources, although com-

mercially processed sheep's wool appears almost never to be an offender.

Tobacco smoke is an acknowledged respiratory irritant containing a remarkable assortment of toxic agents, but none confirmed as allergens. In contrast, plant products such as cottonseed, flaxseed, and castor bean meals are among the most potent sensitizers and are major symptom sources in industry.

For several decades, antihistaminic drugs (i.e., histamine H_1 receptor blockers) have been the most useful agents in the symptomatic (i.e., nonspecific) treatment of allergic nasal disease. Although many antihistaminics also share anticholinergic, antiserotonin, and/or tranquilizing properties, their capacity to compete with histamine for tissue receptors seems to underlie their usefulness in hay fever and so on. These drugs are generally effective when given orally, and they may be administered safely for long periods if necessary. Side effects of older agents are common though seldom severe in normal persons and may include drowsiness, lethargy, mucous membrane dryness, and occasionally, nausea, cramps, or lightheadedness. However, because of these symptoms and frequent impairment of depth perception, activities involving moving vehicles, dangerous machinery, or fine hand-eye coordination in general must be undertaken with care by those taking antihistaminics. Recently, several effective newer agents that do not cross the blood-brain barrier have been shown to produce little or no sedation and are generally preferred. In practice, several antihistaminic agents often must be tried before an optimal (or even a satisfactory) one is identified, and the results of such trials defy prediction at the outset. In choosing drugs for

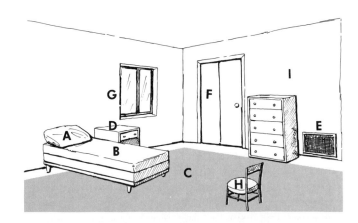

FIG. 9-10   Measures designed to minimize exposure to house dust mites (and other inhalant allergens) as applied to a bedroom. Objectives include covering pillows *(A)* plus mattresses and box springs *(B)* with plastic encasings; maintaining a bare floor *(C)* and uncluttered surfaces *(D)*; applying final filters to warm-air ducts *(E)*; keeping closet doors closed *(F)*; and minimizing window coverings *(G)*, upholstered furnishings *(H)*, and wall decorations *(I)*. These empirically derived measures greatly decrease exposure to mite-derived allergens.

comparison by individuals, it must be recalled that many marketed preparations are merely different forms of a few generic agents (e.g., chlorpheniramine); efficacy trials should compare different chemical species. Patients often report a waning of previous antihistaminic effectiveness, prompting substitution (or addition) of different agents; at times, this reflects suboptimal compliance in drug dosing.

Sympathomimetic amines offer additional benefit in relieving nasal stuffiness and are often marketed in combinations with antihistaminic agents. Drugs including ephedrine, isoephedrine, and phenylpropanolamine act as mucosal decongestants and, by causing more or less psychomotor stimulation, can offset the sedative effects of antihistaminic agents. It is unclear whether oral sympathomimetic drugs significantly affect the release of mediator substances from tissue mast cells, although (opposing) beta- and alpha-adrenergic effects are possible. In addition, these agents produce side effects that may impair ocular, cardiac, GI, and genitourinary function (see Chapter 10). The topical use of sympathomimetic agents as drops, sprays, and vapors is widespread and provides prompt mucosal shrinkage, which is helpful in acute illness such as bacterial sinusitis. Unfortunately, these preparations are easily obtained and often abused. Prolonged overuse results in an irritant effect, so that each dose gives transient decongestion followed by a prolonged obstructive response, prompting further self-medication. In habituated persons, the resulting mucosal inflammation, or *rhinitis medicamentosa,* produces persistent nasal stuffiness and a congested, or edematous, appearance. Complete withdrawal of topical nasal medication is mandatory, and when possible, oral agents are substituted. In some cases a topical nasal corticosteroid spray must be given for several weeks to make this change tolerable. Recently introduced agents, such as beclomethasone and flunisolide, which are both locally effective and rapidly metabolized by the liver, are generally safe and well tolerated.

Intranasal steroids are useful also in suppressing the primary symptoms of allergic rhinitis and are preferred, especially for seasonal periods of exquisite severity. Currently, five agents are available for prescription as Freon-propelled or hand-pumped preparations. In addition, systemic corticosteroids suppress hay fever manifestations when other remedies have failed. However, the widespread side effects of these systemically active agents make their chronic administration for nasal allergy unacceptable.

Except for antibiotics, when indicated, few other drugs offer benefit to rhinitis sufferers. The appropriate topical application of cromolyn sodium (see Chapter 10) also can reduce the symptoms of allergic rhinitis and conjunctivitis. Additional ocular agents (e.g., levocabastine drops) provide benefit when eye symptoms are prominent.

Immunotherapy (hyposensitization) continues to pro-

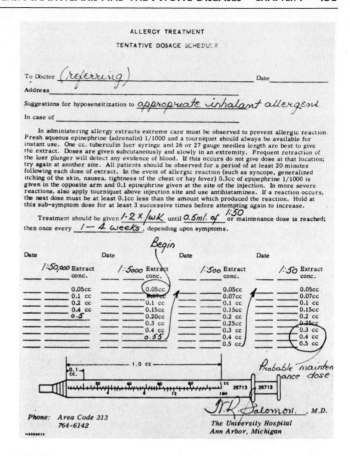

FIG. 9-11 Typical dosage schedule form used at the allergy clinic of the University Hospital, Ann Arbor, for patients whose injection treatment will be administered by their personal physicians. Additional dilutions or dosage volumes may be desirable for specific persons.

vide an important allergen-specific treatment approach for respiratory allergy. In this procedure, incremental doses of extracts of a recognized allergen are injected subcutaneously over prolonged periods so as to modify clinical reactivity. After reaching an empirically indicated "maximum" level, this dosage is maintained, pending evaluation of symptoms, and adjustments in the program are carried out accordingly. Indications for immunotherapy include allergic asthma, as well as allergic rhinitis or conjunctivitis that is inadequately controlled despite optimal avoidance measures and acceptable medication treatment. In each instance, sensitivity to specific, *inhalant* allergens must be confirmed, because any nonspecific benefits of injection treatment are unpredictable; food factors are approached by diet modification exclusively. A typical treatment schedule is illustrated in Fig. 9-11. Properly controlled clinical trials have confirmed the value of immunotherapy for grass and ragweed pollen and strongly suggest that tree pollen, animal dander, *Alternaria* (an important fungus), and dust mite immunotherapy is beneficial. Injection treatment for other materials either has been shown to be valueless (e.g., for respiratory bacterial vaccines) or remains incompletely studied (e.g., for most fungi). Trials of pollen extracts indicate also that (1) optimal symptom suppression is seen when the largest well-tolerated doses are given, (2) symptom suppression caused by treatment may carry over to one or more subsequent years in which injections are withheld, and (3) a placebo, or inert material, given by injection, may decrease symptoms in one third to one half of subjects, which reemphasizes the need for proper controls in evaluating treatment results.

The basis of the efficacy of immunotherapy remains unclear, although several tissue effects that might promote benefit are known. It was initially assumed that the procedure induced active immunization against a pollen toxin, but this rationale was soon discredited. Although immunotherapy might "turn off" specific IgE production, RAST values and skin test positivity often change little during extended successful treatment, and specific IgE values usually rise early in the injection sequence. The appearance in serum of IgG antibodies specific for the injected allergen is well documented, and these factors can compete with IgE for allergen, thus showing "blocking" capabilities. Although a general correlation between blocking antibody titer and clinical improvement is seen, exceptions (e.g., persons with high titers and unabated rhinitis) imply that other factors must also contribute. Recently described elevations, with immunotherapy, of IgG and IgA (blocking) antibodies in respiratory tract secretions suggest an alternative tissue mechanism. In addition, blood basophils from persons receiving high-dose immunotherapy are seen to release progressively less histamine on allergen challenge in vitro, in some cases becoming wholly unresponsive. Current interest also surrounds possible treatment-induced changes in the function of allergen-specific T helper lymphocytes (e.g., decreased lymphokine production). At present, therefore, although the clinical value of hyposensitization for selected allergens is established, the responsible mechanisms are not; several effects, varying among patients, are possible.

Although serious, long-term adverse effects of immunotherapy are not evident, significant transient local or systemic reactions can occur. Redness, whealing, and tender swelling lasting up to 36 hours may develop at treatment sites if dosage is excessive. These reactions usually mandate a reduction in the amount of allergen next injected. However, their severity also may be decreased by wiping the needle with a sterile swab before injection to remove adhering extract and applying firm pressure to the injected site to reduce retrograde oozing of fluid along the needle track. Acute systemic reactions are often preceded by increasingly prominent local

swellings but may occur at any time without warning. A generalized reaction may be anaphylactic or may be accompanied by or confined to rhinitis or asthma symptoms; management has been described previously. In addition, 0.1 to 0.2 ml of epinephrine is usually introduced at the site of the responsible injection to slow allergen absorption. Extract should be given into a site distal enough to allow for a proximal tourniquet. Although adverse reactions may occur capriciously, their risk increases with conditions that elevate cutaneous blood flow, including high environmental temperature, fever, physical exertion, hyperthyroidism, and pregnancy. Human error also is a factor. Mishaps may occur as a result of misreading previously recorded doses or vial labels; confusion of persons with similar names is a common error. Usually, reactions that require treatment have onset within 20 to 30 minutes after injection; therefore most clinics require their patients to remain quietly seated in a well-ventilated room for this period after they receive injections. The low but inescapable risk of systemic reactions and a corresponding need for rapid, complex treatment measures leave no justification for self-injection of extract by any patient. Facilities that administer treatment extracts should be prepared to quickly provide epinephrine, oxygen, and intravenous fluids and have personnel competent in cardiopulmonary support.

At present, skin testing and most injection treatments are carried out with sterile, aqueous extracts containing, usually, an antimicrobial agent such as phenol or thimerosal and a protein stabilizer such as human serum albumin. Attempts to establish standards of biologic activity for these materials have developed slowly, although assays of defined allergens in ragweed and grass pollen extracts are now used as indicators of potency. Other materials typically are rated on a "weight-by-volume" basis. In this system a 1:500 ragweed pollen extract is the solution resulting when 1 g of defatted ragweed pollen is extracted under defined conditions in 500 ml of fluid. Alternative approaches based on assays of total protein or total nitrogen are no more instructive. Comparisons of extract potency based on ability to inhibit standardized RAST assays or skin test potency in panels of sensitive subjects (e.g., "allergy units") also appear feasible. In addition, therapeutic materials suitable for infrequent administration and combining low skin reactivity with prominent immunizing potency remain desired goals. Currently, alum-precipitated aqueous extracts are available with modestly long-acting properties, although local and systemic adverse reactions can occur. Allergens absorbed to other carriers as well as those chemically modified and aggregated by agents such as formalin or glutaraldehyde continue to hold promise.

QUESTIONS

▼ *Answer the following on a separate sheet of paper.*

1. Differentiate between hypersensitivity and sensitization in the context of immunologic events.
2. Contrast angioedema with lymphedema.
3. Describe the pathogenesis of an acute systemic (anaphylactic) reaction.
4. What accounts for differences among species in patterns of an anaphylactic response?
5. What are the necessary conditions for anaphylactic sensitization in humans?
6. List three principal considerations that dominate the management of respiratory allergy as exemplified by allergic rhinitis.
7. What measures should be taken to reduce the risk of an anaphylactic reaction?

▼ *Circle the letter preceding each item below that correctly answers the question or completes the statement. More than one answer may be correct.*

8. Immunologic processes that are most clearly recognized as immunologic disease are reactions of:
   a. Delayed hypersensitivity
   b. Immediate hypersensitivity
   c. Both a and b
   d. Neither a nor b
9. All the following are important characteristics of clinical hypersensitivity (allergy) as an immunologic response *except:*
   a. Specificity—reaction is to a specific, exogenous antigen.
   b. Response usually involves immunologic mechanisms.
   c. Reaction is abnormal (inappropriate or damaging).
   d. Prior contact with a specific substance (allergen) is not necessary to elicit a response.
10. The initial exposure to a vaccine will often principally elicit which of the following responses?
    a. IgE
    b. IgM
    c. IgA
    d. IgG
11. IgE antibody has specific affinity for:
    a. Mast cells
    b. Neutrophils
    c. Basophils
    d. Red blood cells

12. Which of the following characteristics may be associated with IgE?
    a. It is a tissue-fixing antibody associated with allergic rhinitis.
    b. It participates in reactions leading to release of histamine.
    c. It is involved in immunologically induced wheal-and-flare reactions.
    d. All the above are associated with IgE.
13. The Fc fragment (crystallizable fragment) of antibodies is the portion of the immunoglobulin that involves the following activities:
    a. Activation of the complement pathway
    b. Facilitation of the uptake by phagocytes of antigen-bound immunoglobulins
    c. Combination with specific antigenic components
    d. Shared by immunoglobulins of a defined class (isotype)
14. Which of the following immunoglobulin types is most important in the body's defense against pyogenic infections?
    a. IgA
    b. IgE
    c. IgG
    d. IgM
15. Tissue effects of the classic complement pathway include all the following *except:*
    a. Production of direct lesions in cell membranes
    b. Lysis of target cells
    c. Release of transfer factor from sensitized lymphocytes
    d. Attraction of leukocytes
    e. Release of permeability-enhancing factors
16. Characteristics of acute systemic (anaphylactic) reaction include all the following *except:*
    a. Pruritus of the scalp and palms of the hands
    b. Exposure usually from ingesting the offending agent
    c. Severe laryngeal edema and bronchial obstruction
    d. Hypovolemic shock caused by exudation of fluid from the vascular compartment
17. All the following statements about anaphylaxis are true *except:*
    a. It is a condition caused by an immunologic reaction.
    b. It is a potentially fatal condition.

    c. It is thought to be mediated mainly by IgG.
    d. Acute systemic reactions generally begin within minutes after introduction of an allergen.
18. Important considerations to be observed in treating acute anaphylactic reactions include which of the following?
    a. Ensuring a patent airway
    b. Improving vascular or blood vessel integrity or intactness
    c. Supporting the blood pressure
    d. Promoting rapid absorption of the allergen
    e. Administering antipruritic lotions to the skin
    f. Maintaining arterial oxygen levels
19. A 25-year-old man collapses after an intramuscular (IM) penicillin injection; he is unconscious, he has generalized hives, and his blood pressure is 60/20 mm Hg. Initial treatment should be:
    a. IM penicillinase
    b. Intravenous (IV) adrenalin and IM diphenhydramine (Benadryl)
    c. IV corticosteroids in normal saline solution
    d. Subcutaneous adrenalin and IV saline solution
    e. IV corticosteroids and IM diphenhydramine
20. Which of the following immunoglobulin types is involved in mediating atopic disease?
    a. IgA
    b. IgE
    c. IgG
    d. IgM
21. Common characteristics of the atopic state include:
    a. A strong family history of chronic bronchitis and emphysema
    b. The occurrence of typical infantile eczema without evident precipitating allergens
    c. The genetically inherited predisposition to become hypersensitive
    d. Presence of numerous wheal-and-flare reactions on testing the skin with food and pollen extracts
22. The most prevalent atopic condition in North America among young adult populations is:
    a. Allergic asthma
    b. Nasal allergy
    c. Eczema
    d. Gastrointestinal allergy

Continued.

QUESTIONS—cont'd

23. Jane, a 15-year-old female patient, has pruritus, repetitive sneezing, and watery profuse rhinorrhea. Her diagnosis is allergic rhinitis. Which of the following data would be most significant in diagnosing the allergen responsible for this allergic rhinitis?
   a. Positive reaction to an intradermal skin test
   b. Clinical history of symptoms on exposure to a specific allergen in her home
   c. Levels of total serum IgE
   d. Predominance of basophils in nasal or lacrymal secretions

24. A 20-year-old man has a large wheal-and-flare reaction on skin testing with ragweed pollen extract; a comparable test with the diluent is nonreactive. He may be told, with confidence, that:
   a. He has large amounts of IgG-blocking antibody specific for ragweed pollen allergens in his blood.
   b. He has ragweed hay fever.
   c. He is immune to ragweed pollen and will never have difficulty related to it in the future.
   d. He has IgE antibodies specific for ragweed pollen allergens fixed at skin sites.

25. Antihistaminic drugs:
   a. Prevent the release of histamine from mast cells
   b. Prevent the release of histamine from macrophages
   c. Are highly beneficial in treatment of severe asthma
   d. At least partially control symptoms in a majority of patients with hay fever

26. Which of the following drugs should be immediately available when intracutaneous skin tests are being performed with atopic allergens?
   a. Epinephrine
   b. Cortisone tablets
   c. Horse serum
   d. Antihistamine tablets

27. All the following describe recognized effects of immunotherapy *except:*
   a. This causes an immediate decrease in IgE in the blood.
   b. This often causes an increase in IgG that may compete with IgE for antigens.
   c. Decreased histamine release from sensitized mast cells occurs with specific amounts of added allergen.
   d. Treated persons are able to tolerate progressively larger amounts of injected allergen.

28. Injection treatment (immunotherapy) would be most appropriate for:
   a. A 30-year-old mother of three with severe wheezing as a result of a guinea pig present in the home for 3 months
   b. A 60-year-old vice-president of IBM with angioedema following ingestion of abalone (and other snails)
   c. A 30-year-old veterinarian with well-identified asthma caused by dog dander
   d. A 9-month-old infant with severe eczema known to be worsened by egg
   e. A 20-year-old nursing student with grass and ragweed pollen hay fever, readily controlled with an antihistamine-decongestant drug preparation

29. Persons with seasonal allergic rhinitis or hay fever:
   a. Are less likely than normal to have had asthma or atopic dermatitis
   b. Usually have other members in their family with atopic conditions
   c. Develop sensitivity to penicillin in more than 70% of cases
   d. Typically wheeze with exposure to offending allergens in normal seasonal concentrations

30. John, a 19-year-old man, has had severe allergic reactions to insect stings (bee, wasp, hornet, yellow jacket). Which of the following precautions must be followed to avoid a likely systemic reaction?
   a. He must avoid situations favored by stinging insects.
   b. He must always have available and be able to self-administer preloaded syringes of epinephrine.
   c. He must undergo immunotherapy, which includes injecting "whole-body" extracts of incriminated insects.
   d. He should undergo incremental injections of dilutions of purified venoms.

▼ *Circle T if the statement is true and F if it is false. Correct any false statements.*

31. T   F   Individuals normally have minute amounts of IgE present in their blood serum.

32. T   F   The distinctive feature of allergic rhinitis is that compatible symptoms appear or worsen predictably in response to specific exposures.

33. T   F   Strongly positive skin tests eliciting wheal-and-flare reactions provide assurance that symptoms of allergic respiratory conditions do arise from exposure to the allergens in question.

34. T   F   The preferred method of skin testing for clinical evaluation of respiratory allergy is to inject highly concentrated aqueous extracts of allergenic material intracutaneously.

35. T   F   The radioallergosorbent test (RAST) is used to measure allergen-specific IgE using venous blood in vitro.

36. T   F   In vitro procedures such as ELISA and FAST are more sensitive and specific than conventional skin tests.

37. T   F   Dextrans and narcotic analgesics stimulate mediator secretion by mast cells, which may cause a picture resembling anaphylaxis.

CHAPTER 10

Bronchial Asthma
ALLERGIC AND OTHERWISE

WILLIAM R. SOLOMON

Asthma is a clinically defined condition marked by recurrent episodes of reversible bronchial narrowing, often separated by periods of more normal ventilation. These events are readily provoked in asthma-prone subjects by a variety of stimuli, denoting a characteristic state of bronchial hyperreactivity.

Tissue changes in uncomplicated asthma (Fig. 10-1) are confined to bronchial airways and consist of spasm of smooth muscle, mucosal edema and persistent infiltration by inflammatory cells, and hypersecretion of viscid mucus. Mobilization of luminal secretions is compromised by airway narrowing and shedding of ciliated bronchial epithelial cells that normally aid in the clearance of mucus.

FIG. 10-1   Bronchial changes in chronic asthma. This small bronchus shows increased width of the epithelial basement membrane *(arrow)* and partial loss of mucosal cells. The lumen *(A)* is filled with mucus and cellular debris, and the submucosa *(B)* is densely infiltrated with inflammatory cells, including many eosinophils. (From Sheldon JM, Lovel RG, Mathews KP: *A manual of clinical allergy,* ed 2, Philadelphia, 1967, Saunders.)

VENTILATORY DYSFUNCTION

The person experiencing asthma has a fundamental inability to achieve normal rates of airflow during respiration (especially expiration). This is reflected in a lowering of FEV_1, the volume of air produced during the first second of forced expiratory effort, and by related parameters. Fig. 10-2 shows these components in relation to the curve (flattened in asthma), which related total expiratory volume and time. Because many narrowed airways cannot fill and empty quickly enough, there is uneven lung aeration and a loss of the normal spatial matching of ventilation and pulmonary blood flow (Fig. 10-3). Depending on their severity, these defects may produce no symptoms or merely a sense of tracheal irritation; in other cases, respiratory distress may be intolerable. Airstream turbulence and the vibrations of bronchial mucus lead to audible wheezing during asthmatic attacks; however, this

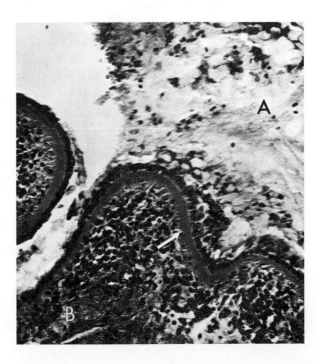

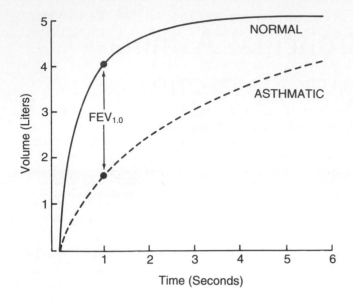

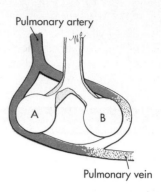

FIG. 10-2   Forced expiratory curves produced by two 20-year-old men—one normal and one with moderately severe asthma. The slope of these curves at any point is equivalent to flow rate. An inability to move air quickly is the major ventilatory defect in asthma, and this is evident most clearly as a prolongation of the forced expiratory time when airways are narrowed.

FIG. 10-3   Mismatching of ventilation and perfusion in asthma. Because of narrowing of its bronchus, alveolus *A* does not properly oxygenate its share of pulmonary artery blood; alveolus *B* functions normally. As a result of these contributions, average oxygen saturation of pulmonary venous blood is abnormally low. In asthma a shift of blood flow from *A*-type to *B*-type alveoli occurs secondarily but is usually incomplete. Furthermore, hyperventilation of *B* with room air cannot compensate for the venous-to-arterial "shunting" at *A*.

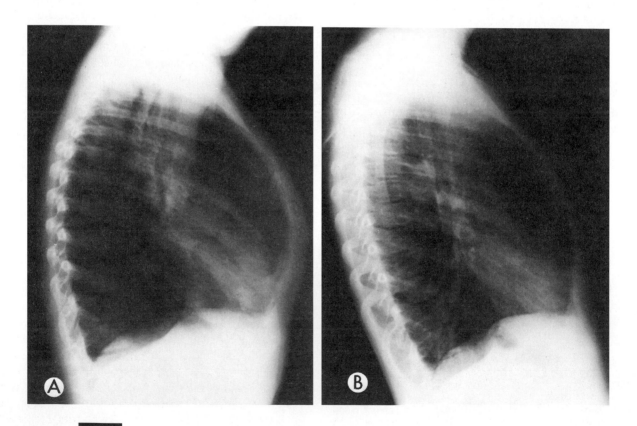

FIG. 10-4   Hyperinflation of the chest of an 8-year-old boy with asthma. **A,** Radiograph taken during a severe status asthmaticus attack that later required mechanical ventilation. (Note especially the broad space between the heart and sternum.) **B,** Radiograph taken during a symptom-free interlude 4 months later, which shows much less severe changes.

physical sign is also prominent in other obstructive airway problems. Distressed asthmatic people usually breathe more rapidly than normal (even though this tends to increase resistance to airflow) and avoid unnecessary activity. In addition, the chest assumes a position of maximum inspiration that is voluntarily achieved at first and dilates the airways. Later this appearance is sustained because of incomplete emptying of alveoli, which results in progressive hyperinflation of the thorax (Fig. 10-4). In uncomplicated asthma, cough typically is prominent only as attacks resolve, when it serves to clear accumulated secretions. Rarely, "dry" cough may be the only evident manifestation of asthma. Between bouts of asthma the patient may be wheeze-free and asymptomatic, although heightened bronchial reactivity and defects in ventilation remain. However, in chronic asthma, symptomless interludes decline, leading to a state of continuous asthma, often with secondary infection.

Asthmatic people as a group, those with and those without allergic mechanisms, share an abnormal bronchial lability that promotes airway narrowing by many factors that have no effect on normal persons. The basis of this tendency remains unclear, but it seems to parallel bronchial inflammatory changes. Functionally, asthmatic airways behave as though their beta-adrenergic innervation (which helps preserve airway patency) is incompetent, and much evidence suggests that, at least functionally, partial blockage of beta-adrenergic receptors exists in typical asthma. Bronchoconstrictor influences, which are normally mediated by parasympathetic (cholinergic) and alpha-adrenergic pathways, therefore tend to predominate. In clinical practice the bronchial lability of asthmatic patients may be confirmed by demonstrating their ready airway obstructive responses to extremely low concentrations of inhaled histamine and methacholine, a substance with activity resembling that of acetylcholine. Related mechanisms probably contribute to the bouts of asthma that often follow inhalation of cold air as well as exposure to diverse mists, dusts, and volatile irritants. Poorly understood nervous pathways also mediate airway closure in response to psychic stimuli. (Asthma solely caused by emotional factors is exceptionally rare, however.) In asthma, reflex pathways promoting bronchospasm with forced chest deflation are activated by maneuvers such as laughing, blowing up a balloon, or providing a full expiration for ventilatory testing.

SUBSETS OF ASTHMA

Asthma must be distinguished from two conditions described in detail in Chapter 38. These are *chronic bronchitis,* marked by continuous bronchial hypersecretion, and *emphysema,* in which loss of supporting lung tissues allows severe airway narrowing to occur with expiration. Although atopy is readily implicated in many instances

of bronchial asthma, a substantial number of asthmatic persons lack demonstrable allergic factors even after exhaustive study. Such persons, including many infants as well as middle-aged and older adults, are often said to have "intrinsic" asthma, although their problem is more properly termed "idiopathic" (i.e, unexplained).

Some adults with idiopathic asthma also manifest nasal polyps, recurrent sinusitis, and severe airway obstructive responses to aspirin in various combinations. Typically, other nonsteroidal antiinflammatory drugs (NSAIDs, e.g., ibuprofen and indomethacin) also precipitate severe attacks in these patients. Moderate asthma is often persistent even when recognized offenders are avoided, however, and prominent (nonallergic) vasomotor rhinitis frequently ushers in the disease. It is essential to accept the patient's report of respiratory distress after aspirin and so on, since no safe confirmatory test is available. In addition, since severe intolerance to aspirin and NSAIDs may begin suddenly, asthmatic adults with polyps and/or sinusitis should recognize the risks associated with these agents.

Flares of asthma frequently accompany viral or bacterial respiratory infections and may progress in severity, ultimately requiring inpatient care. When responsible pathogens have been sought in pediatric asthma patients, rhinovirus and parainfluenza virus infections have been especially implicated. The presence of significant secondary infection may be manifested by fever, purulent expectoration, elevated white blood cell count, or recovery of pathogens from sputum; however, persistent asthma often provides the only signal. Many children with infection-triggered asthma in preschool years go on to develop classic nasal allergy or allergic (atopic) asthma in later life. However, few indications exist that "bacterial allergy" is responsible for asthma accompanying infection. Rather, since invading organisms frequently destroy already compromised ciliated epithelium and localize agents of inflammation in labile bronchi, their adverse effect on asthma is predictable. In addition, animal studies have suggested that microbial substances may further reduce already inadequate beta-adrenergic activity.

Many asthmatic patients experience increased wheezing and *dyspnea* (abnormal shortness of breath) with exertion of any intensity. In addition, a specific form of *exercise-induced asthma* (EIA) often is noted in which, after several minutes of brisk activity and often well after its termination, significant bronchospasm occurs. EIA is most often evident in children and characteristically appears in subjects symptomless before beginning exertion. Although a minimum total energy expenditure is necessary, above this critical level the risk of symptoms varies with the type of activity. Generally, at comparable work levels, sprint running is most and swimming least conducive to EIA. Current evidence suggests airway cooling caused by evaporation of moisture from the mucosa as an important determinant of EIA.

DIFFERENTIAL DIAGNOSIS

Because bronchial asthma is an abnormal pattern of response rather than a discrete disease, differential diagnosis requires attention to the clinical form and major determinants of this syndrome,* as well as to its distinction from other obstructive airway problems. Rarely, persons who overbreathe with psychic stress or children with noisy respiration because of large adenoids, a short neck, or a "floppy" epiglottis are suspected of having asthma; laryngeal muscle dysfunction also can narrow the airway episodically, mimicking (or accompanying) more distal obstruction. In adults, at least, airway hyperactivity often may be excluded by demonstrating a normal test response to inhalation of metacholine, whereas the childhood problems usually are clarified by careful examination, and they may resolve, in time, with developmental changes. At any age, however, the impaction of a foreign body or growth of a localized tumor in the bronchi (or larynx) may lead to diffuse wheezing, simulating asthma. More typical recurrent symptoms may be encountered in certain forms of diffuse vascular inflammation (vasculitis) and with secreting carcinoid tumors when these are metastatic to the liver (see Chapter 42).

Severe airway obstruction, capable of producing respiratory failure and associated with fever, is characteristic of the bronchiolitis of small children. This illness is often recurrent and frequently results from infection with respiratory syncytial virus. Intense local inflammation promotes closure of small, distal airways, although humoral immune mechanisms also may contribute to this process.

A striking picture occasionally occurs in individuals who display symptoms of allergic asthma with growth of the fungus *Aspergillus fumigatus* in their bronchial lumina. Although little or no tissue invasion occurs, this organism excites an intense, apparently immunologically directed, inflammatory response with fever, pulmonary infiltrates (shadows) on chest x-ray films, and prominent tissue and peripheral blood eosinophilia. Affected persons have fatigue, weight loss, severe asthma, and expectoration of bronchial mucus plugs that may show the fungus as minute, dark growth points. Immediate wheal-and-flare skin reactivity to the fungus organism is striking, and total serum immunoglobulin E (IgE) levels are extremely high. IgG-precipitating antibodies with specificity for this organism also are demonstrable in more than 70% of this allergic bronchopulmonary aspergillosis group. Suppression of the disease with adequate doses of adrenocortical steroids (see later in this chapter) is feasible and also essential if irreversible bronchial damage (bronchiectasis) is to be averted (Fig. 10-5).

Especially in older adults, chronic bronchitis and pul-

---

*A syndrome is a set of signs and symptoms that occur together characteristically in an illness or related group of illnesses.

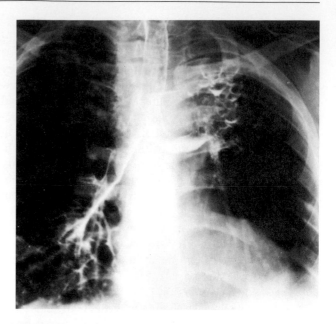

FIG. 10-5 Saccular (saclike) bronchiectasis of the left upper lobe demonstrated by bronchography in an adult with long-standing allergic bronchopulmonary aspergillosis. Bronchi in lower lung fields are essentially uninvolved. (Radiograph courtesy of Terry Silver, MD.)

monary emphysema often require distinction from bronchial asthma when the latter has no evident allergic factors. Chronic bronchitis is a prolonged and often slowly progressive condition of bronchial inflammation and hypersection manifested by cough and sputum production extending over months and years. In addition, a proportion of those with chronic bronchitis also experience episodic bouts of airway obstruction—in effect, a form of idiopathic asthma—late in the disease. Pulmonary emphysema, by contrast, presents prominent, irreversible anatomic changes with diffuse loss of the alveolar walls that normally exert outward traction on bronchi that they surround. Deprived of this source of support, the airways tend to close in expiration wherever pressure outside their walls exceeds that within. Affected persons develop predictable periods of dyspnea and wheezing with any increase (usually exertional) in respiratory effort rather than experiencing spontaneous attacks, typical of asthma, which readily begin at rest or, often, during sleep. The prognosis of emphysema is quite unfavorable, with variably increasing disability the rule, and this diagnosis cannot be proposed lightly. However, since asthmatic individuals with recurrent infection also may acquire chronic bronchitis and severely bronchitic patients ultimately may show emphysema as well, a sharp distinction between these disorders is impossible at times. On the other hand, when chest hyperinflation, evident on radiographic or physical evaluation, is casually (and erroneously) designated "emphysema," a grave stigma may be implied without basis. In fact, the hyperinflation and resulting thoracic deformity of young asthmatic persons may be totally reversed with successful treatment, leaving them anatomically and functionally normal.

LONG-TERM TREATMENT CONSIDERATIONS IN BRONCHIAL ASTHMA

The protracted course typical of asthma and its associated state of bronchial hyperreactivity determine a chronic need for treatment measures. Where IgE-mediated factors are evident, efforts to reduce exposure to and institution of immunotherapy for selected inhalant allergens have established value (see Chapter 9). Avoidance of irritants, especially tobacco smoke, and prompt treatment of unresolved bacterial respiratory infections are beneficial but frequently overlooked.

Perfumes, aerosol cleaners and cosmetics, strong cooking odors, solvents, and paint fumes also pose potentially avoidable risks that must be appreciated. Cold air is an additional bronchoconstrictor influence that may be mitigated by wearing a scarf or gauze mask over the nose and mouth as a heat exchanger. Adding moisture to dry indoor air (to maintain a relative humidity of about 30%) is desirable, although poorly maintained humidifiers can become sources of microbial aerosols. In addition, programs of regular medication can effectively reduce bronchial lability and thereby raise the threshold for obstructive airway responses.

Recent evidence that asthma prevalence and mortality are increasing globally and the promise implicit in newer treatment options have prompted an extensive re-examination of approaches to this condition. The resulting guidelines reflect several increasingly accepted principles:

1. The overall severity of impairment caused by asthma differs widely among individuals and, typically, varies with time in any affected person.
2. Treatment programs of increasing potency (and complexity) are appropriate to control asthma of mounting severity.
3. Antiinflammatory drugs are fundamental treatment for all but the most minimal forms of asthma.
4. Increasing symptom intensity should prompt a *pre-planned* set of remedial behaviors designed to improve the individual's functional status.*

Beta-adrenergic agents (e.g., metaproterenol, pirbuterol, albuterol) remain the most widely used antiasthmatic drugs. These remedies show predominant $beta_2$-adrenergic effects, primarily airway smooth muscle re-laxation with lesser ($beta_1$-adrenergic) tendencies to increase cardiac rate and contractile force. However, the latter effects are not absent from current preparations, and muscle tremor, sleeplessness, and psychomotor stimulation are additional, *intrinsic* $beta_2$-induced events. Direct comparisons readily confirm that inhaled preparations produce more rapid and effective asthma relief, with fewer systemic side effects, than the same agents given orally. This principle, which especially favors beta-adrenergic aerosols, also can be generalized to other drug classes (e.g., corticosteroids, anticholinergics). However, *overuse* of bronchodilator aerosols is potentially harmful and has been variably linked to excess asthma fatalities. Furthermore, since patients readily control and may become habituated to aerosol use, a substantial abuse potential exists. Current guidelines recognize that beta-agonist aerosols alone may suffice for minimal asthma, which occurs at most once or twice a week and may be rapidly reversed by these agents. More frequent or severe symptoms require the addition (or substitution) of anti-inflammatory medications (see following discussion) on a regular schedule. Combined-drug programs increasingly have used inhaled salmeterol, twice daily, for its extended beta-adrenergic effects, although this agent cannot quickly reverse acute asthma. *Oral* $beta_2$-adrenergic drug treatment enjoys less popularity when symptoms are resistant; increased use of antiinflammatory and bronchodilator aerosols usually is preferable. However, $beta_2$-adrenergic syrups often benefit very small children when given for sporadic asthma or specific, short-term circumstances (e.g., respiratory infection, predictable allergen exposure) that provoke symptoms.

Recognition of bronchial inflammation as characteristic of and fundamental to asthma has focused attention increasingly on means to reduce the accumulation and activation of cells in the airway. When these changes follow IgE-mediated mast cell secretion, inhaled cromolyn sodium and nedocromil have shown practical value. The ability of these relatively safe drugs to block airway responses to specific allergens in laboratory provocative challenges may realistically model their potential for clinical benefit. However, it is not clear that IgE-based processes alone are affected, since these agents often can suppress EIA, and additional effects, apparently independent of mast cells, have been suggested.

Whatever the place of cromolyn sodium and nedocromil in drug treatment, inhaled corticosteroids now are broadly accepted as medications indicated for most persons with symptomatic asthma. Several agents, marketed in *metered-dose inhalers* (MDIs), offer topical effectiveness and rapid (hepatic) metabolism of any absorbed drug; some of these permit twice-daily (bid) dosing to promote enhanced compliance. The addition of inhaled corticoids to treatment programs has significantly lessened asthma morbidity, measurable bronchial hyperreactivity, and both the numbers and the activation levels of airway inflammatory cells. These effects are almost

---

*Objective determinations such as patient-determined peak flow values are useful.

certainly interrelated and are routinely achieved without the systemic side effects associated with oral or parenteral corticosteroid use. Despite these safety factors, extrabronchial effects *can* be seen when dosing guidelines are grossly exceeded. In addition, local side effects rarely occur at recommended doses and increase as medication use rises; these include throat irritation, oropharyngeal *Candida* infection, and laryngeal myopathy (muscle dysfunction) producing hoarseness. Patients using corticosteroid inhalers can reduce the risk of these events by briefly washing out their mouths with tap water after drug inhalation.

Atropine and related anticholinergic agents also have demonstrated activity as bronchial muscle relaxants. The inhalation of an aerosolized congener, ipratropium bromide, achieves moderate bronchodilation without the side effects expected of a systemic muscarinic antagonist. Ipratropium is used especially when asthma has complicated chronic bronchitis but can benefit other patients with reactive airway problems. Adverse effects occur infrequently, and efforts to better define indications for this agent continue.

The benefits of administering antiasthmatic drugs by aerosol are now established beyond reasonable doubt. However, realizing their full value requires patient compliance and optimal inhalation technique. Although increasingly potent MDI preparations have been marketed that require fewer inhalations, these devices still are underused by many patients. Even more often, faulty inhalation technique limits drug delivery to the tracheo-

bronchial airways and increases deposition on oropharyngeal mucous surfaces from which systemic absorption readily occurs. The principal errors recognized involve the following:

1. Failure to synchronize inhalation and nebulizer discharge
2. Inadequate time before passive exhalation occurs to permit aerosol mixing and deposition in the airways
3. Interception and effective loss of rapidly moving particles by oropharyngeal "baffles" (e.g., teeth, tongue, uvula)

The box on p. 143 lists points of technique for optimizing lower airway delivery of aerosols. Many of these deficiencies are reduced when MDIs are used with spacers, which are basically reservoirs for aerosol. Such devices are essential for children and many adult users and substantially increase lung deposition (Fig. 10-6).

Although no longer asthma remedies of first choice for ambulatory patients, systemically administered drugs still offer potent options when lesser measures fail to control symptoms. For example, the addition of oral beta-agonists to a program of inhaled agents may suffice to restore comfort during brief or extended periods of need (e.g., respiratory infection). For many patients, however, side effects (noted earlier) preclude effective use of these drugs by mouth; inhalation (of increasing doses) remains the preferred route.

While less often employed, theophylline remains a useful antiasthmatic drug for selected patients. This methylxanthine agent appears to promote bronchodila-

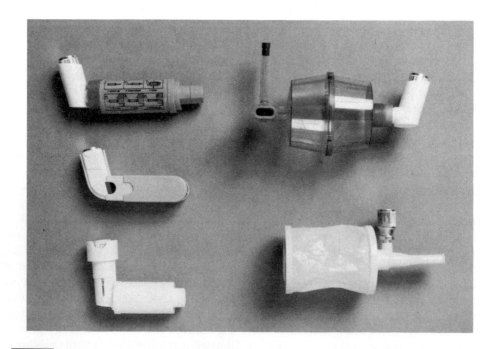

FIG. 10-6 Commercially available "spacing" devices for use with pressurized nebulizers, also called metered-dose inhalers (MDIs). Spacers provide a mixing chamber in which rapidly ejected particles can decelerate, allowing them to be captured more efficiently at the next inspiration.

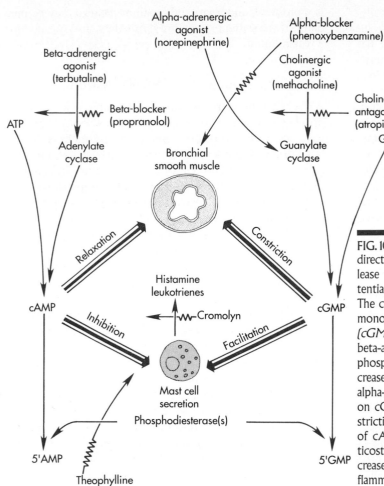

FIG. 10-7   Actions of drugs that affect bronchial patency either directly *(upper portion)* or by modifying mediator substance release from mast cells *(lower portion).* Smooth lines indicate potentiation of an effect; wavy lines signify inhibitory influences. The central importance and opposing effects of cyclic adenosine monophosphate *(cAMP)* and cyclic guanosine monophosphate *(cGMP)* deserve special attention. cAMP levels are increased by beta-agonists acting on adenylate cyclase and by inhibition of phosphodiesterase effect (e.g., theophylline). cGMP levels are increased by cholinergic agents (e.g., methacholine) and possibly by alpha-adrenergic agents. Effects of theophylline and other drugs on cGMP–active phosphodiesterases are not clear. Bronchoconstrictive effects of alpha-adrenergic agents may reflect inhibition of cAMP or promotion of cGMP synthesis. The scope of corticosteroid effects is uncertain, but they are associated with increased responsiveness to beta-adrenergic agents and reduced inflammatory cell movement into airway tissues.

tion by inhibiting airway muscle phosphodiesterase, thereby increasing cyclic adenosine monophosphate (cAMP) levels (Fig. 10-7); however, other effects may contribute. Several marketed preparations are well absorbed and are active for 8 to 12 or as long as 24 hours. Drug effects are closely related to concurrent blood levels, with maximum benefit often achieved in the range from 10 to 18 μg/ml; below 10 μg/ml, lesser responses are expected. Similarly, the risk of toxicity rises as theophylline serum levels increase; values greater than 20 μg/ml generally should be avoided. Individual tolerances vary widely, however, with some patients unable to achieve even the lowest therapeutic levels without discomfort. Intolerance usually manifests as nausea and vomiting, but bowel hypermotility (rarely with bleeding), palpitation, or anxiety may develop. Potentially fatal seizures and cardiovascular collapse can appear as blood levels rise further and, occasionally, may be the first signs of excessive dosage. The latter events are seen especially in older patients, those with liver dysfunction (impairing drug disposition), infants, and others unable to express symptoms (e.g., nausea) of milder toxicity. In addition, several drugs (e.g., macrolide antibiotics, cimetidine) predictably

CONSIDERATIONS FOR USERS OF METERED-DOSE INHALERS (MDIs)

1. Shake the inhaler briefly to mix its contents and invert (so pressurized canister is above mouthpiece) to fill the metering chamber.
2. After complete exhalation, position the mouthpiece two fingerbreadths from the open lips. (NOTE: When a spacer is used, the lips are closed on its exit port instead.)
3. Activate the MDI synchronously, with slow, full inspiration.
4. Hold the breath for a count of 5 or 10; allow passive exhalation; repeat steps 2 to 4 as indicated.
5. If appropriate (i.e., with corticosteroids), rinse out mouth and throat and discard the washings.
6. Record the number of puffs used. Discard the inhaler when the rated total has been reached; drug-free discharge of propellants may still occur after this point.

elevate serum levels of theophylline by impeding its metabolism. With attention to these concerns and the increasingly astute use of serum values, theophylline has remained a useful drug for outpatients who fail initial antiinflammatory/bronchodilator aerosol therapy alone and a continuing aid in emergent treatment.

Corticosteroids provide a variety of antiinflammatory activities that ameliorate asthma but also have the greatest potential for adverse effects with prolonged administration. This paradox can be resolved for most patients by regular use of inhaled agents (e.g., budesonide, beclomethasone, flunisolide, triamcinolone), but "steroid-dependent" asthmatic patients, who require regular oral corticosteroid treatment to maintain acceptable function, are not rare. For these, adequate control of symptoms with the lowest feasible daily dose of a rapidly metabolized agent such as prednisone or methylprednisolone is an appropriate goal. Alternatively, administration of moderate corticosteroid doses *every other day* may be effective while reducing both systemic side effects and suppression of hypothalamic-pituitary-adrenocortical function. The latter benefits must reflect brief periods (beginning more than 36 hours after dosing) when no drug effect remains, since required alternate-day doses often are more than twice those necessary in daily administration.

Persons requiring systemic corticosteroids have special needs for optimization of other drug therapy and of antiallergic management when relevant. In addition, possible contributions to symptom severity by factors such as paranasal sinusitis, gastroesophageal reflux, and vocal cord dysfunction* merit concern.

Because control of asthma may require doses of corticosteroids and other agents that induce unacceptable side effects, an active search for new approaches continues. Fragmentary evidence exists to support the value of investigational lipoxygenase pathway inhibitors, gold compounds, and twice-weekly low-dose methotrexate as "steroid-sparing" antiasthmatic drugs; however, none of these approaches has gained full clinical acceptance.

Antihistamines offer uncertain benefits, even in allergic asthma, and traditionally used agents, by drying secretions, may compound the problem of sputum mobilization. The expectorant properties of iodides and glyceryl guaiacolate (guaifenesin) remain controversial at doses that do not produce uniform gastrointestinal irritation. In addition, unpredictable adverse responses to iodides include painful parotid swelling ("iodide mumps"), prolonged fever, worsening of acne, and the appearance of other skin rashes. Benefits of simple systemic hydration should not be overlooked when sputum mobilization

is a problem, and many mild asthma attacks may be curtailed if the patient sits calmly, breathes slowly, and sips a warm liquid.

Treatment Approach to Severe Asthma

Although proper management can promote a favorable prognosis for most asthmatic persons, flares of the disease occur, requiring more intensive treatment or hospitalization and rarely resulting in fatalities. A sustained increase in symptoms often follows respiratory infection or the sudden withdrawal of a necessary suppressive medication. However, allergen exposure alone rarely precipitates hospitalization.

Medical aid is often sought only after many days of increasing symptoms. During this period, poor fluid and calorie intake coupled with increased respiratory work and fluid loss may produce significant dehydration and metabolic acidosis as well as progressive bronchial mucus plugging. As previously emphasized, the extent of airway obstruction is not uniform, and despite vascular compensation, imperfect matching of ventilation and blood flow in local areas of lung is common. Because of these disparities, portions of the pulmonary blood flow escape aeration, which produces hypoxia and tends to impede carbon dioxide (CO_2) clearance. The deficit for CO_2 is overcome easily by respiratory effort, which can clear this readily diffusible gas by hyperventilating a minority of adequately perfused alveoli. Because hyperventilation typically is an early response to increased airway closure, the partial pressure of CO_2 (P_{CO_2}) in arterial blood is often below the normal value (40 mm Hg) with asthma of mild or moderate severity. A rise to normal or elevated P_{CO_2} levels, therefore, signifies that an advanced and perilous stage of obstruction (and of ventilation-perfusion mismatching) has been reached. Similar compensation is not possible even transiently for deficient oxygen (O_2) uptake; as a result, arterial P_{O_2} values fall progressively as asthma worsens. Substantial increases in respiratory work compound these defects by greatly raising the O_2 cost of breathing and its penalty in CO_2 production. Ultimately, ventilation may not suffice even for the metabolic needs of the respiratory system. Fig. 10-8 summarizes changes observed in several parameters during increasingly severe asthma.

Epinephrine administration remains an appropriate first step in the urgent treatment of asthma, although inhaled beta-adrenergic agents (e.g., metaproterenol, albuterol) often are equally effective, especially if nebulized slowly with a compressor. If substantial improvement is not evident in 1 hour or less, other measures must be substituted. Epinephrine-fast asthma often yields to intravenous aminophylline, although oral theophyllines (including hydroethanolic preparations) rarely suffice. Because many hours of self-medication with ephedrine-like drugs or with theophylline may have occurred, an estimate of residual drug effects is mandatory. When pos-

---

*Episodic, "paradoxical" closure of the vocal cords may simulate asthma or angioedema of the larynx and may complicate otherwise typical asthma. Ventilatory test patterns and direct visualization of the larynx during attacks can be diagnostic. Voluntary control of this problem with speech therapy techniques often provides significant improvement.

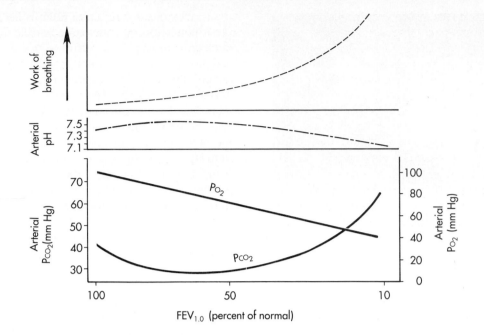

FIG. 10-8   Changes in the work of breathing and in arterial pH, P_{O_2}, and P_{CO_2} observed in asthmatic patients with increasingly severe airway obstruction *(left to right)*. Hyperventilation is adequate to decrease P_{CO_2} and raise pH until airway narrowing and plugging are severe (see text).

sible, rapid determination of theophylline serum levels can be used to predict dosage requirements initially. Persons without theophylline "on board" may receive 5 to 6 mg/kg of the drug intravenously by manual injection over at least 10 minutes, or by a "drip" infusion. Care will minimize instances of vomiting, hypotension, and seizures; however, a treatment facility must be prepared to handle these side effects promptly. Severe asthma that has persisted for at least 24 hours and is not substantially benefited by optimal doses of epinephrine and theophylline is often termed *status asthmaticus*. This condition presents a serious threat to life and should prompt intensive inpatient care with high-dose corticosteroid therapy.

Most hospitalized asthmatic patients require supplementary hydration to replace water deficits that may amount to several liters. The oral route rarely is adequate to achieve this, and a significant risk of aspiration must be faced unless fluids and medication are given parenterally to patients with air hunger. Without supplementary O_2, hypoxemia is present almost uniformly in status asthmaticus and should be corrected to a level of at least 70 mm Hg after initial arterial blood gas determinations. Supplementary humidified oxygen is best provided by 24% or 28% Venturi mask (Fig. 10-9) or, lacking these units, by nasal prongs.

When bronchial unresponsiveness to epinephrine has been confirmed, this agent is withheld initially, although some patients may benefit from regular doses of inhaled adrenergic agents. However, aminophylline remains a mainstay of bronchodilator therapy, and after an initial "priming" dose of 5 to 6 mg/kg, this amount is given by continuous drip during each succeeding 6- to 8-hour period. Appropriate dosage adjustments are facilitated by determining serum theophylline levels. In addition, the need for antibiotic drugs must be decided after appropriate cultures are obtained.

Systemic corticosteroids may be lifesaving in patients with status asthmaticus and are usually begun at or before admission. High doses are also given promptly to those who have required steroids either to terminate previous bouts of severe asthma or, within the previous 6 to 12 months, to use as a regular outpatient medication. Preparations of hydrocortisone or methylprednisolone for intravenous infusion are preferred, although even with these, at least several hours are required for initial therapeutic effects. Often, several days of intensive corticosteroid and other treatment elapse before benefit is evident.

A favorable outcome in status asthmaticus necessitates that competent personnel monitor the patient's condition closely, recognize deterioration promptly, and anticipate problems. Prominent complications can include pneumothorax, pneumomediastinum, aspiration, drug toxicity or idiosyncrasy, and cardiac failure or rhythm disturbance. Widespread plugging of airways may develop rapidly; it is manifested by a decrease in wheezing and by distant breath sounds over affected areas (an ominous combina-

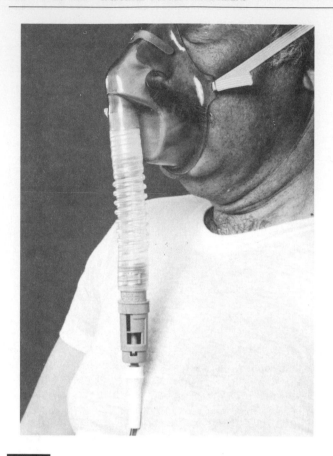

FIG. 10-9 Variable-concentration oxygen mask, using a Venturi effect, helps control O_2 administration. With this particular device, inspired O_2 concentrations between 30% and 55% may be chosen.

tion). Obvious deterioration often is heralded by drowsiness, confusion, and decreased muscle tone, as well as by a flagging of respiratory effort, signaling general physical exhaustion. This situation readily leads to inadequate alveolar ventilation with mounting hypoxia and rising arterial levels of CO_2. The clinical state and arterial P_{CO_2} correlate closely, and an upward trend is disquieting even though the absolute value may be normal (i.e., 40 mm Hg) or only minimally elevated. When P_{CO_2} levels exceed 55 mm Hg, despite a period of optimal treatment, mechanical ventilation must be implemented to reestablish adequate gas transfer. A volume-cycled ventilator is usually chosen for this purpose after placement of a soft, cuffed endotracheal tube; tracheostomy rarely is required. Details of respirator care are beyond the scope of this discussion. Ventilatory assistance in status asthmaticus usually is needed for only 24 to 60 hours, when improvement produced by bronchodilators, steroids, antibiotics, and other agents usually has become evident.

For many inpatients with severe asthma, attaining an audibly clear chest is a realistic and useful predischarge goal, even though ventilatory test results (forced expiratory time, FEV_1, maximum midexpiratory flow rate, etc.) may remain somewhat abnormal; in others, irreversible bronchopulmonary changes may preclude a wheeze-free state. In either case, intensive treatment is continued until the anticipated maximum benefit is manifest, and then preparations are made for an outpatient program. During recovery, bronchial responsiveness to epinephrine and beta-adrenergic aerosols generally reappears. Sputum production often increases during recovery; however, clearance of secretions may remain difficult despite optimal hydration and use of iodides or glyceryl guaiacolate (which have equivocal expectorant properties). Chest physiotherapy (i.e., repetitive manual percussion of the chest with postural drainage) is generally available. This approach appears to promote sputum mobilization and at times can dislodge obstinate bronchial plugs, permitting reexpansion of atelectatic areas.

QUESTIONS

▼ *Answer the following on a separate sheet of paper.*
1. Define bronchial asthma.
2. What is the pattern of ventilatory dysfunction in asthma?
3. What is the relationship of atopy to bronchial asthma?
4. Describe a postulated basis for the abnormal bronchial lability that is characteristic of asthmatic persons. In clinical practice, how is this bronchial lability confirmed?

5. Why do flares of asthma typically accompany viral or bacterial respiratory infection?
6. List the principles that reflect the newer treatment options for asthma.
7. Explain why drugs with intrinsic beta-adrenergic effects continue to be useful for acute and long-term management of asthma.
8. Describe the faulty inhalation techniques associated with administering antiasthmatic drugs by aerosol (metered-dose

inhalers). How could these techniques be improved for optimizing lower airway delivery of these aerosols?
9. Explain the role of corticosteroids in the treatment of asthmatic patients who need to maintain an acceptable level of functioning.

▼ *Circle the letter preceding each item below that correctly answers the question or completes the statement. More than one answer may be correct.*

QUESTIONS—cont'd

10. Which of the following tissue changes are associated with uncomplicated asthma?
    a. Gradual loss of supporting lung tissues
    b. Irreversible anatomic changes with diffuse loss of the alveolar walls
    c. Atrophy of bronchial smooth muscle
    d. Spasm of smooth muscle, mucosal edema
    e. Hypersecretion of viscid mucus

11. Evidence suggests that an important determinant of exercise-induced asthma (EIA) is:
    a. High serum IgG levels in bronchial tree mucus
    b. Airway cooling caused by evaporation of moisture from the mucosa
    c. Decrease in viscid mucus secretion
    d. Dilation of smooth bronchial muscle

12. Which of the following manifestions are typical of distressed asthmatic people?
    a. "Allergic salute" as a result of pruritus of nasal mucosa
    b. Hyperinflation of the thorax
    c. Rhinorrhea
    d. Dyspnea
    e. Prolonged expiration and wheezing

13. The following substances may be responsible for severe airway obstructive responses in some adults with idiopathic asthma:
    a. Aspirin
    b. Corticosteroids
    c. Ibuprofen and other nonsteroidal antiinflammatory agents
    d. All the above

14. Which of the following may precipitate individual attacks of asthma?
    a. Volatile irritants from organic solvents
    b. Exposure to mists and dusts in industrial plants
    c. Inhalation of cold air
    d. Psychic stimuli
    e. All the above

15. In what range (μg/ml) should theophylline blood serum levels be maintained for optimal theapeutic effect in asthma?
    a. 5 to 10   c. 10 to 20
    b. 10 to 18   d. 20 to 30

16. Which of the following are recognized effects of excessive dosing with theophylline?
    a. Headache

b. Nausea
c. Bloody diarrhea
d. Vomiting
e. Hair loss

17. Aminophylline may be given appropriately to treat asthma:
    a. Orally as a liquid or tablets
    b. Intravenously
    c. Rectally as a suppository
    d. By inhalation

18. Which of the following are effective as antiasthmatic drugs?
    a. Prednisone
    b. Metaproterenol
    c. Pirbuterol
    d. Albuterol

19. Jane S. was 6 years old when she had her first asthmatic attack. She was admitted to the hospital emergency room in acute respiratory distress. Jane was anxious and had shortness of breath. Her temperature was 99.2° F rectally, her pulse was 100 beats/min, and her respirations were 30 breaths/min. Chest examination revealed expiratory wheezing and normal resonance. It was thought that she was having an acute attack of asthma. The most appropriate initial treatment would have been:
    a. Phenobarbital, 25 mg orally
    b. Epinephrine subcutaneously
    c. Aminophylline, 50 mg rectally
    d. Albuterol rectally

20. Prominent manifestations of status asthmaticus include all the following *except:*

a. Wheezing evident only on exertion
b. Widespread plugging of airways
c. Hypoxemia
d. Increasing respiratory fatigue

21. In status asthmaticus, when arterial Pco$_2$ levels exceed 55 mm Hg despite a prolonged period of optimal treatment, there is usually need for:
    a. Mechanical ventilation using a soft, cuffed endotracheal tube
    b. A tracheostomy
    c. Both a and b
    d. Neither a nor b

▼ *Circle T if the statement is true and F if it is false. Correct any false statements.*

22. T F   Exercise-induced asthma (EIA) is most often seen in older adults with idiopathic asthma and does not occur unless mild wheezing is present before exertion.

23. T F   Diffuse wheezing is a manifestation characteristic only of asthma.

24. T F   In more than 70% of asthmatic people with allergic aspergillosis, serum precipitins are demonstrable, and almost all patients have elevated IgE levels.

25. T F   In early uncomplicated asthma the patient is usually symptom free between attacks.

26. T F   Ipratropium bromide is an atropine-like anticholinergic agent useful in treating asthma associated with chronic bronchitis.

▼ *Match the disease condition in column A with the appropriate description in column B. More than one letter may be used in column A.*

Column A

27. _____ Chronic bronchitis
28. _____ Pulmonary emphysema
29. _____ Bronchial asthma

Column B

a. Irreversible anatomic changes with loss of supporting lung tissue associated with severe airway narrowing with exertion
b. A prolonged and slowly progressive condition of bronchial inflammation and hypersecretion with or without airway obstruction
c. Predictable periods of dyspnea and wheezing with any increase in respiratory effort
d. Daily cough and increased sputum production extending over months and years
e. Spontaneous attacks of wheezing and dyspnea often occurring at rest; between attacks, patient typically symptom free

CHAPTER 11

Atopic Dermatitis and Urticaria

WILLIAM R. SOLOMON

ATOPIC DERMATITIS

Atopic dermatitis is a familiar, chronic skin disorder (or group of related disorders) seen especially in individuals with allergic rhinitis and asthma, as well as among their family members. High total serum immunoglobulin E (IgE) levels and multiple positive immediate skin test reactions are common with this condition. These associations would seem to classify atopic dermatitis as a de facto "atopic disease." However, the lesions of atopic dermatitis are not readily explained in terms of the transient wheal-and-flare response typical of IgE-mediated reactions. Rather, established skin lesions of atopic dermatitis show edema and variable infiltration with mononuclear cells and eosinophils, as well as fluid collections within the skin (forming clinically evident vesicles). Rupture of numerous tiny blisters leads to crusting and scaling. These changes and severe pruritus, which precedes and accompanies the eruption, are associated with excessively dry skin. Sweating also is impaired in this condition, and sweat retention often leads to prominent heat-induced itching. In addition, sebaceous secretions are deficient, and the skin shows both a low threshold for pruritus-inducing stimuli and an abnormal tendency to *lichenification* (thickening of the skin with accentuation of normal creases).

Atopic dermatitis most often appears in response to scratching in the first year of life (as "infantile eczema") with red, raised, pruritic, scaling areas involving the cheeks, scalp, and/or diaper area. In most children, the condition remits by age 5 but often only after the neck, antecubital and popliteal fossae, wrists, ankles, and waist also have become affected. The latter areas are prominently involved when this problem still is present in late childhood or when, following onset in infancy or adolescence, it persists into adult life (Fig. 11-1).

Intractable itching and painful cracks in the skin are major sources of discomfort for eczematous persons. In addition, the abraded, fissured epidermis is readily infected by bacteria, especially staphylococci, and by viruses that localize in skin. As a result, contact with herpes simplex virus, the "cold sore" agent, may produce a generalized eruption (Fig. 11-2), fever, and toxicity. An even more severe illness, eczema vaccinatum, has followed exposure to vaccinia virus.*

As many as one half of children with eczema may manifest overt respiratory allergy before puberty. Despite this strong association, it is rare to identify allergens that substantially determine the activity of any case of atopic dermatitis.† In persons with strong skin reactivity, factors such as house dust and pets may worsen the rash, appearing to act by direct contact with an abraded epidermis. Foods, especially egg white, cause skin lesions to flare in a minority of children and deserve careful attention. Although the importance of ingestant allergens appears to decline with increasing age, prolonged avoidance of food offenders identified by well-controlled test challenge is clearly justified.

Because no basis for allergen-specific measures is found in most cases, the approach to treatment of atopic dermatitis remains largely symptomatic (i.e., by non-specific symptom suppression). Care to avoid potential irritants and topical sensitizers is essential. Prolonged use of bland, inexpensive lubricants is the foundation of most treatment programs and often keeps the disorder

---

*In the era of compulsory vaccination, the high mortality rate associated with eczema vaccinatum had been substantially reduced by administration of vaccinia immune globulin and by improved supportive care.
†Although sensitivity to staphylococci does not appear to contribute, IgE responses to resident skin yeasts (*Pityrosporum* species) have been demonstrated and may contribute to this chronic inflammatory condition.

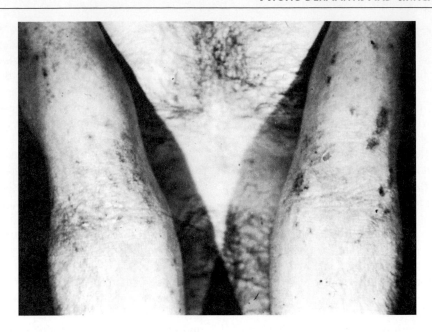

FIG. 11-1 Chronic lesions of atopic dermatitis (atopic eczema) on the flexor surfaces of the arms of a young man; erosions, pigmentary changes, and a deepening of skin creases (lichenification) are evident. Additional typical lesions in a child and an adult are shown in Figs. 78-1 and 78-2, respectively. (From Sheldon JM, Lovell RG, Mathews KP: *A manual of clinical allergy*, ed 2, Philadelphia, 1967, Saunders.)

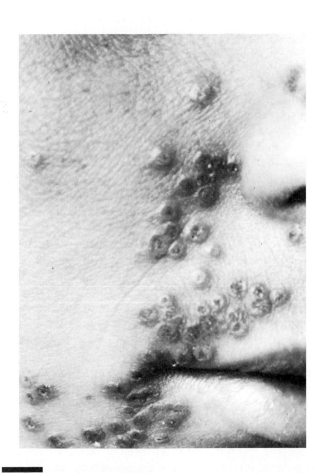

FIG. 11-2 Facial lesions of eczema herpeticum in a young adult with lifelong atopic dermatitis.

quiescent. Oil-in-water emulsions (e.g., water-washable base USP) may be adequate and act as minimally greasy vanishing creams. More effective lubrication can be obtained with water-in-oil emulsions (ointments), including hydrophilic ointment USP, Eucerine®, and Aquaphor®. Inert oils such as petrolatum provide maximum greasiness and protection from drying, but their occlusive properties often promote retention of debris, causing troublesome pruritus.

Topical corticosteroids are widely useful in atopic dermatitis, but these preparations should be employed for their antiinflammatory properties alone rather than for general lubrication. When indicated, topically applied steroids may be covered with an occluding layer of polyethylene to promote penetration of the drug, a strategy especially feasible at night. Steroids have largely replaced the once-popular coal tar preparations as antiinflammatory agents. Tars are still used rarely to reduce lichenification and cracking, although urea-containing ointments are more cosmetically acceptable agents to promote healing, hydration, and restoration of skin texture.

In managing atopic dermatitis, reduction of pruritus is both an end in itself and a means of interrupting the harmful "scratch-itch" cycle. Oral antipruritic agents such as diphenhydramine (Benadryl) and hydroxyzine (Atarax, Vistaril) are especially useful at night when subconscious scratch responses can do serious damage. Fingernails and toenails should be kept as short as possible (consistent with comfort) to minimize trauma, and, for young children, soft, padded mittens or restraint of the extremities may be essential to sustain improvement. Well-washed cotton clothing is generally preferred, and as a rule, fibers such as wool and synthetics that "snag" the skin are best avoided. Chapping because of cold dry air is irritating to eczematous persons, and well-maintained sources of humidification can offset the tendency of the rash to worsen in winter; organic solvents that defat even normal skin also must be scrupulously excluded. A more subtle drying effect is inflicted by the regular use of soap and water or by contact with water alone. This problem may be approached in part by using skin cleaners with low emulsifying activity. In addition, application of topical lubricants after washing or use of emulsified oils in bath water is often helpful. However, frequent bathing by eczematous persons is rarely desirable, and water temperature should be maintained in a tepid range since body heating usually will increase pruritus.

Acute flares of atopic dermatitis are especially frequent in children, with prominent redness, vesicle formation, and oozing. Brief periods of high-dose systemic corticosteroids will usually speed resolution, and antimicrobial agents may be required. In addition, cool soaks will reduce itching and remove cutaneous debris. As acute lesions begin to resolve, topical creams are employed, followed by the progressively greasier applications emphasized in chronic care programs.

URTICARIA

Hives (urticaria) are familiar skin lesions that, at some time, probably affect at least 25% of the population. Many clinical forms of urticaria exist, which suggests that a variety of determinants ultimately will be recognized. At present, it seems clear that *some* types of urticaria reflect immunologic processes, especially those involving IgE, whereas others remain totally unexplained. This practical reality must be faced, since the resemblance of urticarial wheals to IgE-mediated skin reactions often has prompted the false inference that hives per se indicate allergy. Microscopically, most urticarial lesions present only edema, variable dilation of vessels, and occasional neutrophils and eosinophils. In some patients, however, grossly identical lesions show a definite vasculitis with disruption of blood vessel walls and infiltrating phagocytes. The discrete, raised, pruritic, nontender lesions of urticaria appear most often on the trunk and proximal extremities, and individual wheals rarely last more than 36 hours. Angioedema (see Chapter 9) manifested by painless and minimally pruritic swelling of subcutaneous and submucosal tissues may be associated.

Most episodes of urticaria are brief and self-limited, especially in childhood, when hives often are related to respiratory infections. However, in a minority of adults (and rarely children), unexplained hives may persist for many months or years. Such persons should be evaluated for the presence of a serious underlying disease as the factor promoting urticaria; prominent among these are lymphomas, systemic lupus erythematosus, hyperthyroidism, and nonlymphoid neoplasms. Although chronic foci of bacterial infection and intestinal parasites are often sought in these patients, they are rarely shown to cause the chronic hives.

As with anaphylactic reactions, urticaria can result from IgE-mediated responses to protein allergens. In both situations the implicated agents usually are ingestants, especially such foods as egg, fish, diverse shellfish, and nuts, including the peanut. In addition, drugs and drug metabolites that are complete antigens or are capable of stable bonding to proteins (e.g., penicillin derivatives) are prominent factors in systemic or urticarial type I reactions (see Chapter 9). However, many drugs also appear to cause urticaria by mechanisms exclusive of IgE. Aspirin is probably the most frequent offender in this group and has been said also to worsen nonspecifically at least 30% of patients with chronic urticaria.

In some patients with chronic urticaria, environmental influences may play a role; cold is probably most frequently implicated. *Cold urticaria* affects especially young adults and may appear with the most minor degrees of chilling. Hives develop in some as skin temperature falls but generally require rewarming for their appearance. Cold urticaria has been associated with elevated plasma histamine levels (e.g., in venous blood from a chilled extremity), and both headache and hypotension may result. This effect has led to disaster occasionally when affected persons fainted while swimming and subsequently drowned. Urticaria also may be elicited specifically by local heating; the lesions may be immediate in some subjects and delayed as long as several hours in others. Total body heating (e.g., in a warm bath) can also worsen pruritus and whealing of diverse additional causes. Furthermore, *cholinergic urticaria* is a clinically distinct condition in which physical exertion, emotional stress, and environmental warmth elicit crops of tiny wheals, each surrounded by a broad border of redness. Affected persons typically show abnormally large whealing or erythematous responses to intradermal methacholine, although the pathogenetic significance of this reactivity remains unclear. A period of sustained running usually elicits typical wheals, which confirm the diagnosis. Local urtication (hive formation) or angioedema also may follow exposure to sustained pressure, various wavelengths of light, or vibratory stimuli. Some of these rare conditions appear to be familial. Furthermore, in certain examples of heat-, light-, or cold-induced urticaria, local specific reactivity can be conferred on normal subjects by transfer of IgE in the serum of affected persons. At present, it is not clear whether these "passive transfer" phenomena involve classic antigen-antibody reactions or alternative mechanisms.

Urticaria caused by pressure usually occurs in those

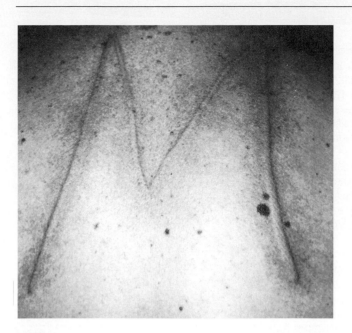

FIG. II-3 Dermographism evident 2 minutes after the patient's back is lightly stroked with a fingernail. The subject had occasional urticarial wheals at the belt line and on the buttocks after prolonged sitting.

with *dermographism* (Fig. 11-3), in whom firm stroking will produce definite whealing responses. Dermographism is longstanding in a small proportion of normal persons but also may be acquired, appearing after adverse drug reactions or in disease states prompting infiltration of the skin by mast cells. Dermographic persons typically develop wheals at pressure points, including the buttocks and soles of the feet, as well as beneath watch straps, belts, and tight underclothing.

Instances of angioedema accompanying acute urticaria are occasionally confused with *hereditary angioedema* (HANE), a familial defect in the control of inflammation. HANE manifests as recurrent bouts of edema involving peripheral structures as well as the larynx and bowel, the last producing intense abdominal pain and often leading to exploratory laparotomies. These episodes rarely appear before age 10 and may recur indefinitely, although their frequency often decreases after the sixth decade of life. Emotional stress or physical trauma (often quite subtle) may precede the edema, but many bouts are unexplained. Laryngeal edema poses a serious threat to life in these patients, and pedigree analysis usually reveals one or more instances in each family where this complication has caused death by asphyxiation. Swelling in this condition develops over many hours, regresses slowly, and is *not* accompanied by urticaria. HANE patients are known to share low activity levels of the factor that normally inhibits the activated first component of the complement system (C1) as well as additional components concerned with clotting, inflammation, and fibrinolysis. As a result

of this deficiency, C1 effects are unopposed, and C1 proceeds to activate and consume the early components of the sequence, C4 and C2, which, on assay, are demonstrably low in this condition. However, which of the factors, normally checked by the C1 inhibitor, may be responsible for the swellings in this condition is unknown. Treatment measures are properly focused on preservation of the airway, avoidance of needless laparotomy when bowel edema occurs, and general support. Currently available drugs contribute little to acute care; however, regular use of either methyltestosterone or other anabolic agents of limited androgenic potency (e.g., danazol, stanozolol) stimulates synthesis of the deficient factor and can greatly reduce frequency of attacks.

A few additional conditions lend confusion to the evaluation of ordinary urticaria and angioedema. IGE-medicated urticaria to rubber latex is increasingly seen, especially in health care personnel. Exposure may also induce respiratory symptoms or overt anaphylaxis. Occasionally, penetrants such as stinging plant hairs or insects produce troublesome whealing reactions. Chronic, pruritic, raised papules, termed *papular urticaria,* often follow insect bites, especially on the legs in childhood, but the persistence and induration (i.e., firm consistency) of these lesions usually sets them apart. Typical urticaria may accompany serious primary disease or may follow trivial viral syndromes, but frequently no cause is evident. Drugs or chemical additives in foods and beverages are often identified as sources of urticaria and should be evaluated carefully, although confirmatory in vitro tests are rarely available. Similarly, a painstaking review of historical details may provide evidence implicating foods, physical agents, or psychogenic factors.

Because bouts of hives generally are self-limited and vary in duration as well as severity, the value of treatment measures for affected individuals often is difficult to evaluate. However, epinephrine speeds the resolution of acute urticaria and angioedema. Agents such as diphenhydramine and hydroxyzine also have value in this condition, although both cause prominent sedation; nonsedating alternatives also are worthy of trial.* These drugs are considered to inhibit a type of histamine receptor termed H_1. A second histamine receptor type (H_2) is blocked by agents that include cimetidine and ranitidine; these may provide additional relief for patients with urticaria. Adrenocortical steroids have been beneficial to persons with severe acute hives but may fail to interrupt longer established disease. In chronic urticaria, optimal antihistaminic medications are of paramount importance with or without sympathomimetic agents. Of the former, hydroxyzine and astemizole (Hismanal) often are especially valuable. Although repeated study of such patients rarely is fruitful, all concerned should remain receptive to clues that may implicate a responsible factor.

---

*Claritin, Hismanal, Seldane, and Zyrtec are often helpful preparations.

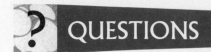

▼ *Answer the following on a separate sheet of paper.*

1. Describe the similarities between anaphylactic reactions and urticaria.
2. Discuss the treatment measures used for acute urticaria and angioedema.
3. What is the prevalence of urticaria (hives)?
4. Why are treatment modalities for urticaria difficult to evaluate?

▼ *Circle the letter preceding each item below that correctly answers the question or completes the statement. More than one answer may be correct.*

5. Patients with atopic dermatitis usually have increased serum levels of:
   a. IgE
   b. IgM
   c. IgG
   d. IgA
6. All the following descriptions are typical of the skin lesions of atopic dermatitis *except:*
   a. Edema
   b. Typical wheal-and-flare response
   c. Crusting and scaling
   d. Infiltration with mononuclear cells and eosinophils
7. Atopic dermatitis occurs with particular frequency among persons manifesting:
   a. Hay fever
   b. Allergic rhinitis
   c. Allergic eczematous contact dermatitis
   d. Bronchial asthma
8. Which of the following are characteristics of infantile eczema?
   a. It usually appears in the first year of life.
   b. It is associated with a great increase in sebaceous activity producing an excessively oily skin.
   c. In most patients it resolves permanently by 5 years of age.
   d. It is associated with red, raised, pruritic, scaling areas involving the cheeks, scalp, and/or diaper area.
9. Eczematous individuals who have contact with the herpes simplex virus may experience which of the following reactions?
   a. Fever
   b. Toxicity
   c. Generalized eruptions
   d. Localized eruptions
10. All the following are potential complications of infantile eczema *except:*
    a. Infection with pyogenic (pus-forming) bacteria

b. Massive hemorrhage into affected skin
    c. Sweat retention and severe itching
    d. Thickening and lichenification of skin
11. In children, acute flares of atopic dermatitis that are characterized by prominent redness, vesicle formation, and oozing may be treated by all the following *except:*
    a. Systemic corticosteroids
    b. Antipruritic agents
    c. Oral coal tar preparations
    d. Antimicrobial agents
12. Most urticarial lesions show microscopically:
    a. Edema
    b. Variable dilation of vessels
    c. Neutrophils and eosinophils
    d. Severe destructive vasculitis
13. Which of the following groups are most often affected by cold urticara?
    a. Infants
    b. Young children
    c. Young adults
    d. Elderly persons
14. The occurrence of cold urticara has been associated with elevated levels of:
    a. IgE
    b. IgG
    c. IgM
    d. Plasma histamine
15. Which of the following characteristics are true of urticaria?
    a. There are pruritic, nontender lesions.
    b. Inflammatory swelling of subcutaneous tissue occurs.
    c. Lesions appear most often on the face, palms, and soles.
    d. Angioedema is always present.
16. The evaluation of persons with unexplained hives that persist for months or years requires exclusion of which of the following diseases?
    a. Hay fever
    b. Lymphomas
    c. Bronchial asthma
    d. Systemic lupus erythematosus
17. In chronic urticaria the systemic medication(s) likely to be beneficial include:
    a. Corticosteroids
    b. Hydroxyzine
    c. Coal tar preparations
    d. Astemizole
18. In the causation of chronic urticaria, which of the following physical factors is probably the most frequently responsible?
    a. Cold
    b. Light
    c. Heat
    d. Vibration

19. All the following factors may elicit generalized cholinergic urticaria *except:*
    a. Physical exertion
    b. Emotional stress
    c. Environmental cold
    d. Intradermal methacholine
20. Hereditary angioedema (HANE):
    a. Involves the same mechanism as angioedema accompanying acute urticaria
    b. Manifests as recurrent bouts of edema involving peripheral structures as well as the larynx and bowel
    c. Produces laryngeal edema, which usually develops in a matter of minutes and is accompanied by urticaria
    d. May be effectively treated by administering C4 to raise the low levels of this complement component

---

▼ *Circle T if the statement is true and F if it is false. Correct any false statements.*

21. T F   In persons with atopic dermatitis, factors such as house dust and animal danders often worsen the rash through inhalant exposure.
22. T F   The approach to the treatment of atopic dermatitis remains largely symptomatic.
23. T F   Topical corticosteroids are used in atopic dermatitis for their general lubricating properties.
24. T F   In atopic dermatitis, oral antipruritic agents such as diphenhydramine and hydroxyzine are especially useful at night when subconscious scratch responses can do serious damage.
25. T F   Coal tar preparations are, at present, the most widely used preparations for reducing lichenification and cracking.
26. T F   To prevent chapping from cold, dry air in eczematous persons, organic solvents should be used.
27. T F   Anaphylactic reactions and urticaria can result from IgE-mediated responses to protein allergens.
28. T F   Hives per se indicate allergy.
29. T F   Local urtication (hive formation) may follow exposure to local body heating.
30. T F   Dermographism in normal persons may appear after adverse drug reactions or in disease states promoting infiltration of the skin by mast cells.

CHAPTER 12

Autoimmune and Immune Complex–Induced Diseases

WILLIAM R. SOLOMON

AUTOIMMUNITY AS FAILURE OF NORMAL IMMUNE MECHANISMS

Although injury is often incidental to immune processes, host tissues are rarely attacked by the body's own antibody or specifically sensitive cells. However, antibodies that bind to autologous tissue components can arise and may provide valuable diagnostic markers.

The lack of reaction to "self" components is normal and contrasts with the brisk response induced by (transplanted) tissues of other individuals and species. Selective unresponsiveness to potential antigens characterizes "immunologic tolerance," which may reflect several mechanisms operating singly or in combination. The tissue components that produce tolerance are the same ones responsible for normal immune reactivity. They include the following:

1. Antigen-presenting cells (usually macrophages and "dendritic" cells in skin and lymph nodes)
2. T_H (helper T) cells, which assist the antibody production by B cells and promote activities of other T cell subgroups

3. T_S (suppressor T) cells, which inhibit the maturation of B cells, from which antibody-forming cells are derived, and the activity of other T cell subgroups

Most antibody responses require that the antigen be processed by an antigen-presenting cell, be presented to a specific T_H cell, and be transferred with "help-promoting" soluble factors to one or more specifically reactive B cells. The latter multiply and mature into antibody-forming cells, which, as plasma cells, secrete immunoglobulins.

Antigen exposure may also result in T_C (cytotoxic T) lymphocytes, which kill other cells that display a sensitizing antigen, such as a virus or a tumor marker. To be effective in host protection, all the component cell types must be present and functionally mature and must participate in the proper sequence. A failure to respond will occur if a cell subset, cell receptor, or normally secreted factor is missing. The resulting immunologic unresponsiveness blocks immune events induced by all or most antigens. However, "tolerance" is antigen-specific, and it implies selective functional inactivity or loss of cells with highly defined reactivity.

Animal studies have shown that tolerance can be established in B cells, in the subsets of T cells, or in both, and it is most easily accomplished in fetal life or shortly after birth. Presentation of antigen at these times may promote specific tolerance. If immature lymphocytes (especially T_H cells) encounter large antigen loads, their function may be suppressed and they may die. With such clonal deletion, the ability to respond to a specific antigen may be permanently lost.

B cells generally require larger amounts of antigens to produce tolerance. However, B cell clones may be deleted, or intense antigenic stimulation may exhaust their ability to secrete antibody for long periods. Tolerance induced in this way may be sustained if antigen continuously binds all the antigen-reactive (immunoglobulin) receptors on clones of specifically responsive B cells. Depending on the amount of antigen present, T_S cells also may develop and restrict reactive T and B cells with the same specificity. Although their roles have not been confirmed, each of these mechanisms appears to contribute to tolerance. Clonal deletion is most easily accomplished in fetal life and is an important function of the thymus. Embryonic T_H and B cells that become constitutively reactive with "self" antigens are lost or their function is eliminated under extended exposure to these antigens. At any rate, the human infant is born tolerant to normal body components, and the developing individual normally remains so.

The appearance of autoantibodies or autoreactive T_C cells implies either an acquired mutation among immunocompetent cells or the activation of cells that had been suppressed but not eliminated. Several mechanisms may result in autoimmunity. With some agents, such as ocular pigment and endocrine gland cell components, the inciting antigens are normally sequestered in closed tissue compartments throughout development; therefore they may remain "foreign" even to mature lymphoid tissues. If injury releases these once locally confined materials into the general circulation, an immune response may occur, with secondary damage to the injured organ and antigenically related structures. This mechanism appears to operate in certain eye conditions (e.g., sympathetic ophthalmia) and in several endocrine deficiency states. Immune responses to host tissue components could also arise after more subtle injury incident to microbial invasion. The possibility that infecting bacteria and viruses may produce limited changes in host tissue components that render them "foreign" to immune surveillance has also been proposed. Antibodies (or sensitized lymphocytes) resulting from this process might have specificities broad enough to permit reaction with native as well as modified tissue determinants. In addition, autoimmune phenomena could result if an invading organism (or other introduced agent) and normal host tissues shared an antigen or closely similar antigenic group as a result of parallel evolution. Although invoked especially with regard to the pathogenesis of poststreptococcal glomerulonephritis and rheumatic fever, this mechanism remains theoretic. Finally, autoaggressive immune reactions may originate with mutant ("forbidden") clones of lymphoid cells programmed to recognize normal host components as "foreign." Alternatively, disease, including viral invasion, may damage T_S cells that normally repress such T and B cell responsiveness with "self" components.

Organ-Specific Autoimmune Disease

Human antibody-dependent, autoimmune disorders most often affect formed elements of the blood, with platelets and red blood cells (RBCs) attacked predominantly. Increasing evidence has linked the disease, *idiopathic thrombocytopenic purpura* (ITP), with circulating immunoglobulin G (IgG) molecules reactive with host platelets. Even when fixed to platelet surfaces, these antibodies do not cause localization of complement proteins or lysis of platelets in the free circulation. However, platelets, bearing IgG molecules, are more readily removed and destroyed by macrophages, bearing membrane receptors for IgG, in the spleen and liver. Evidence supporting this mechanism for thrombocytopenia has come from studies of ITP patients and subjects who have shown severe but brief platelet deficits after receiving ITP patients' serum. *Transient thrombocytopenia*, noted in infants delivered by mothers with ITP, is also consistent with IgG-dependent damage caused by placentally transmitted antibody. ITP may follow infections, especially in childhood, but it often appears without prior event and typically resolves after days or weeks. Persistent ITP usually can be suppressed by corticosteroids, which are thought to reduce platelet removal by the spleen and liver. However, if the disease has lasted 6 or more months, the prospect of prolonged high-dose steroid treatment with its inherent side effects generally prompts a splenectomy. Platelet counts usually rise and may become normal after this procedure, despite continued sequestration by the liver; in either case, lower steroid requirements result in most patients (see Chapter 19). Recently, patients with ITP have been treated with repeated infusions of commercially prepared gamma globulin (human serum immune globulin). This approach usually raises platelet levels for brief (or longer) periods and may avert splenectomy for some patients.

RBC membranes carry hundreds of described antigens, and immunoglobulins reacting with one or more of these are found in ill as well as in otherwise normal persons. Depending on the type, specificity, and number of antibody molecules involved, their fixation to membrane sites may have no effect or may shorten cell life by allowing extravascular removal (e.g., in the spleen) or intravascular lysis. When decreased RBC survival results, signs of increased turnover of heme pigments (see Part Three) usually can be demonstrated, and frank anemia will develop if RBC replacement cannot fully compensate for the losses. Generically, these conditions often are described as *immunohemolytic (IH) processes.* Hemolytic transfusion reactions are a distinctive form of IH process usually occurring when a recipient already sensitized to "foreign" human RBC antigens by pregnancy or prior transfusion receives blood containing these antigens. Much less often, transfused blood contains antibodies reactive with the recipient's erythrocytes. However, most IH processes arise through production of antibodies reactive with the body's own RBCs.

The *Coombs' test* provides information central to the description of IH disorders. In this procedure, antibodies derived from another species (e.g., goat) and directed toward human immunoglobulins and/or complement components are mixed with washed human erythrocytes. If these cells have human immunoglobulin and/or complement factors bound to their surfaces, the foreign antiserum, by reacting with molecules carried on adjacent cells, will tend to link the cells and cause them to clump

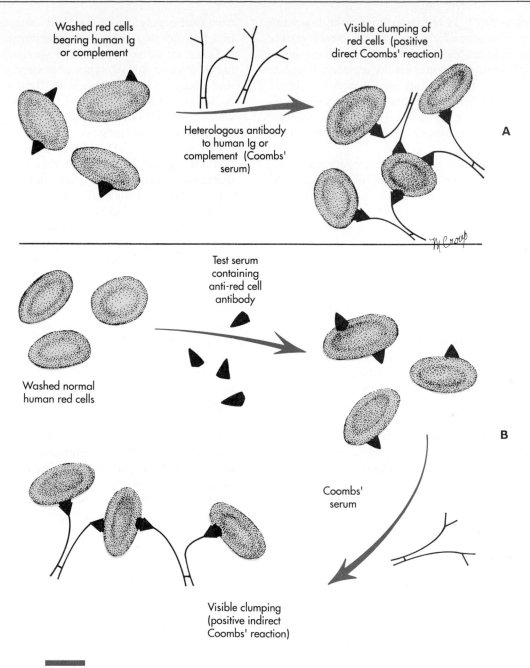

Washed red cells
bearing human Ig
or complement

Visible clumping of
red cells (positive
direct Coombs' reaction)

Heterologous antibody
to human Ig or
complement (Coombs'
serum)

A

Test serum
containing
anti-red cell
antibody

Washed normal
human red cells

B

Coombs'
serum

Visible clumping
(positive indirect
Coombs' reaction)

FIG. 12-1   Reaction sequences in the direct **(A)** and the indirect **(B)** Coombs' test.

visibly (Fig. 12-1). In practice the foreign (Coombs') serum usually is mixed directly with cells from drawn blood. A positive (clumping) reaction in this *direct Coombs' test* indicates that circulating cells with significant numbers of bound immunoreactive molecules are present. At times the direct test is negative, despite the presence in a patient's serum of antibodies reactive with human erythrocyte antigens other than those of the host. These unbound antibodies may be detected by incubating the test serum with human RBCs of compatible ABO and Rh types and then adding Coombs' serum. RBC agglutination in this *indirect Coombs' test* indicates unsuspected serum antibody. Coombs' reactions are often performed with antiserums specific for human IgG or the third component of serum complement (C3).

Hemolytic reactions to transfused blood provide the most dramatic and dangerous IH phenomena observed clinically. These responses almost always appear during infusion of the offending blood and are marked by rapid intravascular lysis of RBCs induced by the circulating antibodies. Those at risk include persons sensitized to RBC antigens by prior pregnancy, transfusion, or unknown factors that may include bacterial or viral infection. Victims of transfusion reactions have chills, fever, and low back pain, occasionally preceded by urticaria or flushing and often by uneasiness and mild air hunger. In addition, when cell lysis is massive, the resulting debris may trigger widespread clotting within small vessels. This process reduces blood flow to tissues and consumes clotting factors faster than they can be replaced. Bleeding from wounds and venipuncture sites typically follows. Survivors of severe acute reactions also share a high risk of acute kidney failure promoted by shock and massive hemoglobinuria (i.e., passage of free hemoglobin into the urine).

Considering these dire consequences, every reasonable measure to prevent or mitigate hemolytic transfusion reactions is justified. It is critical that the source and proper recipient of blood products be identified, and persons receiving blood, especially those whose mobility or awareness is impaired, must be under continual observation. If any evidence suggestive of an incipient reaction should occur, the suspect infusion should be discontinued immediately, intravenous (IV) access should be maintained, and the patient should be closely monitored. A carefully drawn venous sample from the recipient should be checked for serum hemoglobin, a sign of intravascular RBC breakdown, and the compatibility of donor and recipient should be reconfirmed. Without exception, all materials used for transfusion should be saved to facilitate serologic and microbiologic testing. Special precautions to monitor urine output are essential, and examination of serial centrifuged urine specimens for hemoglobin is useful, since clearance of serum hemoglobin is rapid. Maintenance of adequate hydration and urine flow are important in treatment, and osmotic diuresis with cautiously administered IV mannitol may help in achieving this goal. Safe fluid therapy demands precise and regular evaluation of cardiopulmonary and renal function. Measures to combat shock, pulmonary edema, acute renal failure, and defibrination with bleeding may be required.

In addition to manifestations of hemolysis, several adverse reactions may accompany transfusion of blood or blood products. Urticaria alone occurs rarely in recipients and, especially in atopic persons, may reflect trace amounts of food or other allergens in transfused serum. In those requiring blood repeatedly or after multiple pregnancies, antibodies directed to human leukocyte membrane antigens often develop. With subsequent transfusion of "foreign" whole blood, these factors agglutinate leukocytes and, at times, platelets. Such reactions are the most common source of transfusion-associated fever, although vital organs are minimally affected. Suitable blood for those with leukoagglutinins may be obtained by filtration through nylon fibers or reconstitution from the frozen state; both preparations are essentially free of leukocytes. Recipients of serum containing potent leukoagglutinins have developed fever, cough, shortness of breath, and lung shadows on chest radiographs; several days have been required for full resolution. In addition to these problems, personnel supervising transfusion therapy must be alert for possible air embolism, volume overload, septicemia from microbial contamination, chilling from excessively cold blood, and calcium or platelet deficiency after massive blood replacement.

There are three categories of spontaneously developing IH phenomena: (1) types associated with medications (see Chapter 13); (2) types with "warm" RBC autoantibodies reacting at 37° C; and (3) a group of conditions with "cold" antibodies that bind at lower temperatures and often only in a range of 4° to 15° C. Warm autoantibodies are usually of the IgG class and are recognized primarily in middle-age adults. In more than one half of these, a serious primary disease, such as chronic lymphocytic leukemia, lymphoid (and rarely nonlymphoid) tumors, or systemic lupus erythematosus (SLE), will become evident, and these conditions substantially determine the prognosis for affected individuals. The IH disorder may be manifested only as a positive Coombs' test (using antibody to human IgG); rarely it leads to symptoms or fulminant, fatal hemolysis. Usually, however, shortened RBC life promotes chronic pallor, fatigue, and weakness as well as recurrent fever and jaundice; dyspnea arising from heart failure, angina pectoris, and vascular thrombosis also are common. Splenic enlargement is a frequent finding, because this organ is the main site of RBC destruction. Splenic trapping of erythrocytes is most marked when both IgG autoantibody and C3 are present on their surfaces. When treatment is necessary, adrenocortical steroids are a proper first consideration; they induce remissions in more than two thirds of patients, although relapses are common when these drugs are withdrawn. Splenectomy is undertaken when steroids, in acceptable doses, have proved inadequate alone. In addition, immunosuppressive (cytotoxic) agents (e.g., cyclophosphamide, azathioprine) may be helpful in highly selected patients. Since warm hemolysins usually react with cells of essentially all potential normal donors, transfusions pose extreme difficulties and are avoided if possible. When no other choice remains, addition of Coombs' serum after incubation of the patient's serum with panels of cells permits the least incompatible ones to be chosen.

Cold autoantibodies to RBCs generally bind at temperatures well below 32° C; however, these molecules become dissociated at the warmer levels required for the "fixation" (i.e., cell-surface localization) of complement. Because of this, hemolysis may be absent and RBC agglutination minimal despite extremely high levels of autoantibody. Immunoglobulin M (IgM) cold agglutinins frequently are found in infectious mononucleosis and *Mycoplasma pneumoniae* infections, although decreased RBC survival rarely results. Chronic cold-dependent hemolysis is seen, however, in certain elderly persons, many of whom have lymphoid neoplasms and IgM autoantibodies. Besides stigmata of chronic hemolysis, these patients display signs of RBC agglutination (e.g., pain, cyanosis) in the peripheral circulation when they are exposed to cold. Treatment considerations usually focus on the associated malignancy, if present, although

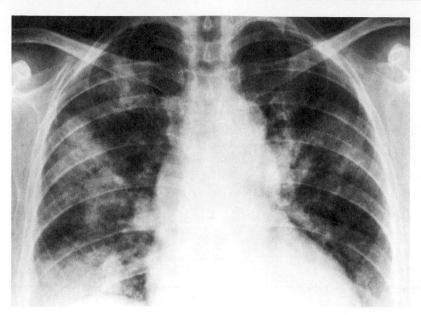

FIG. 12-2   Frontal chest radiograph during active pulmonary involvement in Goodpasture's syndrome. (Radiograph courtesy of Terry Silver, MD.)

corticosteroids or immunosuppressive drugs seem beneficial in individual cases.

General (Non-Organ-Specific) Autoimmune Disease

Goodpasture's syndrome is a rare disorder that exemplifies antibody-mediated human autoimmunity as a cause of major damage to internal organs. The typical clinical picture of recurrent pulmonary hemorrhage (Fig. 12-2) and anemia coupled with progressive kidney failure is described in Part Eight; however, the relative severity of these features varies among patients. Most cases of Goodpasture's syndrome have no *obvious* cause, although the disease has followed viral and chemical insults to the lungs. Circulating antibodies that are reactive with glomerular (kidney) and alveolar (lung) basement membrane glycoproteins, especially collagen, are usually present and, along with complement components, form linear deposits at these sites. The associated tissue damage reflects, in part, complement-mediated cytotoxicity and local effects of recruited neutrophils.*

Antibodies apparently reactive with normal tissue are associated with many additional human diseases, especially those of connective tissue (e.g., dermatomyositis, scleroderma) and thyroid gland inflammations. However, in most of these conditions, antibody-induced damage as such has not been easily demonstrated, although in some instances (e.g., SLE) pathogenic immune complexes are recognized. Complexes that contain antibody to double-stranded deoxyribonucleic acid (DNA) combined with that antigen are important factors in the nephritis of SLE. In addition, antibodies to organ-specific components and to nuclear and cytoplasmic antigens occur in SLE. Since these various serum factors currently are associated more with diagnostic than pathogenetic considerations, they are discussed briefly in chapters treating diseases of major organ systems.

SERUM SICKNESS AND OTHER CONDITIONS INDUCED BY CIRCULATING IMMUNE COMPLEXES (TYPE III DISORDERS)

Serum sickness is considered the prototypic immune complex–induced illness. Originally observed after administration of large volumes of unfractionated equine antiserums for prophylaxis of diphtheria, tetanus, and so on, this condition is most prevalent today after administration of drugs, such as penicillin and sulfonamides. The development of serum sickness requires administration (often by injection) of an antigenic material that will remain in the circulation until a specific antibody response occurs, as shown in Fig. 12-3. At that time the slowly diminishing blood levels of antigen drop sharply, signaling the formation of immune (antigen-antibody) complexes that are rapidly cleared from circulation by macrophage-monocyte scavenging and other mechanisms (i.e., "immune elimination"). Complexes form initially in consid-

---

*Many mononuclear cells have membrane receptors that lead them to sites of IgG deposition. Direct contact with these activated cells causes cytotoxic effects and other tissue damage without complement activation. This process, termed *antibody-dependent cell-mediated cytotoxicity* (ADCC), may play a part in Goodpasture's syndrome and many other hypersensitivity disorders.

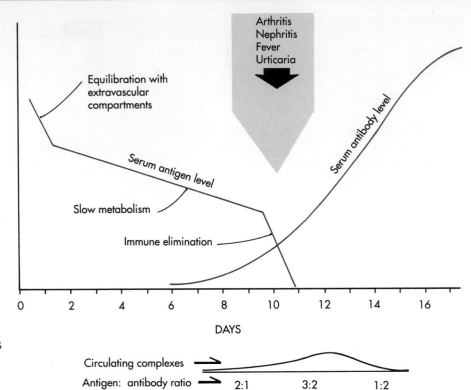

FIG. 12-3   Trends in immune reactants during the course of serum sickness.

erable antigen excess, with small aggregates composing one antibody molecule and two antigen molecules (or determinant groups) predominating. As antibody synthesis and immune elimination of the antigen proceed, a state of antibody excess progressively develops. Between these extremes is a usually brief period when modest antigen excess occurs and somewhat larger complexes with molecular proportions approaching three antigen to two antibody molecules predominate. Such complexes activate complement components and probably other amplification systems that mediate inflammation. Furthermore, because of their physical properties, these complexes are readily deposited in the walls of small vessels in many organs, including the kidneys; inflammatory changes follow at these sites.

After initial exposure to an appropriate sensitizer, manifestations of serum sickness classically appear in 7 to 14 days; shorter latency periods precede second or subsequent attacks if exposure is repeated. Usually the most prominent manifestation is urticaria (Fig. 12-4), which is often severe and confluent, and angioedema, although skin lesions may resemble bruises or the rash of measles. In addition, many persons develop fever, muscle soreness, and malaise. Lymphadenopathy, with enlarged and tender nodes, is often generalized and may be especially striking in those node groups draining the site of introduction of the causative agent. Joint pain (arthralgia) may occur alone, or frank arthritis may affect several large joints together or sequentially. Although genitourinary

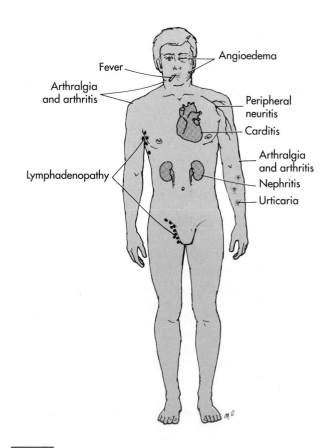

FIG. 12-4   Possible manifestations of serum sickness. Most patients, however, experience only fever with skin or joint problems.

symptoms are rare, urinalysis may reveal excessive excretion of albumin, erythrocytes, and leukocytes. Gastrointestinal complaints of nausea, vomiting, and abdominal pain infrequently dominate the picture, and cardiac and peripheral nerve dysfunction are seen rarely. These diverse manifestations often make it difficult to distinguish serum sickness from certain infectious processes (especially viral) as well as from such conditions as rheumatic fever, sickle cell crisis, glomerulonephritis, and bacterial endocarditis. Laboratory findings offer limited guidance in this differential process, although a modest leukocytosis, elevated RBC sedimentation rate, and transient depression of serum complement activity are characteristic of serum sickness.

As indicated earlier, complement-fixing immune complexes are implicated strongly in the causation of serum sickness. Among the complement system products formed (see Chapter 5) are *anaphylatoxins* (C5a and C3a), which can release histamine and other proinflammatory agents from mast cells. In addition, most affected persons have tissue-fixing antibodies that mediate wheal-and-flare skin reactivity to the implicated antigen and may contribute additionally to clinical urticaria and angioedema.* Furthermore, growing evidence indicates that mast cell–derived mediator substances that increase the permeability of small vessel walls favor the deposition of complement-fixing complexes. In support of this mechanism are data suggesting that prophylactic use of antihistaminic agents may reduce the incidence of clinical serum sickness in high-risk populations—an effect also shown in animal models.

Serum sickness typically is a brief illness and may require no medication. However, discomfort may be relieved with regular doses of aspirin for fever and joint pain, as well as antihistaminic drugs and, if needed, epinephrine to suppress urticaria and angioedema. When these measures do not suffice, especially if urinary tract or neurologic changes are pronounced, a brief course of corticosteroid treatment is justified. Careful prospective avoidance of the implicated antigen is essential, since acute systemic reactions and a more prompt reappearance of serum sickness may develop if exposure recurs.

Prolonged antigen exposure in individuals with only modest antibody responses can promote a chronic condition in which complexes formed in relative antigen excess circulate continuously. This situation may be readily produced in laboratory animals and, in humans, occurs with SLE, bacterial endocarditis, and prolonged infections, including malaria, syphilis, and leprosy. Deposition of immune complexes especially affects the kidney, where antigen as well as host antibody and complement (singly or in combination) may be demonstrated along the glomerular basement membrane or between adjacent

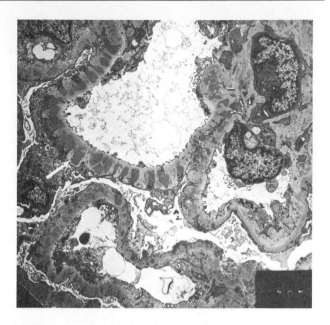

FIG. 12-5   Antigen-antibody complex deposition *(arrow)* in the glomerular basement membrane of a nephritic subject. The irregular "lumps" of material are typical of blood-borne immune complexes in which the antigen is not a kidney component.

capillaries (Fig. 12-5). As an apparent result of these deposits, inflammatory cells accumulate, the basement membranes thicken, and glomerular cells swell and proliferate, obliterating normal nephron structure. Changes in other organs are also recognized, largely because of accumulation of complexes in vascular walls.

A syndrome of fever, arthritis, urticaria, and low serum complement levels has been observed early in the course of hepatitis B and, less often, C infection associated with circulating complexes of viral surface antigen (e.g., HBsAg) and host antibody. As liver involvement becomes manifest, this syndrome clears; its subsidence correlates with rising antibody titers and, usually, disappearance of viral antigen from serum. Additional examples of immune complex–induced systemic vascular damage may be revealed in the future. In addition, effects of locally formed complexes have been implicated increasingly in conditions that include extrinsic allergic alveolitis (hypersensitivity pneumonitis) and rheumatoid synovitis. Although offending antigens remain speculative in many cases, longstanding viral infections and pollutant chemicals deserve special consideration.

CONTACT DERMATITIS: A TYPE IV RESPONSE

Delayed-type hypersensitivity (DTH), mediated by specifically sensitized lymphocytes, provides a major defense against fungi, viruses, and bacteria adapted to in-

---

*Most of these factors are probably IgE; however, in a few cases studied, this activity may have resided in other immunoglobulin classes.

tracellular growth and also deters growth of malignant cells. Inflammation involving these beneficial responses often injures normal host tissues. In certain situations, however, DTH underlies a response that is not substantially protective; the most familiar of these is *allergic eczematous contact dermatitis* (AECD). Indeed, in the North American population as a whole, AECD (especially that caused by poison ivy and its relatives) is the most frequently encountered allergic disorder.

AECD typically presents a pruritic, red, and thickened area of skin that often shows relatively fragile vesicles (Fig. 12-6). Edema of the involved area may be intense at the outset and, if the face, genitalia, or a distal extremity is involved, can mimic angioedema. With chronicity, although pruritus remains, the rash comes to resemble "eczema" of any cause, with prominent lichenification (i.e., thickening with accentuation of skin creases) and scaling. Involved skin shows an influx of mononuclear cells, especially surrounding minute blood vessels, and separation, by edema, of cells in deeper layers of the epidermis (termed *spongiosis*) and the adjacent dermis. In many lesions, mast cells are uniquely prominent in the inflammatory infiltrate. AECD reflects application of a sensitizer to the skin, and the rash typically is confined to the area of exposure. Although any portion of the skin surface may become affected, hairless areas, especially the eyelids, are more often involved. Reactions of contact sensitivity occur rarely on the oral, vaginal, and anal mucous membranes.

Contact sensitizers are highly reactive substances that often have quite simple chemical structures. Studies in laboratory animals suggest that these materials, on application to skin, penetrate to the deeper epidermal layers, where they complex, as *haptens*, with cutaneous proteins. The resulting conjugates are presented to cells of draining lymph nodes, where lymphocytes specifically able to recognize conjugates of the hapten and adjacent portions of the protein carrier are generated. Hapten-protein conjugation recurs with subsequent contact exposures, and sensitized lymphocytes respond, providing direct cytotoxicity and lymphokine-generated inflammation.

AECD should be suspected when highly pruritic eruptions have patterns of distribution that suggest specific topical exposure. Potential offenders are assessed through a comprehensive environmental review with special attention to topical medications, plant oils, cosmetics and perfumes, cleaning supplies, and work-associated materials. Possible sensitizers may be evaluated by attempting to create the disease in miniature through the use of *patch tests*. With this approach, extracts or solid fragments of test materials are placed on unabraded skin, covered with a water-repellant patch, and taped in place. In 48 to 72 hours the sites are uncovered and examined for induration (increased firmness) and vesicle formation (Fig. 12-7). Positive reactions may be intense, and painful skin erosions may result. Subjects should remove patches promptly if itching is severe; offending sites then should be washed thoroughly. In addition, patch testing may worsen ongoing dermatitis and should be deferred until the skin is substantially clear. For many substances, concentrations appropriate for testing may be found by consulting standard references. Tests with other materials must be carried out also on normal (control) subjects, who may be expected to respond comparably to primary

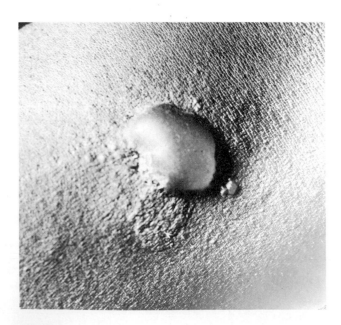

FIG. 12-6 Large vesicles at the site where a crushed leaf of poison ivy had been applied 72 hours previously. The subject had had recurrent poison ivy dermatitis for many years.

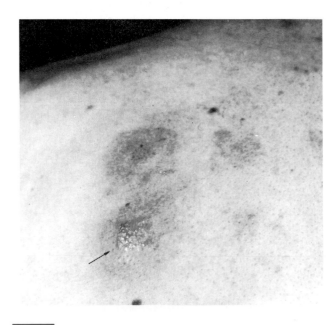

FIG. 12-7 Patch test reactions to procaine applied in several concentrations to the back of a sensitive dentist. Vesicles *(arrow)* denote the strongest grade of reaction.

irritant agents but not consistently to bland but sensitizing materials. Systemic corticosteroid drugs can partially suppress patch reactivity and are withheld, if possible, for at least 24 hours before as well as during testing; antihistaminic drugs and sympathetic agonists appear to have negligible effects. As with wheal-and-flare skin reactions, positive patch tests cannot signify the cause of a dermatitis, especially since contact sensitivity to some substances, such as specific plant oils, may occur in more than one half of exposed persons. However, test results provide essential correlates for use with clinical data in implicating exposure.

Photocontact sensitizers become allergenic after skin to which they have been applied is exposed to visible light or adjacent bands. In the recent past, a family of antimicrobial agents (i.e., halogenated salicylanilides) found in commercial soaps caused widespread skin eruptions in this manner. The resulting "photoallergic" rash—restricted to light-exposed areas—must be distinguished from eruptions caused by wind-borne contact sensitizers (e.g., plant oils) or direct photosensitizers (e.g., tetracyclines, phenothiazines, psoralens), which produce *phototoxic* reactions (Fig. 12-8).

AECD can develop after several years of unabated exposure or, through an unexplained "hardening" process, may diminish or resolve completely despite persistent contact with an offending agent. However, since dermatitis usually follows exposure indefinitely, avoidance of implicated sensitizers remains essential. Health care personnel who work with local anesthetics, penicillins, and aminoglycoside antibiotics, may develop contact sensitivity. Later injection of contact-sensitive persons with these drugs may provoke a severe erythematous or maculopapular rash, with fever and toxicity, progressing occasionally to extensive exfoliation of skin.

Established dermatitis is managed with soaks when open vesicles predominate and subsequently with creams for partially healed lesions. Topical corticosteroids are beneficial, although finite courses of systemic steroids often promote rapid resolution of the dermatitis. At present,

no available means of reducing sensitivity is sufficiently safe and effective enough to justify its recommendation. Patch test reactivity may be reduced during prolonged periods of ingestion or injection of specific agents, such as poison ivy oils. However, the results are usually limited and are rarely worth the time, effort, and expense required for such therapy or the substantial risk of inducing local and/or systemic dermatitis.

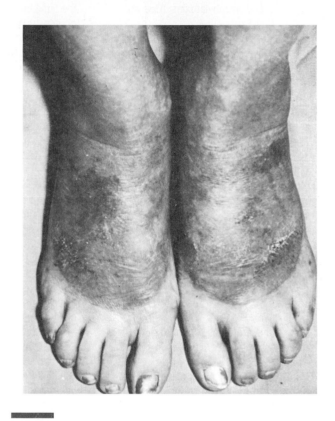

FIG. 12-8 Phototoxic reaction in a subject taking dimethyl-chlortetracycline. An immunologic process is not present here, unlike the case of *photoallergic* reactions. (From Sheldon JM, Lovell RG, Mathews KP: *A manual of clinical allergy,* ed 2, Philadelphia, 1967, Saunders.)

? QUESTIONS

▼ *Answer the following on a separate sheet of paper.*

1. What is the significance of the appearance of autoantibodies?
2. Describe the way in which immune responses to tissue components could arise.
3. Describe Goodpasture's syndrome as an apparent example of antibody-mediated human autoimmunity.
4. What are the usual manifestations (signs and symptoms) of transfusion reactions?

5. Evaluate the measures that must be employed to prevent or mitigate hemolytic transfusion reactions.
6. What reactions can occur when serums containing potent leukoagglutinins have been infused?

▼ *Circle T if the statement is true and F if it is false. Correct any false statements.*

7. T F Human antibody-dependent, autoimmune disorders affect formed elements of the blood,

with neutrophils and eosinophils attacked predominantly.

8. T F Hemolytic transfusion reactions comprise a distinct form of immunohemolytic process and usually occur when a recipient already sensitized to "foreign" human red blood cell (RBC) antigens receives blood containing these antigens.

9. T F Autoaggressive immune reactions may originate with mutant

Continued.

QUESTIONS—cont'd

clones of lymphoid cells programmed to recognize normal host components as foreign.

10. T F The pathogenesis of serum sickness probably involves complement system–derived products called anaphylatoxins (C5a and C3a).

11. T F Viral infection reactions may foster the immune response to "self" antigens by damaging CD4 T helper/promoter lymphocytes.

▼ *Circle the letter preceding each item below that correctly answers the question or completes the statement. More than one answer may be correct.*

12. The pathogenic mechanism of idiopathic thrombocytopenic purpura (ITP) is associated with:
    a. Circulating IgG molecules reactive with platelet surfaces
    b. Activation of the complement cascade
    c. Catastrophic lysis of platelets in the free circulation
    d. Platelets with bound IgG molecules that are more readily removed and destroyed by macrophages in spleen and liver

13. Persistent ITP may be suppressed by:
    a. Corticosteroid therapy
    b. Splenectomy
    c. Both a and b
    d. Neither a nor b

14. Individuals at risk for hemolytic reactions to transfused blood are those sensitized to RBC antigens by prior:
    a. Transfusions
    b. Pregnancy
    c. Bacterial or viral infections
    d. All the above

15. All the following spontaneously developing immunohemolytic (IH) phenomena are characteristic of "warm" RBC autoantibody reactions *except:*
    a. Hemolysis may be absent and RBC agglutination minimal.
    b. Autoantibodies are usually of the IgG class and are recognized primarily in middle-age adults.

c. Hemolysis is evident with rewarming after cold exposure.
d. The IH disorder may be evident only as a positive Coombs' test (with antibody to human IgG).

16. In serum sickness the pathogenicity of the antigen-antibody complex depends on the antigen-antibody ratio. Symptoms occur 10 to 14 days after first administration of an antigenic material when this ratio is such that:
    a. There is a relative antibody excess—three antibody molecules (Ab) to two antigen molecules (Ag).
    b. There is a relative antigen excess—three Ag to two Ab.
    c. The antigen-to-antibody ratio is equal to one.

17. Serum sickness:
    a. Occurs only after the administration of foreign serums to humans
    b. Occurs within a few minutes after administration of the offending antigen
    c. May cause joint pain (arthralgia), lymph node enlargement (lymphadenopathy), and neuritis
    d. Requires many previous periods of exposure to an offending antigen before frank disease is seen

18. Mr. J received an antibiotic injection 12 days before his admission to the emergency room. He has a fever and angioedema and is complaining of pain in his hip, antecubital fossa, and knee joints. His diagnosis is serum sickness. Which of the following is true regarding the pathogenesis of this condition?
    a. It is an immune complex–induced illness.

b. It is only IgE mediated.
c. Circulating antibody-antigen complexes are capable of activating complement components.
d. It is a delayed hypersensitivity reaction.

19. The treatment of serum sickness may require:
    a. No medication
    b. Aspirin for fever and rheumatic complaints
    c. Epinephrine to relieve urticaria and angioedema
    d. High doses of corticosteroids for carditis or neurologic manifestations
    e. All the above

20. Which of the following statements is (are) true of allergic eczematous contact dermatitis (AECD)?
    a. It is exemplified by burns caused by caustic detergents.
    b. It may be studied by patch tests of extracts or solid fragments of test material applied to unabraded skin.
    c. It is exemplified by poison ivy dermatitis.
    d. It is a form of atopic eczema.

21. An obstetric nurse has developed AECD to penicillin ointment. She last received intramuscular penicillin as a high-school student without adverse effect. An injection of penicillin at this time:
    a. Can be given with no fear of adverse reaction
    b. Would almost certainly produce anaphylaxis
    c. Would almost certainly produce serum sickness
    d. Would impose a definite risk of a generalized drug rash

---

▼ *Match the immunologic mechanisms in column B with the conditions to which they correspond in column A.*

Column A	Column B
22. _____ Goodpasture's syndrome	a. Immune complex–induced systemic reaction
23. _____ Serum sickness	b. Non–organ specific autoimmunity disorder
24. _____ Allergic eczematous contact dermatitis (AECD)	c. Organ specific autoimmune disorder
25. _____ Idiopathic thrombocytopenic purpura (ITP)	d. Delayed-type hypersensitivity reaction

CHAPTER 13

Adverse Reactions to Drugs and Related Substances

WILLIAM R. SOLOMON

More than 10% of patients who receive indicated drugs experience unforeseen adverse effects from their medication. This constitutes a substantial public health problem and causes a serious waste of human and material resources.

NONIMMUNOLOGIC REACTIONS

Many adverse responses are unwanted (but recognized) associated effects of drugs, or they represent frank toxicity arising from the dosage employed or its rate of administration. However, the reactions of some individuals are unique and inappropriate; these are called *idiosyncratic reactions*. Personal response patterns and instances of readily induced toxicity may arise from inborn deficiencies in drug-metabolizing capability or related pharmacogenetic defects. Reactions that mimic immunologic events are seen with drugs that cause direct histamine release from human mast cells (Fig. 13-1). Agents such as morphine alkaloids, thiamine, polymyxin, and *d*-tubocurarine share this property and produce whealing at injection sites or, rarely, generalized hives and flushing after injection. A similar mechanism may be responsible for certain adverse events (e.g., flushing, hypotension, urticaria) after intravenous (IV) injection of radiographic contrast media. Local anesthetics often precipitate distressing reactions marked by syncope, hypotension, cardiac rhythm disturbances, and, at times, convulsions. Although reminiscent of anaphylaxis, more likely these

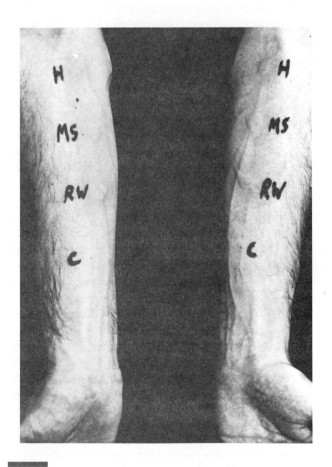

FIG. 13-1 Skin test sites injected intracutaneously with histamine, morphine sulfate (a histamine releaser), ragweed pollen extract, and a saline solution control. Several mechanisms have produced similar wheals in this ragweed-sensitive subject.

reactions generally are a direct toxic effect of the large doses of drug required for local infiltration. High blood levels may result, especially when these agents are injected with some force into restricted tissue compartments, as often occurs for dental procedures. Many reactions involving skin and/or internal organs are not otherwise explained and are often termed *allergic;* however, a causative immunologic process has been established in only a small fraction of these.

IMMUNOLOGIC REACTIONS

Type I reactions, apparently mediated by immunoglobulin E (IgE) antibodies, occur with systemically administered agents, such as foreign sera (e.g., antilymphocyte globulin). These agents act as complete antigens along with those of small molecular size that are capable of stable protein bonding. Adverse reactions to penicillins exemplify the latter mechanism, in which a drug and/or its metabolites serve as haptens. The sensitizing agent may produce anaphylaxis as well as "late" urticaria, with onset after 48 to 72 hours; penicillins may also produce immunohemolytic (IH) reactions, serum sickness, and allergic eczematous contact dermatitis (AECD). IgE responses to *injected* antigens are possible in most persons; therefore the risk of immediate systemic and urticarial reactions is not confined to, or even concentrated among, the atopic population. In human subjects, penicillin metabolism can proceed along several potential pathways, involving many final and intermediate products, some of which are allergenic. Of the resulting substances, the penicilloyl radical appears to be the predominant sensitizer, and antibodies to this particular substance are frequently associated with late urticarial and, at times, acute systemic reactions. By contrast, systemic (anaphylactic) responses with potentially fatal consequences make up a major proportion of the adverse reactions referable to native penicillin G or derivatives that include penicilloic and penilloic acids. Based on the frequency of associated reactions rather than their relative severity, the penicilloyl radical is often designated as the "major determinant" of penicillin allergy and the others as "minor determinants."

In clarifying the antigens responsible for penicillin sensitivity, efforts were directed to identify reactive subjects. This goal was attained, however, only after development of a skin-reactive but nonsensitizing "major determinant" reagent, through conjugation of numerous penicilloyl groups to the synthetic peptide poly-L-lysine. Skin testing with the product, *penicilloyl polylysine* (PPL),* is now widely performed, although minor determinant materials are less readily available. Both materi-

als assist in the evaluation of reported previous reactions and of the future risk of untoward events. In practice, skin tests are performed initially with PPL, a mixture of minor determinants, and saline solution as a control. Penicillin G is applied in a strength of 10,000 units/ml unless extreme sensitivity is suggested, in which case testing is begun at 10 units/ml. Because higher levels may produce skin irritation, 10,000 units/ml is the highest penicillin G concentration employed for testing. If epidermal sites are negative, intracutaneous tests are performed (see Chapter 9) with 0.02 ml portions of PPL, penicillin G, other minor determinants, and the control. Persons who react negatively to all these materials have been shown empirically to tolerate therapeutic doses of penicillin G with essentially no danger of acute systemic reactions. A small portion of nonreactors to PPL may show late urticarial responses or ultimately a picture of serum sickness. In addition, indications suggest that not all persons with positive PPL reactions would have adverse responses to administered penicillin. However, the predictive value of these test procedures is strong, and the high risk associated with positive skin reactivity (especially to minor determinants) is particularly noteworthy. Unfortunately, patterns of skin and systemic reactivity to semisynthetic penicillins (e.g., methicillin, ampicillin, carbenicillin) do not always parallel those to penicillin G and its derivatives. Furthermore, those with previous adverse reactions to penicillin(s) are at increased risk of harm with cephalosporin agents. These issues are especially distressing because only the unmodified, parenteral forms of the newer penicillins and the cephalosporins are available for testing (usually performed at 6 mg/ml). In addition, a single set of negative skin tests cannot predict lifelong freedom from adverse reactivity when that drug is repeated.

An immunologic basis usually can be shown for acute systemic and urticarial reactions to various immunizing biologicals, penicillins, and cephalosporins but rarely for additional agents, including aspirin.

In rare instances, autoimmune phenomena also are clearly related to the administration of specific medications. Several drugs, for example, including hydralazine, procainamide, phenytoin, and certain ovulatory suppressants, may promote formation of antinuclear antibodies. Furthermore, some affected persons manifest symptoms that mimic systemic lupus erythematosus and that recede slowly only after the offending drug has been withdrawn. Additional agents, most notably alpha-methyldopa, in some way induce red blood cell (RBC) autoantibodies that lead to positive direct Coombs' tests and, in a minority of persons, bring on spherocytosis and frank hemolysis. Drug-associated hemolysis also has occurred in persons receiving large IV doses of penicillin because of acquired sensitivity to a penicillin-conjugated RBC substance. Responsible immunoglobulin G (IgG) molecules participate in the direct and indirect Coombs' reactions using, respectively, patients' cells and "penicillinized"

---

*Available as Pre-Pen.

normal cells. Hemolysis characteristically begins 1 to 2 weeks after initiation of high-dose penicillin treatment but ceases shortly after the drug has been stopped.

Although hemolysis is not a feature of classic serum sickness, drug-associated circulating complexes are known to facilitate RBC, leukocyte, and platelet destruction in certain persons. These occurrences have been associated prominently with quinidine, antituberculous drugs (p-aminosalicylic acid and isoniazid), and sulfonamides, although other medications have been implicated. Initially, complexes of host IgG or IgM and drug (or drug-protein conjugate) become attached to one or more blood cell types. Complement components then are localized to these surface sites, and their interaction (see Fig. 5-13) results in discrete membrane lesions or rapid removal of affected cells from the circulation. In this process, blood elements are injured as "innocent bystanders" rather than as direct participants. After fixation of complement factors, the immune complexes initially responsible often dissociate from affected membranes. Such cells may show Coombs' reactivity with antisera specific for human complement (i.e., positive "nongamma" Coombs' tests) alone.*

Many additional forms of adverse drug reactivity are encountered with some frequency; of these, however, only AECD also has a well-defined immunologic basis, that is, in type IV (cell-mediated) hypersensitivity (see Chapter 12). A remarkably high proportion of topically applied agents are known to elicit contact sensitivity; among the foremost offenders are penicillin, aminoglycoside antibiotics, antihistaminic drugs, and local anesthetics.

ADDITIONAL IMMUNOLOGIC REACTIONS OF UNCERTAIN MECHANISM

Fever is a feature of many drug reactions and occasionally is the sole manifestation of an adverse response. Because granulocytes, monocytes, and other cells release substances that indirectly elevate body temperature, it is not surprising that fever accompanies a variety of health problems. Drug-related fever has been noted particularly with penicillin, sulfonamides, iodide, streptomycin, phenytoin (Dilantin), and additional agents.

Nitrofurantoin, a drug often used to treat urinary tract infections, has been associated with distinctive adverse effects centered in the respiratory tract. Affected persons manifest fever, cough, and variable chest discomfort, often with a marked increase in peripheral blood eosinophil numbers. Chest x-ray films obtained during these reactions often are abnormal, showing diffuse lung infiltrates and, at times, fluid in the pleural spaces. These rapidly developing changes are thought to resolve completely if nitrofurantoin is promptly discontinued; however, a chronic increase in lung fibrous connective tissue may occur without acute manifestations in those receiving the drug over long periods.

Many drugs are directly nephrotoxic (i.e., they cause kidney dysfunction and/or damage). In addition, several of the penicillins, especially methicillin, have been implicated in diffuse renal inflammatory reactions, or "interstitial nephritis." Drug-specific antibody responses often are demonstrable, but their significance remains controversial. Kidney damage also has been associated frequently with fever and skin rashes and may result from immune complex deposition.

The liver is a principal site of drug metabolism and often bears the brunt of adverse reactions to therapeutic agents. A spectrum of tissue effects is recognized, with certain agents characteristically leading to cholestasis (a failure of bile transport) with little or no inflammation, whereas others mimic florid viral hepatitis in causing necrosis of liver cells and collapse of supporting tissues. Cholestasis is an infrequent complication of treatment with certain anabolic steroids as well as some oral contraceptives, erythromycin estolate,* chlorpropamide, and so on. Bile stasis and jaundice also occur in reactions to chlorpromazine; however, pathologically, dense infiltration of portal areas with neutrophils, eosinophils, and macrophages is an additional feature, and progression to permanent liver damage is rarely seen. Frank hepatitis has resulted during treatment with isoniazid, alphamethyldopa, phenytoin, thiazide diuretics, and additional drugs, including the anesthetic agents halothane and methoxyflurane. These drugs may be associated with acute fatal reactions or may lead to a picture of chronic liver inflammation and scarring (i.e., a form of cirrhosis). In some instances, evidence of liver involvement may be preceded by fever, joint pains, peripheral blood eosinophilia, and a variety of skin rashes. Although such manifestations have led to increased speculation concerning an "allergic" basis for these reactions, the case for immune causation is preliminary, at best.

By far the largest proportion of familiar adverse drug reactions affect the skin. The resulting lesions generally are transient and not at all distinctive. Most "drug rashes" consist of macules (flat red spots) or papules (raised red spots), which are pruritic and tend to coalesce into a morbilliform (rubeola-like) eruption. In the case of penicillin, maculopapular rashes may be associated with reactions in tissue of drug-specific IgM antibodies; however, similar correlations have not been suggested for other agents. Failure to withdraw the responsible medication may lead to an exfoliative dermatitis, in which the skin effectively

---

*"Nongamma" Coombs' test reactions are obtained using antiserums to human serum components other than the gamma globulin fraction or specific immunoglobulin classes that it comprises.

*But less often other salts of erythromycin.

is shed, leading to serious infection as well as heat and fluid losses. Additional common skin manifestations of an adverse response to systemic medication include eruptions that are erythematous (diffuse flush), eczematous, vesicular (small blisters), bullous (large blisters), petechial (tiny hemorrhagic spots), purpuric (large hemorrhagic patches), and urticarial. Firm hemorrhagic spots often accompany inflammatory lesions of small blood vessels (vasculitis), which can involve diverse organs. Reactions to iodides (and bromides) may consist of pustules or merely worsening lesions of acne vulgaris on the face and upper dorsal area. Skin reactions occasionally are confined to discrete patches of rash (i.e., "fixed drug eruptions"), which become active with each administration of the responsible systemic agent.

PREVENTIVE MEASURES

The prevention of adverse drug reactions is a serious responsibility that all health care personnel share. An effective approach to this problem requires knowledge of the potential complications of medication and a willingness to consider adverse drug reactivity as a possible cause of any unexpected clinical event. Since untoward responses usually are repetitive, no drug should be given without first reviewing the individual's past experience with that agent. Similarly, the clinical data base requires no less than a comprehensive assessment of past drug reactivity. Health care personnel also must be prepared to accept, at face value, reports of previous problems arising from medication until these have been disproved conclusively.

Close surveillance can reveal the earliest stigmata of drug reactions, facilitating prompt withdrawal of the offender and, often, limiting morbidity. Once recognized, adverse reactivity must be clearly indicated in the clinical record (Fig. 13-2); if possible, the sensitivity should be identified for the patient or responsible family members. Documentation is aided, for practical purposes, if the patient can carry a card, bracelet, or medallion indicating medication(s) to be avoided. Careful instruction is also necessary when a risk of reaction from related agents exists or when, as with aspirin, the offender has many readily available and poorly identified sources.

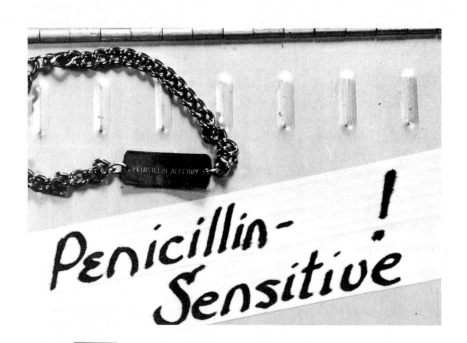

FIG. 13-2   Adverse drug reactivity may be minimized by clearly identifying those at risk. Well-marked health records and personal identification, as shown, complement patient education.

QUESTIONS

▼ *Circle the letter preceding each item below that correctly answers the question or completes the statement. More than one answer may be correct.*

1. Which of the following statements is (are) true regarding adverse drug reactions?
   a. Toxicity may arise through inborn deficiencies in drug-metabolizing capability.
   b. A causative immunologic process has been established in the majority of reactions involving the skin and/or internal organs.
   c. Idiosyncrasy is an adverse drug reaction that is unrelated to the expected pharmacologic effect.
   d. More than 10% of patients·who receive indicated drugs experience adverse reactions from their medication.

2. Wheal-and-flare reactions are readily produced by local:
   a. Injection of histamine into most normal persons
   b. Injection of ragweed pollen extract into most normal persons
   c. Injection of morphine into most normal persons
   d. Application of local anesthetics to the skin of a person with a specific allergic eczematous contact dermatitis to these agents.

3. Type I reactions, apparently mediated by IgE, occur with systemically administered agents that serve as:
   a. Complete antigens
   b. Haptens that are capable of stable protein binding
   c. Both a and b
   d. Neither a nor b

4. Regarding the predictive value of the results of skin testing with penicilloyl polylysine (PPL), which of the following statements is (are) true?
   a. Not all persons with positive PPL reactions have adverse responses to subsequently administered penicillin.
   b. Persons with negative reactions to PPL and other penicillin metabolites have been shown to tolerate therapeutic doses of penicillin G with es-

sentially no danger of fatal systemic reactions.
   c. This test accurately predicts skin and systemic reactions to semisynthetic penicillins.
   d. Persons who experience adverse reactions to penicillin(s) are at increased risk of harm with cephalosporin agents.
   e. A single set of negative skin tests can predict lifelong freedom from adverse reactivity when the drug is administered in repeated doses.

5. An immunologic basis usually can be shown for acute systemic and urticarial reactions to all the following *except:*
   a. Certain biologic substances
   b. Aspirin
   c. Penicillin
   d. Cephalosporins

6. Autoimmune phenomena are clearly related to the administration of which of the following medications that may induce formation of antinuclear antibodies?
   a. Alpha-methyldopa
   b. Aspirin
   c. Hydralazine
   d. Procainamide

7. Adverse drug reactions to nitrofurantoin are manifested by:

   a. Fever
   b. Diffuse lung infiltrates and fluid in the pleural spaces
   c. Decrease in eosinophil leukocytes
   d. Jaundice

8. Drug rashes are characterized by which the following lesions?
   a. Macules
   b. Papules
   c. Morbilliform eruptions
   d. Purpuric manifestations (purpura)

▼ *Circle T if the statement is true and F if it is false. Correct any false statements.*

9. T F The risk of IgE-mediated responses (immediate systemic and urticarial reactions) to injected antigens is usually confined to atopic individuals.

10. T F Drug-associated circulating complexes are known to facilitate red blood cell, leukocyte, and platelet destruction in certain persons.

11. T F Drug-related fever has been associated with penicillin, sulfonamides, iodide, streptomycin, phenytoin (Dilantin), and additional agents.

12. T F Most familiar adverse drug reactions affect the skin.

▼ *Match the medication in column A with its characteristic reaction in column B. More than one item from column B may be used in column A.*

Column A	Column B
13. _____ Morphine alkaloids	a. Bile stasis and jaundice
14. _____ Chlorpropamide	b. Hepatitis
15. _____ Isoniazid	c. Maculopapular rashes
16. _____ Iodides	d. Chronic liver inflammation and scarring
17. _____ Halothane	e. Whealing at injection sites
18. _____ Penicillin	f. Pustules or worsening facial and upper dorsal lesions of acne vulgaris

---

▼ *Answer the following on a separate sheet of paper.*

19. Explain the basis of the adverse reactions observed with drug-associated circulating complexes that affect blood elements.

20. List the reactions typically associated with the administration of local anesthetics. What is the probable mechanism of these reactions?

21. Discuss the considerations that are helpful in reducing the prevalence of adverse drug reactions.

CHAPTER 14

Approaches to Immune Deficiency States

WILLIAM R. SOLOMON

Current views of immune function emphasize the complex integration of antigen-specific components and effector systems required for normal humoral and cellular hypersensitivity. Both inborn and acquired defects have been recognized; the resulting flaws in immune competence may have no clinical consequences or may open the way for catastrophic infection or neoplastic disease. No attempt is made here to describe or catalog the various immunodeficiency disease states. Instead, this chapter focuses briefly on methods of evaluating immune function as they relate to deficiency states of several major types.

Deficits in humoral (i.e., antibody-mediated) immunity frequently undermine defenses against virulent bacteria, many of which are encapsulated and stimulate pus formation. Hosts with impaired antibody function are likely to have recurrent infections of the skin, middle ear, and meninges, as well as of the paranasal sinuses and bronchopulmonary structures. Repeated attacks by bacteria of a single antigenic type are often demonstrable, and, in those with the greatest impairment, naturally acquired viral infections and live viral vaccines also may cause serious disseminated illness.

Assay of serum immunoglobulins by *radial immunodiffusion* (Fig. 14-1) provides a widely available, direct measurement of circulating molecules having potential antibody activity. In this procedure, test serums and samples of known immunoglobulin (Ig) content are placed in separate wells cut into agar that contains antiserum, derived from another species, to human IgA, IgG, IgM, or IgD. As the human serum diffuses outward, a line of precipitation forms at the forward edge, where a favorable ratio of antiserum and specific human Ig is achieved; within this perimeter, an excess of the Ig (here, serving as the antigen) suppresses precipitation. The ring diameter around each well is proportional to the Ig content of the test serum added, and absolute levels* are derived by re-

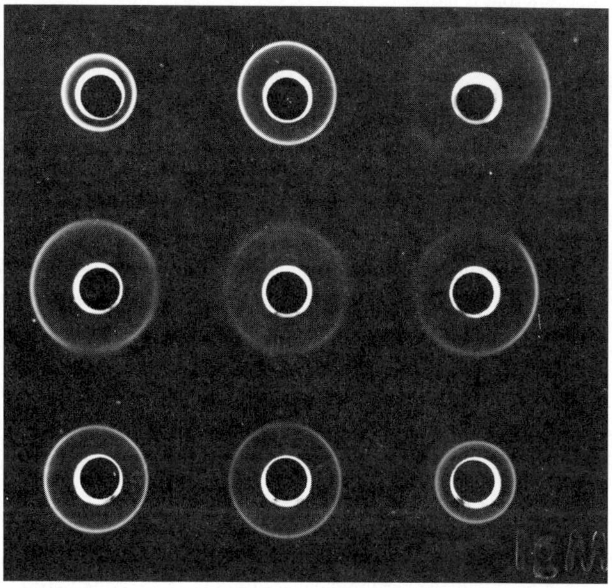

FIG. 14-1   Determination of immunoglobulin (Ig) levels by radial immunodiffusion. The agar plate shown contains goat antihuman IgM. The IgM content of samples added to the wells is evidenced by the diameters of the resulting circles of precipitation. The uppermost row of wells contains known serums of increasing IgM content *[left to right]*, allowing the system to be calibrated.

ferring to assayed "known" samples. (Determination of IgE content requires alternative techniques employing radioactive or other markers because of the lower range in which levels of this Ig fall.) Normal total values for specific Ig classes are indicated in Table 14-1. More discrete deficiencies of one or more of the IgG subclasses (i.e., IgG1 to IgG4) are also recognized to promote bacterial infection.

Several methods are available to evaluate antigen-specific antibody activity associated with one or more Ig classes, including the following:

1. Determination of naturally occurring (IgM) antibodies to ABO blood group substances that are ab-

---

*The traditional approach has been replaced in some laboratories by *nephelometry,* in which test serum and antihuman Ig isotope are reacted in solution and the resulting turbidity measured by light scatter.

TABLE 14-1   Normal Serum Immunoglobulin (Ig) Levels at Various Ages*

Age	IgG (mg/dl)	IgA (mg/dl)	IgM (mg/dl)	IgE (IU/ml†)
At birth	650-1250	1-6	5-35	1-3
1-3	250-1320	15-160	15-115	10-500
5-10	550-1450	20-220	30-135	15-600
10-15	620-1450	30-230	35-150	20-750
Adult	720-1800	60-300	45-160	25-900

*Values are approximations of expected ranges derived from several sources.

†IU (international unit) = 2.3 nanograms (ng) IgE.

sent from subjects' own red blood cells (RBCs). Normal persons consistently demonstrate such iso-hemagglutinins by age 1 year.

2. Schick testing of persons previously immunized with diphtheria toxoid. If adequate levels of specific (IgG) antibody have been produced, tissue breakdown at the site of toxin injection is prevented.

3. Determination of antibody titers before and after nonviable immunizing materials using proteins (tetanus toxoid and influenza vaccine) or pneumococcal polysaccharides (Pneumovax). These determinations generally are available from state or large municipal health departments.

In addition, estimates of circulating B lymphocyte numbers may be made by *immunofluorescent staining* of the Ig molecules that typically are prominent on their cell surfaces. In the blood of normal persons, approximately 15% to 20% of lymphocytes bear such markers, identifying them as B lymphocytes.

In certain immunodeficiency states, early B cell forms showing either *no* surface Ig or IgM and IgD *alone* may be found. The numbers and functional state of T lymphocytes also affect antibody secretion, since antigen recognition by T cells must precede most antibody (humoral) responses. T helper cells that bear the CD4* membrane marker also drive B cell proliferation and development into Ig-secreting plasma cells. Conversely, T suppressor cells (bearing CD8) may act to down-regulate B cell responses. Determining the numbers of these T cell subsets can provide a clue to factors responsible for defective antibody responses as well as impaired cell-mediated immunity (CMI). In acquired immunodeficiency syndrome (AIDS; see Chapter 15) the human immunodeficiency virus type 1 (HIV-1) directly attacks the CD4 molecule and progressively destroys the helper T cells that bear it;

as a result, specific antibody responses and CMI are impaired.

The most frequently encountered form of continuing antibody-dependent immunodeficiency is a selective *deficit of IgA*, which is observed in 1 in every 500 to 1000 persons. Serum levels of IgA are less than 5 mg/dl in this condition, and at mucosal surfaces the normal preponderance of IgA typically is replaced by IgG and IgM. Some affected persons remain free of evident illness, but many manifest recurrent paranasal sinus and pulmonary infections. In addition, increased risks of atopic allergic problems and certain rheumatic and gastrointestinal diseases seem to exist in this condition. Replacement of deficient serum IgA is not feasible, and systemic reactions caused by anti-IgA antibodies may follow transfusion of human blood products containing IgA (see Chapter 12).

Male patients with (Bruton's) *X-linked hypogammaglobulinemia* exhibit the most severe selective deficiency of humoral immune function, with virtual absence of circulating immunoglobulins and B cells. In addition, these individuals have marked reduction in the size and structural organization of lymph nodes and lymphoid tissues of the pharynx and gut (see Chapter 5). Recurrent purulent infections usually begin after 4 to 6 months of age, when transplacentally acquired levels of maternal IgG have been cleared and are no longer protective. Otitis media, bronchitis, pneumonitis, meningitis, and skin infections are prominent and often lead to permanent organ damage, such as bronchiectasis. In addition, viruses, including hepatitis B and attenuated strains present in certain vaccines, may produce severe illnesses, at times with central nervous system damage. Rapidly progressive tooth decay and chronic conjunctivitis often add to patients' discomfort, and an eczematous dermatitis, arthritis resembling rheumatoid disease, and intestinal malabsorption are frequently associated. The administration of commercial gamma globulin by injection controls many of these problems and complements appropriate antibiotic treatment; adequate doses usually approximate 0.2 to 0.4 ml/kg every 2 to 4 weeks. These preparations contain no IgA or IgM and, possibly as a result, fail to control infection in some persons despite maximum doses. Although intramuscular (IM) administration had been the norm, current preparations largely free of molecular aggregates now permit high-dose intravenous (IV) replacement.

Persons of either sex with low Ig levels and infections beginning after infancy are seen with some frequency. This group with acquired, "common, variable immunodeficiency (hypogammaglobulinemia)" often have prominent lymph nodes and intestinal lymphoid aggregates as well as normal numbers of circulating B cells. However, Ig synthesis and/or secretion tends to be deficient. As a result, these persons experience recurrent and sustained sinopulmonary infections as well as intestinal malabsorption, often augmented by infection with the protozoan *Giardia lamblia.* Affected persons and their relatives

---

*The CD ("cluster designation") system is used to define groups (clusters) of cells that bear a particular membrane component as defined by the binding to them of a specific monoclonal antibody. Certain CD-defined specificities may be found on several different types of cells; some are associated with molecules having well-recognized functions.

have an increased risk of autoantibodies and related diseases, including idiopathic thrombocytopenic purpura (ITP), immunohemolytic (IH) anemia, pernicious anemia, systemic lupus erythematosus (SLE), and rheumatoid arthritis. Laboratory evidence of impaired T cell function also has been obtained in some patients. Appropriate antibiotic therapy and Ig replacement provide substantial benefit in most cases.

Humoral immunodeficiency is especially prominent in certain malignant states, such as multiple myeloma and chronic lymphocytic leukemia, and becomes a concern whenever tumor cells infiltrate lymphoreticular structures. Similar infectious problems (with pyogenic bacteria) may develop in persons deficient in one or more serum complement factors as well as with inadequate leukocyte numbers or function. Serum levels of C3 may be assayed by radial immunodiffusion. In addition, overall complement activity is usually estimated from the ability of test serums to facilitate hemolysis of optimally sensitized RBCs; this capacity is expressed as "CH_{50} activity." Granulocyte deficiencies may be inborn or may accompany conditions such as alcoholism or corticosteroid excess. Defects in leukocyte function may affect random movement, directed movement (chemotaxis), phagocytosis, formation of enzymatically active vacuoles, and intracellular killing by white blood cells (WBCs). These modalities can be examined individually with acceptable precision in only a few laboratories. More generally available studies include the WBC count, leukocyte morphology in peripheral blood smears, and peroxidase stain to confirm the content of myeloperoxidase, a leukocyte enzyme required for intracellular killing of certain ingested organisms.

In addition, the quantitative assay of *nitroblue tetrazolium* (NBT) dye reduction provides a valuable clue to the diagnosis of *chronic granulomatous disease* (CGD) (of childhood). Recurrent infection by *Staphylococcus aureus (Micrococcus pyogenes), Pseudomonas* species, and *Escherichia coli* as well as organisms normally of low virulence (e.g., *Serratia, Staphylococcus epidermidis, Candida*) are typical of this X-linked disorder.* Offending organisms are ingested normally but escape death and can multiply intracellularly, ultimately destroying the inept phagocytes; a clinical picture of recurrent abscesses, indolent drainage of lymph nodes, osteomyelitis, pneumonia, and persistent diarrhea results. Defective killing appears to reflect impaired leukocyte metabolism with decreased generation of hydrogen peroxide and related substances that inactivate living microorganisms.† The metabolic defect also precludes the normal reduction of NBT to a readily visible blue-black form, a deficit easily quantitated by colorimetric assay, useful as

a disease marker, and increasingly subject to confirmation by deoxyribonucleic acid (DNA) analysis.

Cell-mediated immune function is inadequate in many disease states either as a "primary defect" or secondary to disorders including sarcoidosis, Hodgkin's disease, certain non-Hodgkin's neoplasms, and uremia; therapy with corticosteroids or cytotoxic drugs (e.g., cyclophosphamide) is also a frequent factor. In addition, CMI may be impaired transiently by viral infections such as rubeola (measles). Of the steadily growing list of conditions associated with abnormalities of T cell function, many also display some aberrant humoral (i.e., B cell–dependent) function. Overall, persons with these disorders are prone to infection by characteristic organisms that include viruses; protozoa, especially *Pneumocystis carinii;* fungi; and bacteria, especially intracellular forms. Lymphoreticular malignancies are common terminal complications of many of these disorders.

Relatively complete absence of T cell function occurs when the thymus fails to develop (as in *DiGeorge syndrome*), and affected infants have been restored immunologically to adequate function with grafts of early fetal thymus tissue. The most compromised individuals have *severe combined immunodeficiency* (SCID), totally lack B cell as well as T cell function, and often succumb within the first year of life. Transplantation of bone marrow from optimally matched donors has permitted survival, and partial reconstitution has been achieved with early fetal liver or thymus grafts. A variety of other conditions with combined defects are recognized; most often observed are the *Wiskott-Aldrich syndrome* (eczema, platelet deficiency, low IgM level) and *ataxia telangiectasia* (ataxia, spontaneous movements, vascular malformations of skin and conjunctiva, mental retardation), both of which are familial. In addition, AIDS presents severe defects in cellular and humoral immunity because of the assault of the HIV-1 retrovirus on CD4-bearing T lymphocytes and other cells (see Chapter 15).

Although numerous correlates and functional components of CMI are recognized, only a few are widely tested at present. T cell defects may be reflected in decreased numbers of peripheral blood lymphocytes (the majority of which are T cells), and counts consistently less than $1200/\mu l$ ($2000/\mu l$ in infancy) suggest cellular immunodeficiency. Reactivity to *delayed-type hypersensitivity* (DTH) skin tests provides a readily available indicator of cellular immune competence. For this purpose, intradermal injections are performed with 0.1 ml portions of substances that elicit DTH and to which a previous sensitizing exposure may be assumed. Frequently used materials include purified protein derivative of the tubercle bacillus (PPD), tetanus toxoid, and antigens from *Candida albicans,* mumps virus, *Histoplasma capsulatum,* and fungi of superficial skin infections. Test sites are observed and palpated after 48 hours, and an indurated area with a diameter of 10 mm or larger generally is regarded as a positive reaction. Using a "battery" of such materials, at least

---

*A variant form in females is known to occur rarely.
†Recently, partial correction of this defect has followed treatment with a lymphokine, gamma interferon.

one positive test should be evident in the vast majority of normal individuals (excluding infants). For nonreactors, the next step has become determination of B and T cell categories using monoclonal antibodies to tag their cell membrane components. Automated approaches to such assays (i.e., by flow cytometry) can estimate levels of helper/inducer, suppressor/cytotoxic and null cells as well as functional subcomponents within these groups. Additional tests reflecting T cell function may include the following:

1. Response of lymphocytes in short-term tissue culture to antigens and nonspecific agents (e.g., phytohemagglutinin) that stimulate cell division and associated nucleic acid synthesis. An increase in the incorporation of added thymidine tagged with tritium normally is observed in response to these agents.

2. Peripheral aggregation of sheep RBCs (i.e., "rosette formation") around human peripheral lymphocytes (T lymphocytes) when the two are mixed and incubated (Fig. 14-2). Normally, more than 60% of lymphocytes demonstrate rosetting, although a teleologic basis for the sheep cell receptor is unknown.

3. Assays of lymphokines produced in response to appropriate antigens added to lymphocyte preparations (see Chapter 5). Currently available monoclonal antibodies provide an expanding variety of specific reagents.

Antigen-specific defects in CMI also are recognized; perhaps the best-studied example is *chronic mucocutaneous candidiasis* (Fig. 14-3). In this condition, indolent *Candida albicans* infection with granuloma formation occurs. Although systemic dissemination is almost unknown, oral candidiasis (thrush), esophageal involvement with dysphagia (difficulty in swallowing), and *Candida* vaginitis may cause severe distress. In addition, affected individuals often show autoantibodies reactive with endocrine tissues and defects in endocrine function (especially adrenal and parathyroid deficiencies) as a possible result. Although CMI to *Candida* is ineffective in this condition, other T cell functions usually are intact. Defective responses to *Candida* antigens vary among patients, being total in some, whereas others show intact lymphocyte mitogenic responses despite negative skin tests at 48 hours; in a few, circulating inhibitors of *Candida*-directed CMI occur. Treatment with newer anti-*Candida* agents has greatly improved the outlook for these patients. Repeated injection of transfer factor (see Chapter 5) prepared from lymphocytes of persons with strong DTH to *Candida* has led to prolonged remissions in some patients but remains an experimental approach.

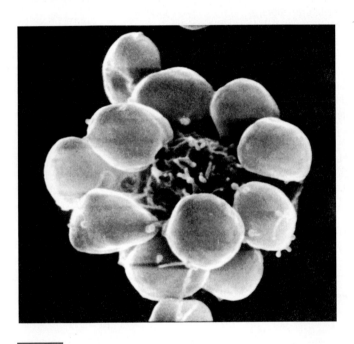

FIG. 14-2   Human T cell rosette. A central T lymphocyte is shown surrounded by adherent sheep red blood cells. This property of mature T cells reflects a specific receptor (CD2) on their cell membranes. (Scanning electron micrograph courtesy of Michael Deegan, MD, and Bertram Schnitzer, MD.)

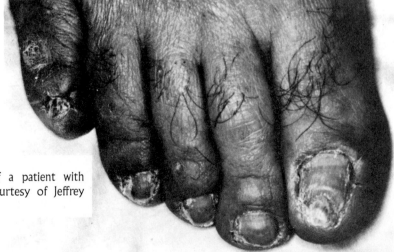

FIG. 14-3   Skin and nail lesions on the foot of a patient with chronic mucocutaneous candidiasis. (Photograph courtesy of Jeffrey Callen, MD.)

QUESTIONS

▼ *Circle the letter preceding each item below that correctly answers the question or completes the statement. More than one answer may be correct.*

1. Deficits in humoral immunity frequently impair defenses against:
   a. Tubercle bacilli
   b. Herpes simplex
   c. *Giardia lamblia*
   d. Virulent pus-forming bacteria
2. Which of the following characteristics is (are) true of acquired, common, variable immunodeficiency hypogammaglobulinemia?
   a. Virtual absence of circulating T cells
   b. Only males involved
   c. Normal number of circulating B cells
   d. Low Ig levels
3. The usual treatment of X-linked hypogammaglobulinemia includes:
   a. The administration of commercial gamma globulin
   b. Appropriate antibiotic therapy
   c. Both a and b
   d. Neither a nor b
4. Cell-mediated immune function is inadequate in or may be impaired transiently by:
   a. Cytotoxic drugs
   b. Viral infections
   c. Adrenal corticosteroids
   d. Streptococcal pharyngitis
5. The most common form of continuing antibody-dependent immunodeficiency is a selective deficit of which of the following immunoglobulins?
   a. IgA
   b. IgE
   c. IgG
   d. IgM

▼ *Circle T is the statement is true and F if it is false. Correct any false statements.*

6. T F Assay of serum immunoglobulins by radial immunodiffusion provides a widely available, direct measurement of circulating molecules having potential antibody activity.
7. T F Deficiencies of one or more of the IgG subclasses (IgG1 to IgG4) are recognized to promote bacterial infection.
8. T F Some persons with a deficit of IgA (level below 5 mg/dl) remain free of evident illness, but most manifest recurrent paranasal sinus and pulmonary infections.
9. T F Humoral immunodeficiency is present most often as an isolated immunologic deficit in non-Hodgkin's lymphoma and uremia.
10. T F Patients with DiGeorge syndrome totally lack B cell as well as T cell function because the thymus fails to develop.
11. T F Chronic mucocutaneous candidiasis is an example of an antigen-specific defect in cell-mediated immunity and is characterized by indolent *Candida* albicans infections of the skin, nails, and mucous membranes with granuloma formation.
12. T F T helper cells bearing the CD8 membrane marker are the principal lymphocyte subset promoting B cell proliferation and development into Ig-secreting plasma cells.

▼ *Answer the following on a separate sheet of paper.*

13. List three methods used to evaluate antigen-specific antibody activity associated with one or more Ig classes.
14. Explain the significance of delayed-type hypersensitivity (DTH) skin tests as an indicator of cellular immune competence.
15. Describe three additional laboratory tests reflecting lymphocyte function.
16. Why is it important to determine the numbers of T cells in subsets that are involved in antibody (humoral) responses?

CHAPTER 15

Human Immunodeficiency Virus / Acquired Immunodeficiency Syndrome (HIV / AIDS)

BETTY J. BEARD

Acquired immunodeficiency syndrome (AIDS) first came to the attention of the health community in 1981 after the unusual occurrence of *Pneumocystis carinii* pneumonia (PCP) and Kaposi's sarcoma (KS) in young homosexual men in California (Gottlieb, 1981; Centers for Disease Control, 1981). Epidemiologic evidence suggested that an infectious agent was involved, and in 1983 the human immunodeficiency virus type 1 (HIV-1) was identified as the cause of the disease (Barre-Sinoussi, 1983; Gallo, 1984). AIDS comprises a set of defined clinical conditions that are the end result of infection with HIV. The actual cases of AIDS reflect mature, longstanding infection with HIV. Today, AIDS is found in nearly every country and is a worldwide pandemic.

ETIOLOGY

Formerly called HTLV-III (human T cell lymphotrophic virus type III) or LAV (lymphadenopathy virus), HIV is a cytopathic human retrovirus of the lentivirus family. *Retroviruses* convert their ribonucleic acid (RNA) to deoxyribonucleic acid (DNA) once they enter the host cell. HIV-1 and HIV-2 are cytopathic lentiviruses, with HIV-1 being the most significant cause of AIDS throughout the world.

The HIV genome codes nine proteins essential for every aspect of the life cycle of the virus (Fig. 15-1). In terms of genomic structure, the viruses differ in that the HIV-1 protein, Vpu, which helps in virus release, appears to be replaced by the protein Vpx in HIV-2. Vpx facilitates infectivity and may be a duplication of another protein, Vpr. Vpr is thought to enhance viral transcription. HIV-2, first recognized in serum from West African (Senegalese) women in 1985, causes clinical disease but appears to be less pathogenic than HIV-1 (Marlink, 1994).

EPIDEMIOLOGY

HIV-2 is more prevalent in many countries in western Africa, but HIV-1 predominates in central and eastern Africa and the rest of the world. According to the World Health Organization's (WHO's) Global Program on AIDS (1995), 1,025,073 cumulative cases of AIDS in adults and children had been reported by the end of 1994. However, WHO believes that, allowing for underdiagnosis, incomplete reporting, underreporting, and based on the available data on HIV infections around the world, the overall estimate of AIDS cases actually approaches 4.5 million people since the pandemic began in the late

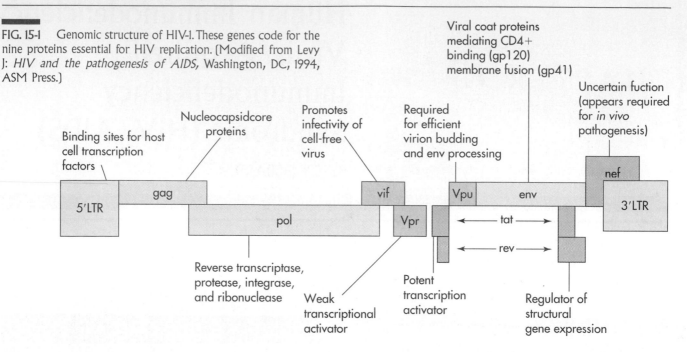

FIG. 15-1   Genomic structure of HIV-1. These genes code for the nine proteins essential for HIV replication. (Modified from Levy J: *HIV and the pathogenesis of AIDS*, Washington, DC, 1994, ASM Press.)

▶ **TABLE 15-1   1993 Revised Classification System for HIV Infection and Expanded Surveillance Case Definition Among Adolescents and Adults***

CD4+ T Cell Categories	Clinical Categories		
	(A) Asymptomatic Acute (Primary) HIV or PGL†	(B) Symptomatic, Not (A) or (C) Conditions	(C) AIDS-Indicator Condition
1. ≥500/μL	A1	B1	C1
2. 200-499/μL	A2	B2	C2
3. <200/μL AIDS indicator T cell count	A3	B3	C3

Modified from *MMWR* 41(RR-17):1-19, December 1992.

*The nine-cell matrix combines the three clinical categories associated with HIV infection and three levels of CD4+ lymphocyte counts (see the boxes on pp. 180 and 181). This system replaces the classification system published in 1987. Persons with AIDS-indicator conditions (C1, C2, C3) and those with CD4+ T cell counts less than 200/μL (A3, B3) have been counted as AIDS cases since Jan. 1, 1993. Before 1993, persons in cells A3 and B3 would not have been reportable as AIDS cases.

†*PGL*, Persistent generalized lymphadenopathy.

1970s/early 1980s. Ninety percent of persons who have developed AIDS have died.

In 1995 WHO estimated that about 18 million adults (Fig. 15-2) and 1.5 million children had been infected with HIV. The developing world is of immediate concern, particularly southern and central Africa and southern Asia (primarily India and Thailand). It is projected that by the year 2000, more than 40 million people worldwide will have been infected with HIV, with the majority living in developing countries.

Worldwide case surveillance is a challenge because there is no current case definition of AIDS that can be used globally (Stanley, Fauci, 1995). In 1993 the U.S. Centers for Disease Control and Prevention (CDC) revised the classification system for HIV infection to

emphasize the clinical importance of the CD4+ T lymphocyte count in the categorization of HIV-related clinical conditions. This classification system, outlined in Table 15-1 and the boxes on pp. 180 and 181, has replaced the system published by the CDC in 1987. The revised system is discussed later in this chapter. The expansion of the surveillance case definition for AIDS initially resulted in a large increase in reported AIDS cases for 1993. This was caused by the inclusion of persons diagnosed with severe immunosuppression, which typically occurs before the onset of the opportunistic diseases associated with AIDS.

By the end of 1994, 441,528 cumulative AIDS cases (since 1981) had been reported in the United States. Among persons for whom risks are reported, the largest

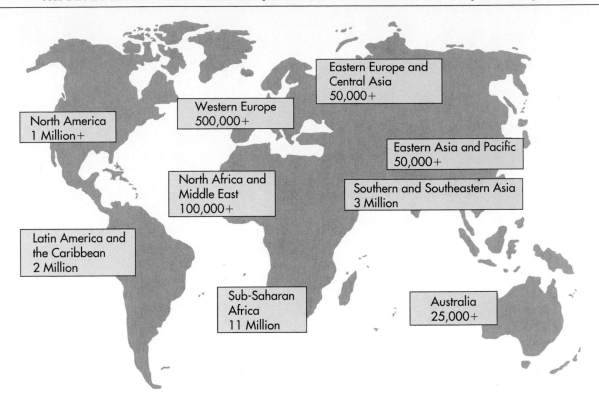

FIG. 15-2   Estimated distribution of total adult HIV infections from late 1970s/early 1980s until late 1994; global total: 18 million. (Data from World Health Organization, 1995.)

decline has been in the proportion of reported cases among homosexual/bisexual men. The greatest increases reported in 1994 were in the proportion of cases accounted for by women, racial/ethnic minorities, and children. The cumulative number of pediatric AIDS cases (children younger than 13 years) reported to the CDC, as of June 1994, was 5734. Because pediatric AIDS is predominantly a reflection of prenatal or perinatal infection (vertical transmission), as the rate of HIV infection in women rises, more infants will acquire HIV.

In 1993 AIDS was the fourth leading cause of death among women ages 25 to 44 years—the primary childbearing and childrearing years. AIDS among women is primarily associated with two modes of transmission: injecting drug use (IDU) and heterosexual contact with an at-risk partner. Heterosexual contact is becoming the most common transmission method for women (CDC, 1995b).

PATHOPHYSIOLOGY

Pathogenesis

Transmission and entry

HIV has been isolated from blood, cerebrospinal fluid, semen, tears, vaginal/cervical secretions, urine, breast milk, and saliva. Transmission occurs most efficiently by means of blood and semen. HIV has also been transmitted via breast milk and vaginal/cervical secretions. The three major means of transmission are blood, sexual contact, and maternal-infant. Once the virus is transmitted, an elaborate series of steps involved in infection begins.

Viral attachment

A mature HIV virion is approximately spherical in shape (Fig. 15-3). Its outer coat, or viral envelope, consists of a lipid bilayer that contains many protein spikes. These spikes include two glycoproteins: gp120 and gp41. Gp refers to the glycoprotein, and the number refers to the mass of the protein in thousands of daltons. Gp120 is the external surface envelope of the spike, and gp41 is the stem or transmembrane portion.

The inner segment of the viral membrane is surrounded by a matrix protein called p17. The core is circumscribed by a capsid protein called p24. Inside the capsid, p24, are two identical strands of RNA. HIV is a retrovirus, so the genetic material is in the form of RNA rather than DNA. *Reverse transcriptase* is the enzyme that transcribes viral RNA into DNA once the virus enters the cell. Other enzymes accompanying the RNA are integrase and protease.

HIV infects cells primarily by binding to the surface of a target cell that has a CD4 membrane receptor molecule (Fig. 15-4). By far, HIV's preferred target is the CD4-positive T helper lymphocyte, or T4 cell (CD4+ lymphocyte). HIV's gp120 binds tightly to the CD4+ lym-

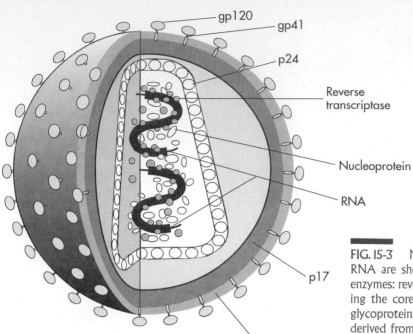

FIG. 15-3 Mature HIV virion structure. Two molecules of viral RNA are shown in the center associated with three important enzymes: reverse transcriptase, integrase, and protease. Surrounding the core is a nucleocapsid composed of p24 proteins. Two glycoproteins, gp120 and gp41, are embedded in the lipid bilayer derived from the cell membrane. (Redrawn from Greene WC: *Sci Am* 269[3]:100, 1993.)

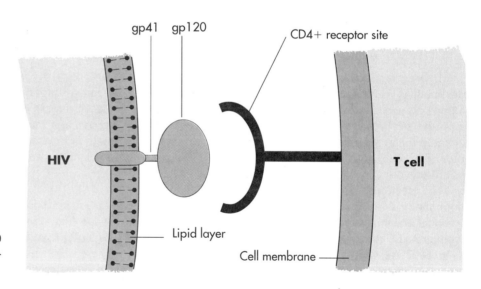

FIG. 15-4 Attachment/binding of gp120 to receptor protein on CD4+ T lymphocyte.

phocyte, allowing the gp41 to mediate in the virus-to-cell membrane fusion.

Other cells that may be susceptible to HIV infection include monocytes and macrophages. Infected monocytes and macrophages can serve as reservoirs for HIV but are not destroyed by the virus. HIV is polytropic and may infect a wide variety of human cells (Levy, 1994), such as CD8 cells, natural killer (NK) cells, B lymphocytes, endothelial cells, epithelial cells, Langerhans' cells, dendritic cells (which are present on the body's mucosal surfaces), microglial cells, and various body tissues.

After fusion of the virus to a CD4+ lymphocyte, a complex series of events occurs that, if not interrupted,

leads to the production of new virus particles from the infected cell. The infected CD4+ lymphocyte may remain latent in a proviral state or may undergo replication cycles producing multiple viruses. Infection of the CD4+ lymphocyte may also lead to cytopathogenicity through a variety of mechanisms, including *apoptosis* (programmed cell death), *anergy* (prevention of further cell division), or formation of *syncytium* (cell fusion).

Viral replication

Once the virus-cell fusion occurs (Fig. 15-5), viral RNA enters the core of the CD4+ lymphocyte's cytoplasm. After uncoating of the nucleocapsid, *reverse tran-*

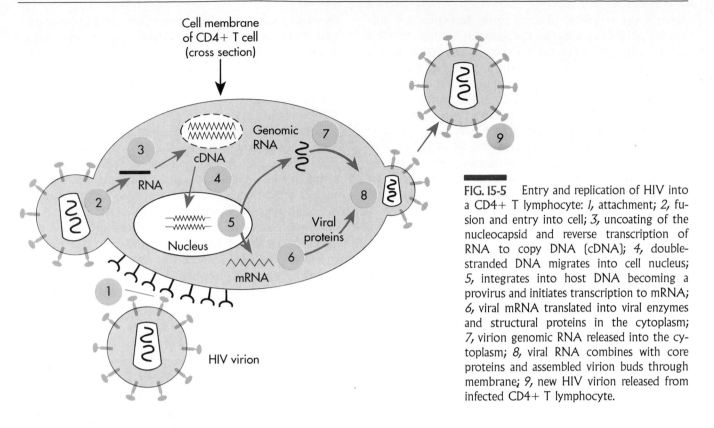

FIG. 15-5 Entry and replication of HIV into a CD4+ T lymphocyte: *1,* attachment; *2,* fusion and entry into cell; *3,* uncoating of the nucleocapsid and reverse transcription of RNA to copy DNA (cDNA); *4,* double-stranded DNA migrates into cell nucleus; *5,* integrates into host DNA becoming a provirus and initiates transcription to mRNA; *6,* viral mRNA translated into viral enzymes and structural proteins in the cytoplasm; *7,* virion genomic RNA released into the cytoplasm; *8,* viral RNA combines with core proteins and assembled virion buds through membrane; *9,* new HIV virion released from infected CD4+ T lymphocyte.

scription occurs from a single strand of RNA to double-stranded copy DNA (cDNA) of the virus. The HIV *integrase* aids in the insertion of the viral cDNA into the host nucleus. When the two strands of DNA are integrated into the host cell's chromosomes, they become a *provirus* (Greene, 1993). The provirus produces viral messenger RNA (mRNA), which leaves the nucleus and enters the cytoplasm. Viral proteins are produced from full-length and spliced mRNA, as genomic RNA is released into the cytoplasm. Viral *protease* is activated as RNA and viral proteins enter the new virion, which buds through the host cell, acquiring a lipid membrane and viral envelope. The host cell is now producing new HIV.

Replication of HIV continues throughout the period of clinical latency, even when minimal viral activity is demonstrated in blood (Embretson et al, 1993; Pantaleo et al, 1993). HIV is found in massive amounts in CD4+ lymphocytes and macrophages throughout the lymphoid system at all stages of infection. Virus particles have also been associated with follicular dendritic cells, which may transmit infection to cells during migration through lymphoid follicles.

Therefore, although low levels of viremia and viral replication may be found in peripheral blood mononuclear cells during clinical latency, a true latency does not exist. HIV is continually accumulating and replicating in the lymphoid organs. Some data suggest that an extraordinarily large number of replications and rapid cell turnovers occur, with the composite half-life of plasma

virus and virus-producing cells being about 2 days (Wei et al, 1995; Ho et al, 1995). This indicates that a persistent battle occurs between the virus and the individual's immune system.

Immune Responses to HIV Infection

For a review of the response of the body to immunologic challenge, see Chapter 5. Both humoral and cell-mediated immune responses are involved in HIV infection.

Soon after a person is exposed to HIV, he or she mounts an intense immune defense. B cells produce specific antibodies against the viral proteins. Neutralizing antibodies to regions of the envelope gp120 and to the external portion of gp41 are found. The detection of antibodies is the basis for various HIV tests (e.g., ELISA). Both the immunoglobulin G (IgG) and the immunoglobulin M (IgM) classes of antibodies appear in the circulation, but as the IgM titer decreases, in most cases the IgG titer remains high throughout infection. IgG antibodies are the principal antibodies used in HIV testing. Antibodies to HIV can appear within 1 month after initial infection and in most HIV-infected persons within 6 months of exposure.

Immunoglobulin production is regulated by the CD4+ lymphocyte. As discussed in Chapter 5, the CD4+ lymphocyte is activated by an antigen-presenting cell (APC) to produce cytokines such as interleukin-2 (IL-2), which help to stimulate B cells to divide and differentiate into plasma cells. These plasma cells then produce immunoglobulins specific to the stimulating antigen. The cytokine IL-2 is just one of many cytokines that influence both humoral and cell-mediated immune responses. The extent of cytokine control, expression, and potential function in HIV infection is still being explored, but it is certain that cytokines are critical in intracellular activities. For example, the addition of the cytokine IL-12 (natural killer cell stimulatory factor) seems to counter the reduction in NK cell activity and function seen in HIV infection. NK cells are important because they normally recognize and destroy virus-infected cells by secreting perforins similar to those produced by CD8 cells.

Recent research supports the cytotoxic and suppressor roles of CD8 cells in HIV infection. The CD8 cell's cytotoxic role involves binding with the virus-infected cell and releasing perforins, which cause cell death. The cytotoxic activities of CD8 cells are vigorous at the beginning of HIV infection. The CD8 cell can also suppress HIV replication in CD4+ lymphocytes. This suppression has been found to be variable not only among individuals, but also within the same person as the disease develops. The antiviral activity of the CD8 cell decreases with disease advancement. As the disease progresses, the number of CD4+ lymphocytes also is depleted. Various hypotheses as to the cause of this gradual loss are discussed later.

What is irrefutable is the essential regulator function of CD4+ lymphocytes in cell-mediated immunity. As discussed earlier and in Chapter 5, CD4+ lymphocytes release cytokines that expedite processes such as production of immunoglobulins and activation of additional T cells and macrophages. Two specific cytokines produced by CD4+ lymphocytes—IL-2 and gamma interferon—are pivotal in cell-mediated immunity. Under normal conditions, CD4+ lymphocyte release of gamma interferon attracts macrophages and intensifies the immune reaction to the antigen. If the CD4+ lymphocyte is not functioning properly, however, gamma interferon production is diminished. IL-2 is important in facilitating not only the production of plasma cells, but also the growth and antiviral activity of CD8 cells and the self-replication of the CD4+ lymphocyte population.

Although the precise mechanism of the CD4+ lymphocyte cytopathogenicity is as yet unknown, arguments could be made for hypotheses such as apoptosis, anergy, syncytia formation, and lysis of the cell. *Antibody-dependent, complement-mediated cytotoxicity* (ADCC) may be one humoral immune effect that helps to remove HIV-infected CD4+ lymphocytes. ADCC is induced by antibodies to the two glycoproteins, gp120 and gp41. Cells such as NK then act to kill the infected cells.

Apoptosis is one of several theories offered to explain the marked loss of circulating CD4+ lymphocytes through the course of HIV disease. Many CD4+ lymphocytes seem to commit cellular suicide when stimulated by an activating agent or by a defect in activation signaling (Gougeon, Montagnier, 1993). CD4+ lympho-

cytes also may fail to divide, resulting in a phenomenon called anergy. Another theory involves the formation of syncytia. In syncytium formation, uninfected CD4+ lymphocytes are fused with infected cells—the "bystander effect" (Weiss, 1993)—thereby eliminating many uninfected cells. Finally, the decrease in numbers of CD4+ lymphocytes may result from the budding of new viruses. They may rupture through the CD4+ lymphocyte membrane, effectively killing it in the process.

No matter which theory supports the loss of CD4+ lymphocytes, depletion of these cells remains a principal feature of HIV infection. The depletion varies among individuals with HIV infection. Some of the factors influencing this variation include function of the host immune system, presence of other host factors (e.g., congenital or metabolic disorders, nutritional deficiencies, additional pathogens), or differences in viral strains (Schattner, Laurence, 1994).

MEASUREMENT OF CD4+ CELLS AND MONITORING LOSS

In an intact immune system the number of CD4+ lymphocytes ranges from 600 to 1200/μL (or mm^3) of blood. Because CD4+ lymphocyte counts can vary even within the same individual, a baseline count is established as soon as possible after exposure to HIV. Immediately after primary virus infection, the CD4+ lymphocyte count drops below the normal level for the individual. The cell number then increases, but to a level somewhat below normal for the individual. A slow decrease in CD4+ lymphocyte count occurs over time and correlates with the clinical course of the disease. External factors such as stress, smoking, drugs, and alcohol can affect hormone and immune functions and may serve as intervening variables. Their effects on CD4+ lymphocyte counts need further evaluation.

In 1993 the CDC expanded the AIDS surveillance case definition to include persons with "AIDS-indicator conditions" and persons with a CD4+ lymphocyte count less than 200/μL (whether asymptomatic or symptomatic) (Table 15-1). Persons with CD4+ lymphocyte counts less than 200 are severely immunosuppressed and are at high risk for malignancies and opportunistic infections. The body becomes nearly defenseless to invaders such as bacteria, viruses, fungi, protozoa, and parasites.

CLINICAL PROGRESSION

Phases of Infection

AIDS is the final stage in a continuum of immunologic and clinical abnormalities known as the "spectrum of

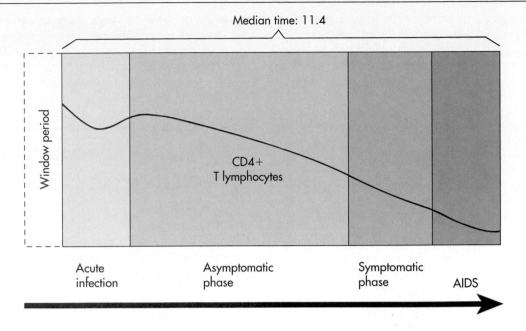

Median time: 11.4

Window period

CD4+
T lymphocytes

Acute
infection

Asymptomatic
phase

Symptomatic
phase

AIDS

FIG. 15-6   Phases of HIV infection. The period of time between HIV seroconversion and the appearance of symptoms may be about 10 years or less. The median time between seroconversion and death is 11.4 years. (Modified from Grimes D, Grimes R: *AIDS and HIV infection,* St Louis, 1994, Mosby.)

HIV infection" (Fig. 15-6 and Table 15-2). The course of disease is initiated when transmission occurs and the person becomes infected. Not every person who is exposed becomes infected. Cofactors to acquisition still need to be identified. After initial infection with HIV, an individual may remain seronegative for several months. However, the individual is infectious during this period and can transmit the virus to others. This is called the "window" period. Clinical manifestations in the infected individual can be present as early as 1 to 4 weeks after exposure.

Acute infection occurs at the point of seroconversion from negative antibody status to positive. Some people have a virus-like or mononucleosis-like ailment that lasts for a few weeks. Symptoms might include malaise, fever, diarrhea, lymphadenopathy, and a maculopapular rash. A few people experience more acute symptoms, such as meningitis and pneumonitis. During this period, high levels of HIV can be detected in the peripheral blood (Levy, 1994). CD4+ lymphocyte levels drop and then return to a level slightly below the original level for that individual.

Within weeks following acute infection, the person enters an *asymptomatic phase*. At the beginning of this phase, CD4+ lymphocyte levels have generally returned to near-normal levels. However, CD4+ lymphocyte levels decrease gradually over time. During this phase of infection, both the virus and the viral antibodies can be found in the blood. As discussed earlier, replication of the virus is taking place in the lymphoid tissue. The virus itself never enters a period of latency even though the phase of clinical infection may be latent.

In the *symptomatic phase* of the disease course, the individual's CD4+ cell counts have usually dropped below

  TABLE 15-2   CDC Classification of HIV Infection Based on Pathophysiology of the Disease as Immune Function Progressively Worsens

Class	Criteria
Group I	1. Acute infection with HIV 2. Flu-like symptoms; resolve completely 3. HIV antibody negative

HIV ASYMPTOMATIC

Class	Criteria
Group II	1. HIV antibody positive 2. No laboratory or clinical indicators of immunodeficiency

HIV SYMPTOMATIC

Class	Criteria
Group III	1. HIV antibody positive 2. Persistent generalized lymphadenopathy

Group IV-A	1. HIV antibody positive
	2. Constitutional disease
	  a. Persistent fever or diarrhea
	  b. Weight loss >10% of normal body weight

Group IV-B	1. Same as group IV-A, and
	2. Neurologic disease
	  a. Dementia
	  b. Neuropathy
	  c. Myelopathy

Group IV-C	1. Same as group IV-B, and 2. CD4+ T lymphocyte count <200/μL 3. Opportunistic infection
Group IV-D	1. Same as group IV-C, and 2. Pulmonary tuberculosis, invasive cervical cancer, or other malignancy

Data from Centers for Disease Control and Prevention, March 1993.

CDC SURVEILLANCE CASE DEFINITION FOR AIDS

For national reporting, a case of AIDS is defined as an illness characterized by one of the following "indicator" diseases. Diseases listed under part A require that the patient have no other cause of immunodeficiency; part B diseases indicate a diagnosis of AIDS regardless of the presence of other causes of immunodeficiency, provided there is laboratory evidence of HIV infection. Laboratory evidence for HIV infection consists of repeated positive reaction to antibody screening tests confirmed with supplementary tests (e.g., ELISA tests confirmed by Western blot tests); direct identification of the virus in host tissues; HIV antigen detection; or a positive result with any other highly specific, licensed test for HIV.

A. Indicator diseases without evidence of HIV infection

1. Candidiasis of the esophagus, trachea, bronchi, lungs
2. Cryptococcosis, extrapulmonary
3. Cryptosporidiosis with diarrhea persisting >1 month
4. Cytomegalovirus disease of any organ, excluding liver, spleen, lymph nodes, in a patient >1 month of age
5. Herpes simplex virus infection causing mucocutaneous ulcer persisting >1 month; or bronchitis, pneumonia, or esophagitis in a patient >1 month of age
6. Kaposi's sarcoma in a patient <60 years old
7. Lymphoma of the brain (primary) in a patient <60 years old
8. Lymphoid interstitial pneumonia and/or pulmonary lymphoid hyperplasia in a child <13 years old
9. *Mycobacterium avium-intracellulare* complex or *M. kansasii* disease (disseminated)
10. *Pneumocystis carinii* pneumonia
11. Progressive multifocal leukencephalopathy
12. Toxoplasmosis of the brain in a patient >1 month of age

B. Indicator diseases with laboratory evidence of HIV infection

1. Bacterial infections (multiple or recurrent) in children <13 years old caused by *Haemophilus, Streptococcus,* or other pyogenic bacteria
2. Coccidioidomycosis, disseminated
3. HIV encephalopathy (also called HIV dementia)
4. Histoplasmosis, disseminated
5. Isosporiasis with diarrhea persisting >1 month
6. Kaposi's sarcoma at any age
7. Non-Hodgkin's lymphoma: Burkitt's or immunoblastic
8. Mycobacterial disease, disseminated, excluding *M. tuberculosis*
9. *Mycobacterium tuberculosis,* disseminated
10. *Salmonella* (nontyphoid) septicemia, recurrent
11. HIV wasting syndrome (>10% weight loss, chronic diarrhea >30 days, weakness, constant or intermittent fever) in the absence of other illness other than HIV infection that could explain findings

C. The 1993 expanded definition includes the following:

1. All HIV-infected persons who have CD4+ T cell counts <200/μL or CD4+ T cells <14% of total T cells
2. Pulmonary tuberculosis
3. Recurrent pneumonia
4. Invasive cervical cancer

Modified from *MMWR* 36(suppl no 1S):3S-9S, 1987; *MMWR* 41(RR-17):1-19, December 1992.

300 cells/μL (Levy, 1994). Symptoms indicating immunosuppression are present and continue until the person develops an AIDS-related condition. Symptomatic conditions for this clinical category are defined by the CDC and are outlined in the box above and the box on p. 181.

The CDC has added a CD4+ lymphocyte count of less than 200/μL as a sole criterion for AIDS diagnosis, regardless of clinical category, asymptomatic or symptomatic. The presence of any of the AIDS-indicator conditions, as defined by the CDC, denotes a reportable AIDS case. When the CDC expanded its definition in 1993, three clinical conditions were added: pulmonary tuberculosis, recurrent pneumonia, and invasive cervical cancer. These conditions joined the 23 others contained in the previous case definition published in 1987.

Clinical Manifestations

AIDS comprises a variety of clinical manifestations in the form of characteristic opportunistic malignancies and infections.

Malignancies

Kaposi's sarcoma (KS) is the most common type of malignancy seen in AIDS patients. KS is believed to originate from the endothelial cell wall and generally develops in a multicentric fashion in asymptomatic nodules. Reddish purple patches occur on the skin, but the color may vary to include violet, dark purple, pink, red, and red-brown (see Color plates 1 to 3). In addition to the skin changes seen in KS, common extraneous sites are the gastrointestinal (GI) tract, lymph nodes, and lungs. KS can cause structural and functional damage, such as lymphedema and malabsorption. When KS is primarily localized to the skin, cryosurgery, laser surgery, and surgical excision have been somewhat successful, but radiotherapy is the treatment of choice for local disease. Chemotherapeutic agents such as vinblastine, vincristine, bleomycin, and doxorubicin have been useful to varying degrees. Of the various immune stimulation agents available, interferon has been the most effective because of its antiviral, antiproliferative, and immunostimulating effects.

1993 REVISED HIV CLASSIFICATION SYSTEM FOR ADOLESCENTS AND ADULTS

,The revised CDC classification for HIV-infected adolescents and adults emphasizes the importance of CD4+ T lymphocyte counts in the clinical management of patients who are infected with HIV. This classification is divided into laboratory and clinical categories. In contrast, the usefulness of the classification in the box on p. 180 is limited to epidemiologic and surveillance purposes.

LABORATORY CATEGORIES

Category 1: >500µL CD4+ T lymphocytes/µL
Category 2: 200-499µL CD4+ T lymphocytes/µL
Category 3: <200µL CD4+ T lymphocytes/µL

CLINICAL CATEGORIES
Category A

Category A consists of one or more of the following conditions in an adolescent or adult (≥ 13 years) with documented HIV infection. Conditions listed under categories B and C must not have occurred.
- Asymptomatic HIV infection
- Persistent generalized lymphadenopathy (PGL)
- Acute (primary) HIV infection with accompanying illness or history of acute HIV infection

Category B

Category B consists of symptomatic conditions occurring in an HIV-infected adolescent or adult that are not listed in category C and meet at least one of the following criteria:
1. The conditions are attributed to HIV infection and/or are indicative of a defect in cell-mediated immunity.
2. The conditions are considered by physicians to have a clinical course or management that is complicated by HIV infection.

Selected examples of conditions include the following:
- Bacterial endocarditis, meningitis, pneumonia, or sepsis
- Candidiasis, oropharyngeal (thrush)
- Candidiasis, vulvovaginal, persistent for >1 month
- Cervical dysplasia, severe or carcinoma
- Constitutional symptoms such as fever or diarrhea >1 month
- Hairy leukoplakia (oral) (see Color plate 8)
- Herpes zoster (shingles), at least two distinct episodes or > one dermatome
- Idiopathic thrombocytopenic purpura
- Listeriosis
- *Mycobacterium tuberculosis* infection, pulmonary
- Pelvic inflammatory disease
- Peripheral neuropathy

Category C

Category C consists of any condition listed in the 1987 surveillance case definition (including the 1993 expansion) affecting an adolescent or adult (see box, p. 180).
- The conditions in category C are strongly associated with severe immunodeficiency, occur frequently in HIV-infected patients, and cause serious morbidity and mortality.
- According to the proposed classification system, HIV-infected patients would be classified on the basis of both the following:
1. The lowest accurate (not necessarily the latest) CD4+ T lymphocyte count
2. The most severe clinical condition diagnosed regardless of the patient's present clinical condition

Modified from *MMWR* 41(RR-17):1-19, December 1992.

Most malignant lymphomas are high-grade pathologic B cell tumors, including small, noncleaved lymphoma and Burkitt's or Burkitt's-like lymphoma (see Color plate 4). A common finding is the occurrence of symptoms that include fever, weight loss, and night sweats, which are probably caused by the malignancy. Patients who have *persistent generalized lymphadenopathy* (PGL) are at significant risk to develop malignant lymphoma.

Initial signs and symptoms of primary central nervous system (CNS) lymphoma include headache, short-term memory loss, cranial nerve palsies, hemiparesis, and personality changes. These impairments may be caused by the location of the tumor, edema, or coexisting diseases. The space-occupying lesion needs to be differentiated from other lesions, especially toxoplasmosis.

Other malignancies have occurred in HIV-infected persons, including multiple myeloma, B cell acute lymphocytic leukemia, T lymphoblastic lymphoma, Hodgkin's disease, carcinoma of the anus, squamous cell carcinoma of the tongue, adenosquamous carcinoma of the lung, adenocarcinoma of the colon and pancreas, and testicular cancer. More research needs to be completed to generalize about the impact of an underlying HIV infection on the course of concurrent malignancies or other chronic illnesses not related to the HIV infection.

Infections

AIDS causes a progressive, presently irreversible destruction of immune functioning. The morbidity and mortality, however, primarily result from the major opportunistic infections that develop because of unsuccessful immune surveillance and action. Patients with AIDS are susceptible to a broad range of protozoal, bacterial, fungal, and viral infections, and some of them are quite rare, such as *Cryptosporidium* and *Mycobacterium avium-intracellulare*. They are persistent, severe, and frequently relapsing. Patients typically have more than one infection at the same time.

Pneumocystis carinii pneumonia (PCP) is the most frequently diagnosed serious infection in AIDS patients. The presentation is frequently atypical when compared with that of PCP in cancer patients. In AIDS the only symptom may be a fever; other symptoms may include exercise intolerance, a dry, nonproductive cough, weakness, and shortness of breath at a gradual, indolent rate. A high degree of suspicion of PCP needs to accompany the clinical evaluation of every HIV-seropositive or suspected positive patient. Prophylactic or suppressive treatment is of the utmost importance because of the severity and frequency of PCP in persons with AIDS. Trimethoprim-sulfamethoxazole (Bactrim, Septra) is the drug of choice.

Infection with *Toxoplasma gondii* is mostly silent in healthy individuals, although some develop lymphadenopathy. No prophylaxis exists. Patients with AIDS have a 30% risk of developing toxoplasmosis over a 2-year period, usually as a reactivation of an earlier infection. Specific agents that determine reactivation are unknown. In AIDS patients, CNS disease develops, marked by multiple or solitary lesions that can be seen on computed tomography (CT) scan (Fig. 15-7).

Cryptosporidium can cause acute, self-limiting diarrheal episodes. Both isosporiasis and microsporiasis are spread by the fecal-oral route; sexual, food, water, or animal contact; and possibly inhalation. Isosporiasis, as with cryptosporidiosis, causes diarrhea, but it is much less severe and occurs less frequently.

Infection with *Mycobacterium avium-intracellulare* (MAI) occurs evenly in all risk groups and is a late complication of AIDS. Most patients die within months. Although it clearly contributes to morbidity, its relationship to mortality is unclear. Symptoms include fever, rigor, diarrhea, and abdominal cramping. Recommended prophylaxis against MAI is controversial, but the drug most often suggested is rifabutin.

Mycobacterium tuberculosis, the cause of tuberculosis (TB), is endemic in certain geographic locations, and most cases of AIDS/TB are reactivations of prior infection. AIDS/TB is usually an early indication of AIDS, occurring when T cells are fairly high ($>200/\mu L$). Its manifestation is similar to normal TB, with 60% to 80% of patients having pulmonary disease. However, extrapulmonary disease develops in 40% to 75% of HIV patients, with lymphatic TB and miliary disease being particularly common. Patients respond well to the traditional drug regimen of isoniazid (INH), rifampin, pyrazinamide, and ethambutol. Patients who are at high risk for TB may benefit from INH prophylaxis. As patients progress to AIDS with decreasing immunocompetence, many HIV-infected persons become anergic; therefore they should be tested early for TB.

Fungal infections include *candidiasis, cryptococcosis,* and *histoplasmosis.* Oral candidiasis is common in patients with AIDS and causes dry mouth and oral irritation (see Color plates 5 to 7). Candidiasis of the bronchi,

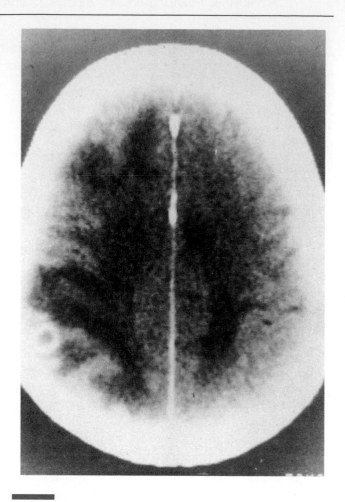

FIG. 15-7 Toxoplasmosis in AIDS patient. Note ring lesion at left. (Courtesy of Bruce Polsky, MD, Memorial Sloan-Kettering Cancer Center.)

lungs, trachea, or esophagus is pathognomonic for an AIDS diagnosis. Rarely do patients develop systemic disease. *Cryptococcus neoformans* infections occur in 7% of AIDS patients, with meningitis being the most common presentation. Treatment with fluconazole provides limited prophylaxis against both oral candidiasis and *Cryptococcus neoformans.* In persons with AIDS, symptoms of infection with *Histoplasma capsulatum* are varied and nonspecific, including fevers, chills, sweats, weight loss, nausea, vomiting, diarrhea, skin lesions, pneumonitis, and bone marrow depressions. Amphotericin B is used for induction therapy, with lower dosages used for maintenance.

Opportunistic infections caused by invasion by viruses are numerous and responsible for further pathology. Infection with *herpes simplex virus* (HSV) in AIDS patients usually manifests as genital or perianal ulcerations that are easily diagnosed by viral cultures. HSV can be spread by direct skin contact. HSV also may manifest as esophagitis and can cause pneumonia and encephalitis. Acyclovir is the drug of choice for both HSV and herpes zoster.

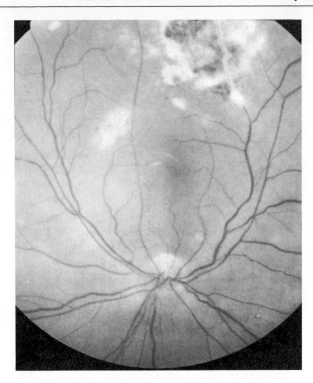

FIG. 15-8   Cytomegalovirus (CMV) retinitis. (Courtesy of Bruce Polsky, MD, Memorial Sloan-Kettering Cancer Center.)

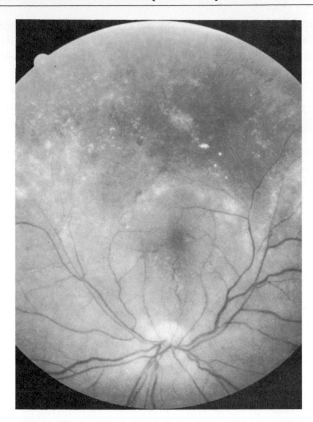

FIG. 15-9   Cytomegalovirus (CMV) retinitis after treatment with gancyclovir (DHPG). (Courtesy of Bruce Polsky, MD, Memorial Sloan-Kettering Cancer Center.)

The development of *herpes zoster (shingles)* may signal progression of illness in an HIV-infected patient. Infections in the skin and eyes may precede opportunistic infections. *Cytomegalovirus* (CMV) is a common finding in AIDS patients. It causes disseminated disease with four clearly defined illnesses: chorioretinitis (Figs. 15-8 and 15-9), enterocolitis, pneumonia, and adrenalitis. Asymptomatic individuals can shed CMV. CMV pneumonia is difficult to distinguish from other pneumonias and may occur simultaneously with another pathogen such as *P. carinii.* Symptoms of adrenal insufficiency may be detected. Treatment with gancyclovir or foscarnet is indicated for CMV-related illnesses (Goldschmidt, Dong, 1995).

Progressive multifocal leukoencephalopathy is a rapidly progressive illness caused by a papovavirus. Clinically the patient has personality changes and motor and sensory deficits. Symptoms may include headache, tremors, coordination and balance difficulties, weakness, and other signs of cerebellar dysfunction. *Epstein-Barr virus* (EBV) is implicated in the development of oral hairy leukoplakia, pneumonitis in children, and lymphomas. It is frequently isolated from the throat washings of AIDS patients.

Testing

Two tests are typically used for detecting antibodies to HIV. The first, *enzyme-linked immunosorbent assay* (ELISA), reacts to the presence of antibodies in serum by demonstrating a more intense color as large quantities of viral antibodies are detected. Since false-positive results could be psychologically devastating, positive ELISA studies are repeated, and if both results are positive, a more specific test, *Western blot,* is performed. The Western blot test is also confirmed twice. This test is less likely to give a false-positive or false-negative reading. Inconclusive tests also can occur, such as when ELISA or Western blot is weakly reactive and somewhat suspicious. This may occur in early HIV infection, in developing infection (until all necessary bands on the Western blot studies are completely present), or in the cross-reactivity to another high retrovirus titer, such as HIV-2 or HTLV-I. Once confirmed, the person is said to be *HIV seropositive.* At this point, additional clinical and immunologic studies are performed to evaluate the extent of the illness and efforts to control infection are initiated.

HIV can also be detected by other tests, which discern the presence of the virus or viral components before ELISA or Western blot can detect antibodies. These procedures include viral culture, measurement of p24 antigen, and measurement of HIV DNA and RNA by means of the *polymerase chain reaction* (PCR). Tests such as these are useful in studies of immunopathogenesis, as disease markers, in early detection of infection, and in neonatal transmission. Infants born to HIV-infected mothers can demonstrate maternal anti-HIV antibodies in their blood for up to 18 months after birth, regardless of whether they actually are infected.

PEDIATRIC AIDS

In the early 1980s, children with hemophilia or those receiving blood or blood products were at high risk for HIV infection. With the testing of the blood supply, however, begun in 1985, this mode of transmission is now almost nonexistent. Today, HIV in children is predominantly a result of *vertical transmission*—acquired prenatally or perinatally. Babies have also acquired HIV postpartally through breast milk.

Infants of HIV-infected women demonstrate antibodies to the virus up to 12 to 18 months after birth because of the transfer of maternal anti-HIV IgG across the placenta. The placenta may be a barrier but is not a perfect one. Therefore testing an infant's serum for IgG antibodies is futile, since the test does not discriminate between the infant's and the mother's antibodies. Most of these babies, over time, will stop demonstrating maternal antibodies and will also fail to develop their own antibodies to the virus, indicating a seronegative status. True HIV infection can be measured in many infants through tests such as viral culture, p24 antigen, or PCR analysis for viral RNA.

The mechanism for transfer of HIV from mother to fetus remains elusive. Infection can occur in utero or during and after the delivery. Although reports have varied regarding infection rates of infants from vertical transmission, generally the rate is considerably less than 50%. The major question is: What mechanism protects those babies who are not infected, especially when such a preponderance of body fluids is exchanged during the birth process (whether vaginal or cesarean birth)? The process may involve the infant's immune system, which could serve a protective function when infected by the virus. Maternal factors such as the level of disease (and CD4+ lymphocyte count), viremia, or characteristics of the maternal viral strain may play a role in infection (Borkowsy et al, 1994). At this time, infection in infants is unstable and unpredictable. Some studies of twins have demonstrated discordant results in each of the twins, further confounding the problem.

It is known that the progression of the disease is accelerated in children. The asymptomatic phase is shorter in children who have contracted the virus through vertical transmission. The median time to onset of symptoms is less in children, and once symptoms appear, progression to death is expedited. In 1994 the CDC revised the classification system for HIV infection in children younger than 13 years. In this system, infected children are classified into categories according to three parameters: infection status, clinical status, and immunologic status. These categories are mutually exclusive.

Similarities and differences exist in the clinical course of HIV disease in children and in adults. B cell dysfunction often occurs in children before changes are seen in the CD4+ lymphocyte number. As a result of these immune system dysfunctions, children are subjected to recurrent bacterial infections (Krasinski, 1994; Rubinstein, Calvelli, 1995). Invasion by these bacterial pathogens results in the clinical syndrome seen in children, such as otitis media, sinusitis, urinary tract infection, meningitis, respiratory infection, GI diseases, and other diseases.

Additional infections seen in children include toxoplasmosis, cryptococcal infection, chronic herpes (simplex and zoster) infection, disseminated cytomegaloviral infection, histoplasmosis, and candidiasis (oral, esophageal, disseminated). About one half of infants and children with AIDS develop PCP. PCP is the most common opportunistic infection seen in HIV-infected children, and their prognosis is typically poor, especially if additional pathogens are present (Rubinstein, Calvelli, 1994).

Infection with the EBV appears related to the *lymphoid interstitial pneumonitis/pulmonary lymphoid hyperplasia* (LIP/PLH) and the generalized lymphadenopathy seen in children. HIV-infected children demonstrate a high incidence of LIP/PLH. In the clinic, lymphadenopathy and parotid swelling, as well as developmental delays, unexplained fever, diarrhea, or failure to thrive, are part of the clinical picture, particularly in older children.

Thrombocytopenia is a common hematologic complication. Progressive encephalopathy is seen in many infants and children and is considered the most severe of the CNS problems associated with HIV infection (Brouwers et al, 1994). KS is rarely seen in children. Malignancies (e.g., lymphomas) in children probably result from the dysfunction in both B and T cells.

Antiretroviral therapy is a part of cancer treatment protocol and can benefit some HIV-infected children. Antiretroviral drugs such as zidovudine (ZDV, formerly known as AZT) have been used with a selected group of HIV-infected pregnant women and their infants. Preliminary reports indicate that ZDV reduced the risk for perinatal HIV transmission with these subjects. ZDV was administered to women throughout pregnancy and intrapartally. It was also administered to infants for 6 weeks after delivery (CDC, 1994c). In their recommendations, the U.S. Public Health Services (USPHS) Task Force cautioned that the results of this study need to be adjusted to the clinical situations of individual persons. Later in 1994, the USPHS published guidelines related to the use of ZDV to reduce perinatal HIV transmission (CDC, 1994d).

ANTIVIRAL THERAPEUTIC INTERVENTION

As discussed earlier, HIV is probably replicating from the time it infects an individual. True viral latency may not exist. Many researchers believe that therapeutic intervention and antiretroviral treatment should be started as early as possible, perhaps even before seroconversion is noted with the detection of anti-HIV antibodies in the blood.

Therapeutic intervention in the life cycle of HIV must deal with HIV's ability to infect macrophages and its capacity to cross the blood-brain barrier and cause neurologic damage. Treatment strategies are evolving rapidly as more is learned about the virus and the pathogenesis of the disease. Current therapies confront the issues of targeting the multiple stages of viral entry and replication, manipulating viral genes to control for production of viral proteins, using cytokine therapy to rebuild the immune system, and finally, combining medications and treatments.

Levy (1994) suggests not only that antiviral/infected cell approaches are effective therapies for HIV infection, but also that interruptions in the steps of the HIV life cycle (e.g., before integration of the provirus, after integration, during viral budding) are significant. In the United States (1995), the only class of drugs approved by the Food and Drug Administration (FDA) for HIV infection include nucleic acid analogs that compete with the viral reverse transcriptase and protease inhibitors. Examples of anti-reverse transcriptase drugs include zidovudine (ZDV, formerly known as AZT), didanosine/dideoxyadenosine (ddI), zalcitabine (ddC), and stavudine (d4T). Researchers continue to develop strategies to address areas such as the development of resistance to and toxicity from these drugs (Volberding, 1994). Treatments for interrupting the life cycle at other stages are being developed. Potential targets include other enzymes such as integrase. Additional targets are the regulatory proteins controlling viral replication; the most promising seem to be Tat (assists in transcription), Rev (regulates viral protein expression), and Nef.

Cytokine therapy has met with some guarded success. Cytokines such as IL-2 and gamma interferon encourage cell-mediated immunity and help prevent immunologic deterioration. In a recent study (Kovacs et al, 1995), the use of IL-2 with persons who were infected with HIV but who had not yet developed AIDS sharply increased the CD4+ lymphocyte count for some. However, a minimum CD4+ lymphocyte count of 400/μL was necessary to benefit from IL-2 intervention.

Controlled clinical trials using cytokines in conjunction with antiretrovirals are being conducted (Johnson, Hoth, 1993). As noted earlier, HIV demonstrates genetic variations not only between individuals, but also within the same person, possibly because of the many replication cycles that occur (Coffin, 1995). Mutations may affect or can be affected by therapeutic agents. Benefits from one regimen might be temporary, and drugs that target only one step in the HIV life cycle might not be effective over time. Therefore constant monitoring of an individual's response to treatment, in addition to combination therapy, is critical.

Genetic mutations can complicate vaccine development, which is a national priority. The ideal vaccine would induce both humoral and cellular immunity. Efficacy trials are being initiated as more information about HIV is being discovered (Bolognesi, 1994). A comprehensive HIV prevention program, however, includes not only vaccine development, but also research and education geared toward preventing transmission of the virus.

QUESTIONS

▼ *Circle the letter preceding each item that correctly answers the question or completes the statement. More than one answer may be correct.*

1. HIV-1 is one of a group of viruses referred to as:
   a. Herpes viruses
   b. Slow viruses
   c. Retroviruses
   d. None of the above
2. The estimated number of persons infected with the AIDS virus in the entire world at the end of 1994 was:
   a. 1 million
   b. 5 million
   c. 10 million
   d. 18 million
3. The groups in whom the problem of HIV infection/AIDS is growing the fastest in the United States are:
   a. Homosexual white males
   b. Racial/ethnic minorities
   c. Women and children
   d. Hemophiliacs
4. The estimated number of persons infected with the AIDS virus in the United States at the end of 1994 was approximately:
   a. 100,000
   b. 200,000
   c. 500,000
   d. More than 1 million
5. In 1995, AIDS was the _____ leading cause of death in women ages 25 to 44 years.
   a. 2nd
   b. 3rd
   c. 4th
   d. 5th
6. HIV is classified as a retrovirus because:
   a. The genome RNA is transcribed into DNA once it enters the host cell.
   b. The promotor region of the genome RNA is in the reverse position.
   c. Pieces of the genome RNA are spliced into a single strand before translation.
   d. The envelope glycoproteins (gp120 and gp41) are in a reverse position.

Continued.

QUESTIONS—cont'd

7. The primary cells affected by HIV infection are:
   a. CD4+ T (helper) cells
   b. CD8 T (cytotoxic) cells
   c. B cells
   d. All white blood cells
   e. CD4+ cells only

8. Which of the following is the *least* accurate statement regarding the nature of HIV?
   a. The genome of HIV contains sequences that enhance the transcription of other genes.
   b. Host cell specificity is determined by the interaction of the envelope glycoproteins of the virus with CD4+ proteins on the surface of cells.
   c. Both the genome of HIV and the antigenicity of its envelope glycoprotein are remarkably stable compared with other retroviruses.
   d. One of the cytopathic effects caused by HIV infection of CD4+ T lymphocytes is the formation of giant cells.

9. Which of the following statements is *true* of the HIV virus?
   a. HIV is an RNA retrovirus that utilizes the enzyme reverse transcriptase to produce DNA in the infected cell.
   b. The virus attaches to the host cell membrane and remains there without entering the cell.
   c. The virus remains in the host for only a limited time and then disappears.
   d. The virus remains quiescent and does not replicate during the asymptomatic phase of HIV disease.
   e. Central nervous system cells are safe from infection because of the blood-brain barrier.

10. All the following statements about the HIV virus are correct *except:*
    a. HIV is an enveloped RNA virus.
    b. The virion contains an RNA-dependent DNA polymerase.
    c. A DNA copy of the HIV genome integrates into the host cell DNA.
    d. Replication of the virus is inhibited by acyclovir.

11. Modes of transmission of HIV include all the following *except·*
    a. Penile-anal
    b. Penile-vaginal
    c. Fecal-oral
    d. Parenteral
    e. Mother to fetus/newborn

12. A HIV-positive woman has just given birth to a baby boy. As her nurse, you would advise her to:
    a. Seek professional counseling to deal with the guilt associated with the almost certain event of transmitting the disease to her infant
    b. Identify all her sexual partners so that they may be reported immediately to the infectious disease department
    c. Have her infant tested immediately, using the ELISA test, to determine if he is infected
    d. Avoid breastfeeding her infant

13. The preferred laboratory method of diagnosing AIDS infection is:
    a. Complement fixation test
    b. Enzyme-linked immunoassay confirmed by Western blot
    c. Hemagglutination followed by immunoelectrophoresis
    d. Polymerase chain reaction
    e. Measurement of p24 antigen

14. Which of the following statements would *not* be appropriate when explaining the significance of positive ELISA and Western blot tests to a patient?
    a. Antibodies to the AIDS virus are present in your blood.
    b. You probably have active virus in your body and should assume that you are capable of passing the virus to others.
    c. You have AIDS.
    d. You have been infected with the AIDS virus, and your body has produced antibodies.

15. The laboratory criterion used for the diagnosis of AIDS is a CD4+ T lymphocyte count of:
    a. 600 to 1200 cells/mm^3
    b. 500 to 1000 cells/mm^3
    c. 200 to 500 cells/mm^3
    d. Less than 200 cells/mm^3

16. In assisting a patient with long-range planning, the nurse should inform the patient that the time between HIV-positive seroconversion (clinical latency period) and the appearance of symptoms may be about:
    a. 6 months
    b. 1 year
    c. 5 years
    d. 10 years

17. Which of the following terms is used to describe the mechanism of programmed cell death in HIV-infected CD4+ T lymphocytes?
    a. Anergy
    b. Apoptosis
    c. Syncytia
    d. Karyolysis

18. Cytopathic mechanisms that may explain a progressive decrease in the CD4+ T lymphocyte count during the course of HIV infectious disease include all the following *except:*
    a. Antibody-dependent complement-mediated mechanisms resulting in the death of HIV-infected T cells
    b. Budding of new HIV viruses causing the death of the host cell
    c. Programmed death of the HIV-infected cell
    d. Fusion of uninfected and HIV-infected cells into giant cells (syncytia)
    e. Suppression of CD6 lymphocytes

19. Chronic signs and symptoms indicating immune dysfunction and the possible presence of AIDS would include:
    a. Unexplained diarrhea
    b. Unexplained night sweats
    c. Unexplained fatigue/malaise
    d. Cutaneous anergy to multiple skin test antigens
    e. All the above

20. When an AIDS patient is infected with *Cryptosporidium* protozoa, his or her presenting problem would be:
    a. Delirium
    b. Severe upper respiratory tract infection
    c. Profuse watery diarrhea
    d. Painful cutaneous lesions

21. The percentage of infants who acquire AIDS from a HIV-infected mother is approximately:
    a. 10%
    b. Less than 50%
    c. More than 75%
    d. Almost 100%

22. AIDS in children differs from that in adults in that:
    a. The disease has a slower progression and is more benign in children.
    b. Evidence of B lymphocyte dysfunction generally precedes a decrease in the CD4+ count in children.
    c. The asymptomatic period is longer in children.
    d. Kaposi's sarcoma is more common in children.

QUESTIONS—cont'd

▼ Match the clinical manifestations in column A with the phase of HIV infection in column B with which they are most likely to be associated.

Column A

23. Generally asymptomatic, but CD4+ T cell count gradually decreased below normal value
24. CD4+ T cell count less than 500/mm³, persistent generalized lymphadenopathy, minor opportunistic infections (e.g., thrush from *Candida,* shingles, oral hairy leukoplakia from Epstein-Barr virus)
25. Mononucleosis-like illness lasting 3 to 6 weeks (e.g., fever, malaise, lymphadenopathy, erythematous maculopapular rash), CD4+ T cell count slightly decreased below normal value
26. Individual infected with HIV but virus cannot be detected using the standard antibody tests; no detectable physiologic response to virus screenings
27. CD4+ T cell count less than 200/mm³, recurrent opportunistic infections such as *Pneumocystis carinii* pneumonia and neoplasms

Column B

a. Incubation phase (window period)
b. Acute HIV syndrome soon after initial infection
c. Clinical latency phase
d. Early symptomatic disease
e. Advanced symptomatic disease

28. Place the following steps in the life cycle of HIV infection in the proper order:
    1. On activation, provirus initiates transcription to messenger RNA (mRNA).
    2. Reverse transcription of viral RNA to copy DNA (cDNA) occurs.
    3. Fusion of HIV with the host cell membrane occurs via gp41, facilitating entry of HIV into cell.
    4. cDNA migrates to host cell nucleus.
    5. cDNA integrated into host cell chromosomes with help of integrase to become a provirus.
    6. gp120 protein binds with CD4+ receptor on target cell.
    7. Viral mRNA is translated into viral enzymes and structural proteins in the cytoplasm.
    8. Assembly of new HIV occurs with release from host cell by budding.

    a. 6, 3, 2, 4, 5, 1, 7, 8   c. 6, 3, 2, 4, 5, 1, 7, 8
    b. 2, 3, 1, 5, 6, 4, 7, 8   d. 3, 6, 2, 5, 4, 1, 8, 7

▼ Match the AIDS-related illnesses in column A with the most appropriate treatment in column B.

Column A

29. *Pneumocystis carinii* pneumonia
30. HIV-positive children and adults (asymptomatic and symptomatic)
31. Kaposi's sarcoma
32. Cytomegalovirus retinitis
33. Herpes simplex abscesses
34. *Mycobacterium* pulmonary tuberculosis

Column B

a. Zidovudine
b. Gancyclovir
c. Bactrim or Septra
d. Acyclovir
e. Local radiation therapy and/or chemotherapy
f. Isoniazid, rifampin, ethambutol, and pyrazinamide

▼ Circle T if the statement is true and F if it is false. Correct any false statements.

35. T F HIV has a bar-shaped nucleoid surrounded by an envelope containing virus-specific proteins, gp120 and gp41.
36. T F The *gag* gene of the HIV genome encodes the internal core proteins, the most important of which is p24, an antigen used in serologic tests.
37. T F The genome of HIV consists of two identical molecules of single-stranded, positive-polarity DNA.
38. T F Only T helper cells can be infected with HIV, since they are the only cells that have CD4+ molecules on their surface.
39. T F The opportunistic infections seen in AIDS are primarily the result of a loss in cell-mediated immunity.
40. T F One of the most common opportunistic infections in individuals with AIDS is *Pneumocystis carinii* pneumonia.
41. T F Kaposi's sarcoma is the most common malignancy seen in AIDS.
42. T F Homosexual contact is the most common mode of HIV transmission worldwide.

BIBLIOGRAPHY ▼ PART II

Barre-Sinoussi F et al: Isolation of a T-lymphocyte retrovirus from a patient at risk for acquired immunodeficiency syndrome (AIDS), *Science* 220:868-871, 1983.

Bierman CW, Pearlman DS: *Allergic disease of infancy, childhood, and adolescence,* Philadelphia, 1980, Saunders.

Bolognesi D: Prospects for an HIV vaccine, *Sci Am Sci Med* 1:44-53, 1994.

Borkowsky W et al: Correlation of perinatal transmission of human immunodeficiency virus type 1 with maternal viremia and lymphocyte phenotypes, *J Pediatr* 125:345-351, 1994.

Brouwers P et al: Central nervous system involvement: manifestations, evaluation, and pathogenesis. In Pizzo P, Wilfert C, editors: *Pediatric AIDS,* Baltimore, 1994, Williams & Wilkins.

Centers for Disease Control: *Pneumocystis* pneumonia—Los Angeles, *MMWR* 30:250-252, 1981.

Centers for Disease Control: 1993 revised classification system for HIV infection and expanded surveillance case definition for AIDS among adolescents and adults, *MMWR* 41 (RR-17):1-19, 1992.

Centers for Disease Control: *HIV/AIDS surveillance report,* Atlanta, Oct. 12, 1994, Document #320200, 1994a, CDC.

Centers for Disease Control: 1994 revised classification system for human immunodeficiency virus infection in children less than 13 years of age, *MMWR* 43 (RR-12):1-7, 1994b.

Centers for Disease Control: Zidovudine for the prevention of HIV transmission from mother to infant, *MMWR* 43(16):285-287, 1994c.

Centers for Disease Control: Recommendations of the US Public Health Service task force on the use of zidovudine to reduce perinatal transmission of human immunodeficiency virus, *MMWR* 43(11):1-20, 1994d.

Centers for Disease Control: Update: acquired immunodeficiency syndrome—United States, 1994, *MMWR* 44(4):64-67, 1995a.

Centers for Disease Control: Update: AIDS among women—United States, 1994, *MMWR* 44(5):81-84, 1995b.

Coffin J: HIV population dynamics in vivo: implications for genetic variation, pathogenesis, and therapy, *Science* 167:483-489, 1995.

Embretson J et al: Massive covert infection of helper T lymphocytes and macrophages by HIV during the incubation period of AIDS, *Nature* 362:359-362, 1993.

Fisher AA: *Contact dermatitis,* ed 3, Philadelphia, 1986, Lea & Febiger.

Gallo RC et al: Frequent detection and isolation of cytopathic retroviruses (HTLV-III) from patients with AIDS and at risk for AIDS, *Science* 224:500-503, 1984.

Goldschmidt R, Dong B: Current report—HIV: treatment of AIDS and HIV-related conditions, 1995, *J Am Board Fam Pract* 8:139-162, 1995.

Gottlieb MS et al: *Pneumocystis carinii* pneumonia and mucosal candidiasis in previously healthy homosexual men, *N Engl J Med* 305:1425, 1981.

Gougeon M, Montagnier L: Apoptosis in AIDS, *Science* 260:1269-1270, 1993.

Greene W: AIDS and the immune system, *Sci Am* 269(3):99-105, 1993.

Grimes D, Grimes R: *AIDS and HIV infection,* St Louis, 1994, Mosby.

Ho D et al: Rapid turnover of plasma virions and CD4 lymphocytes in HIV-1 infection, *Nature* 373:123-126, 1995.

Johnson M, Hoth D: Present status and future prospects for HIV therapies, *Science* 260:1286-1293, 1993.

Kaplan AP, editor: *Allergy,* New York, 1985, Churchill Livingstone.

Kovacs J et al: Increases in CD4 T lymphocytes with intermittent courses of interleukin-2 in patients with human immunodeficiency virus infection, *N Engl J Med* 332:567-575, 1995.

Krasinski K: Bacterial infections. In Pizzo P, Wilfert C, editors: *Pediatric AIDS,* Baltimore, 1994, Williams & Wilkins.

Levy J: *HIV and the pathogenesis of AIDS,* Washington, DC, 1994, ASM Press.

Mallory SB: Allergy contact dermatitis, *Immunol Allergy Clin North Am* 7:407-421, 1987.

Marlink R et al: Reduced rate of disease development after HIV-2 infection as compared to HIV-1, *Science* 265:1587-1590, 1994.

Mathews KP: Urticaria and angioedema, *J Allergy Clin Immunol* 72:1-14, 1983.

Middleton E Jr, Reed CE, Ellis EF: *Allergy: principles and practice,* ed 4, St Louis, 1993, Mosby.

Mudge-Grout C: *Immunologic disorders,* St Louis, 1993, Mosby.

Pantaleo G et al: HIV infection is active and progressive in lymphoid tissue during the clinically latent stage of disease, *Nature* 362:355-358, 1993.

Rubinstein A, Calvelli T: Pediatric acquired immunodeficiency syndrome. In Frank M et al, editors: *Samter's immunologic diseases,* ed 5, Boston, 1995, Little, Brown.

Schattner E, Laurence J: HIV-induced T-lymphocyte depletion, *Clin Lab Med* 14:221-238, 1994.

Stanley SG, Faucie A: Acquired immunodeficiency syndrome. In Frank M et al, editors: *Samter's immunologic diseases,* ed 5, Boston, 1995, Little, Brown.

Stiehm ER, Fulginiti VA: *Immunological disorders in infants and children,* ed 3, Philadelphia, 1989, Saunders.

Volberding P: Perspectives on the use of antiretroviral drugs in the treatment of HIV infection, *Infect Dis Clin North Am* 8:303-318, 1994.

Wei X et al: Viral dynamics in human immunodeficiency virus type 1 infection, *Nature* 373:117-122, 1995.

Weiss R: How does HIV cause AIDS? *Science* 260:1273-1278, 1993.

Williams R: *Immune complexes in clinical and experimental medicine,* Cambridge, Mass, 1980, Harvard University Press.

World Health Organization: *The current global situation of the HIV/AIDS pandemic,* Geneva, 1995, WHO.

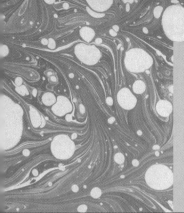

PART THREE
HEMATOLOGIC SYSTEM DISORDERS

Hematology deals with blood and the blood-forming tissues. The hematologic system also includes the monocyte-macrophage (mononuclear phagocyte) system, originally described as the reticuloendothelial system (RES), which is located throughout the body, especially in the spleen, liver, lymph nodes, and bone marrow. It phagocytizes materials ranging from foreign microorganisms to dying red blood cells from the blood and body tissues. Disorders arising from these systems, called *blood dyscrasias*, range from mild and curable to rapidly progressing and lethal diseases. Diagnosis and treatment focus on the accurate interpretation of historical data, careful physical assessment, and laboratory examination.

This section examines the blood-forming tissues, the blood, and its components, with emphasis on alterations relating to red blood cells, white blood cells, platelets, and the clotting factors. ▼

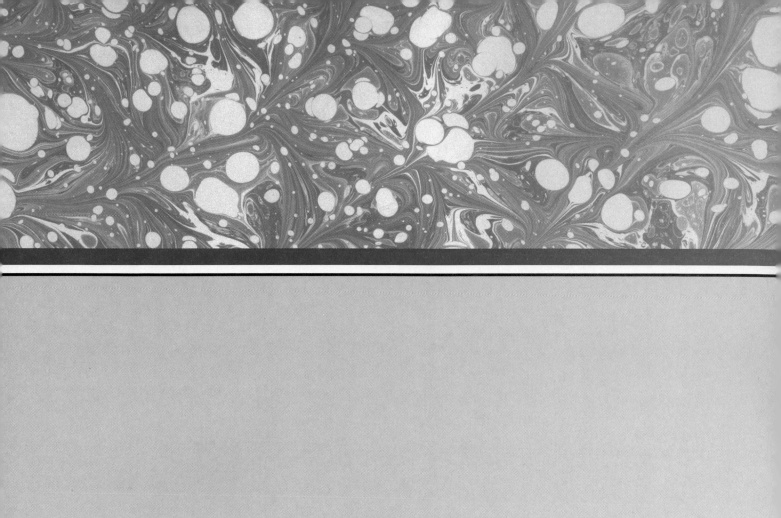

CHAPTER 16

The Composition of Blood and the Monocyte-Macrophage System

CATHERINE M. BALDY

COMPONENTS OF NORMAL BLOOD

Blood is a suspension of particulate material in an aqueous colloid solution containing electrolytes. It serves as a medium of exchange between the fixed cells of the body and the external environment and possesses properties protective to the organism as a whole and to itself in particular.

The aqueous component of blood, called *plasma,* consists of 91% to 92% water as a transport medium and 8% to 9% solids. The solids include proteins such as albumin, globulins, clotting factors, and enzymes; other organic constituents such as nonprotein nitrogenous substances (urea, uric acid, xanthine, creatinine, amino acids), neutral fats, phospholipids, cholesterol, and glucose; and inorganic constituents, including sodium, chloride, bicarbonate, calcium, potassium, magnesium, phosphorus, iron, and iodine. A supernatant remains after the removal of fibrinogen and the clotting factors from plasma. Even though all the elements play a vital role in homeostasis, the plasma proteins are often involved in blood dyscrasias. Of the three major types, albumin formed in the liver accounts for approximately 53% of the serum protein. The major roles of albumin are in the maintenance of blood volume by providing colloid osmotic pressure, in pH and electrolyte balance, and in the trans-port of metal ions, fatty acids, hormones, and drugs. Globulins, accounting for 43% of the protein, are formed in the liver and lymphoid tissues. Antibodies (immunoglobulins) are among the most important globulins. Fibrinogen, accounting for 4% of the protein, is one of the clotting factors.

The cellular component of whole blood consists of red blood cells (erythrocytes, red corpuscles, or RBCs), several different types of white blood cells (leukocytes, white corpuscles, or WBCs), and fragments of cells called platelets (or thrombocytes). RBCs transport or exchange O_2 and CO_2, WBCs are responsible for infection control, and platelets maintain hemostasis. Because these cells have a finite life span, constant production is necessary to maintain levels required to meet tissue needs. This production, called *hematopoiesis* (formation and maturation of blood cells), takes place in the bone marrow of the skull, vertebrae, pelvis, sternum, ribs, and the proximal epiphyses of the long bones. During periods of increased demand, as in hemorrhage or cell destruction (hemolysis), production may resume in all the long bones, as it does in childhood.

On the basis of sophisticated karyotype (chromosomal) studies, all normal blood cells are thought to derive from a single pluripotential stem cell with mitotic capability. Daughters of stem cells can differentiate into either lymphoid or myeloid stem cells, which become progenitor cells. Progenitor cells differentiate along a single pathway. Through a series of divisions and maturational changes, these cells become specific mature cells in the circulating blood (Fig. 16-1). The marrow stem cells continuously replace senescent blood cells and respond to acute changes, such as hemorrhage or infection, by preferentially differentiating into the specific cell lines needed.

The monocyte-macrophage system is a part of the hematologic system and includes circulating monocytes and their precursor cells in the bone marrow. The more mature tissue monocyte is called a *macrophage* (a specific WBC responsible for phagocytosis in the inflammatory reaction). This system is described in Chapter 4.

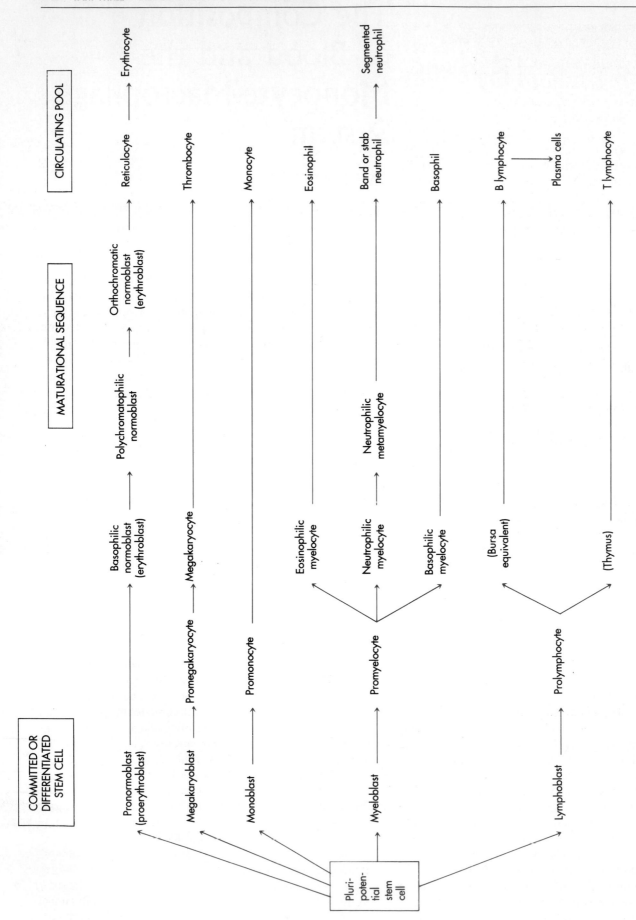

FIG. 16-1   Theory of formation and maturation of blood cells (hematopoiesis).

METHODS FOR STUDYING BLOOD

Inherent in an accurate diagnosis of hematologic disorders (blood dyscrasias) is an in-depth assessment of the individual. This assessment includes a thorough history (i.e., past and current illnesses, drug exposure, bleeding tendencies, nutritional habits, and family history), physical examination, and selective diagnostic studies. Specific studies attempt to quantitate the various constituents of blood and bone marrow. This may be accomplished by examining a specified volume of blood. For the most accurate results, a blood sample obtained by a venipuncture is preferred. However, capillary blood specimens may be obtained by pricking the free margin of the earlobe or the palmar surface of the fingertips.

Descriptive Terms and Methods of Measurement

Blood cell count refers to an actual count of the number of formed elements (i.e., RBCs, WBCs, and platelets) in a specific volume of blood. RBCs must be lysed (destroyed) before the WBCs can be counted. These counts are usually expressed as a number of cells per cubic millimeter (mm^3) of blood. Abnormal cell counts are a reflection of the body's response or lack of response to certain processes.

Differential blood cell count determines the morphologic characteristics, as well as the numbers of the various blood cells. This is done by extracting a drop of capillary blood from the fingertip or the earlobe and carefully spreading a thin film on a glass slide. The slide is stained with Wright's stain, which imparts different colors to the various cell structures according to their pH. Colors range from blue to pink or red. The various types of white blood cells, red blood cells, and platelets can be differentiated according to (1) the color they stain, (2) their size and configuration, (3) the structure of the nuclear chromatin, and (4) the presence or absence of nucleoli within the nucleus. An experienced hematologist, hematopathologist, or laboratory technologist can identify the various cells, their maturities, and other characteristics.

The RBCs visible on smears may be characterized according to variations in size and shape (Color plates 9, 10, and 11). The term *anisocytosis* refers to an abnormal variation in the size of the cells. Abnormal variation in shape is *poikilocytosis* and may denote cells shaped like teardrops, pears, helmets, and ovals. Both poikilocytosis and anisocytosis may reflect defective erythropoiesis (formation and development of RBCs).

Spherocytes have a decreased diameter/thickness ratio. They are spherical instead of having the normal biconcave disk shape. They have increased osmotic fragility and are seen in a congenital hemolytic anemia called *congenital spherocytosis*. Sickle cells are characteristic of hemoglobin S and other sickling forms of hemoglobin. The cells assume a sickle shape on deoxygenation.

Polychromasia is a term used when cells vary in their color distribution. *Normochromia* reflects a normal hemoglobin concentration in cells. *Hypochromia* denotes a cell that is pale, reflecting a decreased hemoglobin concentration as seen in iron-deficiency anemia.

Other variations in RBC structure that can be identified on a stained smear are *siderocytes,* which are cells containing granules of inorganic iron, and *nucleated red blood cells* or *normoblasts* (erythroblasts), which are normally observed in the bone marrow but present in the peripheral blood in response to high erythrocyte demand.

The major component of the RBC is the protein hemoglobin (Hb). Synthesis of hemoglobin in RBCs extends from the normoblast to the reticulocyte stage of development. Hemoglobin's major function is to transport O_2 and CO_2. The hemoglobin concentration of blood is measured by its color intensity, using a photometer, and it is expressed as grams of hemoglobin per hundred milliliters of blood (g/100 ml) or grams per deciliter (g/dl).

The type of hemoglobin can also be identified. Approximately 300 variants of hemoglobin, differing in the genetic code and thus the sequence of aminoacids, have been identified. Although most types are without clinical significance and are functionally normal, some produce marked morbidity and mortality. Hemoglobin electrophoresis identifies the abnormal hemoglobin. The various types move at different characteristic velocities across paper or starch gel, based on their electrical charge. Hemoglobins are identified by letters or by their place of occurrence and discovery:

Hb A: normal adult hemoglobin
Hb F: fetal hemoglobin
Hb S: hemoglobin found in sickle cell disease
Hb Memphis

Another measure, the *hematocrit* (Hct) or packed cell volume, indicates the volume of the whole blood that is composed of RBCs. This measurement is the percentage of RBCs in the whole blood after centrifugation of the specimen and is expressed as cubic millimeters of packed cells per dl of blood or in volumes per dl.

The results of the RBC count, its hemoglobin concentration, and the hematocrit are used to calculate the red cell indices, which reflect the size of the RBC, its hemoglobin content, and its concentration. Dividing the hematocrit by the RBC count gives the *mean corpuscular volume* (MCV). This is a size measurement, expressed as cubic micrometers, with the normal range being 81 to 96 μm^3. RBCs in that range are termed *normocytic,* being of normal cell size. An MCV less than 81 μm^3 indicates cells that are microcytic, because they appear smaller than 7 μm on smears, whereas an MCV greater than 96 μm^3 indicates macrocytic cells that are larger than 8 μm on smears.

The *mean corpuscular hemoglobin concentration* (MCHC) measures the amount of hemoglobin in 100 ml

TABLE 16-1   Methods for Examining Blood

Measurement	Description
Red blood cell (RBC) count	Number of RBCs in 1 mm³ of blood (millions per cubic millimeter)
Hemoglobin concentration	Amount of hemoglobin in a given volume of blood (expressed as g per dl ml)
Hematocrit	Percent of blood made up of RBCs (volume %)
Mean corpuscular volume (MCV)	Volume of each individual RBC (μm³): $$MCV = \frac{\text{Hematocrit (vol \% } \times 10)}{\text{RBC count (millions/mm}^3)}$$
Mean corpuscular hemoglobin concentration (MCHC)	Proportion of each RBC occupied by hemoglobin (concentration measurement): $$MCHC = \frac{\text{Hemoglobin (g/dl } \times 100)}{\text{Hematocrit (vol \%)}}$$
Mean corpuscular hemoglobin (MCH)	Amount of hemoglobin present in each RBC (weight measurement): $$MCH = \frac{\text{Hemoglobin (g/dl } \times 10)}{\text{RBC count (millions/mm}^3)}$$
White blood cell (WBC) count	Number of WBCs in 1 mm³ of blood
Differential count	Percent of the various types of WBCs seen on examination of a peripheral film (granulocytes including PMNs,* Segs,* eosinophils, and basophils; monocytes; and lymphocytes)
Platelet count	Number of platelets in 1 mm³ of blood
Reticulocyte count	Percent of immature nonnucleated RBCs containing residual RNA

*PMN, Polymorphonuclear leukocyte; Segs, segmented neutrophils.

(1 dl) of packed RBCs. Determined by dividing the hemoglobin measurement by the hematocrit, it is expressed in grams per 100 ml (g/dl). The normal range is 30 to 36 g/dl of blood and such blood is termed normochromic; a finding of less than 30/dl is hypochromic because these cells appear pale on the smear. The *mean corpuscular hemoglobin* (MCH) measures the amount of hemoglobin present in a single RBC. It is determined by dividing the amount of hemoglobin in 1000 ml of blood by the number of red cells per cubic millimeter of blood. The MCH is expressed in picograms of hemoglobin per RBC. The normal value is about 27 to 31 pg per RBC.

The *reticulocyte count,* another important determination, reflects bone marrow activity. A reticulocyte is an immature nonnucleated RBC that contains residual RNA in its cytoplasm. Normally only 1% to 2% are seen in the peripheral blood. A peripheral blood smear, taken as just described, is treated with a supravital stain, which imparts a blue color to any RNA within immature RBCs; such cells appear to have a net or "reticulum" inside, hence the name reticulocyte (Table 16-1). The residual RNA disappears within the first day or two that the cell is outside the bone marrow, and the cell becomes a mature RBC. An increased number of circulating reticulocytes indicates increased bone marrow activity, whereas a decrease or absence indicates bone marrow failure.

Normal values for these measurements are given in Table 16-2.

 TABLE 16-2   **Normal Blood Cell Values**

Measurement	Men	Women
Red blood cell (RBC) count (million cells/mm³)	4.7-6.1	4.2-5.2
Hemoglobin (g/dl)	13.4-17.6	12.0-15.4
Hematocrit (vol %)	42-53	38-46
MCV (μm³/RBC)	81-96	
MCHC (g/dl RBC)	30-36	
MCH (pg/RBC)	27-31	
Total white blood cell (WBC) count (cells/mm³)	4000-10,000	
Granulocytes*		
PMNs (%)	38-70	
Eosinophils (%)	1-5	
Basophils (%)	0-2	
Monocytes (%)*	1-8	
Lymphocytes (%)*	15-45	
Platelets (cells/mm³)	150,000-400,000	
Reticulocyte count (%)†	1-2	

*% of total WBCs.
†% of total RBCs.

Study of Bone Marrow

A bone marrow aspiration and biopsy are performed when the preceding studies yield insufficient data or when diseases are suspected that may affect the hematologic system. Aspiration studies are also used to guide the dosages of chemotherapy and radiation therapy in patients with hematologic malignancies.

An accurate bone marrow specimen in an adult can be obtained from the sternum, the spinous processes of the vertebrae, or the anterior or posterior iliac crest. If a biopsy is also required, the latter is the preferred site.

Bone marrow biopsy, as well as aspiration, must be considered a minor surgical procedure and carried out under aseptic conditions. The patient is placed comfortably on his or her side with the back slightly flexed and the knees drawn toward the chest. The posterior iliac crest is cleansed and covered with antiseptic solution. The skin, subcutaneous tissue, and periosteum are anesthetized using 1% to 2% lidocaine (Xylocaine). A 2 to 3 mm incision is made to facilitate penetration with a 14-gauge 2 to 4 cm bone marrow needle and to avoid introducing a skin plug into the marrow cavity. On entry, the stylet is removed from the needle, a 10-ml syringe is attached, and with a swift, short aspiration, approximately 25 μl of bone marrow is withdrawn. Even though the patient experiences tremendous pressure throughout the procedure, he or she must be warned that a sudden sharp but brief pain may be felt because of the negative pressure that occurs with aspiration. Smears are quickly made with the aspirate, and grayish white particulate matter can usually be observed along with fat vacuoles. A portion of the specimen is allowed to clot and is sectioned for further study. Cell counts and differentials are also obtained from the aspirate.

A biopsy is usually indicated in hematologic malignancies. In this procedure a special biopsy needle (a Jamshidi needle, 11 cm long with a 3 mm diameter tapering to a 2 mm cutting edge) is used to obtain a bone spicule. This bone spicule is extruded onto a glass slide using a probe inserted through the cutting edge. Several imprints are made by gently touching the slide with the spicule, which can be stained with Wright's stain, as discussed earlier with the peripheral smear. One or two slides may be stained, with Prussian blue reaction depicting stored iron. The biopsy spicule is placed in Bouin's or Zenker's solution, both of which are fixatives. The specimen is then placed in paraffin blocks, sectioned, stained, and studied microscopically.

The bone marrow biopsy is used to study the marrow cellularity without destroying the architecture. Bone marrow of increased activity is termed *hypercellular* or *hyperplastic;* marrow with decreased activity is *hypocellular* or *hypoplastic.* The ratio of myeloid (bone marrow leukocytes) to erythroid (red blood cell) elements (M/E ratio) is calculated, and the presence of a normal, increased, or decreased number of megakaryocytes (platelet precursors) is noted. Cell distribution, maturation abnormalities, and neoplastic cells can be observed. Status of the bone, such as fibrosis, can also be identified.

Biochemical Studies

Various studies can be used to measure levels of the elements necessary for cell development, especially that of red blood cells. These studies include measurements of serum iron (Fe), total iron-binding capacity (TIBC), vitamin B_{12}, and folic acid levels. The iron-binding capacity measures the ability of plasma transferrin to carry iron from the gastrointestinal tract or iron stores to the bone marrow. It is elevated in iron-deficiency anemia. Other studies related to hematology include the coagulation studies (see Chapter 19).

QUESTIONS

▼ *Answer the following on a separate sheet of paper.*
1. Define hematology.
2. Describe the hematologic system.
3. Describe the three major types of cells found in the cellular component of whole blood.
4. Explain the theory of hematopoiesis.
5. Describe the assessment process applied when diagnosing blood dyscrasias.

▼ *Circle the letter preceding each item below that correctly answers the question or completes the statement. More than one answer may be correct.*
6. The portion of blood in which cellular elements are suspended is referred to as the:
   a. Cytoplasm of cells
   b. Platelets
   c. Plasma
7. The aqueous component of blood is referred to as:
   a. Globulins
   b. Platelets
   c. Plasma
   d. Leukocytes
8. Globulins consist of approximately what percent of the serum protein?
   a. 13   c. 43
   b. 24   d. 53
9. Fibrinogen accounts for what percent of the serum protein?
   a. 1   c. 6
   b. 4   d. 10
10. The purpose of the red cell indices is to measure:
   a. The number of normal platelets
   b. The size of the red blood cell
   c. The hemoglobin concentration of the red blood cell
   d. The morphologic content of the red blood cell

11. Which of the following anatomic sites are used for a bone marrow specimen?
   a. Posterior iliac crest
   b. Sternum
   c. Spinous processes of the vertebrae
   d. Anterior iliac crest

---

12. Which of the following red blood cells is characteristically found in congenital hemolytic anemia:
   a. HbA
   b. Hb Memphis
   c. Spherocytes
   d. Hb F

▼ *Match each descriptive statement in column A with its appropriate measurement in column B.*

Column A	Column B
13. _____ Red cell count	a. Percentage of packed RBCs in a sample of blood (volume percent)
14. _____ Hematocrit	b. Amount of hemoglobin in a given volume of blood (g/dl)
15. _____ Mean corpuscular volume (MCV)	c. Number of WBCs in 1 mm³ of blood
16. _____ Hemoglobin concentration	d. Number of RBCs in 1 mm³ of blood (millions/mm³)
17. _____ Mean corpuscular hemoglobin concentration (MCHC)	e. The proportion of each RBC occupied by hemoglobin (concentration measurement)
18. _____ Reticulocyte count	f. Number of platelets in 1 mm³ of blood
19. _____ White cell count	g. Volume of each individual RBC (μm³)
20. _____ Mean corpuscular hemoglobin (MCH)	h. Percentage of the different types of WBCs seen on examination of a peripheral film
21. _____ Differential count	i. Percentage of immature nonnucleated RBCs containing residual RNA
22. _____ Platelet count	j. Amount of hemoglobin present in each RBC (weight measurement)

▼ *Circle T if the statement is true and F if it is false. Correct any false statements.*
   Approximate normal values:
23. T F   Red cell count (millions/mm³): 3.0 to 4.0 (men); 2.0 to 3.0 (women)
24. T F   Hematocrit (volume percent): 42 to 53 (men); 38 to 46 (women)
25. T F   Hemoglobin (g/dl): 13.4 to 17.0 (men); 12.0 to 15.0 (women)
26. T F   Total white cell count (cells/mm³): 1000 to 3000
27. T F   Platelets (cells/mm³): 50,000 to 100,000

28. T F   Lymphocytes (percent of WBCs): 15 to 45

▼ *Complete the following statements by filling in the blanks.*
29. _____ is an abnormal variation in the shape of cells (teardrops, pears, ovals).
30. _____ denotes a red blood cell that is pale, reflecting decreased hemoglobin in concentration.
31. The major component of the red blood cell is _____.

CHAPTER 17

Red Blood Cell Disorders

CATHERINE M. BALDY

NORMAL STRUCTURE AND FUNCTION

Red blood cells (RBCs), or erythrocytes, are nonnucleated biconcave disks approximately 8 μm in diameter, 2 μm thick at the outer perimeter, and decreasing to 1 μm or less at the center (Fig. 17-1). Because these cells are soft and pliable, they change in configuration during passage through the microcirculation. The outer leaflet of the cell membrane contains the blood group antigens A and B and the Rh factor identifying the individual's blood type. The RBC's major component is the protein hemo-

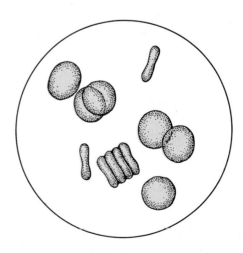

FIG. 17-1   Erythrocytes.

globin (Hb), which transports most of the O_2 and a small fraction of CO_2 and maintains normal pH through a series of intracellular buffers. The Hb molecule consists of two pairs of polypeptide chains (globin) and four heme groups, each one containing an atom of ferrous iron. This configuration allows the most expedient exchange of gases.

There are approximately 5 million RBCs per cubic millimeter of blood in the average adult, and they have an average life span of 120 days. A steady balance is maintained between normal daily losses and replacement. RBC production is stimulated by a glycoprotein hormone, *erythropoietin,* known to originate primarily in the kidney. Erythropoietin production is stimulated by renal tissue hypoxia caused by changes in atmospheric O_2 pressure, decreased O_2 content of arterial blood, and decreased hemoglobin concentration. Erythropoietin stimulates the stem cells to initiate the proliferation and maturation of RBCs. Maturation depends on adequate amounts and proper use of nutrients, such as vitamin B_{12}, folic acid, protein, iron, and copper.

All the steps of hemoglobin synthesis take place in the bone marrow. The late steps continue after the immature RBC is released into the circulation as a reticulocyte.

As the RBC ages, it becomes rigid and fragile and it finally ruptures. The hemoglobin is phagocytosed primarily in the spleen, liver, and bone marrow and is reduced to globin and heme. Globin reenters the amino acid pool. Iron is liberated from heme, and the greater part is transported by the plasma protein transferrin to the bone marrow for RBC production. The remaining iron is stored in the form of ferritin and hemosiderin in the liver and other body tissues for future use (Guyton, 1991). The remaining heme portion is reduced to carbon monoxide (CO) and biliverdin. The CO, carried in the form of carboxyhemoglobin, is excreted via the lungs. The biliverdin is reduced to free bilirubin; this is slowly released into plasma, where it combines with plasma albumin and is transported to the hepatic cells for excretion into the bile canaliculi (Robinson, 1990). In the presence of active red cell destruction, as in hemolysis, the rapid release of large amounts of bilirubin into the extracellular fluids causes the yellowish hue to the skin and conjunctivae called *jaundice* (Guyton, 1991).

ABNORMALITIES OF RED BLOOD CELL PRODUCTION

Alterations of the RBC mass produce two distinct entities. When there are insufficient numbers of RBCs, anemia develops. The opposite condition, too many RBCs, is called polycythemia.

Anemia

By definition, *anemia* is a reduction below the normal level in the number of RBCs, the quantity of hemoglobin, and the volume of packed RBCs (hematocrit) per 100 ml of blood. Anemia is thus not a diagnosis but a reflection of an underlying pathophysiologic alteration revealed by a careful history, physical examination, and laboratory confirmation.

Because all organ systems may be involved, a wide range of clinical manifestations may be seen in anemia, depending on (1) the rate at which the anemia develops, (2) the age of the individual, (3) his or her compensatory mechanism, (4) his or her activity level, (5) the underlying disease state, and (6) the severity of the anemia.

As the effective number of RBCs decreases, less O_2 is delivered to the tissues. Sudden blood loss (30% or more), as in hemorrhage, results in symptoms of hypovolemia and hypoxemia, including restlessness, diaphoresis (cold perspiration), tachycardia, shortness of breath, and rapid progression to circulatory collapse or shock. However, a drop in RBC mass over a period of several months (even a 50% decrease) allows the body's compensatory mechanism to adapt and the patient is usually asymptomatic, except on exertion. The body adapts by (1) increasing the cardiac output and respirations, thereby increasing the delivery of O_2 to the tissues by the RBCs, (2) increasing the release of O_2 by hemoglobin, (3) expanding plasma volume by pulling fluid from the tissue spaces, and (4) redistributing blood flow to vital organs (DeGruchy et al., 1978).

One of the most common signs attributed to anemia is pallor. This generally results from decreased blood volume, decreased hemoglobin, and vasoconstriction to maximize O_2 delivery to major vital organs. Skin color is not a reliable index for pallor because of influences such as skin pigmentation, temperature, and depth and distribution of the capillary bed. Nail beds, palms, and mucous membranes of the mouth and conjunctivae are better indicators for assessing pallor.

Tachycardia and cardiac murmurs (sounds caused by increased velocity of blood flow) reflect the increased cardiac workload and output. Angina (chest pain), especially in older individuals with coronary stenosis, may result from myocardial ischemia. In severe anemia, congestive heart failure may result because the anoxic heart muscle cannot adapt to its increased workload. Dyspnea (difficulty in breathing), shortness of breath, and increased fatigue on exertion are manifestations of decreased O_2 delivery. Headache, dizziness, faintness, and tinnitus (ringing in the ears) may reflect the decreased oxygenation of the central nervous system. Gastrointestinal symptoms such as anorexia, nausea, constipation or diarrhea, and stomatitis (a sore tongue and mouth) may also occur in severe anemia; they are generally associated with deficiency states, such as iron deficiency.

Classification of anemias

Anemias may be classified according to (1) the morphology of the red blood cell and the indices or (2) the etiology.

In the morphologic classification of anemias, *micro-* or *macro-* refers to the size of the RBCs and *chromic* to their color. Three major categories are recognized. In the first, *normocytic, normochromic* anemia, the RBCs are normal in size and shape and contain the normal amount of hemoglobin (MCV and MCHC are normal or low normal). Causes of this type of anemia are acute blood loss, hemolysis, chronic diseases including infections, endocrine disorders, renal disorders, marrow failure, and metastatic infiltrative diseases of the bone marrow.

The second major category is *macrocytic, normochromic* anemia, in which the RBCs are larger than normal but are normochromic because the hemoglobin concentration is normal (MCV increased; MCHC normal) (Fig. 17-2). This results from disordered or interrupted synthesis of DNA as seen in deficiency states of vitamin B_{12} and/or folic acid. It may also occur in cancer chemotherapy because the agents interfere with DNA synthesis.

The third category is *microcytic, hypochromic* ane-

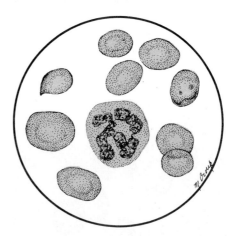

FIG. 17-2 Peripheral blood characteristic of macrocytic anemia. In the upper right, the red blood cells are not as uniformly round (poikilocytosis) as they are in Fig. 17-1, and they are of different sizes (anisocytosis). Most of the cells are either of normal size or too large. The large oval red cells seen in the lower left are called ovalomacrocytes. These cells are characteristic of vitamin B_{12} and folate deficiencies.

mias (Fig. 17-3). Microcytic means small, and hypochromic means containing less than the normal amount of hemoglobin (MCV decreased; MCHC decreased). This generally reflects either insufficient heme synthesis, or lack of iron, as in iron deficiency anemia, sideroblastic states, and chronic blood loss, or impaired globin synthesis, as in thalassemia. Thalassemia involves a mismatch in the amounts of alpha- and beta-chains synthesized, so that the normal tetrameric hemoglobin molecule cannot form.

Anemias may also be classified by etiology. The major causes considered are (1) increased RBC loss and (2) decreased or defective cell production.

Increased RBC loss may be caused by bleeding or by cell destruction. Bleeding may result from trauma or ulcers, or there may be chronic bleeding from polyps in the colon, malignancy, hemorrhoids, or menstruation. Destruction of circulating RBCs, known as *hemolysis,* occurs when a defect in the RBC itself shortens its life or an altered environment leads to its destruction. Conditions in which the RBC itself is defective include the following:

1. Hemoglobinopathies, that is, inherited abnormal hemoglobin, such as sickle cell disease
2. Impaired globin synthesis, such as thalassemia
3. RBC membrane defects, such as hereditary spherocytosis
4. Enzyme deficiencies, such as glucose 6-phosphate dehydrogenase (G6PD) deficiency

The foregoing are hereditary disorders. However, hemolysis can also be caused by problems of the RBC environment, which often entail an immune response. An *isoimmune* response involves different individuals within the same species and results from an incompatible blood transfusion. An *autoimmune* response consists of production of antibodies against the body's own RBCs. Autoimmune hemolytic anemia can occur without known cause after the administration of certain drugs, such as alpha-

methyldopa, quinine, sulfonamides, or L-dopa, or in other disease states, such as lymphoma, chronic lymphocytic leukemia, lupus erythematosus, rheumatoid arthritis, and viral infections. Autoimmune hemolytic anemias are classified according to the temperature at which the antibody reacts with the RBCs—they may be warm antibody type or cold antibody type.

Malaria is a parasitic disease transmitted to humans by the bite of an infected female *Anopheles* mosquito. It results in severe hemolytic anemia when RBCs become infested by a *Plasmodium* parasite, which causes an irregular surface defect in the RBC. The defective RBCs are then rapidly removed from the circulation by the spleen (Beutler, 1990b).

Hypersplenism (enlarged spleen) can also cause hemolysis by markedly increased trapping and destroying of RBCs. Because the enlarged spleen sequesters all types of blood cells, a hypersplenic patient will demonstrate pancytopenia and a normal or hypercellular bone marrow. Severe burns, especially when the capillary bed is disrupted, can also lead to hemolysis.

The second major etiologic classification includes decreased or defective RBC production (dyserythropoiesis). Any condition affecting the bone marrow function falls into this category. Included are (1) metastatic solid tissue malignancies, the leukemias, and multiple myeloma; toxic drugs and chemicals; and irradiation and (2) chronic diseases involving the kidneys and liver, infections, and endocrine deficiencies. Lack of essential vitamins, such as B_{12}, folic acid, and C, and lack of iron can bring about ineffective RBC formation, leading to anemia. To determine the diagnosis of anemia, both the morphologic and etiologic considerations must be incorporated.

Aplastic anemia

Aplastic anemia is a life-threatening disorder of the stem cell in the bone marrow, in which insufficient numbers of blood cells are produced. Aplastic anemia may be congenital, idiopathic (cause unknown), or secondary to industrial or viral causes (Hoffbrand, Pettit, 1993). Individuals with aplastic anemia are pancytopenic (deficient in all types of blood cells). Morphologically the RBCs are normocytic and normochromic, the reticulocyte count is low or absent, and bone marrow biopsy indicates a "dry tap" with marked hypoplasia and replacement with fatty tissue. The idiopathic aplastic anemias are thought to be immunologically mediated, with the patient's T lymphocytes suppressing hematopoietic stem cells.

Secondary causes of aplastic anemia (temporary or permanent) include the following:

1. Antineoplastic or cytotoxic agents
2. Radiation therapy
3. Certain antibiotics
4. Miscellaneous drugs, such as anticonvulsants, thyroid medication, gold compounds, and phenylbutazone
5. Chemicals such as benzene, organic solvents, and in-

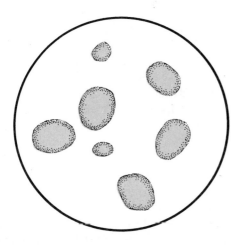

FIG. 17-3 Erythrocytes characteristic of hypochromic anemia.

secticides (agents thought to damage the marrow directly) (Hoffbrand, Pettit, 1993).

Table 17-1 identifies various drugs and their hematologic effects. In addition, aplastic anemia following viral hepatitis is particularly severe and likely to be fatal.

The symptom complex in aplastic anemia relates to the pancytopenia. The signs and symptoms include those of RBC anemia and other symptoms attributable to deficiencies of platelets and WBCs. Platelet deficiency may lead to (1) ecchymoses and petechiae (bleeding into the skin), (2) epistaxis (nosebleeds), (3) gastrointestinal bleeding, (4) genitourinary bleeding, and (5) central nervous system bleeding. Deficiency of WBCs increases susceptibility to infection.

Severe aplasia with a decreased or absent reticulocyte count, a granulocyte count of less than 500/mm³, and a platelet count of less than 20,000 may bring about death from infection and/or bleeding within weeks or months. However, a person less severely affected may live for years. Treatment of aplastic anemia dictates the removal of the causative agent, if known. The major focus of treatment is supportive care until the bone marrow recovers. Since infection and bleeding are the major causes of death, prevention of bleeding and infection becomes essential. Prevention measures may include a protected environment and good hygiene. In the event of bleeding and/or infection, judicious use of blood component therapy (red cells and platelets) and antibiotics becomes essential. Bone marrow–stimulating agents, such as androgens, may induce erythropoiesis, but their efficiency is uncertain. Patients with chronic aplastic anemia adapt well and can be maintained at a hemoglobin level between 8 and 9 g with periodic blood transfusions.

In young individuals with severe aplastic anemia secondary to stem cell damage, transplantation with compatible donors (siblings with matching human histocompatibility leukocyte antigens [HLA]) is indicated. The overall success rate is about 60% to 70% long-term survival. In cases considered to be immunologically mediated, antithymocyte globulin (ATG) containing antibodies against human T cells has been used together with corticosteroids to benefit 50% to 60% of the patients. Response can be expected within months (Hoffbrand, Pettit, 1993).

Iron deficiency anemia

Morphologically this condition is classified as microcytic, hypochromic anemia with a decrease in the quantity of hemoglobin synthesis. Iron deficiency is the major cause of anemia in the world. It is particularly prevalent in women of childbearing age, secondary to menstrual losses and to increased iron demand during pregnancy. Other causes of iron deficiency include (1) inadequate iron intake, for example, infants maintained on milk-only diets for 12 to 24 months and individuals who follow vegetarian dietary habits; (2) impaired absorption after gastrectomy; and (3) persistent blood loss, as with slow gastrointestinal bleeding from polyps, neoplasms, gastritis, esophageal varices, aspirin ingestion, and hemorrhoids.

Normally the average adult body contains 3 to 5 g of iron, depending on sex and size. Nearly two thirds of the iron is found in hemoglobin, and it is released with cell senescence and death and transported via plasma transferrin to the bone marrow for erythropoiesis. With the exception of minute amounts in myoglobin (muscle) and in heme enzymes, the remaining third is stored for further needs in the liver, spleen, and bone marrow as ferritin and hemosiderin.

Although the average diet contains 10 to 20 mg of iron, only about 5% to 10% (1 to 2 mg) is actually absorbed. As iron stores become depleted, more is absorbed from the diet. Ingested iron is converted to ferrous iron in the stomach and duodenum and is absorbed from the duodenum and proximal jejunum. It is then transported by plasma transferrin to the bone marrow for hemoglobin synthesis or to the tissue stores.

Each milliliter of blood contains 0.5 mg of iron. Iron losses generally are minute, from 0.5 to 1 mg/day. However, menstruating women lose an additional 15 to 28 mg/month. Although loss to menses ceases during pregnancy, the daily iron requirement increases to meet the demands of the mother's increased blood volume and the formation of the placenta, umbilical cord, and fetus, as well as to compensate for blood lost during delivery.

In addition to the signs and symptoms presented for anemia, severely iron deficient individuals (plasma iron <40 mg/dl; hemoglobin 6 to 7 g/dl) have brittle, fine hair and nails that are thin, flat, easily broken, and possibly spoon shaped (koilonychia). In addition, the papillae of the tongue atrophy, resulting in a pale, smooth, shiny, beefy-red appearance, and the tongue becomes inflamed and sore. Angular stomatitis, cracking with redness and pain at the corners of the mouth, may also occur.

Examination of the blood reveals a normal or near-normal red cell count and a reduced hemoglobin level. On peripheral smear, the RBCs are microcytic and hypochromic (decreased MCV, decreased MCHC, and decreased MCH) with poikilocytosis and anisocytosis (Color plate 12). The reticulocyte count may be normal or decreased. The iron level is reduced, whereas the total serum iron-binding capacity is increased.

To treat iron deficiency, the underlying cause of the anemia must be identified and resolved. Surgical intervention may be necessary to inhibit active bleeding from polyps, ulcers, malignancies, and hemorrhoids; dietary alterations may be needed for babies fed milk only or for individuals with food idiosyncrasies or who are taking large doses of aspirin. Although dietary modifications may increase the available iron (e.g., by adding liver), supplemental iron is needed to increase the hemoglobin and restore iron stores. Iron is available in parenteral and oral forms. Most patients respond well to oral compounds, such as ferrous sulfate. Parenteral iron prepara-

▶ TABLE 17-1 Hematologic Effects Secondary to Drugs

Generic Name	Trade Name*	Hemolysis	Megalo-blastosis	Aplasia	Leukopenia or Agranulocytosis	Thrombo-cytopenia†	Thrombo-cytopathy†
ANTIBIOTICS							
Chloramphenicol	Chloromycetin	X		XX	X	X	
Erythromycin	Ilosone			X	X	X	
Penicillin	Pen-Vee K	XX		X	X	X	X
Sulfisoxazole	Gantrisin	XX		X	X	XX	
Tetracycline	Sumycin	X		X	X	X	
ANTICONVULSANTS							
Phenytoin	Dilantin	X	X	X	X	X	
Phenobarbital	Luminal	X	X	X		X	
Mephenytoin	Mesantoin	X	X	X	X	X	
ORAL HYPOGLYCEMICS							
Tolbutamide	Orinase	X		XX	X	X	
Chlorpropamide	Diabinese			X	X		
ANTIINFLAMMATORY DRUGS							
Acetylsalicylic acid, aspirin	Colsalide	X		X	X	XX	XX
Colchicine				X	X	X	X
Gold compounds				X	XX	X	
Indomethacin	Indocin	X		X	X	X	XX
Phenylbutazone	Butazolidin			XX	XX	XX	XX
ANTIHYPERTENSIVES AND DIURETICS							
Chlorothiazide	Diuril	X		X	X	X	
Methyldopa	Aldomet	XX		X	X	X	
ANTINEOPLASTICS							
Mechlorethamine hydrochloride	Mustargen			XX	XX	XX	
Cyclophosphamide	Cytoxan			XX	XX	XX	
Cytarabine	Cytosar-U		XX	XX	XX	XX	
Methotrexate	Folex	X	XX	XX	XX	XX	
Mercaptopurine	Purinethol		XX	XX	XX	XX	
TRANQUILIZERS							
Chlordiazepoxide	Librium			X	X		X
Imipramine	Tofranil			X	XX		X
Chlorpromazine	Thorazine	X	X	X	X	X	X

X, Infrequently occurring; *XX*, frequently occurring.
*This list is not all inclusive; other equally effective brands may exist.
†Thrombocytopenia is a decrease in platelet numbers; thrombocytopathy is an alteration in platelet function.

tions are used selectively because they are costly and have a high incidence of adverse reactions.

Megaloblastic anemias

Megaloblastic anemias (large red cells) are classified morphologically as macrocytic normochromic anemias. Megaloblastic anemias are often caused by vitamin B_{12} and folic acid (folate) deficiencies, which result in disordered DNA synthesis. These deficiencies may be secondary to malnutrition, folic acid deficiency, malabsorption, lack of intrinsic factor (as seen in pernicious anemia and postgastrectomy), parasitic infestations, intestinal disease, and malignancies, as well as being caused by chemotherapeutic agents. In individuals with tapeworm infections (with *Diphyllobothrium latum*) secondary to ingestion of infected freshwater fish, the tapeworm competes with its host for the vitamin B_{12} in ingested food, which leads to megaloblastic anemia (Beck, 1990).

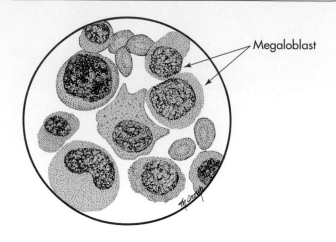

Megaloblast

FIG. 17-4 Bone marrow characteristic of megaloblastic anemia. In the upper left there is one red blood cell precursor that is nearly normal, with a condensed nuclear chromatin pattern. The remaining cells are large and have an open nuclear chromatin pattern. These large cells (two to three times normal size) are also red blood cell precursors. In the lower left is a large white blood cell precursor (metamyelocyte) that is two to three times normal size. This finding indicates that all cell lines develop abnormally in this condition.

Although pernicious anemia typifies megaloblastic anemias, folate deficiency is more commonly encountered in clinical practice. Megaloblastic anemia often is seen as malnutrition in older adults, alcoholics, or teenagers, and in pregnancy where there is an increased demand to meet the needs of the fetus and lactation. This demand is also increased in hemolytic anemias, malignancies, and hyperthyroidism. Celiac disease and tropical sprue also cause malabsorption, and drugs that act as folic acid antagonists interfere with use.

The minimum daily requirement of folate, approximately 50 mg, is easily provided in an average diet. The most abundant sources are red meats, such as liver and kidney, and fresh, leafy green vegetables. However, proper preparation of the food is necessary to ensure adequate nutrition. For example, 50% to 90% of the folate can be lost with cooking in large volumes of water. Folate is absorbed from the duodenum and upper jejunum, weakly bound to plasma proteins, and stored in the liver. In the absence of folate intake, folate stores are usually depleted in approximately 4 months. In addition to the symptoms described for anemias, individuals with megaloblastic anemia secondary to folate deficiency may appear malnourished and experience severe glossitis (inflamed, painful tongue), diarrhea, and loss of appetite. Serum folate levels are also decreased (<4 ng/ml). The bone marrow of a patient with megaloblastic anemia is depicted in Fig. 17-4. Color plate 13 illustrates the peripheral blood findings seen in megaloblastic anemia. The reticulocyte count is usually decreased along with the hematocrit and hemoglobin.

As mentioned previously, treatment depends on identifying and removing the underlying cause. This includes correcting the dietary deficiencies and replacement therapy with folic acid or vitamin B_{12}. Alcoholic patients who are hospitalized often have a "spontaneous" response when given a nutritionally balanced diet.

Sickle Cell Disease
Causes

Sickle cell disease is a hemoglobinopathy resulting from abnormalities in hemoglobin structure. The defect in structure occurs in the globin fraction of the hemoglobin molecule. Recall that globin is constructed of two pairs of polypeptide chains. For example, Hb S differs from normal Hb A in the substitution of valine for glutamic acid in one pair of chains. In Hb C, lysine is in that position. As noted previously, many abnormal hemoglobins exist with varying degrees of symptoms, ranging from none to severe.

Sickle cell disease is a genetic disorder whereby an individual inherits the sickle hemoglobin (hemoglobin S) from both parents (homozygous). Heterozygous individuals (abnormal gene inherited from only one parent) are said to have sickle cell trait. They are generally asymptomatic and have a normal life span. In patients with sickle cell trait, morbidity related to impaired oxygenation, such as that during anesthesia, at high altitudes, and with chronic obstructive pulmonary disease (COPD), has been reported but is extremely rare and not well documented (Beutler, 1990a).

The amino acid substitution in sickle cell disease results in major rearrangement of the hemoglobin molecule when deoxygenation (decreased O_2 tension) occurs. The RBCs then elongate and become rigid and crescent- or sickle-shaped (Fig. 17-5).

Deoxygenation can occur for many reasons. Erythrocytes containing Hb S traverse the microcirculation more slowly than normal erythrocytes, giving more time for deoxygenation. It is postulated that the Hb S erythrocytes adhere to the endothelium, further retarding blood flow. The increased deoxygenation may take the abnormal red blood cells below a critical point and bring on sickling within the microvasculature. Because of their rigidity and irregular membrane, sickle cells clump together, leading to vascular occlusion, pain crisis, and organ infarctions (Hebbel et al., 1980). Repeated episodes of sickling and unsickling cause the cell membranes to become fragile and fragment. The cells are then hemolyzed and removed by the monocyte-macrophage system. The RBC life span is markedly reduced, and an increased demand is put on the bone marrow for replacement. Fig. 17-6 depicts the cycle of sickle cell infarctive crisis.

Sickle cell anemia is the most prevalent form of congenital hemolytic anemia. Affecting about 1 in 600 African Americans, sickle cell anemia is the most common form of sickle cell disease. Hb S accounts for 75%

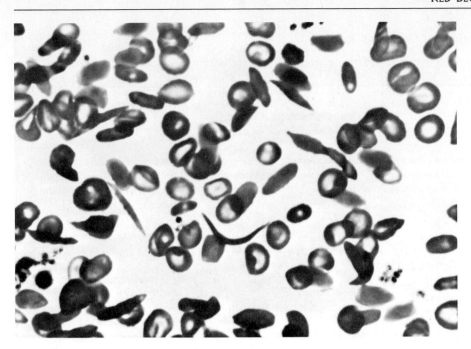

FIG. 17-5   The characteristic sickle- or crescent-shaped red blood cells are shown in a peripheral smear. (Courtesy of Kolchi Maeda, MD, Henry Ford Hospital, Detroit, Mich.)

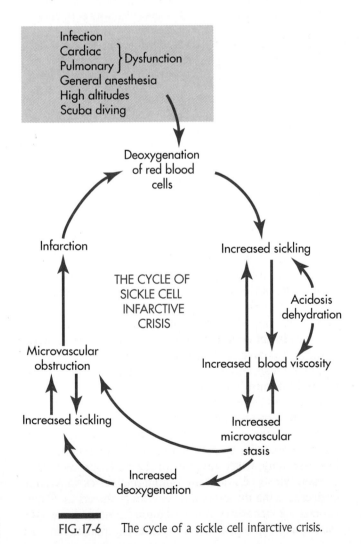

FIG. 17-6   The cycle of a sickle cell infarctive crisis.

to 95% of the hemoglobin; the remainder is Hb F, which accounts for 1% to 20%. The diagnosis is based on the patient's history, physical findings, and a laboratory evaluation. A sickle solubility test is done to confirm the presence of Hb S in the red blood cell. In this test, RBCs are mixed with a reducing agent and the solution becomes turbid. Hemoglobin electrophoresis further delineates the abnormal hemoglobin. The anemia is generally normocytic and normochromic, with hemoglobin levels ranging between 5 and 10 g/dl. Peripheral smear shows anisocytosis and poikilocytosis (irreversibly sickled cells), leukocytosis (increased WBCs), thrombocytosis, and nucleated RBCs (see Fig. 17-5). The reticulocyte count is markedly increased.

Signs and symptoms

Signs and symptoms occur as a result of the vascular occlusions that cause infarcts in various organs, such as kidney, lung, and central nervous system. Infants usually are asymptomatic for 5 to 6 months because of the persistence of fetal hemoglobin (Hb F), which tends to inhibit sickling. Clinical manifestations include failure to thrive, impaired growth and development, and frequent episodes of bacterial infections, especially pneumococcal infections. Initially the spleen is enlarged, but owing to repeated infarcts it becomes atrophied and nonfunctional before the child is 8 years of age. This process is referred to as *autosplenectomy*. Susceptibility to infection persists throughout life.

Swollen, painful, inflamed hands and feet (hand-foot syndrome known as *dactylitis*) are seen in about 20% to 30% of children under 2 years of age. They result from is-

► TABLE 17-2 Clinical Manifestations of Sickle Cell Anemia

System	Complications	Signs and Symptoms	Related To
Cardiac system	Congestive heart failure	Cardiomegaly, systolic ejection murmur, tachycardia, shortness of breath, dyspnea on exertion, restlessness	Anemia, chronic hemolysis
Pulmonary system	Pulmonary infarction, pneumonia (especially *Haemophilus influenzae* and *Streptococcus pneumoniae*), pneumococcal pneumonia	Chest pain, cough, shortness of breath, fever, hemoptysis, restlessness	Infarctive crisis, increased susceptibility to infection, intrapulmonary arteriovenous shunting, functional asplenia
Central nervous system	Cerebral thromboses	Hemiplegia, aphasia, drowsiness, convulsions, headache, bowel and bladder dysfunction	Infarctive crisis
Genitourinary system	Renal dysfunction	Flank pain, hematuria, isothenuria	Renal papillary necrosis secondary to microinfarcts
	Priapism	Penile engorgement and pain	Infarctive crisis and intravascular sickling
Gastrointestinal system	Cholecystitis, hepatic fibrosis, hepatic abscess	Abdominal pain, hepatomegaly, jaundice, fever	Chronic hemolysis, infarctive crisis
Ocular system	Retinal detachment, peripheral vessel disease, hemorrhage	Pain, altered vision, blindness	Microinfarcts
Skeletal system	Aseptic necrosis of femoral or humeral heads, dactylitis (usually in young children)	Pain, decreased mobility, painful and swollen hands and feet	Infarctions, infection, intramedullary infarction with or without periostitis
Skin	Chronic leg ulcers	Pain, open and draining ulcers	Infarctions, impaired circulation in capillaries and venules caused by intravascular sickling

chemia and infarction of the metacarpal and metatarsal bones; the condition is accompanied by fever. Debilitating, recurrent, painful "crises" are the major cause of the morbidity from sickle cell disease. The most frequent sites affected are the abdomen, back, chest, and joints. Crises are exacerbated by infection or dehydration, may mimic other acute illnesses, and last from a few hours to several days. The incidence of the crises decreases with increasing age. Aplastic crisis may also occur, especially in children, with intermittent cessation of bone marrow function and marked decrease in erythropoiesis and reticulocyte count (see Fig. 17-6). Visceral sequestration crisis with sickling and pooling of blood, especially in the chest, is a leading cause of death.

Cardiac signs of anemia, such as tachycardia or murmurs, are usually present. Increased heart size and congestive heart failure may also occur. Renal involvement is evidenced by an impaired ability to concentrate urine, and repeated infarctions can lead to papillary necrosis and hematuria. Repeated pulmonary infections and/or infarctions impair pulmonary function. Central nervous system infarctions ("strokes"), although rare, can lead to varying degrees of hemiplegia. Chronic leg ulcers above the ankle and along the medial aspect of the tibia are encountered. Because of the increased RBC breakdown, the

patients are often icteric (jaundiced) and develop cholelithiasis (gallstones) secondary to increased bilirubin. Physical appearance ranges from the thin asthenic to that of normal development. Table 17-2 depicts the clinical manifestations of sickle cell anemia.

Treatment

Currently there is no known therapy to reverse sickling; therefore treatment is primarily preventive and supportive. Because infections seem to trigger sickle cell crises, emphasis is placed on the prevention, early detection, and prompt treatment of infections. Pneumococcal vaccine (Pneumovax) should be offered prophylactically because it decreases the incidence of pneumococcal infections. Treatment includes prompt and vigorous administration of antibiotics and hydration. Oxygen should be administered only if the patient is hypoxic. Daily folic acid supplements are required to replenish the folate stores depleted as a result of chronic hemolysis. The painful crisis that occurs independently or secondary to infection may affect any part of the body. Prompt intervention with hydration and opioid analgesics may abort or decrease the duration and severity of the crisis. Transfusions are necessary only during aplastic or hemolytic crises or during pregnancy. Exchange transfusions are used for patients with repeated crises or neurologic damage. Iron overload becomes a problem, and these patients need deferoxamine to reduce their iron stores.

Bone marrow transplantation and the use of hydroxyurea to increase Hb F levels are still in the investigation stages (Hoffbrand, Pettit, 1993; Rodgers et al., 1994).

Frequent crises have an impact on the entire quality of life for the patient and the family. Patients are often disabled by chronic recurrent pain and vasoocclusive events. There is a high incidence of drug dependency in this population, as well as school and job difficulties. Ongoing teaching and counseling, including genetic counseling, are essential to the prevention and treatment of sickle cell disease.

Polycythemia

The previous discussion has focused on conditions resulting from insufficient numbers of RBCs. In the condition called polycythemia there are too many RBCs. *Polycythemia* means an excess (poly) of all the cell lines (cythemia), but it is generally used for conditions in which the volume of RBCs exceeds normal. This condition results in increased whole blood viscosity and increased blood volume.

There are relative and absolute forms of polycythemia. Relative polycythemia occurs when the volume of circulating plasma is decreased (hemoconcentration) but the total volume of circulating RBCs is normal. Therefore the hematocrit rises in men to 53% and in women to 46%. The major cause is dehydration. This may be caused by (1) increased fluid losses as seen with diuretic therapy, excessive vomiting, burns, and fever; (2) decreased fluid intake; or (3) redistribution of fluids from plasma to tissues because of a crushing injury (DeGruchy et al., 1978). Another form of relative polycythemia is pseudo or stress polycythemia. Although the exact cause is not known, the incidence of this condition is highest in middle-age, obese, highly anxious men, which makes stress a highly suspected cause. Cigarette smoking seems to exacerbate this state because the chronic carbon monoxide exposure enhances erythrocytosis.

Absolute polycythemia refers to a condition where the actual circulating red cell mass is increased. This may be primary, as in polycythemia vera, or secondary, which results from underlying medical problems that stimulate erythropoietin production, such as cardiopulmonary diseases that decrease arterial O_2 saturation or cardiovascular diseases or renal tumors that decrease renal blood flow. This condition is also seen in individuals who live at high altitudes where atmospheric O_2 is decreased.

In primary or polycythemia vera, the pluripotential stem cell is abnormal. There is marked erythrocytosis, leukocytosis, and thrombocytosis. This is a progressive disease of middle age, equally affecting men and women. The signs and symptoms are secondary to the increased total blood volume and increased blood viscosity. The plasma volume is usually normal, and vasodilation occurs to accommodate the increased RBC volume. The patient presents with a plethoric (brick-red) complexion and "bloodshot" eyes. The symptoms are nonspecific, ranging from a sensation of "fullness in the head" to headache, dizziness, difficulty in concentrating, visual blurring, and postbathing pruritus (itching). The increased blood volume and viscosity (slow blood flow) along with the elevated platelet numbers and abnormal platelet function predispose the individual to thrombosis as well as hemorrhage. The disease progresses over a 10- to 15-year period with complications such as the bone marrow becoming increasingly fibrosed and the liver and spleen increasing in size; it ends with a "spent," nonproductive marrow.

Laboratory studies reveal a persistently elevated hemoglobin (>18 g), hematocrit, and blood volume. The WBC and platelet counts are also elevated. The reticulocyte count is normal or slightly increased.

Treatment modalities for polycythemia vera include periodic phlebotomy (removal of blood by venesection), radioactive phosphorus, and chemotherapeutic agents such as busulfan and hydroxyurea. For secondary polycythemia, treatment depends on the underlying cause.

QUESTIONS

▼ *Answer the following on a separate sheet of paper.*

1. What are the major components and functions of the normal red blood cell?
2. Explain the relationship of erythropoietin to red blood cell production.
3. Define anemia.
4. List the classic signs and symptoms of anemia.
5. State two etiologic factors related to anemia, and give at least two examples of each type.
6. Describe the three morphologic classifications for anemia, and give at least two examples of each type.
7. What are the three major principles to consider when treating anemia?
8. What is polycythemia?
9. Describe the two classifications of absolute polycythemia, and include an example of each type.
10. Draw a normal red blood cell.
11. Explain why deoxygenation can occur in sickle cell disease.
12. Describe aplastic anemia.
13. What are the secondary causes of aplastic anemia?
14. Describe the treatment modality and survival success rate for young individuals with severe aplastic anemia secondary to stem cell damage.

▼ *Circle the letter preceding each item below that correctly answers the question or completes the statement. More than one answer may be correct.*

15. The blood cells that can be described as
Continued.

QUESTIONS—cont'd

nonnucleated, biconcave disks are:
a. Eosinophils
b. Thrombocytes
c. Erythrocytes
d. Monocytes

16. In which of the following sites does hemoglobin production occur through all the maturational stages:
a. Bone marrow
b. Lymphatic tissue
c. Spleen
d. Liver

17. Mr. B., a 20-year-old man, was recently diagnosed as having a fish tapeworm infection *(Diphyllobothrium latum)* after eating infected raw freshwater fish. The type of anemia most likely to be associated with this condition is:
a. Aplastic
b. Iron-deficiency
c. Megaloblastic
d. Hemolytic

18. The development of autoimmune hemolytic anemia can occur secondary to:
a. An incompatible blood transfusion
b. Lymphoma
c. Administration of quinine or methotrexate
d. Hereditary spherocytosis

19. A microcytic, hypochromic anemia usually results from:
a. Acute blood loss
b. Insufficient heme (iron) synthesis
c. Impaired globin synthesis
d. Disordered or interrupted nucleic acid synthesis of DNA
e. Sideroblastic states

20. A macrocytic normochromic anemia is usually caused by a deficiency of:
a. Vitamin B_{12} c. Folic acid
b. Iron   d. Potassium

21. Mrs. B., a 36-year-old woman, was diagnosed as having iron-deficiency anemia. Which one of the following red blood characteristics is most commonly found in anemia resulting from iron deficiency?
a. Normocytic normochromic
b. Microcytic hypochromic
c. Macrocytic normochromic

22. Mr. M., a 65-year-old man, is very depressed since his wife died over 1 year ago. He eats very little—his diet consists mainly of hamburgers. He was referred to a health maintenance organization (HMO) because of weakness and loss of appetite. Physical assessment revealed:
    Pale, emaciated white male
    Pale mucous membranes and nail beds
    Diarrhea
    Severe glossitis
Laboratory data revealed the following:
    Hemoglobin: 6.2
    B_{12}: 343 pg/ml (normal range 200 to 900)
    Folic acid: 3.0 ng/ml (normal range 6 to 20)
    Hematocrit: 17
    Many ovalomacrocytes
The most likely diagnosis is:
a. Megaloblastic anemia secondary to folate deficiency
b. Pernicious anemia
c. Polycythemia
d. Aplastic anemia

23. In sickle cell disease, the most common form of hemoglobin is:
a. Hb C
b. Hb S
c. Hb A
d. Hb F

24. Which of the following describes sickle cell disease?
a. Recessive autosomal-dominant hereditary disease
b. Sex-linked recessive disorder
c. Displays increased deoxygenation within the microvasculature
d. Marked by occurrence of clumping
e. Red blood cells' life span is markedly reduced
f. Most prevalent form of congenital hemolytic anemia

25. A 6-year-old African American girl presents with pale mucous membranes and conjunctival icterus. Further examination revealed lymphadenopathy, cardiac enlargement, ascites, joint swelling, and splenic enlargement. Oval, cigar-shaped sickled cells were seen on a stained blood smear. She is diagnosed as having sickle cell disease. The patient developed severe bone and joint pain in her extremities and an elevated temperature of 102° F (38.9° C) with leukocytosis. This syndrome is referred to as:
a. Chronic sickle cell anemia
b. Sickle cell thalassemia disease
c. Sickle cell crisis
d. Chronic normochromic anemia

26. The principles of treatment for the syndrome described in the above question include:
a. Monitoring of the blood pH
b. Administration of respiratory suppressants
c. Administration of chemotherapeutic agents to reverse the sickling process
d. Prompt intervention with hydration, analgesics, and sedatives
e. Use of exchange transfusions in the initial crisis

▼ *Circle T if the statement is true and F if it is false. Correct any false statements.*

27. T F   Relative polycythemia is characterized by a normal total red blood cell mass.

28. T F   Absolute polycythemia refers to a condition in which the circulating red blood cell mass is increased.

29. T F   Sickle cell disease affects approximately 1 in 300 African Americans.

30. T F   Bone marrow transplantation and the administration of hydroxyurea are the preferred treatment for sickle cell disease.

▼ *Complete the following statements by filling in the blanks.*

31. An anemia in which the MCV is normal and the MCHC is normal is referred to as _____.

32. The leading cause of death in sickle cell disease is _____.

CHAPTER 18

White Blood Cell and Plasma Cell Disorders

CATHERINE M. BALDY

NORMAL STRUCTURE AND FUNCTION

Defense against infection is the major role of leukocytes or white blood cells (WBCs). The normal range for the WBC count is from 4000 to 10,000/mm³. The five types identified in the peripheral blood are (1) neutrophils (50% to 75% of the total WBCs), (2) eosinophils (1% to 2%), (3) basophils (0.5% to 1%), (4) monocytes (6%), and (5) lymphocytes (25% to 33%).

Neutrophils, eosinophils, and basophils are also called *granulocytes,* which means cells with granules in the cytoplasm (Color plates 14 to 16). Granulocytes range in size from 10 to 14 μm in diameter. Their identification depends on the affinity of the granules for certain dyes. Cells whose granules have an eosin affinity, staining red to red-orange, are called *eosinophils,* whereas cells with a blue or basic dye affinity are called *basophils.* The granules of the neutrophils, which are also called *segmented neutrophils* and *polymorphonuclear leukocytes* (PMNs), have little affinity for either eosin or basic dyes and stain a faint pink or blue surrounded by a light pink cytoplasm. All three types of granulocytes (Fig. 18-1) seem to originate from the pluripotential stem cell in the bone marrow.

Although all the regulatory mechanisms for the differentiation and maturation of the WBCs and all the cell lines are not yet fully understood, the identification of several colony-stimulating factors (CSFs) or hematopoietic growth factors has clarified that process. The CSFs are a group of cell-derived glycoproteins that belong to a broader group of WBC regulators called *cytokines.* They are continuously synthesized by a variety of cells, the most important of which are the lymphocyte/macrophage system, fibroblasts, and endothelial cells found in the bone marrow. CSFs have been detected (Robinson, 1990) in various body tissues and in human serum and urine (Barr, Seymore, 1982; Golde, 1983). Detectable levels of CSFs have been found in the serum during periods of inflammation, viral infections, and stress. There seems to be further rapid production after stimulation by various antigens and microorganisms and their products, such as endotoxins (Robinson, 1990).

The CSFs are believed either to act where they are produced or to circulate and attach themselves to specific receptors on the cell surface of the hematopoietic precursors (Robinson, 1990), committing them to differentiation, which, in the case of the WBCs, is to the granulocyte, monocyte, and lymphatic cell lines.

The cells undergo a mitotic (dividing) proliferating phase, followed by a maturation phase. The time required varies for the different leukocytes and ranges from 9 days for the eosinophil to 12 days for the neutrophil. All these phases are accelerated during periods of infection. In the bone marrow, as the cell matures it becomes smaller, and the round or oval nucleus acquires two to five lobes, surrounded by cytoplasm containing small, evenly distributed granules (see Fig. 18-1). These granules contain enzymes (e.g., myeloperoxidase, muramidase, and cationic antibacterial proteins) that, after degranulation of the WBCs, kill and digest bacteria.

The bone marrow contains a constant reserve of about 10 times the quantity of neutrophils produced daily (Schrier, 1979). In the presence of infection, the reserve neutrophils are mobilized and released into the circulation, where they remain for about 6 to 8 hours. This egress from the bone marrow is believed to be regulated by a neutrophil-releasing factor (Quesenberry, 1990).

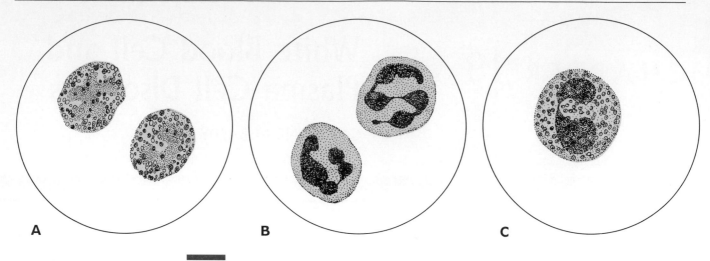

FIG. 18-1   Granulocytes. **A,** Basophils. **B,** Neutrophils. **C,** Eosinophil.

Neutrophils in the circulation are divided between the circulating pool and the marginating pool (WBCs that lie along the capillary wall). With ameboid movements, the neutrophils move by diapedesis from the marginal pool into the tissues and mucous membranes. Neutrophils are the body's primary defense system against bacterial infection; their method of defense is phagocytosis, which is discussed in detail in Chapter 4. A negative feedback system is thought to inhibit neutrophil production and release when large numbers of neutrophils are present (Haeuber, DiJulio, 1989). The overall dynamic feedback mechanism has yet to be clarified and is not within the scope of this chapter.

Eosinophils have a weak phagocytic function that is not clearly understood. They appear to function in antigen-antibody reactions; levels are elevated during asthmatic attacks, drug reactions, and certain parasitic infestations (see Chapter 9). *Basophils* carry heparin and histamine- and platelet-activating factors in their granules to inflamed tissues. Their actual function is poorly defined. Elevated levels of basophils (basophilia) are found in myeloproliferative disorders, that is, proliferative disorders of blood-forming cells.

The *monocyte* (Fig. 18-2 and Color plate 17) is larger than the neutrophil and has a relatively simple monomorphic nucleus. The nucleus is folded or indented and looks lobulated with brainlike convolutions. The cytoplasm appears more abundant in relation to its nucleus and stains dull blue-gray with faint, evenly distributed granules. The differentiation, maturation, and release of monocytes occur over 24 days—a much longer period than for granulocytes.

Monocytes leave the circulation and become tissue macrophages and are a part of the monocyte-macrophage system. The monocyte's life span is weeks to months. Monocytes have phagocytic functions, removing injured and dead cells, cell fragments, and microorganisms (as in bacterial endocarditis).

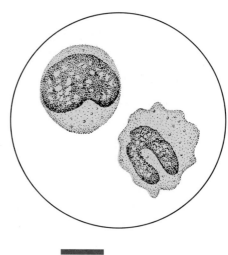

FIG. 18-2   Monocytes.

The other mononuclear (monomorphonuclear) leukocytes in the blood are the lymphocytes. They have a round or oval nucleus surrounded by a narrow rim of blue-staining cytoplasm containing a few granules. The nuclear chromatin pattern is heavily clumped with a network of inner connections. Lymphocytes (Fig. 18-3 and Color plate 18) vary in size from small (7 to 10 μm) to large cells the size of granulocytes. They also appear to originate from a pluripotential stem cell in the bone marrow and migrate to other lymphoid tissues, including the lymph nodes, spleen, thymus, and the mucosal surfaces of the gastrointestinal tract and the respiratory tract. There are two types of lymphocytes: the long-lived, thymus-conditioned, thymus-dependent T lymphocytes and the non–thymus-dependent B lymphocytes. T lymphocytes migrate from the thymus gland to other lymphoid tissue. They are typically located in the paracortex of lymph nodes and the periarteriolar lymphoid sheets of the white pulp of the spleen. B lymphocytes are distributed in the

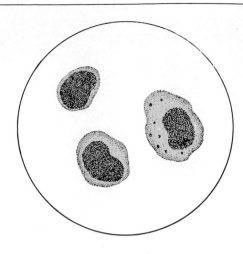

FIG. 18-3   Mature lymphocytes.

follicles of lymph nodes, the spleen, and the medullary cords of the lymph nodes (Sweet, Golomb, 1980). The T lymphocytes are responsible for cellular immune responses through the production of antigen-reactive cells, whereas B lymphocytes, when properly stimulated, differentiate into immunoglobulin-producing plasma cells responsible for the humoral immune response. Chapter 5 contains a complete discussion of the functions and interrelationships of the T and B lymphocytes.

WHITE BLOOD CELL DISORDERS

Disorders of the WBCs can affect any or all of the cell lines and are generally related to production defects or early destruction.

Leukocytosis refers to an increase in the leukocytes generally exceeding 10,000/mm³. *Granulocytosis* refers to an increase in granulocytes but in common usage refers only to an increase in the neutrophils; thus *neutrophilia* is the more accurate term. Leukocytes increase as a physiologic response to protect the body from invading microorganisms. In response to an acute infection or inflammation, neutrophils leave the marginating pool and enter the area of infection; the bone marrow releases its reserves and initiates accelerated granulopoiesis. Because of this increased demand, an increased number of immature forms called *band* (or *stab*) neutrophils enter the circulation, a process referred to as a "shift to the left" (Color plate 19). As the infection subsides, the number of neutrophils decreases and the number of monocytes increases (monocytosis). With progressive resolution, the number of monocytes decreases and mild lymphocytosis (increased lymphocytes) and eosinophilia (increased number of eosinophils) occur. Leukemoid reaction refers to a state of elevated leukocytes, with

an increase in immature forms, reaching levels of 100,000/mm³. This is in response to infectious, toxic, and inflammatory states and also occurs in malignancy, especially in breast, kidney, lung, and metastatic carcinomas (Beck, 1991). Disorders in which there is a general increase in blood-forming cells are called *myeloproliferative disorders*.

Neutrophilia

Neutrophilia also occurs following stresses, such as severe violent exercise or injection with epinephrine. This is a "pseudoleukocytosis" because granulopoiesis in the bone marrow is not accelerated and the number of granulocytes in the body is not actually increased. Rather, granulocytes are mobilized from the marginated pool so that the number of granulocytes that can be drawn into the sampling device is increased. Treatment with corticosteroids also results in a pseudoleukocytosis. Corticosteroids are thought to increase the release of granulocytes from the marrow reserves as well as to inhibit the margination of granulocytes. This results in a greater amount of circulating leukocytes. Eosinophilia occurs with skin disorders such as mycosis fungoides and eczema, allergy states such as asthma and hay fever, drug reactions, and parasitic infestations. Eosinophilia is also seen in malignancies and myeloproliferative disorders, as is basophilia.

Monocytosis is seen during the recuperating phase of infection and in chronic granulomatous diseases such as tuberculosis and sarcoidosis. *Lymphocytosis* refers to an elevated lymphocyte count. Lymphocytes activated by viral or antigenic stimuli are transformed into larger atypical lymphocytes. These cells are present in larger numbers in infectious mononucleosis, infectious hepatitis, toxoplasmosis, measles, mumps, some allergic reactions such as serum sickness, drug sensitivities, and the malignant lymphomas (Schrier, 1979). In addition to lymphocytosis, these patients often have an enlarged liver, spleen, and lymph nodes, all areas of lymphocyte formation.

Leukopenia refers to a decreased number of leukocytes, and *neutropenia* refers to a decrease in the absolute neutrophil count. Because of the role of neutrophils in host defense, an absolute neutrophil count of less than 1000/mm³ predisposes the individual to infection; and counts under 500/mm³ predispose the person to serious, life-threatening infections. Neutropenia may result from ineffective and defective neutrophil production. This is seen in hypoplastic or aplastic anemias secondary to cytotoxic drugs, toxic substances, and viral infection; starvation; and replacement of normal bone marrow by malignant cells, such as in leukemia.

Agranulocytosis is a serious condition characterized by an extremely low leukocyte count and absence of neutrophils. The causative agent is generally a drug that interferes with cell formation or enhances cell destruction.

Drugs commonly implicated are the myelosuppressive (suppress bone marrow) chemotherapeutic agents used to treat hematologic and other malignancies. Increasingly, more commonly used drugs, such as analgesics, antibiotics, and antihistamines, have been identified as capable of causing severe neutropenia or agranulocytosis. This response to the drugs is either dose-related or an idiosyncratic reaction.

Common symptoms of agranulocytosis are infection and feelings of general malaise (discomfort, lassitude, headache, and muscle aches) followed by ulceration of the mucous membranes, fever, and tachycardia. If agranulocytosis is untreated, sepsis and death ensue. Removal of the offending agent will often inhibit and reverse the process with an increased production of the neutrophils and other normal marrow elements.

Leukemia

Classification

Leukemia, originally described by Virchow in 1847 as "white blood," is a neoplastic disease characterized by differentiation and proliferation of malignantly transformed hematopoietic stem cells, leading to suppression of normal cells (Devine, Larson, 1994). The most widely used classification of leukemia is the French-American-British (FAB) classification (see box to the right). This is a morphologic classification based on the differentiation and maturation of the predominant leukemic cells in the bone marrow, as well as on cytochemical studies (Dabich, 1980; Gralnick et al., 1977). Since its early report by Gralnick, further subclassifications have been added (Bennett et al., 1985).

Advances in immunology, cytogenetics, and molecular biology have had a marked impact on distinguishing normal hematopoietic cells from the malignant clone. Immunologic technology has enhanced the classification by identifying the malignant clone as myeloid, B lymphoid, T lymphoid, or biphenotypic (having characteristics of both myeloid and lymphoid cells) (Devine, Larson, 1994). Cytogenetic analysis has yielded vast knowledge of the chromosomal aberrations seen in patients with leukemia. Chromosomal changes can include numeric changes, where whole chromosomes may be added or deleted, or structural changes, including translocations, deletions, inversions, and insertions. In these situations two or more chromosomes exchange genetic material, with the development of altered genes thought to be responsible for the start of abnormal cellular proliferation (Sandberg, 1994). The Philadelphia chromosome (Ph) is an example of a cytogenetic change seen in 85% of patients with chronic myeloid leukemia and in some patients with acute myeloid or lymphoid leukemia. This is a translocation of chromosomes 9 and 22, identified as t(9,22). Molecular studies detecting changes at the DNA level have further delineated the Ph chromosome as varying in the different types of leukemia. More than 90% of children with acute lymphocytic leukemia (ALL) have

FRENCH-AMERICAN-BRITISH (FAB) COOPERATIVE GROUP CLASSIFICATION OF ACUTE LEUKEMIAS

ACUTE LYMPHOBLASTIC LEUKEMIA

L-1   Acute lymphocytic leukemia of childhood: homogeneous cell population

L-2   Acute lymphocytic leukemia seen in adults: heterogeneous cell population

L-3   Burkitt's lymphoma–type leukemia: large cells, homogeneous cell population

ACUTE MYELOBLASTIC LEUKEMIA

M-1   Granulocytic differentiation without maturation

M-2   Granulocytic differentiation with maturation to promyelocytic stage

M-3   Granulocytic differentiation with hypergranular promyelocytes, associated with disseminated intravascular coagulation

M-4   Acute myelomonocytic leukemia: both granulocytic and monocytic cell lines

M-5a   Acute monocytic leukemia: poorly differentiated

M-5b   Acute monocytic leukemia: well differentiated

M-6   Predominance of erythroblasts with severe dyserythropoiesis

M-7   Megakaryocytic leukemia

From Gralnick HR et al: *Ann Intern Med* 87(6):740-753, 1977; and Bennett JM et al: *Ann Intern Med* 103(3):460-462, 1985.

been shown to have one or more chromosomal aberrations. Numerous chromosomal aberrations have been identified and are diagnostic for specific types of leukemia. Identification of these changes is predictive of the clinical course, prognosis, and attainment of a remission or relapse (Sandberg, 1994). These findings have a tremendous impact on treatment modalities and overall prognosis.

Incidence

Although both genders are affected, there is a slight male to female predominance. Acute granulocytic or myelocytic leukemia is seen in adults of all ages, with increases noted after 40 years of age. The mean age is 60 years. Acute lymphocytic leukemia is more prevalent in children under 15 years of age, with a peak between the ages of 2 and 4 years. It is also seen in adults of all ages, with a gradual increase at 60 years of age. Chronic granulocytic or myelocytic leukemia is most frequently seen in middle-age patients with a mean age of 60 years, but it can occur in any age-group. Chronic lymphocytic leukemia is seen in older individuals.

Etiology

Although the basic cause of leukemia is unknown, both genetic predisposition and environmental factors seem to play a role. Familial leukemias are rare, but there seems to be a higher incidence of leukemia in siblings of affected children, with the incidence increasing to 20% in monozygotic (identical) twins. Individuals with chromosomal abnormalities such as Down's syndrome seem to have a twentyfold increased incidence of acute leukemia.

Environmental factors include exposure to high doses of ionizing radiation with manifestations of leukemia occurring years later. Chemicals (e.g., benzene, arsenic, pesticides, chloramphenicol, phenylbutazone, and antineoplastic agents) are being implicated with increased frequency, especially the alkylating agents. The likelihood of leukemia increases in patients treated with both radiation and chemotherapy. Any hypoplastic bone marrow state seems to predispose the individual to leukemia. Patients with myelodysplastic syndrome (stem cell disorder manifested by presence of blasts and pancytopenia seen in older adults) often progress to acute nonlymphocytic leukemia.

Therapy is directed toward elimination of the abnormal cell line; 65% of patients, with resumption of normal hematopoiesis, achieve remission of disease. Table 18-1 lists the chemotherapeutic agents commonly used to treat hematologic malignancies. Most current regimens include the antimetabolite cytosine arabinoside and an anthracycline antibiotic such as idarubicin, mitoxantrone, or daunorubicin hydrochloride. The chemotherapeutic agents selected destroy the cells by various mechanisms, such as interfering with cell metabolism and maturation. The same clinical manifestations of pancytopenia accompanying active disease are present after chemotherapy. Infection remains the leading cause of death in patients with acute leukemia. Supportive care is the key to increasing the survival rate of these patients. Care should include assiduous precautions against infection and bleeding, aggressive antimicrobial therapy in the case of infection, and the judicious use of blood component therapy (e.g., platelets and packed RBCs). Bone marrow transplantation can rescue about 30% of patients in first relapse or second remission.

Acute leukemia

The acute leukemia affecting the myeloid series is termed *acute nonlymphocytic leukemia* (ANLL), *acute myelocytic leukemia* (AML), or *acute granulocytic leukemia* (AGL) (Color plate 20). It seems to be a uniclonal neoplasm that originates with the transformation of a single hematopoietic cell or a few hematopoietic cells. The exact nature of the molecular lesion or lesions responsible for the transformed cell's neoplastic properties is not yet clear, but the critical defect is intrinsic and inheritable by the cell's progeny (Clarkson, 1983; Hoffbrand, Pettit, 1993). Both quantitative and qualitative defects are in all the myeloid cell lines (McGlave, 1988).

ANLL accounts for 80% of the acute leukemias seen in adults. The onset may be abrupt or progressive over a 1- to 6-month period. If untreated, it is fatal in approximately 3 to 6 months. Treatment with combination chemotherapy enables 70% to 85% of the patients to achieve a complete remission. Approximately 25% of the patients achieve a 5-year disease-free survival.

The diagnosis of ANLL can be made on the basis of peripheral blood findings but is verified by a bone marrow examination. The peripheral WBC count may be markedly elevated, normal, or decreased with circulating myeloblasts and a decreased absolute granulocyte count. The platelet count is also decreased, with levels often below 50,000. Moderate anemia may also be seen. The bone marrow is generally hypercellular, with 30% to 90% of myeloblasts containing Auer rods. The remaining cellular elements are suppressed. Cytogenetic studies most often reveal chromosomal abnormalities. Metabolic alterations are seen, with elevations in the uric acid levels caused by the high levels of WBC turnover.

Clinical manifestations are related to the decrease of normal hematopoietic cells, especially the granulocytes and thrombocytes. Patients often present with infections or bleeding at the time of diagnosis. Chills, fever, tachycardia, and tachypnea are frequently presenting symptoms. Infections can involve all organ systems. Cellulitis, pneumonia, oral infections, perirectal abscesses, and septicemia are just a few examples of infections encountered by this patient population.

Thrombocytopenia results in bleeding evidenced by petechiae and ecchymoses (bleeding into the skin), epistaxis (nosebleeds), and hematomas in the mucous membranes, as well as gastrointestinal (GI) and urinary tract bleeding. Bone pain and tenderness may result from bone infarcts or subperiosteal (beneath the periosteum) infiltrates.

Anemia is not an early manifestation because of the long life span of the erythrocyte (120 days). When anemia is present, headaches and symptoms of fatigue and dyspnea on exertion are evident, along with marked palor.

Acute lymphocytic leukemia. Acute lymphocytic leukemia (ALL) is the most common cancer affecting children under the age of 15 years, with a peak incidence between 3 and 4 years of age. There is, however, a 20% incidence in adults with acute leukemia. It is manifested by an abnormal proliferation of lymphoblasts in the bone marrow and extramedullary sites (those outside of the bone marrow, such as lymph nodes and spleen) (Fig. 18-4 and Color plate 21). Diagnosis is established through a complete blood cell count (CBC), differential, platelet count, and bone marrow examination. The WBC count is generally markedly elevated, but it may be normal or low, with a lymphocytosis. The platelet, neutrophil, and RBC counts are generally low. The bone marrow is hypercellular, with infiltrating lymphoblasts. Cytogenetics and immunotyping are also done to elucidate the malignant clone. Because of the recognized incidence of central nervous system (CNS) involvement, an analysis of the spinal fluid is also included.

Diagnosis and classification of acute lymphocytic leukemia are likewise based on morphologic characteristics utilizing the FAB classification (see box, p. 210).

TABLE 18-1   Commonly Used Chemotherapeutic Agents in Hematologic Malignancies

| Drug | | Disease | Administration | Toxicity | |
Generic Name	Trade Name*			Acute	Long-term
ALKYLATING AGENTS					
Mechlorethamine hydrochloride, nitrogen mustard	Mustargen	Hodgkin's lymphoma	IV push	Anorexia; nausea and vomiting: nausea, 30 minutes to 4 hours after injection	Myelosuppression, amenorrhea, male sterility
Cyclophosphamide	Cytoxan, Endoxan	Lymphomas Chronic lymphocytic leukemia Acute leukemia Multiple myeloma Waldenström's macroglobulinemia	PO, IV	Delayed nausea, 6-18 hours	Alopecia, hemorrhagic cystitis, myelosuppression, amenorrhea, male sterility, immunosuppression
Busulfan	Myleran	CGL Polycythemia vera Thrombocythemia	PO	Minimal nausea	Myelosuppression, skin pigmentation, pulmonary fibrosis, addisonian syndrome
Chlorambucil	Leukeran	CLL Hodgkin's lymphoma Lymphomas	PO	Mild anorexia; nausea and vomiting	Myelosuppression
ANTIMETABOLITES					
Methotrexate	A-Methopterin	ALL AGL	PO, IV, IM, IT, IP	Nausea, vomiting	Myelosuppression, stomatitis, diarrhea, alopecia, mucosal ulceration, hepatic-renal dysfunction, immunosuppression
Cytarabine (cytosine arabinoside)	Cytosar-U, Ara-C	AGL Acute myelomonocytic leukemia	IV, SC	Nausea, vomiting	Myelosuppression, GI mucositis, immunosuppression
6-Mercaptopurine	6-MP, Purinethol	ALL AGL	PO, IV	Nausea, vomiting	Myelosuppression, hepatocellular dysfunction, GI mucositis
6-Thioguanine, 6-TG		AGL	PO	Nausea, vomiting	Myelosuppression, photosensitivity, hepatocellular dysfunction
Cladrabine 2-Chlorodeoxyadenosine	Leustatin	Hairy cell leukemia CLL Lymphomas	IV	Mild nausea	Myelosuppression with delayed recovery, especially platelets, rash, fever, malaise, anorexia
Fludarabine hydrochloride	Fludara	B cell CLL	IV	Tumor lysis syndrome, mild nausea	Myelosuppression, mild hair loss, cardiotoxicity and neurotoxicity with high doses, mucositis, malaise
Hydroxyurea	Hydrea	CGL Sickle cell anemia	PO	None	Myelosuppression, anorexia, stomatitis, nausea and vomiting, diarrhea, hallucinations

CGL, Chronic granulocytic leukemia; *CLL,* chronic lymphocytic leukemia; *ALL,* acute lymphocytic leukemia; *AGL,* acute granulocytic leukemia; *IV,* intravenous; *PO,* by mouth; *IM,* intramuscular; *IT,* intrathecal; *IP,* intraperitoneal; *SC,* subcutaneous.
*This list is not all-inclusive. Other equally effective brands may exist.

▶ TABLE 18-1   Commonly Used Chemotherapeutic Agents in Hematologic Malignancies—cont'd

Drug				Toxicity	
Generic Name	Trade Name*	Disease	Administration	Acute	Long-term
NATURAL PRODUCTS, PLANT ALKALOIDS					
Vincristine	Oncovin	ALL AGL Hodgkin's lymphoma	IV	Nausea, local phlebitis	Peripheral neuropathy, myopathy, alopecia
Vinblastine	Velban	Hodgkin's lymphoma Lymphomas	IV	Local phlebitis, mild nausea, stomatitis, glossitis	Leukopenia, rare peripheral neuropathy
Etoposide VP-16	VePesid	AGL	IV	Orthostatic hypotension, mild nausea, vomiting, anorexia	Myelosuppression, alopecia
ANTIBIOTICS					
Doxorubicin	Adriamycin	Acute leukemia Lymphomas	IV	Severe vesicant with tissue necrosis, nausea	Myelosuppression, alopecia Cardiac toxicity with cumulative doses
Daunorubicin (daunomycin)	Cerubidine	Acute leukemia Lymphomas Hodgkin's lymphoma Multiple myeloma	IV	Severe vesicant with tissue necrosis, nausea	Myelosuppression, alopecia Cardiac toxicity with cumulative doses
Bleomycin	Blenoxane	Lymphomas	IV, IM, SC	Fever, possible anaphylaxis, acute pulmonary edema	Pulmonary fibrosis with cumulative doses Minimal myelosuppression, skin and nail discoloration
Idarubicin hydrochloride	Idamycin	ALL AGL Lymphoma	IV	Nausea, vomiting, vesicant with tissue necrosis	Myelosuppression, cardiotoxicity with cumulative doses, alopecia, mucositis
Mitoxantrone hydrochloride	Novantrone	AGL ALL CLL CGL in blast crisis Lymphoma	IV	Nausea, vomiting, vesicant	Myelosuppression, stomatitis, mild congestive heart failure, alopecia
ENZYMES					
L-asparaginase	Elspar	ALL	IV, IM	Hypersensitivity with potential for anaphylaxis Nausea, vomiting, and anorexia	Hyperglycemia, pancreatitis, hepatotoxicity, general malaise, somnolence, depression
ADRENOCORTICOIDS					
Prednisone	Orasone, Deltasone	ALL AGL Lymphomas Multiple myeloma Waldenström's macroglobulinemia	PO	GI distress, water retention	GI distress, chemical diabetes, water retention, osteoporosis, psychosis

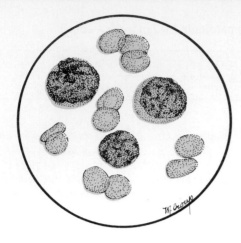

FIG. 18-4   Lymphoblasts.

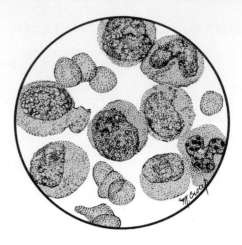

FIG. 18-5   Bone marrow characteristic of chronic granulocytic leukemia.

ALL is further subclassified by immunologic criteria, identifying cells as T cell, B cell, cALLa, or null cell (see Table 18-2). On cytogenetic analysis the majority of children have one or more cytogenetic abnormalities. As in ANLL, the results of these studies provide valuable information for planning treatment programs to maximize the curative potential.

Clinical manifestations of lymphocytic leukemia resemble those of acute granulocytic leukemia, with signs and sumptoms related to suppression of the normal bone marrow elements (Hoelzer, 1994). Therefore infection, bleeding, and anemia are major clinical manifestations. One third of the patients present with infection and bleeding at the time of diagnosis. Malaise, fever, lethargy, weight loss, and night sweats may all be presenting symptoms. Because extramedullary sites are also involved, these patients have lymphadenopathy (enlarged lymph nodes) and hepatosplenomegaly (enlarged liver and spleen). Bone pain and arthralgia, although seen in adults, are more commonly seen in children. Signs and symptoms of CNS involvement (seen most often during relapse) include headaches, vomiting, seizures, and visual disturbances.

The onset of ALL is usually abrupt and rapidly progresses to death if untreated. Improved survival with treatment has been dramatic. Not only do 90% to 95% of children achieve a full remission, but 60% go on to be cured. Eighty percent of adults achieve a complete remission (Devine, Larson, 1994) with one third experiencing long-term survival. This is achieved through aggressive chemotherapy directed at the bone marrow as well as the CNS. Treatment programs use combinations of vincristine, prednisone, L-asparaginase, cyclophosphamide, and an anthracycline such as daunorubicin (see Table 18-1). Because the meninges may harbor leukemia cells, prophylactic intrathecal (into the subarachnoid space) chemotherapy is also included to prevent CNS re-

lapse. Bone marrow transplantation should be considered for adults with aggressive, poor prognosis disease to prolong a disease-free survival. Children with shorter than 18-month remissions should be considered for bone marrow transplantation (Gale, Waldman, 1989).

Chronic leukemias

Chronic granulocytic leukemia. Chronic granulocytic leukemia (CGL) or chronic myelocytic leukemia (CML), accounting for 15% of the leukemias, is seen most frequently in middle-age adults but may occur in any age-group. Unlike AGL, CGL is insidious in its onset; it is often discovered during routine examinations and blood screening. CGL is considered a myeloproliferative disorder because the bone marrow is hypercellular with proliferation of all the cell lines (Fig. 18-5 and Color plate 22). Granulocyte counts generally are greater than 30,000/mm^3. Although maturation is disordered, most of the cells are mature and functional. In 85% of the cases a chromosomal abnormality referred to as the *Philadelphia chromosome* is present. The Philadelphia chromosome is a translocation of the long arm of chromosome 22 to that of 9 (Fig. 18-6). This chromosomal abnormality affects the hematopoietic stem cell and is therefore present in the myeloid cell lines as well as some of the lymphoid lines.

Signs and symptoms are related to a hypermetabolic state—fatigue, weight loss, increased diaphoresis, and heat intolerance. The spleen is enlarged in 90% of the cases, which leads to a sensation of abdominal fullness and early satiety. If anemia is present, the patient may be tachycardic, pale, and short of breath. Bruising may occur secondary to abnormal platelet function. Although some long-term survivals have been reported, the median survival rate, with or without treatment, is about 3 years. Treatment with intermittent chemotherapy is directed toward suppressing the excessive hematopoiesis and reducing spleen size. Invariably the patients progress to a more

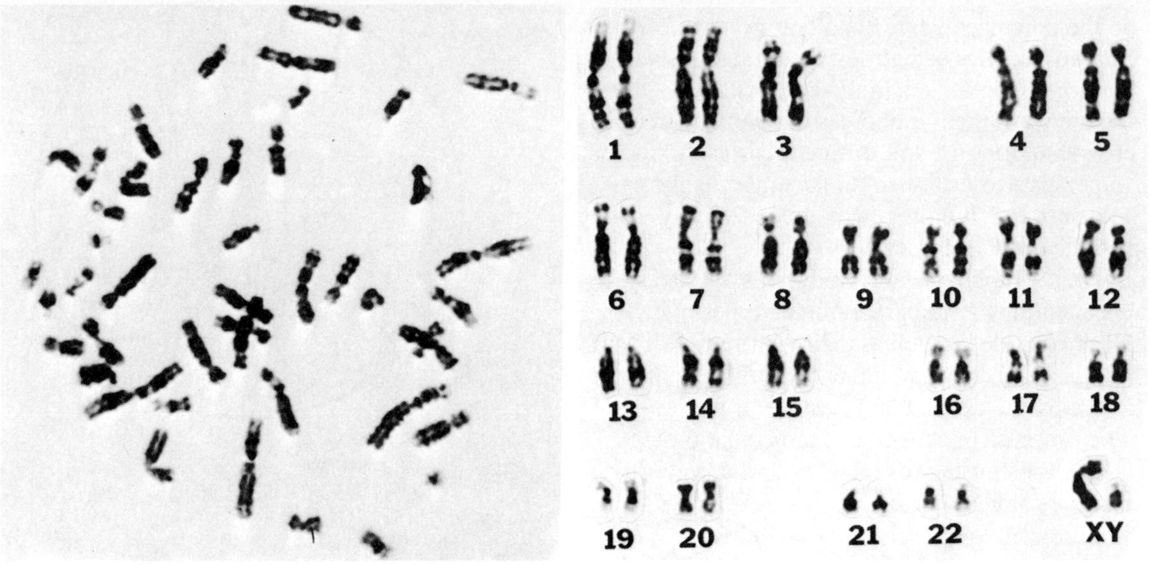

FIG. 18-6   Karyotype of a marrow cell from a male patient with chronic granulocytic leukemia. A fragment has been lost from chromosome 22 and translocated to chromosome 9. The preparation at left is stained with the acetic-saline-Giemsa method 1 to show banding patterns. (Reproduced with permission from Raymond Teplitz, MD.)

aggressive, resistant phase with an overwhelming production of myeloblasts ("blast transformation"). Death occurs within weeks to months after blast transformation. An allogeneic (from another individual) bone marrow transplantation, done while the patient is in the stable, chronic phase of CGL, offers a hope of cure in an otherwise fatal disease. Although the morbidity and mortality remain high during transplantation, it should be considered for all young patients with an HLA-identical sibling.

Chronic lymphocytic leukemia. Chronic lymphocytic leukemia (CLL) is a lymphoproliferative disorder seen in older individuals (median age 60 years) with a 2:1 male predominance (Color plate 23). It is manifested by a proliferation and accumulation of 30% small abnormal mature lymphocytes in the bone marrow, peripheral blood, and extramedullary sites, with levels reaching 100,000+/mm³. In more than 90% of the cases the abnormal lymphocyte is a B lymphocyte, which leads to insufficient immunoglobulin synthesis and depressed antibody response. The onset is insidious and is often discovered during routine blood work showing an elevated absolute lymphocyte count, or because of painless lymphadenopathy and splenomegaly. As the disease progresses, the liver also enlarges. Patients with only lymphocytosis and lymphadenopathy may survive 10 years or longer. Early anemia and thrombocytopenia (low platelet count) reflect a poor prognosis with a median survival of 2 years.

Signs and symptoms, which are similar to those of CGL, reflect a hypermetabolic state. Massive organ enlargement causes mechanical pressure on the stomach with symptoms of early satiety, abdominal discomfort, and bowel irregularities. Infections of the skin and pneumonia complicate the course in more than 75% of the patients. These infections are secondary to the altered immunologic state as well as the neutropenia.

Treatment is directed toward reducing the lymphocytic mass, thus reversing the pancytopenia and relieving the discomfort caused by the organ enlargement. New antimetabolites, corticosteroids, and chemotherapy with alkylating agents are used.

Table 18-2 presents the differential features of the leukemias.

Lymphoma

The lymphomas are classified as lymphoproliferative disorders. The etiology is unknown, but identified risk factors include immunodeficiency states (congenital or acquired), as well as exposure to herbicides, pesticides, and organic solvents such as benzene. The increased incidence of acquired immune deficiency syndrome (AIDS) associated with high-grade lymphomas during recent years implicates immunosuppression as a causative factor (Williams et al., 1994). Viruses have also been implicated, especially the Epstein-Barr virus seen in Burkitt's lymphoma and more recently implicated in the possible pathogenesis of Hodgkin's disease (Weinshel, Peterson, 1994).

The initial tumor formation in lymphoma is in the secondary lymphatic tissues (e.g., the lymph nodes or spleen) where abnormal lymphocytes replace the normal structure.

Two broad categories of lymphomas are identified on the basis of the microscopic histopathology of the involved lymph nodes. The categories are Hodgkin's disease and the non-Hodgkin's lymphomas. Although the signs and symptoms of the lymphomas overlap, the treatment and prognosis for cure are different for each kind. Thus it is imperative to establish an accurate diagnosis. For this, one or more lymph nodes are surgically removed and studied microscopically.

Non-Hodgkin's lymphomas and Hodgkin's disease are differentiated according to the predominant types of cells found in the lymph node, as well as their distribution. The cells may be distributed in a nodular or diffuse manner. These cells destroy the normal architecture of the lymph nodes. Current progress in genetic and molecular biology to identify phenotypic (genetic) markers and chromosomal translocations, along with the clinical features of the disease, differentiates aggressive from indolent lymphomas and guides treatment and progress. B cell lymphomas are noted to be more indolent with long relapse-free survivals, whereas T cell lymphomas of the same histologic type have higher relapse rates with shorter relapse-free survivals (Williams et al., 1994).

One of the major determinants of treatment, as well as the prognosis, is the clinical stage (extent of disease) of the patient at the time of diagnosis (see the box below). After the tissue diagnosis is established, staging procedures must be carried out. These commonly include the following:

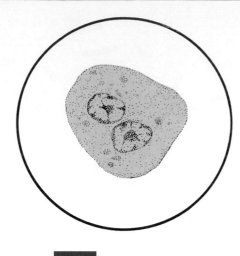

FIG. 18-7   Reed-Sternberg cell.

1. Physical examination with particular attention to the lymphatic system (lymph nodes, liver, and spleen)
2. Routine CBC, differential, and platelet count
3. Chemistries (liver and kidney function; uric acid)
4. Chest x-ray films to look for hilar adenopathy (enlarged bronchial lymph nodes)
5. Computed tomography (CT) scans of the chest, abdomen, and pelvis
6. Bipedal lymphangiograms to check for retroperitoneal and iliac node involvement if the CT scan below the diaphragm is negative
7. A bone scan if there is bone tenderness

A gallium scan done before and after therapy identifies the sites of disease or residual disease in the mediastinum. Bilateral bone marrow biopsies are indicated for patients with systemic symptoms or stage III disease. In the absence of bone marrow involvement, a laparotomy (see Chapter 27) with splenectomy and liver biopsy may be done for accurate diagnosis and treatment in patients with Hodgkin's disease. This is not routinely done in patients with non-Hodgkin's lymphoma.

Hodgkin's disease

Hodgkin's disease is a lymphoma seen predominantly in young adults between the ages of 18 and 35 years and in persons older than 50 years. The etiology to date is unknown, but it may be the culmination to diverse pathologic processes, such as viral infections, environmental exposures, and a genetically determined host response (Weinshel, Peterson, 1994). There is a 3:2 male/female predominance. The Reed-Sternberg cell, which is a malignant, large, binucleated or multinucleated cell containing two or more large nucleoli, is the characteristic finding in Hodgkin's disease (Fig. 18-7 and Color plate 24).

Hodgkin's disease is classified according to the Rye classification based on histology. The classifications and incidence are as follows: lymphocyte predominant (LP), seen in 2% to 10% of the cases; mixed cellularity (MC), seen in 20% to 40% of cases; nodular sclerosis (NS), seen

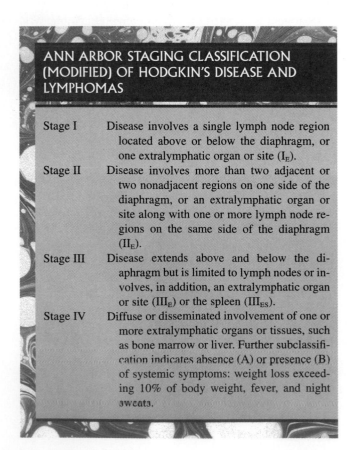

ANN ARBOR STAGING CLASSIFICATION (MODIFIED) OF HODGKIN'S DISEASE AND LYMPHOMAS

Stage I	Disease involves a single lymph node region located above or below the diaphragm, or one extralymphatic organ or site (I_E).
Stage II	Disease involves more than two adjacent or two nonadjacent regions on one side of the diaphragm, or an extralymphatic organ or site along with one or more lymph node regions on the same side of the diaphragm (II_E).
Stage III	Disease extends above and below the diaphragm but is limited to lymph nodes or involves, in addition, an extralymphatic organ or site (III_E) or the spleen (III_{ES}).
Stage IV	Diffuse or disseminated involvement of one or more extralymphatic organs or tissues, such as bone marrow or liver. Further subclassification indicates absence (A) or presence (B) of systemic symptoms: weight loss exceeding 10% of body weight, fever, and night sweats.

▶ TABLE 18-2   Differential Features of the Leukemias

	Acute Myelogenous (Granulocytic) Leukemia	Acute Lymphoblastic (Lymphocytic) Leukemia	Chronic Myelogenous (Granulocytic) Leukemia	Chronic Lymphocytic Leukemia
Incidence (age)	Adult; 10% in children, peak 60 years	Usually in children <15 years; peak 3-4 years; may occur in adults	Ages 20-60 years Peak 40 years May occur in children	Median 60 years
Gender distribution	Slight M/F predominance 3:2	M/F predominance 5:4	Slight M/F predominance	M/F predominance 2:1
Implicated causal factors	High ionizing radiation, chemical exposure, genetic aberrations (e.g., Down's syndrome)	Genetic aberrations (e.g., Down's syndrome), irradiation, virus	Ionizing radiation, chemical exposure	Unknown
Survival	3-6 months without treatment 1-3 years with treatment Some long-term survivors	3-6 months without treatment Low-risk features (>50% 5+ years survival): null cell*; ages 2-10 years High-risk features (±2 years' survival): T and B cell; children <2 years, teens, young adults	1-10 years; mean 3 years	2-25 years
Signs and symptoms	Variable: ecchymoses, gum and nose bleeding, malaise, fatigue, fever, sternal tenderness, occasional hepatosplenomegaly	Variable: hepatosplenomegaly, lymphadenopathy, 10% mediastinal mass, ecchymoses, low-grade fever, weight loss, sternal tenderness, bone and joint pain, malaise, fatigue	Splenomegaly, bone tenderness, pallor, hypermetabolic symptoms, diaphoresis, weight loss, anorexia	Painless lymphadenopathy, hepatosplenomegaly, acquired hypersensitivity to insect bites
Peripheral blood	Elevated, normal, or decreased WBCs with myeloblasts Thrombocytopenia Anemia	Markedly elevated WBCs with lymphocytosis WBC count may be normal or decreased Thrombocytopenia Anemia	Markedly elevated WBCs, mainly mature granulocytes All developmental stages present, including blasts Basophilia Eosinophilia Early thrombocytosis Thrombocytopenia and anemia (end stage)	Moderately elevated small mature lymphocytes; neutrophils Thrombocytopenia Anemia with progressive disease
Bone marrow	Hypercellular (>50% myeloblasts) Auer rods†	Hypercellular with infiltrating lymphoblasts	Hypercellular (<50% blasts, megakaryocytes)	>30% Lymphocytes
Cytogenetics	Nonrandom chromosomal aberrations t(8;21) (q22; q22) +8 t(15;17) (q22; q11)	Variable chromosomal aberrations; 5% Philadelphia chromosome aberrations + 21 t (4;11) (q21; q23) t (9;22) (q34; q11)	85% Philadelphia chromosome aberrations Other chromosomal aberrations t (9;22)	Random unconfirmed chromosomal aberrations t (12;14) t (11;14) t (17;14)
Immunologic identification	Not identified Lack cALLa‡ antigen Lack T and B cell determinants	85% cALLa‡ antigen (lack B or T cell characteristics)	None identified	Majority have B cell markers 1%-3% have T cell markers

t, Translocation.

*Null cell: lymphocyte that lacks B cell (membrane immunoglobulin) or T cell (E-rosette formation) markers.

†Auer rods: red-staining rods seen in cytoplasm of myeloblasts characteristic of acute myelogenous leukemia.

‡cALLa: common ALL antigen—a distinct surface membrane glycoprotein complex carried on 70% of non–T cell leukemia lymphoblasts.

Continued.

▶ TABLE 18-2   Differential Features of the Leukemias—cont'd

	Acute Myelogenous (Granulocytic) Leukemia	Acute Lymphoblastic (Lymphocytic) Leukemia	Chronic Myelogenous (Granulocytic) Leukemia	Chronic Lymphocytic Leukemia
Treatment (see Table 18-1)	Combination chemotherapy including cytosine arabinoside; and daunorubicin, idarubicin or mitoxantrone Blood products and antibiotic support Bone marrow transplant	Combination chemotherapy including vincristine and prednisone; methotrexate; L-asparaginase Blood products and antibiotic support Bone marrow transplant	Generally single alkylating agent; melphalan (Alkeran) or hydroxyurea Bone marrow transplant Alpha-interferon	When symptomatic alkylating agents, corticosteroids, radiation therapy, fludarabine
Complications	Hemorrhage, sepsis, disseminated intravascular coagulation (DIC)	Hemorrhage, sepsis, CNS involvement	Myelofibrosis, pancytopenia, blast transformation, splenic infarction	Pancytopenia, hemolytic anemia, idiopathic thrombocytopenic purpura (ITP) viral infection

in 40% to 80% of cases; and lymphocyte depleted (LD), seen in 2% to 15% of cases (Weinshel, Peterson, 1994).

Although histology has been used to predict prognosis, it correlates with the distribution of the disease. Lymphocyte predominant and nodular sclerosis subtypes are generally stage I or II at presentation, whereas lymphocyte depleted is generally stage III or IV. Hilar and mediastinal involvement are more commonly seen in the nodular sclerosing subtype.

Clinical manifestations vary. The younger patient generally presents with a nontender, rubbery-feeling enlarged lymph node low in the cervical or supraclavicular area or with a dry cough secondary to hilar lymphadenopathy.

The general mode of dissemination is an orderly involvement of contiguous sites. Approximately 25% of patients have unexplained persistent fever or night sweats. Constitutional symptoms such as anorexia, cachexia, weight loss, and fatigue are seen in disseminated disease and have prognostic significance. In certain cases the Pel-Ebstein fever (a cyclic pattern of elevated evening temperatures lasting a few days to weeks) is present. Splenomegaly occurs during the course of the disease in 50% of the patients (Hoffbrand, Pettit, 1993). Defects in immunity are present in all phases of Hodgkin's, both during and after therapy, and the incidence of infections, especially viral and fungal infections, increases. Tuberculosis is also seen. Hematologic manifestations depend on the stage of disease and presence of organ involvement (Weinshel, Peterson, 1994).

Accurate clinical and pathologic staging, with appropriate treatment, has improved the prognosis of Hodgkin's disease. For example, 90% curcs of patients with asymptomatic stages I and II disease are evident, especially of the lymphocyte predominant (LP) or nodular sclerosis (NS) types (see box, p. 216). Treatment, depending on staging, includes extensive radiotherapy (in stage IA or IIA disease), combination of chemotherapy and radiotherapy, or multidrug chemotherapy alone (in stage IIIB or IV).

Non-Hodgkin's lymphomas

The median age of individuals with non-Hodgkin's lymphomas is 50 years. Classification of the non-Hodgkin's lymphomas is in a state of transition. The widely used Rappaport classification (introduced in 1956) is based on the cytology and the architectural arrangement of the malignant lymphocytes in the lymph nodes. It divides lymphomas according to (1) the nodular type (N), where neoplastic cells group in cohesive aggregates that stimulate lymphoid follicles, and (2) the diffuse type (D), where no aggregation occurs.

The advancement of knowledge in the field of immunology and lymphocyte physiology, such as identifying lymphocytes as B cells or T cells, has led to more definitive classification of the non-Hodgkin's lymphomas as reflected in the classification by Lukes and Collins. Lukes and Collins demonstrated that 70% of the lymphomas are of B cell origin. The most current classification, known as the *Working Formulation,* is the result of an international multiinstitutional effort. It is based on immunology, lymphocyte physiology, and morphology as well as the biologic behavior of lymphomas. Three prognostic categories are identified, namely, low-grade, intermediate-grade, and high-grade malignant lymphoma. Table 18-3 presents the Working Formulation, the Rappaport equivalent, the incidence, and median survival rates (Johnson, 1994).

Although constitutional symptoms (fever, weight loss, and night sweats) do occur, the incidence is lower than it is in Hodgkin's disease and does not necessarily influence prognosis. Painless diffuse lymphadenopathy is seen and may affect any or all of the peripheral lymph nodes. Hilar adenopathy is usually not seen; however,

TABLE 18-3   Working Formulation With Rappaport Classification of Malignant Lymphomas

Working Formulation	Non-Hodgkin's Lymphomas (%)	Median Survival (Years)	Rappaport Equivalent
LOW GRADE			
Malignant lymphoma			
Small lymphocytic (SL)	3.6	5.8	Diffuse, well-differentiated lymphocytic (DWDL)
Consistent with CLL			
Plasmacytoid			
Malignant lymphoma, follicular			
Predominantly small cleaved cell (FSC)	22.5	7.2	Nodular, poorly differentiated lymphocytic (NPDL)
Diffuse areas			
Sclerosis			
Malignant lymphoma, follicular			
Mixed, small cleaved and large cell (FM)	7.7	5.1	Nodular, mixed lymphocytic-histiocytic (NM)
Diffuse areas			
Sclerosis			
INTERMEDIATE GRADE			
Malignant lymphoma, follicular			
Predominantly large cell (FL)	3.8	3.0	Nodular histiocytic (NH)
Diffuse areas			
Sclerosis			
Malignant lymphoma, diffuse			
Small cleaved cell (DSC)	6.9	3.4	Diffuse, poorly differentiated lymphocytic (DPDL)
Sclerosis			
Malignant lymphoma, diffuse			
Mixed, small and large cell (DM)	6.7	2.7	Diffuse, mixed lymphocytic-histiocytic (DM)
Sclerosis			
Epithelioid cell component			
Malignant lymphoma, diffuse			
Large cell (DL)	19.7	1.5	Diffuse, histiocytic (DH)
Cleaved cell			
Noncleaved cell			
Sclerosis			
HIGH GRADE			
Malignant lymphoma			
Large cell, immunoblastic (IBL)	7.9	1.3	Diffuse, histiocytic (DH)
Plasmacytoid			
Clear cell			
Polymorphous			
Epithelioid cell component			
Malignant lymphoma			
Lymphoblastic (LBL)	4.2	2.0	Lymphoblastic (LBL)
Convoluted cell			
Nonconvoluted cell			
Malignant lymphoma			
Small noncleaved cell (SNC)	5.0	0.7	Diffuse, undifferentiated (DU)
Burkitt's			Burkitt's
Follicular areas			Non-Burkitt's
MISCELLANEOUS	12.0		
Composite			
Mycosis fungoides			
Histiocytic			
Extramedullary plasmacytoma			
Unclassifiable			
Other			

From Johnson G: Malignant lymphomas. In Mazza J, editor: *Manual of clinical hematology,* Boston, 1994, Little, Brown.

pleural effusions are common. Approximately 20% or more of the patients have symptoms related to retroperitoneal or mesenteric lymph node enlargement and present with abdominal pain or irregularities of bowel movements. Involvement of the stomach and small intestine is common, with symptoms of pain similar to that of peptic ulcer: anorexia, weight loss, nausea, hematemesis (bloody vomiting), and melena. In diffuse (large cell) lymphoma, the tonsillar lymphatic tissue in the oropharynx and nasopharynx (referred to as *Waldeyer's ring*) is also the site of involvement in 15% to 30% of patients (Johnson, 1994).

Patients with non-Hodgkin's lymphomas of the nodular (diffuse, small, cleaved cell), poorly differentiated lymphocytic type tend to present at more advanced stages initially, with about 60% to 80% incidence of bone marrow involvement. Staging laparotomy is generally not indicated in these individuals. In addition to tissue biopsy, cytochemistry, surface marker studies, gene rearrangement, and cytogenetics are invaluable in the accurate diagnosis of non-Hodgkin's lymphomas.

Central nervous system (CNS) diseases, although rare, do occur in the diffuse histiocytic lymphomas (large cell, immunoblastic). The CNS is frequently the site for relapse in patients with stage IV disease, along with the sites of previous involvement.

The treatment of choice for patients with localized extranodal disease is radiation, either localized or extended-field radiotherapy. This treatment is curative in 80% to 90% of the cases with diffuse, aggressive disease. Patients with stage II diffuse disease require a combination of chemotherapy (using three to five drugs) and radiation directed at the local disease. Approximately 50% remission or cure rates are obtained in previously untreated cases. Indolent lymphomas generally respond to nonaggressive single- or two-drug regimens. The median survival rate is 8 to 10 years for this condition (Sweet, Golomb, 1980). The number of cures in the vast majority of patients with non-Hodgkin's lymphomas remains very low. The common chemotherapeutic agents used are listed in Table 18-1 and generally include cytoxan, prednisone, and vincristine.

PLASMA CELL DYSCRASIAS

Plasma cell dyscrasias are a group of disorders manifested by a proliferation of plasma cells in the bone marrow and/or peripheral blood. Plasma cells are lymphoid in origin (B lymphocyte) and are normally responsible for immunoglobulin synthesis. The five main classes of immunoglobulins are IgA, IgD, IgE, IgG, and IgM (see Chapter 5). In plasma cell dyscrasias the plasma cells synthesize and secrete an abnormal, structurally homogeneous immunoglobulin called the *M component*. These proteins are found in serum and/or urine of affected patients (Foerster, 1993).

Multiple Myeloma

Multiple myeloma is a neoplastic plasma cell dyscrasia arising from a single clone (monoclonal) of plasma cells, manifested by the uncontrolled proliferation of immature and mature plasma cells in the bone marrow. The clinical consequences of the abnormal plasma cells include bone destruction and replacement of normal bone marrow elements, leading to anemia, thrombocytopenia, and leukopenia; altered immune function, with an increased risk for infections; hemostatic abnormalities with bleeding manifestations; and cryoglobulinemia and hyperviscosity related to the abnormal protein *M component*. Bence Jones protein is a light-chain monoclonal protein excreted by the kidneys that plays a role in renal failure (Foerster, 1993).

The exact cause of multiple myeloma is unknown. Genetic susceptibility has been considered, as has radiation exposure. The incidence increases with age. The median age at diagnosis is 60 years, and it is rarely seen in individuals younger than 20 years.

The diagnostic workup of a patient with suspected multiple myeloma includes (1) a history; (2) a physical examination; (3) skeletal x-ray films and bone survey; (4) hematologic studies including a bone marrow examination, CBC, and differential; (5) a monoclonal protein evaluation that includes the serum immunoglobulins and a 24-hour urine collection for Bence Jones proteins; and (6) biochemical studies including renal function, albumin, calcium, uric acid, and lactic dehydrogenase (LDH) levels. Positive findings to confirm the diagnosis include the following (Foerster, 1993):

1. Greater than 10% plasma cells in the bone marrow
2. Plasma cells in bone or soft tissue biopsies
3. Presence of the myeloma protein (M component) on plasma or urine immunoelectrophoresis
4. Presence of "punched-out" lytic bone lesions on skeletal x-ray films
5. Peripheral smear containing myeloma cells

Clinical manifestations vary. Infection is a common complication of multiple myeloma and often the cause of death. *Streptococcus, Haemophilus influenzae, Staphylococcus aureus,* bacteremias, and gram-negative urinary tract infections are commonly seen because of the decrease or lack of normal immunoglobulins, as well as the leukopenia secondary to marrow replacement or chemotherapy. Increased levels of abnormal globulins cause increased serum viscosity with visual disturbances, headaches, somnolence, irritability, and confusion. Expanded plasma volume and amyloid infiltration may result in congestive heart failure. The RBCs become coated with proteins, which causes them to stick together like stacks of coins (rouleaux) (Fig. 18-8). Bleeding manifestations occur because the protein interacts with the plasma coagulation factors, as well as interferes with platelet function. One of the globulins (cryoglobulin) precipitates in cold temperatures, causing blanching, pain,

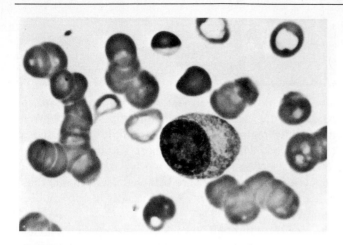

FIG. 18-8   Peripheral blood characteristic of multiple myeloma. Peripheral blood depicting rouleaux formation typically seen in multiple myeloma. The large cell in the center is an immature plasma cell. (Courtesy of Rita C. Pohlod, MT [ASCP], SH, Special Hematology Department, Henry Ford Hospital, Detroit, Mich.)

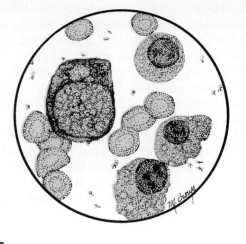

FIG. 18-9   In the upper right field is a normal plasma cell and a plasma cell typical of multiple myeloma; the other cells are malignant plasma cells.

and ulceration in fingertips and toes (Raynaud's phenomenon). A normochromic normocytic anemia is also present. Fig. 18-9 depicts a peripheral blood smear in multiple myeloma, which illustrates malignant plasma cells. (Color plate 25).

Severe disabling bone pain, especially in weight-bearing areas, is common secondary to bone destruction and pathologic fractures. Simple maneuvers such as turning in bed, coughing, or sneezing can result in fractures of the arms and ribs. Compression fractures of thoracic and lumbar vertebrae cause loss of height. Because of the bone destruction, calcium is mobilized, causing hypercalcemia (increased calcium levels). Symptoms include mental confusion, nausea, vomiting, constipation, polydipsia, and polyuria. Neurologic symptoms range from peripheral neuropathy to cord compression. The latter is a medical emergency, and unless treatment is promptly instituted with radiotherapy, chemotherapy, or surgery, the patient will be paralyzed. These patients may have symptoms of renal failure, anorexia, confusion, and coma. If the renal failure is untreated, death occurs. In addition to hypercalcemia, renal impairment may result from the myeloma proteins (referred to as *Bence Jones proteins*), damaging the renal tubules. High uric acid levels secondary to the increased plasma cell turnover may also lead to renal failure. This may result from the primary disease or may be secondary to chemotherapy. Dehydration may precipitate actual renal failure.

Newly diagnosed patients with multiple myeloma who present with a high tumor mass, hemoglobin values below 8.5 g, hypercalcemia, serum IgG above 7 g or IgA above 5 g, and renal failure carry a poor prognosis, whereas those with a low tumor mass have a median survival of 5 to 6 years. Response to therapy is also a good prognostic indicator.

Treatment is aimed at reducing the number of malignant plasma cells and preventing and controlling the complications. Indolent disease is monitored and treatment initiated when there is evidence of progression. A solitary area of plasma cell tumor (plasmacytoma) is treated with local irradiation. Active disease requires combinations of radiotherapy and chemotherapy. Multiple drug combinations using three to five agents are employed; they include prednisone and an alkylating agent such as melphalan (Alkeran). These regimens are administered intermittently every 4 to 6 weeks for approximately 12 to 48 months. Approximately 50% of the patients will show a significant tumor reduction. Autologous bone marrow or stem cell transplantation is used in some cases for long-term remissions.

Impending spinal cord compression (see Chapter 56), localized painful bone lesions, or other tumor masses are treated with irradiation. Because immobility exacerbates bone demineralization and osteoporosis, the patient must maintain a high level of mobility. Supportive garments, walking aids, and judicious use of analgesics are beneficial. Other preventive measures, such as hydration and control of infections and bleeding, will limit most of the previously described complications. Survival averages 2 to 5 years.

Waldenström's Macroglobulinemia

Waldenström's macroglobulinemia is also a plasma cell dyscrasia that predominately affects males older than 50 years. Morphologically it resembles a malignant lymphoma with B lymphocytes, plasma cells, and plasmacytoid lymphocytes (resembling plasmactyes) infiltrating the bone marrow. As the disease progresses, the clinical pattern is that of a lymphoma or chronic lymphocytic leukemia. Hepatic, splenic, and other lymphoid tissue involvements are common, resulting in enlargement of these organs. The malignant cells rarely produce bone destruction but synthesize and release large quantities of IgM into the intravascular space. This causes increased plasma volume and severe hyperviscosity. The immunoglobulin is relatively nonfunctional but may suppress production of normal immunoglobulins.

Patients may experience general malaise, fatigue, weight loss, and bleeding tendencies for years before diagnosis, as the disease progresses (Foerster, 1993). The major clinical manifestations relate to the hyperviscosity syndrome, the abnormal plasma immunoglobulin, and bone marrow infiltration. The symptoms of hyperviscosity are similar to those of multiple myeloma. These include a marked increase in plasma volume, vision disturbances, and segmental dilation of retinal veins and hemorrhages. Cold agglutinin disease (agglutination of RBCs at cold temperature) with hemolytic anemia has been described, as has Raynaud's phenomenon and anemia secondary to bone marrow replacement. Bleeding tendency, which is attributed to coating of the platelets with the macroglobulins and interference with the coagulation factors, is also seen and is further aggravated by thrombocytopenia caused by marrow replacement. Lymphadenopathy and splenomegaly may be present. Patients may present with bruising, oral mucous membrane bleeding, and retinal hemorrhages. Polyneuropathies may also be seen.

Laboratory findings include an increased sedimentation rate and rouleaux formation. Pancytopenia is seen with disease progression. Blood volume and serum viscosity are increased. The bone marrow is often a "dry tap" because of the hypercellularity. The predominant cells are lymphoplasmacytoid. Serum protein electrophoresis depicts an IgM spike.

Treatment of Waldenström's macroglobulinemia is aimed at decreasing the IgM plasma load and bone marrow infiltration and lymphoid tissues. Because IgM is mainly a circulating intravascular protein, plasmapheresis can be used effectively to decrease the globulin and temporarily reduce the hyperviscosity symptoms. Plasmapheresis is a process whereby plasma is removed by means of a cell separator and replaced with volume expanders. In the anemic patient this procedure should be done before RBC infusion because the RBCs add to the hyperviscosity syndrome. Combination chemotherapy with alkylating agents and steroids is used intermittently. Radiation is used to reduce large lymphoid aggregates. Prevention, early detection, and prompt treatment of infections are imperative because of their high incidence and increased mortality from infection. Asymptomatic patients with stable M component and no hyperviscosity or hematologic changes may go for years without treatment. Once the disease progresses, even with appropriate treatment measures, the median survival is only 4 years.

TREATMENT OF HEMATOLOGIC MALIGNANCIES

The hallmark in the treatment of the hematologic malignancies is the use of chemotherapeutic agents. Current therapeutic regimens consist of multiple drugs used in combination, which result in more sustained remission rates. In select cases of Hodgkin's disease and acute lymphocytic leukemia, cures are being attained. In other diseases, such as multiple myeloma, quality of life has been improved.

All cells go through a series of divisions (mitosis) and maturational stages called a *cell cycle.* During the mitotic phase, chromosome replication takes place, followed by the first gap or G_1 phase with RNA and protein synthesis. This is followed by the S or DNA synthesis phase and then the second gap or G_2 phase with resumed RNA synthesis. Mitosis follows, producing two daughter cells (Fischer, Knobf, 1989).

In general, therapeutic regimens are developed to include drugs acting at different stages of the cell cycle. *Phase-specific agents* arrest or kill dividing cells during a specific phase of this cycle. For example, vincristine arrests cell division, and cytarabine (Cytosar) interferes with DNA synthesis during the S phase. *Cycle-specific drugs* such as cyclophosphamide (Cytoxan) kill proliferating cells more effectively than resting cells, and non–cycle-specific agents such as nitrogen mustard and carmustine (BCNU) kill both proliferating and resting cells.

The drugs are further classified according to their mode of action. *Alkylating agents* are substances in which an alkyl radical (hydrocarbon molecule with an absent hydrogen atom) is substituted for a hydrogen atom, causing cross-linking of DNA strands and abnormal base-pairing, thereby interfering with DNA replication. This category includes nitrogen mustard, cyclophosphamide, phenylalanine mustard, and chlorambucil (Fischer, Knobf, 1989). The *antimetabolites,* such as methotrexate, cytosine arabinoside, and 6-mercaptopurine, interfere with the biologic synthesis of DNA and RNA, and thus the cell metabolism, by either blocking the needed developmental enzymes or actually being incorporated into the DNA and/or the RNA.

The *antibiotic agents,* isolated from microorganisms, seem to inhibit DNA and RNA synthesis. Doxorubicin hydrochloride (Adriamycin) and bleomycin are only two of many antibiotic antitumor agents. Natural products—the vinca alkaloids, vincristine, and vinblastine, derived from the periwinkle plant—interfere with the mitotic spindle formation and arrest cell division at the metaphase stage (Fischer, Knobf, 1989).

The *nitrosourates* are lipid-soluble alkylating agents that inhibit nucleic acid synthesis (DNA and/or RNA).

Drugs in this category include lomustine (CCNU) and carmustine (BCNU).

Adrenocorticosteroids are hormone preparations; although their exact action is unclear, they may influence synthetic processes related to RNA and protein synthesis. Prednisone is the one most commonly used in the hematologic malignancies and may be seen in many combinations.

The commonly used chemotherapeutic agents as presented in Table 18-1 are listed according to their classification. Their adverse reactions are divided according to acute or chronic toxicity. Acute toxicity occurs within minutes to hours after administration; chronic toxicity occurs over a longer period and is generally a cumulative, or dose-related, effect.

 QUESTIONS

▼ Match the white blood cells listed in column A with their appropriate function in column B. More than one letter may be used in each space in column A.

Column A	Column B
1. _____ PMNs	a. Involved in phagocytosis of dead red and white corpuscles
2. _____ Eosinophils	b. Chief source of antibody production
3. _____ Basophils	c. Responsible for the humoral immune response
4. _____ Monocytes	d. Present early in the acute phase of an inflammatory reaction
5. _____ B lymphocytes	e. Involved in phagocytosis, killing, and/or digestion of bacteria
6. _____ Plasma cells	f. Involved in the production of antigen-reactive cells
7. _____ T lymphocytes	g. Appear to function in combating acute systemic allergic reactions
	h. Carry histamine and platelet-activating factors
	i. Have phagocytic function, also appear to function in antigen-antibody reactions

▼ Answer the following on a separate sheet of paper.

8. Explain the role of colony-stimulating factor (CSF) or hematopoietic growth factors in the differentiation and maturation of white blood cells.

9. Describe the French-American-British (FAB) classification of leukemia.

10. Cite the importance of the genetic and environmental factors associated with leukemia.

11. Formulate a definition of multiple myeloma.

12. Describe the symptoms associated with Hodgkin's disease.

13. What are the aims of the treatment for multiple myeloma and Waldenström's macroglobulinemia?

▼ Circle T if the statement is true and F if it is false. Correct any false statements.

14. T F T cell lymphomas are more indolent with a long relapse-free survival.

15. T F Granulopoietin is the stimulating factor responsible for leukocyte cell differentiation.

16. T F Plasma cells normally circulate in the peripheral blood.

17. T F Neutropenia is characterized by an extremely low leukocyte count and absence of neutrophils.

18. T F Granulocytes appear to originate from the pluripotential cell in the bone marrow.

19. T F The Lukes and Collins classification of non-Hodgkin's lymphomas demonstrated that 70% of the lymphomas are of T cell origin.

20. T F Cells whose granules have a blue or basic dye affinity are called eosinophils.

▼ Circle the letter preceding each item below that correctly answers the question or completes the statement. More than one answer may be correct.

21. Pseudoleukocytosis occurs because:
a. The number of neutrophils decreases and the number of monocytes increases
b. The leukocyte count is low and neutrophils are absent

c. Granulopoiesis in the bone marrow is not accelerated
d. Granulocytes are mobilized from the marginated pool so that the number of granulocytes drawn into the sampling device is increased

22. The Philadelphia chromosome (Ph) is evidenced in 85% of patients with:
a. Chronic myeloid leukemia
b. Acute myeloblastic leukemia
c. Chronic lymphoblastic leukemia
d. Acute monocytic leukemia

23. The major clinical manifestations of Waldenström's macroglobulinemia include:
a. Abnormal plasma immunoglobulin
b. Bone marrow infiltration
c. Hyperviscosity syndrome
d. Bone pain and arthralgia

24. In multiple myeloma there is an excessive production of which of the following homogeneous immunoglobulin(s):
a. IgD   c. IgE
b. IgG   d. IgA

25. Which of the following are frequent complications encountered in patients with multiple myeloma that must be considered when planning treatment and care?
a. Bone destruction and pathologic fractures
b. Pulmonary infections
c. Hypocalcemia
d. Increased bleeding tendencies

26. Mr. R., a 70-year-old man, has been complaining of severe infections with ulcerations of the mucous membranes and repeated episodes of pneumonia. Laboratory tests indicate that the WBC count is normal with circulating myeloblasts. Bone marrow biopsy revealed myeloblasts containing Auer rods. The most likely diagnosis of Mr. R.'s condition is:
a. Chronic lymphocytic leukemia
b. Lymphoma

Continued.

QUESTIONS—cont'd

c. Multiple myeloma
d. Acute myelocytic leukemia

27. The complications associated with multiple myeloma are the result of:
    a. Decrease or lack of normal immunoglobulins
    b. Leukopenia secondary to bone marrow replacement
    c. Absence of normal hematopoietic cells
    d. Destruction of the normal architecture of the lymph nodes

28. Mr. A., a 62-year-old man, presents with a painless lymphadenopathy. splenomegaly, and slightly enlarged liver. Diagnostic studies revealed small, abnormal, mature B lymphocytes in the bone marrow (>30%) with serum levels at 90,000 cells/mm³. The most likely condition is:
    a. Acute myelogenous (granulocytic) leukemia
    b. Agranulocytosis
    c. Chronic lymphocytic-leukemia
    d. Chronic granulocytic leukemia

29. Which of the following reactions are seen in patients with leukemia?
    a. Growth of leukemic cells in abnormal areas
    b. Destruction of normal bone marrow
    c. Hypermetabolic rate
    d. Production of abnormal protein

30. Your patient is an adult who complains of increasing weakness and fatigue. He has recently noticed abnormal bruising and epistaxis (nosebleeds). On admission, he developed fever and pneumonia. The spleen is not palpable. Laboratory studies reveal immature-appearing cells of the neutrophilic series. The most likely diagnosis is:
    a. Acute lymphocytic leukemia
    b. Acute myelogenous or acute granulocytic leukemia
    c. Chronic granulocytic leukemia
    d. Chronic lymphocytic leukemia

31. Complications associated with chronic lymphocytic leukemia include:
    a. Pancytopenia
    b. Blast transformation
    c. Hemolytic anemia
    d. Splenic infarction

32. Hodgkin's disease, a lymphoproliferative disease, will usually be diagnosed by:
    a. A blood test
    b. A tissue biopsy
    c. Both a and b
    d. Neither a nor b

33. Sites of spread of Hodgkin's disease may include:
    a. Lymph nodes
    b. Liver
    c. Spleen
    d. Bone marrow

34. Stage III Hodgkin's disease is defined as:
    a. Lymphatic involvement on both sides of the diaphragm

b. Localized involvement of more than two adjacent or nonadjacent regions on one side of the diaphragm
c. Diffuse involvement of one or more extralymphatic organs or tissues, such as bone marrow or liver

▼ *Complete the following statements by filling in the blanks.*

35. _____ refers to a neoplastic disease characterized by an abnormal proliferation and impaired functional capability of the hematopoietic cells.

36. The cells characteristic of Hodgkin's disease are called _____.

37. _____ is a decrease below normal in the leukocyte count.

38. Certain abnormal chromosome patterns, such as the Philadelphia chromosome, are encountered in approximately 85% of the cases of _____.

▼ *Fill in the blanks.*

39. List the type of WBC count that is elevated in the following conditions:

Condition		Type of cell
Acute bacterial infection	a.	_____
Allergic rhinitis	b.	_____
Myeloproliferative disorders	c.	_____

▼ *Match the drug in column A with the associated toxic reaction(s) in column B. More than one letter may be used in each space in column A. Items may be used more than once.*

Column A

40. _____ Bleomycin
41. _____ Doxorubicin
42. _____ Cyclophosphamide
43. _____ Methotrexate
44. _____ Vincristine
45. _____ Chlorambucil
46. _____ L-Asparaginase

Column B

a. Alopecia, hemorrhagic cystitis
b. Severe vesicant with tissue necrosis, nausea
c. Mild anorexia, nausea, and vomiting
d. Delayed nausea, 6 to 18 hours
e. Hypercalcemia, pancreatitis, hepatotoxicity
f. Alopecia, peripheral neuropathy, myopathy
g. Myelosuppression
h. Stomatitis, ulceration, diarrhea
i. Pulmonary fibrosis with cumulative doses, minimal myelosuppression
j. Immunosuppression

CHAPTER 19 ▶ Coagulation Disorders

CATHERINE M. BALDY

NORMAL COAGULATION PROCESS AND PLASMA CLOTTING FACTORS

Hemostasis and coagulation refer to a complex series of reactions that lead to the control of bleeding through the formation of a platelet and fibrin clot at the injury site. Clotting is followed by resolution or lysis of the clot and regeneration of the endothelium. In homeostatic states, hemostasis and coagulation protect the individual from massive bleeding secondary to trauma. In abnormal states, life-threatening hemorrhage or thrombosis occluding the vascular tree can occur.

At the time of injury, three major processes are responsible for hemostasis and coagulation: (1) transient vasoconstriction; (2) platelet reaction consisting of adhesion, release reaction, and aggregation of platelets; and (3) activation of the clotting factors (see box below). The initial steps occur at the exposed surfaces of the injured tissue, and subsequent reactions occur on surface phospholipids of the aggregated platelets.

PLASMA CLOTTING FACTORS

I   Fibrinogen: precursor of fibrin (polymerized protein)
II Prothrombin: precursor of the proteolytic enzyme thrombin and perhaps other accelerators of prothrombin conversion
III Thromboplastin: a tissue lipoprotein activator of prothrombin
IV Calcium: necessary for prothrombin activation and fibrin formation
V   Plasma accelerator globulin: a plasma factor that accelerates the conversion of prothrombin to thrombin
VII Serum prothrombin conversion accelerator: a serum factor that accelerates prothrombin conversion
VIII Antihemophilic globulin (AHG): a plasma factor associated with platelet factor III and Christmas factor (IX); activates prothrombin
IX Christmas factor: serum factor associated with platelet factors III and VIII$_{AHG}$; activates prothrombin
X   Stuart-Power factor: a plasma and serum factor; accelerator of prothrombin conversion
XI Plasma thromboplastin antecedent (PTA): a plasma factor that is activated by Hageman factor (XII); accelerator of thrombin formation
XII Hageman factor: a plasma factor; activates PTA (XI)
XIII Fibrin stabilizing factor: plasma factor; produces stronger fibrin clot that is insoluble in urea
—   Fletcher factor (prekallikrein): contact-activating factor
—   Fitzgerald factor (high-molecular-weight kininogen): contact-activating factor

Platelets

Platelets, or thrombocytes, are not cells but are granular, disk-shaped nonnucleated cell fragments. They are the smallest of the bone marrow cellular elements and are vital to hemostasis and coagulation. Platelets are derived from a noncommitted pluripotential stem cell, which on demand and in the presence of a platelet-stimulating factor (Mk-CSF [megakaryocyte colony-stimulating factor]) (Haeuber, DiJulio, 1989), differentiates into the committed stem cell pool to form the megakaryoblast. This cell, through a maturation sequence, becomes a giant megakaryocyte (see Fig. 16-1). Unlike the other cellular elements, megakaryocytes undergo endomitosis, whereby nuclear division occurs within the cell but the cell itself does not duplicate. The cell expands as increased DNA is synthesized. The cell cytoplasm eventually breaks up into individual platelets.

Platelets measure 1 to 4 μm in diameter and have a life span of approximately 10 days. Approximately one third are in the spleen as a reserve pool, and the remainder are in the circulation, numbering between 150,000 and 400,000/mm³. When Wright's stain is used on a peripheral smear, these cells appear light blue with red-purple granules (Color plate 26). Adsorbed on the platelet membrane are factors V, VIII, and IX, the contractile protein actomyosin, or thrombosthenin, and various other proteins and enzymes. The granules contain the potent vasoconstrictor serotonin, the aggregating factor adenosine diphosphate (ADP), fibrinogen, von Willebrand's factor, platelet factors 3 and 4 (heparin-neutralizing factor), and calcium, as well as enzymes. All these factors are released and activated in response to injury.

Clotting Factors

The clotting factors, with the exception of factors III (tissue thromboplastin) and IV (calcium ion), are plasma proteins. They circulate in the blood as inactive molecules. The box on p. 225 identifies the coagulation factors, using the internationally accepted and standardized Roman numerals, gives their synonyms, and summarizes their functions. Prekallikrein and high-molecular-weight kininogen (HMWK), along with factors XII and XI, are called *contact factors*. They are activated at the time of injury by contact with tissue surfaces. They also play a role in the dissolution of clots once they are formed.

Activation of the coagulation factors is believed to occur as an enzyme splits off a fragment of an inactive predecessor form, for this reason called a *procoagulant*. Each activated factor, except for V, VIII, XIII, and I (fibrinogen), is a protein-cleaving enzyme (serine protease), which thus activates the succeeding procoagulant.

The liver is the site of synthesis of all the coagulation factors except factor VIII and possibly XI and XIII. Vitamin K is essential for the synthesis of the prothrombin factors II, VII, IX, and X. The available evidence suggests that factor VIII is really a complex molecule of three distinct subunits: (1) the procoagulant part, which contains the antihemophilic factor, VIII$_{AHG}$, absent in patients with classic hemophilia; (2) another subunit containing an antigenic site; and (3) von Willebrand's factor, VIII$_{VWF}$, necessary for platelet adhesion to vascular walls (Erslev, Gabuzda, 1985).

Phases of Coagulation

Coagulation is initiated in homeostatic states by vascular injury. Vasoconstriction is an immediate response to the injury, followed by adhesion of platelets to collagen in the vessel wall exposed by the injury. Adenosine diphospate (ADP) is released by the platelets, causing them to aggregate. Minute amounts of thrombin (created as described below) also stimulate platelet aggregation, serving to amplify the reaction. Platelet factor III, from platelet membranes, also accelerates plasma clotting. In this way, a platelet plug forms, soon to be strengthened by the filamentous protein known as *fibrin*.

Fibrin production begins with conversion of factor X to Xa, as the activated form of a factor is designated. Factor X can be activated by means of two reaction sequences (Fig. 19-1). One requires tissue factor, or tissue thromboplastin, which is released by the vascular endothelium at the time of injury. Because tissue factor is not in the blood, it is an extrinsic element in coagulation, hence the name *extrinsic pathway* for this sequence.

The other sequence leading to activated factor X is the *intrinsic pathway,* given that name because it employs factors found within the vascular system of plasma. In this sequence, there is a "cascade" of reactions, one procoagulant's activation leading to activation of a successor form. The intrinsic pathway is initiated by plasma exposed to skin or collagen within a damaged vessel. Tissue factor is not required, but platelets adhering to the collagen again play a part. As Fig. 19-1 shows, factors XII, XI, and IX must be activated in succession, and factor VIII must be involved before factor X can be activated. The substances prekallikrein and high-molecular-weight kininogen are participants as well, and calcium ion is needed.

From this point coagulation proceeds along what has been called the *common pathway*. As the illustration shows, activation of factor X takes place as a result of either extrinsic or intrinsic pathway reactions. Clinical experience suggests that both pathways participate in hemostasis (Nossel, 1980).

The next step toward fibrin production is taken when factor Xa, helped by phospholipids from activated platelets, splits prothrombin, creating thrombin. Thrombin in turn cleaves fibrinogen to form fibrin. (Small amounts of thrombin are apparently reserved to amplify platelet aggregation.) This fibrin, at first a soluble gel, is stabilized by factor XIIIa and polymerizes into a tight meshwork of fibrin, platelets, and entrapped blood cells.

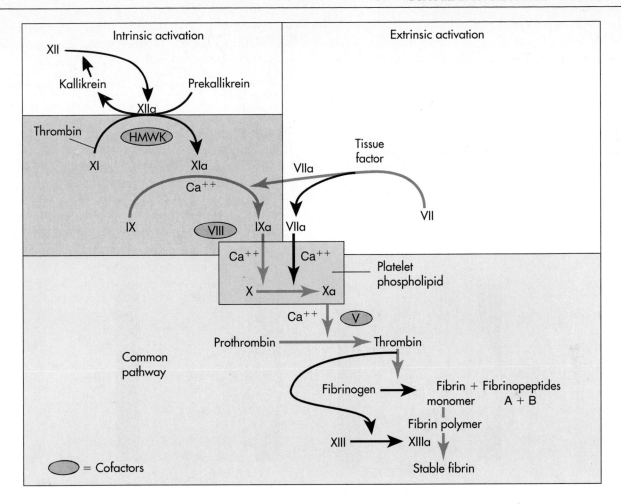

FIG. 19-1   Activation of factor X by the steps in the extrinsic and intrinsic coagulation pathways. [Redrawn from Hoffbrand AV, Pettit JE: *Essential haematology,* ed 3, London, 1993, Blackwell Scientific Publications.]

The fibrin strands then shorten (clot retraction), bringing together the edges of the wounded vessel wall and sealing the site.

Clot Resolution

The fibrinolytic system refers to the sequence whereby fibrin is split by plasmin (also called *fibrinolysin*) into fibrin degradation products, leading to the dissolution of the clot. As seen diagrammatically in Fig. 19-2, several interactions are required to convert the specific inactive circulating plasma proteins into the active fibrinolytic enzyme plasmin. Circulating proteins known as *plasminogen proactivators,* in the presence of kinases (enzymes) such as streptokinase, staphylokinase, and tissue kinase, as well as factor XIIa, are catalyzed to plasminogen activators. In the presence of additional enzymes such as urokinase, the activators convert plasminogen, a plasma protein that has been incorporated within the fibrin clot, into plasmin. Plasmin then splits fibrin and fibrinogen into fragments (fibrin-fibrinogen degradation products), which interfere with thrombin activity, platelet function, and fibrin polymerization, leading to the dissolution of the clot. Macrophages and neutrophils also play a role in fibrinolysis through their phagocytic activities. Fig. 19-3 is a graphic presentation of the sequence of events of the clotting process, as previously discussed.

Diagnostic Approach

It is evident from the preceding discussion that abnormalities can occur at any stage of the hemostatic process. Evaluation then includes an in-depth history and physical and laboratory assessments. A carefully elicited history will often direct one toward the accurate diagnosis and required laboratory studies. This includes family history, coexisting medical problems, medication exposure, prior bleeding episodes (e.g., "spontaneous" or related to surgery or tooth extractions), and the need for blood component therapy.

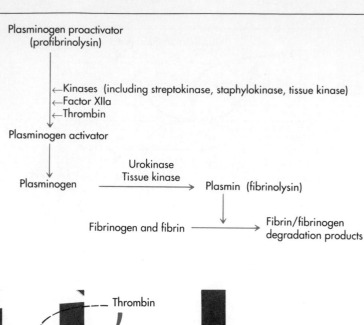

FIG. 19-2   Fibrinolytic system. Antithrombin is a circulating protein that inactivates fibrin and helps maintain blood fluidity.

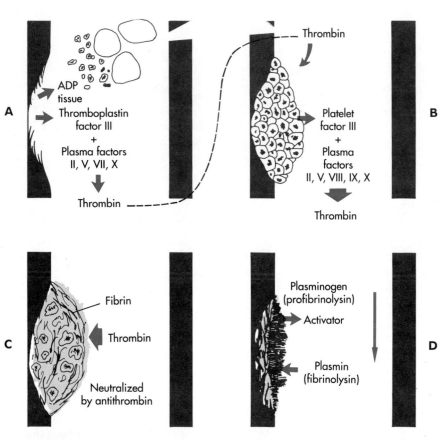

FIG. 19-3   Sequence of events in the clotting process. (Modified from Hiss RG, Penner J: The before and after of blood clotting, *Med Clin North Am* 53[6]:1309-1320, 1969.)

Careful scrutinizing of the skin and mucous membranes with attention to the type of lesions may suggest the abnormality present.

Telangiectasias are dilated capillaries and venules. They are 2 to 3 mm purple to red-purple macular spots that blanch with pressure and bleed with the slightest trauma. They are seen most commonly on the face, lips, mucous membranes, fingertips, and toes. Telangiectasias are seen as birthmarks or in a hereditary hemorrhagic disorder—Osler-Weber-Rendu disease. *Arterial spiders* are bright-red lesions with a pulsatile center and thread-like extensions radiating 5 to 10 mm in length. They are commonly seen in the face and trunk, above the waistline. These likewise blanch if pressed at their center and represent vascular anomalies, often seen in liver disease.

Petechiae are 1 to 4 mm flat, round, nonblanching,

TABLE 19-1   Coagulation Studies

Study	Purpose	Normal Values	Clinical Significance
Bleeding time	Measures platelet and vascular function	2-9½ minutes	Prolonged in thrombocytopenia, thrombocytopathy, von Willebrand's disease, aspirin ingestion, anticoagulant therapy, and uremia
Platelet count	Assesses platelet concentration	150,000-400,000/mm³	Decreased in ITP and bone marrow malignancies Drugs, especially chemotherapeutic agents, may cause prolonged bleeding Elevated in early myeloproliferative disorders After splenectomy, may predispose to later thrombotic episodes
Clot reaction	Assesses platelet adequacy to form fibrin clot	Clot retracts to one-half size in 1 hour, firm clot in 24 hours if undisturbed	Poor clot retraction in thrombocytopenia and polycythemia; lysis of clot in fibrinolysis
Lee-White clotting time (coagulation)	Assesses coagulation mechanism—time required for blood to form a solid clot after exposure to glass	6-12 minutes	Relatively insensitive test Prolonged with severe deficiencies of coagulation factors, in excessive anticoagulant therapy, and with selected antibiotics Decreased with corticosteroid therapy
Prothrombin time (PT)	Measures extrinsic and common coagulation pathway	11-16 seconds	Prolonged in deficiencies of factors VII and X and fibrinogen, excess dicumarol therapy, severe liver disease and disseminated intravascular coagulation (DIC), and vitamin K deficiency
Activated partial thromboplastin time (APTT)	Measures intrinsic and common coagulation pathway	26-42 seconds	Prolonged in deficiencies of factors VIII to XII and fibrinogen, with circulating anticoagulant therapy, in liver disease and DIC, and in vitamin K deficiency Shortened in malignancies (except liver)
Thrombin time (TT) or thrombin clotting time	Measures fibrinogen to fibrin formation	10-13 seconds	Prolonged with low fibrinogen levels, inhibitors, DIC, and liver disease, anticoagulant therapy, and in dysproteinemias
Thromboplastin generation test (TGT)	Measures ability to form thromboplastin	12 seconds or less	Prolonged in thrombocytopenia, with deficiencies of factors VIII to XII, and with circulating anticoagulants
D-Dimer test	Measures breakdown products of plasma fibrin clots	<500	Elevated in DIC, pulmonary emboli, infarcts, thrombolytic therapy, surgery, trauma
Platelet aggregation test	Tests platelet function	Platelets aggregate within a specified time when exposed to substances such as ADP, collagen, epinephrine	Decreased or absent aggregation in thrombasthenia, aspirin ingestion, myeloproliferative disorders, severe liver disease, dysproteinemias, von Willebrand's disease

purplish hemorrhagic lesions, which may coalesce to form larger lesions called *purpura*. These are found in the mucous membranes and skin, especially in the dependent or pressure areas. These generally reflect a platelet abnormality. Hematomas (blood blisters) can also be seen in mucous membranes.

All of these lesions reflect a platelet abnormality, either in the number of platelets or their function.

Ecchymoses, bruises or black-and-blue marks, are large macular areas of extravasated blood in the subcutaneous tissues and skin. Fresh bleeding is blue-black and fades to green-brown and yellow on resolution. Although ecchymoses are commonly seen with trauma, extensive ecchymoses may reflect a platelet abnormality and/or a coagulation defect.

Laboratory Evaluation

Laboratory evaluation will further differentiate and confirm the hemostatic defect. This should always include a peripheral blood smear and a platelet count as previously described. These studies provide morphologic platelet characteristics, as well as numbers.

The *bleeding time* tests both vascular status and platelet number and function, but it does not differentiate between the two. A controlled puncture incision is made in the free-hanging earlobe (Duke method) or on the volar surface of the forearm (Ivy method). The length of time for bleeding to cease is recorded. Normal bleeding time is 3 to 7 minutes. Prolongation, such as 10 minutes, may indicate thrombocytopenia (platelet count of less than 100,000/mm³), thrombocytopathy (abnormal platelet function), or both. Aspirin ingestion can interfere with platelet function for 7 to 10 days and thus should be withheld before testing the bleeding time. Although a battery of tests is available to evaluate the coagulation status, screening tests should include the *prothrombin time* (PT), measuring the extrinsic and common pathway, and the partial *thromboplastin time* (PTT), measuring the intrinsic and common pathway.

In tests of the prothrombin time an aliquot of the patient's citrated plasma is mixed with phospholipid and tissue thromboplastin. Because calcium has been removed coagulation does not occur. Next, calcium is added and the time required for clot formation is recorded. Normal plasma requires 11 to 13 seconds to clot under such conditions. Deficiencies of factors VII, X, and V, prothrombin, and fibrinogen will prolong the PT.

In tests of the PTT, phospholipid is added to the patient's citrated plasma, resulting in clot formation in 60 to 90 seconds. Adding a contact-activating agent such as kaolin reduces the variability of the study as well as the time required for clot formation. This modification gives an *activated partial thromboplastin time* (APTT). The results are compared with the APTT of normal plasma. The normal range is 26 to 42 seconds. Because the PTT measures the intrinsic and common pathways, it is prolonged

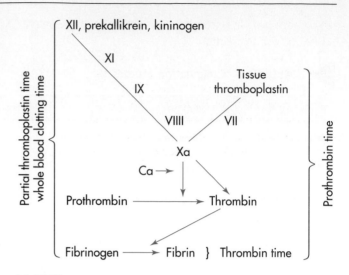

FIG. 19-4   Coagulation tests. (From Nossel HL: Bleeding. In Isselbacher K et al, editors: *Harrison's principles of internal medicine*, ed 9, New York, 1980, McGraw-Hill.)

by deficiencies of prekallikrein, high-molecular-weight kininogen, factors V, VIII, IX, X, XI, and XII, prothrombin, and fibrinogen. If only the PT is prolonged, a deficiency or an inhibitor of factor VII can be assumed. If only the PTT is prolonged, a deficiency or an inhibitor of any intrinsic pathway factor can be assumed. With prolongation of both, a deficiency or inhibitor of the common pathway factors V and X, prothrombin, and fibrinogen can be assumed. Liver disease likewise can cause prolongation of both PT and PTT.

In tests of the *thrombin time* or thrombin clotting time (normal 10 to 13 seconds), exogenous thrombin is added to citrated plasma and clotting time is measured. Because this measures the time for transformation of fibrinogen to fibrin and detects abnormalities in fibrin polymerization or low fibrinogen level, it is used to further delineate the missing clotting factors when both PT and PTT are abnormal. Coagulation tests are depicted in Fig. 19-4 (see also Table 19-1). Heparin, a potent anticoagulant, enhances the neutralizing effects of antithrombin III on factors IXa, Xa, XIa, thrombin, and plasmin and thus prolongs the PT, PTT, and thrombin time.

ABNORMALITIES OF HEMOSTASIS AND COAGULATION

Vascular Defects

A wide variety of abnormalities can occur at any level of the hemostatic mechanism. A patient with defects in the vascular system usually presents with cutaneous hemorrhages, often involving the mucous membranes. The hemorrhages can be classified as either nonallergic or allergic purpuras. In both, platelet function and the coagulation factors are normal.

Many forms of nonallergic purpura exist, that is, diseases where no true allergy is present but where various forms of vasculitis develop. The most common of these is seen in systemic lupus erythematosus. This is a collagen-vascular disease in which the patient develops autoantibodies (see Chapter 72). Vasculitis, or inflammation of vessels, occurs and destroys the integrity of the vessels, resulting in purpura.

Ineffective, deteriorating vascular supportive tissue, as seen with aging, results in *senile purpura*. Cutaneous hemorrhages are seen generally on the dorsum of the hands and forearms and are aggravated by trauma. Except for the cosmetic annoyance, this is a nonthreatening condition. A similar cutaneous manifestation is seen with long-term corticosteroid therapy, believed to result from the protein catabolism in the vascular supportive tissue. Scurvy, related to malnutrition, and alcoholism likewise affect the integrity of the connective tissue of the vascular wall.

An autosomal dominant form of vascular purpura, *hereditary hemorrhagic telangiectasia* (Osler-Weber-Rendu disease), presents with profuse intermittent epistaxis and gastrointestinal (GI) bleeding. Diffuse telangiectasia is found in the buccal mucosa, tongue, nose, and lips and probably extends throughout the GI tract. It generally develops in adulthood. Treatment is mainly supportive.

The Ehlers-Danlos syndrome, another hereditary disease, involves decreased compliance of the perivascular tissues, leading to severe hemorrhage.

The *allergic* or *anaphylactoid purpuras* are thought to result from immunologic damage to the vessels. They are characterized by petechial hemorrhages on dependent portions of the body and also involve the buttocks. Henoch-Schönlein purpura, a triad of purpura and mucosal bleeding, GI symptoms, and arthritis, is a form of allergic purpura that affects primarily children. The mechanism of this disease is not well understood. Its symptoms are often preceded by an infectious state. Patients develop an inflammation of the vascular tree, at the capillary and venous levels, leading to vascular disruption, loss of red blood cells, and bleeding. Glomerulonephritis is a frequent complication. Treatment is supportive, with avoidance of aspirin and its compounds.

Thrombocytosis and Thrombocytopenia

The platelets adhering to the exposed collagen of injured blood vessels, contracting and releasing ADP and platelet factor 3, are important in the initiation of the clotting system. Abnormalities in the numbers and/or functions of the platelets can interfere with blood coagulation. Too many or too few platelets can interfere with blood coagulation. The condition characterized by too many is known as thrombocytosis or thrombocythemia. *Throm-*

bocytosis is generally defined as an increase in the platelet counts above 400,000/mm³ and may be primary or secondary. Primary thrombocytosis is seen in primary thrombocythemia, in which there is an abnormal proliferation of megakaryocytes, with platelet counts exceeding 1 million. It is also seen with other myeloproliferative disorders, such as polycythemia vera or chronic granulocytic leukemia, in which there is an abnormal proliferation of the megakaryocytes, along with other cell lines, in the bone marrow. Both hemorrhage and thrombosis can occur. The pathophysiology is obscure but thought to be related to intrinsic qualitative abnormality in platelet function as well as the consequences of the increased platelet mass. The bleeding time is usually prolonged (Bithell, 1993).

When the platelet count exceeds 1 million or the patient is symptomatic, treatment is initiated and aimed at reducing the bone marrow activity through the use of cytotoxic agents. In the presence of acute bleeding or thrombosis, platelet pheresis offers temporary relief. Antiplatelet agents such as aspirin and anticoagulants have also been used.

Secondary thrombocytosis occurs as a consequence of other underlying causes. It may be seen temporarily after stress or exercise with storage pool release (from the spleen) or may accompany increased bone marrow demand states as with hemorrhage or hemolytic anemia. An increased number of platelets is briefly seen in patients whose spleens have been surgically removed. Because the spleen is the primary site of platelet storage and destruction, removal (splenectomy) without a concomitant decrease in bone marrow production will lead to thrombocytosis, often exceeding 1 million/mm³. Treatment of secondary or reactive thrombocytosis is generally not indicated.

Thrombocytopenia is defined as a platelet count below 100,000/mm³. This is caused by either decreased production or increased destruction of platelets. Clinical manifestations, however, are generally absent until the count falls below 100,000 and are further influenced by other underlying or coexisting conditions such as leukemia or liver disease. Increased ecchymosis and prolonged bleeding with minor trauma are seen with levels under 50,000/mm³. Petechiae are the major manifestations seen with platelet counts below 30,000. Mucosal, deep tissue, and intracranial bleeding can be seen with counts under 20,000 and require immediate intervention to prevent exsanguination and death.

Decreased platelet production, verified by bone marrow aspiration and biopsy, is seen in any condition interfering with or inhibiting bone marrow function. This includes aplastic anemia (Chapter 17), myelofibrosis (replacement of bone marrow elements by fibrous tissue), acute leukemia (Chapter 18), and other metastatic carcinomas that replace the normal marrow elements. Deficiency states, as of vitamin B₁₂ and folic acid, affect megakaryopoiesis with production of large hyperlobulated megakaryocytes. Chemotherapeutic agents (Chapter 18) are particularly toxic to the bone marrow, suppressing platelet production.

In the event of thrombocytopenia with normal platelet production, excessive destruction or sequestration is usually the cause. Any condition causing splenomegaly (markedly enlarged spleen) may be accompanied by thrombocytopenia. This includes such states as hepatic cirrhosis, lymphomas, and myeloproliferative diseases. The spleen normally holds one third of the produced platelets, but with splenomegaly this pool may increase to 80%, decreasing the available circulating pool.

Platelets can also be destroyed by drug-induced antibody production, as seen with quinidine and gold (Table 17-1) or by autoantibodies (antibodies acting against the body's own tissues). These are seen in such disease states as lupus erythematosus, chronic lymphocytic leukemia, certain lymphomas, and idiopathic thrombocytopenic purpura (ITP). The last, seen primarily in young women, is manifested by severe life-threatening thrombocytopenia with platelet counts often below 10,000/mm³. As described in Chapter 12, an IgG antibody is demonstrated on the platelet membrane, resulting in defective platelet aggregation and increased platelet removal and destruction by the macrophage system.

Platelet function can be altered (thrombocytopathy) in various ways, the result being prolonged bleeding. Drugs such as aspirin, indomethacin, and phenylbutazone inhibit platelet aggregation and release reaction, thus causing prolonged bleeding in spite of normal platelet numbers. The effects of a single dose of aspirin may last 7 to 10 days.

Plasma proteins as seen in macroglobulinemia and multiple myeloma coat platelets, interfering with platelet adhesion, clot retraction, and fibrin polymerization. In all these situations, correcting the underlying problem will reverse the abnormal platelet function.

INHERITED PLASMA FACTOR DISORDERS

Hemophilia

Hemophilia is among the most common hereditary or acquired coagulation disorders, manifested by intermittent bleeding episodes. It is an X-linked recessive disease. Therefore all the daughters of hemophiliac males are carriers of the disease, and the sons are not afflicted. Sons of a carrier female have a 50% chance of being hemophiliacs. Homozygous females with hemophilia (father a hemophiliac, mother a carrier) can be seen, but it is extremely rare. Approximately 33% of the patients do not have a family history and are presumably from spontaneous mutations (Hoffbrand, Pettit, 1993).

Two clinically identical major types of hemophilia are (1) classic hemophilia, or hemophilia A, in which antihe-mophilic factor VIII activity is deficient or absent; and (2) Christmas disease, or hemophilia B, in which factor IX activity is deficient or absent. Hemophiliacs are classified as (1) severe, with factor activity levels less than 1%; (2) moderate, with activity levels between 1% and 5%; and (3) mild, if 5% or greater. Spontaneous bleeding is seen with factor activity levels less than 1%. However, with levels of 5% or more, bleeding is generally related to trauma or surgical procedures. Clinical manifestations include bleeding into soft tissues, muscles, and joints, especially the weight-bearing joints, called hemarthrosis (joint bleeding). Repeated bleeding into the joints leads to articular cartilage degeneration with symptoms of arthritis. Retroperitoneal bleeding and intracranial bleeding are life threatening. The degree of bleeding is related to the amount of factor activity and the severity of injury. Bleeding may occur immediately or hours after the injury. Surgical bleeding is common in all hemophiliacs, and any anticipated surgical procedure requires aggressive preoperative and postoperative factor replacement to greater than 50% activity level.

Laboratory diagnosis includes measuring the appropriate factor level: factor VIII for hemophilia A, or factor IX for hemophilia B. Because factors VIII and IX are part of the intrinsic pathway of coagulation, the PTT is prolonged, whereas the PT, which bypasses the intrinsic pathway, is normal. Bleeding time, measuring platelet function, is usually normal, but delayed bleeding may occur because of inadequate fibrin stabilization. The platelet count is normal.

Treatment of hemophilia dictates intervention at the earliest signs or symptoms of bleeding, as well as preoperative factor replacement in preparation for surgical procedures. The treatment is aimed at increasing the deficient factor VIII or IX to a normal level. Severity of the bleeding, anticipated surgical complexity, the patient's weight, and the patient's specific factor level will determine the dosage of the factor replacement. For minor bleeding events, such as early muscle or joint bleeding, a 20% to 50% activity level maintained for a few days may suffice, whereas for major events such as intracranial bleeding or surgery, 100% activity level should be attained and maintained for a minimum of 2 weeks. Currently available, highly purified, recombinant factor VIII products are *Recombinate* and *Kogenate*. *Monoclate* P is a pasteurized monoclonal factor VIII product, and *Mononine* is a highly purified factor IX preparation. Dosages for all the factors are calculated in units per kilogram of body weight and infused on a daily basis. A loading dose of factor is administered, followed by twice daily dosing. A continuous infusion may be utilized in patients with hemophilia undergoing major surgical procedures. The patient is monitored with serum factor level determinations and responsiveness to the prescribed therapy.

There was a marked incidence of human immune virus (HIV) infection in the hemophiliac population starting with the 1980s. In addition, most of the adult population has serologic evidence of hepatitis. Improved donor screening, HIV testing of blood, and the development of virucidal methods and recombinant (genetically engineered) factor preparations, as noted with the above factors, have greatly reduced the risk of transmission of blood-borne infections including acquired immune deficiency syndrome (AIDS) (Andreoli et al., 1993; Bauer et al., 1994). Since 1985 the prophylactic use of the hepatitis vaccination series at the time of diagnosis has further reduced the incidence or eliminated hepatitis B for these patients.

The majority of the patients are now monitored through hemophilia treatment centers where the global needs of patients are addressed and they have the benefit of consultation from a comprehensive health care team. Improved preventive care, physical therapy, and teaching good health habits and self-administration of factor concentrates in the home setting have vastly improved the quality of life for this patient population.

Antibody inhibitors directed against the specific coagulation factor occur in 5% to 10% of patients with factor VIII deficiency and less often in factor IX. Subsequent infusions of the factor stimulate more antibody formation. Immunosuppressive agents, plasmapheresis to remove the inhibitor, and prothrombin complexes that bypass factors VIII and IX inhibitors found in fresh frozen plasma (FFP) are used to treat these patients. A synthetic product, DDAVP (1-deamino 8-D arginine vasopressin) is available for the treatment of mild to moderate hemophilia. Administered by intravenous (IV) infusion, it can induce a threefold to sixfold increase in the factor VIII activity level. Because DDAVP is a synthetic product, the risk of transmitting harmful viruses such as hepatitis or AIDS is alleviated.

von Willebrand's Disease

von Willebrand's disease is the most common inherited coagulation disorder. Various subtypes are identified, but the most common is type I. Except for types II and III, which are autosomal recessive, all are inherited as an autosomal dominant trait, occurring in males and females alike. As in hemophilia, there are cases without a family history and the disorder is thought to occur as a genetic mutation. Depending on the subtype and severity of the disease, the spectrum of bleeding may be infrequent, mild-to-moderate mucocutaneous (skin and mucous membranes) bleeding; bleeding secondary to trauma or surgery; or life-threatening hemorrhage. GI bleeding, epistaxis, and menorrhagia are common. Most patients are asymptomatic. In von Willebrand's disease, decreased activity of both factor VIII_{vWF} and factor VIII_{AHG} exists (Bithell, 1993). von Willebrand's factor is synthesized in endothelial cells and megakaryocytes and is stored in storage organelles. It facilitates platelet adhesion to components in the vascular subendothelium under conditions of high flow and shear stress. It is also the intravascular carrier for factor VIII to sites of active hemorrhage (Bauer et al., 1994; Bithell, 1993). In von Willebrand's disease, the platelets do not adhere to collagen secondary to deficient or defective vWF.

Diagnostic studies for von Willebrand's disease include an assay of the vWF, showing subnormal levels. A prolonged bleeding time in the presence of factor VIII deficiency and defective platelet aggregation with ristocetin (an antibiotic that causes platelet aggregation) are diagnostic for von Willebrand's disease.

The treatment of von Willebrand's disease varies depending on the type and degree of bleeding. Treatment options include cryoprecipitate, factor VIII concentrates, desmopressin (DDAVP), fresh frozen plasma, and estrogens. The goal is to increase the availability of von Willebrand's factor (Bauer et al., 1994). If cryoprecipitate is used, it should be obtained from carefully selected and repeatedly tested donors according to the Medical and Scientific Council of America (MASAC).

Desmopressin (DDAVP) is used in the treatment of types I and IIA of von Willebrand's disease. In most instances it can be used to control minor bleeding, and it is used prophylactically before surgical procedures. It is now available as a nasal spray, and its role is the release of von Willebrand's factor from the storage pools. For the replacement of von Willebrand's factor, the newer generation, virus-inactivated factor VIIIs, known to contain the vWF, are used. Patients scheduled for surgical procedures must be evaluated and prepared in advance of and during their procedure by a qualified hematologist.

ACQUIRED PLASMA FACTOR DEFICIENCIES

Acquired plasma factor deficiencies may be related to decreased production of the coagulation factors, as seen in liver disease or vitamin K deficiency, or increased consumption accompanying disseminated intravascular coagulation (DIC) or fibrinolysis.

Because the liver is the major site of synthesis of factors II, V, VII, IX, and X, severe liver impairment (i.e., cirrhosis) will alter the hemostatic response. There is also a decreased hepatic clearing of the activated coagulation factors. In addition, there is an impaired vitamin K assimilation, which further impairs the synthesis of the K-dependent coagulation factors. Portal hypertension in liver disease results in congestive splenomegaly with thrombocytopenia, as well as esophageal varices. These conditions, together with coagulation defects, can lead to massive hemorrhage. The PT, PTT, and bleeding time are all prolonged.

Vitamin K, which is obtained from diet and bacterial synthesis, is required for the synthesis of factors II, VII, IX, and X. In cases of malnutrition, malabsorption, or GI sterilization by antibiotics, vitamin K is markedly reduced with a resultant decrease in the biologic activity of the coagulation factors (Beck, 1991). Therapy for severe bleeding requires replacement of the coagulation factors with fresh frozen plasma (which supplies factors II, VII, IX, and X), parenteral vitamin K, and resolution of the underlying disease process.

Disseminated Intravascular Coagulation

Disseminated intravascular coagulation (DIC) is a multi-faceted, complex syndrome in which a normally homeo-static and physiologic system of maintaining the fluidity of blood becomes a pathologic system leading to diffuse fibrin thrombi occluding the microvasculature of the body. The fibrinolytic system is likewise activated, resulting in diffuse hemorrhage. DIC is not a disease, but the consequence of an underlying disease process. Alter-ation of any of the components of the vascular system, namely, the vessel wall, plasma proteins, and platelets, can result in a consumptive disorder (Coleman et al., 1993). The introduction of a procoagulant material or ac-tivity into the circulating blood initiates the syndrome. This can occur in any condition where tissue thrombo-plastin is liberated secondary to tissue destruction, with an initiation of the extrinsic clotting pathway. Because the placenta is a rich source of tissue thromboplastin, one of the most common causes of DIC is placental abruption (abruptio placentae, premature separation of the pla-centa). This condition causes retention of the conceptual products (placenta, fetus), leading to necrosis and further tissue damage. Tumor products, burns, and crushing trauma all cause thromboplastin release. In promyelo-cytic leukemia, the granular promyelocytes exhibit thromboplastin-like activity often when chemotherapy is initiated and the granules are released. Initiation of the in-trinsic pathway also occurs with the exposure of intrinsic procoagulants to damaged vascular endothelium as in vasculitis, sepsis, and shock. During the process of coag-ulation, platelets aggregate and, together with the coagu-lation factors, are used and depleted. The resultant fibrin thrombi may or may not occlude the microvasculature. Concomitantly, the fibrinolytic system is activated for the dissolution of the fibrin thrombi, producing large num-bers of fibrin and fibrinogen degradation products that in-terfere with fibrin polymerization and platelet function

(McKay, 1983). This results in the diffuse hemorrhage that is characteristic of DIC.

The clinical manifestations depend on the extent and duration of the fibrin thrombi formation, the organs in-volved, and the resultant necrosis and hemorrhage. The organs most frequently involved include the kidney, skin, brain, pituitary, lungs, and adrenals, and the mucosa of the GI tract. Mucous membrane and deep-tissue bleed-ing, as well as bleeding around sites of injury, venipunc-ture, injection, and every orifice, are seen. Petechiae and ecchymoses are common. Other manifestations include hypotension (shock), oliguria or anuria, convulsions and coma, nausea and vomiting, diarrhea, abdominal pain, back pain, dyspnea, and cyanosis (McKay, 1983).

Diagnostic tests reveal prolonged PT, PTT, and TT and increased fibrin split products. The fibrinogen level and platelet count are depressed. The peripheral blood smear may show erythrocyte fragmentation with a variety of bizarre shapes secondary to damage by fibrin strands.

Management is aimed at correcting the underlying mechanism. This may require use of antibiotics and chemotherapeutic agents, cardiovascular support, and, in the event of retained placenta, emptying the uterine con-tents. Replacement of plasma factors with plasma and cryoprecipitate, as well as platelet and red blood cell transfusions, may be necessary. In the presence of intense bleeding, the role of heparin, a potent antithrombin anti-coagulant, is highly controversial. Heparin neutralizes thrombin activity, thereby inhibiting the consumption of the coagulation factors and fibrin deposition. Increasing the concentration of the clotting factors and platelets with infusions of plasma and platelets should then inhibit the bleeding diathesis. Heparin is indicated whenever re-placement therapy does not enhance the coagulation fac-tors and bleeding persists. It is also indicated in the pres-ence of fibrin deposition resulting in dermal necrosis (Logan, 1994). Low-dose heparin has been successfully used concomitantly with chemotherapeutic agents in the treatment of promyelocytic leukemia, preventing DIC secondary to thromboplastin release by the leukocytic granules.

Hypercoagulable states with an increased incidence of thrombosis also occur. These were discussed in Chapter 7 and will not be addressed here.

QUESTIONS

▼ *Answer the following on a separate sheet of paper.*
1. Explain the maturation sequence of platelet cells when vascular injury oc-curs.
2. List in proper sequence the three ways

that platelets contribute to blood coag-ulation.
3. Which two plasma coagulation factors are shared by both the extrinsic and in-trinsic systems?
4. State the mechanism that causes bleed-

ing in primary and secondary thrombo-cytosis. Cite an example of each.
5. What is von Willebrand's factor? Why is it important in coagulation?
6. What are the treatment options and goal for von Willebrand's disease?

QUESTIONS—cont'd

7. Describe the treatment goals for hemophiliacs.
8. Define disseminated intravascular coagulation (DIC).
9. Describe the role of heparin in the presence of intense bleeding.
10. What preventive measures are currently being used to reduce the risk of transmission of blood-borne infection, including AIDS?

▼ *Circle T if the statement is true and F if it is false. Correct any false statements.*

11. T F Platelets are the primary source of immunoglobulins.
12. T F Treatment of hemophilia A patients is administration of immunosuppressive agents.
13. T F All the coagulation factors circulate in the blood as plasma proteins in a procoagulant form.
14. T F At the time of injury, a deficiency of coagulation factor XI results in clinical bleeding.
15. T F Hemophilia is an X-linked recessive genetic disorder.
16. T F The liver plays a vital role in the synthesis of certain plasma coagulation factors, such as prothrombin and factors I, V, VIII, and X.
17. T F The purpose of blood clotting is to stop bleeding at the site of injury.
18. T F Partial thromboplastin time (PTT) measures the extrinsic coagulation pathway.
19. T F Because all daughters of hemophiliac men are carriers, the son of a carrier woman has a 75% chance of being a hemophiliac.

▼ *Circle the letter preceding each item below that correctly answers the question or completes the statement. More than one answer may be correct.*

20. An abnormal proliferation of megakaryocytes along with other cell lines in the bone marrow best describes:
   a. Osler-Weber-Rendu disease
   b. Primary thrombocytosis
   c. Vasculitis
   d. Secondary thrombocytopenia
21. Which of the following statements describes what occurs in blood clotting?
   a. Tissue thromboplastin is released at the site of vascular injury.
   b. Platelets that have aggregated release factors that stimulate the extrinsic system.
   c. Fibrinolysis causes the release of factor III.
   d. Prothrombin unites with fibrinogen to form fibrin.
22. The key initiating step in the extrinsic system is the release by tissue injury of a substance known as:
   a. Prothrombin
   b. Thrombin
   c. Tissue thromboplastin
   d. Platelet factor
23. What is the normal range of bleeding time, in minutes?
   a. 2 to 4
   b. 2 to 9½
   c. 3 to 10
   d. 4 to 8
24. What is the normal value for a platelet count, in platelets/mm³?
   a. 50,000 to 75,000
   b. 100,000 to 150,000
   c. 125,000 to 300,000
   d. 150,000 to 400,000
25. Thrombocytopenia may result from:
   a. Vitamin K deficiency
   b. Disseminated intravascular coagulation (DIC)
   c. Chronic liver disease
   d. Antiplatelet antibodies
26. Thrombocytopenia may be considered severe and the risk of hemorrhage is great when the platelet count is below:
   a. 20,000/mm³
   b. 10,000/mm³
   c. 125,000/mm³
   d. 250,000/mm³
27. A patient with classic hemophilia A has deficient or absent activity of:
   a. Prothrombin
   b. Factor VII
   c. Christmas factor IX
   d. Factor VIII
28. A hemophiliac person cannot initiate clotting at which of the following levels?
   a. Extrinsic
   b. Intrinsic
   c. Vascular
   d. Platelet
29. In classic hemophilia A, which laboratory findings would you expect?
   a. Normal prothrombin time (PT), abnormal partial thromboplastin time (PTT)
   b. Abnormal PT, normal PTT
   c. Abnormal PT, abnormal PTT
30. Mrs. A., a 23-year-old primipara, was admitted to the hospital as an obstetric emergency with an abruptio placentae. She has been hemorrhaging profusely. Which of the following conditions would you suspect?
   a. Secondary thrombocytosis
   b. Thrombocytopenia
   c. Osler-Weber-Rendu disease
   d. Disseminated intravascular coagulation (DIC)
31. An anticoagulant was ordered for Mrs. A. This treatment is expected to:
   a. Release tissue thromboplastin to prevent the production of thrombin
   b. Block tissue thromboplastin from activating the coagulation process
   c. Inactivate the intrinsic system
   d. Prohibit the consumption of the coagulation factors and fibrin so that the production of plasma factors is increased

---

▼ *Match the normal range for clot formation or clotting time in column B with the appropriate screening test in column A*

Column A	Column B
32. _____ Prothrombin time (PT)	a. 10 to 13 seconds
33. _____ Thrombin time (TT)	b. 26 to 42 seconds
34. _____ Thromboplastin generation test (TGT)	c. 6 to 12 minutes
35. _____ Activated partial thromboplastin test (APTT)	d. 12 seconds or less
	e. 11 to 16 seconds

Andreoli TE et al, editors: *Cecil's essentials of medicine,* ed 3, Philadelphia, 1993, WB Saunders.

Barr RD, Seymore P: Hematologic effects of antineoplastic therapy. In Holland JF, Frei F III, editors: *Cancer medicine,* ed 2, Philadelphia, 1982, Lea & Febiger.

Bauer KA et al: Coagulation/hemostasis. In Beng EJ, McArthur JR, editors: *Hematology education program,* Nashville, 1994, American Society of Hematology (University of Washington), Smith, Bueklin & Associates, Inc.

Beck WS: The megaloblastic anemias. In Williams WJ et al, editors: *Hematology,* ed 4, New York, 1990, McGraw-Hill.

Beck WS: *Hematology,* ed 5, Cambridge, Mass, 1991, The MIT Press.

Bennett JM et al: Criteria for the diagnosis of acute leukemia of M7, *Ann Intern Med* 103(3):460-462, 1985.

Beutler E: Genetic principles. In Williams WJ et al, editors: *Hematology,* ed 4, New York, 1990a, McGraw-Hill.

Beutler E: Hematolytic anemia due to infections with microorganisms. In Williams WJ et al, editors: *Hematology,* ed 4, New York, 1990b, McGraw-Hill.

Bithell TC: Thrombocytosis and hereditary coagulation disorders. In Lee GR et al, editors: *Wintrobe's clinical hematology,* ed 9, Philadelphia, 1993, Lea & Febiger.

Bray GL et al: A multicenter study of recombinant factor VIII, *Blood* 83(9):2428-2435, 1994.

Cheson BD: Recent advances in the treatment of B-cell chronic lymphocytic leukemia, *Oncology* 4(9):71-84, 1990.

Clarkson B: The acute leukemias. In Petersdorg RJ et al, editors: *Harrison's principles of internal medicine,* ed 10, New York, 1983, McGraw-Hill.

Coleman RW et al: *Hemostasis and thrombosis, basic principles and clinical practice,* ed 3, Philadelphia, 1993, JB Lippincott.

Dabich L: Adult acute non-lymphocytic leukemias, *Med Clin North Am* 64(4):683-704, 1980.

DeGruchy GC et al, editors: *Clinical haematology in medical practice,* ed 4, London, 1978, Blackwell Scientific Publications.

Devine SM, Larson RA: Acute leukemia in adults: recent developments in diagnosis and treatment, *CA* 44(6):326-352, 1994.

Dorr RT, VonHoff DD, editors: *Cancer chemotherapy handbook,* ed 2, Norwalk, Conn, 1989, Appleton and Lange.

Erslev A Jr, Gabuzda TG: Pathophysiology and hematologic disorders. In Soderman W Jr, Doseman W: *Pathologic physiology,* ed 7, Philadelphia, 1985, WB Saunders.

Fischer DS, Knobf MT: *The cancer chemotherapy handbook,* ed 3, St Louis, 1989, Mosby.

Foerster J: Waldenstrom's macroglobulinemia and multiple myeloma. In *Wintrobe's clinical hematology,* ed 9, Philadelphia, 1993, Lea & Febiger.

Foon KA et al: Chronic lymphocytic leukemia: new insights into biology and therapy, *Ann Intern Med* 113(7):525-539, 1990.

Gale RP, Waldman A: Clinical advances in acute leukemias. II. Chemotherapy, *Clin Adv Oncol Nurs* 1(3):1-4, 1989.

Golde DW: Neutrophil kinetics: production, distribution and fate of neutrophils. In Williams WJ et al, editors: *Hematology,* ed 3, New York, 1983, McGraw-Hill.

Gralnick HR et al: Classification of acute leukemia, *Ann Intern Med* 87(6):740-753, 1977.

Greenberg PL et al: Myeloproliferative disorders and myelodysplastic syndromes: recent therapeutic, cytogenetic and molecular advances. In Beng EJ, McArthur JR, editors: *Hematology education program,* Nashville, 1994, American Society of Hematology (University of Washington), Smith, Bueklin & Associates, Inc.

Guyton A: *Textbook of medical physiology,* ed 8, Philadelphia, 1991, WB Saunders.

Haeuber D, DiJulio J: Hemopoietic colony stimulating factors: an overview, *Oncol Nurs Forum* 16(2):247-255, 1989.

Hebbel RP et al: Erythrocyte adherence to endothelium in sickle cell anemia, *N Engl J Med* 302(18):992-995, 1980.

Hoelzer D: Treatment of acute lymphocytic leukemia, *Semin Hematol* 31(1):1-15, 1994.

Hoffbrand AV, Pettit JE: *Essential haematology,* ed 3, London, 1993, Blackwell Scientific Publications.

Johnson G: Malignant lymphomas. In Mazza J, editor: *Manual of clinical hematology,* Boston, 1994, Little, Brown.

Larson RA et al: Acute leukemia; biology and treatment. In Beng EJ, McArthur JR, editors: *Hematology education program,* Nashville, 1994, American Society of Hematology (University of Washington), Smith, Bueklin & Associates, Inc.

Logan L: Hemostasis and bleeding disorders. In Mazza J, editor: *Manual of clinical hematology,* ed 2, Boston, 1994, Little, Brown.

Lusher JM: *Mild hemophilia A and mild to moderate type I von Willebrand's disease: continued challenges, but reasons for optimism,* teleconference, 1994.

McGlave P: Acute leukemias in adults. In Mazza J, editor: *Manual of clinical hematology,* ed 2, Boston, 1988, Little, Brown.

McKay DG: Clinical significance of intravascular coagulation, *Bibl Haematol (Basel)* 49:6378, 1983.

Morrison VA: Chronic leukemias, *CA* 44(6):353-377, 1994.

Nossel HL: Bleeding. In Isselbacher KJ et al, editors: *Harrison's principles of internal medicine,* ed 9, New York, 1980, McGraw-Hill.

Oken MM et al: Multiple myeloma. In Beng EJ, McArthur JR, editors: *Hematology education program,* Nashville, 1994, American Society of Hematology (University of Washington), Smith, Bueklin & Associates, Inc.

Quesenberry PJ: The concept of the hematopoietic stem cell. In Williams WJ et al, editors: *Hematology,* ed 4, New York, 1990, McGraw-Hill.

Robinson SH: Degradation of hemoglobin. In Williams WJ et al, editors: *Hematology,* ed 4, New York, 1990, McGraw-Hill.

Rodgers GP et al: Current and future strategies for the management of hemoglobinopathies and thalassemia. In Beng EJ, McArthur JR, editors: *Hematology education program,* Nashville, 1994, American Society of Hematology (University of Washington), Smith, Bueklin & Associates, Inc.

Rose EH, Aledort LM: Nasal spray desmopressin (DDAVP) for mild hemophilia A and von Willebrand's disease, *Ann Intern Med* 114(7):563-568, 1991.

Sandberg AA: Cytogenetics for clinicians, *CA* 44(3):136-159, 1994.

Schrier SL: Hematology. In Rubenstein E, Federman DD, editors: *Scientific American medicine,* New York, 1979, Scientific American Books.

Sweet DL, Golomb HM: The non-Hodgkin's lymphomas, *Curr Probl Cancer* IV(7):entire issue, 1980.

Weinshel EL, Peterson BA: Hodgkin's disease, *CA* 44(6):327-346, 1994.

Williams ME et al: Hodgkin's disease and non-Hodgkin's lymphoma. In Beng EJ, McArthur JR, editors: *Hematology education program,* Nashville, 1994, American Society of Hematology (University of Washington), Smith, Bueklin & Associates, Inc.

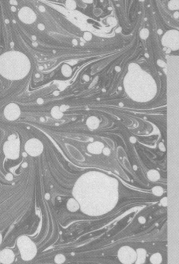

PART FOUR

FLUID AND ELECTROLYTE DISORDERS

All the cells and tissues of the human body are bathed in a fluid similar in chemical composition to sea water, reflecting our evolutionary beginnings. The normal functioning of the cell demands that the composition of this fluid be relatively constant. The dynamic equilibrium or homeostasis of water, electrolyte, and acid-base balance in the body is maintained through complex physiologic mechanisms involving the cooperation of multiple body systems.

Fluid and electrolyte and acid-base disorders are common manifestations of underlying illness and, in turn, produce systemic derangements. Recognition and treatment of these disorders are best enhanced through an understanding of normal fluid and electrolyte physiology and pathophysiologic mechanisms involved in their genesis.

Chapter 20 summarizes fluid and electrolyte balance in health and an approach to the assessment of fluid and electrolyte status. Chapter 21 deals with abnormalities of fluid volume, osmolality, and selected electrolytes. Acid-base disorders are discussed in Chapter 22. Fluid and electrolyte and acid-base disorders are discussed throughout the book in subsequent chapters, as they are associated with various diseases and disorders. ▼

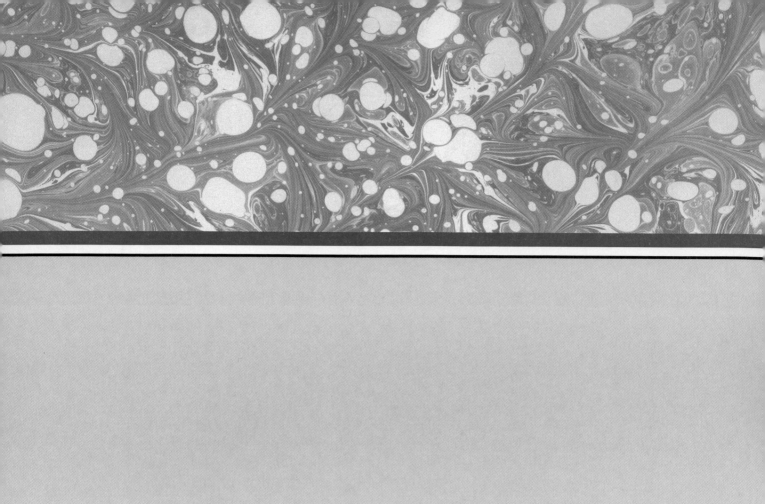

CHAPTER 20

Fluid and Electrolyte Balance and Assessment

LORRAINE M. WILSON

Fluid and electrolyte balance involve the composition and movement of body fluids. Body fluids are solutions composed of water and solutes. Electrolytes are chemical substances that form electrically charged particles called *ions* when they are in solution. Fluids and electrolytes enter the body in food, drink, and intravenous (IV) fluids and are distributed throughout the body compartments. Fluid and electrolyte balance mean that total body water and electrolytes are normal, as is their distribution within body compartments. Fluid and electrolyte balance are interdependent; if one is abnormal, so is the other. Therefore they should be discussed together.

Because fluids and electrolytes constitute the intracellular and extracellular environment for all the cells and tissues of the body, fluid and electrolyte imbalances cut across systemic classifications of disease. Fluid and electrolyte disorders are associated with all major systemic illnesses and even with some minor ones.

This chapter deals with the normal physiology of fluid and electrolytes and their regulatory mechanisms, as well as the assessment of fluid and electrolyte status.

TOTAL BODY FLUID AND ITS DISTRIBUTION

The largest single component of the body is water. It is the solvent in which all solutes in the body are either suspended or dissolved. Total body water (TBW), which is the percentage of total body weight composed of water, varies with gender, age, and body fat content. Water constitutes about 60% of the weight of men and about 50% of the weight of women. In the elderly, TBW accounts for about 45% to 50% of body weight (Narins, 1994). Because fat is essentially water-free, the less fat present, the greater the percentage of body weight that is water. Muscle tissue, on the other hand, has a high water content. Thus an obese person can be expected to have less TBW with respect to body weight than a lean person. Women generally have proportionately more fat and a smaller muscle mass than men, which accounts for their smaller amount of water in relation to TBW. Older adults also have a higher percentage of body fat than younger adults. Finally, TBW is highest in a newborn infant, at 75% of total weight. This percentage decreases rapidly to about 60% at the end of 1 year and then more gradually until

TABLE 20-1   Total Body Water in Percentage of Body Weight*

Age	Percentage of Body Weight
Infant (newborn)	75%
Adult	
Male (20-40 yr)	60%
Female (20-40 yr)	50%
Elderly (60+ yr)	45%-50%

*Data from Maxwell M, Kleeman CR, Narins RG: *Clinical disorders of fluid and electrolyte metabolism,* ed 4, New York, 1987, McGraw Hill.

adult male and female proportions are reached during adolescence (Table 20-1).

Major Compartments of Body Fluid

Various membranes (capillary, cell) separate total body fluids into two major compartments. In the adult about 40% of body weight or two thirds of TBW is within cells or *intracellular fluid* (ICF). The remaining one third of TBW or 20% of body weight is found outside of cells, the *extracellular fluid* (ECF). The extracellular fluid compartment is further divided into the *interstitial-lymph fluid* (ISF) compartment between the cells (15%) and the *intravascular fluid* (IVF) or plasma compartment (5%). In addition to the ISF and IVF, special secretions, such as the cerebrospinal fluid, intraocular fluid, and gastrointestinal secretions, form a small proportion (1% to 2% of body weight) of the extracellular fluid called transcellular fluid. Fig. 20-1 illustrates the volume and distribution of body fluids in a healthy young man.

Major Electrolytes and Their Distribution

The solutes found in body fluids include electrolytes and nonelectrolytes. *Nonelectrolytes* are solutes that do not dissociate in solution and do not carry an electrical charge. Nonelectrolytes include proteins, urea, glucose, oxygen, carbon dioxide, and organic acids. Salts that dissociate in water into one or more charged particles are called *ions* or *electrolytes.* Body electrolytes include sodium (Na^+), potassium (K^+), calcium (Ca^{++}), magnesium (Mg^{++}), chloride (Cl^-), bicarbonate (HCO_3^-), phosphate ($HPO_4^=$), and sulfate ($SO_4^=$). Electrolyte solutions conduct an electric current. Ions that carry a positive charge are called *cations,* and those carrying a negative charge are called *anions.* For example, sodium chloride (NaCl) dissociates in solution into Na^+ (cations) and Cl^- (anions). On the other hand, when glucose is dissolved in water, it does not break down into anything smaller.

The electrolyte concentration of body fluid varies from one compartment to another, and in health it must be in the right compartment in the right amount (Fig. 20-2). The chief cation of the ECF is sodium (Na^+), and the chief anions are chloride (Cl^-) and bicarbonate (HCO_3^-); their concentrations are low in the ICF. In the ICF, potassium (K^+) is the chief cation and phosphate ($HPO_4^=$) is the chief anion, whereas their concentrations are low in ECF. As the most abundant particle in the ECF, sodium plays a major role in controlling total body fluid volume, whereas potassium is important in controlling the volume of the cell. An electrical gradient across the cell membrane is necessary for the generation of nerve and muscle action potentials, and differential K^+ and Na^+ concentrations across the cell membrane are important in its maintenance. Despite the differences in ionic concentration between compartments, the *law of electrical neutrality* states that the sum of negative charges must be equal to the sum of positive charges (measured in milliequivalents) in any particular compartment. The need to maintain electroneutrality is an important determinant of ion transport between the ECF and ICF and in the kidney. Finally, note that the ionic composition of the ISF and IVF is very similar. The main difference is that the ISF contains very little protein as compared with the IVF. The higher amount of protein in plasma plays a significant role in maintaining the volume of the IVF.

Units of Solute Measurement

Terminology plays an important role in the interpretation and management of fluid and electrolyte disorders. Thus understanding the units of measurement commonly used is essential. The concentration of a given solute can be expressed in milligrams/deciliter (mg/dl or mg%), millimoles/liter (mmol/L or mM/L), milliequivalents/liter (mEq/L), milliosmoles/kilogram (mOsm/kg, or milliosmoles/liter (mOsm/L). The box on p. 242 summarizes the definition of each type of measurement and their equivalencies.

The molecular weight of a substance is the sum of the atomic weights of all the elements specified in the formula of that substance. A *mole* (mol) is the molecular (or atomic) weight of a substance expressed in grams, and a millimole is $1/1000$ of a mole, or its weight in milligrams. The terms mole and millimole may be applied to all substances, regardless of whether they are organic or nonorganic or ionized or nonionized, because it is independent of valence. Thus 1 mmol of glucose ($C_6H_{12}O_6$) = 180 mg[6(12) + 12(1) + 6(16) = 180]; 1 mmol of NaCl = 58 mg (23 + 35), whereas 1 mmol of sodium ions (Na^+) = 23 mg.

The term *milliequivalent* is $1/1000$ of an equivalent or the atomic (or molecular) weight in milligrams divided by its *valence* or *electrochemical combining power* in the reaction. The weight of an element in grams that combines with or replaces 1 g of hydrogen ion (as a standard) would be its equivalent weight. The concept of a milliequivalent is important in discussing the composition of body fluids, because ions combine milliequivalent for milliequivalent and not milligram for milligram or mil-

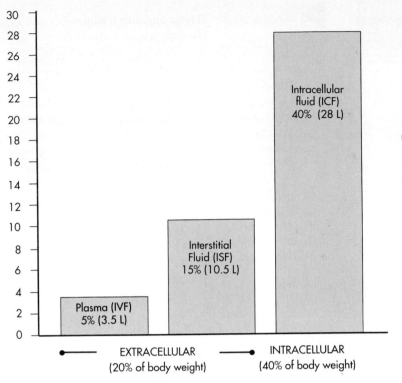

FIG. 20-1   Volume and distribution of body fluids in a healthy young man. Water is 60% of body weight and is distributed in two main compartments: the extracellular and intracellular. The extracellular fluid is subdivided into the interstitial and intravascular (plasma) fluid compartments.

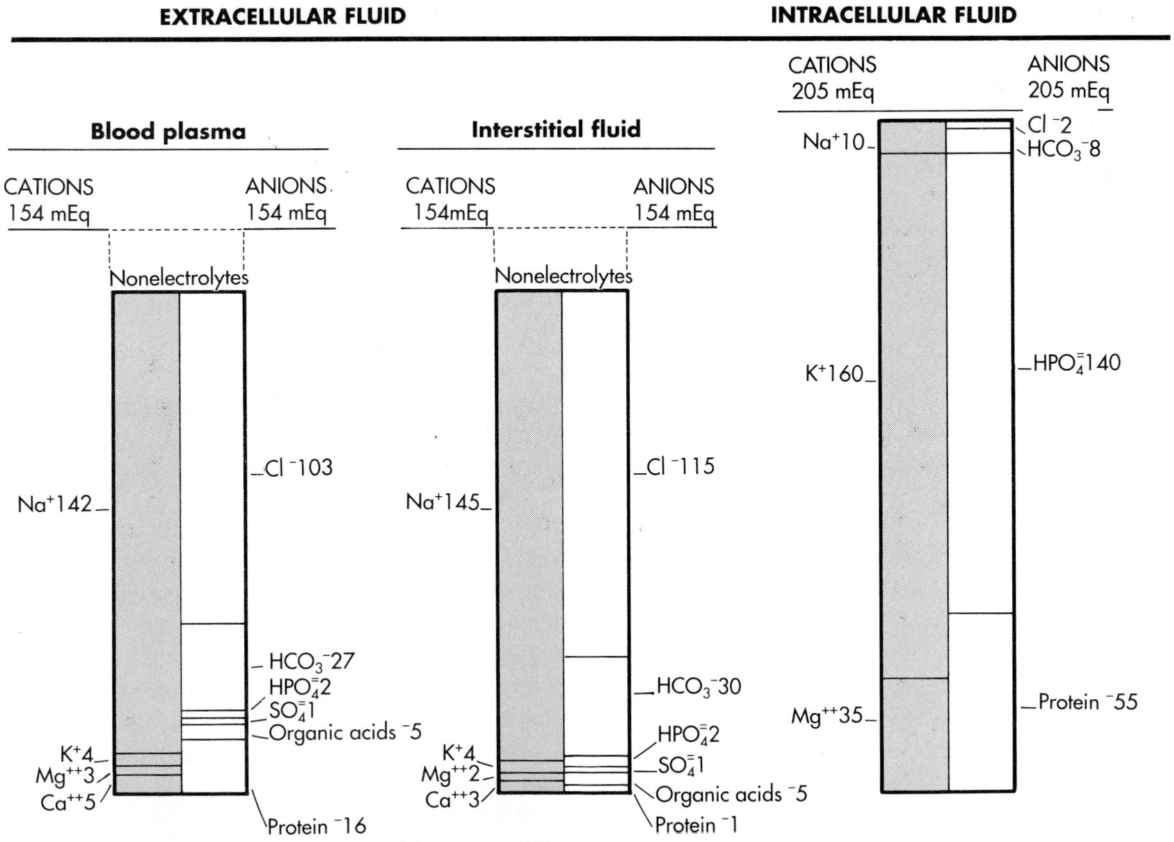

EXTRACELLULAR FLUID

INTRACELLULAR FLUID

CATIONS
205 mEq

ANIONS
205 mEq

Cl⁻2
HCO₃⁻8

Na⁺10

K⁺160

HPO₄⁼140

Mg⁺⁺35

Protein⁻55

Blood plasma

CATIONS
154 mEq

ANIONS
154 mEq

Nonelectrolytes

Na⁺142

Cl⁻103

HCO₃⁻27
HPO₄⁼2
SO₄⁼1
Organic acids⁻5

K⁺4
Mg⁺⁺3
Ca⁺⁺5

Protein⁻16

Interstitial fluid

CATIONS
154 mEq

ANIONS
154 mEq

Nonelectrolytes

Na⁺145

Cl⁻115

HCO₃⁻30

HPO₄⁼2
SO₄⁼1
Organic acids⁻5

K⁺4
Mg⁺⁺2
Ca⁺⁺3

Protein⁻1

FIG. 20-2   Electrolyte content of fluid compartments. (Modified from *Fluids and electrolytes*, 1970, Abbott Laboratories, Abbott Park, Ill, pp 10-11.

UNITS OF MEASURE FOR BODY FLUIDS AND THEIR CONVERSIONS

mg/dl = mg of solute/100 ml solvent
Example:
Serum Ca^{++} = 10 mg/dl

mmol = molecular (or atomic) weight in mg
Examples:
1 mmol Ca^{++} = 40 mg
1 mmol Cl^- = 35.5 mg
1 mmol Na^+ = 23 mg
1 mmol NaCl = 58.5 mg (23 + 35.5 = 58.5)

$$mEq = \frac{mol\ (or\ atomic)\ weight\ in\ mg}{valence}$$

Valence: Na^+ = 1; Ca^{++} = 2
Examples:
Na^+ = 23 mg/l; 23 mg Na^+ = 1 mEq
Ca^{++} = 40 mg/2; 20 mg CA^{++} = 1 mEg
1 mmol Ca^{++} = 2 mEq (2 × 20 mg)

$$mOsm = \frac{mol\ (or\ atomic)\ weight\ in\ mg}{n\ (particles\ exerting\ osmotic\ pressure)}$$

Na^+ = 1 particle in solution
NaCl = 2 particles in solution (Na^+ and Cl^-)
Examples:
mOsm Na^+ = 23 mg/1; 23 mg Na^+ = 1 mOsm
mOsm NaCl = 58.5 mg/2; 29.3 mg NaCl = 1 mOsm
1 mmol NaCl = 2 mOsm

$$mmol/L = \frac{mg/dl \times 10}{mol\ weight}$$

$$mEq/L = \frac{mg/dl \times 10 \times valence}{mol\ weight}$$

Example:

$$Ca^{++}\ in\ mEq/L = \frac{10\ mg/dl \times 10 \times 2}{40\ mg} = 5\ mEq/L$$

mEq/L = mmol/L × valence

$$mOsm/kg = mmol/L \times n = \frac{mg/dl \times 10}{mol\ weight} = \frac{mEq/L \times n}{valence}$$

Examples:
For monovalent ions:
1 mmol Na^+ = 1 mEq = 1 mOsm (1 valence; 1 particle)
1 mmol NaCl = 2 mEq = 2 mOsm (2 valences; 2 particles)
For multivalent ions:
1 mmol $MgSO_4$ = 4 mEq = 2 mOsm (4 valences; 2 particles)
1 mmol Na_2SO_4 = 4 mEq = 3 mOsm (4 valences; 3 particles)

▶ **TABLE 20-2   Plasma and Intracellular Electrolytes**

	Plasma	Intracellular
CATIONS		
Sodium (Na^+)	142 mEq	10 mEq
Potassium (K^+)	4 mEq	160 mEq
Calcium (Ca^{++})	5 mEq	
Magnesium (Mg^{++})	3 mEq	35 mEq
	154 mEq/L	205 mEq/L
ANIONS		
Chloride (Cl^-)	103 mEq	2 mEq
Bicarbonate (HCO_3^-)	27 mEq	8 mEq
Phosphate ($HPO_4^=$)	2 mEq	140 mEq
Sulfate ($SO_4^=$)	1 mEq	
Organic acids	5 mEq	
Proteins	16 mEq	55 mEq
	154 mEq/L	205 mEq/L

limole for millimole. The equivalent weight differs from the gram molecular weight because it considers the valence (combining power) of the electrolyte. Sometimes the clinical laboratory reports are in milligrams per deciliter or 100 ml (mg/dl or mg%). This value may be converted to mEq/L using the conversion formula in the box on the left. A final advantage of expressing ion concentrations in mEq/L is that the total number of cations in mEq/L is always equal to the number of anions in mEq/L, thus preserving electroneutrality (Table 20-2).

A *milliosmole* equals $^1/_{1000}$ of an osmole and is a measure of the number of discrete particles in a solution independent of their valence, electrical charge, or mass. The osmolality of body fluid has a great deal to do with water movement and balance as will be discussed later.

MOVEMENT OF BODY FLUIDS AND ELECTROLYTES

Body fluids and their dissolved substances are in a constant state of mobility. There is a continual intake and output of fluids within the body as a whole, and between the various compartments as the fluids transport nutrients and oxygen to the cells and remove wastes and manufactured substances from the cells. First, oxygen, nutrients, fluids, and electrolytes are picked up by the lungs and gastrointestinal tract, where they become part of the IVF and are transported to various parts of the body via the circulatory system. Second, IVF and its dissolved substances are rapidly exchanged with the ISF through the semipermeable capillary membrane. Third, ISF and its constituents are exchanged with the ICF through the selectively permeable cell membrane. Even though the situation as a whole is one of incessant replacement and exchange, the composition and volume of the fluid are relatively stable, a state called *dynamic equilibrium* or *homeostasis*. The movement of water and solutes between body compartments involves active and passive transport mechanisms. An *active transport* mechanism involves the expenditure of energy, but a *passive transport* mechanism does not. Diffusion and osmosis are passive transport mechanisms.

Movement of Solutes Between Body Fluid Compartments

The primary barrier to the movement of solutes in the body is the cell membrane. The lipid and protein molecules that make up these membranes are arranged so that only certain substances can pass through them. Pores in these membranes allow the passage of water and small water-soluble substances such as ions and glucose, but larger protein molecules do not readily pass. Substances that are lipid-soluble, such as urea, oxygen, and carbon dioxide, can pass directly through the membrane.

Most solutes move by passive transport mechanisms. *Simple diffusion* is the random movement of particles in all directions through a solution or gas. Several factors affect how readily a solute diffuses across capillary and cell membranes, including membrane permeability, concentration, electrical potential, and pressure gradients. *Permeability* refers to the size of the diffusing particles relative to the size of the membrane pores. Small particles, such as water and ions, diffuse through the membrane pores most easily. Large particles, such as glucose and amino acids, must pass through the membrane by a process called facilitated diffusion. In *facilitated diffusion,* a membrane-bound carrier protein combines with the transported molecule, acting as a shuttle in the process. In diffusion, solutes move from an area of higher concentration to one of lower concentration until the concentration is equal on both sides of the membrane. In addition to concentration gradients, the diffusion of charged particles (electrolytes) is affected by the *electrical gradient* or *potential* across the cell membrane. Positively charged particles tend to move to the negative side of the cell membrane (usually the inside of the cell), whereas negatively charged particles tend to move to the positive side (usually the outside of the cell) because like charges repel and opposite charges attract. Concentration and electrical gradients together compose the *electrochemical potential*, which is the force that drives the (passive) movements of electrolytes. The electric potential component, although quite small, is important in excitable tissues. Finally, a *hydrostatic pressure* gradient increases the rate of diffusion of solutes through the capillary membrane (see the discussion of movement of water between the plasma and interstitial fluid).

The movement of solutes across a cell membrane against a concentration and/or electrical gradient is called active transport. *Active transport* differs from passive transport in that it requires the expenditure of energy in the form of adenosine triphosphate (ATP). One of the most widely distributed active transport systems is the *NaK-activated–ATPase system* (also called the *sodium-potassium pump*) located in cell membranes. This single enzyme molecule pumps three Na^+ ions out of the cell in exchange for two K^+, at the expense of one ATP molecule. The NaK-ATPase system plays an important role in maintaining the proper concentrations of Na^+ and K^+ inside and outside the cell, thus maintaining the membrane electropotential. Recall that ECF Na^+ concentration is high (142 mEq/L), whereas ICF Na^+ concentration is low (10 mEq/L), and the reverse is true for K^+ (4 mEq/L in the ECF and 155 mEq/L in the ICF). In addition, the resting cell membrane is selectively permeable to K^+ and quite impermeable to Na^+. The membrane potential is created because K^+ diffuses out of the cell, leaving behind most of the negative ions (primarily proteins and phosphate) that are too large to follow. Na^+ also diffuses into the cell down its concentration gradient but at a much slower rate than K^+ exit. The net diffusion of Na^+ and K^+ is balanced by the active transport of these ions in the opposite direction across the cell membrane. Potassium balance is important clinically because of the life-threatening dysrhythmias that develop when there is either an excess or deficit of this ion.

Movement of Water Between Body Fluid Compartments

Unlike electrolytes and other solutes, water freely crosses all body membranes. The movement of water between the various fluid compartments is controlled by two forces: osmotic and hydrostatic pressures.

Osmotic and hydrostatic pressures

Osmotic pressure refers to the drawing force for water exerted by solute particles. The concept of osmotic pressure is most easily grasped by an illustration. Fig. 20-3 shows a **U**-tube, with each arm separated by a semipermeable membrane. A certain volume of a NaCl solution is placed in one arm (side *B*), with an equal volume of pure water in the other arm (side *A*). Water diffuses freely through the membrane, but both Na^+ and Cl^- ions are nondiffusible. Net water movement is from side *A* (pure water) to side *B* (salt solution) with the final result that the total volume is greater in side *B*. The hydrostatic pressure (compression force of a liquid) that would have to be applied over the solution in side *B* to prevent the net diffusion of water to that side is equal to the osmotic pressure of that solution. *Osmosis* is the process of the net diffusion of water caused by a concentration gradient. Net diffusion of water occurs from an area of low solute concentration (dilute solution) to one of high solute concentration (concentrated solution). To put it another way, water diffuses from an area of higher water activity to one

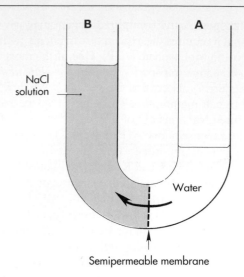

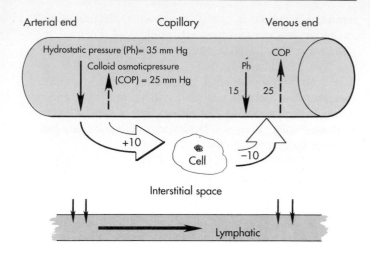

FIG. 20-3 Osmosis. The effect of adding an *impermeable solute* on one side of a semipermeable membrane. Water moves freely from the high solvent on side *A* to the low solvent on side *B*, causing the levels of the fluid columns to become farther apart. A hydrostatic pressure is created on side *B* (measured by the height of this column), which will be equal to the osmotic pressure of this solution at equilibrium. The amount of pressure required to stop osmosis completely is called the *osmotic pressure* of the solution.

FIG. 20-4 Starling's law of the capillaries. Fluid outflow is favored at the arterial end and fluid resorption at the venous end of the capillary.

of lower water activity. The osmotic pressure of body fluids may be measured by freezing point depression (see Chapter 45) and expressed as either osmolality or osmolarity. The terms osmolality and osmolarity are almost but not quite synonymous. *Osmolality* refers to the number of osmols (the standard unit of osmotic pressure) per kilogram of *solvent* (water) (mOsm/kg). *Osmolarity* refers to the number of osmols per liter of *solution* (mOsm/L). In the first case (osmolality), the total volume will be 1 L of water plus the small volume taken up by the solutes; in the second case (osmolarity), the volume of water will be less than 1 L by an amount equal to the volume of the solute. Osmolality is therefore more exact. However, the terms osmolality and osmolarity are used interchangeably in clinical practice because the difference is negligible with dilute body fluids.

The osmotic concentration of a solution depends only on the *number of particles* without regard to their size, charge, or mass. The solute particles may be crystalloids (substances that form a true solution, such as sodium salts) or colloids (substances that do not readily dissolve into true solutions, such as large protein molecules). For a particle to serve as an *effective osmole,* it must be largely confined to one particular compartment. Na^+ (and its anions) contributes most to the osmolality of the ECF, because it is the most numerous particle in the ECF and the cell membrane is relatively impermeable to it. K^+ plays this role in the ICF. Although urea and glucose are solutes in the plasma, they freely diffuse across cell mem-

branes and are not important contributors to the plasma osmolality, except under abnormal circumstances.

Movement of Water Between the Plasma and Interstitial Fluid

Sodium does not play an important role in the movement of water between the plasma and interstitial fluid compartments because the concentration of sodium is nearly the same in both compartments. The distribution of water between these two compartments is determined by the hydrostatic pressure of the capillary blood, produced mainly by the pumping action of the heart, and the counterbalancing *colloid osmotic pressure* (COP) or *oncotic pressure,* produced primarily by serum albumin. Colloids, such as albumin and other high-molecular-weight serum proteins, act as effective osmoles because they are confined to the intravascular space and do not readily cross the capillary membrane. The process of fluid movement from the capillary to the interstitial space is called *ultrafiltration* because water, electrolytes, and other solutes (except plasma proteins and blood cells) readily cross the capillary membrane. Another example of ultrafiltration in the body is the renal corpuscle (glomerulus).

Fig. 20-4 illustrates Starling's law of the capillaries, which states that the rate and direction of fluid exchange between the capillaries and ISF are determined by the hydrostatic and colloid osmotic pressures of the two fluids. At the arterial end of the capillary, the hydrostatic pressure of the blood (pushing fluid out) exceeds the colloid osmotic pressure (holding the fluid in) so that net movement is from the intravascular to the interstitial compartments. At the venous end of the capillary, fluid moves from the interstitial space to the intravascular space because colloid osmotic pressure exceeds the hydrostatic pressure. This process delivers oxygen and nutrients to the cells and removes carbon dioxide and waste products. The interstitial compartment also has hydrostatic and colloid osmotic pressures, but they are generally quite small and so are ignored in this illustration. In cases of inflammation or injury causing plasma proteins to leak into the interstitial space, however, the tissue colloid osmotic pressure increases considerably. The lymphatic system normally returns excess interstitial fluid and protein to the general circulation. In cases of lymphatic blockage or removal (e.g., surgical removal of axillary lymph nodes for treatment of breast cancer), excess ISF may accumulate.

The accumulation of excess fluid in the interstitial spaces is called *edema*. A review of the capillary dynamics just discussed indicates that the following four factors favor edema formation:

1. Increased capillary hydrostatic pressure (as in congestive heart failure with sodium and water retention or venous obstruction)
2. Decreased plasma oncotic pressure (as in nephrotic syndrome or liver cirrhosis, which results in decreased albumin concentration in the plasma)
3. Increased capillary permeability resulting in an increase in interstitial fluid colloid osmotic pressure (as in inflammation or injury)
4. Lymphatic obstruction or increased interstitial oncotic pressure

Movement of Water Between the ECF and the ICF

Movement of water between the ECF and the ICF is determined by osmotic forces. Recall that osmosis is the net transfer of water across a semipermeable membrane to the side with the larger concentration of nondiffusible particles. Sodium chloride in the ECF and potassium and organic solutes in the ICF are the major effective nonpenetrating solutes that determine the water concentration on the two sides of the membrane. (Some Na^+ ions do leak into the cell, and some K^+ ions leak out of the cell, but the Na-K pump transfers them to their proper compartments so that they have the effect of nonpenetrating particles.) Because sodium composes over 90% of the particles in the ECF, it has a major effect on total body water and its distribution, thus the axiom, "water goes where the salt is." Water moves easily and rapidly across most cell membranes until osmotic equilibrium between the two compartments is attained.

The principle of osmosis can be applied in the administration of IV solutions, which are designated as isotonic, hypotonic, or hypertonic, depending on whether their particle concentrations are respectively the same as, less than, or more than the body cell fluids. Basically, an isotonic solution is physiologically isoosmotic with the plasma and cell fluids. The plasma osmolality is normally about 287 mOsm/kg.

When red blood cells (RBCs) are placed in an isotonic

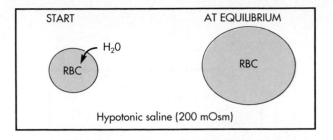

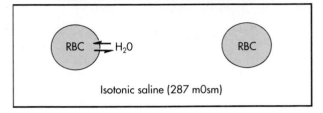

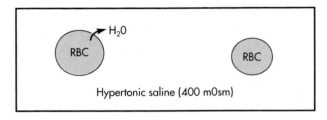

FIG. 20-5   Change of the volume of red blood cells as a result of placing them in hypotonic, isotonic, and hypertonic solutions of sodium chloride (NaCl).

saline (0.9%) solution, they undergo no change in volume (Fig. 20-5). The osmolal concentration of the saline solution is exactly equal to that of the cell contents (isoosmotic) so that net water diffusion in and out of the cell is zero. Placing RBCs in a hypotonic solution, such as 0.45% saline, would cause cell swelling. The solution is hypoosmotic to the RBC so that net diffusion of water is from the solution into the cell. Conversely, placing RBCs in a hypertonic solution, such as 3% saline, would cause the cells to shrink because the solution is hyperosmotic to the cells. Net diffusion of water is from the RBC to the hypertonic solution. These principles dictate that the safe administration of an IV solution requires that it be nearly isoosmotic with body fluids. For example, IV administration of distilled water (osmolality = 0) would cause RBC swelling and hemolysis. To provide free water to the cells, 5% glucose in water (D_5W) may be given. D_5W is isotonic with body fluids when first infused. As glucose enters cells and is metabolized, the glucose molecule is removed from the ECF. Ultimately it contributes only carbon dioxide and water as final metabolites. Thus D_5W, isotonic with body fluids at the time of infusion, becomes hypotonic as carbon dioxide is removed and water retained. A final point must be made about the terms isotonic and isoosmotic when applied to IV solutions. Even though an isotonic IV solution is isoosmotic, the converse may not be true (Rose, 1994). For example, an

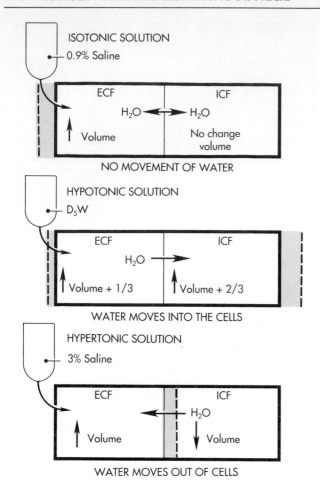

ISOTONIC SOLUTION
0.9% Saline

ECF | ICF
$H_2O \longleftrightarrow H_2O$
↑ Volume | No change volume

NO MOVEMENT OF WATER

HYPOTONIC SOLUTION
D_5W

ECF | ICF
$H_2O \longrightarrow$
↑ Volume + 1/3 | ↑ Volume + 2/3

WATER MOVES INTO THE CELLS

HYPERTONIC SOLUTION
3% Saline

ECF | ICF
$\longleftarrow H_2O$
↑ Volume | ↓ Volume

WATER MOVES OUT OF CELLS

FIG. 20-6   The effect of the intravenous administration of isotonic, hypotonic, and hypertonic solutions on the distribution of water between the body fluid compartments.

TYPICAL DAILY FLUID GAINS AND LOSSES IN HEALTHY ADULTS

INTAKE		OUTPUT	
Ingested liquids	1200 ml	Kidneys (urine)	1500 ml
Solid foods (water)	1000 ml	Intestines (in feces)	200 ml
Food oxidation (water)	300 ml	Lungs (in expired air)	400 ml
Total intake =	2500 ml	Skin (sweat, diffusion)	400 ml
		Total output =	2500 ml

creases. Hypotonic IV solutions are commonly used to provide for maintaining fluid needs and for replacing fluid losses. Finally, if a hypertonic solution of 3% saline is given intravenously, the volume of the ECF compartment increases but the volume of the ICF compartment decreases. NaCl remains in the ECF compartment, increasing osmolality. Water leaves the cells by osmosis until the osmolal concentrations of the ECF and ICF are equal. Thus one indication for administering hypertonic saline is for the treatment of cerebral edema.

Exchange of Water with the External Environment

Total body water (and electrolyte) balance is determined by a balance between intake and output. The normal daily water requirement for healthy adults or infants is about 1500 ml/m² of body surface area. Water and electrolytes enter the body via the digestive tract, both in liquids and in food. Water is also formed from the oxidation of food. The oxidation of each 100 calories of food provides approximately 14 ml water. Thus a diet of 2100 calories/day would produce about 300 ml of water.

Water is normally lost from the body to the external environment by four routes: kidneys (urine), intestines (feces), lungs (water vapor in the expired air), and skin (through evaporation and sweat). The loss of water through vaporization in the airways and from nonsweating skin is known as *insensible water loss*. This type of water loss should not be confused with the loss of water from sweat, which is low in the basal state but can increase markedly during exercise or exposure to a hot environment. Loss of heat by vaporization of sweat helps to regulate body temperature.

According to the cardinal principle of fluid balance, fluid intake equals fluid output. The normal daily fluid requirements for an adult are about 2500 ml (see box above), although this figure can vary considerably and

isoosmotic solution of urea would cause hemolysis of RBCs if given intravenously. Both urea (a penetrating molecule) and water equilibrate across the cell membrane (in contrast to saline and glucose, which do not).

The same principles identified in the experiment with RBCs apply to water distribution between the ECF and ICF compartments. If ECF osmolality increases (becomes hyperosmotic), water shifts from the ICF to the ECF, decreasing cell volume. If the ECF osmolality decreases (becomes hypoosmotic), water shifts from the ECF to the ICF, increasing cell volume.

IV administration of isotonic saline results in no change in the ICF volume or osmolality, and the entire volume remains in the ECF (Fig. 20-6). Consequently, isotonic IV fluids may be the first choice for the treatment of hypovolemic shock for the purpose of ECF volume expansion and restoration of perfusion. IV administration of D_5W (isotonic in the bottle but hypotonic when metabolized) provides free water. The volume of the ECF increases by one third of the volume of D_5W infused; the volume of the ICF increases by two thirds of the infused volume; and the osmolality of both ECF and ICF de-still be considered normal. The minimum water intake is the amount required to replace loss from all body sources, and the maximum intake is the amount that can be excreted by the kidneys. Insensible water loss from the lungs and skin and in the feces (about 1 L) is obligatory. *Obligatory losses* are those fluid losses essential for the excretion of body wastes. There is also an obligatory volume of urine output, which is directly related to solute excretion (mostly urea, Na^+, and K^+). The formula for determining minimum urine output is:

$$\frac{\text{Minimum urine output}}{\text{(L/day)}} = \frac{\text{Osmolar load (mOsm/day)}}{\text{Renal concentrating ability (mOsm/L)}}$$

If 600 mOsm of solute is excreted per day and the maximum renal concentrating ability is 1200 mOsm/L, the minimum obligatory urine output per day is 0.5 L. Fluid intake (from all sources) must equal the total obligatory fluid losses to maintain fluid balance.

PHYSIOLOGIC REGULATION OF FLUIDS AND ELECTROLYTES

A number of homeostatic mechanisms operate to maintain not only the electrolyte and osmotic concentration of body fluids, but also total body fluid volume. Normal body fluid and electrolyte balances are the consequences of dynamic equilibrium among oral fluids and dietary intake and equilibria involving a large number of organ systems. The kidneys, cardiovascular system, pituitary gland, parathyroid glands, adrenal glands, and the lungs are particularly involved.

The kidney mediates the majority of control over fluid and electrolyte levels. TBW and electrolyte concentration are primarily determined by "what the kidney keeps." The kidney, in turn, responds to a number of hormones in its regulatory function.

Sodium and Water

Body water and salt (NaCl) balances are closely related, affecting both the osmolality and volume of the ECF. However, the regulation of sodium and water balances involves different but overlapping mechanisms. Body water balance is primarily regulated by the thirst and antidiuretic hormone (ADH) mechanisms for the purpose of maintaining isoosmotic plasma (near 287 mOsm/kg). Sodium balance, on the other hand, is primarily regulated by aldosterone for the purpose of maintaining the ECF volume and tissue perfusion.

Water balance and osmotic regulation

Osmotic regulation is mediated via the hypothalamus, pituitary, and renal tubules. ADH is a peptide hormone synthesized in the hypothalamus and stored in the pituitary. The hypothalamus also contains osmoreceptors sensitive to the osmolality of the blood, and the thirst center. Fig. 44-18 shows that an increase in plasma osmolality stimulates both thirst and ADH release. Thirst stimulates ingestion of water, and ADH alters the permeability of the renal collecting ducts, increasing water reabsorption. The result is an increase in the volume of body water, which restores plasma osmolality to normal and a smaller volume of hyperosmotic (concentrated) urine. A decrease in plasma osmolality results in the opposite response with suppression of thirst and ADH release. The ADH mechanism is so sensitive that the plasma osmolality does not normally vary more than 1% to 2% from the normal 287 mOsm/kg. A relatively large decline in ECF volume (5% to 10%) is required to stimulate thirst or the release of ADH (Rose, 1994). Thus the ADH mechanism is largely concerned with osmoregulation through controlling water balance and is much less sensitive to volume regulation. Because sodium salts (mainly NaCl) compose 90% of the effective osmoles, hypoosmolality is synonymous with hyponatremia and hyperosmolality is synonymous with hypernatremia. The plasma osmolality may be estimated by multiplying the measured serum sodium by two. Hypernatremia and hyponatremia indicate intracellular water depletion and excess, respectively, because the ICF and ECF are in osmotic equilibrium.

Sodium balance and volume regulation

Maintaining plasma volume, which is essential for tissue perfusion, is closely related to the regulation of sodium balance. The mechanisms that regulate volume balance respond primarily to changes in the effective circulating volume. *Effective circulating volume* is that part of the ECF volume in the vascular space that effectively perfuses the tissues. In healthy persons the ECF volume generally varies directly with the effective circulating volume and is proportional to the total body sodium stores because sodium is the principal solute that holds water within the ECF. Thus renal mechanisms controlling sodium excretion are primarily responsible for volume regulation in the body.

The renin-angiotensin-aldosterone system is a mechanism of primary importance in the regulation of the ECF volume and renal sodium excretion. Aldosterone is a hormone secreted by the zona glomerulosa of the adrenal cortex. The major stimulus for aldosterone production is a reflex initiated by baroreceptors located in the afferent arteriole of the kidney. A decrease in the effective circulating volume is detected by the baroreceptors, which in turn cause the renal juxtaglomerular cells to secrete a protein, *renin*. Renin acts as an enzyme that splits off angiotensin I from the plasma protein angiotensinogen. Angiotensin I is then converted into angiotensin II in the lungs. Angiotensin II stimulates the adrenal cortex to secrete aldosterone. Aldosterone acts on the renal collecting ducts, causing sodium (and water) retention. In addition, angiotensin II causes vasoconstriction of arteriolar smooth muscles. Both mechanisms help to restore the effective circulating volume. A fall in plasma sodium concentration (Na$^+$) of only 4 to 5 mEq/L is another stimulus for aldosterone release, but it does not play an important role in normal subjects because Na$^+$ is held relatively constant by the effects of ADH (Rose, 1994). In fact, even when hyponatremia is present, its effect on aldosterone is often overridden by concomitant changes in the ECF volume. Thus aldosterone secretion is increased in the hyponatremic patient who is volume-depleted but may be reduced in a patient who is volume-expanded because of the retention of water.

Osmoregulation versus volume regulation

The mechanisms regulating plasma osmolality and plasma volume are different. The plasma osmolality (P_{OSM}) is determined by the ratio of solutes to water, whereas the ECF volume is determined by the absolute amounts of sodium and water present.

Changes in P_{OSM} (primarily determined by the ratio of sodium salts to water or P[Na]) are sensed by osmoreceptors in the hypothalamus, which then affect water intake and water excretion by influencing thirst and the release of ADH. ADH causes water retention and increases urine osmolality by enhancing the permeability of the renal-collecting ducts. Thus osmoregulation is achieved by altering water balance, and sodium handling is not affected unless there are concomitant changes in volume.

Volume regulation, on the other hand, is for the purpose of maintaining tissue perfusion. Different sensors and effectors are involved because renal sodium excretion, but not osmolality, is primarily regulated. The only major overlap between these two mechanisms is the hypovolemic stimulus to ADH secretion.

Regulation of ECF Potassium

Aldosterone is a primary control mechanism for potassium secretion by the distal nephron of the kidney. An increase in secretion of aldosterone causes sodium (and water) reabsorption and potassium excretion. Conversely, a decrease in the secretion of aldosterone causes sodium and water excretion and potassium conservation. The primary stimulus for aldosterone secretion is a decrease in the effective circulating volume, a decrease in serum sodium, or an increase in the serum potassium. Hypervolemia, a decrease in serum potassium, or an increase in serum sodium causes a decrease in aldosterone. Potassium excretion is also influenced by acid-base status and flow rate in the distal tubule. In the presence of an alkalosis, K$^+$ excretion is increased and in acidosis it is decreased. Within the distal tubule, H$^+$ ions and K$^+$ ions compete for excretion in exchange for Na$^+$ reabsorption to maintain body electroneutrality. When a metabolic alkalosis exists with a deficit of H$^+$ ions, the tubule exchanges Na$^+$ for K$^+$ to conserve H$^+$ ions. Metabolic aci-

dosis results in an increase in H$^+$ excretion and a decrease in K$^+$ excretion. This mechanism explains why hypokalemia is often associated with alkalosis and hyperkalemia is associated with acidosis. High rates of urine flow in the distal tubule result in an increase in total K$^+$ excretion and a low flow rate in a reduced K$^+$ excretion.

Regulation of ECF Calcium and Phosphate

Normal serum concentrations of calcium and phosphate ions are maintained by three mechanisms: intestinal absorption, exchange between the ECF and bone, and renal excretion. The homeostasis of these ions is interrelated and under hormonal control. Parathyroid hormone (PTH) and 1,25-dihydroxycholecalciferol (active form of vitamin D$_3$) act on the intestine, bone, and kidney to maintain normal serum levels. PTH is secreted by the parathyroid glands, four (or sometimes more) structures resembling wheat grains located on the posterior poles of the thyroid gland. Vitamin D$_3$ is activated by the kidneys. Serum levels of calcium and phosphate are reciprocal, so as levels of one rise, the levels of the other decline. PTH release occurs in response to a decrease in the serum Ca^{++}. It then acts to increase serum Ca^{++} in the following three ways:

1. It stimulates bone reabsorption in the presence of permissive amounts of vitamin D$_3$, resulting in the release of calcium phosphate.
2. It promotes the activation of vitamin D$_3$ by the kidney, which in turn promotes calcium phosphate absorption through the intestinal mucosa.
3. It augments calcium reabsorption in the renal tubule and phosphate excretion in the urine; a rise in the serum Ca^{++} suppresses PTH secretion.

Calcitonin is a hormone produced by the parafollicular cells of the thyroid gland. Calcitonin is released in response to a large increase in serum Ca^{++}. It lowers serum Ca^{++} by inhibiting bone reabsorption. However, Ca^{++} fluctuations in the normal range do not influence the secretion of calcitonin, although they clearly affect PTH secretion.

Regulation of ECF Hydrogen Ion Concentration

The blood buffers, lungs, and kidneys play a major role in maintaining acid-base balance by regulating the hydrogen ion concentration ([H$^+$]) of the ECF. Blood buffers are able to accept or donate H$^+$, thus acting rapidly like sponges to prevent large fluctuations in acid-base balance. The lungs are also vital in maintaining homeostasis. The lungs regulate [H$^+$] by controlling the level of CO$_2$ in the ECF. Metabolic acidosis causes compensatory hyperventilation, resulting in CO$_2$ excretion by the lungs, thus reducing the acidity of the ECF; metabolic alkalosis causes compensatory hypoventilation, resulting in CO$_2$ retention and thus increased acidity of the ECF. Finally, the kidneys play a vital role in acid-base homeostasis by excreting excess H^+ and are able to compensate for respiratory acidosis and alkalosis by increasing or decreasing the reabsorption of bicarbonate.

In summary, it is evident from this brief discussion of the systems that regulate fluids and electrolytes that precise mechanisms exist in the body to maintain homeostasis. The kidneys, more than any other organ, play a critical role in these regulatory processes. Thus renal failure results in multiple fluid and electrolyte disorders (see Part Eight).

ASSESSMENT OF FLUID AND ELECTROLYTE STATUS

History: Clues to Likely Imbalances

The assessment and diagnosis of fluid and electrolyte disturbances require a thorough understanding of normal physiologic mechanisms and conditions likely to cause disturbances. Many illnesses, diseases, and therapeutic modalities may cause fluid and electrolyte disturbances. In addition, many fluid and electrolyte disturbances produce symptoms that are nonspecific or subtle. Therefore a high degree of suspicion is required to recognize them, particularly if the imbalance is mild or in the early stages.

Metheny (1991) has developed an excellent approach to the assessment of fluid and electrolyte status based on correlation and analysis of history, clinical assessment data, and laboratory tests. The box below lists six important questions to consider during history taking. The first question requires knowledge about the most likely fluid

SIX CRITICAL QUESTIONS TO ASK WHEN ASSESSING FLUID AND ELECTROLYTE STATUS

1. Is there a disease process or injury state present that could disrupt fluid and electrolyte balance?
2. Is the patient receiving any medication, parenteral fluid, or other treatment that could disrupt fluid and electrolyte balance? If so, how might this therapy upset fluid balance?
3. Is there an abnormal loss of body fluids and, if so, from what source? What type of imbalance is usually associated with the loss of these fluids?
4. Have any dietary restrictions (e.g., low-sodium diet) been imposed? If so, how might fluid balance be affected?
5. Has the patient taken adequate amounts of water and other nutrients orally or by some other route? If not, how long has the intake been inadequate?
6. How does the total intake of fluids compare with the total fluid output?

From Metheny NM: *Fluid and electrolyte balance: nursing considerations*, ed 2, Philadelphia, 1991, JB Lippincott.

and electrolyte disturbances associated with particular diseases so that the clinician may anticipate them. For example, respiratory acidosis would be an anticipated electrolyte disturbance in a patient with chronic bronchitis and emphysema because of CO_2 retention. In a patient with end-stage renal failure, one would anticipate fluid volume excess, metabolic acidosis, hyperkalemia, and calcium disturbances because of the inability of the kidneys to excrete acid metabolites, potassium, and fluids adequately. Calcium disturbance results from phosphate retention and secondary hyperparathyroidism.

Answers to the second question require knowledge about fluid and electrolyte imbalances likely to result from medications and other treatment. For example, one should expect the use of thiazide diuretics to result in hypokalemia and therefore should monitor for its presence and prevent its development.

Answering the third question requires knowledge of the composition of specific body fluids to anticipate the type of imbalance that is likely to occur with their excessive loss. The gastrointestinal (GI) tract is a common site of abnormal fluid loss. Normally, about 8 L of GI secretions is produced each day, most of which is reabsorbed (about 100 to 200 ml is excreted in the stool). Thus a fluid volume deficit may easily develop in cases of vomiting, gastric suction, diarrhea, or drainage from fistulas or an ostomy. The various GI secretions vary in electrolyte composition, so their loss produces different imbalances in addition to fluid volume deficit. Gastric secretions are very acidic (pH = 1 to 3) and contain considerable amounts of sodium and potassium chlorides. Thus vomiting and prolonged gastric suction are often associated with sodium and potassium deficit and metabolic alkalosis. On the other hand, bile and intestinal and pancreatic secretions are quite alkaline (pH = 8) and are high in sodium, potassium, and bicarbonate. Thus diarrhea, intestinal suction, fistulas, or T-tube drainage of bile after gallbladder surgery is often associated with fluid volume deficits, sodium and potassium deficits, and metabolic acidosis from the loss of bicarbonate. Finally, perspiration, a hypotonic fluid, may cause the loss of water in excess of sodium, resulting in hypernatremia. Losses from perspiration can increase dramatically during heavy exercise and hot environments (up to 1 L/hr). Similarly, water losses in febrile, hyperventilating patients may be higher. Answering all of the six questions should suggest potential fluid and electrolyte disturbances. A detailed list and discussion of the causes of the various imbalances are presented in Chapters 21 and 22.

Clinical Assessment

After a hypothesis is formed about a particular potential fluid and electrolyte imbalance, systematic clinical observations are critical to follow up cues suggested by the history and to arrive at a diagnosis. Systematic clinical observations are also critical for monitoring an actual problem and response to treatment. However, to be valuable these observations must be planned and based on an understanding of the physiology of fluid and electrolyte balance. Table 20-3 presents a brief and general guide for making clinical observations related to fluid and electrolyte disturbances. Signs and symptoms commonly associated with specific disorders are presented in Chapters 21 and 22.

Laboratory Values

Finally, because many fluid and electrolyte disturbances produce nonspecific signs and symptoms, they can be confirmed only through laboratory data. It must be emphasized, however, that laboratory values are rarely suf-

ficient by themselves to interpret fluid and electrolyte disturbances; they must always be correlated with history and clinical observations. It is also important to observe trends in measurements and compare them with the patient's baseline values rather than to ascribe undue importance to a single measurement. The intelligent use of laboratory values in identifying and managing requires a thorough knowledge of pathophysiology and the limitations of individual tests. Table 20-4 presents normal values for frequently used laboratory measurements used in the evaluation of fluid and electrolyte disturbances. Laboratory tests used to evaluate acid-base status are listed in Chapter 22.

TABLE 20-3   Fluid and Electrolyte Clinical Assessment Guide

Observation	Comments
Monitor weight daily	Rapid losses (or gains) indicate changes in total body water (TBW)
	1 kg = 2.2 lb = 1 L
	1 lb = 1 pint ≈ 500 ml
	Body weight unchanged when fluid sequestered in a "third space"
	Most accurate method assessing fluid balance
Loss (or gain)	
2%: mild fluid volume deficit or excess	(2.4 lb in a 120 lb person)
5%: moderate fluid volume deficit or excess	(6.0 lb in a 120 lb person)
8%: severe fluid volume deficit or excess	(9.6 lb in a 120 lb person)
Monitor intake and output (I/O)	Keep accurate records and include all sources of I/O; compare I/O pattern over several days
Observe eyes	
Dry conjunctiva	Fluid volume deficit
Decreased tearing	
Soft eyeballs	
Periorbital edema	Fluid volume excess
Observe lips and oral cavity	
Dry, cracked lips	Fluid volume deficit (or mouth breathing); tongue normally has one longitudinal furrow
Small, multifurrowed tongue	
Observe skin turgor	Pinch skin over sternal area; normally springs back immediately
Decreased skin turgor	Fluid volume deficit
Assess cardiovascular status	
Temperature	Elevated temperature (101°-103° F) increases fluid requirements by 500 ml/day
Tachycardia	Fluid volume deficit
Orthostatic BP drop	Lying/standing systolic BP drop >10 mm Hg sensitive index of fluid volume deficit
Narrow pulse pressure	
Hand veins	Normal filling time 3-5 sec in dependent position; emptying time 3-5 sec when elevated
	(prolonged filling time in fluid volume deficit; prolonged emptying time in fluid volume excess)
Jugular vein distention (JVD)	Built-in CVP manometer reflecting changes in fluid volume
	Normal: JVD 2 cm above sternal angle in 45-degree position
	Fluid volume deficit: flat neck veins in supine position
	Fluid volume excess: JVD may extend to jaw angle in 45-degree position
Central venous pressure (CVP)	Normally 4-11 cm water in vena cava or 0-4 cm water in right atrium
	Low CVP may indicate hypovolemia
	High CVP may indicate hypervolemia
Cardiac dysrhythmias	May indicate excess or deficits of K^+, Mg^{++}, Ca^{++}

▶ TABLE 20-3   Fluid and Electrolyte Clinical Assessment Guide—cont'd

Observation	Comments
Assess respiratory system	
Moist rales, rhonchi	Pulmonary edema; fluid volume excess
Increased respiratory rate	
Dyspnea	
Assess GI system	
Absent bowel sounds	Potassium deficit
Nausea, diarrhea	Potassium excess
Assess renal system	
Oliguria (< 30 ml/hr)	Renal failure; severe fluid volume deficit
	Normal urinary volume = 40-80 ml/hr
Observe extremities/sacrum for edema	Fluid volume excess
	Grade: 1+, barely perceptible, to 4+, pitting edema
Assess neurologic system	
Depressed CNS	Fluid volume deficit
	Acidosis
Increased intracranial pressure (ICP)	Hyponatremia
Seizures	Hypocalcemia, hypomagnesemia
Assess for neuromuscular irritability/hypoactivity	
Hyperactive reflexes	Hypocalcemia, hypomagnesemia, alkalosis
Carpopedal spasm	
Positive Chvostek's sign	
Hypoactive reflexes	Hypercalcemia, hypermagnesemia, hypokalemia, hyponatremia

▶ TABLE 20-4   Selected Laboratory Tests Used to Evaluate Fluid and Electrolyte Status

	Normal Value	Comments
BLOOD TESTS		
Serum potassium	3.5-5.0 mEq/L	Serum K^+ higher in acidosis (because of K^+ shift out of cells) and lower in alkalosis (because of K^+ shift into cells); get repeat measurement if laboratory error suspected; correlate with ECG observations
Serum sodium	135-145 mEq/L	Serum Na^+ usually reflects plasma osmolality because sodium salts provide 90% of ECF solute particles Hyponatremia indicates that body fluids are diluted by an excess of water relative to total solute; it is not equivalent to Na^+ depletion Hypernatremia always indicates that body fluids are hyperosmotic, that there is a deficit of water relative to total solute; rarely due to an absolute sodium excess.
Serum chloride	98-106 mEq/L	Hypochloremia commonly associated with metabolic alkalosis and hypokalemia Hyperchloremia may be associated with some types of metabolic acidosis
Serum calcium	9-10.5 mg/dl (4-5.5 mEq/L)	Interpret in relation to serum albumin and pH, which both affect the ionized (physiologically active) fraction of serum Ca^{++}. Normally about 50% of the total serum calcium is in the ionized form, while the rest is bound to protein, mostly albumin. Total serum calcium drops when the albumin level is decreased, but the ionized fraction does not. Thus symptoms of hypocalcemia rarely develop in the hypoalbuminemic (<4-5 g/dl) patient. Alkalosis can produce symptoms of hypocalcemia even when the total serum calcium is normal, since less calcium is in the ionized form with a high pH.

Continued.

TABLE 20-4   Selected Laboratory Tests Used to Evaluate Fluid and Electrolyte Status—cont'd

	Normal Value	Comments
BLOOD TESTS—cont'd		
Serum phosphate	2.5-4.5 mg/dl (1.8-2.6 mEq/L)	Rises during early stage of chronic renal failure, causing hyperparathyroidism and renal osteodystrophy; soft tissue precipitation of calcium phosphate salts occurs when $Ca \times PO_4$ cross-product exceeds 60 in mg/dl (see Part Eight)
Serum magnesium	1.5-2.5 mEq/L (1.8-3.0 mg/dl)	
Serum glucose	70-100 mg/dl	High values cause osmotic diuresis and fluid volume deficit
Hematocrit	Men: 44%-52% Women: 39%-47%	May be elevated in hypovolemia and depressed in hypervolemia
Blood urea nitrogen	10-20 mg/dl	Elevated in renal failure, conditions of increased catabolism, and with hypovoemia; depressed in hypervolemia
Serum creatinine	0.7-1.5 mg/dl	Elevated in renal failure
Serum osmolality $$P_{OSM} = 2 \times [Na] + \frac{Glucose}{18}$$ $$= 2 \times [Na]$$	280-295 mOsm/kg	Increased in water deficit (hypernatremia) and decreased in water excess (hyponatremia) Effective plasma osmolality may be estimated by either formula on the left or measured by laboratory tests
Serum proteins Total Albumin Globulin	6.0-8.0 g/dl 3.5-5.5 g/dl 2.0-3.5 g/dl	
URINE TESTS		
Urinary sodium	100-260 mEq/24 hr (>40 mEq/L in random specimen)	Varies with intake <10 mEq/24 hr in hyponatremia associated with edema or with volume depletion because of extrarenal causes >20 mEq/24 hr if hyponatremia is caused by syndrome of inappropriate antidiuretic hormone (SIADH), salt wasting renal disease, or adrenal insufficiency
Urinary potassium Na/K = 2:1	25-100 mEq/24 hr	Varies with intake Increased in hyperaldosteronism (Na/K ratio may be reversed) Decreased in adrenal insufficiency (Na/K ratio may be 10:1)
Urinary chloride	110-250 mEq/24 hr	<10 mEq/L in metabolic alkalosis caused by diuretics, vomiting, or gastric suction >20 mEq/L in metabolic alkalosis caused by hyperaldosteronism or severe K^+ depletion
Urine osmolality Rough equivalencies: *Sp. gravity Osmolality* 1.000 0 1.003 100 1.010 300 1.025 800 1.035 1200	50-1400 mOsm	Reflects renal concentrating/diluting ability Fixed near 287 mOsm (or 1.010 specific gravity) in renal failure Osmolality measurement more accurate than specific gravity
Urinary pH	4.5-8	

QUESTIONS

▼ *Answer the following on a separate piece of paper.*

1. Name the three main fluid compartments of the body.
2. List six critical questions to consider in assessing fluid and electrolyte status.
3. Name the three systems that play a large role in maintaining acid-base homeostasis.

▼ *Circle the letter preceding each item below that correctly answers the question or completes the statement. More than one answer may be correct.*

4. The percentage of body water in proportion to body weight is influenced by many factors. Which of the following is true?
   a. In proportion to body weight, the water content of the body decreases with age.
   b. The body of a fat person contains more water than that of a thin person.
   c. In proportion to body weight, an infant will have less water than an older adult.
   d. Gender has no bearing on the amount of water in proportion to body weight.
5. In disease conditions where extracellular fluid is lost, which is the first fluid compartment to be depleted?
   a. The interstitial fluid
   b. The intravascular fluid
   c. The intracellular fluid
   d. None of the above
6. The intracellular fluid volume of a 25-year-old woman weighing 120 lb (TBW = 50% of weight) would be about:
   a. 60 L
   b. 48 L
   c. 24 L
   d. 20 L
7. The 24-hour maintenance fluid requirements for an average-sized adult are about:
   a. 600 ml
   b. 1000 ml
   c. 1500 ml
   d. 2500 ml
8. Which of the following statements about intracellular fluid is true?
   a. It is approximately equal to 40% of the body weight.
   b. It has a lower osmotic concentration than the extracellular fluid.
   c. It has a higher concentration of organic ions than the extracellular fluid.
   d. It is approximately equal to 5% of body weight.

9. A milliequivalent is a unit of:
   a. weight
   b. chemical activity
   c. osmotic concentration
10. Serum electrolyte concentrations are preferably reported in terms of:
    a. mm Hg
    b. mg/dl
    c. mg%
    d. mmol/L
    e. mEq/L
11. The law of body electroneutrality states that:
    a. The absolute numbers of cations and anions in the body must be equal
    b. The sum of the positive and negative charges (measured in mEq) in any particular body compartment and in the body as a whole must be equal
    c. The intravascular protein molecules must be neutral and cannot carry a positive or negative charge
    d. Positively charged sodium ions must always be coupled with negatively charged chloride ions
12. The NaK-activated–ATPase system (Na-K pump) located in the cell membrane helps maintain the electrochemical gradient across the cell membrane by:
    a. Actively moving water out of cells
    b. Actively transporting sodium out of cells
    c. Osmotically moving potassium into cells
    d. Actively transporting potassium into cells
13. Which of the following statements about sodium is *not* true?
    a. It aids in maintaining total body water balance.
    b. It aids in maintaining plasma osmotic concentration.
    c. It is the chief ECF cation.
    d. Renal excretion of sodium is primarily regulated by ADH.
14. The plasma osmolality is primarily determined by:
    a. The plasma sodium concentration
    b. The total ECF sodium stores
    c. The plasma potassium concentration
    d. The total body water (TBW)
15. The pressure exerted by serum protein in holding fluid within the intravascular compartment is known as:
    a. Hydrostatic pressure
    b. Osmotic pressure

c. Ultrafiltration pressure
d. Colloid osmotic pressure
16. Two fluid compartments containing nondiffusible solutes are separated by a semipermeable membrane. The osmotic concentration of compartment A is 300 mOsm and that of compartment B is 800 mOsm. Net movement of water will be:
    a. From compartment A to compartment B
    b. From compartment B to compartment A
    c. Equal in both directions
    d. None of the above
17. What would be the minimum volume of obligatory urine output in a patient with renal insufficiency who must excrete 600 mOsm of solute if the maximum renal concentrating ability is 400 mOsm/L?
    a. 400 ml
    b. 600 ml
    c. 1500 ml
    d. 2000 ml
18. Aldosterone is important in controlling the volume of the ECF because it controls:
    a. Protein metabolism
    b. Sodium (and water) reabsorption
    c. Potassium reabsorption
    d. All of the above
19. Which of the following changes would stimulate the release of ADH?
    a. An increase in the plasma osmolality of 1% to 2%
    b. A decrease in the plasma volume by at least 5% to 10%
    c. Hyponatremia
    d. Hypernatremia
    e. The stress of surgery
20. The organs that play the largest role in maintaining fluid and electrolyte balance in the body as a whole are the:
    a. Adrenal glands
    b. Parathyroid glands
    c. Kidneys
    d. Lungs
21. The choice intravenous solution for the purpose of reducing cerebral edema would be:
    a. Hypertonic (3% saline)
    b. Isotonic (0.9% saline)
    c. Hypotonic (D_5W)
22. Extracellular fluid characteristically contains:
    a. 80 mEq of Cl^-/L
    b. 140 mEq of Na^+/L

Continued.

c. 4 mEq of K$^+$/L
d. 5 mEq of Ca^{++}/L

23. Which of the following signs/symptoms would indicate an ECF volume deficit?
    a. Rales and rhonchi heard over posterior lung fields
    b. Blood pressure 130/80 mm Hg, lying position; 104/76 mm Hg, sitting position
    c. Flat neck veins in the lying position
    d. Oliguria (small amount of concentrated urine)

24. A urine specific gravity measurement of 1.010 indicates that the estimated osmolality is about:
    a. 100 mOsm
    b. 300 mOsm
    c. 600 mOsm
    d. 1200 mOsm

▼ *Circle T if the statement is true and F if it is false. Correct any false statements.*

25. T   F   The movement of solutes across a cell membrane against a concentration or electrical gradient is called simple diffusion.

26. T   F   A subnormal level of the serum albumin in a patient with liver cirrhosis would favor edema formation.

27. T   F   The serum Ca^{++} level is primarily under the hormonal control of parathyroid hormone.

28. T   F   The osmolality (or specific gravity) is an indication of the kidney's ability to concentrate or dilute urine (conserve water when there is a deficit or excrete water when there is an excess).

29. T   F   Increased aldosterone production caused by stress may produce an increased loss of sodium in the urine.

30. T   F   Changes in blood pressure may indicate alterations in the effective circulating fluid volume.

31. T   F   Accurate daily weights are vital in evaluating TBW changes.

32. T   F   A loss of 4 lb of body weight after the administration of a diuretic means that about 4 L of fluid was lost from the body.

33. T   F   ECF excess or deficit can be diagnosed from the electrolyte report alone.

34. T   F   The milliequivalent and millimole measurements are equivalent measures for any given ion, so they can be used interchangeably.

35. T   F   Osmotic concentration is determined by the total number of particles confined to a body fluid compartment.

CHAPTER 21

Disorders of Fluid Volume, Osmolality, and Electrolytes

LORRAINE M. WILSON

Three general categories of changes describe abnormalities of body fluids: (1) volume, (2) osmolality, and (3) composition. Although these disturbances are interrelated, each is a separate entity.

Volume imbalances affect primarily the extracellular fluid (ECF) and involve relatively equal losses or gains of sodium and water leading to an ECF volume deficit or excess. For example, the acute loss of an isotonic ECF fluid, as occurs with diarrhea, is followed by a significant decrease in the ECF volume and little, if any, change in the intracellular fluid (ICF) volume. Fluid will not be transferred from the ICF to the ECF as long as the osmolality in the two compartments remains the same. ECF volume disturbances are generally identified by clinical signs and symptoms.

Osmotic imbalances affect primarily the ICF and involve relatively unequal losses or gains of sodium and water. If water alone is lost or added from the ECF, the concentration of the osmotically active particles will change. Sodium ions and the chloride and bicarbonate ions that electrically balance them together account for 90% of the osmotically active particles in the ECF, and changes in the sodium concentration generally reflect changes in the osmolality of body fluid compartments. If the concentration of sodium in the ECF is decreased, water moves from the ECF to the ICF (causing cell swelling) until osmolality is again equal in the two compartments. Conversely, if the concentration of sodium in the ECF should increase, water moves from the ICF to the ECF (causing cell shrinkage) until osmolality is again equal in the two compartments. Osmotic disturbances are generally associated with hyponatremia and hypernatremia, so serum sodium values are important in their identification.

The concentration of most other ions within the ECF compartment can be altered without significant changes in the total number of osmotically active particles, thus producing a *compositional change*. For example, a rise in the serum potassium concentration from the normal 4 to 8 mEq/L would have a significant effect on myocardial function, but it would not significantly change the osmolality of the ECF. If the kidneys are functioning normally, fluid and electrolyte disturbances are minimized, especially if the loss or addition of solute or water is gradual.

There may be a change in the distribution of body fluids, such as the internal loss of ECF into a nonfunctional space. Examples include the sequestration of isotonic fluid in a burn, ascites, or muscle trauma. The functional loss of ECF is sometimes referred to as *third spacing* (non-ECF, non-ICF). Essentially, changes in the distribution of fluids result in ECF volume deficits or excesses, so they will be considered as subcategories of ECF volume imbalances.

The following discussion focuses on single imbalances of fluids and electrolytes. It is important to realize, however, that in practice a combination of fluid and electrolyte imbalances is far more common than single disturbances.

VOLUME IMBALANCES

Extracellular Fluid (ECF) Volume Deficit

ECF volume deficit or *hypovolemia* is defined as the isotonic loss of body fluids, with relatively equal losses of sodium and water. Isotonic fluid volume deficits are often mistakenly referred to as *dehydration,* a term that should be used only to describe relatively pure water depletion leading to hypernatremia.

Pathogenesis

Fluid volume deficit is a common condition that occurs in a wide variety of clinical circumstances. It is almost al-

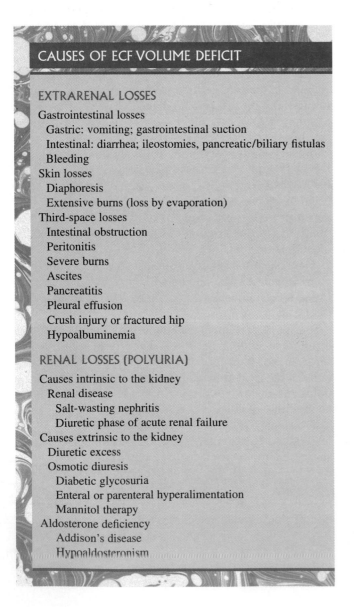

CAUSES OF ECF VOLUME DEFICIT

EXTRARENAL LOSSES

Gastrointestinal losses
 Gastric: vomiting; gastrointestinal suction
 Intestinal: diarrhea; ileostomies, pancreatic/biliary fistulas
 Bleeding
Skin losses
 Diaphoresis
 Extensive burns (loss by evaporation)
Third-space losses
 Intestinal obstruction
 Peritonitis
 Severe burns
 Ascites
 Pancreatitis
 Pleural effusion
 Crush injury or fractured hip
 Hypoalbuminemia

RENAL LOSSES (POLYURIA)

Causes intrinsic to the kidney
 Renal disease
  Salt-wasting nephritis
  Diuretic phase of acute renal failure
Causes extrinsic to the kidney
 Diuretic excess
 Osmotic diuresis
  Diabetic glycosuria
  Enteral or parenteral hyperalimentation
  Mannitol therapy
Aldosterone deficiency
 Addison's disease
 Hypoaldosteronism

ways related to the renal or extrarenal loss of body fluids. Fluid volume depletion occurs more rapidly if the abnormal loss of body fluids is coupled with decreased intake for any reason (see box to the left below).

The most common cause of isotonic fluid volume deficit is the loss of a significant fraction of the 8 L of gastrointestinal (GI) fluids secreted daily. Significant losses may occur through prolonged vomiting, nasogastric suction, massive diarrhea, fistulas, or bleeding. Because the sodium concentration of these fluids is high, their loss causes combined sodium and water deficits. Because gastric secretions also contain large amounts of potassium and hydrogen ion, volume depletion caused by such losses is often combined with metabolic alkalosis and hypokalemia. The loss of lower GI tract secretions, which contain large amounts of bicarbonate in addition to sodium and potassium, often results in fluid volume deficit combined with metabolic acidosis and hypokalemia.

Other common causes of fluid volume deficit include sequestration of fluid in soft tissue injuries, extensive burns, peritonitis, or within an obstructed GI tract. The accumulation of fluid within these non-ECF and non-ICF spaces is called *third spacing*. Third-space fluid loss refers to a distributional loss of fluids into a space that is not easily exchangeable with the ECF. It is essentially trapped fluid that is unavailable for use by the body. Rapid and extensive fluid volume accumulation in such spaces occurs at the expense of the ECF volume and may reduce the effective circulating blood volume. For example, 5 to 10 L of fluid can accumulate within an obstructed bowel; 4 to 6 L of fluid may accumulate in the peritoneal cavity in acute peritonitis; several liters may accumulate in the interstitial space during the first 48 to 72 hours after extensive burns (Rose, 1994).

Sweat is a hypotonic fluid consisting mainly of water, sodium (30 to 70 mEq/L), and chloride. During heavy exercise in hot environments, as much as 1 L of sweat per hour may be lost and contribute to fluid volume deficit if oral intake is inadequate. Large amounts of fluid may be lost in illnesses in which there is fever, diaphoresis, and inadequate fluid replacement. A temperature between 101° and 103° F increases 24-hour fluid requirements by about 500 ml, whereas temperatures above 103° F increase it by at least 1000 ml. Finally, large amounts of fluid may be lost from the skin by evaporation when burns are treated by the open method.

Abnormal losses of sodium and water in the urine may occur in several ways. During the recovery (diuretic) phase of acute renal failure or in certain chronic renal diseases primarily involving the tubules (salt-losing nephritis), large amounts of sodium and water may be lost in the urine. However, the usual problem in renal failure is sodium retention (see Part Eight).

Renal loss of sodium and water in the absence of renal disease occurs in three circumstances, the most common being excessive use of diuretics, especially the thiazides or potent loop diuretics such as furosemide. An obligatory osmotic diuresis is another common cause of sodium and water loss, which occurs during the marked glycosuria of uncontrolled diabetes mellitus (diabetic ketoacidosis [DKA] or hyperglycemic hyperosmolar nonketotic [HHNK] coma). In the case of high-protein enteral or parenteral alimentation, large amounts of urea are formed and may act as an osmotic agent. An iatrogenic cause of diuresis and fluid volume deficit is the use of mannitol for the treatment of cerebral edema or prerenal azotemia. Finally, excessive loss of sodium and water in the urine may occur in Addison's disease and hypoaldosteronism because of a deficiency of aldosterone.

Hemodynamic responses to fluid volume deficit

Regardless of the cause of the fluid volume deficit, contraction of the ECF volume (hypovolemia) impairs

---

ECF VOLUME DEFICIT: CLINICAL FEATURES

SIGNS/SYMPTOMS

Lassitude, weakness, and fatigue (early)
Anorexia
Thirst
Orthostatic hypotension (>10 mm Hg drop in systemic blood pressure)
Tachycardia
Dizziness, syncope
Altered level of consciousness
Decreased body temperature unless infection present
Cold extremities (late)
Prolonged filling time of hand veins (>3-5 seconds)
Flat jugular veins in supine position
Falling central venous pressure (CVP)
Sticky oral mucosa
Dry, furrowed tongue (normally, only one longitudinal furrow in midline)
Poor skin turgor
Oliguria (<30 ml/hr)
Rapid loss of body weight
   2% loss = mild deficit
   5% loss = moderate deficit
   8% loss = severe deficit

LABORATORY FINDINGS

Increased hematocrit
Increased serum protein level
Normal serum Na^+ (usually)
Blood urea nitrogen (BUN)/serum creatinine ratio >20:1 (normal = 10:1)
Urine specific gravity high
Urine osmolality >450 mOsm/kg
Urine Na^+ <10 mEq/L (extrarenal cause)
Urine Na^+ >20 mEq/L (renal or adrenal causes)

---

cardiac output by diminishing venous return to the heart. Clinical manifestations of volume contraction encompass the direct effects of a reduced cardiac output and the secondary effects of homeostatic mechanisms activated to compensate for the falling cardiac output. Because mean arterial pressure = cardiac output × total peripheral resistance (MAP = CO × TPR), it follows that the fall in cardiac output lowers blood pressure. The lowered blood pressure is sensed by the cardiac and carotid baroreceptors and communicated to the vasomotor centers in the brain stem, which then induce a sympathetic response. Sympathetic-induced changes include peripheral vasoconstriction, increased heart rate, and increased cardiac contractility, all of which help to restore cardiac output and perfusion of the coronary, cerebral, and pulmonary vascular beds. Diminished renal perfusion results from renal vasoconstriction, mediated in turn by activation of the sympathetic nervous system. Diminished renal perfusion activates the renin-angiotensin-aldosterone mechanism. Angiotensin II enhances systemic vasoconstriction, and aldosterone increases renal sodium (and water) reabsorption. These changes increase cardiac output by restoring the effective circulating volume and blood pressure toward normal. If the fluid volume deficit is small (500 ml), activation of the sympathetic response is generally adequate to restore cardiac output and blood pressure to near normal, although the heart rate may still be increased.

If the hypovolemia is more severe (1000 ml or more), there is increased sympathetic and angiotensin II–mediated vasoconstriction. Blood is shunted away from the renal, gastrointestinal, muscular, and cutaneous systems, with the relative preservation of coronary and cerebral blood flow. The intense vasoconstriction may be adequate to maintain systemic blood pressure in a recumbent position, but orthostatic hypotension and dizziness result when assuming a sitting or standing posture.

Clinical features

The cause of fluid volume deficit can usually be suspected from the history. However, no specific electrolyte test indicates the presence or development of a deficit. Clinical examination of the patient is the best guide to volume abnormalities.

The signs and symptoms of a fluid volume deficit depend on the rapidity and magnitude of its development. The key findings on physical assessment are interstitial and plasma volume depletion (see box to the left). In the case of a large and rapid loss of volume as in hemorrhage, massive diarrhea, or massive sequestration in a third space, the signs and symptoms are synonymous with circulatory collapse and shock. In most cases, however, the development of a fluid volume deficit occurs more gradually.

General symptoms of moderate-to-severe volume depletion include weakness, lassitude, fatigue, and anorexia. An early sign of plasma volume depletion is orthostatic hypotension, with a decrease in blood pressure of at least 10 mm Hg and an increase in heart rate with postural changes. Tachycardia develops as the heart attempts to maintain tissue perfusion. Arterial pulses are weak and thready. The patient may become dizzy on sitting or standing. The peripheral veins, such as the hand veins, may be collapsed and fill slowly when the hand is held in a dependent position. Other signs of a decrease in the venous volume include flat jugular veins and low central venous pressure, reflecting decreased venous return to the right side of the heart.

Decreased interstitial volume may be recognized by decreased tissue and tongue turgor. Dry mucous membranes, oliguria, and thirst are other signs of fluid volume depletion. The oliguria results from the actions of antidiuretic hormone and of aldosterone, both of which are secreted in response to volume contraction. Weight loss is another cardinal sign of fluid volume deficit, which may be used to estimate the magnitude of the loss, with the exception of third-space sequestration of fluid.

No single diagnostic test confirms fluid volume deficit. Serum laboratory values vary, depending on the underlying cause of the fluid volume deficit. A rise in the BUN, serum proteins, hemoglobin, or hematocrit may indicate hemoconcentration (unless the condition is caused by hemorrhage, which results in decreased hemoglobin and hematocrit since all blood products are lost). These elevations may be difficult to discern, however, unless baseline values are known. It must be emphasized that in isotonic fluid volume losses, the serum sodium concentration will be normal because equal proportions of sodium and water are lost. Deviations of the serum sodium concentration above or below normal levels indicate disproportionate losses or gains of sodium and water and a disturbance in osmolality. Volume imbalances, however, may be combined with osmolality disturbances (see the discussion of osmolality imbalances).

The response of the kidney to volume depletion is to conserve sodium and water. Consequently, a small volume of concentrated urine (high osmolality or high specific gravity) with a low sodium concentration is excreted when the kidneys are functioning normally. In fact, low urine sodium concentration is virtually pathognomonic of reduced tissue perfusion (Rose, 1994). However, a low urine sodium concentration does not necessarily mean that there is true fluid volume deficit, because it may occur in some edematous conditions such as congestive heart failure with a decrease in effective circulating volume. Differentiation between edema states and true volume depletion is easily made from physical assessment. The urinary sodium concentration is helpful in identifying the cause of true fluid volume deficit. With extrarenal losses, urinary sodium is less than 10 mEq/L; the concentration will usually exceed 20 mEq/L when renal or adrenal disorders are at fault.

A final characteristic of moderate to severe fluid volume deficit is a rise in the BUN and plasma creatinine, resulting from decreased renal perfusion and glomerular filtration rate (GFR). BUN tends to rise proportionately more than serum creatinine. This finding is termed *prerenal azotemia.* The disproportionate rise in the BUN reflects enhanced renal tubular reabsorption of urea, which accompanies tubular reabsorption of sodium and water. Azotemia in this setting must be regarded as a physiologic trade-off for homeostatic mechanisms otherwise geared to defend the ECF volume by enhancing sodium and water reabsorption. Prolonged renal hypoperfusion and prerenal azotemia may progress to acute renal failure, so they should be promptly corrected (see Chapter 49).

Treatment

The goal of treatment for an isotonic fluid volume deficit is to restore normovolemia and treat any associated acid-base or electrolyte imbalances. The underlying cause of the fluid volume deficit must also be treated. Bleeding must be controlled. Vomiting may be treated with antiemetics and diarrhea with antidiarrheal drugs.

When there is a mild volume deficit, increasing dietary sodium and water intake in patients not suffering from GI disorders may be sufficient to correct the imbalance. Severe depletion requires therapy with intravenous (IV) solutions. Isotonic saline (0.9%) is the infusion of choice in patients whose serum sodium concentration is approximately normal, because it will expand the plasma volume. As soon as the patient is normotensive, one-half normal saline (0.45%) may be ordered to provide free water to the cells and help eliminate metabolic waste products.

If the patient with severe fluid volume deficit is oliguric, it is necessary to determine if the depressed renal function is the result of reduced renal blood flow and secondary to the fluid volume deficit (prerenal azotemia) or, more seriously, secondary to acute tubular necrosis (a form of acute renal failure) from prolonged renal ischemia. In this situation, an initial bolus of IV fluid is given in a fluid challenge test to determine if urine flow will increase, which indicates normal renal function. In the case of prerenal azotemia and normal renal function, the fluid volume deficit is easier to treat, but the treatment becomes more complicated in the case of acute tubular necrosis (see Chapter 49).

The amount of IV solution to be unfused cannot be determined precisely. However, the history, intake and output record, and record of daily weights provide an estimate of the magnitude of losses. The upper box on p. 259 provides a general guide for the volume of fluid needed for maintenance and replacement based on body surface area and the severity of the deficit (Metheny, Snively, 1979).

The need to correct other concurrent electrolyte abnormalities may alter the composition of the required infusion. For example, potassium may be added to the IV solution when there is concurrent potassium depletion. Lactated Ringer's solution may be given to patients with metabolic acidosis and fluid volume depletion. This solution contains sodium lactate, which is slowly metabolized to sodium bicarbonate in the body, and can help correct the acidosis.

Because numerous factors affect the type and rate of IV infusion (e.g., cardiac and renal status) and the required volume cannot be precisely determined, the best approach is to monitor the patient's response to the IV therapy to avoid fluid overload and pulmonary edema. Metheny (1996) provides detailed guidelines on the care of patients undergoing IV therapy.

Extracellular Fluid (ECF) Volume Excess

Extracellular fluid volume excess develops when both sodium and water are retained in roughly the same proportions. As excessive isotonic fluid accumulates in the ECF (hypervolemia), fluid shifts into the interstitial fluid compartment, causing edema. Fluid volume excess is always secondary to an increase in total body sodium content, which, in turn, causes water retention.

Pathogenesis

Edema is defined as an excessive accumulation of interstitial fluid. Edema may be either localized (as occurs with local inflammation or obstruction) or generalized, so that interstitial fluid accumulates in virtually every tissue of the body. In either case, the proximate cause of the edema is always an alteration in one of the critical Starling forces that govern the distribution of fluid between the capillaries and interstitial spaces. Thus edema may result from increased capillary hydrostatic pressure, decreased colloid osmotic pressure, increased capillary permeability, or obstruction to lymphatic flow (see Chapter 20). This discussion focuses on disorders of fluid volume excess associated with generalized edema.

The presence of generalized edema indicates a disturbance in the normal regulation of the ECF. The three most common conditions resulting in generalized edema are congestive heart failure, cirrhosis of the liver, and the nephrotic syndrome (see lower box on right). Each one of these disorders is characterized by a defect in at least one of the Starling capillary forces and by renal retention of sodium and water. The retention of sodium by the kidney in edema-forming states results from one or two basic mechanisms: the response to effective circulating volume depletion or primary renal dysfunction.

Effective circulating volume is an unmeasurable entity that refers to the intravascular fluid effectively perfusing the tissues. It is generally directly proportional to the cardiac output. Thus, when cardiac output is decreased, the kidney retains sodium and water in an attempt to restore the circulating volume. A decrease in the effective circulating volume is believed to be the mechanism responsible for renal sodium retention in congestive heart failure, liver cirrhosis, and the nephrotic syndrome. In all of these conditions, renal excretory function is intrinsically nor-

---

GUIDELINES FOR IV FLUID REQUIREMENTS

General rules:
1. Provide for maintenance needs and make up for losses
2. Replace concurrent losses volume for volume
3. Administer evenly over 24 hours except in unusual circumstances

24-hour volume needed per square meter of body surface area (BSA):

1. Maintenance	1500 ml/m² BSA
2. Moderate fluid volume deficit + maintenance (acute weight loss <5%)	2400 ml/m² BSA
3. Severe fluid volume deficit + maintenance (acute weight loss >5%)	3000 ml/m² BSA

Body weight to BSA conversions for persons of average build:

Weight		Approximate BSA in m²
kg	lb	
3	6.6	0.20
6	13.2	0.30
10	22.0	0.45
20	44.0	0.80
40	88.0	1.30
50	110.0	1.50
57	125.4	1.60
70	154.0	1.76
85	187.0	2.00

Examples of calculations:
Maintenance needs for a 125-lb woman who is taking nothing by mouth and has no abnormal losses:
24-hour IV fluid needs = 1.60 × 1500 ml = 2400 ml
IV fluid needs for a 70-kg man who has been vomiting for 2 days and has a moderate fluid volume deficit:
24-hour IV fluid needs = 1.76 × 2400 ml = 4224

CAUSES OF ECF VOLUME EXCESS

Altered regulatory mechanisms
  Congestive heart failure
  Cirrhosis of the liver
  Nephrotic syndrome
Renal failure
Cushing's syndrome; corticosteroid therapy
Starvation (hypoalbuminemia)
Rapid infusion of IV saline

mal and enhanced renal reabsorption is presumably initiated by the sympathetic nervous system and the renin-angiotensin-aldosterone system. In other words, the kidneys act as if the ECF volume were truly contracted and retain sodium and water despite massive accumulation of fluid in the interstitial space.

In contrast with these mechanisms of edema, edema associated with advanced renal failure results from intrinsic impairment of renal excretory function. Another condition associated with ECF excess includes Cushing's syndrome or corticosteroid therapy because of increased aldosterone activity. Starvation resulting in hypoproteinemia is also associated with edema. Finally, the rapid administration of IV saline may result in hypervolemia.

Clinical features

The box below lists the signs and symptoms and laboratory values commonly associated with an ECF volume excess. In general, acute weight gain is the best indicator of an ECF volume excess because several liters of fluid can be retained without visible evidence of edema. The distribution of generalized edema is governed largely by gravitational forces that impinge on capillary hydrostatic pressure. Thus edema usually develops where capillary hydrostatic pressure is highest (dependent areas, such as the legs or sacral area in a bedridden patient) or where interstitial pressure is lowest (periorbital, facial, scrotal areas). If the finger is pressed over an area of edema, the indentation will remain briefly as the fluid is pushed to another area; this is called *pitting edema*. Fluid then fills the "pit" gradually. The degree of edema may be classified subjectively on a scale of 1+ to 4+ (barely discernible to pitting edema), based on how long it takes fluid to refill the pit.

Pulmonary edema, indicated by moist rales over the lung fields and other signs of respiratory distress, is one manifestation of ECF volume excess that warrants urgent therapy. It occurs most commonly in patients with left ventricular failure, a condition characterized by elevated hydrostatic pressure within pulmonary capillaries. In edematous disorders mediated by reductions in colloid osmotic pressure (e.g., cirrhosis, nephrotic syndrome), frank pulmonary edema is uncommon in the absence of underlying cardiac disease.

Patients with fluid volume excess may accumulate fluid in body cavities. Patients with cirrhosis, in particular, may accumulate fluid in the peritoneal cavity (ascites) because of increased hydrostatic pressure in the portal vasculature. Other signs of fluid volume overload include increased blood pressure, bounding pulse, and slow emptying of hand veins. Jugular venous distention and a rising central venous pressure are other signs of fluid volume excess.

Laboratory findings are not very helpful in identifying fluid volume excess. Serum sodium concentration is normal unless there is an associated osmolality imbalance. Hematocrit is decreased below the patient's baseline level owing to hemodilution. Urine sodium excretion is usually low (<10 mEq/day) because edematous patients are maximally conserving sodium (Schrier, 1986).

Treatment

Treatment of fluid volume excess and edematous states depends on understanding all the factors, both primary and secondary, that caused the problem and treating the underlying causes if possible. Most treatment plans include the restriction of sodium and fluid intake.

Development of acute pulmonary edema with hypoxemia is a life-threatening situation that requires prompt treatment using measures to reduce preload and restore pulmonary gas exchange as rapidly as possible. These measures include positioning the patient in high Fowler's position and administering morphine, a rapidly acting diuretic such as furosemide, and oxygen. In severe cases of acute pulmonary edema, the use of rotating tourniquets to sequester fluid in the limbs may be helpful. To prevent fluid volume excess and acute pulmonary edema, it is important to monitor carefully the rate of administration of IV fluids and patient response. Patients who are elderly or who have compromised cardiac or renal function are particularly vulnerable to acute pulmonary edema. In situations other than acute pulmonary edema, the reduction of edema fluid should be accomplished more slowly.

Congestive heart failure is generally treated with digitalis, diuretics, and dietary sodium restriction. Cirrhosis

---

ECF VOLUME EXCESS: CLINICAL FEATURES

SIGNS/SYMPTOMS

Jugular venous distention
Elevated CVP (>11 cm H_2O)
Elevated blood pressure
Full, bounding pulse
Slow emptying of hand veins (>3-5 seconds)
Peripheral and periorbital edema
Ascites
Pleural effusion
Acute pulmonary edema (if severe)
  Dyspnea, tachypnea
  Moist rales over lung fields
Rapid weight gain
  2% gain = mild excess
  5% gain = moderate excess
  8% gain = severe excess

LABORATORY FINDINGS

Decreased hematocrit
Low serum proteins
Normal serum Na^+
Low urinary Na^+ (<10 mEq/24 hr)

of the liver is treated with a low-sodium diet and diuretics. Administering corticosteroids to patients with the nephrotic syndrome may diminish proteinuria and thereby correct the hypoalbuminemia, which is the primary mechanism that causes edema. Edema caused by malnutrition responds well to adequate dietary intake, especially with the addition of protein foods. Conservative measures, such as bed rest and support hose, help mobilize edematous fluid.

OSMOLALITY IMBALANCES

In contrast to the volume disturbances just discussed, osmolality imbalances involve the concentration of solutes in the body fluids. Because sodium is the major osmotically active solute in the ECF, in most cases hypoosmolality represents hyponatremia and hyperosmolality represents hypernatremia. One notable exception is the hyperglycemia resulting from uncontrolled diabetes mellitus.

Osmolality imbalances affect the distribution of water between the ECF and ICF compartments because water moves from areas of greater water concentration (i.e., lesser solute concentration, lesser osmolality) to areas of lesser water concentration (i.e., greater solute concentration, greater osmolality). The movement of water between compartments continues until osmotic equilibrium is achieved. Loss or gain of water relative to solute or a loss or gain of solute relative to water causes osmolality imbalances.

Hypoosmolality imbalances are caused by either water excess or sodium depletion. Hyperosmolality imbalances are caused by either a water deficit or an ECF sodium excess. Most osmolality imbalances, however, are caused by a combination of sodium and water excesses and deficits. Hypoosmolality imbalances result in ICF water excess (cell swelling), whereas hyperosmolality imbalances result in ICF water depletion (cell shrinkage).

Osmolality imbalances are identified by history, signs and symptoms, and laboratory values, notably the serum sodium concentration. Treatment of hypoosmolality imbalances involves removal of excess water or sodium replacement; treatment of hyperosmolality imbalances involves replacement of pure water or hypotonic IV solutions or removal of excess sodium or glucose.

Hyponatremia (Hypoosmolality Imbalance)

A serum sodium level less than 135 mEq/L defines hyponatremia (normal serum sodium, 140 ± 5 mEq/L), which may result from two primary mechanisms: water retention or sodium loss. Hyponatremia indicates that the body fluids are diluted by an excess of water relative to total solute. Because sodium is the primary ECF ion, hyponatremia is generally associated with plasma hypoosmolality (<287 mOsm/kg). Low plasma osmolality

CAUSES OF HYPONATREMIA (HYPOOSMOLALITY IMBALANCE)

LOSS OF SODIUM IN EXCESS OF WATER

Prolonged diuretic therapy with low-salt diet
Excessive GI losses (vomiting, diarrhea, nasogastric [NG] suctioning, irrigation of NG tube with tap water, excessive amounts of ice chips given to patients with NG suction)
Replacement of lost body fluids (as from diaphoresis, hemorrhage, or third-space transudation) with only water or other sodium-free fluids
Renal failure with impaired ability to conserve sodium when necessary
Adrenal deficiency (Addison's disease)

GAIN OF WATER IN EXCESS OF SODIUM

Decreased ability to excrete free water
    Effective circulating volume depletion (congestive heart failure, nephrotic syndrome, cirrhosis)
    Renal failure
    Excessive use of diuretics
Excessive IV administration of hypotonic fluids
Excessive administration of tap water enemas
SIADH
Compulsive water drinking (psychogenic polydipsia)
Freshwater drowning

HYPONATREMIA WITHOUT SERUM HYPOOSMOLALITY

Osmotic (hyperglycemia, mannitol)

TYPES OF HYPONATREMIA

Associated with ECF volume depletion (see box, p. 256)
Associated with ECF volume excess and edema (see lower box, p. 259)
Associated with normal ECF volume

results in water movement into the cells. Swelling of brain cells, which causes increased intracranial pressure, is primarily responsible for associated central nervous system symptoms.

Etiology and pathogenesis

The causes of hyponatremia are presented in the box above. Hyponatremia associated with sodium loss is called *depletional hyponatremia* and is characterized by contraction of the ECF volume. Hyponatremia caused by water excess is called *dilutional hyponatremia* or *water intoxication* and is characterized by expansion of the ECF volume.

Sodium loss that causes depletional hyponatremia can result from renal and nonrenal mechanisms. Common renal causes are diuretics and, less commonly, a salt-losing renal disease. Nonrenal salt loss occurs with fluid volume losses as in vomiting, diarrhea, or adrenal deficiency (low aldosterone). The mechanism of the sodium-loss type of hyponatremia involves two steps. First, the loss of sodium lowers the $Na:H_2O$ ratio. Second, and more indirectly, the loss of sodium results in ECF volume contraction and, as a result, antidiuretic hormone (ADH) release from the posterior pituitary. ADH prevents the excretion of a dilute urine and can produce hyponatremia when water is ingested. Hyponatremia per se is usually of little clinical significance in sodium (volume) depletion. Reduction of serum sodium by more than 10 to 15 mEq/L is rare. The major features are those of ECF volume contraction.

Dilutional hyponatremia (water excess) is commonly seen in conditions characterized by a defect in renal free-water excretion with continued intake, particularly of hypotonic fluids. Effective circulating volume depletion, as in congestive heart failure, nephrotic syndrome, and cirrhosis, provides a central stimulus to ADH release, primarily via low pressure (venous) receptors, even in the presence of hypoosmolality so that a dilute urine cannot be excreted. ADH also stimulates thirst (water intake must be present to develop hyponatremia). ADH release in this circumstance (low ECF volume) is considered appropriate because it helps maintain tissue perfusion, albeit at the expense of decreasing plasma osmotic concentration and increasing total body water.

ADH release in the absence of hyperosmolality, decreased effective circulating volume, and other physiologic stimuli is said to be "inappropriate." Thus patients with this type of hyponatremia are said to have a syndrome of inappropriate ADH (SIADH) secretion. SIADH is more common than previously recognized and is associated with a large number of neoplastic, pulmonary, and central nervous system disorders (see box to the right). The autonomous release of ADH can be caused by abnormal stimulation of the hypothalamus by disease, pain, drugs, or central nervous system dysfunction. ADH-like substances may also be produced ectopically in malignancies, especially oat-cell carcinoma of the lung. In addition, SIADH occurs as a complication of therapy with a large variety of drugs. Some of these drugs augment the hypothalamic release of ADH, whereas others enhance the action of ADH on the renal distal tubule and collecting ducts.

Other causes of dilutional hyponatremia include renal failure, in which there is impaired ability to dilute the urine, and the excessive use of diuretics (see box, p. 261). Psychogenic polydipsia is a rare neurotic disorder characterized by compulsive water drinking, sometimes as much as 15 to 20 L/day. Although renal function capacity is normal in psychogenic polydipsia, the large intake of water exceeds the normal excretory capacity, resulting in mild hyponatremia. A similar disorder may also occur in excessive beer drinkers with a poor dietary intake. For example, if the maximum urine diluting ability is 50 mOsm/kg in a person who eats a normal diet (solute par-

ORIGIN OF HIGH ADH IN HYPONATREMIA

INCREASED HYPOTHALAMIC PRODUCTION OF ADH

Central nervous system disorders*
  Head injury, cerebrovascular accidents
  Brain tumors
  Encephalitis
  Guillain-Barré syndrome
Pulmonary disorders
  Pneumonia*
  Tuberculosis
  Mechanical ventilation
Endocrine disorders
  Hypothyroidism
  Addison's disease
Postoperative states* (especially after heart surgery)
Excessive pain (during postoperative period) and vomiting

ECTOPIC (NONHYPOTHALAMIC) PRODUCTION OF ADH

Malignancies, especially oat-cell carcinoma of lung*

EXOGENOUS ADMINISTRATION OF ADH

Vasopressin
Oxytocin* (ADH-like agent) for labor induction, especially if given with sodium-free IV fluids

POTENTIATION OF ENDOGENOUS ADH BY CERTAIN DRUGS

Oral hypoglycemics (chlorpropamide* [Diabinese])
Tricyclic antidepressants (amitriptyline [Elavil])
Morphine/barbiturates
Cholinergic (nicotine)
Antineoplastics (vincristine, cyclophosphamide*)
Anticonvulsant (carbamazepine)
Antilipemic (clofibrate)
Isoproterenol (Isuprel)
Prostaglandin inhibitors (aspirin, indomethacin)

*Most common conditions causing SIADH.

ticles = about 750 mOsm/day), the most urine that person can excrete is 15 L/day (750 mOsm/50 mOsm = 15). However, the daily solute load may be only 250 mOsm in an excessive beer drinker who does not eat well, so that maximum daily urine output would be only about 5 L (250 mOsm/50 mOsm = 5). Finally, dilutional hyponatremia results when a large volume of water enters the lungs and is rapidly absorbed into the intravascular compartment during fresh-water drowning.

Hyponatremia caused by the accumulation of osmotically active solutes in the plasma is the sole exception to the rule that hyponatremia means hypoosmolality. The most common cause of this type of hyponatremia is the hyperglycemia of uncontrolled diabetes and a history of

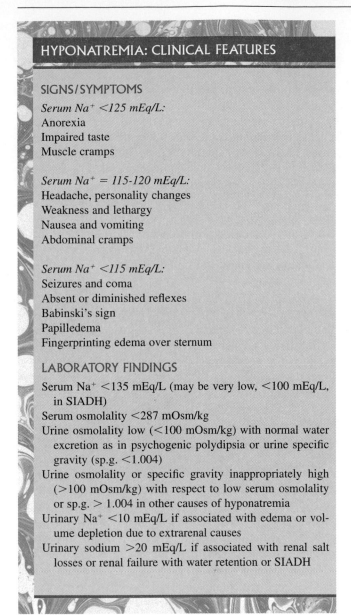

HYPONATREMIA: CLINICAL FEATURES

SIGNS/SYMPTOMS

Serum Na⁺ <125 mEq/L:
Anorexia
Impaired taste
Muscle cramps

Serum Na⁺ = 115-120 mEq/L:
Headache, personality changes
Weakness and lethargy
Nausea and vomiting
Abdominal cramps

Serum Na⁺ <115 mEq/L:
Seizures and coma
Absent or diminished reflexes
Babinski's sign
Papilledema
Fingerprinting edema over sternum

LABORATORY FINDINGS

Serum Na⁺ <135 mEq/L (may be very low, <100 mEq/L, in SIADH)
Serum osmolality <287 mOsm/kg
Urine osmolality low (<100 mOsm/kg) with normal water excretion as in psychogenic polydipsia or urine specific gravity (sp.g. <1.004)
Urine osmolality or specific gravity inappropriately high (>100 mOsm/kg) with respect to low serum osmolality or sp.g. > 1.004 in other causes of hyponatremia
Urinary Na⁺ <10 mEq/L if associated with edema or volume depletion due to extrarenal causes
Urinary sodium >20 mEq/L if associated with renal salt losses or renal failure with water retention or SIADH

recent administration of mannitol. Plasma sodium is diluted by movement of water from the ICF to the ECF along the osmotic gradient produced by the additional solute particles (glucose or mannitol).

Clinical features

A high degree of suspicion is mandatory to detect hyponatremia, because the clinical manifestations are mainly nonspecific during the early period when the serum sodium is greater than about 120 mEq/L. Hyponatremia is a common electrolyte disorder among hospitalized patients. Patients who present one or more risk factors need to be monitored carefully so that hyponatremia may be identified and treated early in its course before it becomes life-threatening.

Signs and symptoms of hyponatremia primarily reflect neurologic dysfunction induced by hypoosmolality. As the serum osmolality falls, water enters brain cells (as well as other cells), causing intracellular overhydration and increased intracranial pressure. The severity of the neurologic symptoms is related to the rapidity and the severity of the reduction of the serum Na⁺ concentration. The box to the left provides a rough correlation between the signs and symptoms and the degree of reduction in the serum Na⁺ concentration. The patient may not have any symptoms with mild hyponatremia (serum Na⁺ levels above 125 mEq/L). The earliest symptoms, including lethargy, anorexia, nausea, and muscle cramps, may occur when the serum Na⁺ is 120 to 125 mEq/L and progress to convulsions and coma with further reductions. When hyponatremia of this magnitude (<120 mEq/L) develops in less than 24 hours, mortality reaches 50%. By contrast, patients remain relatively asymptomatic when the serum Na⁺ is reduced to comparable levels over a period of days to weeks. Slowly developing hyponatremia causes milder symptoms because of the compensatory loss of solutes such as Na⁺, K⁺, and amino acids from brain cells so that the degree of intracellular swelling is lessened (Rose, 1994).

The diagnosis of hyponatremia, as with other fluid and electrolyte imbalances, involves analysis of findings from the history, clinical signs and symptoms, and laboratory tests. Three simple laboratory tests are helpful in diagnosing the cause of hyponatremia: serum osmolality, urine osmolality, and urine Na⁺. Serum osmolality levels will be normal or high when the cause of hyponatremia is renal failure or diabetic hyperglycemia. Urine osmolality level is low (<100 mOsm/kg or sp.g. <1.004) when the cause is primary polydipsia with normal water excretion and high (>100 mOsm/kg or sp.g. >1.004) for other causes of hyponatremia in which water excretion is impaired. Finally, urinary Na⁺ is low (<10 mEq/L) if the hyponatremia is associated with edema or volume depletion caused by extrarenal causes; urinary Na⁺ is high (>20 mEq/L) if renal salt-wasting or SIADH is present.

Treatment

The goals of treatment for patients with hypoosmolality and true hyponatremia is to elevate the serum sodium toward normal and to treat the underlying cause. The two basic treatments are either restricting water or administering sodium, depending on the severity and underlying cause.

Mild hyponatremia (120 to 135 mEq/L) in patients with true volume depletion from GI or renal losses is treated with oral NaCl or normal saline given intravenously. Correction of the hypovolemia suppresses ADH release, leading to renal excretion of excess water and correction of the hyponatremia. Correction of K⁺ depletion is also another important aspect of treatment. In more severe cases of hyponatremia (<120 mEq/L), hypertonic saline may be given at a rate sufficient to raise the serum Na⁺ 0.5 mEq/L per hour until a serum Na⁺ level of about 120 mEq/L is reached and the patient is out of danger. Care must be

CAUSES OF HYPERNATREMIA (HYPEROSMOLALITY IMBALANCE)

INSUFFICIENT WATER INTAKE

Unable to perceive or respond to thirst (e.g., comatose, confused)
Nothing by mouth without sufficient IV maintenance
Unable to swallow (e.g., cerebrovascular accident)

EXCESSIVE WATER LOSS

Nonrenal
  Fever and/or diaphoresis
  Burns
  Hyperventilation
  Prolonged use of mechanical ventilator
  Watery diarrhea
Renal
  Diabetes insipidus (central, nephrogenic)
    Head trauma (especially basal skull fracture)
    Neurosurgery
    Infection (encephalitis, meningitis)
    Brain neoplasm
  Osmotic diuresis
    Glycosuria in uncontrolled diabetes
    Urea diuresis in high-protein tube feedings
    Mannitol

SODIUM GAIN

Sea-water drowning
Excessive use of IV sodium salts
  Hypertonic saline (3% or 5%)
  Excessive IV sodium bicarbonate used to treat cardiac arrest
  Isotonic saline
Accidental replacement of sugar with salt in infant formula
Therapeutic abortion with accidental entry of hypertonic saline into circulation

TYPES OF HYPERNATREMIA

Associated with normal ECF volume
Associated with ECF volume depletion
Associated with ECF volume excess

Water restriction alone is often effective treatment for mild cases of SIADH. Removing the cause of the ADH release, such as discontinuing the offending drug or recovering from the offending disease process, may help to resolve the problem. The treatment of severe cases of hyponatremia may require the administration of a small volume of hypertonic saline in addition to restriction of fluid intake and administration of a loop diuretic. In chronic cases caused by the ectopic production of ADH, demeclocycline, a drug that blocks the effect of ADH on the renal tubule, may be given to treat SIADH.

The treatment of the hyponatremia associated with diabetic hyperglycemic states is not directed toward raising the serum sodium because this condition does not represent a true hyponatremia. Rather, the treatment involves the administration of insulin and glucose.

Hypernatremia (Hyperosmolality Imbalance)

Hypernatremia is defined by the presence of a serum sodium level greater than 145 mEq/L. It is always associated with hyperosmolality because sodium salts are the main determinants of the plasma osmolality. The rise in serum osmolality causes water to shift from the ICF to the ECF, resulting in cell dehydration and shrinkage. The basic causes are water loss in excess of sodium or sodium gain in excess of water.

Etiology and pathogenesis

The box at left lists the major causes of hypernatremia and hyperosmolality. These causes are classified as insufficient water intake with or without loss of water in excess of sodium and sodium gain. The major protective mechanism against hypernatremia is thirst and renal water conservation stimulated by ADH when the serum solute or sodium concentration increases. Hypernatremia rarely occurs except when there is a disturbance in water intake in combination with hypotonic fluid loss. Inadequate water intake is most commonly seen in older adults who have a disturbance in level of consciousness, in the very young who have inadequate access to water, or in a rare person with a primary disturbance in thirst. Hypotonic water losses may be caused by nonrenal or renal losses that are not replaced. Water loss from the respiratory tract and skin (a hypotonic fluid) is normally just under 1 L/day. However, losses may increase dramatically in patients who are febrile and hyperventilating or exposed to a hot environment. Central diabetes insipidus and nephrogenic diabetes insipidus are conditions in which either ADH secretion or its renal effect is impaired, leading to the excretion of large volumes of hypoosmotic urine. Central diabetes insipidus occurs in patients with a central nervous system (CNS) lesion, especially after head injury. Nephrogenic diabetes insipidus is associated with hypokalemia and a number of drugs and disease processes and is not discussed further in this chapter. Osmotic diuresis is another major cause of renal water loss.

---

taken not to raise the serum sodium too rapidly, which could cause central pontine myelinosis and irreversible neurologic damage (Rose, 1994).

In addition to correcting the underlying disorder whenever possible, water restriction constitutes the first line of therapy in patients with dilutional hyponatremia and increased ECF because the administration of sodium worsens the condition. Restricting water intake to less than urine output is usually sufficient to correct the hyponatremia. In more severe cases, hypertonic saline in combination with a loop diuretic can raise the serum sodium more quickly.

Glycosuria in uncontrolled diabetes mellitus is the most common cause of osmotic diuresis. Osmotic diuresis may also be caused by the urea produced from high-protein tube feedings or with mannitol administration.

Hypernatremia caused by an absolute excess of sodium is much less common than that caused by water depletion. Some examples that involve intake of sodium via the lungs, intravenously, or orally include sea-water drowning (a hypertonic saline solution), IV administration of saline solutions, and accidental ingestion of large amounts of salt orally. Therapeutic abortion has caused a death on rare occasions when the hypertonic saline used to induce the abortion entered the maternal bloodstream.

Hypernatremia may be associated with normovolemia (usually caused by insensible water loss), hypovolemia (loss of water in excess of sodium), and hypervolemia (relatively greater gain of sodium than of water).

Clinical features

The most prominent manifestations of hypernatremic and hyperosmotic imbalances are neurologic and result from cellular dehydration, particularly of brain cells (see box at right). Lethargy, agitation, irritability, hyper-reflexia, and spasticity may occur and culminate in coma, seizures, and death. Thirst is the major symptom of hypernatremia, although its absence or the inability to communicate may be an underlying cause. Other clinical findings include dry, sticky mucous membranes; flushed skin; and a dry, rough, red tongue. Oliguria or anuria may be present, and the patient may be febrile.

The morbidity and mortality of acute hypernatremia in children are high; about 45% die, and two thirds of those who survive have serious neurologic sequelae. In adults, acute elevations of the serum sodium above 160 mEq/L are associated with a 75% mortality, whereas mortality in chronic cases is about 60% (Schrier, 1986). The mechanism of brain injury resulting in death is brain hemorrhage from the shrinkage of brain cells, causing tearing of cerebral blood vessels.

The diagnosis of hypernatremia is made from the signs and symptoms and measurement of serum sodium and osmolality. The cause can usually be inferred from the history when it is caused by extrarenal water loss, an osmotic diuresis, or sodium excess. In these cases the urine is hyperosmotic to plasma. The diagnosis of central diabetes insipidus is usually easy to confirm because the patient has a CNS problem plus a history of polyuria (3 to 10 L/day) and polydipsia (excessive thirst, usually preferring cold liquids).

Treatment

The primary goal in the treatment of hypernatremia is to gradually lower serum sodium to the normal range and restore normal serum osmolality. The therapeutic approach depends on the underlying pathophysiologic mechanism causing the hypernatremia. Free water can be given orally or as IV D_5W to the patient who is normo-

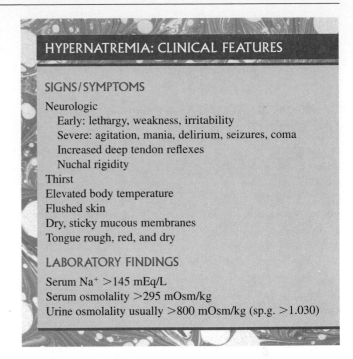

HYPERNATREMIA: CLINICAL FEATURES

SIGNS/SYMPTOMS

Neurologic
   Early: lethargy, weakness, irritability
   Severe: agitation, mania, delirium, seizures, coma
   Increased deep tendon reflexes
   Nuchal rigidity
Thirst
Elevated body temperature
Flushed skin
Dry, sticky mucous membranes
Tongue rough, red, and dry

LABORATORY FINDINGS

Serum Na^+ >145 mEq/L
Serum osmolality >295 mOsm/kg
Urine osmolality usually >800 mOsm/kg (sp.g. >1.030)

volemic and has hypernatremia caused by pure water loss. When the patient is hypovolemic, IV isotonic saline is given to restore normal blood pressure and tissue perfusion, and thereafter hypotonic (0.45%) saline may be infused to provide free water and correct the hypernatremia. When the patient is both hypernatremic and hypervolemic, the goal is to remove the excess sodium. Removal may be achieved either by the concurrent administration of diuretics and D_5W infusion or by dialysis if renal function is impaired. Most authors recommend that the plasma Na^+ concentration be lowered to normal at a maximum rate of 2 mEq/hr. Rapid correction of hypernatremia is hazardous because it can induce cerebral edema, convulsions, permanent neurologic damage, and death (Rose, 1994). These complications occur because the administration of a hypotonic infusion renders the ECF temporarily hypoosmotic so that water moves from the ECF to the ICF, causing cerebral edema. Central diabetes insipidus is treated by administering exogenous ADH (usually dDAVP [Desmopressin] in the form of a nasal spray).

Finally, careful clinical observation of patients at risk for developing hypernatremia must be practiced so that the condition may be detected before serious elevations of the serum Na^+ concentration occur. Serious elevations of serum Na^+ concentration do not usually occur except when the patient is unable to respond to thirst, so special care must be taken to provide adequate water.

POTASSIUM IMBALANCES

Few of the disturbances in fluid and electrolyte metabolism are as frequently encountered or as immediately life-threatening as disturbances in potassium balance. The critical modulating effect of potassium on neuromuscular conduction, particularly cardiac conduction, accounts for the fatalities and near fatalities that accompany either hypokalemia or hyperkalemia.

Physiologic Considerations

Potassium is the major cation of the intracellular fluid. In fact, 98% of the body's stores (3000 to 4000 mEq) is inside cells, and the remaining 2% (about 70 mEq) is located primarily in the ECF compartment. The normal range of serum K^+ is 3.5 to 5.5 mEq/L in contrast with a concentration of about 160 mEq/L inside cells. Because potassium constitutes a large proportion of the intracellular solute, it plays an important role in keeping fluid inside the cell and maintaining cell volume. The ECF potassium, although a small fraction of the total, greatly influences neuromuscular function. The difference in the concentration of potassium in the ICF and that of the ECF compartments is maintained by an active Na-K pump in the cell membrane.

The ratio of the ICF to ECF potassium concentration is the principal determinant of the cell membrane potential in excitable tissues, such as cardiac and skeletal muscle. The resting membrane potential sets the stage for the generation of the action potential that is essential for normal neural and muscular function. Because the concentration of ECF potassium is so much lower than the concentration inside the cell, small changes in the ECF potassium can significantly alter this ratio. Conversely, only large changes in the ICF potassium influence the ratio significantly. One practical consequence of this relationship is that the toxic effects of a severe hyperkalemia can be mitigated as an emergency treatment by inducing the movement of potassium from the ECF to the ICF. In addition to playing a primary role in maintaining normal neuromuscular function, potassium is an important cofactor in a number of metabolic processes.

The homeostasis of potassium in the body is influenced by the distribution between the ECF and ICF, as well as the balance between intake and output. A number of hormonal and nonhormonal factors play a role in its regulation, including aldosterone, catecholamines, insulin, and acid-base variables.

In the healthy adult, the daily dietary intake of potassium is about 50 to 100 mEq. After a meal, virtually all of the absorbed K^+ is first shifted into cells within minutes; thereafter K^+ excretion occurs primarily by the renal route over a period of hours. A smaller proportion (<20%) may be excreted in the sweat and feces. The shift of K^+ into the cells after a meal until renal excretion can occur is an important mechanism to prevent a dangerous hyperkalemia. Renal K^+ excretion is under the influence of aldosterone, distal tubule sodium, and the urine flow rate. The secretion of aldosterone is stimulated by the amount of sodium reaching the distal tubule and an increase in the serum K^+ level above normal and is suppressed when the level decreases. Most of the K^+ filtered by the glomerulus is reabsorbed in the proximal tubule. Increased aldosterone then causes more K^+ to be secreted into the distal tubule in exchange for Na^+ or H^+ reabsorption. The secreted K^+ is then excreted in the urine. Potassium secretion in the distal tubule is also flow dependent, so that increased distal tubule delivery of fluid (polyuria) favors K^+ excretion.

The distribution of potassium between the ICF and ECF is influenced by acid-base balance and hormones. Acidosis tends to shift potassium out of cells, whereas alkalosis favors movement from the ECF to the ICF. The degree of shift is greater in metabolic acid-base disturbances and greater in alkalosis than in acidosis. Several hormones also influence the movement of K^+ between the ICF and ECF. Insulin and epinephrine stimulate K^+ movement into cells. Conversely, alpha-adrenergic agonists impair cellular K^+ uptake. These facts have important clinical implications for the treatment of diabetic ketoacidosis, which is discussed in Chapter 22.

Hypokalemia

Hypokalemia is defined as a serum potassium concentration of less than 3.5 mEq/L. Because only 2% of the body potassium is in the ECF, the serum K^+ value may not always reflect total body potassium. In addition, the blood pH affects the serum K^+ as previously discussed. For every 0.1 unit fall in pH, the serum K^+ increases 0.5 mEq/L; for every 0.1 unit rise in pH, the serum K^+ decreases by 0.5 mEq/L.

Etiology and pathogenesis

The box on p. 267 lists the principal causes of hypokalemia: gastrointestinal and urinary losses, inadequate potassium intake, and K^+ shifts caused by alkalosis or the treatment of diabetic ketoacidosis with insulin and glucose. Moderate hypokalemia may result from potassium-deficient dietary intake alone or contribute to the hypokalemia caused by GI or renal losses. For example, the older adult who exists on tea and toast has little potassium intake. The alcoholic who eats infrequently and poorly may likewise have a deficient potassium intake. All seriously ill patients who are ingesting nothing by mouth should receive K^+ additives in their IV infusions because renal excretion of potassium continues, even though there is no intake.

GI disorders characterized by vomiting, NG suction, diarrhea, or loss of other secretions are perhaps the most frequent causes of hypokalemia. The potassium depletion that occurs with vomiting or NG suction does not occur, primarily because of the potassium lost in the gastric secretions. The potassium content of gastric secretions is only 5 to 10 mEq/L. Rather, the hypokalemia associated with vomiting is primarily the result of increased renal excretion of potassium. The increased renal excretion of

CAUSES OF HYPOKALEMIA

DECREASED DIETARY INTAKE OF K^+

Seriously ill patient NPO several days without K^+ supplement added to IV infusion
Starvation, tea and toast diet
Alcoholism

GASTROINTESTINAL LOSS

Protracted vomiting, NG suction
Diarrhea, chronic laxative abuse
Ileostomy, fistulas
Villous adenoma of colon

RENAL LOSS

Diuretic drugs (thiazides, furosemide)
Some renal diseases
   Diuretic recovery phase of acute renal failure
   Renal tubular acidosis (RTA)
Diabetic acidosis leading to osmotic diuresis
Healing stage of severe burns
Excessive mineralocorticoid effect
   Primary or secondary hyperaldosteronism
   ECF volume deficit (by far, the most common cause)
   Cushing's syndrome; corticosteroid therapy
   Licorice ingestion (aldosterone-like activity)
   Swallowing chewing tobacco (contains large amounts of licorice)
Antibiotics (carbenicillin, aminoglycosides)
Magnesium depletion

INCREASED LOSS IN SWEAT DURING HEAT STRESS

Heavily perspiring individual acclimated to heat

SHIFT OF K^+ INTO CELLS

Metabolic alkalosis
Treatment of DKA with insulin and glucose

---

cause acidosis causes K^+ to shift out of the cells, raising the serum K^+ concentration and obscuring the actual total body deficit. Villous adenomas are potentially malignant tumors of the colon, which are associated with the loss of diarrheal fluid high in potassium content.

The kidney can be a major site of potassium loss. Diuretics are among the most frequent causes of hypokalemia. Thiazides, loop diuretics, and carbonic anhydrase inhibitors all increase potassium loss in the urine. Many patients being treated for a fluid volume excess have cardiac disease and are also receiving digitalis preparations. Hypokalemia augments the effect of digitalis so that toxic effects may result. Thus it is important to encourage eating potassium-rich foods and/or to administer potassium supplements to these patients. Although end-stage renal disease generally results in hyperkalemia, some renal diseases, such as renal tubular acidosis and the diuretic recovery phase of acute renal failure, cause potassium loss and hypokalemia. Potassium excretion is increased during an osmotic diuresis, which leads to potassium depletion in diabetic ketoacidosis. The solutes causing the polyuria are glucose and ketoacid anions. Acidosis and insulin deficiency cause K^+ to shift from the ICF to the ECF so that the serum K^+ may be in the normal range, despite total body potassium depletion. When the diabetic ketoacidosis is corrected by the administration of IV glucose and insulin, a serious hypokalemia may result as the serum K^+ shifts back into the cells. Patients with severe burns in the healing stage may develop hypokalemia because potassium may shift from the cells to the ECF and then is lost in the urine through diuresis.

Patients with primary hyperaldosteronism caused by an adrenal adenoma present with hypokalemia and metabolic alkalosis resulting from renal potassium wasting. ECF volume contraction is probably the most frequent cause of secondary hyperaldosteronism and potassium wasting, as previously discussed. However, patients with cirrhosis, congestive heart failure, and the nephrotic syndrome are usually not hypokalemic, despite secondary hyperaldosteronism (unless they receive diuretics), probably because decreased effective circulating plasma volume causes less sodium and water to be delivered to the distal tubule. High levels of glucocorticoid hormones can exert a mineralocorticoid (aldosterone) effect, causing hypokalemia. Thus hypokalemia may be associated with Cushing's syndrome or the therapeutic administration of exogenous steroids. Finally, some forms of licorice contain a compound with aldosterone-like activity, which may cause hypokalemia with excessive ingestion. This cause of hypokalemia is not generally a problem in the United States, where an artificial licorice flavoring is used. However, chewing tobacco contains large amounts of true licorice, which can cause potassium wasting if swallowed.

Certain antibiotics, such as carbenicillin, can cause hypokalemia by acting as an anion and increasing potas-

---

K^+ appears to involve three mechanisms: (1) loss of gastric acid leads to metabolic alkalosis, which stimulates a shift of K^+ into renal tubular cells; (2) metabolic alkalosis causes more $NaHCO_3$ and fluid to be delivered to the distal tubule and the HCO_3^- (an anion) augments K^+ excretion; and (3) loss of gastric fluid causes ECF volume contraction, which in turn stimulates increased aldosterone secretion via the renin-angiotensin-aldosterone mechanism. Aldosterone stimulates K^+ excretion and helps to maintain the hypokalemia. Large amounts of potassium can be lost directly from the lower GI tract when there is diarrhea. Potassium content in stool is often in the range of 40 to 70 mEq/L. In addition, lower GI tract secretions are high in sodium and bicarbonate. Loss of large amounts of stool results in ECF volume contraction and metabolic acidosis, as well as potassium depletion. The potassium deficit may be difficult to assess be-

HYPOKALEMIA: CLINICAL FEATURES

SIGNS AND SYMPTOMS

Central nervous system and neuromuscular
  Early symptoms are vague: fatigue, "not feeling well"
  Paresthesias
  Diminished deep tendon reflexes
  Generalized muscle weakness
Respiratory
  Weak respiratory muscles, shallow respirations
    (advanced)
Gastrointestinal
  Decreased bowel motility: anorexia, nausea, vomiting,
    ileus
Cardiovascular
  Postural hypotension
  Dysrhythmias (especially if digitalis or heart disease
    present)
  ECG changes
    Broad, progressively flat T waves (sometimes inverted)
    ST segment depression
    Prominent U wave
Renal
  Polyuria, nocturia (concentrating defect)

LABORATORY FINDINGS

Serum K^+ <3.5 mEq/L
Serum pH >7.45; elevated serum bicarbonate (hypokalemia
  often associated with metabolic alkalosis)

---

sium excretion. Magnesium depletion can apparently cause potassium depletion through urinary and fecal losses, although the exact mechanism is not understood. Hypomagnesemia and hypokalemia frequently occur together in alcoholics.

Normally only a small amount of potassium is lost in perspiration. However, the potassium content of sweat may increase in persons acclimated to a hot environment. Several liters of fluid per day may be lost by persons who exercise in a hot environment. Hypokalemia may occur unless potassium intake is appropriately increased.

Clinical features

The box above lists the signs and symptoms and laboratory findings in hypokalemia. The most prominent features of hypokalemia are reflected in the neuromuscular status, and the most serious complication is cardiac arrest, which is more apt to occur if the depletion has been rapid (e.g., treatment of diabetic ketoacidosis with insulin and glucose without potassium additives). Patients with hypokalemia may experience muscle weakness or leg cramps. GI smooth muscle dysfunction results in decreased bowel motility, with progression to paralytic

ileus and abdominal distention. The respiratory muscles may be affected with profound hypokalemia. Paresthesias and diminished deep tendon reflexes are other manifestations. Cardiac dysrhythmias and ECG changes are important manifestations of hypokalemia, which become increasingly abnormal and life-threatening in rough parallel with the severity of potassium depletion. The major effect of hypokalemia on cardiac conduction is prolonged repolarization, resulting in increasingly flattened T waves. The U wave increases in magnitude and ST segment depression occurs with severe hypokalemia (Fig. 21-1). A variety of atrial and ventricular dysrhythmias may occur, especially in patients receiving digitalis because hypokalemia increases sensitivity to this drug. It is important to remember that patients can be asymptomatic, especially if hypokalemia develops over a long period.

The cause of hypokalemia is usually evident from the history. A high degree of vigilance in persons at risk is required to detect hypokalemia. The ECG, signs and symptoms of hypokalemia, and serum potassium levels should be monitored. Initial and repeat serum potassium levels should be obtained to rule out laboratory error.

Treatment

The primary goal with respect to potassium should be to prevent an imbalance. Remember that diuretics, digitalis, and hypokalemia are a potentially lethal combination because many diuretics cause hypokalemia, and hypokalemia enhances the effect of digitalis. Toxic effects of digitalis and hypokalemia may both cause life-threatening dysrhythmias. Thus serum potassium and digitalis levels should be monitored in these patients and adequate potassium intake provided.

When possible, potassium depletion should be corrected by increased dietary intake of potassium-rich foods or supplementation with potassium salts. Foods rich in potassium include fruits (especially bananas, raisins, and citrus fruits), fruit juices, meats, milk, fresh tomatoes, potatoes, and lentils. Potassium chloride is the supplementary salt of choice, especially if the patient is alkalotic. Intravenous administration of potassium is necessary when the patient cannot take potassium orally or when the potassium deficiency is severe. It should be given in a nondextrose solution in a severe deficit because dextrose stimulates insulin release, causing K^+ to shift into the cells. The rate of infusion of potassium should not exceed 20 mEq/hr to avoid a serious hyperkalemia.

Hyperkalemia

Hyperkalemia is defined as a serum potassium concentration of 5.5 mEq/L or greater. Acute hyperkalemia is a medical emergency requiring prompt recognition and treatment to avoid a fatal cardiac dysrhythmia and cardiac arrest.

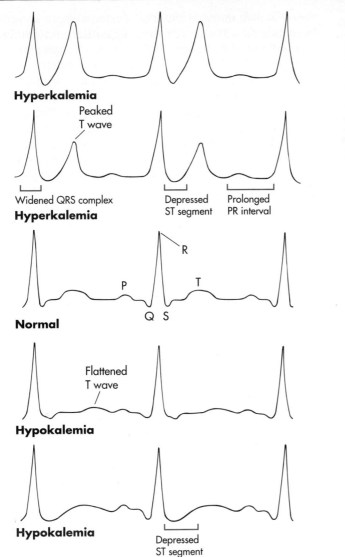

Hyperkalemia

Peaked T wave

Hyperkalemia

Widened QRS complex   Depressed ST segment   Prolonged PR interval

R

P   T

Normal

Q   S

Flattened T wave

Hypokalemia

Hypokalemia

Depressed ST segment

FIG. 21-1   ECG changes in potassium imbalances.

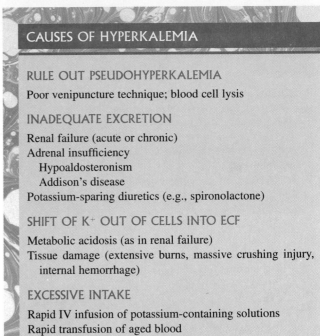

CAUSES OF HYPERKALEMIA

RULE OUT PSEUDOHYPERKALEMIA

Poor venipuncture technique; blood cell lysis

INADEQUATE EXCRETION

Renal failure (acute or chronic)
Adrenal insufficiency
　Hypoaldosteronism
　Addison's disease
Potassium-sparing diuretics (e.g., spironolactone)

SHIFT OF K$^+$ OUT OF CELLS INTO ECF

Metabolic acidosis (as in renal failure)
Tissue damage (extensive burns, massive crushing injury, internal hemorrhage)

EXCESSIVE INTAKE

Rapid IV infusion of potassium-containing solutions
Rapid transfusion of aged blood
Ingestion of salt substitutes in persons with renal failure

Etiology and pathogenesis

The common causes of hyperkalemia are listed in the box above, right. Although a low serum potassium concentration can usually be taken at face value, the report from the laboratory of a high serum potassium concentration does not always represent a true hyperkalemia. A tight tourniquet around an exercising extremity (e.g., opening and closing fist) can elevate the potassium as much as 2 to 3 mEq/L. Hemolysis of the red blood cells also produces a falsely elevated serum potassium concentration because blood cells are high in potassium. Therefore it is important to rule out artifacts that produce a falsely elevated serum potassium or pseudohyperkalemia. Serial measurements should be obtained if there is doubt about the veracity of the laboratory measurement. Alternatively, the plasma concentration of K$^+$ can be measured by obtaining a blood sample in a heparinized tube. The plasma concentration of K$^+$ will be within normal limits and the serum value elevated in

pseudohyperkalemia. Potassium may be falsely elevated with the serum measurement, since the ECF is separated from the red cells *after* clotting has occurred. A small amount of K$^+$ normally moves out of white cells and platelets during coagulation, and the amount may be much greater when there is leukocytosis or thrombocytosis. Consequently, the measured serum K$^+$ exceeds the true level in the plasma.

Hyperkalemia can be used by inadequate excretion, redistribution of potassium in the body, and increased intake. The most common cause of hyperkalemia is inadequate renal excretion. Because 80% to 90% of the potassium is excreted by the kidneys, one would expect renal failure to result in hyperkalemia. However, hyperkalemia does not occur until late in the course of chronic renal failure unless the patient is challenged with a potassium load. This circumstance might occur if a patient with chronic renal failure receives a drug containing potassium or uses a salt substitute (one that contains potassium salts). An endogenous source of potassium overloading might be internal bleeding with the release of K$^+$ during hemolysis of red blood cells. Both Addison's disease and isolated hypoaldosteronism can present with severe hyperkalemia. The latter condition is more common in older adults with renal impairment and diabetes mellitus. Potassium-sparing diuretics, such as spironolactone, can produce severe hyperkalemia, especially if they are administered to patients with renal insufficiency who are also taking potassium supplements.

Acidosis and tissue damage, such as results from burns or a crushing injury, cause potassium to shift from the ICF to the ECF and are other causes of hyperkalemia. Fi-

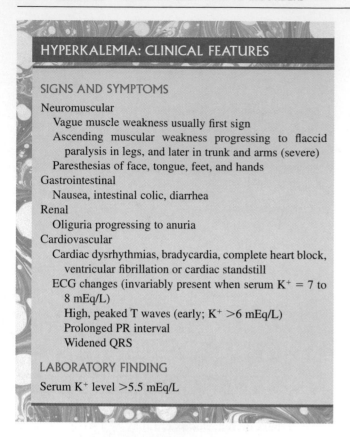

HYPERKALEMIA: CLINICAL FEATURES

SIGNS AND SYMPTOMS

Neuromuscular
  Vague muscle weakness usually first sign
  Ascending muscular weakness progressing to flaccid paralysis in legs, and later in trunk and arms (severe)
  Paresthesias of face, tongue, feet, and hands
Gastrointestinal
  Nausea, intestinal colic, diarrhea
Renal
  Oliguria progressing to anuria
Cardiovascular
  Cardiac dysrhythmias, bradycardia, complete heart block, ventricular fibrillation or cardiac standstill
  ECG changes (invariably present when serum K^+ = 7 to 8 mEq/L)
    High, peaked T waves (early; K^+ >6 mEq/L)
    Prolonged PR interval
    Widened QRS

LABORATORY FINDING

Serum K^+ level >5.5 mEq/L

---

nally, potassium-containing IV solutions must be given slowly to prevent iatrogenic potassium overload. If possible, fresh blood or packed cells should be used for transfusions because potassium is gradually released from red blood cells into the ECF when blood is stored.

A final point must be made about interpreting hyperkalemia. In hypokalemia there is a rough correlation between total body potassium stores and serum potassium, but such a correlation does not exist between total body potassium and the serum potassium in hyperkalemia. In most instances of hyperkalemia, total potassium stores are not increased because the body has little capacity for storing potassium. In fact, body potassium stores may even be reduced in hyperkalemia. In most types of metabolic acidosis (except lactic acidosis), potassium shifts from the ICF to the ECF, giving rise to moderately severe hyperkalemia when potassium stores are normal and to a normalization of the serum potassium when body potassium stores are depleted.

Clinical features

Most patients with hyperkalemia are asymptomatic until there is a marked rise in the serum potassium concentration. The neuromuscular effects of hyperkalemia resemble those of hypokalemia (see box above). Muscle weakness predominates, and symptoms most often begin in the lower extremities and ascend to the trunk and upper extremities. Other signs and symptoms may include listlessness, paresthesias, nausea, intestinal colic, or diar-

rhea. Cardiac arrest is the most feared complication of hyperkalemia. The progressive disturbance in cardiac conduction can be appreciated from the changes that occur in the ECG. The earliest changes are symmetric peaking, or "tenting" of the T waves (serum K^+ >6 mEq/L). Serum levels of 6.5 to 8.0 mEq/L produce more advanced changes, including a prolonged PR interval and widening of the QRS complex. Severe hyperkalemia (serum K^+ >8.0 mEq/L) yields a sine wave pattern, an ominous sign of impending cardiac arrest (see Fig. 21-1). It must be emphasized, however, that the progressive ECG changes may not correlate perfectly with the degree of hyperkalemia. Hypocalcemia, hyponatremia, acidemia, and a rapid rise of serum K^+ enhance the toxic effects of hyperkalemia (a common combination in renal failure). Hypernatremia and hypercalcemia counteract the effects of hyperkalemia on the membrane potential.

The diagnosis of hyperkalemia cannot be made on the basis of clinical signs and symptoms because they are nonspecific and many are identical with those of hypokalemia. Rather, the diagnosis is made on the basis of the serum K^+ and by observing the characteristic ECG changes.

Treatment

Treatment of hyperkalemia varies with the severity of the imbalance. Severe hyperkalemia (>8 mEq/L or advanced ECG changes) requires correction within minutes to bring the serum K^+ down to a safe level. Correction is best accomplished by directly counteracting the cardiac effects with calcium, together with redistribution of the K^+ from the ECF to the ICF. Three methods are used for the emergency treatment of severe hyperkalemia:

1. 10 ml 10% IV calcium gluconate infused slowly over 2 to 3 minutes with ECG monitoring; onset within 5 minutes but effect lasts only about 30 minutes
2. 500 ml 10% glucose with 10 U regular insulin shifts K^+ into cells; onset within 30 minutes and lasts several hours
3. 44 to 88 mEq sodium bicarbonate IV corrects acidosis and shifts K^+ into cells; onset within 30 minutes and lasts several hours

Emergency treatment of hyperkalemia must be followed with treatment methods to permanently reduce the serum K^+. These methods include the use of an exchange resin or dialysis. Sodium polystyrene sulfonate (Kayexalate) is a nonabsorbable ion exchange resin that can be given orally or rectally as an enema. Forty grams given orally in four divided doses will lower the serum K^+ by 1 mEq/L over 24 hours. Enemas should be retained for at least 30 minutes to permit exchange. This treatment is often given to patients with renal failure and moderate hyperkalemia. The best method to remove potassium from the body is by peritoneal dialysis or hemodialysis. Intermittent dialysis is used to treat patients with renal failure and chronic hyperkalemia to maintain the serum K^+ within an acceptable range (see Part Eight).

The most important aspect of preventing hyperkalemia is to recognize the clinical circumstances that predispose to it because hyperkalemia is a predictable consequence of many diseases and the result of the administration of many drugs. Particular care must be taken to avoid rapid infusion of potassium-containing IV solutions.

CALCIUM, PHOSPHATE, AND MAGNESIUM IMBALANCES

Although imbalances of calcium, phosphate, and magnesium are less common than those of potassium and sodium, the consequences can be major. Because abnormalities of these three electrolytes are closely linked, excesses and deficits of these ions will be discussed together.

Calcium Homeostasis

Total body calcium in adults is about 1 to 2 kg. About 99% of body calcium is found in the bones and teeth in the form of calcium phosphate salts, about 1% is found in the ECF, and 0.1% is found within the cytosol. Calcium has two important physiologic roles: maintaining the structural integrity of the skeleton and participating in many vital cellular processes.

Osteoclastic resorption of existing bone and *osteoblastic formation* of new bone are tightly coupled and take place throughout life (Fig. 21-2). Bone resorption always precedes new bone formation, and the length of one replacement sequence is about 4 to 5 months in adults. The three major influences on the equilibrium of bone tissue are (1) mechanical stress stimulating osteoblastic activity, (2) calcium and phosphate levels in the ECF, and (3) hormones and local factors influencing resorption and formation (see below).

In the ECF and cytosol, ionized calcium (Ca^{++}) is essential for a variety of cellular processes. Calcium is an important constituent of cell membranes, affecting their permeability and electrical properties. For example, lowering the ECF Ca^{++} causes increased permeability and excitability of the cell membrane. Calcium also affects neuromuscular activity. A decrease in ECF Ca^{++} increases the excitability of nerve tissue and can stimulate muscle contraction. In fact, Ca^{++} acts as a coupling factor between muscle excitation and contraction of actomyosin. Calcium influences cardiac contractility and automaticity via slow calcium channels in the heart muscle (see Chapter 29). Calcium is involved in the release of preformed hormones from endocrine cells and in the release of acetylcholine at neuromuscular junctions. It also participates in the mechanism of action of hormones within the cells. For example, calcium is an important component in the action of cyclic adenosine monophosphate (cyclic AMP or cAMP), the secondary intracellular

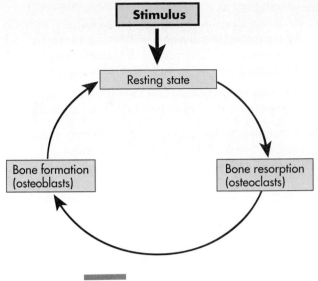

FIG. 21-2   Bone maintenance.

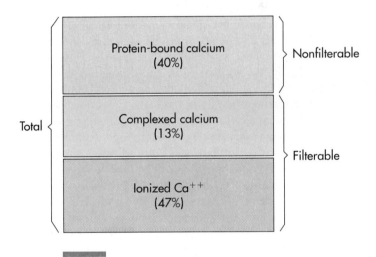

FIG. 21-3   Distribution of calcium in plasma.

messenger. Calcium is important in the property of adhesiveness that binds cells together, in enzyme activity, and in blood coagulation. Because of these various and important functions, the level of ionized calcium in the ECF must be carefully maintained within a narrow range.

The concentration of the total serum calcium is normally 9.0 to 10.5 mg/dl (4.5 to 5.5 mEq/L). The calcium in plasma is in three forms: bound to proteins (principally albumin), complexed with small ligands (phosphate, citrate, and sulfate), and ionized Ca^{++} (Fig. 21-3). The ionized and complexed forms are diffusible, accounting for 47% and 13% of total calcium, respectively, whereas the protein-bound calcium is not. It is the ionized calcium in plasma that is physiologically active and clinically important in defining hypocalcemia and hypercalcemia. Ionized calcium can be measured directly using a calcium-specific electrode, but generally the total serum calcium is measured. When only the total serum calcium measurement is available, it must be evaluated in relation to the serum albumin. A decrease in the serum albumin of 1 g/dl (assuming 4 g/dl as normal) will decrease the total serum calcium by 0.8 mg/dl. A frequently used formula for estimating the total serum calcium is the following:

$$\text{Total serum Ca} = \text{Measured total Ca} + 0.8 \times (4 - \text{measured albumin}) \text{ (g/dl)}$$
$$\text{(mg/dl)} \quad\quad \text{(mg/dl)}$$

For example, if the measured total serum calcium is 8.0 mg/dl (subnormal) and the serum albumin is only 2.0 (subnormal), the corrected total calcium would be 8.0 + (2 × 0.8) = 9.6 mg/dl (normal range). However, this formula is not valid in conditions that alter serum pH. Calcium binding declines with a reduction of pH so that more of the total serum calcium is ionized and less is bound to albumin in conditions of acidosis. Alkalosis (higher pH) produces the converse situation with less Ca^{++} ionized and more bound to albumin. Thus signs and symptoms of hypocalcemia are more likely to occur when associated with alkalosis but are masked when associated with acidosis.

The serum calcium depends on the balance between calcium input and output from the ECF. Calcium input is determined by the amount ingested and the amount mobilized from the skeletal pool. The average intake of calcium for a North American adult is 600 to 1000 mg/day; the major sources are dairy products. Calcium absorption occurs principally in the duodenum and upper jejunum by an active transport process. Generally less than half of the ingested calcium is absorbed. Calcium loss from the ECF occurs through secretion into the GI tract, urinary excretion, and deposition in bone (Fig. 21-4).

The level of ionized calcium in the ECF is homeostatically maintained within the narrow normal range of 9 to 10.5 mg/dl by an effective balance of bone formation and bone resorption, calcium absorption, and calcium excretion. The principal sites of this regulation are in the bones, kidneys, and GI tract under the control of three hormones: parathyroid hormone, calcitonin, and calcitriol or 1,25-dihydroxycholecalciferol (1,25[OH]$_2$D$_3$).

Parathyroid hormone or *parathormone* (PTH) is a polypeptide secreted by the parathyroid glands, which are located in the neck behind the lobes of the thyroid gland. There are four parathyroid glands: one right superior, one left superior, one right inferior, and one left inferior. PTH secretion occurs in response to hypocalcemia, and it is suppressed by hypercalcemia. PTH acts directly on bone and kidney and indirectly on the GI tract through stimulating dihydroxyvitamin D$_3$ synthesis. PTH stimulates osteoclastic bone resorption, thereby releasing both calcium and phosphate into the ECF. It also stimulates increased renal tubular reabsorption of calcium (thus returning it to the blood) and increases the excretion of phosphate. Finally, PTH acts directly on the kidney to modulate the synthesis of 1,25(OH)$_2$ vitamin D$_3$, the most active metabolite of vitamin D, which in turn causes increased calcium and phosphate absorption from the gut. The net effect is that PTH raises the plasma calcium concentration while having little effect on the plasma phosphate concentration, since changes in the phosphate handling in bone, intestine, and kidney tend to balance out. Excessive PTH causes hypercalcemia and hypophosphatemia, and deficiency of PTH causes hypocalcemia and hyperphosphatemia.

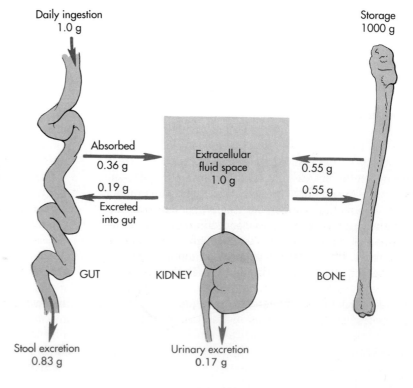

FIG. 21-4   Outline of calcium intake, absorption, excretion, and storage in humans. In conditions of calcium balance, rates of calcium release and uptake into bone are equal and calcium excretion via urine and feces is equal to intake.

Calcitonin is a hormone produced by the C cells, or parafollicular cells, of the thyroid gland. Calcitonin is released in response to hypercalcemia. Its main effect is to lower serum calcium by inhibiting osteoclastic bone resorption. The actual physiologic role of calcitonin in the minute-to-minute regulation of calcium levels has not been clarified. The hypothesis that calcitonin functions to prevent postprandial hypercalcemia and prevents postprandial urinary loss of calcium (especially in the milk-drinking infant) will require further investigation.

Vitamin D and its metabolites are not vitamins but *steroid hormones*. Vitamin D works in concert with PTH in the regulation of serum calcium levels. *Vitamin D₃*, or *cholecalciferol,* is either ingested with the diet* or is synthesized from *7-dehydrocholesterol* in the skin by ultraviolet radiation from the sun. Vitamin D_3 is absorbed in the ileum and jejunum and is subsequently metabolized to its active form, first in the liver and ultimately in the kidney. The metabolism of vitamin D_3 involves sequential hydroxylations. In the liver it is converted to *25-hydroxycholecalciferol* and in the kidney to *calcitriol* or *1,25-dihydroxycholecalciferol* $(1,25[OH]_2D_3)$ (Fig. 21-5). PTH is a potent stimulator of vitamin D_3 activation (as well as hypophosphatemia). The major target sites of $1,25(OH)_2D_3$ are intestine and bone. In the intestine it promotes absorption of ingested calcium and phosphate, and in the bone it acts in concert with PTH to enhance bone resorption, releasing calcium and phosphate into the ECF. The net effect is the elevation of both the serum calcium and phosphate (in contrast to PTH, which only raises the serum calcium). These actions are consistent with the two major functions of $1,25(OH)_2D_3$, which are to ensure the availability of calcium and phosphate for new bone formation and to prevent hypocalcemia and hypophosphatemia. A deficiency of $1,25(OH)_2D_3$ results in inadequate mineralization of bone matrix, called *rickets* in children and *osteomalacia* in adults. The latter condition is common in chronic renal failure (see Chapter 48). Fig. 21-6 illustrates the regulation of calcium and phosphate metabolism by PTH and $1,25(OH)_2D_3$.

Phosphate Homeostasis

Phosphorus is the most abundant constituent of all tissues in the body and is involved in a large number of essential biologic processes. Along with calcium, phosphorus is an essential component of bones and teeth. It is an important constituent of phospholipids that are components of cell membranes. Phosphorus is the primary anion in intracellular fluid, and it is essential in the metabolism of proteins, fats, and carbohydrates. Virtually all metabolic processes require phosphorus, including the provision of high-energy phosphate bonds in the form of adenosine

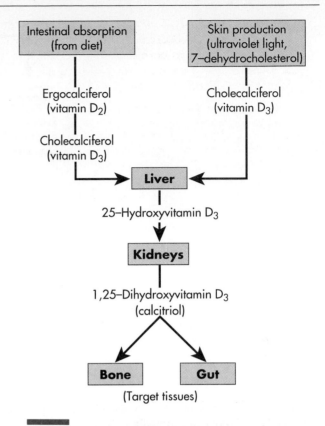

FIG. 21-5 Overview of the metabolism of vitamin D.

triphosphate (ATP). Phosphorus plays an essential role in muscle function, neurologic function, and formation of 2,3-diphosphoglycerate in red blood cells, which facilitate oxygen delivery to the tissues (see Chapter 35). Phosphorus in the form of inorganic phosphate plays a major role in maintaining acid-base balance through its action as a urinary buffer in excreting a large portion of the daily acid load (see Chapter 44).

Of the average 700 g of phosphorus in the body, 85% is in the bones and teeth, 15% is in soft tissues, and 0.1% is in the ECF. Plasma phosphorus exists largely as *inorganic phosphate* ions ($HPO_4^=$ and $H_2PO_4^-$) with only 10% bound to proteins and the remainder freely diffusible and in equilibrium with intracellular and bone phosphorus. Normally the serum phosphate levels range from 2.5 to 4.5 mg/dl (1.8 to 2.6 mEq/L) in an adult. Serum phosphate has a wider physiologic range and varies with age. Infants and young children have higher levels because of the influence of growth hormone and their higher rate of skeletal growth.

The average diet contains 1000 to 1600 mg of phosphorus, and phosphorus is present in a large variety of foods so that it is almost impossible to consume less than is needed. Phosphate absorption occurs largely in the jejunum by passive diffusion and by active transport under the influence of $1,25(OH)_2D_3$. Intestinal absorption varies with intake but can be impaired by certain drugs such as phosphate-binding antacids and by malabsorption syn-

---

*Another source of dietary vitamin D is vitamin D_2 (ergocalciferol), found in irradiated milk, vitamin supplements, fish, and liver.

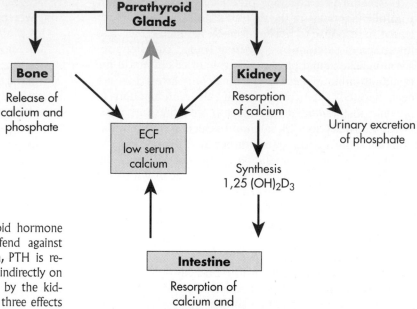

FIG. 21-6 Mechanism of the action of parathyroid hormone (PTH). The principal function of PTH is to defend against hypocalcemia. In response to a low serum calcium, PTH is released, which acts directly on bone and kidneys and indirectly on the gut through stimulating $1,25(OH)_2D_3$ synthesis by the kidneys (most active form of vitamin D hormone). All three effects favor elevation of the serum calcium. PTH secretion is suppressed by elevated levels of serum calcium.

dromes. The major route for phosphate excretion is the kidneys (90%) under the control of PTH. PTH causes increased renal calcium reabsorption and decreased phosphate reabsorption. Because calcium and phosphate interact in a reciprocal relationship, urinary excretion of phosphates increases or decreases in inverse proportion to serum calcium levels. Normally the serum $Ca^{++} \times PO_4$ cross-product (in mg/dl) is maintained at about 30 to 40 (e.g., $9.5 \times 3.5 = 33.25$), allowing precipitation of calcium phosphate salts in the bone but not in the soft tissues. If both the serum calcium and the serum phosphate should rise simultaneously so that their cross-product exceeds 60 to 70, soft tissue deposition of calcium salts, or *metastatic calcification,* can occur. The latter condition is possible when secondary hyperparathyroidism develops in chronic renal failure (see Chapter 47).

Magnesium Homeostasis

Magnesium is the fourth most abundant cation in the body. Like potassium, magnesium is found primarily in the ICF. Magnesium is an important regulator of cellular processes that are essential for life. Its best-defined function is the activation of a wide variety of enzyme systems. For example, all ATPases require magnesium for activation. Magnesium is required for the synthesis of nucleic acids and proteins. Magnesium affects muscle directly by decreasing acetylcholine release at the neuromuscular junction and at sympathetic ganglia, resulting in a curare-like effect. This effect can be antagonized by an excess of calcium or by the simultaneous administration of potassium. Magnesium plays a role in maintaining normal calcium and potassium homeostasis; it facilitates

the transportation of sodium and potassium across the cell membrane (accounting for the secondary hypokalemia that occurs in hypomagnesemia), and it influences intracellular calcium levels through its effect on PTH secretion. Hypomagnesemia interferes with the release of PTH and with its effect on target tissue so that hypocalcemia may develop as a result of hypomagnesemia.

The human body contains about 2000 mEq of magnesium. About 67% of this is in the bones, 31% is intracellular, and less than 2% is in the ECF. The normal serum level of Mg^{++} is 1.8 to 3.0 mg/dl (1.5 to 2.5 mEq/L). Of the total plasma magnesium, about 35% is protein-bound, 55% is free, and 15% is complexed to phosphates, citrates, and other ligands. Only the free ionized Mg^{++} is available for biochemical processes. Normally there is an exchange between ECF Mg^{++} and bone Mg^{++} in response to an excess or deficit of this ion. Mg^{++} exists in two forms inside cells: bound to organic components and in solution, which is in equilibrium with the free Mg^{++} form in plasma. Because most Mg^{++} inside cells is bound to ATP, MgATP is in equilibrium with free Mg^{++} ions. Thus shifts in free Mg^{++} may help to regulate stores of ATP. Because ATP is critical to all metabolic processes, a normal concentration of serum Mg^{++} is essential to maintain stores of this important nucleotide. Considering that magnesium is predominantly an intracellular cation, its serum levels may not always reflect total body stores of magnesium.

The normal diet supplies about 25 mEq of magnesium daily, mostly in meat, green vegetables rich in chlorophyll (a chelator of magnesium), whole grains, and nuts. About 10 mEq of the dietary intake is absorbed in the je-

CAUSES OF HYPOCALCEMIA

PTH DEFICIT

Hypoparathyroidism
  Idiopathic
  Postsurgical*
Hypomagnesemia*

ABNORMAL METABOLISM OF VITAMIN D

Deficiency
  Inadequate intake
  Poor exposure to sunlight
  Malabsorption disease
Impaired 25-hydroxylation in liver
  Alcoholic liver disease
Impaired renal hydroxylation
  Chronic renal failure*
  Hypoparathyroidism
  Hypophosphatemic rickets
  Pseudohypoparathyroidism
  Vitamin D–dependent rickets, type I
Impaired response to $1,25(OH)_2D_3$
  Anticonvulsant drugs
  Vitamin D–dependent rickets, type II

OTHER FACTORS

Alkalosis*
Hypoalbuminemia
Hyperphosphatemia
Neonatal hypocalcemia
Osteoblastic metastases
Medullary thyroid carcinoma
Acute pancreatitis
Drugs
  Chemotherapy
  Phosphates (IV, oral, enema)
  Citrate-buffered blood
  Loop diuretics (e.g., furosemide)
  Magnesium-lowering drugs
  Radiographic contrast media

*Most common conditions causing hypocalcemia.

junum and ileum, an equal amount is excreted in the urine, and the remainder is excreted in the feces. Regulation of magnesium metabolism is not well understood. Under conditions of hypomagnesemia, more magnesium is absorbed in the intestine and less is excreted in the urine. Renal conservation of Mg^{++} is so efficient that the total loss of urinary Mg^{++} can be reduced to only 1 mEq.

Hypocalcemia

Hypocalcemia is defined as a total serum calcium level less than 9 mg/dl (4.5 mEq/L) or ionized calcium less than 4.5 mg/dl. The box above lists some of the causes of hypocalcemia. These include deficiency in the production, secretion, or actions of PTH and/or $1,25(OH)_2D_3$.

Occasionally, hypocalcemia is caused by malabsorption of calcium or hyperphosphatemia. Idiopathic hypoparathyroidism (causing a PTH deficit) is a rare condition that can result from autoimmune destruction of the parathyroid glands. The serum calcium is low, serum phosphate is normal or increased, and $1,25(OH)_2D_3$ is low because of the lack of PTH. Hypoparathyroidism may be secondary to accidental removal of the parathyroid glands with thyroidectomy, but this is less common today since hyperthyroidism is more commonly treated by radioactive iodine ablation rather than surgery. More commonly, hypoparathyroidism follows a subtotal parathyroidectomy although the hypocalcemia is generally only transitory until the remaining parathyroid tissue can increase PTH secretion. A deficiency of magnesium (<1 mg/dl) can cause hypocalcemia by interfering with PTH secretion, as well as its peripheral action.

Hypocalcemia is a common feature of vitamin D deficiency that may occur because of inadequate intake, lack of exposure to sunlight, or malabsorptive disease. Some causes of intestinal malabsorption include sprue, chronic pancreatitis, partial gastrectomy, intestinal bypass surgery for obesity, biliary cirrhosis, and prolonged abuse of laxatives. Alcoholic liver disease may interfere with the 25-hydroxylation of vitamin D_3, and a number of factors may interfere with the final hydroxylation to $1,25(OH)_2D_3$ in the kidney. Chronic renal failure is the most common cause of hypocalcemia. The hypocalcemia is the result of several factors, including hyperphosphatemia (causing a reciprocal drop in serum calcium), impaired sensitivity of the skeleton to the bone-resorbing action of PTH, reduced production of $1,25(OH)_2D_3$ by surviving renal tissue, and decreased intestinal absorption. Patients develop secondary hyperparathyroidism and hyperplasia of the parathyroid glands, and with autonomous parathyroid function they may eventually develop hypercalcemia and metastatic calcification (see Chapter 47). Hypophosphatemic rickets, pseudohypoparathyroidism, and vitamin D–dependent rickets (types I and II) are rare hereditary disorders in which there is either impaired production of $1,25(OH)_2D_3$ or resistance to its effect. Hypocalcemia, rickets, or osteomalacia may occur in patients with epilepsy who are receiving treatment with anticonvulsant drugs, which interfere with the peripheral actions of $1,25(OH)_2D_3$.

Alkalosis can cause symptoms of hypocalcemia as a result of decreased ionized Ca^{++} in the serum although the total serum calcium may be normal. Hypoalbuminemia, as occurs in the nephrotic syndrome or cirrhosis of the liver, results in decreased total serum calcium although the ionized fraction may be normal. Some causes of hyperphosphatemia that lead to hypocalcemia include administration of phosphates and hematologic malignancies either because of high cell turnover as part of the malignancy or because of cell destruction when chemother-

HYPOCALCEMIA: CLINICAL FEATURES

SIGNS/SYMPTOMS

Cardiovascular
ECG changes
Dysrhythmias
Decreased sensitivity to digitalis
Neuromuscular
Paresthesias (circumoral, hands, feet)
Hyperactive reflexes
Tetany
Trousseau's sign
Chvostek's sign
Muscle tics/spasms of face, extremities
Laryngospasm
Central nervous system
Altered mood, impaired memory, confusion
Convulsive seizures
Gastrointestinal
Diarrhea, loose stools
Malabsorption and steatorrhea
Skin
Dry, scaly skin
Coarse, dry hair
Brittle nails
Ocular
Cataracts

LABORATORY FINDINGS

Total serum calcium <8.5 mg/dl
Evaluate serum albumin: suspect ionic hypocalcemia if decreased Ca in presence of normal albumin
Evaluate serum pH: suspect ionic hypocalcemia if normal Ca in presence of severe alkalosis (pH >7.55)
Ionic serum calcium <4.5 mg/dl

Ca^{++} mobilization from bone), and certain radiographic contrast media (form complexes with Ca^{++}).

Clinical features

Symptoms of hypocalcemia depend on the degree, duration, and rate of its development. Hypocalcemia may be asymptomatic. The box at left outlines the clinical manifestations of hypocalcemia that are primarily caused by an increase in neuromuscular irritability. Tetany is the most characteristic sign of hypocalcemia. *Tetany* is characterized by involuntary muscle spasms. It may involve muscles of the upper and lower extremities, causing carpopedal spasms, and paresthesias of the hands and feet and around the mouth. Latent tetany can be demonstrated by testing for Trousseau's sign. A blood pressure cuff is placed on the upper arm and inflated above systolic pressure for 1 to 4 minutes. *Carpopedal spasm* (adducted thumb, flexed wrist and metacarpophalangeal joints, and extended interphalangeal joints with fingers together) indicates a positive *Trousseau's sign*. Latent tetany may also be demonstrated by tapping over the facial nerve just anterior to the ear and observing for ipsilateral contraction of the facial muscles, called *Chvostek's sign* (Fig. 21-7). Hyperactive deep tendon reflexes are additional

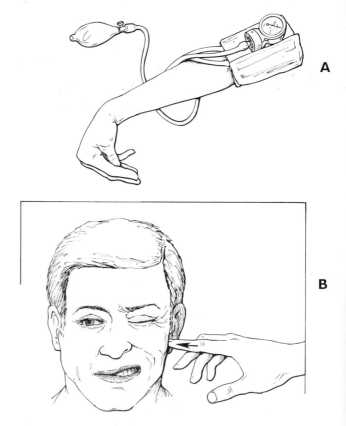

FIG. 21-7 Checking for latent tetany. **A,** Trousseau's sign: carpal spasm induced by inflating a blood pressure cuff above systolic pressure. **B,** Chvostek's sign: contraction of facial muscles induced by a light tap over the facial nerve.

apy is instituted. Hypocalcemia may develop in neonates who are fed cow's milk. The cause has been attributed to two mechanisms: physiologic hypofunction of the parathyroids and hyperphosphatemia from the high phosphate content of cow's milk compared with human milk. Hypocalcemia may develop in patients with malignant neoplasms of the prostate, lung, and breast with osteoblastic (bone-forming) metastases. Medullary thyroid carcinoma may cause hypocalcemia if calcitonin is secreted by the carcinoma. Acute pancreatitis may result in severe hypocalcemia, possibly the result of precipitation of calcium soaps in the abdomen caused by enzymatic fat necrosis. Multiple transfusions of banked blood buffered with sodium citrate may cause hypocalcemia. The excess citrate not only can bind calcium ions, but also may cause alkalosis when it is metabolized to form bicarbonate. Other drugs that can lower serum calcium include loop diuretics (increase Ca^{++} excretion), drugs that lower magnesium such as cisplatin and gentamycin (decrease

signs that may be elicited indicating increased neuromuscular irritability. Severe hypocalcemia may result in convulsive seizures or in laryngospasm.

Patients with hypocalcemia usually experience a variety of neuropsychiatric disturbances including irritability, emotional instability, impairment of memory, and confusion. Patients with hypocalcemia often have diarrhea or loose stools and may even develop intestinal malabsorption and steatorrhea (excess fecal fat). Prolonged hypocalcemia, as seen in idiopathic hypoparathyroidism, may cause changes in the skin, hair, nails, teeth, and lenses. The skin may be coarse, dry, and scaly, and alopecia may develop with patchy or absent eyelashes and eyebrows. The teeth in young children may erupt late and appear hypoplastic. Cataracts may develop within a few years of untreated hypocalcemia.

Hypocalcemia classically produces prolongation of the QT interval and ST segment, which are frequently present when serum calcium is 7 mg/dl and consistently present when serum calcium is 6 mg/dl or less (Chan, Gill, 1990; Fig. 21-8). Heart block and dysrhythmias may develop. The heart may be refractory to digitalis.

Treatment

Treatment of hypocalcemia focuses on correcting the imbalance and the underlying cause. Severe symptomatic hypocalcemia with tetany or seizures is a medical emergency and is treated with 10 ml of 10% calcium gluconate administered intravenously over a 4-minute period followed by an additional calcium infusion (e.g., 30 to 60 ml of 10% calcium gluconate mixed in 1000 ml of D_5W) given over 6 to 12 hours (Kokko, Tannen, 1990). The serum calcium and ECG should be monitored frequently during the treatment to avoid hypercalcemia. The most common situation associated with severe symptomatic hypocalcemia is following parathyroidectomy.

Chronic mild hypocalcemia is treated by administering calcium salts and vitamin D. Calcium salts are available as calcium gluconate, calcium lactate, or calcium carbonate. Giving 10 to 15 g of calcium gluconate or calcium lactate daily is usually necessary. Vitamin D is given in doses of 50,000 to 150,000 units/day. 1,25-Dihydroxycholecalciferol is given in doses of 0.25 μg/day. When patients are treated with the proper combination of calcium and vitamin D, serum calcium can be maintained within the normal range. The treatment of the calcium and phosphate disturbances associated with chronic renal failure is discussed in Chapter 48.

Hypercalcemia

Hypercalcemia exists when the total serum calcium exceeds 10.5 mg/dl (5.5 mEq/L). In 90% of the cases, hypercalcemia is caused by either primary hyperparathyroidism or cancer. The causes of hypercalcemia are outlined in the first box on p. 278.

Many conditions may lead to hypercalcemia, but PTH

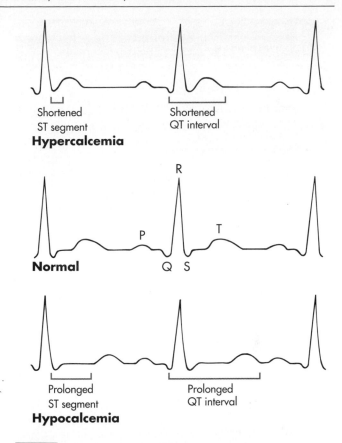

FIG. 21-8   ECG changes in calcium imbalances. In hypocalcemia the QT interval and ST segment may be prolonged. Hypercalcemia causes shortening of the QT interval and ST segment.

excess is by far the most common cause. Excessive production of PTH may result from primary hyperparathyroidism or secretion of a PTH-like peptide by nonparathyroid malignancies. In addition, hypercalcemia may be associated with severe secondary hyperparathyroidism observed in chronic renal failure and after dialysis or renal transplantation. Primary hyperparathyroidism is usually caused by a benign adenoma of the parathyroid glands (but may be caused by hyperplasia of all four glands). The incidence has risen dramatically since the introduction of automated analysis and frequent measurement of calcium by laboratories. The condition occurs more frequently in women than in men, and the occurrence rises with age. Hypercalcemia results from the PTH-mediated mobilization of calcium from bone and the PTH-enhanced renal reabsorption of calcium. Some patients have elevated $1,25(OH)_2D_3$, which in turn causes increased intestinal absorption that may cause *hypercalciuria* (excessive loss of calcium in the urine). PTH causes increased renal phosphate excretion so that patients with primary hyperparathyroidism often have either a low or normal serum phosphate. They also have increased renal cAMP, and measurements of this nucleotide are often used to diagnose primary hyperparathyroidism.

A malignant neoplasm is the single most common cause

CAUSES OF HYPERCALCEMIA

HYPERPARATHYROIDISM

Primary hyperparathyroidism
Secondary hyperparathyroidism
   Chronic renal failure
   Vitamin D malabsorption

MALIGNANCIES

Solid tumors without bone metastasis
   Squamous cell carcinoma of the lung, head, and neck; carcinoma of the ovary, kidney
Solid tumors with bone metastasis
   Carcinoma of the breast
Hematologic malignancies
   Multiple myeloma
   Lymphomas
   Acute leukemia

ABNORMAL VITAMIN D METABOLISM

Sarcoidosis
Tuberculosis

ENDOCRINE

Hyperthyroidism
Adrenal insufficiency

PROLONGED IMMOBILIZATION

DRUGS

Thiazide diuretics
Lithium
Vitamin A intoxication
Vitamin D intoxication
$1,25(OH)_2D_3$ intoxication
Milk-alkali syndrome

HYPERCALCEMIA: CLINICAL FEATURES

SIGNS AND SYMPTOMS

Cardiovascular
  Hypertension
  ECG changes
  Dysrhythmias
    Bradycardia
    Heart block
  Increased sensitivity to digitalis
Neuromuscular
  Generalized muscular weakness
  Depressed deep tendon reflexes
  Metastatic calcification in soft tissues
Central nervous system
  Impaired concentration, confusion
  Altered state of consciousness:
      lethargy → stupor → coma
Gastrointestinal
  Polydipsia
  Anorexia
  Nausea and vomiting
  Weight loss
  Constipation
Renal
  Polyuria
  Nephrolithiasis
  Nephrocalcinosis
  Renal failure
Skeletal (secondary to hyperparathyroidism)
  Bone resorption
  Formation of bone cysts
  Subperiosteal erosion of long bone (Fig. 21-9)
  Osteitis fibrosa cystica
Skin
  Pruritus
Ocular
  Band keratopathy

LABORATORY FINDINGS

Total serum calcium >10.5 mg/dl
  Evaluate serum albumin and calculate true serum calcium

of hypercalcemia, and this complication often occurs during an advanced stage of the disease. Common malignancies associated with hypercalcemia include squamous cell carcinoma of the lung, head, or neck; carcinoma of the kidney, ovary, or pancreas; breast cancer; and hematologic malignancies such as multiple myeloma, lymphomas (especially T cell lymphoma), and acute leukemia. These malignancies can be divided into three classes as shown in the box above: (1) solid tumors without bone metastasis, called *humoral hypercalcemia of malignancy,* (2) solid tumors with bone metastasis, and (3) hematologic malignancies. Two mechanisms causing the hypercalcemia of malignancy are localized bone destruction from osteolytic metastasis and humoral factors that stimulate osteoclastic bone resorption. In the past it was assumed that tumor invasion of the bone with localized destruction was the predominant mechanism causing

the hypercalcemia of malignancy. There is certainly extensive bone destruction in patients with multiple myeloma, lymphomas, and breast cancer with bone metastasis. However, recent research has revealed that humoral factors produced by these tumors play a major role in causing the hypercalcemia of malignancy whether or not there is bone invasion or bone metastasis (Chan, Gill, 1990). Some of these humoral factors include PTH-related peptide (PTHrP), tumor necrosis factor (TNF), transforming growth factors (TGF-alpha and -beta), interleukin-1 (IL-1), prostaglandin E, and lymphotoxin. All of these humoral factors cause increased bone resorption and, when PTHrP is present, increased renal calcium reabsorption. In addition, some lymphoma cells synthesize $1,25(OH)_2D_3$, resulting in both increased osteoclastic bone resorption and increased gut absorption of calcium.

Hypercalcemia occasionally occurs in sarcoidosis and in pulmonary tuberculosis, and the mechanism involves extrarenal synthesis of $1,25(OH)_2D_3$. Hypercalcemia occurs in 8% to 22% of patients with hyperthyroidism, but the serum calcium is only mildly elevated (Chan, Gill, 1990). There is increased bone turnover in hyperthyroidism. PTH secretion is suppressed, as well as $1,25(OH)_2D_3$, accounting for the characteristically high urinary and fecal calcium. Hypercalcemia sometimes occurs in adrenal insufficiency (Addison's disease) caused by glucocorticoid deficiency and ECF volume deficit. Glucocorticoid deficiency stimulates prostaglandin synthesis and increased bone resorption. The ECF volume deficit decreases the glomerular filtration rate so that more of the filtered calcium is reabsorbed. Prolonged immobilization, as occurs in persons with quadriplegia or paraplegia, invariably leads to bone loss and hypercalciuria because of the uncoupling of bone remodeling so that bone resorption exceeds bone formation. Usually the calcium released from bone is excreted in the urine and does not lead to hypercalcemia.

A number of drugs can cause hypercalcemia. Thiazide diuretics act directly to increase calcium release from bone and increase its renal tubular reabsorption. Chronic lithium administration, commonly used to treat manic-depressive illness, is sometimes associated with both mild hypercalcemia and hypermagnesemia. Excess intake of vitamin A results in increased bone resorption. Excess intake of the standard vitamin D_2 (ergocalciferol) or the active $1,25(OH)_2D_3$ (Rocaltrol) can lead to hypercalcemia and hypercalciuria. The milk-alkali syndrome can occur in persons who ingest large amounts of milk and alkali (e.g., sodium bicarbonate or calcium carbonate) to relieve the symptoms of peptic ulcer disease. The syndrome is characterized by alkalosis, hypercalcemia, hyperphosphatemia, soft tissue deposition of calcium salts, and progressive renal failure. Because this form of treatment for peptic ulcers is no longer used, the syndrome is seldom encountered.

Clinical features

Signs and symptoms of hypercalcemia vary greatly, depending on the rapidity of onset and the degree of elevation of calcium levels. In mild cases, patients may be completely asymptomatic and the hypercalcemia is discovered through routine laboratory investigation. On the other hand, in severe cases with marked elevation of serum calcium levels, patients deteriorate rapidly and become dehydrated, confused, and lethargic. The clinical features are summarized in the second box on p. 278.

Hypercalcemia depresses neuromuscular irritability and release of acetylcholine at the myoneural junction, giving rise to symptoms such as muscular weakness,

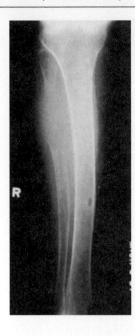

FIG. 21-9 Lesions of osteitis fibrosa cystica in the tibia and fibula of a patient with hyperparathyroidism.

anorexia, nausea, and constipation. Neuropsychiatric signs may be prominent when the serum calcium is greatly elevated (>15 mg/dl), and the patient may show mental confusion, slurred speech, and lethargy progressing to coma. Polyuria and polydipsia, with clinical signs of ECF volume deficit, may accompany excessive urinary loss of calcium, phosphate, and sodium. Renal colic caused by *nephrolithiasis* (kidney stones) is common. Widespread precipitation of calcium salts in the kidney, *nephrocalcinosis,* may lead to obstructive uropathy and renal failure. When bone disease is present, x-ray studies may show a generalized decrease in bone density, fractures, cysts, and subperiosteal bone erosion (Fig. 21-9). Precipitation of calcium salts in the skin may cause *pruritus* (itching) and in the eye, band keratopathy (see Fig. 47-4). Cardiovascular changes in hypercalcemia include systolic hypertension, bradycardia, shortening of the QT interval and the ST segment (see Fig. 21-8), and dysrhythmias. Cardiac arrest may occur when the serum calcium is about 18 mg/dl (hypercalcemic crisis). Hypercalcemia can also precipitate digitalis toxicity, since there is increased sensitivity to its effects.

The diagnosis of primary hyperparathyroidism is based on the demonstration of a high serum level of calcium and a low level of phosphate together with an elevated level of PTH. It is important to measure the serum albumin, since hypoalbuminemia may mask an increase in ionized calcium. PTH radioimmunoassay directed to the intact molecule or its *N*-terminal portion is the most reliable test. In cases other than primary hyperparathyroidism, serum phosphate levels may be elevated and PTH depressed. The urine may show an increased calcium content (normally <275 mg/day in males and <250 mg/day in females), and urinary excretion of cyclic AMP (cAMP) is increased in primary hyperparathyroidism, as well as in some other causes of hypercalcemia.

MANAGEMENT OF HYPERCALCEMIA

GENERAL MEASURES

Hydration
Restriction of calcium intake
Withholding of drugs that potentiate hypercalcemia (vitamin A and D; thiazide diuretics)
Maintenance of weight bearing/avoidance of immobilization
Dialysis

ENHANCE URINARY CALCIUM EXCRETION

IV saline
Diuretics
    Furosemide
    Ethacrynic acid

INHIBIT BONE RESORPTION

Calcitonin
Diphosphonates
Glucocorticoids
Plicamycin (Mithracin)
Gallium nitrate
Phosphates

TREAT UNDERLYING DISEASE

CAUSES OF HYPOPHOSPHATEMIA

DECREASED INTAKE/INTESTINAL ABSORPTION

Deficiency of dietary phosphate
Antacid abuse
Various malabsorption states
Vitamin D deficiency

SHIFT FROM ECF INTO CELLS/BONE

Respiratory alkalosis
Total parenteral nutrition (TPN)
Diabetic ketoacidosis
Glucose/insulin infusion
Nutritional recovery syndrome
Severe burns
Hungry bone syndrome
Alcohol withdrawal

INCREASED URINARY LOSSES

Hyperparathyroidism
Renal tubular disorders

Treatment

When possible, the treatment of hypercalcemia is directed toward reversing the underlying pathogenic disorder. For example, primary hyperthyroidism is usually treated by surgery, and antineoplastic therapy may improve malignancy-related hypercalcemia. Symptomatic or severe hypercalcemia (>14 mg/dl) requires medical treatment as outlined in the box above. Treatment goals are directed toward improving hydration, promoting urinary excretion of calcium, and inhibiting bone resorption. The first priority in severe hypercalcemia is hydration with isotonic saline at the rate of 3 to 4 L/day until ECF volume is restored. The saline also promotes urinary calcium excretion by inhibiting its reabsorption. Once the ECF is restored, a diuretic such as furosemide is given to promote further excretion of calcium. In life-threatening hypercalcemia, especially in persons with renal insufficiency, hemodialysis or peritoneal dialysis with a dialysate containing little or no calcium may rapidly restore serum calcium to normal levels.

A variety of drugs may be used to inhibit bone resorption, the usual source of the excess serum calcium. Calcitonin inhibits bone resorption and increases renal calcium excretion. This drug may be given when a rapid decrease of serum calcium is required. Diphosphonates, such as etidronate or pamidronate, are potent inhibitors of osteoclastic bone resorption and are of great value in the treat-

ment of primary hyperthyroidism and cancer. Gallium nitrate reduces the osteolytic response to PTH and is used to treat cancer-related hypercalcemia. It is a nephrotoxic drug, so the patient must be well hydrated and have adequate renal function before taking this drug. Plicamycin (Mithracin) is a cytotoxic antibiotic that inhibits bone resorption, but it is rarely given because of its high toxicity. Glucocorticoids block bone resorption, decrease intestinal absorption of calcium, and increase its urinary excretion and are quite effective in the treatment of hypercalcemia from a number of causes. Finally, sodium phosphate can rapidly decrease serum calcium when given intravenously but is potentially dangerous, since a fatal hypocalcemia could result. Another danger is metastatic calcification caused by precipitation of calcium phosphate in the soft tissues. These risks are diminished when it is given orally.

Hypophosphatemia

Hypophosphatemia is defined as a serum phosphate level less than 2.5 mg/dl (normal, 2.5 to 4.5 mg/dl) although symptoms do not usually occur until serum phosphate is less than 1.0 mg/dl. A low serum phosphate level does not necessarily indicate a deficiency of total body phosphate since only 1% is in the ECF. Because phosphate is available in so many foods and is easily absorbed, hypophosphatemia is unusual unless there is (1) reduced oral intake, (2) a shift of phosphate from the ECF into the cells/bone, or (3) excessive renal loss of phosphate. Some of the most common causes of hypophosphatemia are listed in the box above.

Phosphate absorption is under the influence of $1,25(OH)_2D_3$, and renal phosphate excretion is under the control of PTH. Thus vitamin D deficiency, intestinal malabsorption, and hyperparathyroidism are causes of hypophosphatemia. Excess ingestion of antacids (e.g., aluminum hydroxide) for the treatment of peptic ulcer disease, for example, can cause hypophosphatemia. The antacids bind phosphate in the gut, after which it is excreted in the feces. Fanconi's syndrome is a descriptive phrase for a group of inherited or acquired renal tubular transport disorders that may result in excess phosphate excretion (as well as bicarbonate, glucose, and amino acids), resulting in hypophosphatemia and metabolic acidosis.

One of the most common causes of severe hypophosphatemia is prolonged, intense hyperventilation causing respiratory alkalosis. Gram-negative bacteremia, alcohol withdrawal, heat stroke, and acute salicylate poisoning are examples of clinical situations leading to respiratory alkalosis. Intracellular alkalosis occurs in respiratory alkalosis, because CO_2 is readily diffusible across the cell membrane but bicarbonate is not. Intracellular alkalosis activates phosphofructokinase and increases phosphorylation of glucose, and serum phosphate moves into the cells to be consumed in the process. Total parenteral nutrition without adequate phosphate replacement, treatment of diabetic ketoacidosis with glucose and insulin, and refeeding persons with severe protein-calorie malnutrition all cause phosphate movement into cells as anabolism occurs and can result in severe hypophosphatemia.

Severe hypophosphatemia is common in patients with extensive burns. Because nearly all severely burned patients hyperventilate, respiratory alkalosis and the resulting accelerated glycolysis are a likely cause.

Increased deposition of calcium phosphate salts in bone following parathyroidectomy, called the *hungry bone syndrome,* is a factor in both the hypophosphatemia and hypocalcemia frequently seen after this surgery.

Finally, hypophosphatemia develops in about half of patients hospitalized for withdrawal from alcohol abuse (Schrier, 1986). Several factors are responsible for the phosphate depletion in alcoholics, including poor dietary intake, vomiting, diarrhea, ingestion of antacids, and hypomagnesemia. Chronic alcoholism causes magnesium deficiency, which in turn may cause phosphaturia. These patients may also be given glucose infusions, causing phosphate to move from the ECF into cells.

Clinical features

Most of the clinical features of hypophosphatemia (see box at right) can be attributed to the deficiency of adenosine triphosphate (ATP) and/or 2,3-diphosphoglycerate (2,3-DPG). A deficiency of ATP impairs active cellular processes that require it as an energy source, and a deficiency of 2,3-DPG impairs oxygen delivery to the tissues.

Hypophosphatemia may be associated with depletion

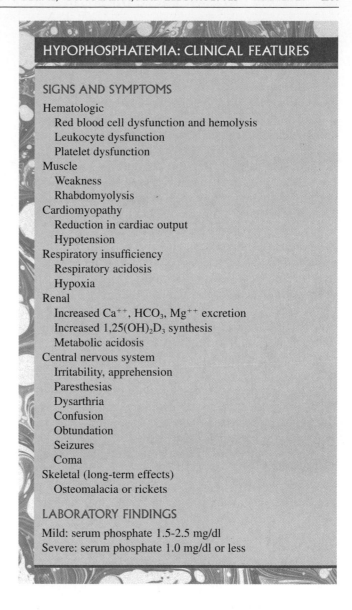

HYPOPHOSPHATEMIA: CLINICAL FEATURES

SIGNS AND SYMPTOMS

Hematologic
  Red blood cell dysfunction and hemolysis
  Leukocyte dysfunction
  Platelet dysfunction
Muscle
  Weakness
  Rhabdomyolysis
Cardiomyopathy
  Reduction in cardiac output
  Hypotension
Respiratory insufficiency
  Respiratory acidosis
  Hypoxia
Renal
  Increased Ca^{++}, HCO_3, Mg^{++} excretion
  Increased $1,25(OH)_2D_3$ synthesis
  Metabolic acidosis
Central nervous system
  Irritability, apprehension
  Paresthesias
  Dysarthria
  Confusion
  Obtundation
  Seizures
  Coma
Skeletal (long-term effects)
  Osteomalacia or rickets

LABORATORY FINDINGS

Mild: serum phosphate 1.5-2.5 mg/dl
Severe: serum phosphate 1.0 mg/dl or less

of ATP in RBCs, WBCs, and platelets, reducing their function and survival time. Leukocyte dysfunction results in impaired chemotaxis, phagocytosis, and intracellular killing, with consequent increased susceptibility to bacterial and fungal infections. Platelet dysfunction may result in a bleeding tendency because of impaired aggregation. The RBC is the only tissue in the body that produces 2,3-DPG. Severe phosphate deficiency can reduce RBC content of 2,3-DPG, causing RBCs to become rigid spherocytes that hemolyze easily and whose shape impairs capillary perfusion. Both ATP and 2,3-DPG facilitate dissociation of oxyhemoglobin in the RBC and promote oxygen delivery to the tissues. Reduced 2,3-DPG and ATP in the RBC enhance affinity of oxygen for hemoglobin and reduce tissue oxygenation.

In the muscles, severe phosphate depletion may be associated with muscle weakness manifested as respiratory insufficiency when the respiratory muscles are affected and as congestive cardiomyopathy when the heart muscle is affected. *Rhabdomyolysis,* disintegration of skeletal muscle fibers with excretion of myoglobin in the urine, may occur in persons with chronic alcoholism who become acutely hypophosphatemic during the course of alcohol withdrawal.

Phosphate depletion has multiple effects on renal function, including increased excretion of urinary calcium, bicarbonate, and magnesium and increased synthesis of $1,25(OH)_2D_3$. Severe hypophosphatemia may also result in metabolic acidosis through two mechanisms. The hypophosphatemia results in decreased urinary phosphate excretion, thereby limiting H^+ excretion as NaH_2PO_4. The conversion of ammonia (NH_3) to ammonium (NH_4), another mechanism for acid excretion, is also depressed in phosphate deficiency.

Central nervous system function may be impaired in hypophosphatemia, with symptoms of irritability, paresthesias, weakness, and encephalopathy progressing from confusion to coma. These symptoms usually occur in the setting of refeeding (e.g., victims of famine in a war-torn country) or hyperalimentation-induced hypophosphatemia that develops over the course of 8 to 10 days (Knochel, 1994).

Hypophosphatemia causes calcium and phosphate to be mobilized from bones and muscle and causes hypercalciuria. A consequence of long-term phosphate depletion includes osteomalacia or rickets.

Treatment

Treatment of hypophosphatemia should be primarily preventive. Adequate phosphate supplements must be given when hyperalimentation containing high glucose concentrations is administered. The treatment of hypophosphatemia varies with the cause. Phosphate depletion is rapidly reversible by correcting the underlying disorder and by phosphate therapy. Milk is an excellent source of phosphorus, supplying about 240 mg per cup. Alternately, sodium and/or potassium phosphate tablets containing 250 mg of inorganic phosphate can be given in divided doses. In rare circumstances, phosphate may be given intravenously for severe hypophosphatemia. However, hypocalcemia and metastatic calcification may result as a complication.

Hyperphosphatemia

In adults, hyperphosphatemia is defined as an elevation of serum phosphate above 4.5 mg/dl. Hyperphosphatemia may be caused by decreased renal phosphate excretion, redistribution from the ICF to the ECF, and increased intake and intestinal absorption. The degree of hyperphosphatemia is a function of the rate of entry of phosphate into the ECF and the renal excretion of phosphate. If renal function is normal, clinically significant hyperphosphatemia seldom occurs. Some of the most common conditions causing hyperphosphatemia are listed in the box at right, above.

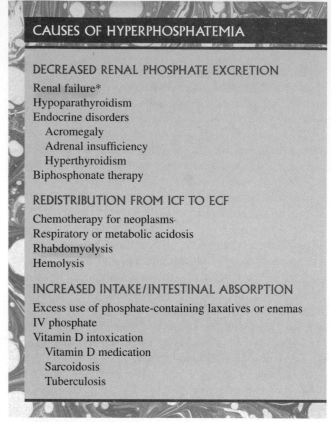

CAUSES OF HYPERPHOSPHATEMIA

DECREASED RENAL PHOSPHATE EXCRETION

Renal failure*
Hypoparathyroidism
Endocrine disorders
   Acromegaly
   Adrenal insufficiency
   Hyperthyroidism
Biphosphonate therapy

REDISTRIBUTION FROM ICF TO ECF

Chemotherapy for neoplasms
Respiratory or metabolic acidosis
Rhabdomyolysis
Hemolysis

INCREASED INTAKE/INTESTINAL ABSORPTION

Excess use of phosphate-containing laxatives or enemas
IV phosphate
Vitamin D intoxication
   Vitamin D medication
   Sarcoidosis
   Tuberculosis

*Most common cause.

Acute or chronic renal failure is by far the most important cause of hyperphosphatemia, and it regularly occurs when the glomerular filtration rate (GFR) falls to 25% to 50% of normal (see Chapter 47). Decreased PTH secretion in hypoparathyroidism results in decreased urinary phosphate excretion. Acromegaly or administration of growth hormone causes modest hyperphosphatemia. Finally, biphosphonate therapy for malignancy-related hypercalcemia may result in hyperphosphatemia as a complication because of increased renal tubular reabsorption of phosphate.

Because phosphate is largely contained within cells, conditions causing transcellular shifts from the ICF to the ECF can result in hyperphosphatemia. Chemotherapy, especially for hematologic malignancies, causes cell lysis and the release of phosphate. Muscle contains large phosphate stores, and the breakdown of muscle in rhabdomyolysis, as sometimes occurs in withdrawal from alcohol, can cause hyperphosphatemia. Acidosis reduces phosphorylation and may cause phosphates to diffuse out of the cell. Phosphate is likewise released from RBCs in hemolysis.

Hyperphosphatemia may be produced from excess intake of phosphate-containing laxatives or enemas (e.g., Sal-Hepatica or Fleet enema) or from IV phosphate administration. Overmedication with vitamin D or the abnormal secretion of vitamin D in sarcoidosis or tuberculosis can cause an increased intestinal absorption of phosphate.

Clinical features

Very few signs and symptoms can be attributed to hyperphosphatemia alone. When symptoms do occur they can usually be attributed to the accompanying hypocalcemia. An acute rise in serum phosphate tends to result in an acute fall in serum calcium because of the reciprocal relationship of these two ions. Symptoms of hypocalcemia include paresthesias, muscle spasms, and tetany (see previous discussion of hypocalcemia). However, renal failure patients rarely have symptoms of hypocalcemia, since they generally have a metabolic acidosis that causes more serum calcium to exist in the ionized form. Long-term consequences of hyperphosphatemia may include precipitation of calcium phosphate salts around joints and in the soft tissues of the body.

Treatment

Therapy for hyperphosphatemia is directed at the underlying cause. The hyperphosphatemia of renal failure is treated by restriction of dietary phosphate and by the administration of calcium carbonate, a phosphate binder. Phosphate-binding antacids such as aluminum hydroxide (Amphojel) or aluminum carbonate (Basaljel) are used less frequently than in the past because of the danger of aluminum toxicity. Magnesium hydroxide (Maalox) should never be used for the treatment of hyperphosphatemia in patients with renal failure since a fatal hypermagnesemia could result.

Hypomagnesemia

Hypomagnesemia is defined as serum magnesium less than 1.5 mEq/L or 1.8 mg/dl, the lower limits of normal. Like other electrolytes that are largely intracellular, serum values of Mg^{++} may not accurately reflect total body deficits or excesses. When symptomatic hypomagnesemia is present, the serum magnesium is usually less than 1 mEq/L. Magnesium deficiency rarely occurs alone. When any of the three major intracellular ions (potassium, magnesium, or phosphate) is lost, losses of the others usually follow. Hypocalcemia also frequently accompanies hypomagnesemia since a magnesium deficit interferes with the release of PTH. The most common cause of hypomagnesemia is chronic alcoholism and alcoholic withdrawal. Studies have shown that hypomagnesemia is also common in critically ill patients, although it has often been overlooked in this population (Duarte, 1990). Hypomagnesemia results from insufficient dietary intake, excessive loss in GI fluids or urine, or movement from the ECF to the ICF (see box at right, above).

It is difficult to produce clinically symptomatic magnesium deficiency by dietary deficiency alone unless other factors such as GI or renal losses occur simultaneously; a subclinical deficiency is more likely. However,

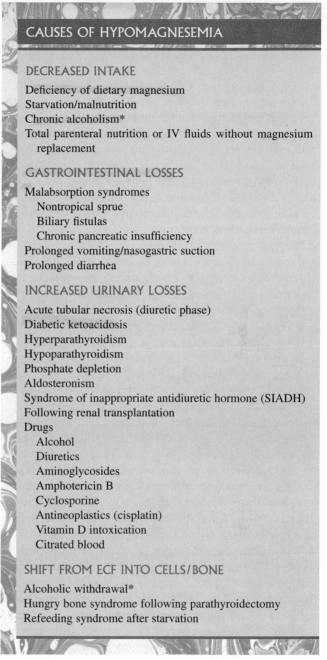

CAUSES OF HYPOMAGNESEMIA

DECREASED INTAKE

Deficiency of dietary magnesium
Starvation/malnutrition
Chronic alcoholism*
Total parenteral nutrition or IV fluids without magnesium replacement

GASTROINTESTINAL LOSSES

Malabsorption syndromes
  Nontropical sprue
  Biliary fistulas
  Chronic pancreatic insufficiency
Prolonged vomiting/nasogastric suction
Prolonged diarrhea

INCREASED URINARY LOSSES

Acute tubular necrosis (diuretic phase)
Diabetic ketoacidosis
Hyperparathyroidism
Hypoparathyroidism
Phosphate depletion
Aldosteronism
Syndrome of inappropriate antidiuretic hormone (SIADH)
Following renal transplantation
Drugs
  Alcohol
  Diuretics
  Aminoglycosides
  Amphotericin B
  Cyclosporine
  Antineoplastics (cisplatin)
  Vitamin D intoxication
  Citrated blood

SHIFT FROM ECF INTO CELLS/BONE

Alcoholic withdrawal*
Hungry bone syndrome following parathyroidectomy
Refeeding syndrome after starvation

*Most common causes.

magnesium deficiency can occur under conditions of prolonged malnutrition (e.g., chronic alcoholics who eat poorly), prolonged starvation, or prolonged administration of magnesium-free parenteral fluids without oral food intake.

Intestinal malabsorption is a common cause of magnesium loss, especially if there is steatorrhea. Both calcium and magnesium form insoluble fatty acid soaps that are then excreted in the feces, resulting in both hypomagnesemia and hypocalcemia. Prolonged diarrhea in inflammatory bowel disease (e.g., Crohn's disease or ulcerative colitis), as well as prolonged vomiting or nasogastric suction, can cause magnesium depletion.

Excess renal loss of magnesium can occur during the diuretic phase of acute tubular necrosis (a type of acute renal failure) or from the diuresis following renal transplantation. Renal transplant patients are also given cyclosporine to prevent organ rejection, and this drug causes increased renal tubular excretion of magnesium. The most common cause of excess urinary loss of magnesium is the prolonged administration of diuretics, especially loop diuretics, such as furosemide or ethacrynic acid. Excessive urinary loss of magnesium also occurs in diabetic ketoacidosis, hyperaldosteronism, primary hyperparathyroidism and other hypercalcemic states, and the syndrome of inappropriate antidiuretic hormone (SIADH). Hypomagnesemia is frequently seen in patients with hypoparathyroidism who have increased loss of Mg^{++} in their urine and feces. Other drugs causing excess renal magnesium wasting include aminoglycosides (e.g., gentamycin, tobramycin), amphotericin B, cisplatin (an antineoplastic drug), and vitamin D overdosage. Transfusion with citrated blood may cause both hypomagnesemia and hypocalcemia because of the formation of complexes with the citrate.

Several factors play a role in the hypomagnesemia associated with chronic alcoholism and alcohol withdrawal. Chronic alcoholics are often malnourished from poor dietary intake and have reduced intake of magnesium-containing foods. Diarrhea is common in alcoholism, resulting in loss of magnesium-rich intestinal fluids. Alcohol has a direct effect on the kidney, causing increased urinary excretion of magnesium. The mild hypomagnesemia associated with chronic alcohol abuse may become severe during alcoholic withdrawal because of a shift of magnesium into the cells superimposed on the net deficit. Respiratory alkalosis and insulin release, stimulated by the administration of IV glucose, act in concert to incorporate phosphate into cells. Increased ATP synthesis as a result of phosphate moving into cells may cause increased magnesium binding and worsen the hypomagnesemia. It is common for hypomagnesemia, hypophosphatemia, and hypokalemia to coexist during alcohol withdrawal. Hypocalcemia may also be present during alcohol withdrawal because a deficit of magnesium interferes with the secretion and action of PTH.

Other situations besides alcohol withdrawal that cause hypomagnesemia because of transcellular shifts of magnesium include refeeding after starvation and the hungry bone syndrome following parathyroidectomy. The rapid deposition of magnesium in the newly formed bone salts following parathyroidectomy or into muscle tissue during the refeeding syndrome causes a reduction in the serum magnesium.

Clinical features

The clinical manifestations of magnesium deficiency are difficult to define because of other electrolyte abnormalities, such as hypokalemia and hypocalcemia, that frequently accompany depletion of this ion. Signs and

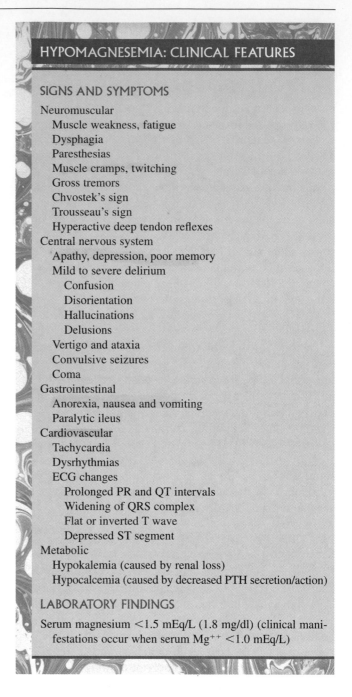

HYPOMAGNESEMIA: CLINICAL FEATURES

SIGNS AND SYMPTOMS

Neuromuscular
  Muscle weakness, fatigue
  Dysphagia
  Paresthesias
  Muscle cramps, twitching
  Gross tremors
  Chvostek's sign
  Trousseau's sign
  Hyperactive deep tendon reflexes
Central nervous system
  Apathy, depression, poor memory
  Mild to severe delirium
    Confusion
    Disorientation
    Hallucinations
    Delusions
  Vertigo and ataxia
  Convulsive seizures
  Coma
Gastrointestinal
  Anorexia, nausea and vomiting
  Paralytic ileus
Cardiovascular
  Tachycardia
  Dysrhythmias
  ECG changes
    Prolonged PR and QT intervals
    Widening of QRS complex
    Flat or inverted T wave
    Depressed ST segment
Metabolic
  Hypokalemia (caused by renal loss)
  Hypocalcemia (caused by decreased PTH secretion/action)

LABORATORY FINDINGS

Serum magnesium <1.5 mEq/L (1.8 mg/dl) (clinical manifestations occur when serum Mg^{++} <1.0 mEq/L)

symptoms usually involve the neuromuscular, central nervous, cardiovascular, and GI systems (see box above).

Magnesium plays an important role in neuromuscular transmission. Consequently, in magnesium depletion signs and symptoms of neuromuscular irritability are prominent and similar to those seen in hypocalcemia (which may also be present). These signs and symptoms include paresthesias (numbness and tingling of fingertips or around the mouth), dysphagia, muscle weakness, cramps and tremors, occasional positive Chvostek's or Trousseau's signs, and hyperactive deep tendon reflexes.

Central nervous system manifestations of magnesium deficit include personality changes such as agitation, ap-

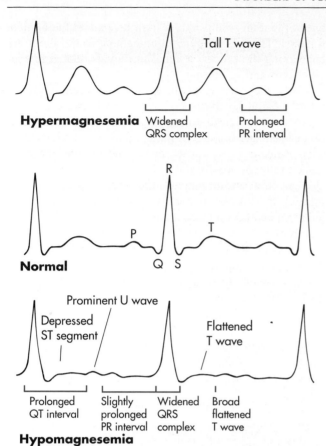

FIG. 21-10   ECG changes in magnesium imbalances. A prolonged PR interval, widened QRS complex, flattened T waves, and ST segment depression are changes that may be seen in hypomagnesemia. A prolonged PR interval, widened QRS complex, and peaked T waves may be seen in mild hypermagnesemia (<9 mEq/L). Complete heart block and cardiac arrest occur at higher levels.

athy, or memory loss. The patient may have vertigo and ataxia and various degrees of delirium, convulsions, and coma. *Delirium tremens,* a term describing the neuromuscular irritability and CNS signs and symptoms, commonly occurs during acute alcohol withdrawal.

GI changes include decreased contractility of smooth muscle, which may lead to anorexia, nausea and vomiting, and even paralytic ileus. The cardiovascular abnormalities observed as a result of magnesium depletion may result from the malfunction of the many enzyme systems activated by magnesium and/or from the hypokalemia and hypocalcemia that are often present. Cardiac dysrhythmias include premature ventricular contractions (PVCs) and atrial or ventricular fibrillation; ECG changes that may be noted include prolonged PR and QT intervals, widened QRS complex, flat or inverted T waves, and ST segment depression (Fig. 21-10). Some of the ECG changes are similar to those seen in hypokalemia and hypocalcemia, which may play a role in

their creation. There is also an increased sensitivity to digitalis that may require a decrease in dosage to avoid toxicity.

A magnesium deficit affects the sodium-potassium pump, often resulting in hypokalemia, and an associated hypocalcemia may occur because hypomagnesemia suppresses PTH secretion and target organ action.

Treatment

Treatment seeks to correct the magnesium imbalance and identify and treat the underlying disorder. One must also look for and correct any associated potassium, calcium, and phosphate deficiencies. It is important to assess renal function before administering magnesium since the dosage should be reduced in the presence of renal insufficiency or failure.

A mild magnesium deficit may be treated by the administration of foods high in magnesium (green vegetables, meat, beans, nuts) and possibly daily oral magnesium salts in liquid or tablet form. Treatment with oral magnesium salts is limited because of the diarrhea it causes. When hypomagnesemia is severe with seizures or cardiac dysrhythmias, magnesium sulfate or chloride can be administered by intramuscular injection or by intravenous infusion. When magnesium is given intravenously, it must be given slowly (maximum infusion rate is 150 mg/min) with careful monitoring of serum electrolytes, vital signs, deep tendon reflexes (e.g., knee jerk), and ECG to detect and prevent hypermagnesemia and possible cardiac arrest.

Hypermagnesemia

Hypermagnesemia is defined as a serum magnesium greater than 2.5 mEq/L (3.0 mg/dl), the upper limit of normal. Hypermagnesemia is uncommon and is caused by either decreased renal excretion or increased intake of magnesium. When hypermagnesemia occurs, it is almost always in patients with renal failure who have ingested magnesium-containing drugs (e.g., antacids, such as Maalox or Riopan, or laxatives, such as milk of magnesia). Patients with renal insufficiency have limited ability to excrete magnesium, and a fatal hypermagnesemia may result. Phosphate-binding antacids administered to patients with chronic renal failure to prevent secondary hyperparathyroidism should be limited to magnesium-free antacids (Amphojel, Basojel, or calcium carbonate). The parenteral administration of magnesium to treat hypomagnesemia or *eclampsia* (toxemia of pregnancy) is another situation that could result in hypermagnesemia if not carefully monitored. Magnesium is a standard form of therapy for preeclampsia and eclampsia and could cause intoxication in both the mother and neonate. Other less common causes of hypermagnesemia include untreated diabetic ketoacidosis, Addison's disease (hypoadrenalism), and hemodialysis using hard water high in magnesium.

▶ TABLE 21-1   Hypermagnesemia: Clinical Features

Serum Mg⁺⁺ (mEq/L)	Signs and Symptoms
1.5-2.5	Normal
3-5	Facial flushing with sensation of heat and thirst Muscular weakness Diminished deep tendon reflexes (DTRs) Nausea and vomiting
5-9	Lethargy, drowsiness Peripheral vasodilation, hypotension Increasing weakness and paralysis of all muscles Respiratory compromise Absent deep tendon reflexes (DTRs) ECG: bradycardia, prolonged PR interval, peaked T waves, widened QRS complex
10-12	Coma
15-20	ECG: Complete heart block Cardiac arrest Respiratory arrest

Clinical features

The predominant clinical manifestations of hypermagnesemia involve the neuromuscular and cardiovascular systems. Magnesium excess produces a sedative effect on the neuromuscular system, causing muscular weakness. The eventual result is ventilatory arrest from paralysis of the respiratory muscles. Magnesium excess produces this effect mainly by suppressing the release of acetylcholine at the myoneural junction, thus blocking neuromuscular transmission and reducing muscle cell excitability. Excess magnesium also reduces the responsiveness of the postsynaptic membrane, displacing calcium from binding sites and preventing its action.

Hypermagnesemia impairs cardiac function by interfering with atrioventricular conduction, producing a variety of disturbances in the ECG that may eventually culminate in complete heart block and cardiac arrest. Magnesium excess causes hypotension by relaxing vascular smooth muscle and reducing vascular resistance by displacing calcium from the vascular wall surface (Duarte, 1990). Table 21-1 depicts a rough correlation be-tween the total serum magnesium levels and the clinical findings. There is no general agreement in the literature concerning the precise magnesium levels related to specific signs and symptoms.

When the serum magnesium is between 3 and 5 mEq/L, facial flushing may be present because of cutaneous vasodilation that may be accompanied by a sensation of heat and thirst. The patient may complain of muscular weakness and nausea and vomiting, and the deep tendon reflexes are diminished.

When the serum magnesium level is about 5 to 9 mEq/L, the patient becomes increasingly drowsy and lethargic and becomes comatose at higher levels. The patient may be hypotensive because of peripheral vasodilation, and DTRs may be completely absent. Increasing weakness and finally a curare-like paralysis of all the muscles occur. Respiratory compromise occurs because of respiratory center depression and involvement of the respiratory muscles. Fig. 21-10 depicts some of the ECG changes that may occur with magnesium excess.

When serum magnesium levels reach 15 to 20 mEq/L, complete heart block and cardiac arrest, as well as respiratory arrest, may occur.

Treatment

Hypermagnesemia should be prevented by avoiding the administration of magnesium-containing medications to persons with renal insufficiency. Patient education is particularly important with respect to achieving this goal. When magnesium is administered parenterally, the nurse must closely monitor the rate of administration and assess the patient frequently for any signs or symptoms of magnesium excess.

When hypermagnesemia is mild, the only treatment that may be necessary is to discontinue magnesium administration. Instituting peritoneal dialysis or hemodialysis with magnesium-free dialysate may be the treatment of choice for patients with renal failure. In patients with normal renal function, saline and furosemide may be given to provide hydration and promote diuresis with elimination of excess magnesium. When cardiac conduction or respiratory effects occur, emergency care is required. Calcium gluconate (a magnesium antagonist) may be given under ECG monitoring to reverse the effects of magnesium temporarily, and the patient may be placed on a ventilator.

? QUESTIONS

▼ *Circle the letter preceding the item below that correctly answers each question or completes the statement. More than one answer may be correct.*

1. ECF volume imbalances are characterized by:

   a. Isotonic body fluid losses/gains
   b. Relatively greater losses/gains of sodium than water
   c. Relatively greater losses/gains of water than sodium
   d. None of the above

2. Sodium ions account for what percentage of the osmotically active particles in the ECF?

   a. 5%   c. 20%
   b. 15%   d. 90%

QUESTIONS—cont'd

3. Which of the following effects would result from a decrease of the serum sodium concentration below the normal range?
   a. Shift of water from the ICF to the ECF, causing cell shrinkage
   b. Shift of water from the ECF to the ICF, causing cell swelling
   c. Shift of water and sodium from the ECF to the interstitial fluid (ISF), causing edema
   d. None of the above

4. Third-space fluid loss:
   a. Is manifested by rapid decrease in body weight
   b. Is the accumulation of fluid in a non-ECF or non-ICF compartment, which is not easily exchangeable with the ECF
   c. May reduce the effective circulating blood volume
   d. Represents a distributional loss of fluids from the ECF

5. The most common condition that causes a fluid volume deficit is:
   a. GI losses (e.g., vomiting, diarrhea) combined with inadequate fluid intake
   b. Third-space losses
   c. Osmotic diuresis
   d. Aldosterone deficiency

6. Which of the following test results indicate an isotonic fluid volume deficit caused by extrarenal losses?
   a. Serum Na⁺ 140 mEq/L
   b. Hematocrit 55%
   c. Urine specific gravity 1.038 (or 1200 mOsm/kg)
   d. Urine Na⁺ <10 mEq/L

7. Somatic compensatory responses to the rapid loss of a large amount of body fluid (e.g., sequestration in intestinal obstruction, bleeding) include:
   a. Sympathetic activation and peripheral vasoconstriction
   b. Diminished renal perfusion
   c. Stimulation of the ADH mechanism, causing thirst and increased renal water reabsorption
   d. Activation of the renin-angiotensin-aldosterone mechanism, causing increased renal sodium (and water) reabsorption
   e. Increased heart rate and contractility to restore cardiac output

8. The most sensitive assessment parameter for the early detection of fluid volume deficit is:
   a. Orthostatic hypotension and tachycardia

   b. Blood pressure of 100/70 mm Hg in the supine position
   c. Lassitude, weakness, and fatigue
   d. Prolonged filling time of the hand veins
   e. Decreased serum Na⁺ concentration

9. A previously healthy 45-year-old man is admitted to the hospital with a history of nausea, vomiting, and diarrhea over 4 days and a diagnosis of gastroenteritis from eating contaminated food in a restaurant. Physical assessment reveals: oral temperature, 97.0° F; pulse, 110 beats/min; respirations, 20 breaths/min; blood pressure, 120/80 mm Hg supine and 90/60 mm Hg sitting; neck veins flat in the supine position; decreased skin and tongue turgor. His weight is 66.0 kg (normal = 70 kg). He is lethargic and weak. Laboratory tests on the blood serum reveal: Na⁺, 143 mEq/L; chlorides, 106 mEq/L; K⁺, 3.3 mEq/L; BUN, 35 g/dl; creatinine, 1.5 mg/dl; hematocrit, 55%. Urinary findings reveal urine output, 25 ml/hr; specific gravity, 1.038; urinary Na⁺, 8 mEq/L. These findings indicate:
   a. The patient has an isotonic fluid volume deficit
   b. The patient has combined hyperosmolality disturbance and fluid volume deficit
   c. The patient has a moderate (5%) fluid volume deficit with the loss of about 4 L of body fluid
   d. The patient has hyperkalemia
   e. The low urinary Na⁺ indicates that the fluid loss is extrarenal

10. Which of the following IV solutions would be preferred initially to help correct the patient's problem in question 9?
    a. Isotonic saline (0.9% NaCl)
    b. Isotonic saline with added 20 mEq KCl/L
    c. Half-normal saline (0.45% NaCl)
    d. D₅W

11. Approximately how much fluid should be given to the patient in question 9 over the next 24 hours?
    a. 1500 ml   c. 3000 ml
    b. 2500 ml   d. 4000 ml

12. In which of the following situations is there a danger of circulatory overload (hypervolemia)?
    a. Administration of a hypertonic IV solution
    b. Congestive heart failure
    c. Acute renal failure
    d. Pyrexia lasting 4 days

13. Rapid administration of IV fluids can result in pulmonary edema because:
    a. Tissue hydrostatic pressure in the lung parenchyma increases
    b. Colloid osmotic pressure in the pulmonary vessels increases
    c. Hydrostatic pressure in the pulmonary vessels increases
    d. Lymphatic clearance in the interstitium increases

14. You are caring for Mr. Brown, a 75-year-old patient with congestive heart failure who is receiving IV fluids. You notice that he is becoming increasingly restless and short of breath. His blood pressure and respiratory rate are increasing and he has a moist-sounding cough. You also note that he has neck vein distention up to the jaw angle in the sitting position. You hear medium rales (crackles) throughout both posterior lung fields. Mr. Brown's symptoms are probably caused by:
    a. Decreased venous return to the right ventricle
    b. Circulatory overload and pulmonary edema
    c. Liver congestion from fluid reflux from the heart
    d. Increased tissue hydrostatic pressure in the alveoli
    e. Decreased hydrostatic pressure in the pulmonary capillaries

15. The best nursing intervention for Mr. Brown would be:
    a. Elevation of the foot of the bed to aid venous return
    b. Slowing down the IV to a keep open rate and notifying physician
    c. Continuing to monitor the vital signs
    d. Encouraging the patient to cough and breathe deeply to improve alveolar ventilation

16. The *first* emergency action in the treatment of severe acute pulmonary edema is:
    a. Positioning the patient in high Fowler's position with the legs lowered to reduce hydrostatic pressure in the chest
    b. Placing the patient in a supine position to aid venous return to the heart
    c. Increasing the IV rate to increase the effective circulating volume
    d. Applying rotating tourniquets

▼ *Answer the following on a separate piece of paper.*

17. What effect would the loss of 3 L of iso-

Continued.

tonic fluid (e.g., diarrhea fluid or gastric fluid) have on the following parameters?

a. Effective circulating blood volume
b. Plasma osmolality
c. Plasma Na⁺ concentration
d. ADH secretion
e. Urine osmolality and specific gravity
f. Thirst
g. Blood pressure

18. What would happen to the plasma osmolality if the patient in Question 17 ingested a large amount of pure water?

19. Compare the effects of the loss of pure water caused by insensible losses (from the lungs because of hyperventilation or renal loss in diabetes insipidus) to the loss of an equal volume of isotonic fluid (as in vomiting or diarrhea) on the following:

a. ECF volume and blood pressure
b. Plasma osmolality
c. Intracellular fluid volume of brain cells

20. Why is normal saline the IV infusion of choice for the treatment of hypovolemic shock rather than D₅W?

▼ *Circle the letter preceding the item below that correctly answers each question or completes the statement. More than one answer may be correct.*

21. Serum osmolality changes represent total body water changes provided that:
a. No solute is lost from the body
b. Only electrolytes are lost from the body
c. Cell membranes are impermeable to water
d. The serum osmolality is corrected for the urea concentration

22. What is the estimated serum osmolality in a patient with a serum sodium concentration of 140 mEq/L and a serum glucose of 100 mg/dl?
a. 280 mOsm/kg
b. 140 mOsm/kg
c. 100 mOsm/kg
d. 240 mOsm/kg

23. The osmolality of urine in a person with normal renal function:
a. Is only lowered to 100 mOsm/kg in water diuresis
b. May be lowered to less than 30 mOsm/kg in water diuresis
c. Is raised only to 900 mOsm/kg in fluid volume deficit
d. Is isoosmotic with the plasma in an isotonic fluid volume deficit

e. Is isoosmotic with the plasma in water diuresis

24. A middle-aged woman is started on a thiazide diuretic for the treatment of hypertension. After taking the drug for 3 weeks, she complains of weakness, muscle cramps, and postural dizziness. She is alert and oriented to time, place, and person. Physical findings include blood pressure, 130/90 mm Hg (previously 170/100 mm Hg); decreased skin turgor; decreased filling time of hand veins; flat neck veins in the supine position. Laboratory serum tests: Na⁺, 115 mEq/L; Cl⁻, 66 mEq/L; K⁺, 2.1 mEq/L; plasma osmolality, 240 mOsm/kg; HCO₃⁻, 32 mEq/L. Urine tests: Na⁺, 4 mEq/L; K⁺, 20 mEq/L; urine osmolality, 540 mOsm/kg. Which of the following has contributed to this patient's hyponatremia?
a. The thiazide diuretic
b. ECF volume depletion
c. Increased ADH secretion
d. Water ingestion and retention
e. Potassium depletion

25. The appropriate treatment for the patient in question 24 should include which of the following:
a. Water restriction alone
b. Rapid administration of D₅W
c. Isotonic (0.9%) saline
d. KCl
e. Half-isotonic (0.45%) saline

26. A 65-year-old man with a 40-year history of heavy cigarette smoking and a recent diagnosis of oat cell carcinoma of the lung is admitted to the hospital with a 2-week history of progressive lethargy and headaches. Physical assessment is within normal limits except for the lethargy, headaches, and diminished deep tendon reflexes. Serum laboratory values show: Na⁺, 105 mEq/L; Cl⁻, 72 mEq/L; K⁺, 4 mEq/L; HCO₃⁻, 23; plasma osmolality, 222 mOsm/kg. Urine laboratory values: urine Na⁺, 78 mEq/L; urine osmolality, 804 mOsm/kg; specific gravity, 1.029. The most likely cause of this patient's problem is:
a. Diabetes insipidus (ADH deficiency)
b. Isotonic ECF volume excess
c. SIADH (ectopic source)
d. Hyperaldosteronism
e. Compulsive water drinking (psychogenic polydipsia)

27. The direct cause of the patient's neurologic symptoms in Question 26 is:
a. Brain cell shrinkage

b. Increased levels of circulating ADH
c. Decreased serum Na⁺ concentration
d. Brain cell swelling and increased intracranial pressure

28. Which of the following is the best treatment for the patient in Question 26?
a. Water restriction alone
b. Isotonic saline alone
c. Hypotonic saline
d. Hypertonic saline and water restriction

29. If hypertonic (3% to 5%) saline is injected intravenously, which of the following will occur?
a. Water will be drawn out of the cells to the ECF compartment
b. Water will shift from the ECF to the ICF compartment
c. The sodium pump will maintain equilibrium
d. Urine output will decrease

30. SIADH may be associated with:
a. Massive edema
b. CNS lesions and injuries
c. Postoperative conditions: cardiac surgery
d. Administration of oxytocin for labor induction
e. Administration of oral hypoglycemics

31. Which of the following conditions associated with hyponatremia causes plasma hyperosmolality rather than hypoosmolality?
a. Acute renal failure
b. SIADH
c. Uncontrolled diabetes mellitus
d. Diuretic excess

32. A 35-year-old male alcoholic was brought to the hospital in a comatose state after being discovered in an alley behind a tavern. The patient's skull was fractured. An indwelling catheter inserted into his bladder revealed a urine output of 175 ml/hr. Serum laboratory tests showed: Na⁺, 170 mEq/L; Cl⁻, 132 mEq/L; K⁺, 4.0 mEq/L; serum glucose, 80 mg/dl; plasma osmolality, 345 mOsm/kg. The urine osmolality was 100 mOsm/kg. After administration of the vasopressin test, the urine output decreased to 90 ml/hr and the osmolality increased to 270 mOsm/kg. His vital signs were: blood pressure 120/84 mm Hg; oral temperature, 99.6° F; pulse, 90 beats/min; respirations, 20 breaths/min. The probable cause of this patient's problem is:
a. Central diabetes insipidus

QUESTIONS—cont'd

b. Nephrogenic diabetes insipidus
c. Osmotic diuresis
d. SIADH

33. Which of the following statements are correct regarding the treatment of the fluid and electrolyte imbalance of the patient in question 32?
   a. The primary goal is to lower the serum sodium gradually to avoid causing cerebral edema.
   b. A hypotonic IV solution (D_5W or D_5/0.2% NaCl) should be given.
   c. Water restriction is the treatment of choice to decrease polyuria.
   d. Chronic treatment consists of administering exogenous ADH.

34. Some iatrogenic causes of hypernatremia include:
   a. High-protein enteral tube feedings with insufficient water intake
   b. Insufficient fluid provided for confused elderly persons
   c. Prolonged use of artificial ventilator
   d. Therapeutic abortion with hypertonic saline entry into circulation

35. Mr. Rogers, a business executive, was in a private airplane accident along an isolated section of the seacoast. While awaiting rescue, he drank large amounts of ocean water. When admitted to a local hospital, his condition was complicated by salt intoxication. Which of the following signs, symptoms, and laboratory values might this patient exhibit?
   a. Hot, flushed skin
   b. Mental confusion and agitation
   c. Hypoactive tendon reflexes
   d. Dry, red tongue and dry, sticky oral mucosa

36. Hypokalemia is associated with all of the following conditions except:
   a. Protracted vomiting or diarrhea
   b. Cushing's syndrome
   c. Administration of IV glucose and regular insulin to correct diabetic ketoacidosis
   d. Mineralocorticoid deficiency in Addison's disease
   e. Metabolic acidosis

37. Hypokalemia associated with protracted vomiting is caused by:
   a. Loss of K^+ in vomitus
   b. Loss of K^+ in the urine
   c. Lowering of serum potassium because of a shift into the cells
   d. All of the above

38. Probably the most frequent cause of hypokalemia is:
   a. Licorice ingestion

b. Diuretic drugs
c. Magnesium depletion
d. Primary hyperaldosteronism

39. Clinical manifestations of hypokalemia include all of the following except:
   a. Fatigue and generalized muscle weakness
   b. Serum K^+ <3.5 mEq/L
   c. Tall, peaked T waves
   d. Decreased bowel sounds
   e. Paresthesias

40. Which statement about hypokalemia is false?
   a. Diuretics, digitalis, and hypokalemia are a particularly dangerous combination.
   b. Hypokalemia can be diagnosed on the basis of clinical signs and symptoms alone.
   c. The rate of K^+ administration should not exceed 20 mEq/hr when it is added to an IV line to correct hypokalemia.
   d. Ingestion of citrus fruits and juices should be encouraged in persons on long-term diuretic therapy.

41. Some causes of hyperkalemia include:
   a. Poor venipuncture technique
   b. Acute and chronic renal failure
   c. Ingestion of salt substitutes in a person with renal insufficiency
   d. Aldosterone deficiency
   e. Tissue damage (e.g., surgery, burns)

42. ECG changes suggesting hyperkalemia include:
   a. High, peaked T waves
   b. Prolonged PR interval
   c. Depressed ST segment
   d. Prolonged QRS intervals

43. When hyperkalemia reaches critical levels (>7 to 8 mEq/L) there is a distinct danger of:
   a. Cardiac dysrhythmias
   b. Cardiac arrest
   c. Hypertensive crisis
   d. Hypovolemic shock
   e. Increased cardiac contractility

44. Hyperkalemia can be treated by all of the following procedures except:
   a. IV calcium gluconate
   b. IV glucose and insulin
   c. IV sodium bicarbonate
   d. Oral or rectal ion exchange resin (Kayexalate)
   e. IV acidic solution

45. Which of the following statements best describes normal calcium homeostasis?
   a. The rate of calcium absorption from

the gut is equal to the urinary excretion of calcium.
   b. The rate of calcium reabsorption from the bone is equal to the amount of serum calcitonin.
   c. The rate of calcium reabsorption by the renal tubules is equal to the rate of phosphate reabsorption by the renal tubules.

46. Body processes affected by the concentration of calcium ion include:
   a. Contraction of cardiac and skeletal muscle
   b. Permeability of the cell membrane to sodium and potassium
   c. Release of neurotransmitters at synaptic junctions
   d. Excitability of nerve tissue
   e. All of the above

47. All of the following statements concerning $1,25(OH)_2D_3$ are true except:
   a. It is the most metabolically active form of vitamin D
   b. It acts in concert with PTH to increase osteoclastic bone activity
   c. It increases the absorption of calcium and phosphate from the gut
   d. PTH stimulates its final hydroxylation in the liver

48. The major effect of calcitonin is to:
   a. Stimulate hydroxylation of cholecalciferol in the liver
   b. Inhibit PTH secretion by the parathyroid glands
   c. Inhibit osteoclastic bone activity
   d. Stimulate hydroxylation of 25-cholecalciferol in the kidney

49. Direct effects of PTH secretion on target organs include all of the following except:
   a. Increased osteoclastic bone resorption of calcium and phosphate
   b. Increased renal tubular calcium reabsorption
   c. Increased renal tubular phosphate reabsorption
   d. Increased serum calcium

50. Which of the following forms of calcium is physiologically active (i.e., plays a role in muscle contraction, nerve conduction, and blood coagulation)?
   a. Ionized calcium
   b. Calcium bound to albumin
   c. Calcium bound to globulin
   d. Calcium complexed with phosphate

51. To accurately assess the total serum calcium concentration in the laboratory report, the examiner must correlate the measurement with:

Continued.

a. Serum sodium level
b. Serum chloride level
c. Serum albumin level
d. Serum potassium level

52. The most common cause of hypoparathyroidism and hypocalcemia is:
    a. Idiopathic
    b. End-organ resistance
    c. Surgical removal of the parathyroids
    d. Postradiation therapy

53. A postoperative complication that results from sudden increased skeletal absorption of calcium and phosphate from the blood is called:
    a. Hungry bone syndrome
    b. Hypercalcemic crisis
    c. Thyroid crisis
    d. Acromegaly

54. Signs and symptoms of hypocalcemia are more likely to be manifested under conditions of:
    a. Metabolic acidosis
    b. Metabolic alkalosis
    c. ECF volume deficit
    d. Hyperphosphatemia

55. To check for Trousseau's sign (indicating latent tetany) a blood pressure cuff is applied to the arm and inflated above systolic pressure for 3 to 5 minutes. A positive response would be:
    a. Paresthesias of the fingers
    b. Bounding pulses in the wrist following removal of the cuff
    c. Spasm of the wrist and finger muscles
    d. Hyperemia of the hand

56. Spasm of the facial muscles induced by tapping the facial nerve in front of the ear (indicating latent tetany) is known as:
    a. Chvostek's sign
    b. Temporomandibular sign
    c. Homans' sign
    d. Brudzinski's sign

57. Hypocalcemia may be treated by giving:
    a. Calcitonin
    b. Calcium gluconate
    c. Vitamin D
    d. Diphosphonates
    e. Plicamycin (Mithracin)

58. The most common cause of hypercalcemia is:
    a. Malignancies
    b. Primary hyperparathyroidism

c. Vitamin D intoxication
d. Adrenal insufficiency

59. Factors important in the development of humoral hypercalcemia of malignancy include all of the following except:
    a. Transforming growth factors such as TGF-alpha
    b. Parathyroid hormone-related peptide (PTHrP)
    c. Lymphotoxin
    d. Osteoclast deactivating factors
    e. Interleukin-1

60. In primary hyperparathyroidism:
    a. Serum levels of PTH are always greater than in persons with hypercalcemia caused by vitamin D_3 intoxication
    b. An adenoma of one or more of the parathyroid glands is often the cause of the PTH hypersecretion
    c. There may be a generalized loss of bone mineralization evident on x-ray examination

61. ECG changes characteristic of hypercalcemia are:
    a. Shortened PR interval
    b. Shortened QT interval
    c. Prolonged QT interval
    d. Sinus tachycardia

62. The treatment of hypercalcemia requires adequate:
    a. Vitamin D intake
    b. Treatment with thiazide diuretics
    c. Protein intake
    d. Hydration with saline followed by giving loop diuretics

63. Asymptomatic patients with malignancy-related hypercalcemia (<12 mg/dl) who are receiving antineoplastic treatment may only require:
    a. Increased oral fluid intake
    b. Restriction of dietary calcium
    c. Limitation of weight-bearing activities
    d. Liberal use of sedatives to ensure a good night's rest

64. Gallium nitrate, used in the treatment of malignancy-related hypercalcemia, exerts a hypocalcemic effect by:
    a. Stimulating an antitumor response
    b. Reducing renal sodium excretion
    c. Blocking PTH-induced bone resorption of calcium

d. Enhancing the action of prostaglandin-synthesis inhibitors

65. Which of the following signs or symptoms would the nurse be most likely to observe when assessing for hypophosphatemia?
    a. Irritability, apprehension
    b. Paresthesias
    c. Diarrhea
    d. Hypertension

66. The most common cause contributing to hypomagnesemia is:
    a. Alcohol abuse
    b. Vitamin D intoxication
    c. Administration of cisplatin
    d. Hyperparathyroidism

67. The effect of hypomagnesemia on the neuromuscular system is:
    a. Decreased excitability
    b. Increased excitability
    c. Significant paralysis
    d. Release of ATP from cells

68. The most common cause of hypermagnesemia is:
    a. Ingestion of magnesium-containing drugs by a patient with renal insufficiency or failure
    b. Diabetic ketoacidosis
    c. Adrenal insufficiency
    d. Hemodialysis using untreated (hard) water

69. Which of the following drugs should the nurse have available for emergency use when magnesium is administered intravenously?
    a. Digoxin
    b. Lidocaine
    c. Potassium chloride
    d. Calcium gluconate

70. The nurse administers injections of magnesium sulfate for the treatment of a patient with toxemia of pregnancy and preeclampsia. Which of the following signs or symptoms observed during assessment would indicate that the patient is developing magnesium toxicity?
    a. Progressively decreased deep tendon reflexes
    b. Hyperactive deep tendon reflexes
    c. Marked fall in blood pressure
    d. Increase in blood pressure
    e. Prolongation of the PR interval

CHAPTER 22 ▶ Acid-Base Disorders

LORRAINE M. WILSON

Disturbances in acid-base balance are common clinical problems that range in severity from mild to life-threatening. This chapter reviews the basic principles of acid-base physiology, the general mechanisms by which abnormalities can occur, and an approach to the clinical assessment of acid-base disturbances. This review is followed by a more detailed discussion of the four primary acid-base disorders—metabolic acidosis, metabolic alkalosis, respiratory acidosis, and respiratory alkalosis—and mixed acid-base disorders.

PHYSIOLOGIC CONSIDERATIONS

Acid-base balance refers to the homeostasis of the hydrogen ion concentration ($[H^+]$) in body fluids. Acids are produced continuously from normal metabolism. Despite the large addition of acids from metabolism, the $[H^+]$ of body fluids is low. The normal H^+ concentration of the arterial blood is 0.00000004 (4×10^{-8}) mEq/L or about one millionth of the concentration of Na^+. Despite this low concentration, the maintenance of a stable $[H^+]$ is required for normal cellular function, because small fluctuations have important effects on the activity of cellular enzymes. Because of these effects on cellular enzymes, only a relatively narrow range of $[H^+]$ is compatible with life.

pH Scale

An increase in the $[H^+]$ makes a solution more acid, and a decrease more alkaline. Because the $[H^+]$ is a small quantity, the pH scale was devised by chemists as a means to express it. The pH is defined as the negative log of the hydrogen ion concentration ($pH = -\log [H^+]$). Thus a $[H^+]$ of 0.0000001 g/L equals 10^{-7} g/L equals pH 7. Thus the pH and the $[H^+]$ are inversely related. As the $[H^+]$ increases, the pH decreases; as the $[H^+]$ decreases, the pH increases. A low pH means that a solution

TABLE 22-1 Relationship Between the pH and the Hydrogen Ion Concentration in the Physiologic Range

pH	[H⁺] nmol/L
7.80	16
7.70	20
7.60	26
7.50	32
7.45	35
7.40	40
7.35	45
7.30	50
7.20	63
7.10	80
7.00	100
6.90	125
6.80	160

is more acidic, whereas a high pH means that a solution is more alkaline or basic. Water, a liquid having a pH of 7, is neutral because at that pH the number of (acid) hydrogen ions (H⁺) is exactly balanced by the number of (basic) hydroxyl ions (OH⁻). An acid solution has a pH less than 7; an alkaline or basic solution has a pH greater than 7. The pH scale ranges from 1 (most acid) to 14 (most alkaline).

The mean pH of the blood or extracellular fluid (ECF) is slightly alkaline at 7.4. The normal range of the blood pH is from 7.38 to 7.42 (1 standard deviation [SD] from the mean) or 7.35 to 7.45 (2 SD from the mean).

Rather than use the pH scale, some medical centers prefer to express the [H⁺] in nanomoles per liter (nmol/L). Table 22-1 contains a pH to nanomoles conversion table. This table illustrates that a log scale such as the pH scale may obscure the magnitude of a change in the [H⁺] if one is not mathematically inclined. For example, it is evident that when the [H⁺] increases from 40 to 80 nmol, a doubling of [H⁺] has occurred, but this may not be evident when the pH changes from 7.4 to 7.1.

Acids

An acid is a substance containing one or more H⁺ ions that can be liberated in solution (proton donor). A strong acid, such as hydrochloric acid (HCl), is almost completely dissociated in solution, thus liberating more H⁺ ions. A weak acid, such as carbonic acid (H_2CO_3), is only partially dissociated in solution so that fewer H⁺ ions are liberated.

Two types of acids are formed by metabolic processes in the body: volatile and nonvolatile. A *volatile acid* can change between liquid and gaseous states. Carbon dioxide—a major end-product in the oxidation of carbohy-

drates, fats, and amino acids—can be regarded as an acid by virtue of its ability to react with water to form carbonic acid (H_2CO_3), which in turn can dissociate to form H⁺ and HCO_3^-:

$$CO_2 + H_2O \rightleftharpoons H_2CO_3 \rightleftharpoons H^+ + HCO_3^-$$

Because carbon dioxide is a gas that can be eliminated by the lungs, it is often called a volatile acid.

All other sources of H⁺ are considered to be *nonvolatile* or *fixed acids*. Nonvolatile acids cannot be converted to a gaseous form to be excreted by the lungs but must be excreted by the kidneys. Nonvolatile acids may be inorganic or organic. Sulfuric acid is the end-product of the oxidation of sulfur-containing amino acids, whereas phosphoric acid is formed from the metabolism of phospholipids, nucleic acids, and phosphoproteins. Because organic acids, such as lactic acid and ketoacids, are formed during the metabolism of carbohydrates and fats and are further oxidized to CO_2 and water, they do not normally affect the body pH. However, these organic acids may accumulate in certain abnormal circumstances. Lactic acid accumulates in the absence of oxygen, as in circulatory shock or cardiac arrest. In uncontrolled diabetes mellitus, ketoacids (acetoacetic and beta-hydroxybutyric acids) may accumulate because of increased lipid metabolism. About 20,000 mmol of carbonic acid and 80 mmol of nonvolatile acids are produced in the body each day and eliminated by the lungs and kidneys, respectively.

Bases

In contrast to an acid, a base is a substance that can capture or combine with hydrogen ions from a solution (proton acceptor). A strong base, such as sodium hydroxide (NaOH), is highly dissociated in solution and reacts strongly with an acid. A weak base, such as sodium bicarbonate ($NaHCO_3$), is only partially dissociated in solution and reacts less vigorously with an acid.

Buffers

The term *buffer* describes a chemical substance that minimizes the pH change in a solution caused by the addition of either an acid or a base. A buffer is a mixture of a weak acid and its alkali salt (or a weak base and its acid salt). A buffer is most effective in defending the [H⁺] against acids or bases when it is 50% dissociated (having an equal amount of undissociated acid and its salt). The pH at which an acid or base is 50% dissociated is known as its pK. The effectiveness of a given buffer is determined by its concentration and its pK relative to the pH of the compartment in which it is active.

Four main buffer pairs or systems in the body help to maintain the constancy of the pH:

1. Bicarbonate/carbonic acid system ($NaHCO_3$ and H_2CO_3)

2. Disodium/monosodium phosphate buffer system (Na_2HPO_4 and NaH_2PO_4)
3. Hemoglobin/oxyhemoglobin buffer system in red blood cells (RBCs) (HbO_2^- and HHb)
4. Protein buffer system (Pr^- and HPr)

The bicarbonate–carbonic acid buffer system is quantitatively the largest in the body and operates in the ECF. It contributes more than half of the buffering capacity of whole blood. The remaining nonbicarbonate buffer systems operate primarily in the intracellular fluid (ICF). The phosphate buffer system is an important buffer in RBCs and in renal tubule cells. The H^+ excreted in the urine buffered by phosphate is referred to as *titratable acid.* Hemoglobin is an effective buffer of hydrogen ions produced within the RBC in the course of transporting carbon dioxide from the tissues to the lungs in the form of bicarbonate. Because reduced hemoglobin has a strong affinity for H^+, most of these ions become bound to hemoglobin. In this manner, only a few H^+ ions remain free, so that the acidity of venous blood is only slightly greater than that of arterial blood. As venous blood passes through the lungs, hemoglobin becomes saturated with oxygen and its ability to bind H^+ ions decreases. The H^+ ions are released, whereupon they react with bicarbonate to give CO_2, which is then expired by the lungs. In effect, the hemoglobin/oxyhemoglobin system actually buffers the bicarbonate–carbonic acid buffer system. The protein buffer system is predominant in tissue cells and also operates in the plasma. More than half of the 70 mmol of H^+ derived from the diet is initially buffered intracellularly.

Regulation of the ECF pH

Because various acids and bases continually enter the blood from absorbed foods and from catabolism of foods, some kind of mechanism is necessary for neutralizing or eliminating these substances. Actually, the constancy of the pH is maintained by the integrated action of the body buffers, lungs, and kidneys. These three regulatory mechanisms vary in the rapidity and effectiveness of defending the constancy of the pH when acids or bases are added or lost from the body.

The immediate response (within seconds) to an increase or decrease in $[H^+]$ is the chemical buffering of H^+ by both the ECF and ICF buffer systems. Buffering, however, is only a temporary measure in restoring normal pH.

A second line of defense that stabilizes the hydrogen ion concentration consists of the respiratory control of the CO_2 level in the body fluids through changes in alveolar ventilation. This response is fairly rapid, taking only minutes to be fully operative.

Ultimately, the restoration of normal pH during acid-base disturbances depends on the renal regulation of the bicarbonate level of body fluids. This response is relatively slow, taking several days to complete the correction.

The carbonic acid–bicarbonate buffer system

The carbonic acid–bicarbonate buffer system is of central importance in understanding the physiologic processes involved in normal acid-base equilibrium and its abnormalities. It is the major ECF buffer, and the assessment of its components provides the basis for the clinical evaluation of the patient's acid-base status. The following equation describes the components of the carbonic acid–bicarbonate buffer system and the relationships among them:

$$\underset{(40\ mm\ Hg)}{CO_2} + H_2O \overset{CA}{\rightleftharpoons} \underset{(1.2\ mEq/L)}{H_2CO_3} \rightleftharpoons \underset{(pH\ 7.4)}{H^+} + \underset{(24\ mEq/L)}{HCO_3^-}$$

The bidirectional arrows indicate that the reaction can proceed in either direction with equal facility, depending on the concentrations of the components in each section of the equation. This reaction readily occurs in RBCs because of the presence of the catalyzing enzyme carbonic anhydrase (CA). Because this enzyme is absent in blood plasma, the reaction is slowed there. It is evident from this equation that the $[H^+]$ is a function of the ECF $[HCO_3^-]$ and the carbon dioxide gas dissolved in the blood (PCO_2). *Acidemia* (an increase in $[H^+]$) occurs when there is either a fall in $[HCO_3^-]$ or an increase in PCO_2 (both displace the equation to the *right,* generating additional H^+). Conversely, *alkalemia* (a fall in the $[H^+]$) occurs when there is either an increase in the $[HCO_3^-]$ or a fall in PCO_2 (both of which displace the equilibrium to the *left*). The $[H^+]$, $[HCO_3^-]$, and PCO_2 are thus the three parameters controlling the acid-base status of the ECF.

The left side of the buffer equation is the respiratory component: $CO_2 + H_2O \rightleftharpoons H_2CO_3$. The respiratory component is controlled primarily by the lungs through variations in alveolar ventilation. If the PCO_2 is above or below normal, the amount of alveolar ventilation is inadequate (hypoventilation) or excessive (hyperventilation). The PCO_2 is regulated by pulmonary function and reflexes in the brain stem, which control respiratory drive (see Chapter 35).

The right side of the equation is the renal-metabolic component: $H_2CO_3 \rightleftharpoons H^+ + HCO_3^-$. The carbonic acid formed by the hydration of carbon dioxide gas dissociates into hydrogen ions and bicarbonate ions. This half of the equation is regulated primarily by the kidneys. They contribute to acid-base balance by regulating the plasma $[HCO_3^-]$ in two ways: (1) by reabsorbing the filtered HCO_3^- and preventing its loss in the urine and (2) by excreting the daily load of excess H^+ produced by metabolism. Two thirds of the excess H^+ is excreted in the form of ammonium ions (NH_4^+); one third is excreted in the form of phosphoric acid (H_3PO_4) or sulfuric acid (H_2SO_4). The latter process results in the generation of new bicarbonate to replace that bicarbonate lost in buffering the daily H^+ load. Thus the kidneys are able to retain or eliminate HCO_3^- as needed, either with Na^+ and K^+, or in exchange for Cl^- (chloride).

Although several buffer systems operate simultaneously in the body, only one of them needs to be measured to analyze acid-base disorders. The *isohydric principle* states that all buffer systems in a solution are in equilibrium with the same hydrogen ions. For practical purposes, then, changes in one buffer system accurately reflect changes in the others. Clinically, the carbonic acid–bicarbonate system is the one chosen for analysis because it is the largest buffer system of the ECF and is easiest to measure.

Henderson-Hasselbalch equation

At equilibrium, the relationship between the reactants of the bicarbonate–carbonic acid buffer system may be expressed by the law of mass action:

$$[H^+] = 24 \times \frac{Pco_2}{[HCO_3^-]}$$

or by the Henderson-Hasselbalch equation:

$$pH = pK + \log \frac{[HCO_3^-]}{[H_2CO_3]}$$

where pK is the carbonic acid dissociation constant, HCO_3^- is the plasma bicarbonate concentration, and H_2CO_3 is the plasma carbonic acid concentration. Because the Pco_2 in the plasma is proportional to the concentration of carbonic acid and dissolved carbon dioxide in the plasma, the Henderson-Hasselbalch equation can be rewritten:

$$pH = pK + \log \frac{[HCO_3^-]}{S \times Pco_2}$$

$$= 6.1 + \log \frac{24 \text{ mEq/L}}{0.03 \times 40 \text{ mm Hg}} = \frac{24}{1.2}$$

$$= 6.1 + \log \frac{20}{1}$$

$$7.4 = 6.1 + 1.3$$

where S is the CO_2 solubility constant and has a value of 0.03. The pK for the bicarbonate–carbonic acid buffer system is a constant with a value of 6.1. Substituting in the normal plasma values for the bicarbonate (24 mEq/L) and Pco_2 (40 mm Hg) and solving the equation, the result is the normal pH of 7.4. This equation shows that the ratio of the bicarbonate to carbonic acid determines the pH. At a body pH of 7.4 the ratio of bicarbonate to carbonic acid must be 20:1 as shown. As long as the 20:1 ratio is maintained, regardless of the absolute values, the pH will be 7.4.

Overview of the primary acid-base imbalances

Fig. 22-1 illustrates the normal range of blood pH near 7.4 and the widest range compatible with life from 6.8 to 7.8 or an interval of one pH unit. The normal range of pH is from 7.38 to 7.42 if one uses the more sensitive value of one standard deviation (1 SD) from the mean of 7.4. Most clinicians, however, use the less sensitive value of 7.35 to 7.45, which is 2 SD from the mean. A blood pH of less than 7.35 is called *acidemia,* and the process causing it is called *acidosis.* A pH of 7.25 or less is life threatening, and a pH of 6.8 is incompatible with life. Similarly, a blood pH greater than 7.45 is called *alkalemia,* and the process causing it is called *alkalosis.* A pH greater than 7.55 is life threatening, and a pH greater than 7.8 is incompatible with life.

The four primary acid-base disturbances and their compensations may be visualized using a simplified version of the Henderson-Hasselbalch equation:

$$pH \propto \frac{[HCO_3^-]}{Paco_2} = \frac{20 \text{ (metabolic component controlled by kidneys)}}{1 \text{ (respiratory component controlled by lungs)}}$$

This equation emphasizes the fact that the ratio of base to acid must be 20:1 to maintain the pH in the normal range. It also emphasizes the ability of the kidneys to alter the base bicarbonate through metabolic processes and

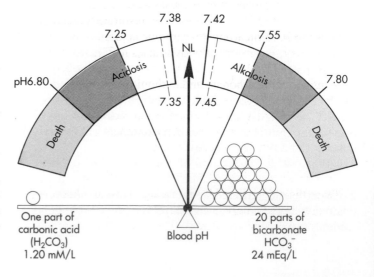

FIG. 22-1 Normal blood pH is 7.40 ± 0.02 (1 standard deviation [SD]) or ± 0.05 (2 SD). Acid-base balance occurs when the ratio of bicarbonate to carbonic acid is 20:1. Any change in this ratio tips the balance and swings the pointer to the acidosis or alkalosis side. A pH below 7.25 or above 7.55 is life-threatening, and the extremes of 6.8 or 7.8 cause death.

▶ TABLE 22-2 Simple Acid-Base Disorders

Acid-Base Disorder	Cause	Bicarbonate–Carbonic Acid Ratio 20:1	Compensation
Respiratory acidosis	Hypoventilation (retained CO_2)	Ratio <20:1	Renal: retention of HCO_3^-; excretion of acid salts; increased ammonia formation
Respiratory alkalosis	Hyperventilation (excessive loss of CO_2)	Ratio >20:1	Renal: excretion of HCO_3^-; retention of acid salts; decreased ammonia formation
Metabolic acidosis	Retention of fixed acids Loss of base bicarbonate	Ratio <20:1	Lungs: hyperventilation Renal: as in respiratory acidosis
Metabolic alkalosis	Loss of fixed acids Gain of base bicarbonate K^+ depletion	Ratio >20:1	Lungs: hypoventilation Renal: as in respiratory alkalosis

the ability of the lungs to alter the Pa_{CO_2} (partial pressure of CO_2 in the arterial blood) through respiration.

Metabolic imbalances are those in which the primary disturbance is in the concentration of bicarbonate. Because bicarbonate appears in the numerator of the Henderson-Hasselbalch equation, an increased bicarbonate concentration causes increased pH, which is called *metabolic alkalosis*. A decrease in the bicarbonate concentration causes a decrease in the pH, which is called *metabolic acidosis*. Respiratory imbalances are those in which the primary disturbance is in the concentration of carbon dioxide (carbonic acid). The carbon dioxide concentration appears in the denominator of the Henderson-Hasselbalch buffer equation. An increase in the Pa_{CO_2} lowers the pH and is called *respiratory acidosis* (also referred to as alveolar hypoventilation, or hypercapnia). A decrease in the Pa_{CO_2} raises the pH and is called *respiratory alkalosis* (also referred to as alveolar hyperventilation or hypocapnia). Note that the 20:1 bicarbonate–carbonic acid ratio is altered in each of the four primary acid-base imbalances, which causes a deviation in the pH from the normal 7.4. Metabolic or respiratory acidosis lowers the 20:1 bicarbonate–carbonic acid ratio, whereas metabolic or respiratory alkalosis raises it. Thus all of the four primary acid-base disturbances may be identified by looking at the bicarbonate and carbonic acid relationship in the Henderson-Hasselbalch equation. Various combinations of the primary acid-base disturbances are called *mixed acid-base disturbances*. An example would be respiratory acidosis and metabolic acidosis.

Compensatory responses to alterations in pH

Once the pH is altered by a primary acid-base disorder, the body immediately uses compensatory responses to bring the pH back to normal. There are three compensatory responses as discussed previously: (1) ECF and ICF buffering; (2) respiratory alteration of the Pa_{CO_2} by hypoventilation or hyperventilation, and (3) renal alteration of the $[HCO_3^-]$ or $[H^+]$. ECF and ICF buffering may involve the shift of H^+ into or out of the cells in exchange for K^+ and is discussed later. The respiratory and renal compensatory responses are easily analyzed in terms of the Henderson-Hasselbalch equation.

A primary metabolic acidosis (decreased $[HCO_3^-]$) is compensated by respiratory hyperventilation, thus reducing the Pa_{CO_2} and restoring the pH toward normal. Primary metabolic alkalosis (increased $[HCO_3^-]$) is compensated by respiratory hypoventilation, thus increasing the Pa_{CO_2} and restoring the pH toward normal. The respiratory compensatory response occurs within minutes. In contrast, the kidneys compensate for primary respiratory acidosis (increased Pa_{CO_2}) or alkalosis (decreased Pa_{CO_2}) by retention or excretion of HCO_3^- or H^+ ion. However, renal compensation is slower so no effects are noticeable for about 24 hours. Full compensation takes about 2 to 3 days. Thus respiratory acidosis is classified as *acute* if renal compensation has not yet occurred and the HCO_3^- is still normal; when renal compensation has occurred and the HCO_3^- is increased, it is classified as *chronic*. Primary respiratory alkalosis may also be classified as acute or chronic, depending on whether renal compensation is partial or complete. In terms of the Henderson-Hasselbalch equation, when the numerator increases, the denominator must increase to maintain the 20:1 ratio and minimize deviations of the pH from the normal. Compensation always involves a compensatory change in the numerator (or denominator) that is in the same direction as the primary disturbance. Table 22-2 presents a simplified overview of the four primary acid-base disorders.

ASSESSMENT OF ACID-BASE IMBALANCE

Diagnosis and treatment of acid-base disorders require a thorough understanding of the pathogenesis and pathophysiology of these disturbances. Many authors have developed various methods to simplify the interpretation of the respiratory and metabolic components of the arterial blood gas values to identify the primary major imbalance (whether acute or compensated) or a mixed disorder. These methods include the use of acid-base nomograms and the use of standard bicarbonate, with the base excess and base deficit as a method of identifying metabolic disorders. It must be pointed out, however, that none of these methods are foolproof and all are subject to misinterpretation. The acid-base nomogram uses confidence bands to identify the acute and compensated primary acid-base disorders, with mixed disorders falling between the confidence bands. It is possible for the pH to be normal in the presence of an acid-base disturbance such as a mixture of respiratory acidosis and metabolic alkalosis. This mixture, in turn, would be hard to differentiate from a well-compensated chronic respiratory acidosis without the appropriate clinical information.

The standard bicarbonate and base deficit/excess is another popular method devised to assist interpretation of acid-base disturbances. The standard bicarbonate is supposed to represent a measure of the true plasma bicarbonate in place of the classic carbon dioxide content measure. The latter contains the respiratory or carbonic acid component (although small).

The base excess/deficit may be calculated from the standard bicarbonate and is supposedly a sure way of evaluating the metabolic component of an acid-base disorder. Many authors, however, have severely criticized the use of the standard bicarbonate and base excess/deficit values (Rose, 1994; Schwartz, Relman, 1963). These authors point out that the standard bicarbonate is also an estimate of the true plasma bicarbonate and offers no advantage over the carbon dioxide content measure. They do not recommend using the base deficit or excess because these values may be misleading.

A final warning about the interpretation of laboratory values in the diagnosis of acid-base disturbances needs to be emphasized. The $PaCO_2$ cannot be regarded solely as an indicator of a respiratory disturbance nor can the HCO_3^- be viewed exclusively as an index of metabolic disorders. A low $PaCO_2$ may indicate a primary respiratory alkalosis or may result from the expected respiratory compensation for a metabolic acidosis. Similarly, an increased $[HCO_3^-]$ may reflect the presence of a primary metabolic alkalosis or may be a compensatory response to chronic respiratory acidosis. To further complicate the picture, most acid-base disturbances are partially compensated when first detected and mixed disorders occur frequently. In summary, there are no easy shortcuts to the accurate assessment of acid-base disorders. The acid-base laboratory variables cannot stand alone but must be interpreted in the context of a thorough knowledge of the clinical situation, experience, good judgment, and a sound understanding of acid-base physiology.

With these caveats in mind, the box on p. 297 presents a systematic guide for the assessment of acid-base disorders. Assessment begins with a high degree of clinical suspicion because acid-base disorders may be difficult to detect unless severe, and signs and symptoms tend to be vague and nonspecific. The clinical history, signs and symptoms, and other laboratory data that suggest a disease process associated with an acid-base disorder are noted. The common causes and symptoms of the specific acid-base disorders are discussed later.

Next, one confirms clinical suspicions with a systematic examination of the acid-base variables. Table 22-3 presents the normal values of the arterial blood parameters used in analyzing acid-base disorders, as well as some useful formulas. The first step is to examine the pH to determine whether acidemia or alkalemia is present and, if so, its magnitude. The second step is to examine the $PaCO_2$ and $[HCO_3^-]$ in relationship to the pH in an attempt to characterize the disturbance as a primary respiratory or metabolic or mixed acid-base imbalance. The Henderson-Hasselbalch equation or an acid-base nomogram (Fig. 22-2) may be helpful in making a tentative decision. Knowledge of the clinical situation is essential in making a decision. The third step is to estimate the expected compensatory response to the primary acid-base disorder. Table 22-4 may be helpful in this regard, as well as suggesting possible mixed acid-base disorders when the compensatory response is less than or greater than expected. The acid-base nomogram may also be helpful. One should also calculate the anion gap to determine if a metabolic acidosis is the result of the retention of fixed acids associated with an increased anion gap. Actually, an anion gap does not exist in reality because an equal number of positive and negative ions are required for body electroneutrality. Rather, the anion gap represents unmeasured anions because the sum of the plasma chloride plus bicarbonate concentrations is less than the serum sodium concentration:

$$140 \text{ mEq/L} - (104 \text{ mEq/L} + 24 \text{ mEq/L}) = 12 \text{ mEq/L}$$
$$= \text{Normal anion gap}$$

The increase in the anion gap should also be compared with the decrease in the $[HCO_3^-]$ to detect a mixed disorder such as a metabolic alkalosis combined with the metabolic acidosis. A reduced anion gap provides an index to certain other disorders. For example, the serum sodium may remain normal while the serum bicarbonate and chlorides increase. This occurs most commonly in hypoalbuminemia.

The final step in the assessment of an acid-base disorder is identifying the primary imbalance and characterizing it as acute or chronic (compensated) or as a mixture

A SYSTEMATIC APPROACH TO THE ASSESSMENT OF ACID-BASE DISTURBANCES

BEGIN WITH A HIGH DEGREE OF CLINICAL SUSPICION

1. Examine the *clinical history* for disease processes that may lead to simple acid-base disorders.
   a. This requires knowledge of the pathogenesis of the various acid-base disorders.
   b. For example, one might expect a person with advanced chronic obstructive pulmonary disease to develop respiratory acidosis.
2. Note *clinical signs and symptoms* that suggest an acid-base disorder.
   a. Unfortunately, many of the signs and symptoms of an acid-base disorder are subtle or nonspecific.
   b. For example, Kussmaul respirations in a diabetic patient may represent respiratory compensation for metabolic acidosis.
3. *Examine laboratory reports of the electrolytes and other data* that suggest disease processes associated with acid-base disorders.
   a. For example, hypokalemia is often associated with metabolic alkalosis.
   b. For example, an elevated serum creatinine level indicates renal insufficiency, and renal insufficiency and failure are usually associated with metabolic acidosis.

EVALUATE ACID-BASE VARIABLES TO IDENTIFY THE TYPE OF DISORDER

1. First, *examine the arterial blood pH* to determine the direction and magnitude of the acid-base disturbance.
   a. If decreased, the patient has acidemia with two potential causes: metabolic acidosis or respiratory acidosis.
   b. If increased, the patient has alkalemia with two potential causes: metabolic alkalosis or respiratory alkalosis.
   c. It is helpful to note that the renal and respiratory compensations rarely return the pH to normal so that a normal pH in the presence of changes in the $PaCO_2$ and HCO_3^- suggests a mixed disorder; for example, a person with a combined respiratory acidosis and metabolic alkalosis might have a normal pH.
2. *Examine the respiratory ($PaCO_2$) and metabolic (HCO_3^-) variables in relation to the pH* to tentatively characterize the primary disturbance as a respiratory, metabolic, or mixed disorder.
   a. Is the $PaCO_2$ normal (40 mm Hg), increased, or decreased?
   b. Is the HCO_3^- normal (24 mEq/L), increased, or decreased?
      (1) Optional: Is there a base excess or deficit?
   c. In a simple acid-base disorder, the $PaCO_2$ and HCO_3^- are always altered in the same direction.
   d. Deviation of the $PaCO_2$ and HCO_3^- in opposite directions indicates the presence of a mixed acid-base disorder.
   e. Make a tentative decision about the primary disturbance by correlating the findings with the clinical situation.
3. *Estimate the expected compensatory response to the primary acid-base disorder.*
   a. Use Table 22-4 to determine the expected respiratory or metabolic compensatory response to the primary disorder.
   b. If the compensatory response is greater or less than expected, a mixed acid-base disorder is suggested (an acid-base nomogram may also be used to help identify a mixed acid-base disorder).
   c. Calculate the plasma anion gap.
      (1) If increased (>16 mEq/L), metabolic acidosis is most likely.
   d. Compare the magnitude of fall in plasma $[HCO_3^-]$ with the increase in the anion gap; these should be similar in magnitude.
      (1) If the anion gap has risen < the fall in $[HCO_3^-]$, this suggests that a component of the metabolic acidosis is due to HCO_3^- loss.
      (2) If the increase in anion gap is much greater than the fall in $[HCO_3^-]$, there is a coexistent metabolic alkalosis.
4. *Make the final interpretation.*
   a. Simple acid-base disorder
      (1) Acute (uncompensated) or
      (2) Chronic (partially or fully compensated)
   b. Mixed acid-base disorder
   c. Normal or wide anion gap: metabolic acidosis

▶ TABLE 22-3   Arterial Blood Parameters Used for the Analysis of Acid-Base Status

Parameter	Normal Value	Definition and Implications

Pao_2	80-100 mm Hg	Partial pressure of oxygen in arterial blood (decreases with age)
		In adults <60 yr:
		   60-80 mm Hg = mild hypoxemia
		   40-60 mm Hg = moderate hypoxemia
		   <40 mm Hg = severe hypoxemia

pH	7.40 ($\pm$0.05 [2 SD])
	
	7.40 ($\pm$0.02 [1 SD])
		Identifies whether there is acidemia or alkalemia; the value using
		  2 standard deviations (SD) from the mean is the common clin-
		  ical value.
		pH <7.35 = acidosis; pH >7.45 = alkalosis

$[H^+]$	40 ($\pm$2) nmol/L or nEq/L	The hydrogen ion concentration may be used instead of the pH
$Paco_2$	40 ($\pm$5.0) mm Hg	Partial pressure of CO_2 in the arterial blood Pco_2 <35 mm Hg = respiratory alkalosis Pco_2 >45 mm Hg = respiratory acidosis

CO_2 content	25.5 ($\pm$4.5) mEq/L	Classic method of estimating $[HCO_3]$; measures HCO_3^- + dis-
		  solved CO_2 (latter is generally quite small except in respira-
		  tory acidosis)

Standard HCO_3^-	24 ($\pm$2) mEq/L	Estimated HCO_3^- concentration after fully oxygenated arterial
		  blood has been equilibrated with CO_2 at a Pco_2 of 40 mm Hg
		  at 38° C; eliminates the influence of respiration on the plasma
		  HCO_3^- concentration.

Base excess	0 ($\pm$2) mEq/L	Reflects pure metabolic component Base excess = 1.2 × deviation from 0 Negative in metabolic acidosis Positive in metabolic alkalosis Misleading in respiratory and mixed acid-base disturbances Not essential for interpretation of acid-base disturbances

Anion gap	12 ($\pm$4) mEq/L	Anion gap (or delta) reflects the difference between the unmea-
		  sured cations (K^+, Mg^{++}, Ca^{++}) and unmeasured anions (al-
		  bumin, organic anions, HPO_4^-, $SO_4^=$); useful in identifying
		  types of metabolic acidosis; value > 16-20 indicates acidosis
		  is caused by retention of organic acids (for example,
		  diabetic ketoacidosis)

USEFUL FORMULAS

Plasma anion gap = $[Na^+] - ([HCO_3^-] + [Cl^-])$

Calculation of third acid-base parameter when two are known:

$$[H^+] = 24 \times \frac{Paco_2}{[HCO_3^-]}$$

Conversion of pH into $[H^+]$ (use conversion in Table 22-1 or formulas below):

pH of 7.4 = $[H^+]$ of 40 mEq/L

For every 0.1 increase in pH above 7.4, multiply 40 × 0.8

For every 0.1 decrease in pH below 7.4, multiple 40 × 1.25

For example, pH of 7.60 = 40 × 0.8 × 0.8 = $[H^+]$ of 26 mEq/L

▶ TABLE 22-4   Expected Compensatory Responses in Primary Acid-Base Disorders

Disorder	Expected Response	Possible Mixed Disorder
Metabolic acidosis	For every 1 mEq decrease in HCO_3^-, 1.2 mm Hg decrease in Pa_{CO_2}	Fall in Pa_{CO_2} > expected Superimposed respiratory alkalosis + metabolic acidosis Fall in Pa_{CO_2} < expected Superimposed respiratory acidosis + metabolic acidosis
Metabolic alkalosis	For every 1 mEq increase in HCO_3^-, 0.7 mm Hg increase in Pa_{CO_2}	Rise in Pa_{CO_2} > expected Superimposed respiratory acidosis + metabolic alkalosis Rise in Pa_{CO_2} < expected Superimposed respiratory alkalosis + metabolic alkalosis
Respiratory acidosis		
Acute	For every 10 mm Hg increase in Pa_{CO_2}, 1 mEq/L increase in HCO_3^-	Rise in HCO_3^- > expected Secondary metabolic alkalosis + respiratory acidosis
Chronic	For every 10 mm Hg increase in Pa_{CO_2}, 3.5 mEq/L increase in HCO_3^-	Rise in HCO_3^- < expected Superimposed metabolic acidosis + respiratory acidosis
Respiratory alkalosis		
Acute	For every 10 mm Hg decrease in Pa_{CO_2}, 2 mEq/L decrease in HCO_3^-	Fall in HCO_3^- > expected Secondary metabolic acidosis + respiratory alkalosis
Chronic	For every 10 mm Hg decrease in Pa_{CO_2}, 5 mEq/L decrease in HCO_3^-	Fall in HCO_3^- < expected Secondary metabolic alkalosis + respiratory alkalosis

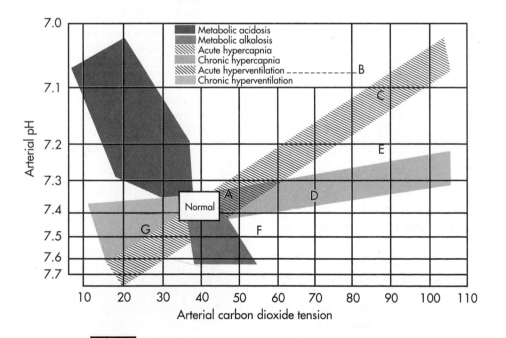

FIG. 22-2   Nomogram for acid-base disturbances. This graph displays the quantity and direction of changes in pH and Pa_{CO_2} in various types of acid-base disturbances. The shaded areas represent the range of variability in persons with pure acid-base disorders. See text in Chapter 41 for explanation of lettered points. [Modified from Burrows B, Knudson RJ, Kettel LJ: *Respiratory insufficiency,* Chicago, 1975, Mosby.]

of two or more disturbances. Metabolic acidosis should be classified as a normal or an increased anion gap.

METABOLIC ACIDOSIS

Metabolic acidosis (HCO_3^- deficit) is a systemic disorder characterized by a primary decrease in the plasma bicarbonate concentration that results in a decrease of the pH (increase in the [H^+]). The ECF [HCO_3^-] is less than 22 mEq/L, and the pH is less than 7.35. Respiratory com-

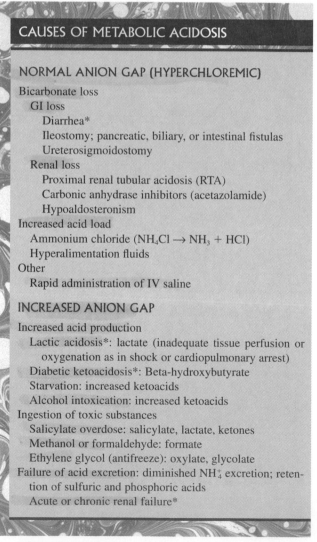

FIG. 22-3   Classification of metabolic acidosis arrived at by using the anion gap. Values are given in milliequivalents per liter. The bar on the left shows the normal relationship of the unmeasured anions (A^-) to the plasma electrolytes. To maintain electroneutrality, the number of cations and anions must be equal. Normally, the number of sodium (Na^+) ions exceeds the number of chloride (Cl^-) and bicarbonate (HCO_3^-) ions, called the anion gap (normally 12). The anion gap is made up of anions such as sulfate and organic acids such as ketones not normally measured in routine laboratory tests. The anion gap is significant because it gives the level of unmeasured anions. The bar in the middle depicts hyperchloremic (or normal anion gap) acidosis usually caused by renal or GI loss of bicarbonate, with a compensatory increase in chloride ions to preserve electroneutrality. The bar on the right depicts normochloremic (or high anion) acidosis caused by an increase in unmeasured anions as, for example, in diabetic ketoacidosis or lactic acidosis.

pensation begins immediately to lower the $Paco_2$ by hyperventilation so that metabolic acidosis seldom develops acutely.

Causes and Pathogenesis

The basic causes of metabolic acidosis are either gains of fixed (noncarbonic) acid, failure of the kidneys to excrete the daily acid load, or a loss of base bicarbonate. The causes of metabolic acidosis are commonly divided into two groups according to whether the anion gap is normal or increased. As stated previously, the anion gap is calculated by subtracting the sum of the plasma concentrations of Cl^- and HCO_3^- from the Na^+ concentration. The normal value is 12. The cause of high anion gap metabolic acidosis is an increase in unmeasured anions such as sulfate, phosphate, lactate, and other organic acids. If the acidosis is caused by the loss of bicarbonate (e.g., diarrhea) or gain of a chloride acid (e.g., administration of ammonium chloride), the anion gap will be normal. Conversely, if the acidosis is caused by increased production

CAUSES OF METABOLIC ACIDOSIS

NORMAL ANION GAP (HYPERCHLOREMIC)

Bicarbonate loss
  GI loss
    Diarrhea*
    Ileostomy; pancreatic, biliary, or intestinal fistulas
    Ureterosigmoidostomy
  Renal loss
    Proximal renal tubular acidosis (RTA)
    Carbonic anhydrase inhibitors (acetazolamide)
    Hypoaldosteronism
Increased acid load
  Ammonium chloride ($NH_4Cl \rightarrow NH_3 + HCl$)
  Hyperalimentation fluids
Other
  Rapid administration of IV saline

INCREASED ANION GAP

Increased acid production
  Lactic acidosis*: lactate (inadequate tissue perfusion or oxygenation as in shock or cardiopulmonary arrest)
  Diabetic ketoacidosis*: Beta-hydroxybutyrate
  Starvation: increased ketoacids
  Alcohol intoxication: increased ketoacids
Ingestion of toxic substances
  Salicylate overdose: salicylate, lactate, ketones
  Methanol or formaldehyde: formate
  Ethylene glycol (antifreeze): oxylate, glycolate
Failure of acid excretion: diminished NH_4^+ excretion; retention of sulfuric and phosphoric acids
  Acute or chronic renal failure*

*Most common causes.

of an organic acid (e.g., lactic acid in circulatory shock) or the retention of sulfuric or phosphoric acid (e.g., in renal failure), the concentration of unmeasured anions (anion gap) increases (Fig. 22-3).

The box on p. 300 lists some of the common causes of metabolic acidosis. In normal anion gap metabolic acidosis, bicarbonate loss may occur via the gastrointestinal (GI) tract or kidneys. Diarrhea, small bowel fistula, and ureterosigmoidostomy cause significant losses of bicarbonate, whereas renal reabsorption of bicarbonate is decreased in proximal renal tubular acidosis or in persons taking carbonic anhydrase inhibitors such as acetazolamide. Because chloride combines with sodium in competition with bicarbonate, it is related to the acid-base balance of the body. When bicarbonate is lost from the body, reducing the serum [HCO_3^-], the plasma [Cl^-] rises in compensation because the total number of anions and cations in the ECF must be equal to maintain electroneutrality. The result is *hyperchloremic metabolic acidosis.* Administration of excess chloride salts (e.g., NH_4Cl) also causes hyperchloremic metabolic acidosis. The acidosis caused by the rapid administration of IV saline is usually mild and temporary and is called *dilutional acidosis.*

Conditions associated with high anion gap metabolic acidosis are listed in the box on p. 300. The most common condition is shock or inadequate tissue perfusion from any number of causes, resulting in the accumulation of large amounts of lactic acid. Diabetic ketoacidosis (DKA), starvation, and ethanol intoxication cause elevation of the anion gap because of the formation of ketoacids; renal failure causes such elevation by the retention of sulfuric and phosphoric acids. Poisoning by salicylate overdose, methanol, or ethylene glycol produces increased anion gaps by elevation of their organic acid counterparts (salicylate, formate, oxylate).

Compensatory Response to Acid Load in Metabolic Acidosis

The immediate response to the H^+ load in metabolic acidosis is ECF buffering by bicarbonate, thus reducing the plasma [HCO_3^-]. Excess H^+ also enters the cells and is buffered by proteins and phosphates (which provide 60% of the buffering). To maintain electroneutrality, the entry of H^+ into cells is accompanied by movement of K^+ out of the cells into the ECF. Thus the serum K^+ rises in conditions of acidosis. When a patient with acidosis has normokalemia or hypokalemia, K^+ depletion is present and must be corrected along with the acidosis.

The second mechanism activated within minutes in metabolic acidosis is respiratory compensation. The increased arterial [H^+] stimulates chemoreceptors in the carotid bodies, which in turn stimulate increased alveolar ventilation (hyperventilation). Consequently, the $Paco_2$ is lowered and the pH restored toward 7.4.

The renal compensatory response provides the final

means of correcting the metabolic acidosis, although it is slower and may require several days. This takes place by several mechanisms. Excess H^+ is secreted into the tubule and excreted as NH_4^+ or as titratable acid (H_3PO_4). Increased NH_4^+ excretion is accompanied by increased HCO_3^- resorption, but H_3PO_4 excretion results in the formation of new bicarbonate. Renal insufficiency or failure decreases the effectiveness of H^+ elimination.

Clinical Features and Diagnosis

Signs and symptoms of metabolic acidosis tend to be vague, and the patient may be asymptomatic unless the serum [HCO_3^-] falls below 15 mEq/L. Kussmaul breathing (deep, rapid respirations indicating compensatory hyperventilation) may be more prominent in the acidosis of diabetic ketoacidosis than in that of renal failure. The major signs and symptoms of metabolic acidosis are manifested as abnormalities in cardiovascular, neurologic, and bone function. If the pH is less than 7.1, there is a reduction of cardiac contractility and the inotropic response to catecholamines. Peripheral vasodilation may be present. These effects may lead to hypotension and cardiac dysrhythmias.

Neurologic symptoms range from lethargy to coma related to the fall in pH of the cerebrospinal fluid. Nausea and vomiting may be present. Neurologic symptoms are less severe in metabolic acidosis than in respiratory acidosis because the lipid-soluble CO_2 crosses the blood-brain barrier more rapidly than the water-soluble HCO_3^-.

The buffering of H^+ by bone bicarbonates in the metabolic acidosis of chronic renal failure retards growth in children and may lead to a variety of bone disorders (renal osteodystrophy).

The diagnosis of metabolic acidosis is made on the basis of clinical features and confirmed by laboratory measurement of the pH, $Paco_2$, and HCO_3^- using a systematic approach as outlined previously. The pH is less than 7.35, HCO_3^- is less than 22 mEq/L, and the $Paco_2$ is less than 40 mm Hg but rarely falls to less than 12 mm Hg. The expected degree of compensation should be calculated to determine if a mixed acid-base disorder exists.

Treatment

The treatment goal for metabolic acidosis is to raise the systemic pH to a safe level and treat the underlying cause of the acidosis. Only a small increase in the plasma pH to 7.20 or 7.25 is necessary to restore the patient to a safe range. The HCO_3^- must be less than 15 mEq/L and the pH less than 7.20 to cause serious disruption of physiologic processes. The metabolic acidosis should be corrected slowly to avoid the following complications of IV $NaHCO_3$ administration:

1. Increased pH of cerebrospinal fluid (CSF) and suppressed respiratory drive, resulting in less respiratory compensation.
2. Respiratory alkalosis because patients tend to hyper-

ventilate for several hours after the ECF acidosis is corrected.

3. Shift of the oxyhemoglobin dissociation curve to the left in the event of a complicating respiratory alkalosis, which increases the affinity of oxygen for hemoglobin and possibly reduces oxygen delivery to the tissues.

4. Metabolic alkalosis (because there is no loss of potential bicarbonate and the ketoacids can be metabolized back to lactate) in a patient with diabetic ketoacidosis (DKA). Insulin alone will usually restore acid-base balance; however, it is important to monitor the serum K^+ while the acidosis is being corrected because the acidosis may be masking K^+ deficit.

5. Serious metabolic alkalosis as a result of overcorrection of lactic acidosis resulting from cardiac arrest. Some investigators found that the serum pH reached 7.9 and the serum bicarbonate 60 to 70 mEq/L with the indiscriminate infusion of $NaHCO_3$ during CPR (Mattar et al., 1974).

6. Functional hypocalcemia from administering IV $NaHCO_3$ to a renal failure patient with severe metabolic acidosis (the acidosis may be masking a hypocalcemia because Ca^{++} is more soluble in an acid medium; Ca^{++} is less soluble in an alkaline medium), resulting in tetany, convulsions, and death. Hemodialysis is the usual treatment for renal metabolic acidosis.

7. Serious circulatory overload (hypervolemia) in patients who already have an ECF fluid volume excess, such as those with congestive heart failure or renal failure.

IV lactated Ringer's solution is generally the fluid of choice to effect the correction of normal anion gap metabolic acidosis and the ECF fluid volume deficit that often accompany this condition. The sodium lactate is slowly metabolized to $NaHCO_3$ in the body and corrects the acidosis slowly.

Treatment of high anion gap metabolic acidosis is generally directed toward correcting or ameliorating the causative factor. Treatment of the acidosis itself is required only if it causes serious organ dysfunction (HCO_3^- <10 mEq/L). In these cases sufficient $NaHCO_3$ is given to raise the HCO_3^- to 15 mEq/L and a pH of about 7.20 over a period of 12 hours (Schrier, 1986).

METABOLIC ALKALOSIS

Metabolic alkalosis (HCO_3^- excess) is a systemic disorder characterized by a primary increase in the plasma bicabonate concentration, resulting in an increase in the pH (decrease in the [H^+]). The ECF [HCO_3^-] is greater than 26 mEq/L and the pH is greater than 7.45. Metabolic alkalosis is frequently accompanied by ECF volume contraction and hypokalemia. Respiratory compensation consists of raising the $Paco_2$ by hypoventilation; how-

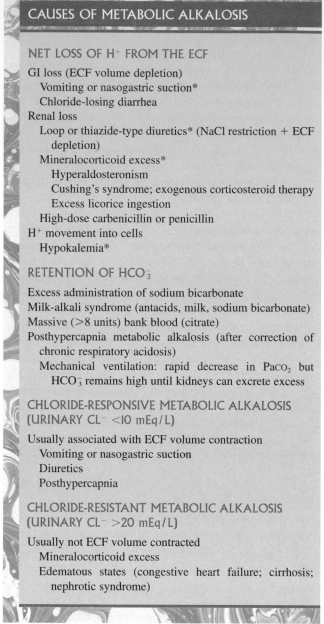

CAUSES OF METABOLIC ALKALOSIS

NET LOSS OF H^+ FROM THE ECF

GI loss (ECF volume depletion)
    Vomiting or nasogastric suction*
    Chloride-losing diarrhea
Renal loss
    Loop or thiazide-type diuretics* (NaCl restriction + ECF depletion)
    Mineralocorticoid excess*
        Hyperaldosteronism
        Cushing's syndrome; exogenous corticosteroid therapy
        Excess licorice ingestion
    High-dose carbenicillin or penicillin
H^+ movement into cells
    Hypokalemia*

RETENTION OF HCO_3^-

Excess administration of sodium bicarbonate
Milk-alkali syndrome (antacids, milk, sodium bicarbonate)
Massive (>8 units) bank blood (citrate)
Posthypercapnia metabolic alkalosis (after correction of chronic respiratory acidosis)
    Mechanical ventilation: rapid decrease in $Paco_2$ but HCO_3^- remains high until kidneys can excrete excess

CHLORIDE-RESPONSIVE METABOLIC ALKALOSIS (URINARY CL^- <10 mEq/L)

Usually associated with ECF volume contraction
    Vomiting or nasogastric suction
    Diuretics
    Posthypercapnia

CHLORIDE-RESISTANT METABOLIC ALKALOSIS (URINARY CL^- >20 mEq/L)

Usually not ECF volume contracted
    Mineralocorticoid excess
    Edematous states (congestive heart failure; cirrhosis; nephrotic syndrome)

*Most common causes.

ever, the degree of hypoventilation is limited because respiration continues to be driven by hypoxia.

Causes and Pathogenesis

The box above lists common causes of metabolic alkalosis, which are net loss of H^+ (and chloride ions) or excess retention of HCO_3^-. HCL may be lost from the GI tract, as in prolonged vomiting or nasogastric suction, or in the urine because of the administration of loop or thiazide diuretics. Sustained metabolic alkalosis caused by the oral or parenteral ingestion of bicarbonate is rare because the bicarbonate load is excreted in the urine unless there is also a chloride deficit.

The pathogenesis of metabolic alkalosis is best understood as occurring in three stages: generation, maintenance, and recovery. It is generated by the net loss of H^+ from the body with the consequent elevation of the ECF HCO_3^- (or by the addition of exogenous HCO_3^-). The maintenance of a sustained metabolic alkalosis occurs because the base excess cannot be excreted. A variety of factors (Cl^- and K^+ deficit, ECF volume [Na^+ and water] depletion, and aldosterone excess) may cause this condition. Cessation of the event that caused the metabolic alkalosis (e.g., vomiting) is not necessarily accompanied by resolution and recovery from the alkalosis. The specific therapy required is evident by understanding the factors that maintain alkalosis.

The depletion of chlorides is crucial, both in the generation and the maintenance of *hypochloremic metabolic alkalosis*. Na^+ is the primary cation in the ECF, balanced by an equal number of anions, mainly Cl^- and HCO_3^-. In addition, Cl^- and HCO_3^- have a reciprocal relationship: a decrease in Cl^- results in an increase in HCO_3^-, and an increase in Cl^- causes a decrease in HCO_3^-. The purpose of this relationship is to balance the total negative and positive charges to maintain ECF electroneutrality. Thus, when HCL is secreted into the stomach, an equimolar amount of HCO_3^- is secreted into the ECF. Metabolic alkalosis is commonly initiated by vomiting or nasogastric suction, with the consequent loss of fluids rich in chlorides (HCl) and deficient in HCO_3^-. KCl and NaCl and water are lost as well. The result is an increase in the serum HCO_3^-, potassium depletion, and fluid volume depletion.

The immediate compensatory response to metabolic alkalosis is intracellular buffering. H^+ exits the cells to buffer the excess ECF HCO_3^-. K^+ moves into cells in exchange for the H^+. There is also a small increase in lactic acid production within cells to produce more H^+. Consequently, there is a paradoxic ICF acidosis and an ECF alkalosis.

The increased pH is sensed by the chemoreceptors in the carotid bodies, which in turn cause a reflex decrease in alveolar ventilation. However, the magnitude of the respiratory compensation is generally quite small. The degree of hypoventilation and rise in the $Paco_2$ is limited by the need for oxygen and rarely exceeds 50 to 55 mm Hg.

The final renal correction of metabolic alkalosis requires the excretion of the excess HCO_3^-. It is difficult to produce a sustained metabolic alkalosis from the ingestion of bicarbonate because the kidneys normally have a great capacity to excrete HCO_3^-.

Research findings by Galla and Luke (1987) suggest that chloride depletion plays the major role in preventing the renal excretion of HCO_3^-. In contrast to previous theories positing a major role for ECF volume depletion and secondary hyperaldosteronism, these authors claim that intrarenal mechanisms responsible for chloride depletion can account for the maintenance of metabolic alkalosis, regardless of the status of the ECF volume. According to the findings of Galla and Luke, Cl^- depletion stimulates the renin-angiotensin-aldosterone mechanism, increased renal K^+ and H^+ excretion, and increased reabsorption of HCO_3^- independent of the sodium. In addition to chloride depletion as a cause of the perpetuation of metabolic alkalosis, fluid volume depletion stimulates the renin-angiotensin-aldosterone mechanism. Aldosterone causes increased Na^+ and water reabsorption in an effort to restore the ECF volume. Protection of the ECF volume takes precedence over correction of the alkalosis, because this would require the excretion of Na^+ along with HCO_3^-. When there is Cl^- depletion, not enough Cl^- is available to absorb with Na^+, so that more Na^+ is reabsorbed in exchange for H^+, both in the proximal and the distal tubule (via aldosterone). In fact, H^+ secretion can increase to the point where all of the filtered HCO_3^- is reabsorbed and additional HCO_3^- is generated. The result of the increased H^+ secretion is a paradoxically acid urine in the presence of an alkalosis. Aldosterone also stimulates K^+ excretion. K^+ depletion, in turn, promotes H^+ excretion and accelerated HCO_3^- reabsorption. In summary, Cl^- depletion, fluid volume depletion, hyperaldosteronism, and K^+ depletion all contribute to the maintenance of metabolic alkalosis.

Clinical Features and Diagnosis

There are no specific signs and symptoms in metabolic alkalosis. The disorder should be suspected in patients with a history of vomiting, nasogastric suction, or diuretic therapy or patients recovering from hypercapneic respiratory failure. Signs and symptoms of hypokalemia and fluid volume deficit, such as muscle cramps and weakness, may be present. Severe alkalemia (pH >7.6) can cause cardiac dysrhythmias in normal persons and particularly in those with cardiac disease. If the patient is hypokalemic, especially if digitalized, ECG abnormalities or a cardiac dysrhythmia may develop. Occasionally tetany may occur in a patient if the serum Ca^{++} is borderline low and the alkalosis has developed rapidly. Ca^{++} is more closely bound to albumin in an alkaline pH, and the drop in ionized Ca^{++} may be sufficient to produce tetany or a seizure.

Diagnosis of metabolic alkalosis is made on the basis of the history and appropriate laboratory studies. Plasma pH is elevated above 7.45, and the HCO_3^- is greater than 26 mEq/L. The $Paco_2$ may be normal or slightly elevated; the expected compensatory rise is 0.7 mm Hg for every 1 mEq increase in the HCO_3^-. The serum K^+ will usually be less than 3.5 mEq/L, and the serum chlorides may be less than 98 mEq/L (hypokalemic hypochloremic metabolic alkalosis). Measurement of the urinary chlorides helps determine the cause and appropriate treatment. Patients with *chloride-responsive metabolic alkalosis* and ECF volume depletion have a urinary chloride of less than 10 mEq/L. Those with urinary chlorides greater than

20 mEq/L are not usually fluid volume depleted and have *chloride-resistant metabolic alkalosis* (see box, p. 302). The latter type of alkalosis is much less common and is associated with aldosterone excess.

Treatment

Mild *chloride-responsive metabolic alkalosis* may be corrected by replacing the ECF deficit with parenteral isotonic saline with added KCl. The provision of chloride allows increased Na^+ reabsorption in the proximal tubule, with less Na^+ presented to the distal tubule. As the amount of Na^+ reabsorbed in the distal tubule decreases, the alkalosis begins to resolve because less H^+ is secreted and less HCO_3^- is generated. In addition, H^+ secretion is decreased further as hypokalemia is corrected because more K^+ is now available to exchange with Na^+. A dilute HCl IV solution (100-200 mEq/L) may be given if the alkalosis is severe and life-threatening (pH >7.55) and there is an immediate need for correction. Other acidifying agents that are occasionally administered for severe alkalosis include IV NH_4Cl (ammonium chloride) or arginine HCL.

    Chloride-resistant metabolic alkalosis caused by excess adrenal steroids in hyperaldosteronism or Cushing's syndrome is corrected by treating the underlying disorder. Acetazolamide, a carbonic anhydrase inhibitor that enhances bicarbonate excretion, may be given to patients who have a fluid volume excess (e.g., a patient with congestive heart failure who is taking diuretics). KCl is also helpful for treating and preventing alkalosis and hypokalemia in these patients.

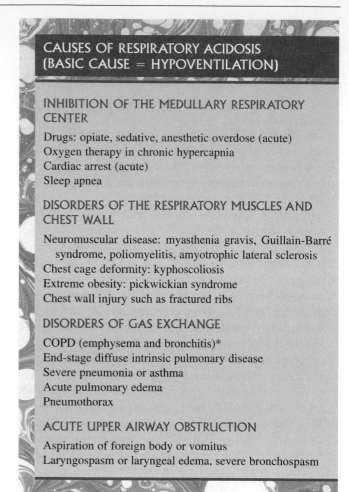

CAUSES OF RESPIRATORY ACIDOSIS (BASIC CAUSE = HYPOVENTILATION)

INHIBITION OF THE MEDULLARY RESPIRATORY CENTER

Drugs: opiate, sedative, anesthetic overdose (acute)
Oxygen therapy in chronic hypercapnia
Cardiac arrest (acute)
Sleep apnea

DISORDERS OF THE RESPIRATORY MUSCLES AND CHEST WALL

Neuromuscular disease: myasthenia gravis, Guillain-Barré syndrome, poliomyelitis, amyotrophic lateral sclerosis
Chest cage deformity: kyphoscoliosis
Extreme obesity: pickwickian syndrome
Chest wall injury such as fractured ribs

DISORDERS OF GAS EXCHANGE

COPD (emphysema and bronchitis)*
End-stage diffuse intrinsic pulmonary disease
Severe pneumonia or asthma
Acute pulmonary edema
Pneumothorax

ACUTE UPPER AIRWAY OBSTRUCTION

Aspiration of foreign body or vomitus
Laryngospasm or laryngeal edema, severe bronchospasm

*Most common cause of chronic respiratory acidosis.

RESPIRATORY ACIDOSIS

Respiratory acidosis (carbonic acid excess) is characterized by a primary rise in the Pa_{CO_2} (hypercapnia), resulting in a decrease of the pH. The Pa_{CO_2} is greater than 45 mm Hg and the pH is less than 7.35. Renal compensation results in a variable increase in the serum HCO_3^-. Respiratory acidosis may be acute or chronic. Hypoxemia (low Pa_{O_2}) invariably accompanies respiratory acidosis if the patient is breathing room air.

Causes and Pathogenesis

The fundamental cause of respiratory acidosis is alveolar hypoventilation, a term virtually synonymous with CO_2 accumulation. Normally, 15,000 to 20,000 mmol of CO_2 are produced each day by tissue metabolism and eliminated by the lungs. Most of the CO_2 is transferred to the lungs in the form of blood HCO_3^- (see the bicarbonate/buffer equation). When tissue CO_2 enters the blood, it causes an increase in the H^+ ion concentration, which in turn stimulates the respiratory center, resulting in increased ventilation. Normally, this process is so efficient that the Pa_{CO_2} and pH are kept within a normal range. CO_2 accumulation is nearly always caused by impairment of the rate of alveolar ventilation rather than overproduction of CO_2 from hypermetabolism.

    The box above lists some common causes of respiratory acidosis. Acute respiratory acidosis usually stems from acute airway obstruction as in laryngospasm, foreign body aspiration, or central nervous system (CNS) depression of the medullary respiratory center, such as that from barbiturate or opiate overdose. In severe acute respiratory acidosis, as in asphyxia or cardiopulmonary arrest, the resulting respiratory acidosis is worsened by an accompanying metabolic acidosis from the rapid accumulation of lactic acid produced during cellular anaerobic glycolysis. High concentration oxygen therapy may depress the respiratory drive, particularly in persons with chronic hypercapnia. Other causes of acute respiratory acidosis include disorders of the respiratory muscles or chest wall injury. The terminal stage of respiratory failure because of any number of causes always involves hypercapnia in addition to hypoxemia.

    The most common cause of chronic respiratory acidosis by far is chronic obstructive pulmonary disease

(COPD). In such patients, acute respiratory failure is often superimposed on chronic CO_2 retention when they develop an acute bronchitis secondary to a viral or bacterial lung infection. Kyphoscoliosis, the pickwickian syndrome, and sleep apnea are other causes of chronic respiratory acidosis. All of these conditions are discussed in detail in Part Seven.

The arterial pH and plasma HCO_3^- are different in acute and chronic respiratory acidosis. In response to acute respiratory acidosis, only the cellular buffering defense has time to be used because the renal compensatory mechanism will not be significant for 12 to 24 hours. ECF buffering is provided by plasma proteins, but this is minor. (Because the increased H_2CO_3 is a member of the major ECF buffer pair HCO_3^-/H_2CO_3, the pair does not directly participate in the buffer defense in respiratory acidosis.) Hemoglobin provides the major ICF buffering. As CO_2 enters the RBCs (producing H^+), HCO_3^- moves out in exchange for Cl^-. The expected rise of the serum HCO_3^- is about 1 mEq/L for every 10 mm Hg rise in the CO_2. Cellular buffering alone is ineffective in restoring a normal pH. Thus acute respiratory acidosis is poorly compensated and the pH is seriously reduced.

Chronic respiratory acidosis, in contrast to acute respiratory acidosis, is well compensated because the renal compensatory mechanism has had time to become operational. The kidneys increase secretion and excretion of H^+, accompanied by the resorption and generation of new HCO_3^-. The compensatory increase in plasma HCO_3^- requires 2 to 3 days for complete expression. Conversely, there is a 2- to 3-day lag time in renal HCO_3^- excretion, resulting in posthypercapnia metabolic alkalosis, as discussed previously. Thus patients with respiratory acidosis, which is relatively well compensated, as evidenced by a nearly normal pH, should not be treated overzealously. Lowering their $PaCO_2$ too rapidly leaves them with a sizable bicarbonate excess and shifts their acid-base balance into acute alkalosis. The expected compensatory rise of the plasma HCO_3^- in chronic respiratory acidosis is 3.5 mEq/L for every 10 mm Hg rise in the $PaCO_2$ above 40 mm Hg.

Clinical Features and Diagnosis

The signs and symptoms of CO_2 retention are nonspecific and, in general, have an unpredictable relationship to the level of the $PaCO_2$. In addition, because both acute respiratory acidosis and chronic respiratory acidosis are always accompanied by hypoxemia, it is the hypoxemia itself that is responsible for many of the clinical characteristics of CO_2 retention. In general, the greater the magnitude and the faster the rate of rise in $PaCO_2$, the more severe the symptoms. An acute rise in the $PaCO_2$ to 60 mm Hg or above results in somnolence, mental confusion, stupor, and eventually coma. Because a high $PaCO_2$ produces a kind of metabolic brain syndrome, asterixis (flapping tremor) and myoclonus (muscle jerking) may be present. Because CO_2 retention causes cerebral vasodila-

tion, the consequent cerebral vascular congestion leads to increased intracranial pressure (ICP). Increased ICP may be manifested as papilledema (swelling of the optic disc visible on examination with the ophthalmoscope). The laboratory findings in acute respiratory acidosis reveal a low PaO_2, pH below 7.35, and $PaCO_2$ above 45 mm Hg, with a small compensatory rise of the HCO_3^- (less than 30 mEq/L). Of course, in acute airway obstruction, respiratory distress symptoms related to hypoxemia may completely dominate the clinical picture.

Chronic respiratory acidosis appears to be tolerated much better than acute respiratory acidosis. There may be few signs and symptoms related to the CO_2 retention and acidosis unless the $PaCO_2$ is greater than 60 mm Hg. The $PaCO_2$ is greater than 45 mm Hg and the HCO_3^- is greater than 30 mEq/L, indicating renal compensation. The serum pH may be normal or slightly decreased in a well-compensated chronic respiratory acidosis. A compensatory polycythemia commonly occurs in states of chronic hypercapnia. Hemoglobin levels may reach 16 to 22 g/L. The signs and symptoms of COPD, with or without cor pulmonale, generally predominate (see Part Seven). Acute respiratory acidosis and chronic respiratory acidosis are differentiated on the basis of the history and analysis of the arterial blood gases.

Treatment of Acute and Chronic Respiratory Acidosis

Treatment of acute respiratory acidosis is restoration of effective ventilation as soon as possible by administering oxygen therapy and treating the underlying cause. The PaO_2 must be raised to a minimum level of 60 mm Hg and the pH above 7.2 to avoid the development of cardiac dysrhythmias. High concentration oxygen (>50%) may be given safely to patients for 1 to 2 days if there is no history of chronic hypercapnia. When patients with chronic hypercapnia develop an acute rise in the $PaCO_2$, attention should be directed toward identifying factors, such as pneumonia or pulmonary embolism, that may have aggravated the underlying disorder and precipitated the crisis. Mechanical ventilation may be necessary to deal with the crisis. Great caution must be exercised in administering oxygen to patients with chronic hypercapnia. In these patients, hypoxia replaces hypercapnia as the major stimulus for respiration. Thus, if the oxygen therapy raises the PaO_2 above the person's normal level, it will remove the hypoxic drive to respiration and result in even further reduction in alveolar ventilation. Consequently, the correct approach in treating these patients is to start with the lowest possible concentration of oxygen (24% to 28%) to raise the PaO_2 to 60 to 70 mm Hg. Arterial blood gases must be monitored carefully during the treatment to detect signs of increasing $PaCO_2$ and deterioration of alveolar ventilation. The $PaCO_2$ is lowered, but achievement of a normal value is not the goal.

RESPIRATORY ALKALOSIS

Respiratory alkalosis (carbonic acid deficit) is characterized by a primary decrease in the Pa_{CO_2} (hypocapnia), resulting in an increase in the pH. The Pa_{CO_2} is less than 35 mm Hg, and the pH is greater than 7.45. Renal compensation consists of decreased excretion of H^+ and consequently less absorption of HCO_3^-. The serum HCO_3^- is reduced in varying amounts, depending on whether the condition is acute or chronic.

Causes and Pathogenesis

The fundamental cause of respiratory alkalosis is alveolar hyperventilation or excess excretion of CO_2 in expired air. Hyperventilation should not be confused with an increased respiratory rate (tachypnea), which may or may not be associated with hyperventilation. Hyperventilation can occur with a normal respiratory rate if tidal volume is increased. Hyperventilation can be positively identified only by a decreased Pa_{CO_2}. Respiratory alkalosis may well be the most common acid-base imbalance, although it is often not recognized. Hyperventilation may be difficult to recognize clinically, and the diagnosis is often made only by blood gas determination.

The box below lists some of the common causes of respiratory alkalosis. Respiratory alkalosis may occur as a result of stimulation of the medullary respiratory center.

CAUSES OF RESPIRATORY ALKALOSIS (BASIC CAUSE = HYPERVENTILATION)

CENTRAL STIMULATION OF RESPIRATION

Psychogenic hyperventilation caused by emotional stress*
Hypermetabolic states: fever, thyrotoxicosis
CNS disorders
Head trauma or vascular accidents
Brain tumors
Salicylate intoxication (early)

HYPOXIA

Pneumonia, asthma, pulmonary edema
Congestive heart failure
Pulmonary fibrosis
High-altitude residence

EXCESSIVE MECHANICAL VENTILATION

UNCERTAIN MECHANISM

Gram-negative sepsis
Hepatic cirrhosis

EXERCISE

*Most common cause.

The most common cause by far is functional hyperventilation caused by anxiety and emotional stress (hyperventilation syndrome or psychogenic hyperventilation). When one considers all the stressful life situations that humans encounter, both within a hospital environment (e.g., pain, awaiting a potential diagnosis of a malignancy) and in the community, it is not surprising that the hyperventilation syndrome is common. Nearly everyone has experienced it at some time during his or her life. Other conditions causing stimulation of the respiratory center include hypermetabolic conditions caused by fever or thyrotoxicosis and CNS lesions, such as cerebral vascular accidents, meningitis, head trauma, or brain tumors. Salicylates are the most important drugs that cause respiratory alkalosis, presumably by direct stimulation of the medullary respiratory center. Hypoxia is a common cause of primary hyperventilation in association with pneumonia, pulmonary edema or fibrosis, or congestive heart failure. In general, a reduction of the Pa_{O_2} below 60 mm Hg is necessary to stimulate ventilation. Correction of the tissue hypoxia results in rapid resolution of the respiratory alkalosis. Chronic hyperventilation occurs in the acclimation response to high altitudes (low ambient oxygen tension). Respiratory alkalosis is commonly produced iatrogenically by mechanical ventilation with a volume-cycled or pressure-cycled ventilator. Respiratory alkalosis is commonly associated with gram-negative sepsis and hepatic cirrhosis. Finally, although hyperpnea is an adaptive response to increased oxygen demand during physical exercise, it may occasionally produce transitory respiratory alkalosis.

The immediate response to an acute reduction in the Pa_{CO_2} is intracellular buffering. H^+ is released from the intracellular tissue buffers, which minimizes the alkalosis by lowering the plasma HCO_3^-. Acute alkalosis also stimulates lactic acid and pyruvate production within the cells and helps to provide more H^+ for release into the ECF. Extracellular buffering by plasma proteins is minor. The effect of ECF and ICF buffering is a small decrement in the plasma HCO_3^-. When hypocapnia is sustained, renal adjustments yield a much larger decrement in plasma HCO_3^-. Renal tubular reabsorption and generation of new HCO_3^- are inhibited. As in respiratory acidosis, compensation for chronic respiratory alkalosis is much more complete than for the acute condition. In the acute condition, the expected fall in plasma HCO_3^- is 2 mEq/L for every 10 mm Hg fall in the Pa_{CO_2}; the expected decrease of HCO_3^- is 5 mEq/L for every 10 mm Hg fall in the Pa_{CO_2} in the chronic condition.

Clinical Features and Diagnosis

The breathing pattern in anxiety-induced hyperventilation syndrome varies from an apparently normal respiratory pattern to obviously frequent, deep, sighing respirations. Often, frequent yawning may be observed. Patients are surprisingly unaware of their hyperventilation. When symptoms are referable to respirations, the complaint is usually "unable to get enough air" or "unable to catch my breath," despite the fact that unimpaired overbreathing is taking place. Other prominent symptoms include "light-headedness," circumoral paresthesias, numbness and tingling of the fingers and toes, and if the alkalosis is sufficiently severe, manifestations of tetany such as carpopedal spasm. The patient may complain of chronic exhaustion, palpitations, anxiety, dry mouth, and sleeplessness. The palms of the hands and soles of the feet may feel cold and clammy to the examiner's touch and may indicate emotional tension. Severe respiratory alkalosis may be associated with inability to concentrate, mental confusion, and syncope.

The basis of the neuromuscular signs and symptoms may be attributed to the alkalosis, as it directly enhances neuromuscular irritability. In addition, less calcium is ionized in an alkaline medium so that a functional hypocalcemia may contribute to manifestations of tetany. CNS symptoms may be related to cerebral hypoxia. Alkalosis not only shifts the oxyhemoglobin dissociation curve to the left (causing hemoglobin to have a greater affinity for oxygen), but also reduces cerebral blood flow. Both of these mechanisms may induce cerebral hypoxia. Cerebral blood flow is reduced approximately 40% at a $PaCO_2$ of 20 mm Hg. In fact, hyperventilation and acute hypocapnia are such a potent producer of cerebral vasoconstriction that they are deliberately induced on a mechanical ventilator as a treatment for cerebral vascular congestion and increased intracranial pressure. Although some cerebral hypoxia may be induced, the benefits of reducing the cerebral edema outweigh this adverse effect.

As stated previously, laboratory findings in acute respiratory alkalosis consist of a pH above 7.45 and a $PaCO_2$ below 35 mm Hg. If the $PaCO_2$ should rapidly drop to 20 mm Hg, for example, the drop in plasma HCO_3^- should be no greater than about 4 mEq/L because of cellular buffering. In chronic metabolic alkalosis, the plasma HCO_3^- would be expected to drop about 10 mEq/L with the same degree of hypocapnia. A greater than expected fall in the plasma HCO_3^- suggests coexistent metabolic acidosis; if the fall is less than expected, a coexistent metabolic alkalosis may be present. Other laboratory findings may include a reciprocal hyperchloremia and a hypokalemia. The diagnosis of respiratory alkalosis is made on the basis of the history, signs, and symptoms and confirmed by evidence of the laboratory findings.

Treatment

The only successful treatment for respiratory alkalosis is elimination of the underlying cause. Hyperventilation with mechanical ventilators may be corrected by reducing minute ventilation when excessive or by adding dead space. If this cannot be achieved without compromising oxygenation, a gas mixture containing 3% CO_2 may be used for a short time (Schrier, 1986).

When severe anxiety produces the hyperventilation syndrome, air rebreathing with a paper bag held tightly around the nose and mouth generally terminates the acute attack. These patients may need stress management counseling.

MIXED ACID-BASE DISORDERS

Mixed acid-base disorders are conditions in which two or more of the more simple acid-base disturbances coexist. Given the large number of pathophysiologic processes that can alter the $PaCO_2$ or HCO_3^-, it is not surprising that one acid-base disorder does not preclude the existence of another that has independent effects on acid-base balance. In fact, the existence of some acid-base disturbances increases the likelihood that another will develop. Mixed acid-base disturbances frequently occur in the presence of complex medical problems so that the clinical features are difficult to distinguish from the underlying illness.

Table 22-5 lists four combinations of the primary acid-

TABLE 22-5   Common Mixed Acid-Base Disorders

Dual Mixed Disorder	Common Causes
ADDITIVE EFFECT ON pH CHANGE	
Metabolic acidosis + Respiratory acidosis $PaCO_2$ too high HCO_3^- too low pH very low	Cardiopulmonary arrest Patient with COPD goes into shock Chronic renal failure with fluid volume excess and pulmonary edema Patient with DKA receives potent opiate or barbiturate
Metabolic alkalosis + Respiratory alkalosis $PaCO_2$ too low HCO_3^- too high pH very high	Patient with previously compensated respiratory acidosis caused by COPD overventilated on mechanical respirator Hyperventilating patient with CHF or hepatic cirrhosis who is vomiting or is treated with potent diuretics or nasogastric suction Head trauma patient with hyperventilation treated with diuretics
OFFSETTING EFFECT ON pH CHANGE	
Metabolic acidosis + Respiratory alkalosis $PaCO_2$ too low HCO_3^- too low pH near normal	Lactic acidosis complicating septic shock Hepatorenal syndrome Salicylate intoxication
Metabolic alkalosis + Respiratory acidosis $PaCO_2$ too high HCO_3^- too high pH near normal	COPD patient who is vomiting or who is treated with NG suction or potent diuretics Adult respiratory distress syndrome

base disorders and examples of diseases and clinical situations implicated in their pathogenesis. These mixed disturbances include (1) metabolic acidosis and respiratory acidosis, (2) metabolic alkalosis and respiratory alkalosis, (3) metabolic acidosis and respiratory alkalosis, and (4) metabolic alkalosis and respiratory acidosis. Any of the simple acid-base disturbances may be superimposed on another or may follow each other in sequence. It is evident from the combinations of mixed acid-base imbalances that the individual components may have either additive or offsetting effects on the plasma acidity so that the resulting change in pH may be profoundly severe or deceptively mild.

Metabolic Acidosis and Respiratory Acidosis

The most common situation leading to metabolic acidosis and respiratory acidosis is untreated cardiopulmonary arrest. Respiratory arrest with absent alveolar ventilation results in the rapid accumulation of CO_2, and the tissue hypoxia from lack of oxygenation results in activation of anaerobic metabolism with the consequent accumulation of lactic acid. Another example is a person with COPD (chronic respiratory acidosis) who goes into shock (metabolic acidosis). A third example is a patient with chronic renal failure (metabolic acidosis) complicated by respiratory insufficiency secondary to fluid overload and pulmonary edema. Patients with chronic renal failure often find that compliance with their sodium-restricted diet is difficult and may indulge in a pizza binge, with resulting fluid overload and pulmonary edema. A less obvious situation that produces this mixed disorder is a patient with diabetic ketoacidosis who receives an opiate or a potent sedative, which causes depression of the respiratory center.

In each of these examples, the respiratory disorder prevents a compensatory fall in the $Paco_2$ for the metabolic acidosis and the metabolic disorder prevents buffering and renal mechanisms from raising the HCO_3^- in response to the respiratory acidosis. Consequently, the laboratory data show an increased $Paco_2$ and a decreased HCO_3^-, with a profound drop in the plasma pH. The clue to recognizing this mixed disorder is that the respiratory and metabolic components of the buffer equation change in opposite directions. The clinical history provides obvious clues to the diagnosis in the case of cardiopulmonary arrest, but recognition of this mixed disorder may not be so obvious in the case of a person with COPD (chronic respiratory acidosis) who develops diabetic ketoacidosis.

Therapy for mixed respiratory and metabolic acidosis is directed toward treatment of each of the underlying disorders. In the case of cardiopulmonary arrest, the goal is to restore tissue perfusion and oxygenation by restoring heart and lung function. It may be necessary to give a small amount of $NaHCO_3$ to raise the pH to a more optimal level (7.2) so that cardiac function will respond to resuscitation efforts.

Metabolic Alkalosis and Respiratory Alkalosis

The combination of metabolic and respiratory alkalosis is one of the most common mixed acid-base disorders according to Schrier (1986). A common clinical example is a person with COPD (compensated respiratory acidosis with increased HCO_3^-) who is hyperventilated on a respirator. The respiratory acidosis is thus rapidly converted to a respiratory alkalosis, which combines with the metabolic alkalosis produced by the original compensatory rise in HCO_3^-. Another example is a person with congestive heart failure who is hyperventilating (respiratory alkalosis) and treated with potent diuretics (metabolic alkalosis and hypokalemia) or has prolonged vomiting or nasogastric suction. The same aggravating factors in a person with hepatic cirrhosis who is hyperventilating might produce similar consequences. Another example is a person with central neurogenic hyperventilation of brain stem trauma who receives diuretics.

Each acid-base disorder blocks the appropriate compensatory response of the other when alkalotic acid-base disturbances are combined. Consequently, there is a marked increase in the pH. The $Paco_2$ and the HCO_3^- deviate from the normal range in opposite directions. In addition to the history, other laboratory findings that provide clues to recognition of this mixed disorder include hypokalemia.

In the case of the person placed on a ventilator, great care must be taken in adjusting the ventilation and oxygen concentration so that the Pao_2 is kept at a minimally safe level of about 60 to 70 mm Hg, and at the same time the $Paco_2$ is reduced very slowly, giving the kidneys time to reduce the elevated HCO_3^-. Patients with chronic hypercapnia depend on a hypoxic stimulus for breathing and are relatively insensitive to CO_2 as a stimulus. Thus raising oxygen tension and lowering carbon dioxide tension to normal values in patients with COPD may depress the respiratory drive, resulting in a deterioration of their condition. The other mixed disorders mentioned previously are treated with $NaCl$ and KCl to reduce the HCO_3^- and restore a safe pH level because it would be difficult, if not impossible, to direct attention toward elevating the $Paco_2$.

Metabolic Acidosis and Respiratory Alkalosis

A mixed metabolic acidosis and respiratory alkalosis can be identified when plasma HCO_3^- and $Paco_2$ are both low and the pH is normal or nearly normal, because these two disorders tend to offset each other.

Primary respiratory alkalosis can coexist with various types of metabolic acidosis. It occurs commonly with lactic acidosis complicating septic shock. The latter condition is associated with hyperventilation. It also occurs with renal acidosis in the hepatorenal syndrome and with organic acidosis in salicylate intoxication.

In a mixed metabolic acidosis and respiratory alkalosis, the drop in the $Paco_2$ is greater than would be expected as a compensation for a primary metabolic acidosis and the drop in HCO_3^- is greater than would be expected as a compensation for primary respiratory alkalosis. The treatment must be directed at the specific entities causing the mixed acid-base imbalance because the pH is normal or nearly normal.

Metabolic Alkalosis and Respiratory Acidosis

A diagnosis of mixed respiratory acidosis and metabolic alkalosis can be made when the plasma HCO_3^- and the $Paco_2$ are both elevated and the pH is normal or nearly normal. This mixed disorder is quite common and occurs most often when patients with COPD (chronic respiratory acidosis) are treated with potent diuretics or have other conditions causing metabolic alkalosis, such as vomiting, nasogastric suction, or steroid therapy. This dual acid-base disturbance also occurs in adult respiratory distress syndrome (ARDS).

It is important to detect even small degrees of metabolic alkalosis in patients with COPD and chronic hypercapnia because their respiratory drive depends in part on the accompanying acidosis. Thus any reduction in H^+ (increase in pH) from an accompanying elevated HCO_3^- will depress ventilation and cause a further rise in the $Paco_2$ and a fall in the Pao_2. In such cases, treatment of the alkalosis can significantly improve ventilation. Increasing dietary chlorides or KCl therapy will help lower the plasma HCO_3^-.

OTHER MIXED ACID-BASE DISTURBANCES

Although the four possible dual mixed acid-base disturbances have been reviewed, it is important to keep in mind another common imbalance, *acute-on-chronic respiratory acidosis.* Common precipitating factors are intercurrent pulmonary infection or administration of sedative in a patient with COPD and chronic hypercapnia. This situation causes a marked acute rise in the $Paco_2$ and a seriously low pH. $Paco_2$ levels above 70 mm Hg may depress respirations and cause stupor, coma (CO_2 narcosis), and hypoxemia. Treatment is directed at the factors causing the respiratory failure. Mechanical ventilation may be necessary to correct the hypercapnia, acidosis, and more important, the hypoxemia. On the other hand, care must be taken to gradually lower the $Paco_2$ so that a posthypercapnic metabolic alkalosis is not precipitated.

In summary, acid-base disturbances can be complex. A thorough understanding of acid-base physiology and pathophysiology, coupled with a systematic approach as outlined at the beginning of this chapter, is a necessary prerequisite for recognizing them. In particular, recognizing offsetting mixed acid-base disorders requires an accurate history and ancillary laboratory data.

QUESTIONS

▼ *Answer the following on a separate sheet of paper.*

1. Why does the body maintain a critical pH range?
2. Define the following terms: pH, acid, base, pK, buffer.
3. Differentiate between a volatile and a nonvolatile acid. Name some. How are they excreted?
4. Name the four major blood buffer systems. Which are intracellular, and which are extracellular?
5. List the two main functions of the kidneys in maintaining acid-base balance.
6. What is the role of the lungs in maintaining acid-base balance? Define hypoventilation and hyperventilation.
7. What is the anion gap? How is it calculated? What is its significance in describing an acid-base imbalance?
8. What is the isohydric principle, and what is its significance?
9. How do the CO_2 content, $Paco_2$, and standard bicarbonate differ? What are their normal values? What is base excess?
10. Outline the steps in the systematic assessment of acid-base status.
11. How is calculation of the expected compensatory response of a primary acid-base disturbance helpful in assessment?
12. Describe several hazards of rapidly correcting metabolic acidosis or chronic respiratory acidosis by $NaHCO_3$ administration.

▼ *Circle the letter preceding each item that correctly answers the question or completes the statement. More than one answer may be correct.*

13. Acid-base balance in the human body is maintained by controlling the concentration of:
    a. Blood
    b. Hydrogen ions
    c. Carbon dioxide
    d. Oxygen
14. An acid can best be explained as:
    a. An anion
    b. A cation
    c. A chemical that is able to donate a hydrogen ion
    d. A chemical that combines with a hydrogen ion to form an acid
15. The normal pH of the blood serum indicates that the serum is:
    a. Neutral
    b. Slightly acid
    c. Slightly alkaline
    d. None of the above
16. Normally the pH of human blood serum is:
    a. 7.38 to 7.42
    b. 7.31 to 7.42
    c. 7.35 to 7.48
    d. 7.35 to 7.55
17. The normal $[H^+]$ of the blood is:
    a. 16 mEq/L
    b. 35 mEq/L
    c. 40 mEq/L
    d. 63 mEq/L
18. Which of the following are classified as blood buffers?
    a. Bicarbonate–carbonic acid system

Continued.

? QUESTIONS—cont'd

b. Hemoglobin
c. Phosphate
d. Protein

19. The Henderson-Hasselbalch equation reveals that maintaining a normal pH requires that the ratio of base bicarbonate to carbonic acid must be:
    a. 20:1   c. 2:20
    b. 1:20   d. 30:2

20. Three body systems act to maintain the blood pH near 7.4 and defend against large deviations. Choose the series below that lists these three systems in order, from the fastest acting to the slowest acting.
    a. Kidneys, lungs, blood buffers
    b. Blood buffers, lungs, kidneys
    c. Blood buffers, kidneys, lungs
    d. Lungs, blood buffers, kidneys

21. The lowest limit of blood pH at which a person can live more than a few minutes is about:
    a. 6.0
    b. 6.8
    c. 7.2
    d. 7.3

22. The first step in the assessment of the acid-base status is:
    a. Review the clinical history for disease processes that might lead to an acid-base disturbance
    b. Examine the Pa_{CO_2}
    c. Look at the laboratory report of the base excess because it always leads to the right conclusion about acid-base disturbances
    d. Calculate the anion gap

23. The clues to a mixed acid-base disturbance are:
    a. Undercompensation or overcompensation of a primary acid-base disorder
    b. Failure to balance the expected compensation formula
    c. The change in the anion gap does not equal the change in the bicarbonate
    d. A large anion gap

▼ Renal mechanisms compensate for respiratory insufficiency, and, conversely, respiratory mechanisms partially compensate for metabolic acid-base disturbances. Tell how this mechanism works in each of the following cases by filling in the blanks with the correct word(s).

24. When respiratory acidosis occurs, the kidneys compensate by increasing excretion of _____ and conserving _____.

25. When respiratory alkalosis occurs, the kidneys compensate by decreasing excretion of _____ and increasing excretion of _____.

26. When metabolic acidosis occurs, the lungs are able to compensate by _____ _____.

27. When metabolic alkalosis occurs, the lungs are able to partially compensate by _____ _____.

▼ Match the type of primary acid-base disturbance in column A with a likely cause in column B.

Column A	Column B
28. _____ Hyperchloremic metabolic acidosis	a. Diarrhea
29. _____ High anion gap metabolic acidosis	b. NG suction or vomiting
30. _____ Metabolic alkalosis	c. Renal failure
31. _____ Acute respiratory acidosis	d. Laryngospasm
32. _____ Chronic respiratory acidosis	e. Loop or thiazide diuretic
33. _____ Respiratory alkalosis	f. Uncontrolled diabetes
	g. Starvation
	h. Secondary hyperaldosteronism
	i. COPD
	j. Emotional stress
	k. Salicylate poisoning
	l. Mechanical ventilation

▼ Match the type of mixed acid-base disturbance in column A with a likely cause in column B.

Column A	Column B
34. _____ Metabolic acidosis and respiratory acidosis	a. COPD patient receiving NG suction
35. _____ Metabolic alkalosis and respiratory alkalosis	b. Hyperventilating chronic heart failure patient treated with diuretics
36. _____ Metabolic acidosis and respiratory alkalosis	c. Cardiopulmonary arrest
37. _____ Metabolic alkalosis and respiratory acidosis	d. COPD patient placed on mechanical ventilator
38. _____ Acute-on-chronic respiratory acidosis	e. Salicylate intoxication
	f. COPD patient who develops pneumonia

QUESTIONS—cont'd

▼ *Circle the letter preceding each item that correctly answers the question or completes the statement. More than one answer may be correct.*

39. The rapid or prolonged administration of normal saline may cause:
    a. Metabolic alkalosis
    b. Metabolic (chloride) acidosis
    c. Dehydration
    d. Hypoventilation

40. Diarrhea from a colostomy will cause metabolic acidosis. The primary reason that this acid-base imbalance occurs is a:
    a. Primary bicarbonate deficit
    b. Primary bicarbonate excess
    c. Primary carbonic acid excess
    d. Primary carbonic acid deficit

41. The primary defect in respiratory acidosis is:
    a. Primary bicarbonate deficit
    b. Primary bicarbonate excess
    c. Primary carbonic acid excess
    d. Primary carbonic acid deficit

42. A person who has a condition in which there is an increase in the production of endogenous organic acids (e.g., diabetic ketoacidosis) above the normal level will develop:
    a. Respiratory acidosis
    b. Respiratory alkalosis
    c. Metabolic alkalosis
    d. Normal anion gap metabolic acidosis
    e. High anion gap metabolic acidosis

43. A not uncommon method of providing a feeling of euphoria, often expressed as "being high," is to deliberately hyperventilate. Hyperventilation causes an acid-base imbalance called:
    a. Respiratory acidosis
    b. Respiratory alkalosis
    c. Metabolic acidosis
    d. Metabolic alkalosis

44. Indiscriminate administration of oxygen can be deadly for the patient with chronic obstructive pulmonary disease (chronic bronchitis and emphysema). Which of the following sequences describes the progression of adverse effects?
    1. Hypoventilation
    2. Depression of the respiratory center
    3. CO_2 retention
    4. CO_2 narcosis (coma)
       a. $1 \rightarrow 2 \rightarrow 3 \rightarrow 4$
       b. $2 \rightarrow 1 \rightarrow 3 \rightarrow 4$

       c. $3 \rightarrow 4 \rightarrow 2 \rightarrow 1$
       d. $4 \rightarrow 3 \rightarrow 1 \rightarrow 2$

45. To reduce the risk of metabolic alkalosis, nasogastric suction tubes should be irrigated with:
    a. Tap water
    b. Normal saline

46. A 30-year-old man was admitted to the hospital in a coma with a diagnosis of brain tumor. A tracheostomy was performed on the day of admission and pressure-controlled mechanical ventilation given continuously. His temperature has ranged between 102° and 103.4° F. On the fifth day after admission you note that he has carpopedal spasms of the hands when you check his blood pressure. Which of the following statements best explains this phenomenon?
    a. The patient's elevated temperature has induced a neuromuscular irritability and a febrile convulsion is imminent.
    b. Serum pH has decreased because of respiratory acidosis produced by hypoventilation. The decreased pH in turn caused irritability of the nervous system.
    c. Serum pH has increased because of respiratory alkalosis produced by hyperventilation. The alkalosis directly stimulates the nervous system and in addition causes a decrease in ionized serum Ca^{++}. Consequently, hyperirritability of the nervous system occurred.
    d. Total serum calcium has decreased because of the patient's immobility and its consequent loss in the urine.

47. A 60-year-old widow has been in the hospital for several days for a complete medical check-up. She is very worried that she may have cancer, even though all tests have been negative. Her physician has diagnosed her case as an anxiety reaction following the death of her husband (from cancer). In the middle of the night, she calls the nurse into her room complaining of muscle cramps in her feet and a prickling sensation in her fingers and toes. The nurse notes that she sighs frequently. Her hands are cold and clammy to the touch and have a slight tremor. The probable difficulty is:
    a. Respiratory alkalosis
    b. Respiratory acidosis
    c. Metabolic acidosis
    d. Metabolic alkalosis

48. Intervention(s) that might help relieve the symptoms of the patient in question 47 include:
    a. Offering her the antacid of her choice
    b. Elevating the head of her bed to improve ventilation
    c. Having her breathe into a paper bag
    d. Offering her reassurance and allowing her to discuss her fears with you

49. The IV fluid of choice to treat a patient with metabolic alkalosis and a fluid volume deficit secondary to vomiting over several days is:
    a. Lactated Ringer's solution (metabolized to bicarbonate)
    b. D_5W
    c. Normal saline
    d. Normal saline with added KCl

50. Factors that contribute to the maintenance of metabolic alkalosis include:
    a. K^+ depletion
    b. NA^+ excess
    c. Cl^- depletion
    d. Fluid volume deficit and secondary hyperaldosteronism

▼ *Analyze data from the following cases by answering the following questions used in the systematic assessment presented at the beginning of the chapter. You may use the acid-base nomogram to assist if desired.*
    a. What acid-base disturbance is suggested by the history?
    b. What do the signs and symptoms suggest?
    c. Analyze $Paco_2$ and HCO_3^- in relation to the pH. What primary acid-base disorder is suggested?
    d. What is the expected compensation for this disorder?
    e. Calculate the anion gap.
    f. What is your final conclusion?

51. A 36-year-old woman is seen after several days of severe diarrhea. She complains of weakness and postural dizziness. Her blood pressure is 100/60 mm Hg when recumbent and 80/50 mm Hg when standing. Her resting pulse is 100 beats/min and regular. Her neck veins are flat in the recumbent position. Skin turgor is poor, and mucous membranes are dry. Laboratory data included: plasma Na^+, 142 mEq/L; K^+, 3.9 mEq/L; Cl^-, 118; pH, 7.27; HCO_3^-, 12 mEq/L; $Paco_2$, 28 mm Hg; urine Na^+, 4 mEq/L.

Continued.

QUESTIONS—cont'd

52. A 40-year-old woman has chronic renal failure. The following laboratory data were obtained: plasma Na^+, 137 mEq/L; K^+, 6.0 mEq/L; Cl^-, 102; pH, 7.14; HCO_3^-, 8 mEq/L; $Paco_2$, 24 mm Hg; creatinine, 9.6 mEq/dl; BUN, 110 mg/dl.

53. A previously stable patient with chronic renal failure was admitted to the hospital renal unit in a moribund state. The chest radiograph and lung auscultation were suggestive of pulmonary edema. The patient had skipped the last two hemodialysis sessions while on a vacation trip. Weight gain was 10 lb since the last dialysis. The following laboratory data were obtained: plasma pH, 7.02; HCO_3^-, 15 mEq/L; $Paco_2$, 60 mm Hg; Pao_2, 40 mm Hg.

▼ A 67-year-old man is admitted to the hospital because of severe dyspnea. The man has a history of heart disease treated with digoxin and occasional diuretics. The following laboratory data were obtained over the next 7 days:

	Day 1	Day 3	Day 4	Day 7
Serum pH	7.30	7.34	7.42	7.53
$Paco_2$	54	60	58	40
HCO_3^-	27	34	38	36
Na^+	139	138	140	137
K^+	5.8	5.2	4.6	4.6
Cl^-	100	96	93	90
Anion gap	12	8	9	11
BUN	15	15	24	24

54. What acid-base disturbance is present on day 1?
55. What has occurred between day 1 and day 3?
56. What has occurred between day 3 and day 4?
57. What was the acid-base disturbance on day 7?
58. Explain the probable cause of each disturbance.

▼ Circle T is the statement is true and F if it is false. Correct any false statements.

59. T F Chloride-responsive metabolic alkalosis is caused most often by vomiting or diuretics, and urine chlorides are <10 mEq/L.

60. T F Bicarbonate and chlorides have a direct relationship: when bicarbonate increases chlorides also increase.

61. T F The basic cause of respiratory acidosis is hyperventilation.

62. T F Laboratory values alone are usually sufficient to recognize acid-base disturbances.

63. T F Kussmaul breathing in a patient with metabolic acidosis indicates that the lungs are attempting to compensate for the disturbance.

BIBLIOGRAPHY ▼ PART IV

Chambers JK, editor: Common fluid and electrolyte disorders, *Nurs Clin North Am* 22:749-871, 1987.

Chan JCM, Gill JR: *Kidney and electrolyte disorders,* New York, 1990, Churchill Livingstone.

Cohen J: Acid-base disturbances. In Thier S, Cohen S, Relman A, editors: *American College of Physicians Annual Session,* Boston, 1978.

Duarte CG: Disorders of magnesium metabolism. In Chan JCM, Gill JR, editors: *Kidney and electrolyte disorders,* New York, 1990, Churchill Livingstone.

Galla JH, Luke RG: Pathophysiology of metabolic alkalosis, *Hosp Pract* 22:123-146, 1987.

Goldberger E: *A primer of water, electrolyte, and acid-base syndromes,* ed 7, Philadelphia, 1986, Lea & Febiger.

Knochel JP: Disorders of phosphorus and magnesium metabolism. In Wilson JD et al, editors: *Harrison's principles of internal medicine,* ed 13, New York, 1994, McGraw-Hill.

Kokko J, Tannen R: *Fluids and electrolytes,* ed 2, Philadelphia, 1990, WB Saunders.

Mattar JO, Weil MH, Shubin H, Stein L: Cardiac arrest in the critically ill, *Am J Med* 56:162-167, 1974.

McCurdy DK: Mixed metabolic and respiratory acid-base disturbances; diagnosis and treatment, *Chest* 62(suppl):35, 1972.

Metheny NM: *Fluid and electrolyte balance: nursing considerations,* ed 3, Philadelphia, 1996, JB Lippincott.

Metheny NM, Snively WD: *Nurses' handbook of fluid balances,* ed 3, Philadelphia, 1979, JB Lippincott.

Narins RG: *Maxwell and Kleeman's clinical disorders of fluid and electrolyte metabolism,* ed 5, New York, 1994, McGraw-Hill.

Rose BD: *Clinical physiology of acid-base and electrolyte disorders,* ed 3, New York, 1994, McGraw-Hill.

Schrier RW: *Renal and electrolyte disorders,* ed 3, Boston, 1986, Little, Brown.

Schwartz WB, Relman AS: A critique of the parameters used in the evaluation of acid-base disorders: "whole blood buffer base" and "standard bicarbonate" compared with blood pH and plasma bicarbonate concentration, *N Engl J Med* 268:1382, 1963

CHAPTER 23 ► Disorders of the Esophagus

LORRAINE M. WILSON

ANATOMY AND PHYSIOLOGY

The esophagus is a hollow cylindric organ about 25 cm long and 2 cm in diameter that extends from the hypopharynx to the cardiac portion of the stomach. It lies posterior to the heart and trachea, anterior to the vertebrae, and passes through a hiatus in the diaphragm just anterior to the aorta. The primary function of the esophagus is to transport ingested material from the pharynx to the stomach.

Each end of the esophagus is guarded by a sphincter. The *cricopharyngeus muscle* forms the *upper esophageal sphincter* (UES) and consists of skeletal muscle fibers. It is normally in a tonic or contracted state except during swallowing. The *lower esophageal sphincter* (LES), although not anatomically distinct, behaves as a sphincter and serves as a barrier to reflux of stomach contents into the esophagus. It is normally closed except when food passes into the stomach or during belching or vomiting (Fig. 23-1).

The wall of the esophagus, as with other parts of the gastrointestinal (GI) tract, consists of four layers: mucosa, submucosa, muscularis, and adventitia (outer layer). The inner *mucosal layer* is made up of stratified squamous epithelium that is continuous with the pharynx at the upper end; it undergoes a sharp transition at the esophagogastric junction (Z line) to form the simple columnar epithelium of the stomach. The esophageal mucosa is normally alkaline and cannot tolerate the highly acid contents of the stomach. The *submucosal layer* contains secretory cells that produce mucus. The mucus facilitates the passage of food during swallowing and protects the mucosa from chemical injury. The *muscle layer* is arranged in outer longitudinal and inner circular layers. The muscles of the upper 5% of the esophagus are striated, and those of the lower half are smooth. The intervening portion of the esophagus consists of a mixture of both striated and smooth muscles. Unlike the remainder of the GI tract, the *adventitia,* or outer layer, of the esophagus, has no serosa or peritoneal covering. Rather, it is made up of loose connective tissue that joins it to adjacent structures. This lack of serosa may contribute to the more rapid spread of tumor cells (in the case of esophageal cancer) and to the increased chance of leakage after surgical resection.

The major innervation of the esophagus is supplied by the parasympathetic and sympathetic fibers of the autonomic nervous system. The parasympathetic fibers are carried by the vagus nerve, which is considered to be the motor nerve of the esophagus. The function of the sympathetic fibers is poorly understood.

In addition to the extrinsic innervation, an intrinsic intramural meshwork of nerve fibers *(Auerbach's plexus)* exists between the circular and longitudinal muscle layers and appears to be involved in coordinating normal esophageal peristalsis. A second intrinsic nerve meshwork *(Meissner's plexus)* exists in the submucosa of the GI tract but is sparse in the esophagus.

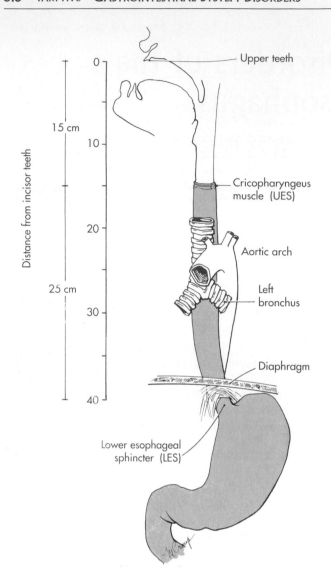

FIG. 23-1   Gross structure and anatomic relationships of the esophagus.

Blood distribution to the esophagus follows a segmental plan. The upper portion is supplied by branches from the inferior thyroid and subclavian arteries. The midportion is supplied by segmental branches from the aorta and from bronchial arteries, and the subdiaphragmatic portion is supplied by the left gastric and inferior phrenic arteries.

Venous drainage also follows a segmental pattern. The cervical esophageal veins drain into the azygos and hemiazygos veins, and below the diaphragm the esophageal veins enter the left gastric vein. Communication between the portal and systemic veins allows for bypass of the liver in cases of portal hypertension. Collateral flow through the esophageal veins causes the formation of *esophageal varices* (varicose veins of the esophagus). These enlarged veins may rupture, causing hemorrhage that may be fatal. This complication is common in pa-

tients with cirrhosis of the liver and is discussed in detail in Chapter 27.

Swallowing

Swallowing is a complex physiologic act whereby food or liquid passes from the mouth to the stomach. It is a highly coordinated muscular sequence initiated by a voluntary movement of the tongue and completed by a series of reflexes in the pharynx and esophagus. The afferent side of this reflex arc involves fibers in the fifth, ninth, and tenth cranial nerves. A swallowing, or *deglutition,* center is present in the medulla. Under the coordination of this center, impulses pass outward in a flawlessly timed sequence via the fifth, tenth, and twelfth cranial nerves to the muscles of the tongue, pharynx, larynx, and esophagus.

Although swallowing is a continuous process, it occurs in three phases: oral, pharyngeal, and esophageal. During the *oral phase* of swallowing, a mouthful of chewed food, called a *bolus,* is thrown backward against the posterior wall of the pharynx by a voluntary movement of the tongue. The impact of the bolus against the pharynx is the stimulus that sets off the reflex movements of swallowing.

During the *pharyngeal phase,* the soft palate and uvula reflexively close off the nasal cavity; at the same time the larynx is elevated and the *glottis* is closed off, keeping food from entering the trachea. Contractions of the pharyngeal constrictor muscles move the bolus past the *epiglottis* to the lower pharynx and into the esophagus. Retroversion of the epiglottis over the laryngeal orifice further protects the respiratory pathway, but is is primarily the closure of the glottis that prevents food from entering the trachea. Respirations are simultaneously inhibited to decrease the possibility of aspiration. In fact, it is almost impossible to inhale and swallow voluntarily at the same time.

The *esophageal phase* begins as the cricopharyngeus muscle relaxes briefly and allows the bolus to enter the esophagus. After this brief relaxation, a *primary peristaltic wave,* beginning in the pharynx, is transmitted to the cricopharyngeus, causing it to contract. The peristaltic wave continues throughout the body of the esophagus, propelling the bolus to the LES, which relaxes briefly to allow entry into the stomach. The primary peristaltic wave moves at the rate of 2 to 4 cm/second, so that swallowed food reaches the stomach within 5 to 15 seconds. Beginning at the level of the aortic arch, a *secondary peristaltic wave* occurs if the primary wave fails to empty the esophagus. It is triggered by distention of the esophagus from remaining food particles. The primary peristaltic wave is essential for conveying food and liquids through the upper esophagus but is less important in the lower esophagus. The upright posture and the force of gravity facilitate lower esophageal transport, but peristalsis makes it possible to drink water while standing on one's head.

During swallowing, pressure changes occur within the esophagus that reflect its motor function. In the resting state, pressure in the body of the esophagus is slightly below atmospheric pressure, reflecting intrathoracic pressure. In the regions of the UES and LES, areas of high pressure exist. These high-pressure zones prevent aspiration and reflux of the gastric contents. The pressure decreases when each sphincter area relaxes during swallowing and then increases when the peristaltic wave passes through.

It is evident that the complex series of movements that make up the act of swallowing may be upset by a number of pathologic processes. These processes involve interference either with transport or with the prevention of gastric reflux.

SYMPTOMS OF ESOPHAGEAL DISORDERS

Dysphagia, or the subjective awareness of an impairment in the active transport of ingested material from the pharynx, is a major symptom of disease of the pharynx or esophagus. Dysphagia should not be confused with *globus hystericus* (the feeling of a "lump in the throat"), which may be emotional in origin and occurs without swallowing.

Dysphagia occurs in nonesophageal disorders that result from muscular or neurologic disease. These diseases include cerebrovascular accidents (CVAs, strokes), myasthenia gravis, muscular dystrophy, and bulbar poliomyelitis.

Esophageal dysphagia may be of obstructive or motor origin. Obstructive causes include esophageal stricture and tumors extrinsic or intrinsic to the esophagus, resulting in narrowing of the lumen. Motor causes of dysphagia may result from diminished, absent, or disordered peristalsis or dysfunction of the UES or LES. Common motor disorders that produce dysphagia are achalasia, scleroderma, and diffuse esophageal spasm.

Pyrosis (heartburn) is another common symptom of esophageal disease. It is characterized by a hot, burning sensation usually felt high in the epigastrium or behind the xiphoid process and radiates upward. Heartburn may be caused by reflux of gastric acid or bile secretions into the lower esophagus; both of these are irritating to the mucosa. Persistent reflux is caused by incompetence of the LES and may occur with or without hiatus hernia or esophagitis. Heartburn is a common complaint during pregnancy.

Odynophagia is defined as pain induced by swallowing and may occur with dysphagia. It may be experienced as a sensation of tightness or as a burning pain, indistinguishable from heartburn, in the midchest. It may result from esophageal spasm induced by acute distention, or

it may be secondary to inflammation of the esophageal mucosa.

Regurgitation refers to the backflow or welling up of gastric or esophageal contents into the oral cavity. It differs from vomiting in that it is effortless and not accompanied by nausea. It is felt in the throat as a sour or bitter-tasting hot liquid. This effortless regurgitation is quite common in infants as a result of incomplete development of the LES. In adults, regurgitation reflects both LES incompetence and failure of the UES to serve as a regurgitation barrier. *Waterbrash* is reflex salivary hypersecretion in response to peptic esophagitis and should not be confused with regurgitation.

DIAGNOSTIC PROCEDURES

In addition to taking a careful history and performing a physical examination, special diagnostic measures helpful in detecting esophageal disease include barium radiologic studies, esophagoscopy with biopsy and possibly cytologic studies, manometric or motility studies, and acid reflux tests.

Barium Radiologic Studies

Radiologic examination of the esophagus as a routine is usually combined with that of the stomach and duodenum (upper GI tract radiologic series) using barium sulfate in a liquid or creamy suspension that is swallowed. The swallowing mechanism may be directly visualized by fluoroscopy, or the radiographic image may be recorded using motion picture techniques (cineradiography). When esophageal disease is suspected, the radiologist may place the patient in various positions to bring out in greater detail alterations in form and function. Tumors, polyps, diverticulitis, strictures, hiatus hernia, large esophageal varices, uncoordinated swallowing, and weak peristalsis may all be detected using this method.

Esophagoscopy

Direct inspection of the esophageal mucosa is important in diagnosing esophageal disorders. Flexible fiberoptic instruments have made this procedure much simpler and safer for the patient. Inflammation, ulcers, tumors, and esophageal varices may be visualized, photographed, and biopsied. Cell washings may be obtained for cytologic studies, which can be highly accurate in diagnosing esophageal carcinoma.

Preparation for esophagoscopy includes 6 hours of fasting and various forms of premedication, such as spraying the throat with a local anesthetic. Endoscopic examinations of the esophagus, stomach, and duodenum are often combined in one examination.

Motility Studies

Motor function of the esophagus may be studied by placing three pressure-sensitive catheters or miniature balloons in the stomach and then drawing them back incrementally. Pressures are then transmitted to a transducer located outside the patient. Measurements of pressure changes in the esophagus and stomach at rest and during swallowing have greatly increased understanding of esophageal activity both in health and in disease.

Fig. 23-2, *A* and *B*, shows normal motility in a recording of the esophagus in the resting state and during swallowing. The function of the LES is of particular interest to the gastroenterologist. Normally a zone of high pressure (15 to 30 cm H_2O above that of the intragastric pressure) exists in this region; this prevents reflux of gastric contents into the esophagus. Reflux may occur if the sphincter fails to maintain a pressure above the intraabdominal pressure.

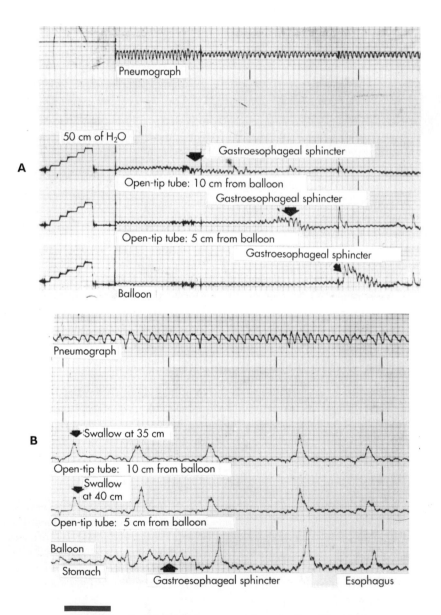

FIG. 23-2   **A,** Esophageal manometric recordings. The pressure is recorded by three catheters spaced 5 cm apart. The catheters are pulled from the stomach into the esophagus. Note the zone of high resting pressure at the junction between the stomach and the esophagus (LES). **B,** Normal swallowing. Swallowing produces a single contraction; at the same time, the sphincter zone relaxes.

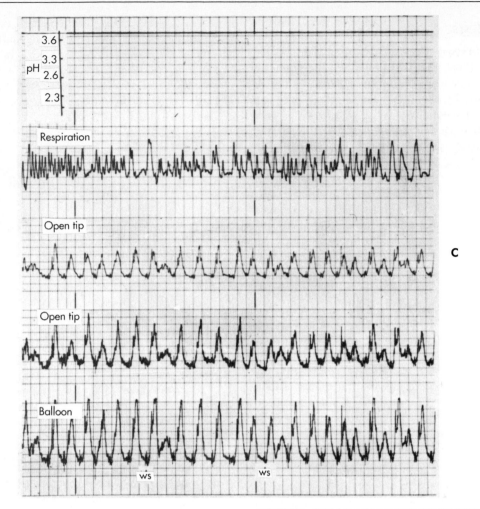

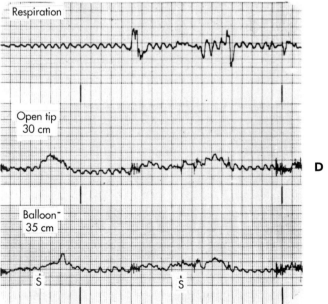

FIG. 23-2, cont'd.   **C,** Diffuse esophageal spasm. Repetitive non-progressive contractions independent of water swallowing *(ws)* occur. **D,** Scleroderma. The contractions produced by swallowings *(S)* are low in amplitude.

Acid Reflux Tests

The *acid perfusion test (Bernstein test)* is used to differentiate between chest pain that is cardiac in origin and pain resulting from acid-induced esophageal spasm, since the symptoms may be identical.

In the acid perfusion test, 0.1 *N* hydrochloric acid (HCl) is permitted to drip through a catheter at 6 to 15 ml/minute into the distal esophagus (the HCl is of the same concentration as normal gastric acid). If the patient has esophageal pain or heartburn, the test result is positive. Rapid cessation of the pain after instillation of a neutral or alkaline solution confirms that the esophageal mucosa is the site of acid-induced pain. The most common finding in a positive result is reflux esophagitis, but any disease that causes a break in mucosal continuity could cause a positive result. The person with chest pain of cardiac origin is unable to distinguish between saline and acid perfusion.

Other reflux tests include monitoring of the pH within the esophagus to detect the reflux of acid contents from the stomach, fluoroscopic observation of the esophagus to detect the reflux of barium from the stomach into the esophagus, and fluoroscopic observation of the esophagus during the ingestion of a mixture HCl and barium to detect momentary disorders in peristaltic activity. All the currently available tests for acid reflux have possible false-positive and false-negative results; therefore a combination of two or more of these studies is used to make a diagnosis in difficult cases.

DISORDERS OF ESOPHAGEAL MOTILITY

Achalasia

Achalasia, formerly called cardiospasm, is an uncommon hypomotility disorder characterized by weak and uncoordinated peristalsis or aperistalsis within the body of the esophagus, elevated LES pressure, and failure of the LES to relax completely during swallowing. Consequently, food and fluids accumulate in the lower esophagus and then slowly drain as the hydrostatic pressure increases. The body of the esophagus loses its tone and may become greatly dilated (Fig. 23-3).

The exact etiology of achalasia is unknown, but evidence suggests that degeneration of Auerbach's plexus causes the loss of neurologic control. As a result, primary peristaltic waves do not reach the LES to stimulate relaxation. *Primary* idiopathic achalasia accounts for most of the cases seen in the United States. *Secondary* achalasia may be caused by gastric carcinoma invading the esophagus, by irradiation, and by certain toxins and drugs.

Achalasia is more common in adults than in children. The onset is usually insidious, and the most prominent symptom is dysphagia for liquid and solid foods. Meals

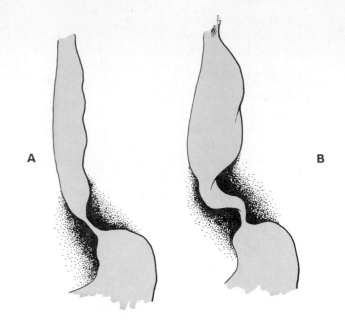

FIG. 23-3   Esophageal achalasia. **A,** Early stage, showing tapering of lower esophagus. **B,** Advanced stage, showing dilated, tortuous esophagus.

may be interrupted by the necessity to regurgitate. Nocturnal regurgitation may result in aspiration, resulting in chronic pulmonary infections or sudden death. The stasis of food in the esophagus may lead to inflammatory changes, erosions, and in some cases, cancer of the esophagus, although this is usually a late complication.

The diagnosis is made on the basis of the history and the characteristic radiographic appearance. When barium is swallowed, the peristaltic wave is weak and the collection of barium in the lower esophagus gives it a funnel-like appearance. The administration of small doses of a cholinergic or parasympathomimetic drug causes marked contraction and emptying of the esophagus and confirms the diagnosis. Esophageal motility studies may be helpful in the early diagnosis of achalasia. Manometric measurements in these studies reveal that the LES fails to relax with swallowing. The resting pressure of the LES is usually elevated (35 mm Hg versus the normal pressure of 15 to 30 mm Hg).

Treatment of achalasia is palliative and consists of measures to relieve the obstruction of the lower esophagus. There is no known method of restoring normal peristalsis to the body of the esophagus. Two forms of therapy that effectively relieve the symptoms are dilation of the LES and esophagomyotomy. Dilation may be achieved by passing a mercury-filled tube called a *bougie* (procedure is *bougienage*) or, more often, by placing a pneumatic bag in the area of the LES and forcefully dilating it. When dilation fails to relieve the symptoms, surgical intervention may be indicated.

The surgery most frequently performed for achalasia

or esophageal stricture is the *Heller esophagomyotomy,* which consists of dividing the muscle fibers of the gastroesophageal junction. A *pyloroplasty* (enlargement of gastric outlet) frequently accompanies this procedure to allow rapid emptying of stomach contents and prevent reflux into the esophagus (Fig. 23-4).

Drug therapy is currently reserved for patients who are not considered suitable for either pneumatic dilation or surgery. Isosorbide (long-acting nitrate) and nifedipine (calcium channel antagonist) lower LES pressure and have been used with some success to treat achalasia.

Other helpful measures to minimize symptoms include slow eating and avoidance of alcohol and hot, cold, or spicy foods. Patients should be instructed to sleep with the head elevated to avoid aspiration.

Diffuse Esophageal Spasm

Diffuse esophageal spasm is a fairly common condition characterized by uncoordinated, nonpropulsive contractions (tertiary peristalsis) of the esophagus in response to swallowing. It is most prominent in the lower two thirds of the organ but may involve the entire esophagus. The two sphincters operate normally. It is a disease of unknown cause and is seen more frequently in older patients. Similar motility disturbances may be secondary to reflux esophagitis or obstruction of the lower esophagus, as in carcinoma (usually, results of manometric studies in early carcinoma are normal).

Primary diffuse spasm of the esophagus usually occurs in patients over 50 years of age. Nonperistaltic responses to swallowing are common findings on barium radiologic studies and increase with aging. These radiologic findings are referred to as "corkscrew esophagus," "rosary bead esophagus," "curling," and a variety of other descriptive names that are usually of little clinical significance.

The pathogenic basis for the diffuse spasm is poorly understood. It may represent a degeneration of local neurons, since some patients have a positive response to cholinergics, as occurs in achalasia.

Diffuse esophageal spasm is usually asymptomatic, but in a few cases the contractions may give rise to symptoms. The most common symptoms include intermittent dysphagia and odynophagia, which are aggravated by ingestion of cold foods and large boluses and by nervous tension. When the patient has intermittent chest pain, diffuse esophageal spasm may be confused with angina pectoris, especially if the symptoms are not associated with eating. To add to this confusion, the pain caused by diffuse spasm is often relieved by nitroglycerin. Consequently, some patients with diffuse esophageal spasm have been misdiagnosed as having cardiac disease.

Motility studies reveal a hypermotile pattern of nonperistaltic contractions and aid in the diagnosis (Fig. 23-2, *C*).

Treatment consists of dietary manipulations (small

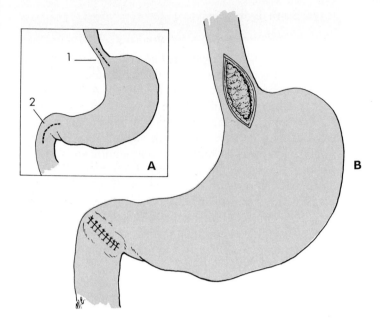

FIG. 23-4   Surgical treatment of esophageal achalasia. **A,** Longitudinal incision for Heller esophagomyotomy, *1,* and pyloroplasty, *2.* **B,** The esophageal incision is made through the muscle layers to allow pouching of the mucosa, thus relieving the esophageal obstruction. A gastric drainage procedure (pyloroplasty) often accompanies the esophagomyotomy to prevent esophageal reflux. The pyloric incision is sutured in the opposite direction to enlarge the gastric outlet.

meals, avoidance of cold foods), antacids, sedatives, and nitroglycerin to relieve the spasm. If symptoms are persistent and distressing, esophageal dilation may be recommended. As a last resort, a longitudinal myotomy of the distal esophagus may be performed.

Scleroderma

Esophageal motor dysfunction occurs in more than two thirds of patients with *progressive systemic sclerosis (scleroderma).* The basic abnormality in the GI tract is atrophy of the smooth muscle of the lower portion of the esophagus.

The diagnosis is suspected on barium swallow radiographic examination but is confirmed by manometric findings. Aperistalsis or weak peristalsis of the distal one half to two thirds of the esophagus and diminished pressure of the LES characterize scleroderma (Fig. 23-2, *D*).

Incompetence of the LES often leads to reflux esophagitis with subsequent stricture formation in the lower esophagus. Although gastroesophageal reflux and esophagitis occur often with scleroderma, heartburn is not a common symptom. Dysphagia becomes a prominent symptom when esophagitis has led to stricture formation (see following discussion).

ESOPHAGITIS

Inflammation of the esophageal mucosa may be acute or chronic and is seen in a variety of circumstances, including the motility disorders just discussed. An innocuous type of esophagitis follows the ingestion of hot liquids. The substernal burning sensation is usually of short duration and may be associated with superficial edema and esophagospasm. The most common significant form of esophagitis is caused by acid reflux from the stomach, often in association with hiatus hernia. There are also infectious forms of esophagitis, including those caused by *Candida albicans* (thrush) or the herpesviruses. Infectious esophagitis is common in persons with severe immunodeficiency, such as in acquired immunodeficiency syndrome (AIDS).

An acute, severe form of esophagitis follows the ingestion of strong alkalis or acids. Strong alkalis are typically found in most households in the form of drain cleaners, which will produce a severe liquefying necrosis of the mucosa if ingested. Accidental ingestion of these substances occurs most often in small children, but occasionally these substances are used in suicide attempts. Immediate symptoms include severe odynophagia, fever, toxicity, and possible esophageal perforation with consequent infection of the mediastinum and death. Long-term effects include scarring and esophageal stricture that requires periodic dilation with bougies for the remainder of the patient's life. Treatment must be prompt and vigorous and includes the use of antibiotics, steroids, intravenous fluids, and possibly surgery.

Chronic Reflux Esophagitis and Hiatus Hernia

Chronic reflux esophagitis is the most common form of esophagitis encountered clinically. It is caused by incompetence of the LES and reflux of acid gastric or alkaline intestinal juice into the esophagus over a long period. The sequelae of reflux are inflammation, ulcer formation, bleeding, and scarring with stricture formation. Chronic reflux esophagitis is often associated with hiatus hernia. Little correlation exists between the severity of symptoms and the degree of esophagitis. Some patients with heartburn have minimal evidence of esophagitis, whereas others with chronic reflux may be asymptomatic until stricture formation develops.

Mechanisms preventing reflux

Fig. 23-5 illustrates the mechanisms that normally prevent reflux of gastric contents into the esophagus. The high-pressure zone at the gastroesophageal junction (or LES) is probably the most important mechanism for preventing reflux. The tone of this sphincter is affected not only by a variety of drugs, but also by influences of hormones such as gastrin and secretin, which may play an important role in maintaining the integrity of the sphincter. The importance of the anatomic configuration of the esophagogastric junction is not known at present. The acute angle between the esophagus and stomach may be an important mechanism for preventing reflux, since this creates an arrangement similar to a flap valve, which would prevent material from regurgitating. It has also been suggested that the short segment of the esophagus below the diaphragm is kept closed by intraabdominal pressure. Displacement of this lower esophageal segment into the chest, as occurs in hiatus hernia, would eliminate this barrier to reflux and may explain why an association seems to exist with reflux esophagitis. However, the role of a sliding hiatus hernia is not thought to be as important as once thought.

Hiatus hernia

Hiatus hernia is defined as a herniation of a portion of the stomach into the chest through the esophageal hiatus of the diaphragm. There are two distinct types of hiatus

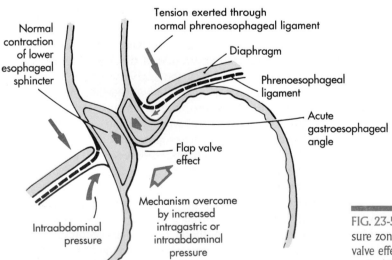

FIG. 23-5 Mechanisms preventing esophageal reflux: high-pressure zone at the LES; acute gastroesophageal angle causing a flap valve effect; and phrenoesophageal (PE) ligament causing a pinchcock valve effect.

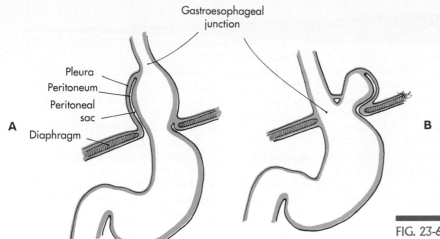

FIG. 23-6   **A,** Sliding or direct hiatus hernia. **B,** Rolling or paraesophageal hiatus hernia.

hernia (Fig. 23-6). The most common form is the *direct* or *sliding hiatus hernia,* in which the gastroesophageal junction slides into the thoracic cavity, especially when the patient assumes a supine position. The competency of the LES may be destroyed, resulting in reflux esophagitis. Often it is asymptomatic and is discovered only accidentally during a search for the cause of a variety of epigastric symptoms or on routine GI tract radiographs.

In *paraesophageal* or *rolling hiatus hernia,* part of the gastric fundus rolls through the hiatus and the gastroesophageal junction remains below the diaphragm. There is no insufficiency of the LES mechanism, and consequently, reflux esophagitis does not occur. The major complication of paraesophageal hernia is strangulation.

Sliding and rolling hiatus hernias are diagnosed radiographically or endoscopically. The important clinical question is whether there is esophageal reflux, since this has serious consequences, including esophagitis with ulceration and stricture, asthma, and aspiration pneumonia. Continuous monitoring of esophageal pH with a miniaturized pH meter has been helpful in demonstrating reflux and correlating reflux with symptoms.

Treatment of sliding hiatus hernia is directed toward prevention of reflux, neutralizing refluxate, and protecting the esophageal mucosa. The patient is instructed to eat small, frequent meals and to take antacids. H₂ blockers such as ranitidine and a protective agent such as sucralfate may be helpful. If overweight, the patient is instructed to reduce. Calcium channel blockers and anticholinergic drugs should not be given because they delay gastric emptying and relax the LES. Metoclopramide, a derivative of procainamide, increases the tone of the LES and is useful in the treatment of selected cases of reflux. Omeprazole, a drug that suppresses gastric acid secretion, may be given to patients with resistant conditions. Nicotine, which decreases LES tone, should be avoided. The patient should avoid activities that involve stooping forward, especially after meals. The head of the bed generally should be elevated during sleep to prevent reflux.

Surgical repair may be indicated if medical treatment fails and if there is evidence of persistent reflux esophagitis or stricture formation.

TUMORS

Benign tumors of the esophagus are rare. The most common type, however, is a *leiomyoma* (smooth muscle tumor). Leiomyomas may occasionally bleed but are usually of little clinical significance and are discovered incidentally.

Cancer of the esophagus, however, is not rare. It caused approximately 2% of all cancer deaths in the United States in 1995 and 9% of those involving the digestive organs. (American Cancer Society, 1995). Men between ages 50 and 70 years are affected most frequently. Predisposing factors include heavy smoking, alcohol abuse, and esophageal obstruction. *Squamous cell carcinoma* is the most common type of tumor and is highly malignant. Tumors can occur in any part of the esophagus, but most develop in the lower two thirds.

Barium radiologic and cytologic studies and esophagoscopy with biopsy are important in the diagnosis. The 5-year survival rate is less than 10%. The reason for the poor prognosis is the early lymphatic spread and the late development of symptoms. The first symptom is generally dysphagia, but this does not generally occur until the tumor involves the entire circumference of the esophagus.

Irradiation and surgical resection are the major forms of treatment. Lesions in the upper portion of the esophagus may be impossible to resect and are treated by irradiation. Bougies may be passed to dilate the lumen, or a plastic prosthesis may be inserted to enable the patient to continue eating. A newer form of palliation is the use of a laser beam to vaporize the core of the obstructing tumor and thus reestablish the lumen and allow passage of food.

QUESTIONS

▼ *Answer the following on a separate sheet of paper.*

1. Describe the function of the esophagus.
2. Why is regurgitation more common in infants than in adults?
3. What are esophageal varices and why are they often associated with cirrhosis of the liver? Why is this condition important?
4. What is an esophagomyotomy? What is a pyloroplasty? Why are these two procedures often combined? What condition is often treated by esophagomyotomy and pyloroplasty?
5. What kind of instructions would you give to patients with the following conditions to minimize symptoms and prevent complications: diffuse esophageal spasm, scleroderma, and sliding hiatus hernia?
6. Sketch the anatomic relations of the gastroesophageal junction, and briefly describe the three mechanisms preventing reflux.
7. Describe the consequences of chronic esophageal reflux.
8. Why do patients with achalasia and sliding hiatus hernia often have chronic pulmonary infections?
9. Why is chronic reflux esophagitis sometimes difficult to identify? What test is used to assist in the diagnosis?

▼ *Circle the letter preceding each item that correctly answers the question or completes the statement. Only one answer is correct unless otherwise noted.*

10. Which of the following statements concerning anatomy of the esophagus is *false?*
    a. It passes through the esophageal hiatus of the diaphragm.
    b. It lies posterior to the heart.
    c. Its length is about 25 cm.
    d. An anatomically distinct sphincter is present at the gastroesophageal junction.
11. The muscle that functions as the UES is the:
    a. Palatopharyngeus
    b. Phrenoesophageal
    c. Cricopharyngeus
    d. Palatine
12. The LES is:
    a. A well-differentiated zone of muscle
    b. A zone of high pressure near the gastroesophageal junction
    c. Normally located above the level of the diaphragm

d. A diaphragmatic muscle band externally compressing the esophagus

13. Which of the following types of epithelium is present throughout most of the length of the esophagus?
    a. Simple columnar
    b. Pseudostratified ciliated columnar
    c. Stratified squamous
14. The extrinsic motor nerve that coordinates esophageal peristalsis is the:
    a. Vagus
    b. Auerbach's
    c. Hypoglossal
15. The normal pH of esophageal secretions is:
    a. Slightly acidic
    b. Slightly alkaline
    c. Identical with the pH of gastric secretions
16. The terminal one third of the tunica muscularis of the esophagus is composed of:
    a. Smooth muscle fibers
    b. Skeletal muscle fibers
    c. Both skeletal and smooth muscle fibers
17. The second stage of swallowing is characterized by (more than one answer may be correct):
    a. Inhibition of respiration
    b. Being under voluntary control
    c. Closure of the vocal cords
    d. Relaxation of the cricopharyngeus muscle
18. All the following cranial nerves are involved in the control of swallowing *except:*
    a. Third   d. Tenth
    b. Fifth   e. Twelfth
    c. Ninth
19. Transportation of a bolus of food through the esophagus is a function of:
    a. Primary peristaltic wave
    b. Secondary peristaltic wave
    c. Tertiary peristaltic wave
    d. All the above
20. After being swallowed, food or liquids normally enter the stomach within:
    a. 5 to 15 seconds
    b. 30 to 40 seconds
    c. 60 seconds
    d. 2 minutes
21. Which of the following are required for the diagnosis of achalasia (more than one answer may be correct)?
    a. Findings of weak, uncoordinated peristalsis on motility study
    b. "Rosary bead esophagus" on barium x-ray study

c. Positive response to cholinergics
d. Narrowed gastroesophageal junction

22. Achalasia is thought to be caused by:
    a. Stress and nervous tension
    b. Degeneration of Auerbach's plexus
    c. Gastric reflux
    d. Failure of the cricopharyngeus muscle to relax
    e. Infection with a parasite (filaria)
23. Which of the following is the treatment of choice in achalasia?
    a. Dilation with bougies (bougienage)
    b. Pneumatic dilation
    c. Heller esophagomyotomy
    d. Anticholingeric drugs
    e. Psychotherapy
24. Which of the following tests is most helpful in differentiating cardiac and esophageal pain?
    a. Electrocardiogram
    b. Relief of pain by nitroglycerin confirms cardiac origin of pain
    c. Mecholyl test
    d. 0.1 *N* HCl acid perfusion test
25. The portion of the esophagus primarily affected in scleroderma is the:
    a. Body   c. LES
    b. Upper one third   d. UES
26. The most effective early treatment measures for an alkali burn of the esophagus include (more than one answer may be correct):
    a. Corticosteroid drugs
    b. Immediate induction of vomiting
    c. Broad-spectrum antibiotics
    d. Immediate pneumatic dilation
27. Which of the following statements about hiatus hernia is *true?*
    a. There are two distinct types.
    b. The paraesophageal type is the most common.
    c. All require surgery.
    d. All are associated with gastric reflux.
28. Which of the following statements concerning sliding hiatus hernia is *true?*
    a. Most frequent complication is strangulation.
    b. Presence of gastric reflux is principal indication for surgery.
    c. It should always be treated by surgery
    d. Gastric fundus rolls through the hiatus, and gastroesophageal junction remains below the diaphragm.
29. All the following statements concerning chronic reflux esophagitis are true *except:*
    a. Associated with hiatus hernia

QUESTIONS—cont'd

b. Caused by irritating gastric secretions
c. Often accompanied by projectile vomiting
d. May lead to columnar metaplasia of the lower esophagus
e. May result in esophageal ulcers

30. Which of the following statements concerning cancer of the esophagus are *true* (more than one answer may be correct)?
   a. Rare form of cancer
   b. More common in men
   c. Associated with alcohol abuse and heavy smoking

d. More often located in the upper esophagus
e. Prognosis generally good

▼ *Circle T if the statement is true and F if it is false. Correct any false statements.*

31. T F Nonperistaltic responses to swallowing increase with age.

32. T F Secondary peristalsis is important in removing food particles that remain in the esophagus after the primary peristaltic wave has passed.

33. T F The aid of gravity is essential to swallowing of liquids.

34. T F Cell washings for cytologic study is one of the most accurate ways to identify early cancer of the esophagus.

35. T F Endoscopic examination of the esophagus with a fiberoptic instrument requires general anesthesia.

36. T F Tertiary peristalsis consists of uncoordinated, nonpropulsive contractions of the esophagus.

37. T F Long-term effects of lye ingestion may include esophageal stricture and the necessity of periodic bougienage.

▼ *Match each of the following symptoms in column A with its proper definition or description in column B.*

Column A	Column B
38. _____ Dysphagia	a. Hot, burning sensation usually felt high in the epigastrum
39. _____ Regurgitation	b. "Lump in the throat" present during the absence of swallowing
40. _____ Odynophagia	c. Subjective awareness of difficulty in swallowing
41. _____ Pyrosis	d. Pain in midchest induced by swallowing
42. _____ Globus hystericus	e. Effortless welling up of esophageal or gastric contents into the mouth

▼ *Match each of the following esophageal motor disorders in column A with its common findings in motility studies in column B.*

Column A	Column B
43. _____ Diffuse esophageal spasm	a. Loss of contractile power in lower distal portion of esophagus
44. _____ Achalasia	b. Characterized by a hypermotile pattern of ineffective contractions
45. _____ Scleroderma	c. Absence of peristalsis in body of esophagus and incomplete relaxation of the LES
	d. Characterized by resting pressure lower than normal at the LES
	e. Characterized by resting pressure higher than normal at the LES

CHAPTER 24

Disorders of the Stomach and Duodenum

LORRAINE M. WILSON
GLENDA N. LINDSETH

ANATOMY

The stomach lies obliquely from left to right across the upper abdomen directly beneath the diaphragm. When empty, the stomach resembles a J-shaped tube and, when full, a giant pear. The normal capacity of the stomach is 1 to 2 L. Anatomically, the stomach is divided into the *fundus,* the *body,* and the *pyloric antrum,* or *pylorus* (Fig. 24-1). The concave *lesser curvature* forms the upper right border of the stomach, and the convex *greater curvature* forms the left and lower borders. Sphincters at each end of the stomach regulate inflow and outflow. The *cardiac sphincter,* or lower esophageal sphincter (LES), allows food to flow into the stomach and prevents the reflux of gastric contents into the esophagus. The area of the stomach into which the cardiac sphincter opens is known as the *cardiac region.* The terminal *pyloric sphincter* relaxes to permit food to enter the duodenum, and when contracted, it prevents backflow of intestinal contents into the stomach.

The pyloric sphincter is of particular clinical interest because obstructive narrowing (stenosis) may occur as a complication of peptic ulcer disease. Abnormalities of the pyloric sphincter may also occur in infants. *Pyloric stenosis* or pylorospasm results when hypertrophied or spastic muscle fibers surrounding the opening fail to relax sufficiently to permit food to pass easily from the stomach to the duodenum. The infant vomits the food instead of digesting and absorbing it. These conditions may be corrected by surgery or by adrenergic drugs that relax the muscle fibers.

The stomach is composed of four layers. The *serosa,* or outer layer, is a part of the visceral peritoneum. The two layers of the visceral peritoneum come together at the lesser curvature of the stomach and duodenum and extend upward to the liver, forming the *lesser omentum.* Peritoneal folds reflected from one organ to another are distinguished as ligaments. Thus the lesser omentum (also known as the hepatogastric and hepatoduodenal ligaments) suspends the stomach along its lesser curvature to the liver. At the greater curvature, the peritoneum continues downward as the *greater omentum,* draping over the intestines like a large apron. The lesser omental sac is a common site for the accumulation of fluid (pancreatic pseudocyst) as a complication of acute pancreatitis.

Unlike other areas of the digestive tract, the stomach's *muscularis* is composed of three rather than two layers of smooth muscle: an outer longitudinal layer, a middle circular layer, and an inner oblique layer. This unique

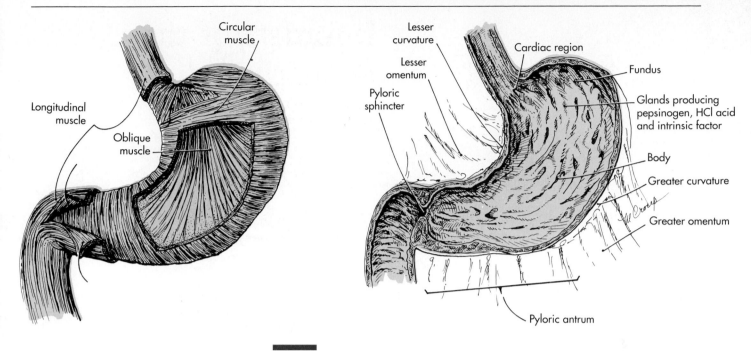

FIG. 24-1   Anatomy of the stomach.

arrangement of fibers provides the variety of contractions necessary to break food into small particles, churn and mix it with gastric juices, and propel it into the duodenum.

The *submucosa* is composed of loose areolar tissue that connects the muscularis and mucosal layers. It permits the mucosa to move with peristaltic motion. This layer also contains the nerve plexuses, blood vessels, and lymph channels.

The *mucosa,* the inner layer of the stomach, is arranged in longitudinal folds called *rugae,* which allow for distention as the stomach becomes filled with food. Several types of glands are located in this layer and are categorized according to the anatomic portion of the stomach in which they are located. *Cardiac glands* lie near the cardiac orifice and secrete mucus. The *fundic* or *gastric glands* are located in the fundus and over the greater part of the body of the stomach. Gastric glands have three main types of cells. *Zymogenic* or *chief cells* secrete *pepsinogen.* Pepsinogen is converted into *pepsin* in an acid environment. *Parietal cells* secrete hydrochloric acid (HCl) and intrinsic factor. *Intrinsic factor* is necessary for the absorption of vitamin B_{12} in the small intestine. A lack of intrinsic factor results in pernicious anemia. *Mucous (neck) cells* are found in the neck of the fundic glands and secrete mucus. The hormone *gastrin* is produced by G cells located in the pyloric region of the stomach. Gastrin stimulates the gastric glands to produce HCl and pepsinogen. Other substances secreted in the stomach include enzymes and various electrolytes, especially sodium, potassium, and chloride ions.

The stomach receives its extrinsic nerve supply entirely from the autonomic nervous system. The parasympathetic nerve supply for the stomach and duodenum is conveyed to and from the abdomen through the vagus nerves (Fig. 24-2). Gastric, pyloric, and celiac branches emerge from the vagal trunks. It is especially important to understand this anatomy, because selective vagotomy is of primary importance in the surgical treatment of duodenal ulcers. It is discussed in greater detail later in this chapter.

Sympathetic innervation is supplied via the greater splanchnic nerves and the celiac ganglia. The afferent fibers conduct pain impulses stimulated by distention, muscle contraction, and inflammation and are felt in the epigastric region of the abdomen. Efferent sympathetic fibers inhibit gastric motility and secretion. The *myenteric* (Auerbach's) and the *submucosal* (Meissner's) *nerve plexuses* form the intrinsic innervation within the wall of the stomach and coordinate its motor and secretory activity.

The entire blood supply of the stomach and pancreas (as well as the liver, gallbladder, and spleen) is derived mainly from the celiac artery or trunk, which gives off branches supplying the lesser and greater curvatures. Two arterial branches of particular clinical significance are the *gastroduodenal* and the *pancreaticoduodenal* (retroduodenal) *arteries,* which course along the posterior duodenal bulb (Fig. 24-3). Ulcers of the posterior duodenal wall may erode into these arteries and cause hemorrhaging. The venous blood from the stomach and duodenum, as well as that from the pancreas, spleen, and the remainder of the gastrointestinal (GI) tract, is conveyed to the liver by the portal vein.

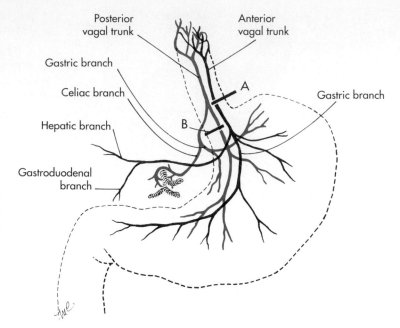

FIG. 24-2 Parasympathetic (vagal) innervation of the stomach. It is possible to sever the vagal nerve branches supplying the stomach at points *A* and *B,* leaving intact those branches supplying other abdominal structures (selective vagotomy). Selective vagotomy is an important aspect of the surgical treatment of duodenal ulcers.

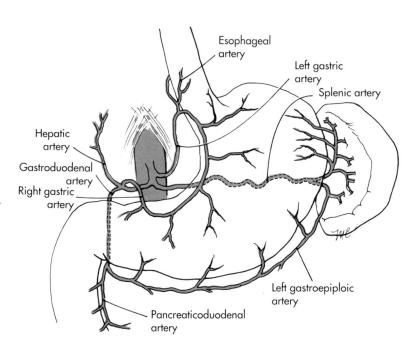

FIG. 24-3 Blood supply of the stomach and duodenum.

PHYSIOLOGY

The digestive and motor functions of the stomach are summarized in the box on p. 329. The types of secretions have already been discussed. Motor functions include storing, mixing, and emptying *chyme* (a semifluid mass of partly digested food mixed with gastric secretions) into the duodenum. Understanding the regulation and control of gastric secretions is essential for a rational understanding of the pathogenesis and treatment of peptic ulcer disease.

Control of Gastric Secretion

Gastric secretion may be divided into three phases: cephalic, gastric, and intestinal. The *cephalic phase* occurs even before food enters the stomach. It results from the site, smell, thought, or taste of food. It is mediated entirely by the vagus nerve and is eliminated by vagotomy. Neurogenic signals causing the cephalic phase may originate in the cerebral cortex or in the appetite center. Efferent impulses are then transmitted via the vagus nerves to the stomach. As a result, the gastric glands are stimulated to secrete HCl, pepsinogen, and increased amounts

FUNCTIONS OF THE STOMACH

MOTOR FUNCTIONS

Reservoir function: stores food until it can be partially digested and moved on in GI tract; adapts to increased volume without an increase in pressure by receptive relaxation of the smooth muscle; this is mediated by the vagus nerve and induced by gastrin.

Mixing function: breaks food into small particles and mixes it with gastric juice through contractions of muscular coat; peristaltic contractions are controlled by a basic intrinsic electrical rhythm.

Gastric emptying function: controlled by opening of pyloric sphincter, which is influenced by viscosity, volume, acidity, osmotic activity, and physical state, as well as by emotions, drugs, and exercise; gastric emptying is controlled by nervous and hormonal factors.

DIGESTIVE AND SECRETORY FUNCTIONS

Digestion of protein by pepsin and HCl is begun; digestion of starches and fats by gastric amylase and lipase is of little importance in the stomach.

Gastrin synthesis and release are affected by ingestion of protein, distention of the antrum, alkalinization of the antrum, and vagal stimuli.

Intrinsic factor secretion enables the absorption of vitamin B_{12} from the distal small bowel to occur.

Mucus secretion forms a protective shell for the stomach and contributes to lubrication of food for easier transport.

Bicarbonate secretion, along with mucous gel secretion, seems to act as a barrier from luminal acid and pepsin.

TABLE 24-1   Actions of Gastrin

Actions	Physiologic Significance
Stimulates acid and pepsin secretion	Promotes digestion
Stimulates secretion of intrinsic factor	Promotes vitamin B_{12} absorption in small intestine
Stimulates pancreatic enzyme secretion	Promotes digestion
Stimulates increase in flow of hepatic bile	Promotes digestion
Stimulates release of insulin	Promotes glucose metabolism
Stimulates gastric and intestinal motility	Promotes mixing and propulsion of ingested food
Promotes receptive relaxation of stomach	Stomach can greatly increase volume without increasing pressure
Increases resting tone of LES	Prevents gastric reflux during active mixing and churning
Inhibits gastric emptying	Allows time for thorough mixing of gastric contents before delivery to intestine

of mucus. The cephalic phase of secretion accounts for about 10% of the gastric secretions normally associated with a meal.

The *gastric phase* is initiated by the presence of food in the pyloric antrum. Distention of the antrum can also result in the mechanical stimulation of receptors in the wall of the stomach. Impulses travel to the medulla over vagal afferents and return to the stomach over vagal efferents; these impulses stimulate the release of the hormone gastrin and also directly stimulate the gastric glands. Gastrin is released from the antrum and is then carried by the bloodstream to the gastric glands, causing secretion. Gastrin release is also stimulated by an alkaline pH, by bile salts in the antrum, and especially by protein foods and alcohol. Parietal cell membranes in the fundus and body of the stomach contain receptors for gastrin, histamine, and acetylcholine, which stimulate the acid secretion. After meal consumption, gastrin can act on the parietal cells directly for acid secretion and can also stimulate release of histamine from the enterochromaffin cells of the mucosa for acid secretion. Table 24-1 lists the effects of gastrin.

The gastric phase of secretion accounts for more than two thirds of the total gastric secretion after a meal is eaten and thus accounts for most of the total daily gastric secretion of about 2000 ml. The gastric phase can be affected by surgical resection of the pyloric antrum, since this is the site of gastrin production.

The *intestinal phase* is initiated by the movement of chyme from the stomach to the duodenum. This phase of gastric secretion is believed to be largely hormonal. The presence of partially digested proteins in the duodenum apparently stimulates the release of enteric gastrin, a hormone that causes the stomach to continue to secrete small amounts of gastric juice. However, the role of the small intestine as an inhibitor of gastric secretion is of much greater importance.

Distention of the small intestine initiates the *enterogastric reflex,* mediated through the myenteric plexus, sympathetic nerves, and vagus nerve, which inhibits gastric secretion and emptying. The presence of acid (pH less than 2.5), fat, and protein breakdown products causes the release of several intestinal hormones. *Secretin, cholecystokinin* (CCK), and *gastric-inhibiting peptide* (GIP) all have inhibitory effects on gastric secretions.

During the *interdigestive period,* when digestion is not occurring in the gut, HCl secretion continues at the low rate of 1 to 5 mEq/hour. This is called the *basal acid output* (BAO) and may be measured by analysis of gastric secretions after a 12-hour fast. The normal gastric secretions during the interdigestive period are mainly composed of mucus and contain little pepsin and acid. Strong emotional stimuli, however, can increase the BAO via the parasympathetic (vagus) nerves and are believed to be one of the factors in the development of peptic ulcers.

DIAGNOSTIC PROCEDURES

Diagnostic procedures that help identify gastric and duodenal disease include barium radiologic studies, gastric analysis, and endoscopy using a flexible fiberoptic gastroscope. Photography, biopsy, and exfoliative cytology may be performed through the gastroscope. *Exfoliative cytology,* or collection of cells by lavage with normal saline solution, is a valuable technique for identifying malignancies that may not be directly visible through the gastroscope. Malignant cells exfoliate (slough off) more readily than normal cells. The collected solution should be placed on ice and taken to the laboratory immediately for analysis. Delay will result in destruction of the exfoliated cells by the digestive enzymes. Cytologic washings are about 90% accurate in the diagnosis of stomach cancer.

Gastric analysis of acid secretion is another important technique in the diagnosis of gastric disease. A nasogastric tube is inserted into the stomach, and the fasting contents are aspirated for analysis. The *basal analysis* measures BAO in the absence of stimulation. This test is valuable in the diagnosis of *Zollinger-Ellison syndrome,* in which a tumor of the pancreas secretes large amounts of gastrin, which in turn causes marked hyperacidity and multiple recurrent peptic ulcers. Duodenal ulcers are usually associated with a high BAO, whereas the BAO is normal to low in gastric ulcer and carcinoma.

Stimulation analysis may be performed by measuring *maximum acid output* (MAO) after administration of a drug that stimulates acid secretion, such as histamine; betazole hydrochloride (Histalog), a histamine analogue; or pentagastrin, a synthetic, gastrinlike peptide. *Achlorhydria* is defined as a lack of acid secretions after administering a maximum dose of one of the stimulating drugs, provided the analysis is accurate and no reflux of duodenal contents has occurred into the stomach, which would neutralize the acid. If a patient is achlorhydric and has a gastric ulcer, the ulcer probably represents cancer and is not related to acid secretions. Patients with pernicious anemia are also achlorhydric as a result of atrophy of the secretory cells in the stomach. Without intrinsic factor, vitamin B_{12} absorption is impaired and the serum levels of vitamin B_{12} will be low.

NAUSEA AND VOMITING

Nausea and vomiting are common signs and symptoms accompanying GI disorders as well as many other illnesses. Several theories concerning the cause of nausea and vomiting have evolved, but no agreement exists on a definitive cause or treatment. Nausea and vomiting can be considered a phenomenon that occurs in three stages: (1) nausea, (2) retching, and (3) vomiting. The first stage, *nausea,* may be described as a very disagreeable feeling experienced in the back of the throat and the epigastrium, often resulting in vomiting. Various changes in digestive tract activity have been associated with nausea, such as increased salivation, decreased gastric tone, and peristalsis. An increase in duodenal and jejunal tone results in a reflux of duodenal contents into the stomach. However, no evidence suggests that these events cause nausea (Lang, 1990). Signs and symptoms of nausea often include pallor, increased salivation, queasiness, faintness, and tachycardia.

Retching, an involuntary attempt to vomit, often follows nausea and precedes vomiting. It consists of spasmodic respiratory movements against the glottis and inspiratory movements of the chest wall and diaphragm. Expiratory abdominal muscle contractions control the inspiratory movements. The distal antrum and pylorus contract while the fundus relaxes.

The last stage, *vomiting,* is defined as a reflex causing the forceful expulsion of the contents of the stomach and/or intestine through the mouth. The vomiting center receives input from the cerebral cortex, vestibular organs, *chemoreceptor trigger zone* (CTZ), and afferent fibers, including those of the GI system (Chin, 1988). Vomiting is the result of stimulation of the *emetic center,* which is located in the area postrema of the medulla in the floor of the fourth ventricle. It can be stimulated through the afferent neural pathways by vagal and sympathetic nerve stimulation or by an emetic stimulus that leads to vomiting by activating the CTZ. The efferent pathways relay the signals that lead to the coordinated respiratory, GI, and abdominal muscle expulsive movements and accompanying emetic epiphenomena called vomiting. Because the vomiting center is anatomically near the salivation and respiratory centers, hypersalivation and respiratory movements often occur with vomiting.

Vomiting is considered important because it can be an indicator of various conditions, such as intestinal obstruction, infections, pain, metabolic diseases, pregnancy, labyrinthine and vestibular disorders, exogenous emetic substances such as poisons, uremia or kidney failure, radiation sickness, psychologic conditions, migraines, myocardial infarction, and circulatory syncope. Because nausea and vomiting can result from many different illnesses, it is important to distinguish among characteristics of the symptoms. Symptoms that have been present for a few hours or days may indicate an acute infection, inflammatory conditions, or pregnancy. Nausea and vomiting that have been present for weeks may indicate obstructive, carcinogenic, or psychogenic origins. Factors that should be considered include timing of the nausea and vomiting, relationship to meals, content and odor of the vomitus, and associated symptoms such as pain, weight loss, fever, menstruation, abdominal mass, jaundice, headache, and other factors that may influence the patient's diagnosis and care. Vomiting can also lead to life-threatening complications because of its relationship with the autonomic and sympathetic nervous systems, as well as the impact of nausea and vomiting on the body's fluid and electrolytes.

GASTRITIS

Gastritis is an inflammation or hemorrhagic condition of the gastric mucosa that may be acute, chronic, diffuse, or localized. The two most common types of gastritis are acute superficial and chronic atrophic.

Acute Superficial Gastritis

Acute gastritis is a common, usually benign, and self-limiting disease that represents the response of the gastric mucosa to a variety of local irritants. Bacterial endotoxins (after the ingestion of contaminated food), caffeine, alcohol, and aspirin are common offending agents. *Helicobacter pylori* is more frequently being considered a cause of acute gastritis. The organism attaches to gastric epithelium and destroys the protective mucosal layer, leaving areas of denuded epithelium. Other drugs, such as nonsteroidal antiinflammatory drugs (NSAIDs; e.g., indomethacin, ibuprofen, naproxen), sulfonamides, steroids, and digitalis, have also been implicated. Bile acids, pancreatic enzymes, and ethanol are also known to disrupt the gastric mucosal barrier. Gastric irritation may be caused by alcohol, caffeine, and strong spices such as chili powder, pepper, or garlic.

When alcohol is ingested in combination with aspirin, the effect is more deleterious than the effect of either taken alone. *Diffuse hemorrhagic erosive gastritis* is known to occur with heavy alcohol and aspirin use and may lead to the necessity of gastric resection. This serious condition is considered with stress ulcers, since many similarities exist between the two. Destruction of the gastric mucosal barrier is believed to be the pathogenic mechanism responsible for the injury and is considered later.

In superficial gastritis the mucosa is reddened and edematous and covered with adherent mucus; small erosions and hemorrhages are common. The degree of inflammation is highly variable.

Clinical manifestations of acute gastritis may range from vague abdominal complaints, such as anorexia, eructation (belching), or nausea, to more severe symptoms, such as epigastric pain, vomiting, bleeding, and hematemesis. In some patients, when symptoms are prolonged and resistant to treatment, additional diagnostic measures, such as endoscopy, mucosal biopsy, and gastric analysis, may be needed to clarify the diagnosis.

Acute superficial gastritis usually resolves when the offending agent is removed. Antiemetic drugs may help relieve the nausea and vomiting. If vomiting persists, it may be necessary to correct fluid and electrolyte imbalances with intravenous (IV) infusions. The use of H_2 blockers (e.g., ranitidine) to decrease acid secretion, antacids to neutralize secreted acid, and sucralfate to coat inflamed or ulcerated areas may facilitate healing.

Chronic Atrophic Gastritis

Chronic atrophic gastritis is characterized by progressive atrophy of the glandular epithelium with loss of parietal and chief cells. Consequently, there is decreased production of HCl, pepsin, and intrinsic factor. The gastric wall becomes thin, and the mucosa has an unusually smooth surface. This form of gastritis is frequently seen in association with pernicious anemia, gastric ulcer, and cancer.

Chronic atrophic gastritis is now thought to be caused primarily by *H. pylori*. It occurs more often in elderly persons. Heavy alcohol intake, hot tea, and smoking may predispose to the development of atrophic gastritis.

In the case of pernicious anemia the pathogenesis may be related to a disturbance of immunologic mechanisms. Most of these patients have circulating antibodies against parietal cells and, more specifically, have antibodies to intrinsic factor as well.

Chronic atrophic gastritis may predispose the patient to the development of gastric ulcers and carcinoma. The incidence of gastric cancer is particularly high in patients with pernicious anemia (10% to 15%).

Symptoms of chronic gastritis are generally varied and vague; they may include a feeling of fullness, anorexia, and vague epigastric distress. The diagnosis is suspected when the patient has achlorhydria or a low BAO or MAO, and the diagnosis is confirmed by the typical histologic changes on biopsy.

The treatment of chronic atrophic gastritis varies, depending on the suspected cause of the disorder. If duodenal ulcer lesions are present, antibiotics may be given to eliminate *H. pylori*. However, lesions are not typically present with chronic gastritis. Alcohol and drugs known to irritate the gastric mucosa are avoided. Iron deficiency anemia (caused by chronic bleeding), if present, is corrected. Vitamin B_{12} and other appropriate therapy are given in the case of pernicious anemia.

PEPTIC ULCER DISEASE

Peptic ulcers are circumscribed breaks in the continuity of mucosa, extending below the epithelium. Strictly speaking, breaks in the mucosa not extending below the epithelium are called *erosions*, although they are often referred to as "ulcers" (e.g., stress ulcers). *Chronic ulcers*, as opposed to acute ulcers, have scar tissue at the base (Fig. 24-4).

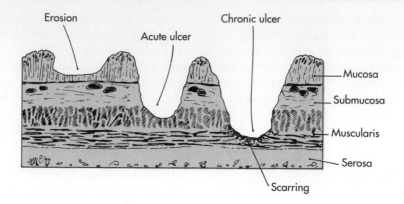

FIG. 24-4   Peptic ulcers, illustrating an erosion, an acute ulcer, and a chronic ulcer. Acute and chronic ulcers may penetrate the entire wall of the stomach.

▶ **TABLE 24-2**   Differentiating Features of Duodenal, Gastric, and Stress Ulcers

	Duodenal Ulcer	Gastric Ulcer	Stress Ulcer
Incidence	Peak age: 40 years Duodenal/gastric ulcer: 4:1 Prevalence: 10% of population Men/women: 1:1	Peak age: 50-60 years Men/women: 2.5:1 Lifetime prevalence: 10%	Related to severe stress, trauma, sepsis, burns, head injuries No gender difference
Pathogenesis	Hyperacidity important factor Gastric colonization with *Helicobacter pylori* reported in 90%-95% of patients Associated diseases: hyperparathyroidism, chronic pulmonary disease, chronic pancreatitis, alcoholic cirrhosis Ulcerogenic drugs, alcohol, tobacco Blood group O: higher frequency Psychosocial stress and chronic anxiety possible factors in exacerbations	Disruption of mucosal barrier seems important factor Normal to low HCl production Presence of *H. pylori* gastritis Ulcerogenic drugs, alcohol, tobacco Chronic bile reflux Not related to blood group More common in laboring groups Familial predisposition	Head injuries: hypersecretion of HCl All others: ischemia of gastric mucosa, disruption of mucosal barrier, back diffusion of HCl, acute gastritis Hemorrhagic gastric erosions possibly drug induced; alcohol and aspirin most common offenders
Pathology	90% in duodenal bulb	90% in antrum and lesser curvature	Usually multiple, diffuse erosions; more often located in stomach, especially fundus
Complications	About 10% of patients; most respond to medical therapy	More common than with duodenal ulcer	
Hemorrhage	Common in posterior wall of duodenal bulb	25% occurrence	Most frequent complication; high mortality
Perforation	More common when located in anterior wall of duodenum	More common in anterior wall of stomach	Common
Obstruction	Common	Rare	
Malignancy	Almost never	Incidence about 4%	
Clinical features	Pain-food-relief pattern of pain Patient usually well nourished Seasonal exacerbations Night pain possible	Food-pain pattern of pain Anorexia, weight loss common Night pain possible	May be asymptomatic until serious complication such as hemorrhage or perforation

By definition, peptic ulcers can be located in any part of the GI tract exposed to the acid-pepsin gastric juice, including the esophagus, stomach, duodenum, and after gastroenterostomy, the jejunum. Although the peptic digestive activity of gastric juice is an important etiologic factor, evidence indicates that many factors are important in the pathogenesis of peptic ulcer disease, including *Helicobacter pylori* gastritis, mucosal bicarbonate secretions, genetic characteristics, and stress. Because many similarities and differences exist between gastric and duodenal ulcers, some aspects of these two entities are considered together for convenience, and special problems relating to each are discussed separately. Gastric erosions or stress ulcers are considered last. Table 24-2 lists some of the differences between the various types of peptic ulcers.

Pathogenesis

Because pure acid gastric juice is capable of digesting all living tissues, one of the major questions is, "Why doesn't the stomach digest itself?" Two factors seem to protect the stomach from autodigestion: the gastric mucus and the epithelial barrier.

Gastric mucosal barrier

According to Hollander's *two-component mucus barrier* theory, the thick, tenacious layer of gastric mucus constitutes the first line of defense against autodigestion. It provides protection against mechanical trauma and chemical agents. NSAIDs, including aspirin, produce qualitative changes in the gastric mucus that may facilitate its degradation by pepsin. Prostaglandins are present in abundant quantities in the gastric mucus and appear to play an important role in gastric mucosal defense.

Davenport (1978) emphasized the importance of a gastric mucosal barrier. Although the exact nature of this barrier is not understood, it probably involves the mucous lining, the lumen of the columnar epithelial cells, and the tight junctions at the apices of these cells. Normally this mucosal barrier allows very little back diffusion of H^+ from the lumen to the blood, even though there is a large concentration gradient (gastric acid with a pH of 1.0 versus blood with a pH of 7.4).

Destruction of gastric mucosal barrier

Aspirin, alcohol, bile salts, and other substances injurious to the gastric mucosa alter the permeability of the epithelial barrier, which allows back diffusion of HCl with resultant injury to underlying tissues, especially blood vessels (Fig. 24-5). Histamine is liberated, which stimulates further acid and pepsin secretion and increased capillary permeability to proteins. The mucosa becomes edematous, and large amounts of plasma proteins may be lost. The mucosal capillaries may be damaged, resulting in interstitial hemorrhage and bleeding. The mucosal barrier is unaffected by vagal inhibition or atropine, but back diffusion is inhibited by gastrin.

Destruction of the gastric mucosal barrier is believed to be an important factor in the pathogenesis of gastric ulcers. It is known that the antral mucosa is more susceptible to back diffusion than that of the fundus, which explains why gastric ulcers are often located in the antrum. It has also been suggested that the low level of acid recovered in gastric analysis of patients with gastric ulcer is caused by increased back diffusion, not lower production. This pathogenic mechanism may also be important in patients with acute hemorrhagic gastritis caused by alcohol, aspirin, and severe stress.

The resistance of the duodenum to peptic ulceration is believed to be a function of *Brunner's glands* (submucosal duodenal glands in the intestinal wall), which produce a highly alkaline, viscid, mucoid secretion that neutralizes the acid chyme. Patients with duodenal ulcers often have excessive acid secretion, which seems to be the most important pathogenic factor. The normal mucosal defense mechanisms may be overwhelmed. The factor of decreased tissue resistance is implicated in both gastric and duodenal ulcers, although it seems to be more important in gastric ulcers.

In addition to the mucosal and epithelial barriers, tissue resistance also depends on an abundant vascular supply and continued, rapid regeneration of epithelial cells (normally replaced every 3 days). Failure of this mechanism may also play a role in the pathogenesis of peptic ulcer.

Other factors

Although the incidence of duodenal ulcers is decreasing, currently about 500,000 new cases occur each year, with 10% to 12% of the population affected. Duodenal ulcers generally occur in a much younger age-group than do gastric ulcers. The lower incidence of peptic ulcers in women seems to indicate a gender-linked influence.

It has been suggested that certain drugs, such as aspirin, alcohol, indomethacin, phenylbutazone, and corticosteroids, may have a direct irritating effect on the gastric mucosa and produce ulceration. If they do have an effect, it may be caused by a disruption of one of the protective barriers in the stomach. Other drugs, such as caffeine, increase acid production. Emotional stress has long been thought to have a role in ulcer development, although recent studies show that it is not more stress but rather how patients with ulcers perceive their "stressful" life events. Emotional conflict for these patients is often perceived more negatively and precedes the disease by many months or years. Exposure to these stressful life events leads to ulcer development through the repeated stimulation of acid and pepsin secretion and decreased mucosal defense.

Most peptic ulcers occur "downstream" from the source of acid secretion. More than 90% of duodenal ul-

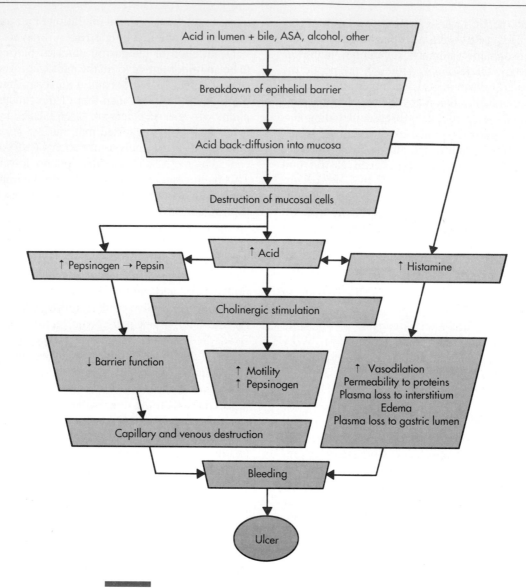

FIG. 24-5 Pathophysiologic consequences of back diffusion of acid through the damaged mucosal barrier.

cers are located on the anterior or posterior wall of the first part of the duodenum, within 3 cm of the pyloric ring. Although gastric ulcers may occur anywhere in the stomach, 90% are situated along the lesser curvature and in the pyloric gland region.

Approximately 40% to 60% of patients with ulcers have a family history of ulcer disease. Individuals with certain blood groups (e.g., group O) also seem to be more susceptible to duodenal ulcers.

A number of diseases seem to be associated with peptic ulcer formation, including alcoholic liver cirrhosis, chronic pancreatitis, chronic lung disease, hyperparathyroidism, and Zollinger-Ellison syndrome.

Abnormal pyloric sphincter function resulting in bile reflux has been proposed as a pathogenic mechanism in the development of gastric ulcer. The bile disrupts the gastric mucosal barrier, causing gastritis and increased susceptibility to ulcer formation. The damaged mucosa is ultimately eroded and digested by the action of acid and pepsin.

Clinical Features

The principal clinical feature of peptic ulcer is chronic, intermittent epigastric pain typically relieved by food or antacids. Pain usually occurs 2 or 3 hours after a meal or at night when the stomach is empty. Peptic ulcer pain is often described as gnawing, burning, or nagging in nature. About one fourth of patients with ulcers experience bleeding, although it is more common with duodenal ulcer. Signs and symptoms may also include vomiting, red or "coffee-ground" emesis, nausea, anorexia, and weight loss. Persistent upper abdominal pain is rarely a symptom of peptic ulcers; exacerbation and remissions are more

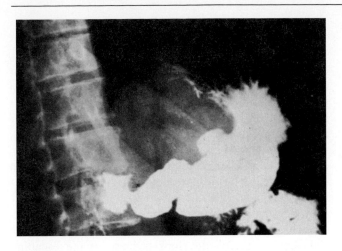

FIG. 24-6   Barium radiographic appearance of gastric ulcer. Note the large, nodular-shaped protrusion on the lesser curvature of the stomach.

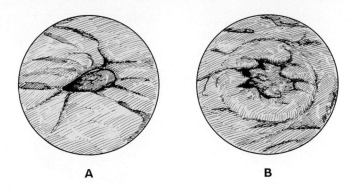

A   **B**

FIG. 24-7   Gastroscopic appearance of, **A,** a benign gastric ulcer and, **B,** a malignant gastric ulcer (carcinoma). The benign ulcer has a sharp, well-defined margin. The malignant ulcer has an irregular margin that fades into the surrounding tumor mass.

characteristic of peptic ulcers. The pain-food-relief pattern may not be typical with gastric ulcers. In fact, with gastric ulcers, food sometimes aggravates the pain.

Diagnosis

The most important criterion in the diagnosis of duodenal ulcer is a history of the typical *pain-food-relief pattern.* The history is not as informative in patients with gastric ulcer, since vague symptoms of epigastric distress occur more often. Usually it is not possible to distinguish between gastric and duodenal ulcers on the basis of history alone.

The diagnosis of peptic ulcer is usually confirmed by barium meal radiography (Fig. 24-6). When barium radiography fails to reveal an ulcer in the stomach or duodenum but characteristic symptoms persist, endoscopic examination is indicated. Serum gastrin levels may be assayed if Zollinger-Ellison syndrome is suspected.

Benign versus malignant ulcers

Although duodenal ulcers are almost never malignant, about 4% of gastric ulcers turn out to be carcinoma of the stomach. It is therefore important for the gastroenterologist to differentiate between a benign and a malignant gastric ulcer. In general, malignant ulcers have a shaggy, necrotic base, whereas benign ulcers have a smooth, clean base with a distinct margin (Fig. 24-7). Biopsy and cytologic studies are also helpful in distinguishing a benign from a malignant ulcer.

Medical Treatment

The primary objective in the medical treatment of peptic ulcer is to inhibit or buffer acid secretions to relieve symptoms and promote healing. Measures that achieve these ends are antacids, dietary management, anticholin-

ergics, H₂ blockers (cimetidine, ranitidine, famotidine), antimicrobial therapy, and physical and emotional rest.

Antacids are given to neutralize the acid gastric contents by keeping the pH high enough so that pepsin is not activated, thus protecting the mucosa and relieving the pain. The most widely used antacid preparations are mixtures of aluminum hydroxide and magnesium hydroxide. Small, frequent meals are also important in neutralizing the gastric contents. Stimulants of acid secretion, such as alcohol and caffeine, are avoided. Anticholinergic drugs, such as propantheline bromide (Pro-Banthine) and atropine (from *Atropa belladonna*), inhibit the direct effect of the vagus nerve on the acid-secreting parietal cells. Anticholinergics also inhibit gastric motility and emptying time, and therefore many physicians do not prescribe this type of drug for patients with gastric ulcers. H₂ blockers have rapidly become the most common drugs used to treat duodenal ulcers because of their ability to reduce acid secretion by 70%. Another drug, sucralfate, not only forms an acid-impermeable membrane that adheres to injured mucosa, but also accelerates mucosal cell production (a cytoprotective effect).

Physical and emotional rest are promoted by providing a quiet environment, listening to the patient's problems, and offering emotional support. Small doses of sedatives may be prescribed.

About 80% to 90% of patients with duodenal ulcer have a benign course interrupted by the necessity for medical therapy. An unknown number of patients undoubtedly treat themselves successfully with diet and antacids available without a prescription. The response of gastric ulcers to traditional medical therapy (diet and antacids) is not quite as successful, but using the newer histamine receptor antagonists for 12 weeks results in healing of 80% to 90% of gastric ulcers. Close monitoring of progress is required because drugs may relieve the symptoms of malignant gastric ulcers, thus masking the symptoms that lead to a diagnosis. Ulcers caused by *H. pylori* have been treated with some success through a combination of ther-

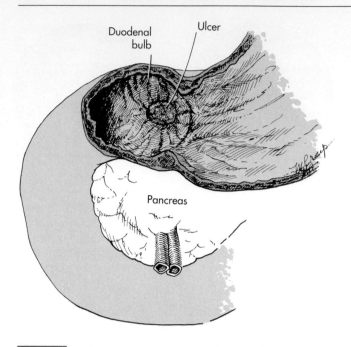

FIG. 24-8 Duodenal ulcer of the posterior wall, penetrating into the head of the pancreas and resulting in a walled-off perforation.

apies using bismuth salts, antimicrobial agents, and H_2 blockers (Hosking et al, 1994). Eradication rates of 65% to 98% have been reported (de Boer, 1995).

Complications

Complications of peptic ulcer disease include hemorrhage, perforation, pyloric obstruction, and intractability. Any of these complications is an indication for surgical treatment.

Hemorrhage

Bleeding is the most frequent complication of peptic ulcer and occurs in 15% to 20% of patients at some time during the course of the disease. Although ulcers in any site may bleed, the most common site of hemorrhage is in the posterior wall of the duodenal bulb, since erosion into the pancreaticoduodenal or gastroduodenal artery may occur in that location.

The symptoms associated with bleeding ulcer depend on the rapidity of blood loss. Mild, chronic blood loss may lead to iron deficiency anemia. The stools may be positive for occult blood (positive guaiac test) or may be black and tarry (melena). Massive bleeding may lead to *hematemesis* (vomiting blood) and the development of shock and may require blood transfusions and emergency surgery. Relief of pain often follows bleeding as a result of the buffering effect of blood. The mortality in these patients ranges up to 10%, with patients over age 50 years having a higher mortality rate. This represents about 20% to 25% of the total deaths attributable to ulcer disease.

Perforation

Approximately 5% of all ulcers perforate, and this complication accounts for about 65% of deaths from peptic ulcer disease (see Fig. 4-11). The ulcers are usually on the anterior wall of the duodenum or stomach. The primary cause of perforation is thought to be excess acid secretion and often is a result of ingestion of NSAIDS, which deplete the cells of adenosine triphosphate (ATP), rendering them vulnerable to oxidant stress. This delayed cellular repair leads to perforation.

Most patients with perforation present in a characteristically dramatic fashion. There is a sudden onset of excruciating pain in the upper abdomen. Within minutes a chemical peritonitis develops because of the escaping gastric acid, pepsin, and food, and this causes intense pain. The patient fears to move or breathe. The abdomen becomes silent to auscultation and assumes a boardlike rigidity to palpation. Acute perforation can usually be diagnosed on the basis of the symptoms alone. The diagnosis is confirmed by the presence of free gas within the peritoneal cavity, presenting as a translucent crescent between the liver and diaphragm shadows; the air has entered the peritoneal cavity through the perforated ulcer. The treatment is immediate surgery with gastric resection or simple suture of the perforation, depending on the patient's condition.

Occasionally a gastric or duodenal ulcer breaks through the wall but remains sealed off by a contiguous structure and is called a *penetrating ulcer.* A classic example of a penetrating ulcer is a duodenal ulcer of the posterior wall that penetrates into the pancreas and is walled off (Fig. 24-8). Clinically, the pain becomes intractable and may radiate to the back. The patient may present with pancreatitis.

Obstruction

Obstruction of the gastric outlet as a result of inflammation and edema, pylorospasm, or scarring occurs in about 5% of patients with peptic ulcer. It occurs more often in patients with duodenal ulcer but occasionally occurs when a gastric ulcer is located close to the pyloric sphincter.

Anorexia, nausea, and bloating after eating are common symptoms; weight loss often results. When the obstruction becomes severe, pain and vomiting may occur.

Treatment is directed toward restoring fluids and electrolytes, decompressing the stomach by insertion of a nasogastric tube, and surgically correcting the obstruction (pyloroplasty).

Intractability

Another complication of peptic ulcer is intractability, which simply means that medical therapy fails to control the symptoms adequately, resulting in frequent, rapid recurrences. Patients may have their sleep interrupted by pain, lose time from work, require frequent hospitalization, or just be unable to follow a medical regimen. Surgery is typically recommended for intractability. Malignant transformation is not an important consideration in either gastric or duodenal ulcer. About 4% of gastric ulcers that start out benign are later diagnosed as malignant.

Surgical Treatment

Patients who do not respond to medical therapy or who develop other complications such as perforation, hemorrhage, or obstruction are treated surgically by one of two procedures, vagotomy or gastrectomy, or sometimes by both. Many variations of these two procedures exist, and the type of surgery elected depends on many factors, including the nature of the pathology and the patient's age and general condition.

The common aim in the surgical treatment of duodenal ulcers is to reduce permanently the stomach's capacity to secrete acid and pepsin. This can be achieved in at least four ways:

1. *Vagotomy* is the division of the vagus nerve branches to the stomach, thus eliminating the cephalic phase of gastric secretion. *Conventional truncal vagotomy* not only diminishes gastric secretions, but also decreases gastric motility and emptying. Consequently a "drainage" procedure is required to prevent gastric retention—either a gastrojejunostomy or pyloroplasty. Truncal vagotomy also denervates the hepatobiliary tract, pancreas, small intestine, and proximal colon. Two other types of vagotomy, selective and superselective, are being used with increasing frequency. With *selective vagotomy,* only the branches of the vagus nerve that supply the stomach are transected, resulting in more complete vagotomy, less ulcer recurrence, and fewer postvagotomy complications. Because the antrum and pylorus are denervated, a drainage procedure is still required. *Superselective* or *parietal cell vagotomy* denervates only the acid-secreting portion of the stomach, sparing the branches that supply the antrum, which makes a gastric drainage procedure (e.g., pyloroplasty) unnecessary. More recently the posterior truncal vagotomy and anterior lesser curve *seromyotomy* have come into use as a surgical treatment for chronic duodenal ulcer. The procedure results in denervation of the entire lesser curvature of the stomach while reducing acid secretion rates with no alteration in gastric emptying. This procedure is also gaining popularity because it can be performed using laparoscopic technique, making this surgery a minimally invasive procedure.

2. *Antrectomy* is the removal of the entire antrum of the stomach, thus eliminating the hormonal or gastric phase of gastric secretion.

3. *Vagotomy plus antrectomy* eliminates both the cephalic and the gastric phases of gastric secretion. Thus neural stimulation is interrupted, drainage is enhanced, and the major site of gastrin production is removed. It is thought to be superior to some of the more extensive surgical procedures.

4. *Partial gastrectomy* is the removal of the distal 50% to 75% of the stomach, thus removing a substantial portion of the acid-secreting and pepsin-secreting mucosa. After gastric resection, GI continuity may be restored by anastomosing the gastric remnant to the duodenum (*gastroduodenostomy,* or *Billroth I procedure*) or to the jejunum (*gastrojejunostomy,* or *Billroth II procedure*).

Fig. 24-9 illustrates some of the common surgical procedures for treating peptic ulcers.

Most surgeons treat gastric ulcer by partial gastrectomy and a gastroduodenal anastomosis. The line of resection is usually proximal to the gastric ulcer. A vagotomy usually is not performed, since these patients have normal to low gastric acid production.

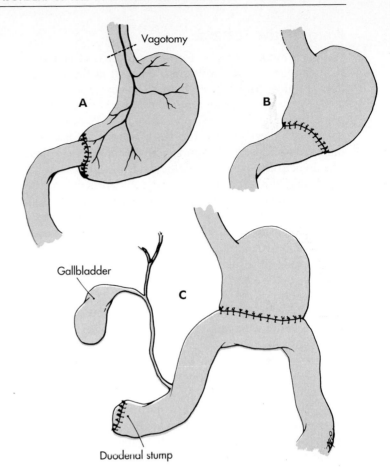

FIG. 24-9   Common surgical procedures for treating peptic ulcers. **A,** Vagotomy plus antrectomy (removal of pyloric antrum). **B,** Billroth I procedure (gastroduodenostomy anastomosis after resection). **C,** Billroth II procedure (gastrojejunostomy anastomosis after resection).

Postoperative Sequelae

Although modern surgery for peptic ulcer is effective in the treatment of ulcer complications and in the prevention of ulcer recurrence, numerous postoperative sequelae may occur. *Dumping syndrome* is a complication that occurs after eating in approximately 20% of patients after peptic ulcer surgery. It is believed to result from the rapid emptying of hyperosmotic chyme into the intestine. The hypertonic contents of the intestine then cause a rapid fluid shift from the vascular compartment into the intestinal lumen. The decrease in plasma volume results in hypotension, which causes dizziness and weakness. The hypotension initiates reflex tachycardia, diaphoresis, and vasoconstriction of the skin, resulting in pallor. Feelings of fullness, nausea, vomiting, and diarrhea are common. Symptoms usually occur during or within minutes after a meal.

Hypoglycemia may occur within 2 to 3 hours after eating as a result of increased insulin secretion in response to eating soups, fluids, or high-carbohydrate meals. The hyperosmolar material in the proximal intestine causes excessive release of enteroglucagon, which sensitizes the beta cells of the pancreatic islets so that they release large amounts of insulin. This, in turn, overcorrects the hyperglycemia, resulting in hypoglycemia and related symptoms. Treatment consists of eating frequent, small meals that are low in carbohydrate and high in protein and restricting liquids at mealtimes. Restricting fluids at mealtimes delays the emptying time of stomach contents into the small intestine. The stomach empties more rapidly after gastric resection because of decreased acid-secreting activity. For patients who have had gastric surgery, gastric emptying and limiting the hyperosmolarity of food intake are ongoing problems that often correct themselves over time. Antimuscarinic medications have been used for patients who fail to benefit from diet therapy.

Other sequelae after peptic ulcer surgery include recurrent ulcer caused by incomplete vagotomy or incomplete antrectomy; bile reflux gastritis; diarrhea, especially after truncal vagotomy; megaloblastic anemia caused by vitamin B_{12} malabsorption; osteomalacia and osteoporosis caused by malabsorption of calcium and vitamin D; general malabsorption and weight loss; and increased incidence of stomach cancer.

Acute Stress-Induced and Drug-Induced Ulcers

The term *stress ulcer* has been used to describe gastric or duodenal erosions that occur as a sequela to prolonged psychologic or physiologic stress. The stress may take many forms, such as hypotensive shock after traumatic injury and major surgery, sepsis, hypoxia, severe burns (Curling's ulcers), or cerebral trauma (Cushing's ulcers). Any seriously ill patient in an intensive care setting is susceptible to the development of a stress ulcer. Acute erosive and hemorrhagic gastritis induced by an alcoholic bout, aspirin or other ulcerogenic drugs, and bile reflux are often grouped with stress ulcers, since the lesions are similar.

Acute stress ulcers are usually shallow, irregular, punched-out lesions that may be large and multiple and often are located in the stomach. The lesions may bleed slowly, causing melena, and often are asymptomatic or are overshadowed by the serious illness in the patient. Because these lesions are superficial, they are not usually evident on radiographic examination.

Stress ulcers are clinically apparent when there is massive gastric hemorrhage or perforation. In fact, stress ulcers account for 5% of all cases of peptic ulcer bleeding. Massive bleeding resulting from alcohol-induced acute erosive gastritis is also a common problem.

Pathogenesis

Stress ulcers are generally divided into two different groups, based on probable pathogenic mechanisms. *Cushing's ulcers* associated with serious brain injury are characterized by marked hyperacidity, which is possibly mediated by vagal stimulation (cerebral injury → vagal stimulation → hyperacidity → acute peptic ulcer).

On the other hand, stress ulcers associated with *shock, sepsis, burns,* and *drugs* are not characterized by gastric acid hypersecretion. Studies have suggested that disruption of the mucosal barrier function of the stomach, especially in the presence of ischemia resulting from poor vascular perfusion, may be important in the pathogenesis (Fig. 24-10).

Treatment

Recent studies reveal that the presence of erosive gastritis (stress ulcers) is a common finding in critically ill patients. About 80% of severely burned patients have evidence of occult blood in their stools. Other studies have revealed an even higher incidence of stress ulcers identified by gastroscopy in critically ill patients. Most of these patients do not have symptoms until there is massive bleeding, which occurs in about 5%. This has led to the prophylactic treatment of high-risk patients with H_2 blockers or antacids. The other 95% heal with little or no residual effects.

When bleeding is serious, some patients have been treated successfully by continuous intraarterial perfusion with vasopressin, a powerful vasoconstrictor. Vasopressin infusion is accomplished by inserting a catheter into an artery supplying the bleeding site and thereby controlling arterial bleeding. Vasopressin may also be infused into a peripheral vein to control bleeding from varices. The bleeding site is identified by arteriography, after which a vasopressin infusion is started. Thermal devices have been tested and are being used for hemostasis. Methods using these coagulation devices include electrocoagulation and photocoagulation (laser coagulation).

When these conservative methods of treatment fail,

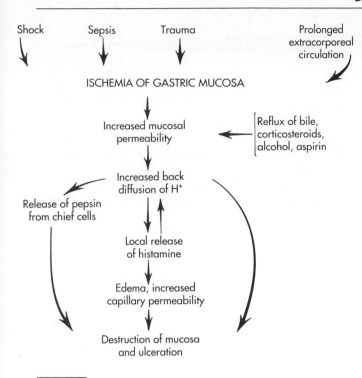

Shock   Sepsis   Trauma   Prolonged extracorporeal circulation

ISCHEMIA OF GASTRIC MUCOSA

Increased mucosal permeability ← Reflux of bile, corticosteroids, alcohol, aspirin

Increased back diffusion of H⁺

Release of pepsin from chief cells

Local release of histamine

Edema, increased capillary permeability

Destruction of mucosa and ulceration

FIG. 24-10   Pathogenesis of "stress" ulcers. (Modified from Silen W, Skillman JJ: *Advances in internal medicine,* Vol 19, Chicago, 1974, Mosby.)

surgery may be the only method of treatment, even though these patients are critically ill and poor surgical risks. The most effective surgical procedure is total gastrectomy, since these erosions are multiple or diffuse and tend to rebleed.

STOMACH CANCER

Carcinoma of the stomach is the third most common form of GI neoplasm and accounts for about 2.7% of all cancer deaths (American Cancer Society, 1995). Men are more frequently affected, and most cases occur after age 40.

The cause of stomach cancer is unknown, but certain predisposing factors are recognized. Genetic factors seem to be important, since gastric cancer is more common in persons with blood group A. Geographic or environmental factors also appear to be important, since gastric cancer is common in Japan, China, Thailand, Finland, Ireland, and Columbia. For unknown reasons, gastric cancer has been declining in the United States during the past 60 years. It occurs more often in lower socioeconomic

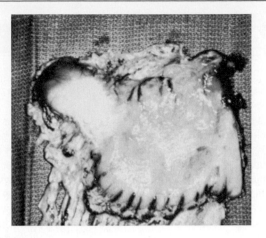

FIG. 24-11   Surgical specimen of gastric infiltrative carcinoma. The entire wall is cartilaginous and stiff.

groups. One of the most important predisposing factors is the presence of atrophic gastritis or pernicious anemia, as previously discussed. *Helicobacter pylori* infection is becoming more accepted as a factor in chronic atrophic gastritis and, in turn, is being associated with the increased risk of gastric cancer.

About 50% of gastric cancers are located in the pyloric antrum. The remainder of the lesions are distributed throughout the body of the stomach.

There are three general forms of gastric carcinoma. *Ulcerating carcinoma* is the most common type and must be differentiated from a benign gastric ulcer. *Polypoid carcinoma* appears as a cauliflower-like mass protruding into the lumen and may arise from an adenomatous polyp. *Infiltrating carcinoma* may penetrate the entire thickness of the stomach wall and is responsible for the inflexible "leather bottle stomach" *(linitis plastica)* (Fig. 24-11).

Carcinoma of the stomach is seldom diagnosed in an early stage because symptoms develop late or are vague and indefinite. Early symptoms may include a mild feeling of discomfort in the upper abdomen or a feeling of fullness after eating. Eventually the patient has anorexia and weight loss. When the tumor is located near the cardia, dysphagia may be the first major symptom. Vomiting from pyloric obstruction may occur when the tumor is near the gastric outlet.

Radiologic studies, exfoliative cytology, and endoscopy with biopsy are all important methods in the diagnosis of gastric cancer. Surgical excision is the only effective therapy. Because of the usually late diagnosis, the prognosis is poor, with a 10% 5-year survival rate..

QUESTIONS

▼ *Answer the following on a separate sheet of paper.*

1. Sketch the stomach and indicate the location of the following: fundus, body, pyloric antrum, pyloric sphincter, cardiac region, lesser curvature, greater curvature and glands secreting HCl and pepsin, intrinsic factor, and gastrin.
2. What are the lesser and greater omenta? Where are they located?
3. What are rugae and what is their purpose in the stomach?
4. How is pepsinogen activated in the stomach? What is the action of pepsin?
5. Describe the extrinsic and intrinsic innervation of the stomach and the function of each.
6. Name the truncal artery and its major branches supplying the stomach.
7. Why is hemorrhage a more frequent complication in duodenal ulcers of the posterior wall?
8. List three motor functions of the stomach.
9. What is the normal capacity of the adult stomach? What prevents an increase in intragastric pressure during a moderate-sized meal?
10. Why do patients become anemic when there is a deficiency or absence of intrinsic factor?
11. What controls the mixing and emptying activities of the stomach?
12. What prevents the stomach from digesting itself? Explain your answer using the theories of gastric mucosal defense formulated by Hollander and Davenport. What drugs or chemicals may alter mucosal defense? What protects the duodenum from the actions of acid and pepsin?
13. List five effects of gastrin and the physiologic significance of each.
14. What is acute superficial gastritis? Do you think you have ever had this condition? What are the symptoms?
15. Explain how gastric secretions are controlled during the three phases of gastric secretion.

▼ *Circle the letter preceding each item below that correctly answers the question or completes the statement. Only one answer is correct unless otherwise noted.*

16. Gastrin is a hormone produced by the:
    a. Pancreas
    b. Brunner's glands
    c. Duodenum

d. Gastric antrum
e. Gastric fundus

17. Which of the following agents have been associated with an increased incidence of ulcer disease (more than one answer may be correct)?
    a. Aspirin
    b. Ethyl alcohol
    c. High doses of corticosteroids
    d. Phenylbutazone
18. Achlorhydria or hypochlorhydria is often seen in (more than one answer may be correct):
    a. Pernicious anemia
    b. Zollinger-Ellison syndrome
    c. Atrophic gastritis
    d. Carcinoma of the stomach
19. Which of the following is known to cause an elaboration of gastrin from the gastric antrum (more than one answer may be correct)?
    a. Distention of the antrum
    b. Alkalinization of the antrum
    c. Acidification of the antrum
    d. Distention of the fundus
    e. Stimulation of the vagus
20. Which of the following phases accounts for the largest volume of gastric acid secretion?
    a. Cephalic
    b. Gastric
    c. Intestinal
    d. Interdigestive
21. The enterogastric reflex (more than one answer may be correct):
    a. Is mediated via the myenteric nerve plexus
    b. Stimulates gastric emptying
    c. Inhibits gastric emptying
    d. Inhibits gastric secretion
22. The gastric secretory pattern in duodenal ulcer is usually in which range?
    a. Achlorhydria
    b. Normal to low
    c. Normal to high
    d. Marked hyperacidity
23. Which of the following foods has the greatest acid secretory effect?
    a. Proteins
    b. Fats
    c. Carbohydrates
24. Theories regarding the pathogenesis of gastric ulcers include (more than one answer may be correct):
    a. Overactivity of the vagus
    b. Hypersecretion of acid
    c. Impaired mucosal resistance
    d. Reflux of bile into the stomach

25. Duodenal ulcer disease is:
    a. More common in women than in men
    b. Always responsive to medical treatment
    c. Common, affecting more than 10% of the population
    d. Associated with blood group A
26. When bleeding complicates peptic ulcer disease, pain:
    a. No longer responds to antacids
    b. Radiates to the back
    c. Becomes more severe
    d. Usually disappears
27. Signs, symptoms, and findings indicating acute perforation of a peptic ulcer include (more than one answer may be correct):
    a. Boardlike rigidity of abdomen to palpation
    b. Relief from pain
    c. Severe pain in upper abdomen
    d. Subphrenic air bubble evident radiographically
28. Which of the following contiguous structures would most likely be involved in a confined perforation of a peptic ulcer?
    a. Liver
    b. Gallbladder
    c. Pancreas
    d. Lesser omentum
29. Recurrent ulcer after peptic ulcer surgery (more than one answer may be correct):
    a. Is related to the preoperative level of gastric acid secretion
    b. Occurs most often after gastric ulcer
    c. Is less common if vagotomy is performed
30. Which of the following statements applies to the surgical treatment of duodenal ulcer?
    a. Billroth I procedure is the surgery of choice.
    b. Billroth II procedure is the surgery of choice.
    c. A vagotomy and 75% gastric resection should be performed.
    d. Some form of vagotomy should be performed.
31. Which of the following mechanisms would be the most probable to explain the development of stress ulcers in a patient who developed hypotensive shock after cardiac surgery?
    a. Excess vagal stimulation hyperacidity

QUESTIONS—cont'd

b. Gastric ischemia
c. Disruption of gastric mucosal barrier
d. Increased back diffusion of HCl

32. Carcinoma of the stomach (more than one answer may be correct):
   a. Is most frequent after age 40
   b. Is more common in persons with pernicious anemia
   c. Generally has a good prognosis
   d. Most often presents as an ulcerative lesion
   e. May infiltrate the stomach wall, causing it to become inflexible

33. Methods of treating acute hemorrhagic gastritis include:
   a. Electrocoagulation
   b. Local intraarterial vasopressin infusion
   c. Laser coagulation
   d. Total gastrectomy
   e. All the above

34. Signs and symptoms that precede vomiting indicating autonomic nervous system discharge include:
   a. Nausea
   b. Increased rate
   c. Increased salivation
   d. Retching
   e. All of the above

35. Helicobacter pylori infection has been implicated in the etiology of:
   a. Acute gastritis
   b. Chronic gastritis
   c. Gastric ulcers
   d. Crohn's disease

▼ *Circle T if the statement is true and F if it is false. Correct any false statements.*

36. T F The chief cells of the stomach secrete HCl.

37. T F The neck cells of the gastric glands secrete mucus.

38. T F Chronic ulcers, as opposed to acute ulcers, have scar tissue at their base.

39. T F A break in the gastric mucosa that does not extend beyond the mucosal layer is called an erosion.

40. T F Prostaglandins are believed to play an important role in gastric mucosal defense.

41. T F *Helicobacter pylori* is thought to be a primary cause of gastritis and gastric ulceration.

▼ *Match the following gastric acid analysis tests in column A with their diagnostic value in column B.*

Column A	Column B
42. _____ Basal acid output (BAO)	a. Especially useful in the diagnosis of Zollinger-Ellison syndrome
43. _____ Maximum acid output (MAO)	b. May be used to determine if true achlorhydria is present

▼ *Match the following differentiating features of gastric and duodenal ulcers in column B with the type of peptic ulcer in column A.*

Column A	Column B
44. _____ Gastric ulcer	a. Symptomatic improvement with antacids
45. _____ Duodenal ulcer	b. Nocturnal pain possible
	c. Always should be treated surgically
	d. Obstruction an infrequent problem
	e. More common in persons with blood type O
	f. Higher frequency in persons subjected to stress

CHAPTER 25

Disorders of the Small Intestine

LORRAINE M. WILSON
GLENDA N. LINDSETH

ANATOMY

The small intestine is a complex, folded tube extending from the pylorus to the ileocecal valve. It is about 12 feet (3.6 m) long in life (almost 22 feet (6.6 m) in the cadaver as a result of relaxation) and is contained in the central and lower part of the abdominal cavity. The proximal end is about 1½ inches (3.8 cm) in diameter, but the diameter gradually diminishes to about 1 inch (2.5 cm) at the lower end.

The small intestine is divided into the duodenum, jejunum, and ileum. This division is rather imprecise and is based on slight modifications in structure and relatively more important differences in function. The *duodenum* is about 25 cm long and extends from the pylorus to the jejunum. The division between the duodenum and jejunum is marked by the *ligament of Treitz,* a musculofibrous band that originates from the right crus of the diaphragm near the esophageal hiatus and attaches to the junction of the duodenum and jejunum, acting as a suspensory ligament. Approximately two fifths of the remaining intestine is the jejunum, and the terminal three fifths is the ileum. The *jejunum* lies in the left midabdominal region, and the *ileum* tends to lie in the right lower abdominal region. Entry of chyme into the small intestine is controlled by the *pyloric sphincter,* and exit of digested materials into the large intestine is controlled by the *ileocecal valve.* The ileocecal valve also prevents reflux of contents of the large intestine into the small intestine.

The *vermiform appendix* is a blind tube about the size of the little finger located in the ileocecal region at the apex of the cecum. Inflammation or rupture of this structure is an important cause of morbidity in young persons, although it is a less frequent cause of death now than in the preantibiotic era.

The wall of the small intestine is composed of four basic layers. The outer, or serous, coat is formed by the peritoneum. The *peritoneum* has a visceral and a parietal layer, and the potential space between these layers is called the *peritoneal cavity.* The peritoneum is reflected over and almost completely envelops the abdominal viscera.

Special names have been given to the folds of the peritoneum. The *mesentery* is a broad, fanlike fold of peritoneum that suspends the jejunum and ileum from the posterior abdominal wall and allows considerable motion of the bowel. The mesentery supports the blood and lymph vessels supplying the intestine. The *greater omentum* is a double layer of peritoneum that hangs from the greater curvature of the stomach and descends in front of the abdominal viscera like an apron. The omentum usually contains fat in considerable amounts and lymph nodes, which aid in protecting the peritoneal cavity against infection. The *lesser omentum* is the fold of peritoneum that extends from the lesser curvature of the stomach and upper duodenum to the liver, forming the hepatogastric and hepatoduodenal suspensory ligaments. One of the important functions of the peritoneum is to prevent friction between contiguous organs by secreting a serous fluid that acts as a lubricant. Inflammation of the peritoneum is called *peritonitis* and may be a serious sequela to inflammation or perforation of the bowel. *Adhesions* (fibrous bands) may develop after peritonitis or abdominal surgery, sometimes causing obstruction of the bowel.

The muscular coat of the small intestine has two layers: an outer, thinner layer of longitudinal fibers and an inner one of circular fibers. This arrangement aids the peristaltic action of the small intestine. The submucosal layer is composed of connective tissue, and the inner mucosal layer is thick, vascular, and glandular.

The small intestine is characterized by three structural features that greatly increase its surface area and aid in its primary function of absorption. The mucosal and submucosal layers are arranged in circular folds called *valvulae conniventes* (Kerckring's folds), which project into the lumen of the tube about 3 to 10 mm. These folds are prominent in the duodenum and jejunum and disappear near the mid-ileum. They are responsible for the feathery appearance of the small intestine on barium radiographs. The *villi* are fingerlike projections of mucosa numbering about 4 or 5 million and are present in the entire length of the small intestine (see Fig. 6-2). The villi are 0.5 to 1.5 mm long (just visible to the naked eye) and account for the velvetlike appearance of the mucosa. The *microvilli* are fingerlike projections about 1.0 μ in length along the outer surface of each individual villus. They are visible by electron microscopy and appear as a *brush border* on light microscopy. If the lining of the small intestine were smooth, the surface area would be about 2000 cm². The valvulae conniventes, villi, and microvilli together increase the total absorbing surface to 1.6 million cm², which is about a 1000-fold increase. Diseases of the small intestine (e.g., sprue) that cause atrophy and flattening of the villi greatly reduce the surface area for absorption, resulting in malabsorption.

Structure of the Villus

Fig. 25-1 illustrates the structure of a villus, which is the functional unit of the small intestine. Each villus consists

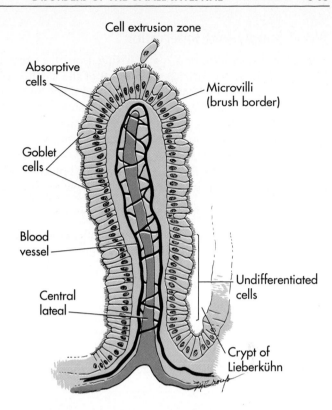

Cell extrusion zone

Absorptive cells

Microvilli (brush border)

Goblet cells

Blood vessel

Undifferentiated cells

Central lateal

Crypt of Lieberkühn

FIG. 25-1   Structure of a villus of the small intestine.

of a central lymph channel called a *lacteal,* surrounded by a network of blood capillaries held together by connective tissue. This in turn is surrounded by columnar epithelial cells. After food has been digested, it passes into the lacteals and capillaries of the villi. The villous epithelium consists of two cell types: *goblet cells,* which produce mucus, and *absorptive cells* (with microvilli projecting from the surface), which are responsible for absorption of nutrients. Enzymes are located on the brush border and complete the process of digestion as absorption is taking place.

Surrounding each villus are several small pits called the *crypts of Lieberkühn.* These crypts are intestinal glands that produce secretions containing digestive enzymes. Undifferentiated cells in the crypts of Lieberkühn proliferate rapidly and migrate upward toward the tip of the villus, where they become absorptive cells. At the tip of the villus, they are shed into the intestinal lumen. Maturation and migration from the crypts to the tip of the villus require only 5 to 7 days. It is estimated that 20 to 50 million epithelial cells are extruded into the intestinal lumen each minute. Because of this high cell-turnover rate (fastest in the body), the intestinal epithelium is especially vulnerable to alterations in cell proliferation. Cytotoxic drugs given to treat cancer or leukemia inhibit cell division, resulting in mucosal atrophy and shortening of both crypts and villi. Patients receiving these drugs often develop ulcerations of the gastrointestinal (GI) mucosa. Villi may be flattened or absent in sprue.

Blood Supply and Innervation

The *superior mesenteric artery,* arising from the aorta just below the celiac artery, supplies all of the small intestine except the duodenum, which is supplied by the gastroduodenal artery and its branch, the superior pancreaticoduodenal artery. Blood is returned by the superior mesenteric vein, which unites with the splenic vein to form the portal vein.

The small intestine is innervated by both branches of the autonomic nervous system. Parasympathetic impulses stimulate secretory activity and motility and those of the sympathetic system relay pain, whereas those of the parasympathetic regulate intestinal reflexes. The intrinsic nerve supply, which initiates motor function, passes through Auerbach's plexus in the muscular layer and Meissner's plexus in the submucosal layer.

PHYSIOLOGY

The small intestine has two primary functions: digestion and absorption of ingested nutrients and water. All other activities either regulate or facilitate this process. The digestive process is initiated in the mouth and stomach by the actions of ptyalin, hydrochloric acid (HCl), pepsin, mucus, renin, and gastric lipase on the ingested food. The process is continued in the duodenum primarily by the action of pancreatic enzymes, which hydrolyze carbohydrates, fats, and proteins into simpler substances. The presence of bicarbonate in the pancreatic secretion helps neutralize the acid and provide an optimum pH for the action of the enzymes. Mucus also provides some protection from the acid. The secretion of bile from the liver aids the digestive process by emulsifying fats so that a

▶ TABLE 25-1   Principal Digestive Enzymes

Enzyme	Source	Substrate	Products	Optimal pH	Volume of Secretion* (Daily)
Salivary amylase (ptyalin)	Salivary glands	Starch	Maltose (a disaccharide and smaller carbohydrate polymer; minor physiologic role)	6 to 7	1 to 1.5 L
Pepsin	Chief cells of stomach	Protein	Proteoses, peptones	1.5 to 2.5	2 to 4 L
Gastric lipase	Stomach	Fat	Fatty acids, glycerides (minor physiologic role)	—	
Enterokinase	Duodenal mucosa	Trypsinogen	Tripsin		
Trypsin	Exocrine pancreas	Denatured proteins and polypeptides	Small polypeptides (also activates chymotrypsinogen to chymotrypsin)	8	0.6 to 0.8 L
Chymotrypsin		Proteins and polypeptides	Small polypeptides	8	
Carboxypeptidases		Polypeptides	Smaller polypeptides (removes C-terminal amino acid)	—	
Nucleases		Nucleic acids	Nucleotides	—	
Pancreatic lipase		Fat	Glycerides, fatty acids, glycerol	8	
Pancreatic amylase		Starch	Disaccharides	6.7 to 7	
Bile acids (not an enzyme)	Liver	Unemulsified fats	Emulsified fats (formation of micelles; action is physical)	7.5	0.8 to 1 L
Aminopeptidases	Intestinal glands	Polypeptides	Smaller polypeptides (removes N-terminal amino acid)	8	2 to 3 L
Dipeptidase		Dipeptides	Amino acids	—	
Maltase		Maltose	Glucose	5 to 7	
Lactase		Lactose	Glucose + galactose (all monosaccharides)		
Sucrase		Sucrose	Glucose + fructose		
Intestinal lipase		Fat	Glycerides, fatty acids, glycerol	8	
Nucleotidase		Nucleotides	Nucleosides, phosphoric acid	8	

*All secretions are reabsorbed, except about 100 ml water normally excreted in stool per day.

greater surface area is presented for the action of pancreatic lipase.

The action of bile results from the detergent properties of conjugated bile acids, which solubilize lipid material by the formulation of micelles. *Micelles* are aggregates of bile acids and fat molecules. Fats form the hydrophobic core, and the bile acids, being polar molecules, form the surface of the micelles, with the hydrophobic end pointing inward and the hydrophilic end pointing outward toward the aqueous medium. The center of the micelle also dissolves fat-soluble vitamins and cholesterol. Thus free fatty acids, glycerides, and fat-soluble vitamins are kept in solution until they can be absorbed by the epithelial cell surface.

The process of digestion is completed by a number of enzymes present in the intestinal juice (succus entericus). Many of these enzymes are located on the brush border of the villi, and they digest food substances as they are being absorbed. Table 25-1 lists the principal digestive enzymes.

Two hormones are important in the regulation of intestinal digestion. Fat, in contact with the duodenal mucosa, causes the gallbladder to contract; this is mediated by the action of *cholecystokinin.* Products of partially digested proteins and fatty acids in contact with the duodenal mucosa stimulate the secretion of pancreatic juice rich in enzymes; this is mediated by the action of *pan-*

creozymin. Pancreozymin and cholecystokinin are considered to be the same hormone having two different effects; it is called *CCK* (some textbooks still refer to this hormone as CCK-PZ). This hormone is produced by the duodenal mucosa.

Gastric acid in contact with the intestinal mucosa causes the release of another hormone, *secretin,* and the amount released is proportional to the amount of acid flowing through the duodenum. Secretin stimulates the secretion of the bicarbonate-containing juice from the pancreas and bile from the liver and also potentiates the action of CCK.

Segmental movements of the small intestine mix ingested materials with pancreatic, hepatobiliary, and intestinal secretions, and peristaltic movements propel the contents from one end to the other at a rate suitable for optimal absorption and continuing entry of gastric contents.

Absorption

Absorption is the transfer of the end products of carbohydrate, fat, and protein digestion (simple sugars, fatty acids, and amino acids) across the intestinal wall to the vascular and lymphatic circulation for use by the body cells. In addition, water, electrolytes, and vitamins are absorbed. Absorption of the various substances takes place by both active and passive transport mechanisms that are for the most part poorly understood.

Although many substances are absorbed throughout the entire length of the small bowel, there are principal sites of absorption for specific nutrients. Knowledge of these absorption sites is necessary to understand how disease of the intestine may cause specific nutritional deficiencies (Fig. 25-2).

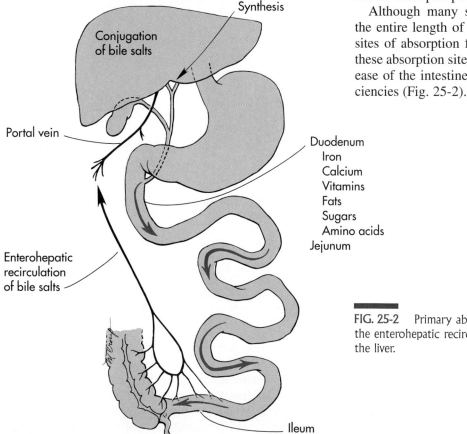

FIG. 25-2   Primary absorption sites of the major nutrients and the enterohepatic recirculation of bile salts for reconjugation by the liver.

The absorption of sugars, amino acids, and fats is largely complete by the time the chyme reaches the mid-jejunum. Iron and calcium are primarily absorbed in the duodenum and jejunum, and absorption of calcium requires vitamin D. Absorption of the fat-soluble vitamins (A, D, E, K) is facilitated by bile acids and occurs in the duodenum and upper jejunum. Most water-soluble vitamins are absorbed in the upper small intestine. The absorption of vitamin B_{12} takes place in the terminal ileum by a special transport mechanism requiring gastric intrinsic factor. Most of the bile acids released by the gallbladder into the duodenum to aid in the digestion of fats are reabsorbed in the terminal ileum and recirculated to the liver. This circuit is termed the *enterohepatic circulation of bile salts* and is important in maintaining the bile pool. The bile acids or salts thus perform their action in relation to fat digestion many times before being excreted in the feces. Disease or resection of the terminal ileum may thus cause deficiency of bile salts and interference with fat digestion. The entry of large amounts of bile salts into the colon causes colonic irritation and diarrhea.

MALABSORPTION

Diseases of the small intestine are often accompanied by alterations in function manifested by the malabsorption syndrome. *Malabsorption* is the condition in which intestinal mucosal absorption of single or multiple nutrients is impaired, resulting in inadequate movement of digested food from the small intestine into the blood or lymphatic system.

It is important to distinguish between malabsorption and maldigestion, since increased loss of nutrients in the stool may be a reflection of either process. *Maldigestion* refers to a breakdown of the chemical processes of digestion that take place in the intestinal lumen or at the brush border of the intestinal mucosa, resulting in a failure to absorb nutrients.

Causes

The box at right lists some of the more common causes of the malabsorption syndrome. The basic causes of maldigestion are included in the first three categories. Gastrectomy, especially the Billroth II procedure, causes poor mixing of chyme with gastric secretions. Hepatobiliary disease may result in insufficiency of intraluminal bile acids. Failure of the pancreas to produce or release sufficient enzymes may result from a number of pancreatic disorders. Failure of release of CCK, which stimulates pancreatic secretion, may occur in Zollinger-Ellison syndrome as a result of excessive acidification of the duodenum or may result from disease of the intestinal mucosa itself, as in sprue. Disease of the terminal ileum or

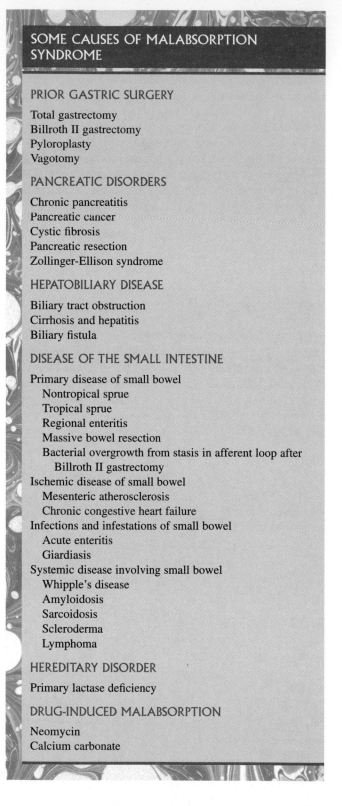

SOME CAUSES OF MALABSORPTION SYNDROME

PRIOR GASTRIC SURGERY

Total gastrectomy
Billroth II gastrectomy
Pyloroplasty
Vagotomy

PANCREATIC DISORDERS

Chronic pancreatitis
Pancreatic cancer
Cystic fibrosis
Pancreatic resection
Zollinger-Ellison syndrome

HEPATOBILIARY DISEASE

Biliary tract obstruction
Cirrhosis and hepatitis
Biliary fistula

DISEASE OF THE SMALL INTESTINE

Primary disease of small bowel
    Nontropical sprue
    Tropical sprue
    Regional enteritis
    Massive bowel resection
    Bacterial overgrowth from stasis in afferent loop after
      Billroth II gastrectomy
Ischemic disease of small bowel
    Mesenteric atherosclerosis
    Chronic congestive heart failure
Infections and infestations of small bowel
    Acute enteritis
    Giardiasis
Systemic disease involving small bowel
    Whipple's disease
    Amyloidosis
    Sarcoidosis
    Scleroderma
    Lymphoma

HEREDITARY DISORDER

Primary lactase deficiency

DRUG-INDUCED MALABSORPTION

Neomycin
Calcium carbonate

ileal resection for treatment of regional enteritis may cause a deficiency of bile salts by interfering with ileal resorption. Bacterial overgrowth in the duodenal stump (blind or afferent loop created in the Billroth II procedure) causes vitamin B_{12} malabsorption by using this vitamin and causes fat maldigestion by deconjugating bile salts. Unconjugated bile salts are to a lesser extent effective in forming micelles and are absorbed less in the ileum. Lack of intrinsic factor causes inability to absorb vitamin B_{12}; lack of B_{12} causes pernicious anemia. A hereditary lack of lactase causes selective malabsorption of lactose (a milk disaccharide) and is common in Hispanics, African Americans, and Southeast Asian populations. Mesenteric atherosclerosis (abdominal angina) may cause malabsorption and is a source of discomfort in older persons, but it is infrequently diagnosed. Chapter 27 deals with pancreatic and hepatobiliary disorders, and this chapter discusses a few of the more common intestinal disorders associated with malabsorption.

Signs and Symptoms

The signs and symptoms of malabsorption may be divided into two groups: those resulting from abnormal content in the intestinal lumen and those resulting from deficiency of dietary nutrients. Weight loss, diarrhea, steatorrhea, flatulence, and nocturia are the most common signs and symptoms and all are caused by abnormal intestinal luminal content. Table 25-2 lists the signs and symptoms of malabsorption and their pathophysiologic basis.

Detection

Most of the tests useful in the diagnosis of malabsorption indicate the presence of either malabsorption or maldigestion. Only a few of the tests distinguish between these two entities.

Stool fat

The oldest and most reliable test for documenting the presence of steatorrhea, and thus malabsorption, is the quantitative determination of stool fat. Qualitatively, the stool can be examined for neutral fat, split fats, and undigested muscle fibers. This can be a reliable screen for steatorrhea and a means of differentiating between celiac sprue and pancreatic insufficiency. Normal persons excrete less than 6 g of fat in the stool per day. Fat excretion in excess of 6 g is considered excessive and is termed *steatorrhea.* In severe cases the stools are abnormal to the naked eye and appear pale, greasy, and frothy and may float. They may stick to the side of the toilet and not flush away easily.

A 72-hour stool collection for quantitative fat determination is routinely used to eliminate errors resulting from daily variations. Testing stools for fat is essential in the diagnosis of nontropical sprue, after extensive gastrectomy, and in other malabsorptive disorders. This test does not differentiate between maldigestion as in pancreatic disorders and malabsorption caused by an intestinal disease such as nontropical sprue. However, there is a marked increase in undigested meat fibers in the stool in

 TABLE 25-2   Signs and Symptoms of Malabsorption Syndrome

Sign or Symptom	Pathophysiology
Weight loss and generalized malnutrition	Impaired absorption of carbohydrate, fat, and protein leading to loss of calories
Diarrhea	Excess load of fluids and electrolytes introduced into colon, which may exceed its absorptive capacity; bile acids and fatty acids in colon cause decreased colonic absorption of sodium and water and laxative effect from colonic irritation
Steatorrhea (bulky, frothy, voluminous stools)	Excess fat content of feces
Flatulence, abdominal distention	Undigested lactose $\rightarrow$ fermentation $\rightarrow$ gas formation
	Undigested lactose $\rightarrow$ osmotic effect $\rightarrow$ shift of extracellular fluid into gut $\rightarrow$ diarrhea (may be caused by primary lactase deficiency or secondary damage to brush border from intestinal lesions)
Nocturia	Delayed absorption and excretion of water (may be pooled in gut during day)
Weakness and easy fatigability	Anemia; electrolyte depletion caused by diarrhea (hypokalemia, hypomagnesemia)
Edema	Impaired absorption of amino acids $\rightarrow$ protein depletion $\rightarrow$ hypoproteinemia
Amenorrhea	Protein depletion $\rightarrow$ secondary hypopituitarism
Anemia	Impaired absorption of iron, folic acid, and vitamin B_{12}
Glossitis, cheilosis	Deficiency of iron, folic acid, vitamin B_{12}, and other vitamins
Peripheral neuropathy	Deficiency of vitamin B_{12}, thiamine
Bruising, bleeding tendency	Vitamin K malabsorption, hypoprothrombinemia
Bone pain, skeletal deformities, fractures	Calcium malabsorption $\rightarrow$ hypocalcemia; protein depletion $\rightarrow$ osteoporosis; vitamin D malabsorption $\rightarrow$ impaired calcium absorption
Tetany, paresthesias	Calcium malabsorption $\rightarrow$ hypocalcemia; magnesium malabsorption $\rightarrow$ hypomagnesemia and hypokalemia
Eczema	Cause uncertain

pancreatic insufficiency that is not usually present in non-tropical sprue.

D–Xylose absorption test. D-Xylose is a relatively inert pentose that is absorbed in the proximal bowel without digestion, passes through the liver, and is then excreted by the kidneys. Measurement of the amount of D-xylose excreted in the urine therefore gives an indication of the absorptive capacity of the small intestinal mucosa. This test is useful to assess for carbohydrate absorption.

The test is carried out after the patient has fasted for 12 hours. At least 20% of a 25 g dose of D-xylose given orally should be excreted in the urine in 5 hours, provided renal function is normal. Excretion of less than this amount or blood levels of D-xylose lower than 30 mg/dl indicates malabsorption. Abnormal D-xylose test results are found most frequently in disorders affecting the proximal bowel, such as sprue. The results are normal in maldigestive disorders such as chronic pancreatitis.

Schilling test for vitamin B_{12} absorption

The Schilling test is a valuable measure of vitamin B_{12} absorption and is frequently carried out in stages to determine the specific cause of the malabsorption. If urine collection is adequate, low excretion of ^{60}Co-tagged vitamin B_{12} indicates impaired absorption as a result of a lack of intrinsic factor (pernicious anemia), bacterial overgrowth in the proximal small bowel after Billroth II gastrectomy, diseased ileal mucosa as in regional enteritis, or pancreatic insufficiency. Correction of the malabsorption with intrinsic factor confirms intrinsic factor deficiency, which causes pernicious anemia. If the Schilling test returns to normal after antibiotic therapy, this helps confirm the diagnosis of malabsorption as a result of bacterial overgrowth in the proximal bowel after Billroth II gastrectomy (the bacteria take up vitamin B_{12}, thus preventing its absorption). Malabsorption of vitamin B_{12} as a result of pancreatic insufficiency may be corrected by the administration of pancreatic enzymes. Vitamin B_{12} malabsorption resulting from regional enteritis involving the terminal ileum is not corrected by any of the measures just mentioned.

Culture of duodenal and jejunal contents

The most reliable test for confirming the presence of bacterial overgrowth in the proximal bowel is aspiration and culture of the contents. The proximal small bowel normally contains less than 10^5 organisms/ml, and these are generally of the oropharyngeal variety. The most important mechanisms keeping the proximal bowel bacteriologically sterile is the normal peristalsis that sweeps bacteria distally, the gastric acid, and the secretion of immunoglobulin A (IgA) into the gut. Consequently, any condition that causes stasis of proximal intestinal contents, such as the blind loop after Billroth II surgery, may result in macrocytic anemia (because of use of vitamin B_{12} by organisms), diarrhea, and steatorrhea (because of deconjugation of bile salts by bacteria). Gastric achlorhydria and hypogammaglobulinemia are other conditions that may cause bacterial overgrowth.

Gastrointestinal barium radiologic studies

The radiographic appearance of the small bowel may be nonspecific or diagnostic. Characteristic features in the malabsorption syndrome are the loss of the feathery pattern of the barium and increased flocculation of the barium with segmentation and clumping. This finding is common in sprue but is also found in other malabsorptive disorders. In regional enteritis, the ileal lumen may be narrowed (i.e., the "string sign").

Biopsy of the small intestine

The biopsy is a useful test to examine abnormalities in diseases such as sprue because a biopsy of the intestinal mucosa can reveal atrophy of villi. The biopsy may be performed through the use of a sighted endoscope or suction capsule endoscope along with radiography to identify mucosal lesions.

Breath tests

The human body does not normally produce hydrogen gas (H_2), which is, however, a normal by-product of bacterial carbohydrate metabolism. The fasting patient normally has a low baseline concentration of expired H_2. This principle has been used to design several noninvasive breath tests that assist in the diagnosis of various malabsorption disorders.

The *lactose breath test* is a sensitive test for detecting lactase deficiency (see later discussion). Fifty grams of lactose is given by mouth, and the patient's breath H_2 is monitored. Normally the lactose is absorbed and, in the absence of bacterial overgrowth of the small intestine, the patient's breath H_2 does not increase significantly. Malabsorption of lactose produces high peaks of H_2 excretion caused by colonic fermentation. The *lactulose breath test* and the *^{14}C-cholyglycine (bile acid) breath test* are used to detect bacterial overgrowth within the small bowel. Ingestion of lactulose (a nonabsorbable disaccharide) normally produces a sharp increase in H_2 when it arrives in the cecum, and it is sometimes used in this way to estimate the intestinal transit time. An earlier peak of breath H_2 after lactulose ingestion suggests small bowel bacterial overgrowth. In the bile acid breath test, ^{14}C-labeled bile acid is given by mouth and normally is absorbed intact and undergoes enterohepatic circulation. Consequently, little $^{14}CO_2$ is released in the breath. If it is degraded by bacteria, the ^{14}C is metabolized and eventually exhaled as $^{14}CO_2$. An early peak of breath $^{14}CO_2$ is typical of a patient with proximal bowel bacterial overgrowth, although raised levels also occur with bile salt malabsorption (as in regional enteritis) as a result of degradation by colonic bacteria.

PRIMARY SMALL INTESTINAL DISORDERS ASSOCIATED WITH MALABSORPTION

Nontropical Sprue (Celiac Disease)

Idiopathic steatorrhea in adults and celiac disease in children are the most important causes of severe malabsorption in nontropical areas. Both of these conditions are considered phases of the same disease. Sprue is characterized by marked atrophy of the villi in the proximal small intestine, induced by ingestion of gluten-containing foods.

Pathophysiology

Gluten is a high-molecular-weight protein found in rye, oats, barley, and especially wheat. It is found in bread, bread products, beer, and many other processed foods. Gluten and/or gluten breakdown products (especially gliadin) are toxic to patients with this disease. Symptoms disappear when gluten is withdrawn from the diet and reappear when it is reintroduced. The characteristic lesion of the bowel mucosa induced by gluten is blunting or loss of the villi and elongation of the crypts, which cause the mucosa to appear flat. The loss of villi causes a marked reduction of absorptive surface.

Although the mechanism of gluten toxicity is not understood, it has been suggested that these patients lack a specific peptidase that would normally detoxify a noxious peptide of gluten. This hypothesis is supported by the fact that there is a strong familial and genetic tendency in occurrence. It has also been proposed that gluten or its metabolites cause a hypersensitivity reaction in the intestinal mucosa. This theory is supported by the fact that circulating antibodies to gliadin have been found in patients with this disease and that partial improvement of symptoms is provided by corticosteroid therapy.

Clinical features

Patients with nontropical sprue are presumably born with the disease tendency but may not develop symptoms for many years, even though they include gluten in the diet. Factors that precipitate the clinical onset are unknown. The onset generally occurs in infants between ages 6 months and 2 years and in adults between ages 20 and 50 years. The symptoms seldom begin during childhood or adolescence.

In infants, anorexia, irritability, and diarrhea with pale, bulky stools are soon followed by weight loss. If the infant is not treated, failure to grow is soon obvious. Diarrhea, lassitude, weakness, and steatorrhea are the most common symptoms in adults, but patients may present with any of the signs and symptoms of malabsorption syndrome listed in Table 25-2. Adults frequently have a history suggesting sprue during childhood.

The diagnosis is established by evidence of malabsorption, typical small-bowel biopsy changes, and clinical improvement on a gluten-free diet.

Treatment

The treatment of nontropical sprue by a gluten-free diet is generally successful, provided the patient adheres to the diet. Response to the gluten-free diet is noted by the return of normal color to the stools, disappearance of diarrhea, and increase in weight. The minority of patients who do not respond to a gluten-free diet may respond to corticosteroids; however, those who do not may have a dismal prognosis. Mortality was 20% before discovery of the gluten-free dietary treatment during World War II, but it is now almost nil in gluten-sensitive cases.

Tropical Sprue

Tropical sprue occurs in tropical regions such as Puerto Rico, India, and southwestern Asia. The signs and symptoms are similar to those of nontropical sprue, and the biopsy changes are similar but less severe. It is a malabsorptive disorder with the cause not really known. Malabsorption of at least two nutrients is considered essential for the diagnosis. Patients are usually deficient in iron as well as vitamin B_{12} and folate. Most patients improve after combined treatment with folic acid and a broad-spectrum antibiotic, such as tetracycline.

Lactase Deficiency

As indicated in the previous discussion, hydrolysis of disaccharides to monosaccharides occurs within the brush border of the intestinal mucosa. Deficiency of specific enzymes that hydrolyze disaccharides may be present as a result of a genetic defect or may be secondary to a wide variety of GI diseases that damage the mucosa of the small intestine.

Lactase deficiency is the most common type of the disaccharide deficiency syndromes. Lactase is an enzyme that normally splits lactose (a disaccharide) into glucose and galactose (monosaccharides) at the intestinal brush border so that absorption may take place. Since lactose is the principal carbohydrate in milk, many persons showing milk intolerance prove to be lactase deficient. Significant racial variation exists in primary lactase deficiency. It appears that about 5% to 10% of the Caucasian population is lactase deficient but that the incidence is as high as 80% to 90% among African Americans, Hispanics, Asians, and Bantus. Although lactase deficiency appears to be hereditary, milk intolerance may not become clinically apparent until adolescence. Secondary lactase deficiency is associated with a large number of conditions that cause intestinal mucosal injury, such as nontropical and tropical sprue, regional enteritis, viral and bacterial infections of the intestinal tract, giardiasis, cystic fibrosis, and ulcerative colitis.

Typical symptoms of lactase deficiency are abdominal cramps, bloating, and diarrhea after milk ingestion. The pathogenic mechanism explaining the diarrhea is as follows. When unhydrolyzed lactose enters the large intestine, it produces an osmotic effect, causing the entry of water into the colonic lumen. Colonic bacteria also ferment the lactose, producing lactic and fatty acids that are irritating to the colon. The result is increased motility which is caused by colonic irritation, and an explosive diarrhea.

A history of intolerance to milk or milk products and a decreased fecal pH of 6.0 (normal pH 7.0 to 7.5) is strongly suggestive of lactase deficiency. The diagnosis is confirmed by the lactose breath test, as described earlier, or by the lactose tolerance test. The *lactose tolerance test* consists of giving 50 g of lactose and then measuring the blood glucose level as for a glucose tolerance test; in lactase deficiency, the blood sugar fails to rise more than 20 mg/dl above the fasting level.

Treatment consists of eliminating milk and milk products from the diet. However, patients are often able to tolerate yogurt because it contains bacterial-derived lactases.

Postgastrectomy Malabsorption

Malabsorption and weight loss are well-recognized features after a gastrectomy. They are the rule after total gastrectomy, common after the Billroth II procedure, and rare after the Billroth I procedure. Increased fat loss in the stools occurs in many patients after the Billroth II procedure, especially if the duodenal stump (afferent or blind loop) is long. The principal causes of the steatorrhea are the following: (1) poor mixing of food and enzymes because of rapid emptying of the gastric remnant (low concentration of digestive secretion and food particles too large for the enzymes); (2) reduced pancreatic output because the duodenum is bypassed and has less stimulation by the acid chyme to release secretin and CCK; (3) stasis of intestinal contents in the afferent loop, resulting in abnormal bacterial proliferation, which uses up vitamin B_{12} and deconjugates bile salts; and (4) the loss of stomach reservoir function, which may result in a more rapid intestinal transit time with resultant diarrhea.

If malabsorption is severe, the patient may be at risk to develop symptoms as a result of the nutritive deficiencies listed in Table 25-2. Identification of the mechanism responsible for the malabsorption is essential for optimal treatment of postgastrectomy malabsorption. Broad-spectrum antibiotics such as tetracycline may be given when the cause is bacterial overgrowth. Pancreatic enzyme therapy may be helpful with functional pancreatic deficiency (a condition of insufficient production of pancreatic enzymes that are required for protein digestion). Smaller meals that are low in carbohydrates and taken without fluids may help delay rapid gastric emptying (dumping syndrome).

Regional Enteritis (Crohn's Disease)

Regional enteritis, ileocolitis, or *Crohn's disease* is a chronic, relapsing granulomatous inflammatory disease of the intestinal tract. Classically the terminal ileum is affected, although any portion of the GI tract may be involved. It usually develops in young adults and affects men and women about equally.

The etiology of regional enteritis is unknown. Although no autoantibodies have been demonstrated, it has been speculated that regional enteritis may represent a hypersensitivity reaction or may be caused by an infectious agent that has not yet been identified. These theories are suggested by the granulomatous lesions, which are similar to those found in fungal and tubercular lesions of the lung.

Some interesting similarities exist between regional enteritis and ulcerative colitis. Both are inflammatory diseases, although the lesions of each are distinct. Both diseases have extragastrointestinal manifestations, including uveitis, arthritis, and skin lesions that are identical. Some of these similarities and differences are discussed in Chapter 26.

Pathology

The terminal ileum is involved in regional enteritis in about 75% of the cases. In about 35% of the cases, lesions occur in the colon. The esophagus and stomach are less frequently affected. In some instances, "skip" lesions occur; that is, portions of diseased bowel are separated by areas of normal bowel a few inches or several feet long.

Lesions are believed to begin in the bowel wall or in the lymph nodes next to the small bowel, with eventual obstruction of the lymphatic channels of drainage. The submucosal coat of the intestine becomes greatly thickened as a result of the hyperplasia of the lymphoid tissue and lymphedema. With progress of the pathologic process, the affected segment of the bowel becomes thickened to such a degree that it is as stiff as a garden hose (Fig. 25-3). The lumen of the bowel may become greatly narrowed, so that it admits only a thin stream of barium, giving rise to the "string sign" seen radiographically. The entire wall of the bowel is involved. The mucosa is usually inflamed and ulcerated with grayish white exudate.

Clinical Features

The signs and symptoms of regional enteritis vary a great deal according to whether the disease is early or late and according to what parts of the GI tract are involved. Mild intermittent diarrhea, colicky pain in the lower abdomen, and malaise increasing over years are typical symptoms. Patients with more severe forms of the disease may have frequent liquid stools with blood and pus. Some patients develop steatorrhea, weight loss, anemia, and other manifestations of malabsorption. Low-grade fever is common.

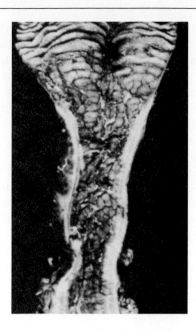

FIG. 25-3   Regional enteritis (Crohn's disease). The gut wall has been thickened by inflammation and scarring, causing marked narrowing of the lumen. The mucosa at the top is more normal looking. Extending downward are longitudinal ulcers that cross the transverse folds, giving the mucosa a cobblestone appearance. (Courtesy of Henry D. Appleman, MD, Associate Professor of Pathology, University of Michigan.)

Certain complications are typical of regional enteritis. The development of stenosis may cause symptoms of vomiting and other signs of intestinal obstruction. An ulcerous lesion may perforate through the intestinal wall, causing peritonitis. More often the perforation is closed, and fistulas are formed between loops of bowel, or less often it involves the bladder or vagina. Ulcers, abscesses, and fistulas often occur in the perianal and perirectal regions. External fistulas to the anterior abdominal wall may also occur. High fever is usually associated with extensive inflammation or complications such as fistulas and abscesses.

Extragastrointestinal manifestations of the disease, such as arthritis, uveitis, and skin lesions, occur but are less frequent than they are in ulcerative colitis.

The diagnosis is established on the basis of the clinical presentation, the characteristic radiographic changes, and in the case of colonic or rectal involvement, biopsy changes showing granulomatous lesions. Laboratory examination usually is not used in diagnosis as much as for measurement of malabsorption and extent of the inflammatory process (Glickman, 1994).

Treatment and prognosis

No specific or curative treatment exists for regional enteritis. The initial management of most patients is medical, supportive, and palliative, aimed at attaining remission of the disease. Corticosteroid, azathioprine (Imuran), 6-mercaptopurine (6-MP), and sulfasalazine (Azulfidine) are used to promote remission and control suppurative complications. Anticholingeric drugs, such as propantheline bromide (Pro-Banthine), and antidiarrheal drugs, such as diphenoxylate with atropine (Lomotil), may help reduce cramping, abdominal pain, and diarrhea. These drugs are contraindicated if there is bowel obstruction. Nutrient deficiencies and steatorrhea are treated by the appropriate replacements and a low-fat, low-residue diet.

Surgical treatment is generally avoided because recurrence and spread of the lesion is usual after surgical resection. Nevertheless, surgical intervention is usually necessary sometime during the course of the disease to treat complications.

When regional enteritis is characterized by an acute onset, as many as 90% of the patients can achieve remission. However, regional enteritis has an insidious onset in most patients. Approximately 75% of the patients experience relapses. Mortality as a direct result of the disease is low.

APPENDICITIS

Appendicitis is the most common major surgical disease. Although it may occur at any age, it is most common in adolescents and young adults. Before the era of antibiotics, the mortality from this disease was high.

Pathogenesis

The *vermiform appendix* is the remnant of the apex of the cecum and has no known function in humans. It is a long, narrow tube (about 6 to 9 cm). It contains the appendicular artery, which is an end artery.

In the usual position, the appendix is located on the abdominal wall under McBurney's point. *McBurney's point* is located by drawing a line from the right anterior superior iliac spine to the umbilicus. The midpoint of this line locates the root of the appendix (Fig. 25-4).

Appendicitis is an inflammation of the appendix involving all layers of the wall of the organ. The primary pathogenic hallmark is obstruction of the lumen, usually by a *fecalith* (hardened stool typically formed around vegetable fibers). Obstruction of the outflow of mucous secretions then results in swelling, infection, and ulceration. The increased intraluminal pressure may cause occlusion of the appendicular end artery. If the condition is allowed to progress, necrosis, gangrene, and perforation usually result. Current research indicates that appendicitis begins with ulceration of the mucosa in about 60% to 70% of the cases, rather than luminal obstruction. The cause of the ulceration is unknown, but a viral origin has been speculated. An infection by the *Yersinia enterocolitica* is the most recently speculated cause.

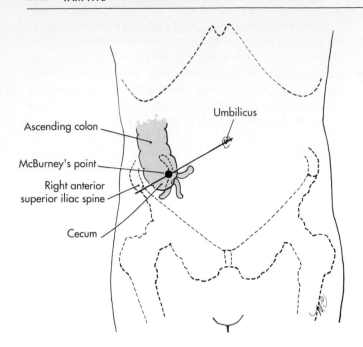

FIG. 25-4   McBurney's point and several common positions of the appendix.

Clinical Features

In the classic case of acute appendicitis, the initial symptoms are mild periumbilical pain or discomfort. These symptoms generally develop over 1 or 2 days. Within hours the pain shifts to the lower right quadrant, followed by anorexia, nausea, and vomiting. Tenderness to palpation over McBurney's point may also be present. Later, muscle spasm and rebound tenderness may be present. A low-grade fever and moderate leukocytosis are usual findings. When rupture of the appendix occurs, signs of the perforation may include pain, tenderness, and spasm. This often follows a brief dramatic relief from pain.

Diagnostic Problems

The diagnosis of even the classic case of appendicitis is complicated because many disorders present a similar clinical picture of an acute abdominal condition and must be differentiated from acute appendicitis. Some of these conditions include the following:
1. Acute gastroenteritis (probably the most common)
2. Mesenteric lymphadenitis in children
3. Ruptured ectopic pregnancy
4. Mittelschmerz (pain caused by rupture of ovarian follicle during ovulation)
5. Pelvic inflammatory disease
6. Regional enteritis
7. Inflammation of Meckel's diverticulum (persistence of a duct that, in the fetus, extends from the ileum to the umbilicus; this condition is rare)

Further diagnostic difficulties result from the fact that some individuals, particularly infants and older persons, deviate from the classic presentation. When doubt exists, it is usually safer to perform surgery, since the penalty of delay may be a ruptured appendix and peritonitis. Hospitalization is then prolonged, and some patients may die from the peritonitis.

Treatment

Once the diagnosis of appendicitis is made, the patient is prepared for surgery and the appendix is promptly removed at any time of the day or night. If surgical removal is carried out before rupture and before the signs of peritonitis occur, the postsurgical course is generally uncomplicated. The time until the patient is discharged from the hospital depends on how early the appendicitis was diagnosed, the degree of inflammation, and whether a laparoscopic or open surgical method was used.

PERITONITIS

Inflammation of the peritoneum is a serious complication that may occur in both acute and chronic forms. The condition usually results from spread of infection from abdominal organs (e.g., appendicitis, salpingitis), from perforation of the alimentary tract, or from penetrating abdominal wounds. The most common infecting organisms are the colon group (in the case of a ruptured appendix) that might include *Escherichia coli* or *Bacteroides*. Other organisms such as staphylococci or streptococci are often introduced from outside sources.

The initial reaction of the peritoneum to invasion by bacteria is the outpouring of a fibrinous exudate. Pockets of pus (abscesses) form between the fibrinous adhesions, which glue together the surrounding surfaces and thus localize the infection. The adhesions usually disappear when the infection disappears but may persist as fibrous bands that may later lead to intestinal obstruction.

If the infecting material is distributed widely over the surface of the peritoneum or if the infection spreads, generalized peritonitis may result. As generalized peritonitis develops, peristaltic activity diminishes until a state of paralytic ileus results; the intestine then becomes atonic and distended. Fluids and electrolytes are lost into the lumen of the bowel, leading to dehydration, circulatory embarrassment, oliguria, and possibly shock. Adhesions may form between the distended loops of intestine and may impede the return of intestinal motility and result in intestinal obstruction.

Symptoms vary with the extent of the peritonitis, its severity, and the type of organisms responsible. The principal symptoms are abdominal pain (usually continuous), vomiting, and a tense, rigid, tender, and rebound abdomen; bowel sounds are often absent. In chronic peritonitis, little or no rebound tenderness is found. Fever and leukocytosis are typically seen.

The prognosis is good in localized and mild forms of peritonitis and grave in generalized peritonitis caused by virulent organisms.

The general principles of treatment include administration of a suitable antibiotic, decompression of the GI tract by nasogastric or intestinal suction, intravenous repletion of fluid and electrolyte losses, bedrest in a medium Fowler's position, removal of the septic focus (appendix, etc.) or other cause of inflammation, if possible, and measures to relieve pain.

INTESTINAL OBSTRUCTION

Intestinal obstruction may be defined as an interference (from whatever cause) with the normal flow of intestinal contents through the intestinal tract. Intestinal obstruction may be acute or chronic, partial or complete. Chronic bowel obstruction usually involves the colon as a result of a carcinoma or tumor growth and is slow in development. Most obstructions involve the small bowel. Com-

plete obstruction of the small bowel is a grave condition that requires early diagnosis and emergency surgical intervention if the patient is to survive.

There are two types of intestinal obstruction: (1) *nonmechanical* (e.g., *paralytic ileus* or *adynamic ileus*), in which intestinal peristalsis is inhibited as a result of toxic or traumatic affectation of autonomic control of motility; and (2) *mechanical,* in which there is intraluminal obstruction or mural obstruction caused by extrinsic pressure.

Mechanical obstruction is further classified as *simple mechanical obstruction,* in which only one point of obstruction exists, and *closed-loop obstruction,* in which there are at least two points of obstruction. Because a closed-loop obstruction cannot be decompressed, there is a rapid increase in intraluminal pressure, leading to compression of blood vessels, ischemia, and infarction (strangulation). Fig. 25-5 illustrates some of the mechanical causes of bowel obstruction.

Etiology

Nonmechanical obstruction or adynamic ileus typically follows abdominal surgery in which reflex inhibition of

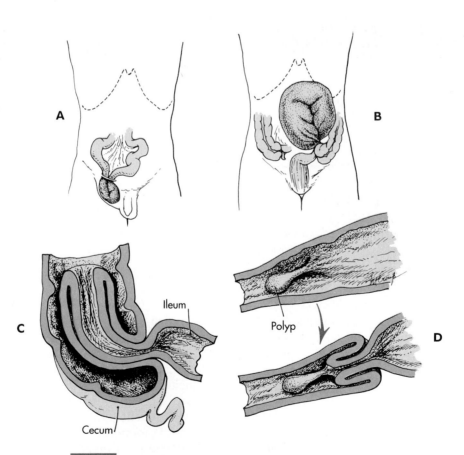

FIG. 25-5   Mechanical causes of bowel obstruction. **A,** Strangulated inguinal hernia. **B,** Volvulus of the sigmoid colon. **C,** Ileocecal intussusception. **D,** Enteroenteric intussusception caused by pedunculated polyp.

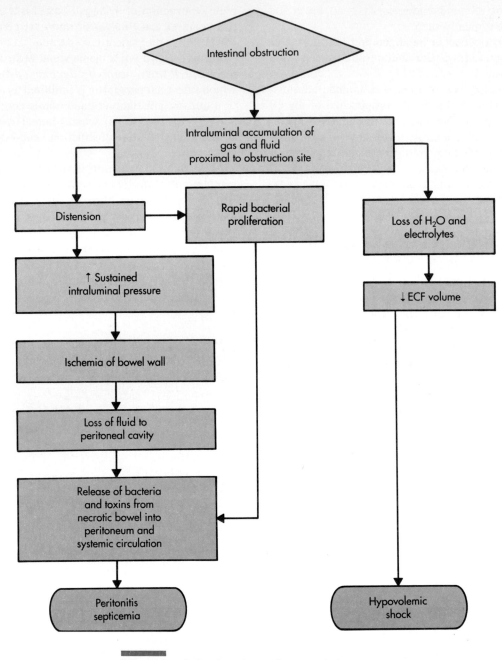

FIG. 25-6   Pathophysiology of intestinal obstruction.

peristalsis results from handling of the abdominal viscera. This reflex inhibition of peristalsis is often called *paralytic ileus,* although there is not complete paralysis of peristalsis. Another condition that is a common cause of adynamic ileus is peritonitis. Intestinal atony and gaseous distention accompany a wide variety of traumatic conditions; they especially may follow rib fracture, concussion of the spinal cord, or fracture of the spine.

The causes of mechanical obstruction are related to the age-group affected and the site of the obstruction. About 50% of all obstructions occur in adults and result from adhesions from previous surgery. Malignant tumors, diverticulitis, and volvulus are the most common causes of

obstruction of the large intestine in middle-age and older people; they account for about 90% of the obstructions. *Volvulus* is twisting of the intestine on itself. It occurs most frequently in elderly men and usually involves the sigmoid colon. Incarceration of a loop of bowel in an inguinal or femoral hernia is a common cause of small bowel obstruction. *Intussusception* is invagination of one section of the intestine into the next section and is a cause of obstruction encountered almost exclusively in infants and young children. A common site for intussusception is invagination of the terminal ileum into the cecum. Foreign bodies and congenital anomalies are the other common causes of obstruction in infants and children.

Pathophysiology

The pathophysiologic events that occur after intestinal obstruction are similar, whether they result from mechanical or functional causes. The main difference is that in paralytic obstruction, peristalsis is inhibited from the start, whereas in mechanical obstruction, peristalsis is accentuated at first, is then intermittent, and is finally absent.

The major pathophysiologic alterations that occur in intestinal obstruction are presented in Fig. 25-6. The wall of the intestine proximal to the obstructed segment is progressively distended by the accumulation of liquid and gas (70% from swallowed air) in the lumen. Severe distention of the wall reduces the flux of water and ions from the intestinal lumen into the blood. Because about 8 L of fluid are secreted into the GI tract each day, nonabsorption can lead to rapid intraluminal accumulation. Vomiting and intestinal suction after treatment has begun are major sources of fluid and electrolyte loss. The net effect of these losses is contraction of the extracellular fluid compartment leading to shock, that is, hypotension, reduced cardiac output, decreased tissue perfusion, and metabolic acidosis. Continuing bowel distention results in a vicious cycle of decreased fluid absorption and increased fluid secretion into the bowel. The local effects of bowel distention are ischemia from distention and increased permeability caused by necrosis, with absorption of bacterial toxins into the peritoneal cavity and systemic circulation.

Signs and Symptoms

The cardinal symptoms of small bowel obstruction are abdominal distention, pain, vomiting, and absolute constipation. Pain is usually cramping and midabdominal (typically paraumbilical) and becomes more severe when the obstruction is higher. The abdomen may also be tender. The frequency of vomiting varies with the site of obstruction. If the obstruction is high in the small bowel, vomiting is more prevalent than if the obstruction is in the ileum or large intestine. Absolute constipation is likely to occur early in large bowel obstruction, but flatus and feces may be passed early during the course of small bowel obstruction.

The abdominal radiograph is extremely important in the diagnosis of intestinal obstruction. Mechanical obstruction of the small bowel is characterized by air in the small intestine but not in the colon, whereas colonic obstruction is characterized by gas throughout the colon but with little or no gas in the small intestine. When the plain films are inconclusive, a barium radiograph may be performed to locate the site of obstruction.

Treatment

Treatment principles for bowel obstruction include correction of fluid and electrolyte imbalances, relief of distention and vomiting by intubation and decompression, control of peritonitis and shock if present, and removal of the obstruction to restore normal bowel continuity and function.

Many cases of adynamic ileus are cured by tubal decompression alone. A small bowel obstruction is much more serious and rapid in development than colonic obstruction. Mortality for nonstrangulating obstruction is 5% to 8%, provided surgical intervention occurs soon enough. Delay in surgical intervention or the development of strangulation or other complications raises the mortality to about 35% to 45%.

QUESTIONS

▼ *Answer the following on a separate sheet of paper.*

1. Why is the gastrointestinal mucosa especially vulnerable to side effects such as ulceration and bleeding from the administration of such cytotoxic drugs as cyclophosphamide (Cytoxan) and mercaptopurine?
2. Describe the function of bile in the digestion and absorption of fats and fat-soluble vitamins.
3. Differentiate between maldigestion and malabsorption.
4. Describe the appearance and characteristics of stool from a patient that would cause you to suspect steatorrhea.
5. What are the characteristics of regional enteritis that have led theorists to suspect that hypersensitivity might be responsible in its pathogenesis?
6. Name the three structures that greatly increase the absorptive surface area of the small bowel.
7. List four causes of steatorrhea in a patient following total gastrectomy or gastrojejunostomy.
8. Describe the pathophysiologic events leading to death from small bowel obstruction. Explain why early diagnosis and surgical intervention are important in mechanical obstruction of the small bowel.

▼ *Fill in the blanks with the correct word(s).*

9. The major artery supplying the small bowel (except the duodenum) is the _____ artery.
10. The _____ sphincter controls the entry of chyme into the small bowel, and the _____ valve controls the exit of digested material into the large intestine.

Continued.

QUESTIONS—cont'd

11. The fanlike fold of peritoneum that suspends the jejunum and ileum from the posterior abdominal wall is called the _____.

12. The fold of peritoneum that drapes over the small bowel like an apron is called the _____ _____. This structure has sometimes been called the policeman of the abdomen because one of its important functions is to localize _____.

13. The musculofibrous band extending from the diaphragm to the duodenojejunal juncture and that acts as a support for this portion of the small bowel is called the _____ of _____.

14. The structures responsible for giving the barium radiograph of the small bowel a feathery appearance are the _____.

15. The structures that account for the velvetlike appearance of the small bowel are the _____.

16. Several small pits surrounding each villus are the _____ of _____.

17. The lymphatic channel of the villus where fat absorption takes place is called the _____.

18. McBurney's point is located at the midpoint on a line between the _____ and the anterior superior _____ spine. It is the point where the _____ is normally located.

▼ *Circle the letter preceding each item below that correctly answers the question or completes the statement. Only one answer is correct, unless otherwise noted.*

19. Which of the following hormones has the primary effect of stimulating the bicarbonate component of the pancreatic juice?
    a. Gastrin
    b. Cholecystokinin
    c. Pancreozymin
    d. Secretin

20. Hydrolysis of lactose into glucose and galactose takes place:
    a. In the stomach
    b. Along the brush border
    c. Within the lumen of the duodenum
    d. Within the lumen of the jejunum

21. Mechanisms that normally keep the proximal bowel relatively sterile include which of the following (more than one answer may be correct)?
    a. Peristalsis
    b. Acid chyme entering duodenum
    c. Alkalinity of the pancreatic bicarbonate secretion
    d. Secretion of IgA into the gut

22. The length of the small bowel in the living person is about:
    a. 22 feet   c. 10 feet
    b. 12 feet   d. 6 feet

23. The greatest portion of gastrointestinal gas (air) is derived from:
    a. Food breakdown
    b. Bacterial fermentation
    c. Swallowed air

24. The diagnosis of gluten-induced enteropathy must include:
    a. History of weight loss
    b. Steatorrhea
    c. Abnormal small bowel biopsy
    d. Abnormal D-xylose excretion

25. Administration of intrinsic factor caused the Schilling test to return to normal after an initial low value in a 56-year-old woman. The probable cause of this patient's problem is:
    a. Bacterial overgrowth in the proximal small bowel
    b. Regional enteritis
    c. Chronic pancreatitis
    d. Atrophic gastritis

26. The afferent loop syndrome is characterized by (more than one answer may be correct):
    a. Malabsorption of vitamin B_{12}
    b. Megaloblastic anemia
    c. Heavy growth of colonic bacteria
    d. Amelioration with administration of broad-spectrum antibiotics

27. The earliest sign on examination in acute appendicitis is:
    a. Periumbilical hyperesthesia
    b. Abdominal distention
    c. Localized tenderness in the lower right quadrant
    d. Rebound tenderness

28. Which of the following conditions may present difficulties in differentiation from acute appendicitis (more than one answer may be correct)?
    a. Acute gastroenteritis
    b. Ruptured ectopic pregnancy
    c. Regional enteritis
    d. Inflammation of Meckel's diverticulum
    e. Mittelschmerz

29. Bile salts are conjugated in the liver and deconjugated by bacteria in conditions of duodenal stasis.
    a. First statement is true but second is false.
    b. First statement is false but second is true.
    c. Both statements are true.
    d. Both statements are false.

30. Lactase deficiency is (more than one answer may be correct):
    a. Always congenital
    b. Only found in the western hemisphere
    c. Common in African Americans
    d. Less common in Caucasians
    e. Common in Asians

31. The secretion of CCK is stimulated by (more than one answer may be correct):
    a. Contact of the acid chyme with the duodenal mucosa
    b. Fat in contact with the duodenal mucosa
    c. Alkaline chyme in contact with duodenal mucosa
    d. Amino acids in contact with the duodenal mucosa

32. Which of the following may be a cause of intestinal malabsorption (more than one answer may be correct)?
    a. Acute enteritis
    b. Chronic hepatitis
    c. Whipple's disease
    d. Mesenteric atherosclerosis

QUESTIONS—cont'd

▼ Match each of the following enzymes in column A with its secretory source in column B and with its substrate in column C.

Column A	Column B	Column C
33. _____ Lactase	a. Duodenal mucosa	e. Denatured proteins
34. _____ Ptyalin	b. Exocrine pancreas	and polypeptides
35. _____ Enterokinase	c. Salivary glands	f. Lactose
36. _____ Trypsin	d. Intestinal glands	g. Starch
		h. Trypsinogen

▼ Match each of the following nutrients in column A with its major site of absorption in column B. (Items may be used more than once.)

Column A	Column B
37. _____ Iron	a. Stomach
38. _____ Vitamin B_{12}	b. Duodenum
39. _____ Sugars	c. Duodenum and jejunum
40. _____ Fats	d. Duodenum, jejunum, and ileum
41. _____ Amino acids	e. Terminal ileum
42. _____ Bile salts	f. Large intestine

▼ Match each of the following symptoms of malabsorption in column A with its pathophysiologic basis in column B.

Column A	Column B
43. _____ Edema	a. Impaired absorption of amino acids
44. _____ Peripheral neuropathy	b. Vitamin K malabsorption
45. _____ Bleeding tendency	c. Deficiency of vitamin B_{12}
46. _____ Diarrhea	d. Bile salts in colon
47. _____ Tetany, paresthesias	e. Lactase deficiency
48. _____ Nocturia	f. Calcium malabsorption
	g. Delayed absorption of fluid in gut

▼ Match each of the following terms related to bowel obstruction in column A with the proper descriptive statements in column B.

Column A	Column B
49. _____ Adhesions	a. Twisting of a loop of bowel on itself
50. _____ Volvulus	b. Only one point of obstruction
51. _____ Simple bowel obstruction	c. Fibrous bands that form as a result of a fibrinous exudate from peritoneum
52. _____ Strangulated hernia	d. Obstruction of the blood supply to a loop of bowel protruding through muscle wall
53. _____ Intussusception	e. Almost exclusively a condition of infants and young children
	f. Often occurs in the sigmoid colon in elderly men
	g. Telescoping of the bowel
	h. Most common cause of bowel obstruction in adults

▼ Match each of the following descriptions in column A with the correct entity in column B.

Column A	Column B
54. _____ Usually responds to broad-spectrum antibiotics	a. Nontropical sprue (celiac disease)
55. _____ During exacerbation is associated with very low D-xylose excretion	b. Tropical sprue
56. _____ Usually responds to gluten withdrawal	c. Both
57. _____ Characterized by atrophy and flattening of villi	d. Neither

▼ Circle T if the statement is true and F if it is false. Correct any false statements.

58. T F The lumen of the bowel is open and the obstruction is functional in paralytic ileus.

59. T F Parasympathetic fibers supplying the small bowel relay pain.

60. T F The daily total volume of the digestive secretions is about 8 L.

61. T F Most of the enzymes of the succus entericus would be inactivated by a pH of 5.

62. T F Two factors that account for frequent obstruction and ischemic necrosis of the appendix are its narrow lumen ending in a blind pouch and its blood supply from an end artery.

CHAPTER 26

Disorders of the Large Intestine

LORRAINE M. WILSON
GLENDA N. LINDSETH

ANATOMY AND PHYSIOLOGY

The large intestine or colon is a hollow muscular tube about 5 feet (1.5 m) in length, extending from the cecum to the anal canal. The diameter of the large intestine is noticeably larger than that of the small intestine. Its average diameter is about 2.5 inches (6.5 cm), but its diameter decreases toward the lower end of the tube.

The large intestine is divided into the cecum, colon, and rectum, as illustrated in Fig. 26-1. The *cecum,* containing the ileocecal valve and with the appendix attached to its apex, constitutes the first 2 or 3 inches of the large intestine. The ileocecal valve controls the flow of chyme from the ileum into the cecum and prevents backflow of fecal material from the large intestine into the small intestine. The colon is subdivided into the *ascending, transverse, descending,* and *sigmoid* colon. The points at which the colon makes a sharp turn at the right and left

upper abdomen are called the *hepatic* and *splenic flexures,* respectively. The sigmoid colon begins at the level of the iliac crest and describes an **S**-shaped curve. The lower part of the curve bends toward the left as it joins the rectum and is the anatomic reason for placing a patient on the left side when giving an enema. In this position, gravity aids the flow of water from the rectum into the sigmoid flexure. The last major portion of the large intestine is called the *rectum* and extends from the sigmoid colon to the *anus* (opening to the outside of the body). The terminal inch of the rectum is called the *anal canal* and is guarded by internal and external sphincter muscles. The length of the rectum and anal canal is approximately 5.9 inches (15 cm).

Throughout most of its length the large intestine exhibits the four morphologic layers seen in the remainder of the gut. Several features, however, are peculiar to the large intestine. The longitudinal muscle coat is incomplete, being collected into three bands called the *taenia coli.* The taenia coalesce in the distal sigmoid, so the rectum has a complete longitudinal muscle coat. The taenia are shorter than the intestine, causing it to pucker and form small sacs called *haustra.* The *epiploic appendages* are small, fat-filled sacs of peritoneum attached along the taenia. The mucosal layer of the large intestine is much thicker than that of the small intestine and contains no villi or rugae. The crypts of Lieberkühn (intestinal glands) are deeper and have more goblet cells than those of the small intestine.

The large intestine is clinically divided into right and left halves, based on the blood supply. The *superior mesenteric artery* supplies the right half (cecum, ascending colon, and proximal two thirds of the transverse colon), and the *inferior mesenteric artery* supplies the left half (distal one third of the transverse colon, descending and sigmoid colon, and proximal part of the rectum). Additional blood supply to the rectum is provided by the middle and inferior hemorrhoidal arteries, which arise from the abdominal aorta and internal iliac arteries.

Venous return from the colon and superior rectum is via the superior and inferior mesenteric veins and superior hemorrhoidal veins, which become a part of the portal system delivering blood to the liver. The middle and inferior hemorrhoidal veins drain into the iliac veins

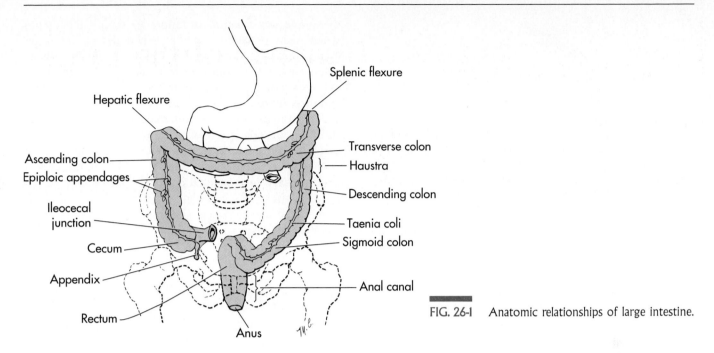

FIG. 26-1   Anatomic relationships of large intestine.

and consequently are part of the systemic circulation. Anastomoses exist between the superior and the middle and inferior hemorrhoidal veins, so increased portal pressure may cause backflow into these veins, resulting in hemorrhoids.

The nerve supply to the large intestine is provided by the autonomic nervous system, with the exception that the external sphincter is under voluntary control. Parasympathetic fibers travel via the vagus nerve to the mid-transverse colon, and pelvic nerves of sacral origin supply the distal part. Sympathetic fibers leave the sympathetic trunk via the splanchnic nerves. These fibers synapse in the celiac and aorticorenal ganglia, from which postganglionic fibers reach the colon. Sympathetic stimulation causes inhibition of secretion and contraction and stimulates the rectal sphincter, whereas parasympathetic stimulation has the opposite effect.

The large intestine has a variety of functions, and all are related to the final processing of intestinal contents. The most important function is the absorption of water and electrolytes, which is largely completed in the right side of the colon. The sigmoid colon is a reservoir for the dehydrated fecal mass until defecation takes place.

The colon absorbs about 800 ml of water/day compared with about 8000 ml absorbed by the small intestine. The absorption capacity of the large intestine, however, is about 1500 to 2000 ml/day. When this amount is exceeded by excessive delivery of fluid from the ileum, diarrhea results. The final daily excreted feces weighs about 200 g, of which about 80% to 90% is water. The remainder is made up of nonabsorbed food residue, bacteria, desquamated epithelial cells, and unabsorbed minerals.

The small amount of digestion that occurs in the large intestine results from bacterial rather than enzymatic action. The large intestine secretes an alkaline mucus that contains no enzymes. The mucus lubricates and protects the mucosa (see Fig. 6-3).

The bacteria of the large intestine synthesize vitamin K and several vitamins of the B group. Bacterial putrefaction of remaining proteins to amino acids and simpler substances results in the formation of peptides, indole, skatole, phenol, and sulfur compounds. When fatty acids and hydrochloric acid (HCl) are neuralized by bicarbonate, carbon dioxide (CO_2) is produced. The formation of NH_3, CO_2, H_2, H_2S, and CH_4 contributes to flatus (gas) in the colon. Some of these substances are expelled with the feces, and others are absorbed and carried to the liver, where they are changed to less toxic compounds and excreted in the urine.

Bacterial fermentation of the remaining carbohydrates with the release of CO_2, H_2, and CH_4 also contributes to flatus in the colon. About 1000 ml of flatus is normally expelled each day. An excess of gas occurs with *aerophagia* (excessive swallowing of air) and with an increase in intraluminal gas frequently related to the diet. "Gassy foods" such as navy beans have a high content of indigestible carbohydrates.

In general, the movements of the large intestine are slow. A movement characteristic of the large intestine is *haustral churning*. The pouches or haustra become distended, and from time to time the circular muscles contract and cause them to empty. The movements are not progressive but cause the contents to move back and forth in a kneading action, thus allowing time for absorption. There are two types of propulsive peristalsis: (1) slow, irregular contractions that arise in a proximal segment and move forward, obliterating a few haustra; and (2) *mass peristalsis,* which is a contraction involving a large segment of the colon. Mass peristalsis moves the fecal mass forward, eventually stimulating defecation. It occurs two

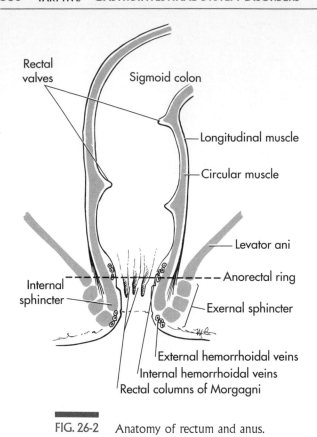

Rectal valves

Sigmoid colon

Longitudinal muscle

Circular muscle

Levator ani

Anorectal ring

Internal sphincter

Exernal sphincter

External hemorrhoidal veins

Internal hemorrhoidal veins

Rectal columns of Morgagni

FIG. 26-2   Anatomy of rectum and anus.

or three times a day and is stimulated by the gastrocolic reflex after eating, particularly after the first meal of the day.

Propulsion of feces into the rectum results in distention of the rectal wall and stimulation of the *defecation reflex.* Fig. 26-2 illustrates the basic anatomy of the rectum and anus. Defecation is controlled by the internal and external anal sphincters. The internal sphincter is controlled by the autonomic nervous system, and the external sphincter is under voluntary control. The defecation reflex is integrated in the second to fourth sacral segments of the spinal cord. Parasympathetic fibers reach the rectum via the pelvic splanchnic nerves and are responsible for contraction of the rectum and relaxation of the internal sphincter. As the distended rectum contracts, the levator ani muscle relaxes, causing the anorectal ring and angle to disappear. The internal and external sphincter muscles relax as the anus is pulled up over the fecal mass. Defecation is facilitated by an increase in intraabdominal pressure brought about by voluntary contraction of the chest muscles on a closed glottis and simultaneous contraction of the abdominal muscles (Valsalva's maneuver or straining). Defecation can be inhibited by voluntary contraction of the levator ani and external sphincter muscles. The rectal wall gradually relaxes, and the urge to defecate passes.

The rectum and anus are the sites of some of the most common disorders known to humans. A common cause of simple constipation is failure to empty the rectum when mass peristalsis occurs. When defecation is not completed, the rectum relaxes and the desire to defecate disappears. Water continues to be absorbed from the fecal mass, causing it to become hard, so subsequent defecation is more difficult. Excessive straining at the stool causes congestion of the internal and external hemorrhoidal veins and is one of the important causes of hemorrhoids (varicose veins of the rectum). Incontinence of stool may result from damage to sphincter muscles or from damage to the spinal cord. The anorectal area is a frequent site of abscesses and fistulas. The colon and rectum are the most frequent sites of cancer of the gastrointestinal (GI) tract.

DIAGNOSTIC PROCEDURES

Diagnosis of pathology associated with the large intestine relates mainly to symptoms associated with elimination. Constipation, diarrhea, alteration in size or color of stool, and the presence of blood in the stools are all important symptoms that focus attention on the colon and rectum. Pain of colonic origin is lateralized to the left or right side of the abdomen, as opposed to pain of small intestinal origin, which is usually paraumbilical.

The history and the physical examination are important diagnostic procedures. Abdominal masses may be palpated, and digital examination is important, since about 15% of all rectal carcinomas are within reach of the examiner's finger. Examination of the stools, sigmoidoscopy, colonoscopy, and radiologic examination are required for a complete assessment in cases of suspected colonic disease.

The *barium enema radiograph* is a common test carried out on patients for identification of disorders of the colon. Preparation or prior cleansing of the intestine is important for a proper examination, but in the presence of an obstructing lesion or active ulcerative colitis, the use of strong cathartics may be hazardous or life-threatening to the patient. Neoplasms, strictures, diverticulosis, and polyps may all be visualized. The cecum and ascending colon may be visualized 3 to 5 hours after a barium swallow. The barium enema radiograph should always precede the barium swallow.

Direct visualization of the terminal 25 cm of the large intestine is possible through the *rigid proctosigmoidoscope.* Sixty percent of all the tumors of the large intestine can be visualized directly with this instrument. In addition to visual inspection of the area, bacteriologic, parasitologic, and cytologic studies can be made on washings through the instrument, and biopsy of suspicious lesions is easy to perform. The *flexible fiberoptic colonoscope* allows visualization and biopsy of lesions of the entire colon. Experienced examiners may be able to insert the instrument as far as the terminal ileum.

DIVERTICULAR DISEASE OF THE COLON

Diverticulosis is a condition of the colon characterized by herniation of the mucosa through the muscularis to form flask-shaped saccules. If one or more of the saccules become inflamed, the condition is called *diverticulitis*.

Pathophysiology

The overall incidence of diverticulosis is high; it affects about 10% of the population, according to most necropsy studies. It is rare in those younger than 35 years but increases with age, so that at age 85 two thirds of the population are afflicted. The most common site for diverticula to occur is in the sigmoid colon, which is involved in about 90% of the cases.

Although the etiology of diverticulosis is unknown, recent motility and pressure studies have done much to support the possibility that diverticular disease may result from a disordered motility pattern of the colon. Fig. 26-3 illustrates the normal motility pattern in the colon and the proposed pathogenic mechanism of diverticulosis. Diverticula-bearing zones of the colon are prone to strong contractions of the circular muscles, which build up high intraluminal pressures. It seems likely that these high pressures are responsible for herniations of the mucosa through the muscle coat, which become diverticula. The usual position for the diverticula is at the mesenteric attachment of the colon, where the entry of blood vessels weakens the wall. The pressure changes in diverticular disease are similar to those found in spastic or irritable colon syndrome, which is believed by many to have a basis in anxiety and emotional tension.

A factor of even greater importance in the etiology of diverticular disease relates to the amount of roughage in the diet. Diverticulosis is rare in those who eat a diet high in roughage but is common in Europeans and North Americans (of all races) who eat a low-roughage diet. The tension or strain on the wall of a hollow organ is related to the pressure within and to the diameter of the organ. If a tube such as the colon is habitually of narrow bore (as the result of a low-fiber diet), the strain on the wall from a buildup of pressure is greater than if it were filled with feces.

Clinical Features and Complications

Most patients with diverticulosis have no symptoms, and the problem remains unidentified unless a barium enema radiographic or endoscopic study is performed in the investigation of some unrelated condition. When diverticula are discovered, it is important for the physician to rule out carcinoma. This differentiation is made by the radiographic appearance, colonoscopic examination, and biopsy. A barium enema radiographic study is dangerous during an attack of acute diverticulitis because of the danger of perforation.

In many patients, symptoms are mild and consist of flatulence, intermittent diarrhea or constipation, and discomfort in the lower left quadrant of the abdomen. These symptoms can usually be attributed to the irritable colon syndrome that may precede the development of diverticulosis in some patients.

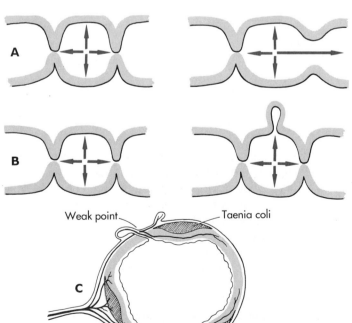

FIG. 26-3   Pathogenesis of diverticular disease. **A,** Normal motility pattern. **B,** Abnormal motility pattern in which there is failure of relaxation and buildup of high intraluminal pressure, resulting in the formation of a diverticulum. **C,** Cross section of colon showing that the weak point in the circular muscle is where a blood vessel pierces the muscle. Herniation of the lining mucosa and the formation of diverticuli develop at these points.

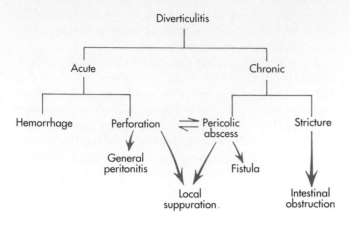

FIG. 26-4   Complications of diverticulitis.

The complications of diverticular disease are the result of acute or chronic diverticulitis, which may result in bleeding, perforation and peritonitis, abscess and fistula formation, or intestinal obstruction from stricture (Fig. 26-4).

In the case of acute diverticulitis, fever, leukocytosis, and pain and tenderness in the lower left quadrant of the abdomen are present. During a bout of acute inflammation, bleeding may occur from vascular granulation tissue and is usually minor. In rare instances, bleeding may be massive as a result of erosion of the large penetrating blood vessel next to the diverticula. Bleeding is usually treated conservatively, but on rare occasions a bowel resection is necessary.

Sometimes, acutely inflamed diverticula rupture. If the perforation is small, the result may be abscess formation next to the perforated diverticulum. If the perforation is large, fecal material may enter the peritoneum and cause a most severe form of peritonitis with a high mortality. Symptoms of perforation are similar to those of a perforated ulcer except that pain, rigidity, and tenderness are most marked in the lower left quadrant.

The term *chronic diverticulitis* applies to a bowel subjected to repeated attacks of inflammation. The result may be fibrosis and adhesions of the surrounding structures. When chronic inflammation has caused significant narrowing of the lumen, chronic incomplete bowel obstruction may result, giving rise to symptoms of constipation, ribbonlike stools, intermittent diarrhea, and abdominal distention. The final obstructive picture may be precipitated by a superimposed acute attack, leading to a pericolic abscess that narrows the already occluded lumen. A fistula may also form as a complication of a pericolic abscess. The most common type is the vesicosigmoid fistula. The flow is usually from the colon to the bladder, and the complaint is *pneumaturia,* or the passage of air bubbles (gas) in the urine. The fistula may also lead to the small bowel or peritoneum.

Treatment

If diverticula are discovered incidentally and the patient is asymptomatic, they are not generally treated. However, 90% of patients with diverticulitis are treated medically. Those with mild cases without signs of perforation are treated with a liquid diet or intravenous (IV) fluids, stool softeners, bedrest, and a broad-spectrum antibiotic. Antibiotics effective against gram-negative anaerobic bacteria may be given to patients with suspected perforation or abscess. Incision and drainage of abscesses may be necessary. After the acute phase, a high-residue diet is indicated.

Surgical intervention is needed only for severe and extensive disease or in the event of complications. The essential surgical treatment is resection of the diseased colon with anastomosis to restore continuity. In the absence of complications, the surgery may be carried out in one stage. In other cases the surgeon may perform a temporary colostomy (diversion of the colon to the abdominal surface). Anastomosis and closure are then carried out at a later date.

INFLAMMATORY DISEASE OF THE LARGE INTESTINE

Chronic inflammatory disease of the large bowel is divided into two major entities: nonspecific ulcerative colitis and Crohn's disease of the large bowel (granulomatous colitis). Although these two conditions have many features in common, enough differences exist to separate them into two distinct clinical entities. Table 26-1 lists the differentiating features of these two diseases. There are enough overlapping features to lead some investigators to believe that both these diseases may represent variations in response to the same etiologic agent.

Ulcerative Colitis

Ulcerative colitis is a nonspecific inflammatory disease of the colon generally following a prolonged course characterized by alternating periods of remissions and exacerbations. Abdominal pain, diarrhea, and rectal bleeding are the cardinal signs and symptoms. The essential lesion is an inflammatory reaction of the subepithelial zone developing at the base of the crypts of Lieberkühn, which may eventually produce ulceration of the mucosa (Color plate 27). The peak onset of the disease is between ages 15 and 40 years, and the disorder is equally distributed between the genders. The incidence of ulcerative colitis is about 1 per 10,000 white adults per year. Crohn's disease is about one fourth as common. Both diseases are less common in nonwhites.

▶ TABLE 26-1   Differentiating Features of Ulcerative Colitis and Crohn's Disease

Characteristic Feature	Ulcerative Colitis	Crohn's Disease
Depth of involvement	Mucosa and submucosa	Transmural
Granulomatous inflammatory response	Rare	Common
Rectal involvement	95%	50%
Small bowel involvement	Usually normal	80%
Right colon involvement	Occasional	Frequent
Distribution of lesion	Continuous with rectum	Discontinuous "skip" lesions
Inflammatory mass	Rare	Usually palpable
Diarrhea	Common	Common
Rectal bleeding	Common, continuous	Rare
Internal fistulas	Rare	Common
Anal abscesses	Occasional	Common
Anorectal fissures and fistulas	Rare	Common
Cobblestone appearance of mucosa	Unusual (pseudopolyps, granular, shaggy)	Common
Toxic megacolon	Occasional	Rare
Malignant potential	High after 10 years	Low
Extragastrointestinal manifestation (e.g., arthritis, eye and skin involvement)	Occasional	Less frequent than in ulcerative colitis
Strictures	Occasional, mild	Common
Finger clubbing	Rare	Common
Relative frequency	Three to four times more common than Crohn's disease	
Familial and Jewish association	Yes	Yes
Autoantibodies	Frequent	Not found

Etiology and pathogenesis

The etiology of ulcerative colitis, as with that of Crohn's disease, is unknown. Genetic factors seem to be involved in the etiology, since a definite familial relationship exists among ulcerative colitis, Crohn's disease, and ankylosing spondylitis.

Evidence also suggests that autoimmunity is involved in the pathogenesis of ulcerative colitis. Humoral antibodies to colon cells have been found in the serum of patients with this disease. However, studies do not indicate that patients with ulcerative colitis have more immune complexes present (Glickman, 1994).

The psychologic aspects of ulcerative colitis have been the subject of much controversy. It now seems that psychologic stress is not related to the etiology of ulcerative colitis.

The initial pathologic lesion is confined to the mucosal layer and consists of abscess formation in the crypts, as opposed to Crohn's disease, which involves the entire thickness of the bowel wall. Early in the disease, edema and congestion of the mucosa occur. The edema may lead to extreme friability, so that bleeding occurs from any minor trauma, such as the surface being lightly rubbed.

In more advanced stages of the disease, the crypt abscess breaks through the wall of the crypt and spreads in the submucosa, undermining the mucosa. The mucosa is then shed into the bowel lumen, leaving areas of denuded mucosa (ulcers). Ulceration is at first scattered and shallow, but at a later stage the mucosal surface is lost over wide areas, leading to considerable loss of tissue, protein, and blood.

Clinical features

The three common clinical types of ulcerative colitis are related to frequency of symptoms. The *acute fulminating* ulcerative colitis is characterized by an abrupt onset, with severe, bloody diarrhea, nausea, vomiting, and fever, which causes a rapid depletion of fluids and electrolytes. The entire colon may be involved, with undermining and stripping of the mucosa, causing loss of considerable blood and mucus. This type of colitis occurs in about 10% of the patients. The prognosis is poor, and toxic megacolon is a frequent complication.

Most patients with ulcerative colitis have the *chronic intermittent (recurrent)* type of colitis. The onset tends to be insidious, occurring over months to years. The mild form of the disease is characterized by short attacks occurring at intervals of months to years and lasting 1 to 3 months. There may be little or no fever or constitutional symptoms, and usually only the distal colon is affected. Fever and systemic symptoms may accompany the more severe form, and the attack may last 3 or 4 months, sometimes passing into the *chronic continuous* type of disease. In the chronic continuous disease, the patient continues to have diarrhea after the initial attack. As compared with the intermittent type, more of the colon tends to be involved and complications are more frequent.

In mild forms of ulcerative colitis, diarrhea may be mild and bleeding is intermittent and slight. In severe disease, there are more than six stools per day with considerable blood and mucus. The chronic loss of blood and mucus may lead to anemia and hypoproteinemia. Severe, colicky pain may be present in the lower abdomen and is relieved somewhat by defecation. Few deaths occur directly from this disease, but it may be mildly or severely disabling.

The diagnosis of ulcerative colitis is usually straightforward. There is diarrhea with passage of blood, and sigmoidoscopy reveals a friable and intensely inflamed mucosa with exudate. In 95% of the cases the rectosigmoid area of the colon is involved. The disease may extend from this area but always in a continuous fashion, in contrast to Crohn's disease, which tends to skip. Barium radiographic studies of the colon aid in determining the extent of more proximal changes but should not be done during an acute attack, since they may precipitate toxic megacolon and perforation. Colonoscopy and biopsy can often differentiate ulcerative colitis from granulomatous colitis.

Complications

Complications of ulcerative colitis may be local or systemic. Rectal fistulas, fissures, and abscesses are not as common as in granulomatous colitis. Occasionally a rectovaginal fistula forms. A few patients may have narrowing of the bowel lumen as a result of fibrosis, which is generally mild as compared with Crohn's disease.

One of the more serious complications is *toxic dilation,* or *megacolon,* in which there is paralysis of the motor function of the transverse colon, with rapid dilation of that segment of the bowel. Toxic megacolon is most frequently associated with pancolitis. The mortality is about 30%, and perforation of the bowel frequently results. The treatment for this complication is emergency colectomy. Massive hemorrhage is another complication sometimes requiring emergency colectomy.

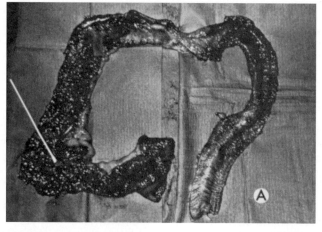

FIG. 26-5   Some complications of ulcerative colitis. **A,** Hemorrhage: surgical specimen of large intestine removed from a patient with ulcerative colitis to control bleeding. The probe is at the site of a small perforation. **B,** Toxic megacolon: the large, dilated colon protruding through a surgical incision. **C,** Pyoderma gangrenosum: a necrotic skin ulcer found in association with inflammatory bowel disease. (Courtesy of Daniel J. Fall, MD, St. Joseph Mercy Hospital, Ypsilanti, Mich.)

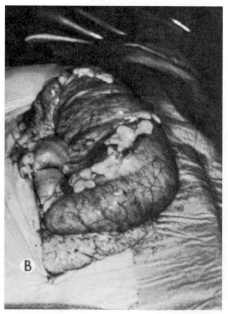

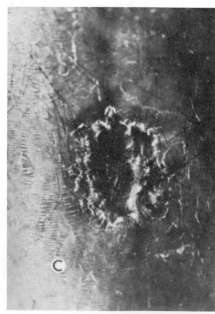

Another significant complication is carcinoma of the colon, which occurs with increasing frequency after the patient has had the disease for more than 10 years. After patients have had total colon involvement with ulcerative colitis for 25 years, the probability of cancer is increased to 40%.

The systemic complications are diverse, and it is difficult to relate some of them causally to the colonic disease. These include pyoderma gangrenosum, episcleritis, uveitis, arthritis, and ankylosing spondylitis. Disordered hepatic function is common in ulcerative colitis. The presence of severe systemic complications may be an indication for surgical treatment of the colitis, even when the colonic symptoms are mild (Fig. 26-5; Color plate 28).

Treatment

No cure or specific medical treatment exists for ulcerative colitis. The aims of therapy are to control the inflammation, maintain the patient's nutritional status, give symptomatic relief, and prevent infection and other complications.

Corticosteroid drugs are given to reduce inflammation and induce clinical remission. Sulfonamide drugs are given, but their mechanism of action is poorly understood. A low-residue diet causes diminution in the number of stools and thereby makes the patient more comfortable. The diet must also be high in protein to compensate for that lost in the exudative lesions; the diet should be high in vitamins as well. During exacerbations, tincture of opium and paregoric are sometimes given to control diarrhea. Anticholingeric drugs may also help relieve the abdominal cramps and diarrhea. Agents to control diarrhea should be used with caution to avoid precipitating colonic dilation and toxic megacolon. Emotional support and reassurance are important aspects of treatment.

When medical management fails and when the condition becomes intractable, surgical intervention is indicated. The most common procedure performed is total colectomy and the creation of a permanent ileostomy. Some physicians also recommend a colectomy for all patients who have had total colon involvement for several years, since the incidence of carcinoma of the colon in these patients is so high. Colon cancer is difficult to diagnose in these patients, since such symptoms as weight loss or bloody stools may be regarded as another exacerbation of the ulcerative colitis rather than as signs of cancer.

NEOPLASMS OF THE LARGE INTESTINE

Neoplasms of the colon and rectum may be benign or malignant. True benign neoplasms (lipomas, carcinoid tumors, and leiomyomas) are rare in the colon. Colonic polyps, however, are common and occupy an intermediate position between benign and malignant neoplasms.

Colonic Polyps

A *polyp* is a growth that arises from a mucosal surface and extends outward. There are three recognized patterns of colonic polyps: pedunculated adenomas, villous adenomas, and familial polyposis.

Pedunculated adenomas (also called adenomatous polyps or polypoid adenomas) are globelike structures attached to the mucous membrane by a thin stalk. This type of polyp occurs in both genders and in all age-groups, although they become increasingly common with advancing age. Autopsy and sigmoidoscopy studies indicate that about 9% of the population over age 45 years are afflicted. Although pedunculated polyps may occur in any part of the colon, they are more frequently located in the distal 10 to 12 inches (25 to 30 cm). Pedunculated polyps may be singular or multiple; they are usually ⅕ to ⅖ inch (0.5 to 1 cm) in diameter but may be as large as 1⅗ to 2 inches (4 or 5 cm). Histologically, these polyps consist of proliferating glands. The relationship of adenomatous polyps to cancer of the colon is a subject of great controversy, since they have much the same distribution in the colon as cancer and are often associated with cancer. The prevailing opinion is that they are harmless. However, if the polyps are multiple or if the head is greater than 1 cm in diameter, the chances of malignancy are higher.

Another form of pedunculated polyp occurring most frequently in children younger than 10 years is the *juvenile polyp*. Juvenile polyps are often large and vascular and have long pedicles. They are believed to be inflammatory in origin and may present by bleeding or prolapse through the anus. Juvenile polyps occasionally occur in adults.

The *villous adenoma* (villous papilloma, sessile adenoma), in contrast to the pedunculated adenoma, is a sessile (broad-based) tumor. The surface is distinctly papillary to the naked eye and appears as a nodular mass. Histologically, the lesion is composed of fingerlike (villous) projections. It is usually solitary and located in the sigmoid colon or rectum. Villous adenomas are generally large (greater than 5 cm) and are about one eighth as frequent as pedunculated adenomas. Malignancy is much more likely to occur in these tumors (with a 25% chance) than in the pedunculated adenomas.

Familial polyposis is a rare disorder transmitted genetically as a dominant trait and characterized by the presence of hundreds of adenomatous polyps, both pedunculated and sessile, throughout the entire large intestine. Both genders are equally affected. The polyps are not present at birth but usually appear about the time of puberty. The probability of the development of cancer increases with age and is almost 100% by age 40.

Clinical features

Most adenomatous polyps are asymptomatic and are found incidentally on examination by sigmoidoscopy, by barium enema, or on autopsy. When polyps do give rise to symptoms, these generally consist of overt or occult bleeding. Occasionally a large polyp may initiate an intussusception and cause bowel obstruction (see Fig. 25-5, *D*). Diarrhea and mucus discharge may be associated with large villous adenomas and familial polyposis.

Treatment

The treatment of colonic polyps is influenced by the debate concerning their malignant potential. Because there is no question about the malignant potential in familial polyposis, this condition is treated by total proctocolectomy and permanent ileostomy or subtotal resection with ileorectal anastomosis. When the rectum is preserved, it is examined periodically for cancer.

The guidelines for the treatment of pedunculated or villous adenomas are not as clear. In general, polyps that are greater than 2 cm in diameter, multiple, or villous are regarded with a high degree of suspicion and should be removed. Polyps that are pedunculated, singular, and less than 1 cm in diameter are rarely malignant and can be observed periodically.

Polyps may be excised from below through the sigmoidoscope or colonoscope. Larger lesions and villous adenomas are treated by laporotomy and segmental resection.

Carcinoma of the Colon and Rectum

The colon (including the rectum) is the most common site for malignancy of the GI tract. Cancer of the colon is the third most common cause of all cancer deaths in both men and women in the United States (American Cancer Society, 1995). Cancer of the large intestine is usually a disease of older people, with peak incidence in the 50- and 60-year-olds. It is rare in those younger than 40 years, except in persons with a history of ulcerative colitis or familial polyposis. The genders are affected about equally. Approximately 60% of all the cancers of the bowel occur in the rectosigmoid portion, so they may be either palpated during a rectal examination or viewed with a sigmoidoscope. The cecum and ascending colon are the next most common sites. The transverse colon and flexures are least likely to be affected.

The tumor may present as a *polypoid,* bulky, fungating mass projecting into the lumen and quickly becoming ulcerated. It may extend around the bowel as an *annular* (ringlike) stricture. Annular lesions are more common in the rectosigmoid portion of the bowel, whereas polypoid flat lesions are more common in the cecum and ascending colon. Histologically, almost all the large bowel cancers are *adenocarcinomas* (composed of glandular epithelium) and may secrete mucus to a varying degree. The tumor may spread (1) by direct infiltration of adjacent structures, as into the bladder; (2) by lymphatics to the pericolic and mesocolic lymph nodes; and (3) by the bloodstream, usually to the liver, since the colon is drained by the portal system. The prognosis is relatively favorable when the lesion is confined to the mucosa and submucosa at the time of surgical resection and much less favorable when lymph node metastasis has occurred.

Etiology

Although the causes of cancer of the large bowel, as with other cancers, have not been established, certain predisposing factors have been identified. The relationship between ulcerative colitis, certain types of colonic polyps, and cancer of the bowel has already been discussed.

Another important predisposing factor may relate to dietary habits, since cancer of the bowel (as with diverticulosis) is about 10 times more common in Western populations, who eat foods high in refined carbohydrates and low in roughage, than in emerging populations (e.g., in Africa), who eat foods high in roughage. Burkitt (1971) proposed that a low-fiber, highly refined carbohydrate diet leads to alterations in fecal flora and changes in the degradation of bile salts or of the breakdown products of protein and fat, some of which may be carcinogenic. A low-fiber diet allows concentration of these potential carcinogens into a smaller volume of stool. In addition, the transit time is increased. The net result is prolonged contact time of potential carcinogens with the bowel mucosa.

Screening

Because colorectal cancer causes approximately 60,000 deaths per year in the United States, some organizations (e.g., National Cancer Institute, American Cancer Society, American College of Physicians) have endorsed guidelines for screening so that colorectal cancer can be detected at a curable stage to help reduce morbidity and mortality of this disease. Strategies for screening of asymptomatic persons are recommended as follows: (1) men and women over 40 years of age should receive annual digital rectal examinations, and (2) persons over 50 years of age should have a fecal occult blood test annually and a sigmoidoscopy examination every 3 to 5 years after two initial examinations a year apart. Persons at high risk because of family history should also have the total colon examined by either a air-contrast barium enema or colonoscopy every 3 to 5 years. Other organizations have found that insufficient evidence exists to do occult blood tests or sigmoidoscopy examinations in asymptomatic persons; however, they suggest offering screening to persons 50 years of age and older with known risk factors for colorectal cancer.

Clinical features

The most common symptoms of cancer of the bowel are changes in bowel habits, bleeding, pain, anemia, anorexia, and weight loss. The signs and symptoms vary according to the location and are usually divided into those affecting the right and left halves of the large bowel.

Carcinoma of the left colon and rectum tends to cause

a change in bowel habits as a result of irritation and reflex responses. Diarrhea, crampy pain, and distention are common. Because lesions of the left colon tend to encircle, obstruction is a common problem. Stool may be narrow and ribbonlike in shape. Both mucus and gross blood are often visible on the feces. Anemia may result from chronic blood loss. A sigmoid or rectal growth may involve nerve roots, lymphatics, or veins, producing symptoms in the legs or perineum. Hemorrhoids, low back pain, rectal urgency, or urinary frequency may develop as a result of pressure on these structures.

Carcinoma of the right colon, where the bowel contents are liquid, tends to remain occult until far advanced. There is little tendency to obstruct, since the bowel lumen is larger and the feces are liquid. Anemia caused by bleeding is common, but the blood is occult and can be detected only by a guaiac test (a simple test that may be performed on the clinical unit). Because bleeding may be intermittent, an endoscopic or full-bowel radiographic examination may be indicated when anemia persists. Mucus is likewise not visible because it is well mixed in the stool. In the thin person, a tumor of the right colon may sometimes be palpated, but this is not typical at an early stage. The patient may have vague abdominal discomfort that is sometimes epigastric.

Treatment

The treatment of carcinoma of the colon and rectum is surgical removal of the tumor and its lymphatic drainage. The most common procedures performed are the right hemicolectomy, transverse colectomy, left hemicolectomy or anterior resection, and abdominoperineal resection. The results of surgical tumor resection are fairly good compared with results with cancer in other areas of the body. The overall 5-year survival rate is approximately 50%.

ANORECTAL DISORDERS

Hemorrhoids

Hemorrhoids, or "piles," are varicose veins of the anal canal. They are divided into two classes, internal and external. *Internal hemorrhoids* are varices of the superior and middle hemorrhoidal veins, and *external hemorrhoids* are varices of the inferior hemorrhoidal veins. As the terms imply, external hemorrhoids appear external to the sphincter ani muscles, and the internal hemorrhoids appear above (or alternately, proximal to) the sphincter.

Both types of hemorrhoids are common and are present in about 35% of the population over age 25 years. Although the condition is not life-threatening, it may cause considerable discomfort.

Hemorrhoids result from venous congestion caused by interference with venous return from the hemorrhoidal veins. Several etiologic factors have been implicated, including constipation or diarrhea, straining, pelvic congestion associated with pregnancy, enlargement of the prostate, uterine fibroids, and tumors of the rectum. Chronic liver disease associated with portal hypertension frequently results in hemorrhoids, since the superior hemorrhoidal veins drain into the portal system (see Fig. 27-2). In addition, the portal system is valveless, so backflow readily occurs.

External hemorrhoids are classified as acute or chronic. The *acute* form presents as a bluish, rounded swelling at the anal verge and is actually a hematoma, although it is referred to as an acute external thrombosed hemorrhoid. These are often quite painful and pruritic because the nerve endings in the skin are pain receptors. Sometimes it is necessary to evacuate the clot under local anesthesia, or it may be treated by hot sitz baths and analgesics. A *chronic* external hemorrhoid or *skin tag* is usually the sequela to an acute hematoma. Anal skin tags consist of one or more folds of anal skin composed of connective tissue and a few blood vessels.

Internal hemorrhoids are classified as first, second, and third degree. *First-degree (early)* internal hemorrhoids do not protrude through the anal canal and can be detected only by proctoscopy. They are usually located in the right and left posterior and right anterior positions, following the distribution of the tributaries of the superior hemorrhoidal vein, and appear as globular reddish swellings. *Second-degree* hemorrhoids may prolapse through the anal canal after defecation; they may recede spontaneously or can be reduced manually. *Third-degree* hemorrhoids are permanently prolapsed. The most common symptom of internal hemorrhoids is painless bleeding, since no pain fibers exist in this area. Most cases of hemorrhoids are of the mixed variety rather than being strictly internal or external.

The most common complications of hemorrhoids are bleeding, thrombosis, and strangulation. A strangulated hemorrhoid is a prolapsed one in which the blood supply is cut off by the anal sphincter.

Diagnosis of hemorrhoids is made by inspection, digital examination, and viewing through a proctoscope or anoscope. It is important to rule out carcinoma when hemorrhoids occur in the middle and later years.

Most patients with hemorrhoids need not undergo surgery. Medical treatment includes sitz baths, or other forms of moist heat, bed rest, stool softeners to prevent constipation, high-roughage diet, and the use of soothing suppositories. Surgical excision may be indicated when there is persistent bleeding, prolapse, or intractable pruritus and anal pain.

Anal Fissure (Fissure in Ano)

An *anal fissure (fissure in ano)* is a crack in the lining of the anus caused by stretching from the passage of hard fecal matter; therefore constipation is a common cause. It is also caused by diarrhea and the persistent tightening of the anal canal as a result of emotional stress. The most prominent symptom is severe burning pain after defecation, and the bowel movement is usually accompanied by a small amount of bright-red blood. These patients are nearly always constipated; since the bowel movement is so painful, the constipation becomes progressively worse because they fear to have a bowel movement. Anal fissures are often seen in association with the skin tags of external hemorrhoids. Treatment is surgical excision of the tract if local dilations, ointments, and cleansing do not help.

Anorectal Abscess and Fistula in Ano

An *anorectal abscess* is a localized infection, with the collection of pus in the anorectal area. The infecting organisms are usually *Escherichia coli,* staphylococci, or streptococci. A *fistula in ano* is a chronic granulomatous tract that proceeds in a linear path from the anal canal to the skin outside the anus or from an abscess to the anal canal or the perirectal area. An anorectal fistula is often preceded by abscess formation. Fig. 26-6 illustrates the sites of abscess and fistula formation. The perianal abscess is the most common type of anorectal abscess, followed by the ischiorectal, submucous, and pelvirectal locations. The perianal abscess is usually obvious as a red, painful swelling close to the anal verge. The pain is aggravated by sitting or coughing. A submucous or ischiorectal abscess may be palpated as a swelling on rectal examination. A pelvirectal abscess may be more difficult to identify. Discharge of pus from an anorectal fistula may be the first sign. Sometimes a fistula may be palpated or its course determined by the gentle passage of a probe from the external opening, with a finger of the other hand in the anal canal.

Anorectal abscesses typically begin as an inflamma-

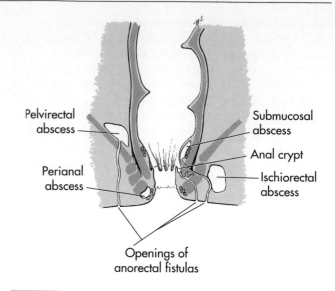

FIG. 26-6   Common sites of anorectal abscesses and fistulas. Inflammation often begins in the anal crypts.

tion of the anal crypts, which are located at the lower end of the columns of Morgagni (see Fig. 26-2). The anal glands open into these crypts. Obstruction or trauma to their ducts gives rise to stasis and predisposes to infection. Mucosal tears from hard, constipated stools may be a predisposing factor. In a few cases a predisposing local lesion such as an ulcerated hemorrhoid or anal fissure may be present.

When symptoms of diarrhea are associated with recurrent anorectal fistulas, Crohn's disease must be suspected, since as many as 50% of patients with Crohn's disease develop a fistula in ano.

The treatment of anorectal abscesses and fistulas is incision and drainage of the abscess and excision of any associated fistulas.

QUESTIONS

▼ *Answer the following on a separate sheet of paper.*

1. Draw a picture of the large intestine in the abdominal and pelvic cavities and label the parts with the following terms: appendix; cecum; ascending, transverse, descending, and sigmoid colon; rectum; anal canal; anus; hepatic and splenic flexures; haustra; and taenia coli.
2. What are the most important functions of the large bowel?
3. Discuss the differences in structure between the small and large bowel. How do these lead to differences in function?
4. Briefly summarize the mechanical operation of the large bowel (haustral churning, mass peristalsis).
5. List five common anorectal disorders.
6. List the most common diagnostic procedures used for the detection of disease of the large bowel. What can be detected with each?
7. Do all cases of acute diverticulitis require surgical intervention? If not, what is the medical treatment for acute diverticulitis?
8. Identify three predisposing factors in the pathogenesis of cancer of the colon or rectum.
9. What is Burkitt's hypothesis concerning the relationship of diet to the development of cancer of the bowel?
10. Why are hemorrhoids a frequent manifestation of hepatic cirrhosis and portal hypertension?
11. Define fissure in ano and fistula in ano. Is there any relationship between these two disorders and hemorrhoids? What disease of the gastrointestinal tract is often associated with anorectal fistulas?

QUESTIONS—cont'd

▼ *Circle the letter preceding each item that correctly answers the question or completes the statement. Only one answer is correct, unless otherwise noted.*

12. The right half of the colon receives its blood supply from the:
    a. Superior mesenteric artery
    b. Splenic artery
    c. Inferior mesenteric artery
    d. Left colic artery

13. The superior hemorrhoidal veins are part of the:
    a. Portal circulation
    b. Systemic circulation

14. The major reservoir for feces is in which segment of the large bowel?
    a. Cecum
    b. Transverse colon
    c. Ascending colon
    d. Descending colon
    e. Sigmoid colon

15. In which segment of the colon is the greatest amount of water absorbed?
    a. Cecum and ascending colon
    b. Descending and sigmoid colon
    c. Rectum

16. Which of the following statements are true about colonic mucus (more than one answer may be correct)?
    a. It is under autonomic control.
    b. Parasympathetic stimulation causes an increase in mucus production.
    c. The colonic mucosa maintains a layer of mucus on its surface.
    d. The presence of visible mucus in the stools indicates overproduction.

17. Variations in intestinal gas normally depend on (more than one answer may be correct):
    a. How much air is swallowed
    b. Variations in diet
    c. Type of intestinal bacteria
    d. Weight of the individual

18. The desire to defecate is initiated by:
    a. Contraction of the external anal sphincter
    b. Contraction of the internal anal sphincter
    c. Contraction of the rectum
    d. Distention of the sigmoid colon
    e. Distention of the rectum

19. Substances produced by bacterial putrefaction in the large intestine are:
    a. Indole
    b. Skatole
    c. Phenol
    d. Amino acids and fatty acids
    e. All of these

20. The cecum and ascending colon may be visualized radiographically within how many hours after a barium meal?
    a. ½
    b. 1 to 2
    c. 3 to 5
    d. 10 to 12

21. Approximately what percentage of rectal and large bowel tumors may be visualized or palpated on rectal digital or proctosigmoidoscopic examination?
    a. 100%
    b. 60% to 70%
    c. 25% to 35%
    d. 10% to 20%

22. Which of the following statements concerning diverticulosis is true (more than one answer may be correct)?
    a. It is a common condition in persons over the age of 50 years in the United States.
    b. It occurs more frequently in Africans, who eat a high-fiber diet.
    c. It is frequently associated with or preceded by the irritable colon syndrome.
    d. Disordered colonic motility with generation of high intraluminal pressures in the colon is important in the pathogenesis.
    e. Diverticula of the colon form most frequently at the point where arterioles penetrate the muscularis.

23. Diverticula are most common in which segment of the colon?
    a. Cecum
    b. Ascending colon
    c. Transverse colon
    d. Descending colon
    e. Sigmoid colon

24. The most common symptom of an attack of acute diverticulitis is:
    a. Pain in the lower left quadrant of the abdomen
    b. Pain in the lower right quadrant of the abdomen
    c. Vomiting
    d. Massive bleeding from the rectum

25. The most common complications of acute or chronic diverticulitis are (more than one answer may be correct):
    a. Massive bleeding requiring emergency colectomy
    b. Perforation
    c. Stricture causing partial bowel obstruction
    d. Vesicosigmoid fistula

26. The most common site of fistula formation as a result of a perforated diverticulum is the:
    a. Peritoneum
    b. Small intestine
    c. Urinary bladder
    d. Vagina

27. Which of the following is the most common clinical course of ulcerative colitis?
    a. Acute fulminating
    b. Acute onset with full recovery
    c. Chronic continuous
    d. Chronic continuous with full recovery after 5 to 10 years
    e. Chronic intermittent (relapsing-remitting course)

28. Patients with ulcerative colitis may reveal abnormalities in which of the following organ systems (more than one answer may be correct)?
    a. Joints
    b. Heart
    c. Eyes
    d. Lungs
    e. Skin

29. The rectosigmoid segment of the large bowel is involved in what percentage of cases of ulcerative colitis?
    a. 15%
    b. 25%
    c. 75%
    d. 95%

30. Which of the following statements are true concerning toxic megacolon (more than one answer may be correct)?
    a. It is often associated with pancolitis.
    b. The motor function of a bowel segment is paralyzed.
    c. The transverse colon is frequently affected.
    d. It is usually treated medically.
    e. It is associated with a high mortality.

31. A cardinal symptom or sign of ulcerative colitis is:
    a. Constipation
    b. Diarrhea with blood and mucus in the stool
    c. Ribbon-shaped stools
    d. Periumbilical pain

32. Some of the known extracolonic manifestations of ulcerative colitis are (more than one answer may be correct):
    a. Uveitis
    b. Pyoderma gangrenosum
    c. Episcleritis
    d. Arthritis
    e. Ankylosing spondylitis

33. Skin manifestations are associated with

Continued.

? QUESTIONS—cont'd

which of the following disorders (more than one answer may be correct)?
a. Diverticulosis
b. Ulcerative colitis
c. Cancer of the colon
d. Granulomatous colitis
e. Regional enteritis

34. The role of adrenal steroid drugs in the treatment of ulcerative colitis is to:
a. Cure the active disease
b. Induce clinical remission
c. Prevent recurrence completely

35. The most common surgical treatment for intractable ulcerative colitis is:
a. Right hemicolectomy
b. Left hemicolectomy
c. Total colectomy with permanent ileostomy
d. Cecostomy

36. Cancer of the bowel involving which of the following sites is frequently diagnosed late in its course?
a. Cecum
b. Descending colon
c. Sigmoid colon
d. Rectum

37. The most common cause of death secondary to gastrointestinal cancer in the United States is from cancer of the:
a. Esophagus
b. Stomach
c. Small intestine
d. Colon and rectum

38. The most common symptom of cancer of the right colon is:
a. Change in bowel habits
b. Pain
c. Constipation
d. Gross blood in the stools
e. Diarrhea

39. Symptoms that frequently accompany cancer of the left colon include (more than one answer may be correct):
a. Change in bowel habits
b. Melena
c. Back pain
d. Abdominal cramps

40. Which statements are true with respect to adenomatous polyps (more than one answer may be correct)?

a. It is the most common type of benign tumor in the colon.
b. They are most frequently located in the distal 25 to 30 cm of the bowel.
c. They are familial.
d. They occur more frequently in patients with cancer of the large bowel.
e. They are generally benign when singular or less than 1 cm in diameter.

41. Familial polyposis of the colon is characterized by (more than one answer may be correct):
a. Densely packed polyps throughout the colon
b. An inheritable recessive trait
c. Marked predisposition to cancer of the large bowel
d. Alopecia

42. The most common site of malignant lesions of the large bowel is:
a. Rectosigmoid area
b. Descending colon
c. Cecum
d. Transverse colon

▼ *Fill in the blanks with the correct word(s) or circle the correct option.*

43. _____ is a condition in which there is herniation of the mucosa through the muscularis of the large bowel to form flask-shaped saccules. The condition is called _____ when the saccules become inflamed.

44. _____ adenoma or adenomatous polyp is a globelike structure on a pedicle arising from a mucosal surface. _____ polyps have very long pedicles and often occur in children.
A _____ adenoma is a broad-based tumor composed of villous projections. _____ _____ is a hereditary disease characterized by the presence of hundreds of polyps throughout the colon.

45. An encircling or _____ form of cancer growth is more common in the left colon, whereas the shape is more likely to be _____ in the cecum.

46. Three routes of spread of cancer of the bowel are _____, _____, and _____.

47. Internal hemorrhoids are varicosities of the _____ and _____ hemorrhoidal veins and are located (inside or outside) the anal sphincters. The _____ hemorrhoidal veins are involved in external hemorrhoids.

48. Three common complications of hemorrhoids are _____, _____, and _____.

QUESTIONS—cont'd

▼ *Match each of the following characteristic features of inflammatory bowel disease in column A with the correct disorder in column B.*

Column A

49. _____ Caused by a specific infectious agent
50. _____ Granulomatous inflammation
51. _____ Familial and Jewish association
52. _____ Transmural lesion common
53. _____ Internal fistulas common
54. _____ Lesions continuous with rectum
55. _____ High malignant potential after 10 years
56. _____ Most often associated with toxic megacolon
57. _____ More common disease of the two
58. _____ "Skip" lesions common
59. _____ May represent an immunologic disorder
60. _____ Anorectal abscesses, fissures, and fistulas common complications

Column B

a. Crohn's disease
b. Ulcerative colitis
c. Both
d. Neither

61. Rank the following types of colonic polyps according to malignant potential, with 1 being the highest:
   a. Villous adenoma
   b. Familial polyposis
   c. Pedunculated polyp less than 1 cm in diameter

_____

▼ *Circle T if the statement is true and F if it is false. Correct any false statements.*

62. T   F   Fecal incontinence results from destruction of the second to fourth sacral segments of the spinal cord.

63. T   F   The external anal sphincter is under autonomic nervous control.

64. T   F   Diverticulitis almost always requires surgical resection.

65. T   F   Vitamin D is synthesized in the large bowel by the action of colonic bacteria.

66. T   F   Normally, about 1000 ml of flatus is expelled from the anus daily.

67. T   F   Barium enema radiographic studies are generally contraindicated during acute diverticulitis because of the danger of perforation.

68. T   F   First-degree internal hemorrhoids are permanently prolapsed.

69. T   F   Second-degree hemorrhoids prolapse occurs after straining at the stool but recedes spontaneously or can be reduced manually.

70. T   F   Approximately 5% of the population over age 25 years have hemorrhoids.

71. T   F   The perianal and ischiorectal areas are the most common sites of anorectal abscess formation.

72. T   F   The formation of an anorectal abscess or fistula is often preceded by anal cryptitis initiated by a mucosal tear from hard feces.

73. T   F   Successful treatment of anorectal abscess or fistula usually requires surgery.

74. T   F   Medical treatment of hemorrhoids includes stool softeners, moist heat, and the use of suppositories.

CHAPTER 27

Disorders of the Liver, Gallbladder, and Pancreas

LORRAINE M. WILSON
GLENDA N. LINDSETH

ANATOMY AND PHYSIOLOGY

The liver, biliary tract, and pancreas all develop as off-shoots of the fetal foregut in a region that later becomes the duodenum; all are intimately associated with the physiology of digestion. It is reasonable to consider these structures together because of their anatomic proximity, their closely related functions, and the similarity of the symptom complexes induced by many of their disorders.

Liver

The liver is the largest gland in the body, averaging about 1500 g, or 2% of the body weight in a normal adult (Fig. 27-1). It is a soft, plastic organ that is molded by the surrounding structures. The superior surface is convex and lies beneath the right dome and part of the left dome of the diaphragm. The lower portion of the liver is concave and provides a roof over the right kidney, stomach, pancreas, gallbladder, and intestines. There are two principal lobes, the right and the left. The *right lobe* is divided into anterior and posterior segments by the right segmental fissure, not seen from the exterior. The *left lobe* is divided into medial and lateral segments by the externally visible falciform ligament. The *falciform ligament* passes from the liver to the diaphragm and the anterior abdominal wall. The surface of the liver is covered by visceral peritoneum, except for a small area on the posterior surface that is attached directly to the diaphragm. Several ligaments that are reflections of the peritoneum help support the liver. Beneath the peritoneum is a dense connective tissue layer called the *capsule of Glisson*, which covers the surface of the entire organ with the thickest parts around the porta hepatis, forming a framework for the branches of the portal vein, hepatic artery, and bile ducts. The *porta hepatis* is the fissure of the liver where the portal vein and hepatic artery enter and the hepatic duct leaves.

372

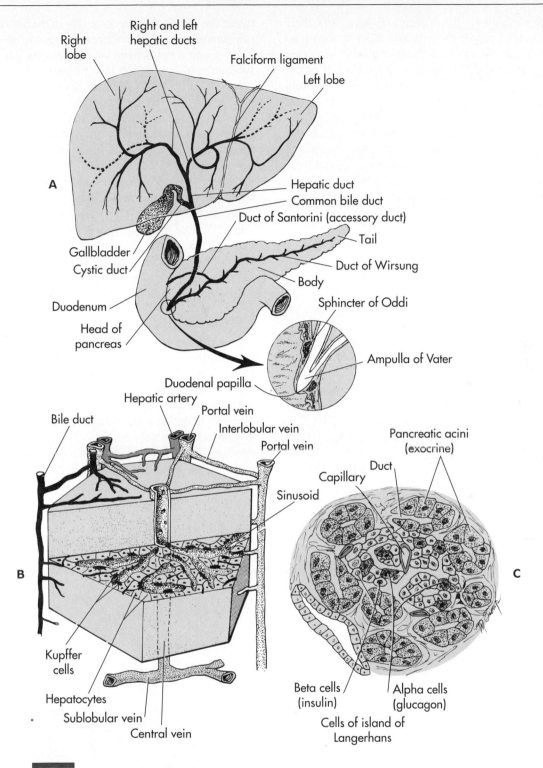

FIG. 27-1   **A,** Liver, gallbladder, and pancreas. **B,** Microscopic structure of hepatic functional unit (liver lobule). **C,** Pancreatic acinar units.

Microscopic structure

Each lobe of the liver is divided into structures called *lobules,* which are the microscopic and functional units of the organ (Fig. 27-1, *B*). Each lobule is a hexagonal body composed of plates of cuboidal hepatic cells arranged radially around a central vein that drains the lobule. Between the plates of hepatic cells are capillaries called *sinusoids,* which are branches of the portal vein and hepatic artery. The sinusoids, unlike other capillaries, are lined with phagocytic, or Kupffer, cells. *Kupffer cells* belong to the monocyte-macrophage system, and their main function is to engulf bacteria and other foreign particles in the blood. As many as 50% of all macrophages are found in the liver as Kupffer cells; thus it is one of the principal organs of defense against bacterial invasions and toxic agents. In addition to branches of the portal vein and hepatic artery encircling the periphery of the liver lobule, bile ducts are also present. The interlobular bile ducts form small bile capillaries called *canaliculi* (not shown), which course within the center of the liver cell plates. Bile formed in the heptaocytes is excreted into the canaliculi, which join to form larger and larger bile ducts until the common bile duct is reached.

Circulation

The liver has a dual blood supply: from the digestive tract and the spleen via the *hepatic portal vein* and from the aorta via the *hepatic artery.* About one third of the incoming blood is arterial, and about two thirds is venous from the portal vein. A total volume of 1500 ml passes through the liver each minute and is drained via the right and left *hepatic veins,* which empty into the inferior vena cava (Fig. 27-2).

The portal vein is unique in that it is interposed between two capillary beds, one in the liver and the other in the digestive area that it drains. On entering the liver, the portal vein divides into branches that come into contact with the circumference of the liver lobules. These branches then give off interlobular veins, which run be-

tween the lobules. These give rise to the sinusoids, which run between the plates of hepatocytes to enter the central veins. Central veins from several lobules join to form the sublobular veins, which in turn join to form the hepatic veins (see Fig. 27-1, *B*). The finest branches of the hepatic artery also empty into the sinusoids, making the blood composition unique in that it is a mixture of arterial blood from the hepatic artery and venous blood from the portal vein. Fig. 27-2 illustrates the origin of blood flowing into the portal system; increased pressure in this system is a common manifestation in liver disorders, with serious consequences involving the vessels in which the portal blood originates. Several points of portacaval anastomosis are of clinical significance. In cases of obstruction to flow in the liver, portal blood may be shunted around the liver to the systemic venous system. The consequences of portal hypertension and shunting are discussed in greater detail later in this chapter.

Liver function

In addition to ranking first in size as a parenchymal organ, the liver also ranks first in the number, complexity, and variety of its functions. The liver is essential for the maintenance of life, is involved in almost every metabolic function of the body, and is specifically responsible for more than 500 separate activities. Fortunately, it has a large reserve capacity and needs only 10% to 20% functioning tissue to sustain life. Complete destruction or removal of the liver results in death in less than 10 hours.

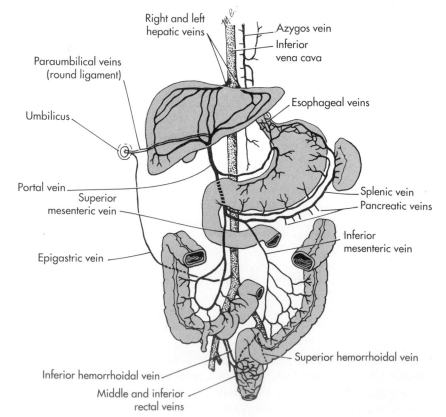

FIG. 27-2   Hepatic portal system. Blood is carried from the stomach, intestines, spleen, and pancreas into the liver sinusoids. Hepatic veins convey blood to the inferior vena cava. Clinically significant sites of anastomosis between the hepatic and systemic circulations are (1) the esophageal veins (portal tributary), which anastomose with the azygos veins (systemic tributary); (2) the paraumbilical veins in the round ligament, which originate in the left branch of the portal vein and connect with the superficial veins of the anterior abdominal wall (systemic tributaries) in the area of the umbilicus; (3) the superior rectal or hemorrhoidal veins (portal tributaries), which anastomose with the middle and inferior rectal veins (systemic tributaries); and (4) the portal tributaries to the intestines, pancreas, and liver, which anastomose with the phrenic, renal, and lumbar veins (systemic tributaries not shown). In portal hypertension and chronic liver disease, blood may be backed up in these veins and shunted around the liver through the points of anastomosis.

▶ TABLE 27-1   Major Functions of the Liver

Function	Comments
Formation and excretion of bile	
Bile salts metabolism	Bile salts are essential for the digestion and absorption of fats and fat-soluble vitamins in the intestine.
Bile pigment metabolism	Bilirubin, the main bile pigment, is a metabolic end product from the processing of old red blood cells; it is conjugated in the liver and excreted in bile.
Carbohydrate metabolism	The liver plays an important part in maintaining the normal blood glucose level and providing energy for the body; carbohydrates are stored in the liver as glycogen.
Glycogenesis	
Glycogenolysis	
Gluconeogenesis	
Protein metabolism	Serum proteins synthesized by the liver include albumin and the alpha and beta globulins (not gamma globulin).
Protein synthesis	Blood-clotting factors synthesized by the liver include fibrinogen (I), prothrombin (II), and factors V, VII, IX, and X; vitamin K is a necessary cofactor in the synthesis of all these factors except V.
Urea formation	Urea is formed exclusively in the liver from ammonia (NH_3), which is then excreted in the urine and feces; NH_3 is formed from deamination of amino acids and action of intestinal bacteria on amino acids.
Protein (amino acid) storage	
Fat metabolism	Triglycerides, cholesterol, phospholipids, and lipoproteins (absorbed from intestine) are hydrolyzed to fatty acids and glycerol.
Ketogenesis	
Cholesterol synthesis	The liver plays major role in cholesterol synthesis, most of which is excreted in the bile as cholesterol or cholic acid.
Fat storage	
Vitamin and mineral storage	Fat-soluble vitamins (A, D, E, K) are stored in the liver, as are vitamin B_{12}, copper, and iron.
Steroid metabolism	The liver inactivates and excretes aldosterone, glucocorticoids, estrogen, progesterone, and testosterone.
Detoxification	The liver is responsible for biotransformation of substances that are potentially harmful (e.g., drugs) into harmless substances that are then excreted by the kidneys.
Flood chamber and filter action	Liver sinusoids provide a depot for blood backed up from venae cavae (right-sided heart failure); the phagocytic action of Kupffer cells removes bacteria and debris from blood.

The liver has an impressive regenerative ability. In most patients, partial surgical removal will stimulate hepatocyte growth to replace the dead or diseased cells. The regeneration process is essentially complete in 4 to 5 weeks. In some persons, normal liver mass has been restored within 6 months.

Table 27-1 lists the major functions of the liver. Understanding these functions is a prerequisite to understanding liver pathophysiology.

The formation and excretion of *bile* represent a major function of the liver; the bile ducts transport and the gallbladder stores and releases bile into the small intestine as needed. The liver secretes about 500 to 1000 ml of yellow bile each day. The basic components of bile are water (97%), electrolytes, bile salts, phospholipids (mainly lecithin), cholesterol, inorganic salts, and bile pigments (mainly conjugated bilirubin). *Bile salts* are essential for fat digestion and absorption in the small intestine. After being acted on by bacteria in the small intestine, most of the bile salts are reabsorbed in the ileum, recirculated to the liver, and reconjugated and resecreted (see Chapter 25). Although *bilirubin* (bile pigment) is a metabolic end product and has no physiologically active role, it is nonetheless important as an indicator of liver and biliary tract disease, since it tends to color the tissues and fluid with which it comes in contact. Most bilirubin conjugates are waste products and are fecally excreted. Normal bilirubin metabolism and jaundice as a sign of disease are discussed later in this chapter.

The liver plays an essential role in the metabolism of three types of foodstuffs delivered by the portal vein after absorption from the intestines: carbohydrates, proteins, and fats. Monosaccharides from the small intestine are converted into glycogen and stored as such in the liver *(glycogenesis)*. The release of glucose from this storage depot of glycogen *(glycogenolysis)* is varied in a controlled manner so as to meet the body's changing requirements for glucose. Some of the glucose is metabolized in the tissues to produce heat and energy, and the remainder is converted either into glycogen and stored in the muscles or into fat and stored in the subcutaneous tissues. The liver is also capable of synthesizing glucose from proteins and fat *(gluconeogenesis)*. The role of the liver in protein metabolism is essential to survival. The plasma proteins, except gamma globulin, are synthesized by the liver. These include albumin, which is necessary for the maintenance of the colloid osmotic pressure, and prothrombin, fibrinogen, and other clotting factors. In addition, most degradation of amino acids begins in the liver with *deamination,* or the removal of an amino group (NH_2). The ammonia (NH_3) released is then synthesized into urea and excreted by the kidneys and intestines. NH_3 formed in the gut by the action of bacteria on protein is also converted to urea in the liver.

Other metabolic functions of the liver include fat metabolism; vitamin, iron, and copper storage; the conjugation and excretion of adrenal and gonadal steroids; and the detoxification of numerous endogenous and exogenous substances. The important detoxification function is accomplished by liver enzymes that oxidize, reduce, hydrolyze, or conjugate the potentially harmful substance, rendering it physiologically inactive. Endogenous substances, such as indol, skatol, and phenol, which are produced by the action of bacteria on amino acids in the large intestine, and exogenous substances, such as morphine, phenobarbital, and other drugs, are detoxified in this manner.

Finally, the liver functions as a "flood chamber" and "filter" because of its strategic position between the intestinal and general circulation. In cases of right-sided heart failure, the liver may become passively congested with a large amount of blood. The Kupffer cells in the sinusoids filter bacteria and other injurious materials from the portal blood by phagocytosis.

Gallbladder

The gallbladder is a pear-shaped hollow sac resting directly beneath the right lobe of the liver (see Fig. 27-1). Bile, which is secreted continuously by the liver, enters the small bile ducts within the liver. The small bile ducts join to form two larger ducts, which emerge from the undersurface of the liver as the *right* and *left hepatic ducts* but which immediately join to form the *common hepatic duct.* The hepatic duct merges with the *cystic duct* from the gallbladder, forming the *common bile duct.* In many persons the common bile duct merges with the pancreatic duct to form the *ampulla of Vater* (dilated portion in common channel) before opening into the small intestine. The terminal parts of both ducts and the ampulla are surrounded by circular muscle fibers known as the *sphincter of Oddi* (see Fig. 27-1, *A,* inset).

The principal function of the gallbladder is the storage and concentration of bile. It is capable of holding about 40 to 60 ml of bile. Hepatic bile may not immediately enter the duodenum; instead, after passing down the hepatic duct, it may be diverted into the cystic duct and gallbladder. In the gallbladder the lymphatics and blood vessels absorb water and inorganic salts, so gallbladder bile is up to five times as concentrated as hepatic bile. At intervals the gallbladder contents are emptied into the duodenum by simultaneous contraction of the muscular coat and relaxation of the sphincter of Oddi. The hormone cholecystokinin (CCK), released from duodenal cells in response to the presence of digestive products from dietary lipids and proteins, stimulates gallbladder contraction.

Pancreas

The pancreas is a long, slender organ about 6 to 8 inches (15 to 20 cm) in length and 1½ inches (3.8 cm) in width. It lies retroperitoneal and is divided into three major segments: the head, body, and tail (see Fig. 27-1). The head lies in the concavity formed by the duodenum, and the tail touches the spleen.

The pancreas is made up of two basic types of cells having entirely different functions (see Fig. 27-1, *C*). The *exocrine cells,* clustered into groups called *acini,* produce the components of the pancreatic juice (see Table 25-1). The *endocrine cells,* or *islets of Langerhans,* produce the endocrine secretions insulin and glucagon, which are important for carbohydrate metabolism.

The pancreas is a compound tubuloalveolar gland. As a whole it resembles a bunch of grapes, the branches of which are the ducts terminating into the main pancreatic duct *(duct of Wirsung).* Small ducts from each acinus empty into the main ducts. The main duct, extending throughout the length of the gland, often joins the common bile duct at the ampulla of Vater before entering the duodenum. An accessory duct, the *duct of Santorini,* is frequently found extending from the head of the pancreas into the duodenum, about 1 inch (2.5 cm) above the duodenal papilla.

OVERVIEW

Pathologic changes in diseases of the liver, gallbladder, and pancreas may be broadly categorized into three types: *inflammatory, fibrotic,* and *neoplastic changes.* Hepatitis, cholecystitis, and pancreatitis show evidence of acute or chronic inflammation of the involved tissues. Gallstones and biliary tract obstruction are frequently associated with cholecystitis and pancreatitis. Fibrotic changes occur with cirrhosis of the liver and in chronic inflammatory conditions. Primary tumors of the liver, pancreas, or gallbladder, whether benign or malignant, are rare. Widespread destruction of parenchymal cells resulting from inflammation, fibrosis, neoplasms, or obstruction interferes with secretory and excretory functions. *Jaundice* (yellow coloration of the body tissues) is a common symptom and results from interference with the excretion of bilirubin. Portal hypertension, ascites, esophageal varices, and hepatic encephalopathy are common complications in advanced cirrhosis and hepatic failure.

DIAGNOSTIC TESTS

Table 27-2 lists some of the most common diagnostic tests used to detect disordered function of the liver, biliary system, and pancreas. It should be emphasized that no single test or procedure is capable of measuring the total function of the liver, since it is involved in almost every metabolic process in the body and has a large functional reserve. Usually a battery of diagnostic tests is used.

Table 27-3 summarizes radiologic methods useful in the diagnosis of disorders of the liver, biliary system, and pancreas. Other diagnostic methods include *esophagoscopy,* which allows direct visualization of esophageal varices; *duodenoscopy,* which allows visualization of the papilla of Vater and involves insertion of a catheter to in-

▶ TABLE 27-2   Liver, Biliary, and Pancreatic Function Tests

Test	Normal	Clinical Significance
BILIARY EXCRETION		Measures ability of liver to conjugate and excrete bile pigment.
Direct serum bilirubin (conjugated)	0.1-0.3 mg/dl	Elevated when excretion of conjugated bilirubin is impaired.
Indirect serum bilirubin (unconjugated)	0.2-0.7 mg/dl	Elevated in hemolytic conditions and Gilbert's syndrome.
Total serum bilirubin	0.3-1.0 mg/dl	Both direct and total serum bilirubin elevated in hepatocellular disease.
Urine bilirubin	0	Conjugated bilirubin excreted in urine when elevated in serum, suggesting liver cell or biliary tract obstruction; urine appears brown; foam appears yellow when shaken (simple bedside test).
Urine urobilinogen	1.0-3.5 mg/24 hr	Decreased when bile excretion is impaired, as in liver damage, biliary obstruction, or inflammation; increased when amount produced exceeds ability of liver to reexcrete it, as in hemolytic jaundice.
DYE EXCRETION		
Sulfobromophthalein sodium (Bromsulphalein, BSP) clearance test	<5% retention in 45 minutes	Rate of intravenously administered sulfobromophthalein clearance from plasma is used in evaluating liver function; excretion depends on functional liver cells, patent biliary ducts, and hepatic blood flow; BSP test is a sensitive index of liver function, useful in detecting early liver cell damage and recovery from infectious hepatitis, but because of occasional toxic reactions, it is not widely used.
PROTEIN METABOLISM		
Total serum protein Serum albumin Serum globulin	6-8 g/dl 3.2-5.5 g/dl 2.0-3.5 g/dl	Most of serum proteins and coagulation proteins are synthesized by liver and are therefore decreased in a variety of liver impairments.
Prothrombin time	11-15 seconds	Increased with decreased prothrombin synthesis resulting from liver cell damage or decreased vitamin K absorption in biliary obstruction; vitamin K is essential for prothrombin synthesis.
Blood ammonia (NH_3)	80-100 μg/dl	Liver converts NH_3 to urea; level increases in hepatic failure or large portal-systemic shunts.
CARBOHYDRATE METABOLISM		
Serum amylase	60-180 Somogyi units/dl	Obstruction and inflammatory disease of pancreas interfere with normal flow of amylase into intestinal tract and result in increased serum levels; value increases greatly in acute pancreatitis; also increases in parotid gland disease and other conditions.
Urine amylase	35-260 Somogyi units/hr	Urine amylase remains high longer than serum amylase (1 week); values >300 indicate pancreatitis.

Continued.

▶ TABLE 27-2   Liver, Biliary, and Pancreatic Function Tests—cont'd

Test	Normal	Clinical Significance
FAT METABOLISM		
Serum lipase	<1.5 units/ml (Cherry-Crandall method)	Pancreatic digestive enzymes are released into blood with breakdown of acinar cells in obstructive or inflammatory conditions of pancreas.
Serum cholesterol	<200 mg/dl	Increased in bile duct obstruction, decreased in liver cell damage; values >200 increase risk for coronary heart disease.
SERUM ENZYMES		
AST (SGOT)	5-35 units/ml (Frankel)	Aspartate aminotransferase (AST), formerly serum glutamic-oxaloacetic transaminase (SGOT), alanine aminotransferase (ALT), formerly serum glutamic-pyruvic transaminase (SGPT), and lactic dehydrogenase (LDH) are intracellular enzymes concentrated in the heart, liver, and skeletal tissue; released from damaged tissue (necrosis or altered cell permeability); increased in liver cell damage and in other conditions, especially myocardial infarction.
ALT (SGPT)	5-35 units/ml (Frankel)	
LDH	200-450 units/ml (Wrobleski)	
Alkaline phosphatase	30-120 IU/L *or* 2-4 units/dl (Bodansky)	Manufactured in bone, liver, kidneys, and intestine and excreted into bile; level increases in biliary obstruction, as well as bone disease and liver metastasis.
IMMUNOLOGIC TESTS		Key diagnostic tests are for viral hepatitis (see Table 27-5).

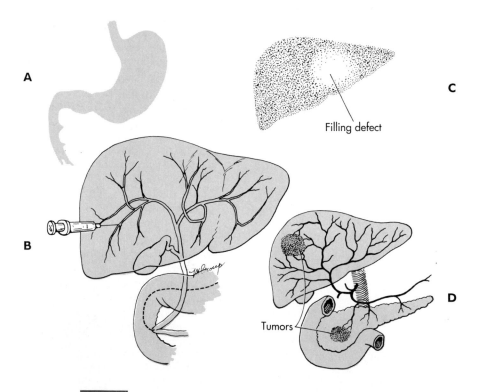

FIG. 27-3   Tests useful in the diagnosis of liver, biliary, and pancreatic disorders. **A,** Barium radiograph of the gastrointestinal tract. **B,** Transhepatic cholangiogram in which contrast material is injected percutaneously. The hepatic or pancreatic ductal systems may also be approached from below by inserting a catheter into the papilla of Vater and injecting contrast material (endoscopic retrograde cholangiopancreatography, (ERCP). **C,** Liver scan. **D,** Selective celiac axis angiography.

▶ TABLE 27-3   Radiologic Methods in Diagnosis of the Liver, Biliary, and Pancreatic Disorders

Test	Comments
Plain radiograph of abdomen	May reveal calcific densities in gallbladder, biliary tree (gallstones), pancreas, and liver; may also reveal splenomegaly or gross ascites.
Ultrasonography	Preferred method for detecting gallstones; reliable in detecting dilated bile ducts and cystic and solid masses of liver and pancreas; noninvasive and inexpensive.
Computed tomography (CT)	Provides high-resolution images of liver, gallbladder, pancreas, and spleen; reveals stones, solid masses, cysts, abscesses, and structural abnormalities; often used with contrast media.
Magnetic resonance imaging (MRI)	Same applications as CT scan but greater sensitivity; can also detect blood flow and blood vessel patency; noninvasive but expensive.
Barium swallow/meal (see Fig. 27-3, A)	Reveals esophageal varices in more than 70% of cases; tumors often produce displacement of duodenum (reverse-3 sign common).
Oral cholecystography	Conjugation and excretion of dye by liver allow visualization of gallbladder and bile ducts, thus revealing gallstones; poor or no visualization of contrast medium may be caused by liver cell disease or biliary obstruction; often used with extracorporeal shock wave lithotripsy and dissolution therapy for cholelithiasis treatment.
Percutaneous transhepatic cholangiogram (THC) (see Fig. 27-3, B)	Dye given by percutaneous puncture and blind probing for a bile duct into which dye is injected; may help to distinguish intrahepatic ducts and causes of biliary obstruction or cholestasis; hazards involve bile leakage, hemorrhage, and sepsis.
Endoscopic retrograde cholangiopancreatography (ERCP) (see Fig. 27-3, B)	Endoscopic insertion of a catheter into duodenal papilla and injection of contrast medium through catheter into pancreatic or biliary ductules allow visualization of these structures.
Technetium-99m (^{99m}Tc) biliary radioisotope scan	Reveals cholestasis, acute or chronic obstruction, bile leaks, fistulas, and cysts.
Radioisotope liver scan with radio-tagged blood cells, ^{99m}Tc-labeled sulfur colloid, or gallium scanning (see Fig. 27-3, C)	Reveals anatomic changes in liver tissue; lesions appear as filling defects (tumors, cysts, abscesses).
Selective celiac axis angiography (see Fig. 27-3, D)	Visualization of pancreatic, hepatic, and portal circulation possible; reveals tumor masses, disruption as in cirrhosis, and portal collateral circulation including hepatic lesions.
Portal pressure measurement (see Fig. 27-3, E)	Principal procedures are by direct measurement through portal vein catheterization or indirectly by intrasplenic pressure or wedge hepatic pressure determinations; portal pressure elevated in cirrhosis; procedures often combined with injection of contrast medium.
Splenoportogram (see Fig. 27-3, E)	Demonstrates size and patency of portal and splenic collaterals.

FIG. 27-3, cont'd   E, Splenoportogram and measurement of portal pressure. F, Liver biopsy. (See Table 27-3 and text for explanation of tests.)

ject contrast medium directly into the biliary or pancreatic system; *peritoneoscopy*, which involves insertion of a peritoneoscope through an abdominal stab wound and allows direct visualization of the anterior surface of the liver and gallbladder; and *electroencephalography*, which may reveal abnormal patterns in hepatic encephalopathy. Finally, percutaneous liver biopsy is a common procedure performed at the bedside.

Percutaneous liver biopsy is a valuable method of diagnosing diffuse parenchymal diseases, such as cirrhosis, hepatitis, and lymphoma. Before performing the procedure, the patient's capacity to clot blood is evaluated, and cross-matched blood is provided in case of need. The procedure itself is brief. The skin is cleansed and anesthetized. As a patient holds his or her breath in expiration to bring the liver and diaphragm to the highest position, the needle is inserted into the liver in the eighth or ninth intercostal space or subcostally and withdrawn (Fig. 27-3, F). The specimen is then expelled into formalin for later histologic examination. It is vitally important that patients understand that they are to hold their breath and not move during the procedure, to prevent laceration of the liver. The procedure is contraindicated in patients who cannot meet this requirement. For patients at high risk or those who cannot hold their breath, a transvenous liver biopsy may be performed. This involves placement of an intravenous (IV) catheter transjugularly into the hepatic vein.

After the procedure the patient lies on the right side for several hours to splint the chest and remains in bed for 24 hours. Although rare, complications of liver biopsy may be dangerous. The chief danger is intraperitoneal hemorrhage (0.4% of cases), which results from penetration of a large blood vessel. Bile peritonitis is a rare but serious complication that requires immediate surgical intervention. Vital signs are checked every 15 minutes until stable and then every 1 or 2 hours for the first 24 hours after the procedure. The dressing is checked frequently for local bleeding, and a pressure dressing is applied if necessary. Severe abdominal pain may indicate bile peritonitis and should be carefully evaluated. A "directed" rather than a "blind" liver biopsy may be performed with the use of computed tomography (CT) scan or ultrasonography. The use of new and improved noninvasive diagnostic methods such as ultrasound and CT scan has obviated the need for biopsy in many circumstances. Fig. 27-3 illustrates some of the diagnostic procedures useful in liver, biliary, and pancreatic disorders.

BILIRUBIN METABOLISM AND JAUNDICE

The accumulation of bile pigments in the body causes yellow discoloration of the tissues called *jaundice*. Jaundice can usually be detected in the sclerae (whites of eyes) or skin or by a darkening of the urine when the serum bilirubin reaches 2 to 3 mg/dl. The normal serum bilirubin is 0.3 to 1.0 mg/dl. Surface tissues richest in elastin, such as the sclerae and the undersurface of the tongue, usually become stained first.

A consideration of the mechanisms of jaundice involves an understanding of the formation, transportation, metabolism, and excretion of bilirubin.

Normal Bilirubin Metabolism

In the normal individual, bilirubin formation and excretion proceed smoothly through the steps outlined in Fig. 27-4. About 80% to 85% of the bilirubin is produced by the breakdown of senescent red blood cells (RBCs) in the monocyte-macrophage system. The average life span of an RBC is 120 days. Each day about 50 ml of blood is destroyed, and 250 to 350 mg of bilirubin is produced. It is now known that about 15% to 20% of total bile pigment does not depend on this mechanism but is derived from destruction of maturing erythroid cells in the bone marrow (ineffective hematopoiesis) and from other hemoproteins, notably those in the liver.

In the catabolism of hemoglobin (largely occurring in the spleen), globin is first dissociated from heme, after which the heme is converted to biliverdin. Unconjugated bilirubin is then formed from biliverdin. *Biliverdin* is a greenish pigment formed by oxidation of bilirubin. Unconjugated bilirubin is lipid soluble, water insoluble, and incapable of being excreted in the bile or the urine. Unconjugated bilirubin, bound to albumin in a water-soluble complex, is transported in the blood to the liver cells. Hepatic metabolism of bilirubin involves three steps: uptake, conjugation, and excretion. Uptake by the liver cell involves two hepatic proteins, designated Y and Z (Fig. 27-4). Conjugation of bilirubin with glucuronic acid is catalyzed by the enzyme *glucuronyl transferase* in the endoplasmic reticulum. Conjugated bilirubin is lipid insoluble, water soluble, and capable of being excreted in both the bile and the urine. Transport of conjugated bilirubin across the cell membrane into the bile by an active process is the final step in hepatic bilirubin metabolism. Unconjugated bilirubin is not excreted into the bile except after photooxidation or photoisomerization (see following discussion).

Intestinal bacteria reduce conjugated bilirubin to a series of compounds called *stercobilin* or *urobilinogen*. These substances account for the brown color of stool. About 10% to 20% of the urobilinogen undergoes enterohepatic circulation, and a small fraction is excreted in the urine.

Pathophysiologic Mechanisms in Jaundice States

There are four general mechanisms by which hyperbilirubinemia and jaundice can occur:
1. Excess production of bilirubin
2. Impaired hepatic uptake of unconjugated bilirubin
3. Impaired conjugation of bilirubin
4. Decreased excretion of conjugated bilirubin into bile because of either intrahepatic or extrahepatic factors that may be functional or caused by mechanical obstruction

The first three mechanisms result in predominantly unconjugated hyperbilirubinemia, whereas the fourth results in predominantly conjugated hyperbilirubinemia.

Excess bilirubin production

Hemolytic disease, or an increased rate of RBC destruction, is the most common cause of excess bilirubin production. The resultant jaundice is customarily called *hemolytic jaundice*. Conjugation and transfer of bile pigment proceed normally, but the supply of unconjugated bilirubin is greater than the liver can handle. Consequently, the level of unconjugated bilirubin in the blood rises. The serum bilirubin level, however, rarely exceeds 5 mg/dl in patients with severe hemolysis, and the jaun-

RETICULOENDOTHELIAL SYSTEM

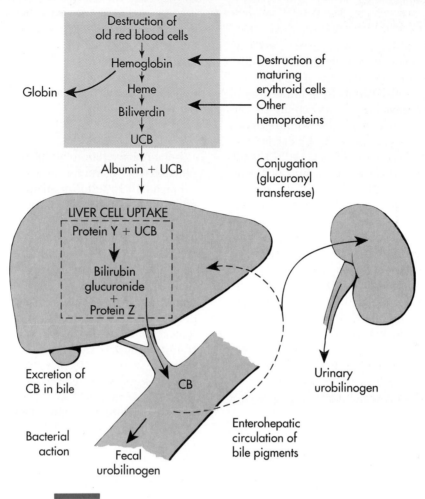

FIG. 27-4   Normal bilirubin metabolism. *CB,* Conjugated bilirubin; *UCB,* unconjugated bilirubin.

dice is a mild pale yellow. Because unconjugated bilirubin is water insoluble, it cannot be excreted in the urine and bilirubinuria does not occur. There is, however, increased production of urobilinogen (caused by the increased bilirubin load presented to the liver and increased conjugation and excretion), which in turn results in increased fecal and urinary excretion. The urine and stool may thus be darker.

Some common causes of hemolytic jaundice are abnormal hemoglobins (hemoglobin S in sickle cell anemia), abnormal RBCs (hereditary spherocytosis), antibodies in the serum (Rh or transfusion incompatibility or as a result of autoimmune hemolytic disease), administration of some drugs, and increased hemolysis. Sometimes hemolytic jaundice can result from a process referred to as *ineffective erythropoiesis.* Essentially this process increases destruction of RBCs or their precursors in the bone marrow (thalassemia, pernicious anemia, porphyria).

In the adult, chronic overproduction of bilirubin may lead to the formation of gallstones predominantly composed of bilirubin; otherwise the mild hyperbilirubinemia is not generally harmful. Treatment is directed toward correction of the hemolytic disease. In infancy, however, unconjugated bilirubin levels greater than 20 mg/dl may lead to kernicterus (see following discussion).

Impaired uptake of bilirubin

The uptake of albumin-bound unconjugated bilirubin by liver cells involves the dissociation and binding of bilirubin to acceptor proteins. Only a few drugs have been shown to influence the uptake of bilirubin by the liver: flavaspidic acid (used to treat tapeworms), novobiocin, and some cholecystographic dyes. The unconjugated hyperbilirubinemia and jaundice usually disappear when the offending drug is withdrawn. Previously, neonatal jaundice and some cases of Gilbert's syndrome were believed to involve a deficiency of acceptor protein and a defect in hepatic uptake. In most of these cases, however, a deficiency of glucuronyl transferase has been demonstrated, so these conditions are best considered as a defect in bilirubin conjugation.

Impaired conjugation of bilirubin

The mild unconjugated hyperbilirubinemia (less than 12.9 mg/dl) that develops between the second and fifth days of life is called *physiologic jaundice of the newborn.* This normal neonatal jaundice results from immaturity of the enzyme glucuronyl transferase. The activity of glucuronyl transferase normally increases within several days to 2 weeks after birth, and the jaundice disappears.

When unconjugated bilirubin levels exceed 20 mg/dl in the newborn, a condition called kernicterus develops. This condition could occur when a hemolytic process (e.g., erythroblastosis fetalis) is superimposed on the normal glucuronyl transferase deficiency in the newborn. *Kernicterus,* or bilirubin encephalopathy, results from the deposition of unconjugated bilirubin in the lipid-rich basal ganglia. If untreated, death or serious neurologic damage occurs. The current treatment approach to unconjugated hyperbilirubinemia in the newborn is phototherapy. *Phototherapy* involves the application of intense fluorescent or blue light (wavelength of 430 to 470 nm) on the infant's exposed skin. Exposure to the light leads to a structural change in the bilirubin (photoisomerization) to water-soluble polarized isomers that are rapidly excreted in the bile without the prior need for conjugation.

Three hereditary conditions represent progressive deficiency of glucuronyl transferase: Gilbert's syndrome and type I and type II Crigler-Najjar syndrome. *Gilbert's syndrome* is considered to be a benign familial condition characterized by mild (2 to 5 mg/ml) and chronic unconjugated hyperbilirubinemia and jaundice. Current research has identified two forms of Gilbert's syndrome. One group includes patients with evidence of hemolysis and increased bilirubin turnover. The other has decreased bilirubin clearance and no hemolysis. Both forms can occur at the same time in the same patient (Podolsky, Isselbacher, 1994). In Gilbert's syndrome the degree of jaundice fluctuates and is often aggravated by prolonged fasting, infection, stress, surgery, and excessive alcohol intake. The onset is most common during adolescence. Gilbert's syndrome is common and may affect up to 5% of the male population. Liver function tests and fecal and urinary urobilinogen levels are normal. Bilirubinuria is absent. Studies reveal that these patients have a partial deficiency of glucuronyl transferase. The condition may be treated by the administration of phenobarbital, which stimulates glucuronyl transferase enzyme activity.

Type I *Crigler-Najjar syndrome* is a rare hereditary disorder caused by a recessive gene in which there is a complete absence of glucuronyl transferase from birth. Because conjugation of bilirubin cannot take place, the bile is colorless and unconjugated bilirubin levels exceed 20 mg/dl, resulting in kernicterus. Phototherapy may temporarily reduce the unconjugated hyperbilirubinemia, but infants generally die within the first year of life. Type II Crigler-Najjar syndrome represents a milder form of the disease transmitted as a dominant genetic trait in which there is only a partial deficiency of glucuronyl transferase. Serum unconjugated bilirubin levels are lower (6 to 20 mg/dl) and jaundice may not be manifested until adolescence. Phenobarbital, which induces increased glucuronyl transferase activity, often causes jaundice to disappear in these patients.

Decreased excretion of conjugated bilirubin

Impaired excretion of bilirubin, whether caused by functional or obstructive factors, results in predominantly conjugated hyperbilirubinemia. Because conjugated bilirubin is water-soluble, it is excreted in the urine and gives rise to bilirubinuria and dark urine. Fecal and urinary urobilinogen are commonly decreased, so the stools are pale. Elevated conjugated bilirubin levels may be accompanied by other evidence of hepatic excretory failure, such as elevated serum levels of alkaline phosphatase, aspartate aminotransferase, cholesterol, and bile salts. The presence of elevated bile salts in the blood adds the new dimension of itching to the jaundice. Jaundice resulting from conjugated hyperbilirubinemia is usually deeper than that resulting from unconjugated hyperbilirubinemia. The color change ranges from a mild or deep orange-yellow to a yellow-green in cases of complete obstruction of biliary outflow. These changes are evidence of *cholestatic jaundice,* which is another name for *obstructive jaundice.* Cholestasis may be either *intrahepatic* (involving the liver cell, canaliculi, or cholangioles) or *extrahepatic* (involving bile ducts outside the liver). Similar biochemical disturbances are present in both.

The most common causes of intrahepatic cholestasis are *hepatocellular diseases* in which the hepatic parenchymal cells are damaged by viral hepatitis or the various types of cirrhosis. In these diseases, swelling and disorganization of the liver cells can compress and block the canaliculi or cholangioles. Hepatocellular disease usually interferes with all phases of bilirubin metabolism—uptake, conjugation, and excretion—but since excretion is usually impaired to the greatest extent, conjugated hyperbilirubinemia predominates. Other less common causes of intrahepatic cholestasis include certain drugs and the rare hereditary disorders of the Dubin-Johnson and Rotor's syndromes. In these conditions, there appears to be interference with transfer of bilirubin across the hepatocyte membrane, causing a retention of bilirubin within the cell. Common offending drugs include halothane (anesthetic), oral contraceptives, estrogens, anabolic steroids, isoniazid, and chlorpromazine.

The most common causes of extrahepatic cholestasis are impaction of a gallstone, usually at the lower end of the common bile duct; carcinoma of the head of the pancreas, producing extrinsic pressure on the bile duct; and carcinoma of the ampulla of Vater. Less common causes are strictures from previous inflammation or surgery and

▶ TABLE 27-4   Differentiating Features of Hemolytic, Hepatocellular, and Obstructive Jaundice

Feature	Hemolytic	Hepatocellular	Obstructive
Skin color	Pale yellow	Mild or deep orange-yellow	Mild to deep yellow-green
Urine color	Normal (may darken with urobilin)	Dark (conjugated bilirubin)	Dark (conjugated bilirubin)
Stool color	Normal or dark (more stercobilin)	Pale (less stercobilin)	Clay colored (no stercobilin)
Pruritus	None	Not persistent	Usually persistent
Serum bilirubin, indirect or unconjugated	Increased	Increased	Increased
Serum bilirubin, direct or conjugated	Normal	Increased	Increased
Urine bilirubin	Absent	Increased	Increased
Urine urobilinogen	Increased	Slight increase	Decreased

enlarged lymph nodes in the porta hepatis. Intrahepatic lesions such as a hepatoma may sometimes obstruct the right or left hepatic duct.

Intrahepatic versus extrahepatic cholestasis. The most important diagnostic decision for the physician and surgeon in conjugated hyperbilirubinemia is to determine whether the obstruction to bile flow is intrahepatic or extrahepatic. Patients with extrahepatic cholestasis may benefit from surgery, whereas surgery on those with hepatocellular disease (intrahepatic cholestasis) may exacerbate the illness and even lead to death. The differentiation is not easy, since all forms of cholestasis produce the same clinical syndrome of jaundice, itching, increased transaminases, increased alkaline phosphatase, defective excretion of cholecystographic dyes, and nonvisualization of the gallbladder. Although the ultimate judgment is a clinical one, making the differentiation is facilitated by evaluating the degree of obstruction. Intrahepatic obstruction is seldom as complete as extrahepatic obstruction. Consequently, intrahepatic cholestasis generally results in only moderate elevations of alkaline phosphatase, and small amounts of pigment appear in the stools or urobilinogen in the urine compared with these values in extrahepatic cholestasis. Liver biopsy or duodenal or transhepatic cholangiography may be used to clarify difficult cases. Table 27-4 lists some of the differentiating features of the common types of jaundice.

VIRAL HEPATITIS

Acute viral hepatitis is an infectious disease that is generalized in its distribution within the body, although the predominant effect is on the liver. Five categories (and possibly a sixth category) of viral agents have been identified as causal agents, as follows:
1. Hepatitis A virus (HAV)
2. Hepatitis B virus (HBV)
3. Hepatitis C virus (HCV)
4. Hepatitis D virus (HDV)
5. Hepatitis E virus (HEV)

Although these five viruses are discernible through their antigenic markers, they produce clinically similar illnesses, ranging from subclinical asymptomatic infections to fatal acute infections.

The best known forms of the disease are HAV and HBV. These terms are preferred to the former terminology of "infectious" and "serum" hepatitis, since both may be transmitted through parenteral and nonparenteral routes. The differential features of HAV and HBV are listed in Table 27-5 and are discussed later.

Viral hepatitis that could not be designated as A or B by serology were formerly called non-A, non-B hepatitis (NANBH) and more recently, hepatitis C (Dienstag, 1990). With the discovery of two non-A, non-B agents, one parenterally transmitted and the other enterically transmitted, these were further designated as PT-NANBH and ET-NANBH, respectively (Bradley, 1990; Centers for Disease Control, 1990). More recently, proposed nomenclature would designate PT-NANBH as hepatitis C and ET-NANBH as hepatitis E.

Delta virus, or hepatitis D (HDV), is a defective ribonucleic acid (RNA) virus that causes infection only in the presence of HBV. HDV may occur as a coexistent infection with HBV or as a superinfection in an HBV carrier.

Viral hepatitis is an important public health problem not only in the United States, but also throughout the world. It ranks third among reportable communicable diseases in the United States, following venereal disease and varicella, and is epidemic in much of the Third World. The Centers for Disease Control and Prevention (CDC) estimates that approximately 200,000 primary HBV infections occur each year in the United States. Although mortality from viral hepatitis is low, exten-

TABLE 27-5   Differential Features of Hepatitis A Virus (HAV) and Hepatitis B Virus (HBV)*

Feature	HAV	HBV
Virus	Hepatitis A virus RNA virus	Hepatitis B virus Double-shelled DNA virus
Synonym	Infectious hepatitis	Serum hepatitis
Transmission mode	Fecal-oral, parenteral (rare), sexual (possible)	Parenteral, sexual, perinatal
Incubation period	15 to 45 days (shorter) Average: 30 days	50 to 180 days (longer) Average: 60 to 90 days
Age	Children, young adults	Any age
Transmission risks	Poor sanitation, overcrowded areas such as day-care centers and mental institutions, infected food handlers, health care workers	Homosexual activity, multiple sexual partners, injectable drug use, chronic hemodialysis, health care workers, blood transfusion (rare now because of routine testing)
Carrier state chronicity	No	Yes
Laboratory tests	Anti-HAV IgM: acute infection Anti-HAV IgG: past infection, immune to HAV	HBsAg: acute infection, chronic infection if present longer than 6 months Anti-HBs: immune to HBV HBcAg (in hepatocytes): no test available Anti-HBc IgM: recent infection Anti-HBc IgG: past infection beyond 6 months HBeAg: correlates with high infectiousness Anti-HBe: resolution of acute infection
Prophylaxis	Immune globulin (IG) Vaccine	HBV immune globulin (HBIG) Vaccine

*Hepatitis D virus (HDV, delta virus) causes infection only in the presence of HBV and is diagnosed by HDV antigen during early infection and by antibody to HDV during or after infection. Hepatitis C and hepatitis E viruses were formerly non-A, non-B hepatitis (NANBH), or hepatitis C. Now two viruses are identified: blood-borne NANB (proposed name, hepatitis C, HCV) and enterically transmitted NANB (proposed name, hepatitis E, HEV).

sive morbidity and economic loss are associated with the disease.

Etiology and Epidemiology

Hepatitis A

The hepatitis A virus (HAV) is a small RNA virus 27 nm in diameter that can be detected in the liver, bile, feces, and blood during the late incubation and preicteric phase of the illness. With the onset of jaundice, antibody to HAV (anti-HAV) becomes measurable in the serum. Initially the level of anti-HAV antibody of the immunoglobulin M (IgM) class rises sharply, making it an accurate and simple diagnostic measure of HAV infection. After acute illness, anti-HAV antibody of the immunoglobulin G (IgG) class predominates and persists indefinitely, indicating past HAV infection and immunity. A carrier state has not been demonstrated.

HAV is the most common type of viral hepatitis in the United States. In 1988, 50% of the cases of hepatitis reported in this country were attributed to HAV infection. It is common among children and young adults. A seasonal increase in the incidence of the disease occurs in autumn and winter.

HAV is primarily transmitted through oral ingestion of fecally contaminated material. Transmission by blood

transfusion has been reported but occurs infrequently (Centers for Disease Control, 1990). The disease is typically spread among children or from contact with an infected individual through the fecal contamination of food or water or by ingestion of inadequately cooked shellfish that may harbor the virus. Sporadic cases occur, and epidemics may arise from the spread of the disease in overcrowded areas such as day-care centers and mental institutions. Travelers to highly endemic areas such as Southeast Asia, North Africa, and the Middle East are at greater risk if they bypass the usual tourist routes. Transmission is facilitated by poor sanitation, poor personal hygiene, and intimate (intrahousehold or sexual) contact. The average incubation period is 30 days. Greatest infectivity is during the 2-week period immediately before the onset of jaundice.

A newly approved HAV vaccine can be given for use by international travelers. It provides long-term protection compared with immune globulin, which provides protection for approximately 5 months, depending on the dosage (Marwick, 1995).

Hepatitis B

The hepatitis B virus (HBV) is a 42 nm, double-shelled deoxyribonucleic acid (DNA) virus that possesses a surface coat and an inner core (Fig. 27-5). The typical sero-

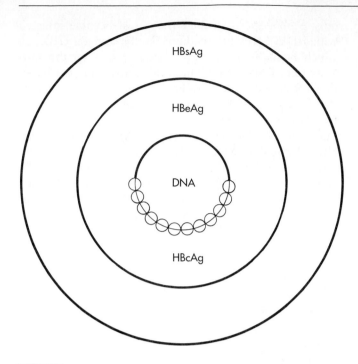

FIG. 27-5   Components of the hepatitis B virus (HBV). Diagram shows that HBV has an incomplete ring of circular DNA within a core particle (HBcAg) surrounded by a surface protein coat (HBsAg). The virus also contains the "e" antigen (HbeAg).

logic markers associated with HBV are listed in Table 27-5. The first serologic marker used to identify HBV is the surface antigen (HBsAg, formerly called the "Australia antigen" [HAA]), which is positive for approximately 2 weeks before the onset of clinical symptoms and generally disappears during early convalescence but may persist for 4 to 6 months. In approximately 1% to 5% of patients with chronic hepatitis, HBsAg persists for more than 6 months, and these patients are said to be "carriers" for HBV (Dienstag, 1990). The presence of HBsAg means that the patient can transmit HBV to others and infect them.

The next marker to appear is usually the antibody to "core" antigen (anti-HBc). The core antigen itself (HBcAg) is not detectable routinely in the serum of patients with HBV infection because it is sequestered within the HBsAg coat. Anti-HBc becomes detectable soon after the appearance of clinical hepatitis and persists indefinitely; it is the clearest marker of immune status acquired from HBV infection (not vaccination). Anti-HBc may be further fractionated into IgM and IgG portions. IgM anti-HBc appears early during infection and persists longer than 6 months. It is a reliable marker of current or recent infection. Predominance of IgG anti-HBc indicates either recovery from HBV in the remote past (6 months) or chronic HBV infection.

The next antibody to appear is that to surface antigen (anti-HBs). Anti-HBs develops after a resolved infection and is responsible for long-term immunity. After vaccination (which immunizes only to surface antigen), im-

munity is assessed by measuring the anti-HBs level. Immunity from a spontaneous infection is best ascertained by measurement of anti-HBc levels.

The "e" antigen (HBeAg) represents a soluble portion of HBV. It appears concurrently or shortly after HBsAg and disappears a few weeks before HBsAg disappears. HBeAg is present in all acute infections and indicates viral replication and that the patient is highly infectious to others. Its persistence may indicate chronic replicative infection. Antibody to HBeAg (anti-HBe) develops in most HBV infections and correlates with the loss of replicating virus and with lower infectiousness.

Finally, an HBV carrier is defined as a person who either tests positive for HBsAg on at least two occasions at least 6 months apart or tests positive for HBsAg and negative for IgM anti-HBc when a single specimen is tested (Centers for Disease Control, 1990). The degree of infectiousness is best correlated with testing positive for HBeAg. Carrier status is thought to be directly related to the person's age when HBV is acquired. For example, in endemic areas, HBV is often acquired early in childhood by vertical transmission from the carrier mother or by horizontal transmission through contact with open wounds. In low endemic areas, however, only a small percentage of those acquiring HBV after 6 years of age become chronic carriers.

HBV infection is a major cause of acute and chronic hepatitis, cirrhosis, and liver cancer throughout the world. It is endemic in the Far East, most Pacific islands, most of Africa, parts of the Middle East, and in the Amazon basin. It is not very endemic in the United States, with infection occurring primarily during adulthood. The CDC estimates that 200,000 to 300,000 persons, primarily young adults, are infected with HBV each year. Only about 25% of these become jaundiced, 10,000 require hospitalization, and about 1% to 2% die with fulminant disease. The estimated number of carriers in the United States is about 800,000 to 1 million. About 25% of these carriers develop chronic active hepatitis, which often progresses to cirrhosis. In addition, the risk of developing primary cancer of the liver increases significantly in carriers. An estimated 25% to 40% of persons who have had acute HBV are at substantial risk for cirrhosis and hepatocellular carcinoma.

The main route for the transmission of HBV is parenteral and across mucous membranes, especially by sexual intercourse. The average length of the incubation period is 120 days. HBsAg has been found in almost every body fluid from infected persons: blood, semen, saliva, tears, ascites, breast milk, urine, and even feces. At least some of these body fluids, especially blood, semen, breast milk, and saliva, have been shown to be infectious. Sources from the CDC state that body fluids such as urine, saliva, ascites, and tears become infectious when they contain blood (Williams, 1995).

Although HBV infection occurs infrequently in the general adult population, certain groups and those with certain life-styles carry a high risk, including the following:

1. Immigrants from areas where HBV is endemic
2. IV drug users who share common needles and syringes
3. Persons who engage in heterosexual activity with multiple partners or infected persons
4. Sexually active homosexual men
5. Patients in custodial institutions for developmentally disabled persons
6. Male prisoners
7. Hemodialysis patients and hemophiliac patients receiving certain plasma-derived products
8. Household contacts of HBV carriers
9. Health care workers, especially those in frequent contact with blood
10. Newborn infants of infected mothers, who can acquire infection during or soon after birth.

HBV-related blood transfusions are no longer a major problem, since all blood is tested before administration.

Hepatitis C (formerly non-A, non-B hepatitis)

The existence of a non-A, non-B form of infectious hepatitis has been known since 1975. In 1988, after years of intense research, the causal agents were identified. There are two forms of non-A, non-B viral hepatitis, one blood borne and the other enterically transmitted. Now these two distinct viruses are known as hepatitis C virus (HCV) and hepatitis E virus (HEV).

HCV is a linear, single-stranded RNA virus about 50 to 60 nm in diameter. A second-generation enzyme immunoassay has been used to detect antibodies to HCV (anti-HCV) but has resulted in many false-negative tests; therefore a supplemental recombinant assay (RIBA) is also being used. Anti-HCV was introduced as a blood donor test in May 1990 and has lowered the rate of transfusion-related HCV significantly. Since HCV has been cloned, work on a vaccine is a goal.

HCV, as with HBV, is believed to be transmitted primarily by the parenteral route and is attributable primarily to IV drug use and blood transfusions. Risk of sexual transmission is controversial but appears low. The incubation period ranges from 15 to 160 days, with an average of 50 days. HCV accounts for about 90% of blood transfusion–related cases of hepatitis. Chronic hepatitis develops in about 50% of infected individuals, and 20% to 40% of these eventually develop cirrhosis of the liver. Chronic HCV is also strongly associated with the development of primary liver cancer. Research has confirmed the existence of a carrier state for HCV, which may be present in about 1% to 6% of volunteer blood donors.

Hepatitis D

The hepatitis D virus (HDV, delta virus) is a 35 to 37 nm RNA virus that is unusual in that it requires HBsAg to serve as the outer shell of the infectious particle. Thus only patients positive for HBsAg can become infected with HDV. Serologic markers for the antigen (HDAg), which indicates acute early infection, and for the antibody (anti-HDV), which indicates present or past infection, are commercially available. Transmission is primarily by serum, and in the United States the disease occurs mainly among IV drug users. One third or two thirds of those who are HBV positive also are positive for the anti-HDV. In Mediterranean countries, HDV infection is endemic with HBV. The incubation period is believed to be similar to that of HBV, about 1 to 2 months. HDV may present itself as an acute infection, chronic infection, or coinfection or superinfection with HBV.

Hepatitis E

The hepatitis E virus (HEV) is a small, 32 to 34 nm, nonenveloped, single-stranded RNA virus. HEV is a water-borne type of "non-A, non-B" hepatitis that is enterically transmitted by the fecal-oral route. Currently, serologic testing for HEV can be done using a specially encoded enzyme immunoassay. This method has been effective in discriminating antibody to HEV (anti-HEV) activity in sera. HEV infection is rarely encountered in the United States and is much more prevalent in India and the Indian subcontinent. To date, cases in Western countries have been related to travel to endemic areas. Young to middle-age adults are most often affected, with an approximate mortality of 1% to 2% in the general population and an unusually high (20%) mortality among pregnant women. The incubation period is approximately 6 weeks.

Possible hepatitis F

Sporadic cases of acute liver failure (formerly termed non-A non-B hepatitis) may be attributed to "candidate hepatitis F" (Fagan, 1994). Through more comprehensive diagnoses of hepatitis non-A, non-B, and possibly non-C, non-D, and non-E hepatitis, researchers are attempting to demonstrate that a possible hepatitis F is caused by hepatitis B (HBV) variants (Uchida et al, 1994). However, research is ongoing, and an official identification of hepatitis F is premature (Centers for Disease Control and Prevention, 1995).

Pathology

The morphologic changes in the liver are often similar for the various categories of viral hepatitis agents. In the classic case the liver appears normal in size and color but is sometimes slightly edematous, enlarged, and "tender edged" to palpation. Histologically, hepatocellular disarray, varying degrees of liver cell injury and necrosis, and periportal inflammation are present. These changes are completely reversible when the acute phase of the disease subsides. In a few cases, submassive or massive necrosis may lead to fulminant hepatic failure and death.

Clinical Features

Infection with a hepatitis virus can result in a range of effects, from fulminant hepatic failure to anicteric subclinical hepatitis. The latter is more common in HAV infections, and the patient often mistakes it for the "flu." HBV infections tend to be more severe than HAV infections, and the incidence of massive necrosis and fulminant hepatic failure is more common.

The vast majority of HAV and HBV infections are mild with complete recovery, and the clinical features are similar. *Prodromal symptoms* occur in all patients and may be present 1 or 2 weeks before the onset of jaundice (although not all patients develop jaundice). The main features at this time are malaise, lassitude, anorexia, headache, low-grade fever, and for smokers the loss of desire to smoke. Many patients experience arthralgias, arthritis, urticaria, and transient skin rashes. These extrahepatic manifestations of viral hepatitis may represent a syndrome similar to serum sickness and may be caused by circulating immune complexes. In addition, the patient may have discomfort in the right upper quadrant, usually attributed to stretching of the liver capsule.

The prodromal phase is followed by the *icteric phase* and the onset of jaundice. This phase usually lasts 4 to 6 weeks but may start to subside within a few days. A few days before the jaundice, the patient generally has an improved feeling of well-being. The patient's appetite returns after a couple of weeks. As the fever subsides, the urine becomes darker and the stools somewhat paler. The liver is moderately enlarged and tender, and the spleen is palpably enlarged in about one fourth of patients. A tender lymphadenopathy is often present.

The earliest biochemical abnormality is an elevation of aspartate aminotransferase (AST) and alanine aminotransferase (ALT) levels, which precedes the onset of jaundice by 1 or 2 weeks. Urine examination at the onset reveals the presence of bilirubin and an excess of urobilinogen. The bilirubinuria persists throughout the illness, but the urine urobilinogen may disappear temporarily if there is an obstructive phase caused by cholestasis; later in the course of the illness, a secondary rise in urine urobilinogen may occur.

The icteric phase is associated with hyperbilirubinemia (both conjugated and unconjugated fractions), which is usually less than 10 mg/dl. The serum alkaline phosphatase level is usually normal or only moderately elevated. Atypical lymphocytes are common in acute viral hepatitis, and the prothrombin time may be prolonged. HBsAg is found in the serum during the prodromal phase and definitely establishes HBV hepatitis.

In the uncomplicated case, recovery begins 1 or 2 weeks from the onset of jaundice and lasts 2 to 6 weeks. Easy fatigability is a common complaint. The stools rapidly regain their normal color, the jaundice lessens, and urine color lightens. Splenomegaly, if present, subsides rapidly, but hepatomegaly may resolve only after several weeks. Abnormal laboratory findings and liver function tests may persist for 3 to 6 months.

Complications

Not every patient with viral hepatitis has an uneventful course. A few patients (less than 1%) show rapid clinical deterioration after the onset of jaundice as a result of fulminant hepatitis and massive liver necrosis. *Fulminant hepatitis* is characterized by signs and symptoms of acute liver failure: shrinking liver size, rapidly rising serum bilirubin levels, marked prolongation of prothrombin time, and hepatic coma. The outcome is death in 60% to 80% of these patients. Death may occur within days in some patients, and others may survive for weeks if the damage is less extensive. HBV accounts for more than 50% of the cases of fulminant hepatitis and is often associated with HDV infection. The delta agent (HDV) is able to cause hepatitis when it is present in the body along with the HBsAg. Fulminant hepatitis is less frequently a complication of HCV and is rarely associated with HAV.

The most common complication of viral hepatitis is a more prolonged course that can range from 2 to 8 months. This is called *chronic persistent hepatitis* and occurs in 5% to 10% of patients. Despite the delayed convalescence in chronic persistent hepatitis, patients almost always recover.

Approximately 5% to 10% of patients with viral hepatitis have a relapse after recovering from the initial episode. This may be associated with individuals who are in high-risk categories (e.g., substance abusers, carriers). Usually the jaundice is not as marked, and the liver function tests do not show the same degree of abnormality. Further bed rest is usually followed by an uneventful recovery.

After acute viral hepatitis, a few patients may develop *chronic active* or *aggressive hepatitis,* in which piecemeal destruction of the liver occurs and cirrhosis develops. The condition is distinguished from chronic persistent hepatitis by liver biopsy. Corticosteroid therapy may retard the progression of hepatic injury, but the prognosis is poor. Death often occurs within 5 years in more than half of these patients as a result of hepatic failure or the complications of cirrhosis. Chronic active hepatitis may develop in as many as 50% of patients with HCV; a much smaller proportion (about 1% to 3%) of patients with HBV develop these complications after successful therapy. In contrast, chronic hepatitis does not occur as a complication of HAV or HEV. Not all cases of chronic active hepatitis follow acute viral hepatitis. Drugs may be involved in the pathogenesis of this disorder. Specific drugs implicated include alpha-methyldopa (Aldomet), isoniazid, sulfonamides, and aspirin.

Finally, a significant late complication of hepatitis is the development of primary hepatocellular carcinoma.

Although uncommon in the United States, primary liver cancer is quite common in many developing countries. Two major causal factors have been implicated in the pathogenesis: chronic HBV infection and related cirrhosis. HCV-related cirrhosis and chronic HCV infection also have been associated with primary liver cancer.

Treatment

No specific treatment exists for viral hepatitis. Bed rest during the acute phase is important, and a diet low in fat and high in carbohydrates is generally the most palatable for these patients. IV feeding may be necessary during the acute phase if the patient has persistent vomiting. Some limitation of physical activity is usually necessary until symptoms have subsided and the liver function tests return to normal.

Prevention

Because effective treatment of viral hepatitis is limited, emphasis is placed on prevention through immunization. Currently, passive and inactive immunization are available for HAV and both passive and active immunization for HBV. Recommendations for preexposure and postexposure immunization practices have been published by the CDC (Centers for Disease Control, 1990, 1991).

In February 1995 the first vaccine against HAV was approved for licensure by the U.S. Food and Drug Administration (FDA). The inactivated vaccine is being marketed under the name Havrix. The virus for the vaccine is cultivated on human cells and inactivated with formaldehyde solution, and aluminum hydroxide is used as the adjuvant (Marwick, 1995). A second vaccine against HAV is also under investigation.

The vaccine is being distributed with recommendations for a two-dose administration schedule for adults 18 years of age and older and for the second dose to be given 6 to 12 months after the first. Children over age 2 years and adolescents are given three doses; the second dose is given 1 month after the first dose, and the third dose is given 6 to 12 months later. Children under age 2 years are not vaccinated. Route of administration is by intramuscular (IM) injection in the deltoid muscle.

Immune globulin (IG), formerly called immune serum globulin, is administered to provide protection before or after exposure to HAV. All preparations of IG contain anti-HAV. Preexposure prophylaxis is recommended for international travelers to countries where HAV is endemic. When such travel lasts less than 3 months, a single IM dose of IG (0.2 ml/kg body weight) is given; if longer travel is anticipated, 0.06 ml/kg should be given every 4 to 6 months.

The postexposure use of IG is effective in preventing or decreasing the severity of HAV infection. A dose of 0.02 ml/kg is given as soon as possible or within 2 weeks after exposure. Inoculation with IG is indicated for household members, day-care center staff, workers at custodial institutions, and travelers to tropical and developing countries.

Both high-titer HBV immune globulin (HBIG) and a vaccine are available to prevent and treat HBV. Preexposure prophylaxis is recommended for persons at risk for developing HBV, including the following:

1. Health care workers
2. Clients and staff of custodial institutions for developmentally disabled persons
3. Hemodialysis patients
4. Sexually active homosexual men
5. IV drug users
6. Recipients of blood products on a chronic basis
7. Household or sexual contacts of HBsAg carriers
8. Sexually active heterosexuals with multiple partners
9. International travelers to areas where HBV is endemic
10. Adoptees or refugees from areas where HBV is endemic

The original 1982 HBV vaccine derived from HBV carriers has been largely replaced by the newer, genetically engineered vaccine made from recombinant DNA. The vaccine contains noninfectious HBsAg particles. A series of three injections produces antibodies to HBsAg in 95% of those vaccinated but has no effect on people who are carriers.

HBIG is the drug of choice for short-term postexposure prophylaxis. Concurrent HBV vaccine may be given to provide long-term immunity, depending on the circumstances of the exposure. The CDC recommends that both HBIG and HBV vaccine be given within 12 hours after birth to infants with HBsAg-positive mothers. They further recommend routine HBsAg prenatal testing of all pregnant women in the future, since pregnancy may result in severe disease for the mother and chronic infection for the newborn. Infants born to HBsAg-positive and HBeAg-positive mothers have a 70% to 90% risk for HBV infection; 80% to 90% of infected infants become chronic HBV carriers, and more than 25% of these carriers die from primary hepatocellular carcinoma or cirrhosis of the liver. An estimated 18,000 births to HbsAg-positive mothers occurred in 1987 (Centers for Disease Control, 1990).

HBIG (0.06 ml/kg) is the treatment of choice for preventing HBV infection after percutaneous (needle stick) or mucosal exposure with HBsAg-positive blood. HBV vaccine should also be initiated within 7 to 14 days if the exposed person has not been vaccinated. Exposed persons who have already been vaccinated should have their anti-HBs antibody level measured. If the anti-HBs antibody level is adequate, no treatment is necessary; if inadequate, a booster dose of vaccine should be given.

Personnel engaged in high-risk contact, as in hemodialysis, exchange transfusions, and parenteral therapy, need to exercise great care in the handling of equipment and the avoidance of needle puncture.

Community measures important in the prevention of hepatitis include the provision of a safe food and water supply as well as effective sewage disposal. Careful attention to general hygiene, handwashing, and safe disposal of the urine and feces of infected patients are important. The use of disposable catheters, needles, and syringes eliminates an important source of infection. All blood donors should be screened for the presence of HAV, HBV, and HCV before being accepted on the donor panel.

CIRRHOSIS

Cirrhosis is a chronic disease of the liver characterized by distortion of the normal hepatic architecture by bands of connective tissue and by nodules of regenerating liver cells unrelated to the normal vasculature. The regenerating nodules may be small (micronodular) or large (macronodular). Cirrhosis may interfere with intrahepatic blood circulation, and in far-advanced cases it causes gradual failure of liver function.

The incidence of this disease has increased significantly since World War II, establishing cirrhosis as one of the most prominent causes of death in men. This increase is partly the result of a corresponding increase in the incidence of viral hepatitis but more significantly to an enormous increase in the intake of alcohol. Alcoholism is the single most important cause of cirrhosis.

Etiology, Pathology, and Pathogenesis

Although the etiology of many forms of cirrhosis is poorly understood, three characteristic patterns account for the majority of cases: Laennec's, postnecrotic, and biliary cirrhosis.

Laennec's cirrhosis

Laennec's cirrhosis (also called alcoholic, portal, and nutritional cirrhosis) is a peculiar pattern of cirrhosis associated with chronic abuse of alcoholic beverages. It accounts for about 50% or more of the cases of cirrhosis.

The exact relationship between alcohol abuse and Laennec's cirrhosis is not known, although a clear and unmistakable association exists. The first change in the liver caused by alcohol is the gradual accumulation of fat within the liver cells (fatty infiltration) (see Fig. 3-3). A similar pattern of fatty infiltration is also seen in *kwashiorkor* (a disorder common in developing countries as a result of severe protein deficiency), hyperthyroidism, and diabetes. Most authorities agree that alcoholic beverages exert a direct toxic effect on the liver. The accumulation of fat reflects a number of metabolic disturbances, including excess formation of triglycerides, the decreased export of triglycerides from the liver, and decreased oxidation of fatty acids from inhibition of the citric acid cy-

cle. The person ingesting excessive amounts of alcohol also may not eat properly. The primary cause of liver damage appears to be the direct effect of alcohol on the liver cell, which is increased by malnutrition. These patients may have several nutritional deficiencies, including thiamin, folic acid, pyridoxine, niacin, ascorbic acid, and vitamin A. Bone loss often occurs from decreased calcium intake and faulty metabolism. Vitamin K, iron, and zinc intakes also tend to be deficient in these patients. Protein-calorie deficiencies are also common.

Uncomplicated fatty degeneration of the liver, as might be seen in early alcoholism, is reversible provided the person ceases ingestion of alcohol; few cases of this relatively benign condition progress to cirrhosis. Grossly the liver is enlarged, fragile, and greasy in appearance and may be functionally deficient because of the large accumulation of fat.

If the habit of alcohol abuse persists, particularly when it becomes more severe, something may occur (although there is still uncertainty as to what causes it) to tip the whole process in favor of widespread scar formation. Some authorities believe that the critical lesion in the development of cirrhosis of the liver may be alcoholic hepatitis. *Alcoholic hepatitis* is characterized histologically by hepatocellular necrosis, ballooned cells, and polymorphonuclear neutrophil leukocyte (PMN) infiltration of the liver. However, not all patients who develop the lesion of alcoholic hepatitis progress to full-blown cirrhosis of the liver.

In far-advanced cases of Laennec's cirrhosis, thick fibrous bands form at the periphery of many lobules, partitioning the parenchyma into fine nodules. These nodules may enlarge somewhat as a result of regenerative activity as the liver attempts to replace damaged cells. The liver appears to consist of tightly packed nests of degenerating and regenerating liver cells encased in thick, fibrous capsules. On this basis, the condition is often referred to as *fine nodular cirrhosis*. In the final stages the liver is shrunken, hard, and almost devoid of normal parenchyma, which results in portal hypertension and hepatic failure. Persons with Laennec's cirrhosis have an increased risk of developing primary liver cell (hepatocellular) carcinoma.

Postnecrotic cirrhosis

Postnecrotic cirrhosis presumably follows patchy necrosis of liver tissue. Hepatocytes are surrounded and partitioned by scar tissue, with excessive loss of liver cells and interspersion with normal liver parenchyma. About 75% of the cases tend to progress and result in death within 1 to 5 years. Postnecrotic cirrhosis accounts for about 10% of the cases of cirrhosis. About 25% to 75% of the cases have a prior history of viral hepatitis. Many patients have positive test results for HBsAg, indicating that chronic active hepatitis may be an essential event. HCV accounts for about 25% of cirrhosis cases. A small percentage of cases stem from documented intoxication with industrial chemicals, poisons, or drugs, such as yellow phosphorus, oral contraceptives, methyldopa, arsenicals, and carbon tetrachloride.

A peculiar feature of postnecrotic cirrhosis is that it appears to predispose the patient to the occurrence of a primary hepatic neoplasm of the liver (hepatocellular carcinoma).

Biliary cirrhosis

Liver cell destruction that begins around the bile ducts gives rise to a pattern of cirrhosis known as *biliary cirrhosis*. It accounts for about 2% of deaths from cirrhosis.

The most common cause of biliary cirrhosis is posthepatic biliary obstruction. Stasis of bile causes its accumulation within the liver substance with destruction of liver cells. Fibrous bands begin forming around the periphery of the lobule, but they rarely transect a lobule as in the pattern of Laennec's cirrhosis. The liver is enlarged, firm, and finely granular and has a green hue. Jaundice is always an early and primary part of the syndrome, as are pruritus, malabsorption, and steatorrhea.

Primary biliary cirrhosis presents a pattern somewhat similar to the secondary biliary cirrhosis just described, but it is much more rare. The cause of this condition, which is associated with lesions of the intrahepatic bile ductules, is unknown. The bile capillaries and ductules contain bile plugs, and the liver cells frequently contain a green pigment. The extrahepatic biliary tract is not involved. Portal hypertension as a complication is rare. Osteomalacia occurs about 25% of the time in patients with primary biliary cirrhosis.

Clinical Manifestations

The clinical features and complications of cirrhosis are common to all forms of the disease regardless of the cause, although individual types of cirrhosis may have additional distinctive clinical and biochemical features. The period during which cirrhosis presents as a clinical problem is generally only a small fraction of the total life history of the disease. Cirrhosis is latent for many years, the pathologic changes progressing slowly until major symptoms induce awareness of the disease. During the long latency period, gradual deterioration of liver function occurs.

Early symptoms are vague and nonspecific and include lassitude, anorexia, dyspepsia, flatulence, a change in bowel habits (either constipation or diarrhea), and slight weight loss. Nausea and vomiting, especially in the morning, are common. A dull ache or heavy feeling in the epigastrium or right upper quadrant is present in about half the patients. In most cases the liver is hard and palpable regardless of whether it is enlarged or atrophied.

Liver failure and portal hypertension are two major manifestations of cirrhosis that develop late in the disease process. Hepatocellular failure is evidenced by jaundice, peripheral edema, bleeding tendencies, palmar erythema (red palms), spider angiomas, hepatic fetor (a mousy odor to the breath when there is liver impairment), and hepatic encephalopathy. Portal hypertension often results in splenomegaly, esophageal and gastric varices, and other evidence of abnormal collateral circulation. Ascites (fluid in the peritoneal cavity) can be considered as a manifestation of both hepatocellular failure and portal hypertension. Fig. 27-6 illustrates the primary clinical manifestations of cirrhosis discussed next.

Manifestations of hepatocellular failure

Jaundice occurs in at least 60% of patients at some time during the course of cirrhosis and is usually minimal. Hyperbilirubinemia without jaundice is more common. The patient may become jaundiced during a phase of decompensation with reversible deterioration of liver function. For example, the patient with cirrhosis may become jaundiced after a heavy drinking bout. Intermittent jaundice is a characteristic feature of biliary cirrhosis and occurs with active inflammation of the liver bile ductules *(cholangitis)*. Patients dying from hepatic failure are usually jaundiced.

Endocrine disturbances are common in cirrhosis. Hormones of the adrenal cortex, testes, and ovaries are metabolized and inactivated by the normal liver. Spider angiomas are seen on the skin, particularly around the neck, shoulders, and chest. Spider angiomas consist of a central arteriole from which many small vessels radiate. Spider angiomas, testicular atrophy, gynecomastia, pectoral and axillary alopecia, and palmar erythema are all considered to be caused by an excess of circulating estrogen. Increased pigmentation of the skin is believed to result from excessive activity of melanocyte-stimulating hormone (MSH).

Hematologic disorders common in cirrhosis include bleeding tendencies, anemia, leukopenia, and thrombocytopenia. Nosebleeds, gingival bleeding, heavy menstrual bleeding, and easy bruising may occur, and the prothrombin time may be prolonged. These manifestations are the result of decreased hepatic production of the clotting factors. The anemia, leukopenia, and thrombocytopenia are believed to result from hypersplenism. Not only is the spleen enlarged *(splenomegaly)*, but it is also more active in the removal of blood cells from the circulation. Other mechanisms contributing to the anemia include folate deficiency, vitamin B_{12} deficiency, iron deficiency secondary to blood loss, and increased hemolysis of RBCs. The patient is also more susceptible to infection.

The peripheral edema that generally occurs after the development of ascites may be explained by the hypoalbuminemia and abnormal salt and water retention. The failure of the liver cells to inactivate aldosterone and antidiuretic hormone (ADH) contributes to sodium and water retention.

Hepatic fetor is a musty, sweetish odor that may be detected on the patient's breath, especially in hepatic coma,

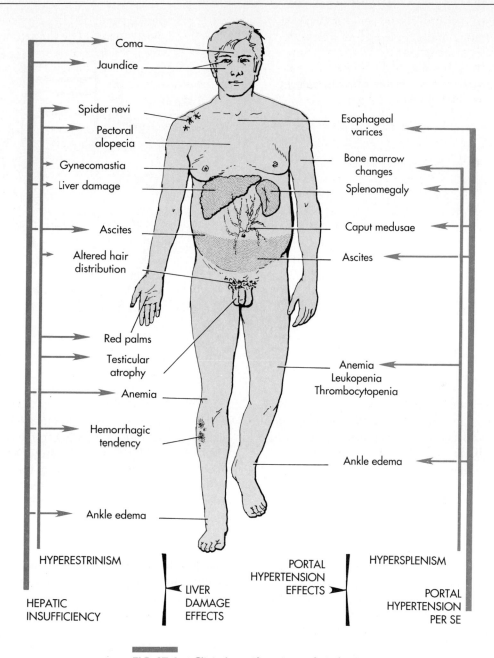

Coma
Jaundice

Spider nevi
Pectoral alopecia
Gynecomastia
Liver damage
Ascites
Altered hair distribution

Red palms
Testicular atrophy
Anemia
Hemorrhagic tendency

Ankle edema

Esophageal varices
Bone marrow changes
Splenomegaly
Caput medusae
Ascites

Anemia
Leukopenia
Thrombocytopenia

Ankle edema

HYPERESTRINISM

PORTAL HYPERTENSION EFFECTS

HYPERSPLENISM

HEPATIC INSUFFICIENCY

LIVER DAMAGE EFFECTS

PORTAL HYPERTENSION PER SE

FIG. 27-6   Clinical manifestations of cirrhosis.

and is believed to result from the liver's inability to metabolize methionine.

The most serious neurologic disorder in advanced cirrhosis is *hepatic encephalopathy* (hepatic coma). It is believed to result from abnormalities in the metabolism of ammonia and increased cerebral sensitivity to toxins. The development of hepatic encephalopathy is often a terminal event in cirrhosis and is discussed in greater detail later.

Manifestations of portal hypertension

Portal hypertension is defined as a sustained elevation of pressure in the portal vein above the normal level of 6 to 12 cm H_2O. The primary mechanism for inducing por-

tal hypertension, regardless of the disease, is increased resistance to blood flow through the liver. In addition, there is usually an increase in splanchnic arterial flow. The two factors of decreased outflow through the hepatic vein and increased inflow combine to overload the portal circuit. This overload of the portal circuit stimulates the development of collateral channels (varices), which circumvent the hepatic obstruction. The back pressure in the portal system causes splenomegaly and is partly responsible for the accumulation of ascites.

Ascites is an intraperitoneal accumulation of watery fluid containing small amounts of protein. Key factors in the pathogenesis of ascites are the increased hydrostatic pressure in the intestinal capillary bed (portal hyperten-

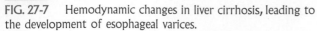

FIG. 27-7 Hemodynamic changes in liver cirrhosis, leading to the development of esophageal varices.

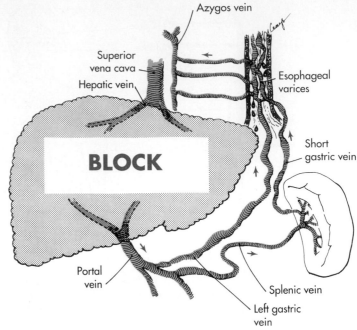

sion) and the decreased colloid osmotic pressure from hypoalbuminemia. Other contributing factors include abnormal sodium and water retention and increased synthesis and flow of hepatic lymph (see later discussion).

The important collateral channels that develop as a result of cirrhosis and portal hypertension are found in the lower esophagus. The shunting of blood through this circuit to the venae cavae causes dilation of these veins *(esophageal varices)*. These varices occur in about 70% of patients with advanced cirrhosis. Bleeding from these varices is a common cause of death (Fig. 27-7).

The collateral circulation also involves the superficial veins of the abdominal wall, and its development leads to dilated veins around the umbilicus (caput medusae). Because the rectal venous system helps decompensate portal pressure, the veins dilate and may lead to the development of internal hemorrhoids (see Fig. 27-2 to review points of anastomoses). Serious hemorrhage from the rupture of hemorrhoids does not usually occur, since the pressure is not as high there as in the esophagus because of the greater distance from the portal vein.

Splenomegaly in cirrhosis can be explained on the basis of chronic passive congestion as a result of backup and higher pressure of blood in the splenic vein.

Treatment and Complications

The treatment of cirrhosis is unsatisfactory. No pharmacologic agents arrest or reverse the fibrotic process. Therapy first deals with the underlying cause, such as alcohol abuse or bile duct obstruction, and then treats the various complications, including gastrointestinal (GI) bleeding, ascites, and hepatic encephalopathy.

Gastrointestinal bleeding

The most common and the most serious cause of GI bleeding in cirrhosis is bleeding from esophageal varices, which accounts for about one third of all deaths from cirrhosis. Other causes of bleeding include acute gastric erosions, a generalized bleeding tendency as a result of prolonged prothrombin and thrombocytopenia, and less often, gastric and duodenal ulcers.

The patient presents with either melena or hematemesis. Occasionally a sign of bleeding is hepatic encephalopathy. Depending on the amount and rapidity of the blood loss, the patient may have hypovolemia and hypotension.

A variety of measures have been used for the immediate control of bleeding. Tamponade with apparatuses such as the Sengstaken-Blakemore (triple-lumen) tube (Fig. 27-8) and Minnesota (quadruple-lumen) tube can temporarily stop the hemorrhage. The veins can be visualized with fiberoptic instruments and injected with a solution that will cause a clot to form in the vein, thus stopping the hemorrhage. Most clinicians believe this has a temporary effect and is not effective for long-term management. Vasopressin (Pitressin) has been used to control bleeding. The drug decreases portal pressure by decreasing splanchnic blood flow, although the effect is only temporary. The overall mortality rate of bleeding varices is about 35% because of liver failure and complications (Way, 1994).

If the patient recovers from the bleeding, a portacaval shunt procedure may be performed to reduce the portal pressure by anastomosing the portal vein (high pressure) to the inferior vena cava (low pressure). The shunt procedure represents drastic therapy for this major compli-

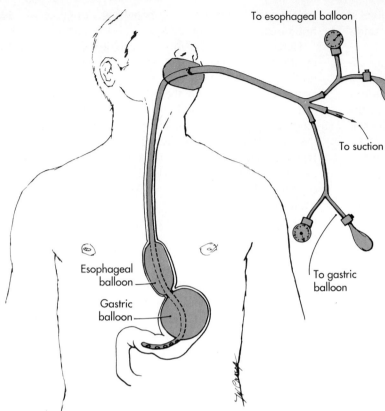

To esophageal balloon

To suction

Esophageal balloon

Gastric balloon

To gastric balloon

FIG. 27-8 Sengstaken-Blakemore tube in place for the emergency treatment of hemorrhage from esophageal varices. The tube has three openings for (1) gastric aspiration, (2) inflating the esophageal balloon, and (3) inflating the gastric balloon. The esophageal balloon is inflated to a pressure of 20 to 40 mm Hg (monitored by attachment to a gauge or a sphygmomanometer) that compresses the esophageal veins. The gastric balloon, inflated with 250 cc of air, applies pressure to the fundal veins when slight traction is applied.

cation of cirrhosis. It lessens the chance of further esophageal bleeding, but at the price of an increased risk of hepatic encephalopathy. The procedure does not increase the patient's life expectancy, which is still determined by the progress of the liver disease.

GI bleeding is one of the important precipitating causes of hepatic encephalopathy. The encephalopathy results when ammonia (NH_3) and other toxins enter the systemic circulation. The source of NH_3 is the bacterial breakdown of protein in the GI tract. Hepatic encephalopathy will follow if the blood is not removed by gastric aspiration, saline cathartics, and cleansing enemas and if the bacterial breakdown of the blood protein is not prevented by the administration of neomycin or a similar antibiotic. These measures are discussed in more detail later.

Ascites

As mentioned earlier, ascites is the accumulation of serous fluid within the peritoneal cavity. Ascites is a cardinal manifestation of cirrhosis and other severe forms of liver disease. Several factors are involved in the pathogenesis of ascites in liver cirrhosis: (1) portal hypertension, (2) hypoalbuminemia, (3) increased production and flow of hepatic lymph, (4) sodium retention, and (5) impaired water excretion. The primary mechanism for inducing portal hypertension, as previously described, is resistance to blood flow through the liver. This causes an

increase in the hydrostatic pressure in the intestinal vascular bed. Hypoalbuminemia develops because of its reduced synthesis by impaired liver cells. Hypoalbuminemia results in decreased colloid osmotic pressure. The combination of increased hydrostatic pressure and decreased colloid osmotic pressure in the intestinal vascular bed favors transudation of fluid from the intravascular space to the interstitial space according to the law of Starling forces (the peritoneal space in the case of ascites). The portal hypertension further increases the production of hepatic lymph, which "weeps" from the liver into the peritoneal cavity. These mechanisms may contribute to the high protein content in the ascitic fluid, thus raising the colloid osmotic pressure in the peritoneal cavity fluid and promoting the transudation of fluid from the intravascular space to the peritoneal space. Finally, sodium retention and impaired water excretion are important factors in perpetuating ascites. Sodium and water retention are caused by secondary hyperaldosteronism (decreased effective circulating volume activates the renin-angiotensin-aldosterone mechanism). Decreased hepatic inactivation of circulating aldosterone also may occur because of hepatocellular failure.

A sign of ascites is increased abdominal girth. More pronounced accumulation of fluid may cause shortness of breath because of the elevated diaphragm. As peritoneal fluid accumulates, amounts greater than 500 ml can be demonstrated during a physical assessment by shifting dullness, a fluid wave, and bulging flanks. Smaller quantities may be revealed by ultrasound examination or paracentesis.

Salt restriction is the primary method of treating ascites. Diuretics may also be used in conjunction with a low-sodium diet. Various diuretics and diuretic programs are available, but the essential feature is to introduce the diuretics gradually to avoid too brisk a diuresis. A loss of no more than 1.0 kg/day of fluid is recommended if ascites and peripheral edema are present. Electrolyte imbalance must be avoided, and even then diuretics may precipitate hepatic encephalopathy.

Paracentesis is the insertion of a cannula into the peritoneal cavity to remove ascitic fluid. In the past, paracentesis was a common form of treatment for ascites but is no longer considered desirable because of its deleterious effects. There is danger of inducing hypovolemia, hypokalemia, hyponatremia, hepatic encephalopathy, and renal failure. Because ascitic fluid may contain 10 to 30 g of protein/L, serum albumin is further depleted, promoting hypotension and reaccumulation of the ascitic fluid. Therefore IV replacement of albumin may be given during paracentesis to avoid these complications. Paracentesis is usually performed only for diagnostic purposes and when ascites causes prominent respiratory difficulty as a result of a large volume of fluid. Some patients with ascites also develop pleural effusions, especially in the right hemithorax. The fluid is thought to enter the chest through tears that develop in the tendinous portion of the diaphragm because of the increased abdominal pressure.

Hepatic encephalopathy

Hepatic encephalopathy (hepatic coma) is a neuropsychiatric syndrome in a patient with severe liver disease. It is characterized by mental confusion, muscle tremors, and a peculiar flapping tremor called *asterixis*. The mental changes may begin with alterations in personality, memory loss, and irritability and may progress to death in a deep coma. Hepatic encephalopathy ending in coma is the mechanism of death in about one third of the fatal cases of cirrhosis.

Pathogenesis. In simplest terms, hepatic encephalopathy can be described as a form of cerebral intoxication caused by intestinal contents that have not been metabolized by the liver. This condition may occur when there is either liver cell damage or shunting (pathologic or surgically created) that permits large amounts of portal blood to reach the systemic circulation without traversing the liver.

The metabolites responsible for the encephalopathy have not been identified with certainty. The basic mechanism appears to be intoxication of the brain by breakdown products of protein metabolism produced by bacterial action in the gut. These products are able to bypass the liver because of liver cell disease or shunting. NH_3, normally converted into urea by the liver, is one of the

known toxic substances and is believed to interfere with brain metabolism (Fig. 27-9).

Hepatic encephalopathy is usually precipitated by events such as GI bleeding, excessive protein intake, diuretics, paracentesis, hypokalemia, acute infections, surgery, azotemia, and the administration of morphine, sedatives, or NH_3-containing drugs. *Azotemia* is the retention of nitrogenous substances (e.g., urea) in the blood that are normally filtered by the kidneys. The harmful effects of many of these can be traced to mechanisms that cause large amounts of NH_3 to form in the bowel. Encephalopathy that follows potassium depletion or paracentesis is probably related to excessive NH_3 formed by the kidneys and acid-base balance alterations. Table 27-6 summarizes factors that may precipitate hepatic encephalopathy and the possible physiologic mechanisms involved.

Clinical features. Clinical signs and symptoms of hepatic encephalopathy may arise quickly and progress to coma when hepatic failure occurs in a patient with fulminating hepatitis. In cirrhotic patients the progress usually is much slower and is reversible in the early stages if detected in time. Progression of hepatic encephalopathy to coma is usually divided into four stages.

The signs in *stage I* are subtle and may be easily missed. Danger signals include slight personality and behavioral changes, including an unkempt appearance, vacant stare, slurred speech, inappropriate laughter, forgetfulness, and inability to concentrate. Patients may appear to be perfectly rational but uncooperative or disrespectful at times. Careful observation may reveal that they are more lethargic or sleep more than usual or that their sleep rhythms are reversed. Because of close association with such a patient, the nurse is in a strategic position to notice these changes and should enlist the help of the family to detect subtle personality changes.

The signs in *stage II* are more prominent and are easily detected. Behavior may be inappropriate, and sphincter control is not maintained. Generalized muscle twitching and asterixis are characteristic findings. *Asterixis,* or flapping tremor, is elicited by having the patient raise both arms with forearms fixed, wrists hyperextended, and fingers separated. This maneuver causes involuntary rapid flexion and extension movements of the wrists (flapping) and metacarpophalangeal joints. Asterixis is a peripheral manifestation of impaired cerebral metabolism. It may also occur in the uremic syndrome. During this stage the lethargy and personality and behavioral changes become more marked.

Constructional apraxia is another prominent feature of hepatic encephalopathy. The patient cannot write clearly or draw figures such as stars or houses. A serial record of handwriting or figure construction is a useful method of determining the progress of the encephalopathy.

In *stage III* the patient may have pronounced confusion and inappropriate behavior. If the patient is given a sedative at this time rather than treatment to reverse the

TABLE 27-6   Common Factors That May Precipitate Hepatic Encephalopathy (HE)

Precipitating Factor	Possible Mechanisms Leading to HE
INCREASED NITROGENOUS LOAD	
Gastrointestinal (GI) bleeding Excess dietary protein Azotemia (increased blood urea nitrogen [BUN]) Constipation	Excess blood in GI tract (10 to 20 g protein/dl) or excess dietary protein provides substrate for increased ammonia (NH_3) production. Action of gut bacteria on protein produces NH_3, which is absorbed and normally detoxified in the liver by conversion to urea. Increased NH_3 enters the systemic circulation when there is *hepatocellular failure* or *portosystemic shunting*. NH_3 (and possibly other toxic metabolites) readily crosses the blood-brain barrier, where it has a direct toxic effect on the brain. Impaired renal function and increased BUN causes more urea to diffuse into the gut, where it is converted to NH_3 by gut bacteria. Constipation favors increased production and absorption of NH_3 because of prolonged contact of protein substrates with gut bacteria.
ELECTROLYTE IMBALANCES	
Alkalosis Hypokalemia Hypovolemia	Alkalosis and hypokalemia, often caused by hyperventilation and vomiting, favor the diffusion of NH_3 from extracellular fluid to intracellular fluid, including brain cells, where it exerts a toxic effect. In alkalosis, more of the NH_3 produced from glutamine in the kidney reenters the systemic circulation rather than being excreted as ammonium ions (NH_4^+). Hypovolemia, caused by GI hemorrhage, excessive use of diuretics, or paracentesis, may precipitate HE by causing renal failure and azotemia, which in turn lead to increased blood NH_3.
MEDICATIONS	
Diuretics Tranquilizers, narcotics, sedatives, anesthetics	Overzealous use of diuretics can cause electrolyte imbalances, including alkalosis, hypokalemia, and hypovolemia. Thus potassium-depleting diuretics in particular should be avoided. Sedatives and other drugs that cause central nervous system depression act synergistically with NH_3. Impaired metabolism of these drugs also occurs from hepatocellular failure.
MISCELLANEOUS	
Infection Surgery	Infection or surgery causes increased tissue catabolism, leading to increased BUN and NH_3 production. Hyperthermia, dehydration, and impaired renal function may potentiate NH_3 toxicity.

Modified from Greenberger NJ: *Gastrointestinal disorders: a pathophysiologic approach,* ed 4, St Louis, 1989, Mosby.

toxic process, the encephalopathy will probably progress to coma and the outcome may be fatal. Hyperventilation and hypothermia may be seen before the onset of coma. During this stage the patient may sleep much of the time. The electroencephalogram (EEG) begins to change in stage II and is definitely abnormal in stages III and IV.

In *stage IV* the patient fades into a coma from which he or she cannot be aroused. Hyperactive reflexes and a positive Babinski's sign appear. At times a musty, sweetish odor (hepatic fetor) may be detected on the patient's breath or by just entering the room. Hepatic fetor is a grave prognostic sign, and the intensity of the odor correlates well with the degree of somnolence and confusion. Elevation of the blood NH_3 level is an additional laboratory finding that may be helpful in the detection of encephalopathy.

Treatment. The steps in treatment of hepatic encephalopathy have been suggested in discussing the mechanisms that cause it. It is most important to look for any precipitating factors, such as GI bleeding or overenthusiastic diuretic therapy, and provide corrective treatment.

The initial treatment is to exclude all protein from the diet and inhibit the action of bacteria on protein substances in the bowel, since the breakdown of protein in the bowel is the source of NH_3 and other nitrogenous substances. Neomycin, a minimally absorbed antibiotic, is usually the drug of choice for the inhibition of gut bacteria. The usual dosage is about 4 to 12 g/day for adults. Intestinal bacteria may also be lowered through use of lactulose.

Lactulose also lowers stool pH when it is fermented to organic acids by colonic bacteria. The lowered pH traps NH_3 in the colon as nondiffusible ammonium ions (NH_4^+), which are then excreted in the stool. If the patient has had recent GI bleeding (source of protein), magnesium sulfate or enemas may be given to purge the bowel. It is important to correct fluid and electrolyte imbalance, especially hypokalemia, which exacerbates encephalopathy. Sedatives, tranquilizers, and diuretics are avoided, and the use of diuretics is minimized, especially potassium-depleting diuretics. Nourishment is given in the form of sweetened fruit juices or IV glucose. These measures are usually successful if instituted early in the course of precoma and if the liver damage is not too far advanced.

Several measures are used to prevent encephalopathy in the patient who has a portacaval shunt or who has re-

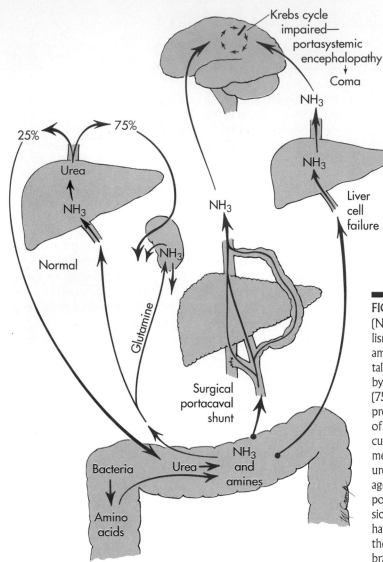

FIG. 27-9 Normal and abnormal circulation of ammonia (NH_3). The left side of the diagram shows the normal metabolism of NH_3. Ingested proteins are transformed into NH_3 and amines by the action of gut bacteria, are absorbed into the portal venous system, and are detoxified by conversion into urea by the hepatocytes. Urea is mostly excreted by the kidney (75%), but 25% is excreted into the intestine. The kidney also produces varying amounts of NH_3, largely by the deamination of glutamine. Normally, very little NH_3 enters the systemic circulation. The right side of the diagram shows the two major mechanisms causing hyperammonemia in liver cirrhosis: (1) failure of the liver to form urea as a result of hepatocellular damage and (2) portosystemic shunting (bypassing the liver) via portosystemic collaterals in the presence of portal hypertension. A portocaval surgical shunt as shown in the diagram can have the same effect. Excess NH_3 in the blood readily crosses the blood-brain barrier, where it causes a toxic effect on the brain called hepatic encephalopathy or hepatic coma.

covered from encephalopathy. These measures include a diet with modest amounts of protein, maintenance doses of neomycin, avoidance of potassium-depleting diuretics and NH_3-containing medications, avoidance of sedatives and narcotics, avoidance of constipation, and prohibition of all dietary protein if the symptoms should recur.

CHOLELITHIASIS AND CHOLECYSTITIS

The two most prominent diseases of the biliary tree, from the standpoint of frequency, are stone formation (*cholelithiasis*) and an associated chronic inflammation (*cholecystitis*). Although either of these conditions may occur alone, they are usually associated and are discussed together.

Pathology

Gallstones are essentially precipitates of one or more components of bile: cholesterol, bilirubin, bile salts, calcium, protein, fatty acids, and phospholipids (see Fig. 3-10). Of these substances, cholesterol is nearly insoluble in water and bilirubin is poorly soluble. Gallstones are divided by composition into primarily three types: pigment, cholesterol, and mixed stones. *Pigment stones* are composed of calcium salts and one of four of the following anions: bilirubinate, carbonate, phosphate, or long-chain fatty acids. They tend to be small, multiple, and black to brown in appearance. Black pigment stones are associated with chronic hemolysis and brown pigment stones with chronic biliary infection. These gallstones are less common. "Pure" *cholesterol stones* usually present a large, solitary, round or oval structure that is pale yellow in color and often contain some calcium and pigment. *Mixed cholesterol stones* constitute a larger category and are the most common. They have features of both cholesterol and pigment stones and are multiple and dark brown in color. Gallstones of mixed composition are frequently visible radiographically, whereas those of pure composition may not be.

Etiology and Pathogenesis

Gallstones are unusually common in the United States, with as many as 20% of the population (16 to 20 million people) affected (Way, 1994). Each year, several hundred thousand of these patients undergo biliary tract surgery. Although gallstones are relatively uncommon during the first two decades of life, women who take oral contraceptives or who are pregnant are at increased risk for gallstones, even in the teen years and 20s. Racial and familial factors seem to be associated with a higher incidence of gallstones. Native Americans have an unusually high incidence, followed by Caucasians and then African Americans. Pathologic conditions associated with a higher incidence of gallstones include diabetes, cirrhosis of the liver, pancreatitis, cancer of the gallbladder, and ileal disease or resection. Other risk factors correlating with gallstone occurrence include obesity, multiparity, increasing age, female gender, and the sudden ingestion of low-fat or low-calorie (fasting) diets.

Gallstones are almost invariably formed in the gallbladder and rarely in other parts of the biliary tree. The etiology of gallstones is still incompletely understood, but the most important predisposing factors appear to be metabolic disturbances causing changes in the composition of bile, bile stasis, and gallbladder infection.

Changes in the composition of bile are probably the most important factor in gallstone formation. A number of studies have indicated that the liver of patients with cholesterol gallstone disease secretes bile that is supersaturated with cholesterol. This excess cholesterol is precipitated (in a manner that is not yet fully understood) to form gallstones.

Stasis of bile in the gallbladder can lead to progressive supersaturation, changes in the chemical composition, and precipitation of the constituents. Disordered contractility of the gallbladder, spasm of the sphincter of Oddi, or both could cause stasis. Hormonal factors, especially during pregnancy, may be related to delayed gallbladder emptying and may account for the higher incidence in this group.

Bacterial infection within the biliary tract can play a role in stone formation. Mucus increases the viscosity of bile, and the cellular elements or bacteria may serve as a nidus for precipitation. However, infection probably is more often a result of the formation of gallstones than a cause of them.

Clinical Features

Patients with gallstones often have symptoms of acute or chronic cholecystitis. The acute form is characterized by

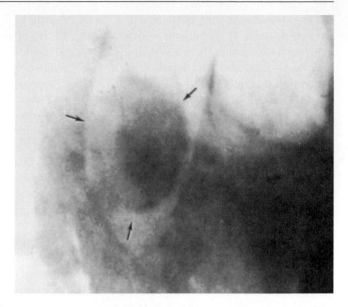

FIG. 27-10   Gallstone.

the sudden onset of agonizing pain in the epigastrium or right upper quadrant; it may radiate to the back and right shoulder. The patient may break out in a profuse sweat or walk the floor or roll from side to side in the bed. Nausea and vomiting are common, and a fever may be present. The pain may last for several hours or may recur after a partial remission. As the pain subsides, tenderness may be noted over the gallbladder region. Acute cholecystitis is often associated with impaction of a stone in the cystic duct and is frequently referred to as *biliary colic.*

The symptoms of chronic cholecystitis are similar to those of acute cholecystitis, but the severity of the pain and the presence of physical signs are less marked. Often the patient has a history of vague dyspepsia, fat intolerance, heartburn, or flatulence over a prolonged time.

Once formed, gallstones may lie quietly in the gallbladder and cause no trouble or they may cause complications. The most common complications are inflammation of the gallbladder (cholecystitis) and obstruction of the cystic or common bile ducts by a stone. Such obstruction may be temporary, intermittent, or permanent. Rarely, stones may penetrate through the wall of the gallbladder and cause severe inflammation, often leading to peritonitis, or may cause the gallbladder walls to become thin and rupture.

Diagnosis and Treatment

The diagnosis of both the acute and the chronic forms of cholecystitis and cholelithiasis often relies on ultrasound or cholecystography to reveal the presence of stones or malfunctioning of the gallbladder (Fig. 27-10).

Palliative treatment for these patients is the avoidance

of offending foods, such as those with high fat content. In the acute phase, many patients with cholecystitis initially achieve remission with rest, IV fluids, nasogastric suction, analgesia, and antibiotics. Oral bile acids may be used to dissolve cholesterol of mixed gallstones. According to studies, partial or complete dissolution of these stones has been successful about 50% to 60% of the time. Through a method called *lithotripsy,* gallstones may be fragmented by extracorporeal shock waves generated by electromagnetic types of devices in patients with (1) biliary colic, (2) radiolucent stones, (3) functioning gallbladder with normal emptying, (4) up to a maximum of three stones, and (5) absence of complications, such as infection, obstruction, and pancreatitis.

The common treatment of cholecystitis and cholelithiasis is surgical removal of the gallbladder *(cholecystectomy)* or removal of stones from the common bile duct *(choledocholithotomy),* which can be expected to effect a cure in about 95% of patients. In patients who have acute cholecystitis with severe symptoms and suspicion of pus formation, some surgeons perform surgery at once, whereas others do so only if improvement does not occur within a few days. Currently the traditional open method of abdominal surgery is used about 20% of the time, with a laparoscopic method of abdominal surgery used for cholecystectomies about 80% of the time (Milamed, Hedley-Whyte, 1994). In cases of empyema or if the patient is in poor condition, the gallbladder may not be removed but merely drained *(cholecystotomy).*

PANCREATITIS

The pancreas is unusual in that this organ functions as both an endocrine and an exocrine gland. A primary endocrine disorder of the pancreas is diabetes (see Chapter 63). The exocrine products of the pancreas contain powerful enzymes that normally digest proteins, fats, and carbohydrates in ingested food. However, these potent enzymes that are so effective in digestion in the lumen of the small intestine may also serve as a source of great danger to the organism if they are activated within the substance of the pancreas itself. The autodigestion theory suggests that this is essentially what happens in pancreatitis. Pancreatitis is typically divided into acute and chronic forms.

Acute Pancreatitis

Acute pancreatitis is an acute inflammatory process involving the pancreas and characterized by varying degrees of edema, hemorrhage, and necrosis of the acinar cells and blood vessels. The mortality and clinical symptoms vary with the degree of the pathologic process. In 85% to 90% of patients with acute pancreatitis, symptoms usually cease 3 to 7 days after treatment is started.

The mortality rate with acute pancreatitis is 10%, whereas the rate with severe necrotizing pancreatitis is about 50%. Surgery seems to decrease mortality rates.

Etiology and pathogenesis

The main etiologic factors in acute pancreatitis are biliary tract disease and alcoholism. Less common causes include trauma (especially bullet or knife wounds), penetrating duodenal ulcer, hyperparathyroidism, hyperlipidemia, viral infection, and certain drugs such as sulfonamides and thiazide diuretics. Often a precipitating cause cannot be found.

Pancreatitis is quite common in adults but is rare in children. In men it is more frequently associated with alcoholism, and in women it is associated more often with gallstones.

Virtually universal agreement exists that the common pathogenetic mechanism in pancreatitis is *autodigestion,* but the process by which the pancreatic enzymes become activated is not clear. In the normal pancreas a number of protective mechanisms safeguard against inadvertent activation of enzymes and autodigestion. First, the enzymes that digest protein are secreted as inactive precursors (zymogens) that must be activated by trypsin. *Trypsinogen,* the inactive form of trypsin, is normally converted into trypsin by the action of enterokinase in the small intestine. Once *trypsin* is formed, it is the key that activates all the other proteolytic enzymes. Tripsin inhibitors are present in the plasma and in the pancreas; they can bind and inactivate any trypsin inadvertently produced, so that proteolytic digestion is unlikely to occur in the normal pancreas.

Reflux of bile and duodenal contents into the pancreatic ducts has been proposed as a possible mechanism for the activation of pancreatic enzymes. This could occur when a common channel is present and a gallstone becomes impacted at the ampulla of Vater. Atony and edema of the sphincter of Oddi might permit duodenal reflux. Obstruction of the pancreatic ducts and pancreatic ischemia may also play a role.

The two activated enzymes believed to play a critical role in pancreatic autodigestion are elastase and phospholipase A. *Phospholipase A* may be activated by trypsin or bile acids and digests the phospholipids of cell membranes. *Elastase* is activated by trypsin and digests the elastic tissue of blood vessel walls, causing hemorrhage. The activation of *kallikrein* by trypsin is believed to play a role in the development of local damage and systemic hypotension. Kallikrein causes vasodilation, increased vascular permeability, invasion of white blood cells, and pain.

Clinical features

The most prominent symptom of acute pancreatitis is severe abdominal pain that is sudden in onset and continuous. It is usually felt in the epigastrium but may be accentuated to the right or left of the midline. Radiation of the pain to the back is common, and the patient may obtain some relief by sitting forward. Nausea, vomiting, sweating, and weakness often accompany the pain. The pain is usually severe for about 24 hours and then decreases over a period of days.

Physical examination may reveal varying degrees of shock, tachycardia, leukocytosis, and fever. There is tenderness and guarding of the abdominal muscles, with distention, rigidity, and other evidence of peritonitis occurring when the inflammation involves the peritoneum. Bowel sounds may be reduced or absent. Severe retroperitoneal bleeding may manifest as bruising in the flanks or around the umbilicus.

The diagnosis of acute pancreatitis is usually established by the finding of an increased serum amylase level. The serum amylase level is elevated during the first 24 to 72 hours, and values are often over two times greater than normal. Urinary amylase levels are elevated as much as 2 weeks after an episode of acute pancreatitis. Other biochemical changes include elevation of the serum lipase level, hyperglycemia, hypocalcemia, and hypokalemia. Hypocalcemia is a common finding caused by marked fat necrosis with the formation of calcium soaps. It may be severe enough to cause tetany.

Complications of acute pancreatitis include the development of diabetes mellitus, severe tetany, pleural effusion (especially in the left hemithorax), and a pancreatic abscess or pseudocyst. *Abscesses* are defined as collections of liquid secretory and necrotic products within the pancreas, whereas collections that occur outside the gland are called *pseudocysts.* A *phlegmon,* a solid mass of swollen, inflamed pancreas, often containing patchy areas of necrosis, may be present for 1 to 2 weeks after onset.

Pancreatic abscesses and pseudocysts often occur during the second or third week after the onset of pancreatitis. A common site of a pancreatic pseudocyst is within the lesser omental sac. Secondary infection of these collections of fluid are frequently seen.

The most common sequelae of acute pancreatitis are recurrent acute attacks and the development of chronic pancreatitis.

Treatment

The primary early treatment of acute pancreatitis is medical, with surgery limited to treatment of biliary obstruction or specific complications such as a pancreatic pseudocyst. Treatment objectives include relief of pain, reduction of pancreatic secretions, prevention and treatment of shock, restoration of fluid and electrolyte balance, and treatment of secondary infection. Shock and hypovolemia are treated with plasma and electrolyte infusions using the hematocrit, central venous pressure, and urine output as indexes of adequate volume replacement. Meperidine (Demerol), rather than opiates, is used to relieve the pain because it causes less spasm of the sphincter of Oddi. Elimination of all oral intake and constant gastric suction reduce intestinal distention and pre-

vent acid contents from entering the duodenum and stimulating pancreatic secretion. Antibiotic treatment of established infection is essential to minimize the risks of secondary infections. According to more recent studies, treatment of acute pancreatitis routinely with antibiotics has been found to be ineffective (Greenberger, Toskes, Isselbacher, 1994).

Pancreatic abscesses are treated by surgical drainage through the anterior abdominal wall or flank. Pseudocysts are managed by internal drainage between the anterior wall of the cyst and the posterior wall of the gastric antrum.

Once the acute phase of the illness subsides, oral feedings may be started. As bowel sounds return, clear liquids are given and the patient progresses to a low-fat, high-carbohydrate diet so that pancreatic secretions are minimally stimulated. Attempts are made to determine the cause of the inflammation. The patient is advised against consuming alcohol for at least 3 months, and if the pancreatitis is believed to be alcohol induced, abstinence should be permanent and total.

Chronic Pancreatitis

Chronic pancreatitis is characterized by progressive destruction of the gland, with fibrotic replacement that may result in stricture and eventual calcification. The etiologic factors are the same as those in acute pancreatitis, although in the United States about 75% of patients with chronic pancreatitis are alcoholics. The clinical course may be one of recurrent episodes of acute pain, each leaving the patient with a lower-functioning pancreatic mass, or may be a slow advance. Steatorrhea, malabsorption, weight loss, and diabetes are manifestations of advanced destruction. Chronic pancreatitis may follow acute pancreatitis, but in many patients it begins insidiously.

The most sensitive test for detecting chronic pancreatitis is the determination of *bicarbonate concentration and output* in the duodenum after stimulation with secretin. Other useful diagnostic measures include fecal fat determination, fasting blood glucose levels to determine islet cell damage, and arteriography and radiographic examinations to detect fibrosis and scattered calcification. Unfortunately, invasive pancreatic carcinoma can produce the same pathophysiologic findings as those produced by chronic pancreatitis and thus presents a major problem for the physician in the differential diagnosis.

The treatment of chronic pancreatitis is taxing and unsatisfactory. Relief of pain is difficult and may require large and frequent doses of analgesics. Narcotic addiction becomes a serious problem. Sometimes local resection of the pancreatic gland may relieve the pain. Pancreatic enzymes have also been effectively used in selected patients to decrease the abdominal pain of chronic pancreatitis. Steatorrhea is managed with a low-fat diet and oral administration of fat-soluble vitamins and pancreatic enzymes. Diabetes requires control with either oral hypoglycemic agents or insulin. Alcohol ingestion is contraindicated.

CANCER OF THE LIVER, GALLBLADDER, AND PANCREAS

Primary cancer of the liver and gallbladder are relatively uncommon tumors in the United States. However, primary cancer of the liver is quite common in Africa and Japan. Both of these malignancies have a poor prognosis.

Malignant tumors primary to the liver arise from either parenchymal cells or bile duct epithelium. The former, known as *hepatocellular carcinoma,* makes up 80% to 90% of primary liver malignancies; the latter is *cholangiocarcinoma.* About 75% of patients who develop hepatoma have underlying cirrhosis of the liver, primarily the alcoholic and postnecrotic types. The most important diagnostic cues are unexplained deterioration in a cirrhotic patient and rapid enlargement of the liver.

The most common neoplasm of the liver is a malignant tumor that has metastasized from some other site. Metastasis to the liver can be detected in more than 50% of all cancer deaths. This is particularly true of GI malignancies, but many others also show this tendency (e.g., cancers of the breast, lung, ovaries, and pancreas) (see Fig. 8-8).

Most cancers of the gallbladder are *adenocarcinomas,* and as many as 90% of these patients have gallstones. Diagnosis is generally late, since the early symptoms are insidious and resemble those of chronic cholecystitis and cholelithiasis.

Cancer of the pancreas is a relatively common tumor. Approximately 27,000 persons died of pancreatic cancer in 1995, making it the fifth most common cause of cancer-related mortality. Smoking is the major risk factor; incidence is more than twice as high for smokers versus nonsmokers; the disease is more common in men than in women; and it occurs more often in African Americans than in white Americans (American Cancer Society, 1995). The peak incidence is in the advanced years. About 60% arise in the head of the pancreas, usually obstructing the biliary tract and causing jaundice and a palpably enlarged gallbladder. Those arising in the body and tail often remain silent until far advanced. Other signs and symptoms include abdominal pain, weight loss, anorexia, and nausea. Differential diagnosis from chronic pancreatitis may be difficult. Because of the difficulties in diagnosis, the tumor is usually not discovered until it has already spread beyond hope of local resection.

The average life expectancy is less than 1 year after the diagnosis of cancer of the liver, gallbladder, or pancreas is established.

? QUESTIONS

▼ *Answer the following on a separate sheet of paper.*

1. Explain why blood circulation through the liver is unusual.
2. Briefly describe the structure and function of the gallbladder and pancreas. What hormones control the release of bile and the exocrine pancreatic secretions?
3. List the eight major functions of the liver. Why is the liver a major organ of defense? Why is the liver called a flood chamber? How does the liver perform its detoxification functions (mechanisms involved)? What is the role of the liver in carbohydrate, fat, and protein metabolism?
4. List the four general pathogenetic mechanisms of jaundice.
5. What is kernicterus? What is its significance?
6. Why do newborns often have a slight transient jaundice during the first few days after birth?
7. Does immune globulin (IG) have any value in the treatment of existing hepatitis? Why or why not?
8. Enumerate measures that might help prevent the spread of viral hepatitis in the community, in the home, and in the clinical unit.
9. What percentage of liver destruction is still compatible with life? How long could you live after a total hepatectomy?

▼ *Fill in the blanks with the correct words or circle the correct word option when indicated.*

10. a. The liver is roughly _____ in shape, weighs about (150) or (1500) g, and is located in the _____ quadrant of the abdomen.
    b. The right lobe forms a roof over the right _____ and _____.
    c. The left lobe forms a roof over two important digestive organs, the _____ and the _____.
    d. The _____ ligament divides the medial and lateral segments of the left lobe of the liver and is attached to the anterior abdominal wall.
    e. The liver is enveloped by dense connective tissue called the _____, and the stretching of this capsule in cases of hepatic enlargement is believed to cause tenderness or dull pain.

QUESTIONS—cont'd

11. a. The chief excretory product of the liver is _____, which exits from the liver through the right and left _____ ducts, which immediately merge to form the common _____ duct.
    b. Bile enters the gallbladder through the _____ duct and enters the duodenum through the common _____ duct.
    c. This terminal bile duct joins with the main _____ duct before entering the duodenum through the ampulla of _____.
    d. The sphincter of _____ encircles the common channel and controls the entry of secretions into the duodenum.

12. a. Blood is supplied to the liver by the _____ artery and the _____ vein; it is drained by the right and left _____ veins, which enter the inferior _____.
    b. The paraumbilical veins form a potential pathway from the umbilicus to the _____ vein, allowing passage of a catheter and direct measurement of pressure in this vein.
    c. In cases of right-sided heart failure, blood may back up through the _____ veins, causing passive congestion of the liver but rarely cirrhosis.
    d. When blood flow through the liver is blocked in cirrhosis, blood may back up in the splenic vein, causing enlargement of the _____; blood may be shunted around the liver through the _____ veins, causing varices; or blood may be shunted through the _____ veins, causing hemorrhoids.

13. a. The structural and functional unit of the liver is called the _____; it is hexagonal in shape and composed of plates of liver cells.
    b. Mixed arterial and portal venous blood flows through liver capillaries called _____, which are lined with phagocytic cells called _____ cells, and drains into a central vein at the center of the structural unit.
    c. Bile capillaries course between the hepatocytes and are called _____.

▼ *Circle the letter preceding each item below that correctly answers the question or completes the statement. Only one answer is correct unless otherwise noted.*

14. Which of the following clotting factors is not synthesized by the liver?
    a. Prothrombin   d. Factor VII
    b. Factor IV   e. Factor X
    c. Factor V

15. All the following serum proteins are synthesized by the liver *except:*
    a. Albumin
    b. Alpha globulins
    c. Beta globulins
    d. Gamma globulins
    e. Fibrinogen

16. Which of the following hormones are catabolized by the liver (more than one answer may be correct)?
    a. Estrogen   c. Cortisone
    b. Testosterone   d. Aldosterone

17. Which of the following is *not* a basic liver function?
    a. Synthesis of albumin
    b. Detoxification of chemicals by oxidation, reduction, and conjugation
    c. Synthesis of urea from ammonia
    d. Catabolism of bile

    e. Phagocytosis of bacteria in portal blood

18. Which of the following functions is evidence that the liver plays a central role in lipid metabolism (more than one answer may be correct)?
    a. Chief site of bile formation
    b. Synthesis of fatty acids from carbohydrate
    c. Cholesterol synthesis
    d. Phospholipid formation
    e. Lipoprotein hydrolysis

19. The greatest value of liver scanning is in the detection of:
    a. Hepatitis
    b. Cirrhosis
    c. Circumscribed hepatic lesions
    d. Portal hypertension

20. Which of the following statements is *not* true concerning percutaneous liver biopsy?
    a. The procedure is contraindicated in persons with a prolonged prothrombin time.
    b. The patient must hold his or her breath and not move during needle insertion.

    c. The patient must lie on the left side for several hours after procedure.
    d. Postbiopsy care includes frequently monitoring vital signs.
    e. Significant hemorrhage is a rare complication.

21. Direct measurement of portal vein pressure may be achieved by:
    a. Percutaneous measurement of intrasplenic pressure
    b. Catheterizing the hepatic vein and measuring wedge pressure
    c. Passing a catheter through the umbilical vein to the left branch of the portal vein
    d. Percutaneous measurement of pressure in the liver ductules

22. The chief source of bilirubin is:
    a. Senescent red blood cells
    b. Red blood cell precursors in the bone marrow
    c. Hemoproteins from the liver
    d. Spleen

23. Bilirubin is formed in the monocyte-macrophage system by the reduction of:
    a. Hemoglobin   c. Biliverdin
    b. Globin   d. Urobilinogen

24. The primary site of free (unconjugated) bilirubin formation is:
    a. Liver
    b. Kidneys
    c. Spleen
    d. Gastrointestinal tract

25. Unconjugated bilirubin is transported in the blood to the liver bound to:
    a. Globulins
    b. Red blood cell membranes
    c. Fibrinogen
    d. Albumin

26. The enzyme responsible for the final step in bilirubin conjugation is:
    a. Glucuronyl transferase
    b. Aspartate aminotransferase
    c. Alkaline phosphatase
    d. Lactate dehydrogenase

27. Conjugated bilirubin is (more than one answer may be correct):
    a. Excreted in the bile
    b. Water soluble
    c. Characterized by its great affinity for lipids
    d. Capable of being excreted in the urine

28. A 21-year-old male college student is seen with the chief complaint of jaundice. His friend, a nursing student, noticed that his eyes were yellow, al-

Continued.

QUESTIONS—cont'd

though he had been completely asymptomatic. He also remembered that a younger brother had been icteric on several occasions. The physical examination was negative. AST, alkaline phosphatase, CBC, and liver scan were all normal. The test for urine bilirubin was negative. Total serum bilirubin was 4.8 mg/dl (conjugated portion, 0.5 mg/dl). His most likely problem is:
a. Viral hepatitis
b. Infectious mononucleosis
c. Hemolytic anemia
d. Gilbert's syndrome

29. The prognosis for the condition in question 28 is:
a. Poor
b. Good

30. The most likely pathogenetic mechanism causing the condition in question 28 is:

a. Transport failure of bilirubin caused by defective binding to albumin
b. Excessive load of bilirubin presented to liver as a result of hemolysis
c. Impaired excretion of conjugated bilirubin
d. Impaired conjugation of bilirubin by hepatocyte

31. Ms. B. has been admitted to the hospital for evaluation of her jaundice. Additional findings include clay-colored stools, dark urine that forms a yellow-tinted foam when shaken, pruritus, and predominantly conjugated hyperbilirubinemia. These findings are compatible with:
a. Hemolytic jaundice
b. Intrahepatic cholestasis
c. Extrahepatic cholestasis
d. Only b or c
e. All the above

32. In hemolytic jaundice, increased direct bilirubin will not be present because the unconjugated bilirubin is greater.
a. Both statement and reason are true.
b. Statement is true; reason is false.
c. Both statement and reason are false.
d. Statement is false; reason is true.

33. Pathologic changes common to diseases of the liver, gallbladder, and pancreas include:
a. Fibrosis
b. Inflammation
c. Neoplasms
d. All the above

34. Common findings during the prodromal phase of hepatitis include (more than one answer may be correct):
a. Malaise
b. Icterus
c. Anorexia and loss of desire to smoke
d. Periportal inflammation revealed by biopsy
e. Low-grade fever

▼ Match each of the features in column B with the types of hepatitis or their serologic markers in column A.

Column A
35. _____ Hepatitis A
36. _____ Hepatitis B
37. _____ Hepatitis C
38. _____ Hepatitis D
39. _____ HB$_s$Ag
40. _____ Anti-HB$_s$
41. _____ Anti-HB$_c$
42. _____ HB$_e$Ag

Column B
a. It is major cause of blood transfusion–related hepatitis.
b. It requires the presence of another virus.
c. Positive test identifies persons previously infected, except for carriers.
d. Positive test identifies persons previously infected (carriers and noncarriers) but cannot differentiate between the two.
e. It is transmitted primarily by fecal-oral route.
f. It is especially common in IV drug abusers.
g. Serum level indicates the degree of infectivity.
h. It forms outer protein coat of virus.

▼ Answer the following on a separate sheet of paper.

43. What is alcoholic hepatitis and what is its significance in relation to cirrhosis of the liver?

44. Why is cirrhosis of the liver usually not diagnosed until it is advanced?

45. What is portal hypertension? What is the basic mechanism involved in its development?

46. Describe two emergency methods of treatment for bleeding esophageal varices. Why is it so important to remove the blood from the gastrointestinal tract? Describe the surgical treatment of esophageal varices to prevent recurrent bleeding. Why does the patient often develop hepatic encephalopathy after this type of surgery?

47. What is hepatic encephalopathy? How is it related to portosystemic shunting and liver cell failure? Why is it impor-

tant to detect hepatic encephalopathy in its early stages?

48. What is asterixis? How is it tested for?

49. What is constructional apraxia and what is its significance?

50. Make a table that outlines the four progressive stages of hepatic encephalopathy and gives the major clinical features of each stage.

51. Compare the clinical features of acute and chronic cholecystitis.

52. Why is the liver such a common site of metastasis of malignant tumors?

▼ Circle the letter preceding each item below that correctly answers the question or completes the statement. More than one answer may be correct.

53. Pathologic changes present in cirrhosis of the liver include:
a. Distortion of the liver architecture
b. Fibrosis

c. Necrosis
d. Regenerative nodules
e. Fatty infiltration

54. The single most important cause of cirrhosis in the United States is:
a. Cholecystitis
b. Cholestasis
c. Chronic alcoholism
d. Viral hepatitis

55. The major body site for the metabolism of alcohol is:
a. Gastrointestinal tract
b. Kidneys
c. Brain
d. Liver

56. The first morphologic change in the liver associated with alcohol abuse is:
a. Fatty infiltration   c. Necrosis
b. Cholestasis   d. Fibrosis

57. The hepatic lesion in severe kwashiorkor is:
a. Cirrhosis of the postnecrotic type

QUESTIONS—cont'd

b. Laennec's cirrhosis
c. Hepatitis-like picture
d. Fatty infiltration

58. Possible pathogenic mechanisms accounting for fatty infiltration of the liver include:
a. Excess formation of triglycerides
b. Excess formation of urea by the liver cell
c. Decreased oxidation of fatty acids by the liver cell
d. Decreased synthesis of lipoproteins

59. The two most serious consequences of liver cirrhosis are (choose two):
a. Hepatocellular failure
b. Fatty infiltration of the liver
c. Portal hypertension
d. Increased production of alcohol dehydrogenase

60. The most common cause of biliary cirrhosis is:
a. Chronic active hepatitis
b. Posthepatic biliary obstruction
c. Alcoholism
d. Primary inflammatory disease of the bile ductules

61. Postnecrotic cirrhosis is characterized by:
a. Prior intoxication with chemicals in a few cases
b. A pattern of patchy necrosis
c. An enlarged firm liver with a green hue
d. An increased incidence of hepatoma

62. The incidence of esophageal varices in advanced Laennec's cirrhosis is:
a. 20%   c. 70%
b. 50%   d. 100%

63. Possible causes of anemia associated with some cases of cirrhosis include:
a. Blood loss
b. Folate and vitamin B_{12} deficiency
c. Increased hemolysis in the spleen
d. All the above

64. Common physical signs in cirrhosis include:
a. Ascites
b. Vascular spiders
c. Palmar erythema
d. Prominent superficial abdominal veins
e. All the above

65. What is the overall mortality rate of bleeding from esophageal varices?
a. 15%   c. 50%
b. 35%   d. 70%

66. The most important source of ammonia in the human body is the:
a. Kidney

b. Liver
c. Digestive tract
d. Central nervous system

67. In hypokalemia, there is increased production of ammonia by the:
a. Liver
b. Kidney
c. Digestive tract
d. Central nervous system

68. Asterixis may be seen in:
a. Hypoglycemic states
b. Hyperglycemic states
c. Hepatic encephalopathy
d. Uremia

69. Characteristics of hepatic encephalopathy include all the following *except:*
a. Mental confusion
b. Deterioration of ability to write and construct figures
c. Abnormal EEG
d. Increased blood urea nitrogen

70. The treatment of hepatic encephalopathy usually includes:
a. High-protein diet
b. Oral neomycin
c. Intravenous penicillin
d. Corticosteroids

71. Hepatic fetor has been related to the metabolism of:
a. Bilirubin
b. Cholic acid
c. Methionine
d. Alpha-ketoglutaric acid

72. Hepatic encephalopathy may be precipitated by:
a. Vigorous diuretic therapy
b. Infection
c. Constipation
d. Paracentesis
e. Gastrointestinal bleeding

73. Prominent veins across the lateral walls of the abdomen suggest:
a. Portal hypertension
b. Inferior vena caval obstruction
c. Hepatic vein thrombosis
d. Thrombosis at the bifurcation of the iliac veins

74. Marked elevation of serum amylase (fivefold) almost invariably signifies:
a. Parotitis
b. Cancer of the pancreas
c. Intestinal obstruction
d. Pancreatitis

75. Pancreatitis may be caused by:
a. Chronic alcohol abuse
b. Common duct gallstones
c. Excess coffee ingestion
d. Trauma to the pancreas

76. Mechanisms that protect the normal

pancreas from autodigestion include:
a. Proteolytic enzymes secreted in inactive form
b. Key enzyme trypsin activated by enterokinase
c. Trypsin inhibitors present in plasma
d. Secretion of bicarbonate

▼ *Circle T if the statement is true and F if it is false. Correct any false statements.*

77. T F Ascites is the accumulation of fluid within the pleural cavity.

78. T F Reflux of bile and/or duodenal contents into the pancreatic ducts causing activation of enzymes within the pancreas is a possible mechanism in the development of pancreatitis.

79. T F Hemorrhagic pancreatitis may be characterized by shock, hypovolemia, paralytic ileus, and tetany.

80. T F Chronic pancreatitis is most frequently associated with cholelithiasis and cholecystitis in men.

81. T F Abdominal pain is the most prominent symptom of pancreatitis.

82. T F Kallikrein, when activated within the pancreas, causes vasodilation, increased vascular permeability, and pain.

83. T F Mixed cholesterol gallstones are frequently associated with hemolytic disorders.

84. T F A pancreatic pseudocyst is a collection of liquid secretory and necrotic products that form within the pancreas during the course of acute pancreatitis.

85. T F Cancer of the liver and gallbladder are common tumors in the United States, are generally detected in the early stages, and have a good prognosis.

86. T F Most patients with cancer of the gallbladder have gallstones.

87. T F Cancer of the head of the pancreas may be difficult to differentiate from chronic pancreatitis.

88. T F Steatorrhea, malabsorption, weight loss, and diabetes are manifestations of advanced destruction of the pancreas.

89. T F Surgical removal of the gallbladder is called choledocholithotomy.

Continued.

QUESTIONS—cont'd

▼ *Match each of the following altered laboratory tests of liver, biliary, and pancreatic function in column A with its possible clinical significance in column B.*

Column A

90. _____ Marked increase in serum amylase
91. _____ Marked increase in serum alkaline phosphatase
92. _____ Prolonged prothrombin time
93. _____ Hypoalbuminemia
94. _____ Increased blood ammonia
95. _____ BSP test
96. _____ Urine bilirubin
97. _____ Hyperbilirubinemia (unconjugated)
98. _____ Urine urobilinogen

Column B

a. Hepatic failure or large portosystemic shunt may be present.
b. May indicate biliary obstruction; also increased in bone disease
c. Results in increased bleeding tendency; may indicate liver cell damage
d. Common in acute pancreatitis
e. Normally absent from urine; presence indicates hepatocellular disease or biliary obstruction.
f. Possible hemolytic process
g. Sensitive index of liver function
h. Decreased in biliary obstruction
i. Related to edema formation in hepatic insufficiency

▼ *Match each of the following clinical features of cirrhosis in column A with the most likely causative mechanism in column B.*

Column A

99. _____ Peripheral edema
100. _____ Jaundice
101. _____ Spider angiomas
102. _____ Leukopenia
103. _____ Clotting abnormalities
104. _____ Hemorrhoids

Column B

a. Increased circulating levels of estrogens caused by failure of liver cell to inactivate them
b. Hypersplenism
c. Impaired uptake, conjugation, and excretion of bilirubin
d. Portal hypertension → increased flow and pressure through points of portosystemic anastomoses
e. Decreased hepatic production of factor V, fibrinogen, and other vitamin K–dependent clotting factors
f. Liver cell failure → hypoalbuminemia → decreased colloid osmotic pressure; increased sodium and water retention

▼ *Answer the following on a separate sheet of paper.*

105. Describe the pathogenesis, signs and symptoms, and treatment of ascites.

BIBLIOGRAPHY ▼ PART V

American Cancer Society: Cancer statistics, 1995, *CA* 45(1):8-30, 1995.

Berne RM, Levy MN: Digestion and absorption. In Berne RM, Levy MN: *Physiology,* ed 3, St Louis, 1993, Mosby.

Bradley DW: Hepatitis non-A, non-B viruses become identified as hepatits C and E viruses, *Prog Med Virol* 37:101-135, 1990.

Burkitt DP: Epidemiology of colon and rectum cancer, *Cancer* 28:3-13, 1971.

Centers for Disease Control and Prevention: Personal communication with I. Wiliams, Epidemiologist, Division of Hepatitis and Infectious Diseases, Centers for Disease Control and Prevention, Altanta, Ga, February 1995.

Centers for Disease Control: Public Health Service inter-agency guidelines for screening donors of blood, plasma, organs, tissues, and semen for evidence of hepatitis B and hepatitis C, *MMWR* 40 (RR-4):1-17, 1991.

Centers for Disease Control: Protection against viral hepatits: recommendations of the Immunization Practices Advisory Committee (ACIP), *MMWR* 39 (No. RR2):1-26, 1990.

Chin R: Low birth weight and hyperemesis gravidarum, *Eur J Obstet Gynecol Reprod Biol* 28:179-183, 1988.

Davenport HW: *A digest on digestion,* ed 2, Chicago, 1978, Mosby.

BIBLIOGRAPHY ▼ PART V

Davis GJ, Lake-Bakaar GB, Grahame-Smith DG, editors: *Nausea and vomiting: mechanisms and treatment,* 1986, Heidelberg, Germany, Springer-Verlag.

de Boer W, Driesen W, Jansz H, Tytgat G: Effect of acid suppression on efficacy of treatment for *Helicobactor pylori* infection, *Lancet* 345(8953):817-820, 1995.

Dienstag JL: Hepatitis non-A, non-B: C at last, *Gastroenterology* 99(4):1177-1180, 1990.

Eastwood GL: Gastritis and other gastric diseases. In Stein JH et al, editors: *Internal medicine,* ed 4, St Louis, 1994, Mosby.

Fagan EA: Acute liver failure of unknown pathogenesis: the hidden agenda, *Hepatology* 19(5):1307-1312, 1994 (editorial).

Friedman LS, Knouer MK: Liver, biliary tract and pancreas. In Tierney LM, McPhee IJ, Papadakis MA: *Current medical diagnosis and treatment,* East Norwalk, Conn, 1994, Appleton & Lange.

Ganong WF: *Review of medical physiology,* East Norwalk, Conn, 1993, Appleton & Lange.

Glickman RM: Inflammatory bowel disease (ulcerative colitis and Crohn's disease). In Isselbacher HJ et al, editors: *Harrison's principles of internal medicine,* ed 13, New York, 1994, McGraw-Hill.

Goldenschmiedt M, Feldman M: Gastric secretion. In Stein JH et al, editors: *Internal medicine,* ed 4, St Louis, 1994, Mosby.

Goyal RK: Diseases of the esophagus. In Isselbacher KJ et al, editors: *Harrison's principles of internal medicine,* ed 13, New York, 1994, McGraw-Hill.

Grant M: Symptom distress: nausea, vomiting, and anorexia, *Semin Oncol Nurs* 3:277-286, 1987.

Greenberger NJ: *Gastrointestinal disorders: a pathophysiologic approach,* ed 4, St Louis, 1989, Mosby.

Greenberger NJ, Toskes PP, Isselbacher KJ: Acute and chronic pancreatitis. In Isselbacher HJ et al, editors: *Harrison's principles of internal medicine,* ed 13, New York, 1994, McGraw-Hill.

Hayllar J, MacPherson A, Bjarnason I: Gastroprotection and non-steroidal antiinflammatory drugs (NSAIDS): rationale and clinical implications, *Drug Safety* 7:86-105, 1992.

Hosking SW et al: Duodenal ulcer healing by eradication of *Helicobacter pylori* without antacid treatment: randomized controlled trial, *Lancet* 343:508-510, 1994.

Huether SE: Structure and function of the digestive system. In McCance KL, Huether SE: *Pathophysiology: the biological basis for disease in adults and children,* ed 2, St Louis, 1994, Mosby.

Kaplan LM, Isselbacher KJ: Jaundice. In Isselbacher HJ et al, editors: *Harrison's principles of internal medicine,* ed 13, New York, 1994, McGraw-Hill.

Keusch GT, Bart KJ: Immunization principles and vaccine use. In Isselbacher HJ et al, editors: *Harrison's principles of internal medicine,* ed 13, New York, 1994, McGraw-Hill.

Kurtz RC: Incidence and epidemiology of gastric adenocarcinoma. In Stein JH et al, editors: *Internal medicine,* ed 4, St Louis, 1994, Mosby.

LaBrecque DR: Acute and chronic hepatitis. In Stein JH et al, editors: *Internal medicine,* ed 4, St Louis, 1994, Mosby.

Lang IM: Digestive tract motor correlates of nausea and vomiting, *Can J Physiol Pharmacol* 68:242-253, 1990.

Lemon SM, Shapiro CN: The value of immunization against hepatitis A, *Infect Agents Dis* 3(1):38-49, 1994.

Lutz CA, Prztulski KR: *Nutrition and diet therapy,* Philadelphia, 1994, Davis.

Marwick C: Hepatitis A vaccine set for 2-year-olds to adults, *JAMA* 273(12):906-907 1995.

Mayer R: Colorectal cancer. In Isselbacher HJ et al, editors: *Harrison's principles of internal medicine,* ed 13, New York, 1994, McGraw-Hill.

Mayer R: Pancreatic cancer. In Isselbacher HJ et al, editors: *Harrison's principles of internal medicine,* ed 13, New York, 1994, McGraw-Hill.

McGuigan JE: Peptic ulcer and gastritis. In Isselbacher KJ et al, editors: *Harrison's principles of internal medicine,* ed 13, New York, 1994, McGraw-Hill.

McQuaid KR, Isenberg JI: Medical therapy of peptic ulcer disease, *Surg Clin North Am* 72(2):285-316, 1992.

Milamed D, Hedley-Whyte J: Contributions of the surgical sciences to a reduction of the mortality rate in the United States for the period 1968 to 1988, *Ann Surg* 219(1):94-102, 1994.

Peterson WL, Richardson CT: Peptic ulcer disease. In Stein JH et al, editors: *Internal medicine,* ed 4, St Louis, 1994, Mosby.

Podolsky DK, Isselbacher KJ: Derangements of hepatic metabolism. In Isselbacher HJ et al, editors: *Harrison's principles of internal medicine,* ed 13, New York, 1994, McGraw-Hill.

Purcell RH: *Update testing in the blood bank: blood-borne non-A, non-B hepatitis,* vol 2, no 2, Raritan, NJ 1990, Ortho Diagnostic Systems.

Ransohoff DF, Lang CA: Screening for colorectal cancer, *N Engl J Med* 325(1):37-41, 1991.

Richter JE: Motility disorders of the esophagus. In Yamanda T, editor: *Textbook of gastroenterology,* Philadelphia, 1991, Lippincott.

Robinson WS: Biology of human hepatitis viruses. In Zakim D, Boyer T, editors: *Hepatology: a textbook of liver disease,* Philadelphia, 1990, Saunders.

Sherman DJ, Finlayson ND: *Disease of the gastrointestinal tract and liver,* New York, 1989, Churchill Livingstone.

Silen W: Acute intestinal obstruction. In Isselbacher HJ et al, editors: *Harrison's principles of internal medicine,* ed 13, New York, 1994, McGraw-Hill.

Spense AP, Matson EB: *Human anatomy and physiology,* ed 4, St Paul, Minn, 1992, West.

Stabile BE: Current surgical management of duodenal ulcers, *Surg Clin North Am* 72(2):335-356, 1992.

Sugawa C, Joseph AL: Endoscopic interventional management of bleeding duodenal and gastric ulcers, *Surg Clin North Am* 72(2):317-334, 1992.

Thomas CL: *Taber's cyclopedic medical encyclopedia,* ed 17, Philadelphia, 1993, FA Davis.

Uchida T et al: "Silent"–hepatitis B virus mutants are responsible for non-A, non-B, non-C, non-D, non-E hepatitis, *Microbiol Immunol* 38(4):281-285, 1994.

Way LW: *Current surgical diagnosis and treatment,* East Norwalk, Conn, 1994, Appleton & Lange.

Whitehead R: *Mucosal biopsy of the gastrointestinal tract,* ed 4, Philadelphia, 1990, Saunders.

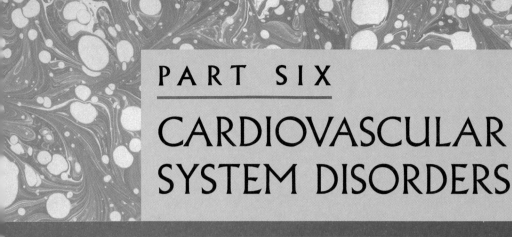

PART SIX

CARDIOVASCULAR SYSTEM DISORDERS

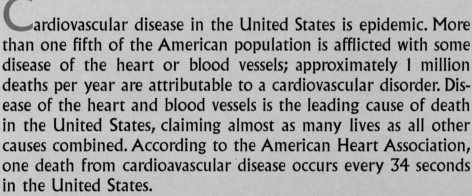

Cardiovascular disease in the United States is epidemic. More than one fifth of the American population is afflicted with some disease of the heart or blood vessels; approximately 1 million deaths per year are attributable to a cardiovascular disorder. Disease of the heart and blood vessels is the leading cause of death in the United States, claiming almost as many lives as all other causes combined. According to the American Heart Association, one death from cardioavascular disease occurs every 34 seconds in the United States.

Heart attack is the major cause of cardiovascular mortality and morbidity. Approximately 500,000 deaths per year are attributable to heart attacks; many of these deaths are of middle-age men. Of great concern is that heart attack often occurs with little or no warning; the incidence of sudden death is high. More than half the deaths from myocardial infarction occur during the first few hours after the onset of symptoms and before reaching the hospital. With the advent of coronary care units in the early 1960s, the hospital mortality rate from lethal disturbances of the cardiac rhythm has decreased significantly. Efforts to assist the ventricle mechanically and reduce the size of the infarct are currently under investigation.

Additional cardiovascular diseases with significant morbidity and mortality include rheumatic heart disease, cerebrovascular accident (stroke), hypertension, congenital heart disease, and congestive heart failure. The major therapeutic thrust for the control of cardiovascular disease must be primary prevention. Although the precise pathogenesis of many cardiovascular diseases remains unknown, control of risk factors by effective screening and public education can effect a substantial reduction in cardiac morbidity and mortality. The emphasis must be on prophylaxis rather than on treatment of established disease; the lethal and disabling sequelae of cardiovascular disease are too pronounced to await evidence of disease.

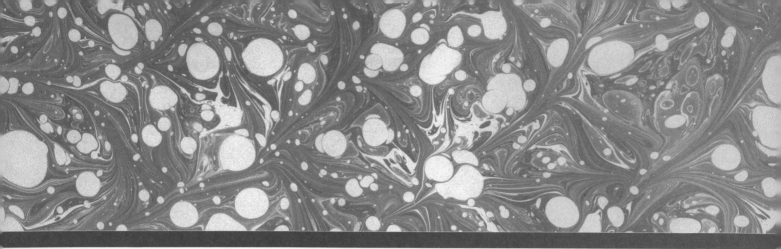

The subsequent chapters present a detailed discussion of coronary atherosclerotic disease, valvular heart disease, heart failure, and peripheral vascular disease. Hypertension, hyperlipidemia, and rheumatic fever as they relate to these disease entities are also considered. Techniques of circulatory assistance and cardiac transplantation are also introduced. ▼

CHAPTER 28

Anatomy of the Cardiovascular System

PENNY FORD CARLETON
MARJORIE A. BOLDT

The apparent simplicity in the design of the cardiovascular system belies the intricate, yet logical, interdependence of circulatory structure and function in health and disease. Each portion of the cardiovascular system is uniquely adapted to contribute to highly integrated cardiovascular responses to disease processes. Therefore an understanding of cardiovascular anatomy is prerequisite to the examination of cardiovascular disease mechanisms and the capabilities and limitations of circulatory compensatory responses.

ANATOMIC RELATIONSHIPS

The heart lies within the mediastinal space of the thoracic cavity between the lungs. The pericardium encloses the heart and is composed of two layers: the inner layer, or *visceral pericardium,* and the outer layer, or *parietal pericardium.* The two pericardial layers are separated by a small amount of lubricating fluid, which reduces the friction created by the pumping action of the heart. The parietal pericardium is attached anteriorly to the sternum, posteriorly to the vertebral column, and inferiorly to the diaphragm; the visceral pericardium is in direct contact with the surface of the heart. The heart itself is composed of three layers: the outer layer, or *epicardium;* the middle, muscular layer, or *myocardium;* and the inner, endothelial layer, or *endocardium* (Fig. 28-1).

The upper chambers of the heart, the *atria,* and the great vessels, the aorta and pulmonary artery, form the base of the heart. The atria are anatomically separated from the lower chambers, the *ventricles,* by a fibrous ring in which the four cardiac valves are situated and to which both the valves and the musculature attach. Functionally, the heart is divided into right-sided and left-sided pumps, which propel venous blood into the pulmonary circulation and oxygenated blood into the systemic circulation, respectively. This functional division facilitates conceptualization of the anatomic sequence of blood flow: venae cavae, right atrium, right ventricle, pulmonary artery, lungs, pulmonary veins, left atrium, left ventricle, aorta, arteries, arterioles, capillaries, venules, veins, and back to the venae cavae (Fig. 28-2).

However, the schematic conception of the right and left sides of the heart shown in Fig. 28-2 is anatomically misleading. The heart actually is rotated to the left, with its apex tilted anteriorly. This rotation places the right side of the heart anteriorly beneath the sternum, with the left side of the heart relatively posterior. The apex of the

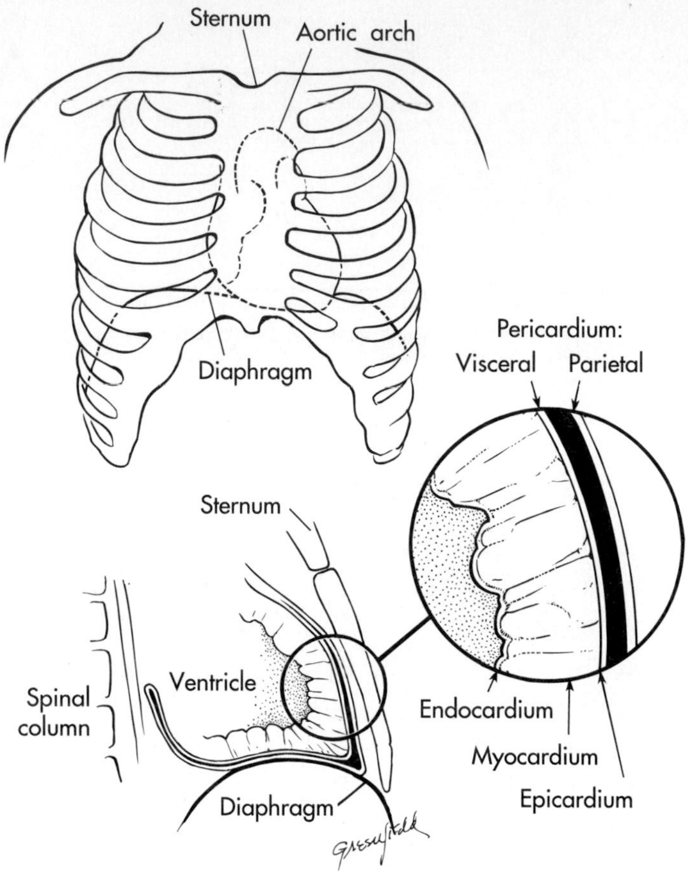

FIG. 28-1   Anatomic relation of the heart to the surrounding structures. Inset shows the layers of the heart and pericardium.

heart can be palpated at the midclavicular line at the fourth or fifth intercostal space (Fig. 28-3).

Right Atrium

The thin-walled right atrium (RA) functions as a reservoir and a conduit for systemic venous blood flowing to the right ventricle (RV). Venous blood enters the RA via the superior vena cava, the inferior vena cava, and the coronary sinus. No true valves are within the orifices of the venae cavae; only rudimentary valvular folds or muscular bands separate the venae cavae from the atrial chamber. Therefore elevation in right atrial pressure as a result of right-sided congestion is reflected backward into the systemic venous circulation.

Approximately 80% of the venous return to the RA flows passively into the RV through the tricuspid valve. An additional 20% of ventricular filling occurs during atrial contraction; this active contribution to ventricular filling is called the *atrial kick*. Loss of the atrial kick in certain cardiac dysrhythmias can reduce ventricular filling and consequently decrease ventricular output.

Right Ventricle

During ventricular contraction, each ventricle must generate adequate force to propel the blood received from the atrium into either the pulmonary or systemic circulation.

The RV has a unique crescent-shaped design and generates a low-pressure, bellowslike contraction that propels blood into the pulmonary artery. The low-pressure pulmonary circulation offers much less resistance to blood flowing into it from the RV than does the high-pressure systemic circulation encountered by the left ventricle (LV). Thus the workload of the RV is much less than that of the LV. Consequently, the wall thickness of the RV is only one-third that of the LV (Fig. 28-4).

In the face of gradually increasing pulmonary pressures, as with progressive pulmonary hypertension, the RV undergoes muscular hypertrophy to increase its pumping force to overcome the elevated pulmonary resistance to ventricular emptying. However, in the event of an acute elevation in pulmonary resistance (e.g., in massive pulmonary embolization), the pumping capability of the RV can be overwhelmed, and death may result.

Left Atrium

The left atrium (LA) receives oxygenated blood from the lungs via the four pulmonary veins. No true valves separate the pulmonary veins from the LA. Therefore alterations in left atrial pressure are readily reflected retrograde into the pulmonary vasculature and acute elevations in left atrial pressure will cause pulmonary congestion. The LA is a thin-walled, low-pressure chamber. Blood flows from the LA into the LV through the mitral valve.

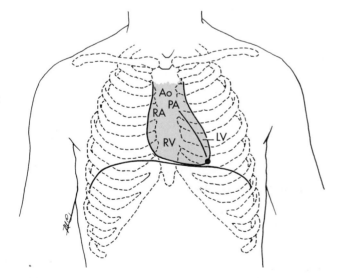

Pulmonary circulation

Aorta

Pulmonary
artery

Pulmonary
veins

Venae cavae

RA

LA

RV

LV

Vein

Artery

Arteriole

Venule

Capillary

FIG. 28-2   Schematic representation of blood flow through the cardiovascular system. *RA,* Right atrium; *LA,* left atrium; *RV,* right ventricle; *LV,* left ventricle.

Left Ventricle

The LV must generate high pressures to overcome the resistance of the systemic circulation and sustain blood flow to peripheral tissues. The thick musculature and circular configuration of the LV facilitate the development of high pressure during ventricular contraction. Even the interventricular septum separating the ventricles contributes to the powerful compression exerted by the entire ventricular chamber during contraction.

Left ventricular pressure exceeds right ventricular pressure approximately fivefold during contraction; if an abnormal communication exists between the ventricles, as with rupture of the interventricular septum after myocardial infarction, blood will be shunted from left to right through the defect. As a result, normal forward blood flow from the LV through the aortic valve to the aorta will be decreased.

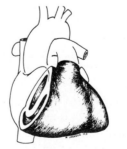

Ao
PA
RA

LV

RV

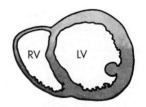

RV   LV

FIG. 28-3   Orientation of the heart within the thorax. *Ao,* Aorta; *RA,* right atrium; *PA,* pulmonary artery; *RV,* right ventricle; *LV,* left ventricle. The black dot marks the normal location of the apical impulse in the fifth left intercostal space near the midclavicular line.

FIG. 28-4   Schematic drawings of the heart to illustrate the differences in shape of the right ventricle *(RV)* and the left ventricle *(LV)*. *Left,* Ventricles in approximate anatomic positions. *Right,* Cross section illustrating the greater wall thickness and nearly circular shape of the left ventricle.

CARDIAC VALVES

The four cardiac valves function to maintain unidirectional blood flow through the chambers of the heart. These valves are of two types: the *atrioventricular (AV) valves,* which separate the atria from the ventricles, and the *semilunar valves,* which separate the pulmonary artery and the aorta from the coresponding ventricles. The valves open and close passively in response to pressure and volume changes within the cardiac chambers and vessels.

Atrioventricular Valves

The leaflets of the AV valves are delicate but durable. The *tricuspid valve,* located between the RA and RV, contains three leaflets. The *mitral valve,* separating the LA and LV, is a bicuspid valve with two valve cusps, or leaflets.

The cusps of both valves are attached to thin strands of fibrous tissue called *chordae tendineae.* The chordae tendineae extend to *papillary muscles,* which are muscular projections arising from the ventricular wall (Fig. 28-5). The chordae tendineae support the valves during ventricular contraction to prevent eversion of the valve cusps into the atria. Rupture or malfunction of the chordae tendineae or papillary muscles supporting a valve would permit backflow or regurgitation of blood into the atrium during ventricular contraction.

Semilunar Valves

Both semilunar valves are of similar configuration; they consist of three symmetric cuplike cusps secured to a fibrous ring. The *aortic valve* is situated between the LV and the aorta, whereas the *pulmonic valve* is positioned between the RV and the pulmonary artery. The semilunar valves prevent backflow from the aorta or pulmonary artery into the ventricles during ventricular relaxation.

Immediately above the cusps of the valves are outpouchings of the aortic and pulmonary walls called the *sinuses of Valsalva* (Fig. 28-6). The orifices to the coronary arteries are located within the outpouchings of the aortic wall. These sinuses protect the coronary orifices from occlusion by the valve leaflets when the aortic valve opens.

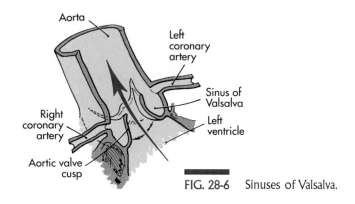

FIG. 28-6 Sinuses of Valsalva.

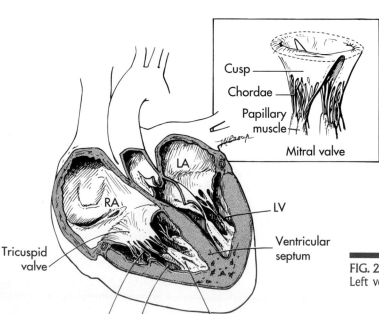

FIG. 28-5 Anatomy of the atrioventricular (AV) valves. *LV,* Left ventricle; *RV,* right ventricle.

CONDUCTION SYSTEM

The fibrous ring between the atria and ventricles isolates these chambers electrically as well as anatomically. To ensure rhythmic and synchronized excitation and contraction of the heart muscle, specialized conduction pathways exist within the myocardium. This conduction tissue exhibits the following properties:

1. *Automaticity:* the ability to generate impulses spontaneously
2. *Rhythmicity:* the regularity of impulse generation
3. *Conductivity:* the ability to transmit impulses
4. *Excitability:* the ability to respond to stimulation

Because of these properties, the heart spotaneously and rhythmically initiates impulses that are transmitted throughout the conduction system to excite the myocardium and stimulate muscular contraction.

The cardiac impulse normally originates in the *sinoatrial (SA) node.* The SA node therefore is referred to as the "natural pacemaker" of the heart. The SA node is located in the posterior wall of the RA near the entrance of the superior vena cava.

The cardiac impulse then spreads from the SA node to specialized atrial conduction pathways and to the atrial muscle. An interatrial pathway, Bachmann's bundle, facilitates impulse spread from the RA to the LA. Internodal pathways—the anterior, middle, and posterior pathways—connect the SA node with the atrioventricular node.

The electrical impulse then reaches the *atrioventricular (AV) node,* which is positioned at the top of the interventricular septum in the RA near the opening of the coronary sinus. The AV node is the normal route for impulse transmission between the atria and ventricles and performs two critical functions. First, the cardiac impulse is delayed here for 0.08 to 0.12 second to allow for ventricular filling during atrial contraction. Second, the AV node controls the number of atrial impulses reaching the ventricles; normally, no more than 180 impulses per minute are permitted to reach the ventricles. This protective effect is critical during certain abnormal cardiac rhythms in which atrial rates can exceed 400 beats per minute (bpm). If the ventricles were not protected from this excessive impulse bombardment, the ventricles would have inadequate time to fill, and cardiac output would fall dramatically. Excessive delay or failure of impulse transmission at the AV node is known as *heart block.*

The wave of electrical excitation spreads from the AV node to the *bundle of His,* a thick bundle of fibers extending down the right side of the interventricular septum. The bundle divides into the *right bundle branch* and the *left bundle branch,* which descend on opposite sides of the interventricular septum. The left bundle branch bifurcates into a thin anterior and a thick posterior division. The bundle branches terminate in a complex branching

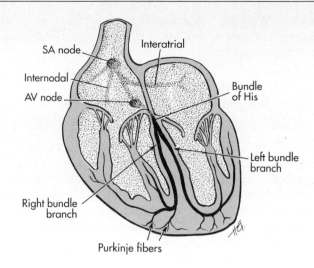

FIG. 28-7   The conduction system of the heart. *SA,* Sinoatrial; *AV,* atrioventricular

network of fibers, the *Purkinje system,* which spreads throughout the inner surface of both ventricles. Spread of the wave of excitation through the Purkinje fibers is extremely rapid.

Although these specialized conduction pathways speed the transmission of the cardiac impulse throughout the heart, the arrangement of myocardial cells outside the conduction system further ensures rapid impulse spread. Adjacent cells are separated by structures called *intercalated disks.* Within these disks are points of close intercellular membrane approximation referred to as *nexi.* These nexi facilitate rapid cell-to-cell transmission of electrical excitation, resulting in virtually simultaneous activation and contraction of the myocardial cells.

Therefore the normal sequence of excitation through the conduction system is as follows: SA node, atrial pathways, AV node, bundle of His, bundle branches, and Purkinje fibers (Fig. 28-7).

Anomalous anatomic connections bypassing portions of the conduction system have been identified in some individuals. These "bypass tracts" or connections can produce premature excitation of the ventricles by bypassing the intrinsic delays in conduction within the normal pathways of the conduction system. The Wolff-Parkinson-White (WPW) syndrome is an example of a preexcitation syndrome produced by impulse conduction via a bypass pathway directly connecting the atria and ventricles and bypassing the AV node.

Excitation normally originates in the SA node because the SA node exhibits the fastest intrinsic rate of impulse generation, approximately 60 to 100 bpm. However, in the event of SA node failure or its inability to generate impulses at an adequate rate, other sites can assume the role of pacemaker. The AV node is capable of generating impulses at a rate of approximately 40 to 60 bpm, and ventricular sites in the Purkinje system can generate impulses at rates of approximately 20 to 40 bpm. These lower, or "escape," pacemakers serve a critical function in the prevention of cardiac standstill (asystole) if the natural pacemaker fails.

SYSTEMIC CIRCULATION

The structural characteristics of each portion of the systemic vasculature determine its physiologic role in the integration of cardiovascular function. The vessel wall consists of three layers: the outer layer, or *adventitia;* the muscular middle layer, or *medial layer;* and the inner layer, or *tunica intima.* The systemic circulation can be subdivided into five anatomic and functional categories: (1) arteries, (2) arterioles, (3) capillaries, (4) venules, and (5) veins (Fig. 28-8).

Arteries

The walls of the aorta and large arteries are composed of much elastic tissue and some smooth muscle. The LV

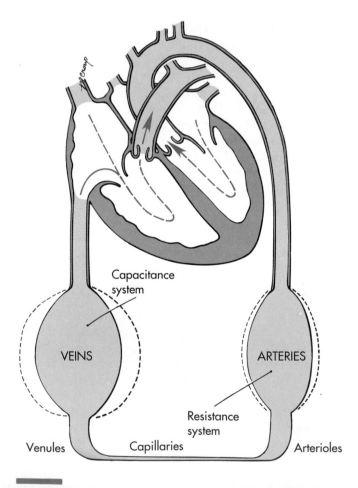

FIG. 28-8 Schematic illustration of the systemic circulation. The arterial system may be considered as a resistance circuit (low volume, high pressure), whereas the venous system may be considered as a capacitance circuit (high volume, low pressure).

ejects blood into the aorta under high pressure. This sudden expulsion of blood distends the elastic arterial walls; during ventricular relaxation the elastic recoil of the walls propels blood forward throughout the circulatory system. Peripherally, the branches of the arterial system proliferate and subdivide into smaller vessels.

The arterial bed contains approximately 15% of the total blood volume at one time. Therefore the arterial system is considered a low-volume, high-pressure circuit. Because of these volume-pressure characteristics, the arterial tree is called a *resistance circuit.*

Arterioles

At the arteriole level, the vascular wall is primarily smooth muscle with some elastic fiber. The muscular wall of the arteriole is highly responsive and can significantly alter the radius of the vessel, resulting in either constriction or dilation. When constricted, the arterioles are the major sites of resistance to flow in the arterial tree. Fully dilated, the arteriole offers almost no resistance to blood flow. The change in flow of blood from pulsatile to steady facilitates the exchange of nutrients at the capillary level. At the junction between the arterioles and capillaries of some tissues is a *precapillary sphincter,* which is subject to intricate physiologic control.

Capillaries

The capillary wall is thin, consisting of a single layer of endothelial cells. Nutrients and metabolites diffuse across this thin, semipermeable membrane from areas of high concentration to areas of lower concentration. Oxygen and nutrients therefore leave the vessel to enter the interstitial space and the cell; carbon dioxide and metabolites diffuse in the opposite direction. Net fluid movement between the blood vessel and the interstitial space depends on the relative balance between hydrostatic and osmotic pressures at the capillary bed.

Venules

The venules function as collecting tubules and are composed of a relatively weak but responsive muscle wall. At the juncture between the capillary and venule, there is a *postcapillary sphincter.*

Veins

The veins are relatively thin-walled conduits for transport of blood from the capillary bed through the venous system to the RA. Venous flow to the heart is unidirectional as a result of valves strategically located within the venous channels. The veins can accommodate large volumes of blood under relatively low pressure. Because of these low-pressure, high-volume characteristics, the venous system is referred to as a *capacitance system.* Approximately 65% of the blood volume lies within the venous system at rest. However, the capacity of the venous bed can be altered. Venoconstriction reduces the capacity of the venous bed, forcing blood forward to the heart and thereby increasing venous return. The movement of blood from the capillary bed toward the heart is influenced by three factors: (1) venous compression by skeletal muscles, (2) sympathetically induced venoconstriction, and (3) alterations in thoracic and abdominal pressures during respiration. Venoconstriction is crucial in maintaining venous return during upright posture and exercise. The venous system terminates in the inferior and superior venae cavae.

CORONARY CIRCULATION

The efficiency of the heart as a pump depends on adequate oxygenation and nourishment of the heart muscle. The coronary circulation courses over the surface of the heart, carrying oxygen and nutrients to the myocardium via small intramyocardial branches. The distribution of the coronary arteries to the heart muscle and to the conduction system must be understood to recognize the consequences of coronary heart disease. The morbidity and mortality associated with myocardial infarction depend on the degree of both mechanical and electrical dysfunction.

Coronary Arteries

The coronary arteries are the first branches of the systemic circulation. The coronary orifices are located within the sinuses of Valsalva in the aorta immediately above the aortic valve. The coronary circulation consists of the *right coronary artery* and the *left coronary artery.* The left coronary artery has two major branches: the *left anterior descending artery* and the *left circumflex artery* (Fig. 28-9).

The arteries course around the heart in two external anatomic grooves: the *atrioventricular groove,* encircling the heart between the atria and ventricles, and the *interventricular groove,* separating the two ventricles. The juncture of these two grooves on the posterior surface of the heart is a critical anatomic landmark known as the *crux of the heart.* The AV node is located at this juncture; therefore whichever vessel crosses the crux nourishes the AV node. The terms *right dominance* and *left dominance* simply designate whether the right or the left coronary artery crosses the crux.

The right coronary artery courses laterally around the right side of the heart in the right atrioventricular groove. In 90% of all hearts, on reaching the posterior surface of the heart, the right coronary artery extends to the crux, then descends toward the apex of the heart in the posterior interventricular groove. The main left coronary artery branches shortly after its origin from the aorta. The left circumflex artery extends laterally around the left side of the heart in the left atrioventricular groove. This circumferential distribution corresponds to its designation as the "circumflex" artery. Similarly, the term "left anterior descending artery" (LAD) describes the anatomic pathway of this arterial branch. The LAD courses down the surface of the heart in the anterior interventricular groove. It crosses the apex of the heart, reversing direction and extending upward along the posterior surface of the interventricular groove to meet the distal branches of the right coronary artery.

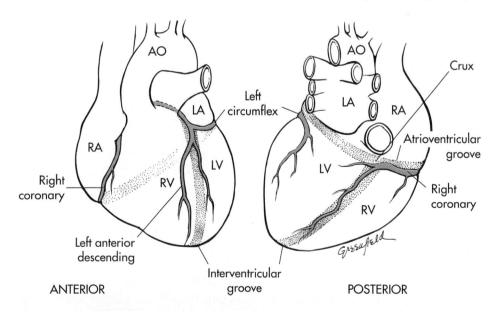

FIG. 28-9   Coronary arteries supplying the anterior and posterior aspects of the heart *Ao,* Aorta; *RA,* right atrium; *LA,* left atrium; *RV,* right ventricle; *LV,* left ventricle.

Each major vessel gives off characteristic epicardial and intramyocardial branches. The LAD gives rise to *septal* branches supplying the anterior two thirds of the septum and *diagonal* branches coursing over the anterolateral surface of the LV. The posterolateral surface of the LV is supplied by *marginal* branches of the circumflex artery.

The anatomic pathways result in the following correlations between coronary arteries and nutrient supply of cardiac muscle. Basically, the right coronary artery supplies the RA, RV, and inferior wall of the LV. The left circumflex artery supplies the LA and the lateral and posterior walls of the LV. The LAD nourishes the massive anterior wall of the LV.

The nutrient supply of the conduction system is another critical correlation determined by anatomic pathways. The SA node, despite its position in the RA, is supplied in 55% of individuals by the right coronary artery and in 45% by a branch of the left circumflex artery. The AV node, supplied by the artery crossing the crux, is nourished in 90% of individuals by the right coronary artery and in 10% by the left circumflex artery.

These correlations have significant clinical implications. For instance, a lesion of the right coronary artery would be expected to be associated with the highest incidence of AV nodal conduction disturbances, whereas a lesion of the LAD would be more likely to interfere with the pumping function of the LV.

Anastomoses between arterial branches exist within the coronary circulation. These intercoronary channels are not functional in the normal circulation but are critically important as potential routes for collateral or alternative circulation to nourish myocardial regions deprived of flow by lesions obstructing normal pathways in the coronary vasculature (Fig. 28-10).

Cardiac Veins

The distribution of the coronary veins essentially parallels that of the coronary arteries. There are three subdivisions of the venous system of the heart:

1. The *thebesian veins* compose the smallest venous system and connect the cardiac chambers with capillary beds, other cardiac veins, and other thebesian veins, thereby providing a conduit through which a portion of the right atrial and right ventricular myocardium is drained.
2. The *anterior cardiac veins* are intermediate in importance, emptying a large portion of the right ventricular venous drainage directly into the RA.
3. The *coronary sinus and its branches* compose the largest, most significant venous system, draining the

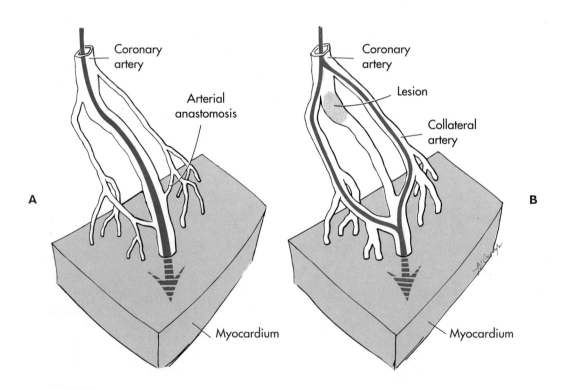

FIG. 28-10   Collateral circulation to the myocardium. **A,** The bulk of blood flow to an area of myocardium is through the coronary blood vessel, with minimal flow through arterial anastomoses. **B,** A lesion (e.g., atherosclerotic plaque) in the coronary artery causes the development of increased collateral circulation, which may allow an adequate blood supply to the compromised area of the myocardium.

bulk of myocardial venous return into the RA through the coronary sinus ostium beside the orifice of the inferior vena cava.

LYMPHATIC CIRCULATION

The lymphatic capillary network in the interstitial spaces collects excess fluid and protein filtered through the systemic capillaries. This capillary filtrate is then returned to the systemic circulation via collecting vessels located in close approximation to the veins. Lymph is propelled upward through unidirectional valves by a combination of two dynamic influences: (1) external compression by muscles and arterial pulsations and (2) intrinsic peristalsis. The terminal thoracic duct and right lymphatic duct empty into the subclavian veins.

PULMONARY CIRCULATION

The pulmonary circulation is described in depth in Part Seven. However, significant differences between the systemic and the pulmonary circulation warrant mention. The pulmonary vasculature has thinner walls and less smooth muscle. The pulmonary circuit therefore is more distensible and offers less resistance to flow. Pressure in the pulmonary circuit is approximately one-fifth that in the systemic circuit. The walls of the pulmonary vasculature are much less reactive to autonomic and humoral influences, whereas alterations in oxygen and carbon dioxide content of the blood and alveoli profoundly alter flow through the pulmonary vasculature. These differences make the pulmonary circuit particularly well suited to fulfill its physiologic function of oxygen uptake and carbon dioxide removal.

INNERVATION OF THE CARDIOVASCULAR SYSTEM

The cardiovascular system is richly innervated by fibers of the autonomic nervous system (ANS). The two divisions of the ANS are the *parasympathetic system* and the *sympathetic system,* which exhibit opposite effects and operate reciprocally to effect changes in heart rate. For instance, stimulation of the sympathetic system is usually coupled with inhibition of the parasympathetic system; conversely, parasympathetic stimulation and sympathetic inhibition are typically concurrent events. This reciprocal action increases the precision of neural regulation by the ANS.

ANS regulation of the cardiovascular system requires the following components: (1) sensors, (2) afferent path-

ways, (3) an integration center, (4) efferent pathways, and (5) receptors.

There are two primary groups of sensors: the baroreceptors and the chemoreceptors. The *baroreceptors* (or pressoreceptors), located in the aortic arch and carotid sinus, are sensitive to the stretch or distortion of the vessel wall caused by alterations in arterial pressure. Stimulation of these receptors by elevation of arterial pressure signals the cardioregulatory center to inhibit cardiac activity; conversely, reduction of arterial pressure initiates reflex augmentation of cardiac activity. The *chemoreceptors,* located in the carotid body and aortic arch, are stimulated by reduction in arterial oxygen concentration, elevation of carbon dioxide tension, and elevation in hydrogen ion concentration (reduced blood pH). Activation of the chemoreceptors stimulates the cardioregulatory center to augment cardiac activity. Other receptors, which are sensitive to stretch resulting from alterations in blood volume, are located at the juncture between the great veins and atria. Two reflex responses occur on stimulation of these receptors: an increase in heart rate (Bainbridge reflex) and diuresis.

Afferent pathways in the vagus and glossopharyngeal nerves carry the neural impulses from the receptors to the brain. The *integration center,* or *cardioregulatory center,* is located in the upper medulla and lower pons. The cardioregulatory center receives impulses from the baroreceptors and chemoreceptors and transmits impulses to the heart and vessels via the parasympathetic and sympathetic nerve fibers. Higher centers of the brain, such as the cerebral cortex and hypothalamus, can also influence ANS activity via the medulla. The efferent pathway from the cardioregulatory center to the heart is mainly through the vagus nerves for the parasympathetic fibers, whereas the sympathetic fibers travel by way of the cardiac nerves. Receptors are located in the conduction system of the heart, the myocardium, and the smooth muscle of the blood vessels. Stimulation of the receptors alters the heart rate, the strength of myocardial contraction, and the diameter of blood vessels.

The parasympathetic fibers innervate the SA node, the atrial musculature, and the AV node via the vagus nerves. Parasympathetic fibers also extend to the ventricular muscle, but the functional significance of these pathways seems limited. Stimulation of parasympathetic fibers causes the release of acetylcholine. *Acetylcholine* mediates the transmission of the neural impulse to the cardiac receptors. Parasympathetic stimulation restrains cardiac action by reducing the heart rate, the speed of impulse conduction through the AV node, and the force of atrial and perhaps ventricular contraction. This response to parasympathetic stimulation is also referred to as a *cholinergic response* or a *vagal response.*

The sympathetic fibers extend to the entire conduction system and myocardium, as well as to the smooth muscle of the vasculature. *Norepinephrine* is the sympathetic neurotransmitter. Sympathetic stimulation causes the release of epinephrine and some norepinephrine from the adrenal medulla. Sympathetic stimulation accelerates the heart by increasing heart rate and the speed of impulse conduction through the AV node, as well as increasing the force of myocardial contraction. This sympathetic response is also called the *adrenergic response*. The response of the heart to sympathetic stimulation is mediated by cardiac receptors called *beta-receptors*. The vasculature contains two types of receptors, alpha- and beta-receptors. Sympathetic stimulation of vascular *alpha-receptors* results in vasoconstriction; vascular beta-receptor stimulation results in vasodilation. The cardiac and vascular beta-receptors are distinguished as $beta_1$ and $beta_2$, respectively. Selective stimulation of these receptors, combined with variations in the intensity of sympathetic activity, regulates the degree of vasocon-

striction, thereby controlling the capacity of the vascular bed and influencing the vascular resistance to blood flow and thus arterial pressure. For example, arterial constriction would increase arterial pressure and the peripheral resistance to blood flow. Venoconstriction would reduce the capacity of the venous bed and increase venous return to the heart.

This *cardiovascular reflex arc* operates to stabilize arterial pressure and cardiac output and to mediate alterations relative to body needs. Cardiac output and arterial pressure can be increased by sympathetic stimulation and parasympathetic inhibition, resulting in an elevation of heart rate, increased force of contraction, and vasoconstriction. Conversely, abnormal elevations in blood pressure will result in reflex slowing of heart rate, reduced contractility, and vasodilation.

QUESTIONS

▼ *Answer the following on a separate sheet of paper.*

1. Trace the anatomic sequence of blood flow through the cardiovascular system, naming the structures traversed.
2. Describe the two critical functions of the atrioventricular (AV) node.
3. Discuss the differences in the wall thickness of the right and left ventricles in terms of function. Relate the relative wall thickness to differences in the systemic and pulmonary circulations.
4. What is the function of the chordae tendineae and papillary muscles?
5. How many valve cusps are there on the valve between the left ventricle and aorta? Name this valve. Name the outpouchings above the valve cusps. What is the function of these outpouchings?
6. Identify the layers of the pericardium. What does the space between the layers contain, and what is its function?
7. How is lymph propelled in lymphatic vessels?
8. Contrast the vascular effects of sympathetic stimulation of the alpha-receptors and beta-receptors. Differentiate between $beta_1$- and $beta_2$-receptors.

▼ *Circle the letter preceding each item below that correctly answers the question or completes the statement. Only one answer is correct unless otherwise noted.*

9. The portion of the heart lying directly beneath the sternum is the:
   a. Cardiac apex
   b. Left atrium
   c. Crux of the heart
   d. Right ventricle
10. The apex of the heart is normally palpated in the:
    a. Fifth intercostal space to the right of the sternum at the midclavicular line
    b. Fifth intercostal space to the right of the sternum at the anterior axillary line
    c. Fifth intercostal space to the left of the sternum at the midclavicular line
    d. Fifth intercostal space to the left of the sternum at the anterior axillary line
11. All the valves of the heart have three cusps *except:*
    a. Pulmonic   c. Mitral
    b. Aortic   d. Tricuspid
12. Oxygenated blood is contained within the:
    a. Pulmonary artery
    b. Pulmonary veins
    c. Superior vena cava
    d. Inferior vena cava
13. To generate high pressure to propel blood through the systemic circulation, the configuration of the left ventricle is:
    a. Crescent shaped
    b. Circular
    c. Elliptic
14. The outermost layer of the wall of a blood vessel is called the:
    a. Intima   c. Adventitia
    b. Media   d. Serosa
15. Blood flow through the capillary beds is *directly* controlled by:
    a. The systemic arterial pressure

b. Oxygen demand of the tissues
   c. The balance between the hydrostatic and osmotic pressures
   d. The precapillary sphincter
16. The sinoatrial (SA) node is the pacemaker of the heart because:
    a. It is the only structure capable of spontaneously generating impulses.
    b. It is richly innervated by sympathetic nerves.
    c. It has the fastest intrinsic rate of impulse generation.
    d. It is anatomically the point of impulse origin.
17. Cardiac impulse conduction is slowest through the:
    a. Purkinje fibers
    b. Interatrial pathways
    c. Bundle branches
    d. AV node
18. At any given time, most of the blood in the circulatory system is in the:
    a. Arteries   c. Capillaries
    b. Veins   d. Heart
19. An increase in the mean arterial pressure causes (more than one answer may be correct):
    a. Activation of baroreceptors
    b. Decreased sympathetic outflow to the heart
    c. Increased parasympathetic outflow to the heart
    d. Increased sympathetic outflow to vascular receptors
20. The response resulting from the answer to question 19 would be (more than one answer may be correct):

? QUESTIONS—cont'd

a. A decrease in the blood pressure
b. An increase in the total peripheral resistance
c. A decrease in the heart rate
d. Reduced contractility of the heart

21. Which of the following statements concerning the cardiovascular chemoreceptors is *not* true?
   a. They are located in the carotid body and aortic arch.
   b. Afferent impulses from the chemoreceptors are carried to the cardioregulatory center via the glossopharyngeal and vagus nerves.
   c. Chemoreceptors are stimulated by a reduction in the arterial oxygen concentration.
   d. Chemoreceptors are stimulated by an elevation of carbon dioxide tension.
   e. Activation of the chemoreceptors stimulates the cardioregulatory center to increase parasympathetic outflow to the heart.

22. Arrange the following structures to represent the normal sequence of cardiac conduction:
   a. Bundle of His
   b. Purkinje fibers
   c. SA node
   d. Bundle branches
   e. Interatrial pathways
   f. AV node

▼ *Match each of the coronary arteries in column A with appropriate items in column B.*

Column A	Column B
23. _____ Right coronary artery	a. Divides into two main branches
24. _____ Left coronary artery	b. One of its branches supplies the anterior wall of the left ventricle
	c. Supplies the AV node in 90% of individuals
	d. Supplies the SA node in more than 50% of individuals

▼ *Match each of the cardiovascular structures in column A with its location in column B.*

Column A	Column B
25. _____ Chordae tendineae	a. Separates right and left ventricles into two chambers
26. _____ Interventricular septum	b. Is the muscular layer of heart
27. _____ Endocardium	c. Attaches to AV valve leaflets on one end and to papillary muscles at the other end
28. _____ Epicardium	d. Is the outer layer of the heart
29. _____ Myocardium	e. Is the inner layer of the myocardial wall
30. _____ Sinuses of Valsalva	f. Contains orifices of coronary arteries

▼ *Fill in the blanks with the correct word or phrase.*

31. The conduction tissue of the heart exhibits the following properties: _____ _____, the ability to spontaneously generate impulses; _____, the ability to respond to stimulation; _____, the ability to transmit impulses; _____, the regularity of impulse generation.

32. Elevations of right atrial pressure or left atrial pressure readily result in neck vein distention and pulmonary congestion, respectively, because the venae cavae and pulmonary veins, unlike most systemic veins, have no true _____.

33. In cases of coronary artery occlusion, _____ circulation may protect the involved muscle tissue from ischemia or necrosis.

34. Lesions of the _____ artery are associated with the highest incidence of AV nodal conduction disturbances. Lesions of the _____ artery are more apt to interfere with the pumping function of the left ventricle.

35. The intrinsic rate of the SA node is _____; the rate of the AV node is _____; and the ventricular rate is _____.

CHAPTER 29

Physiology of the Cardiovascular System

PENNY FORD CARLETON
MARJORIE A. BOLDT

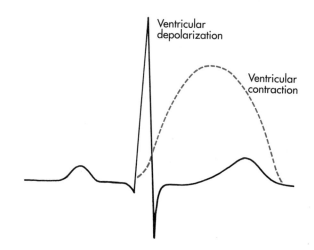

FIG. 29-1 Correlation between ventricular depolarization and ventricular contraction.

CARDIAC CYCLE

Each cardiac cycle consists of a sequence of interdependent electrical and mechanical events. The wave of electrical excitation spreading from the sinoatrial (SA) node through the conduction system and to the myocardium stimulates muscular contraction. This electrical excitation is referred to as *depolarization;* it is followed by electrical recovery, or *repolarization.* The mechanical responses are *systole,* or muscular contraction, and *diastole,* or muscular relaxation. Fig. 29-1 illustrates the correlation between ventricular depolarization and ventricular contraction.

The electrical activity of the cell, recorded graphically via intracellular electrodes, exhibits a characteristic configuration, the *action potential* (Fig. 29-2, *A*). The summated electrical activity of all myocardial cells can be visualized in an *electrocardiogram* (ECG) (Fig. 29-2, *B*). The waves on the ECG reflect the spread of electrical excitation and recovery through the atrial and ventricular myocardium. The significance of the waveforms is discussed in subsequent sections.

Electrophysiology

The electrical activity of the heart is the result of alterations in cell membrane permeability, which permit ionic movement across the cell membrane and change the relative electrical charge along the membrane. Ions are believed to flow through ion-specific channels situated along the membrane. These channels, described as "slow" channels or "fast" channels, are distinguished by the rate of ionic flow and the mechanism activating the different channels. Three ions are of particular importance in cellular electrophysiology: potassium (K^+), sodium (Na^+), and calcium (Ca^{++}) ions. *Potassium* is the dominant intracellular cation, whereas *sodium* and *calcium* ion concentrations are highest extracellularly.

Action potential

Recording an intracellular action potential from a typical myocardial cell produces the distinctive configura-

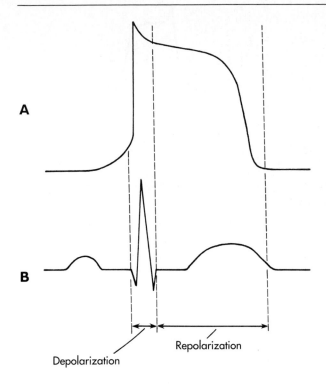

Repolarization

Depolarization

FIG 29-2   Electrical activity of the heart. **A,** Recording of the intracellular potential of a single cardiac cell during a complete cardiac cycle. **B,** Standard electrocardiographic (ECG) recording from the body surface, representing the summated electrical activity of all the myocardial cells. The time periods within the dashed lines represent depolarization and repolarization of the ventricles.

tion illustrated in Fig. 29-2, *A.* This action potential consists of five discrete phases corresponding to distinct electrophysiologic events (Fig. 29-3), as follows:

1. *Resting phase—phase 4.* In the resting state, the cardiac cell exhibits a difference in electrical potential or voltage across the cell membrane. The inside of the cell is relatively negative, and the outside of the cell is relatively positive; thus the cell is polarized. This difference results from the relative permeability of the cell membrane to surrounding ions, particularly the positively charged sodium and potassium ions. In the resting state the cell membrane is more permeable to potassium than to sodium. Therefore small amounts of potassium ions diffuse out of the cell from areas of high potassium concentration into the extracellular fluid, where the potassium concentration is lower. This intracellular loss of positive potassium ions leaves the inside of the cell relatively negative in electrical charge (Fig. 29-3, *A*).

2. *Rapid depolarization—phase 0 (upstroke).* Depolarization of the cell is the result of greatly increased membrane permeability to sodium. Extracellular sodium ions rush into the cell through fast channels, propelled by the sodium concentration gradient. This influx of positive sodium ions reverses the relative

charge across the cell membrane; the outside of the cell becomes negative, and the inside becomes positive (Fig. 29-3, *B*).

3. *Partial repolarization—phase 1 (spike).* Immediately on this reversal of charge, when the inside of the cell has become positive relative to the outside, the "fast" sodium channels close and the potassium channels open. Less sodium enters the cell and more potassium leaves, each along its concentration gradient. The result is a net flux of positive charge out of the cell (Fig. 29-3, *C*).

4. *Plateau—phase 2.* A sustained plateau, corresponding to the absolute refractory period of the myocardium, follows. During this period, no net change in electrical charge across the membrane occurs. A balance is maintained between the influx and efflux of positively charged ions. A slow inward flow of calcium ions is primarily responsible for this plateau; some inward movement of sodium through slow channels also contributes. This inward movement of positive charge is countered by an outward movement of potassium ions (Fig. 29-3, *D*).

5. *Rapid repolarization—phase 3 (downstroke).* During rapid repolarization, the slow inward currents of calcium and sodium cease, and the membrane permeability to potassium increases greatly. Potassium moves out of the cell, reducing the positive charge within the cell; eventually the inside of the cell regains its relative negativity and the outside of the cell its relative positivity (Fig. 29-3, *E*). The distribution of ions in the cell at rest is maintained by the continuous action of the sodium-potassium pump, which actively transports sodium out of the cell and potassium into it.

The action potential configuration just described is characteristic of that found in nonspecialized myocardial fibers located in the atria and ventricles and in specialized conducting fibers located in the atria and ventricles and in specialized conducting fibers of the atrial tracts and His-Purkinje system. This type of action potential is referred to as the *fast response.* A second type of action potential, known as the *slow response,* is observed during intracellular recordings from the specialized fibers of the SA node and the atrioventricular (AV) node. Fig. 29-4 illustrates the configurations of both action potentials. The slow-response configuration is more gradual than that of the fast response. Depolarization of the fast-response action potentials primarily depends on sodium ions, whereas slow-channel depolarization depends primarily on calcium ions.

Action potential and physiologic properties

The physiologic properties of the specialized cells in the SA and in AV node differ distinctly from those of the conducting pathways and myocardium because of differences in behavior between slow and fast action potentials. The property of *automaticity,* the ability to generate impulses spontaneously, results from automatic changes

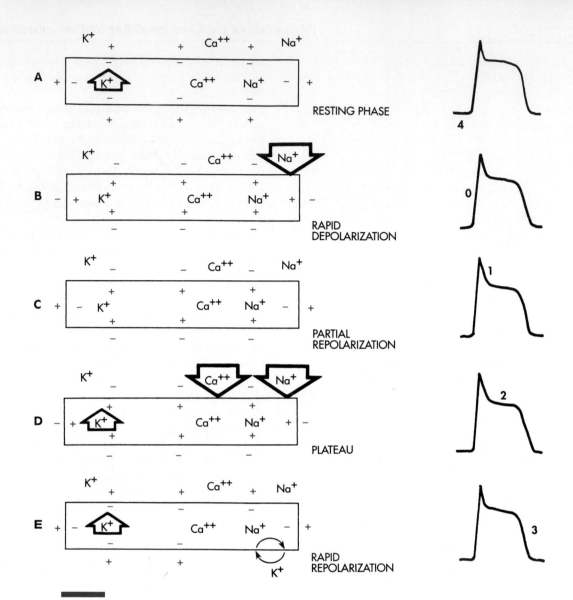

FIG 29-3 Cellular electrophysiology. **A,** Resting phase. **B,** Rapid depolarization. **C,** Partial repolarization. **D,** Plateau. **E,** Rapid repolarization. K+, *Potassium*; Ca++, calcium; Na+, sodium.

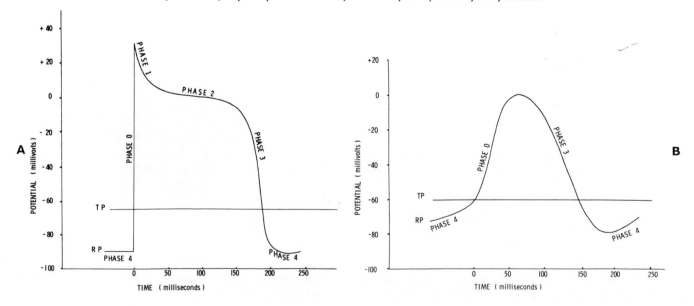

FIG 29-4 Configuration of action potential. **A,** Fast response. **B,** Slow response. (From Hurst JW et al: *The heart,* ed 4, New York, 1978, McGraw-Hill.)

that occur during the resting phase of the slow-response action potential. Note in Fig. 29-4, *B,* that as soon as repolarization is complete, the cell slowly and spontaneously begins to depolarize toward threshold. As soon as threshold is reached, the cell will automatically fire. This behavior is described as the *all-or-none phenomenon;* until threshold is reached, depolarization will not generate an action potential, but once that critical level is attained, a complete depolarization-repolarization cycle results. The sinus node spontaneously depolarizes at the fastest intrinsic rate, approximately 60 to 100 beats per minute (bpm), thereby functioning as the "natural pacemaker" of the heart.

Conduction velocity is also directly attributable to the type of action potential. Slower conduction through the AV node, in contrast to rapid conduction through the Purkinje fibers, results from differences in the configuration of the slow-response and fast-response action potentials. This conduction delay across the AV node allows for ventricular filling during atrial contraction and exerts a protective effect during rapid atrial dysrhythmias.

Excitability is also determined by the action potential. Immediately after myocardial depolarization, a brief interval occurs, known as the *effective* or *absolute refractory period,* during which the myocardium is incapable of responding to any stimulus. A *relative refractory period* follows, during which the myocardium responds only to a stimulus of greater-than-normal intensity. Tetanic contracture of the myocardium as a result of repetitive stimulation therefore is impossible. The effective refractory period in the fast action potential lasts from depolarization through the plateau phase to the middle of phase 3. During this period the fast sodium channels are inactivated. The relative refractory period extends from the middle of phase 3 to the onset of phase 4; some of the channels can be activated during this period.

Muscle Ultrastructure

The *sarcomere* is the basic contractile unit of the myocardium (Fig. 29-5). It is composed of two sets of overlapping myofilaments: the thick *myosin* filament and the thin *actin* filament. Cross-bridges or linkages form between these myofilaments at regular intervals. In addition to the actin and myosin proteins, the sarcomere contains *troponin* and *tropomyosin* proteins. In the resting state, the troponin-tropomyosin complex inhibits cross-bridge formation.

The relationship between electrical excitation of the cell and the mechanical response is referred to as *excitation-contraction coupling.* The action potential is propagated over the surface of the cell along the *cell membrane,* or *sarcolemma,* and into the *T tubules,* which are invaginations in the cell membrane. The action potential is conducted from cell to cell through the intercalated disks (Fig. 29-6).

The concentration of free intracellular calcium deter-

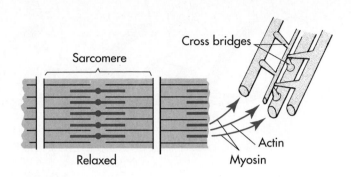

FIG 29-5 Muscle ultrastructure. The myofibrils are composed of thick myosin filaments and thin actin filaments. Cross-bridges are observed at regular intervals between the actin and myosin filaments, forming linkages during muscle contraction. The amount of overlap between the actin and myosin filaments is decreased during muscle relaxation and increased during contraction. This causes a corresponding increase or decrease in the sarcomere length.

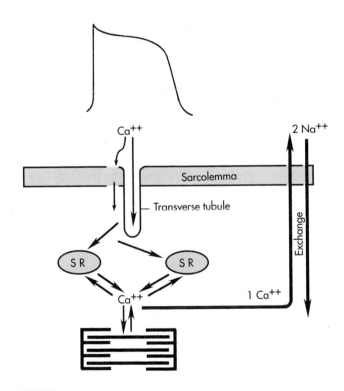

FIG 29-6 Movement of calcium in excitation-contraction coupling in cardiac muscle. The influx of calcium ions (Ca^{++}) from the interstitial fluid during excitation (plateau of action potential) triggers the release of Ca^{++} from the sarcoplasmic reticulum *(SR).* The free cytoplasmic Ca^+ activates contraction of the myofilaments (systole). Relaxation (diastole) occurs as a result of Ca^{++} uptake by the SR and the extrusion of intracellular Ca^{++} by sodium-calcium exchange. (From Berne RM, Levy MN: *Cardiovascular physiology,* ed 6, St Louis, 1991, Mosby.)

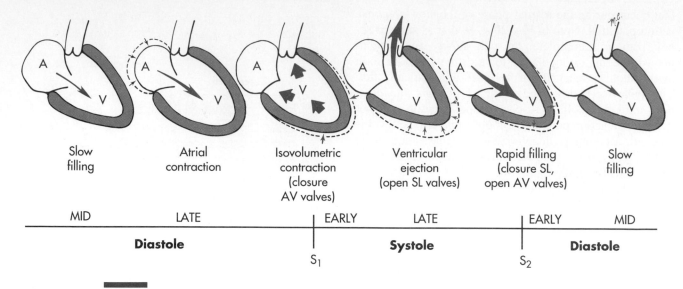

Slow filling	Atrial contraction	Isovolumetric contraction (closure AV valves)	Ventricular ejection (open SL valves)	Rapid filling (closure SL, open AV valves)	Slow filling
MID	LATE	EARLY	LATE	EARLY	MID

Diastole | | **Systole** | | **Diastole**

S_1 S_2

FIG 29-7   Phases of the cardiac cycle. *A,* Atria; *V,* ventricles; S_1, first heart sound; S_2, second heart sound.

mines the contractile state of the myocardium. The electrical excitation of the myocardial cell initiates muscular contraction by stimulating the release of calcium from the *sarcoplasmic reticulum* and other cellular sources. As illustrated in Fig. 29-6, the permeability of the sarcolemma to calcium increases during the plateau phase of the action potential. Calcium diffuses through the T tubules and calcium channels in the sarcolemma. This calcium stimulates the release of additional calcium from intracellular stores in the sarcoplasmic reticulum. Calcium then binds to the troponin protein, inactivating the inhibitory effect of the troponin-tropomyosin system on the contractile proteins, actin and myosin. The actin and myosin myofilaments then interact to form linkages or cross-bridges that generate force to slide these overlapping myofilaments past each other, thereby shortening the sarcomere (see Fig. 29-5). The shortening of multiple sarcomere units produces muscular contraction. Relaxation of the muscle is the result of calcium uptake by the sarcoplasmic reticulum, which dissociates the actin-myosin cross-bridges. Calcium ionic balance is then restored by the exchange of positive sodium ions for calcium ions.

The force of myocardial contraction depends on the interaction between sarcomere myofilaments. Administration of calcium can increase contractile force by increasing calcium availability to the sarcomere. Conversely, overstretching the sarcomere would reduce contractile force by reducing the amount of overlap and subsequent linkage formation between the actin and myosin filaments.

Phases of the Cardiac Cycle

The mechanical events of the cardiac cycle, *systole* or ventricular contraction and *diastole* or ventricular relax-

ation, consist of five distinct phases. The phases of the cardiac cycle can most easily be conceptualized in the following sequence (Fig. 29-7):

1. *Middiastole.* This is the phase of slow ventricular filling, or *diastasis*. The atrial and ventricular chambers are relaxed. Blood entering the atria through venous channels flows passively into the ventricles through the open AV valves. The semilunar valves are closed.
2. *Late diastole.* The wave of depolarization spreads through the atria and pauses at the AV node. The atrial muscle contracts, contributing an additional 20% to 30% to the ventricular volume.
3. *Early systole.* Depolarization spreads from the AV node through the bundle branches to the ventricular myocardium. As ventricular contraction begins, the pressure within the ventricles rises above that of the atria, causing the AV valves to close, which generates the first heart sound (S_1). The ventricular chambers continue to develop higher pressures; however, during this phase the pressures within the aorta and pulmonary artery exceed the ventricular pressures, keeping the semilunar valves closed. This is termed *isovolumetric contraction* because the ventricular volumes remain constant.
4. *Late systole.* As soon as the ventricular pressures exceed the pressures within the blood vessels, the semilunar valves open and ventricular ejection into the pulmonary and systemic circulation occurs. This ejection phase can be divided into a brief, initial phase of "rapid ejection" and a subsequent, more sustained phase of "reduced ejection."
5. *Early diastole.* The wave of repolarization then spreads through the ventricular myocardium, and the ventricular chambers relax. As the muscle relaxes, the ventricular pressures drop below the arterial pres-

sures, causing the semilunar valves to close, which produces the second heart sound (S$_2$). Relaxation continues until the ventricular pressures drop below that of the atrial pressures, causing the AV valves to open. The period between semilunar valve closure and opening of the AV valves is referred to as *isovolumetric relaxation* because ventricular volumes remain constant despite continued reduction in ventricular pressure. As the AV valves open, the ventricles fill rapidly with the venous blood that has accumulated in the atria. Approximately 70% to 80% of ventricular filling occurs during this rapid filling phase.

CARDIAC OUTPUT

Definitions

The result of the synchronized, rhythmic myocardial contraction is the ejection of blood into the pulmonary and systemic circulations. The volume of blood ejected by each ventricle per minute is the *cardiac output*. An average cardiac output is 5 L/min. However, cardiac output varies to meet the needs of the peripheral tissues for oxygen and nutrients. Because cardiac output requirements also vary according to body size, a more accurate indicator of cardiac function is the cardiac index. The *cardiac index* is the cardiac output divided by body surface area; it ranges from 2.8 to 3.6 L/min/m^2 of body surface.

Stroke volume is the volume of blood ejected by each ventricle per beat. Approximately two thirds of the volume of blood in the ventricle at the end of diastole *(end-diastolic volume)* is ejected during systole. This portion of blood ejected is known as the *ejection fraction;* the residual ventricular volume at the end of systole is referred to as the *end-systolic volume*. Depression of ventricular function impairs the ability of the ventricle to empty, thereby reducing stroke volume and the ejection fraction with a consequent elevation of residual ventricular volumes.

Determinants of Cardiac Output

Cardiac output depends on the relationship between two variables—heart rate and stroke volume:

Cardiac output = Heart rate × Stroke volume

Despite alterations in one variable, cardiac output can be held remarkably constant by compensatory adjustments in the other variable. For instance, if the heart rate slows, the period of ventricular relaxation between heartbeats is longer and ventricular filling time is thereby increased. Consequently, ventricular volumes are greater and more blood can be ejected per beat. Conversely, if stroke volume drops, cardiac output can be stabilized by increasing the heart rate. These compensatory adjustments can only

maintain cardiac output within limits. The alteration and stabilization of cardiac output depend on control mechanisms regulating heart rate and stroke volume.

Control of heart rate

Heart rate is largely under the extrinsic control of the autonomic nervous system; parasympathetic and sympathetic fibers innervate the SA node and the AV node, influencing the rate and speed of impulse conduction. Stimulation of the parasympathetic fibers decreases the heart rate, whereas sympathetic stimulation increases it. In the normal resting heart, the influence of the parasympathetic system seems to dominate in maintaining the heart rate at approximately 60 to 80 bpm. If all neural and hormonal influences on the heart were blocked, the intrinsic rate would be about 100 bpm. However, in the presence of heart disease, the sympathetic system predominates in the control of heart rate and the maintenance of cardiac compensation. Norepinephrine stored in cardiac sympathetic nerve terminals augments the catecholamine supply available from neural sympathetic fibers and the adrenal medulla. The norepinephrine in these cardiac nerve terminals eventually becomes depleted in chronic heart failure.

Control of stroke volume

Stroke volume depends on three variables: (1) preload, as explained by Starling's law of the heart, (2) contractility, and (3) afterload.

Starling's law of the heart states that stretching the myocardial fibers during diastole by increasing end-diastolic volume will increase the force of contraction during systole (Fig. 29-8). An analogous example is that of increasing the stretch on a rubber band to increase the force of elastic recoil on release. Myocardial fibers can be stretched by increasing ventricular diastolic volumes. The degree of stretch is expressed in terms of *preload* (i.e., diastolic fiber length before contraction).

The degree of fiber stretch or preload is determined by the ventricular volume. The volume of blood contained within the ventricles during diastole depends on the amount of venous return. Venous return is influenced primarily by circulating blood volume and the venous tone. Increasing venous return, and thus ventricular volumes, stretches the myocardial fibers. Stretching the sarcomere maximizes the number of interaction sites available for actin-myosin linkage by increasing the overlap between the myofilaments. Consequently, the force of contraction rises.

Typically, the sarcomere is stretched to 2.0 μm during diastole (Fig. 29-9, *A*). The optimal sarcomere length is 2.2. μm (Fig. 29-9, *B*). Therefore a reserve in sarcomere length and resultant force of contraction exists. Starling's law is functional within limits determined by the myocardial ultrastructure described earlier. Stretching the sarcomere to more than 2.4 μm would reduce the strength of contraction by reducing the number of available interac-

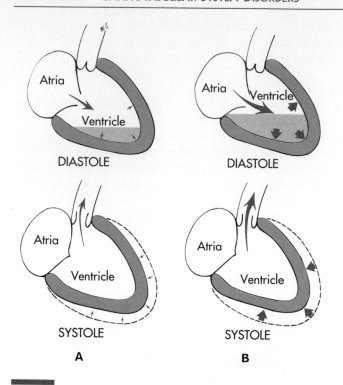

FIG 29-8   Starling's law of the heart. **A,** Normal filling during diastole causes normal fiber stretch and normal contractile force and stroke volume. **B,** Increased filling during diastole causes increased fiber stretch, increased force of contraction, and increased stroke volume.

tion sites (Fig. 29-9, *C*). Fortunately, the myocardial sarcomeres are extremely resistant to overstretching.

The relationship between myocardial fiber length and force of contraction is referred to as the *ventricular function curve* (Fig. 29-10). Increasing ventricular end-diastolic volumes initially increases force of contraction and stroke volume. Thus the curve demonstrates an initial ascending limb of improved function. Eventually the curve flattens, or plateaus, indicating that additional increments in ventricular volume will not improve function further; optimal fiber stretch has been achieved. The normal heart operates on the ascending limb of the ventricular function curve. Considerable cardiac reserve exists to move beyond that point with further improvements in cardiac function. In summary, up to a point, increased preload will increase the force of contraction and consequently the volume of blood ejected from the ventricle.

There is a "family" of ventricular function curves. A shift of the curve upward and to the left reflects an improvement in ventricular function, whereas a shift downward and to the right represents a deterioration in function. Alterations in the position of the ventricular function curve reflect changes in *contractility* or *inotropic state,* the second determinant of stroke volume. Contractility refers to changes in the developed force of contraction that occur independent of changes in myocardial fiber length. Increased contractility is the result of intensification of the interactions at the actin-myosin cross-bridges in the sarcomere. The intensity of these interactions relates to the intracellular concentration of free calcium

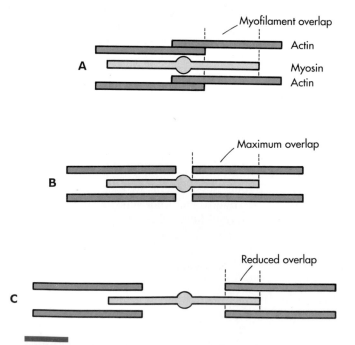

FIG 29-9   Effect of sarcomere length on myofilament overlap. **A,** Usual sarcomere length of 2.0 μm. **B,** Optimal sarcomere length of 2.2 μm. **C,** Excessive sarcomere length of 2.5 μm.

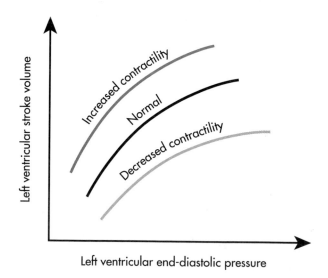

FIG 29-10   Ventricular function curve. The solid black line represents the normal ventricular function curve. Note that increasing end-diastolic volume increases stroke volume up to a point. Displacement of the curve upward and to the left represents improved ventricular function, as would be seen with sympathetic nervous system stimulation. Displacement of the curve downward and to the right represents myocardial depression, as would be seen with acidosis, hypoxia, or cardiac failure.

ions. Myocardial contractility is directly proportional to the amount of intracellular calcium present. Increased contractility elevates stroke volume by increasing ventricular emptying during systole. Factors depressing myocardial function, such as acidosis or hypoxia, shift the curve downward and to the right.

Afterload, the third determinant of stroke volume, is the resistance to ventricular ejection reflected from the systemic arterial tree when the aortic valve opens. It is primarily a function of intraventricular pressure, intraventricular size or radius, and ventricular wall thickness. The relationship between wall tension, pressure, radius, and wall thickness is expressed in this simplified version of the Laplace relationship:

$$\text{Wall tension} = \frac{\text{Intraventricular pressure} \times \text{Radius}}{\text{Ventricular wall thickness}}$$

The *Laplace equation* indicates that a direct relationship exists between intraventricular pressure and chamber size and the amount of tension the ventricle must generate to eject blood during systole. An increment of either intraventricular pressure or intraventricular size elevates the amount of tension the ventricle must develop to eject blood. For example, elevation of arterial pressure increases the resistance to ventricular ejection, thereby necessitating the development of increased intraventricular pressure and wall tension to overcome the resistance. Similarly, as the ventricular radius or chamber size increases, the ventricle must develop more tension during systole to generate a given pressure and eject blood. In other words, a dilated ventricle must develop more tension than a normal ventricle to generate the same systolic pressure (Fig. 29-11). Thus an increase in afterload can be produced by either increased arterial pressure or ventricular dilation. Excessive increases in afterload may ad-

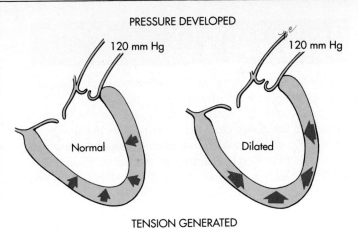

PRESSURE DEVELOPED

120 mm Hg   120 mm Hg

Normal   Dilated

TENSION GENERATED

FIG. 29-11   Effect of ventricular size on afterload. The dilated ventricle on the right must generate more tension than the normal ventricle on the left to generate the same systolic pressure of 120 mm Hg.

versely affect ventricular emptying, reducing stroke volume and consequently cardiac output.

Increases in wall thickness, or myocardial hypertrophy, decrease wall tension or afterload according to the Laplace relationship. In other words, as the ventricle hypertrophies, proportionally less wall tension must be developed by the ventricle to generate pressure and eject blood because of the increase in muscle mass.

In summary, the integration of the mechanisms controlling heart rate and stroke volume determine ventricular function and cardiac output. Heart rate is primarily under extrinsic neural control. Control of stroke volume is a function of the interaction of three variables: preload, contractility, and afterload (Fig. 29-12).

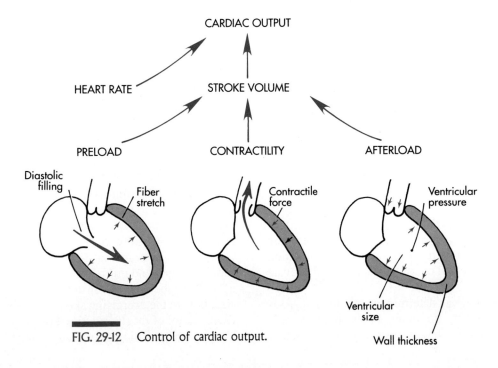

FIG. 29-12   Control of cardiac output.

BLOOD FLOW TO THE PERIPHERY

The dynamics of peripheral blood flow is perhaps the most critical element of circulatory physiology for two reasons. First, the distribution of the cardiac output within the periphery depends on properties of the vascular bed. Second, the volume of cardiac output depends on the amount of blood returning to the heart. Essentially, the heart ejects a volume of blood equivalent to its venous return.

Principles of Blood Flow

Blood flow depends on two opposing variables: (1) the pressure propelling blood and (2) the resistance to flow. Blood flow increases as the pressure that propels blood increases; inversely, flow decreases as resistance increases.

A pressure difference or *pressure gradient* must exist between two points for blood to flow between the points. The greater the pressure gradient, the greater is the flow. Blood flows throughout the entire circulation from the arterial to the venous end in response to pressure gradients. The *mean-arterial pressure* reflects the average blood volume and compliance in the arterial system and is approximately 100 mm Hg. Capillary pressure averages 25 mm Hg. Pressure at the venous end of the circulation or right atrium *(right atrial pressure)* is close to 0 mm Hg. Thus pressure progressively declines throughout the systemic circulation. The pressure gradient between the arterial and venous ends of the systemic circulation is approximately 100 mm Hg (mean arterial pressure minus right atrial pressure or central venous pressure). Alterations in either the mean arterial pressure or the right atrial pressure will influence blood flow by changing the pressure gradient between the two points.

Mean arterial pressure (MAP) changes if either the vascular contents (cardiac output, CO) or the vascular capacity (total peripheral resistance, TPR) is altered:

$$MAP = CO \times TPR$$

For example, either massive hemorrhage or extensive vasodilation (as in gram-negative sepsis) can profoundly reduce arterial pressure. However, the pressure alteration is sensed by the baroreceptors, and reflex-compensatory responses mediated by the autonomic nervous system ensue to stabilize arterial pressure. Right atrial pressure depends on the balance between venous return to the atrium and the ability of the right atrium to empty. Disease of the tricuspid valve and impaired right ventricular function can both reduce right atrial output and abnormally elevate right atrial pressure.

Resistance, the second determinant of blood flow, is primarily determined by the radius of the blood vessel. Other factors, such as blood viscosity and vascular length, also alter resistance to flow. However, because these properties are relatively constant, their influence is normally insignificant. Resistance is extremely sensitive to alterations in the lumen of the blood vessel. *Poiseuille's law* demonstrates that resistance *(R)* is inversely proportional to the fourth power of the radius *(r)* of the blood vessel:

$$R \propto \frac{1}{r^4}$$

Therefore reduction of the radius by one-half will increase the resistance to flow sixteenfold. The arteriole is the major site of vascular resistance. Alterations in the smooth muscle tone of the arteriolar wall regulate resistance to flow and consequently the amount of flow to the capillary bed.

In summary, flow *(F)* is directly proportional to the pressure gradient (ΔP) and inversely proportional to the vascular resistance:

$$F = \frac{\Delta P}{R}$$

The pressure gradient is determined by pressures at the arterial and venous ends of the circulation. Resistance is primarily a function of the radius of the blood vessels, altered most significantly at the arteriolar level.

Velocity of Blood Flow

The velocity of blood flow throughout the vascular system depends on the cross-sectional area of the blood vessels. Velocity *(V)* of blood flow *(F)* decreases as the cross-sectional area *(A)* increases. This inverse relationship is expressed as follows:

$$V = \frac{F}{A}$$

As blood flows into the peripheral arterial system, velocity decreases because of the progressive branching and relative increase in cross-sectional area of the vascular tree. At the capillary level, a profound increase in cross-sectional area occurs, significantly reducing flow velocity. This slowing facilitates the eventual exchange of nutrients and metabolites at the capillary level.

Distribution of Blood Flow

Blood flow is distributed among the multiple organ systems according to the metabolic needs and functional demands of the tissues. Because tissue needs are continually changing, blood flow must continually be readjusted. As tissue metabolism increases, blood flow must increase to supply oxygen and nutrients and to remove the end products of metabolism. For instance, during strenuous exercise, flow to the exercising skeletal muscle must increase. Dual control of the distribution of cardiac output is possible through extrinsic and intrinsic regulatory mechanisms.

Extrinsic control

Blood flow to a given organ system can be increased either by increasing cardiac output or by shunting blood from a relatively inactive organ system to the more active organ. The activity of the sympathetic nervous system can produce both responses. First, sympathetic stimulation augments cardiac output by increasing heart rate and force of contractility. Second, sympathetic adrenergic fibers also extend to the peripheral vasculature, particularly the arteriole. Selective alterations in sympathetic discharge will stimulate alpha-receptors and beta-receptors, preferentially constricting some arterioles and dilating others to redistribute blood to capillary beds according to need. Within any capillary bed, considerable reserve exists for increased flow because only a portion of the capillaries are perfused at a given time. Therefore flow can be increased by opening nonperfused capillaries and by further arteriolar dilation of perfused capillaries.

Skeletal muscle vasculature is uniquely capable of vasodilation because sympathetic cholinergic fibers originating in the cerebral cortex innervate these vessels. These fibers release acetylcholine, resulting in relaxation of vascular smooth muscle. Parasympathetic cholinergic fibers innervate only selected, small portions of the peripheral vasculature; therefore parasympathetic activity does not significantly influence the distribution of cardiac output or total peripheral resistance.

In addition to neural control, an extrinsic influence on peripheral resistance and flow is exerted by humoral agents. The adrenal medulla secretes the catecholamines epinephrine and norepinephrine in response to sympathetic activity. These hormones elicit sympathetic responses in the peripheral vasculature. Other blood-borne agents—vasopressin, angiotensin, serotonin, bradykinin, and histamine—are currently under investigation to establish their role in peripheral vascular control.

Intrinsic control

Local control of blood flow at the tissue level occurs through autoregulation. *Autoregulation* permits readjustment of blood flow relative to tissue metabolic activity. The precise mechanism for local changes in vascular resistance and blood flow is unclear. It has been suggested that tissue metabolites released when oxygen demand exceeds oxygen supply mediate this response. Tissue ischemia is an extremely potent stimulus for vasodilation. The logic of this compensatory response is obvious, although the exact mechanism is unclear. The vasodilation may be a direct response to the oxygen lack, or the lack may trigger the release of chemical vasodilators, such as adenosine or prostaglandins. The direct vasodilatory effect of metabolites, such as carbon dioxide and lactic acid, is another possibility.

The relative strength of extrinsic and intrinsic control mechanisms varies among organ systems. In vital, flow-dependent organs, such as the heart and brain, the intrinsic mechanisms predominate, whereas in other areas, such as the skin, autonomic control predominates.

In addition to these control mechanisms designed to increase oxygen delivery to the tissues, the tissues can increase oxygen supply by extracting more oxygen from the arterial blood. In most organs, with the notable exception of the heart, only a small proportion of the oxygen available in the arterial blood is extracted by the tissue. When an oxygen deficit develops in the tissues, the concentration gradient of oxygen between the arterial blood and the tissue increases. This causes more oxygen to diffuse from the intravascular to the extravascular space, thereby increasing oxygen delivery to the cells.

When compensatory mechanisms are unable to sustain adequate peripheral perfusion, as in shock, flow must be distributed according to priority. Blood will be shunted away from less metabolically active areas, such as the skin and kidney, to maintain perfusion of the brain and heart. Consequently, early signs of shock or inadequate tissue perfusion are decreased urine output and cold, pale skin. Significant alterations in mentation and cardiac function occur much later in the shock state, when flow is compromised even to the vital organs.

CARDIAC RESERVE

Normally the heart possesses the ability to increase its pumping capacity significantly above resting levels. This cardiac reserve enables the normal heart to increase output approximately fivefold. The increase in cardiac output can occur through increments in heart rate or stroke volume (cardiac output = heart rate × stroke volume).

Heart rate can normally increase from resting levels of 60 to 100 bpm to approximately 180 bpm, primarily through sympathetic stimulation. Rates greater than this can be deleterious for two reasons. First, as heart rate increases, the duration of diastole shortens and ventricular filling time is reduced; eventually stroke volume falls, negating the advantage of further rate increments. Second, rapid heart rates can adversely affect myocardial oxygenation because cardiac work is increased while the diastolic period, during which most coronary flow occurs, is reduced.

Stroke volume can increase either by increased ventricular emptying caused by increased contractility or by increased diastolic filling and a subsequent rise in ejection volume. However, both increased force of contraction and increased ventricular volumes will elevate cardiac work and oxygen demand. In addition, the effect of increased diastolic filling on contractility and stroke volume is limited by the degree of myocardial fiber stretch.

If the heart is subjected to chronic volume or pressure overload, the ventricular muscle may *dilate* to increase contractile force, according to Starling's law, or *hypertrophy* to increase muscle mass and pumping force. Both responses, although compensatory in nature, eventually contribute to further cardiac decompensation. According to *Laplace's law,* dilation increases cardiac work because a distended heart requires more energy to maintain the same stroke volume. As ventricular diastolic pressure in- creases, the sarcomere's ability to adapt may be exceeded and contractile force decreased. Hypertrophy increases the muscle mass requiring a nutrient supply, thereby in- creasing oxygen demand.

 ## QUESTIONS

▼ *Answer the following on a separate sheet of paper.*

1. What are the two major mechanical phases of the cardiac cycle, and what does each represent? What does an elec- trocardiogram represent, and how is it different from an action potential? What is the relationship between the electrical and mechanical events of the cardiac cycle?

2. State Starling's law of the heart. What is the relationship between Starling's law and the ventricular function curve?

3. State Poiseuille's law as it applies to blood circulation. How would you cal- culate the systemic blood pressure gra- dient?

4. Hemodynamic measurements on a 46- year-old woman with a body surface area of 1.5 m^2 reveal the following data: car- diac output (CO), 4.5 L/minute; left ven- tricular end-diastolic volume (EDV), 100 ml; left ventricular end-systolic volume (ESV), 30 ml. What is her left ventricular stroke volume (SV)? What is her cardiac index (CI) and left ventricular ejection fraction (EF)? Are these values normal?

▼ *Circle the letter preceding each item that correctly answers the question or com- pletes the statement. Only one answer is correct unless otherwise noted.*

5. The rapid depolarizing phase of an action potential in heart muscle is caused by a:
   a. Sudden increase in permeability of the membrane to sodium.
   b. Decrease in permeability of the mem- brane to potassium
   c. Decrease in the sodium pumping rate
   d. Sudden increase in permeability of the membrane to potassium.

6. Which of the following substances is re- leased from the sarcoplasmic reticulum and diffuses to the sarcomere to produce myocardial contraction?
   a. Sodium ions (Na^+)
   b. Potassium ions (K^+)
   c. Calcium ions (Ca^{++})
   d. ATPase

7. Expected changes resulting from sever- ing both vagi include (more than one an- swer may be correct):

a. Interruption of the afferent pathways from the aortic arch baroreceptors
b. Increase in heart rate to approxi- mately 100 bpm
c. Increase in cardiac output
d. Increase in mean arterial pressure

8. When a patient was given a certain drug, the mean arterial pressure increased and the total peripheral resistance de- creased. This drug probably caused:
   a. Vasoconstriction and an increase in cardiac output
   b. Vasoconstriction and a decrease in cardiac output
   c. Vasodilation and an increase in car- diac output
   d. Vasodilation and a decrease in car- diac output

9. Within limits, an increase in the end- diastolic volume of the ventricle will (more than one answer may be correct):
   a. Increase stroke volume of the ven- tricle
   b. Decrease stroke volume of the ven- tricle
   c. Increase force of contraction
   d. Decrease cardiac work

10. An increase in cardiac contractility re- sults in an increased stroke volume or stroke work force for a given left ven- tricular end-diastolic volume and is re- flected by a shift of the ventricular func- tion curve to the:
    a. Left
    b. Right

11. Cardiac muscle cannot be tetanized be- cause:
    a. The refractory period lasts through- out the period of contractions.
    b. The impulse spread through the con- duction system is too rapid.
    c. The muscle fibers are relatively is- chemic after each contraction.
    d. Intracardiac calcium levels are too low.

12. The volume of blood ejected by the ven- tricle depends on (more than one an- swer may be correct):
    a. Preload
    b. Afterload
    c. Contractile state

13. Which of the following statements con- cerning Laplace's relationship between wall tension, intraventricular pressure, and ventricular radius is true (more than one answer may be correct)?
    a. The ventricle must generate in- creased tension to eject if ventricular size increases.
    b. The ventricle must generate in- creased tension if the ventricular size decreases.
    c. The ventricle must generate in- creased tension if arterial pressure increases.
    d. The ventricle must generate in- creased tension if arterial pressure decreases.

14. The most important extrinsic control mechanism affecting the distribution of cardiac output is:
    a. The parasympathetic system
    b. The sympathetic system
    c. Circulating neurohormones
    d. Tissue ischemia

15. Distribution of blood flow to vital or- gans such as the heart and brain is pre- dominantly controlled by:
    a. Extrinsic mechanisms such as neural control and humoral agents
    b. Intrinsic mechanisms or autoregu- lation

16. The primary reason that blood flow through the capillaries is slow is that:
    a. Capillaries are small.
    b. Capillary pressure is low.
    c. Precapillary resistance is high.
    d. Total capillary cross-sectional area is great.

17. Coronary perfusion takes place:
    a. Primarily during systole
    b. Primarily during diastole
    c. Equally during systole and diastole

18. Stretching myocardial fibers to the opti- mal sarcomere length increases the force of contraction by:
    a. Increasing the overlap of the myofil- aments
    b. Intensifying the cross-bridge interac- tions
    c. Increasing the volume of blood to be ejected

QUESTIONS—cont'd

19. Factors that affect cardiac output include (more than one answer may be correct):
    a. Circulating levels of hormones
    b. Stimulation of the cardiac sympathetic nervous system
    c. Exercise
    d. Stroke volume
20. Arrange the mechanical events of the cardiac cycle in the proper time sequence beginning with (a), AV valves close.
    a. AV valves close.
    b. AV valves open.
    c. Semilunar valves close.
    d. Semilunar valves open.
    e. Ventricular filling occurs.
    f. Ventricular ejection occurs.
    g. Ventricular relaxation occurs.
    h. First heart sound occurs.
    i. Second heart sound occurs.

▼ Match each of the hemodynamic parameters in column A with its equivalent in column B.

Column A

21. _____ Cardiac output
22. _____ Mean arterial pressure
23. _____ Stroke volume
24. _____ Ejection fraction
25. _____ Cardiac indexes
26. _____ Blood flow

Column B

a. End-diastolic volume − End-systolic volume

b. $\dfrac{\text{Cardiac output}}{\text{Body surface area}}$

c. Cardiac output × Total peripheral resistance

d. Heart rate × Stroke volume

e. $\dfrac{\text{Stroke volume}}{\text{End-diastolic volume}}$

f. $\dfrac{\text{Mean arterial pressure} - \text{central venous pressure}}{\text{Resistance}}$

▼ Fill in the blanks with the correct word or phrase or circle the correct option.

27. The _____ period is that time during the cardiac cycle when the myocardium will not respond to any stimulus. The myocardium is capable of responding to a strong stimulus during the _____ refractory period.
28. In the resting state the inside of the cell is _____ charged with respect to the outside. During the repolarization of a cell the sodium-potassium pump moves _____ into the cell and _____ out of the cell.
29. During the ventricular filling phase of the cardiac cycle the AV valves are (open) or (closed) and the semilunar valves are (open) or (closed).
30. During the ventricular ejection phase of the cardiac cycle the AV valves are (open) or (closed) and the semilunar valves are (open) or (closed).
31. During the phase of ventricular filling the cardiac impulse is delayed at the _____.

▼ Circle the letter preceding each item below that correctly answers the question or completes the statement.

32. Choose the *false* statement concerning the slow-response action potential in cardiac tissue:
    a. It is the characteristic intracellular recording from the SA node.
    b. Inward currents of Ca⁺⁺ and Na⁺ are responsible for the unstable resting phase.
    c. The stable resting phase results from an influx of Ca⁺⁺ ions via slow channels.
    d. Characteristics of this type of action potential account for the relatively slower conduction time through the AV node.
33. Automaticity of cardiac tissue may be defined as:
    a. Ability to transmit impulses
    b. Ability to generate impulses spontaneously
    c. Ability to respond to stimulation
    d. Regularity of impulse generation
34. A pacemaker cell in the SA node:
    a. Has a stable phase 4 potential
    b. Has a phase 0 potential primarily caused by a "fast current"
    c. Has a distinct and prolonged phase 1 and 2 potential
    d. Has a phase 0 depolarization, which is much slower than that in nonpacemaker cardiac cells

▼ Match each of the phases of the fast-response action potential in column A with the appropriate descriptive phrase(s) in column B.

Column A

35. _____ Phase 0
36. _____ Phase 1
37. _____ Phase 2
38. _____ Phase 3
39. _____ Phase 4

Column B

a. Slow influx of Ca⁺⁺ is primarily responsible for the plateau during this phase.
b. Rapid decrease in electronegativity of the cell membrane is caused by change of permeability to Na⁺ and its rapid influx into cell.
c. Partial repolarization is caused by abrupt inactivation of fast sodium channels.
d. This phase corresponds to the absolute refractory period.
e. The inside of the cell is negative with respect to the outside, and the ionic concentrations of Na⁺ and K⁺ on either side of the cell membrane are maintained at a steady state by the Na-K pump.
f. Rapid repolarization is caused by cessation of inward currents of Ca⁺⁺ and Na⁺ and rapid efflux of K⁺ from the cell.

CHAPTER 30

Diagnostic Procedures in Cardiovascular Disease

CYNTHIA C. SENERCHIA
PENNY FORD CARLETON

Increasingly sophisticated diagnostic techniques are available to detect heart disease and its clinical sequelae. However, the use of these techniques and the interpretation of test results are adjuncts to the systematic clinical assessment of the patient, not substitutes for a thorough history and physical examination. Thus a brief overview of the systematic bedside assessment of the patient with heart disease must precede a description of common diagnostic procedures.

The authors acknowledge the contribution of Kalon K.L. Ho, MD, MSc, Instructor in Medicine, Harvard Medical School, Boston, Mass., in the preparation of this chapter.

CLINICAL ASSESSMENT

A systematic clinical assessment includes a complete history and physical examination using the techniques of inspection, palpation, percussion, and auscultation. Examination of the cardiovascular system must include the heart and the peripheral vascular system. A detailed discussion of the peripheral vascular examination and related diagnostic tests is presented in Chapter 34.

History

The history must include an assessment of the individual's life-style and the impact of heart disease on the activities of daily living if the patient rather than the disease is to be treated. The patient's history should also include a history of the family and the incidence of cardiovascular disease in the first-degree relatives (parents and siblings). The following signs and symptoms of heart disease are typically elicited during the history of the patient with heart disease:

1. *Angina,* or chest pain, resulting from a lack of myocardial oxygen, or ischemia. Some patients deny chest "pain" and describe a tightness, squeezing, pressure, or heaviness in their chest without pain per se. Angina may present as *referred pain,* or pain that the body interprets as coming from the jaw, upper arms, or middle of the back. Angina may also be "silent" and without discomfort but associated with a feeling of weakness and fatigue
2. *Dyspnea,* or an uncomfortable awareness of breathing, caused by increased respiratory effort associated with pulmonary vascular congestion and alterations in lung distensibility; *orthopnea,* or difficulty in breathing in the recumbent position; *paroxysmal nocturnal dyspnea,* or dyspnea that occurs during sleep because of left ventricular failure and is relieved by sitting up on the side of the bed
3. *Palpitations,* or an awareness of the heartbeat, caused by changes in the rate, regularity, or force of cardiac contraction
4. *Peripheral edema,* or swelling caused by fluid accu-

NEW YORK HEART ASSOCIATION PATIENT CLASSIFICATION GUIDELINES

Class I	Asymptomatic with ordinary physical exertion
Class II	Symptomatic with ordinary physical exertion
Class III	Symptomatic with less than ordinary physical exertion
Class IV	Symptomatic at rest

CANADIAN CARDIOVASCULAR SOCIETY ANGINA CLASSIFICATION

Class 0   Patient does not experience angina or angina-equivalent symptoms.

Class I   Ordinary physical activity (e.g., walking, climbing stairs) does not cause angina or angina-equivalent symptoms. Symptoms occur only with strenuous, rapid, or prolonged exertion at work or recreation.

Class II   Patient experiences slight limitation of ordinary activity because of angina. For example, symptoms are provoked with the following:

ACTIVITY	SETTING
Walking Climbing one flight of stairs	Walking/climbing rapidly After meals In cold weather In wind Under emotional stress During first few hours after awakening
Walking more than two blocks on level ground Walking uphill Climbing more than one flight of stairs	At a normal pace

Class III   Patient experiences marked limitation of activity because of angina. For example, symptoms are provoked with walking one to two blocks on level ground or climbing one flight of stairs or less in normal conditions and at a normal pace.

Class IV   Patient develops angina at rest or with any physical activity.

mulation in the interstitial spaces, usually noted in dependent areas as a result of the effect of gravity, and preceded by weight gain

5. *Syncope,* or transient loss of consciousness, a result of inadequate cerebral blood flow

6. *Fatigue and weakness,* often a consequence of low cardiac output and reduced peripheral perfusion

Factors that precipitate and relieve symptoms must be determined. Angina is usually precipitated by exertion and relieved by rest. Dyspnea is typically associated with exertion; however, changes in body position and the consequent redistribution of body fluid by gravity may precipitate dyspnea. Orthopnea can be relieved by elevation of the trunk with pillows. In addition, the degree of disability associated with the elicited symptoms must be determined. The New York Heart Association has developed guidelines for the classification of patients according to the level of physical activity required to produce symptoms (see box above). The categories range from class I patients, asymptomatic with ordinary physical exertion, to class IV patients, symptomatic at rest. The *New York Heart Association classification* is most often used to determine the effects of congestive heart failure on physical exertion. The Canadian Cardiovascular Society Angina Classification is most often used to determine the degree of angina (see box at right).

Physical Examination

Simple inspection yields a wealth of information regarding the patient's physical and psychologic status. Observations such as color, body build, respiratory pattern, work of breathing, and general appearance must all be incorporated into the clinical picture. Palpation, coupled with inspection, furthers and substantiates the cumulative database. Skin temperature, turgor, and moistness can be evaluated. Severity of edema can be quantified on a scale of 1+ to 4+ according to persistence of the indentation left by the palpating finger in the edematous area (1+ indicates a slight depression that disappears rapidly; 4+ indicates a deep depression that disappears slowly). Capillary refill can be evaluated by depressing the tip of the nailbed until blanching is observed, then releasing the pressure and noting the length of time required for color to return. Normally, immediate refill is observed. The following structures are systematically examined: arteries, veins, and anterior chest wall.

Arterial pulse and pressure

The arterial pulse is palpated to elicit the following information: (1) rate, (2) regularity, (3) amplitude, and (4) quality. Certain cardiac dysrhythmias can be detected by alterations in the *rate* or *regularity* of the arterial pulse. Irregularities of cardiac rhythm are associated with variability in pulse *amplitude.* If the interval between cardiac impulses is irregular, the ventricular filling time and thus the stroke volume vary with each beat. For instance, shortening the interval between beats reduces filling time and stroke volume; consequently, the amplitude of the peripheral arterial pulsation is reduced for that beat. For

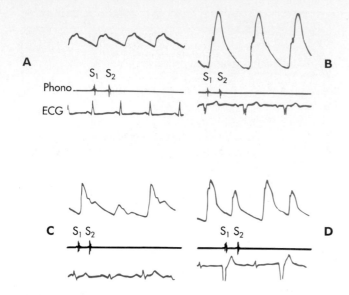

FIG. 30-1   Characteristic arterial pulse wave sphygmograms with simultaneously recorded phonogram and electrocardiogram (ECG). **A,** Anacrotic pulse. **B,** Waterhammer pulse. **C,** Pulsus alternans. **D,** Pulsus bigeminus. S_1, First heart sound; S_2, second heart sound. (From Sana JM, Judge RD: *Physical appraisal for nursing practice*, ed 2, Boston, 1982, Little, Brown.)

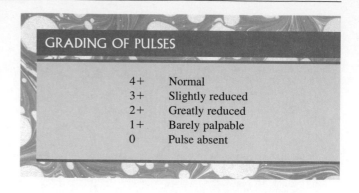

GRADING OF PULSES

4+	Normal
3+	Slightly reduced
2+	Greatly reduced
1+	Barely palpable
0	Pulse absent

this reason, irregular rhythms are occasionally associated with a "radial pulse deficit," or a palpated radial rate slower than the auscultated apical rate. This simply indicates that the ventricular filling time was so short that the volume of blood ejected into the periphery for some beats was too small to be palpated in the peripheral bed.

The *quality* of the arterial pulses is an important index of peripheral perfusion. A consistently weak, thready pulse may indicate a low stroke volume or increased peripheral vascular resistance. Conversely, a forceful, bounding pulse correlates with high stroke volumes and reduced peripheral resistance. The contour of the arterial pulse can be appreciated best by light palpation of the carotid artery. Palpation of a small pulse with a slow upstroke would characterize aortic stenosis—a lesion that impedes blood flow through the aortic valve. This pulse is described as an *anacrotic pulse* (Fig. 30-1); the slow upstroke is also referred to as *pulsus tardus*. The valvular lesion of aortic regurgitation produces a bounding, rapidly rising and collapsing pulse referred to as a *waterhammer pulse*.

Pulsus alternans and pulsus bigeminus are both characterized by alternating strong and weak pulsations at regular intervals. *Pulsus alternans* occurs at regular intervals and reflects left ventricular failure, whereas *pulsus bigeminus* is produced by alteration in pulse volume caused by a bigeminal (every second beat) pattern of premature beats in the cardiac rhythm (Fig. 30-1). *Pulsus paradoxus* is an exaggerated fall in systolic pressure greater than 10 mm Hg during inspiration. Normally, sys-

tolic pressure falls slightly on inspiration because the reduction in intrathoracic pressure is transmitted to the pulmonary vasculature and produces a slight increase in pulmonary blood volume and a corresponding decrease in venous return to the left side of the heart. Cardiac tamponade or constrictive pericarditis can compromise cardiac filling further and exaggerate this inspiratory fall, producing the paradoxical pulse.

An impression of the consistency of the arterial wall can be obtained best by rolling a peripheral artery under the examining fingers; hardening or thickening of the walls can be detected. A full cardiovascular examination includes palpation of arterial pulsations for quality and equality at multiple sites: (1) dorsalis pedis, (2) posterior tibialis, (3) popliteal, (4) femoral, (5) radial, (6) brachial, and (7) carotid. Pulses at each site should be compared with the contralateral pulse. The quality of peripheral pulses is graded on a scale of 0 to 4+ (see the box above). Auscultation over arterial sites for bruits may be indicated if localized narrowing is suspected.

Auscultation of blood pressure for systolic and diastolic components concludes the arterial examination. Arterial blood pressure is measured by listening for the onset and disappearance of sounds referred to as *Korotkoff sounds* (sometimes spelled Korotkov) in an artery occluded by a blood pressure cuff (Fig. 30-2). The timing of these sounds is correlated with pressure readings on a mercury manometer. Initially the pressure in the cuff is increased to exceed systolic pressure in the artery so that no flow through the artery occurs and no sound is heard. To assist in the determination of systolic pressure, the brachial pulse should be palpated as the bladder of the cuff is rapidly inflated. The level at which the pulse disappears and subsequently reappears as the cuff is deflated should be noted to provide a preliminary approximation of the blood pressure. This technique will avoid underinflation of the cuff in the case of auscultatory gap or overinflation in those with low blood pressure (Perloff et al, 1993). As pressure in the cuff is gradually reduced below systolic pressure, flow begins. However, the flow is turbulent because it occurs through a constricted lumen; turbulent flow produces sound. The onset of turbulent flow is heard as the first Korotkoff sound and correlates with systolic pressure. Further reductions in cuff pressure

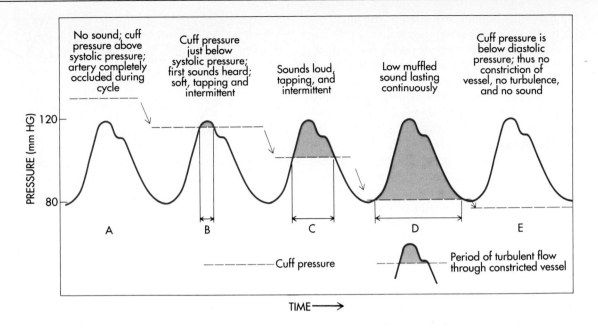

FIG. 30-2   Korotkoff sounds. Systolic blood pressure is recorded at *B* when the first sounds are heard during a blood pressure measurement. Diastolic pressure is recorded at the point of sound muffling or disappearance, *D* or *E*. (From Vander AJ, Sherman JH, Luciano DS: *Human physiology,* ed 2, New York, 1975, McGraw-Hill.)

produce characteristic alterations in the sound as flow increases through the arterial lumen, until the sound disappears. Either abrupt muffling or disappearance of sound correlates with diastolic pressure. The American Heart Association (AHA) recommends reporting both diastolic values.

Pressures should be recorded in both arms. If postural hypotension is suspected, measurements should be compared in the supine, sitting, and standing positions. The normal arterial blood pressure is approximately 120/80 mm Hg. In general, *hypertension* is designated as a diastolic pressure over 90 mm Hg or a systolic pressure over 140 mm Hg (see Chapter 31). *Hypotension,* for a given individual, is best evaluated in terms of adequacy of peripheral perfusion. In elderly persons or patients with chronic hypertension, hypotension may be manifested as altered brain function resulting from decreased cerebral blood flow (e.g., confusion, dizziness, lethargy). Early signs of inadequate peripheral perfusion may be a decreased urine output and cold, pale skin with reduced peripheral pulses. The kidneys and skin are less metabolically active organs; therefore, as arterial pressure falls, blood is shunted from these organs to the more vital organs, the heart and brain.

The *pulse pressure* is the difference between the systolic and diastolic blood pressure. For example, a blood pressure of 120/80 mm Hg corresponds to a pulse pressure of 40 mm Hg. If arterial pressure falls and sympathetic compensatory vasoconstriction occurs, the pulse pressure is reduced or narrowed. A fall in pressure to

105/90 mm Hg narrows the pulse pressure to 15 mm Hg. The pulse pressure is influenced most significantly by stroke volume and peripheral resistance. A narrow pulse pressure indicates a low stroke volume or a high peripheral resistance or both. A falling blood pressure and narrowing pulse pressure is an ominous sign of left ventricular dysfunction. *Mean arterial pressure* (MAP) is the average peripheral perfusion pressure. This value is not simply the average of the diastolic and systolic pressures because the duration of diastole exceeds the duration of systole at normal heart rates. Consequently, mean arterial pressure is estimated by doubling the diastolic pressure, adding the systolic pressure, and dividing the total by three.

Venous pressure and pulsations

Jugular venous pressure and pulsations reflect the function of the right side of the heart. The internal jugular veins are examined to estimate central venous pressure and to analyze pulsations. To estimate *central venous pressure,* the internal jugular veins are examined with the trunk elevated approximately 15 to 30 degrees. Normally the highest point of venous pulsation ascends no more than 3 cm above the sternal angle, or angle of Louis (i.e., juncture between manubrium and body of the sternum). Abnormal elevation of the venous pressure, as in failure of the right side of the heart, can be estimated by measuring the vertical distance between the level of jugular venous pulsation and the sternal angle. With extreme elevations of pressure, usually greater than 25 cm

H_2O, the jugular veins remain distended to the angle of the jaw with trunk elevations of 90 degrees.

Venous pressure normally fluctuates with respiration; inspiration produces a fall in venous pressure because intrathoracic pressure decreases, favoring venous return to the heart. A paradoxical increase in venous pressure with inspiration, known as *Kussmaul's sign,* indicates an impediment to venous return to the right side of the heart, as in severe right heart failure.

The *hepatojugular reflux test* is an important diagnostic clue to the pressure of right heart failure. Manually sustained pressure is applied for approximately 30 to 60 seconds over the right upper quadrant of the abdomen; the neck veins are observed simultaneously. The abdominal pressure increases venous return to the heart. The normal heart is able to adapt and immediately accept the increased venous return. However, the failing right side of the heart is unable to readily accept this increased load; therefore the distention of the jugular veins increases and the level of venous pulsations rises in the neck. This response of the jugular veins is referred to as a *positive* hepatojugular reflux test.

The anatomic basis for the hepatojugular reflux test may be understood by recalling that the liver functions as a "flood chamber" in its strategic location between the intestinal and general circulation. The liver sinusoids hold a large amount of blood, which is forced into the inferior vena cava through the hepatic veins when pressure is applied over the liver during the reflux test (see Fig. 27-2 and Table 27-1).

The pulsations of the jugular veins are also analyzed to evaluate function of the right side of the heart. At normal venous pressures, maximal venous pulsation can best be observed with trunk elevation of approximately 15 to 30 degrees. The venous waves are gentle and undulating, with three positive components: the *a*, *c*, and *v* waves (Fig. 30-3, *A*). The *a* wave is produced by atrial contraction; the *c* wave correlates with the onset of ventricular contraction and seems to result from the bulging of the tricuspid valve into the right atrium; and the *v* wave corresponds to the period of atrial filling during ventricular ejection before the tricuspid valve opens. The *c* wave is difficult to distinguish in the jugular veins because of its low amplitude.

Predictable alterations in waveform configuration result from tricuspid valve disease. Tricuspid stenosis impedes the blood flow from the right atrium into the right ventricle, forcing the right atrium to generate more pressure during contraction and creating "giant *a* waves" (Fig. 30-3, *B*). Tricuspid valvular regurgitation during ventricular systole produces a retrograde flow wave distorting the *c* and *v* waves, referred to as a "significant *v* wave" (Fig. 30-3, *C*). Certain cardiac dysrhythmias also alter the configuration of the venous waves by disrupting the sequential, synchronized contraction of the atria and ventricles.

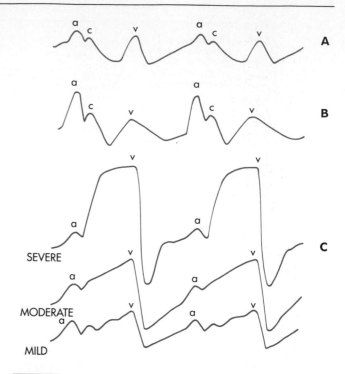

FIG. 30-3 Jugular venous waveforms. **A,** Normal waves, low amplitude and undulating. The *a* wave is produced by atrial contraction; the *c* wave is produced by ventricular contraction and the consequent bulging of the tricuspid valve into the right atrium; and the *v* wave is produced during atrial filling before the opening of the tricuspid valve. **B,** Giant *a* waves seen in tricuspid stenosis. **C,** Mild, moderate, and severe tricuspid regurgitation; the *c* and *v* waves summate into huge *v* waves. (Modified from Hurst JW: *The heart,* ed 3, New York, 1974, McGraw-Hill.)

Precordial movements

Physical examination of the anterior chest involves inspection and palpation of the precordium. Because of the anatomic rotation of the heart in the thorax, the right ventricle lies immediately beneath the sternum (see Fig. 28-3). The thoracic movements are inspected for symmetry and visible pulsations. The chest is then palpated for normal and abnormal pulsations. The apical impulse, produced by the thrust of the left ventricular apex against the chest wall during systole, is located. Normally the *point of maximal impulse* (PMI) can be palpated as a rhythmic, brief tap approximately 1 cm in diameter, located in the fifth intercostal space at the midclavicular line.

With left ventricular hypertrophy, the apical impulse becomes more sustained, more forceful, and larger. The PMI is displaced laterally to the left and downward. Right ventricular hypertrophy characteristically produces a *substernal heave*, or a systolic lift of the sternum, as the contractile force of the anterior right ventricle increases. Abnormal pulsations are also noted with coronary atherosclerotic disease; damaged myocardial fibers with limited or absent contractile force bulge passively outward during systole, creating paradoxical precordial movements. In addition, the turbulent flow associated with heart murmurs can create palpable precordial vibrations known as "thrills."

Heart sounds

Auscultation of the chest permits identification of normal heart sounds, abnormal heart sounds, murmurs, and extracardiac sounds. Normal heart sounds result from vibrations of the blood volume and the surrounding chambers with valve closure. The first and second heart sounds correlate with closure of the atrioventricular (AV) valves and the semilunar valves, respectively. Thus the *first heart sound* (S$_1$) is heard at the onset of ventricular systole, as ventricular pressures rise above atrial pressures and close the mitral and tricuspid valves. An abnormal accentuation of S$_1$ is noted in mitral stenosis as a result of the stiffening of the valve leaflets.

The *second heart sound* (S$_2$) is audible at the beginning of ventricular relaxation as ventricular pressure falls below the pressure within the pulmonary artery and aorta, closing the pulmonic and aortic valves. Typically, right ventricular ejection lasts slightly longer than does left ventricular ejection, resulting in asynchronous valve closure. Therefore the aortic valve closes before the pulmonic valve, producing a normal physiologic splitting or separation of the valve closure sounds. Inspiration accentuates physiologic splitting because venous return to the right side of the heart increases, thus producing an increment in the volume of right ventricular ejection. During expiration, splitting becomes less pronounced or disappears.

Abnormal *paradoxical splitting* signifies closure of the pulmonic valve before closure of the aortic valve. A paradoxical response to respiration is noted; that is, splitting is most pronounced with expiration and subsides with inspiration. Paradoxical splitting is observed during delayed activation of the left ventricle, as in left bundle branch block, or with prolonged left ventricular ejection, as in aortic stenosis.

Two additional heart sounds can occasionally be heard during ventricular diastole. The *third and fourth heart sounds* (S$_3$, S$_4$) can be physiologic manifestations but are usually heard in conjunction with heart disease; the pathologic appearance of S$_3$ or S$_4$ is referred to as a *gallop rhythm*. This term is applicable because the addition of another heart sound simulates the rhythm of a horse's gallop. S$_3$ occurs during the period of rapid ventricular filling and is consequently referred to as a *ventricular gallop* when it is abnormal. This sound can occur normally in children and young adults. However, it is usually a pathologic finding produced by cardiac dysfunction, particularly ventricular failure.

S$_4$ occurs during atrial systole and is referred to as an *atrial gallop*. Normally it is faint or inaudible, occurring immediately before S$_1$. The atrial gallop is audible when

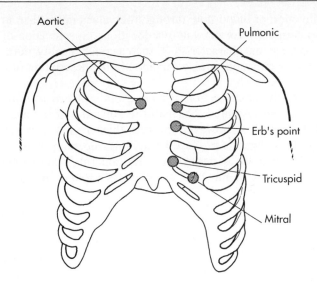

FIG. 30-4 Positions for auscultation of heart sounds: (1) aortic area (second right interspace close to sternum); (2) pulmonic area (second left interspace close to sternum); (3) third left interspace close to sternum, sometimes called Erb's point, where murmurs of both aortic and pulmonic origin may be heard; (4) tricuspid area (fifth left intercostal space close to sternum); and (5) mitral (apical) area (fifth left intercostal space just medial to the midclavicular line).

ventricular resistance to atrial filling increases, as a result of either reduced ventricular wall distensibility or increased ventricular volumes.

Heart murmurs are the result of turbulent flow within the cardiac chambers and vessels. Turbulent flow is produced either by flow through structural abnormalities (narrowed valvular orifices, incompetent valves, dilated arterial segments) or by high-velocity flow through normal structures. Murmurs are described according to (1) timing relative to cardiac cycle, (2) intensity, (3) location or region of maximum audibility, and (4) characteristics.

Diastolic murmurs occur after S$_2$ during ventricular relaxation. The murmurs of mitral stenosis and aortic regurgitation occur during diastole. *Systolic murmurs* are designated as either ejection murmurs, occurring during midsystole after the early phase of isovolumetric contraction, or regurgitant murmurs, occurring throughout systole. Murmurs occurring throughout systole are referred to as *pansystolic* or *holosystolic*. The murmur of aortic stenosis typifies an ejection murmur, whereas mitral regurgitation produces a pansystolic murmur.

The loudness of a murmur is graded on a scale of I to VI, with grade I representing a faint murmur and grade VI representing a murmur audible with the stethoscope off the chest wall. Five standard areas of the chest wall, illustrated in Fig. 30-4 as aortic, tricuspid, pulmonic, and mitral (or apical) regions and Erb's point, are typically used to localize the region of maximum murmur audibility. The murmur is loudest in regions that lie in the direction of blood flow through the valves rather than in anatomically correct valvular locations. Specification of unique sound characteristics, such as pitch, quality, duration, or radiation, is also included in the description of a heart murmur.

Finally, identification and description of *extracardiac sounds* are essential. Normally the opening of the heart valves is silent; however, the stiff, thickened valve cusps in mitral stenosis produce an audible "opening snap" in early diastole. A pericardial "friction rub," caused by pericardial inflammation, is audible as a rough sandpaper sound.

NONINVASIVE DIAGNOSTIC PROCEDURES

Surface Electrocardiogram

The electrocardiogram (ECG) is the graphic recording of the heart's electrical activity. Characteristic waveforms on the ECG, arbitrarily designated as P wave, QRS complex, and T wave, correlate with the spread of electrical excitation and recovery through the conduction system and myocardium (Fig. 30-5, *A*). These waves are recorded on graph paper with a horizontal time scale and a vertical voltage scale (Fig. 30-5, *B*). The significance of the waveforms and intervals on the ECG is as follows:
1. *P wave.* The P wave corresponds to atrial depolariza-

tion. The normal stimulus for atrial depolarization originates in the sinus node; however, the magnitude of electrical current associated with excitation of the sinus node is too small to be visualized on the ECG. The P wave is normally gently rounded and upright in most leads. Atrial enlargement may increase the amplitude or width of the P wave and alter its configuration. Cardiac dysrhythmias can also change the P wave configuration. For instance, rhythms originating near the AV junction may cause inversion of the P wave because the direction of atrial depolarization is reversed.
2. *PR interval.* The PR interval is measured from the beginning of the P wave to the onset of the QRS complex. This interval includes impulse transmission time through the atria and the delay of the impulse at the AV node. The normal interval is 0.12 to 0.20 second. Abnormal prolongation of the PR interval is indicative of an impulse conduction disturbance, referred to as *first-degree heart block.*
3. *QRS complex.* The QRS complex represents ventricular depolarization. The amplitude of this wave is great as a result of the large muscle mass traversed by the electrical impulse. However, impulse spread is rapid; normally the duration of the QRS complex is 0.06 to 0.10 second. Prolongation of impulse spread through the bundle branches, known as *bundle branch block,* widens the ventricular complex. Abnormal cardiac rhythms originating in the ventricles, such as ventric-

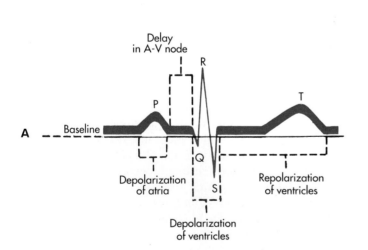

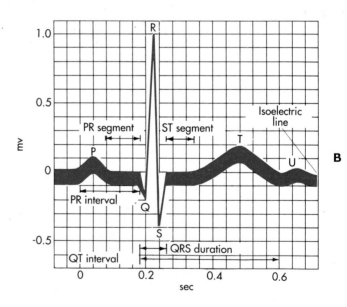

FIG. 30-5   **A,** Correlation between waves of the electrocardiogram (ECG) and impulses that spread through the heart. **B,** Normal recording of ECG on graph paper. Amplitude (in millivolts) is represented on the vertical axis while the horizontal axis represents time (in seconds). Each small square represents 0.04 second, with five small squares equaling 0.2 second. Normal intervals are PR, 0.12 to 0.20 second; QRS, 0.06 to 0.10 second; and QT, 0.36 to 0.44 second. The ventricular rate may be calculated by counting the number of R waves in 6 seconds and multiplying by 10 or counting the number of small squares between two complexes (R to R) and dividing this number into 1500.

ular tachycardia, also widen and distort the QRS complex because the specialized pathways that speed impulse spread through the ventricles are bypassed. Ventricular hypertrophy increases the amplitude of the QRS complex as the muscle mass enlarges.

Atrial repolarization occurs during the period of ventricular depolarization. However, the magnitude of the QRS complex obscures any ECG evidence of atrial recovery.

4. *ST segment.* This interval is interposed between the wave of ventricular depolarization and repolarization. The initial phases of ventricular repolarization occur during this period; however, the changes are too subtle to be apparent on the ECG. Abnormal depression or elevation of the ST segment is associated with myocardial ischemia and infarction, respectively. Digitalis administration characteristically produces sagging of the segment.

5. *T wave.* Ventricular repolarization generates the T wave. Normally the T wave is slightly asymmetric, rounded, and upright in most leads. Inversion of the T wave is associated with myocardial ischemia. Hyperkalemia, or serum potassium elevation, causes peaking and elevation of the T wave.

6. *QT interval.* This interval is measured from the beginning of the QRS complex to the end of the T wave, encompassing ventricular depolarization and repolarization. The average QT interval ranges from 0.36 to 0.44 second and varies with heart rate. The QT interval is prolonged with the administration of certain antidysrhythmic drugs, such as quinidine, as well as other medications such as Hismanal (astemizole) and Seldane (terfenadine).

The electrical currents generated within the heart during depolarization and repolarization are conducted to the body surface, where they can be recorded by electrodes in contact with the skin. By convention, nine recording electrodes are placed on the extremities and chest wall with a ground electrode, used to reduce electrical interference, attached to the right leg. Varying combinations of these electrodes produce 12 standard leads. Each of the 12 leads records the electrical events of the entire car-

diac cycle. However, each lead views the heart from a slightly different perspective; therefore waveforms look slightly different in each lead. Three categories of leads are typically designated (Fig. 30-6) as follows:

1. *Standard limb leads (leads I, II, III).* These leads measure the difference in electrical potential between two points; thus the leads are bipolar, with one negative and one positive pole. Electrodes are placed on the right arm, left arm, and left leg. Lead I views the heart from the axis connecting the right arm and left arm, with the left arm as the positive pole; lead II, from the right arm and left leg, with the left leg positive; and lead III, from the left arm and left leg, with the left leg positive (Fig. 30-6, *A*).

2. *Augmented limb leads (leads aVR, aVL, aVF).* These leads are electrically adjusted to measure the absolute electrical potential at one recording site, that of a positive electrode placed on the extremities, creating, in essence, a unipolar lead. This is accomplished by electrically canceling out the effect of the negative pole and establishing an "indifferent" electrode at zero potential. Adjustments are made automatically within the ECG machine to join the other limb electrodes, creating a common indifferent electrode with essentially no effect on the positive recording electrode. The voltage recorded from the positive electrode is then amplified or "augmented" to produce a selected, unipolar limb lead tracing. There are three augmented limb leads: aVR, recording from the right arm; aVL, from the left arm; and aVF, from the left leg (the aVF location can be easily remembered by associating the "F" with "foot") (Fig. 30-6, *B*).

3. *Precordial or chest leads (leads V_1 to V_6).* These leads are unipolar leads recording the absolute electrical potential of sites on the anterior chest wall, or precordium. Identification of the following landmarks facilitates accurate placement of the precordial electrodes: (1) angle of Louis, the sternal protuberance at the juncture between the manubrium and body of the sternum; (2) the second intercostal space, adjacent to the angle of Louis; (3) the left midclavicular line; and (4) the anterior and midaxillary lines (Fig. 30-6, *C*).

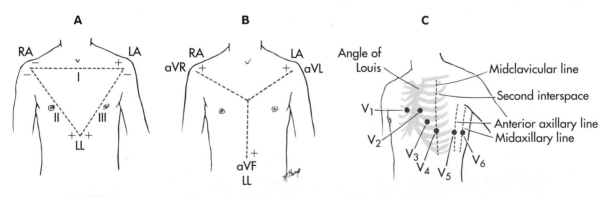

FIG. 30-6   Electrode positions for the standard 12-lead electrocardiogram. **A,** Standard limb leads (I, II, III). **B,** Augmented limb leads (aVR, aVL, aVF). **C,** Precordial leads (V_1 to V_6).

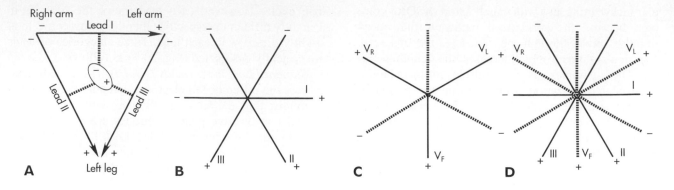

FIG. 30-7   Derivation of the hexaxial reference system. **A,** Einthoven's triangle, showing the axes of the standard limb leads with the heart at the center of the triangle. **B,** The axes of the limb leads are moved to the center of the triangle, forming a triaxial reference system. **C,** The axes of the augmented (unipolar) limb leads. **D,** The axes of the standard and unipolar limb leads are superimposed, forming a hexaxial reference system.

Electrodes are placed sequentially on the chest wall at six different sites, as follows:

V_1: located in the fourth intercostal space to the right of the sternum

V_2: located in the fourth intercostal space to the left of the sternum

V_3: located midway between V_2 and V_4

V_4: located in the fifth intercostal space in the midclavicular line

V_5: horizontal to V_4 in the anterior axillary line

V_6: horizontal to V_5 in the midaxillary line

The standard limb leads and augmented limb leads view the heart in the frontal plane. The relative perspective of each lead is conceptualized most easily using a schematic diagram, known as the *hexaxial reference system.* This reference system is derived in the following manner (Fig. 30-7):

1. Connecting the lead axes of leads I, II, and III forms an equilateral triangle, referred to as *Einthoven's triangle.* The heart is considered the electrical center of the triangle.
2. Positioning the lead axes so that each radiates from the center of the triangle creates a second diagram, known as the *triaxial reference system.*
3. Combining the triaxial reference system diagram with the schematic representation of the augmented limb leads radiating from the electrical center of the thorax produces the hexaxial reference system.

The hexaxial reference system is an invaluable aid to ECG interpretation, permitting calculation of the average direction of electrical activity within the heart. The average direction of electrical activation calculated from the ECG is referred to as the *electrical axis* of the heart.

Other modified leads are often used in special situations. A modified lead V_1 (MCL$_1$) is frequently used for bedside monitoring to facilitate dysrhythmia detection and analysis. This lead is a bipolar lead, with the positive electrode positioned in the standard V_1 position (fourth intercostal space to the right of the sternum) and the negative electrode positioned near the left shoulder beneath the clavicle.

The waveform configurations apparent in each lead depend on the orientation of the particular lead relative to the path of cardiac electrical activity. The leads of the hexaxial reference system view the heart in the frontal plane; the six precordial leads offer another perspective from the horizontal plane. Waves will be positive (i.e., deflected upward) if the electrical activity of the heart approaches the positive electrode of a given lead. For example, in Fig. 30-8 the P wave and QRS complex of lead II are positive because the wave of depolarization approaches the positive left leg electrode of lead II. Conversely, the same waves in lead aVR are negative because the path of electrical activity is moving away from the positive right arm electrode. In addition, the amplitude of waves varies among leads. As a rule, wave amplitude will be greatest in a lead lying parallel to the path of depolarization. Notice that lead II in Fig. 30-8 demonstrates the greatest wave amplitude, indicating that lead II most closely parallels the path of depolarization in this ECG. The ECG permits detection of abnormalities in cardiac rate and rhythm, chamber enlargement, myocardial ischemia or infarction, drug and electrolyte effects, and shifts in the direction of electrical activation.

Conventional bedside monitoring techniques have been extended to ambulatory monitoring *(telemetry)* and continuous 24-hour ECG recording *(Holter monitoring).*

Relative Merits of Imaging Techniques

Multiple noninvasive and invasive imaging techniques are available for diagnosing cardiovascular disease. Each type of study allows varying amounts of information to be obtained for each type of pathology. In addition, an-

▶ TABLE 30-1   Relative Merits of Imaging Techniques

Disorder	CXR	Echo/Doppler	Angio	Radionuclides	RCT	MRI
Ischemic	1	2	4*	3	2	2
Valvular	2	4*	4*	2	3	3
Congenital	2	4*	4*	2	3	3
Traumatic	2	2	3*	2	2	2
Cardiomyopathy	1	4*	3	2	3	3
Pericardial	1	3	2	0	4*	4*
Endocarditis	1	4*	2	0	2	3
Masses	0	4*	3	0	4*	3

From Skorton DJ et al: In Baunwald E: *Heart disease,* ed 4, Philadelphia, 1992, Saunders.
CXR, Chest x-ray film; *Echo,* echocardiography; *Angio,* angiography; *RCT,* rapid computed tomography; *MRI,* magnetic resonance imaging.
Range of information provided by test: 0, no information, to 4(*), best test.

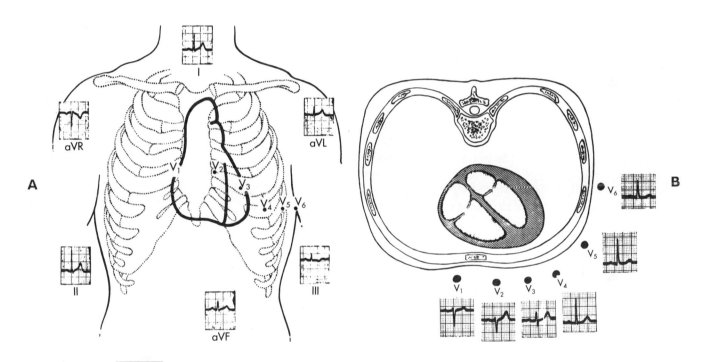

FIG. 30-8   **A,** Normal ECG patterns in the frontal plane (standard leads I, II, and III and augmented unipolar leads aVR, aVL, and aVF). **B,** Normal ECG patterns in the horizontal plane (precordial leads V_1 to V_6). (From Goldman MJ: Principles of clinical electrocardiography, ed 9, Los Altos, Calif, 1976, Lange.)

giography also carries risks to the patient associated with the procedure that the noninvasive studies do not. Table 30-1 presents the strengths and weaknesses of each type of study in diagnosing various types of cardiovascular disease. The ultimate decision of which test to use is influenced by the amount of information obtained versus the risks involved in the test. The diagnostic tools are discussed next.

Echocardiography

Echocardiographic procedures use ultrasound as the examination medium. A transducer emitting ultrasonic waves, or high-frequency sound waves beyond the audible range, is applied to the chest wall and directed at the heart (Fig. 30-9). As the ultrasonic beam traverses the heart, ultrasonic waves are reflected back to the transducer whenever the beam crosses a boundary between tissues of different densities or acoustic impedances. The mechanical energy from these reflected sound waves, or cardiac "echoes," is converted to electrical energy by the transducer and displayed in the form of a cardiac image on an oscilloscope or strip chart recorder.

Echocardiography provides significant information about the structure and movement of the heart chambers, valves, and any unusual masses. The test has over-

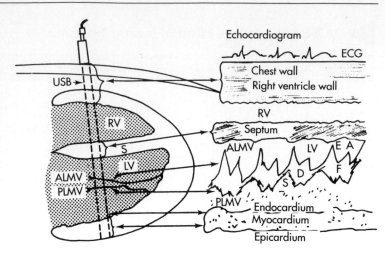

FIG. 30-9 Normal echocardiogram. Path of ultrasound beam *[USB]* is shown schematically on the left. On the right is a diagram of the corresponding echocardiogram for this direction of the transducer. *RV,* Right ventricle; *S,* septum; *LV,* left ventricle; *ALMV,* anterior leaflet of the mitral valve; *PLMV,* posterior leaflet of the mitral valve; *S,* systole; *D,* diastole; *E,* peak of rapid anterior opening of mitral valve during beginning of diastole; *A,* peak of anterior movement of leaflet into the ventricle produced by atrial systole; *F,* position of leaflet during rapid ventricular filling. [From Gazes PC: *Clinical cardiology,* Chicago, 1975, Mosby.]

come the previous limitations with the addition of two-dimensional echocardiography, Doppler flow imaging, and the transesophageal approach to the heart, which virtually eliminates the positioning problems associated with obesity, chest trauma, chronic lung disease, and mechanical or calcified valves. The *M mode* is the most common of the display modes. In the M mode, the echoes are displayed as undulating lines composed of dots of varying intensity (Fig. 30-9). The movement of the lines corresponds to the motion of each structure. The lines are arranged sequentially in layers on the screen. These layers correspond to the anatomic structures traversed by the ultrasonic beam.

M-mode echocardiography

M-mode echocardiography provides an "icepick" view of the dimensions and motion of the tissues in the path of the ultrasonic beam. The ECG is typically displayed with the echocardiogram on a horizontal time axis, permitting correlation of the electrical and mechanical events of the cardiac cycle. The precordium can be scanned by moving the transducer in several directions. Fig. 30-9 illustrates one standard M-mode view.

M-mode echocardiography is of particular value for evaluation of chamber volumes and regional abnormalities, such as the abnormal mitral valve leaflet motion characteristic of mitral stenosis. Fig. 30-10 illustrates the normal motion of the anterior and posterior mitral valve cusps relative to the restricted motion of stenotic, diseased mitral leaflets. However, the application of the M-mode technique in the evaluation of global cardiac function is limited by the one-dimensional scanning path.

Two-dimensional echocardiography

Two-dimensional (2-D) echocardiography captures an image of a pie-shaped wedge of the heart (Fig. 30-11). During this procedure, the ultrasonic transducer on the chest rapidly sweeps along a predetermined examination plane. As the beam scans multiple sites (approximately 30 per second), images from the reflected echoes at each

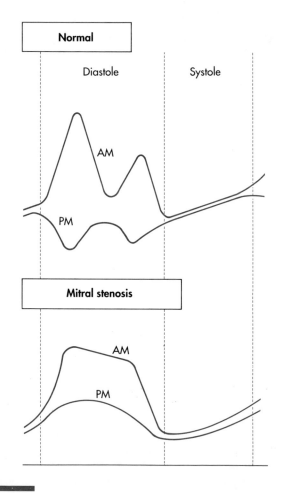

FIG. 30-10 Mitral valve echocardiogram. *Above,* Normal leaflet motion. *Below,* Abnormal leaflet motion with mitral stenosis. *AM,* Anterior mitral valve leaflet; *PM,* posterior mitral valve leaflet. [Modified from Duchak JM, Chang S, Feigenbaum H: *Am J Cardiol* 29:631, 1972.]

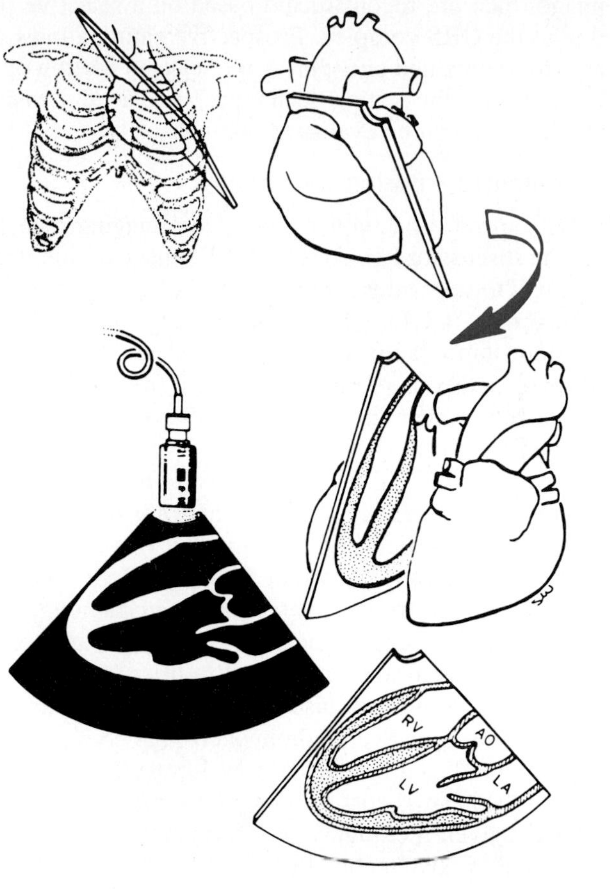

FIG. 30-11   Two-dimensional (2-D) echocardiogram. In contrast to the M-mode, one-dimensional "ice pick" view, 2-D echocardiography simultaneously detects all cardiac structures lying within the plane of examination, displaying the image on a video screen. *AO*, Aorta; *LV*, left ventricle; *RV*, right ventricle; *LA*, left atrium. (From Ream AK, Pogdall RP, editors: *Acute cardiovascular management: anesthesia and intensive care*, Philadelphia, 1982, Lippincott.)

site are stored. After the scan is completed, the composite echoes are displayed on a video screen and valve movement, ventricular contraction, and any abnormalities (e.g., thrombus) may be seen in real time. The resultant image is a full transverse section of the heart. A complete 2-D echocardiogram includes images obtained in multiple planes. This 2-D ultrasonic imaging technique can be coupled with Doppler blood flow studies to obtain information about the velocity and direction of blood flow within the cardiovascular system.

Doppler echocardiography

The technique for Doppler studies is similar to that for echocardiographic studies. Ultrasonic waves of known frequency are directed at the heart through the chest wall. As the beam strikes the tissue interfaces, reflected waves echo back to the transducer. In addition to analyzing the amplitude of the echo as with conventional echocardiography, the frequency of the reflected signal is evaluated

and compared with that of the emitted signal. The frequency of the reflected wave is different from that of the emitted wave if the targeted structure is moving. This change in wave frequency is known as a *Doppler shift*. The direction of the shift (i.e., increased or decreased wave frequency) depends on the direction that the target is moving relative to the transducer.

Red blood cells (RBCs) are the primary ultrasound targets for *Doppler blood velocity studies*. The movement of RBCs can be distinguished from the motion of cardiac structures because the signals reflected by blood and tissue differ in frequency and amplitude. The signals reflected by the tissues can be filtered out so that blood flow can be analyzed selectively. Consequently, the velocity and direction of flow can be determined from the Doppler shift. Doppler measures are of particular interest in the evaluation of valvular regurgitation and intracardiac shunts.

The reflected ultrasound generates an audible signal, which varies with changes in the frequency of the reflected signal. The amplitude and frequencies of the signal can also be displayed on a strip chart recording, monitor, or video screen. The video display can be color-coded to distinguish the direction or magnitude of flow.

Doppler flow imaging is the superimposition of Doppler information on a 2-D echocardiographic image. Doppler and 2-D echo information are obtained simultaneously from multiple sites in the plane of examination by rapid computerized scanning. The data are stored, and the Doppler information is superimposed on the pie-shaped 2-D image at the completion of the scan. The addition of color to this technique creates *color flow mapping*.

Transesophageal echocardiography

In some instances, high-quality echocardiographic images cannot be obtained when the ultrasound transducer is applied to the chest wall. This is most frequently seen when a patient is obese or has chronic obstructive pulmonary disease, since the ultrasound waves are not able to penetrate the heart. Other circumstances that may limit transthoracic echocardiography include limited access because of chest trauma, inability of patients to lie on their left side, and during interventional cardiac procedures or cardiac surgery. In these instances, transesophageal echocardiography (TEE) may be performed by placing the ultrasound transducer into the esophagus in a procedure similar to an endoscopy. Extremely high-quality images are obtained, which often permit improved detection of heart valve vegetations and better visualization of the atrial septum, thrombi, tumors, and atrial intimal tears (Seward et al, 1992) (Fig. 30-12).

Computed Tomography

Tomo- is a Greek word element meaning "section or cutting." Consequently, a *tomograph* is an image of a cross-

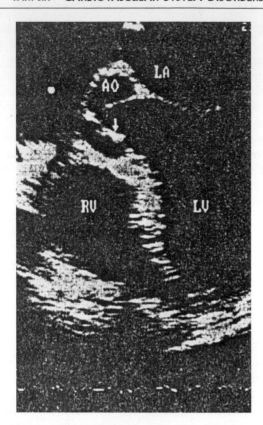

FIG. 30-12   Transesophageal echocardiogram of a patient with a small vegetation *(arrow)* on the aortic valve. *AO,* Aorta; *LA,* left atrium; *RV,* right ventricle, *LV,* left ventricle. (From Braunwald E: *Heart disease,* ed 4, Philadelphia, 1992, Saunders.)

sectional slice of the body. A 2-D echocardiogram is an example of a tomograph. Computed tomography (CT) has extended cardiac imaging from 2-D to three-dimensional (3-D) imaging. To construct this 3-D image, a camera rotates in a 360-degree arc around the chest, recording 2-D images at multiple angles. X-rays are transmitted through the body to detectors on the opposite side. Each x-ray image captures a thin anatomic slice of the body. A composite 3-D image is constructed from these x-ray images by a computer. A small amount of contrast material, usually containing iodine, is injected via a peripheral site to heighten the contrast between the cardiac structures and the blood.

Rapid computed tomography

Rapid CT of the heart usually requires technique modifications because of the motion of the heart. Standard CT may be useful for the evaluation of the aorta, wall thickness, myocardial mass, pericardium, paracardiac or intracardiac tumors, and patency of arterial bypass grafts. To evaluate cardiac motion, quantitative dimensions, or ejection fraction, however, the CT images must be "gated" with the ECG. Gating can be performed retrospectively or prospectively. During retrospective gating, CT data and the ECG are recorded simultaneously, and

images then are reconstructed based on a selective portion of the QRS complex. Prospective gating allows images to be obtained only during the selected portion of the ECG. Using the gating technique, cardiac dimensions and function can be evaluated noninvasively.

Computed emission tomography

CT can be used with radionuclide imaging (see following discussion) to construct 3-D images. This application of tomography is referred to as computed *emission* tomography (CET) as opposed to the computed (transmission) tomography just described. The CET image is based on detection of radiation emitted from decaying radionuclides rather than detection of x-rays transmitted through the body.

Two forms of CET are used: *single-photon emission computed tomography* (SPECT) and *positron emission tomography* (PET). SPECT is simply CT in combination with thallium or technetium imaging. Both these radionuclides are *single-photon emission* radionuclides, meaning that a single packet of energy, or photon, is emitted for each atomic decay. *Positrons,* or positively charged electrons, can also be emitted and detected as atoms decay. However, radionuclides that emit positrons must be produced on site in a cyclotron. Consequently, PET of the heart is cost-prohibitive for most centers, particularly given the quality of information available with other noninvasive techniques.

Radionuclide Imaging
Basic principles

The *nucleus* of an atom is composed of positively charged *protons* and electrically neutral *neutrons*. Negatively charged *electrons* orbit the nucleus. *Radionuclides* are nuclei that are inherently unstable and tend to decay to a more stable form, emitting radiation in the process. The energy emitted during the decay of atoms can be detected and counted by gamma cameras.

Radionuclide imaging of the cardiovascular system involves the intravenous injection of small quantities of radioactive isotopes into a peripheral vein. The isotope either binds to blood elements or is selectively taken up by normal myocardium or infarcted myocardium, thereby acting as a radioactive tracer. The isotope's affinity for either blood or myocardium depends on the properties of the radioactive substance selected.

Three radionuclide techniques are currently used:
1. *Myocardial perfusion imaging* with thallium-201 (^{201}Tl) or technetium-99m–(^{99m}Tc-)sestaMIBI or ^{99m}Tc-teboroxime to evaluate myocardial perfusion
2. *Infarct-avid imaging* with ^{99m}Tc–indium-111 (^{111}In) leukocytes, or ^{111}In antimyosin, to detect acute myocardial necrosis
3. *Blood pool scanning* with ^{99m}Tc to evaluate ventricular function

The distribution of radioactive tracers can be detected by

gamma cameras from the radiation emitted as the radionuclides decay.

Myocardial perfusion imaging

The radioactive isotopes just mentioned are currently being used to measure myocardial perfusion and detect ischemia. Each of these radioactive isotopes accumulates within the myocardium in proportion to myocardial blood flow. The most appropriate use of these isotopes is in conjunction with stress testing for evaluation of ischemic heart disease. During stress testing, myocardial blood flow is decreased in areas of the heart supplied by stenosed blood vessels. At peak exercise the radioactive isotope is injected. The tracer is carried to the myocardium by blood, and areas of decreased perfusion will be supplied with less isotope than areas with adequate blood flow. These areas are detected as "cold spots" on the images. Ischemia is detected by all three isotopes. However, ischemia can be differentiated from infarction only by using ^{201}Tl. After ^{201}Tl is injected, the isotope equalizes into viable (live) tissue and does not perfuse into necrotic (dead) tissue. If the defect "reperfuses" after resting, the area is ischemic but not necrotic. ^{99m}Tc-sestaMIBI and ^{99m}Tc-teboroxime remain relatively fixed, and no significant redistribution occurs.

Infarct imaging

Infarct imaging can be performed using three isotopes: ^{99m}Tc Sn-pyrophosphate, indium-111 antimyosin, and indium-111 leukocytes. Imaging with ^{99m}Tc Sn-pyrophosphate differs from that with thalium because ^{99m}Tc accumulates selectively in acutely damaged myocardium, permitting identification of the site and evaluation of the extent of necrosis. Areas of concentrated uptake appear as "hot spots" on the scan. The patterns of tracer uptake can be observed within 12 to 72 hours after infarction and persist for 10 to 14 days.

Indium-111 antimyosin is a monoclonal antibody specific for intracellular use. The radioactive antibodies attach themselves to cardiac myosin, which becomes exposed as myocardial cellular membrane integrity is destroyed during progressive myocardial ischemia. This methodology offers advantages over other infarct-imaging agents in that these antibodies are thought to be necrosis-specific and therefore allow more accurate quantification of infarct size. Similarly, indium-111 leukocytes are useful in detecting infarct size 2 to 3 days after a myocardial infarction when white blood cell migration occurs.

Blood pool scanning with technetium

Blood pool scanning can be used to evaluate ventricular function and to detect and evaluate coronary artery disease. Abnormalities in ventricular function may appear with exercise if coronary artery disease is present. This technique involves labeling RBCs or albumin with technetium so that the blood volume or blood pool can be visualized, as outlined by the cardiac chambers and vessels.

First-pass blood pool scanning is used to record the initial passage of the radioactive tracer through the heart. This technique is useful to detect and quantify degrees of valvular regurgitation and intracardiac shunting.

Equilibrium imaging involves recording multiple images after the distribution of the radioactive tracer has equilibrated. This technique is referred to as the *multi-gated blood pool scan* (GBS or MUGA). With this method of scanning, images are recorded over multiple cardiac cycles and then summated or superimposed to improve the resolution of the nuclear image (Fig. 30-13). To synchronize the camera accurately with the cardiac cycle, the camera is *gated* or *triggered* by the ECG. The GBS permits noninvasive determination of ejection fraction, ventricular volumes, and regional patterns of wall motion.

Digital Subtraction Angiography

Digital subtraction angiography (DSA) is used to enhance angiographic images obtained after injection of contrast material into a peripheral or central vein. An image, referred to as the *mask image,* is recorded and stored before the injection of contrast material. Multiple images are then obtained as the contrast material passes through the heart. These images are developed into a composite image.

All fluoroscopic images are converted to a digital form. In other words, the intensity of light (in shades of gray) for each point on the image is converted to numbers or digits. The intensity of the signal in digital form is displayed on a video screen composed of a matrix of picture elements, or pixels. This conversion of the image to digital form allows the mask to be subtracted from the composite image. The subtraction process removes background structures, such as bone or soft tissue, from the image, leaving only the opacified chambers and vessels. Thus the image is electronically enhanced.

Magnetic Resonance Imaging

Magnetic resonance imaging (MRI), previously referred to as "nuclear magnetic resonance" (NMR), is a tomographic imaging technique that does not require the administration of radionuclides. This technique is based on analysis of the magnetic behavior of nuclei. Certain types of nuclei possess an inherent *spin*. As the charged nucleus spins, a magnetic field is generated around the atom.

During MRI the body is surrounded by an external magnet. The interactions between the external magnetic field and the magnetic fields of the nuclei shift from random positions to alignment with or against the external magnetic field. An average direction for the magnetic field of the nuclei, or a *magnetization vector,* can be determined.

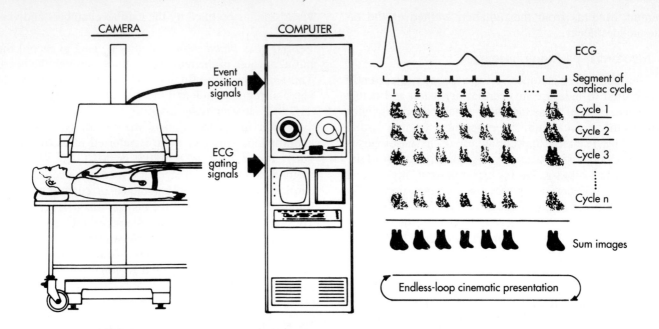

FIG. 30-13 Multigated blood pool imaging uses a computer in association with the scintillation camera to sort the scintillation information into multiple time segments. Although any number of time segments *(n)* can be recorded, the cycle is usually divided into less than 30. In any one cycle the amount of scintillation information is too little to permit an adequate view of the heart to be recorded. By recording data for *n* cycles, however, the quality of the image may build up to a point where sufficient detail can be seen to observe small wall motion abnormalities. (From Johnson RA, Haber E, Austen WG: *The practice of cardiology,* Boston, 1980, Little, Brown.)

Pulses of energy, in the form of *radiofrequency* waves, are then applied. These pulses disturb the magnetization vector. As the pulses are turned off, signals are emitted as the atoms return to resting positions within the external magnet. MRI has been shown to be effective and useful in the diagnosis of a wide variety of cardiovascular diseases. Gating the images to the ECG (similar to CT scanning) is essential to minimize artifacts caused by myocardial contraction. MRI is useful in determining ventricular mass, global and regional wall motion, and valvular insufficiency. In addition, MRI is useful in evaluating extracardiac disease (e.g., aortic aneurysm or dissection) and pericardial thickening. Recently, MRI has been used to evaluate native coronary artery stenosis and quantify coronary blood flow. With further software and hardware improvements, MRI may prove to be a comprehensive noninvasive diagnostic tool (Manning, Edelman, 1993).

Exercise Testing

Exercise testing with a treadmill or bicycle ergometer permits evaluation of exercise-induced symptoms or ECG changes. Multiple ECG leads are monitored continuously, and blood pressure is measured frequently during the test. Patients are instructed to report any symptoms immediately. If the exercise test is abnormal but nondiagnostic for coronary artery disease, thallium exercise testing, or *stress imaging,* is indicated. Combining radionuclide imaging with exercise testing is significantly more accurate for the diagnosis of coronary disease than exercise testing alone. Comparisons are made between the nuclear image obtained at rest and the one obtained during exercise.

Pharmacologic stress tests

If a patient is unable to exercise or if diagnostic images are required during stress testing, adenosine or dipyridamole may be administered to produce an ischemic response during nuclear studies or cardiac catheterization. Adenosine and dipyridamole produce a vasodilatory effect in normal arteries. Myocardial areas perfused by stenotic vessels are hypoperfused because the vessels cannot dilate. Thus ischemia is produced. Pharmacologic studies are most frequently performed with the addition of radioactive isotopes to quantify blood flow to ischemic areas.

Stress echocardiography

A *"stress echo"* may be performed to evaluate the effect of ischemia on left ventricular function. During stress testing, echocardiography is performed and left ventricular wall abnormalities are detected at peak exercise and after resting. The decrease in contractility is related to significant narrowing of the coronary arteries.

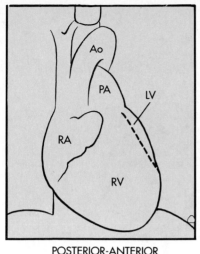

POSTERIOR-ANTERIOR

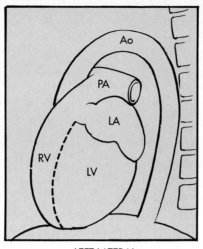

LEFT LATERAL

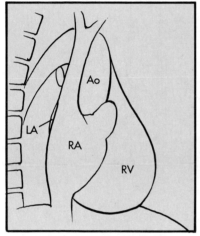

RIGHT ANTERIOR OBLIQUE

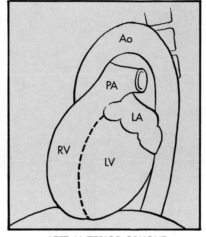

LEFT ANTERIOR OBLIQUE

FIG. 30-14   Orientation of the heart in four standard positions for cardiac radiography. In the posterior-anterior position the borders of the right atrium *(RA)* and left ventricle are displayed. The right ventricle *(RV)* and left atrium are not visible on the borders of the silhouette. *Ao,* Aorta; *PA,* pulmonary artery. In the left lateral position the silhouette of the RV is seen anteriorly and the left atrium *(LA)* posteriorly. *LV,* Left ventricle. In the right anterior oblique position the RV and the LA are again seen in silhouette. In the left anterior oblique position the RV and LV are seen in silhouette. The LA can be discerned in this projection. (Modified from Rushmer RF: *Cardiovascular dynamics,* ed 3, Philadelphia, 1976, Saunders.)

Chest Radiography

A series of chest radiographs in four standard positions is useful in the cardiac diagnostic workup (Fig. 30-14): (1) posterior-anterior or frontal position; (2) left lateral position with left side forward; (3) right anterior oblique position with the body rotated approximately 60 degrees to the left, which places the right shoulder anterior; and (4) left anterior oblique position with the left shoulder anterior. In each position a different anatomic perspective of the heart is visible. The contour of the heart contrasts with the radiolucent air-filled lungs.

The following findings can be detected on the chest radiograph: (1) generalized cardiac enlargement, or cardiomegaly; (2) localized chamber enlargement; (3) calcification in valves or coronary arteries; (4) pulmonary venous congestion; (5) interstitial or alveolar edema; and (6) enlargement of the pulmonary artery or dilation of the ascending aorta.

An impression of generalized cardiac enlargement can be noted in chest radiographs; however, precise estimation of the degree of enlargement is of questionable accuracy. In contrast, chamber enlargement distinctly alters

the contour of the heart, permitting specification of the involved chamber. In the posterior-anterior position the right border of the heart consists of the superior vena cava with the right atrium below. An angle appears at the juncture between the two. The structures comprising the left border, from top to bottom, are the aorta, pulmonary artery, and left ventricle. This projection permits identification of right atrial, left ventricular, and pulmonary arterial enlargement. Right atrial enlargement, for example, displaces the right boundary outward to the right, rounding the curvature of the cardiac contour.

In the left lateral position the anterior border is primarily the right ventricle, with the posterior border consisting of the left atrium superiorly and the posterior wall of the left ventricle inferiorly. The esophagus lies behind the posterior boundary. Right ventricular and left atrial enlargement are best appreciated in this view. Outlining the esophagus with swallowed barium facilitates the diagnosis of left atrial enlargement, which produces an esophageal indentation with posterior displacement.

Radiologic examination of the lungs demonstrates the effects of cardiac dysfunction on the pulmonary vasculature. Left heart failure or mitral valve disease increases pulmonary venous congestion, dilating the pulmonary veins in characteristic patterns. Excessive elevation of venous pressure results in transudation of fluid into the interstitial space and eventually into the alveoli. Fluid seepage from the intravascular space, or pulmonary edema, produces a clouding, or haziness, of the vascular shadows, progressively whitening the normally dark shadows of the radiolucent lungs.

Characteristic findings typify particular cardiac lesions. For example, in mitral stenosis (a lesion impeding blood flow from the left atrium to the left ventricle) left atrial enlargement and pulmonary venous congestion would be noted. Valvular calcification might also be observed.

INVASIVE DIAGNOSTIC PROCEDURES

Electrophysiology Studies

Intracardiac ECG techniques, or *electrophysiology* (EP) *studies,* permit a more detailed analysis of the mechanisms of cardiac impulse formation and conduction than do standard ECG recordings. As the action potential sweeps through the conduction system and the myocardium, the body surface ECG records the summated signals of atrial and ventricular activation, represented by the P wave and QRS complex, respectively. The amplitude of signals generated by specific sites in the conduction system, such as the sinus node or the bundle of His, is too small to be detected on the body surface. An intracardiac ECG can record deflections from these sites via recording electrodes positioned close to the regions of interest in the conduction system or myocardium. Fig. 30-15 compares the body surface and intracardiac ECGs.

EP studies are used for the following purposes: (1) to assess sinus node function, (2) to evaluate AV node conduction, (3) to analyze complex atrial and ventricular tachycardias, and (4) to determine the efficacy of pharmacologic or pacemaker therapy for refractory dysrhythmias. (EP testing for refractory ventricular dysrhythmias is discussed in Chapter 31.)

Several catheters, usually two to five, with multiple electrodes are advanced through peripheral veins under fluoroscopic guidance to the desired intracardiac sites. The sites selected depend on the purpose of the study. Fig. 30-16 illustrates a common catheter placement. These electrodes can be used for intracardiac recording or stimulation. Electrical stimulation of the atria or ventricles with an external programmable pulse generator may be indicated to induce or terminate tachydysrhythmias or to evaluate sinus or AV node responses.

Fig. 30-15 illustrates the use of an intracardiac recording to localize the site of AV block. For this study a recording catheter with multiple electrodes is positioned

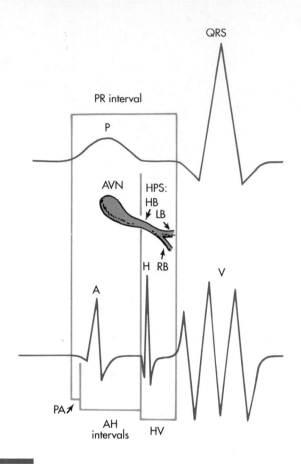

FIG. 30-15 Surface versus intracardiac ECG. Depicted are simultaneously recorded surface *(top)* and intracardiac *(bottom)* ECGs along with the anatomic structures of the atrioventricular (AV) specialized conduction system involved in normal impulse transmission. The surface ECG shows a P wave (atrial muscle depolarization) and a QRS complex (ventricular muscle depolarization). A PR interval can be measured and represents the following conduction times: intraatrial; AV nodal *(AVN)*, His bundle *(HB)*, right bundle *(RB)*, and left bundle *(LB)* branches; and Purkinje fiber. In contrast, the single intracardiac tracing from the AV junction shows three deflections: *A* (low atrial muscle depolarization), *H* (bundle of His activation), and *V* (ventricular muscle depolarization). Three intervals can be measured when the surface and intracardiac ECGs are compared: (1) the PA interval—measure of intraatrial conduction time, as impulse traverses from its exit from the sinus node (near superior vena cava) to the intracardiac recording site low in the right atrium at the AV junction; (2) the AH interval—approximation of AVN conduction time (penetration of the AVN is assumed to occur simultaneously with the arrival of the impulse at the low right atrium, anatomic site of the AVN); and (3) the HV interval—measure of conduction time through the His-Purkinje system (*HPS,* bundle of His, right and left bundles, and Purkinje network) to its exit at the ventricular muscle. From the aforementioned three intervals, conduction delays that exhibit as first-degree AV block (prolonged PR interval) can be differentiated as resulting from delay in the atria, AVN, or HPS. Sites of higher degrees of AV block can also be determined and isolated to one of those areas. (From Gilber CJ, Masgood A: *Heart Lung* 9(1):85-92, 1980.)

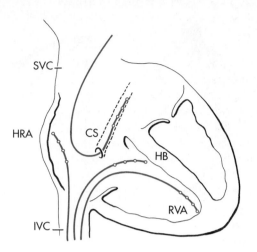

FIG. 30-16   Catheter placement for electrophysiologic (EP) testing. Quadripolar catheters to the high right atrium *(HRA)*, the right ventricular apex *(RVA)*, and the bundle of His *(HB)* are usually inserted via the femoral veins and inferior vena cava *(IVC)*. Left atrial recording and stimulation are usually performed with a catheter in the coronary sinus *(CS)*. *SVC,* Superior vena cava.

across the tricuspid valve beside the membranous interventricular septum. The electrodes record deflections as the wave of electrical activation moves from the atria through the AV node to the bundle of His and right ventricle. The site of delays in conduction can be localized by comparing the conduction time as the impulse moves through the AV node to the bundle of His (AH interval) with that from the bundle of His through the ventricular Purkinje fibers (HV interval).

Cardiac Catheterization

Cardiac catheterization is the insertion of catheters into the cardiovascular system to study the anatomy and function of the heart in the presence of suspected or documented heart disease. Depending on the location of a suspected lesion and the degree of myocardial dysfunction, selected studies are performed, including (1) measurement of pressures in the cardiac chambers and vessels, (2) analysis of the waveform configuration of recorded pressures, (3) sampling of the oxygen content in selected regions, (4) opacification of the cardiac chambers and/or coronary arteries with contrast material, and (5) determination of cardiac output. Fig. 30-17

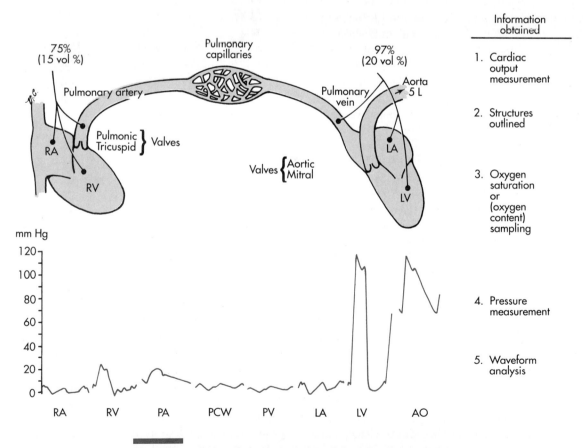

FIG. 30-17   Data obtained during cardiac catheterization. *RA,* Right atrium; *RV,* right ventricle; *PA,* pulmonary artery; *PCW,* pulmonary capillary wedge pressure; *PV,* pulmonary vein; *LA,* left atrium; *LV,* left ventricle, *AO,* aorta.

illustrates normal pressures, waveform configurations, and oxygen contents.

Two general approaches to the heart are currently used: right-sided heart catheterization and left-sided heart catheterization. *Right-sided heart catheterization* requires insertion of a catheter into the venous system, usually via an antecubital vein in the right arm or the femoral vein. The catheter is progressively advanced through the peripheral venous system to the vena cava and into the right atrium, right ventricle, and pulmonary artery. Advancing the catheter further into a distal segment of the pulmonary arterial bed eventually produces a "wedging," or lodging, of the catheter tip in the vessel lumen. This wedge position is referred to as the *pulmonary capillary position* and reflects pressures in the cardiovascular system from the left atrium. Left-sided heart catheterization involves the retrograde passage of the catheter through the arterial system to the aorta, across the aortic valve, and into the left ventricle. The catheter is usually inserted into either the brachial or femoral artery. Passage of the catheter into the aorta also permits selective cannulation and study of the coronary arteries.

Catheterization in coronary atherosclerotic disease

Coronary angiography, or injection of contrast material into the coronary arteries, is most often used to determine the location, extent, and severity of blockages within the coronary arteries. Additional indications for coronary angiography include evaluation of atypical angina and coronary revascularization results. The catheterization procedure involves the opacification of both coronary arteries, followed by a left ventriculogram, or injection of the contrast medium into the left ventricle, to evaluate left ventricular function (Fig. 30-18).

Coronary angiography provides the following information: (1) location of the lesion or lesions, (2) degree of obstruction, (3) presence of collateral circulation, (4) extent of disease in the distal arterial bed, and (5) type of lesion morphology. Once the location and extent of disease are determined, the most appropriate intervention can be planned. Certain lesions identified at the time of catheterization are considered high-risk lesions. One example of a high-risk lesion is significant stenosis of the main left coronary artery, which may require relatively urgent surgical intervention. Single, discrete lesions within the coronary artery may be best treated with percutaneous transluminal coronary angioplasty (PTCA), with coronary bypass surgery reserved for disease in three major vessels or in the left main coronary artery (see Chapter 31).

The evaluation of left ventricular function is an important adjunct to coronary angiography. Injection of contrast material into the left ventricle permits visualization of ventricular wall movement and chamber size; areas of absent motion *(akinesis),* reduced motion *(hypokinesis),* or asynchronous contraction *(dyskinesis)* or bulging are noted. Rupture of a necrotic interventricular septum after

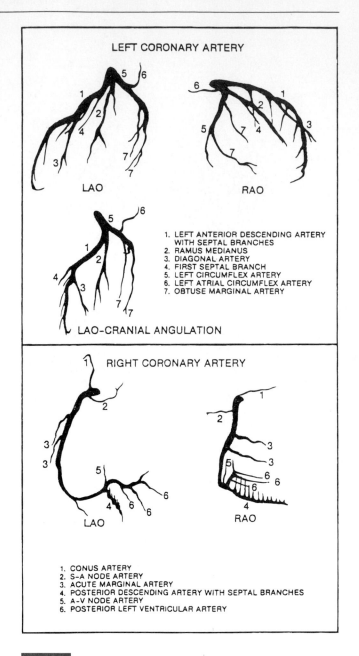

FIG. 30-18 Detailed anatomy of the normal coronary vasculature revealed by angiography. (From Braunwald E: *Heart disease,* ed 4, Philadelphia, 1992, Saunders.)

myocardial infarction would also be detected during left ventriculography. Because the pressures are higher on the left side of the heart than on the right, blood would be shunted through the interventricular defect, opacifying the right ventricle. In addition, oxygen sampling would demonstrate abnormal elevation of oxygen content in the right ventricle as a result of the recirculation of oxygenated blood through the defect. Measurement of left ventricular pressure, arterial pressure, cardiac output, and ejection fraction completes the overall assessment of left ventricular function.

Catheterization in valvular heart disease

Catheterization is useful to confirm the presence of valvular stenosis or regurgitation, to estimate the severity of the disease, and to establish or exclude the presence of associated pathology. The approach to diagnosing these two pathologic conditions—*stenosis* (valvular obstruction to blood flow) and *regurgitation* (backward blood flow through the valve)—differs.

Valvular regurgitation is documented by injection of contrast material into the chamber beyond the diseased valve; if regurgitation is present, opacification of the chamber proximal to the valve will occur when the valve fails to close securely. For example, with mitral regurgitation, the contrast medium injected into the left ventricle would appear in the left atrium during the next ventricular contraction as blood and contrast material flow backward through the diseased valve. The severity of the regurgitation is estimated according to the degree of left atrial opacification and the time required for the contrast material to disappear from the left atrium. Aortic regurgitation is detected by injection of contrast material into the ascending aorta, with subsequent opacification of the left ventricle during ventricular relaxation.

Regurgitation is also associated with abnormalities in the pressures within the cardiac chambers and alterations in waveform configuration. Mitral regurgitation creates a volume overload for the left atrium, elevating left atrial and pulmonary pressures. In addition, the typical low-amplitude undulating left atrial waveform exhibits an abrupt increase in amplitude during ventricular contraction as blood flows backward through the valve.

Valvular stenosis can be visualized by injecting contrast material into the chamber proximal to the diseased valve; as the opacified blood flows through the restricted orifice, the valve boundaries are outlined. Typical alterations in pressures and waveforms are seen with valvular stenosis. For instance, the aortic pressure tracing associated with aortic stenosis demonstrates a slow upstroke and delayed peak as a result of the resistance to ventricular ejection into the aorta (Fig. 30-19). Elevations in pressure in the chambers proximal to a stenotic lesion also occur. For example, mitral stenosis elevates left atrial and pulmonary venous pressures. These pressure elevations are reflected retrograde through the lungs and detected most easily via a catheter in the wedge position in the pulmonary artery. This pressure measurement is known as the *pulmonary capillary wedge pressure* (PCWP) and reflects left atrial pressure.

Valvular stenosis produces a *pressure gradient,* or difference in pressure, between the chambers on either side of the valve. The pressure gradient results because the chamber proximal to the stenotic valve must generate increased pressure to force blood through the obstructed valve. Fig. 30-20 shows an example of a pressure gradient resulting from severe aortic stenosis. Notice the large pressure discrepancy, with the left ventricle generating

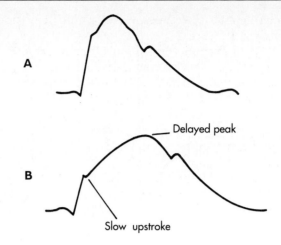

FIG. 30-19   Carotid artery pressure tracing. **A,** Normal. **B,** Aortic stenosis.

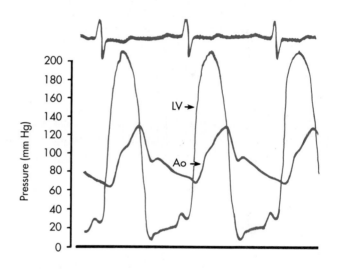

FIG. 30-20   Left ventricular *(LV)* and aortic *(Ao)* pressure tracings in severe aortic stenosis. (Modified from Grossman W: *Cardiac catheterization and angiography,* Philadelphia, 1980, Lea & Febiger.)

pressures up to 210 mm Hg to force blood through the aortic valve to sustain an aortic systolic pressure of 130 mm Hg. The pressure gradient in this example is 80 mm Hg; normally the pressure gradient is less than 5 mm Hg.

In addition to the measurement of the pressure gradient, it is necessary to use a formula to calculate the area of the valve orifice. Determining the pressure gradient across the valve and estimating the valve area are the two most critical indicators of the severity of stenosis.

Hemodynamic monitoring

Bedside monitoring of selected intracardiac and intravascular pressures permits ongoing evaluation of cardiovascular status. The following hemodynamic parameters can be monitored in critical care units: (1) right atrial

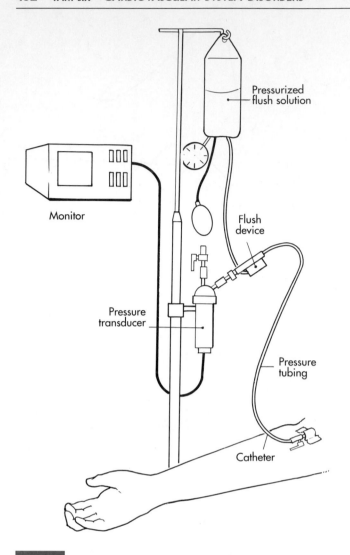

FIG. 30-21   Basic components of pressure monitoring system. [Modified from Boldt MA: *Acute coronary care,* New York, 1983, John Wiley & Sons.]

or central venous pressure (RAP or CVP) and left atrial pressure (LAP), (2) right ventricular pressure (RVP) and (indirectly) left ventricular end-diastolic pressure (LVEDP), (3) pulmonary artery pressure (PAP) and pulmonary capillary wedge pressure (PCWP), (4) arterial pressure, and (5) cardiac output (CO).

The basic components of the pressure monitoring system (Fig. 30-21) include (1) intravascular catheter, (2) fluid-filled extension tubing and stopcocks, (3) continuous flush device, (4) pressure transducer, and (5) pressurized flush solution. Depending on the pressure(s) to be monitored, the catheter may be either of a single-lumen design, such as a radial arterial catheter, or of a multiple-lumen design, such as the Swan-Ganz balloon-tipped pulmonary arterial catheter.

The most frequently used pulmonary arterial catheter contains four separate lumens (Fig. 30-22). One lumen is for the inflation of the balloon at the tip of the catheter, which is used for positioning the catheter. The distal and proximal lumens are used for the monitoring of PAP or PCWP and the RAP, respectively. The final lumen is for CO measurement.

The catheter is connected to the pressure transducer by stopcocks and a noncompliant pressure tubing filled with fluid. The hemodynamic pressures and pulsations are transmitted through this fluid column to the pressure transducer. The pressure transducer converts the mechanical pulsation to an electrical signal, which can be displayed on the bedside monitor.

To maintain the patency of the catheter, a continuous flush device is interposed between the catheter and the transducer. The continuous flush device is designed in a Y configuration to permit simultaneous pressure recording via the transducer and continuous flushing with solution. The device is connected to a bag of heparinized saline solution surrounded by an inflatable bag used to

FIG. 30-22   Pulmonary artery catheter. *RAP,* Right atrial (central venous) pressure; *CO,* cardiac output; *PAP,* pulmonary artery pressure; *PCWP,* pulmonary capillary wedge pressure.

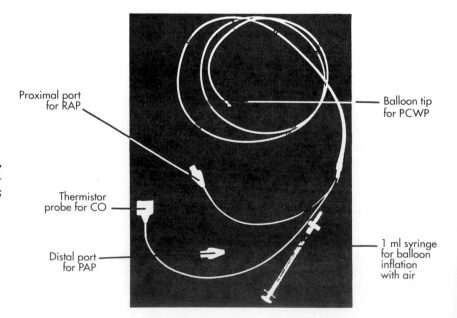

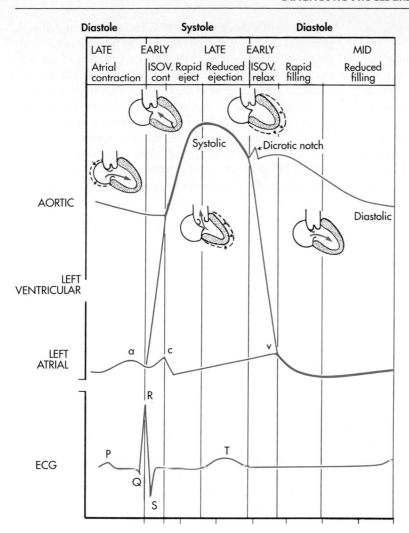

FIG. 30-23   Correlation between the events of the cardiac cycle and waveforms observed in hemodynamic and ECG tracings.

pressurize the solution so that it can flow against the higher intravascular or intracardiac pressures.

To interpret the significance of recorded hemodynamic pressures and waveform configurations, it is necessary to refer back to the electrical and mechanical events of the cardiac cycle discussed in depth in Chapter 29. Fig. 29-1 illustrates the interdependent relationship between electrical stimulation of the myocardium and the mechanical response. The five mechanical phases of the cardiac cycle are also reviewed there. Each of these mechanical phases produces characteristic alterations in the contour of the waveforms recorded within the cardiovascular system. Fig. 30-23 summarizes the relationship between the phases of the cardiac cycle and the characteristic waveforms of the left side of the heart.

Atrial waveforms are normally of low amplitude, given the low pressures generated by these chambers. RAPs average from 0 to 10 mm Hg, with LAPs approximating 3 to 15 mm Hg. Left heart pressures normally exceed right heart pressures because of the higher resistance to ejection posed by the systemic circuit relative to the pulmonary circulation. Direct measurement of left atrial pressure is usually restricted to postoperative cardiac surgical intensive care units.

Atrial pressures reflect changes in the volume status of the heart as well as alterations in cardiac function and structure. A reduction in atrial pressure is produced by hypovolemia; conversely, hypervolemia elevates atrial pressure. Atrial pressures are also valuable in assessing ventricular function, in the absence of AV valve dysfunction. As the ventricles fill during diastole, the atrial and ventricular chambers are in direct communication. At the end of diastole the pressures between these two chambers have equilibrated; therefore atrial pressures are equal to ventricular pressures at the end of diastole. Right or left ventricular failure produces increases in right ventricular end-diastolic pressure (RVEDP) or LVEDP as residual ventricular volumes rise because of impaired ventricular function. A change in ventricular end-diastolic pressure is immediately reflected backward to the atrium, where a corresponding rise in atrial pressure is observed.

Atrial waveforms are characterized by three positive components—the a, c, and v waves—corresponding to three events in the mechanical cycle that increase atrial pressure (see Fig. 30-3). The a wave corresponds to atrial contraction, the c wave is produced by the backward bulging of the AV valve with the onset of isovolumetric contraction, and the v wave results from atrial filling during ventricular ejection (note that the AV valves normally remain closed at this time).

Predictable alterations in the atrial configuration are observed with changes in cardiac function and structure, as discussed earlier in this chapter. For example, loss of atrial contraction during atrial fibrillation is manifested as loss of *a* waves. Asynchronous contraction of the ventricles and atria, as with complete heart block, intermittently superimposes the *a* wave on the *c* and *v* waves, producing large "cannon" *a* waves (Fig. 30-24). Increased resistance to atrial contraction, as with AV valve stenosis or ventricular failure, increases the size of the *a* wave. Regurgitation of blood through an incompetent AV valve during ventricular systole superimposes an abnormal pulsation on the *c* and *v* waves referred to as a "significant *v* wave" (see Fig. 30-3). The characteristic changes of AV valve dysfunction will be apparent in either the right atrial or the left atrial trace, depending on whether the tricuspid or mitral valve is affected.

Ventricular pressures and waveforms are not routinely monitored at the bedside. In certain settings, such as right ventricular failure secondary to chronic obstructive lung disease, a multilumen pulmonary artery catheter with a right ventricular lumen rather than the right atrial lumen described earlier can be inserted for direct RVP monitoring. However, familiarity with the RVP trace is required during monitoring with the pulmonary artery catheter so that backward displacement of the catheter into the ventricle can be detected immediately (Fig. 30-25).

PAPs and PCWPs are measured with the balloon-tipped multiple-lumen catheter described earlier. The catheter is advanced into the pulmonary artery via a peripheral vein

and the right side of the heart. With the balloon deflated, pressures in the pulmonary artery can be measured. Periodically the balloon is inflated. With inflation of the balloon, blood flow propels the catheter distally into the pulmonary vasculature until the tip "wedges" in a small arterial branch. In this position the pressure transmitted backward from the left side of the heart through the pulmonary vasculature is sensed by the catheter tip. Therefore the PCWP reflects left atrial and, consequently, LVEDP (Fig. 30-26). This relationship is distorted by mitral valve or pulmonary vascular abnormalities.

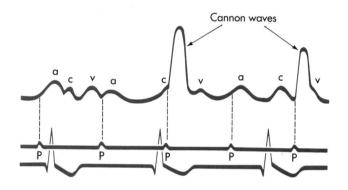

FIG. 30-24   Cannon waves in complete heart block, schematic jugular venous and heart sound tracings, and ECG. Note the irregularly occurring cannon waves produced by atrial systole when atrial contraction occurs with the tricuspid valve closed by ventricular systole. When atrial systole occurs during the rapid phase of ventricular filling, the *a* waves are smaller than usual. [From Hurst JW et al, editors: *The heart*, ed 4, New York, 1978, McGraw-Hill.]

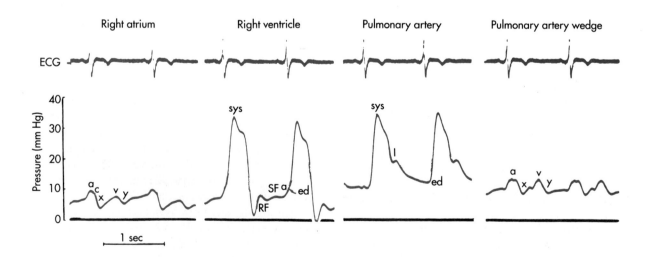

FIG. 30-25   Intracardiac pressure waveforms recorded from a fluid-filled catheter. Right side of the heart and pulmonary artery wedge pressures are on the borderline of being elevated, but the contours are normal. *sys*, Peak systolic pressure; *ed*, end-diastolic pressure; *RF*, rapid-filling wave; *SF*, slow-filling wave; *I*, incisura. Also shown are *a*, *c*, and *v* waves and the *x* and *y* descents. [From Braunwald E, editor: *Heart disease: a textbook in cardiovascular medicine*, Philadelphia, 1980, Saunders.]

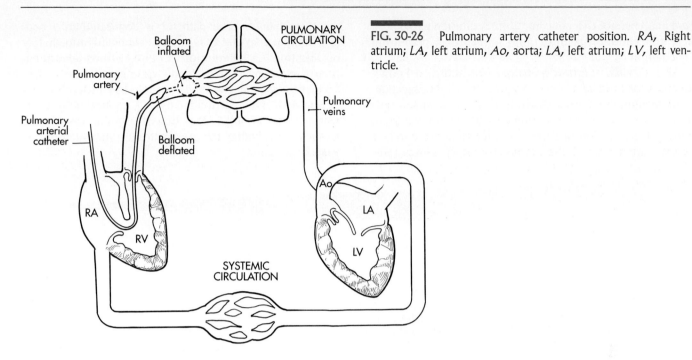

FIG. 30-27   Cardiac output measurement techniques. *RA,* Right atrium; *LA,* left atrium; *AO,* aorta; *RV,* right ventricle; *LV,* left ventricle; *PA,* pulmonary artery.

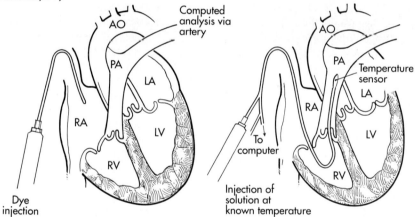

Pulmonary artery pressures average 25/10 mm Hg. Pulmonary hypertension may be observed in conditions such as chronic obstructive lung disease, chronic mitral valve disease, left ventricular failure, and pulmonary emboli. As mentioned, PCWP approximates LAP. The contour of the PCWP trace is similar to that of the LAP trace, although the low-amplitude *c* wave may be more difficult to visualize.

Arterial pressures are usually monitored via the radial artery, although femoral lines may be used. Brachial, axillary, pedal, or temporal sites can also be used. Constant monitoring of arterial pressure is particularly valuable during the intravenous administration of vasoactive drugs, such as sodium nitroprusside, nitroglycerine, or dopamine, which are used to regulate blood pressure.

In addition to recording systolic and diastolic blood pressures, mean arterial pressure (MAP) is measured. This pressure represents the average driving pressure perfusing the tissues. MAP is a function of CO and total peripheral resistance (TPR).

The following alterations in the arterial pulse have been discussed earlier in this chapter: (1) pulsus tardus produced by aortic stenosis, (2) waterhammer pulse associated with aortic regurgitation, (3) pulsus alternans caused by ventricular failure, (4) pulsus bigeminus caused by premature beats in a bigeminal rhythm, and (5) pulsus paradoxus associated with cardiac tamponade.

CO can be measured at the bedside by two techniques: dye dilution or thermal dilution (Fig. 30-27). The *dye dilution technique* involves the injection of a known quantity and concentration of dye into the venous end of the circulation, usually via a central venous line. The dye mixes with the blood and is progressively diluted. A sample of arterial blood is gradually withdrawn downstream and analyzed for dye concentration. A dilution curve (i.e., dye concentration against time) is recorded, permitting calculation of CO.

The *thermal dilution technique* substitutes a known quantity of fluid at a given temperature as the injectate. This technique requires insertion of the four-lumen pulmonary artery catheter. A lumen opens into the right atrium for injection of a cold solution, and a thermistor at the catheter tip in the pulmonary artery senses temperature changes. The catheter is connected to a bedside computer so that COs can be calculated immediately on injection. Calculation of CO also permits determination of pulmonary or systemic vascular resistance (i.e., systemic vascular resistance equals the difference between MAP and RAP divided by CO, multiplied by a correction factor of 80). Calculation of systemic vascular resistance is valuable for administering vasodilators and vasoconstrictors.

QUESTIONS

▼ *Answer the following on a separate sheet of paper.*

1. Mr. H. is a 59-year-old accountant who has been diagnosed as having atherosclerotic heart disease. Recently he found it necessary to resign from the manufacturing firm where he worked because of weakness, fatigue, and inability to climb the stairs to his second-floor office without precipitating an episode of chest pain. At home, Mr. H. is able to perform light housework but experiences shortness of breath and/or chest pain if he attempts to mow the lawn with a power mower. How would this patient's heart disease be categorized according to the New York Heart Association guidelines?

2. Palpation of the carotid arteries on a 68-year-old woman with a blood pressure of 178/100 mm Hg reveals that the left carotid pulse has a much lower amplitude than does the right. Explain the possible significance of this finding. What is this patient's mean arterial pressure?

3. How is the hepatojugular reflux test performed? How would you determine if the test were positive? What is the possible significance of a positive test?

4. What is a hexaxial reference system and how is it derived?

5. Discuss the type of data and evaluation of the cardiovascular status that may be obtained from cardiac catheterization.

6. List the indications for performing coronary angiography.

▼ *Circle the letter preceding each item below that correctly answers the question or completes the statement. Only one answer is correct unless otherwise noted.*

7. The symptoms of weakness and easy fatigability in patients with myocardial failure are probably a consequence of:
   a. Low cardiac output
   b. Increased contractility of the heart muscle
   c. Decreased peripheral perfusion
   d. Only a and c
   e. All the above

8. Hypertension in the adult is defined as blood pressure greater than:
   a. 120/80 mm Hg
   b. 130/80 mm Hg
   c. 140/90 mm Hg
   d. 160/85 mm Hg

9. A decreased pulse pressure may indicate (more than one answer may be correct):
   a. Decreased stroke volume
   b. Decreased peripheral resistance
   c. Increased peripheral resistance
   d. Decreased blood viscosity

10. A slow-rising and sustained carotid pulse is characteristic of:
    a. Mitral stenosis
    b. Aortic stenosis
    c. Mitral regurgitation
    d. Aortic regurgitation

11. A quick-rising and collapsing (water-hammer) pulse is characteristic of:
    a. Mitral stenosis
    b. Aortic stenosis
    c. Mitral regurgitation
    d. Aortic regurgitation

12. Jugular venous distention to the level of the jaw angle in a person sitting with the trunk elevated 90 degrees correlates with a central venous pressure of at least:
    a. 10 cm H_2O c. 20 cm H_2O
    b. 15 cm H_2O d. 25 cm H_2O

13. In the normal adult lying with the trunk elevated 30 degrees, the pulsation within the jugular vein should rise above the sternal angle no more than:
    a. 1 to 2 cm   c. 5 to 6 cm
    b. 2 to 3 cm   d. 7 to 8 cm

14. A large, early *v* wave in the jugular venous pulse is most likely to be present in:
    a. Mitral regurgitation
    b. Tricuspid regurgitation
    c. Mitral stenosis
    d. Tricuspid stenosis

15. A giant *a* wave in the jugular venous pulse is most likely to be present in:
    a. Mitral regurgitation
    b. Tricuspid regurgitation
    c. Mitral stenosis
    d. Tricuspid stenosis

16. In the cardiovascular examination the chest is inspected and palpated for (more than one answer may be correct):
    a. Apical impulse
    b. Thrills
    c. Symmetry of thoracic movements
    d. Lifts or heaves

17. A thrill is a palpable:
    a. Pericardial friction rub
    b. Heart sound
    c. Apical impulse
    d. Murmur

18. The apical impulse is normally located:
    a. At the fifth intercostal space near the left midclavicular line
    b. Adjacent to the angle of Louis
    c. At the lower left sternal border in the fourth intercostal space
    d. At the fourth intercostal space at the anterior axillary line

19. In cases of left ventricular hypertrophy, the point of maximum impulse will (more than one answer may be correct):
    a. Comprise an area less than 2 to 3 cm in diameter
    b. Comprise an area greater than 2 to 3 cm in diameter
    c. Shift laterally to the left and downward
    d. Shift to the mediastinal area, producing a substernal heave

20. The precordium refers to the area of the chest overlying the:
    a. Lungs   c. Heart
    b. Sternum   d. Mediastinum

21. A lift or heave is the rise with each heartbeat of the:
    a. Precordium   c. Sternum
    b. Cardiac apex d. Rib cage

22. A heart sound that occurs in early dias-

QUESTIONS—cont'd

tole and is considered normal in children and young adults but pathologic in older adults is the:
a. First heart sound
b. Second heart sound
c. Third heart sound
d. Fourth heart sound

23. Sounds occurring early in systole are most likely:
a. Atrial gallops
b. Ventricular gallops
c. Systolic ejection murmurs
d. Opening snaps of the mitral valve

24. The heart sound normally heard best over the aortic area is the:
a. First heart sound
b. Second heart sound
c. Third heart sound
d. Fourth heart sound

25. Murmurs occurring in diastole follow the:
a. First heart sound
b. Second heart sound

26. During auscultation of the blood pressure, systolic pressure correlates with the:
a. Onset of sound in the occluded artery
b. Abrupt muffling of sound
c. Disappearance of sound
d. Persistent tapping

27. The ECG monitor strip represents:
a. Mechanical activity of the heart
b. Electrical activity of the heart
c. Both a and b
d. Neither a nor b

28. Normally, ventricular depolarization:
a. Occurs at the T wave
b. Occurs after ventricular contraction
c. Indicates ventricular diastole
d. Stimulates ventricular contraction

29. By convention, a positive wave on the ECG indicates the path of electrical activity is:
a. Approaching a negative electrode
b. Approaching a positive electrode
c. Moving away from a negative electrode

d. Moving away from a positive electrode

30. The ECG leads measuring the horizontal plane of the heart are the:
a. Standard limb leads
b. Augmented limb leads
c. Precordial leads
d. Bipolar leads

31. In standard lead II of the ECG the electrical potential difference is recorded between the:
a. Right arm and left leg
b. Right arm and left arm
c. Right arm and right leg
d. Left arm and right leg

32. Which of the following leads is *not* unipolar?
a. aVR   c. V_6
b. aVF   d. II

33. A normal QRS electrical axis is characterized by:
a. Large, positive QRS deflections in leads II, III, and aVF
b. Large, positive QRS deflections in lead aVR
c. Large, negative QRS deflections in leads II, III, and aVF
d. Large, positive QRS deflections in leads I and aVL

34. A catheter wedged in a branch of the pulmonary artery measures a pressure correlating most directly with:
a. Right atrial pressure
b. Right ventricular pressure
c. Left atrial pressure
d. Pulmonary arterial pressure

35. Which of the following vessels is usually used for right-sided heart catheterization?
a. Femoral artery
b. Brachial artery
c. Jugular vein
d. Antecubital vein

36. The correct identification of the aortic and pulmonic components of the second heart sound on the phonocardiogram is aided by the simultaneous recording of the:

a. Electrocardiogram
b. Jugular venous pulse
c. Carotid arterial pulse
d. Radial pulse

37. Echocardiography utilizes the principle of:
a. Hydrodynamics
b. Ultrasound
c. Radioemission
d. Electromagnetic force

38. A noninvasive procedure for analyzing cardiac structures and wall motion is:
a. Phonocardiography
b. Electrocardiography
c. Echocardiography
d. Vectorcardiography

▼ *Circle T if the statement is true and F if it is false. Correct any false statements.*

39. T F The dorsalis pedis pulse may be palpated at the back of the knee.

40. T F Left atrial enlargement is detected best in the lateral view of the chest radiograph.

41. T F Kussmaul's sign is a decrease in the central venous pressure during inspiration.

42. T F A patient with an apical heart rate of 78 and a radial rate of 70 has a pulse deficit.

43. T F Physiologic splitting of the second heart sound is caused by asynchronous closure of the aortic and pulmonic valves and is always considered pathologic.

44. T F Paradoxical splitting of the second heart sound is heard on expiration and disappears on inspiration and may be caused by left bundle branch block.

45. T F Korotkoff sounds are produced by turbulent blood flow through the aortic valve during blood pressure measurement.

46. T F Paroxysmal nocturnal dyspnea is a symptom of left ventricular failure.

▼ *Match each of the terms in column A with its definition in column B.*

Column A	Column B
47. _____ Angina	a. Awareness of increased breathing effort
48. _____ Palpitations	b. Difficulty in breathing in the recumbent position
49. _____ Orthopnea	c. Chest pain caused by myocardial ischemia
50. _____ Syncope	d. Heartbeats sensed by the patient
51. _____ Dyspnea	e. Accumulation of fluid in the interstitial spaces
52. _____ Edema	f. Transient loss of consciousness
	g. Abnormal chest pulsations noticed by the patient

Continued.

QUESTIONS—cont'd

▼ *Match each of the jugular venous waveforms in column A with its cause in column B.*

Column A

53. _____ *a* wave
54. _____ *v* wave
55. _____ *c* wave

Column B

a. Produced by bulging of the tricuspid valve into the right atrium during ventricular contraction
b. Produced by increased right atrial pressure during atrial filling before the opening of the tricuspid valve
c. Produced by atrial contraction

▼ *Match each of the abnormal heart sounds in column A with its probable cause in column B.*

Column A

56. _____ Midsystolic murmur
57. _____ Pansystolic murmur
58. _____ Middiastolic murmur
59. _____ Opening snap in early diastole

Column B

a. May be produced by aortic stenosis
b. May be produced by pulmonic regurgitation
c. May be produced by mitral stenosis
d. May be produced by mitral regurgitation

▼ *Match each area of transmission of the cardiac valvular sounds in column A with its anatomic location on the chest in column B.*

Column A

60. _____ Mitral
61. _____ Tricuspid
62. _____ Aortic
63. _____ Pulmonic

Column B

a. Second intercostal space, left sternal border
b. Second intercostal space, right sternal border
c. Fifth intercostal space, midclavicular line
d. Lower left sternal border

▼ *Match the ECG waveform in column A with the electrical events in column B.*

Column A

64. _____ P wave
65. _____ QRS complex
66. _____ T wave

Column B

a. Ventricular repolarization
b. Atrial depolarization
c. Ventricular depolarization
d. Atrial repolarization

▼ *Match each of the ECG intervals in column A with its normal duration in column B.*

Column A

67. _____ PR interval
68. _____ QRS complex
69. _____ QT interval

Column B

a. 0.36 to 0.44 second
b. 0.12 to 0.20 second
c. 0.06 to 0.10 secod

▼ *Match each ECG abnormality in column A with its possible cause in column B.*

Column A

70. _____ Depression of the ST segment
71. _____ Elevation of the ST segment
72. _____ Inversion of the P wave
73. _____ Inversion of the T wave
74. _____ Peaking of the T wave
75. _____ Prolonged PR interval
76. _____ Prolonged QT interval

Column B

a. Slow conduction time through the AV node
b. Myocardial ischemia
c. Hyperkalemia
d. Myocardial necrosis
e. AV nodal dysrhythmia
f. Quinidine effect

QUESTIONS—cont'd

▼ *Match each of the cardiac diagnostic techniques in column A with its purpose in column B.*

Column A

77. _____ Flow-directed balloon-tipped catheter
78. _____ Electrophysiology study
79. _____ Multigated blood pool scan
80. _____ M-mode echocardiography
81. _____ Thermodilution pulmonary artery catheter
82. _____ Catheter tip lies in the right atrium or superior vena cava inserted via an antecubital vein
83. _____ Chest radiograph
84. _____ Thallium stress test

Column B

a. Test records intracardiac electrical impulses to evaluate mechanisms of impulse generation and conduction.
b. Noninvasive method that determines ejection fraction and ventricular volumes.
c. CO may be calculated at the bedside with data obtained.
d. Technique is more accurate for diagnosing coronary artery disease than exercise testing alone.
e. Abnormal valve motion may be detected.
f. PWP may be measured.
g. CVP may be measured.
h. Enlargement of the heart and great vessels may be detected.

▼ *Fill in the blanks with the correct word or phrase.*

85. During cardiac catheterization, contrast material is injected into the heart chamber distal to the diseased valve to confirm the diagnosis of valvular _____.
86. The pressure gradient between the left ventricle and the aorta is normally less than _____. A large pressure gradient indicates _____.
87. Heart murmurs are the result of _____ blood flow within the cardiac structures.

CHAPTER 31

Coronary Atherosclerotic Disease

CYNTHIA C. SENERCHIA
PENNY FORD CARLETON

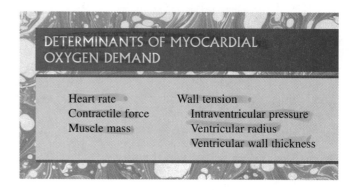

DETERMINANTS OF MYOCARDIAL OXYGEN DEMAND

Heart rate	Wall tension
Contractile force	Intraventricular pressure
Muscle mass	Ventricular radius
	Ventricular wall thickness

A critical balance exists between myocardial oxygen supply and demand; oxygen supply must equal demand (Fig. 31-1). A reduction in oxygen supply or an increase in oxygen demand can disturb this balance and threaten myocardial function.

There are four major determinants of myocardial oxygen demand: heart rate, contractile force, muscle mass, and ventricular wall tension (see box above, right). Wall tension, or *afterload,* is a function of variables identified in the Laplace equation: intraventricular pressure, ventricular radius, and ventricular wall thickness. Therefore cardiac work and oxygen demand are elevated by tachycardia (rapid heart rates), increased force of contraction, hypertension, ventricular dilation, and hypertrophy.

If myocardial oxygen demand increases, oxygen supply must increase concurrently. To significantly increase oxygen supply, coronary flow must increase because myocardial oxygen extraction from the arterial blood is almost maximal under resting conditions. The most potent stimulus to dilating the coronary arteries and increasing coronary flow is local tissue hypoxia. The normal coronary vasculature can dilate and increase flow approximately five to six times above resting levels. However, because stenotic, diseased vessels are unable to dilate, a state of oxygen deficit can result when oxygen demand exceeds the capacity of the vasculature to increase flow. *Ischemia* is a transient, reversible state of inadequate blood flow, which can result in insufficient oxygen delivery to the tissues. Prolonged ischemia will lead to tissue death, or *necrosis.* Clinically, ischemic death of the myocardium is referred to as *myocardial infarction* (MI).

The left ventricle is the chamber most susceptible to myocardial ischemia and infarction because of its unique myocardial oxygenation characteristics. First, left ventricular oxygen demand is great as a result of the high systemic resistance to ejection and the large muscle mass. In addition, coronary flow is phasic in nature. The branches of the coronary arteries are deeply embedded in the myocardium. During systole, these intramyocardial branches are compressed, which increases the resistance to flow. Coronary flow, therefore, occurs primarily during diastole. Contraction of the thick left ventricular wall essentially terminates systolic flow through its intramyocardial branches, especially in the innermost or subendocardial region; some systolic flow continues in the vessels of the thinner-walled right ventricle.

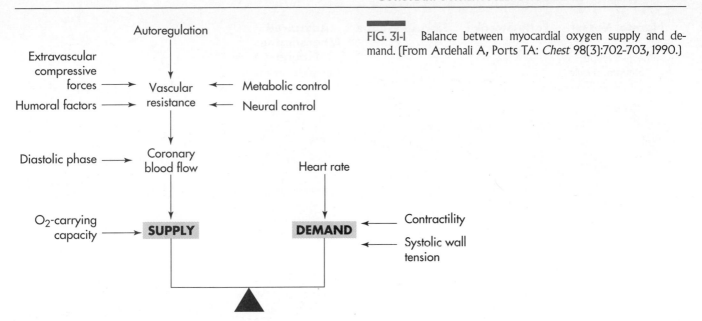

FIG. 31-1   Balance between myocardial oxygen supply and demand. (From Ardehali A, Ports TA: *Chest* 98(3):702-703, 1990.)

PATHOGENESIS AND PATHOLOGY

Coronary atherosclerosis is the most common cause of coronary artery disease (CAD). It has recently been recognized that the first change associated with atherosclerosis is a stiffening of the vessel wall, which impedes the artery's ability to dilate. This loss of dilatory response occurs before significant narrowing resulting from fatty deposits. Atherosclerosis causes a localized accumulation of lipid and fibrous tissue within the coronary artery, progressively narrowing the lumen of the vessel. As the lumen narrows, resistance to flow increases and myocardial blood flow is compromised. As the disease progresses, the luminal narrowing is accompanied by vascular changes that impair the diseased vessel's ability to dilate. Thus the balance between myocardial oxygen supply and demand becomes precarious, threatening the myocardium beyond the lesion.

Considerable research has been performed concerning the pathogenesis of atherosclerosis. The lesions are typically classified as fatty streaks, fibrous plaques, and complicated lesions (Fig. 31-2), as follows:

1. *Fatty streaks* develop as an early sign of atherosclerosis. Fatty streaks are characterized by an accumulation of lipid-filled smooth muscle cells and macrophages (mainly cholesterol oleate) in focal areas of the tunica intima (innermost layer of artery). They are flat and nonobstructive and may be visible to the naked eye as yellowish patches on the endothelial surface of the vessel. Fatty streaks are usually present in the aorta by age 10 years and in the coronary arteries by age 15 years. Some fatty streaks regress, but others develop into fibrous plaques.

2. *Fibrous plaques* (or atheromatous plaques) are palpably elevated areas of intimal thickening that represent the most characteristic lesion of advancing atherosclerosis and are not usually seen until the third decade of life. Typically, a fibrous plaque is dome shaped with an opaque, glistening surface that bulges into the lumen, causing obstruction. It consists of a central core of lipids and necrotic cell debris covered by a fibromuscular cap containing many smooth muscle cells and collagen. Fibrous plaques typically occur where arteries bifurcate, curve, or narrow.

3. *Complicated* or *advanced lesions* occur if the fibrous plaque becomes altered over time by calcification, cellular necrosis, hemorrhage, thrombosis, or ulceration and may lead to MI.

Despite this progressive luminal narrowing and the concurrent loss of vascular responsiveness, clinical manifestations of disease do not appear until the atherogenic process is well advanced. This preclinical phase can last 20 to 40 years. Clinically significant lesions producing myocardial ischemia and dysfunction usually obstruct more than 75% of the vessel lumen. The final step in the pathologic process can occur in the following ways: (1) progressive luminal narrowing by plaque enlargement; (2) hemorrhage into the atheromatous plaque, producing intralesional thrombi arising from the vasa vasorum; (3) thrombus formation within the lumen of the artery initiated by platelet aggregation; (4) embolization of a thrombus or plaque fragment within the vessel; or (5) coronary artery spasm. Despite the variety of causes leading to acute coronary occlusion, autopsy studies suggest intraluminal thrombosis as the major causative event, superimposed on preexisting atherosclerotic lesions. Whether thrombotic occlusion is a primary or secondary event has yet to be determined. Some investigators believe that coronary arterial spasm superimposed on an atherosclerotic plaque increases intraplaque pressure with subsequent

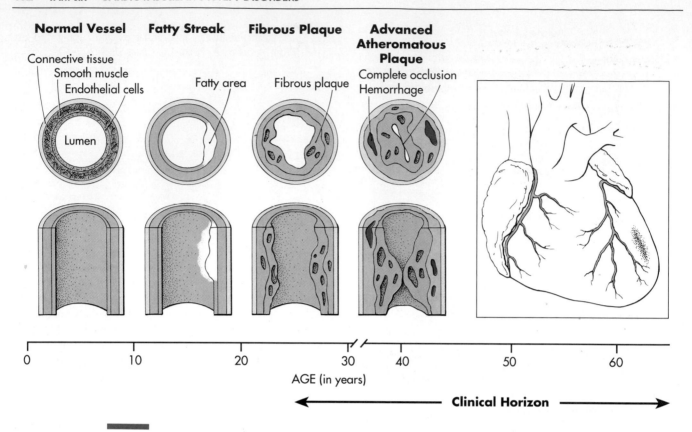

Normal Vessel   **Fatty Streak**   **Fibrous Plaque**   **Advanced Atheromatous Plaque**

Connective tissue
Smooth muscle
Endothelial cells

Fatty area

Fibrous plaque

Complete occlusion
Hemorrhage

Lumen

AGE (in years)

← Clinical Horizon →

FIG. 31-2   Progressive pathologic changes in coronary atherosclerotic disease. Fatty streaks are found as one of the earliest lesions of atherosclerosis. Many fatty streaks regress, whereas others progress to fibrous plaques and eventually to atheromas. These may then become complicated by hemorrhage, ulceration, calcification, or thrombosis and may produce myocardial infarction.

rupture and thrombosis. Still others believe that a combination of mechanisms mentioned previously results in the final occlusive process.

Notably, atherosclerotic lesions usually develop in the proximal, epicardial segments of the coronary artery at sites of abrupt curvature, branching, or attachment. The lesions tend to be localized and focal in distribution; in advanced disease, however, areas of diffuse involvement become pronounced.

RISK FACTORS

It is no longer contended that atherosclerosis is simply a result of the aging process. The appearance of "fatty streaks" in the coronary arterial wall as early as childhood is a natural phenomenon and does not necessarily progress to atherosclerotic lesions. It is now believed that many factors interact to accelerate the atherogenic process. A number of so-called risk factors have been identified that increase susceptibility to the development of coronary atherosclerosis in a given individual (see box, p. 463).

There are three nonmodifiable biologic risk factors: age, male gender, and family history. Susceptibility to coronary atherosclerosis increases with age; the development of significant disease before age 40 is unusual. However, the correlation between age and disease onset may simply reflect the longer duration of exposure to other atherogenic factors. Women seem relatively immune until after menopause and then become as susceptible as men. The protective effect of estrogen has been postulated as an explanation for early female immunity. African Americans are more vulnerable to atherosclerosis than are whites. Finally, a positive family history for CAD (i.e., siblings or parents developing disease before age 50) increases the likelihood of the premature development of atherosclerosis. The relative contribution of genetic and environmental influences is unknown. A genetic component can be linked with some pronounced, accelerated forms of atherosclerosis, as in familial lipid disorders. However, family history may also reflect a strong environmental component, perhaps a life-style that produces tension or obesity.

Additional risk factors are amenable to modification, potentially retarding the atherogenic process. Major modifiable risk factors are elevated serum lipid levels, hyper-

RISK FACTORS FOR CORONARY ATHEROSCLEROSIS*

NONMODIFIABLE

Age (males ≥45 years; females ≥55 years or premature menopause without estrogen replacement therapy)

Male gender

Family history of coronary artery disease (myocardial infarction in father or brother before 55 years or in mother or sister before 65 years)

MODIFIABLE

Hyperlipidemia (low-density lipoproteins: borderline to high, 130-159 mg/dl; high, ≥160 mg/dl

Hypertension (≥140/90 mm Hg or on antihypertensive drug)

Current cigarette smoking

Diabetes mellitus (insulin or noninsulin dependent)

Obesity, especially abdominal

Physical inactivity

Modified from *Second Report of the Expert Panel on Detection, Evaluation and Treatment of High Blood Cholesterol in Adults (Adult Treatment Panel II),* NIH Pub No 93-3095, National Heart, Lung, and Blood Institute, Washington, DC, 1993, National Institutes of Health.

*Race is no longer considered a nonmodifiable risk factor, although coronary artery disease death rates for African Americans are 3% to 70% higher than for Caucasians up through age 74 years. Genetic factors may play an indirect role in atherogenesis because of such factors as the increased incidence of hypertension in African Americans, and efforts should be directed toward reducing it and all modifiable risk factors.

tension, cigarette smoking, diabetes mellitus, sedentary life-style, and obesity, especially the abdominal type.

Hyperlipidemia

The plasma lipids—cholesterols, triglycerides, phospholipids, and free fatty acids—are derived from exogenous dietary sources and endogenous lipid synthesis. Cholesterol and triglyceride are the two lipids of major clinical significance relative to atherogenesis. Because lipids are insoluble in plasma, lipids are bound to proteins as a mechanism for serum transport. This bonding produces four major classes of lipoproteins: (1) chylomicrons, (2) very-low-density lipoproteins (VLDLs), (3) low-density lipoproteins (LDLs), and (4) high-density lipoproteins (HDLs). The relative concentrations of lipid and protein vary among classes. Of the four lipoprotein classes, LDL contains the highest concentration of cholesterol, whereas the chylomicrons and VLDL are richest in triglyceride. HDL contains the largest proportion of protein.

The association between serum cholesterol elevation and increased prematurity and severity of atherosclerosis is well established. Data from the Multiple Risk Factor Intervention Trial showed that as cholesterol levels increased above 180 mg/dl, the risk of CAD rose exponentially, with much higher rates for values greater than 240 mg/dl. Recent epidemiologic evidence suggests a correlation between atherogenesis and distinct patterns of cholesterol elevation. LDL cholesterol elevation is associated with increased coronary risk, whereas high levels of HDL cholesterol seem to act as a protective factor against CAD. Conversely, low levels of HDL appear atherogenic.

The term *hyperlipidemia* denotes an elevation of serum cholesterol or triglycerides above normal limits. Hyperlipidemia can be caused by high dietary fat intake or a genetic metabolic deficiency in ability to clear lipids through the liver, or it may be secondary to another underlying condition, such as hypothyroidism or poorly controlled diabetes mellitus. Lipoprotein elevations, or *hyperlipoproteinemias,* are described according to specific patterns of elevation. Five patterns or types have been identified: I, II (A and B), III, IV, and V; each corresponds to a characteristic elevation of one or more lipoprotein. These patterns are not specific indicators of particular lipid disorders; however, the type of elevation is used as a therapeutic guide. Only three types of hyperlipoproteinemia—II, III, and IV—are associated with premature atherosclerosis.

The term *familial hyperlipoproteinemia* is used to describe a group of primary lipid disorders resulting from inborn abnormalities in lipid metabolism. The following are four disorders known to be associated with coronary atherosclerosis:

Familial hypercholesterolemia

Familial hypertriglyceridemia

Familial combined hyperlipidemia (multiple lipoprotein-type hyperlipidemia)

Familial dysbetalipoproteinemia

Untreated familial hypercholesterolemia carries a particularly ominous prognosis: a 50% probability of developing premature atherosclerosis before 50 years of age.

The therapy of acquired or secondary hyperlipidemia is directed at correcting the underlying cause. Evidence from the Lipid Research Clinics Primary Prevention Trial has demonstrated that for every 1% lowering of cholesterol, there is a corresponding 2% decrease in cardiovascular risk. Therapeutic guidelines established by the National Cholesterol Education Program aim to lower LDL levels to less than 130 mg/dl for people with two or more coronary risk factors and to less than 160 mg/dl for people without risk factors (see box, p. 464).

Initial therapy consists of dietary management. A reduction of serum cholesterol can usually be accomplished with restriction of dietary cholesterol and saturated fat intake. Consumption of cholesterol-rich foods, such as organ meats and egg yolks, and of saturated ani-

GUIDELINES FOR THE TREATMENT OF HIGH BLOOD CHOLESTEROL IN ADULTS

PRIMARY PREVENTION

- For patient *without coronary atherosclerotic disease,* the goal for low-density lipoprotein (LDL) cholesterol depends on the risk status (see box on coronary artery disease [CAD] risk factors). The goals are as follows:

    <160 mg/dl if fewer than two other CAD risk factors are present

    <130 mg/dl if two or more CAD risk factors are present
- Dietary therapy and increased physical activity should begin when LDL cholesterol levels are as follows:

    ≥160 mg/dl in patients who have fewer than two risk factors

    ≥130 mg/dl in patients who have two or more risk factors
- Drug therapy may be considered after an adequate trial of dietary therapy when LDL cholesterol levels are as follows:

    ≥190 mg/dl in patients who have fewer than two risk factors

    ≥160 mg/dl in patients who have two or more risk factors

SECONDARY PREVENTION

- For the patient *with coronary atherosclerotic disease* or other clinical atherosclerotic disease, the goal for LDL cholesterol is as follows:

    ≤100 mg/dl using maximal dietary therapy and, if necessary, drug therapy

Modified from *Second Report of the Expert Panel on Detection, Evaluation, and Treatment of High Blood Cholesterol in Adults (Adult Treatment Panel II),* NIH Pub No 93-3095, National Heart, Lung, and Blood Institute, Washington, DC, 1993, National Institutes of Health.

mal fats should be reduced; substitution of lean meats, fish, poultry, and polyunsaturated vegetable fats should be encouraged. Whole-milk dairy products and tropical oils should be avoided. If triglycerides are elevated, restriction of alcohol consumption and weight normalization are essential.

If dietary therapy is unsuccessful or lipid elevations are severe, hypolipemic drugs are recommended. For hypercholesterolemia, cholestyramine or colestipol is indicated with the addition of nicotinic acid or clofibrate if necessary. A new class of drugs called HMG CoA-reductase inhibitors, such as lovastatin, show great promise for lowering LDL cholesterol levels. These drugs inhibit 3-hydroxy-3-methylglutaryl coenzyme A (HMG CoA) reductase, an enzyme in the cholesterol biosynthetic pathway. Consequently, LDL cholesterol synthesis is decreased and its clearance by the liver enhanced. Hyper-

triglyceridemia is usually most sensitive to clofibrate or nicotinic acid. For highly selected patients, partial ileal bypass surgery has been recommended to reduce serum cholesterol levels secondary to bile acid depletion.

Routine lipid screening tests must be recommended for relatives of individuals with familial hyperlipidemia or premature atherosclerotic heart disease so that appropriate therapy can be instituted to retard atherogenesis and its consequences.

Hypertension

Hypertension is recognized as the leading cause of death in the United States. Approximately one fourth of the adult population is hypertensive, and the incidence is greater among African Americans at every age beyond adolescence. The risk of developing not only cardiac disease but also neurologic, renal, and vascular disease is significantly increased among hypertensive individuals. The higher the blood pressure, the greater is the risk.

Hypertension is defined as an abnormal elevation of systolic and/or diastolic blood pressure. The traditional terms "mild" and "moderate" hypertension fail to convey the major impact of high blood pressure on the risk of cardiovascular disease. Thus a new classification was developed by the Joint National Committee on Detection, Evaluation, and Treatment of High Blood Pressure (Table 31-1).

The course of hypertensive disease is particularly insidious; hypertensive individuals can remain asymptomatic for many years. This latent period masks disease progression until significant organ damage occurs. Symptoms, if present, are typically nonspecific, such as headache or dizziness. If hypertension remains undetected and untreated, death results from heart failure, MI, cerebrovascular accident (CVA, stroke) or renal failure. However, early detection and effective treatment of hypertension can significantly decrease associated morbidity and mortality. Consequently, routine blood pressure screening is of paramount importance in hypertension control.

The cause of hypertension is unknown in approximately 95% of the cases. This idiopathic form of hypertension is referred to as *primary* or *essential* hypertension. The precise pathogenesis appears to be extremely complex with interaction of multiple variables. A genetic predisposition may exist. Other proposed mechanisms include alterations in the following: (1) renal excretion of sodium and water, (2) baroreceptor sensitivity, (3) vascular responsiveness, and (4) renin secretion. The remaining 5% of hypertensive disease is secondary to some other underlying disease process, such as renal parenchymal disease or primary aldosteronism.

The mechanism by which hypertension produces disability and death relates directly to its effect on the heart and blood vessels. The elevation in systemic blood pressure increases the resistance to left ventricular ejection;

TABLE 31-1   Classification of Blood Pressure for Adults Aged 18 Years or Older*

Category	Systolic (mm Hg)	Diastolic (mm Hg)
Normal	<130	<85
High normal	130-139	85-89
Hypertension†		
Stage 1 (mild)	140-159	90-99
Stage 2 (moderate)	160-179	100-109
Stage 3 (severe)	180-209	110-119
Stage 4 (very severe)	≥210	≥120

Modified from *Fifth Report of the Joint National Committee on Detection, Evaluation, and Treatment of High Blood Pressure,* NIH Pub No 93-1088, National Heart, Lung, and Blood Institute, Washington, DC, 1993, National Institutes of Health.

*Not taking antihypertensive drugs and not actuely ill. When systolic and diastolic pressures fall into different categories, the higher category should be selected.

†Based on the average of two or more readings taken at each of two or more visits after an initial screening.

consequently, cardiac workload is increased. In response, the ventricle hypertrophies to increase the force of contraction. However, the ability of the ventricle to sustain cardiac output via compensatory hypertrophy is eventually exceeded, and cardiac dilation and failure result. The heart is further compromised by an associated acceleration of coronary atherosclerosis. As coronary atherosclerosis progresses, myocardial oxygen supply is reduced. Angina or MI can result because a concurrent rise in myocardial oxygen demand occurs secondary to the ventricular hypertrophy and increased cardiac work. Approximately one half of hypertensive deaths are caused by MI or myocardial failure.

Hypertensive vascular damage is apparent throughout the periphery. Retinal vascular changes, easily observed and quantified during ophthalmoscopic examination, are useful in both the evaluation of disease progression and response to therapy. Accelerated atherosclerosis and medial necrosis of the aorta predispose to the formation of aneurysms and dissections. Structural changes in the small arteries and arterioles cause progressive occlusive vascular disease. As the vascular lumen narrows, arterial flow is compromised and tissue microinfarction can result. The consequences of these vascular changes are most striking in the brain and kidneys. Cerebrovascular occlusion or rupture accounts for approximately one third of hypertensive deaths. Progressive sclerosis of the renal vasculature with resultant organ dysfunction and renal failure can also be fatal. Approximately 10% to 15% of an untreated hypertensive population will develop renal failure (see also Parts Eight and Nine).

The goal of treating patients with essential or idiopathic hypertension is to prevent the morbidity and mortality associated with the disorder in the least intrusive manner. The primary goal is to achieve a blood pressure of

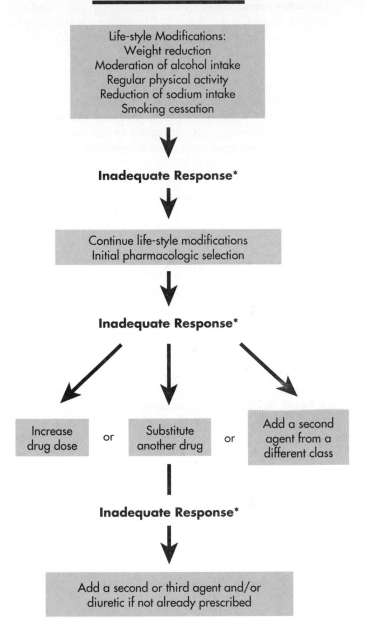

TREATMENT ALGORITHM

FIG. 31-3   Treatment algorithm for hypertension. *Adequate response** means patient achieved goal blood pressure or is making considerable progress toward this goal. [Redrawn from *Fifth Report of the Joint National Committee on Detection, Evaluation, and Treatment of High Blood Pressure,* NIH Pub No 93-1088, National Heart, Lung, and Blood Institute, Washington, DC, 1993, National Institutes of Health.

less than 140/90 mm Hg and control any other cardiovascular risk factors through life-style changes (Fig. 31-3). If life-style changes are inadequate to attain the blood pressure desired, drug therapy should be initiated. A single drug should be prescribed initially. The primary medication may be a diuretic, beta-adrenergic receptor blocker, calcium channel blocker, angiotensin-converting enzyme

(ACE) inhibitor, or alpha-adrenergic receptor blocker, depending on multiple patient considerations, including (1) cost (diuretics are generally the least expensive drug), (2) demographic characteristics (in general, African Americans are more responsive to diuretics and calcium channel blockers than to beta-blockers or ACE inhibitors), (3) concurrent diseases (beta-blockers may worsen asthma, diabetes mellitus, and peripheral ischemia but may improve angina, certain cardiac dysrhythmias, and migraine headache), and (4) quality of life (some antihypertensive drugs may cause undesirable side effects, such as impairment of sexual function). Secondary hypertension (i.e., hypertension caused by a specific organ defect, such as renal disease, Cushing's syndrome, pheochromocytoma, or primary hyperaldosteronism) is treated by attempting to reverse the underlying disease process.

Other Modifiable Factors

The risk of cigarette smoking is related to the number of cigarettes smoked per day, not to the length of time that the patient has smoked. An individual smoking more than a pack a day is twice as susceptible to coronary atherosclerotic disease as a nonsmoker. The effect of nicotine on catecholamine release by the autonomic nervous system seems to be the mechanism responsible. The effect, however, is noncumulative; exsmokers seem to revert to the low risk of nonsmokers.

There tends to be a greater prevalence, prematurity, and severity of coronary atherosclerosis among diabetic patients. The mechanism is as yet unresolved, but perhaps an abnormality in lipid metabolism or a predisposition to vascular degeneration associated with the impaired glucose tolerance is responsible. The typical American diet—high in calories, total fat, saturated fat, sugar, and salt—contributes to the development of hyperlipoproteinemia and obesity. Obesity increases cardiac work and oxygen demand and contributes to a sedentary life-style.

The list of contributing risk factors expands as additional biologic-environmental correlates with coronary heart disease are identified. At present, psychosocial stress seem contributory. An interesting relationship between the so-called type A behavior pattern and accelerated atherogenesis has been popularized by Rosenman and Friedman. The type A personality manifests intense competitiveness, ambition, aggressiveness, and a sense of time urgency. It is typically acknowledged that catecholamine release accompanies stress; however, the question arises as to whether stress is atherogenic or simply precipitates the attack. A theory of stress-induced atherogenesis might postulate neuroendocrine influences on circulatory dynamics, serum lipids, or blood clotting.

Atherosclerosis is a multifactorial disease, and substantiated evidence indicates certain risk factors accelerate atherogenesis. The complexity of the process is highlighted by the fact that in the presence of more than one risk factor, the susceptibility to atherogenesis is not simply additive; the factors are synergistic. The interaction of multiple factors significantly accelerates the disease process.

PATHOPHYSIOLOGY

Ischemia

Oxygen demand in excess of the capacity of the diseased vessels to supply oxygen results in localized *myocardial ischemia*. Transient ischemia causes reversible changes at the cellular and tissue levels, depressing myocardial function.

The lack of oxygen forces the myocardium to shift from aerobic metabolism to anaerobic metabolism. *Anaerobic* metabolism via glycolytic pathways is a much less efficient means of energy production than is *aerobic* metabolism via oxidative phosphorylation and the Krebs cycle; the production of high-energy phosphate is reduced considerably. The end product of anaerobic metabolism, lactic acid, accumulates, reducing cellular pH.

The combination of hypoxia, reduced energy availability, and acidosis rapidly impairs left ventricular function. The strength of contraction in the affected myocardial region is reduced; the fibers shorten inadequately with less force and velocity. In addition, the wall motion of the ischemic segment is abnormal; the segment passively bulges outward with each ventricular contraction (Fig. 31-4).

The reduced contractility and impaired wall motion alter hemodynamics. The hemodynamic response is variable, depending on the size of the ischemic segment and the degree of reflex compensatory response by the auto-

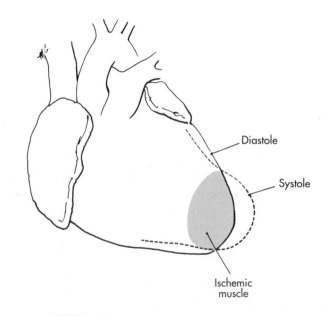

FIG. 31-4 Ischemic wall bulging during systole.

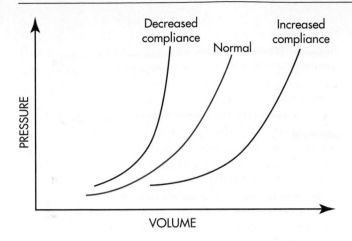

FIG. 31-5   Ventricular compliance, or the pressure-volume relationship of the ventricles. The line in the center indicates the typical relationship between pressure and volume. As volume is increased initially, only a small rise in pressure occurs. As volume increase continues, the rise in pressure is greater. The other lines indicate an alteration in pressure-volume relationships: decreased compliance on the left and increased compliance on the right. This represents a greater or lesser degree of stiffness of the ventricle in relation to the filling volume. Ventricular compliance is a dynamic phenomenon, and this property can change rapidly.

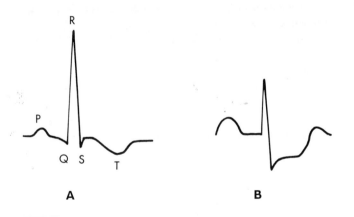

FIG. 31-6   Classic ECG changes with ischemia. **A,** T wave inversion. **B,** ST segment depression.

nomic nervous system. Depression of left ventricular function may lower cardiac output (CO) by reducing stroke volume (SV, the amount of blood ejected per beat). Reduction in systolic emptying increases ventricular volumes. As a result, left-sided pressures—the left ventricular end-diastolic pressure (LVEDP) and pulmonary capillary wedge pressure (PCWP)—rise. This pressure elevation is magnified by changes in wall compliance or distensibility induced by ischemia. A reduction in compliance occurs, accentuating the elevation in pressure for a given ventricular volume (Fig. 31-5).

During ischemia the manifest hemodynamic pattern is usually that of mild increments in blood pressure and

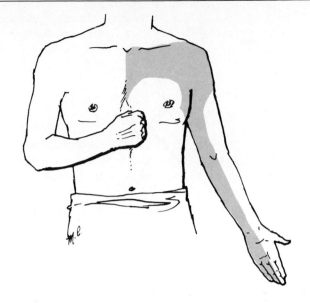

FIG. 31-7   Typical pattern of referred pain in angina pectoris.

heart rate before the onset of pain. Apparently, this pattern represents a sympathetic compensatory response to the depression of myocardial function. With the onset of pain, further sympathetic activation occurs. A depression of blood pressure would suggest ischemic involvement of a large area of myocardium or a vagal response.

Myocardial ischemia is typically associated with two characteristic electrocardiographic (ECG) changes resulting from alterations in cellular electrophysiology: T wave inversion and ST segment depression (Fig. 31-6). A variant form of angina, *Prinzmetal's angina,* is associated with ST segment elevation.

Ischemic attacks usually subside within minutes if the imbalance between oxygen supply and demand is corrected. The metabolic, functional, hemodynamic, and ECG changes are reversible.

Angina pectoris is the chest pain associated with myocardial ischemia. The exact mechanism by which ischemia produces pain is unclear. It seems that neural pain receptors are stimulated by the accumulated metabolites, by an unidentified chemical intermediary, or by local mechanical stress resulting from abnormal myocardial contraction. Typically, the pain is described as a substernal pressure, occasionally radiating down the medial aspect of the left arm. A clenched fist placed on the sternum graphically illustrates the classic pattern (Fig. 31-7). However, many patients never experience typical angina; anginal pain may mimic indigestion or a toothache. Classically, angina is precipitated by activities increasing myocardial oxygen demand, such as exercise, and is relieved within minutes by rest or nitroglycerin. The less common Prinzmetal's angina typically occurs at rest rather than during exertion and is caused by a localized spasm of an epicardial artery. The etiologic mechanism remains unclear.

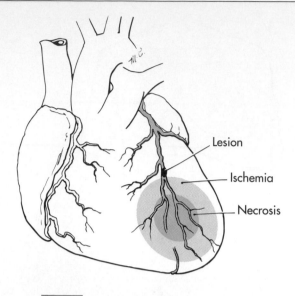

FIG. 31-8   Zones of necrosis and ischemia.

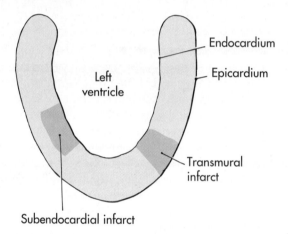

FIG. 31-9   Transmural and subendocardial infarction.

Infarction

Prolonged ischemia longer than 30 to 45 minutes causes irreversible cellular damage and muscle death or necrosis. Permanent cessation of contractile function occurs in the necrotic or infarcted area of the myocardium. The infarct is surrounded by a zone of ischemic, potentially viable tissue (Fig. 31-8). The ultimate size of the infarct depends on the fate of this ischemic zone; necrosis of this marginal area extends the infarct size, whereas reversal of the ischemia minimizes the residual necrosis.

MI usually affects the left ventricle. A *transmural infarction* involves the full thickness of the wall; a *subendocardial infarction* is limited to the inner half of the myocardium (Fig. 31-9). Infarctions are described further according to location on the ventricular wall (Fig. 31-10). For instance, an anterior MI involves the anterior wall of the left ventricle. Other common infarct sites are designated as inferior, lateral, posterior, and septal. Extensive infarctions involving large portions of the ventricle would be described accordingly, that is, as anteroseptal, anterolateral, or inferolateral. MI of the posterior wall of the right ventricle is also observed in approximately one fourth of left ventricular inferior wall infarctions. Biventricular compromise should be anticipated in this situation.

The infarct location correlates with disease in a particular region of the coronary circulation (Table 31-2). For example, anterior wall infarctions result from lesions in the left anterior descending artery. Knowing the coronary anatomy and the location of the infarct is of critical importance in the anticipation of complications associated with MI. For example, inferior wall infarction, usually the result of right coronary artery lesions, can be associated with variable degrees of heart block. This result is to be expected because the atrioventricular (AV) node re-

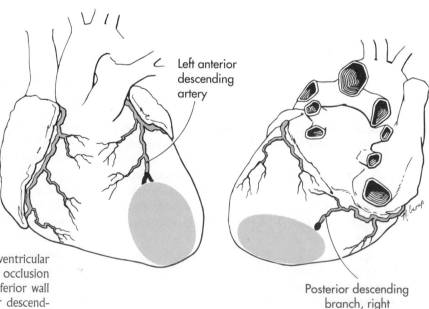

FIG. 31-10   Localization of infarcts on the ventricular wall. *Left,* Infarct of the anterior wall caused by occlusion of the left anterior descending artery. *Right,* Inferior wall infarction caused by occlusion of the posterior descending branch of the right coronary artery.

▶ TABLE 31-2   Correlation Among Ventricular
Surfaces, ECG Leads, and
Coronary Arteries

Surface of Left Ventricle	ECG Leads	Coronary Artery Usually Involved
Inferior	II, III, aVF	Right coronary
Lateral	I, aVL	Left circumflex
Anterior	V_2-V_4	Left anterior descending
Septal	V_1-V_2	Left anterior descending
Apical	V_5-V_6	Left anterior descending
Posterior	V_1-V_2 (reciprocal changes)	Left circumflex

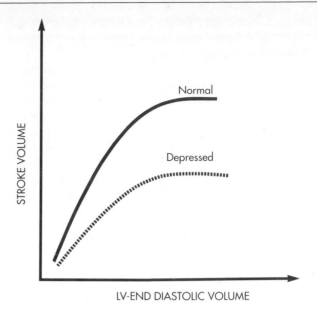

FIG. 31-11   Depression of the ventricular function curve. Normal curve *(solid line)* represents the relationship of stroke volume to left ventricular end-diastolic volume for the normal heart shown in Fig. 29-10. The failing heart *(depressed curve)* must increase the end-diastolic volume to maintain stroke volume. Therefore cardiac dilation occurs.

ceives its nutrient supply from the same vessel that nourishes the inferior wall of the left ventricle.

The infarcted muscle undergoes a sequence of changes during the healing process. Initially the infarcted muscle appears bruised and cyanotic as a result of regional stagnation of blood. Cellular edema and an inflammatory response with leukocytic infiltration ensue within 24 hours. Cardiac enzymes are released from the cells. Tissue degradation and removal of all necrotic fibers begin by the second or third day. During this phase, the necrotic wall is relatively thin. By about the third week, scar formation begins. Gradually, fibrous connective tissue replaces the necrotic muscle and undergoes progressive thickening. By the sixth week the scar is well established.

MI significantly depresses ventricular function as a result of the loss of contracility in the necrotic muscle and the impaired contractility in the surrounding ischemic muscle. Functionally, MI results in changes similar to those noted with ischemia: (1) reduced contractility, (2) abnormal wall motion, (3) altered ventricular wall compliance, (4) reduced SV, (5) diminished ejection fraction, (6) elevated ventricular end-systolic and end-diastolic volumes, and (7) increased LVEDP.

A wide spectrum of left ventricular dysfunction is apparent after MI. The degree of functional impairment depends on a number of factors, including the following:

1. *Infarct size.* Infarcts of more than 40% of the myocardium are associated with a high incidence of cardiogenic shock.
2. *Infarct location.* Anterior wall infarction is more likely to significantly depress mechanical function than inferior wall damage.
3. *Function of uninvolved myocardium.* Old infarcts would compromise residual myocardial function.
4. *Collateral circulation.* Collateral circulation, via either preexisting arterial anastomoses or new channels, can develop in response to chronic ischemia and regional hypoperfusion, improving blood flow to the threatened myocardium.

5. *Cardiovascular compensatory mechanisms.* Reflex compensatory mechanisms operate to maintain CO and peripheral perfusion.

Reflex sympathetic augmentation of the heart rate and contractility can improve ventricular function. Generalized arteriolar constriction increases total peripheral resistance (TPR), thereby increasing mean arterial pressure (MAP). Venoconstriction reduces venous capacity, increasing venous return to the heart and ventricular filling. Increased ventricular filling elevates the force of contraction and subsequent ejection volumes up to a point, beyond which the curve flattens. This process is best illustrated by comparing the normal ventricular function curve with that of the compromised myocardium (Fig. 31-11). With depression of ventricular function, higher diastolic filling pressures are necessary to maintain SV. Elevation of diastolic filling pressure and ventricular volume stretches myocardial fibers, increasing the force of contraction according to Starling's law. Circulatory filling pressures can be increased further by renal retention of sodium and water. As a result, MI is often associated with transient left ventricular enlargement caused by compensatory cardiac dilation. If necessary, compensatory cardiac hypertrophy can also occur to increase the force of contraction and ventricular emptying.

In summary, a battery of reflex responses are available to forestall deterioration of CO and perfusion pressure: (1) augmentation of heart rate and contractility, (2) generalized vasoconstriction, (3) sodium and water retention, (4) ventricular dilation, and (5) ventricular hypertrophy.

However, all compensatory responses can eventually contribute to further myocardial deterioration by increasing myocardial oxygen demand.

The hemodynamic presentation after MI is maintained at normal levels. Heart rate is usually not persistently elevated unless extensive myocardial depression occurs. Blood pressure is a function of the interaction between myocardial depression and autonomic reflexes. The autonomic response to MI is not always the predictable sympathetic support of the compromised circulation. Pain or stimulation of parasympathetic ganglia in the myocardium, especially in the inferior wall, complicates the hemodynamic response. Parasympathetic stimulation, most often seen in inferior MI, reduces the heart rate and blood pressure, adversely affecting CO and peripheral perfusion. This type of response is known as *vasovagal*.

MI is classically associated with a characteristic diagnostic triad. First, the typical clinical picture consists of severe, prolonged chest discomfort (often described as pressure, heaviness, or fullness) frequently associated with sweating, nausea, vomiting, and a sense of impending doom. However, between 20% and 60% of nonfatal MIs are "silent" or asymptomatic. Approximately half of these are truly silent rather than atypical in presentation

and are diagnosed only as the result of a routine ECG or postmortem examination.

Second, serum levels of the cardiac enzymes released by the necrotic myocardial cells are elevated. The released enzymes include creatine phosphokinase, or creatine kinase (CK, or CPK), aspartate aminotransferase (AST; formerly serum glutamic-oxaloacetic transaminase, SGOT), and lactic dehydrogenase (LDH). Although a valuable adjunct to diagnosis, enzyme interpretation is limited because the measured enzyme elevations are not specific indicators of myocardial damage; coexisting processes can produce misleading enzyme elevations. Measurement of isoenzymes, enzyme fractions specifically released by the damaged myocardium, increases diagnostic accuracy. The two isoenzymes most helpful in the diagnosis of acute MI are CK-MB and LDH_1 and LDH_2 because they are specifically concentrated in cardiac muscle. CK-MB rises first after an acute MI but returns to normal within 2 to 3 days. LDH rises later than CK, so it is useful when CK has not been measured within 24 hours after an acute MI. Normally, serum levels of LDH_2 are greater than LDH_1. However, after an acute MI, the ratio reverses, producing the *LDH flip pattern* (LDH_1/LDH_2 ratio greater than 1.0). SGOT (AST)

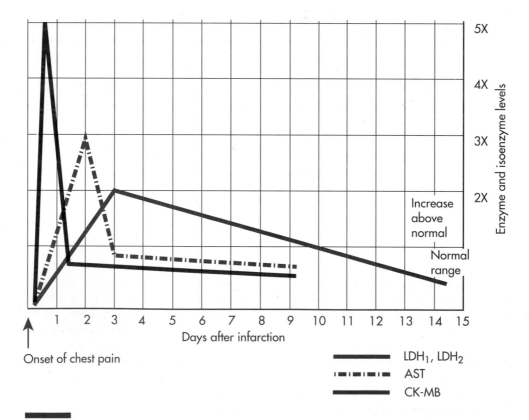

FIG. 31-12 Serum enzyme and isoenzyme levels after acute myocardial infarction (MI). CK-MB rises within 6 to 8 hours after acute MI, peaks in 12 to 24 hours, and returns to normal within 48 to 72 hours. LDH_1 and LDH_2 rise within 12 to 48 hours after acute MI, peak in 2 to 5 days, and return to normal within 7 to 10 days. The time course for AST (SGOT) is intermediate between CK-MB and LDH. *CK,* Creatine kinase; *LDH,* lactic dehydrogenase; *AST,* aspartate aminotransferase.

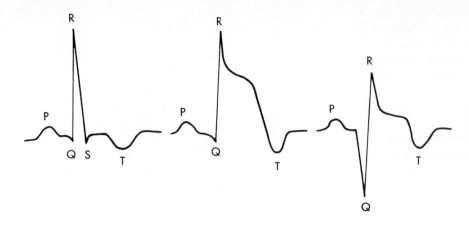

FIG. 31-13   ECG changes overlying an area of MI. T wave inversion *(left)*, ST segment elevation *(middle)*, and pronounced Q waves *(right)*. Q waves may develop early in an infarct, and if they are truly indicative of necrosis, they are irreversible. The ST segment and T wave changes result from the ischemic injury and disappear over time.

was used in the diagnosis of acute MI for many years but has fallen out of favor because of its lack of tissue specificity and because its time course of elevation is intermediate between CK and LDH, thus offering little advantage. Fig. 31-12 depicts the characteristic time courses of the elevation of these enzymes after an acute MI.

Finally, ECG changes, consisting of pronounced Q waves, ST segment elevation, and inverted T waves, are evident during acute infarction (Fig. 31-13). These changes are apparent in the leads overlying the area of myocardial necrosis. Over time the ST segment and T wave changes revert to normal; only the abnormal Q waves persist as ECG evidence of a previous infarction. However, only one half to two thirds of patients manifest this classic ECG evolution of an acute MI. In 30% of patients diagnosed with an infarct, no Q waves develop. Furthermore, the correlation between the presence of a Q wave and transmural infarction is poor. Nearly 50% of nontransmural infarctions produce Q waves. As a result, use of Q wave and non–Q wave infarction is favored over transmural and nontransmural (or "subendocardial").

Complications of Ischemia and Infarction
Congestive heart failure

Congestive heart failure is a state of circulatory congestion produced by myocardial dysfunction. The location of the congestion depends on the ventricle involved. Left ventricular dysfunction, or left heart failure, produces pulmonary venous congestion, whereas right ventricular dysfunction, or right heart failure, results in systemic venous congestion. Failure of both ventricles is referred to as *biventricular failure*. Failure of the left side of the heart is the most common mechanical complication after MI, occurring approximately 50% of the time.

MI compromises myocardial function by reducing contractility, producing abnormal wall motion, and altering chamber compliance. As the ability of the left ventricle to empty effectively lessens, SV falls and residual ventricular volumes rise. Consequently, left ventricular pressures rise. This pressure elevation is transmitted

backward into the pulmonary venous circuit. If the hydrostatic pressure in the pulmonary capillary bed exceeds the vascular oncotic pressure, fluid transudation into the interstitium results. Further elevation of pressure eventually causes pulmonary edema because of fluid seepage into the alveoli.

The fall in SV elicits a compensatory sympathetic response. Heart rate and contractile force increase to maintain CO. Peripheral vasoconstriction occurs to stabilize arterial pressure and redistribute blood flow away from the nonvital organs, such as the kidney and skin, to maintain perfusion of the vital organs. Venoconstriction increases venous return to the right side of the heart, further augmenting contractile force according to Starling's law of the heart. Activation of the renin-angiotensin-aldosterone system in response to the fall in renal blood flow and glomerular filtration rate results in renal retention of sodium and water. This further increases venous return.

The clinical manifestations of heart failure reflect the degree of myocardial compromise and the efficacy and magnitude of compensatory responses. The following findings are frequently noted during left heart failure:

1. *Signs and symptoms:* dyspnea, oliguria, weakness, fatigue, pallor, weight gain
2. *Auscultation:* rales, third heart sound (caused by dilation and noncompliance of the ventricle during rapid filling)
3. *ECG:* tachycardia
4. *Chest radiograph:* cardiomegaly, pulmonary venous congestion, vascular redistribution to the upper lobes

Failure of the left side of the heart can progress to failure of the right as pulmonary vascular pressures rise, stressing the right ventricle. In addition to this indirect route of compromise via the pulmonary vasculature, left ventricular dysfunction directly affects right ventricular function via shared anatomic and biochemical features. The two ventricles share a common wall, the interventricular septum, and lie within the pericardium. In addition, biochemical changes, such as depletion of myocardial stores of norepinephrine during failure, can adversely affect both ventricles. Finally, infarction of the right ventricle can occur, particularly in association with inferior wall infarction of the left ventricle. Right ventricular infarction obviously predisposes the right side of the heart to failure. The systemic venous congestion produced by right heart failure is manifested by findings such as engorged neck veins, hepatomegaly, and peripheral edema.

Cardiogenic shock

Cardiogenic shock results from profound left ventricular dysfunction after massive infarction, usually involving more than 40% of the left ventricle. A vicious, self-perpetuating cycle of progressively irreversible hemodynamic changes ensues: (1) reduced peripheral perfusion, (2) reduced coronary perfusion, and (3) increased pulmonary congestion. Hypotension, metabolic acidosis, and hypoxemia further depress myocardial function. The incidence of cardiogenic shock is 10% to 15%. The associated mortality is approximately 80% to 90% (see Chapter 33 for a detailed discussion).

Papillary muscle dysfunction

Closure of the mitral valve during ventricular systole depends on the functional integrity of the left ventricular papillary muscles and chordae tendineae. Ischemic dysfunction or necrotic rupture of a papillary muscle impairs mitral valve function and permits varying degrees of leaflet eversion into the atria during systole (Fig. 31-14). Valvular incompetence results in retrograde flow from the left ventricle into the left atrium with two consequences: a reduction in forward aortic flow and an elevation in left atrial and pulmonary venous congestion. The volume of regurgitant flow depends on the extent of papillary muscle disease; ischemia typically causes mild to moderate congestive heart failure. However, papillary muscle necrosis and rupture is a catastrophic event with rapid deterioration into pulmonary edema and shock. Although much less common, papillary muscle rupture may also occur in the right ventricle. Severe tricuspid regurgitation and right ventricular failure would result.

Ventricular septal defect

Necrosis of the interventricular septum can result in rupture of the septal wall, which creates a ventricular septal defect. Because the septum receives a dual blood supply from arteries descending the anterior and posterior surfaces of the interventricular groove, septal rupture indicates extensive CAD involving more than one artery.

Essentially, the rupture establishes a second outflow tract from the left ventricle. During each ventricular contraction, competitive outflow occurs through the aorta and the septal defect (Fig. 31-15). Because pressures on the left side of the heart are much greater than pressures on the right side, blood will be shunted through the defect from left to right, from the area of greater pressure to the area of lesser pressure. Great volumes of blood can be shunted over to the right side of the heart, reducing the amount of blood available to be ejected via the aorta. Sig-

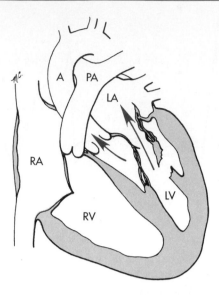

FIG. 31-14 Papillary muscle rupture. *A,* Aorta; *PA,* pulmonary artery; *LA,* left atrium; *RA,* right atrium; *LV,* left ventricle; *RV,* right ventricle.

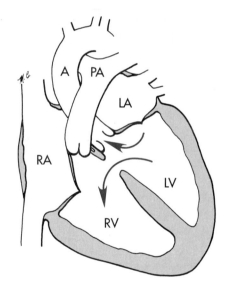

FIG. 31-15 Ventricular setpal defect. (See Fig. 31-14 for abbreviations.)

nificant reductions in CO with concurrent elevations in right ventricular work and pulmonary congestion result.

Cardiac rupture

Although rare, rupture of the ventricular free wall may occur early in the course of transmural infarction during the phase of necrotic tissue removal before scar formation. The thin, necrotic wall ruptures, resulting in massive bleeding into the pericardial sac. The relatively inelastic pericardial sac is unable to distend. Thus the blood-filled pericardial sac compresses the heart, producing *cardiac tamponade* (Fig. 31-16). Cardiac tamponade reduces ve-

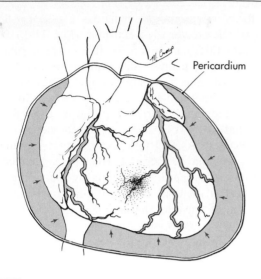

FIG. 31-16   Cardiac tamponade (blood within pericardial space).

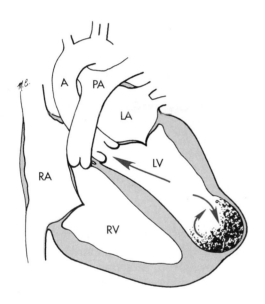

FIG. 31-17   Ventricular aneurysm. (See Fig. 31-14 for abbreviations.)

nous return and CO. Death usually occurs within a few minutes unless the condition is quickly recognized and relieved by needle tap.

Ventricular aneurysm

Transient paradoxical bulging of the ischemic myocardium is common, and a sustained ventricular aneurysm occurs in approximately 15% of patients. The aneurysm is usually on the anterior or apical surface of the heart. Ventricular aneurysms balloon outward with each systole, passively distended by a portion of what should have been the SV (Fig. 31-17). Ventricular aneurysms can produce three problematic consequences: (1) chronic congestive

heart failure, (2) systemic embolization of mural thrombi, and (3) refractory ventricular dysrhythmias.

Thromboembolism

Necrosis of the ventricular endothelium roughens the endothelial surface, predisposing to thrombus formation. A fragment of an intracardiac mural thrombus can dislodge and embolize systemically. A second potential site of thrombus formation is the systemic venous system. Venous embolization, a potential complication of bed rest after MI, would cause pulmonary embolism, a complication discussed in Part Seven.

Pericarditis

Transmural infarction can roughen the epicardial layer in contact with the pericardium, irritating the pericardial surface and resulting in an inflammatory reaction. Rarely, a pericardial effusion, or fluid accumulation between the layers, occurs. Fluid accumulation is rarely significant enough to cause cardiac tamponade. Pain associated with pericarditis may be severe.

Dressler's syndrome

This post-MI syndrome is a benign inflammatory response with pleuropericardial pain. It is postulated that Dressler's syndrome might represent a hypersensitivity reaction to the necrotic myocardium.

Dysrhythmia

A disturbance of cardiac rhythm, or dysrhythmia, is the most common complication during MI, with an incidence of approximately 90%. Dysrhythmias result from alterations in myocardial cellular electrophysiology. The electrophysiologic alteration is manifested by a change in the configuration of the action potential, which is the graphic recording of cellular electrical activity. For instance, sympathetic stimulation increases the slope of spontaneous depolarization, thereby increasing the heart rate (Fig. 31-18). Clinically, dysrhythmia diagnosis is based on interpretation of the ECG.

Multiple predisposing factors account for the high incidence of dysrhythmias in the setting of coronary atherosclerotic disease: (1) tissue ischemia, (2) hypoxemia, (3) autonomic nervous system influences (e.g., parasympathetic stimulation that decreases heart rate), (4) metabolic derangements (e.g., lactic acidosis caused by compromised tissue perfusion), (5) hemodynamic abnormalities (e.g., reduction in coronary perfusion associated with hypertension, (6) drugs (e.g., digitalis toxicity), and (7) electrolyte imbalance (e.g., hypokalemia with excessive diuresis).

Cardiac rhythm abnormalities can be categorized according to the following basic mechanisms: abnormal automaticity, abnormal conduction, or a combination of the two.

The normal heart rate (HR) is between 60 and 100 beats per minute (bpm). An HR less than 60 bpm is re-

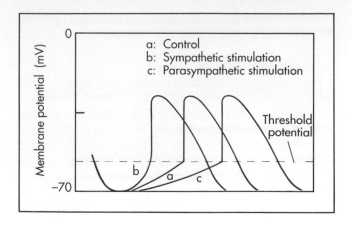

FIG. 31-18 Effects of sympathetic and parasympathetic stimulation on the slope of the action potential of a sinoatrial node cell. (From Vander AJ, Sherman JH, Luciano DS: *Human physiology*, New York, 1970, McGraw-Hill.)

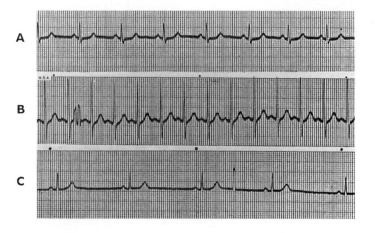

FIG. 31-19 **A,** Normal sinus rhythm (NSR), heart rate of 69. **B,** Sinus tachycardia, heart rate of 125. **C,** Sinus bradycardia, heart rate of 41.

ferred to as a *bradycardia,* whereas a *tachycardia* indicates an HR greater than 100 bpm (Fig. 31-19). Both rate abnormalities can adversely affect cardiac function. Because HR is a primary determinant of CO (cardiac output = heart rate × stroke volume), extreme increments or reductions in HR can lower CO. Tachycardias lower it by reducing ventricular filling time and SV, and bradycardias lower it by reducing the frequency of ventricular ejection. As CO falls, arterial pressure and peripheral perfusion decrease. Furthermore, tachycardias can aggravate myocardial ischemia by increasing myocardial oxygen demand while simultaneously reducing the duration of diastole, the period of greatest coronary flow, thereby compromising coronary oxygen supply.

Any cardiac impulse originating outside of the sinus node is considered abnormal and is referred to as an *ectopic beat.* Ectopic beats can originate in the atria, the AV junction, or the ventricles under two conditions: (1) failure or excessive slowing of the sinus node, or (2) premature activation of another cardiac site. Ectopic beats resulting from sinus node failure serve a protective function by initiating a cardiac impulse before prolonged cardiac standstill can occur (Fig. 31-20). These beats are called *escape beats.* If the sinus node fails to resume normal function, the ectopic site will assume the role of pacemaker and sustain the cardiac rhythm. This is referred to as an *escape rhythm.* After the sinus node resumes normal function, the escape focus is suppressed.

Premature activation of cardiac sites other than the sinus node disrupts the normal cardiac cycle, impulses occur prematurely before the sinus node recovers sufficiently from one beat to initiate another (Fig. 31-21). These beats are referred to as *premature beats.* Premature beats are produced by two basic mechanisms: (1) increased automaticity or (2) reentry, a form of abnormal conduction. Reentry is by far the more common mechanism. During *reentry,* illustrated in Fig. 31-22, a single cardiac impulse reenters and excites a myocardial region previously activated, producing a premature beat. These

FIG. 31-20 Escape beats. A period of cardiac asystole may result when the sinoatrial (SA) node fails to send impulses to the atria unless the lower pacemakers, or escape pacemakers, take over to maintain the cardiac rhythm. If the first beat after the sinus arrest originates in the AV node, it is called a junctional or nodal escape beat. If the impulse after sinus arrest originates in the ventricles, it is called a ventricular escape beat.

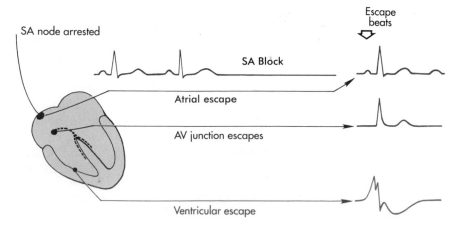

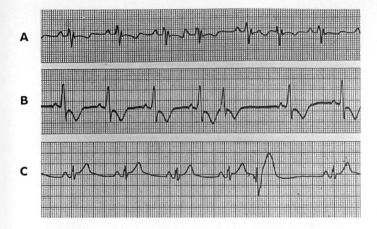

FIG. 31-21   Premature beats. **A,** This is NSR with two premature atrial beats (the fourth and sixth P waves are premature and obviously not sinus-conducted beats). **B,** Junctional premature beat (fifth complex). **C,** This is NSR with one premature ventricular complex (PVC) followed by a full compensatory pause. (From Conover MB: *Understanding electrocardiography,* ed 6, St Louis, 1994, Mosby.)

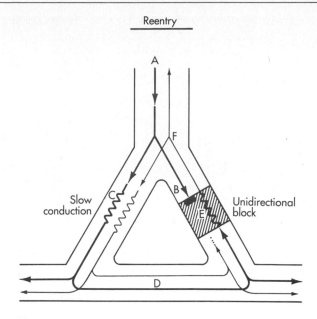

Reentry

FIG. 31-22   Features of reentry. An impulse is shown entering both limbs of an available circuit at point *A.* The impulse encounters antegrade (unidirectional) block in the shaded area at point *B* because the effective refractory period of this region exceeds that of the tissue in region *C.* The impulse is conducted with delay through region *C,* traverses region *D* distal to the site of unidirectional block, and retrogradely penetrates in region E, resulting in completion and perpetuation of the reeentry circuit. Slow conduction in regions *C* or *E* allows sufficient time for recovery of excitability to occur in region *F,* following its previous depolarization by the initiating (antegrade) impulse. A delicate balance of conduction delay and differential refractoriness must coexist in two limbs of the circuit for reentry to be initiated and sustained. Exit into and excitation of the surrounding myocardium by the reentrant impulse may occur at any point in the circuit. The rate of the resulting dysrhythmia is determined both by the conduction time within the reentry circuit and by the refractory period of the surrounding myocardium. (From Johnson RA, Haber E, Austen WG: *The practice of cardiology,* Boston, 1980, Little, Brown.)

sites can produce isolated premature beats or sustained tachycardias; dysrhythmias can develop in the atria, AV junction, or ventricles and are designated accordingly. For instance, an atrial premature beat originates in the atria, whereas ventricular tachycardia is ventricular in origin.

Ventricular premature beats are the most common form of dysrhythmia (Fig. 31-23, *A* and *B*). However, ventricular irritability can degenerate into life-threatening ventricular tachycardia or ventricular fibrillation. *Ventricular tachycardia* severely reduces CO as a result of the rapid rate, usually greater than 120 bpm, and the loss of mechanical synchrony between atrial and ventricular contraction (Fig. 31-23, *C*). *Ventricular fibrillation* results in the abrupt cessation of effective ventricular contraction; the ventricles quiver without coordination (Fig. 31-23, *D*).

Atrial dysrhythmias can be conceptualized along a continuum of rate acceleration associated with progressive reduction in atrial function: (1) *premature atrial beat,* (2) *atrial tachycardia*—atrial rate approximately 150 bpm, (3) *atrial flutter*—atrial rate approximately 300 bpm, and (4) *atrial fibrillation*—quivering, uncoordinated atrial activity (Fig. 31-24). To protect the ventricles from responding to extremely rapid atrial stimulation, the AV node does not normally conduct atrial impulses at rates greater than 180 bpm. For instance, in atrial flutter with an atrial rate of 300 bpm, only every second or third atrial impulse is conducted; consequently the ventricular rate is 100 to 150 bpm. The hemodynamic response to atrial dysrhythmias depends on the ventricular rate and the efficacy of atrial contraction. For instance, in atrial fibrillation, the atrial musculature is unable to contract ef-

fectively and actively contribute to ventricular filling; thus CO may fall.

Heart block is a delay or interruption in impulse conduction between the atria and the ventricles. The cardiac impulse normally spreads from the sinus node along internodal pathways to the AV node and ventricles within 0.20 second (normal PR interval); ventricular depolarization occurs within 0.10 second (normal QRS duration). Heart block occurs in three progressively severe forms. In *first-degree heart block,* all impulses are conducted through the AV junction; however, conduction time is abnormally prolonged. In *second-degree heart block,* some impulses are conducted to the ventricles but some impulses are blocked. There are two types of second-degree heart block. Wenckebach (Mobitz I) is characterized by repetitive cycles of progressively lengthening AV con-

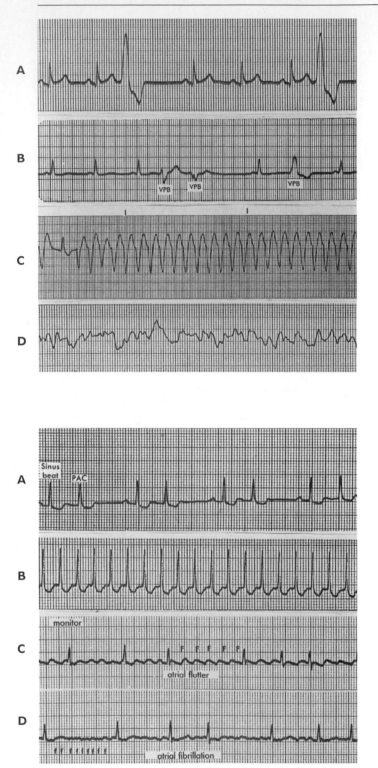

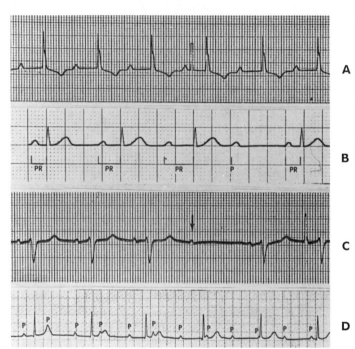

FIG. 31-23 Ventricular dysrhythmias. **A,** Unifocal ventricular premature beats or premature ventricular complexes (*VPBs* or PVCs); since the VPBs are similar in shape, they originated from the same ectopic focus. **B,** Multifocal VPBs have different shapes in the same lead. **C,** Sustained ventricular tachycardia (VT). **D,** Ventricular fibrillation (VF). (From Goldberger AL, Goldberger E: *Clinical electrocardiography,* ed 5, St Louis, 1994, Mosby.)

FIG. 31-25 Heart block. **A,** First-degree heart block with uniform prolonged PR intervals of 0.38 second. **B,** Second-degree heart block—Wenckebach or Mobitz I. The PR interval lengthens progressively with successive beats until one P wave is not conducted at all. **C,** Second-degree heart block—Mobitz II. **D,** Third-degree or complete heart block characterized by independent atrial *(P)* and ventricular (QRS) activity. The PR intervals are completely variable. (From Goldberger AL, Goldberger E: *Clinical electrocardiography,* ed 5, St Louis, 1994, Mosby.)

FIG. 31-24 Atrial dysrhythmias. **A,** Atrial bigeminy. Each sinus beat is followed by an atrial premature beat or premature atrial complex *(PAC).* **B,** Paroxysmal atrial complex (PAC). **B,** Paroxysmal atrial tachycardia (PAT). **C,** Atrial flutter. Note the sawtooth flutter *(F)* waves. **D,** Atrial fibrillation. Note the fine fibrillatory *(f)* waves. (From Goldberger AL, Goldberger E: *Clinical electrocardiography,* ed 5, St Louis, 1994, Mosby.)

duction time, culminating in the nonconduction of one beat. The second type, Mobitz II, involves conduction of some impulses with a constant AV conduction time and nonconduction of other impulses. In *third-degree heart block,* no impulses are conducted to the ventricles. Unless *escape pacemakers,* either junctional or ventricular in origin, begin to function, cardiac standstill results (Fig. 31-25). *Bundle branch block* is an interruption of conduction in the bundle branches that prolongs ventricular depolarization time beyond 0.10 second.

THERAPEUTIC INTERVENTION

Primary Prevention

The most critical therapeutic intervention in the setting of coronary atherosclerosis is the primary prevention of the disease. Disease prevention is essential for many reasons, including the following:

1. Clinically apparent disease is preceded by a long latent period with silent progression of disease, apparently in early adulthood. Lesions considered to be precursors of atherosclerotic disease have been identified in the coronary arterial walls of children and young adults.
2. No curative therapy exists for coronary atherosclerotic disease. Once the disease is recognizable clinically, therapy is essentially palliative, undertaken to minimize the severity of clinical sequelae and potentially to slow disease progression.
3. The consequences of coronary atherosclerosis can be catastrophic. MI often occurs with little or no warning; the incidence of sudden death is high. More than half of the deaths associated with MI occur during the first few hours of infarction, before hospitalization.
4. Coronary atherosclerosis is the leading cause of death in the United States. According to the American Heart Association, approximately 480,170 deaths were attributable to coronary heart disease in the United States in 1992.

Because the precise pathogenesis of atherosclerosis is still undefined, the control of risk factors known to increase susceptibility to atherogenesis is the crux of disease prophylaxis. The risk factors amenable to modification are (1) hyperlipidemia, (2) hypertension, (3) smoking, (4) obesity, (5) sedentary life-style, (6) diabetes mellitus, and (7) psychosocial stress. Measures should be initiated to eliminate or control these risk factors in every individual, with major emphasis on the first three.

When should risk factor surveillance and control be initiated? Currently, the concept of disease prophylaxis has been applied primarily to "coronary-prone" adults, those with identified risk factors, and individuals with evidence of disease. However, control of risk factors earlier in life seems more likely to prevent atherogenesis or retard disease progression so that a substantive reduction in cardiac morbidity and mortality can be achieved. The emphasis must be on health education with early detection and control of risk factors rather than on treatment of the clinical sequelae of established disease.

Treatment

Ischemia and infarction

The therapeutic aim with myocardial ischemia is to correct the imbalance between myocardial oxygen demand and oxygen supply. Restoration of oxygen balance can be accomplished by two mechanisms: reducing oxy-

MEDICAL THERAPY OF MYOCARDIAL INFARCTION/ISCHEMIA

REDUCTION OF OXYGEN DEMAND

Pharmacologic reduction in cardiac work
- Nitroglycerin
- Beta-adrenergic blockers
- Angiotensin-converting enzyme (ACE) inhibitors
- Diuretics
- Vasodilators
- Sedatives or analgesics if agitation or ischemic pain is unrelieved by nitroglycerin
- Calcium channel blockers

ELEVATION OR REESTABLISHMENT OF OXYGEN SUPPLY

- Supplemental oxygen
- Nitroglycerin
- Antidysrhythmics
- Anticoagulants, antiplatelet aggregants
- Thrombolytic agents if total thrombotic occlusion present
- Calcium channel blockers

gen demand and elevating or reestablishing oxygen supply (see box above). (American College of Cardiology/American Heart Association Task Force, 1990; Reeder and Gersh, 1993).

To reduce oxygen demand, the physiologic variables determining myocardial oxygen requirements must be controlled. Three major determinants of oxygen demand are amenable to therapy: (1) heart rate (HR), (2) contractile force, and (3) afterload (arterial pressure and ventricular size). Reducing HR, force of contraction, arterial pressure, and ventricular size reduces cardiac work and oxygen demand. The effects of certain drugs used to manipulate these variables and thereby reduce myocardial ischemia are depicted in Fig. 31-26 and are discussed next.

Nitroglycerin, the therapeutic mainstay for reversal of ischemia, relieves angina (1) primarily by peripheral vasodilation of the arterial and venous beds, which decreases preload, and (2) secondarily by improving the distribution of coronary blood flow to ischemic areas by dilating epicardial arteries and increasing collateral blood flow to ischemic myocardium. Arterial vasodilation reduces arterial pressure, thereby decreasing the systemic resistance to ventricular ejection and afterload. Dilation of the veins increases the capacity of the venous blood with pooling of blood in the periphery. As a result, venous return to the heart falls, decreasing ventricular volume and size. Consequently, oxygen demand is reduced. Intravenous (IV) and long-acting nitrates exhibit similar effects and are useful for reducing ischemia. In the pa-

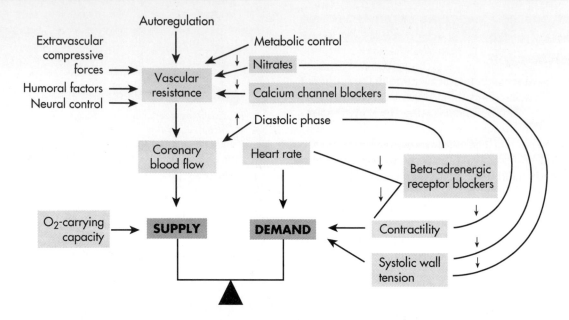

FIG. 31-26   The effects of nitrates, beta-adrenergic receptor blockers, and calcium channel blockers on myocardial oxygen supply and demand. (Modified from Ardehali A, Ports TA: *Chest* 98(3):702, 1990.)

tient with acute MI, sublingual nitroglycerin should be given initially unless the systolic blood pressure is less than 90 mm Hg. If the patient continues to have ischemic pain, the sublingual nitroglycerin may be repeated until an IV line has been inserted. IV nitroglycerin is then given and titrated to control the patient's pain and blood pressure. Administration of nitrates is not generally recommended in patients with right ventricular infarction because of the resultant decrease in venous return and consequent decrease in right ventricular filling pressure and stroke volume (SV).

Beta-adrenergic blocking agents interrupt ischemia by selectively inhibiting the effects of the sympathetic nervous system on the heart; these effects are mediated by beta-receptors. Beta-receptor stimulation increases HR and force of contraction. Beta-blocking agents block these effects, reducing HR and force of contraction, thereby reducing myocardial oxygen requirements. The reduced contractile force does produce a mild increment on ventricular size by lowering SV. However, in the absence of heart failure, this slight increment in oxygen demand is greatly outweighed by the reduced demand prompted by blockade of the sympathetic effects on HR and contractility. If sinus tachycardia and hypertension occur in the setting of an acute MI, IV metoprolol tartrate (Lopressor) has been used to decrease myocardial oxygen demand, thereby limiting infarct size and decreasing ischemic pain. Contraindications for the use of beta-blocking agents in the treatment of acute MI include the following: HR less than 60 bpm, systolic blood pressure less than 100 mm Hg, moderate to severe left ventricular failure, AV block; and severe chronic obstructive pulmonary disease.

Other pharmacologic interventions similarly act on the determinants of myocardial oxygen demand to correct the oxygenation imbalance. Diuretics reduce blood volume and venous return to the heart, thereby reducing ventricular volume and size. Vasodilators, ACE inhibitors, and calcium channel blockers all decrease arterial pressure and resistance to ventricular ejecton. Consequently, afterload is reduced. ACE inhibitors act by selectively suppressing renin-angiotensin I to angiotensin II; dilation of arterial and venous vessels occurs. Calcium channel blockers act by inhibiting calcium ion reflux across the cell membrane in cardiac and smooth muscle, thus producing relaxation and vasodilation of coronary and peripheral arteries. Sedatives can also reduce angina produced by stress.

Thrombolytic therapy. Based on the premise that acute MI is caused by coronary thrombosis in most patients, interventions have been aimed at dissolving coronary thrombosis soon after the onset of acute MI to salvage myocardium, reducing the ultimate size of the infarction. Initiation of treatment within 3 to 6 hours from the onset of symptoms has been widely accepted as a limiting factor for the application of thrombolytic therapy because myocardial necrosis will occur if coronary reperfusion is not carried out before irreversible damage occurs. Recently, however, several large trials of thrombolytic therapy have shown a significant decrease in mortality of patients with ongoing ischemia treated up to 24 hours after initiation of symptoms.

The mainstay of acute coronary reperfusion rests with a group of agents called *fibrinolytics*. The agents include drugs such as streptokinase, urokinase, tissue plasminogen activator (TPA), and anisoylated plasminogen streptokinase activator complex (APSAC). These agents activate the fibrinolytic system, thereby producing clot lysis. By various mechanisms, these agents promote conversion of plasminogen to plasmin, a proteolytic enzyme capable of lysing fibrin clot. By fibrin degradation by plasmin, clot lysis occurs and flow is reestablished to the acutely occluded coronary artery. After fibrinolytic therapy, anticoagulation with heparin and antiplatelet therapy with aspirin are usually carried out to prevent thrombosis. Angioplasty may also be performed to reduce the likelihood of rethrombosis.

Primary angioplasty. Angioplasty as a primary treatment for MI has recently been investigated. The Primary Angioplasty in Myocardial Infarction Trial (PAMI) found a significant decrease in mortality compared with thrombolytic therapy. Although this therapy is not available for most patients experiencing MI and treated in a community hospital where acute cardiac catheterization is not available, it may be lifesaving in specific cases when thrombolytic therapy is contraindicated (see later discussion).

Two potential consequences of myocardial dysfunction that can further the reduction in myocardial oxygen supply are hypoxemia and hypotension. In the setting of *hypoxemia,* oxygen administration can increase the oxygen content of arterial blood and, consequently, myocardial oxygen delivery. *Hypotension* reduces coronary perfusion pressure. This result is particularly worrisome because diseased coronary vessels, unable to dilate to increase flow, are "pressure dependent" to maintain flow. A reduction in coronary perfusion pressure can perpetuate the ischemic imbalance. Therefore, in cases complicated by cardiogenic shock, vasopressors to maintain arterial pressure or volume administration to maintain adequate ventricular filling pressures and SV may be indicated. Dysrhythmias can also adversely affect coronary perfusion by reducing cardiac output (CO) and arterial pressure; therefore antidysrhythmics (primarily IV lidocaine) may be helpful.

The use of oral anticoagulation after MI has gone in and out of favor with the medical community throughout the years. Aspirin therapy, used as an antiplatelet aggregant, is begun after MI whether or not patients have been treated with thrombolytics. Data from the Second International Study of Infarct Survival (ISIS-2) trial (Fig. 31-27) show that aspirin alone was able to reduce mortality after MI when compared with a placebo. A multicenter trial currently underway has enrolled about 9000 patients to test the effectiveness of using warfarin (Coumadin) alone or both aspirin and warfarin together to prevent reinfarction. The Coumadin Aspirin Study (CARS) is randomly assigning patients to receive either 180 mg aspirin per day or a combination of 80 mg aspirin and 3 mg Coumadin per day. The results of the CARS study should be available within a few years and will clarify the effectiveness of anticoagulation in the prevention of repeat MI.

After MI, rest with monitored return to daily activities

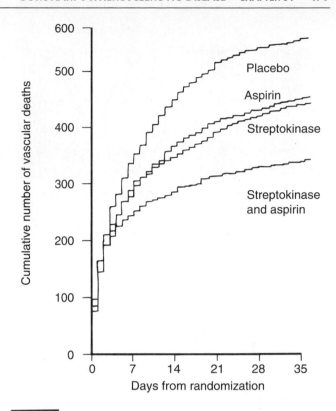

FIG. 31-27 Cumulative vascular mortality of 17,187 patients during the first 5 weeks after MI randomly assigned to four treatment groups: placebo (control) group, aspirin group, streptokinase group; and aspirin plus streptokinase group. Both aspirin alone or streptokinase alone significantly reduced mortality, but the reduction was greatest when these two drugs were given in combination. Deaths in the placebo group were 13.2% (568/4300), 10.7% in the aspirin group (461/4295), 10.4% in the streptokinase group (448/4300), and 8% in the aspirin plus streptokinase group (343/4292). (Redrawn from ISIS-2 [Second International Study of Infarct Survival] Collaborative Group: *Lancet* 8607:354, 1988.)

through a cardiac rehabilitation program is the primary therapy, allowing the infarcted tissue to heal, thus reducing the incidence of complications, and salvaging the ischemic zone surrounding the infarct, thereby reducing the ultimate size of the infarct.

Coronary revascularization

Blood flow to myocardium beyond an atherosclerotic lesion in the coronary artery can be improved by either surgically redirecting flow around the obstruction with a bypass graft or increasing flow in the native vessel by mechanical splitting and compression or pharmacologic lysis of the lesion. The first *coronary artery bypass graft* (CABG) was performed in 1969 by Favaloro. For almost a decade, cardiac surgical bypass techniques were unrivaled as the preferred method for myocardial revascularization. In 1977, however, Gruentzig performed the first nonsurgical dilation of the coronary arteries with the introduction of *percutaneous transluminal coronary angioplasty* (PTCA). These techniques for coronary revascu-

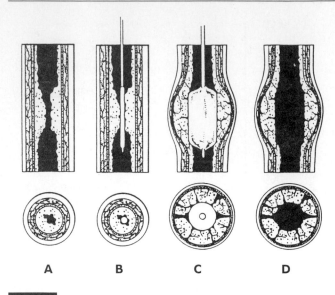

FIG. 31-28 Percutaneous transluminal coronary angioplasty (PTCA). Serial panels show the baseline stenosis **(A)**, passage of the deflated balloon catheter **(B)**, balloon inflation **(C)**, and the postdilation appearance **(D)**, as drawn in longitudinal and cross-sectional views. Balloon inflation **(C)** is associated with fracture and outward displacement of the atherosclerotic plaque, as well as stretching of the media and adventitia. The result **(D)** is enlargement of the lumen because of the expansion of the entire vessel wall rather than compaction of the atherosclerotic material. (From Castaneda-Zuniga WR et al: *Radiology* 135:565, 1980.)

larization are discussed in greater detail in the next section. It should be noted here, however, that the relative indications for these interventions, either alone or in combination, are constantly evolving as technology changes and as results of outcome studies are known.

Angioplasty. PTCA offers an alternative to CABG surgery for selected patients with significant atherosclerotic narrowing resulting in ischemia resistant to medical therapy. Angioplasty is performed in the cardiac catheterization laboratory under fluoroscopy. A small catheter is passed through the skin (percutaneous) over a guide wire into the narrowed section of the artery (transluminal) via the aorta. Inflation of the balloon at the catheter tip compresses and splits the atherosclerotic plaque on the intimal layer of the vessel. Stretching and partial disruption of the medial and adventitial layers of the arterial wall also occurs (Fig. 31-28). The overall diameter of the vessel increases. Angiography is routinely used before and after dilation to determine the degree of stenosis and the effect of dilation.

Initially, PTCA was recommended only for patients with single-vessel disease. Improved catheter technology and growing experience with the procedure, however, have enabled patients with accessible multivessel disease also to be considered acceptable candidates for PTCA in some centers. An estimated 300,000 angioplasty procedures were performed in the United States in 1990. If the procedure fails because dilations were unsuccessful or complications occurred, emergency surgical vasculariza-

tion or placement of a metal scaffold (known as a stent) is necessary to control the dissected coronary artery. Because of this risk, all patients undergoing PTCA must be able to tolerate the rigors of cardiac surgery and should be candidates for CABG surgery (described later). In approximately 20% to 30% of patients undergoing PTCA, clinical *restenosis* or narrowing of the vessel may recur within 6 months; the incidence may be even higher, depending on the location of the stenosis (higher in left anterior descending [LAD] and ostial lesions) or the presence of cardiovascular risk factors, such as elevated LDL cholesterol or diabetes mellitus. Restenosis can usually be treated with a second PTCA.

Among the advances now available with angioplasty are stents, atherectomies, and laser angioplasty. *Stents* are delicate mesh structures that can be placed in an artery to prevent reclosure. Two major clinical trials (the STRESS and BENE Stent studies) have shown that stents significantly decrease the incidence of restenosis compared with simple PTCA procedures. The *atherectomy catheter* has a blade that cuts the plaque. The plaque is then pushed into the nose cone of the catheter and removed from the vessel with the catheter. In *laser angioplasty,* the heat of the laser beam destroys the plaque. This change in the plaque, combined with the pressure of the balloon, increases the diameter of the vessel lumen.

With angioplasty, patients are treated more quickly, at a lower cost, and without the risks and complications of open-heart surgery. However, patients with left main coronary artery disease or complex diffuse narrowing in more than two major epicardial arteries are probably best treated by CABG surgery.

Surgical revascularization. The standard conduits for CABG procedures are the greater saphenous vein from the leg and the left internal mammary artery from the chest (LIMA). With saphenous vein bypass grafting, one end of the vein segment is anastomosed to the ascending aorta and the other end is attached beyond the site of vessel obstruction (Fig. 31-29, *A*). Therefore a vascular conduit is created to shunt blood around the lesion to the myocardium at risk. With LIMA grafting, the origin of the left internal mammary artery at the subclavian artery usually remains intact and the distal end of the vessel is sectioned and anastomosed to the coronary artery (Fig. 31-29, *B*).

Each procedure offers distinct advantages and disadvantages. The saphenous vein bypass graft provides higher flow rates because of the larger vessel caliber. It is easily accessible from the leg and can be positioned with greater latitude on the surface of the heart. However, a significant incidence of late graft closure is caused by fibrous overgrowth of the intimal wall of the vein. The late patency rate of the internal mammary bypass grafts is superior to that of the saphenous vein. Other advantages of this procedure include the absence of a leg incision and the need for one, rather than two, anastomoses. However, internal mammary artery bypass grafting is technically more complex than that for the saphenous vein and is as-

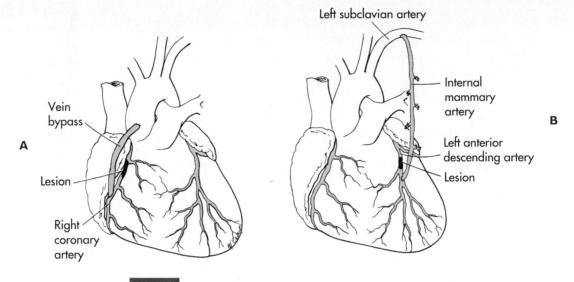

FIG. 31-29 Coronary artery revascularization procedures. **A,** Saphenous vein is sutured to the ascending aorta and to the right coronary artery at a point distal to the blockage so that flow distal to the blockage is again established. **B,** The internal mammary artery is anastomosed to the anterior descending branch of the left coronary artery, bypassing the lesion.

sociated with a slightly higher rate of postoperative complications. Given its anterior location, the internal mammary artery is most frequently used to bypass the left anterior descending artery, and saphenous vein segments are used for lesions of the right and circumflex coronary arteries and their branches.

Current indications for elective surgical revascularization include the following: (1) anginal symptoms uncontrolled or poorly controlled by medical therapy, (2) significant triple-vessel coronary artery stenosis, and (3) significant left main coronary artery occlusion. Surgery is considered whenever there is documented evidence of large territories of myocardium at risk for infarction. Single- and double-vessel coronary artery disease may be an indication if PTCA is not technically possible or has failed to ensure long-term patency of the arteries. Patients with ischemia-induced failure, but not those with chronic ventricular failure, are candidates for surgery.

Urgent surgical revascularization is considered for patients with unstable angina or postinfarction angina who are not PTCA candidates. Surgery is the treatment of choice if coronary artery disease has led to either significant mitral valve dysfunction, ventricular septal rupture, or ventricular aneurysm. Revascularization is performed in conjunction with repair of the mechanical defect.

Complications

General principles

Early detection and prevention of complications are essential after treatment of coronary disease. Two categories of complications must be anticipated: electrical instability or dysrhythmias and mechanical dysfunction or

pump failure. ECG monitoring is initiated immediately. Dysrhythmia management follows logical principles, as outlined below:

1. Tachycardias are decelerated by parasympathetic stimulation (e.g., carotid sinus massage), antidysrhythmic drugs (e.g., verapamil), or electrical cardioversion, if necessary. Bradycardias, if they compromise perfusion, can be accelerated by drugs that inhibit parasympathetic effects (e.g., atropine). Electrical pacing may be indicated if drugs are ineffective.

2. Escape beats, which result from sinus node failure, must be differentiated from premature beats to effectively treat rhythm disturbances originating in sites other than the sinus node. To treat escape rhythms, drugs are administered to speed the normal pacemaker, the sinus node; drugs must not be given to suppress the escape pacemaker, since cardiac standstill could result.

   Ventricular dysrhythmias associated with ischemia usually respond best to lidocaine (Xylocaine); otherwise, procainamide is the drug of choice. Ventricular fibrillation requires immediate defibrillation with cardiopulmonary resuscitative maneuvers. The management of refractory ventricular dysrhythmias is reviewed later.

   Atrial dysrhythmias are best controlled by administering an antidysrhythmic drug. Procainamide is now the antidysrhythmic drug of choice for treating atrial fibrillation. Verapamil administration is used with atrial tachycardias to slow conduction through the AV node and control the ventricular rate response. A combination of drugs may be used to convert the abnormal rhythm to a normal one. Electrical cardioversion may

TABLE 31-3 The North American Society of Pacing and Electrophysiology/British Pacing and Electrophysiology Group Generic Pacemaker Code*

Position I: Chamber Paced†	Position II: Chamber Sensed	Position III: Mode of Response	Position IV: Programmable Functions; Rate Modulation	Position V: Antitachydysrhythmia Functions
V = Ventricle	V = Ventricle	T = Triggers pacing	P = Programmable rate and/or output	P = Antitachydysrhythmia
A = Atrium	A = Atrium	I = Inhibits pacing	M = Multiprogramability of rate, output, sensitivity, etc.	S = Shock
D = Double	D = Double	D = Triggers/inhibits pacing	C = Communicating functions (telemetry)	D = Dual (P + S)
O = None	O = None	O = None	O = None	O = None

From Bernstein AD et al: *PACE* 10:794, 1987.

*Letter positions I to III are used exclusively for antibradydysrhythmia pacing. Although the last two letters contain pertinent information, a pacemaker is typically referred to by the first three letters. For example, with a VVI pacemaker, only the ventricles are paced when the unit discharges an impulse, and the unit is inhibited from firing when intrinsic ventricular activity is sensed.

†Manufacturers use S for single chamber (atria or ventricles).

be indicated to restore the normal rhythm if the dysrhythmia persists and is poorly tolerated. It is especially important to administer loading doses of procainamide before cardioversion.

3. Therapy of heart block is directed at restoring or simulating normal conduction, either by administering drugs to speed conduction and HR, such as atropine or isoproterenol (Isuprel), as a bridge to pacing, or by electrical pacing.

Mechanical dysfunction produces a clinical spectrum ranging from mild congestive heart failure to cardiogenic shock. *Congestive heart failure* prompts efforts to (1) reduce intravascular volume and congestion and associated fluid transudation, (2) improve myocardial function, and (3) reduce cardiac work. Mild to moderate congestive heart failure is managed with oxygen; restricted fluid and salt intake; and diuretics, digitalis, and rest. The development of pulmonary edema requires more aggressive treatment. Morphine, in addition to its sedative and respiratory depressant effects, dilates the periphery with pooling of blood in the veins and reduction in venous return. Administration of vasodilators, such as nitroglycerin or sodium nitroprusside (Nipride), decreases preload by allowing pooling of blood in the venous system and causing a decrease in afterload via peripheral vasodilation. ACE inhibitors may also be prescribed to decrease afterload. Both of these medications decrease the amount of work the failing heart must generate during systole. ACE inhibitors cause a reduction in peripheral systemic vascular resistance and blood pressure (afterload), pulmonary vascular resistance, and capillary wedge pressure. The Survival and Ventricular Enlargement (SAVE) Study, which administered the ACE inhibitor captopril to patients 3 to 16 days after acute MI, found a decrease in mortality in patients with asymptomatic ventricular dysfunction (ejection fractions of 40% or less with no signs of overt heart failure). ACE inhibitors have now become an integral medication to prevent left ventricular remodeling (dilating) after infarction. Aminophylline can be administered to relieve associated bronchospasm and secondarily to increase CO by increasing contractile force. Administration of oxygen and possibly mechanical ventilation are required to correct hypoxemia.

Progression of left ventricular failure to *cardiogenic shock,* characterized by inadequate tissue perfusion, is an ominous development. This syndrome, with a mortality rate approaching 100%, remains a therapeutic dilemma. Efforts are directed at maintaining tissue perfusion and the simultaneous reduction of cardiac work. Vasopressors are frequently needed to maintain arterial pressure. Metabolic acidosis, caused by lactic acid accumulation, must be reversed by the administration of sodium bicarbonate. Emergency intraaortic balloon pumping may be indicated.

Pacing therapy

The use of pacemakers has become increasingly sophisticated. Both temporary and permanent implantable pulse generators have been developed with a variety of pacing characteristics. Current pulse generators are capable of pacing either the atria or the ventricles or pacing both atria and ventricles sequentially. Pacing stimuli can be delivered in demand or fixed-rate modes. *Demand pacing* can be further classified according to two modes of response: (1) inhibited and (2) triggered. In the *inhibited* mode, the pacer shuts off when an intrinsic cardiac impulse is sensed. In the *triggered* mode, the pacer fires during the refractory period of the sensed beat, without generating a paced beat. By contrast, *fixed-rate pacing* delivers a stimulus at a predetermined, fixed rate. An international classification system has been developed to standardize pacemaker coding (Table 31-3). Temporary pacing may be performed transcutaneously if necessary after an acute MI. Skin pads with leads to the pacemaker are placed on the patient's chest in the anterior and posterior positions, and the ECG is sensed through these leads and conveyed to the pulse generator of the pacemaker. If the ventricular heart rate falls below a preset limit (40 bpm), the pulse generator will deliver an electrical stimulus through the skin pads to produce a ventricular contraction.

Management of refractory ventricular dysrhythmias

The presence of recurrent, malignant ventricular dysrhythmias unresponsive to standard pharmacologic therapy is an indication for *electrophysiologic* (EP) *evaluation*. Such dysrhythmias are usually seen in the setting of chronic ischemic heart disease. Ventricular aneurysms or previous ventricular surgery may predispose to the development of refractory ventricular dysrhythmias. Before the initial EP study, all antidysrhythmic drugs are discontinued if possible. Catheters with multiple electrodes are then positioned within the heart under fluoroscopic guidance (see Fig. 30-16 for catheter placement). A stimulation protocol is followed to induce ventricular tachycardia; this programmed stimulation can consist of progressively more premature ventricular stimuli, double-ventricular extrastimuli, or bursts of rapid ventricular pacing. Intracardiac recordings of the dysrhythmia are obtained. The dysrhythmia is terminated with another burst of rapid ventricular pacing or countershock if required.

The purposes of EP testing are (1) to diagnose the type of dysrhythmia and its mechanism, (2) to localize and map the site of the dysrhythmia, and (3) to determine the best course of treatment, depending on the previous information. The options for treatment include (1) pharmacologic; (2) device implantation—antitachycardia pacing and/or implantable cardiac defibrillators (ICDs); (3) radiofrequency ablation using a transvenous or transarterial approach; and (4) surgical ablation.

Once the dysrhythmia has been diagnosed, the first antidysrhythmic drug trial may be performed at the end of the diagnostic procedure. Procainamide usually is the first medication tested. Once this drug is loaded, another series of programmed stimulations is carried out to determine its effectiveness. If the first drug is found to be ineffective in preventing or slowing the dysrhythmia, the catheter is removed and the patient returned to the hospital room. Loading of a second antidysrhythmic drug is begun, and depending on the patient's stability, he or she may be discharged or may remain in the hospital until a steady state for the second drug has been attained. At that time the patient may return for a second EP study. The three most common drugs used to treat tachydysrhythmias are procainamide, sotalol, and amiodarone. Amiodarone is used very cautiously because of its toxic effects on the liver, kidneys, lungs, and thyroid. Additional drugs

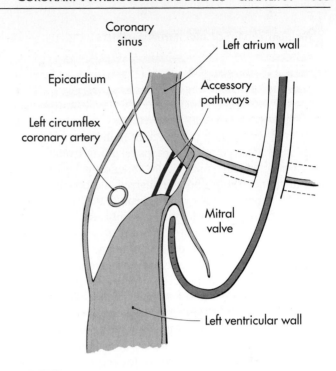

FIG. 31-30   Procedure for radiofrequency catheter ablation of an accessory pathway that is causing a refractory dysrhythmia. A cross section of the left ventricular wall is shown at the level of the atrioventricular groove. (Redrawn from Wagshal AB, Pires LA, Huang SK: *Arch Intern Med* 155:142, 1995.)

that may be used alone or in combination include mexiletine, quinidine, and propranolol and rarely flecainide.

If drug trials are ineffective in treating the dysrhythmia, alternate therapies such as electrical therapy or surgery are considered. Radiofrequency catheter ablation (Fig. 31-30) or ICDs may be used in selected patients.

Electrical therapy for ventricular tachycardia or fibrillation is now available in the form of a programmable antitachycardia device. EP testing is performed to determine the most effective mode of therapy before device implantation. The currently available devices offer antitachycardia pacing. If the dysrhythmia is responsive to pace termination, the device can be programmed for the following two types of termination methods:

1. *Ramp pacing.* The cycle length of the stimulus is "captured" or "paced" for a predetermined time. Pacing is then terminated with the hope that the mechanism of the tachycardia is interrupted and normal sinus rhythm restored.
2. *Burst pacing.* A rapid sequence of pacing is initiated to interrupt and terminate the dysrhythmia.

The device is capable of being programmed to sense ongoing or recurrent ventricular tachycardia and will cardiovert the heart with the lowest amount of electrical stimulation possible to depolarize a critical mass of myocardium. If the stimulus is ineffective, countershocks are delivered until a successful countershock is given or the programmed number of shocks has been delivered.

Surgical repair of mechanical defects

Aneurysmectomy is the removal of the noncontractile, paradoxically bulging scar. There are three indications for aneurysm resection: (1) chronic congestive heart failure, (2) systemic embolization of mural thrombi, and (3) recurrent ventricular dysrhythmias. Aneurysms are associated with a high incidence of malignant, refractory ventricular dysrhythmias, perhaps resulting from the persistent mechanical strain at the boundary between the normal myocardium and the scarred, outpouching segment. The aneurysm is excised through the left ventricular scar with removal of mural thrombi. Removal of the aneurysm and subsequent reduction of ventricular size improves the mechanical efficiency of the heart. Intraoperatively, the site causing recurrent ventricular dysrhythmias can be localized and excised or sectioned.

A *ventricular septal defect* can be repaired either by simple closure of the hole in the septum or by insertion of a patch graft; access to the septum is gained via the infarct in the ventricle. On closure of the left ventricular incision, a portion of the noncontractile left ventricular scar is frequently excised, a procedure referred to as *infarctectomy.*

Dysfunction of the mitral valve resulting from papillary muscle rupture or malfunction necessitates *mitral valve replacement* with excision of the papillary muscles.

Cardiac transplantation can be lifesaving for patients considered inoperable or unsalvageable with less aggressive surgical intervention. Patients with end-stage heart disease are considered for transplantation. The procedure involves removal of the diseased heart and replacement with a normal donor heart. Technically, the surgery is uncomplicated, requiring reanastomoses of the separated vessels with the donor heart. Cardiac transplantation is discussed in more detail in Chapter 33.

Rehabilitation

The ultimate goal of therapeutic intervention in coronary atherosclerotic disease is to restore the cardiac patient to a productive and satisfying life-style. The long-term consequences of MI—physical, psychologic, social, and vocational invalidism—have long been ignored with devastating impact. The complications of myocardial disease are not restricted to the hospital setting, and the responsibility of health professionals for the ultimate well-being and coping ability of patients does not terminate on their discharge from the hospital. As early as clinically feasible, patients should be enrolled in an inpatient cardiovascular rehabilitation program that will continue after hospital discharge within an outpatient setting.

Cardiac rehabilitation, as defined by the American Heart Association and the Task Force on Cardiovascular Rehabilitation of the National Heart, Lung, and Blood Institute, is the process of restoring and maintaining the physical, psychologic, social, educational, and vocational potentials of the patient.

Patients must be assisted to progressively resume a level of activity consistent with physical limitations and to be relatively unhampered by psychologic stressors. Many patients can resume all normal activities. Explicit, individualized patient and family education about diet; medications; activity progression, especially regarding resumption of sexual relations; and risk factor reduction/modification is essential. Every patient and family require guidance and education during the transition from the dependence of illness to the independence of health.

QUESTIONS

▼ *Answer the following on a separate sheet of paper.*

1. Explain why the left ventricle is most vulnerable to ischemia and infarction.
2. What are the most common sites of coronary arterial occlusion?
3. Name five factors affecting the degree of functional impairment after an acute myocardial infarction (MI).
4. What is a vasovagal response, and what might cause this response after an acute MI? How does it affect the compensatory response?
5. Name three important diagnostic findings associated with MI.
6. Explain hemodynamically why either tachycardias or bradycardias may impair cardiac function.
7. Identify three hemodynamic factors that may be modified to reduce oxygen demand in the treatment of myocardial ischemia.
8. Explain why medical efforts to treat myocardial ischemia by increasing coronary blood flow and oxygen supply are of little value.
9. State the primary objective of rest in the treatment of acute MI.
10. Describe the treatment of congestive heart failure, pulmonary edema, and cardiogenic shock.
11. Why is rehabilitation an important aspect of the treatment of patients with atherosclerotic heart disease?

▼ *Circle the letter preceding each item below that correctly answers the question*

or completes the statement. Only one answer is correct unless otherwise noted.

12. The most potent stimulus to increasing coronary blood flow is:
    a. Systemic lactic acidosis
    b. Local myocardial hypoxia
    c. Sympathetic stimulation
    d. Increased arterial pressure
13. In the normal heart, how many times can coronary blood flow increase above resting levels?
    a. 1 to 2   c. 8 to 10
    b. 5 to 6   d. 15 to 20
14. The earliest pathologic change apparent in the coronary blood vessel in the development of coronary atherosclerosis is:
    a. Fibrous encapsulation of the lesion
    b. Fatty streaks in the adventitia

QUESTIONS—cont'd

c. Fatty streaks in the intima
d. Accumulation of beta-lipoprotein in the media

15. MI may result from (more than one answer may be correct):
   a. Hemorrhage into the coronary atheromatous plaque
   b. Platelet aggregates in the coronary blood vessel
   c. Coronary artery spasm
   d. Embolization of a thrombus or plaque fragment

16. Major modifiable risk factors for coronary atherosclerotic disease include all the following *except:*
   a. Hyperlipidemia
   b. Hypertension
   c. Family history
   d. Cigarette smoking

17. Optimal serum LDL cholesterol levels should be no greater than what level to reduce the risk of coronary atherosclerotic disease?
   a. 50 mg/dl   c. 160 mg/dl
   b. 120 mg/dl   d. 200 mg/dl

18. A form of angina in which there is ST segment elevation is:
   a. Preinfarction angina
   b. Prinzmetal's angina
   c. Dressler's angina
   d. Unstable angina

19. Which of the following changes does *not* usually occur before or during an attack of angina pectoris?
   a. An increase in blood pressure
   b. A decrease in heart rate
   c. An increase in myocardial oxygen demand
   d. An increase in left ventricular end-diastolic pressure
   e. A decrease in myocardial wall compliance

20. Depressed left ventricular function resulting from an area of ischemia or necrosis always necessitates:
   a. An increase in end-diastolic volume to maintain stroke volume
   b. A decrease in end-diastolic volume to maintain stroke volume
   c. An increase in heart rate to maintain cardiac output
   d. An increase in blood pressure to maintain tissue perfusion

21. Complete occlusion of the left anterior descending coronary artery would result in:
   a. Anterior wall infarct
   b. Inferior wall infarct

c. Complete heart block
d. Posterior wall infarct

22. Which of the following functional changes would be least expected in patients with acute MI?
   a. A decrease in cardiac output
   b. A decrease in left ventricular end-diastolic pressure
   c. An increase in pulmonary wedge pressure
   d. An increase in the central venous pressure

23. Impending left-sided heart failure after MI can be detected earliest by monitoring the:
   a. Systemic blood pressure
   b. Central venous pressure
   c. Pulmonary wedge pressure
   d. Pulse pressure

24. The earliest stage of lung involvement in left ventricular failure is:
   a. Interstitial edema
   b. Alveolar edema
   c. Pleural effusion
   d. Pulmonary congestion

25. In patients who develop cardiogenic shock, the percentage of left ventricular mass that is infarcted is generally at least:
   a. 10%   c. 40%
   b. 20%   d. 60%

26. Characteristic hemodynamic abnormalities in cardiogenic shock include (more than one answer may be correct):
   a. Decreased peripheral perfusion
   b. Decreased coronary perfusion
   c. Hypotension
   d. Decreased cardiac output

27. Left ventricular papillary muscle rupture after MI results in (more than one answer may be correct):
   a. Mitral regurgitation
   b. A systolic murmur
   c. A diastolic murmur
   d. Death in a high percentage of cases
   e. Pulmonary congestion

28. Which of the following statements about ventricular rupture is *not* correct?
   a. The peak incidence is during the healing phase of necrotic tissue removal.
   b. Rupture is a complication of transmural MI.
   c. The peak incidence is about 6 weeks after MI.
   d. Rupture is associated with cardiac tamponade.

29. The major effect of cardiac tamponade is to:
   a. Produce atelectasis
   b. Distend the pericardium
   c. Compress the heart
   d. Increase the pulse pressure

30. The myocardial scar that develops after MI is well established after approximately:
   a. 3 weeks   c. 3 months
   b. 6 weeks   d. 6 months

31. A ventricular aneurysm may give rise to:
   a. Chronic congestive heart failure
   b. Systemic emboli
   c. Refractory ventricular dysrhythmias
   d. All the above

32. The most frequent complication after MI is:
   a. Congestive heart failure
   b. Cardiogenic shock
   c. Left ventricular papillary muscle dysfunction
   d. Dressler's syndrome
   e. Dysrhythmias

33. Factor(s) predisposing to the development of dysrhythmias in coronary atherosclerotic disease is(are) (more than one answer may be correct):
   a. Myocardial ischemia
   b. Lactic acidosis
   c. Hypokalemia
   d. Digitalis toxicity

34. An ectopic beat may originate in all the following sites *except:*
   a. Atria
   b. Ventricles
   c. Atrioventricular junctional tissue
   d. Sinoatrial node

35. Which of the following dysrhythmias is most often associated with MI?
   a. Atrial tachycardia
   b. Atrial fibrillation
   c. Ventricular premature beats
   d. Ventricular fibrillation
   e. Left bundle branch block

36. Left bundle branch block results in:
   a. Absence of all P waves
   b. Absence of every other P wave
   c. Prolongation of the PR interval
   d. Widening of the QRS complex

37. Which of the following drugs used for the treatment of myocardial ischemia improve(s) cardiac function by decreasing arterial resistance to ventricular ejection (more than one answer may be correct)?
   a. Propranolol

Continued.

QUESTIONS—cont'd

b. Digitalis
c. Diuretics
d. ACE inhibitors
e. Nitroglycerin

38. Which sign or symptom would occur latest in the course of left-sided heart failure?
    a. Orthopnea
    b. Lung congestion
    c. Decreased urine output
    d. Distended neck veins

39. Factors that result from and compound the problem of myocardial ischemia include (more than one answer may be correct):
    a. Hypoxemia   c. Dysrhythmias
    b. Hypotension   d. Acidosis

40. Which of the following statements about atherosclerotic heart disease is *not* true?
    a. Lesion precursors may be found in children and young adults.
    b. The disease begins abruptly in susceptible middle-age adults.
    c. It is the leading cause of death in the United States.
    d. Hypertension, hyperlipidemia, and smoking are major predisposing factors.

41. The dysrhythmia with the least effective ventricular action is:
    a. Atrial flutter
    b. Ventricular tachycardia
    c. Ventricular fibrillation
    d. Complete heart block

42. Which of the following ECG monitor strip tracings is typical of second-degree heart block?
    a. P waves without a QRS complex
    b. PR interval longer than 0.2 second
    c. Widening of the QRS complex
    d. Inversion of the T wave

43. Pacemakers are *not* used to:
    a. Suppress ventricular ectopic beats
    b. Suppress sinus tachycardia
    c. Treat third-degree heart block
    d. Treat sinus bradycardia

44. Coronary bypass surgery is generally indicated for patients with:
    a. Preinfarction angina
    b. Cardiogenic shock
    c. Stable angina pectoris
    d. Acute MI
    e. Ventricular aneurysm

45. The removal of an atherosclerotic plaque in coronary atherosclerotic disease is called:
    a. Infarctectomy
    b. Endarterectomy
    c. Septal defect repair
    d. Aneurysmectomy

▼ *Circle T if the statement is true and F if it is false. Correct any false statements.*

46. T F Atherosclerotic heart disease is more common in diabetic than in nondiabetic persons.

47. T F In post-MI syndrome (Dressler's syndrome), the pain is characteristic of pericarditis rather than of infarction.

48. T F An internal mammary artery bypass graft is associated with a significant incidence of subintimal fibrous hyperplasia.

49. T F Ventricular hypertrophy decreases myocardial oxygen demand.

50. T F Escape beats are caused by myocardial tissue irritability.

▼ *Fill in the blanks with the correct word or circle the correct word.*

51. In MI, an area of _____ surrounds the area of infarction.

52. A reduction in ventricular wall compliance (increases) (decreases) pressure for a constant ventricular volume.

53. Arrange in correct order the following changes that occur after an acute MI.
    a. Removal of necrotic tissue
    b. Bruised and cyanotic tissue
    c. Scar formation
    d. Polymorphonuclear neutrophil infiltration

▼ *Match the characteristics in column A with the disorders in column B.*

Column A	Column B
54. _____ ST segment depression typical	a. Myocardial ischemia
55. _____ ST segment elevation typical	b. Myocardial infarction (MI)
56. _____ Deep Q waves	
57. _____ Pain relieved by nitroglycerin	
58. _____ Muscle death	
59. _____ Muscle hypoxia	
60. _____ If prolonged, results in necrosis	
61. _____ Reversible	
62. _____ Irreversible	

▼ *Match the type of heart block in column A with the ECG pattern in column B.*

Column A	Column B
63. _____ First-degree heart block	a. No impulses conducted
64. _____ Wenckebach or Mobitz I block	b. All impulses conducted with prolonged PR interval
65. _____ Mobitz II block	c. Some impulses nonconducted in repetitive pattern with progressive prolongation of PR interval
66. _____ Complete heart block	d. Some impulses nonconducted but conducted impulses have constant PR interval

QUESTIONS—cont'd

▼ *Match each of the dysrhythmias in column A with its possible therapeutic intervention in column B.*

Column A	Column B
67. _____ Sinus bradycardia	a. Carotid sinus massage
68. _____ Atrial tachycardia	b. Defibrillation
69. _____ Multiple premature ventricular beats	c. Lidocaine
70. _____ Ventricular fibrillation	d. Atropine

▼ *Match each of the drugs used to treat coronary atherosclerotic disease in column A with its effect in column B.*

Column A	Column B
71. _____ Propranolol	a. Suppression of ventricular irritability
72. _____ Lidocaine	b. Increased heart rate
73. _____ Atropine	c. Decreased heart rate and force of contraction
74. _____ Nitroglycerin	d. Increased force of myocardial contraction
75. _____ Digitalis	e. Vasodilation of coronary collaterals and peripheral vessels

▼ *Circle the letter preceding each item below that correctly answers the question or completes the statement. Only one answer is correct unless otherwise noted.*

76. A decreased risk of developing coronary heart disease is believed to be associated with an elevation of:
   a. LDL
   b. HDL
   c. VLDL
   d. Chylomicrons

77. In untreated familial hypercholesterolemia the probability of developing premature atherosclerosis before age 50 years is approximately:
   a. 10%
   b. 30%
   c. 50%
   d. 70%

78. Patterns or types of hyperlipoproteinemias associated with premature atherosclerosis include which of the following (more than one answer may be correct)?
   a. I
   b. II
   c. III
   d. IV
   e. V

79. Initial treatment of primary hyperlipidemia will most likely include all the following measures *except:*
   a. Restriction of alcohol
   b. Restriction of saturated fats
   c. Clofibrate
   d. Weight reduction

80. Which of the following statements is *not* true regarding hypertension?
   a. Approximately 25% of the adult population is hypertensive.
   b. A lower prevalence of hypertension is found among African Americans.
   c. A clear-cut increase in the risk of coronary heart disease is associated with hypertension.
   d. The usual course of hypertensive disease involves an asymptomatic latent period of many years', duration.

81. All the following statements concerning the pathophysiology of essential hypertension are true *except:*
   a. The primary hemodynamic alteration in essential hypertension is an increased vascular resistance.
   b. Left ventricular ejection pressure is increased secondary to the increased vascular resistance.

   c. Myocardial hypertrophy increases myocardial oxygen demand.
   d. Excessive salt intake has been demonstrated to have no significant role in the development of essential hypertension.

82. An elevation of which of the following enzymes is the most specific indication of an MI?
   a. AST (SGOT)
   b. CK
   c. LDH
   d. MB-CK

83. All the following functional changes would be expected after a transmural MI of the anterior myocardial wall *except:*
   a. Increased left ventricular end-systolic and end-diastolic volume
   b. Increased left ventricular end-diastolic pressure
   c. Increased ejection fraction
   d. Decreased contractility

84. Which of the following statements is *false* concerning the reentry phenomenon?
   a. Reentry is the most common mechanism producing a premature beat.
   b. The reentry mechanism refers to increased automaticity.
   c. One or more areas in the heart where the refractory period is longer than others may account for the reentry phenomenon.
   d. The reentry mechanism explains the temporal dependence of certain ectopic beats.

85. Thrombolytic therapy would be most applicable as a means of reestablishing myocardial perfusion in a patient who has:
   a. Symptoms of chronic angina
   b. Significant triple-vessel coronary artery disease
   c. Stenosis of a bypass graft
   d. MI within 6 hours of onset of symptoms

CHAPTER 32 Valvular Heart Disease

PENNY FORD CARLETON
MADELINE M. O'DONNELL

Valvular disease causes abnormalities in blood flow across the cardiac valves. Normal valves demonstrate two critical flow characteristics: unidirectional flow and unimpeded flow. The valves open when the pressure in the chamber proximal to the valve exceeds the pressure in the chamber or vessel beyond the valve. Closure occurs when the pressure beyond the valve exceeds pressure in the proximal chamber. For instance, the atrioventricular valves open when atrial pressures exceed ventricular pressures and close when ventricular pressures exceed atrial pressures. The valve leaflets are so responsive that even a slight pressure difference (less than 1 mm Hg) between chambers will open and close the leaflets.

A diseased valve can produce two types of functional derangements: (1) *valvular regurgitation*—the valve leaflets fail to close securely, permitting backward flow (*valvular insufficiency* and *valvular incompetence* are synonymous terms); and (2) *valvular stenosis*—the valve orifice becomes restricted, impeding forward flow. Regurgitation and stenosis can occur together in the same valve as a "mixed lesion," or either one can occur alone as a "pure lesion."

Valvular dysfunction increases cardiac work. Valvular regurgitation forces the heart to pump the additional regurgitant volume of blood, thus producing an increment in *volume work*. Valvular stenosis necessitates the generation of increased pressure to overcome the increased resistance to flow, thereby elevating *pressure work*. The characteristic myocardial responses to increased volume work and pressure work are chamber dilation and muscular hypertrophy, respectively. Myocardial dilation and hypertrophy are compensatory mechanisms intended to increase the pumping capability of the heart.

PATHOGENESIS

Valvular heart disease was once considered to be almost entirely rheumatic in origin. Despite the declining incidence of rheumatic fever, rheumatic damage is still a common cause of valvular deformity requiring surgical correction. *Acute rheumatic fever* is a sequela of a group A beta-hemolytic streptococcal pharyngitis. Rheumatic fever develops only if a significant immunologic or antibody response to the antecedent streptococcal infection occurs. Approximately 3% of pharyngeal streptococcal infections are followed within 2 to 4 weeks by attacks of rheumatic fever. Initial attacks of rheumatic fever are typically observed during childhood and the early teenage years. The incidence of streptococcal infection, and therefore of rheumatic fever, is directly related to factors predisposing to the development and transmission of infection; socioeconomic factors, such as living conditions and access to medical care and antibiotic therapy, are foremost in this regard.

The precise pathogenesis of rheumatic fever is unknown. Two possible mechanisms are (1) a hyperimmune response, either autoimmune or allergic in nature, and (2) a direct effect of the streptococcal organisms or its toxins. An immunologic explanation is considered most plausible, although the latter mechanism cannot be entirely ruled out. An autoimmune reaction to a streptococcal infection would hypothetically produce tissue damage, or manifestations of rheumatic disease, as follows:

1. Group A streptococcus would produce pharyngeal infection.
2. Streptococcal antigen would result in antibody production in a hyperimmune host.
3. Antibodies would react with the streptococcal antigen and with host tissues that are antigenically similar to streptococcus (i.e., antibodies are unable to distinguish streptococcal antigen from cardiac tissue antigen).
4. Autoantibodies reacting with host tissues would produce tissue damage.

Whatever the pathogenesis of this disease, the presentation of acute rheumatic fever is that of a diffuse, inflammatory process affecting the connective tissue of many organs, particularly the heart, joints, and skin. Signs and symptoms are nonspecific and include fever, migratory arthritis, arthralgia, skin rash, chorea, and tachycardia. Cardiac involvement is most significant for two reasons: (1) mortality during the acute phase, although extremely low, is attributed exclusively to cardiac failure; and (2) residual disability results primarily from valvular deformity.

Acute rheumatic fever can produce inflammation of all cardiac layers, referred to as *pancarditis*. Endocardial inflammation typically involves the valvular endothelium, causing leaflet swelling and erosion of the cusp edges. Beadlike vegetations are deposited along the leaflet borders (Fig. 32-1). These acute changes may interfere with effective valve closure, producing valvular regurgitation; stenosis is not encountered as an acute lesion. The appearance of a murmur is the most common clinical manifestation of acute valvular involvement.

With myocardial involvement, characteristic nodular lesions, referred to as *Aschoff's bodies*, appear in the cardiac walls. Myocarditis may result in cardiac enlargement or congestive heart failure; however, clinical progression to failure is unusual during initial attacks. When present, failure is usually associated with concomitant valvular involvement. Pericarditis, usually observed with myocarditis and valvulitis, occurs infrequently. An exudative pericarditis with thickening of the pericardial layers is characteristic of acute rheumatic fever. Pericarditis typically presents with a friction rub, although pericardial effusions may develop. Progression to cardiac tamponade is rare.

Initial attacks of rheumatic carditis usually subside with little residual damage. However, recurrent attacks produce progressive valvular deformity. The pathologic changes of chronic rheumatic valvular disease are the product of healing with scar formation, recurrent inflammatory insults, and progressive deformity with hemodynamic stress and aging.

Given the gradual progression of chronic rheumatic

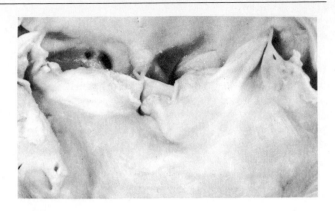

FIG. 32-1 Acute rheumatic endocarditis of the aortic valve. The vegetations form a beadlike row of deposits that tends to conform to the line of closure. (From Hurst JW: *The heart,* ed 3, New York, 1974, McGraw-Hill.)

valvular disease, symptoms generally do not appear for years after the initial attack; this latent period can last into the third, fourth, or fifth decade of life. The eventual deformity producing valvular stenosis is characterized by cusp thickening and leaflet fusion along the commissures (the junction between the leaflets). These changes narrow the valvular orifice and reduce leaflet motion, thus producing an obstruction to forward blood flow. The chordae tendineae of the atrioventricular (AV) valves may also thicken and fuse (Fig. 32-2), creating a fibrous tunnel below the cusps and further impeding flow.

The lesion associated with valvular regurgitation consists of shrunken, retracted cusps that inhibit cusp contact and shortened, fused chordae tendineae that restrain the AV valve leaflets (Fig. 32-3). These changes impair valve closure, thereby permitting backward flow through the valve.

Calcification and sclerosis of valvular tissue with aging contribute to the ultimate deformity in valves with rheumatic malformation. Chronic disease with ventricular failure and enlargement can also disrupt the function of the AV valves. As the ventricular shape alters, the ability of the papillary muscles to approximate the valvular leaflets during valve closure is reduced. In addition, the valve orifice can enlarge, further compromising valve closure. Valvular regurgitation can result. This type of valvular regurgitation occurring secondary to chamber enlargement is known as *functional regurgitation.*

The incidence of valvular disease is highest in the mitral valve, followed by that in the aortic valve. The predominance of left-sided valvular disease is attributed to the relatively greater hemodynamic stress experienced by these valves. It is postulated that hemodynamic stress increases the degree of acquired valvular deformity. The incidence of tricuspid disease is relatively low. Pulmonic disease is rare. Disease of the tricuspid or pulmonic valves is usually associated with other valvular lesions, whereas aortic or mitral disease is frequently seen as an isolated lesion.

In addition to rheumatic disease, other causes of valvular deformity and malfunction are being recognized with increasing frequency. Other significant causes of valvular heart disease are (1) valve destruction by infective endocarditis, (2) inborn defects of connective tissue, (3) dysfunction or rupture of the papillary muscles as a result of coronary atherosclerosis, and (4) congenital malformations.

Infective endocarditis can be caused by many organisms, including bacteria, fungi, and yeast. Bacterial infections are the most common; consequently, the entity is frequently referred to as *bacterial endocarditis.* Endocarditis may present in an acute or subacute form. *Acute* endocarditis is caused by infection with a highly virulent organism, such as staphylococci, and typically follows a rapidly fulminating course with early valvular destruction. Normal valves may be affected. *Subacute* bacterial endocarditis (abbreviated SBE if bacterial in origin) is caused by organisms of less virulence, such as streptococci, and has a more gradual presentation and course. Nonspecific signs and symptoms, including fever, joint pain, myalgias, and skin manifestations, are frequently reported. Typically, valves with preexisting abnormalities or mechanical prosthetics are involved. Endocarditis produces vegetations along the cusp edges; vegetations may extend to involve the valve and even the myocardium. Subsequently, the cusps may fibrose, erode, or perforate, causing typically regurgitant valvular dysfunction.

Mitral valve prolapse is a congenital syndrome characterized by redundancy of the valve leaflets and elongation of the chordae tendineae. The cusps prolapse or balloon into the atrium to varying degrees during ventricular systole; mitral regurgitation may result. These functional changes are caused by alterations in the collagen structure of the cusp. The exact incidence of mitral valve prolapse is estimated to be 5% to 10%. The course of this syndrome can be benign, although endocarditis prophylaxis is usually indicated.

Papillary muscle dysfunction or rupture can lead to a wide spectrum of valvular dysfunction. Papillary muscle abnormalities may be intermittent, may be secondary to ischemia, and may produce only episodic mild regurgitation. However, if rupture of a necrotic papillary muscle occurs after myocardial infarction, acute mitral regurgitation results.

Congenital malformations can occur in any valve. For example, approximately 1% to 2% of aortic valves are bicuspid rather than tricuspid.

Certain valvular lesions strongly suggest the underlying cause of dysfunction. For example, isolated mitral stenosis is usually rheumatic, whereas isolated aortic stenosis usually results from premature calcification and degeneration of a congenitally bicuspid valve. Isolated tricuspid or pulmonic disease is almost invariably a congenital defect. Combined valvular lesions suggest rheumatic causation.

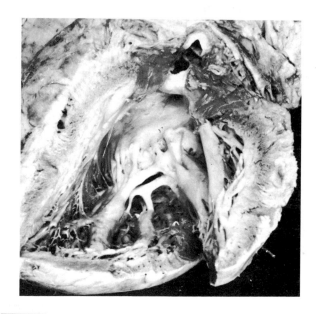

FIG. 32-2   Mitral valve viewed from below in a case of mitral valve stenosis. The valve is converted into a funnel-shaped structure, the apex of which is in the left ventricle. (From Hurst JW: *The heart,* ed 3, New York, 1974, McGraw-Hill.)

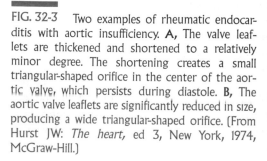

FIG. 32-3   Two examples of rheumatic endocarditis with aortic insufficiency. **A,** The valve leaflets are thickened and shortened to a relatively minor degree. The shortening creates a small triangular-shaped orifice in the center of the aortic valve, which persists during diastole. **B,** The aortic valve leaflets are significantly reduced in size, producing a wide triangular-shaped orifice. (From Hurst JW: *The heart,* ed 3, New York, 1974, McGraw-Hill.)

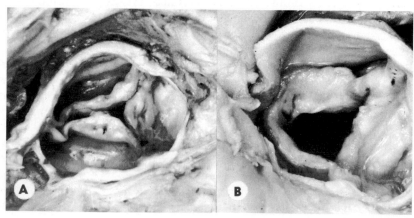

PATHOPHYSIOLOGY

Mitral Stenosis

Mitral stenosis impedes blood flow from the left atrium to the left ventricle during ventricular diastole (Fig. 32-4). To adequately fill the ventricle and maintain cardiac output, the left atrium must generate more pressure to propel blood beyond the valvular obstruction. Therefore the pressure difference, or *pressure gradient,* between the chambers rises; normally the pressure gradient is minimal.

The left atrial musculature hypertrophies to increase its pumping force. The active contribution of atrial contraction to ventricular filling becomes increasingly important. The primary function of the left atrium ceases to be that of a passive reservoir and conduit for blood flowing to the ventricle. Atrial dilation occurs as the left atrial volume rises, because of the inability of the chamber to empty normally.

The rise in left atrial pressure and volume is reflected backward into the pulmonary vasculature—pressure in the pulmonary veins and capillaries rises. A spectrum of pulmonary congestion results, ranging from mild venous congestion to interstitial edema with occasional fluid transudation into the alveoli.

Eventually, pulmonary arterial pressure must rise in response to the chronic elevation of pulmonary venous resistance. This response ensures an adequate pressure gradient for blood flow through the pulmonary vasculature. However, pulmonary hypertension increases the resistance to right ventricular ejection into the pulmonary artery. The right ventricle responds to this increased pressure work with muscular hypertrophy.

The pulmonary vasculature may undergo anatomic changes apparently designed to protect the pulmonary capillaries from excessively high right ventricular pressures and pulmonary flow. Structural changes—medial hypertrophy and intimal thickening—occur in the walls of the small arteries and arterioles. The mechanism mediating this anatomic response is unclear. These changes narrow the vessel lumen, elevating pulmonary vascular resistance. This arteriolar constriction, or *reactive pulmonary hypertension,* significantly elevates pulmonary arterial pressure. Pulmonary pressure can progressively climb to excessive levels approximating systemic pressure.

The right ventricle is poorly suited to perform as a high-pressure pump over long periods. Therefore it eventually fails. Right ventricular failure is reflected backward into the systemic circulation, producing systemic venous congestion and peripheral edema. The right-sided failure can be compounded by functional regurgitation of the tricuspid valve as a result of right ventricular enlargement.

Over a period of years the lesion of mitral stenosis narrows the valve orifice. Symptoms characteristically do

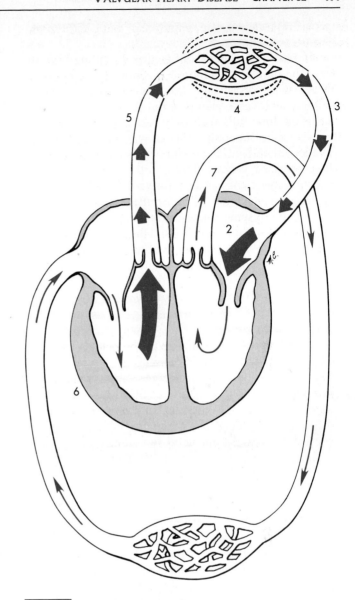

FIG. 32-4   Pathophysiology of mitral stenosis: *1,* left atrial hypertrophy; *2,* left atrial dilation; *3,* pulmonary venous congestion; *4,* pulmonary congestion; *5,* pulmonary hypertension; *6,* right ventricular hypertrophy; *7,* fixed cardiac output.

not appear until the valve orifice has been reduced by more than 50% from a normal area of 4 to 6 cm^2 to less than 1.5 cm^2. With this degree of valvular restriction, left atrial pressure rises to maintain ventricular filling and cardiac output; consequently, pulmonary venous pressure rises, producing dyspnea. A diastolic heart murmur, indicative of abnormal flow through the restricted orifice, is usually noted much earlier in the course of the disease. Valvular dimensions of less than 1 cm^2 reflect critical mitral stenosis.

The clinical picture can differ depending on the underlying hemodynamics; however, the earliest symptom is usually *dyspnea on exertion.* Two hemodynamic changes associated with exertion are poorly tolerated in mitral stenosis: (1) tachycardia (rapid heart rate) and (2) elevated left atrial pressure. Tachycardia reduces the duration of diastole, the period of ventricular filling from the atria. The duration of diastole is critically important in mitral stenosis because the lesion itself impairs ventricular filling and, consequently, atrial emptying. As ventricular filling time falls with tachycardia, cardiac output is reduced further and pulmonary congestion increases. The elevation of left atrial pressure with exertion resulting from increased venous return further compounds pulmonary congestion. Because forward flow is restricted, the pressure elevation is transmitted backward to the lungs. Thus dyspnea on exertion is the result of pulmonary congestion. Weakness and fatigue are also prominent early symptoms as a result of the fixed, and eventually reduced, cardiac output.

As the disease progresses, respiratory symptoms become more pronounced. Susceptibility to pulmonary infection is high. Orthopnea and paroxysmal nocturnal dyspnea at rest may be noted. Transmission of the elevated pulmonary vascular pressures to the bronchial capillaries may result in capillary or bronchial vein rupture and mild hemoptysis. Eventually the lungs become fibrotic and noncompliant. The distribution of blood flow within the lungs shifts. Normally there is relatively greater perfusion of the lower lobes than of the upper lobes because of the effect of gravity on blood flow. In mitral stenosis, flow predominates in the upper lobes, presumably as a result of greater pulmonary vascular disease and interstitial edema in the lower lobes.

Atrial fibrillation frequently develops as a result of chronic atrial hypertrophy and dilation. With the onset of atrial fibrillation, severe exacerbation of symptoms can occur. The quivering atrial musculature is incapable of coordinated muscular contraction. This loss of the active atrial kick reduces ventricular filling. Ventricular filling is further reduced by the rapid ventricular response to atrial fibrillation (heart rates approximate 150 beats per minute [bpm] unless treated). The abrupt onset of rapid atrial fibrillation can result in low cardiac output and pulmonary edema. Hemodynamic adaptation occurs, usually with pharmacologic assistance (e.g., with digoxin). However, the onset of atrial fibrillation exacerbates the risk of thrombus formation and systemic embolization because of stasis of blood in the left atrium proximal to the stenotic valve. Palpitations may also be noted with atrial fibrillation.

End-stage mitral stenosis is associated with right heart failure with consequent systemic venous engorgement, hepatomegaly, peripheral edema, and ascites. Right heart failure and chamber dilation can result in functional tricuspid regurgitation. However, mitral stenosis need not progress to this extreme. With the onset of symptoms, the disease can be managed medically, with eventual surgical correction.

The following findings are typically noted in mitral stenosis:

1. *Auscultation:* low-frequency diastolic murmur (rumble) and accentuated first heart sound (AV valve closure) and opening snap resulting from the loss of leaflet pliability

2. *Electrocardiogram:* left atrial enlargement (widened and notched P wave, most prominent in lead II, known as "P mitrale"), if rhythm is normal sinus; right ventricular hypertrophy; atrial fibrillation common but not specific for mitral stenosis

3. *Chest radiograph:* left atrial and right ventricular enlargement; pulmonary venous congestion; interstitial pulmonary edema; pulmonary vascular redistribution to the upper lobes; mitral valve calcification.

4. *Hemodynamic findings:* elevated pressure gradient across the mitral valve; elevated left atrial pressure and pulmonary capillary wedge pressure with prominent *a* waves; elevated pulmonary artery pressure; low cardiac output; elevated right-sided heart pressures and jugular venous pressure with significant *v* waves in right atrial trace or jugular veins if tricuspid regurgitation present.

Mitral Regurgitation

Mitral regurgitation permits retrograde blood flow from the left ventricle to the left atrium as a result of incomplete valve closure (Fig. 32-5). During systole the ventricle simultaneously ejects blood forward into the aorta and backward into the left atrium. The volume work of both the left ventricle and the left atrium must increase to preserve cardiac output.

The left ventricle must pump a sufficient volume of blood to maintain a normal forward flow into the aorta and the regurgitant flow through the mitral valve. For instance, the normal ventricular output per beat (stroke volume) is 70 ml. If the regurgitant flow is 30 ml/beat, the ventricle must pump 100 ml/beat to maintain a normal stroke volume. The additional volume load created by the regurgitant valve prompts ventricular dilation. According to Starling's law of the heart, ventricular dilation increases myocardial contractility. Eventually the ventricular wall hypertrophies to further increase contractile force.

In the early stages of chronic mitral regurgitation, the left ventricle is able to compensate for the increased volume load. Even though total ventricular output (including both forward and regurgitant flows) increases, the afterload or amount of wall tension the ventricle must develop during systole to eject blood is reduced. Afterload reduction occurs because the ventricle ejects a portion of the stroke volume into the low-pressure left atrium. Paradoxically, this reduction in afterload via regurgitant flow improves the ventricular compensatory ability to maintain forward flow. Eventually, however, the ventricle begins to fail, reducing cardiac output and increasing residual ventricular volumes and regurgitant flow.

Regurgitation creates a volume load not only for the left ventricle, but also for the left atrium. The left atrium dilates to accommodate the increased volume and to in-

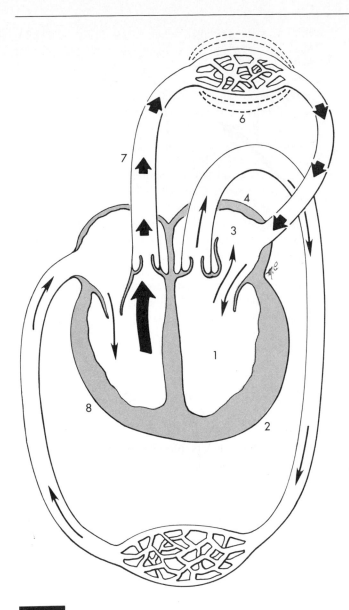

FIG. 32-5 Pathophysiology of mitral regurgitation: *1,* left ventricular dilation; *2,* left ventricular hypertrophy; *3,* left atrial dilation; *4,* left atrial hypertrophy; *5,* pulmonary venous congestion; *6,* pulmonary congestion; *7,* pulmonary artery hypertension; *8,* right ventricular hypertrophy.

crease the force of atrial contraction. Subsequently, the atrium hypertrophies to further increase atrial contractile force and output. Initially, increased left atrial compliance permits accommodation of increased volume without significant pressure elevation. Thus, for a while, the left atrium buffers the effect of the regurgitant volume, protecting the pulmonary vasculature and limiting pulmonary symptoms.

However, mitral regurgitation is a self-perpetuating lesion. As ventricular volumes and dimensions increase, valve function worsens. Chamber enlargement increases the degree of regurgitation by displacing papillary muscles and dilating the mitral orifice, thus reducing leaflet contact during valve closure.

As the lesion worsens, the ability of the left atrium to

distend and protect the lungs is exceeded. Left ventricular failure is usually the prelude to accelerated cardiac decompensation. The left ventricle becomes overburdened, and forward flow through the aorta falls, with a simultaneous rise in backward congestion. Gradually the predictable sequence of pulmonary and right heart involvement ensues: (1) pulmonary venous congestion, (2) interstitial edema, (3) pulmonary arterial hypertension, and (4) right ventricular hypertrophy. These changes are less pronounced than changes with mitral stenosis. Mitral regurgitation can culminate in right heart failure, although less frequently than does mitral stenosis.

The course of the disease is profoundly altered if the onset of mitral regurgitation is acute; as in papillary muscle rupture after myocardial infarction, rather than chronic. Acute mitral regurgitation is poorly tolerated. Normally, the left atrium is relatively noncompliant and therefore unable to abruptly distend and accommodate the regurgitant volume (Fig. 32-6). Thus the sudden increase in volume and pressure is transmitted directly to the pulmonary vasculature. Within hours, fulminating pulmonary edema and shock can develop.

The earliest symptoms of mitral regurgitation are (1) weakness and fatigue caused by the reduction in forward flow, (2) exertional dyspnea, and (3) palpitations. Severe symptoms are precipitated by left ventricular failure with consequent low cardiac output and pulmonary congestion. The following findings are typically associated with chronic, severe mitral regurgitation:

1. *Auscultation:* murmur throughout systole (holosystolic or pansystolic murmur)
2. *Electrocardiogram:* left atrial enlargement (P mitrale), if rhythm is normal sinus; atrial fibrillation; left ventricular hypertrophy
3. *Chest radiograph:* left atrial enlargement; left ventricular enlargement; variable pulmonary vascular congestion
4. *Hemodynamic findings:* increased left atrial pressure with significant *v* waves; elevated left ventricular end-diastolic pressure; variable elevations of pulmonary pressures

Aortic Stenosis

Aortic stenosis obstructs blood flow from the left ventricle into the aorta during ventricular systole. As the resistance to ventricular ejection increases, the pressure work of the left ventricle rises. In response, the left ventricle hypertrophies to generate more pressure and maintain peripheral perfusion; a marked pressure gradient develops between the left ventricle and the aorta (Fig. 32-7). Hypertrophy reduces ventricular wall compliance, and the wall becomes relatively stiff. Thus, despite the maintenance of normal cardiac output and ventricular volumes, ventricular end-diastolic pressure is slightly elevated.

The reserve pumping capability of the left ventricle is considerable. For instance, the left ventricle, which normally generates a systolic pressure of 120 mm Hg, can

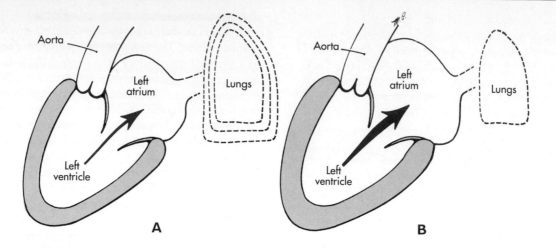

FIG. 32-6   **A,** Acute, and **B,** chronic mitral regurgitation. Note that in chronic mitral regurgitation, greater dilation and hypertrophy of the left atrium and ventricle occur. Acute mitral regurgitation causes greater pulmonary congestion because the left atrium is less pliable or distensible.

develop pressure up to approximately 300 mm Hg during ventricular contraction. To compensate and maintain cardiac output, the left ventricle not only generates higher pressure, but also prolongs the duration of ejection. Therefore, despite the progressive restriction of the aortic orifice and a consequent elevation of ventricular work, the mechanical efficiency of the heart is maintained for long periods. Eventually, however, the adaptive ability of the left ventricle is overwhelmed. The onset of progressive symptoms heralds a critical point in the course of aortic stenosis. Critical aortic stenosis corresponds to a reduction in valvular orifice from 3 to 4 cm^2 to less than 0.5 cm^2; generally a pressure gradient does not develop across the valve until this orifice is reduced by approximately 50%

A characteristic triad of symptoms is associated with aortic stenosis: (1) angina, (2) syncope, and (3) left ventricular failure. If unheeded, these symptoms indicate a poor prognosis, with an average survival of less than 5 years. The onset of *left ventricular failure,* indicating cardiac decompensation, is particularly ominous. *Angina* is produced by an imbalance in myocardial oxygen supply and demand; demand increases with hypertrophy and increased myocardial work, whereas supply is potentially reduced by the powerful systolic compression of the coronary arteries by the hypertrophied muscle. In addition, with myocardial hypertrophy the ratio of capillaries to muscle fiber mass may be reduced. The oxygen diffusion distance therefore is increased, potentially limiting myocardial oxygen availability. The subendocardial layer of the left ventricle is the most vulnerable. Death may ensue within 5 years after the onset of angina. *Syncope* occurs primarily with exertion, as a result of either dysrhythmias or an inability to increase the cardiac output sufficiently to maintain cerebral perfusion. Survival after the onset of syncope has been estimated at 3 to 4 years.

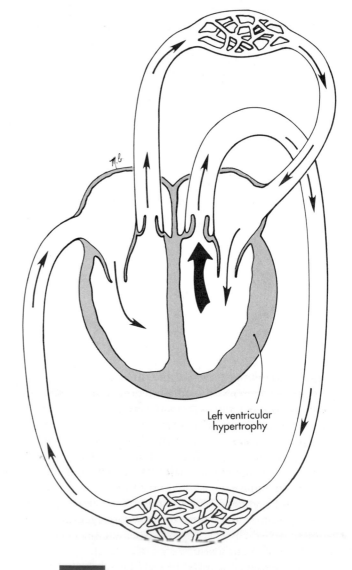

Left ventricular hypertrophy

FIG. 32-7   Pathophysiology of aortic stenosis.

Progressive ventricular failure impairs ventricular emptying. Cardiac output falls, and ventricular volumes rise. Ventricular dilation, occasionally associated with functional mitral regurgitation, ensues. Advanced aortic stenosis is associated with severe pulmonary congestion. Right ventricular failure and systemic venous congestion are indicative of end-stage disease. Aortic stenosis infrequently progresses to this extreme. The infrequent occurrence of right heart failure is probably the result of the high mortality rate associated with left heart failure earlier in the course of the disease. In addition, there is a significant incidence of sudden death in symptomatic patients with severe aortic stenosis. The pathogenesis of sudden death is controversial but is usually precipitated by strenuous exertion.

The prominent signs of severe aortic stenosis are as follows:

1. *Auscultation:* harsh systolic ejection murmur; paradoxical splitting of second heart sound; ejection click
2. *Electrocardiogram:* left ventricular hypertrophy; conduction defects
3. *Chest radiograph:* poststenotic dilation of the ascending aorta (resulting from local trauma from blood ejected under high pressure and striking the aortic wall); valvular calcification (best seen on lateral or oblique views)
4. *Hemodynamic findings:* significant aortic gradient (50 to 100 mm Hg); elevated left ventricular end-diastolic pressure; delayed carotid upstroke

Aortic Regurgitation

Aortic regurgitation produces a reflux of blood from the aorta into the left ventricle during ventricular relaxation (Fig. 32-8). In essence, the peripheral bed competes with the left ventricle for the blood ejected by the ventricle during systole. The magnitude of forward flow, or "runoff," into the periphery relative to retrograde flow into the ventricle depends on the degree of valve closure and the relative resistance to flow between the periphery and the ventricle. Characteristically, peripheral vascular resistance is low in aortic regurgitation, apparently as a compensatory mechanism to maximize forward flow. However, late in the course of the disease, peripheral resistance rises, increasing retrograde flow through the aortic valve and accelerating the disease progression.

The clinical course of chronic aortic regurgitation is the least understood and the most variable of the valvular lesions. However, the disease obviously imposes a severe volume load on the left ventricle. With each contraction, the ventricle must eject a quantity of blood equal to the normal stroke volume plus the regurgitant volume. The left ventricle dilates greatly and eventually hypertrophies, assuming a distinctive globular shape. An associated increase in wall compliance enables the ventricle to tolerate increased diastolic volumes without abnormal pressure elevations.

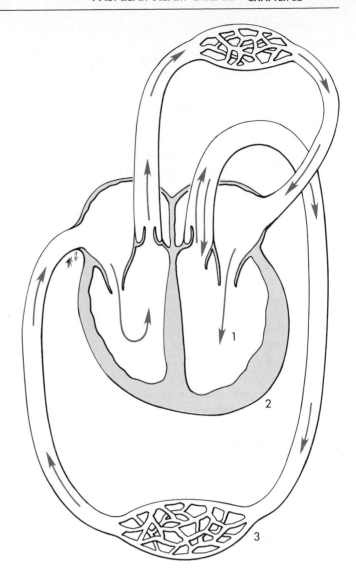

FIG. 32-8   Pathophysiology of aortic regurgitation: *1*, left ventricular dilation; *2*, left ventricular hypertrophy; *3*, hyperdynamic peripheral circulation.

The marked left ventricular compensatory ability in combination with a competent mitral valve maintains ventricular function for a long time. Symptoms rarely develop until left ventricular decompensation occurs, which is occasionally compounded by functional mitral regurgitation. Irreversible left ventricular damage, resulting from the prolonged ejection of the volume overload against systemic resistance, can be sustained. The point of significant deterioration is poorly defined. Early symptoms are palpitations, fatigue, and dyspnea on exertion. Angina may also be noted with left ventricular hypertrophy and low arterial diastolic pressures, which increase oxygen demand and decrease oxygen supply, respectively. However, substernal pain unrelated to myocardial ischemia may occur. Heart failure precipitates a downhill course of falling cardiac output and rising ventricular volume with retrograde left atrial and pulmonary congestion.

The following signs are associated with chronic aortic regurgitation:

1. *Auscultation:* diastolic murmur; characteristic Austin Flint murmur or diastolic rumble; systolic ejection click caused by increased ejection volume
2. *Electrocardiogram:* left ventricular hypertrophy.
3. *Chest radiograph:* left ventricular enlargement; dilation of proximal aorta
4. *Hemodynamic findings:* rapid upstroke and collapse of arterial pulse; widened pulse pressure with elevated systemic and lowered diastolic pressures
5. *Cardiac catheterization:* opacification of the left ventricle during injection of contrast material into the aortic root.

Characteristic findings are noted in the peripheral circulation as a result of the hyperdynamic myocardial action and the low peripheral resistance. The forceful, high-volume, left ventricular ejection followed by the rapid forward runoff of blood into the periphery and backward into the left ventricle through the diseased valve creates a rapid distention of the vasculature followed by a sudden collapse. These cardiovascular dynamics can be manifested by (1) waterhammer pulses (or *Corrigan's pulse*), characterized by a rapid rise and collapse of the arterial pulse; (2) pistol-shot pulses (or *Diroziez's murmur*), audible on auscultation of the femoral artery; (3) *Quincke's capillary pulsation,* visible as alternating flushing and paling of the nailbed capillaries; and (4) systolic head bobbing as the collapsed neck vessels fill rapidly (or *de Musset's sign*).

Tricuspid Valve Disease

Stenosis of the tricuspid valve restricts blood flow from the right atrium into the right ventricle during diastole. This lesion is usually associated with disease of the mitral and aortic valves secondary to severe rheumatic heart disease. Tricuspid stenosis increases the work of the right atrium, forcing the chamber to generate more pressure to maintain flow across the obstructed valve. The right atrium has a limited ability to compensate and thus dilates rapidly. As right atrial volumes and pressures rise, systemic venous engorgement and pressure elevation result (Fig. 32-9).

The classic findings of right heart failure ensue: (1) venous distention with large *a* waves, (2) peripheral edema, (3) ascites, (4) hepatic enlargement, and (5) nausea and anorexia resulting from gastrointestinal engorgement. The following signs are associated with tricuspid stenosis:

1. *Auscultation:* diastolic murmur
2. *Electrocardiogram:* right atrial enlargement (tall, peaked P waves known as *P pulmonale*)
3. *Chest radiograph:* right atrial enlargement
4. *Hemodynamic findings:* pressure gradient across the tricuspid valve and elevated right atrial and central venous pressures with large *a* waves.

Pure tricuspid regurgitation is usually the consequence of advanced left heart failure or severe pulmonary hypertension, resulting in right ventricular deterioration. As the right ventricle fails and enlarges, functional regurgitation of the tricuspid valve is produced. Tricuspid regurgitation is associated with right heart failure and the following findings:

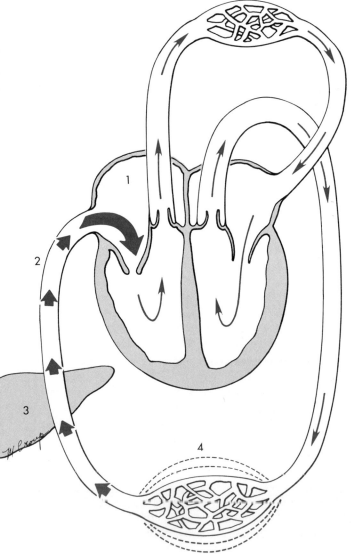

FIG. 32-9   Pathophysiology of tricuspid stenosis: *1,* right atrial dilation; *2,* venous congestion; *3,* hepatomegaly; *4,* systemic congestion.

1. *Auscultation:* murmur throughout systole
2. *Electrocardiogram:* right atrial enlargement (tall and narrow P wave, or P pulmonale), if rhythm is normal sinus; atrial fibrillation; right ventricular hypertrophy
3. *Chest radiograph:* right atrial and ventricular enlargement
4. *Hemodynamic findings:* elevated right atrial pressure with significant *v* waves.

Pulmonic Valve Disease

The incidence of pulmonic valvular lesions is extremely low. Pulmonic stenosis is usually congenital rather than rheumatic. Stenosis of the pulmonic valve increases right ventricular pressure work, producing right ventricular hypertrophy. Symptoms result when right ventricular failure occurs, producing systemic venous engorgement and its clinical sequelae.

Functional pulmonic regurgitation can occur as a sequela to left-sided valvular dysfunction with chronic pulmonic hypertension and dilation of the pulmonic valve orifice. However, this lesion is rarely seen.

Compound Valvular Disease

Mixed lesions, consisting of stenosis and regurgitation in the same valve, frequently occur. This is to be expected because a stenotic, immobile valve is often unable to close completely. *Combined lesions,* or multivalvular disease, are often seen because rheumatic heart disease typically affects multiple valves.

Mixed lesions and combined lesions compound the valvular dysfunction described for isolated or *pure lesions,* altering to a variable degree the physiologic consequences. Compound lesions can either magnify or buffer a physiologic consequence of a pure lesion. For instance, mixed mitral regurgitation and aortic stenosis increase the volume load and pressure work of the left ventricle and greatly intensify the left ventricular strain. As a result, this combination is associated with a rapidly progressive downhill course.

However, the combination of aortic stenosis and mitral stenosis, in essence, protects the left ventricle from the magnitude of left ventricular strain associated with isolated aortic stenosis. This protective effect results from the reduction in left ventricular filling caused by the restriction to blood flow through the mitral valve. Diminished ventricular filling reduces the volume of the blood that the left ventricle must force through the restricted aortic orifice.

THERAPEUTIC INTERVENTION

Rheumatic fever and subacute bacterial endocarditis are two disease processes that can be prevented, thus reducing the incidence or severity of acquired valvular lesions. Rheumatic fever can be prevented by early detection and treatment of group A beta-hemolytic streptococcal infections with penicillin. Early diagnosis and treatment of acute rheumatic fever are also essential. The diagnosis of acute rheumatic fever can be complicated because no single clinical or laboratory finding is pathognomonic for this disease; many of the findings are nonspecific. The modified Jones criteria are useful in the diagnosis of acute rheumatic fever (see box, p. 498). These criteria are designated as major or minor according to their relative importance as diagnostic indicators. The presence of two major criteria or one major and two minor criteria indicates a high probability of acute rheumatic fever. Evidence of an antecedent streptococcal infection is also prerequisite to the diagnosis; elevated antistreptolysin levels (ASO) are frequently used to establish the presence of streptococcal antibodies.

Treatment of acute rheumatic fever is palliative and includes (1) antibiotics, such as penicillin or erythromycin, to eliminate any residual streptococcal organisms; (2) anti-inflammatory agents, such as salicylates or corticosteroids; (3) analgesics, if indicated for arthritic pain; and (4) restriction of physical activity according to the degree of carditis. Associated cardiac failure might necessitate salt restriction, digoxin, and diuretics.

After the initial attack of rheumatic fever, susceptibility to recurrent attacks is extremely high. Consequently, antibiotic prophylaxis must begin as soon as the diagnosis is established. Single monthly injections of penicillin are effective and offer a distinct advantage over daily oral therapy in terms of patient compliance. Antibiotic prophylaxis must continue at least into adulthood to avoid potentially crippling deformity of heart valves produced by recurrent attacks of rheumatic fever. Emphasis must be on prevention rather than treatment of streptococcal infections because recurrent rheumatic fever is frequently preceded by asymptomatic streptococcal infection. In addition, difficulty is often encountered in preventing recurrent attacks after the onset of infection.

Heart valves with congenital malformations or acquired deformity are particularly vulnerable to infection, or endocarditis, from systemic infections or even from the transient septicemia associated with minor surgical procedures (e.g., dental extractions). Appropriate prophylactic antibiotic coverage during substantiated or potential systemic infection is critical to prevent further valvular deterioration. Once valvular damage has been sustained, the course of the disease and medical therapy vary according to the site and severity of the lesion.

Mitral valve disease produces symptoms earlier than aortic valve disease because the diseased mitral valve imposes a burden primarily on the left atrium, whereas the diseased aortic valve burdens the left ventricle. The thin-walled left atrium is poorly suited to maintain its pumping capability in the face of an ever-increasing pressure or volume load. In addition, since no true valves separate

GUIDELINES FOR DIAGNOSIS OF INITIAL ATTACK OF RHEUMATIC FEVER (JONES CRITERIA, 1992 UPDATE)*

MAJOR MANIFESTATIONS

1. Carditis
2. Polyarthritis
3. Chorea
4. Erythema marginatum
5. Subcutaneous nodules

MINOR MANIFESTATIONS

Clinical findings

1. Arthralgia
2. Fever

Laboratory findings

1. Elevated levels of acute-phase reactants
   a. Erythrocyte sedimentation rate (ESR)
   b. C-reactive protein (CRP)
2. Prolonged PR interval

SUPPORTING EVIDENCE OF ANTECEDENT GROUP A STREPTOCOCCAL INFECTION

1. Positive throat culture or rapid streptococcal antigen test results
2. Elevated or rising streptococcal antibody titer (ASO titer)

From The Special Writing Group of the Committee on Rheumatic Fever, Endocarditis, and Kawasaki Disease of the Council on Cardiovascular Disease in the Young of the American Heart Association, *JAMA* 268(15):2070, 1992.

*If supported by evidence of preceding group A streptococcal infection, the presence of two major manifestations or of one major and two minor manifestations indicates a high probability of acute rheumatic fever.

the pulmonary veins from the left atrium, left atrial congestion is readily transmitted retrograde to the lungs, producing pulmonary symptoms. With aortic valve disease, the left ventricle compensates well for a long time, resulting in a long asymptomatic phase. The left atrium is protected from the left ventricular strain as long as the mitral valve remains competent and the left ventricular pumping capability is sustained.

Medical Therapy
Mitral valve disease

The clinical progression of mitral valve disease is gradual and prolonged. Dyspnea is usually the most prominent and disabling symptom. However, symptoms are initially responsive to medical therapy consisting of (1) *diuretics* to reduce congestion; (2) *digoxin* to increase contractile force in the presence of mitral regurgitation or

to reduce ventricular response to atrial fibrillation; if the ventricular rate is not slowed, a beta-adrenergic blocking agent or calcium channel blocker is added; (3) *antidysrhythmics* if atrial fibrillation occurs; (4) *vasodilator therapy* in the presence of mitral regurgitation to reduce afterload, thereby decreasing regurgitant flow and increasing forward blood flow; (5) *anticoagulants* if systemic embolization becomes a threat; (6) *antibiotics* for endocarditis prophylaxis; and (7) catheter balloon *valvotomy* (valvulotomy) in select patients. Eventually, surgical intervention is necessary to control the progressively disabling symptoms. Occasionally, surgical intervention is precipitated by an abrupt deterioration associated with dysrhythmias, embolization, or pulmonary infection.

Aortic valve disease

The management of aortic valve disease is in distinct contrast to that of mitral valve disease. The onset of significant symptoms—angina, syncope, and failure—usually correlates with left ventricular decompensation, signaling a need to consider surgical intervention. The risk of surgery for most symptomatic patients is less than the risk of prolonged medical therapy. Once the patient is symptomatic, the course of aortic disease is progressively downhill. Severe aortic stenosis is a potentially unpredictable, lethal entity; sudden death can occur. Aortic regurgitation poses somewhat of a therapeutic dilemma; the timing of surgery is less well defined. Close surveillance of patients with aortic valve disease is essential to detect early signs of clinical deterioration. As with patients with mitral valve disease, bacterial endocarditis prophylaxis is necessary.

Surgical Therapy
Mitral valve disease

Techniques for correcting deformities of the mitral valve have been expanded in recent years. Patients may have (1) *mitral valvotomy* (valvulotomy), (2) mitral valve replacement, or (3) mitral valve repair.

Mitral valvotomy, or opening of the mitral valve, is considered for select patients with pure mitral stenosis when their symptoms have progressed to functional class II heart disease (i.e., symptomatic with ordinary physical exertion). A stenotic mitral valve can be dilated via a transventricular surgical approach or a percutaneous approach. The surgical transventricular procedure splits the valve leaflets at the point of fusion along the commissures. Balloon valvuloplasty involves threading either one or two balloon-tipped catheters through a peripheral vessel under fluoroscopic guidance into the right atrium, advancing the catheter across the atrial septum into the left atrium, and placing the balloon tip within the valve orifice. In a noncalcified pliable valve, inflation of the balloon should result in separation of the fused commissures. Candidates for either the percutaneous or the surgical approach are usually younger patients without atrial fibrillation, mitral regurgitation, a calcified valve, or history of prior surgical commissurotomy.

Mitral valve replacement is generally considered for mitral regurgitation and for mitral stenosis when symptoms have progressed to functional class III heart disease (i.e., symptoms with less than ordinary physical exertion) despite medical therapy, although with improvements in surgical technique and valve design, surgery may be recommended earlier. Further disease progression to functional class IV is associated with higher surgical mortality and morbidity rates as a result of residual myocardial and pulmonary dysfunction. Systemic embolization or significant pulmonary hypertension are also indications for surgery. Mitral valve replacement involves excision of the valve, chordae tendinae, and papillary muscles. A prosthetic valve designed to simulate normal valve function is inserted (see later section for description of available prosthetics).

Reconstructive surgical techniques may be used to repair the mitral valve, particularly in the setting of degenerative, nonrheumatic disease. Repair of the valve, or *valvuloplasty,* can involve lengthening or shortening the chordae tendinae, repositioning the chordae, or resecting valve leaflets. A prosthetic ring is usually inserted in the valve annulus to stabilize and repair the valve orifice, a technique referred to as *annuloplasty.*

Aortic valve disease

Valve replacement is recommended for aortic regurgitation and calcific aortic stenosis. Percutaneous aortic valvulotomy is considered for older, high-risk patients with aortic stenosis or for younger patients with noncalcific aortic stenosis.

Valve prosthetics

There are two basic types of valves—mechanical valves and tissue valves. Each has distinct advantages and disadvantages. The *mechanical valves,* although noteworthy for durability, are thrombogenic, and patients require long-term anticoagulation. Three types of *tissue valves* are available: (1) porcine heterograph, (2) bovine pericardial heterograph, and (3) homographs, or human heart valves (usually aortic or pulmonic), which have been cryopreserved. *Porcine and bovine valves* are nonthrombogenic but are less durable than mechanical valves. They tend to be recommended for older patients or when anticoagulation is contraindicated. *Homographs* are limited in supply, but over the long term, they may have both the necessary durability and the nonthrombogenic characteristics.

Fig. 32-10 illustrates examples of prosthetic valves. All valves open and close in response to pressure changes on either side of the valve. For example, with the disk valve in the mitral position, the disks are perpendicular to the annulus during ventricular relaxation, permitting blood flow from the atrium to the ventricle. During ventricular contraction, as ventricular pressure exceeds atrial pressure, the disks go into a horizontal position to seal the mitral orifice, preventing backward flow.

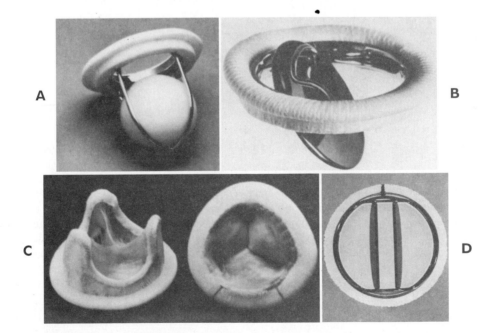

FIG. 32-10   Prosthetic valves. **A,** Starr-Edwards (caged ball) valve. **B,** Björk-Shiley (tilting disk) valve. **C,** Carpentier-Edwards (tissue) valve. **D,** St. Jude Medical (bileaflet) valve in open position. (**A** courtesy of American Edwards Laboratories, Division of American Hospital Supply, Santa Ana, Calif; **B** and **C** from Johnson RA, Haber E, Austen WG: *The practice of cardiology,* Boston, 1980, Little, Brown; **D** from Weiland AP: *Heart Lung* 12(5):500, 1983.)

QUESTIONS

▼ *Answer the following on a separate sheet of paper.*

1. List and briefly describe five causes of valvular heart disease.

2. What is functional AV regurgitation?

3. Comment on the following statement: "Before rendering any treatment that may result in even the slightest release of bacteria into the bloodstream, one is obligated to make absolutely sure that the patient is not affected by any kind of heart deformity. If it is known or suspected that the patient has a deformity of the heart, it is absolutely necessary to administer prophylactic antibiotics."

4. What is the medical treatment for each of the following problems associated with mitral valve disease: pulmonary congestion, atrial fibrillation, and systemic emboli?

5. What is a mitral valvulotomy?

6. List the revised Jones criteria. What is their purpose? Illustrate.

▼ *Circle the letter preceding each item below that correctly answers the question or completes the statement. Only one answer is correct unless otherwise noted.*

7. Mitral valve closure occurs when:
   a. Left ventricular pressure exceeds left atrial pressure
   b. Left atrial pressure exceeds left ventricular pressure
   c. Left ventricular pressure exceeds aortic pressure
   d. Left atrial pressure equals left ventricular pressure

8. Arrange the heart valves in correct order according to relative frequency of involvement in valvular heart disease.
   a. Pulmonic
   b. Aortic
   c. Mitral
   d. Tricuspid

9. The organism that precedes the development of rheumatic heart disease is:
   a. Group A beta-hemolytic streptococcus
   b. *Streptococcus viridans*
   c. *Staphylococcus aureus*
   d. *Staphylococcus albus*

10. Progressive valvular lesions in rheumatic fever are primarily a result of:
    a. A single episode of rheumatic carditis
    b. Chronic infective carditis
    c. Recurrent episodes of rheumatic carditis
    d. Subacute bacterial endocarditis

11. The primary site of vegetations in rheumatic carditis is:
    a. On the papillary muscles
    b. Diffuse distribution over the endocardium
    c. Along the chordae tendineae
    d. Along the valve leaflets at their lines of contact

12. Morphologic changes that characterize pure rheumatic valvular stenosis include all the following *except:*
    a. Leaflet fusion along the commissures
    b. Shrunken, retracted cusps
    c. Thickening of the chordae tendineae
    d. Thickening of valvular cusps

13. Morphologic changes that characterize pure rheumatic valvular regurgitation include all the following *except:*
    a. Shrunken, retracted cusps
    b. Shortened, fused chordae tendinae
    c. Rupture of the papillary muscles
    d. Enlargement of the valvular orifice

14. Dilation and hypertrophy of the left atrium are the initial compensatory response in:
    a. Aortic stenosis
    b. Tricuspid stenosis
    c. Mitral stenosis
    d. Acute rheumatic fever

15. Dilation and hypertrophy of the left ventricle occur in:
    a. Mitral stenosis
    b. Mitral regurgitation
    c. Tricuspid regurgitation
    d. Pulmonary stenosis

16. Which of the following is the earliest symptom in patients with mitral stenosis?
    a. Palpitations
    b. Dyspnea on exertion
    c. Orthopnea
    d. Angina

17. Symptoms with mild exertion appear when the orifice of the mitral valve (normally 4 to 6 cm²) is reduced to:
    a. 3 to 4 cm²
    b. 2 to 3 cm²
    c. 1 to 2 cm²
    d. Less than 1 cm²

18. Which of the following disorders is *least* likely to result in left ventricular strain?
    a. Systemic hypertension
    b. Aortic regurgitation
    c. Mitral stenosis
    d. Ventricular aneurysm

19. Atrial fibrillation complicating mitral stenosis creates the following problem(s) (more than one answer may be correct):
    a. Loss of atrial contraction
    b. Potential systemic embolization
    c. Potential right ventricular failure
    d. Decreased ventricular filling time

20. Chronic mitral stenosis may result in all the following *except:*
    a. Enlargement of the left atrium
    b. Increased pressure in the left ventricle
    c. Redistribution of pulmonary blood flow to the upper lobes
    d. A fixed cardiac output
    e. Pulmonary hypertension

21. Mitral valve insufficiency will result in blood regurgitating from the:
    a. Right ventricle back to the right atrium
    b. Pulmonary artery back to the right ventricle
    c. Left ventricle back to the left atrium
    d. Right atrium back to the superior and inferior venae cavae

22. The most likely cause of acute mitral regurgitation would be:
    a. Recurrent episodes of rheumatic endocarditis
    b. Chest trauma
    c. Bacterial endocarditis
    d. Ruptured papillary muscle complicating myocardial infarction

23. In differentiating acute mitral regurgitation from chronic mitral regurgitation, all the following statements are correct *except:*
    a. Fulminating pulmonary edema is more common in acute mitral regurgitation.
    b. Left ventricular hypertrophy is common in chronic mitral regurgitation.
    c. A dilated left atrium is common in acute and chronic mitral regurgitation.
    d. Atrial fibrillation is common in chronic mitral regurgitation, but normal sinus rhythm is more likely in the acute form.

24. Isolated aortic stenosis usually results from:
    a. A congenital bicuspid valve
    b. Rheumatic valvular disease
    c. Atherosclerotic heart disease
    d. Progressive calcification with aging

25. The primary response to aortic stenosis is:
    a. Right ventricular hypertrophy
    b. Left ventricular hypertrophy

? QUESTIONS—cont'd

c. Pulmonary hypertension
d. Enlargement of the left atrium

26. Atrial fibrillation is *least* likely to be associated with:
   a. Mitral regurgitation
   b. Mitral stenosis
   c. Aortic stenosis
   d. Coronary atherosclerotic disease

27. Which of the following findings would *not* be expected in a patient with severe aortic stenosis?
   a. Paradoxical splitting of the second heart sound
   b. Poststenotic dilation of the aorta on chest radiograph
   c. Enlarged and sustained apical impulse on palpation
   d. A pressure gradient of 100 mm Hg between the aorta and left ventricle on cardiac catheterization
   e. A widened pulse pressure

28. Potential symptoms and signs in moderate aortic stenosis include all the following *except:*
   a. Angina pectoris
   b. Effort syncope
   c. Peripheral edema
   d. Paroxysmal noctural dyspnea

29. In aortic stenosis, life expectancy after the onset of significant symptoms averages:
   a. Less than 5 years
   b. 5 to 8 years
   c. 9 to 11 years
   d. 12 to 15 years

30. Characteristic signs of severe aortic regurgitation include (more than one answer may be correct):
   a. Pistol-shot pulses heard over the femoral artery
   b. Corrigan's (waterhammer) pulse
   c. Austin Flint murmur
   d. Systolic head bobbing
   e. Alternating flushing and paling of nailbed capillaries (Quincke's capillary pulsation)

31. Which of the following statements about tricuspid stenosis is *not* true?
   a. There is an increased pressure gradient between the right ventricle and right atrium on cardiac catheterization.
   b. Electrocardiographic findings include tall, peaked P waves and right atrial enlargement.
   c. Central venous pressure is usually normal.

d. There is accentuation of the *a* wave of the jugular venous pulse.
   e. Hepatomegaly and ascites are common findings on physical examination.

32. Pure tricuspid regurgitation is usually:
   a. Associated with rheumatic heart disease
   b. A functional disorder associated with right heart failure
   c. Associated with acute myocardial infarction
   d. A functional disorder associated with left ventricular hypertrophy

33. Which of the following is *not* associated with tricuspid regurgitation?
   a. Positive hepatojugular reflux test
   b. Waterhammer pulse
   c. Prominent *v* wave of the jugular venous pulse
   d. Distended neck veins
   e. Opacification of the right atrium when the right ventricle is injected with contrast media

34. Which of the following combinations of valvular disease would probably be the most lethal?
   a. Aortic stenosis + mitral stenosis
   b. Tricuspid regurgitation + mitral stenosis
   c. Aortic regurgitation + mitral regurgitation
   d. Aortic regurgitation + aortic stenosis

35. The radiographic findings of right ventricular hypertrophy in the absence of pulmonary arterial hypertension are suggestive of:
   a. Tricuspid stenosis
   b. Mitral stenosis
   c. Pulmonic stenosis
   d. Aortic regurgitation

36. Pulmonic stenosis is usually the result of:
   a. Rheumatic fever

b. Coronary atherosclerotic disease
   c. Congenital deformity of the valve
   d. None of the above

37. Subacute bacterial endocarditis in a susceptible host may be prevented by (more than one answer may be correct):
   a. Replacement of diseased valves
   b. Use of antibiotics before and after dental surgery
   c. Antibiotic prophylaxis throughout adolescence
   d. Antibiotic prophylaxis for genitourinary tract instrumentation

38. Replacement of the mitral valve is indicated when the patient's disability is classified, according to the New York Heart Association, as:
   a. Class I
   b. Class II
   c. Class III
   d. Class IV

39. A suitable candidate for mitral commissurotomy is a patient with a mitral valve that is:
   a. Heavily calcified
   b. Stenotic and regurgitant
   c. Stenotic and flexible
   d. Stenotic and immobile

40. Which of the following criteria is an indication for consideration of imminent aortic valve replacement in aortic stenosis?
   a. Arterial pulse pressure of 50 mm Hg
   b. Aortic valve calcification on chest radiograph
   c. Onset of symptoms of angina pectoris, effort syncope, and left heart failure
   d. An increased left ventricular end-diastolic pressure at cardiac catheterization

▼ *Match the functional valvular disorder in column A with its effects in column B.*

Column A	Column B
41. _____ Valvular regurgitation	a. Increased cardiac volume work
42. _____ Valvular stenosis	b. Increased cardiac pressure work
	c. Backward flow
	d. Resistance to forward flow
	e. Chamber dilation
	f. Muscle hypertrophy

Continued.

QUESTIONS—cont'd

▼ *Circle the letter preceding each item below that correctly answers each question or completes the statement. More than one answer may be correct.*

43. An indication of active rheumatic carditis is the presence of:
    a. Valvular stenosis
    b. Aschoff's bodies
    c. Calcification of vascular tissue
    d. Perivascular fibrosis of the myocardium

44. Possible causes of valvular heart disease include:
    a. Rheumatic fever
    b. Rupture of the papillary muscle secondary to coronary atherosclerosis
    c. Congenital malformations
    d. Bacterial endocarditis

45. Which of the following would be considered major manifestations of acute rheumatic fever according to the revised Jones criteria?
    a. Polyarthritis
    b. Fever
    c. Erythema marginatum
    d. Abnormal erythrocyte sedimentation rate
    e. Carditis

CHAPTER 33

Cardiac Mechanical Dysfunction and Circulatory Support

PENNY FORD CARLETON
MADELINE M. O'DONNELL

There is a wide spectrum of cardiac mechanical dysfunction, ranging from mild, compensated heart failure to cardiogenic shock. This chapter provides an overview of

The authors acknowledge the contribution of Sally Keck, MS, RN, Massachusetts General Hospital, in the preparation of this chapter.

this spectrum and an introduction to the techniques of circulatory assistance and cardiac transplantation.

Heart failure poses a surprising paradox: it is relatively straightforward as a clinical syndrome yet extremely variable and complex as a pathophysiologic state. Because heart failure can be caused by a wide variety of disease entities, this contributes to its complexity. This discussion focuses on the common form of heart failure that occurs as a complication of ischemic heart disease.

Cardiac mechanical dysfunction and methods of circulatory support are considered relative to their effects on the three primary determinants of myocardial function: preload, contractility, and afterload. This framework is used because heart failure and the associated compensatory responses produce abnormalities in each of these determinants.

CONGESTIVE HEART FAILURE

Fundamental Concepts

Preload

Preload is the degree of myocardial fiber stretch at the end of ventricular filling or diastole. Increasing preload, up to a point, optimizes the overlap between actin and myosin filaments, increasing the force of contraction and cardiac output. This relationship is expressed by *Starling's law;* that is, stretching the myocardial fibers during diastole increases the force of contraction during systole (see Fig. 29-8). Preload is increased by elevation of ventricular diastolic volume, as occurs with fluid retention; a reduction of preload results from diuresis.

The relationship between increasing ventricular end-diastolic volume (EDV) and improved ventricular performance is illustrated in Fig. 33-1 as the *ventricular function curve*. The normal curve exhibits an initially steep, ascending limb where increments in volume and fiber stretch produce a corresponding improvement in ventricular function and cardiac output. The normal ventricle operates along the steep ascending limb where considerable reserve exists for improving ventricular function.

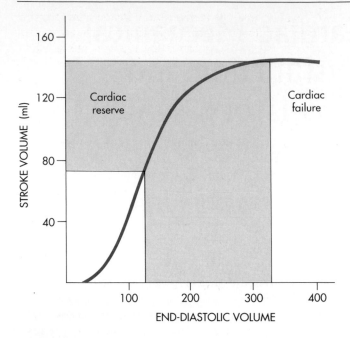

FIG. 33-1   Starling's law of the heart. As the end-diastolic volume increases, so does the force of ventricular contraction. Thus the stroke volume becomes greater, up to a critical point, after which it decreases. (From Langley LF: *Review of physiology*, ed 3, New York, 1971, McGraw-Hill.)

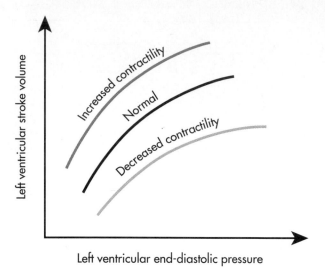

FIG. 33-2   Ventricular function curve. The solid black line represents the normal ventricular function curve. Note that increasing end-diastolic volume increases stroke volume up to a point. Displacement of the curve upward and to the left represents improved ventricular function, as would be seen with sympathetic nervous system stimulation. Displacement of the curve downward and to the right represents myocardial depression, as would be seen with acidosis or hypoxia or with cardiac failure.

At the summit of the curve, a plateau or flattening is observed where additional increments in ventricular volume are not associated with improved performance. This physiologic limit results from the rise in ventricular end-diastolic pressure produced by the increased volume. Excessive pressure elevation produces pulmonary or systemic congestion and edema from fluid transudation, negating the value of further increments in volume and pressure.

The ventricular function curve characteristic of the failing ventricle is depressed and flattened (Fig. 33-2). Depression of the curve signifies that the failing ventricle requires higher volumes to achieve the same improvement of ventricular and cardiac output that the normal ventricle achieves with lower ventricular volumes. In other words, a given increment in ventricular volume is not associated with as great an improvement in ventricular function in the failing ventricle as would be expected in the normal ventricle.

In addition, the pronounced flattening of the curve seen with failure indicates limited cardiac reserve; once the curve flattens, no further improvement of function can be achieved with elevations of volume and pressure. It is presumed that the ventricular function curve in the failing heart flattens suddenly because the distended, hypertrophied ventricle is relatively noncompliant.

A useful analogy for understanding the effect of *chamber compliance* on the volume and pressure relationships is that of blowing up a child's balloon. Initially, balloons are extremely noncompliant and difficult to inflate; one

must generate high pressures to inflate the balloon with even small volumes of air. However, once the balloon has been repeatedly inflated and deflated, it becomes more compliant and easily distensible. One can then easily inflate the balloon with high volumes without exerting much pressure.

Similarly, the precise relationship between a change in intracardiac volume and the resultant change in pressure depends on the compliance or distensibility of the cardiac chambers (Fig. 33-3). An extremely compliant or distensible cardiac chamber can accommodate relatively large changes in volume without significantly increasing pressure; conversely, in the noncompliant, failing ventricle, small increases in volume result in significant pressure elevation and development of congestion and edema.

Contractility

Contractility, the second determinant of myocardial function, refers to changes in the force of contraction or inotropic state that occur independent of changes in fiber length. Changes in contractile function shift the position of the ventricular function curve (see Fig. 33-2). The administration of positive inotropic drugs, such as catecholamines or digoxin, enhances contractility, shifting the curve upward and to the left. Factors depressing contractility, such as hypoxia and acidosis, shift the curve downward and to the right. As indicated, in most forms of heart failure, the ventricular function curve is depressed; this downward shift of the curve represents a depression of myocardial contractility.

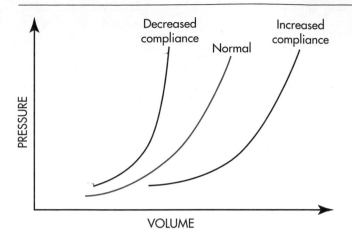

FIG. 33-3   Ventricular compliance, or the pressure-volume relationship of the ventricles. The line in the center indicates the typical relationship between pressure and volume. As volume is increased initially, only a small rise in pressure occurs. As volume increase continues, the rise in pressure is greater. The other lines indicate an alteration in pressure-volume relationships: decreased compliance on the left and increased compliance on the right. This represents a greater or lesser degree of stiffness of the ventricle in relation to the filling volume. Ventricular compliance is a dynamic phenomenon, and this property can change rapidly.

Afterload

Afterload is the amount of wall tension the ventricle must develop during systole to eject blood. According to *Laplace's law,* three variables affect wall tension: intraventricular size or radius, intraventricular systolic pressure, and ventricular wall thickness:

$$\text{Wall tension} = \frac{\text{Intraventricular systolic pressure}}{\text{Ventricular wall thickness}} \times \text{Radius}$$

Factors increasing the pressure the ventricle must generate during systole (e.g., arterial vasoconstriction, which increases the resistance to ventricular ejection) or increasing the ventricular radius (e.g., fluid retention) increase afterload. The failing heart is particularly sensitive to the increased workload imposed by an increase in afterload because of its limited cardiac reserve. Reduction of afterload can be achieved with interventions such as the administration of vasodilators. Ventricular hypertrophy, another consequence of heart failure, also decreases afterload according to Laplace's law. The increased muscle mass facilitates the work of ejection.

Definitions

Heart failure or *cardiac failure* is the pathophysiologic condition in which the heart as a pump is unable to meet the metabolic requirements of the tissues for blood. The critical features of this definition are (1) failure is defined relative to the metabolic needs of the body, and (2) emphasis is placed on the overall failure of the heart's pumping function. The term *myocardial failure* refers specifi-

cally to abnormalities in myocardial function; myocardial failure often leads to heart failure, but circulatory compensatory mechanisms can delay or even prevent progression to failure of the heart as a pump.

The expression *circulatory failure* is even more general than the term heart failure. Circulatory failure refers to the inability of the cardiovascular system to perfuse the tissues adequately. This definition encompasses any abnormality of the circulation responsible for the inadequacy in tissue perfusion, including alterations in blood volume, vascular tone, and the heart. *Congestive heart failure* is the state of circulatory congestion resulting from heart failure and its compensatory mechanisms. Congestive heart failure is defined in contradistinction to the more general term *circulatory congestion,* which is simply circulatory overload caused by excess blood volume from cardiac failure or from noncardiac causes, such as overtransfusion or anuria.

Etiology

Heart failure is the most common complication of virtually all forms of acquired and congenital heart disease. Physiologic mechanisms producing heart failure include conditions that (1) increase preload, (2) increase afterload, or (3) reduce myocardial contractility. States that increase preload include aortic regurgitation and ventricular septal defect; afterload is increased by conditions such as aortic stenosis and systemic hypertension. Myocardial contractility can be depressed by myocardial infarction and cardiomyopathies. In addition to these three physiologic mechanisms causing heart failure, other physiologic factors can cause the heart to fail as a pump. Factors interfering with ventricular filling, such as atrioventricular (AV) valve stenosis, can produce failure. Conditions such as constrictive pericarditis and cardiac tamponade produce failure by a combination of physiologic effects, including impairment of ventricular filling and ventricular ejection. It should be apparent that no single physiologic mechanism or combination of mechanisms is responsible for the development of heart failure; the effectiveness of the heart as a pump can be compromised by any number of pathophysiologic states (see box, p. 506).

Similarly, no unifying biochemical explanation can be identified as the fundamental mechanism producing heart failure. The precise defect that produces the impairment in myocardial contractility is unknown. It is postulated that an abnormality in the delivery of calcium within the sarcomere or in the synthesis or function of the contractile proteins may be responsible.

Factors that can precipitate the development of heart failure by acutely stressing the circulation include (1) dysrhythmias, (2) systemic and pulmonic infection, and (3) pulmonary embolism. Dysrhythmias interfere with the mechanical function of the heart by altering the electrical stimulus initiating the mechanical response; an ef-

CAUSES OF OVERALL HEART PUMP FAILURE

A. Mechanical abnormalities
   1. Increased pressure load
      a. Central (aortic stenosis, etc.)
      b. Peripheral (systemic hypertension, etc.)
   2. Increased volume load (valvular regurgitation, shunts, increased preload, etc.)
   3. Obstruction to ventricular filling (mitral or tricuspid stenosis)
   4. Pericardial tamponade
   5. Endocardial or myocardial restriction
   6. Ventricular aneurysm
   7. Ventricular dyssynergy
B. Myocardial (muscular) abnormalities
   1. Primary
      a. Cardiomyopathy
      b. Myocarditis
      c. Metabolic abnormalities
      d. Toxicity (alcohol, cobalt, etc.)
      e. Presbycardia
   2. Secondary dysdynamic abnormalities (secondary to mechanical abnormalities)
      a. Oxygen deprivation (coronary heart disease)
      b. Metabolic abnormalities
      c. Inflammation
      d. Systemic disease
      e. Chronic obstructive lung disease
C. Altered cardiac rhythm or conduction sequence
   1. Standstill
   2. Fibrillation
   3. Extreme tachycardia or bradycardia
   4. Electrical asynchrony, conduction disturbances

From Hurst JW et al, editors: *The heart,* vol 1, ed 7, New York, 1990, McGraw-Hill.

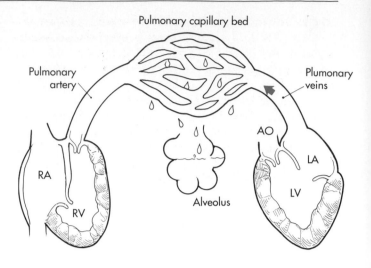

FIG. 33-4   Pulmonary edema in left heart failure. *RA,* Right atrium; *RV,* right ventricle; *AO,* aorta; *LA,* left atrium; *LV,* left ventricle. (Modified from Crawford MV, Spense MI: *Commonsense approach to coronary care,* ed 6, St Louis, 1994, Mosby.)

fective synchronized mechanical response cannot occur without a stable cardiac rhythm. The body's response to infection stresses the heart by increasing metabolic demands on an already compromised circulation. Pulmonary embolism acutely increases the resistance to right ventricular ejection, precipitating right heart failure. Effective management of heart failure requires recognition and treatment of not only the underlying physiologic mechanism and disease state, but also any factors precipitating heart failure.

Pathophysiology

Basic mechanisms

The intrinsic defect in myocardial contractility characteristic of heart failure in ischemic heart disease impairs the ability of the ventricle to empty effectively. Depressed contractility of the left ventricle reduces stroke volume and elevates residual ventricular volumes. As ventricular EDVs rise, there is a corresponding increase in left ventricular end-diastolic pressure (LVEDP). The degree of pressure elevation depends on the compliance of the ventricle. As LVEDP rises, there is a corresponding elevation of left atrial pressure (LAP) because the atrium and ventricle communicate directly during diastole. The increase in LAP is transmitted backward into the pulmonary vasculature, elevating pulmonary venous and pulmonary capillary pressures. If hydrostatic pressure in the pulmonary capillary bed exceeds the vascular oncotic pressure, fluid transudation into the interstitium occurs. When the rate of fluid transudation exceeds the rate of lymphatic drainage, interstitital edema results. Further elevation of pressure may cause fluid seepage into the alveoli and the development of pulmonary edema (Fig. 33-4). (See also Chapter 40 for a discussion of pulmonary edema.)

Pulmonary arterial pressure may rise in response to chronic elevation of pulmonary venous pressure. Pulmonary hypertension increases the resistance to right ventricular ejection. A sequence of events parallel to that affecting the left side of the heart can then result, culminating in systemic congestion and edema.

Development of systemic or pulmonary congestion and edema can be exacerbated by the development of functional regurgitation of the tricuspid or mitral valves, respectively. Functional regurgitation can result from dilation of the AV valve annulus or changes in the orientation of the papillary muscles and chordae tendinae secondary to chamber dilation.

Compensatory response

In response to heart failure, three primary compensatory mechanisms are observed: (1) increased sympathetic adrenergic activity, (2) increased preload secondary to activation of the renin-angiotensin-aldosterone system, and (3) ventricular hypertrophy. All three compensatory responses represent attempts to maintain cardiac output. These mechanisms may be sufficient to maintain cardiac output at normal or near-normal levels early in the course of failure and in the resting state. Typically, however, some degree of abnormality in ventricular performance and cardiac output appears in the failing heart during exercise. As the failure progresses, compensation becomes less effective.

Increased sympathetic adrenergic activity

The decrease in stroke volume with heart failure elicits a compensatory sympathetic response. The increased activity of the sympathetic adrenergic system stimulates release of catecholamines from cardiac adrenergic nerves and the adrenal medulla. Heart rate and contractile force increase to augment cardiac output. Peripheral arterial vasoconstriction occurs to stabilize arterial pressure and redistribute blood volume away from the metabolically less active organs, such as the skin and kidney, to maintain perfusion to the heart and brain. Venoconstriction increases venous return to the right side of the heart, further augmenting contractile force according to Starling's law.

As would be expected, the level of circulating catecholamines is elevated in heart failure, particularly during exercise. The heart becomes increasingly dependent on circulating catecholamines to maintain ventricular performance. Eventually, however, the myocardial response to sympathetic stimulation lessens; the catecholamines have less effect on ventricular performance. This change can best be conceptualized by referring to the ventricular function curve (see Fig. 33-2).

Normally, catecholamines produce a positive inotropic effect on the ventricle, shifting the curve upward and to the left. As the failing ventricle becomes less responsive to catecholamine stimulation, the degree of shift in response to stimulation lessens. This change may be related to the observation that the myocardial stores of norepinephrine become depleted with chronic heart failure.

Increased preload through activation of the renin-angiotensin-aldosterone system

Activation of the renin-angiotensin-aldosterone system results in renal retention of sodium and water, increasing ventricular volume and fiber stretch. This increase in preload augments myocardial contractility according to Starling's law. The exact mechanism responsible for activation of the renin-angiotensin-aldosterone system in heart failure is unclear. However, a number of factors have been implicated, including sympathetic adrenergic stimulation of beta-receptors within the juxtaglomerular apparatus, macula densa receptor response to changes in sodium delivery to the distal tubule, and baroreceptor responses to changes in circulating blood volume and pressure.

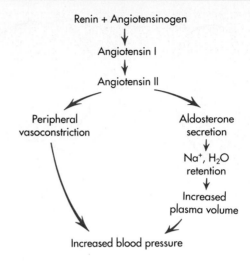

FIG. 33-5   Renin-angiotensin-aldosterone system.

Whatever the precise mechanism, the decrease in cardiac output with heart failure initiates the following events: (1) fall in renal blood flow and eventually of glomerular filtration rate, (2) release of renin from the juxtaglomerular apparatus, (3) renin interaction with circulating angiotensinogen to produce angiotensin I, (4) conversion of angiotensin I to angiotensin II, (5) stimulation of aldosterone secretion from the adrenal gland, and (6) retention of sodium and water in the distal tubule and collecting duct (Fig. 33-5). Angiotensin II also produces a vasoconstrictive effect that contributes to the elevation of blood pressure.

In severe heart failure, the combination of systemic venous congestion and diminished perfusion of the liver impairs hepatic metabolism of *aldosterone,* increasing circulating levels of aldosterone. *Antidiuretic hormone* (ADH) levels are also elevated in severe heart failure, which increases the absorption of water in the collecting ducts.

The role of *atrial natriuretic factor* (ANF) in heart failure is currently under investigation. ANF is a hormone synthesized in the atrial tissue. Atrial distention is believed to stimulate ANF secretion, and patients with heart failure have increased ANF levels. The hormone exerts natriuretic and diuretic effects and relaxes smooth muscle. However, the natriuretic and diuretic effects are overwhelmed by the stronger compensatory factors producing retention of salt and water and vasoconstriction.

Ventricular hypertrophy

The final compensatory response to failure is myocardial hypertrophy or increased wall thickness. Hypertrophy increases the number of sarcomeres within the myocardial cell; depending on the type of hemodynamic load producing the failure, sarcomeres develop either in parallel or in series. For example, a pressure load, as caused by aortic stenosis, is associated with increased numbers of sarcomeres arranged in parallel producing an increase in

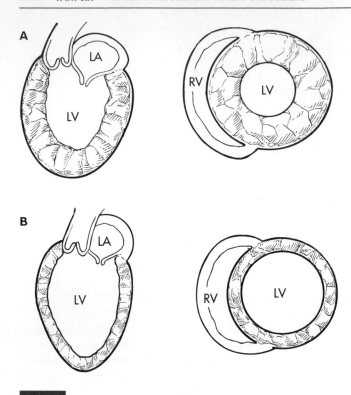

FIG. 33-6 Patterns of ventricular hypertrophy. **A,** Concentric hypertrophy secondary to a pressure load is characterized by increased wall thickness. **B,** Eccentric hypertrophy secondary to a volume load is characterized by a proportional increase in wall thickness and chamber size. *LA,* Left atrium; *LV,* left ventricle; *RV,* right ventricle. (Modified from Rushmer, RF: *Cardiovascular dynamics,* ed 4, Philadelphia, 1976, Saunders.)

wall thickness without increasing the internal chamber size. The myocardial response to volume loads, as in aortic regurgitation, is characterized by dilation as well as increased wall thickness. This combination is believed to result from increased numbers of sarcomeres arranged in series. These two patterns of hypertrophy are referred to as *concentric hypertrophy* and *eccentric hypertrophy* (Fig. 33-6). Whatever the precise sarcomere arrangement, myocardial hypertrophy increases the force of ventricular contraction.

Additional compensatory mechanisms

Additional mechanisms operate at the tissue level to facilitate the delivery of oxygen to the tissues. Plasma levels of 2, 3-diphosphoglycerate (2,3-DPG) increase, reducing the affinity of hemoglobin for oxygen. As a result, the oxygen-hemoglobin dissociation curve shifts to the right, facilitating the release and uptake of oxygen by the tissues. (See Part Seven for further discussion of the oxyhemoglobin dissociation curve.) Oxygen extraction from the blood is increased to maintain oxygen supply to the tissues in the presence of a low cardiac output.

Negative effects of compensatory responses

Initially the compensatory response of the circulation is beneficial; eventually, however, the compensatory mechanisms can produce symptoms, increase cardiac work, and worsen the degree of failure. The fluid retention intended to augment contractile force causes pulmonary and systemic venous congestion and edema formation. Arterial vasoconstriction and redistribution of blood flow impair tissue perfusion in the affected vascular beds and produce signs and symptoms such as decreased urine output and weakness. Arterial vasoconstriction also increases afterload by increasing the resistance to ventricular ejection; afterload is also increased by dilation of the cardiac chambers. Consequently, cardiac work and myocardial oxygen demand or consumption ($M\dot{V}o_2$) increase. Myocardial hypertrophy and sympathetic stimulation further increase $M\dot{V}o_2$. If the increase in $M\dot{V}o_2$ cannot be met by a corresponding increase in myocardial oxygen supply, myocardial ischemia and further myocardial compromise can result. The end result of these interrelated events is an increased myocardial burden and perpetuation of the underlying failure.

Clinical Features

Conceptual framework

Two methods of conceptualizing failure are used in the description of clinical manifestations: (1) forward versus backward failure and (2) right heart failure versus left heart failure. *Forward failure,* "high-output failure," is characterized by a cardiac output that is above normal for the person's age, gender, and size but still inadequate for the body's need for oxygenated blood. *Backward failure,* "low-output failure," is characterized by a cardiac output that is absolutely reduced below what is normal for a person of the same age, gender, and size. Easy fatigability, weakness, and mental confusion result from the marked decrease in cardiac output, the hallmark of forward failure, whereas pulmonary congestion and edema indicate the backup of blood resulting from the failing ventricle, the hallmark of backward failure.

The terms *right heart failure* and *left heart failure* imply that the ventricles function as independent pumps. Although this distinction may be useful as a means of categorizing symptoms, the interdependence of the ventricles must be noted. The ventricles are anatomically interdependent in that they share a common wall, the *interventricular septum,* and the muscle fibers composing the ventricular walls are continuous, encircling both ventricles. Not only does anatomic interdependence exist between the ventricles, but functional interdependence exists as well, in that the ventricles are components of a continuous circuit, and the volume of blood ejected from each ventricle depends on the volume received by that ventricle. It is physiologically impossible for the ventricular stroke volumes to be imbalanced for a prolonged period. For example, the left ventricle cannot sustain an increase in cardiac output unless a corresponding increase occurs in cardiac output in the right ventricle. Impaired function of one ventricle eventually interferes with function of the other ventricle. In fact, left heart failure is rec-

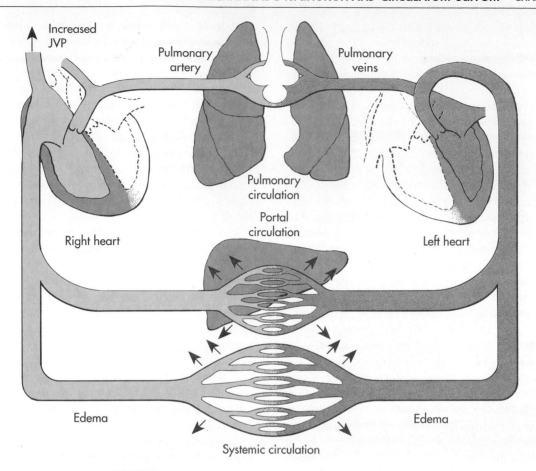

FIG. 33-7   Hemodynamic manifestations of right ventricular failure. *JVP,* Jugular venous pressure.

ognized as the most common cause of right heart failure because of the phenomenon of backward failure described previously.

Because both ventricles are enclosed within the pericardium, physiologic interaction increases; extreme dilation of one ventricle progressively compresses the other ventricle within the pericardium. In addition, the ventricles share common biochemical changes in failure; for example, the depletion of norepinephrine stores mentioned earlier does not seem to be isolated to a single chamber. In sum, the interdependence of the ventricular pumps must be recognized. However, the terms right and left heart failure may be used to refer to a complex of symptoms corresponding to failure of a particular ventricle. For example, right heart failure produces systemic venous congestion and edema (Fig. 33-7), whereas left heart failure produces pulmonary venous congestion and edema (see Fig. 33-4).

Signs and symptoms

The clinical manifestations of heart failure should be considered relative to the degree of physical exertion associated with the appearance of symptoms. Initially, symptoms typically appear only with exertion; however, as failure progresses, exercise tolerance diminishes and

symptoms are manifested earlier with lesser degrees of activity. The *New York Heart Association* (NYHA) *functional classification* is typically used to express the relationship between onset of symptoms and degree of physical exertion (see box, p. 433).

Dyspnea, or the sensation of difficulty in breathing, is the most common manifestation of heart failure. Dyspnea results from the increased work of breathing produced by pulmonary vascular congestion, which reduces lung compliance. Increased airway resistance also contributes to dyspnea. Just as a spectrum of pulmonary congestion exists, ranging from pulmonary venous congestion to interstitial edema and finally to alveolar edema, dyspnea presents in progressively more serious forms. *Dyspnea on exertion* (DOE) represents an early presentation of left heart failure. *Orthopnea,* or dyspnea in the recumbent position, is caused primarily by the redistribution of blood volume from the dependent portions of the body to the central circulation. Reabsorption of interstitial fluid from the lower extremities contributes further to the pulmonary vascular congestion. *Paroxysmal nocturnal dyspnea* (PND), or sudden awakening with dyspnea, is precipitated by the development of interstitial pulmonary edema. It is a more specific manifestation of left ventricular failure than either dyspnea or orthopnea.

A nonproductive cough may also occur secondary to the pulmonary congestion, especially in the recumbent position. Development of *rales* as a result of pulmonary fluid transudation is characteristic of heart failure; initially, rales are audible over the lung bases because of the effects of gravity. All of these signs and symptoms may be ascribed to backward failure of the left side of the heart. *Hemoptysis* may result from bronchial vein bleeding secondary to venous distention. Distention of the left atrium or pulmonary vein may lead to esophageal compression and *dysphagia,* or difficulty swallowing.

Backward failure of the right side of the heart produces signs and symptoms of systemic venous congestion. Elevation of jugular venous pressure (JVP) is noted; the neck veins become engorged. Central venous pressure (CVP) can rise paradoxically during inspiration if the failing right heart is unable to accommodate the inspiratory increase in venous return to the heart. This inspiratory rise in CVP is referred to as *Kussmaul's sign.* If tricuspid valve regurgitation develops, pulsatile *v* waves may be apparent in the jugular vein. A *positive hepatojugular reflux test* can be elicited; manual compression of the right upper quadrant of the abdomen produces jugular venous pressure elevation because, again, the failing right side of the heart is unable to accommodate the associated increase in venous return. *Hepatomegaly,* or liver enlargement, appears; liver tenderness may be noted because of the stretching of the hepatic capsule. Other *gastrointestinal (GI) symptoms,* such as anorexia, fullness, or nausea, may result from hepatic and intestinal congestion.

Peripheral edema develops secondary to fluid accumulation in the interstitial spaces. The edema is initially apparent in dependent regions of the body and is greatest at the end of the day; *nocturia,* or diuresis at night, may occur, lessening the degree of fluid retention. Nocturia results from fluid redistribution and reabsorption in the recumbent position as well as a reduction in the degree of renal vasoconstriction at rest. Advanced failure may be associated with the development of *ascites* or *anasarca* (generalized body edema). Although the signs and symptoms of fluid accumulation in the systemic venous circuit noted earlier are classically considered to be secondary to right heart failure, the earliest manifestations of systemic congestion are usually caused by fluid retention rather than overt right heart failure. All the manifestations described here are typically preceded by weight gain, which simply reflects the retention of sodium and water.

Forward failure of the left ventricle produces signs of diminished organ perfusion. Because blood is shunted from nonvital organs to maintain perfusion of the heart and brain, the earliest manifestations of forward failure reflect diminished perfusion of organs such as the skin and skeletal muscles. Skin pallor and coolness result from peripheral vasoconstriction; further reductions in cardiac output associated with increased oxygen extraction and elevated levels of reduced hemoglobin produce cyanosis. The cutaneous vasoconstriction interferes with

the body's ability to lose heat; therefore a low-grade fever and excessive sweating may be noted. Underperfusion of the skeletal muscles produces weakness and fatigue. These symptoms can be exacerbated by fluid and electrolyte imbalances or anorexia. Further reduction in cardiac output can be associated with changes in mental status, such as the development of insomnia, restlessness, or confusion. With severe chronic failure, progressive weight loss with poor health and malnutrition, or *cardiac cachexia,* may develop. A combination of factors may be responsible, including low cardiac output and anorexia from visceral congestion, drug toxicity, or an unappealing diet.

Examination of the arterial pulse during heart failure reveals a rapid, weak pulse. The rapid heartbeat, or *tachycardia,* represents a response to sympathetic nervous stimulation. A significant fall in stroke volume and the associated peripheral vasoconstriction reduces pulse pressure (the difference between systolic and diastolic pressure), producing a weak or thready pulse. Systolic hypotension is noted with more severe heart failure. In addition, severe left ventricular failure may be associated with the development of *pulsus alternans,* an alteration in the strength of the arterial pulse. Pulsus alternans indicates severe mechanical dysfunction with a repetitive beat-to-beat variation in stroke volume.

Common findings on auscultation of the chest are rales, as noted earlier, and a *ventricular gallop,* or *third heart sound* (S_3). The development of an S_3 is the auscultatory hallmark of left ventricular failures. The ventricular gallop occurs during the early diastolic period and results from rapid ventricular filling of the noncompliant and distended ventricle. A *substernal heave,* or systolic lift of the sternum, may result from right ventricular enlargement. Chest radiography reveals the following: (1) pulmonary venous congestion, progressing to interstitial or alveolar edema with more severe failure; (2) vascular redistribution to the upper lobes of the lung; and (3) cardiomegaly. The electrocardiogram (ECG) frequently reveals asymptomatic ventricular premature beats and runs of nonsustained ventricular tachycardia. Bradycardic events (asystole or heart block) are usually associated with progressively worsening heart failure. The significance of these dysrhythmias is unclear, but sudden death is a common terminal event in patients with heart failure.

Characteristic changes in blood values are also apparent. For example, alterations in fluid and electrolyte concentrations are reflected in serum levels. Typically, dilutional hyponatremia is observed; potassium levels may be normal or reduced secondary to diuretic therapy. Hyperkalemia may occur late in the course of heart failure because of renal impairment. Similarly, blood urea nitrogen (BUN) and creatinine levels may be elevated secondary to changes in glomerular filtration rate. Urine is concentrated, with a high specific gravity and reduced sodium content. Abnormalities in liver function may produce minor prolongation of prothrombin time. Elevations of bilirubin and the liver enzymes aspartate amino-transferase (AST, formerly SGOT), and serum alkaline phosphatase (ALP) may be noted, particularly with acute failure.

Treatment

Heart failure is treated by instituting general measures to reduce cardiac work and by selectively manipulating the three primary determinants of myocardial function, either alone or in combination: (1) preload, (2) contractility, and (3) afterload, as well as heart rate and rhythm. Treatment is usually initiated when symptoms appear with ordinary physical exertion (NYHA functional class II). The treatment regimen is progressively intensified until the desired clinical response is obtained. Acute exacerbations of failure or the development of severe heart failure might necessitate hospitalization and more aggressive treatment. The general measures usually employed to treat chronic congestive heart failure are outlined in the box at right.

Reduction of cardiac work

Restriction of strenuous physical activity constitutes the simplest and earliest intervention in the management of heart failure. Care must be taken, however, not to impose unnecessary restrictions on activity to avoid skeletal muscle deconditioning. The potential contribution of muscle deconditioning to progressive exercise intolerance in heart failure is now recognized, and many patients are able to tolerate graduated exercise training three to five times per week. Sedentary activities and bedrest also predispose to the development of phlebothrombosis. Anticoagulation may be indicated if severe restrictions of activity are necessary to control symptoms.

Reduction of preload

Restriction of dietary salt intake reduces preload by decreasing fluid retention. If symptoms persist with moderate sodium restrictions, oral diuretics are added to counter the retention of sodium and water. Typically the diuretic regimen is maximized before imposing extreme restrictions of sodium intake. A diet of unpalatable food can lead to loss of appetite and poor nutrition.

Vasodilation of the venous bed can also reduce preload through redistribution of blood from the central to the peripheral circulation. Venodilation produces pooling of blood in the periphery and a reduction of venous return to the heart. In extreme situations, physical removal of fluid through hemofiltration or hemodialysis may be necessary to support myocardial function.

Fig. 33-8, A, illustrates the improvement in ventricular function associated with a reduction in preload. As noted earlier, the failing ventricle operates on a depressed and flattened ventricular function curve. As EDV is reduced with diuretics and sodium restriction, the point on the curve corresponding to the ventricular function shift from

OUTLINE OF TREATMENT OF CHRONIC CONGESTIVE HEART FAILURE

1. Restriction of physical activity
   a. Discontinue strenuous sports and heavy labor.
   b. Discontinue full-time work or equivalent activity; introduce rest periods during the day.
   c. Confine to house.
   d. Confine to bed or chair.
2. Restriction of sodium intake
   a. Eliminate salt shaker at table (Na = 1.6 to 2.8 g).
   b. Eliminate salt in cooking and at table (Na = 1.2 to 1.8 g).
   c. Institute a and b + low-sodium diet (Na = 0.2 to 1.0 g).
3. Digitalis glycoside
   a. Usual maintenance dose
   b. Maximum tolerable dose
4. Diuretics
   a. Moderate diuretics (e.g., thiazides)
   b. Loop diuretic (e.g., furosemide)
   c. Loop diuretic and distal tubular (potassium-sparing) diuretic
   d. Loop diuretic, thiazide, and distal tubular diuretic
5. Vasodilators
   a. Captopril, enalapril, or combination of hydralazine and isosorbide dinitrate
   b. Intensification of oral vasodilator regimen
   c. Intravenous nitroprusside
6. Other inotropic agents: dopamine, dobutamine, amrinone
7. Special measures
   a. Consider cardiac transplantation.
   b. Administer dialysis.
   c. Provide assisted circulation: intraaortic balloon pump (IABP), left ventricular assist device (LVAD), or artificial heart.

From Braunwald E, editor: *Heart disease: a textbook in cardiovascular medicine,* ed 3, Philadelphia, 1988, Saunders.

A to B. Note that the symptoms of congestion would be relieved as EDV falls. However, stroke volume and cardiac output would remain stable with optimal preload therapy because the shift occurs along the flat portion of the curve.

Augmentation of contractility

Inotropic drugs increase the force of myocardial contraction. The precise mechanisms that produce this positive inotropic effect are not clear. However, the common denominator seems to be an increase in the availability of intracellular calcium to the contractile proteins, actin and myosin. As noted earlier, the calcium ion is critical to the development of cross-bridges between the contractile proteins and subsequent muscle contraction.

Two classes of inotropic drugs can be used: (1) digi-

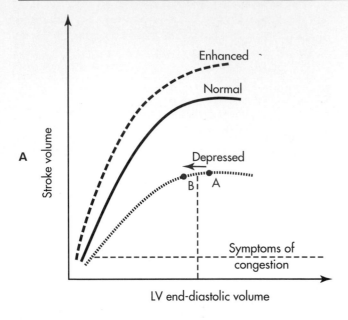

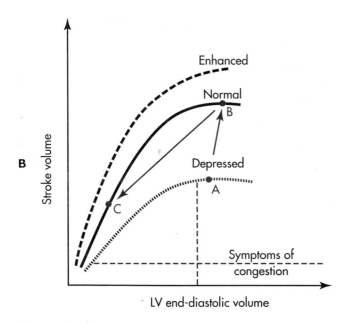

FIG. 33-8   A, Effect of preload therapy on congestive heart failure. The failing ventricle operates on a depressed and flattened ventricular function curve. As end-diastolic volume is reduced with diuretics and sodium restriction, the point on the curve corresponding to ventricular function shifts from *A* to *B,* so symptoms of congestion are relieved. Stroke volume and cardiac output remain stable, since the shift occurs on the flattened part of the curve. **B,** Effect of contractility augmentation on congestive heart failure. Inotropic drugs improve ventricular function by shifting the entire ventricular function curve upward and to the left, so cardiac output is higher for a given end-diastolic volume and pressure. In addition, as the force of contraction increases, stroke volume increases. As end-diastolic volume decreases, an optimal point *[C]* on the ventricular function curve is reached where congestive symptoms are relieved and cardiac output is maintained. *LV,* Left ventricular.

talis glycosides and (2) nonglycoside agents. *Nonglycoside agents* include sympathomimetic amines, such as epinephrine and norepinephrine, and phosphodiesterase inhibitors, such as amrinone and enoximone. *Sympathomimetic amines* increase contractility directly by stimulating the adrenergic beta-receptors on the myocardium. *Phosphodiesterase* (PDE) is an enzyme that causes the breakdown of a substance, cyclic adenosine monophosphate (cAMP), that promotes the movements of calcium into the cell through the slow calcium channels. Inhibition of PDE increases the level of cAMP and therefore of intracellular calcium. PDE inhibitors also cause vasodilation.

Inotropic drugs improve ventricular function by shifting the entire left ventricular function curve up and to the left (Fig. 33-8, *B*) so that cardiac output is higher for a given end-diastolic volume and pressure. In addition, as the force of contraction increases, stroke volume increases. The increase in forward flow produces a corresponding decrease in residual ventricular volumes. As EDV decreases, an optimal point on the ventricular function curve, point C on Fig. 33-8, *B,* is reached where symptoms are relieved and cardiac output is maintained.

Reduction of afterload

Two of the compensatory responses to heart failure, activation of the sympathetic nervous system and of the renin-angiotensin-aldosterone system, produce vasoconstriction and consequently increase the resistance to ventricular ejection and afterload. As afterload rises, cardiac work increases and cardiac output falls. Arterial vasodilators counter these negative effects. The common vasodilators produce dilation of the vasculature by two primary mechanisms: (1) direct dilation of vascular smooth muscle or (2) inhibition of angiotensin-converting enzyme (ACE). Direct vasodilators include drugs such as hydralazine and nitrates. *Hydralazine* exerts a greater dilatory effect on the arterial bed, thereby reducing afterload, whereas *nitrates* produce proportionally more venodilation, reducing preload as described earlier.

ACE inhibitors include enalapril and captopril that block the conversion of angiotensin I to angiotensin II. This action prevents angiotensin-induced vasoconstriction and also inhibits aldosterone production and the associated retention of fluid. ACE inhibitors have demonstrated great promise in the management of all grades of overt heart failure. Consequently, therapy with oral vasodilators is now being instituted earlier in the progression of failure, for NYHA class II rather than class III or IV failure.

Arterial vasodilators reduce the resistance to ventricular ejection. As a result, the ventricle can eject more easily and more completely. In other words, cardiac work is reduced and cardiac output rises. Arterial pressure usually does not fall significantly with optimal management because the increase in cardiac output offsets the potential fall in pressure that would result from vasodilation alone.

SHOCK

Shock does not constitute a single disease entity. It is a complex clinical syndrome encompassing a group of conditions with variable hemodynamic manifestations; however, the common denominator is the *inadequacy of tissue perfusion.* This state of hypoperfusion compromises the delivery of oxygen and nutrients and the removal of metabolites at the tissue level. Tissue hypoxia shifts metabolism from oxidative pathways to anaerobic pathways with a consequent production of lactic acid. Progressive metabolic derangements perpetuate the shock state, culminating in cellular deterioration and multisystem failure.

The nature of shock is progressive and self-perpetuating. A vicious cycle of progressive deterioration will result if shock is not treated aggressively early in its course. Shock may be characterized according to three progressively severe stages: (1) stage I, the *compensated,* or *nonprogressive, stage* during which compensatory responses, outlined earlier in the congestive heart failure section, stabilize the circulation, forestalling further deterioration; (2) stage II, the *progressive stage,* characterized by systemic manifestations of hypoperfusion and worsening organ function; and (3) stage III, the *refractory,* or *irreversible, stage* during which profound cellular derangements inevitably culminate in death.

Fundamental Concepts

The basic relationship governing the perfusion or flow of blood to the tissues is the following:

$$MAP = CO \times TPR$$

Mean arterial pressure (MAP) is the pressure head driving blood to perfuse the tissues. However, tissue perfusion can be compromised even in the face of normal arterial pressure if cardiac output (CO) is inadequate or if the resistance to blood flow is high. Most shock states are characterized by low CO and increased total peripheral resistance (TPR). However, shock can also occur with a normal, or even elevated, CO if TPR falls abruptly, as with acute vasodilation, and CO does not rise proportionally to maintain an adequate perfusion pressure. (See Chapter 29 for the fundamentals of blood flow.)

Etiology

Shock can result from a variety of conditions, which may be categorized according to four basic etiologic mechanisms: (1) cardiogenic mechanisms, (2) obstructive mechanisms, (3) alterations in circulatory volume, and

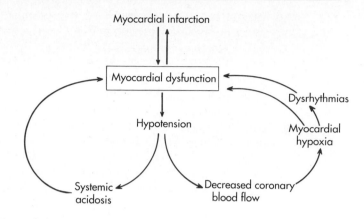

FIG. 33-9   Self-perpetuating cycle of cardiogenic shock. (Reproduced with permission of the American Heart Association from Dunkman WB et al: *Circulation* 46:474, 1972.)

(4) alterations in circulatory distribution (see box, p. 514). This section focuses on cardiogenic shock after myocardial infarction (MI) as illustrative of the shock state.

Cardiogenic shock is characterized by left ventricular dysfunction, leading to severe impairment of tissue perfusion and oxygen delivery to the tissues. Cardiogenic shock caused by acute MI is typically associated with a loss of 40% or more of the left ventricular myocardium. In addition to massive loss of the left ventricular musculature, focal areas of necrosis also may be found throughout the ventricle. Focal necrosis is thought to result from the sustained imbalance in myocardial oxygen supply and demand. The diseased coronary vessels are unable to increase flow adequately in response to the increase in cardiac work and oxygen demand associated with compensatory responses such as sympathetic stimulation.

As a result of the infarction process, left ventricular contractility and performance may be severely impaired. The left ventricle fails as a pump and does not provide adequate cardiac output to maintain tissue perfusion. A self-perpetuating cycle then ensues (Fig. 33-9). The cycle begins with the MI and subsequent myocardial dysfunction. Profound myocardial dysfunction leads to reduced cardiac output and arterial hypotension. Metabolic acidosis and reduced coronary perfusion result, further impairing ventricular function and predisposing to the development of dysrhythmias. As can be deduced, this cycle of cardiogenic shock must be interrupted early in the shock state to salvage left ventricular myocardium and prevent progression to an irreversible stage, which is incompatible with survival.

Mechanical defects caused by MI can also produce significant myocardial dysfunction and shock. These defects include the following:

1. *Acute mitral regurgitation* caused by rupture of a necrotic papillary muscle (see Fig. 31-14). This produces large amounts of backward or regurgitant blood flow into the left atrium and pulmonary circuit and a

ETIOLOGIES OF SHOCK

CARDIOGENIC SHOCK

A. Secondary to dysrhythmias
  1. Bradydysrhythmias
  2. Tachydysrhythmias
B. Secondary to cardiac mechanical factors
  1. Regurgitant lesions
    a. Acute mitral or aortic regurgitation
    b. Rupture of interventricular septum
    c. Massive left ventricular aneurysm
  2. Obstructive lesions
    a. Left ventricular outflow tract obstruction, such as congenital or acquired valvular aortic stenosis and hypertrophic obstructive cardiomyopathy
    b. Left ventricular inflow tract obstruction, such as mitral stenosis, left atrial myxoma, and atrial thrombus
C. Myopathic
  1. Impairment of left ventricular contractility, as in acute myocardial infarction or congestive cardiomyopathy
  2. Impairment of right ventricular contractility caused by right ventricular infarction
  3. Impairment of left ventricular relaxation or compliance, as in restrictive or hypertrophic cardiomyopathy

OBSTRUCTIVE SHOCK*

A. Pericardial tamponade
B. Coarctation of aorta
C. Pulmonary embolism
D. Primary pulmonary hypertension

OLIGEMIC SHOCK

A. Hemorrhage
B. Fluid depletion or sequestration resulting from vomiting, diarrhea, dehydration, diabetes mellitus, diabetes insipidus, adrenocortical failure, peritonitis, pancreatitis, burns, ascites, villous adenoma, or pheochromocytoma

DISTRIBUTIVE SHOCK

A. Septicemic
  1. Endotoxic
  2. Secondary to specific infection, such as dengue fever
B. Metabolic or toxic
  1. Renal failure
  2. Hepatic failure
  3. Severe acidosis or alkalosis
  4. Drug overdose
  5. Heavy metal intoxication
  6. Toxic shock syndrome (possibly caused by a staphylococcal exotoxin)
  7. Malignant hyperthermia
C. Endocrinologic
  1. Uncontrolled diabetes mellitus with ketoacidosis or hyperosmolar coma
  2. Adrenocortical failure
  3. Hypothyroidism
  4. Hyperparathyroidism or hypoparathyroidism
  5. Diabetes insipidus
  6. Hypoglycemia secondary to excess exogenous insulin or a beta-cell tumor
D. Microcirculatory, caused by altered blood viscosity
  1. Polycythemia vera
  2. Hyperviscosity syndromes, including multiple myeloma, macroglobulinemia, and cryoglobulinemia
  3. Sickle cell anemia
  4. Fat emboli
E. Neurogenic
  1. Cerebral
  2. Spinal
  3. Dysautonomic
F. Anaphylactic

From Braunwald E, editor: *Heart disease: a textbook in cardiovascular medicine,* ed 2, Philadelphia, 1984, Saunders.
*Caused by factors extrinsic to cardiac valves and myocardium.

corresponding reduction in forward blood flow or cardiac output.
2. *Acquired ventricular septal defect* resulting from rupture of an infarcted septum (see Fig. 31-15). Shunting the blood from the high-pressure left ventricle to the lower-pressure right ventricle reduces forward flow into the aorta.
3. *Ventricular aneurysms* secondary to weakening and bulging of the infarcted region (see Fig. 31-17). Large left ventricular aneurysms reduce left ventricular output by becoming a reservoir for blood during ventricular ejection. The portion of ventricular volume ejected, or the ejection fraction, is reduced, compromising cardiac output.

Pathophysiology and Systemic Effects

Cardiogenic shock may be viewed as a severe form of left ventricular failure. The pathophysiologic events and compensatory responses parallel that of failure, but they have progressed to a more severe form. The depression of cardiac contractility reduces cardiac output and increases left ventricular volumes and end-diastolic pressure, leading to pulmonary congestion and edema.

As systemic arterial pressure falls, stimulation of the baroreceptors in the aorta and the carotid sinus occurs. Sympathoadrenal stimulation produces reflex vasoconstriction, tachycardia, and increased contractility to augment cardiac output and stabilize blood pressure. Contractility is augmented further according to Starling's law by renal retention of sodium and water. Thus the depressed contractility of cardiogenic shock elicits compensatory responses, increasing afterload and preload. Although these protective mechanisms initially enhance arterial blood pressure and tissue perfusion, their effect on the myocardium is deleterious because of the increase in cardiac work and myocardial oxygen demand. Because coronary flow is inadequate, as evidenced by the MI, the imbalance between myocardial oxygen supply and demand increases. Further myocardial dysfunction ensues secondary to ischemia and focal necrosis, perpetuating a vicious cycle of myocardial compromise. As left ventricular performance continues to deteriorate, the shock state rapidly progresses until such profound circulatory failure exists that every major organ system is affected.

The systemic effects of the shock state contribute to its eventual irreversibility. Some organs are affected quickly and more profoundly than others. As noted, the myocardium undergoes deleterious effects early in the shock state. In addition to the increases in myocardial work and oxygen demand, other significant changes occur. Because of the anaerobic metabolism induced by the shock state, the myocardium cannot maintain its normal level of high-energy phosphate (adenosine triphosphate) stores, and ventricular contractility is further impaired. *Hypoxia* and *acidosis* inhibit energy production and contribute to further destruction of myocardial cells. These two factors also shift the ventricular function curve downward and to the right, depressing contractility further.

Respiratory compromise develops secondary to the shock state. A potentially lethal complication is profound respiratory failure. Pulmonary congestion and intraalveolar edema lead to hypoxia and deterioration of arterial blood gases. Atelectasis and pulmonary infection may also occur. These factors predispose to the development of shock lung, now frequently referred to as adult respiratory distress syndrome (see Chapter 41). Tachypnea, dyspnea, and moist rales are noted, as well as other symptoms described earlier as manifesting backward heart failure.

Reduced renal perfusion results in oliguria with a urine output generally less than 20 ml/hour. With further reductions in cardiac output, an associated fall in urine output usually occurs. Because of the compensatory retention of sodium and water, urine sodium levels are reduced. Along with the reduction in glomerular filtration rate, an increase in BUN and creatinine is noted. With prolonged, severe hypotension, acute tubular necrosis with ensuing acute renal failure may result (see Chapter 49).

Shock of prolonged duration results in *hepatic cellular dysfunction*. Cellular damage may be localized to isolated zones of hepatic necrosis, or massive hepatic necrosis may occur with profound shock. Marked derangements of liver function become apparent and are usually manifested by elevations of the liver enzymes AST and alanine aminotransferase (ALT, formerly SGPT). Hepatic

hypoxia appears to be the etiologic mechanism that initiates these complications.

Prolonged *ischemia of the GI tract* typically results in hemorrhagic necrosis of the bowel. Bowel injury may exacerbate the shock state by sequestration of fluid in the gut and by absorption of bacteria and endotoxins into the circulation. A decrease in GI motility is almost always noted in association with shock.

Normally, cerebral blood flow displays the property of autoregulation of flow, with dilation occurring in response to diminished flow or ischemia. Cerebral autoregulation fails to maintain adequate flow and perfusion when the mean arterial pressure falls below 60 mm Hg. During profound periods of hypotension, symptoms of *neurologic deficit* may be observed. These deficits are not usually sustained if recovery from the shock state occurs, unless a concomitant cerebrovascular accident (CVA, stroke) has resulted.

During sustained shock, intravascular aggregation of cellular components of the hematologic system may occur, increasing peripheral vascular resistance further. Disseminated intravascular coagulation (DIC) may occur during the shock state, further compromising the clinical situation.

Hemodynamic Profile

Criteria for the diagnosis of cardiogenic shock have been established by the Myocardial Infarction Research Units of the National Heart, Lung, and Blood Institute. Cardiogenic shock is characterized by the following:

1. Systolic arterial pressure less than 90 mm Hg or 30 to 60 mm Hg below the previous baseline level
2. Evidence of decreased blood flow to major organ systems:
   a. Urine output less than 20 ml/hour, usually with decreased sodium content
   b. Peripheral vasoconstriction associated with cold, clammy skin
   c. Impaired mental function
3. Cardiac index* less than 2.1 L/min/m^2
4. Evidence of left-sided heart failure with LVEDP/pulmonary capillary wedge pressure (PCWP) greater than 18 to 21 mm Hg

These criteria reflect severe left-sided heart failure with evidence of forward and backward failure. The systolic hypotension and evidence of impaired tissue perfusion are characteristic of the shock state. Extreme depression of the cardiac index to less than 0.9 L/min/m^2 may be observed with profound cardiogenic shock.

In cardiogenic shock with acute mitral regurgitation, the regurgitant flow significantly increases LAP and PCWP. The development of severe pulmonary edema is

---

*Cardiac index is the cardiac output in liters per minute per square meter of body surface area (BSA). The normal resting average is 2.8 L/min/m^2. Average BSA for a 150-pound man is 1.75 m^2.

common in the setting of acute mitral regurgitation. With the development of a ventricular septal defect (VSD), shunting and mixing of blood occur between the left and right ventricles. Consequently, the oxygen content of the blood in the right ventricle increases. Pressures of the right side of the heart also rise because of recirculation of blood through the right side of the heart and pulmonic circuit. Insertion of a pulmonary artery catheter is indicated to detect these alterations through blood sampling and pressure measurement in the right side of the heart. Measurement of cardiac output by dye dilution (see Chapter 30) is useful to document the presence and degree of shunting with VSD or of regurgitant flow with mitral regurgitation, as well as to measure the cardiac output.

Calculated systemic vascular resistance (i.e., the difference between MAP and CVP, divided by CO and multiplied by 80) is markedly increased in cardiogenic shock because of the intense peripheral vasoconstriction.

Treatment

The mortality rate from cardiogenic shock treated with conventional pharmacologic measures to optimize preload, afterload, and contractility approaches 80%. Early, aggressive intervention to interrupt the shock cycle is critical. Survival depends on the efficacy of measures to limit the extent of MI by salvaging myocardium at risk, thereby reducing the potential magnitude of ventricular dysfunction. Therapy for cardiogenic shock has evolved steadily over the last two decades as newer techniques for myocardial salvage have emerged.

In the late 1960s, mechanical support of the circulation with the intraaortic balloon pump, described in the next section, was added to the standard pharmacologic regimen in an attempt to reduce cardiac work and improve coronary and peripheral perfusion. Despite an initial hemodynamic improvement during balloon pumping, however, the overall shock mortality rate did not change. Consequently, in the late 1970s, emergency coronary revascularization was recommended after stabilization of the circulation with intraaortic balloon pumping. This therapeutic combination improved the shock mortality rate significantly, to approximately 50%. The advent of thrombolytic therapy and angioplasty to recanalize occluded vessels promises to further reduce the mortality rate from this lethal shock state.

Invasive monitoring of the cardiovascular system is generally performed to provide continuous information about blood pressure and intracardiac filling pressures. Placement of an indwelling arterial catheter and a Swan-Ganz pulmonary arterial catheter is usually accomplished soon after admission to an intensive care unit.

Initial measures to stabilize the circulation include the intravenous administration of agents to augment contractility as well as efforts to reduce preload and afterload and the initiation of intraaortic balloon pumping. Defini-

tive, aggressive treatment must be instituted within hours of the onset of the shock state, at the same time that specific diagnostic testing and definitive interventions are performed.

Positive inotropic agents, such as dobutamine and amrinone, are used to augment contractility. Preload is decreased by reduction of intravascular volume with diuretics and vascular redistribution of volume with *venodilators,* such as nitroglycerin. Nitroglycerin also exerts a positive vasodilatory effect on the coronary circulation, improving coronary blood flow. PCWP, the clinical measure of LVEDP, is used to guide the administration of diuretics and vasodilators.

Arterial vasodilators or *vasopressors* may be indicated to reduce afterload or increase arterial pressure, respectively. However, both categories of drugs must be used with caution in cardiogenic shock. Arterial vasodilators, such as sodium nitroprusside, dilate the smooth muscle of the arterial system, reducing the resistance to ventricular ejection and thereby improving cardiac output. However, arterial pressure will fall and compromise tissue perfusion further if the increase in cardiac output is not large enough to offset the fall in peripheral resistance with arterial vasodilation (MAP = CO × TPR).

The deleterious effects of vasopressors result from the effects of sympathetic alpha- and beta-receptor stimulation. Alpha-receptor stimulation produces vasoconstriction, which increases arterial pressure and the resistance to ventricular ejection. Beta-receptor effects include augmentation of contractility. Elevation of arterial pressure and improvement in contractility are beneficial to the extent that the circulation is stabilized. However, both effects significantly increase oxygen demand, jeopardizing myocardium at risk for infarction. Agents with beta-receptor activity also are potentially dysrhythmogenic, which further hinders myocardial performance. The use of vasopressors is usually limited to those patients whose hypotension is so profound that no other means of therapy provides blood pressure support.

Vasopressor agents, such as epinephrine, norepinephrine (Levophed), and dopamine, stimulate both alpha-receptors and beta-receptors, although to varying degrees. Dopamine is the vasopressor of choice for cardiogenic shock. In low doses, dopamine exerts a selective vasodilatory effect on the renal vasculature.

Dysrhythmias, hypoxia, and acidosis can perpetuate the shock state. The administration of *antidysrhythmic drugs* may be indicated. Restoration of sinus rhythm generally improves cardiac output and blood pressure. Oxygenation is supported with the administration of supplemental oxygen and the initiation of mechanical ventilation if indicated. Treatment of acute pulmonary edema involves reduction of preload with vasodilators and diuretics as described and the administration of morphine sulfate. Correction of metabolic acidosis is accomplished with adjustment of ventilation or the administration of sodium bicarbonate.

Rapid institution of the conventional measures described previously, combined with intraaortic balloon pumping, typically permits hemodynamic stabilization, allowing for cardiac catheterization and emergency revascularization or repair of mechanical defects, if indicated, under more controlled conditions. The role of thrombolytic therapy and angioplasty in shock therapy is currently under clinical investigation. In some centers, *thrombolytic therapy* is initiated within hours of the MI to recanalize the affected vessel and salvage myocardium. If the thrombolytic drugs are ineffective in dissolving the clot, myocardial revascularization with either angioplasty or coronary artery bypass surgery is considered.

The use of thrombolytic therapy in the hours immediately after infarction seems to reduce not only the mortality rate from cardiogenic shock, but also the incidence of shock. The incidence of cardiogenic shock after MI has remained constant, complicating approximately 5% to 15% of MIs. Thrombolysis and early reperfusion may be most beneficial in preventing the development of shock.

The role of left heart assist devices and cardiac replacement with the artificial heart is being investigated for shock refractory to conventional measures, including intraaortic balloon pumping. Both forms of circulatory assistance are discussed in the next section.

METHODS OF CIRCULATORY ASSISTANCE

Circulatory assistance devices can be used either to support ventricular function or to replace the failing heart. Support devices include cardiopulmonary bypass, intraaortic balloon pumping, and ventricular assist devices (VADs). Alternatively, an artificial heart or transplant can be used to replace the heart.

Cardiopulmonary Bypass

Circulatory assistance was used initially for cardiopulmonary support during cardiac surgical procedures in the early 1950s. During open-heart surgery, the oxygenation and systemic circulation of blood is sustained by a heart-lung machine, referred to as *cardiopulmonary bypass* (Fig. 33-10). Catheters or cannulae are inserted into the superior vena cava and inferior vena cava to shunt venous blood away from the right side of the heart into the cardiopulmonary bypass machine. Additional blood is returned to the bypass machine by a mediastinal "sucker," which is placed in the operative field to collect blood lost during the surgical procedure. The bypass machine performs the following functions: (1) oxygenation of blood, (2) cooling of blood to induce systemic hypothermia and reduce tissue oxygen demand, and (3) filtration of blood to remove air and particulate matter. The blood is then

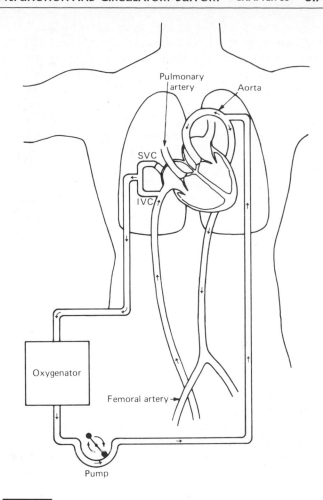

FIG. 33-10   Total cardiopulmonary bypass. Venous blood is shunted from the right atrium to the assist device via catheters inserted into the superior vena cava *(SVC)* and inferior vena cava *(IVC)*. The blood is oxygenated by the device and returned to the arterial system through a cannula in the aorta. (From Kinney M, editor: *AACN's clinical reference for critical care nurses,* New York, 1981, McGraw-Hill.)

pumped into the arterial circulation via a cannula positioned in either the aoritc arch or the femoral artery. Just before weaning from cardiopulmonary bypass, the heat exchanger in the bypass unit rewarms the blood. *Partial cardiopulmonary bypass* can be initiated rapidly via percutaneous cannulation of the femoral vein and femoral artery. This technique has been used for resuscitation at the bedside. *Extracorporeal membrane oxgenation* is a form of partial cardiopulmonary bypass currently used for neonatal respiratory failure.

Intraaortic Balloon Pumping

The intraaortic balloon is positioned in the descending thoracic aorta just distal to the left subclavian artery. It is inserted via either a percutaneous approach or a femoral arteriotomy and is threaded retrograde through the descending abdominal aorta. The balloon is inflated and de-

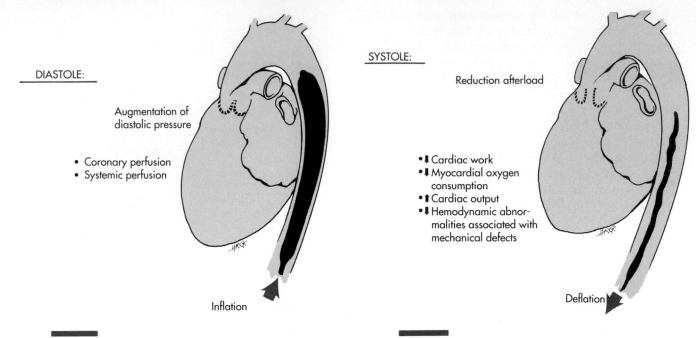

Augmentation of
diastolic pressure

• Coronary perfusion
• Systemic perfusion

Inflation

FIG. 33-11   Effect of intraaortic balloon inflation.

SYSTOLE:

Reduction afterload

• ↓ Cardiac work
• ↓ Myocardial oxygen
  consumption
• ↑ Cardiac output
• ↓ Hemodynamic abnor-
  malities associated with
  mechanical defects

Deflation

FIG. 33-12   Effect of intraaortic balloon deflation.

flated in synchrony with the mechanical events of the cardiac cycle. During left ventricular ejection or systole the balloon must be deflated. During ventricular diastole the balloon is inflated.

Inflation of the balloon with gas occurs just as the aortic valve closes at the end of systole; balloon inflation raises aortic volume, elevating aortic pressure. This effect is referred to as *augmentation of diastolic pressure*. The physiologic effect of diastolic augmentation is twofold (Fig. 33-11): (1) the perfusion pressure at the coronary orifices is increased during diastole, the period of greatest coronary flow, potentially increasing coronary flow; and (2) systemic perfusion also improves through elevation of mean arterial pressure.

Balloon deflation occurs rapidly, immediately before ventricular ejection, just before the aortic valve opens. As gas is removed from the balloon, intraaortic volume is lowered, thereby reducing aortic pressure. This reduction lowers the resistance against which the left ventricle must eject; consequently, ventricular wall tension developed during systole is lower. In other words, balloon deflation reduces afterload. The physiologic effects are as follows (Fig. 33-12): (1) reduction in cardiac work, (2) reduction in oxygen demand and $M\dot{V}o_2$, and (3) increase in cardiac output.

The intraaortic balloon pump is frequently used for cardiogenic shock and for failure to wean from cardiopulmonary bypass. Balloon pumping is particularly effective in the reversal of cardiogenic shock resulting from mechanical defects, such as VSD and mitral regurgitation. Initiation of balloon pumping in these patients reduces aortic pressure and resistance to ejection, thereby increasing forward flow through the aorta and reducing

abnormal flow through the defect. Refractory myocardial ischemia is also responsive to balloon pumping; the intrathoracic balloon pump can influence both the supply and the demand determinants of the myocardial oxygenation balance. Coronary blood flow increases with diastolic augmentation, and myocardial oxygen demand falls as a result of the reduction of afterload. The balloon is also used to maintain organ perfusion in patients with class IV heart failure awaiting transplantation.

Ventricular Assist Devices

Ventricular assist devices (VADs) were originally used for the sole support of the left ventricle. These *left heart assist devices* bypassed the left ventricle, temporarily supporting the circulation. However, once the incidence of right heart failure, either coexistent in left heart failure or in isolation, was recognized, the design of VADs was extended to the right ventricle.

The indication for VAD is usually cardiogenic shock or failure to wean from bypass. Shock must be refractory to conventional pharmacologic therapy and to intraaortic balloon pumping. Ventricular assistance is intended to stabilize the circulation as the myocardium recovers. These devices are also used in highly selective patients as a bridge to transplantation. Once a donor heart becomes available, VAD support is discontinued.

The basic design of the current VADs shunts blood from either atrium through a pneumatic or roller pump into the aorta or pulmonary artery, bypassing the affected ventricle (Fig. 33-13). Alternately, a cannula may be placed in the ventricular apex for inflow into the VAD. The VAD is stabilized externally on the anterior abdomi-

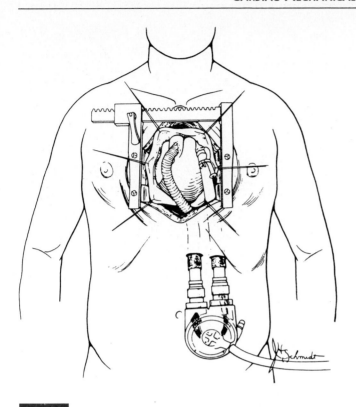

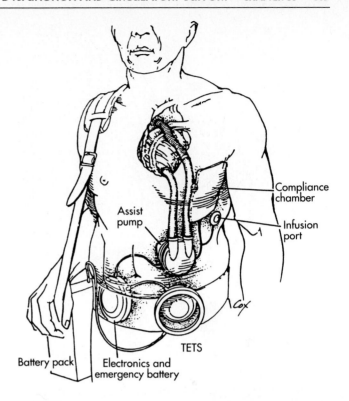

FIG. 33-13   Pneumatically powered ventricular assist pump. Blood is removed from the left atrium and pumped into the ascending aorta. (From Pierce WS et al: *N Engl J Med* 305(27):1606-1610, 1981.)

FIG. 33-14   Proposed placement of the permanent left ventricular assist pump. The pump is positioned in the preperitoneal space in the abdomen, fills from the left ventricular apex, and ejects into the ascending aorta. The energy is provided by a battery pack and is transmitted through the skin by a transcutaneous energy transmission system (TETS). The electronic control system, emergency battery pack, and air system (infusion port and compliance chamber) are necessary components. (From Pierce WS et al: *J Am Coll Cardiol* 14(2):265-275, 1989.)

nal wall. An oxygenator is not required because flow through the lungs is preserved; the device assumes only the work of pumping for the ventricle. If biventricular assist is required, separate circuits are maintained for each ventricle.

Permanent left heart assist devices are under development for patients who are not eligible for cardiac transplantation. Fig. 33-14 illustrates the design of one permanent device.

Artificial Heart

Artificial replacement of the heart has been of interest since the late 1950s. Since then, many advances have made the artificial heart clinically applicable to humans. In 1969 the artificial heart was used in Texas by Cooley for circulatory support before transplantation. The first permanent implantation of the total artificial heart was performed in 1982 at the University of Utah for Dr. Barney Clark. Fig. 33-15 illustrates one artificial heart design, the Jarvik heart. Currently the artificial heart is used almost exclusively as a bridge to transplantation in patients unresponsive to intraaortic balloon pumping or VADs. Development is continuing on the artificial heart to improve long-term survival and reduce morbidity.

Attachment of the artificial heart is accomplished by

excising the recipient's ventricular chambers just above the AV valves and anastomosing the atria and great vessels to the artificial device. The right and left ventricular chambers are separate, permitting individual control of ventricular dynamics. An external heart-drive console is connected to the ventricular drive lines. Air is "pulsed" into the ventricular chamber by the control console. The ventricular chamber is divided into air-filled and blood-filled compartments by a diaphragm. As air moves into the ventricular chamber, this diaphragm is forced upward, propelling blood on the other side of the diaphragm forward into the arterial circuit. Air is then withdrawn from the chamber. As the diaphragm moves downward, the artificial ventricle fills with blood.

The pneumatic mechanism controlling pump dynamics is cumbersome, limiting patient mobility and restricting widespread application of the device. Some centers are investigating the use of portable, electrically driven hearts to circumvent this limitation. Fig. 33-16 illustrates a proposed design of an implantable electric artificial heart.

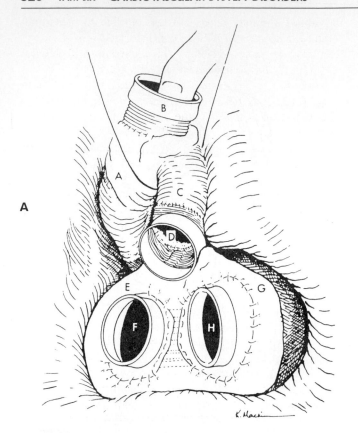

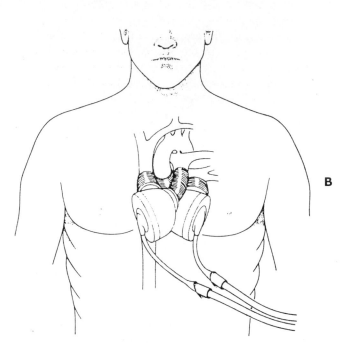

FIG. 33-15   Jarvik-7 total artificial heart. **A,** Four "quick connects" of artificial heart are sequentially sewn into place. *A,* Aorta; *B,* aortic quick connect; *C,* pulmonary artery; *D,* pulmonary aterial quick connect; *E,* right atrium; *F,* right atrial cuff and quick connect; *G,* left atrium; *H,* left atrial cuff and quick connect. **B,** The artificial ventricles of the Jarvik-7 are then secured to the four quick connects. [**A** from Quaal SJ: *Comprehensive intra-aortic balloon pumping,* St Louis, 1983, Mosby; **B** from Smith SL, editor: *Tissue and organ transplantation: implications for professional nursing practice,* St Louis, 1990, Mosby.]

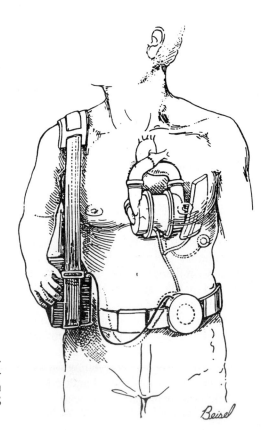

FIG. 33-16   Proposed placement of the electrical artificial heart within the thorax. To obviate the problems of percutaneous tubes, the design will use a transcutaneous energy transmission system with the primary coil positions and use of a belt. The patient will carry a case containing rechargeable batteries. [From Pierce WS et al: *J Am Coll Cardiol* 14(2):265-275, 1989.]

CARDIAC TRANSPLANTATION

The first human cardiac transplant was performed in 1967 by Barnard in South Africa. After an initial period of enthusiastic response, interest waned because of poor long-term success. Rejection seemed an insurmountable problem. Over the years, refinements in immunosuppressive therapy, immunologic monitoring techniques, and organ preservation techniques have resulted in significant improvements in patient survival. Thus the procedure is no longer considered experimental. In 1986 Medicare patients became eligible for federal reimbursement for cardiac transplants. The most extensive clinical and laboratory experience with cardiac transplantation is in the United States at Stanford University in California. According to the Registry of the International Society for Heart Transplantation, approximately 3000 cardiac transplants and 200 cardiopulmonary transplants were performed worldwide in 1993.

Indications

Cardiac transplantation is considered for end-stage heart disease refractory to conventional medical and surgical therapy. Class III and IV heart failure must be evident. The two most common conditions producing such myocardial compromise are congestive cardiomyopathy and advanced coronary disease. These entities combined account for 80% to 90% of all cardiac transplants.

Coronary artery disease is discussed in Chapter 31. *Cardiomyopathies* are diseases of the heart muscle of unknown origin. The key to distinguishing cardiomyopathies from other cardiac disorders is that the underlying abnormality involves the ventricular myocardium as opposed to any other myocardial structure, such as the valves or coronary arteries. Cardiomyopathies may be classified according to three types of abnormalities in structure and function: (1) congestive (dilated), (2) restrictive or obliterative, or (3) hypertrophic (Fig. 33-17).

Congestive cardiomyopathy is characterized by a grossly dilated and hypodynamic ventricle. There may be a lesser degree of myocardial hypertrophy. The hypodynamic ventricle contracts poorly, producing the predictable sequence of forward and backward failure described earlier. It is noteworthy that all four chambers become dilated secondary to increased volumes and pressures. Thrombus frequently develops within these chambers as a result of blood pooling and stasis; thus embolization is a threat. Typically, the onset of the disease is insidious; however, progression to end-stage refractory heart failure can result. The prognosis for refractory heart failure is extremely poor and may lead to consideration for heart transplantation. The exact cause of congestive cardiomyopathy is unknown; however, autoimmune and viral causes have been suggested. Multifactorial causation is probably the most plausible explanation.

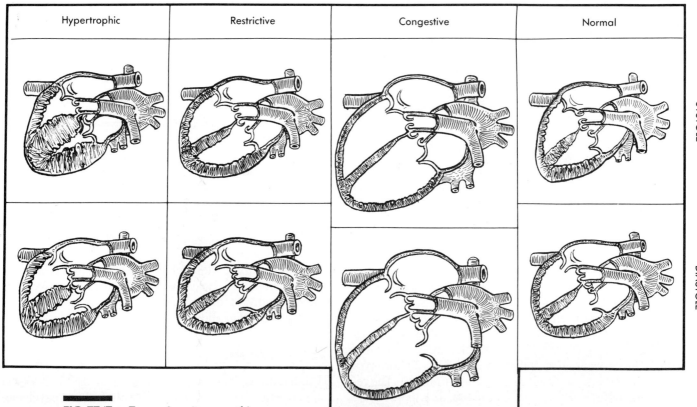

FIG. 33-17   Types of cardiomyopathies.

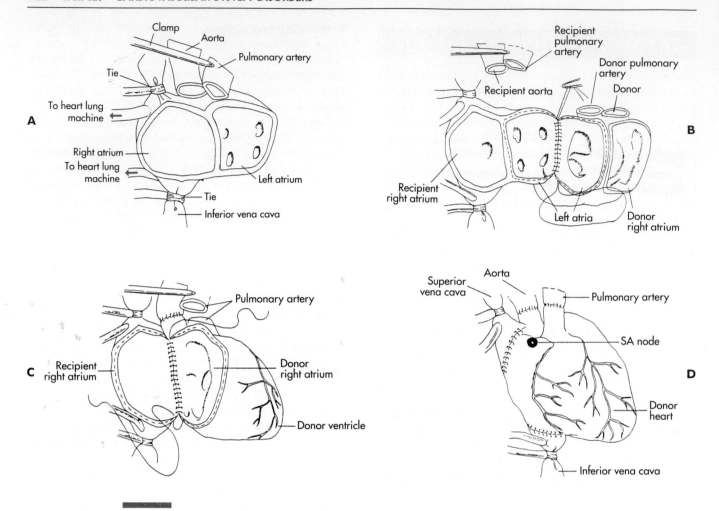

FIG. 33-18   Technique of cardiac transplantation. The procedure is performed as a conventional open-heart procedure with the usual equipment and instrumentation. It does not present any particular mechanical difficulties. The patient is routinely prepared and a median sternotomy performed. The patient is then connected to a cardiopulmonary bypass machine after systematic heparinization. The donor heart is removed after arrest is achieved by infusion of cold cardioplegia solution. It is then placed in cold saline solution for transfer to the recipient's operating room. The heart of the recipient is removed simultaneously. **A,** The aorta and pulmonary artery are divided immediately above their respective valves. Atrial walls and the interatrial septum are divided near the atrioventricular groove, leaving two large right and left atrial cuffs. **B,** Orthotopic graft is performed by anastomosing recipient and donor atrial walls and interatrial septum. **C** and **D,** Major vessels of donor and recipient. The aorta and pulmonary artery are trimmed and sutured, reestablishing anatomic continuity. The cardiac transplantation procedure is terminated as in any conventional open-heart procedure, with great care to prevent hemostasis and to eliminate entrapped air in the graft. The donor heart often starts beating spontaneously in sinus rhythm when perfusion is reestablished and rewarming is achieved. *SA,* Sinoatrial. (From Kern LF: In Michaelson CR, editor: *Congestive heart failure,* St Louis, 1983, Mosby.)

Hypertrophic cardiomyopathy, in contrast to congestive cardiomyopathy, is characterized by a hypertrophied and hyperdynamic heart. The increase in muscle mass is not associated with significant myocardial dilation. A genetic basis is suspected. *Restrictive cardiomyopathy* represents an impairment in ventricular filling caused by reduced ventricular compliance. Endocardial or myocardial fibrosis can result in restriction to filling. The restriction reduces cavity size; progression to a more severe form of cavity restriction is referred to as *obliterative*

cardiomyopathy. Although hypertrophic and restrictive cardiomyopathies can cause heart failure, congestive cardiomyopathy is the most significant entity relative to cardiac transplantation.

Selection Criteria

Cardiac transplant recipients who meet medical criteria for selection undergo an extensive clinical and psychosocial evaluation. As the procedure becomes better established and more widely available, decisions about which individuals are eligible for transplantation become more controversial. Donor availability continues to be a major limiting factor. Consequently, once a decision to perform a transplant has been made, establishing the individual's priority relative to others becomes a problem. Determining the relative priority of individuals with VADs and artificial hearts implanted as bridges to transplantation is a particularly complex question.

In general, however, factors that would complicate the postoperative course or affect long-term survival must be ruled out. These factors include active systemic infection or disease, pulmonary hypertension with fixed pulmonary vascular resistance (greater than 4 Wood units),* pulmonary emboli or infarction, active peptic ulcer disease, insulin-dependent diabetes mellitus with secondary end-organ disease, irreversible liver or renal failure, and active drug addiction or alcoholism. Intangible factors, such as motivation for rehabilitation, family support structure, and psychosocial state, are also considered. As insurance coverage becomes broader, personal financial resources become less significant to the selection process. If no contraindications are identified, a search for a potential donor is undertaken.

Potential donors are typically young trauma victims with no evidence of cardiac damage or disease and no systemic infection. Tissue matching of the donor to the recipient includes matching of the ABO system. An appropriate size match is also important; 20% body weight difference is considered to be an acceptable discrepancy.

Procedure

The surgical technique for cardiac transplantation is relatively straightforward, as illustrated in Fig. 33-18. A portion of both atria remain in situ for anastomosis to the donor heart. The region of the right atria near the superior vena cava is left intact to preserve sinus node function. The donor heart is then sutured to the recipient's atria and to the pulmonary artery and aorta. This procedure, in which the transplant is substituted for the recipient's

---

*Wood units equal pulmonary vascular resistance divided by 80.

heart, is referred to as *orthotopic transplantation.* This is in contrast to *heterotopic,* or "piggyback," *transplantation,* which is considered in some centers if pulmonary vascular resistance is extremely high and the high afterload in the pulmonary artery is likely to lead to refractory right ventricular failure in a transplanted heart. It is reasoned that the native right ventricle has adapted to this high afterload state and therefore should remain in situ. Alternately, some centers are performing cardiopulmonary transplants for primary pulmonary hypertension or pulmonary vascular disease secondary to congenital heart disease.

Rejection and Infection

The greatest challenge in transplantation is the management of rejection. The body's attempt to reject foreign tissue is a fundamental biologic process. The advent of cyclosporin A and monoclonal antibody preparations has significantly improved survival after transplantation. Immunosuppressive therapy with cyclosporin A may be initiated preoperatively. Triple-drug immunosuppressive therapy with azothioprine, cyclosporin A, and steroids is continued indefinitely after surgery. Close immunologic monitoring for signs of rejection is instituted. Transvenous endomyocardial biopsies are the "gold standard" for the detection and diagnosis of rejection. Biopsies are performed at regular intervals and as indicated. (Noninvasive methods to detect rejection, including magnetic resonance imaging and echocardiography, are under investigation). *Endomyocardial biopsy technique* involves the insertion of a biopsy catheter, or *bioptome,* through the right jugular or subclavian vein into the right ventricle to remove several portions of the endocardium for analysis. Results are then graded by a standardized cardiac biopsy grading system. Immunosuppressive therapy can then be adjusted accordingly. Antithymocyte globulin (ATG), antilymphocyte globulin (ALG), or monoclonal OKT3 antibodies may also be added to treat rejection (see Chapter 48). In addition to potential rejection, infection is a significant problem, because of immunosuppressive therapy. Appropriate prophylactic and therapeutic measures are used.

QUESTIONS

▼ *Circle the letter preceding each item below that correctly answers the question or completes the statement. Only one answer is correct unless otherwise noted.*

1. The relationship between left ventricular end-diastolic volume and left ventricular performance is illustrated in the:
   a. Cardiac output curve
   b. Ratio of dp/dt
   c. Frank-Starling curve
   d. Arterial-alveolar gradient

2. The ventricular function curve characteristic of the failing heart is usually:
   a. Depressed and flattened
   b. Elevated and curved
   c. Gradually sloping
   d. None of the above

3. The primary compensatory responses to a reduction in stroke volume include all the following *except:*
   a. Increased sympathetic activity
   b. Increased afterload
   c. Increased preload
   d. Ventricular hypertrophy

4. Which myocardial substance may become depleted during chronic heart failure?
   a. Epinephrine
   b. Myocardial lactate
   c. 2,3-Diphosphoglycerate
   d. Norepinephrine

5. Deleterious effects of compensatory mechanisms include (more than one answer may be correct):
   a. Reduced preload
   b. Increased cardiac work
   c. Improvement of heart failure
   d. Worsening of heart failure

6. A classic symptom of forward heart failure would be:
   a. Weakness and fatigue
   b. Pulmonary edema
   c. Anemia
   d. Hypovolemia

7. A classic symptom of backward heart failure would be:
   a. Weakness and fatigue
   b. Pulmonary edema
   c. Anemia
   d. Hypovolemia

8. Backward failure of the right side of the heart may produce all the following *except* (more than one answer may be correct):
   a. Elevated jugular venous pressure
   b. Rales and rhonchi
   c. Peripheral edema
   d. Weight gain
   e. Hepatomegaly
   f. Ascites
   g. Orthopnea

9. The typical chest radiograph of heart failure reveals all the following *except:*
   a. Cardiomegaly
   b. Retrocardiac densities
   c. Pulmonary venous congestion
   d. Upper lobar vascular redistribution

10. Which of the following laboratory findings may be useful in the diagnosis and management of heart failure (more than one answer may be correct)?
    a. Serum electrolytes
    b. Platelet count
    c. BUN and creatinine
    d. Urine electrolytes
    e. Serum lipids
    f. Liver function tests

11. All the following may precipitate heart failure *except:*
    a. Dysrhythmias
    b. Infection
    c. Disseminated intravascular coagulation (DIC)
    d. Pulmonary embolism

12. Measures to improve myocardial contractility may include all the following *except:*
    a. Digitalis glycosides
    b. Intraaortic balloon pumping
    c. Amrinone
    d. Dobutamine

13. Measures to reduce cardiac work include all the following *except:*
    a. Arterial vasodilators
    b. Digitalis glycosides
    c. Intraaortic balloon pumping
    d. Venodilators

14. The incidence of cardiogenic shock after acute myocardial infarction is approximately:
    a. 5%
    b. 30% to 35%
    c. 80% to 90%
    d. None of the above

15. Conventional medical management of cardiogenic shock is associated with a mortality rate approaching:
    a. 25%
    b. 50%
    c. 75%
    d. 100%

16. Cardiogenic shock may be secondary to (more than one answer may be correct):
    a. Atrial fibrillation
    b. Acute myocardial infarction
    c. Acute mitral regurgitation
    d. Pericarditis
    e. Ventricular septal defect
    f. All the above

17. The effects of cardiogenic shock on the myocardium include (more than one answer may be correct):
    a. Decreased coronary blood flow
    b. Dysrhythmias
    c. Increased afterload
    d. Systemic acidosis
    e. Hypoxia
    f. All the above

18. The hemodynamic profile of cardiogenic shock is characterized by all the following *except:*
    a. Cardiac index less than 2.1 L/min/m²
    b. Evidence of organ hypoperfusion
    c. Left ventricular end-diastolic pressure less than 18 mm Hg
    d. Hypotension

19. The following interventions all reduce preload *except:*
    a. Vasodilators
    b. Vasopressors
    c. Diuretics

20. The following interventions all reduce afterload *except:*
    a. Vasodilators
    b. Vasopressors
    c. Intraaortic balloon pumping

21. Which of the following agents does *not* increase contractility?
    a. Calcium
    b. Digitalis glycosides
    c. Dobutamine
    d. Propranolol

22. During intraaortic balloon pumping, the balloon is (more than one answer may be correct):
    a. Deflated during ventricular systole
    b. Inflated during ventricular systole
    c. Inflated during ventricular diastole
    d. Deflated during ventricular diastole

23. Physiologic effects of the intraaortic balloon include all the following *except:*
    a. Decreased myocardial oxygen demand
    b. Increased cardiac output
    c. Decreased cardiac work
    d. Increased afterload

24. The artificial heart is used primarily to:
    a. Offer temporary support of the circulation
    b. Treat end-stage heart disease

25. The two most common causes of end-stage heart disease in which cardiac transplantation may be considered are:
    a. Congestive cardiomyopathy
    b. Papillary muscle rupture
    c. Lown-Ganong-Levine syndrome
    d. Advanced coronary artery disease

QUESTIONS—cont'd

26. The form of end-stage cardiomyopathy most frequently considered for cardiac transplantation is:
    a.   Hypertrophic
    b.   Restrictive
    c.   Congestive
    d.   All the above

▼ *Circle the correct word(s) within the parentheses or fill in the blank with the correct word or phrase for each statement.*

27. Congestive heart failure is the state of (pulmonary) or (circulatory) congestion resulting from failure of the heart as a (reservoir) or (pump).

28. An increase in left ventricular end-diastolic pressure usually causes a concomitant increase in (right atrial pressure) or (left atrial pressure), which in turn increases (pulmonary venous) or (systemic venous) pressures, which leads to (pulmonary edema) or (hepatomegaly).

29. The most common mechanical complication of acquired and congenital heart disease is

    _____ _____.

30. Cardiogenic shock is typically associated with approximately _____ percent loss of ventricular myocardium.

31. During circulatory support with assist devices for the left side of the heart, venous blood is oxygenated by the (machine) or (patient). Oxygenated blood flows into the left side of the heart, which acts as a (pump) or (reservoir).

32. During cardiopulmonary bypass, venous blood flows through catheters placed in the _____. This venous blood is diverted to the _____, where diffusion of gases takes place. The oxygenated blood is returned to the body by a catheter placed in the _____ or _____.

33. Arrange the following events in correct chronologic order:
    _____ Renin release from the juxtaglomerular apparatus
    _____ Conversion of angiotensin I to angiotensin II
    _____ Sympathetic activation
    _____ Sodium and water retention in the distal tubule and collecting duct
    _____ Reduced renal blood flow and reduced glomerular filtration rate
    _____ Interaction of renin with circulating angiotensinogen to produce angiotensin I
    _____ Adrenal secretion of aldosterone

34. An increased pressure load, such as occurs in aortic stenosis, would result in a _____ pattern of ventricular hypertrophy, whereas an increased volume load, such as occurs in aortic regurgitation, would result in a _____ pattern of ventricular hypertrophy and chamber _____.

▼ *Match each clinical syndrome in column A with its corresponding symptoms in column B.*

Column A	Column B
35. _____ Right heart failure	a. Rales
36. _____ Left heart failure	b. Dependent edema
	c. Pulmonary edema
	d. Third heart sound
	e. Increased jugular venous pressure
	f. Hepatomegaly

▼ *Match each symptom in column A with its definition in column B.*

Column A	Column B
37. _____ Paroxysmal nocturnal dyspnea (PND)	a. Difficulty in breathing
	b. Sudden awakening with shortness of breath
38. _____ Cardiac asthma	c. Shortness of breath in the recumbent position
39. _____ Dyspnea on exertion	d. Auscultatory findings of pulmonary congestion
40. _____ Dyspnea	e. PND with wheezing
41. _____ Orthopnea	f. Shortness of breath with physical exertion
42. _____ Rales	

Continued.

QUESTIONS—cont'd

▼ Match the following types of cardiomyopathy in column A with their corresponding structural abnormalities in column B.

Column A	Column B
43. _____ Hypertrophic	a. Grossly enlarged, hypodynamic ventricle
44. _____ Congestive or dilated	b. Impeded ventricular filling
45. _____ Restrictive or obliterative	c. Increased ventricular muscle mass

▼ Match the following interventions in column B with their primary physiologic effect(s) in column A.

Column A	Column B
46. _____ Reduced preload	a. Venodilators
47. _____ Reduced afterload	b. Inotropic agents
48. _____ Increased contractility	c. Intraaortic balloon pumping
49. _____ Change in vascular tone	

▼ Circle the letter preceding each item below that correctly answers the question or completes the statement. Only one answer is correct unless otherwise noted.

50. Mean arterial pressure (MAP, pressure head driving blood to perfuse the tissues) is equal to:
a. CO × TPR (cardiac output multiplied by total systemic peripheral resistance)
b. CO/TPR (cardiac output divided by total peripheral resistance)
c. EDP − ESP (end-diastolic − end-systolic blood pressure)
d. Diastolic blood pressure plus one-third pulse pressure

51. TPR equals:

a. $\dfrac{MAP - CVP \times 80}{CO}$ (CVP, central venous pressure)

b. CO/BSA (BSA, body surface area)
c. MAP × CVP × CO
d. Systolic plus diastolic blood pressure

52. The underlying pathology of shock regardless of the type is:
a. Decreased cardiac output
b. Low blood pressure
c. Inadequate tissue perfusion
d. Peripheral vasoconstriction

53. The vasopressor of choice for the treatment of cardiogenic shock is:
a. Low-dose dopamine
b. Norepinephrine (Levophed)
c. Epinephrine
d. Sodium nitroprusside

54. The chronic compensatory mechanisms involved in mitral regurgitation associated with chronic volume overload include all the following *except:*
a. Ventricular chamber dilation
b. Increase in ventricular wall stress
c. Increase in myocardial oxygen demand
d. Eccentric hypertrophy
e. Concentric hypertrophy

55. The chronic compensatory mechanisms involved in systemic hypertension associated with chronic pressure overload include all the following *except:*
a. Minimal change in ventricular chamber volume
b. Increase in ventricular wall stress
c. Increase in myocardial oxygen demand
d. Eccentric hypertrophy
e. Concentric hypertrophy

CHAPTER 34 ▸ Vascular Disease

PATRICIA HENRY FOLCARELLI
PENNY FORD CARLETON

Disease processes can affect both the peripheral arteries and the peripheral veins, impairing either tissue perfusion or venous return to the heart. This chapter describes common arterial and venous diseases. The arterial section emphasizes atherosclerotic disease of the aorta and its major branches; occlusive and aneurysmal presentations of atherosclerosis are described in detail. Aortic dissection is also discussed. The venous section focuses on four major disease presentations: (1) superficial thrombophlebitis; (2) deep venous thrombosis, both acute and recurrent; (3) varicose veins; and (4) postthrombotic syndrome. The pathophysiology of superficial thrombophlebitis and deep venous thrombosis is considered under the broader heading of venous thromboembolic disease.

ARTERIAL DISEASE

Anatomy
Arterial wall

The arterial wall consists of three layers: the outer layer, or adventitia; the middle layer, or media; and the inner layer, or intima. The *adventitia* contains the nerve fibers and blood vessels that supply the arterial wall. It is composed of connective tissue and provides the total strength of the arterial wall. The *media* contains collagen, smooth muscle fibers, and elastin and is largely responsible for regulating the diameter of the vessel by dilation and constriction. The *intima* is a smooth layer of endothelial cells providing a nonthrombotic surface for blood flow. The intima and the media are nourished by a process of diffusion from arterial flow. The adventitia and outer portion of the media receive nutrients from the *vasa vasorum*, "vessel of vessels," whose small vessels penetrate the outer arterial wall.

Aorta and its major branches

The aorta traverses the thoracic and abdominal cavities, and its segments are distinguished accordingly. The *thoracic aorta* is divided into the following anatomic segments: (1) ascending thoracic aorta, (2) transverse aortic arch, and (3) descending thoracic aorta. The ascending aorta originates at the aortic valve and extends to the orifices of the vessels supplying the head, neck, and upper extremities. These vessels, collectively referred to as *brachiocephalic vessels,* arise from the aortic arch. As illustrated in Fig. 34-1, the brachiocephalic vessels include the innominate artery (brachiocephalic trunk), the left common carotid artery, and the left subclavian artery. The innominate artery divides into the right common carotid and right subclavian arteries. The axillary arteries arise from the subclavian arteries and extend to the brachial arteries, which branch into the radial and ulnar arteries. The vertebral arteries arise from the subclavian arteries bilaterally.

The descending thoracic aorta begins distal to the left subclavian artery and extends to the diaphragm. The *ab-*

527

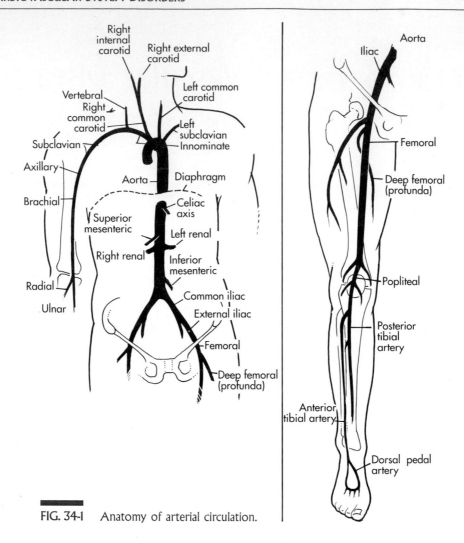

FIG. 34-1 Anatomy of arterial circulation.

dominal aorta begins beneath the diaphragm and branches within a few centimeters to supply the abdominal organs. This portion of the aorta lies posterior to the lungs, diaphragm, duodenum, spleen, stomach, and intestines. The major visceral branches of the abdominal aorta are illustrated in Fig. 34-1 and include the celiac axis, superior mesenteric artery, and renal arteries. The inferior mesenteric artery branches off the aorta below the renal arteries. The abdominal aorta extends to the aortic bifurcation at the level of the pelvis. The *terminal aorta* is the aortic segment between the renal arteries and the bifurcation; the inferior mesenteric artery is the major branch of the terminal aorta.

The aorta bifurcates into the common iliac arteries. The common iliac arteries divide into the external iliac arteries and the hypogastric or internal iliac arteries. The external iliac arteries become the common femoral arteries. The common femoral gives off multiple branches, including the superficial femoral artery and the deep femoral artery, or profunda femoris. The superficial femoral artery extends to the popliteal artery, which in turn branches into the posterior tibial artery, the peroneal artery, and the anterior tibial artery. The anterior tibial artery extends to the dorsal pedal artery.

In the event of obstruction within the arterial system, important collateral networks develop to bypass the involved segment and maintain blood flow. These networks are generally enlarged, preexisting arteries that develop in the presence of stenosis or total occlusion. Collateral vessels are usually a network of smaller and more numerous vessels; however, their size and number are related to the size and the duration of the occlusion or stenosis. Arteries particularly important as potential routes for collateral flow to the lower extremities include the inferior mesenteric artery and the deep femoral artery. For example, the inferior mesenteric artery becomes enlarged to provide collateral flow in the setting of bilateral occlusion of the common iliac arteries (Fig. 34-2).

Etiology and Pathology
Atherosclerotic causes

Atherosclerosis is the most common disease affecting the arterial vasculature. Atherosclerosis is characterized initially by lipid deposition in the intimal layer of the artery. Subsequently, calcification, fibrosis, thrombosis, and hemorrhage can occur, contributing to the development of a complex atherosclerotic plaque, or *atheroma*.

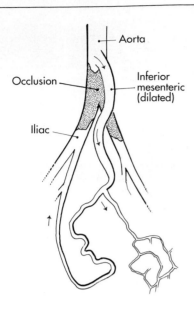

FIG. 34-2   Collateral blood flow via inferior mesenteric artery resulting from bilateral occlusion of common iliac arteries.

Eventually the media begins to degenerate. Necrosis of the fat-filled smooth muscle cells also occurs. These pathologic processes progressively occlude the vessel lumen and weaken the arterial wall. (See Chapter 31 for a discussion of theories of atherogenesis and risk factors.)

The clinical manifestations of atherosclerosis result either from *vascular occlusion* or *stenosis,* caused by intimal deposition or embolization, or from *aneurysm formation,* caused by medial degeneration. The most common course of atherosclerotic disease in the peripheral vasculature is vessel occlusion, whereas in the aorta, aneurysmal presentations are more common. Arterial occlusive and aneurysmal disease caused by atherosclerosis are discussed in subsequent sections.

Given the diffuse and progressive nature of the atherosclerotic process, however, one must remember that peripheral vascular disease is usually associated with cerebral and coronary disease. Management of aortic or peripheral vascular disease without regard for potential consequences resulting from vascular compromise in the coronary or cerebral beds could be catastrophic. (See Chapters 31 and 53 for discussions of coronary and cerebral atherosclerotic disease.)

Nonatherosclerotic causes

The primary nonatherosclerotic causes of arterial disease are (1) cystic medial necrosis; (2) arterial inflammation or arteritis; (3) vasospastic disorders; and (4) fibromuscular dysplasia. Others include infection, trauma, and congenital anomalies.

Cystic medial necrosis. Cystic medial necrosis is a pathologic process that produces degenerative changes in the medial layer of the artery. The cause of this degeneration is unknown. The incidence of cystic medial necrosis is highest in younger men. Medial degeneration can lead to aneurysm formation, aortic dissection, or spontaneous arterial rupture. A variety of conditions can produce cystic medial necrosis, including *Marfan's syndrome,* an inherited disorder of the connective tissue.

Arterial inflammation. Inflammatory disorders of the aorta or peripheral arteries can result in arterial occlusion. *Thromboangiitis obliterans,* or *Buerger's disease,* is a chronic occlusive disease of the medium-size and small arteries and veins. The inflammation and subsequent healing and thrombosis of lesions produce vascular obstruction. A recurring migratory pattern of superficial thrombophlebitis is not uncommon. Smoking appears directly related to the etiology and course of this disease.

Vasospastic conditions. Vasospastic conditions can also produce transient arterial occlusion. *Raynaud's syndrome* is produced by vasospasm of the small cutaneous and subcutaneous arteries and arterioles. The two forms of Raynaud's syndrome are (1) primary or idiopathic *(spastic Raynaud's)* and (2) secondary *(obstructive Raynaud's).* No identifiable cause exists for primary Raynaud's syndrome, and no vascular obstruction is present. The occurrence of vasospasm appears to relate to the local dynamics of the arterial wall. This condition is also called *Raynaud's disease.* Secondary Raynaud's syndrome results from diffuse obstructive disease caused by associated conditions, such as scleroderma.

The vasospasm of Raynaud's syndrome affects the fingers and, less often, the feet and toes. The syndrome is characterized by phasic changes in skin color, usually precipitated by exposure to cold or emotional upset. An initial phase of pallor caused by vasoconstriction is followed by a cyanotic phase and finally by a phase of rubor from reactive vasodilation. During the vasospastic episode, numbness or difficulty with fine motor movement and a sensation of coldness may be noted.

The course of primary Raynaud's syndrome is typically benign because of the intermittent nature of the vasospasm. Treatment is directed at eliminating precipitating factors, such as exposure to cold or smoking. Vasodilation with calcium channel blocking drugs, such as nifedipine, may be beneficial in select patients.

Fibromuscular dysplasia. Fibromuscular dysplasia is characterized by abnormalities in the fibrous connective tissue of the arterial wall. This disorder most frequently affects the renal arteries of women under 40 years of age and results in renovascular hypertension (see Figs. 45-11 and 46-15). In most patients this disorder appears angiographically as a "string of beads" caused by medial fibroplasia. This condition may be treated surgically.

Other causes. Arterial infection typically results from septicemia. Sources of infection include bacterial endocarditis, gastroenteritis (particularly caused by *Salmonella* species), and vascular infection from intravenous drug abuse. Arterial infection tends to localize on roughened endothelial surfaces, such as atherosclerotic plaques. Vascular trauma and congenital anomalies, such as coarctation of the aorta, are also major nonatherosclerotic causes of vascular abnormality.

THREE PULSE-SCORING SYSTEMS*

0 = Pulse absent	0 = Absent	0 = Absent
1 = Pulse present but markedly reduced	1 = Pulse present but barely palpable	1 = Pulse present but diminished
2 = Pulse present but moderately reduced	2 = Pulse normal	2 = Pulse normal
3 = Pulse present but slightly reduced	3+ = Pulse normal, easily palpable	
4 = Pulse present and normal	4+ = Abnormal pulsation (as in aneurysm)	

*The grading of pulses is subjective, and scoring systems to evaluate pulse strength differ among institutions.

Diagnostic Procedures

Physical examination techniques

Physical examination yields much information relative to the degree of arterial disease. Initial visual inspection is for color, hair distribution, edema, atrophy, varicosities, ulcerations, nail condition, and skin integrity. Palpation begins by checking skin temperature at all levels. Auscultation for bruits then follows. Pulses are palpated at multiple sites for presence, strength, and equality relative to the contralateral limb. The grading of pulse strength is subjective and varies among institutions. (Three currently used systems for grading pulses are listed in the box above.) Pulses may be compared before and after exercise; pulses distal to an obstructive lesion typically diminish with exercise.

Leg elevation and dependency tests are extremely useful for evaluating arterial occlusive disease because flow across obstructive lesions is pressure dependent and therefore extremely sensitive to the effects of gravity. Elevation of the extremity produces pallor, followed by redness or rubor with dependency. Elevation pallor is the result of gravitational effects, which reduce arterial pressure and consequently lower the blood volume in the capillary bed. As the extremity is lowered beneath heart level and perfusion pressure increases, color returns. Rubor results from a reactive hyperemia or maximal vascular dilation in response to tissue hypoxia.

The degree of occlusion is estimated according to the length of time required for elevation pallor and dependent rubor to occur; normally no pallor is observed during 60 seconds of leg elevation, and color returns within 10 seconds. Venous filling time in the dependent position is also determined because the veins of the dependent leg also take longer to fill because of the interference with arterial inflow. Normal venous filling time is less than 15 seconds.

Sensation, muscle strength, and skin temperature are also evaluated. Bruits and trophic changes are noted. The results of the physical examination are subjective by nature; therefore noninvasive tests may be indicated for further evaluation. A more complete discussion of signs and symptoms is included in subsequent sections.

Doppler ultrasound

Vascular Doppler studies use ultrasound as the examination medium (see Chapter 30). A Doppler probe contains a piezoelectric crystal that transmits ultrasonic waves of a known frequency. When positioned over a segment of artery or vein, this beam strikes the red blood cells and the back-scattered or reflected wave is shifted in frequency, depending on the direction and velocity of the moving cells. This difference between the transmitted frequency and the reflected frequency is known as the *Doppler shift.* Frequency changes can be used to interpret direction of flow. Flow moving toward the probe has a higher frequency than flow transmitted from cells moving away from the probe.

There are two basic types of Doppler ultrasound. *Continuous-wave ultrasound* transmitters are generally small, portable units. In this type, a continuous signal is emitted from one crystal in the probe and reflected frequencies are received by another crystal within the probe. The second type, *pulsed-wave ultrasound,* is more frequently found in laboratory-based ultrasound devices. A signal crystal alternately sends and receives signals in a pulsing mode. The delay in time from emission to reception allows for sampling at specific depths, adding information to the signal. The Doppler signal can be interpreted audibly as well as through the technique of spectral analysis. A spectral analyzer visually displays all frequencies of the back-scattered signal. Time is displayed on the horizontal axis and frequency on the vertical axis. This analysis allows for less subjectivity than the audible-only analysis.

Duplex scanning

The techniques of pulsed Doppler and spectral analysis have been combined with B-mode ultrasound imaging in a system called duplex scanning. *B mode,* or *brightness mode, ultrasound* allows for a two-dimensional image of the blood vessel in real time. The contrast between the bright vessel wall and the fluid-filled lumen of the vessel affords the examiner the ability to image vascular morphology, including irregularities in the lumen of the vessel caused by atherosclerotic plaque and aneurysmal dilation

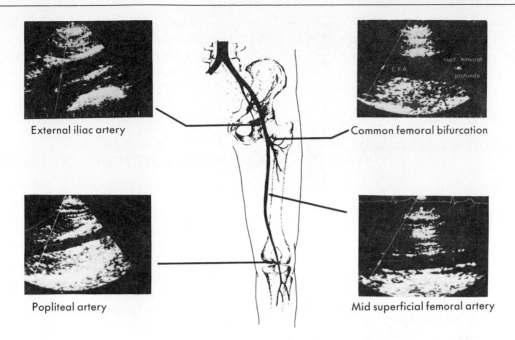

External iliac artery

Common femoral bifurcation

Popliteal artery

Mid superficial femoral artery

FIG. 34-3   B-mode image of distal external iliac artery, common femoral artery *(CFA)* bifurcation, superficial femoral artery, and popliteal artery of a healthy volunteer. Axis of Doppler beam, angle of incidence, and a sample volume placement are displayed. (From Bernstein EF: *Vascular diagnosis,* ed 4, St Louis, 1993, Mosby.)

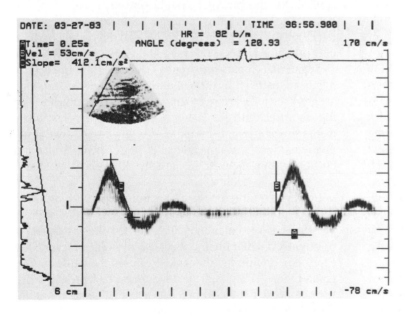

FIG. 34-4   Doppler signal is analyzed by real-time fast Fourier transform (FFT) spectrum analyzer and displayed with time on the horizontal axis, velocity (cm/sec) on vertical axis, and amplitude as shades of gray. *A,* Measurement of time: time of systolic forward flow (0.25 seconds); *B,* velocity parameters: systolic peak velocity (53 cm/sec); *C,* slope: deceleration = peak systolic velocity divided by pulse decay time = 412.1 cm/sec^2. (From Bernstein EF: *Vascular diagnosis,* ed 4, St Louis, 1993, Mosby.)

(Fig. 34-3). Both vessel wall and residual lumen can be visualized, allowing for determination of the percentage of diameter reduction or total occlusion. Duplex scanning allows the examiner to position a pulsed Doppler signal in the midstream of the visualized vessel. The received frequencies are then subjected to spectral analysis (Fig. 34-4). In some systems, color displays of the flow velocities allow for a real-time display of velocities of flow in the vessel lumen. Arterial disease produces distinctive abnormalities in flow velocity and flow patterns. Normal arterial flow is laminar in nature, with higher-frequency (higher-velocity) flow in the midstream of the vessel and lower-frequency (lower-velocity) flow along the walls of the vessels (Fig. 34-5). In areas of narrowing, the velocity increases throughout the narrowest segment. Flow distal and proximal to the stenosed segment is turbulent, with many frequencies displayed on the spectral analysis. Frequency and turbulence increase proportionally with the degree of stenosis, whereas totally occluded vessels have no obtainable flow signal.

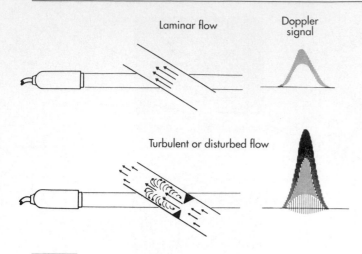

FIG. 35-5 Doppler signals recorded from laminar flow and turbulent or disturbed flow. With laminar flow, all the velocities are similar. The Doppler signal produces a relatively thin waveform with minimal spectral broadening. When blood flows across an area with a significant change in the caliber of the blood vessel, flow with multiple velocities in different directions is produced. Such disturbed flow produces a Doppler signal with multiple frequencies and marked spectral broadening. (From Feigenbaum H: *Echocardiography*, ed 4, Philadelphia, 1986, Lea & Febiger.)

Computed tomography

A tomograph is an image of a cross-sectional slice of the body. B-mode ultrasound, as described earlier, is an example of a tomograph. Computed tomographic (CT) scanning has extended vascular imaging from two-dimensional (2-D) to three-dimensional (3-D) imaging. To construct this 3-D image, a camera rotates in a 360-degree arc around the region of interest, recording 2-D images at multiple angles. X-rays are transmitted through the body to detectors on the opposite side. Each x-ray image captures a thin anatomic slice of the region of interest. A composite 3-D image is constructed from these 2-D x-ray images by a computer. A small amount of contrast material, usually containing iodine, is injected via a peripheral site to heighten the contrast between the vessel wall and the blood.

CT scanning provides direct depiction of the vessel wall, making it an ideal diagnostic tool for assessing the size of aneurysms as well as the structure around vessels that indicate disease (e.g., hematoma, fluid).

Magnetic resonance imaging

Magnetic resonance imaging (MRI) equipment consists of a magnet that supplies the main magnetic field within the bore of a scanner, transmitter, and receiver coils, which deliver the radiofrequency pulses that excite the nuclei of the cells and receive the signals arising from the tissue nuclei. Spatial localization of the MR signal is then obtained. Imaging of perfusion for vascular studies is obtained through the use of contrast agents. This promis-

ing technique for the imaging of the vascular system is suitable because flowing blood produces a unique signal during the MRI process. The MR images portray the morphologic features of the vessel and identify patterns of hemodynamically significant stenosis. MR angiography (MRA) can be used in the evaluation of obstructive disease in the carotid arteries, renal arteries, and peripheral circulation.

Segmental plethysmography

Segmental plethysmography measures changes in pulse volume. Pneumatic cuffs are placed around the upper thigh, lower thigh, and ankle. The cuffs are automatically or manually inflated to approximately 65 mm Hg to ensure optimal cuff contact. A transducer senses changes in cuff pressure during systole as the blood volume in the vessel fluctuates. A pulse volume recording is generated for each site, and the cuffs are deflated.

In the vascular laboratory this technique is usually performed simultaneously with *segmental extremity pressure measurement*. First, the brachial systolic blood pressure is measured to establish a baseline. Then a pneumatic blood pressure cuff is wrapped around the lower extremity with a stethoscope or Doppler flow probe over the arterial pulse. The pneumatic cuff is sequentially inflated on the ankle, upper thigh, and lower thigh to a pressure above the brachial systolic pressure and then deflated. The onset of flow during systole at each site is detected by the stethoscope or probe, and the corresponding cuff pressure is recorded (Fig. 34-6).

Segmental plethysmography and pressure measurements are usually performed during rest and immediately after exercise. Exercise evaluation usually involves walking on a treadmill for 5 minutes or for as long as tolerated. Flow abnormalities increase with exercise, resulting in a reduction or disappearance of pulses distal to the occlusion and an increase in pressure differences or gradients across the occlusion.

Lower-extremity pressures are compared with brachial systolic pressure and with each other. An ankle-to-arm pressure ratio is calculated. The normal ratio is equal to or slightly greater than 1 because systolic pressures at each site, including the ankle, should be equal to or greater than the brachial systolic pressure. A pressure difference greater than 30 mm Hg between segments indicates disease. Severely diseased segments may have an ankle/brachial index (ABI) of less than 4.0. These measurements are limited to those patients with severe calcification of arterial walls, as frequently seen in the diabetic population. Distal pressure in these patients may be elevated to greater than 300 mm Hg, making these pressures meaningless without concomitant segmental plethysmography. A pressure difference of 20 to 30 mm Hg between a lower-extremity site and the contralateral pulse is indicative of arterial occlusion. Analysis of pulse volume recordings and pressure relationships permits estimation of disease severity. Fig. 34-7 illustrates the abnormalities

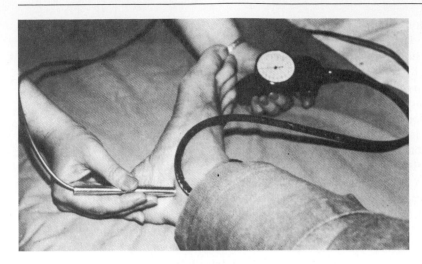

FIG. 34-6   Method of recording ankle systolic pressure. (From Yao JST: In Bernstein EF: *Vascular diagnosis,* ed 4, St Louis, 1993, Mosby.)

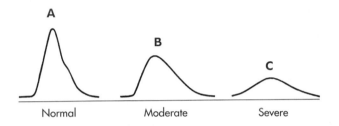

FIG. 34-7   Pulse volume recordings. **A,** Normal; **B,** moderate stenosis; **C,** severe stenosis.

in pulse volume recordings observed with moderate and severe vascular occlusion.

Chest radiography

Chest radiographs are useful in the evaluation of aortic aneurysms and dissections. A thoracic aneurysm or aortic dissection may be detected as mediastinal widening on a chest radiograph. Anteroposterior and lateral abdominal radiographs are useful to confirm clinical suspicions of an abdominal aneurysm.

Arteriography

Arteriography, or opacification of the artery with contrast material, is rarely, if ever, necessary for diagnosis of occlusive arterial disease. However, if surgical correction is indicated, arteriography is required to determine the precise location and extent of disease. Collateral circulation and the condition of the proximal and distal vasculature can also be evaluated.

Arteriography is performed on a selective basis for aneurysm evaluation, particularly if suprarenal extension or involvement of the visceral vessels is suspected. However, arteriography can underestimate aneurysm size because the contrast material opacifies only the blood-filled portion of the aneurysm and mural thrombi, which can occupy a significant portion of the aneurysm, will not be detected. With aortic dissections, *aortography,* or arteriography of the aorta, is indicated to determine the location and extent of dissection.

Occlusive Arterial Disease

The term *chronic occlusive arterial disease* encompasses disorders that cause ischemia as a result of arterial obstruction. As indicated earlier, the most common cause of occlusive disease is atherosclerosis. Atherosclerotic lesions tend to develop at points of branching, bifurcation, abrupt curvature, or vascular narrowing. Turbulent flow in these regions is thought to contribute to atherogenesis, perhaps through traumatic disruption of the endothelial lining.

Lesions occur more frequently in the lower extremities than in the upper extremities and tend to be localized, involving segments of the artery. Common sites of involvement include (1) aortoiliac vessels, (2) femoropopliteal vessels, (3) popliteal-tibial vessels, and (4) combinations of these. The *Leriche's syndrome* is progressive occlusion of the terminal aorta, including the bifurcation and iliac arteries, from atherosclerosis and thrombosis.

Pathophysiology

Chronic arterial occlusive disease progressively narrows the arterial lumen, increasing the resistance to blood flow. As the resistance to flow increases, blood flow to the tissue beyond the lesion is reduced. If the oxygen needs of the tissue exceed the vessel's ability to supply oxygen, tissue ischemia results. A single lesion must reduce the vessel lumen by approximately 50% in diameter or 75% in cross-sectional area to produce clinically significant interference with blood flow. However, multiple stenoses occurring in sequence, as frequently occurs with atherosclerosis, compound the interference with flow; in other words, in combination, less significant lesions can seriously impair flow.

The severity of ischemia distal to an obstructive lesion depends not only on the site and extent of occlusion but also on the degree of collateral flow around the lesion.

Fortunately, the tendency of atherosclerotic lesions to be localized and to enlarge gradually favors the development of collateral circulation. With localized lesions, the distal artery remains patent; thus alternative routes of arterial flow can bypass the lesion to perfuse the tissue beyond. As resistance to flow increases at the site of obstruction, pressure increases proximal to the lesion with a proportionate drop in pressure distal to the lesion. This pressure gradient across the obstruction promotes flow through collateral vessels. These collateral vessels gradually enlarge. Increased velocity of flow through the collateral vessels also stimulates collateral development. Severe ischemia can result from acute occlusion because collateral networks have not had time to develop. The adequacy of collateral flow is also compromised by disease in collateral vessels.

Acute arterial occlusion is primarily a complication of another disease process. Most frequently, these occlusions occur in the lower extremities, but upper extremities can also be affected. Acute arterial occlusion can be produced by thrombosis or embolization. *Thrombosis* is the formation of a blood clot, or thrombus, within the vascular system. Arterial thrombosis usually occurs at the site of an atherosclerotic plaque or within an arterial aneurysm. Detachment of a thrombus into the bloodstream is referred to as *embolization.* The embolus is propelled downstream to lodge in the smaller branches of the arterial system, occluding the vascular lumen.

Most arterial thromboemboli originate in the left side of the heart. Mitral stenosis and atrial fibrillation interfere with left atrial emptying, predisposing to the development of atrial thrombi. Transmural myocardial infarction roughens the endothelial surface of the left ventricle, potentiating the formation of mural ventricular thrombi. Embolization can also result from detachment of mural thrombi from a ventricular aneurysm. Depending on the size and destination of the clot, dislodgement of thrombi from the cardiac chambers is potentially catastrophic. Emboli tend to lodge in regions of bifurcation or branching. The term *saddle embolus* refers to acute occlusion of the aortic bifurcation and iliac arteries.

A condition referred to as *spontaneous atheroembolism* is being recognized with increasing frequency. Thrombi originating in a vascular atherosclerotic plaque may become detached and propagate distally. These emboli may contain remnants of the atheromatous plaque as well as the thrombus. Microemboli, consisting of platelet aggregates or cholesterol fragments, can also occur, presenting as acute occlusion of a digit.

Clinical features

The clinical manifestations of chronic arterial occlusive disease progress slowly over a period of years. The signs and symptoms result from tissue underperfusion and ischemia. The primary symptom is *intermittent claudication* caused by muscle ischemia. Typically, intermittent claudication occurs with exercise, when metabolic demands increase, and subsides with rest within minutes. The location of the pain correlates closely with the site of arterial disease; the arterial segment involved is always proximal to the region of ischemic muscle. For example, intermittent claudication of the hips would correlate with aortoiliac disease, whereas disease of the external iliac or common femoral vessels would be associated with thigh or calf pain. Bilateral claudication is consistent with occlusion at or above the aortic bifurcation.

Pain occurring at rest is indicative of advanced occlusive disease. Ischemic rest pain typically occurs distally in the feet and toes as a combination of aching discomfort and paresthesia. However, the pain can be severe and unremitting. Pain typically occurs in the supine position and may be particularly intense at night, awakening patients from sleep. This intensification of pain occurs because flow across the obstructive lesion is pressure dependent and therefore extremely sensitive to the effects of gravity. Venous return also improves with elevation of the legs, thereby reducing the time for oxygen extraction from the blood in the capillary beds of the lower extremities. In addition, the reduction in sympathetic tone with sleep lowers heart rate and arterial pressure, further impairing peripheral perfusion. Leg dependency or walking may provide some relief. The increased hydrostatic pressure in the dependent position may dilate collateral vessels, increasing flow distally. Ischemic neuropathy occasionally results, particularly in diabetic patients, producing shocklike pain in the foot and leg.

Pulses below the occlusion are diminished or absent. The change in pulses is magnified by exercise because the vasodilation induced by exercise and ischemia increases the pressure gradient across the lesion. A *bruit,* indicative of turbulent flow, may be audible over the diseased arterial segment.

Significant arterial disease of the lower extremities is characterized by *postural changes in skin color.* Elevation of the extremity produces pallor, followed by redness or rubor with dependency. The elevation pallor is the result of gravitational effects that reduce arterial pressure and consequently lower the blood volume in the capillary bed. As the extremity is lowered beneath heart level and perfusion pressure increases, color returns. The rubor results from a reactive hyperemia or maximal vascular dilation in response to tissue hypoxia. The veins of the dependent leg also take longer to fill, because of the interference with arterial inflow.

The following tissue changes result from severe, chronic ischemia of the lower extremities: (1) trophic changes of the skin and nails, with thickening of the nails and drying of the skin; (2) loss of hair, particularly on the dorsum of the feet and toes; (3) development of a temperature gradient between colder regions of poor perfusion and warmer regions of adequate perfusion; and (4) wasting of the leg muscles and soft tissues. Changes in sensation and muscle strength may be noted.

Severe ischemia culminates in ulceration and gangrene. Ischemic ulcers usually begin on the toes or heel and progress proximally. Gangrene represents tissue death or necrosis. Gangrene can be characterized as dry gangrene or wet gangrene, depending on the degree of compromise in perfusion and the resultant necrosis. *Dry gangrene* results from a total cessation of flow with necrosis of the entire region. If the obstruction is not total, areas of necrosis are intermingled with regions of edema and inflammation, resulting in *wet gangrene.*

The constellation of clinical manifestations noted with progressive occlusion of the terminal aorta (Leriche's syndrome) includes absent or diminished femoral pulses; intermittent claudication in the buttock, hip, or thigh; and a loss of sexual potency.

Typically, the manifestations of acute occlusion, which result in sudden ischemia, differ greatly in magnitude from those of chronic ischemia. The typical manifestations are pain, pallor, pulselessness, *poikilothermia* (coolness) paresthesia, and paralysis. In some patients however, the presentation may be more gradual and less dramatic.

Treatment

Medical therapy. Control of risk factors is important to the treatment of arterial occlusive disease. Smoking should be stopped, given its strong association with occlusive disease, particularly with Buerger's disease. Medical therapy of associated diabetes, hypercholesterolemia, and hypertension is indicated. Dietary measures are stressed.

The pain of intermittent claudication usually subsides with rest. Ischemic rest pain can be relieved somewhat by dependency of the extremity or elevation of the head of the bed. Leg dependency increases perfusion pressure, thus relieving ischemia; elevation of the extremity is contraindicated because arterial flow would be further compromised. Analgesics may be necessary for pain control.

A progressive exercise program should be developed and maintained. Physical exercise seems to afford the greatest benefit in the treatment of intermittent claudication. Therapeutic response to physical exercise sustained over time is probably caused primarily by increased collateral development.

Foot care is crucial in the setting of lower-extremity vascular disease to prevent infection and traumatic ulceration. Measures include meticulous attention to cleanliness and nail care and avoidance of trauma and temperature extremes. Preventive measures to avoid injury are important because the ability to heal is retarded by the arterial insufficiency. In addition, susceptibility to injury is increased because sensory function may be impaired.

Management of ischemic ulcers and gangrene is problematic. In addition to the measures described previously, topical antibiotic agents may be indicated. Pressure points should be padded to avoid further breakdown. Bed rest, with elevation of the head of the bed, can reduce oxygen demand and improve flow. Bed cradles are help-

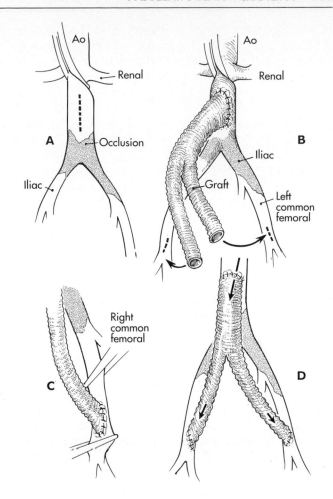

FIG. 34-8   Aortobifemoral bypass graft. **A,** Aortic incision; **B,** proximal anastomosis; **C,** distal anastomosis; **D,** completed graft. *Ao,* Aorta. (Modified from Chung E: *Quick reference to cardiovascular disease,* ed 2, Philadelphia, 1983, Lippincott.)

ful to prevent bedclothes from touching the extremity. Arterial reconstruction or amputation may be necessary.

Surgical therapy. In general, surgery is considered for chronic occlusive disease if symptoms become disabling or threaten limb viability and are unresponsive to medical therapy. The precise indications for surgery and the choice of procedure vary according to the site of disease. Surgical intervention is discussed relative to the following anatomic sites: (1) aortoiliac disease with patent femoropopliteal arteries, (2) aortoiliac with femoropopliteal disease, and (3) femoropopliteal disease.

Surgery for *chronic aortoiliac disease with patent femoropopliteal vessels* is usually performed for disabling intermittent claudication and rest pain. Given the patency of the vessels distal to the site of disease, collateral networks develop around the aortoiliac vessels, preserving limb viability. Surgical correction involves either placement of a bypass graft to shunt blood around the obstruction or endarterectomy to remove atheromatous plaque (Figs. 34-8 and 34-9).

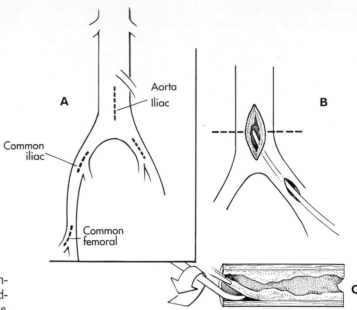

Cross section of aorta

FIG. 34-9 Endarterectomy. **A**, Arteriotomy; **B** and **C**, technique for circumferential dissection and removal of plaque. (Modified from Gaspar M, Barker W: *Peripheral arterial disease,* Philadelphia, 1981, Saunders.)

Bypass grafting with a knitted polyester (Dacron) bifurcation graft is the most common procedure; bifurcation grafts divide into two limbs to be sutured to both extremities. The proximal end of the graft is anastamosed to the side of the abdominal aorta beneath the renal arteries. The distal ends are anastamosed to either the external iliac or the common femoral arteries, depending on the extent of the disease. This aortobifemoral graft shunts blood around the diseased aortoiliac system to the lower extremities (Fig. 34-8).

Endarterectomy consists of dissection and removal of the atheromatous plaque from the arterial lumen, as illustrated in Fig. 34-9. This procedure is performed through an arteriotomy in the vessel wall. Endarterectomy of localized disease may be performed in conjunction with aortobifemoral bypass grafting. Generally, bypass grafting is preferred to endarterectomy, since endarterectomy offers no distinct advantage and is complicated and time-consuming.

Combined aortoiliac and femoropopliteal disease necessitates a combination of interventions. In this setting, surgery is usually indicated for limb salvage given the extent of disease and the severity of ischemia. The proximal aortoiliac lesion must be corrected first to ensure adequate arterial inflow into the femoropopliteal region. Aortobifemoral grafting is usually indicated. Subsequently, the distal femoropopliteal disease requires either endarterectomy or bypass grafting to obtain good flow to the distal vessels.

Despite controversy about the efficacy of *sympathectomy,* this procedure may be performed simultaneously to reduce sympathetic tone to the lower extremities and produce peripheral vasodilation. It is hoped that blood flow through the grafts will thereby be improved.

In highly select patients, transluminal angioplasty may be attempted to dilate the iliac vessels. *Transluminal angioplasty* is a technique used to treat shorter segments of stenosis of the aortoiliac or femoropopliteal vessels. In some patients, angioplasty is used in conjunction with surgical treatment to dilate stenosed inflow arteries before distal reconstruction. A balloon-tipped catheter is advanced into the iliac system via the femoral artery under fluoroscopic and pressure guidance. The balloon is inflated within the diseased segment to compress the lesion and dilate the vessel. The inflated balloon causes a fracture of the intima, separation of the plaque from the media with stretching and rupture of the muscle fibers, and stretching of the adventitial layer. The damaged intimal surface heals within several hours. The role of angioplasty in vascular disease is still being defined. Angioplasty can be particularly useful if surgery is contraindicated or if the disease is restricted to short, isolated arterial segments.

Arterial reconstruction for *femoropopliteal disease* is usually performed for limb salvage. Occasionally, disabling intermittent claudication requires surgery. Bypass grafting is usually preferred over endarterectomy; however, concomitant endarterectomy may be used for localized disease. The graft of choice is the autogenous saphenous vein because of high graft failure rates with prosthetic materials such as Dacron in the lower extremity. The endothelial lining of the native vein provides an antithrombogenic surface, reducing the incidence of graft failure.

Two surgical techniques are used. With the initial technique, a segment of vein is removed from the leg and reversed before arterial anastomosis so that the venous valves do not impede flow through the vein graft. The

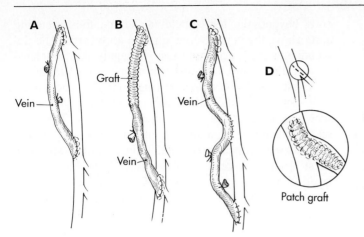

FIG. 34-10   Femoropopliteal bypass graft. **A,** Saphenous vein graft; **B,** composite graft; **C,** sequential femoropopliteal-tibial graft; **D,** profundaplasty with patch graft. [Modified from Gaspar M, Barker W: *Peripheral arterial disease,* Philadelphia, 1981, Saunders.]

proximal end of the reversed graft is anastamosed to the side of the common femoral artery (Fig. 34-10, *A*) and the distal end to the vessel beyond the obstruction, ideally to a branch of the popliteal artery. This approach is referred to as a *reversed saphenous vein technique.*

A more recent technique uses a vein segment left in place (in situ). The vein is severed from the native vessels, venous valves are removed, and the vein segment is sutured proximally and distally into the adjacent artery, replacing the diseased arterial segment. This *vein in situ technique* is preferred because it minimizes trauma to the vein, thereby preserving the integrity of venous endothelium. Preoperative evaluation of the saphenous vein segment via noninvasive techniques, such as B-mode ultrasound, is essential to determine the suitability of the vessel as a vascular conduit.

Distal bypass and in situ grafting to regions beneath the popliteal artery are not as successful because of the smaller caliber of the vessel, poor flows, and the mechanical effects of knee bending and potential graft compression.

If the saphenous vein is not long enough to extend around the diseased segment, composite grafts of vein and prosthetic material can be used (Fig. 34-10, *B*). Sequential grafting may be used to provide flow at multiple points for branches of an extensively diseased segment (Fig. 34-10, *C*).

If femoropopliteal disease involves the deep femoral artery, or profunda femoris, *profundaplasty* is performed in conjunction with bypass grafting. This procedure usually involves endarterectomy through an arteriotomy. If necessary, a patch graft may be inserted within the vessel wall to dilate the vessel (Fig. 34-10, *D*). Profundaplasty is important because of the profunda's importance as a collateral network for the lower extremities. In high-risk patients, profundaplasty may be performed alone under local anesthesia as a palliative procedure.

Amputation is considered in chronic occlusive disease for irreversible gangrene or uncontrolled pain. Amputation is performed as far distally as possible to minimize resultant disability.

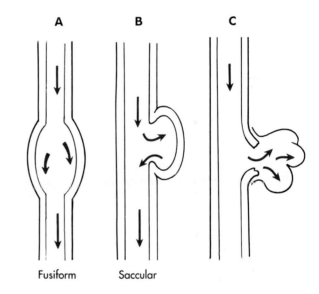

FIG. 34-11   Aneurysm types. **A,** True fusiform aneurysm; **B,** true saccular aneurysm; **C,** false aneurysm.

Acute aortoiliac occlusion necessitates immediate intervention. Anticoagulation is initiated to prevent loss of collateral circulation and further propagation of emboli. Intraarterial thrombolytic agents, such as streptokinase or urokinase, may be administered. Patients receiving this mode of therapy require intensive care monitoring because of the serious risk of hemorrhage or repeat embolization. *Thrombectomy* via a femoral arteriotomy is another method of treatment.

Aneurysmal Arterial Disease

An *aneurysm* is a localized dilation of the arterial wall (Fig. 34-11). A *true aneurysm* results from atrophy of the medial layer of the artery. The arterial wall dilates but remains intact although distorted and composed primarily of fibrous tissue. True aneurysms can be fusiform or saccular in shape. The more common atherosclerotic *fusiform aneurysm* is a uniform, circumferential dilation, whereas the *saccular aneurysm* is a saclike outpouching connected to the arterial wall by a narrow neck. A *false aneurysm* is an extravascular accumulation of blood with disruption of all three vascular layers; the wall of the false aneurysm is thrombus and adjacent tissue. Aneurysms can occur anywhere in the aorta or peripheral vessels. Aortic aneurysms are classified as abdominal, thoracic, or thoracoabdominal, depending on their location. Aortic dissection is discussed in the next section.

Pathophysiology

Aneurysm formation results from degeneration and weakening of the medial layer of the artery. Medial degeneration can result from either acquired or congenital conditions, such as atherosclerosis, or Marfan's syndrome. Vascular dilation can also result from the jet effect of blood streaming across an obstructive vascular plaque, creating turbulence distal to the lesion; this poststenotic dilation weakens the arterial wall.

In addition to these identifiable causes of aneurysms, the interaction of multiple other factors can predispose to aneurysm formation. Turbulence of flow at regions of bifurcation may contribute to the higher incidence of aneurysms in specific regions. It has also been proposed that blood supply to the blood vessels through the vasa vasorum may become compromised with advancing age, weakening the media and predisposing to aneurysm formation.

Whatever the cause, the aneurysm becomes progressively larger according to Laplace's law. Wall tension or stress is directly related to the radius of the vessel and the intraarterial pressure. As the vessel dilates and the radius enlarges, the wall tension rises, further dilating the vessel. Thus aneurysm rupture rates rise with increased size. In addition, the vast majority of individuals with aneurysms are hypertensive, further contributing to wall stress and aneurysm enlargement.

The potential contribution of arterial size to aneurysm formation is also being considered. Individuals with large main arteries, or *arteriomegaly,* and larger body surface areas tend to have an increased incidence of aneurysms. It has been suggested that increased aortic blood flow may affect the development of aneurysms.

Aneurysms typically develop layers of clot along their walls because of stagnant flow. Mural thrombi are a potential source of emobli and spontaneous aneurysm thrombosis.

Etiology and common sites

The most common site for aneurysm formation is the abdominal aorta. *Abdominal aortic aneurysms* typically originate beneath the renal arteries and extend to the aortic bifurcation, occasionally involving the iliac arteries. Rarely does the aneurysm extend above the renal arteries to involve the major visceral branches of the aorta. Most abdominal aneurysms are atherosclerotic in origin.

Thoracic aneurysms can affect the descending thoracic aorta beyond the left subclavian artery, the ascending aorta above the aortic valve, and the aortic arch. The descending aorta is affected most frequently. Atherosclerosis and trauma are the most common causes. Trauma to the chest, usually sustained during a motor vehicle accident, can rupture the intimal and medial layers of the descending aorta at the ligamentum arteriosus. The ligamentum arteriosus stabilizes the aorta at one point, whereas the thoracic structures move forward when the chest abruptly decelerates; this may shear the vascular layers. Consequently, this type of injury is referred to as *deceleration trauma.* The adventitial layer may remain intact, although rupture or the development of false aneurysms may result. Disease of the arch is usually caused by atherosclerosis. Cystic medial necrosis, as in Marfan's syndrome, is most severe in the ascending aorta and frequently results in aneurysm formation.

Multiple aneurysms occur frequently and may involve the peripheral and visceral arteries. The popliteal is the most frequently affected peripheral artery; visceral aneurysms are rare. Most peripheral and visceral aneurysms are atherosclerotic in origin; however, trauma and infection are also etiologic factors.

Clinical features

Aneurysms are frequently asymptomatic. The first sign of disease may be a serious, potentially life-threatening complication, such as rupture, acute thrombosis, or embolization. Abdominal aneurysms may be detected during an abdominal examination as a palpable, expansile abdominal mass usually located in the umbilical region to the left of midline. The appearance of symptoms is usually ominous, indicating aneurysm expansion, chronic retroperitoneal bleeding, or impending rupture. Severe abdominal or back pain may be noted. Duodenal obstruction from large aneurysms may present as epigastric discomfort or difficulties with digestion. If orifices of major visceral branches are involved, impotence may be reported, and infrequently, visceral dysfunction may be noted. Bruits may be audible but are of little diagnostic value. Femoral pulses are diminished in some patients.

Thoracic aneurysms must be quite large to produce symptoms; consequently, aneurysms may be discovered incidentally by chest radiography. Symptoms, when they do occur, are usually caused by expansion and compression of adjacent structures. Esophageal compression, although rare, produces dysphagia; recurrent laryngeal nerve compression presents as hoarseness; neck vein distention and edema of the head and arms may indicate compression of the superior vena cava. The pain associated with thoracic aneurysms occurs in the chest. Aneurysms may cause pain as a result of erosion of the vertebral column and compression of the spinal nerves.

Aneurysm rupture is catastrophic and associated with a poor prognosis. Rupture into the pericardial cavity results in exsanguination; however, rupture is usually into the retroperitoneal space, where adjacent structures exert a tamponade effect. Rupture typically presents with acute abdominal or back pain occurring in association with signs of hemorrhagic shock. A pulsatile abdominal mass may be palpable, although after rupture, detection may not be possible. Immediate surgical resection is necessary.

Treatment

Small, asymptomatic abdominal aneurysms may not warrant immediate surgical intervention. The size of these aneurysms is monitored carefully at regular intervals using palpation, abdominal radiographs, ultrasound, and CT scans. Aneurysmal enlargement to 6 cm is considered an indication for elective aneurysm resection. If the aneurysm becomes symptomatic, surgery is considered on a more urgent basis.

The technique and type of graft used for abdominal aneurysm repair depend on the extent of the vascular involvement. If the aneurysm is confined to the aortic region below the renal arteries and above the aortic bifurcation, a tube graft is used. The aneurysm is resected (Fig. 34-12, *A*), preserving its external layer (Fig. 34-12, *B*); the tube graft is then anastomosed to the aorta

(Fig. 34-12, *C*). If collateral flow to the inferior mesenteric artery is inadequate, it is implanted into the side of the tube graft (Fig. 34-12, *D*). The aneurysmal shell is then wrapped around the graft to minimize blood loss. If the aneurysm extends below the bifurcation or if the iliac arteries are diseased, a bifurcation graft is used. The distal limbs of the bifurcation graft can be anastomosed end to end or end to side to the distal vessels, as shown in Fig. 34-13. Endarterectomy may be necessary.

Thoracic aneurysms require surgical correction. If the aneurysm is large or compressing adjacent structures, surgery is considered on an urgent basis. The grafting technique is similar to that of abdominal aneurysm repair and involves aneurysmal resection and replacement with a tube graft placed within the aneurysmal wall. Involvement of the arch necessitates reimplantation of the brachiocephalic vessels into the graft or use of aortic patch grafts. Ascending aortic aneurysms may involve the aortic valve, requiring replacement or resuspension of the aortic valve. Peripheral perfusion is maintained during thoracic aneurysm resections by cardiopulmonary bypass, bypass of the left side of the heart, or a vascular shunt (Fig. 34-14).

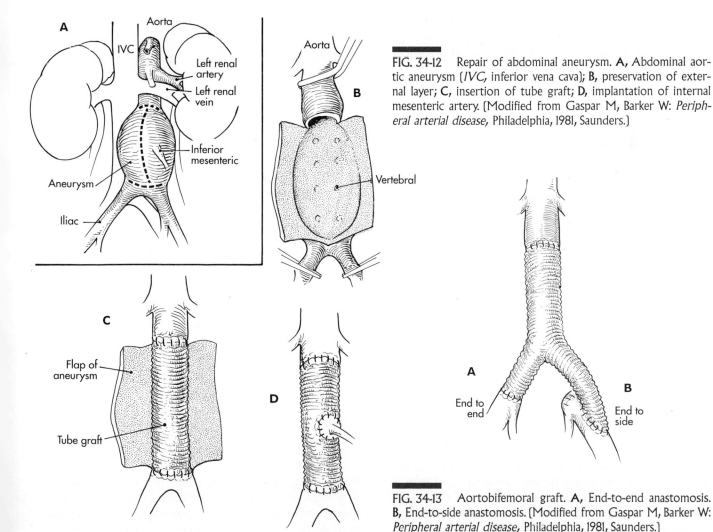

FIG. 34-12 Repair of abdominal aneurysm. **A,** Abdominal aortic aneurysm (*IVC,* inferior vena cava); **B,** preservation of external layer; **C,** insertion of tube graft; **D,** implantation of internal mesenteric artery. (Modified from Gaspar M, Barker W: *Peripheral arterial disease,* Philadelphia, 1981, Saunders.)

FIG. 34-13 Aortobifemoral graft. **A,** End-to-end anastomosis. **B,** End-to-side anastomosis. (Modified from Gaspar M, Barker W: *Peripheral arterial disease,* Philadelphia, 1981, Saunders.)

FIG. 34-14 Repair of aortic dissection. Upper panel illustrates repair of a distal aortic resection. **A,** The dissection has been isolated. A heparinized shunt extending from the apex of the left ventricle to the femoral artery is used to bypass the dissected segment and to support the circulation distal to the dissection during the repair. **B,** After resection of the dissected segment, the dissected ends of the aorta are oversewn with Teflon felt backing on the inside and outside of the aorta, both proximally and distally. **C,** A low-priority Dacron graft is sutured in the descending thoracic aorta. Lower panel illustrates the repair of a proximal aortic dissection. **A,** The patient is on total cardiopulmonary bypass. **B,** Dissection and intimal tear. **C,** Aortic valve is excised and coronary ostia is mobilized. A composite-woven Dacron graft including an attached Björk-Shiley valve is inserted because of proximal disease. **D,** The graft is sewn to the patient's aortic annulus proximally and to the distal aorta. The coronary arteries are reattached to the composite graft above the prosthetic valve. (Modified from Eagle KA et al: *The practice of cardiology,* ed 2, Boston, 1989, Little, Brown.)

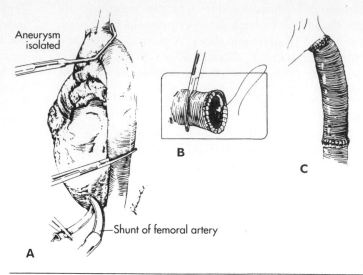

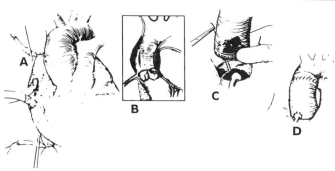

FIG. 34-15 Aortic dissection. **A,** Separation of vascular layers; **B,** classification of aortic dissection.

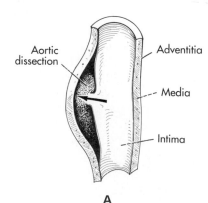

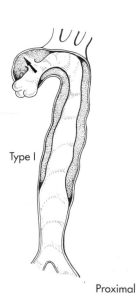

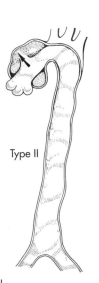

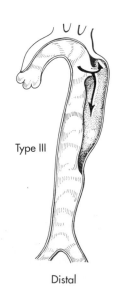

Aortic Dissection

Aortic dissection is separation of the vascular layers by a column of blood (Fig. 34-15, *A*). This vascular separation creates a false arterial lumen, which communicates with the true lumen via a tear in the intima. The dissection does not extend around the circumference of the vessel; rather, it extends along the length of the vessel. This extension can partially or totally occlude any vessel in the path of the dissection by separating the vessel orifice from the true arterial lumen. Occasionally, the dissecting column of blood may recenter the true lumen or terminate; however, rapid progressive dissection is usually observed. Eventually the false lumen may produce aneurysmal enlargement of outer vascular layers; however, aneurysm formation does not characterize the early phase of dissection. The term "dissecting aneurysm" therefore

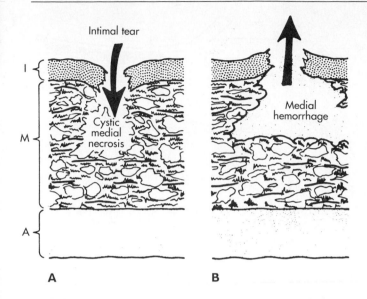

FIG. 34-16   Diagram illustrating the two possible mechanisms for the pathogenesis of aortic dissections. **A,** Primary intimal tear followed by dissection of the aorta into the media *[M]*. **B,** Primary event is hemorrhage into the aortic media followed by rupture of the overlying intima *[I]*. *A,* Adventitia. (From Eagle KA et al: *The practice of cardiology,* ed 2, Boston, 1989, Little, Brown.)

is a misnomer, even though it is used frequently as a synonym for aortic dissection.

Occasionally an intimal tear cannot be demonstrated. In such cases, rupture of the vasa vasorum with subsequent medial hemorrhage is suspected. Consequently, the relationship between the intimal tear and the development of aortic dissection is a subject of debate. Fig. 34-16 illustrates both mechanisms for the development of aortic dissection.

Aortic dissections are characterized according to age and anatomic location. Dissections that are recognized within 2 weeks of onset are categorized as *acute dissections;* if more than 2 weeks have elapsed between onset and recognition of the aneurysm, these are considered *chronic dissections.* Because the mortality rate of untreated aneurysms is highest in the first 2 weeks, the prognosis for chronic dissection is much better than for acute dissection.

The DeBakey classification system is frequently used for anatomic categorization of dissections. This system distinguishes three types of dissections according to site of origin and extent of dissection (Fig. 34-15, *B*). *Type I aneurysms* originate in the ascending aorta just above the aortic valve and extend distally into the abdominal aorta. *Type II aneurysms* are confined to the ascending aorta. *Type III aneurysms* begin in the descending aorta just distal to the left subclavian artery and can extend distally to the aortic bifurcation. Another common system for anatomic classification of aneurysms simply groups type I and II aneurysms together as *proximal aneurysms* orig-

inating in the ascending aorta and distinguishes type III aneurysms as *distal aneurysms* beginning in the descending aorta.

Proximal dissections are frequently associated with cystic medial necrosis, as in Marfan's syndrome. Atherosclerosis is common with distal dissections. Deceleration trauma, as mentioned earlier with aortic aneurysms, can also cause aortic dissections by disrupting the intimal and medial layers, allowing blood to enter the vessel wall.

Clinical features

The clinical manifestations vary, depending on the site and extent of dissection; however, onset tends to be sudden and intense. Typically, severe, tearing pain is experienced. The pain can localize initially in the chest, abdomen, or back; however, as the dissection extends, the pain radiates to the back and distally toward the lower extremities. Signs of shock often develop, even though arterial pressure tends to be elevated because of underlying hypertension.

Retrograde dissection toward the aortic valve can produce aortic regurgitation manifested by a diastolic murmur and signs of congestive heart failure. As the dissection progresses, arterial branches become occluded with loss of pulses and signs of organ dysfunction; anuria may result from renal artery involvement, or lower extremity ischemia may result from iliac occlusion. Rupture is the most frequent cause of death.

Treatment

Early surgical intervention is usually indicated for proximal dissections originating in the ascending aorta and arch. Distal dissections originating in and limited to the descending aorta are usually treated medically first to control the dissection and stabilize the patient. Surgery is indicated if the dissection progresses or if complications such as arterial occlusion or hemodynamic instability arise.

Medical therapy involves the reduction of arterial pressure with drugs, such as trimethaphan camsylate (Arfonad) or sodium nitroprusside, to reduce stress on the aortic wall. The force of left ventricular contraction is reduced by administering drugs such as propranolol in an attempt to lower the velocity of ventricular ejection. Pain is controlled with analgesics and sedation. Hemodynamics and peripheral pulses are monitored carefully to detect complications. Serial chest radiography is performed to monitor the size of the dissection.

Surgical repair usually involves the resection of the involved segment and replacement with a graft. Other surgical techniques include repair and reconstruction of the aorta with sutures or patch grafts. Repair of an ascending aortic dissection may involve aortic valve replacement or annuloplasty and valve resuspension. As with aneurysm repair, the peripheral circulation can be supported with total or partial cardiopulmonary bypass or vascular shunts (see Fig. 34-14).

VENOUS DISEASE

Anatomy

In comparison with arteries, veins are thinner walled and distensible. Approximately 70% of the blood volume is contained within the venous circuit under relatively low pressure. The low-pressure, high-volume venous circuit functions as a *capacitance circuit,* in contrast to the high-pressure, low-volume resistance circuit of the arterial side. The capacity and volume of the venous circuit is an important determinant of cardiac output because the volume of blood ejected by the heart depends on its venous return.

The venous system in the lower extremities (Fig. 34-17) is divided into three subsystems: (1) the superficial venous subsystem, (2) the deep venous subsystem, and (3) the perforating (communicating) subsystem. The *superficial veins* are situated in the subcutaneous tissues of the leg and receive venous flow from smaller vessels within the skin, subcutaneous tissue, and feet. The superficial system consists of the greater saphenous vein and the lesser saphenous vein. The greater saphenous is the longest vein in the body; it extends from the malleolus of the ankle, up the inner aspect of the calf and thigh, emptying into the femoral vein just below the groin. The point of juncture between the two veins, the *saphenous junction,* is an important anatomic landmark. The greater saphenous vein drains the anteromedial aspects of the calf and thigh. The lesser saphenous vein extends along the lateral aspect of the calf from the ankle to the knee, draining the posterolateral aspects of the calf and emptying into the popliteal vein. The junction between the saphenous and the popliteal veins is the *saphenopopliteal junction.* Multiple anastomoses exist between the greater and lesser saphenous veins; these anastomoses are important potential routes of collateral flow in the event of venous obstruction.

The *deep venous system* carries the greater part of the venous blood in the lower extremities and is situated within the muscle compartments. The deep veins receive flow from small venules and intramuscular vessels. The deep venous system tends to parallel the arterial vessels of the lower leg, and many vessels are named accordingly. Consequently, the system includes the anterior and posterior tibial veins, peroneal vein, popliteal vein, femoral vein, profunda femoris vein, and unnamed calf vessels. The iliac veins are also included in the deep venous system of the lower extremity because venous drainage from the legs to the vena cava depends on the patency and integrity of these vessels. The left common iliac vein crosses beneath the right common iliac artery in its path toward the vena cava, where it has the potential to be compressed by the artery. This crossover accounts for the 2:1 preponderance of left-sided deep venous thrombosis over right-sided thrombosis.

The superficial and deep venous subsystems are connected by vascular channels referred to as *perforating*

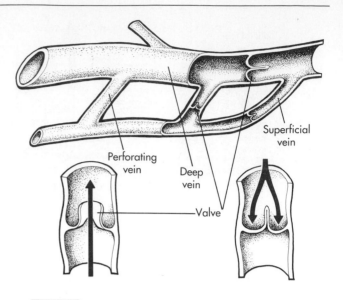

FIG. 34-17   Anatomy of the venous system of the leg.

veins. The perforating veins make up the communicating subsystem of the lower extremities. Flow is normally shunted from the superficial veins to the deep veins and subsequently to the inferior vena cava.

One-way semilunar valves are distributed throughout the venous system of the lower extremities. The valves are folds of the intimal layer of the vessel and consist of endothelium and collagen. These venous valves prevent retrograde flow and direct flow proximally from the lower extremities to the vena cava and from the superficial system to the deep system via the perforators. The competency of these valves is critical because the flow of blood from the extremities to the heart is against gravity.

The physiology of venous flow against gravitational forces involves the interaction of multiple factors referred to as the *venous pump.* There are peripheral and central components to the venous pump. The peripheral venous pump depends on compression of venous channels during muscle contraction. Muscle contraction propels flow forward within the deep venous system; the venous valves prevent retrograde flow or reflux of blood during muscle relaxation. In addition, small valveless venous sinuses, or *venules,* located deep within the soleus and the gastrocnemius muscles function as reservoirs of blood and empty into the deep veins during muscle contraction. The contribution of these intramuscular channels is particularly important to venous return. Central forces that promote venous return include the reduction in intrathoracic pressure with inspiration and the fall in right ventricular and right atrial pressure after ventricular ejection.

Diagnostic Procedures

Because of the unreliability of clinical signs in venous disease, noninvasive and invasive methods of evaluation are of great importance. The objectives of the testing are to detect and evaluate venous obstruction or venous reflux through incompetent valves.

Physical examination

Venous valve incompetence can be evaluated clinically by tests of venous filling time. The *Brodei-Trendelenburg test* involves emptying the saphenous vein by leg elevation and reducing arterial inflow by occlusion. With valve incompetence, rapid venous filling is noted on release of occlusion pressure and assumption of the standing position. Another technique is the *manual compression test,* which involves proximal compression of the vein as the vein is palpated distally to evaluate retrograde venous filling resulting from valve reflux.

Doppler ultrasound

Doppler techniques are used to determine blood flow velocity and flow patterns within the superficial and deep venous systems. Venous flow can be distinguished from arterial flow because venous flow is nonpulsatile and varies with respiration. Normal venous flow patterns are characterized by an increase in flow in the lower extremities during expiration and a decrease during inspiration. With venous obstruction, these phasic respiratory variations are blunted. In veins with total obstruction of the lumen by a thrombus, the signal is absent. In partially thrombosed veins, the pitch of the signal is higher because of increased velocity of flow through the narrowed segment. In addition, thrombosis decreases the phasicity of flow. The examiner also compresses the limb distal to the Doppler probe, listening for augmentation of the signal as venous return increases. Finally, as the patient performs the Valsalva maneuver, the signal should cease as competent venous valves prevent the backflow of blood. With valvular incompetence, such as in the postphlebotic syndrome, the flow continues throughout the Valsalva maneuver.

Doppler techniques provide a qualitative assessment of valve competence in the deep, communicating, and perforating vessels. Superficial and deep venous obstruction can be detected, although Doppler ultrasound is more sensitive to proximal vein thrombosis than to calf vein thrombosis. This technique is inexpensive and portable; however, a high degree of technical skill and experience is required to ensure accurate results.

Duplex ultrasonic scanning

The application of real-time duplex ultrasonic scanning (described earlier in the section on arterial diagnostic techniques) to venous imaging is generating much interest. This technique combines the intravascular Doppler blood flow information with ultrasonic imaging of vein morphology. With this technique, venous obstruction and valve reflux can be detected and localized. While visualizing the vein in real time, the examiner samples for venous flow throughout the vessel lumen. Absence of flow indicates total occlusion by a thrombus. The examiner also attempts to compress the segment of vein by pressing the probe on the visualized segment. An inability to compress the visualized vein may also indicate the presence of a thrombus within the lumen.

Venous plethysmography

Plethysmographic techniques detect changes in the venous blood volume in the leg. Venous obstruction and valve reflux alter normal patterns of venous filling and emptying into the extremities. Common plethysmographic techniques include (1) impedance plethysmography, (2) strain gauge plethysmography, (3) air plethysmography, and (4) photoplethysmography. The techniques differ relative to the method used to detect the changes in blood volume.

In the most common technique, *impedance plethysmography* (IPG), weak electrical currents are transmitted through the extremity and the impedance or resistance to the passage of this current is measured. Because blood is a good conductor of electricity, the impedance falls when the blood volume in the extremity increases during venous filling. Impedance is measured by electrodes on a band encircling the limb. With *strain gauge plethysmography* (SGP), changes in the mechanical strain on electrodes reflects changes in blood volume. *Air plethysmography* detects volume changes via corresponding changes in pressure within an air-filled cuff encircling the limb. As the venous volume increases, the pressure within the cuff increases. *Photoplethysmography* (PPG) is the newest technique and relies on the detection of reflected light from an infrared beam transmitted across the extremity. The proportion of the light reflected back to the transducer depends on the venous blood volume in the cutaneous bed.

Venous reflux and venous obstruction can be evaluated with plethysmographic techniques. The venous blood flow response to respiration is one measure of venous obstruction. Venous flow in the extremities is typically increased during expiration and decreased during inspiration when the increase in intraabdominal pressure impedes venous return. With venous obstruction, these normal phasic flow variations with respiration are blunted. Temporary occlusion of the extremity, with a pneumatic cuff pressurized to a level above venous pressure but below arterial pressure, is typically used to evaluate venous outflow from the extremity. Cuff inflation increases venous filling and volume beyond the cuff because venous outflow is impeded while arterial inflow through the capillary bed continues. Venous reflux would produce abnormal patterns of filling during this period of venous hypertension. When the cuff is deflated, venous outflow is evaluated. Venous obstruction would slow the rate of venous emptying. Plethysmography is more sensitive for detection of proximal vein thrombosis than for calf vein thrombosis.

Radionuclide imaging

Imaging or scanning of the veins with radioactive fibrinogen may be indicated to complement other techniques. *Fibrinogen iodine-125 testing* can be used to detect developing thrombi, particularly below the knee. Iodine-125 is a radioisotope used to tag fibrinogen, which is then incorporated into the growing thrombus. This test, although sensitive for calf thrombi, is not sensitive for groin or pelvic thrombi, which are more serious in nature. This technique is not used often because it is expensive and time-consuming, and the advancement of the noninvasive techniques has replaced its use.

Venography

In the setting of venous disease, venography, or *phlebography,* is the standard to which all other techniques are compared. A bolus of contrast material is injected into the venous system to opacify the veins of the lower extremity and pelvis. Descending venography with injection of contrast into the femoral vein is used to assess the extent of retrograde flow in patients with chronic venous insufficiency. Venography is considered the most reliable technique for the evaluation of the location and extent of venous disease. However, the disadvantages of invasive testing relative to noninvasive testing include greater expense, discomfort, and potential risk. Given the high correlation between combined noninvasive measures of venous obstruction—including Doppler ultrasound, plethysmography, and venous imaging techniques—and invasive venographic techniques, noninvasive tests are used with increasing frequency. Venography may still be used in cases of equivocal noninvasive findings or when surgical interruption of the vena cava for pulmonary embolus is planned.

Thromboembolic Venous Disease

The term *thromboembolic disease* reflects the relationship between thrombosis, the process of blood clot formation, and the ever-present risk of embolization. Frequently, the first sign of venous thrombosis is *pulmonary embolism.* Given the morbidity and mortality associated with pulmonary embolism (see Chapter 40), the primary emphasis in the treatment of deep venous thrombosis is on prevention of embolization. Consequently, the two processes are intertwined.

A distinction used to be made between thrombophlebitis and phlebothombosis, based on the degree of inflammation accompanying the thrombotic process. *Thrombophlebitis* was characterized by acute inflammatory signs. *Phlebothrombosis* referred to venous thrombosis without overt inflammatory signs and symptoms. The distinction was considered important in determining the risk of pulmonary embolism because inflammation was believed to increase the adherence of the clot to the vessel wall, thereby reducing the risk of pulmonary embolism. It is now recognized that a clear distinction between these terms cannot be made; inflammation occurs to some degree with thrombosis. Therefore these states simply represent different degrees of an underlying process. In ad-

dition, pulmonary embolism is always a risk, even when the presentation of venous thrombosis is silent.

The term *superficial thrombophlebitis* is the preferred term for inflammation of the superficial veins. The term *deep venous thrombosis* is preferred for thromboembolic disease of the deep veins of the lower extremity (rather than deep thrombophlebitis). The thromboembolic process in the superficial veins is more inflammatory in character and presentation than that in the deep venous system. Superficial thrombophlebitis and deep venous thrombosis are described in subsequent sections.

Pathophysiology

The precise mechanism that initiates thrombosis is poorly understood. Three categories of contributing factors, referred to as the *Virchow triad,* are usually recognized: (1) stasis of blood flow, (2) endothelial injury, and (3) hypercoagulability of blood. The relative contributions of each factor and the interrelationships among them are debated.

Stasis, or sluggish blood flow, predisposes to thrombosis and appears to be a contributing factor in the setting of immobilization or prolonged limb dependency. Immobilization, such as occurs during the perioperative period or with paralysis, eliminates the effect of the peripheral venous pump, promoting stagnation and pooling of blood in the lower extremities. It is proposed that blood stasis behind venous valve cusps may predispose to platelet and fibrin deposition, precipitating the development of venous thrombosis.

Although *endothelial injury* is known to initiate thrombus formation, overt endothelial lesions cannot always be demonstrated. However, subtle endothelial changes caused by chemical changes, ischemia or anoxia, or inflammation may be implicated. Overt causes of endothelial damage include direct trauma to the vessel, such as fractures and soft tissue injury, and intravenous infusion of irritating substances, such as potassium chloride, chemotherapy, or high-dose antibiotics.

Blood hypercoagulability depends on complex interactions between a multitude of variables, including the vascular endothelium, platelets and clotting factors, and the composition and flow characteristics of blood. In addition, the intrinsic fibrinolytic system balances the coagulation system by lysis and dissolution of clot to maintain vascular patency (see Chapter 19). Hypercoagulable states result from alterations in any of these variables. Hematologic disorders, malignancies, trauma, estrogen therapy, or a surgical event can contribute to coagulation abnormalities.

Venous thrombosis, whatever the underlying stimulus, increases the resistance to venous outflow from the lower extremities. As resistance increases, venous emptying is impaired, resulting in elevation of venous blood volume and venous pressure. Thrombosis can involve the valve pockets and disrupt valve function. Valve dysfunction or incompetence promotes stasis and pooling of blood within the extremity.

The thrombus becomes more organized and adherent to the vessel wall as it matures. Consequently, the risk of embolization is greatest in the earliest phases of thrombosis, although the tail of the clot can still be detached and embolize during the organization phase. In addition, extension of the thrombus can produce a long, free-floating tail that can fragment and embolize into the pulmonary circulation. Progressive extension also increases the degree of venous obstruction and involves additional regions of the venous system. Ultimately, some degree of patency of the lumen may be reestablished (referred to as *recanalization*) by clot retraction and lysis via the endogenous fibrinolytic system. However, residual damage may persist. Most patients have an open lumen but scarred, unclosable valve leaflets, resulting in bidirectional venous flow.

Superficial thrombophlebitis

Superficial thrombophlebitis involves the subcutaneous vessels of the upper and lower extremities. The most common cause of upper extremity thrombophlebitis is intravenous infusions, particularly of acidotic or hypertonic solutions. Superficial thrombophlebitis of the lower extremities is typically caused by varicose veins or trauma. If no obvious cause of superficial thrombophlebitis can be determined, the possibility of underlying disease processes, such as Buerger's disease or malignancy, should be considered.

The course of superficial thrombophlebitis is usually benign and self-limiting. Pulmonary embolization is unusual; however, thrombus extension into the deep venous system can occur, particularly if the thrombus is close to major communicating channels or to the junctions between the saphenous veins and the popliteal or femoral veins.

Clinical presentation. The typical presentation of superficial thrombophlebitis is acute, with aching or burning pain and superficial tenderness. Superficial thrombophlebitis is typically more painful than deep venous thrombosis because of the proximity of the cutaneous sensory nerve endings to the inflammatory process. The skin may be erythematous and warm along the length of the vein. Slight swelling may be noted. The vein may be palpable. This firmness is sometimes called a *subcutaneous cord.* Systemic manifestations of inflammation, such as fever and malaise, may occur.

Treatment. Treatment of superficial thrombophlebitis consists of elevation of the affected extremity and the application of warm, moist heat. Antiinflammatory agents, such as aspirin, may help to reduce discomfort and promote antithrombosis. Compression stockings or elastic bandages reduce stasis and promote venous return of the lower extremities. Any intravenous catheter in the affected area should be removed if it is a contributing factor to the superficial thrombophlebitis. If extension into a major vessel of the deep venous system is threatened, ligation or interruption of the involved superficial vein at the saphenofemoral junction may be indicated.

Acute deep venous thrombosis

Deep venous thrombosis (DVT) involves the vessels of the deep venous system. The initial episode is referred to as *acute deep venous thrombosis.* A history of acute deep venous thrombosis predisposes to the development of *recurrent deep venous thrombosis.* Episodes of DVT can produce long-term disability as a result of the destruction of deep venous valves. Postthrombotic syndrome is discussed in the next section. Pulmonary embolism is a significant risk with deep venous thrombosis.

Most deep venous thrombi originate in the lower extremities; many resolve spontaneously, and others propagate or embolize. One or more veins may be involved; the calf veins are affected most frequently. Thromboses of the popliteal, superficial femoral, and iliofemoral vein segments are also common. The overwhelming majority of pulmonary emboli are caused by DVT of veins of the pelvis and lower extremity.

Major risk factors include the following: (1) marked immobility, (2) dehydration, (3) advanced malignancy, (4) blood dyscrasias, (5) history of DVT, (6) varicose veins, and (7) leg or pelvic trauma or surgery. Other predisposing factors include use of estrogen contraceptives, pregnancy, chronic congestive heart failure, and obesity.

Clinical features. DVT is a particularly insidious problem because it is typically asymptomatic; pulmonary embolism may be the first clinical indication of thrombosis. Thrombus formation in the deep venous system may not be clinically apparent because of the large capacity of the venous system and the development of collateral circulation around obstructions. The diagnosis is particularly troublesome in that the clinical signs and symptoms associated with DVT are nonspecific and their severity does not correlate with the extent of disease.

The most reliable signs are swelling and edema of the involved extremity. Swelling results from the increased intravascular volume caused by venous pooling of blood; edema reflects fluid seepage across the capillary membrane into the interstitium because of elevated hydrostatic pressure. The superficial veins may also be dilated because of the obstruction of flow into the deep system or shunting of blood from the deep to the superficial systems. Although unilateral swelling is typically noted, iliofemoral obstruction can produce bilateral swelling.

Pain is the most common symptom; it is typically described as aching or throbbing and may be severe. Walking may aggravate the pain. Tenderness of the involved extremity may be noted. Two techniques for eliciting limb tenderness are dorsiflexion of the foot and inflation of an air-filled cuff over the extremity. Calf tenderness on dorsiflexion of the foot is referred to as *Homans' sign* and is considered an unreliable sign of DVT; calf or thigh pain with cuff inflation is called *Lowenburg's sign.* Other signs include increased tissue turgor with swelling, increased skin temperature with dilation of superficial veins, mottling and cyanosis caused by stagnant flow, increased oxygen extraction, and reduction of hemoglobin.

Two types of venous thrombosis are rare but bear mentioning because of their severity. The first is *phlegmasia alba dolens,* a form of iliofemoral thrombosis. This thrombosis involves such a severe perivenous inflammatory reaction that the periarterial nerve fibers are affected, causing distal arterial spasm. The resultant decrease in arterial inflow gives the limb a pale, swollen appearance, and pulses in the arterial system are not palpable. The second type is *phlegmasia cerulea dolens* and is an even more serious iliofemoral occlusion. In this case the sudden occlusion of venous outflow from the limb produces such rising pressure in the extremity that arterial inflow is occluded. This may lead to gangrene of the extremity. One might see this sequela in caring for those patients who are terminally ill from a malignancy.

Treatment. Given the morbidity and mortality associated with DVT and pulmonary embolism, the therapeutic emphasis is on recognition of high-risk settings and institution of appropriate prophylaxis. Once DVT is suspected, the therapeutic objective is to avoid further extension of clot and embolization.

Physical methods to minimize venous stasis are typically used for prophylaxis in high-risk settings. External support with compression stockings or elastic bandages is recommended to reduce venous stasis. However, caution must always be exercised with all types of stockings and bandages to avoid a tourniquet effect as a result of poor fit or careless application. Venous return to the heart can also be improved by active and passive leg exercises and early ambulation after surgery. Elevation of the foot of the bed above heart level and periodic elevation of the lower extremities are simple maneuvers to reduce venous hydrostatic pressure and facilitate venous emptying.

Devices are available to simulate or stimulate the mechanical pumping action of the calf muscles. *External pneumatic compression* of the lower extremities is accomplished by enclosing the calves in air-filled plastic boots, which are periodically inflated and deflated. Pneumatic boots have been used most extensively in the neurosurgical setting and postoperatively after major abdominal surgery.

Anticoagulant therapy with low-dose heparin is advocated by some for high-risk prophylaxis. Lower doses of heparin are thought to minimize the risk of complications while permitting adequate anticoagulation. The efficacy of this practice is controversial.

Anticoagulant and *fibrinolytic therapy* are the therapeutic mainstays of treatment for established DVT. The goal of anticoagulation therapy is to prevent thrombus extension, propagation, or embolization. The anticoagulant of choice during the acute phase of DVT continues to be heparin. Typically, heparin is administered by continuous infusion for approximately 7 to 10 days. A loading dose of 5000 to 10,000 units (U) of heparin, with continuous infusion of approximately 1000 U/hour, is initially given. Oral anticoagulation with warfarin (Coumadin) is added several days before cessation of heparin and in some patients is immediately added to the therapy. The average length of oral anticoagulation is 3 to 6 months but depends on the patient's condition.

The administration of *fibrinolytic agents,* such as streptokinase and urokinase, to dissolve clots is becoming more popular to treat DVT. These drugs are administered during the early stages of acute DVT to activate the endogenous fibrinolytic system. The fibrinolytic system is responsible for clot lysis and dissolution. Ideally, fibrinolytic therapy should be initiated within 24 to 48 hours of the onset of DVT because the mature clot is more resistant to lysis. Contraindications to fibrinolytic therapy include recent surgery or gastrointestinal bleeding. The primacy of fibrinolytic therapy versus anticoagulation therapy in the treatment of DVT is controversial.

The role of *antiplatelet drugs* in the therapy of DVT is still being investigated. Because platelet adhesion and aggregation are the basis for developing the primary hemostatic plug in the coagulation schema, antiplatelet agents, such as aspirin, are administered by some to retard thrombosis.

Treatment of established DVT incorporates the physical principles noted earlier with slight modification. Bed rest is indicated initially to allow time for clot organization and adherence to the vessel wall; it is hoped that bed rest will minimize the risk of pulmonary embolization. The foot of the bed should be elevated slightly to maximize venous drainage; external compression at knee or groin level from the bed or pillows should be avoided. Bed rest is typically continued until signs and symptoms, particularly edema, subside. External compression stockings or bandages may be used for treatment of edema after the first day. Progressive ambulation with external compression stockings is instituted after signs and symptoms subside.

Surgical intervention in DVT involves either venous thrombectomy or vena caval interruption to prevent pulmonary embolism. *Thrombectomy* is indicated for selected cases of massive iliofemoral DVT or extensive DVT that threatens limb survival. Thrombectomy involves insertion of a balloon-tipped Fogarty catheter through a venotomy. The balloon is then inflated, and the catheter is withdrawn, removing the clot.

A variety of techniques have been used to prevent passage of lower-extremity emboli through the vena cava to the heart. Venous flow through the inferior vena cava can be either totally or partially interrupted with specially designed clips (Fig. 34-18, *A*) or suturing techniques (Fig. 34-18, *B*). With total interruption, venous return is then shunted around the obstructed vena cava via smaller collateral networks; this reduction in vessel caliber limits the potential size of an embolus reaching the heart. Vena caval clips or sutures divide the vessel into smaller compartments, preventing passage of large emboli. Devices can also be inserted transvenously to interrupt flow through the inferior vena cava. The designs of the Modin-Uddin umbrella, the Greenfield filter, and the Hunter bal-

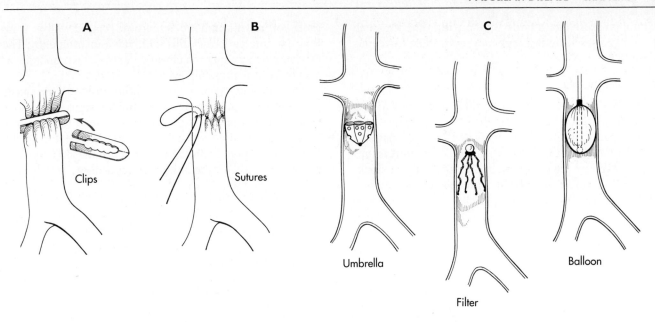

FIG. 34-18 Vena caval interruption techniques. **A,** Clipping; **B,** suturing; **C,** transvenous devices. (Modified from Moore W: *Vascular surgery: a comprehensive review,* Orlando, Fla, 1983, Grune & Stratton.)

loon are illustrated in Fig. 34-18, *C.* The Greenfield filter is used most frequently because it has the lowest incidence of complications.

Varicose Veins

The term *varicose veins* signifies venous dilation, which typically is accompanied by vessel elongation and tortuosity (Fig. 34-19). The exact cause of varicose veins is unknown. Varicosities are distinguished as primary or secondary. The cause of *primary varicosities* appears to be inherent structural weakness in the vessel wall. Dilation can be accompanied by venous valve incompetence because of inability of the valve cusps to overlap and prevent reflux of blood. Primary varicosities tend to involve the superficial veins because of the lack of external support or resistance within the subcutaneous tissue.

Secondary varicosities are caused by acquired or congenital pathology of the deep venous system, which produces dilation of superficial veins, perforators, or collateral channels. For example, destruction of the venous valves of the deep venous system interferes with blood return to the heart; the resultant stasis and pooling of blood result in deep venous hypertension. If the venous valves in the perforating (or communicating) vessels are incompetent, the pressure elevation in the deep venous circuit will reverse blood flow through the perforating vessels. Venous blood will be shunted to the superficial vessels from the deep vessels, predisposing to the development of secondary varicosities in the superficial veins. In this situation, the superficial vessels function as collat-

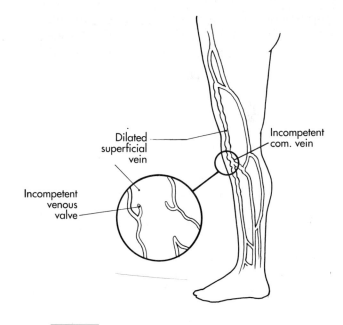

FIG. 34-19 Varicose veins. *Com;* Communicating.

eral vessels for the deep venous system, shunting blood flow from the diseased region.

Predisposing factors

A number of factors predispose to the development of primary varicose veins. A familial tendency has been documented; it is possible that the inherent wall weakness is inherited. In addition, factors increasing the hydrostatic pressure and blood volume within the leg, such as prolonged standing or pregnancy, contribute to venous dilation.

Clinical features

The most common clinical manifestation of varicose veins is *cosmetic disfigurement.* Primary varicosities may be associated with mild, dull aching of the legs, particularly pronounced at the end of the day. Discomfort is typically relieved by leg elevation and elastic support stocking. The discomfort associated with secondary varicosities tends to be more severe. The diagnosis of varicose veins is straightforward and based on observation and palpation of dilated veins.

Complications are unusual. Superficial thrombophlebitis or hemorrhage with ecchymoses may occur. Secondary varicosities may lead to the development of edema, stasis dermatitis, or ulceration.

Treatment

Physical methods described earlier, such as elastic support, to reduce venous stasis should be used to treat varicose veins. Injection of a sclerosing agent may be considered for small, asymptomatic varices; however, sclerotherapy currently has a limited role. Surgery may be indicated to improve appearance of the lower extremity, relieve discomfort, or avoid recurrent superficial thrombophlebitis. Surgery usually involves high ligation and stripping of the greater or lesser saphenous veins. The affected vein is ligated at either the saphenofemoral or the saphenopopliteal junction, and an intraluminal stripper is inserted to remove the entire vessel.

Postthrombotic Syndrome
Pathophysiology

Postthrombotic syndrome (previously called chronic venous insufficiency, or CVI) is usually produced by extensive DVT and venous valve insufficiency; it can develop months or years after the initial episode. Milder degrees of postthrombotic syndrome can develop from longstanding varicose veins with valve insufficiency. The common denominator is chronic venous stasis and elevation of venous pressures.

The chronic elevation of venous pressure produces characteristic and progressive clinical signs of venous stasis. The increased hydrostatic pressure at the capillary level results in fluid transudation into the interstitium and edema formation. Pathologic changes in the skin and subcutaneous tissue of the ankle and leg follow.

Clinical features

The initial presentation is persistent edema of the lower extremities. Subsequently, pathologic tissue changes produce development of a brown pigmentation because of hemosiderin deposition, induration from subcutaneous fibrosis, and dermatitis with eczematous, scaly skin. Tissue ulcerations and necrosis may occur, particularly around the medial malleolus. The extremity is swollen and painful, especially after prolonged dependency.

Treatment

As with thromboembolic venous disease, prevention is more readily accomplished than treatment of established postthrombotic syndrome. Prevention is directed at adequate treatment of acute thrombophlebitis, DVT, and varicose veins. Control of edema is particularly important because the presence of edema indicates elevated venous pressure. The medical treatment of postthrombotic syndrome includes the physical methods described earlier, including elastic support, leg elevation, and bed rest. In addition, one should remember that the tissue is extremely vulnerable to trauma; the foot should be protected whenever possible.

Antibiotic ointments may be necessary to treat the dermatitis and local inflammation or infection. Stasis ulcers are particularly difficult to treat; continual compression with the premedicated Unna's boot may be indicated. On occasion, skin grafting is necessary in conjunction with vein ligation and stripping.

QUESTIONS

1. Label the diagrams on the right by matching the number of the structure on the diagram with the appropriate term from the list.
   Vessel names
   a. _____ Ascending aorta
   b. _____ Aortic arch
   c. _____ Aortic bifurcation
   d. _____ Iliac arteries
   e. _____ Descending aorta
   f. _____ Popliteal arteries
   g. _____ Innominate artery
   h. _____ Femoral arteries

▼ *Answer the following on a separate piece of paper.*

2. What are varicose veins and what causes them? Where are they generally located? What are some possible complications?
3. Which is potentially more serious, deep venous thrombosis or superficial vein thrombosis? Why? Why do the superficial veins often become dilated when there is deep vein thrombosis?
4. List several recommendations for preventing recurrent thrombophlebitis.
5. What is an aneurysm and what causes it? What are the dangers of an aneurysm?
6. What causes brownish pigmentation around the ankles and feet in patients with chronic venous insufficiency?
7. List three major conditions predisposing to venous thrombosis and embolism.

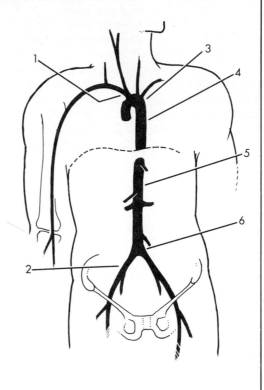
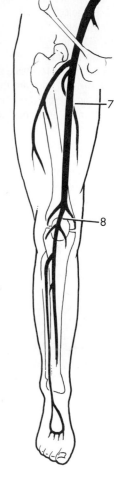

▼ *Circle the letter preceding each item below that correctly answers the question or completes the statement. Only one answer is correct unless otherwise noted.*

8. Which of the following is usually the earliest sign or symptom of chronic occlusive arterial disease in the extremities?
   a. Intermittent claudication
   b. Muscle atrophy
   c. Loss of hair over dorsum of foot
   d. Digital ulceration of the involved extremity
   e. Gangrene of the toes
9. Intermittent claudication resulting from chronic occlusive disease of the superficial femoral arteries commonly causes pain in the:
   a. Arch of the foot
   b. Calf
   c. Thigh
   d. Buttocks

10. A delayed venous filling time when a leg is moved from an elevated to a dependent position occurs with which of the following conditions?
    a. Varicose veins
    b. Chronic venous insufficiency
    c. Peripheral arterial insufficiency
    d. Lymphedema
11. Which of the following physical findings is *not* present in patients with sudden arterial occlusion?
    a. Absence of one or more arterial pulses
    b. Loss of muscular strength
    c. Decreased skin temperature in the extremity
    d. Dilated superficial veins
    e. Pallor and mottling of skin
12. Which of the following is the most common source of arterial emboli?
    a. Pulmonary artery
    b. Aorta

c. Right atrium
d. Left atrium
e. Peripheral artery
13. A stimulus for the development of collateral circulation is:
    a. Hypertension
    b. Peripheral vasodilation
    c. Mild chronic ischemia
    d. Inflammation of the arteries
14. Which of the following statements are *true* concerning true and false aneurysms (more than one answer may be correct)?
    a. False aneurysms are caused by entry of blood between the intima and medial layers of the blood vessel, causing separation.
    b. A true aneurysm is a dilation enclosed by an intact arterial wall.
    c. A false aneurysm consists of a localized area of clot and blood caused by a gap in the arterial wall.

Continued.

d. True aneurysms form only in the aorta.

15. The formation of a blood clot within the vascular system is called:
    a. Embolization
    b. Embolus
    c. Thrombus
    d. Thrombosis

16. Which of the following signs and symptoms might indicate that a postoperative patient has thrombophlebitis of the leg (more than one answer may be correct)?
    a. Decreased hair growth over involved area
    b. Aching of extremity
    c. Positive Homans' sign
    d. Pain and tenderness along course of superficial vein
    e. Oral temperature at 103°F

17. The initial treatment of an acute thrombophlebitis generally consists of (more than one answer may be correct):
    a. Bed rest with the feet elevated
    b. Leg exercises
    c. Venous thrombectomy
    d. Warm moist compresses to the extremity
    e. Anticoagulant therapy

18. Which of the following statements about Raynaud's phenomenon is *incorrect?*
    a. It results from episodic vasoconstriction of the small arteries in an extremity.
    b. Symptoms are more frequent in a warm environment.
    c. Changes in skin color caused by pallor, cyanosis, and hyperemia occur sequentially during an episode.
    d. Ulceration and gangrene of the digits may occur.

19. The presence of deep venous thrombosis can be detected noninvasively by:
    a. Thermography
    b. Impedance measurements
    c. Venography
    d. Monitoring blood pressure along the affected limb
    e. Monitoring skin color changes

▼ *Fill in the blank with the correct word.*

20. _____ means inflammation of the vein accompanied by the formation of a clot; _____ means the formation of a clot in a vein in which there is little or no inflammation.

21. An arterial disease that starts in the smaller arteries of the hands and feet and has an intense inflammatory component is _____.

▼ *Match each of the terms in column A with its best description in column B.*

Column A	Column B
22. _____ Atherosclerosis	a. Episodic attacks of vasoconstriction of the arteries and arterioles in response to cold and emotional stimuli.
23. _____ Raynaud's syndrome	
24. _____ Cystic medial necrosis	b. Degenerative changes in the medial layer of the artery
25. _____ Thromboangiitis obliterans	c. Chronic occlusive disease of the medium and small arteries and veins caused by inflammation and thrombosis
	d. Focal intimal accumulation of lipids, carbohydrates, blood products, fibrous tissue, and calcium

▼ *Match each of the diagnostic methods in column A with the most appropriate statement in column B.*

Column A	Column B
26. _____ Arteriography	a. Noninvasively measures the velocity of flow in a vessel
27. _____ Doppler ultrasound detector	
28. _____ Segmental plethysmography	b. Visualization of arterial anatomy by injection of contrast material directly into an artery
29. _____ Radioactive fibrinogen scanning	c. Measures pulse volume
	d. Injection intravenously of radioactive isotope, which is detected by a counter at the site of actively forming thrombi

▼ *Match each of the blood vessel disease processes in column A with the most appropriate surgical treatment in column B.*

Column A	Column B
30. _____ Abdominal aortic aneurysm	a. Aortobifemoral bypass graft
31. _____ Complete aortoiliac occlusion	b. Saphenous vein graft
32. _____ Femoropopliteal occlusion	c. Aortic tube graft insertion
33. _____ Deep femoral arterial occlusion	d. Profundaplasty

▼ *Match the types of arterial dissection in column B with the appropriate category of the DeBakey classification in column A.*

Column A	Column B
34. _____ Type I	a. Aneurysms beginning beyond left subclavian and extending distally
35. _____ Type II	b. Aneurysms confined to the ascending artery
36. _____ Type III	c. Aneurysms originating in the ascending aorta above aortic valve and extending distally

▼ *Circle T if the statement is true and F if it is false. Correct any false statements.*

37. T F The insertion of a balloon-tipped catheter into a blood vessel to remove a blood clot is called an endarterectomy.

38. T F Patients with arterial occlusive disease of the lower extremities should keep the extremities slightly elevated to improve circulation.

39. T F The superficial veins are connected to the deep veins by perforating or communicating veins.

40. T F Detachment of a blood clot into the arterial circulation is called arterial thrombosis.

BIBLIOGRAPHY ▼ PART VI

Acar J et al: Indications of surgery in mitral regurgitation, *Eur Hear J* 12 (suppl B):52-54, 1991.

Akins CW et al: Mitral valve reconstruction versus replacement for degenerative or ischemic mitral regurgitation, *Ann Thorac Surg* 58:668-676, 1994.

American College of Cardiology/American Heart Association Task Force: Guidelines for the early management of patients with acute myocardial infarction: a report of the ACC/AHA Task Force on Assessment of Diagnostic and Therapeutic Cardiovascular Procedures, *J Am Coll Cardiol* 16:249-292, 1990.

American Heart Association: *Heart facts: 1989,* New York, 1988, American Heart Association.

American Heart Association: *Research facts: update 1994,* Dallas, Texas, 1994, American Heart Association.

Ardehali A, Ports TA: Myocardial oxygen supply and demand, *Chest* 98(3):702-703, 1990.

Ballard D et al: *Abdominal aneurysm surgery: a literature review and ratings of appropriateness and necessity,* Santa Monica, Calif, 1991, Rand.

Bates B: *A guide to physical examination,* ed 6, Philadelphia, 1995, Lippincott.

Bengtson JR et al: Prognosis in cardiogenic shock after acute myocardial infarction in the interventional era, *J Am Coll Cardiol* 20:1482-1489, 1992.

Berne R and Levy M: *Cardiovascular physiology,* ed 6, St Louis, 1991, Mosby.

Bernstein AD et al: The NASPE/BPEG generic pacemaker code for antibradyarrhythmias and adaptive-rate pacing and antitachyarrhythmic devices, *PACE* 10:794, 1987.

Bernstein E: *Vascular diagnosis,* ed 4, St Louis, 1993, Mosby.

Bittl JA: Mitral valve balloon dilatation: long-term results, *J Card Surg* 9:213-217, 1994.

Blank C, Irvin G: Peripheral vascular disorders, *Nurs Clin North Am* 25(4):777-797, 1990.

Block PC et al: Percutaneous mitral valve valvotomy, *Cardiol Clin* 9:271-287, 1991.

Boldt M: *Acute coronary care,* New York, 1983, Wiley.

Braunwald E, editor: *Heart disease: a textbook in cardiovascular medicine,* ed 4, Philadelphia, 1992, Saunders.

Bright L, George S: Peripheral vascular disease: is it arterial or venous? *Am J Nurs* 92(9):34-43, 1992.

Burge DJ: DeHoratius RJ: Acute rheumatic fever, *Cardiovasc Clin* 23:3-24, 1993.

Carabello BA: Timing of surgery in mitral and aortic stenosis, *Cardiol Clin* 9:229-238, 1991.

Conover MB: *Understanding electrocardiology,* ed 6, St Louis, 1992, Mosby.

Crawford MV, Spence MI: *Commonsense approach to coronary care,* 6 ed, St Louis, 1994, Mosby.

Daily EK, Schroeder JS: *Bedside techniques in hemodynamic monitoring,* ed 5, St Louis, 1994, Mosby.

Delahave JP et al: Natural history of severe mitral regurgitation, *Eur Heart J* 12 (suppl B):5-9, 1991.

DeWeese J et al: Practice guidelines: lower extremity revascularization, *J Vasc Surg* 18:279-291, 1993.

Dhalla NS et al: Pathophysiology of cardiac dysfunction in congestive heart failure, *Can J Cardiol* 9:873-887, 1993.

Eagle KA et al, editors: *The practice of cardiology,* ed 2, Boston, 1989, Little, Brown.

Edelman R, Warach S: Magnetic resonance imaging, *N Engl J Med* 32(10):708-716, 1993.

Epstein FH: The pathogenesis of coronary artery disease and the acute coronary syndrome, *N Engl J Med* 326:342-349, 1992.

Eton D, Ahn S: Trends in endovascular surgery, *Crit Care Nurs Clin North Am* 9(3):535-549, 1991.

Fahey VA: *Vascular nursing,* ed 2, Philadelphia, 1994, Saunders.

Fahey VA, Riegal BJ: Advances in diagnostic testing for vascular disease, *Cardiovasc Nurs* 25(3):13-18, 1989.

Feigenbaum H: *Echocardiography,* ed 5, Philadelphia, 1994, Lea & Febiger.

Folders M: The role of duplex and color Doppler imaging in the operating room, *J Vasc Nurs* 12(4):105-110, 1993.

Follman DF: Aortic regurgitation: identifying and treating acute and chronic disease, *Postgrad Med* 93(6):83-92, 1993.

Francis GS: Determinants of prognosis in patients with heart failure, *J Heart Lung Transplant* 13:S113-S116, 1994.

Fraser CD et al: Repair of insufficient bicuspid aortic valves, *Ann Thorac Surg* 58:386-390, 1994.

Frazier OH, Marcris MP: Progress in cardiac transplantation, *Surg Clin North Am* 74:1169-1182, 1994.

Gacioch GM et al: Cardiogenic shock complicating acute myocardial infarction: the use of coronary angioplasty and the integration of the new support devices into patient management, *J Am Coll Cardiol* 19:647-653, 1992.

Ganong WF: *Review of medical physiology,* ed 16, East Norwalk, Conn, 1993, Appleton & Lange.

Goldberger AL, Goldberger E: *Clinical electrocardiography,* ed 5, St Louis, 1994, Mosby.

Greenberg BH: Medical therapy for patients with aortic insufficiency, *Cardiol Clin* 9:255-270, 1991.

Greene HL: Clinical significance and management of arrhythmias in the heart failure patient, *Clin Cardiol* 15(suppl 1):113-121, 1992.

Griffith BP et al: Temporary use of the Jarvik-7 total artificial heart before transplantation, *N Engl J Med* 316:130-134, 1987.

Grossman W, editor: *Cardiac catheterization and angiography,* ed 4, Philadelphia, 1991, Lea & Febiger.

Guyton AC: *Textbook of medical physiology,* ed 8, Philadelphia, 1991, Saunders.

Haimovici H: *Vascular surgery: principles and techniques,* ed 3, East Norwalk, Conn, 1989, Appleton-Century-Crofts.

Hallett JW, Brewster DC, Darling RC: *Patient care in vascular surgery,* ed 2, Boston, 1987, Little, Brown.

Harley JR: Preventing diabetic foot disease, *Am J Primary Health Care* 10:37-44, 1993.

Hart BP: Vascular consequences of smoking and benefits of smoking cessation, *J Vasc Nurs* 11(2):48-51, 1993.

Higgins C: The potential role of magnetic resonance imaging in ischemic vascular disease, *N Engl J Med* 326(24):1624-1625, 1992.

Hosenpud JD et al: The registry of the International Society of Heart and Lung Transplantation: eleventh official report—1994, *J Heart Lung Transplant* 13:561-570, 1994.

Hurst JW, editor: *The heart,* ed 7, New York, 1990, McGraw-Hill.

ISIS-2 (Second International Study of Infarct Survival) Collaborative Group: Randomized trial of intravenous streptokinase, oral aspirin, both or neither among 17,187 cases of suspected acute myocardial infarction, *Lancet* 8607:354, 1988.

Continued.

BIBLIOGRAPHY ▼ PART VI

Johnson RA, Haber E, Austen WG: *The practice of cardiology,* Boston, 1988, Little, Brown.

Kannel WB, D'Agostino RB, Belanger AC: Fibrinogen, cigarette smoking, and the risk of cardiovascular disease, Insights from the Framingham Study, *Am Heart J* 114:1006, 1987.

Kern MJ et al: Enhanced coronary blood flow velocity during intraaortic balloon counterpulsation in critically ill patients, *J Am Coll Cardiol* 21:359-368, 1993.

Kostis JB et al: Nonpharmacologic therapy improves functional and emotional status in congestive heart failure, *Chest* 106:996-1001, 1994.

Kubo SH: Vasodilator therapy in heart failure, *J Heart Lung Transplant* 13:S122-S125, 1994.

Kuyvenhoven JP et al: Prosthetic valve endocarditis: analysis of risk factors for mortality, *Euro J Cardiothorac Surg* 8:420-424, 1994.

Lovell M, Harris K: Abdominal aortic aneurysms, *J Vasc Nurs* IX(1):12-15, 1991.

Lovell MB et al: The management of chronic venous disease, *J Vasc Nurs* 11(2):43-47, 1993.

Magovern JA et al: Operation for congestive heart failure: transplantation, coronary artery bypass, and cardiomyoplasty, *Ann Thorac Surg* 56:418-424, 1993.

Manning WJ, Edelman RR: Magnetic resonance coronary angiography, *Magn Reson Q* 9(3):131-151, 1993.

Marico H et al: Prevalence of Raynaud's phenomenon in the general population, *J Chron Dis* 39:423-427, 1986.

Mattioli AV et al: Symptomatic achievements with diuretics in congestive heart failure, *Cardiology* 84(suppl 2):131-134, 1994.

McCarthy PM et al: Implantable left ventricle assist device: approaching an alternative for end-stage heart failure (Implantable LVAD Study Group), *Circulation* 90:1183-1186, 1994.

McGoon DC, editor: Cardiac surgery, *Cardiovasc Clin* 17(3):entire issue, 1987.

Moore W: *Vascular surgery: a comprehensive review,* ed 4, Philadelphia, 1993, Saunders.

Moosvi AR et al: Early revascularization improves survival in cardiogenic shock complicating acute myocardial infarction, *J Am Coll Cardiol* 19:907-914, 1992.

National Institutes of Health: *Fifth Report of the Joint National Committee on Detection, Evaluation, and Treatment of High Blood Pressure,* National Heart, Lung, and Blood Institute, NIH Pub No 93-1088, Washington, DC, 1993, National Institutes of Health.

National Institutes of Health: *Detection, evaluation, and treatment of high blood cholesterol (Adult Treatment Panel II),* NIH Pub No 93-3075, Washington, DC, National Heart, Lung, and Blood Institute, 1993, National Institutes of Health.

National Institutes of Health: *Second Report of the Expert Panel on Detection, Evaluation, and Treatment of High Blood Cholesterol in Adults (Adult Treatment Panel II),* NIH Pub NO. 93-3095, National Heart, Lung, and Blood Institute, Washington, DC, 1993, National Institutes of Health.

O'Mara C: Noninvasive evaluation of lower extremity arterial disease, *Surg Rounds* 10:57-68, 1989.

Palumbo P et al: Progression of peripheral occlusive arterial disease in diabetes mellitus. what factors are predictive, *Arch Intern Med* 151(4):717-721, 1991.

Pardo-Mindan FJ et al: Pathology of heart transplant through endomyocardial biopsy, *Semin Diagn Pathol* 9:238-248, 1992.

Parmley WW: Pathophysiology of congestive heart failure, *Clin Cardiol* 15:5-12, 1992.

Patterson JH, Adams EF Jr: Pathophysiology of heart failure, *Pharmacotherapy* 13:73S-81S, 1993.

Perloff D et al: Human blood pressure determination by sphygmomanometry, *Circulation* 88:2460-2467, 1993.

Prevost D: Diagnostic arteriography and percutaneous transluminal angioplasty of the lower extremities, *J Vasc Nurs* VIII(4):6-12, 1990.

Quaal SJ, editor: *Comprehensive intra-aortic balloon pumping,* ed 2, St Louis, 1993, Mosby.

Reeder GS, Gersh BJ: Modern management of acute myocardial infarction, *Curr Probl Cardiol* XVIII(2):81-156, 1993.

Roberts WC: Valvular heart disease of congenital origin, *Cardiovasc Clin* 23:34-46, 1993.

Ronoyne R: Acute lower limb ischemia: a case study, *J Vasc Nurs* X(3):14-17. 1992.

Ross R: The pathogenesis of atherosclerosis, *N Engl J Med* 314:488-497, 1986.

Rudalphi D: Renovascular hypertension, diagnosis to discharge: a case study, *J Vasc Nurs* VII(2):6-10, 1990.

Ruttley MS: The chest radiograph in adult heart valve disease, *J Heart Valve Dis* 2:205-217, 1993.

Schreiber TL et al: Management of myocardial infarction shock: current status, *Am Heart J* 117:435-443, 1989.

Schroder JS, Kiess E: *Techniques in bedside hemodynamic monitoring,* ed 3, St Louis, 1985, Mosby.

Schlant RC, Alexander RW: *Hurst's the heart,* ed 8, New York, 1994, McGraw-Hill.

Seward JB et al: Transesophageal echocardiography, *J Am Coll Cardiol* 20(2):506, 1992.

Shaver JA, editor: Cardiomyopathies: clinical presentation, differential diagnosis, and management, *Cardiovasc Clin* 19(1):entire issue, 1988.

Skorton DJ et al: Relative merits of imaging techniques. In Braunwald E: *Heart disease,* ed 4, Philadelphia, 1992, Saunders.

Special Writing Group of the Committee on Rheumatic Fever, Endocarditis, and Kawasaki Disease of the Council on Cardiovascular Disease in the Young of the American Heart Association: Guidelines for the diagnosis of rheumatic fever: Jones criteria, 1992 update, *JAMA* 268(15):2069-2073, 1992.

Turi ZG: Valvuloplasty, *Cardiovasc Clin* 23:293-315, 1993.

Wagshal AB, Pires LA, Huang SK: Management of cardiac arrhythmias with radiofrequency catheter ablation, *Arch Intern Med* 155:142, 1995.

Way LW, editor: *Current surgical diagnosis and treatment,* ed 7, Los Altos, Calif, 1985, Lange.

Weber KT et al: The contractile behavior of the heart and its functional coupling to the circulation, *Prog Cardiovasc Dis* 24:375-397, 1984.

Weiland WP: A review of cardiac valve prostheses and their selection, *Heart Lung* 12(5):500, 1983.

Wolf GL, Marcus ML: Relative merits of imaging techniques. In Braunwald E: *Heart disease,* ed 4, Philadelphia, 1992, Saunders.

Young JB: Angiotensin-converting enzyme inhibitors in heart failure: new strategies justified by recent clinical trials, *Int J Cardiol* 43:151-163, 1994.

Zaret BL, Wackers FJT, Soufer R: *Nuclear cardiology: state of the art and future directions,* St Louis, 1993, Mosby.

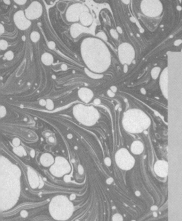

PART SEVEN

RESPIRATORY SYSTEM DISORDERS

Disorders of the respiratory system are a major cause of morbidity and mortality. Respiratory tract infections occur more frequently than infections of any other organ system and range from the common cold, with its relatively mild symptoms and inconvenience, to a fulminant pneumonia. In 1995 approximately 157,400 persons died from lung cancer. Since the mid-1950s, lung cancer has been the most common cause of cancer mortality in men, and in 1987 it overtook breast cancer to become the most common cause of cancer mortality in women. It has increased at an alarming rate and is now about 25 times more prevalent than it was 50 years ago. The incidence of chronic respiratory disease, notably chronic pulmonary emphysema and bronchitis, has also been increasing and is now a leading cause of chronic disability among men. Because of the physical, social, and economic impact of respiratory diseases on the population as a whole, the prevention, diagnosis, and treatment of respiratory disorders are of paramount importance.

This part includes a brief review of respiratory tract anatomy and physiology, a discussion of the common diagnostic tests used to detect respiratory dysfunction, cardinal signs and symptoms of respiratory disease, manifestations of respiratory insufficiency and failure, and a discussion of the common respiratory diseases. ▼

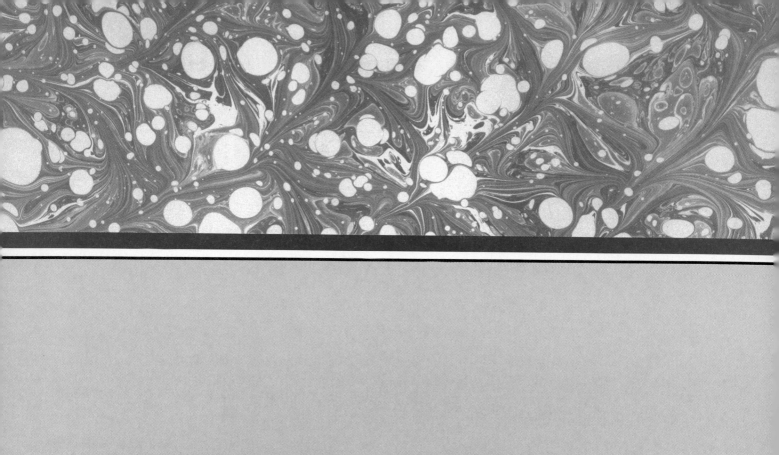

CHAPTER 35

Anatomy and Physiology of the Respiratory System

LORRAINE M. WILSON

ANATOMIC CONSIDERATIONS

Respiration means literally the movement of oxygen (O_2) from the atmosphere to the cells and the return of carbon dioxide (CO_2) from the cells to the environment. O_2 consumption and CO_2 elimination are necessary for normal cellular function within the body; however, most of our billions of cells cannot exchange these gases directly with the air because they are far too distant from it. Therefore they need special structures both for exchange and for transport.

The respiratory process consists of several steps, with the respiratory, central nervous, and cardiovascular systems playing pivotal roles. Essentially, the respiratory system consists of a series of air passages that bring outside air into contact with the *alveolocapillary membrane,* the interface between the respiratory and cardiovascular systems. The movement of air in and out of the air passages is called *ventilation* or *breathing*. The central nervous system provides the inherent rhythmic drive to breathe and reflexly stimulates the thoracic and diaphragm muscles, which provide the driving force for the movement of air. The diffusion of O_2 and CO_2 across the alveolocapillary membrane is often referred to as *external respiration*. The cardiovascular system provides the pump, conduits, and blood essential for the transport of gases between the lungs and cells. An adequate amount of functioning hemoglobin is essential for the transportation of gases. The final transportation phase of gas transport involves the diffusion of O_2 and CO_2 between the body capillaries and cells. *Internal respiration* refers to the intracellular chemical reactions in which O_2 is used and CO_2 is produced, as the cells metabolize carbohydrates and other substances to generate adenosine triphosphate (ATP) and release energy.

Adequate functioning of all these interrelated systems is essential for cell respiration. Malfunction of any of these components can disrupt gas exchange and transport and can seriously compromise these life processes. An understanding of the respiratory process is necessary to assess and treat clients with respiratory disorders. This chapter and Chapter 36 lay the groundwork for this understanding.

Anatomy of the Respiratory Tract

The air-conducting passages that bring air into the lungs are the nose, pharynx, larynx, trachea, bronchi, and bronchioles (Fig. 35-1). The respiratory tract from the nose to the bronchioles is lined with ciliated mucous membranes. As air enters the nasal cavity, it is filtered, warmed, and humidified. These three processes are primarily functions of the respiratory mucosa, which consists of pseudostratified, ciliated, columnar epithelium and goblet cells (see inset *B,* Fig. 35-1). The epithelial surface is covered by a mucous blanket, which is secreted by both the goblet cells and the serous glands. Coarse dust particles are filtered by hair in the nares, and fine particles are trapped in the mucous blanket. Ciliary action propels the mucous blanket posteriorly in the nasal cavity and superiorly in the lower respiratory tract toward the *pharynx,* from which it is swallowed or expectorated. Water for humidification is given up by the mucous blanket, and heat is supplied to the inspired air by a rich underlying vascular

FIG. 35-1   Respiratory system. Inset **A,** Acinus, or pulmonary functional unit. Inset **B,** Ciliated mucous membrane.

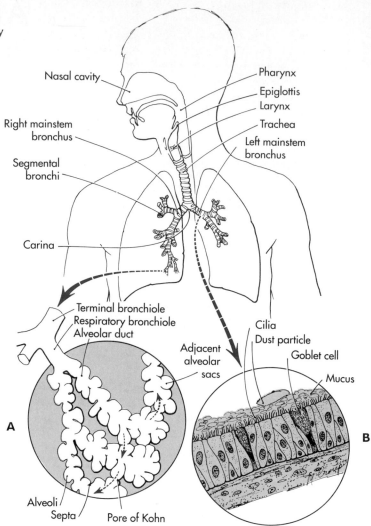

network. Inspired air is thus conditioned so that it reaches the pharynx nearly dust free, at body temperature, and 100% humidified.

Air passes from the pharynx into the larynx, or voice box. The *larynx* consists of a series of cartilaginous rings united by muscles and contains the vocal cords. A triangular space between the vocal cords, the *glottis,* opens into the trachea and forms the division between the upper and lower respiratory tracts. Although the larynx has been thought of chiefly in relationship to phonation, its protective functions are much more important. During swallowing the rising action of the larynx, the closure of the glottis, and the doorlike action of the leaf-shaped *epiglottis,* at the entrance of the larynx, all serve to guide food and fluids into the esophagus. If foreign substances do get beyond the glottis, the cough function of the larynx assists in expelling these substances as well as secretions from the lower respiratory tract.

The *trachea* is supported by horseshoe-shaped cartilaginous rings and is about 12.5 cm (5 inches) long. The structure of the trachea and bronchi is analogous to a tree and is therefore called the *tracheobronchial tree.* The posterior surface of the trachea is flattened rather than round because its cartilaginous rings are incomplete, and it lies immediately in front of the esophagus. Consequently, when a round, rigid endotracheal (ET) tube with inflated cuff is inserted during mechanical ventilation, erosion may occur posteriorly through the membrane to form a tracheoesophageal fistula. Anterior erosion through the cartilaginous rings may also occur but is less common. Swelling and damage to the vocal cords are also complications of ET tube use. The point where the trachea branches into the right and left mainstem bronchi is known as the *carina.* The carina is heavily innervated and can produce severe bronchospasms and coughing when stimulated.

The right and left mainstem bronchi are not symmetric (Fig. 35-1). The *right mainstem bronchus* is shorter and wider and continues from the trachea in a nearly vertical course. In contrast, the *left mainstem bronchus* is longer and narrower and continues from the trachea at a more acute angle. This anatomic peculiarity has important clinical implications. An ET tube that has been placed to secure a patent airway may easily slip down into the right mainstem bronchus unless well secured at the mouth or nose. If it did slip, air would not be able to enter the left lung, which would collapse *(atelectasis).* However, the more vertical course of the right bronchus makes it easier to introduce a catheter for deep suctioning. Also, aspirated foreign bodies are more apt to lodge in the right bronchial tree because of its vertical course.

The right and left mainstem bronchi divide to become the *lobar bronchi* and then the *segmental bronchi.* This branching in ever-decreasing sizes continues down to the *terminal bronchioles,* the smallest airways that do not contain alveoli (air sacs). Terminal bronchioles are about 1 mm in diameter. Bronchioles are not supported by cartilaginous rings but are surrounded by smooth muscle, which allows alterations in size. All the airways down to the level of the terminal bronchioles are called *conducting airways* because their main function is to serve as air conduits to the gas-exchanging areas of the lung.

Beyond the terminal bronchiole is the *acinus,* which is the pulmonary functional unit where gas exchange takes place (see inset *A,* Fig. 35-1). The acinus consists of (1) *respiratory bronchioles,* which have occasional small air sacs or alveoli arising from their walls; (2) *alveolar ducts,* completely lined with alveoli, and (3) *terminal alveolar sacs,* the final structures of the lung. The acinus, or *primary lobule* as it is sometimes called, is about 0.5 to 1.0 cm ($\frac{1}{5}$ to $\frac{2}{5}$ inch) in diameter. There are about 23 generations of branching from the trachea to the terminal alveolar sac. The individual alveolus (in the grape-like cluster of alveolar sacs that make up the terminal sac) is separated from its neighbor by a thin wall, or *septum.* Small openings in the septum, called the *pores of Kohn,* allow communication or airflow between terminal alveolar sacs. The alveolus has only one layer of cells, which is less than the diameter of a red blood cell in thickness. There are about 300 million alveoli in each lung, with a surface area about the size of a tennis court.

Fig. 35-2 shows the microscopic structure of an alveolar duct and the surrounding alveoli, which are polygonal in shape. Because the alveolus is essentially a gas bubble surrounded by a capillary network, the liquid-gas interface creates a surface tension, which tends to resist expansion on inspiration and favors collapse on expiration. The alveoli, however, are lined with a lipoprotein substance called *surfactant,* which lessens the surface tension, lowers the resistance to expansion on inspiration, and prevents collapse of the alveoli on expiration. The production and release of surfactant from the alveolar lining (type II) cells depend on several factors, including maturity of the alveolar cells and their biosynthetic enzyme systems, a normal surfactant turnover rate, adequate ventilation, and blood flow to the alveolar walls. Surfactant is formed relatively late in fetal life; therefore infants born with inadequate amounts (usually premature births) may develop infant respiratory distress syndrome. Surfactant is synthesized rapidly from fatty acids extracted from the blood, and its turnover rate is rapid; thus,

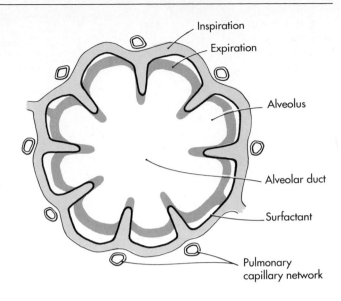

FIG. 35-2   Structural changes in the terminal alveolar sac (cross section) during the respiratory cycle. (Modified from Gluck L: *Hosp Pract* 6(11):45-56, 1971.)

if blood flow to an area of the lung is interrupted (e.g., by a pulmonary embolism), the surfactant in that area may be depleted. The production of surfactant is stimulated by active ventilation, adequate tidal volumes, and periodic hyperventilation (sighing) and is inhibited by high concentrations of O_2 in the inspired air. Thus it follows that prolonged administration of high O_2 concentrations or failure to periodically deep-sigh a patient receiving mechanical ventilation will cause decreased surfactant production and subsequent alveolar collapse (atelectasis). A deficiency of surfactant is believed to be an important factor in the pathogenesis of a number of lung diseases, including adult respiratory distress syndrome (ARDS) (see Chapter 41).

The Thoracic Cavity

The lungs are elastic, cone-shaped organs that lie within the thoracic cavity, or chest. They are separated by the central *mediastinum,* which contains the heart and great vessels (Fig. 35-3). Each lung has an apex (top of lung) and a base. Pulmonary and bronchial blood vessels, bronchi, nerves, and lymphatics enter each lung at the hilus to form the root of the lung. The *right lung* is larger than the left and is divided into three lobes by the interlobar fissures. The *left lung* is divided into two lobes.

Lobes are further divided into segments corresponding to the segmental bronchi. The right lung is divided into 10 segments and the left lung into 9 (Fig. 35-3). Pathologic processes such as atelectasis and pneumonia are often localized to individual lobes and segments. Knowledge of the segmental anatomy of the lung is important not only for the radiologist, bronchoscopist, and thoracic

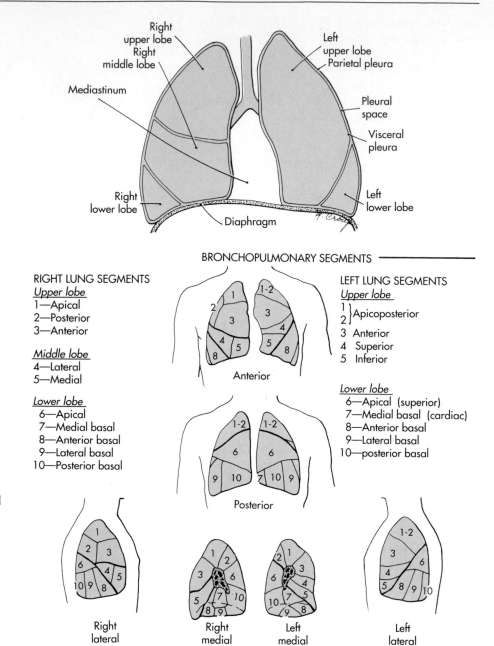

FIG. 35-3 Thoracic cavity and bronchopulmonary segments.

surgeon, but also for the nurse and respiratory therapist, who must know with accuracy the location of the lesion to apply their skills.

A continuous thin sheet of collagen and elastic tissue, known as the *pleura,* lines the thoracic cavity *(parietal pleura)* and encases each lung *(visceral pleura).* Between the parietal and visceral pleura is a thin film of pleural fluid that allows the two surfaces to glide over each other during respiration and prevents the separation of the thorax and lungs, as when two glass slides are stuck together with water: the slides can glide over each other, but they cannot easily be pulled apart.

The same is true of the pleural fluid between the lungs and thorax. Because no actual space separates the parietal and visceral pleurae, the so-called pleural spaces or cavities are potential spaces only. The pressure within the

pleural space is less than that of the atmosphere and thus prevents the collapse of the lung. In disease, the pleura may become inflamed or air or fluid may enter the pleural space, causing compression or collapse of the lung.

Three factors maintain this normal negative pressure. First, the *elastic tissue* of the lungs exerts a continuous force that tends to pull the lungs away from the thoracic cage; for example, the lungs tend to recoil to their smaller original size before the first expansion after birth. However, the visceral and parietal pleural surfaces in contact with each other cannot separate, so the continuous force that tends to separate them persists. This force is popularly known as the *negative pressure* of the pleural space. Intrapleural pressures vary continuously throughout the respiratory cycle (see Fig. 35-8) but are always negative.

The second major factor in maintaining negative intrapleural pressure is the *osmotic forces* exerted across the pleural membranes. Fluid normally moves from the capillaries in the parietal pleura into the pleural space and then is reabsorbed through the visceral pleura. The movement of the pleural fluid is believed to be governed by Starling's law of transcapillary exchange (Light, 1984); that is, fluid movement depends on a net gradient between the hydrostatic pressure of the blood tending to push fluid out and the oncotic pressure of the plasma proteins tending to hold the fluid within. Because the net gradient for pleural fluid absorption through the visceral pleura is greater than the net gradient for fluid formation by the parietal pleura and because the surface area of the visceral pleura is greater than that of the parietal pleura, the pleural space normally contains only a few milliliters of fluid.

The third factor that supports a negative intrapleural pressure is the force of the *lymphatic pump*. A small amount of protein normally enters the pleural space but is removed by the lymphatics in the parietal pleura; the accumulation of protein in the intrapleural space would upset the normal osmotic balance without lymphatic removal.

These three factors therefore regulate and maintain the normal negative and intrapleural pressure. The *diaphragm* is a dome-shaped muscle that forms the floor of the thoracic cavity and separates it from the abdominal cavity.

Pulmonary Circulation

The blood supply to the lungs is unique in several respects. First, the lung has a dual blood supply from the bronchial and pulmonary arteries. The *bronchial circulation* provides oxygenated blood from the systemic circulation and serves to meet the metabolic needs of the lung tissue. The bronchial arteries arise from the thoracic aorta and travel along the posterior walls of the bronchi. The larger bronchial veins empty into the azygos system, which empties into the superior vena cava and returns blood to the right atrium. The smaller bronchial veins drain into the pulmonary veins. Because the bronchial circulation does not take part in gas exchange, the unoxygenated blood accounts for a shunt, which is normally about 2% to 3% of cardiac output.

The *pulmonary artery* arising from the right ventricle provides mixed venous blood to the lungs, where the blood is involved in gas exchange. A vast network of *pulmonary capillaries* surrounds and envelops the alveoli, providing the intimate contact necessary for the exchange of gases between the alveoli and the blood. Oxygenated blood is then returned through the *pulmonary veins* to the left ventricle, which distributes it to the cells via the systemic circulation. Fig. 35-4 shows the functional position of the lungs in the pulmonary circulation.

Another feature of the pulmonary circulation is that it is a low-pressure, low-resistance system compared with

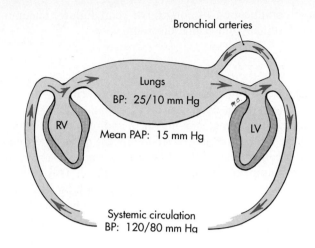

FIG. 35-4   Functional position of the lungs in the pulmonary circulation. *BP,* Blood pressure; *PAP,* pulmonary arterial pressure; *RV,* right ventricle; *LV,* left ventricle.

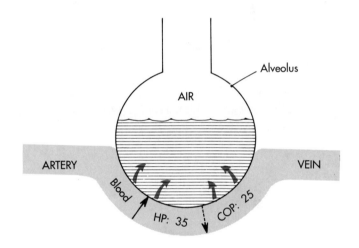

FIG. 35-5   Pathogenesis of pulmonary edema. *HP,* Hydrostatic pressure; *COP,* colloid osmotic pressure.

the systemic circulation. Systemic blood pressure is about 120/80 mm Hg, whereas pulmonary blood pressure is about 25/10 mm Hg, with a mean pressure of about 15 mm Hg. These features of the pulmonary circulation have several important consequences. The great distensibility and low resistance of the pulmonary vascular beds allows the workload of the right ventricle to be much lighter than that of the left and also allows a great increase in pulmonary blood flow during exercise without significantly increasing the pulmonary blood pressure.

As shown in Fig. 35-5, if the normal mean pulmonary hydrostatic pressure of about 15 mm Hg should exceed the colloid osmotic pressure of the blood of about 25 mm Hg, fluid would leave the pulmonary capillaries and enter the interstitium or alveoli, causing pulmonary edema. *Pulmonary edema* interferes with gas exchange by increasing the length of the diffusion pathway between the alveolus and the capillary. Pulmonary edema is a common complication of congestive heart failure, pneumonia, and many other lung disorders.

Control of Respiration

A number of mechanisms contribute to bringing air into the lungs so that exchange of gases can occur. The mechanical function of moving air in and out of the lungs is termed *ventilation* and is accomplished by several interacting components. Of particular importance is a reciprocating pump called the *respiratory bellows*. This bellows has two volume-elastic components: the lung itself and the chest wall surrounding the lung. The chest wall consists of the skeleton and tissues of the thoracic cage, as well as the diaphragm, abdominal contents, and abdominal wall. The respiratory muscles, which are a part of the thoracic wall, provide the driving force for the operation of the bellows. The diaphragm (assisted by those muscles that elevate the ribs and sternum) is the principal muscle involved in increasing the volume of the lung and thoracic cage during inspiration; expiration is a passive process during quiet breathing. The mechanics of ventilation are discussed in greater detail in Chapter 36.

The respiratory muscles are controlled by the *respiratory center,* which is composed of neurons and receptors located in the pons and medulla (Fig. 35-6). The respiratory center is the part of the nervous system that controls all aspects of breathing. The prime factor in the control of breathing is the response of the central chemoreceptors in the respiratory center to the partial pressure (or tension) of carbon dioxide ($Paco_2$) and the pH of the arterial blood. An increase in the $Paco_2$ or a decrease in the pH stimulates breathing.

A decrease of the partial pressure of oxygen in the arterial blood (Pao_2) can also stimulate ventilation. Peripheral chemoreceptors located in the carotid bodies at the bifurcation of the common carotid arteries and in the aortic bodies at the aortic arch respond to decreases in Pao_2 and pH and increases in $Paco_2$. The Pao_2, however, must fall from the normal level of about 90 to 100 mm Hg to a level of about 60 mm Hg before ventilation is significantly stimulated.

Other mechanisms control the amount of air taken into the lungs. As the lung is inflated, these receptors signal the respiratory center to stop further inflation. Signals from the stretch receptors cease at the end of expiration when the lung is deflated and the respiratory center is free to initiate another inspiration. This mechanism, known as the *Hering-Breuer reflex,* was once thought to play a major role in the control of ventilation; however, more recent work shows that the reflex is largely inactive in an adult unless tidal volume exceeds 1 L, as in exercise. It may be more important in newborn babies. Movements of joints and muscles (e.g., during exercise) also stimu-

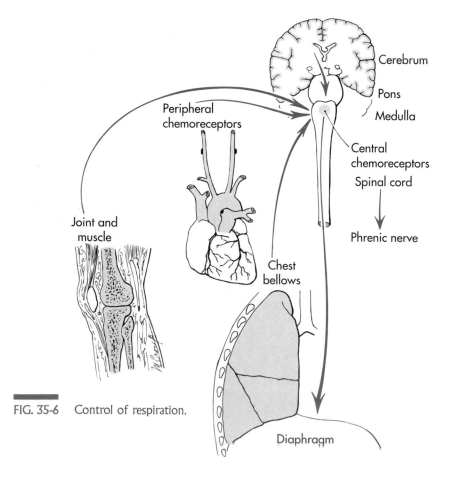

FIG. 35-6　Control of respiration.

late an increase in ventilation. Voluntary control input from the cerebrum can modify output from the respiratory centers, thus allowing interruption of the normal breathing cycle for laughing, crying, and speaking. The pattern and rhythmic control of breathing are exercised through the interaction of the respiratory centers located in the pons and medulla. Final motor output is transmitted via the spinal cord and phrenic nerve, which supplies the diaphragm, the principal muscle of ventilation. Other major nerves involved are the spinal accessory and thoracic intercostal nerves, which supply the accessory muscles of respiration and the intercostal muscles.

Defenses of the Respiratory Tract

The large surface area of the lung, which is separated only by a thin membrane from the circulatory system, makes a person theoretically vulnerable to invasion by foreign bodies (dust) and bacteria in the inhaled air; however, the lower respiratory tract is normally sterile. Several defense mechanisms maintain this sterility. The swallowing or gag reflex, which prevents entry of food or fluid into the trachea, and the action of the "mucociliary escalator," which traps dust and bacteria and transports them to the throat, have already been mentioned. Furthermore, the mucous blanket contains factors that may be effective in defense, including immunoglobulins (especially IgA), polymorphonuclear leukocytes, and interferon. The cough reflex provides another, more forceful mechanism to expel secretions upward so that they may be swallowed or expectorated. The *alveolar macrophage* provides the final and most important defense against bacterial invasion of the lung. The alveolar macrophage is a phagocytic cell with unique migratory and enzymatic

characteristics. It moves freely over the alveolar surface and engulfs inert particulate matter and bacteria. After a microbial particle is engulfed, reactive O_2 metabolites, such as hydrogen peroxide within the macrophage, kill and digest the microorganism without producing any obvious inflammatory reaction. The dust particle or microorganism is then transported by the macrophage to the lymphatics or to the bronchioles, where it is removed by the mucociliary escalator. Alveolar macrophages can clear the lung of inhaled bacteria with amazing speed. Ethyl alcohol ingestion, cigarette smoking, and corticosteroid drugs interfere with this defense mechanism.

PHYSIOLOGIC CONSIDERATIONS

The physiologic process of respiration by which O_2 is transferred from the air to the tissues and CO_2 is excreted in the expired air may be divided into three main stages, as illustrated in Fig. 35-7. The first stage is *ventilation,* which is the flow of a mixture of gases into and out of the lungs. The second stage, *transportation,* must be considered from several aspects: (1) the diffusion of gases between the alveolus and pulmonary capillary (external respiration) and between the systemic blood and tissue cells, (2) the distribution of blood in the pulmonary circulation and its match with the distribution of air in the alveoli, and (3) the chemical and physical reactions of O_2 and CO_2 with the blood. Cell respiration, or internal respiration, is the final stage of respiration, during which substrates are oxidized to obtain energy and CO_2 is produced as a waste product of cell metabolism and excreted by the lungs.

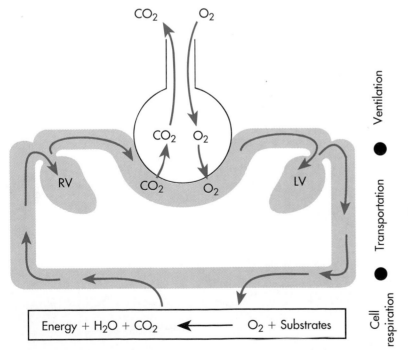

FIG. 35-7   Principal stages of the respiratory process. *RV,* Right ventricle; *LV,* left ventricle.

Ventilation

Air moves in and out of the lungs because pressure gradients are created between the atmosphere and the alveoli by muscular mechanical means. As mentioned previously, the thoracic cage functions as a bellows. The changes in the intrapleural and intrapulmonary (airway) pressures and lung volumes during ventilation may be followed on the graph in Fig. 35-8. During inspiration the volume of the thorax increases because of the descent of the diaphragm and the elevation of the ribs caused by the contraction of several muscles. The sternocleidomastoid muscles lift upward on the sternum, whereas the serratus, scalene, and external intercostal muscles all are involved in elevation of the ribs. The thorax enlarges in three directions: anteroposteriorly, laterally, and vertically. This increase in volume causes the intrapleural pressure to decrease from about -4 mm Hg (relative to atmospheric pressure) to about -8 mm Hg as the lungs are pulled to a more expanded position during inspiration. At the same time, intrapulmonary or airway pressure decreases to about -2 mm Hg (relative to atmospheric pressure) from 0 mm Hg at the beginning of inspiration. The pressure gradient between the airways and the atmosphere causes air to flow into the lungs until airway pressure at the end of inspiration is again equal to atmospheric pressure.

During quiet breathing, expiration is a passive movement produced by the elastic recoil of the chest wall and lungs. As the external intercostal muscles relax, the rib cage is lowered and the dome of the diaphragm ascends into the thoracic cavity, causing the volume of the thorax to decrease. The internal intercostal muscles may forcefully pull the ribs downward and inward during active forceful expiration, coughing, defecating, or vomiting. In addition, the abdominal muscles may contract, increasing the intraabdominal pressure and pushing the diaphragm upward. This decrease in volume of the thorax causes both intrapleural and intrapulmonary pressures to increase. The intrapulmonary pressure now rises to about 1 or 2 mm Hg above that of the atmosphere. The pressure gradient between the airways and the atmosphere is now

reversed, causing gas to flow out of the lungs until airway and atmospheric pressure are again equal at the end of expiration. Note that intrapleural pressure is always below atmospheric pressure during the respiratory cycle. Alterations in ventilation are assessed by pulmonary function tests. The alterations, their significance, and additional complexities of mechanical ventilation are discussed in Chapter 36.

Transportation
Diffusion

The second stage in the respiratory process involves the diffusion of gases across the thin (less than 0.5 μm thick) alveolocapillary membrane interface. The driving force for this transfer is the partial pressure gradients between the blood and gas phases. The partial pressure of oxygen (P_{O_2}) in the atmosphere at sea level is about 159 mm Hg (21% of 760 mm Hg). By the time O_2 is inspired and reaches the alveoli, P_{O_2} is reduced to about 103 mm Hg. This decrease in P_{O_2} occurs because inspired air is mixed with old anatomic dead-space air from the conducting airways and with water vapor. The anatomic dead space normally holds a volume of about 1 ml of air per pound of body weight (e.g., 150 ml per 150-pound man). Only the fresh air that reaches the alveolus is effective ventilation. As seen in Fig. 35-9, the partial pressure of oxygen in the mixed venous blood ($P_{\bar{V}O_2}$) in the pulmonary capillary is about 40 mm Hg. Because the P_{O_2} in the capillary is less than that in the alveolus ($P_{A_{O_2}}$ = 103 mm Hg), O_2 diffuses readily into the bloodstream. A much smaller pressure gradient (6 mm Hg) between the blood and alveolar carbon dioxide ($P_{A_{CO_2}}$) causes CO_2 to diffuse into the alveolus. The CO_2 is then expired into the atmosphere, where its concentration is essentially zero. The CO_2 gradient between blood and alveolus, even though very small, is adequate, since it diffuses about 20 times more readily than O_2 across the alveolocapillary membrane because of its greater solubility in lipid.

Under normal resting conditions, diffusion and equilibration occur between O_2 in the pulmonary capillary

FIG. 35-8   Changes in intrapleural and intrapulmonary (airway) pressures during inspiration and expiration.

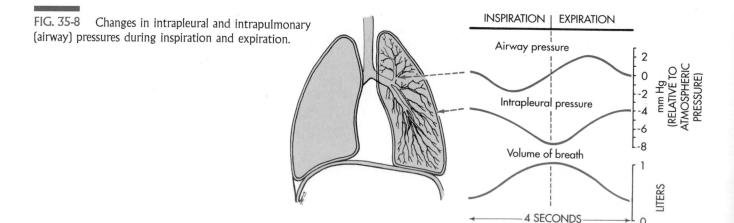

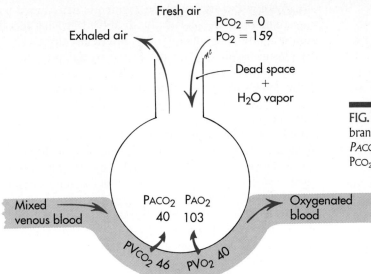

FIG. 35-9   Diffusion of gases across the alveolocapillary membrane. P_{CO_2}, P_{O_2}, Partial pressure of carbon dioxide, oxygen; P_{ACO_2}, P_{AO_2}, alveolar P_{CO_2}, P_{O_2}; P_{VCO_2}, P_{VO_2}, mixed venous P_{CO_2}, P_{O_2}.

blood and alveolus in about 0.25 second of the total contact time of 0.75 second, suggesting that the normal lung has much diffusion time in reserve. In some diseases (e.g., pulmonary fibrosis) the blood-gas barrier may be thickened and diffusion so slowed that equilibrium may be incomplete, especially during exercise when total contact time is reduced. Thus diffusion block may contribute to hypoxemia, but it is not believed to be a major factor. CO_2 elimination is not thought to be affected by diffusion abnormalities.

Ventilation-perfusion relationships

The effective transfer of gas between the alveolus and pulmonary capillary bed requires an even distribution of air in the lungs and perfusion (blood flow) in the capillaries. In other words, the ventilation and perfusion of a pulmonary unit must be evenly matched. In the normal upright person at rest, ventilation and perfusion are nearly evenly matched except at the apex of the lung. The low-pressure, low-resistance pulmonary circulation results in a greater flow of blood at the base of the lung than at the apex as a result of the influence of gravity. Ventilation, however, is fairly evenly distributed. The mean value for the ratio of ventilation to perfusion ($\dot{V}/\dot{Q}$) is 0.8. This figure is obtained by taking the ratio of the normal rate of alveolar ventilation (4 L/minute) and dividing it by the normal cardiac output (5 L/minute). Fig. 35-10 illustrates the normal state of evenly matched ventilation and perfusion in the lung, which is near unity, at 0.8.

Ventilation-perfusion inequalities occur in most respiratory diseases. Fig. 35-11 illustrates three theoretic abnormal respiratory units. Fig. 35-11, *A*, depicts a *dead-space unit* in which there is normal ventilation but no perfusion, causing ventilation to be wasted ($\dot{V}/\dot{Q}$ = infinity). The second abnormal respiratory unit (Fig. 35-11, *B*) is a *shunt unit* in which there is normal perfusion but no ventilation, so perfusion is wasted ($\dot{V}/\dot{Q}$ = 0). The last unit

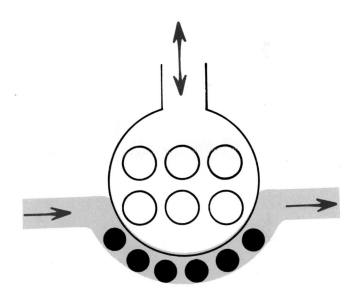

FIG. 35-10   Even match of ventilation and perfusion in an ideal respiratory unit (normal $\dot{V}/\dot{Q}$ = 0.8).

(Fig. 35-11, *C*) is a *silent unit* in which there is neither ventilation nor perfusion. Variations occur between the three extremes depending on the overall balance between ventilation and perfusion in the lungs. Lung diseases and functional respiratory disorders may be classified physiologically according to whether they are largely shunt-producing ($\dot{V}/\dot{Q}$ less than 0.8) or dead-space-producing ($\dot{V}/\dot{Q}$ greater than 0.8) diseases.

Oxygen transport in the blood

Oxygen can be transported from the lungs to the tissues via two routes: physically dissolved in the plasma or chemically combined with hemoglobin (Hb) as *oxyhemoglobin* (HbO$_2$). The chemical combination of O$_2$ with Hb is reversible, and the actual amount carried in this form is related in a nonlinear fashion to the PaO$_2$ (partial pressure of oxygen in the arterial blood), which is determined by the amount of O_2 physically dissolved in the blood plasma. In turn, the amount of O_2 physically dissolved in the plasma is directly related to the partial pressure of oxygen in the alveolus (P_{AO_2}). It also depends on the solubility of O_2 in plasma. The amount of physically dissolved O_2 is normally very small because of its low solubility in plasma. Only about 1% of the total O_2 transported to the tissues is transported in this manner. This method of transport is not sufficient to support life even at rest. The great bulk of O_2 is carried by Hb, which is located inside the red blood cells. Under certain circumstances (e.g., carbon monoxide poisoning or massive hemolysis with insufficient Hb), sufficient O_2 to support life may be transported in physical solution by subjecting the patient to O_2 under greater than atmospheric pressure *(hyperbaric oxygen chamber)*.

Fig. 35-12 illustrates the relationships involved in oxyhemoglobin transportation. A gram of Hb can combine with 1.34 ml O_2. Because the average Hb concentration in the blood for the adult male is about 15 g/dl, 1 dl of blood can carry 20.1 (15×1.34) ml of O_2 when it is completely saturated (S_{AO_2} = 100%). However, a small amount of mixed venous blood from the bronchial circulation is added to the oxygenated blood leaving the pulmonary capillaries (see Fig. 35-9). This dilution accounts for only about 97% of the blood leaving the lungs being saturated and 19.5 (0.97×20.1) volume percent being carried to the tissues.

At the tissue level, O_2 dissociates from Hb into the plasma and diffuses from the plasma into the tissue cells to supply tissue needs. Although tissue needs are highly variable, normally about 75% of Hb is still combined with O_2 when it returns to the lungs as mixed venous blood. Thus only about 25% of the O_2 in the arterial blood is used to supply the tissues. Hb that has dissociated from O_2 at the tissue level is called *reduced hemoglobin*. Reduced Hb is purple in color and accounts for the bluish color of venous blood, which is observed in the superficial veins, as in the hands, whereas oxyhemoglobin (Hb combined with O_2) is bright red in color and accounts for the color of arterial blood.

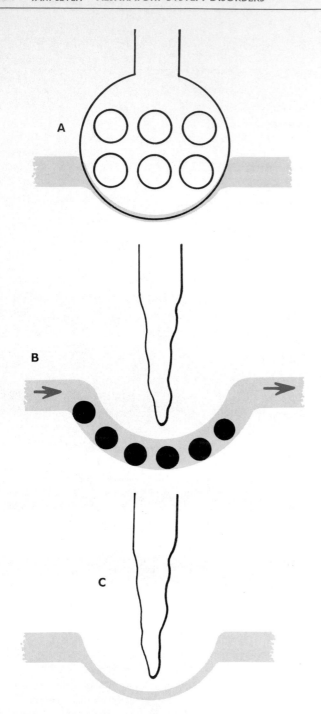

FIG. 35-11   Three theoretic respiratory units. **A,** Dead-space unit: normal ventilation but no perfusion. **B,** Shunt unit: normal perfusion but no ventilation. **C,** Silent unit: no ventilation and no perfusion.

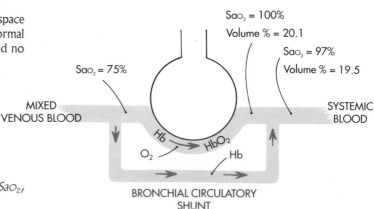

FIG. 35-12   Oxyhemoglobin *[HbO₂]* transportation. *SaO₂,* Oxygen-saturation; *Hb,* hemoglobin.

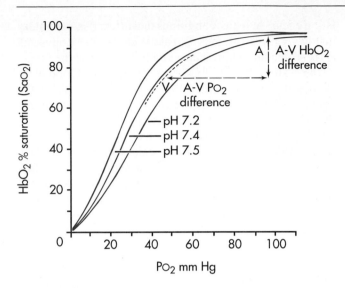

FIG. 35-13   Oxyhemoglobin (HbO₂) dissociation curve. A, Arterial; V, venous.

Oxyhemoglobin dissociation curve

A clear understanding of O_2 carrying capacity requires that one understand the affinity of hemoglobin for oxygen because tissue O_2 supply, as well as pulmonary O_2 uptake, depends critically on this relationship. This knowledge is necessary to interpret blood gas measurements correctly and to apply therapeutic measures for respiratory insufficiency. If whole blood is exposed to different partial pressures of O_2 and the percent saturation of Hb is measured, an S-shaped curve is obtained when these two measurements are plotted. This curve is known as the *oxyhemoglobin dissociation curve* and demonstrates the affinity of Hb for O_2 at various partial pressures. In Fig. 35-13 the middle curve represents the affinity relation between O_2 and Hb under normal conditions of body temperature (98.6° F) and a blood pH of 7.4.

One fact of great physiologic importance to be noted about the curve is that there is a flat upper portion, known as the *arterial portion* (A), and a lower, steeper *venous portion* (V), which is shifted slightly to the right. At the flat upper portion of the curve, large changes in P_{O_2} are associated with very small changes in oxyhemoglobin saturation. This implies that relatively constant quantities of O_2 can be supplied to the tissues even at high altitudes where the P_{O_2} may be 60 mm Hg or less. It also implies that the administration of O_2 in high concentrations (normal air = 21%) to patients with mild hypoxemia (P_{aO_2} = 60 to 75 mm Hg) is wasted because oxyhemoglobin can be increased by only a small amount. In fact, the administration of high O_2 concentrations may be toxic to the lung tissues and may produce other harmful effects. The release of O_2 to the tissues is augmented by the relation of the P_{O_2} to oxygen saturation (S_{aO_2}) on the steep venous portion of the curve, where large changes in oxyhemoglobin saturation are associated with small changes in the

TABLE 35-1   Factors Affecting Oxyhemoglobin (HbO₂) Affinity

HbO₂ Dissociation Curve	
Shift to Left (Decreased P_{50})	Shift to Right (Increased P_{50})
1 ↑ pH	1 ↓ pH
2 ↓ P_{CO_2}	2 ↑ P_{CO_2}
3 ↓ Temperature	3 ↑ Temperature
4 ↓ 2,3-DPG	4 ↑ 2,3-DPG

P_{50}, Oxygen tension required to produce 50% saturation; P_{CO_2}, carbon dioxide partial pressure; *2,3-DPG*, 2-3-diphosphoglycerate.

P_{O_2}. The normal differences in oxyhemoglobin saturation and P_{O_2} between arterial and mixed venous blood are indicated by the arrows on Fig. 35-13.

The affinity of Hb for O_2 is influenced by many other factors that accompany tissue metabolism and that may be modified by disease. Table 35-1 lists some of these factors and their effect on the affinity of Hb for O_2.

The oxyhemoglobin curve is shifted to the right (Fig. 35-13) in cases of a decrease in blood pH or a rise in the P_{CO_2}. In this state, Hb has less affinity for O_2 at a given P_{O_2}, so less O_2 can be transported in the blood. Pathologic conditions that cause metabolic *acidosis,* such as shock (production of excess lactic acid from anaerobic metabolism) or the retention of CO_2 (as in many pulmonary diseases), cause a shift of the curve to the right. A slight shift of the curve to the right, represented by the venous portion of the normal curve (pH 7.38), assists the release of O_2 to the tissues. This shift is called the *Bohr effect.* The slight increase in acidity results from the effect of CO_2 being released from the tissues. Other factors causing a shift of the curve to the right are an increase in temperature and increased 2,3-diphosphoglycerate (2,3-DPG), which is an organic phosphate in red blood cells that binds Hb and decreases its affinity for O_2. Red blood cell 2,3-DPG is increased in conditions of anemia and chronic hypoxemia. It is important to appreciate that although the O_2-carrying capability of Hb is decreased with a rightward shift of the curve, Hb release of O_2 to the tissues is facilitated. Therefore, in conditions of anemia and chronic hypoxemia, the rightward shift of the curve is compensatory. A rightward shift of the curve with a rise in temperature, reflecting increased cell metabolism and a greater need for O_2, is also adaptive and causes more O_2 to be released to the tissues for a given blood flow.

Conversely, an increase in blood pH *(alkalosis)* or a decrease in P_{CO_2}, temperature, and 2,3-DPG causes a leftward shift in the oxyhemoglobin dissociation curve (Fig. 35-13). The shift to the left causes Hb to have a greater affinity for O_2. Thus increased O_2 uptake occurs in the lung with a leftward shift, but release of O_2 to the tissues is impaired. Therefore it is theoretically possible to have hypoxia (insufficient tissue O_2 to meet metabolic needs) in severe conditions of alkalosis, especially if accompanied by hypoxemia. This condition could occur during mechanical overventilation with a respirator or at high altitudes as a result of hyperventilation. Because hyperventilation is also known to decrease cerebral blood flow as a result of the decrease in the $PaCO_2$, cerebral ischemia might also account for symptoms of lightheadedness common under such conditions. Stored blood loses 2,3-DPG activity and causes a greater affinity of Hb for O_2. Therefore patients who receive transfusions of massive amounts of stored blood may also have impaired O_2 release to the tissues because of the leftward shift in the oxyhemoglobin dissociation curve.

The affinity of Hb is popularly defined by the PO_2 required to produce 50% saturation (P_{50}) and is readily measured in modern laboratories. Normally, P_{50} is about 27 mm Hg. It is evident that P_{50} will be increased with the shift of the dissociation curve to the right (decreased Hb affinity for O_2) and reduced with a shift of the curve to the left (increased Hb affinity for O_2).

Hb has an affinity for carbon monoxide (CO) that is about 250 times greater than that for O_2. When this gas is inhaled, it combines with Hb to form carboxyhemoglobin. When O_2 combines with carboxyhemoglobin, the reaction is not reversible, so the amount of Hb available for O_2 transport is reduced. In addition, there is a leftward shift of the remaining normal Hb, resulting in deficient unloading of O_2 to the tissues.

Carbon dioxide transport in the blood

CO_2 homeostasis is also a necessary aspect of respiratory sufficiency. The transportation of CO_2 from the tissues to the lungs for elimination is accomplished in three ways. About 10% of the CO_2 is physically dissolved in plasma because CO_2, unlike O_2, is highly soluble in plasma. About 20% of the CO_2 is combined with the amino groups on Hb (carbaminohemoglobin) in the red blood cell, and about 70% is transported as plasma bicarbonate (HCO_3^-). CO_2 combines with water as shown in the following reaction:

$$CO_2 + H_2O \rightleftharpoons H_2CO_3 \rightleftharpoons H^+ + HCO_3^-$$

This reaction is reversible and is known as the *bicarbonate–carbonic acid buffer equation.* The acid-base balance of the body is greatly affected by pulmonary function and CO_2 homeostasis. In general, *hyperventilation* (alveolar ventilation in excess of metabolic needs) causes alkalosis (increases in blood pH above the normal 7.4) as a result of the excess excretion of CO_2 from the lungs; *hypoventilation* (alveolar ventilation insufficient to meet metabolic needs) causes acidosis (decrease of the blood pH below the normal 7.4) as a result of the retention of CO_2 by the lungs. It is evident from examining the buffer equation that lowering the PCO_2, as in hyperventilation, causes the reaction to proceed to the left, with consequent lowering of the H^+ concentration (elevated pH), and that raising the PCO_2 causes the reaction to proceed to the right, producing an increase in H^+ (decreased pH). Hypoventi-

lation occurs in many conditions that affect the respiratory bellows. CO_2 retention is also associated with emphysema and chronic bronchitis caused by trapped air in the lungs.

Just as the amount of O_2 transported in the blood is related to the PO_2 to which the blood is exposed, so the amount of CO_2 in the blood is related to the PCO_2. Unlike the S-shaped oxyhemoglobin dissociation curve, the CO_2 dissociation curve is nearly linear in the physiologic range of PCO_2. (See Fig. 41-1, which compares the CO_2 and oxyhemoglobin dissociation curves.) This means that the CO_2 content of the blood is directly related to the PCO_2. In addition, there is never any significant barrier to CO_2 diffusion. Therefore the $PaCO_2$ provides a good index of the adequacy of ventilation.

ASSESSMENT OF RESPIRATORY STATUS

It is important to point out that knowledge of the blood gases (PO_2, PCO_2, and pH of arterial blood) alone does not give enough information about the transport of O_2 and CO_2 to be sure that a patient's tissues are being oxygenated properly. Many other factors are involved in the transport process, such as the adequacy of cardiac output and tissue perfusion, as well as diffusion of gases at the tissue level. For example, in shock tissue perfusion may be inadequate as a result of shunting of blood past the tissue cells, stagnation of blood caused by pooling, and inadequate cardiac output. Tissue edema may also interfere with the diffusion pathway at the tissue level. Consequently the detection of tissue hypoxia must always involve clinical observations as well as the interpretation of blood gases.

Other important information needed for the assessment of a patient's respiratory status is the Hb concentration, as well as the percent saturation of that Hb. The correlation among PaO_2, SaO_2, and oxyhemoglobin in volume percent for a patient with anemia (Hb = 10 g/dl), one with a normal Hb of 15 g/dl, and another with polycythemia (Hb = 20 g/dl) is shown in Fig. 35-14. All the information illustrated is necessary for a proper assessment of O_2 transport. Note that the percent saturation of Hb is independent of the Hb concentration, whereas the O_2 content in volume percent is directly related to Hb concentration. The volume percent reveals how much O_2 can be delivered to the tissues at a given PaO_2. For example, at a PaO_2 of 100 mm Hg and 100% saturation of Hb with O_2, the polycythemic patient can transport 26.8 ml of O_2 in every 100 ml blood (O_2 content = 26.8 vol %), whereas the anemic patient can deliver only 13.4 ml at the same PaO_2 and SaO_2. This is a two-fold variation and illustrates that knowledge of the blood gases alone is insufficient information for respiratory assessment. Hb concentration, SaO_2, and cardiac status are also vital data.

From the previous discussion of the structure and function of the respiratory system, one can see that adequate respiration can be inhibited on a number of levels. For

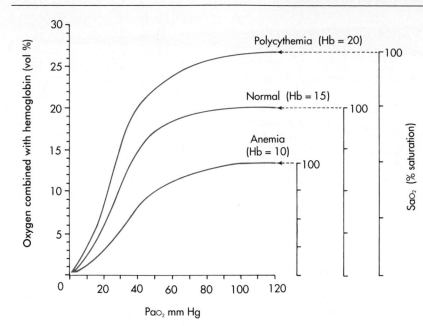

FIG. 35-14   Relationship of hemoglobin *(Hb)* content (g/dl) to oxygen content of blood at various arterial oxygen tensions *(PaO$_2$).* (From Slonim NB, Hamilton LH: *Respiratory physiology,* ed 3, St Louis, 1976, Mosby.)

example, brain injury or barbiturate overdose in an attempted suicide may interfere with control by the respiratory centers in the central nervous system. A decrease in the Po$_2$ of inspired air as a result of high altitudes or airway obstruction interferes with respiration. Neuromuscular diseases and skeletal deformities of the chest result in inadequate bellows performance. Respiratory difficulty occurs at the alveolocapillary interface when there is thickening of the diffusion pathway, as in pulmonary fibrosis or edema. Transport of gases in the blood may be interfered with in many respects, including the limiting factor of the amount of Hb. The pulmonary, cardiovascular, and hematologic systems are thus intimately associated with tissue oxygenation.

QUESTIONS

▼ *Answer the following on a separate sheet of paper.*

1. List three disorders of the respiratory system that are a major source of morbidity and mortality.
2. Define respiration.
3. Draw and label the epithelial surface of the airways, and discuss the function of the mucosal lining in respiration (see inset *B* of Fig. 35-1 if you have forgotten the structure of the mucosal lining of the airways).
4. Why are foreign bodies, when aspirated, usually found in the right mainstem bronchus?
5. What would happen if the pressure within the pleural space were to become equal to that of the atmosphere?
6. Sketch the position of the lungs in the circulatory system, and describe some of the unique features of blood supply to the lungs. (Review Fig. 35-4 if you have forgotten the functional position of the lungs in the circulation.)
7. If the mean pulmonary artery pressure is 30 mm Hg and the colloid osmotic pressure of the blood is 20 mm Hg, is pulmonary edema likely to occur? Why or why not?

▼ *Complete the following statements by filling in the blanks.*

8. The structure that forms the division between the upper and lower respiratory tracts is the _____.
9. The alveoli are lined by a lipoprotein substance called _____. During inspiration, expansion is facilitated, and during expiration, collapse is prevented as this substance functions to lower the _____.
10. The movement of air in and out of the lungs is called _____. To accomplish this function, the thoracic cage and lungs have been compared to a reciprocating pump or _____. The muscle that provides the main driving force during inspiration is the _____.
11. A reflex that controls the amount of air taken into the lungs is known as the _____ reflex.
12. Centers that control the pattern and rhythmicity of breathing are located in the _____ and _____ of the brain.

Continued.

? QUESTIONS—cont'd

▼ *Circle the letter preceding each item below that correctly completes the statement. Choose the one best answer.*

13. Respiration is most affected by:
    a. Body heat
    b. pH
    c. Pa_{CO_2}
    d. Pa_{O_2}
    e. Reflexes from moving limbs

14. The tracheobronchial tree divides repeatedly in a dichotomous fashion and in ever-decreasing sizes until the final pulmonary functional unit is reached. The generations of subdivisions involved number:
    a. 64
    b. 32
    c. 23
    d. 10

15. The right lung has:
    a. 10 lobes
    b. 8 lobes
    c. 3 lobes
    d. 2 lobes

16. Each bronchus divides into functional subunits that include:
    a. Lobar bronchi
    b. Segmental bronchi
    c. Terminal bronchioles
    d. Respiratory bronchioles
    e. All the above

17. The functional unit of the lung (acinus) consists of all the following *except:*
    a. Terminal bronchioles
    b. Respiratory bronchioles
    c. Alveolar duct
    d. Alveolar sac
    e. Alveoli

18. The pores of Kohn:
    a. Are located between pulmonary capillaries
    b. May provide collateral ventilation
    c. Are artifacts and do not really exist
    d. Provide a communication between right and left lungs

19. Alveolar macrophages:
    a. Move freely over the alveolar surface
    b. Are phagocytic cells
    c. Contain lytic enzymes
    d. Are inhibited by cigarette smoking, alcohol ingestion, and corticosteroid drugs
    e. All the above

20. The left mainstem bronchus is:
    a. Symmetric with the right
    b. Shorter and broader than the right

c. Nearer to the vertical in its course than the right
    d. More angulated than the right

21. All the following structures are closely associated with the larynx *except* the:
    a. Epiglottis
    b. Glottis
    c. Carina
    d. Vocal cords

22. Protective functions of the larynx include all the following *except:*
    a. Swallowing reflex
    b. Cough
    c. Major role in humidification of inspired air

23. Match the number of the structure in Fig. 35-15 with the appropriate term from the following list:
    a. Diaphragm   h. Mainstem
    b. Carina   bronchus
    c. Epiglottis   i. Segmental
    d. Mediastinum   bronchus
    e. Pharynx   j. Apex of lung
    f. Larynx   k. Visceral pleura
    g. Trachea   l. Parietal pleura

24. Match the number of the structure in Fig. 35-16 with the appropriate term from the following list:
    a. Pores of Kohn   e. Acinus
    b. Alveolar duct   f. Alveolus
    c. Respiratory   g. Septum
       bronchiole
    d. Terminal bronchiole

25. Functions of the upper airway include all the following *except:*
    a. Removal of dust particles
    b. Humidification of air
    c. Participation in gas exchange
    d. Warming of inspired air

26. The normal range of intrapleural pressure relative to atmospheric pressure is about:
    a. 0 to +2 mm Hg
    b. −4 to −8 mm Hg
    c. +4 to +8 mm Hg
    d. −4 to +4 mm Hg

27. Respiratory distress syndrome in the newborn:
    a. Is related to decreased or absent surfactant

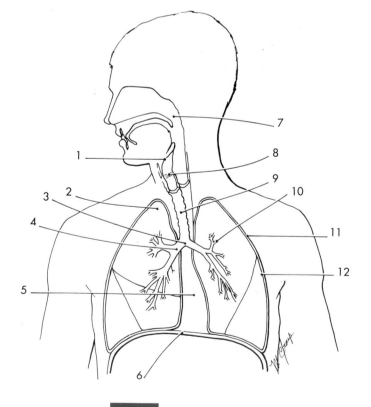

FIG. 35-15   Respiratory tract.

QUESTIONS—cont'd

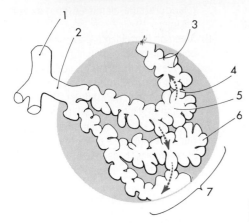

FIG. 35-16   Pulmonary functional unit.

b. Is caused by aspiration of amniotic fluid in utero
c. Most often occurs in full-term infants
d. Is the result of low alveolar surface tension

28. Conditions that may cause a deficiency in the production and release of surfactant and subsequent atelectasis include all the following *except:*
   a. Constant tidal volume breathing in a patient on a ventilator
   b. Shallow breathing in a bedridden patient
   c. Periodic deep breathing (sighing) administered to a patient on a ventilator
   d. Prolonged high concentrations of oxygen (O_2) administered to a patient
   e. Obstruction of blood flow to type II alveolar cells, as in a patient with a pulmonary embolism

29. The oxyhemoglobin dissociation curve illustrates:
   a. The amount of O_2 carried dissolved in blood plasma
   b. The amount of O_2 carried in the blood to the tissues per minute
   c. The ability of hemoglobin (Hb) to bind with O_2
   d. The ability of O_2 to diffuse from the alveolus into the blood

30. What is the clinical significance of a shift of the oxyhemoglobin dissociation curve to the right?
   a. Hb binds O_2 more tightly.
   b. O_2 is more readily dissociated from Hb.
   c. 2,3-DPG levels will be depleted.
   d. Respiratory alkalosis is present.

▼ *Answer the following on a separate sheet of paper.*

31. Why is the alveolar P_{O_2} as low as 103 mm Hg when it is 159 mm Hg in the inspired air?
32. What is the volume of your own anatomic dead space?
33. What is the chief mechanism of gas movement in the respiratory zone of the lung? What provides the driving force?
34. Are ventilation and perfusion perfectly matched in the healthy person at rest in the upright position? Why or why not?
35. If alveolar ventilation is 3 L/minute and cardiac output (perfusion) is 6 L/minute, what is the $\dot{V}/\dot{Q}$ ratio? Is this value normal, or does a person with this value have dead-space-producing or shunt-producing disease?
36. What advantage would be gained, if any, by placing a patient with severe hemolytic anemia in a hyperbaric chamber?
37. If a patient is breathing fresh air at sea level, the alveolar P_{O_2} is about 103 mm Hg, the arterial blood is 97% to 98% saturated with O_2, and the O_2 content is 20 vol %, will it be advantageous to increase the O_2 concentration of the inspired air? Why or why not?
38. Explain why the P_{O_2} can vary over a wide range and have little effect on the Hb saturation.
39. What is the Bohr effect? What is its significance in terms of tissue oxygenation?
40. When a person hyperventilates, why is there no significant increase in the O_2

content of the arterial blood, but a significant decrease in the arterial P_{CO_2}? Explain this phenomenon in terms of the O_2 and CO_2 dissociation curves.
41. Why does an elevated arterial P_{CO_2} never result from impaired diffusion?
42. Does knowledge of the blood gases alone provide all the information necessary to assess accurately the respiratory status? If not, what other data are necessary?
43. Beginning with inspired air, list at least three altered mechanisms or conditions that may interfere with normal respiration.
44. The respiratory process may be divided into three stages. List and describe each briefly.
45. Which muscles are used during normal quiet breathing? During breathing of maximum effort?
46. How many milliliters of O_2 are used by tissue cells each minute if the Hb concentration is 12.0 g/dl blood, there is 100% saturation of Hb, cardiac output is 5000 ml/minute, and 25% of O_2 delivered is used? (1.34 ml O_2 combines with each gram of Hb. Ignore the O_2 that is transported physically dissolved in blood plasma.)
47. Account for the fact that Hb is 100% saturated with O_2 on leaving the pulmonary capillary bed but is 97% to 98% saturated in the systemic arteries.
48. If alveolar ventilation doubles and CO_2 production remains constant, what are the effects on arterial P_{CO_2} and the blood pH? What happens to the oxyhemoglobin dissociation curve, and what are the consequences?
49. What is the P_{O_2} in the inspired air of a climber on the summit of Mount Everest if the atmospheric pressure is 247 mm Hg and water vapor pressure at body temperature is 47 mm Hg? Do you think the mountain climber could walk very far?

▼ *Circle the letter preceding each item below that correctly answers the question. More than one answer may be correct.*

50. In what form is most of the CO_2 carried in the venous blood?
   a. Bicarbonate
   b. Physically dissolved in the plasma
   c. Carbaminohemoglobin

Continued.

QUESTIONS—cont'd

51. Which of the following shift the oxyhemoglobin dissociation curve to the left?
    a. Decrease in temperature
    b. Increase in pH
    c. Decrease in 2,3-DPG
    d. Increase in P_{CO_2}
52. During normal quiet breathing, what will the intrapleural pressure be?
    a. Equal to atmospheric pressure
    b. Below atmospheric pressure
    c. Above atmospheric pressure

▼ *Circle the word that correctly completes each sentence.*

53. During inspiration, muscular contraction causes the size of the thorax to (increase) (decrease). This size change causes a(n) (increase) (decrease) in the intrapleural pressure. Because pressure in the alveoli is (less) (more) than atmospheric pressure, air moves (into) (out of) the lungs.

54. During expiration, when the diaphragm muscle relaxes, the diaphragm (ascends) (descends), thus (increasing) (decreasing) the volume of the thoracic cavity.

55. During normal quiet expiration, the size change in the thoracic cavity causes a(n) (increase) (decrease) in the intrapleural pressure. Because pressure in the alveoli is now (more) (less) than atmospheric pressure, air moves (into) (out of) the lungs.

56. A person is accidentally exposed to carbon monoxide, which combines with half the Hb in the arterial blood. The Pa_{O_2} will be (normal) (high) (low). The Sa_{O_2} will be (normal) (high) (low). The arterial O_2 content will be (normal) (high) (low).

57. In general, hyperventilation causes a(n) (increase) (decrease) in the P_{CO_2} and a(n) (increase) (decrease) in the blood pH, resulting in a condition of (alkalosis) (acidosis).

58. A P_{50} of 34 mm Hg means that the oxyhemoglobin curve is shifted to the (right) (left) and there is a(n) (decreased) (increased) Hb affinity for O_2.

CHAPTER 36

Diagnostic Procedures in Respiratory Disease

LORRAINE M. WILSON

MORPHOLOGIC METHODS

Diagnostic procedures used for the detection of pulmonary disease may be classified as primarily morphologic or physiologic. *Morphologic* methods include radiologic techniques, endoscopy, biopsy studies, and sputum studies. Blood gas measurements and ventilatory function tests reveal *physiologic* function.

Radiologic Techniques

The thorax is an ideal region for a radiologic examination. The aerated lung parenchyma offers little resistance to the passage of x-rays and therefore produces very radiant shadows. The soft tissues of the chest wall, the heart and great vessels, and the diaphragm do not permit the rays to pass through as readily as the lung parenchyma and thus appear denser on the radiograph. The bony structures of the thorax, including the ribs, sternum, and vertebrae, are even less readily penetrated, and their shadows are even denser. Radiologic methods typically used to detect pulmonary disease include routine chest radiography, computed tomography, fluoroscopy, bronchography, angiography, and perfusion and ventilation lung scanning.

Routine chest radiography

The routine chest radiograph is taken at a standard distance after maximum inspiration and breath holding to stabilize the diaphragm. Radiographs are taken from the posteroanterior perspective and sometimes from the lateral and oblique perspectives. These radiographs provide the following information:

1. The status of the thoracic cage, including the ribs, the pleura, and the contour of the diaphragm and of the upper airway as it enters the chest
2. The size, contour, and position of the mediastinum and hilus of the lung, including the heart, aorta, lymph nodes, and root of the bronchial tree
3. The texture and degree of aeration of the lung parenchyma
4. The size, shape, number, and location of pulmonary lesions, including cavitation, fibrous markings, and zones of consolidation

The appearance of the normal chest radiograph varies somewhat according to gender and age in different subjects and to varying conditions of respiration in the same subject. Interpreting a chest radiograph is a skill that takes considerable time to acquire. It is an invaluable aid to the physician when correlated with other observations.

Computed tomography

Computed tomography (CT) is a radiographic technique by which a series of radiographs, each representing a "slice of the lung," is taken so that a detailed image can be built up. Many more shades of gray are visible with CT than with the routine chest radiograph; also, less of a problem exists in detecting abnormalities because of obscuration by normal structures as with the routine chest radiograph. CT is of particular value for identifying abnormalities in configuration of the trachea or major bronchi, defining lesions and anatomy of the pleura or mediastinum (nodes, tumors, vascular structures), and in general, revealing the nature and extent of abnormal shadows in the lungs and other tissues of the thorax. Because it is noninvasive, mediastinal CT is often used for the assessment of mediastinal lymph node size in the staging of lung cancer, although it is not as accurate as mediastinoscopy (see Chapter 42).

Fluoroscopy

Fluoroscopy enables the radiologist to view the thorax and all its contents in motion. Information can be obtained about how various zones of the lung behave during the respiratory cycle. The diaphragm can be studied particularly well using this method. Despite its usefulness, this type of study is discouraged because of the radiation hazards to the patient and the examiner.

Bronchography

A radiograph of the chest taken after radiopaque material is introduced into the tracheobronchial tree is called a *bronchogram.* Substances typically used as radiopaque material are iodized oils and, more recently, tantalum, which is inhaled as a fine powder with the help of positive-pressure equipment. The bronchogram reveals in great detail the size and appearance of the tracheobronchial tree and therefore is a particularly useful technique for confirming the diagnosis of bronchiectasis and for detecting other forms of bronchial distortion. Postoperative care is the same as after bronchoscopy (see following discussion). In addition, percussion and postural drainage should be used to assist in the evacuation of the contrast medium.

Angiography of pulmonary vessels

The pulmonary arterial pattern and flow can be demonstrated by injecting radiopaque fluid through a catheter inserted via an arm vein into the right atrium and right ventricle and then into the main pulmonary artery. This technique is used to locate the site of a massive embolism or to determine the extent of a pulmonary infarction. Anomalies, such as aneurysms and alterations in vascularity common in emphysema, are also detectable. However, simpler diagnostic techniques are preferred for the detection of pulmonary disease whenever possible. The major risk during angiography is the development of cardiac dysrhythmia as the catheter is passed through the heart chambers.

Lung scan

The isotope lung scan, although a less reliable method for the detection of pulmonary embolism, is a safer procedure. Pulmonary perfusion and sometimes ventilation scanning are performed. A *perfusion scan* is obtained by the injection of albumin microspheres, usually labeled with technetium-99m, into a peripheral vein; these particles appear as transient emboli in the pulmonary capillaries in proportion to the active blood flow. The radioactivity distribution is counted with a scintiscanner and the image recorded with a camera. The pattern is almost always abnormal in embolism (area with absent radioactivity) but is not highly specific because abnormalities also occur in other conditions, such as emphysema and pneu-

monia. The *ventilation scan* uses the inhalation of a bolus of radioactive gas, usually xenon-133. The scan is usually normal in embolism but abnormal in infarction, pneumonia, and emphysema.

Bronchoscopy

Bronchoscopy is a technique that allows direct visualization of the trachea and its major subdivisions. It is used most frequently to confirm the diagnosis of bronchogenic carcinoma, but it can be used to remove a foreign body. The conventional bronchoscope is a hollow metal tube containing a lighted mirror-lens system, which is passed readily into the tracheobronchial tree after administration of local anesthesia. The newer *fiberoptic bronchoscope* is a flexible instrument that can transmit light and a clear image around corners. Because of its flexibility and smaller diameter, its use causes much less trauma than the conventional metal bronchoscope. The fiberoptic bronchoscope allows inspection of the smaller bronchial subdivisions and also may be passed through the nose. Tissue biopsy can be obtained by using a tiny forceps or flexible brush at the tip of the bronchoscope. Secretions for culture and cytologic studies may be obtained via suction tubes passed through the bronchoscope. The fiberoptic bronchoscopy can be performed at the bedside, although the location of choice is the operating room.

After bronchoscopy, food and fluids are withheld for 2 or 3 hours until the gag reflex returns; otherwise the patient may aspirate material into the tracheobronchial tree. The return of the gag reflex can be tested by touching a cotton applicator to the back of the patient's throat. When this causes the patient to gag, swallowing may be permitted. Other complications are bleeding and pneumothorax caused by a ruptured bronchus.

Common procedures after bronchoscopy to detect these complications are the monitoring of vital signs for several hours, a chest radiograph, and the collection of all sputum for 24 hours. The nurse should also be aware that laryngeal spasm or edema may be a delayed complication and may require endotracheal intubation and the administration of oxygen.

Biopsy Studies

Tissue specimens for biopsy study may be obtained from the upper or lower airways by endoscopic techniques using either the laryngoscope or the bronchoscope. Biopsy specimens of the pleura or lung tissue may also be obtained by either open or closed techniques. The *open technique* consists of a limited thoracotomy; a small intercostal incision is made after administration of anesthesia, and a tissue specimen is excised under direct visualization. A cylinder of tissue can also be obtained by the newer techniques of *percutaneous needle biopsy* using an air-turbine drill. The main value of the lung biopsy is in diffuse lung disease not diagnosable by other means.

Pneumothorax and bleeding are encountered in a substantial number of patients after this procedure.

Biopsy of the lymph nodes in the mediastinum is accomplished during *mediastinoscopy*. This procedure involves the insertion of a lighted mirror-lens system through an incision at the base of the anterior portion of the neck. The instrument is advanced under visual control into the mediastinum, where inspection and biopsy can be accomplished. Mediastinoscopy is the major preoperative method for pathologic evaluation of regional spread to the hilar lymph nodes in patients with lung cancer.

Sputum Studies

Gross, microscopic, and bacteriologic examinations of the sputum are important in the etiologic diagnosis of many respiratory diseases. The color, odor, and presence of blood provide valuable clues. Microscopic examination may reveal the causative organism in many bacterial pneumonias, in tuberculosis, and in some fungal infections. Exfoliative cell studies of the sputum may also be helpful in the diagnosis of lung carcinoma. The best time for collection of sputum is shortly after awakening because abnormal bronchial secretions tend to accumulate during sleep. Sometimes it is necessary to induce sputum production by the use of a nebulizer. Considerable quantities of sputum are also unknowingly swallowed; the gastric contents may then be aspirated to obtain sputum. This procedure is carried out shortly after the patient awakens in the morning after a period of fasting.

PHYSIOLOGIC METHODS: PULMONARY FUNCTION TESTS

During the past generation, numerous tests and techniques related to the study of respiratory physiology have evolved. These pulmonary function tests (PFTs) fall into two broad categories: those related to ventilatory function of the lungs and chest wall and those related to diffusion of alveolar gases. *Ventilatory* function tests include measurements of lung volumes under static and dynamic conditions as well as pressure measurements. Tests related to diffusion of alveolar gases include analysis of gases in the expired air and in the blood. *Arterial blood gas measurements* (ABGs) typically include arterial oxygen (PaO_2) and arterial carbon dioxide ($PaCO_2$) partial pressures (tensions) and pH and reflect cardiopulmonary physiology.

PFTs are becoming an increasingly important part of routine clinical evaluation and are taking their place among other diagnostic aids such as the chest radiograph and electrocardiogram. It is important to realize, however, that these tests show only the effects of disease on function and cannot be used to give a diagnosis on the basis of a pathologic change. Some diseases, however, have a characteristic pattern of disordered function, and it is possible to distinguish an obstructive pattern of ventilatory abnormality from a restrictive pattern. *Obstructive* ventilatory disorders affect the ability to exhale, whereas *restrictive* disorders affect the ability to inhale. Two major patterns of functional disorders that also emerge from ABGs are disorders in which there is increased *dead space* or disorders in which there is increased *shunting*.

It is essential to realize that no single PFT can measure all possible attributes. Nevertheless, PFTs give valuable information. Ventilatory function tests give quantitative data so that the progress of a lung disease, as well as response to treatment, may be followed. In cases of pulmonary disability in which surgery is planned, such tests help to assess the patient's ability to tolerate anesthetics, narcotics, or removal of lung tissue and to prescribe the postoperative care needed. Because only one aspect of pulmonary function may be altered by some diseases, PFTs occasionally assist in establishing the diagnosis. ABGs are an invaluable aid in assessing the severity of respiratory insufficiency and guiding the appropriate therapy. This chapter focuses on those PFTs that are most widely used and most helpful in patient management.

Ventilatory Function Tests
Static lung volumes

Lung volumes and capacities are anatomic measurements that are affected by exercise and disease. There are four lung volumes and four lung capacities. Lung capacities always consist of two or more lung volumes. Fig. 36-1 shows the relationship between these measurements and the average values for a young, healthy, adult man. Table 36-1 lists the abbreviations and provides a description of the lung capacities and volumes. The following five lung capacities and volumes (designated by the abbreviations listed in the table) can be measured directly on an instrument called the spirometer: V_T, IRV, ERV, VC, and IC. The FRC is measured by indirect means using helium or nitrogen washout methods or by using the body plethysmograph. The TLC and RV are then derived arithmetically (i.e., TLC = FRC + IC and RV = TLC − VC).

A *spirometer* is a simple instrument containing a bellows or bell that is displaced as the patient breathes into it through a valve and connecting tube, as shown in Fig. 36-2. As the spirometer is used, a graphic record of the measurement is made on a rotating drum with a recording pen. Computed bedside spirometry is commonly performed.

Measurements of the static lung volumes in practice are used to reflect the elastic properties of the lungs and thorax. The most useful measurements are the VC, TLC, FRC, and RV. These volumes are reduced by diseases that limit lung expansion (restrictive disorders). In contrast, diseases that cause airway obstruction almost always

▶ TABLE 36-1 Lung Capacities and Volumes

Measurement	Symbol	Adult Male Average Value (ml)	Definition
Tidal volume	V_T	500	Amount of air inhaled or exhaled with each breath (value listed is for resting conditions)
Inspiratory reserve volume	IRV	3100	Amount of air that can be forcefully inhaled after a normal tidal volume inhalation
Expiratory reserve volume	ERV	1200	Amount of air that can be forcefully exhaled after a normal tidal volume exhalation
Residual volume	RV	1200	Amount of air left in the lungs after a forced exhalation
Total lung capacity	TLC	6000	Maximum amount of air that can be contained in the lungs after a maximum inspiratory effort: $TLC = V_T + IRV + ERV + RV$; $TLC = VC + RV$
Vital capacity	VC	4800	Maximum amount of air that can be expired after a maximum inspiration: $VC = V_T + IRV + ERV$ (should be 80% TLC)
Inspiratory capacity	IC	3600	Maximum amount of air that can be inspired after a normal expiration: $IC = V_T + IRV$
Functional residual capacity	FRC	2400	Volume of air remaining in the lungs after a normal tidal volume expiration: $FRC = ERV + RV$

From Comroe JH Jr et al: *The lung,* ed 2, Chicago, 1962, Mosby.

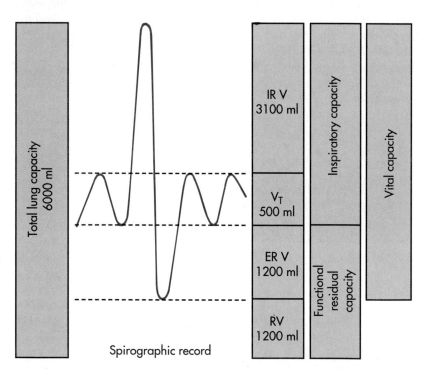

FIG. 36-1 Relationships among the lung volumes and capacities (see Table 36-1 for explanation of abbreviations).

cause an increase in RV and FRC as a result of hyperinflation of the lungs. TLC may be normal or increased, and VC is often decreased. In lung diseases in which RV is increased because of air trapping, VC must decrease by an equal amount, since TLC is relatively stable (unless part of the lung is surgically removed) and since TLC = RV + VC.

Dynamic lung volumes and work of breathing

Much more information can be obtained about the ventilatory status if the rate of air movement into and out of

the lungs is considered as well as the work of breathing. The following definitions are useful in the discussion of effective ventilation:

- *Minute volume,* or *minute ventilation* ($\dot{V}_E$), is the volume of gas collected during expiration over a 1-minute period. It may be calculated by multiplying the V_T by the respiratory rate. At rest, $\dot{V}_E$ is about 6 or 7 L/minute. The $\dot{V}_E$ is measured by collecting the expired air in a large rubber balloon and dividing the volume collected by the number of minutes taken to collect the sample. The subscript E in the symbol for

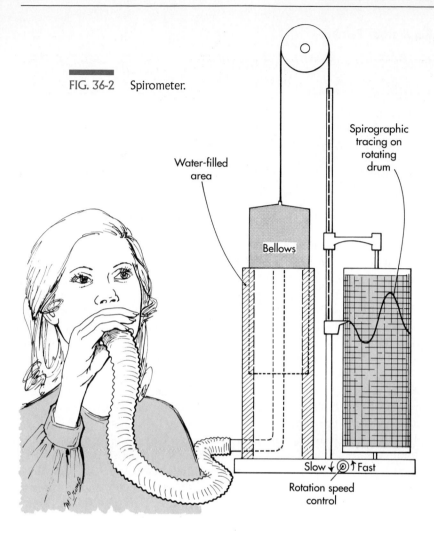

FIG. 36-2   Spirometer.

minute volume means that the measurement is made during the expiratory phase of the V_T, and the dot over the V indicates that it is a timed measurement.

- *Respiratory frequency* (f) or *rate* is the number of breaths taken per minute. At rest the respiratory rate is about 15 breaths/minute.

- *Tidal volume* (V_T) is the amount of air inhaled or exhaled with each breath. The V_T is about 500 ml at rest but may increase to 3000 ml during exercise when deep breaths are taken. It is obtained by dividing the $\dot{V}_E$ by the respiratory rate.

- *Physiologic dead space* (V_D) is the volume of inspired air that does not exchange with pulmonary blood; it may be regarded as wasted ventilation. V_D is composed of *anatomic dead space* (the volume of air in the conducting airways, about 1 ml per pound of body weight), *alveolar dead space* (alveoli being ventilated but not perfused; alveolar dead space is highly variable), and *ventilation in excess of perfusion*. In healthy persons, V_D is only slightly greater than the anatomic dead space, but it may be increased if ventilated alveoli are underperfused or not perfused at all, as in pulmonary embolism. The ratio of dead space to tidal volume (V_D/V_t) reflects the portion of the V_T that does not ex-change with pulmonary blood. In other words, V_D/V_T is a measurement of the percentage of V_T that is physiologic dead space. This ratio is calculated from data collected by measuring the carbon dioxide tension (P_{CO_2}) in the expired air and the P_{CO_2} in the arterial blood. The larger the difference between these two measurements, the greater is the V_D. The V_D/V_T ratio does not exceed 30% to 40% in the healthy person. This ratio is frequently used to follow the course of patients receiving mechanical ventilation.

- *Alveolar ventilation* ($\dot{V}_A$) is the volume of fresh gas entering the alveoli each minute that exchanges with pulmonary blood; it is the effective ventilation. $\dot{V}_A$ is normally about 4.2 L/minute at rest and is calculated by either of the following formulas:

$$\dot{V}_A = (V_T - V_D) \times f$$

$$\dot{V}_A = \dot{V}_E - \dot{V}_D$$

$\dot{V}_A$ is a better index of ventilation than $\dot{V}_E$ or V_T because it takes into account the volume of air wasted in ventilating the V_D. The calculations in Table 36-2 illustrate the relationship among $\dot{V}_E$, breathing pattern, and effective $\dot{V}_A$. The V_D for each of the three patients is assumed to be constant at 150 ml, but the rate and depth of breathing vary.

Patient	V_D (ml)	V_T (ml)	f (breaths/min)	$\dot{V}_E$ ($V_T \times f$) (L/min)	$\dot{V}_A$ [($V_T - V_D$) $\times$ f] (L/min)	V_D/V_T (%)
Patient A (rapid, shallow breathing)	150	250	40	10	4	60
Patient B (normal rate and depth)	150	500	20	10	7	30
Patient C (slow, deep breathing)	150	1000	10	10	$8\frac{1}{2}$	15

See text for abbreviations.

Several deductions can be made from the data in Table 36-2. In each case the total amount of air entering and leaving the lungs is the same ($\dot{V}_E$), although there is great variation in the percentage of the V_T that is physiologic dead space and in the effective ventilation. It is evident that rapid, shallow breathing results in less effective ventilation as more is wasted in dead-space volume. This fact becomes obvious if one considers the formula for the calculation of $\dot{V}_A$. As V_T approaches V_D (150 ml), effective ventilation approaches zero, regardless of the rapidity of the respiratory rate (0 $\times$ f = 0). The percentage of the V_T that is physiologic dead space also approaches 100% as the V_T approaches the V_D. Considering that total V_D (anatomic and alveolar) can vary greatly with disease, it is obvious that clinical observation of ventilatory adequacy has great limitations, even though some gross qualitative judgments can be made.

For air to move in and out of the lungs, the body must work to overcome the combined resistances of the thorax, lungs, and abdomen. The work (in the form of energy expenditure to move the chest bellows) is referred to as the *work of breathing*. The work of breathing can be expressed as the amount of O_2 consumed by the respiratory muscles. In the normal person at rest, this is a small fraction (less than 5%) of the total body O_2 consumption, but in disease the proportion may be much greater.

Expenditure of energy is required to overcome two types of resistance: elastic and nonelastic. The *elastic resistance* is the resistance to stretch caused by the elastic properties of the lungs and thorax. The elastic properties of the thorax result from the stretching properties of the tendons, muscles, and connective tissue. The elastic properties of the lungs are produced by the surface tension of fluid lining the alveoli and by the elastic fibers throughout the lung itself. *Nonelastic resistance* is the frictional resistance to airflow in the airways and, to a small degree, resistance resulting from the viscosity of the lung tissues. The work of breathing increases if there is an increase in either the elastic resistance (e.g., "stiff lungs" as in pulmonary fibrosis) or the nonelastic resistance (e.g., turbulent airflow in emphysema as a result of narrowing of the airways).

Compliance (C) is a measure of the elastic properties (distensibility) of the lungs and thorax and is defined as the change in volume per unit change in pressure under static conditions. Total compliance (compliance of the lungs and thorax) or lung compliance alone can be determined. Two manometers are used to measure pressure changes: one is connected to the mouth or nostrils (to measure alveolar pressure or the total pressure exerted by the lung-thorax system) and the other to an esophageal balloon (to measure intrapleural pressure). Volume and pressure changes (ΔV, ΔP) are then measured under various degrees of lung inflation and breath holding. Compliance is estimated by calculating the slope of the pressure-volume curve, which is plotted from the data. Normal lung compliance and thoracic cage compliance over the V_T range are each 0.2 L/cm H_2O, and total compliance (lungs and thoracic cage) is about 0.1 L/cm H_2O:

$$C = \frac{\Delta V \text{ (change in lung volume in liters)}}{\Delta P \text{ (change in pressure in centimeters of water)}}$$

Compliance is reduced in restrictive patterns of pulmonary disease that increase the stiffness of the lung or thorax and limit expansion. In these patients a greater force (ΔP) than normal is required to give the same increase in volume (ΔV), causing the compliance to be smaller. Common causes of decreased lung compliance are atelectasis (collapse of alveoli), pulmonary edema, pneumonia, and pulmonary fibrosis. When pulmonary surfactant is decreased, compliance is also decreased because the lung becomes stiffer as a result of the increase in surface tension (surfactant normally reduces surface tension). Chest wall compliance is reduced in obesity, abdominal distention, and bony deformities of the chest cage such as kyphoscoliosis.

The *nonelastic airway resistance* (R_{AW}) can be measured by placing the subject in an airtight box (body plethysmograph) and measuring the pressure around the body (which reflects the change in alveolar pressure); at the same time the rate of flow of air at the mouth is measured (Fig. 36-3). The R_{AW} reflects the nonelastic resistance of the upper airways (first to twelfth generations of the tracheobronchial tree) and is approximately 1.8 cm

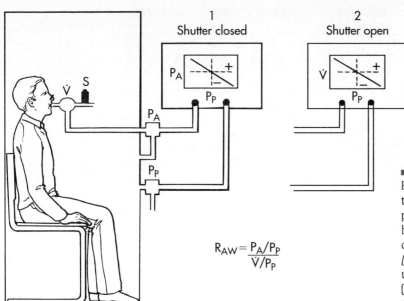

$$R_{AW} = \frac{P_A/P_P}{\dot{V}/P_P}$$

FIG. 36-3   Measurement of airway resistance (R_{AW}) in the body plethysmograph. The ratio between mouth pressure (P_A) (identical to alveolar pressure) and the box pressure (P_P) is determined with the shutter (S) closed. Then the relationship between P_P and airflow $(\dot{V})$ is estimated while the patient pants through the unobstructed pneumotachograph. Now $R_{AW} = P_A/\dot{V}$. (Redrawn from Cherniack RM: *Pulmonary function testing*, Philadelphia, 1977, Saunders.)

H_2O/L/sec of airflow. In patients with obstructive airway disease (e.g., emphysema), R_{AW} is increased and may be greater than 5 cm H_2O/L/sec.

More frequently, however, nonelastic resistance is estimated by measuring forced expiratory volumes and flow rates. This measurement is made on a spirometer or by a portable hand unit that can be used at the bedside. The volumes of air measured by the spirometer are as follows:

* *Forced vital capacity* (FVC) is the vital capacity measurement performed with expiration as forceful and rapid as possible. This volume of air is normally about the same as the VC but may be significantly reduced in patients with airway obstruction because of premature closure of the small airways and the consequent trapping of air.
* *Forced expiratory volume* (FEV) is the volume of air that can be exhaled in a standard time period during the FVC maneuver. Usually the FEV is measured during the first second of the forced exhalation; this is termed FEV_1. The FEV is a very useful index of the impairment of ventilatory capacity, and values of less than 1 L during the first second indicate severe impairment of ventilatory function.

The FEV should always be related to the FVC or VC. Normal persons can expire about 80% of their VC in 1 second, expressed as the FEV_1/FVC ratio. It makes little difference whether the FVC or VC is used for the ratio; the result is about the same. This ratio is of great value in differentiating between diseases that cause airway obstruction and those that cause restriction of lung expansion. In obstructive diseases, such as chronic bronchitis and emphysema, there is a greater reduction in FEV_1 than in VC (VC may be normal), so the FEV_1/FVC ratio is less than 80%. In a restrictive disease of the lung parenchyma such as sarcoidosis, both the FEV_1 and the FVC or VC

are reduced in about the same proportion, and the FEV_1/FVC ratio remains at about 80% or more.

The *maximum midexpiratory flow rate* (MMFR) is an important index of airway obstruction, which may be derived from a forced expiration. It is the flow rate for the middle two quarters of the FVC. The MMFR appears to be independent of effort and thus may be a more sensitive index of airway obstruction in early chronic obstructive lung disease than the FEV_1 (Fig. 36-4).

It is important to understand that these routine PFTs can detect only moderate to advanced obstructive disease involving the large airways, which account for 80% of the resistance. They are not sensitive enough to detect obstruction of the small peripheral airways (bronchioles less than 1 mm in diameter) because these airways contribute only a small fraction of the resistance (less than 20%). Obstructive respiratory disease is believed to begin in the peripheral airways. For these reasons, new techniques have been devised for detecting early airway dysfunction.

One technique is the *single-breath nitrogen test* to detect uneven distribution of gas in the lung and an increased closing volume. During this test the subject fully exhales, takes a single VC inspiration of 100% O_2, and then slowly exhales to the RV. During the last expiration the nitrogen (N_2) concentration in the expired air (now diluted with inspired O_2) is measured with a rapid N_2 analyzer and recorded along with the expired volume.

A number of important parameters may be derived from the N_2 curve (Fig. 36-5) including anatomic dead space, RV, VC, TLC, closing volume, closing capacity, and the slope of the alveolar plateau. *Closing volume* (CV) represents a lung volume at which the small airways in the lowest part of the lung begin to close. It is usually expressed as a percentage of the expired vital capacity (CV/VC). *Closing capacity* (CC) consists

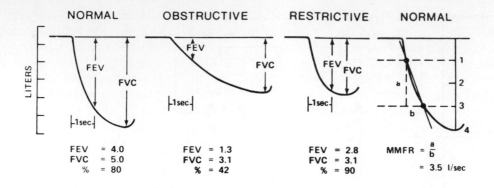

FIG. 36-4   Measurement of the forced expiratory volume *(FEV₁)* and maximum midexpiratory flow rate *(MMFR)*. The patient takes a full inspiration and exhales as hard and as fast as possible. The pen moves down as the patient exhales. The FEV_1 is the volume exhaled in 1 second. The MMFR is the mean flow rate over the middle half of the forced vital capacity *(FVC)*. Note the differences among the normal, obstructive, and restrictive patterns. (From West JB: In Pertersdorf, editor: *Harrison's principles of internal medicine,* ed 11, New York, 1987, McGraw-Hill.)

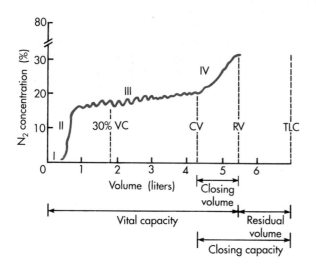

FIG. 36-5   Measurement of the closing volume *(CV)* by the single-breath nitrogen *(N₂)* method. If a vital capacity *(VC)* inspiration of 100% O_2 is followed by slow exhalation to residual volume *(RV)*, four phases of the N_2 concentration measured at the lips can be recognized. Initially there is no N_2 in the expired gas because it is gas from the dead space filled with O_2 (phase I). This is followed by a rapid rise in N_2 (phase II) in which alveolar gas mixes with dead-space gas and the curve is S shaped. From then on, N_2 reaches a plateau with a gradual rise (phase III) followed by an abrupt rise (phase IV), signaling closure of the small airways in the dependent zones of the lung. Phase IV represents closing volume, and closing capacity is the volume of gas left in the lung at the point of onset of phase IV (CV + RV). (Redrawn from Cherniack RM: *Pulmonary function testing,* Philadelphia, 1977, Saunders.)

of the CV plus the RV and is expressed as a percentage of total lung capacity (CC/TLC). The CV/VC ratio is age-dependent and may be as low as 10% in young healthy persons and 40% at age 65 years.

An increase in the CV/VC or CC/TLC ratio suggests premature closure of the small peripheral airways resulting from narrowing or loss of elastic recoil, as in chronic bronchitis and emphysema. An increased CV has been found in apparently healthy cigarette smokers. A rising slope of the alveolar plateau of the N_2 washout curve indicates uneven alveolar gas distribution in the lung and occurs in obstruction of the airways. Excellent and detailed descriptions of these and other PFTs may be found in Cherniack (1977) and West (1995).

The overall effects on alterations in the elastic and nonelastic properties of the lungs can be assessed by a simple test that measures the *maximum breathing capacity* (MBC), or *maximum voluntary ventilation* (MVV). The MVV (or MBC) can be estimated directly by having the patient breathe as rapidly and deeply as possible for 15 seconds and collecting the expired air in a Douglas bag. This volume is multiplied by 4 to determine the $\dot{V}_E$ in liters per minute. This test, used extensively for years, has been largely replaced by the FEV_1 test, which is less demanding and gives essentially the same information. The MBC may be approximated as the product of $FEV_1 \times 30$. The MBC can be affected by changes in compliance because of the increased muscular effort required. It is also affected by changes in airway resistance because of the increased turbulence resulting from airway collapse when breathing at rapid rates. The healthy young male adult can move as much as 170 L air/minute, compared with a $\dot{V}_E$ of about 6 L/minute at rest. The difference represents the *pulmonary reserve*, which is large in the healthy young adult. The pulmonary reserve is reduced in restrictive and obstructive diseases, but much more in the latter.

As already stated, less than 5% of the total O_2 consumption is expended for the work of breathing in the normal person at rest. The O_2 cost of breathing is greatly increased in both obstructive and restrictive patterns of pulmonary disease. The patient with emphysema (increased airway resistance) or the person who is very obese (restriction of chest movement) may consume 25% or more of the total inspired O_2 for the work of breathing. In severe disease, fatigue may be an important factor in the development of respiratory failure because of the increased muscular effort required for the work of breathing.

A relationship exists also between the mechanical work of breathing and the respiratory pattern (rate and depth of breathing). Respiratory physiologists have demonstrated that for any given $\dot{V}_A$, there is an optimum respiratory rate and V_T at which the total work of breathing is minimal. The graphs in Fig. 36-6 show the relationship between the mechanical work of breathing, including the total work and its two components (elastic and nonelastic), expressed in kilogram-meters (kgM), and the respiratory frequency. The principle illustrated is applied to normal persons as well as to those with pulmonary disease. The total work is the sum of the elastic and nonelastic work. (As you will recall, elastic work is expended to overcome the elastic resistances of the lungs and thorax and nonelastic work is expended to overcome flow resistance and tissue viscous resistance.) In the normal person at rest, at a particular $\dot{V}_A$, the total work of breathing is least at about 15 breaths/minute (illustrated by the solid lines in Fig. 36-6). At the same $\dot{V}_A$, rapid, shallow breathing results in the least amount of work for the patient with a restrictive pulmonary disorder (increased elastic work) such as pneumonia or obesity (long dashed lines in Fig. 36-6). This pattern probably occurs because small increments in V_T greatly increase the elastic resistance. However, if the pattern of breathing becomes too rapid and shallow, the V_D becomes disproportionately high. On the other hand, the person with an obstructive pulmonary disorder (increased nonelastic work), such as might occur in emphysema, adopts a slow, deep pattern of respiration (short dashed lines in Fig. 36-6). This pattern is adopted because a higher flow rate is likely to increase the amount of work needed to overcome resistance to airflow. In fact, if the patient with obstructive disease should voluntarily hyperventilate to blow off more CO_2, the Pco_2 might actually rise as a result of its increased production from the increased mechanical work of breathing.

Blood Gas Analysis

To assess respiratory function adequately, it is necessary to look beyond the lung to the volume and distribution of gas transport by the circulatory system. The factors that affect gas transport and removal between the lungs and tissue cells are discussed in Chapter 35, and a systematic approach to the assessment of acid-base disorders is pre-

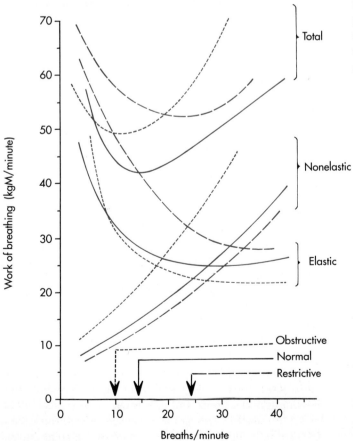

FIG. 36-6 Relationship between the mechanical work of breathing and the respiratory pattern in health and in pulmonary disease. (Modified from Cherniack M, Cherniack L, Naimark A: *Respiration in health and disease*, ed 3, Philadelphia, 1983, Saunders.)

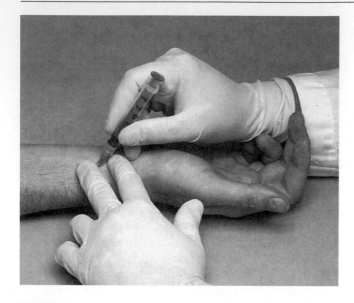

FIG. 36-7 Radial artery puncture technique for obtaining blood to test for arterial blood gas (ABG) levels. (From Potter PA, Perry AG: *Fundamentals of nursing: concepts, process, and practice,* ed 3, St Louis, 1993, Mosby.)

TABLE 36-3 Normal Values for Arterial Blood Gases

Blood Gas Measurement	Abbreviation	Normal Value
Carbon dioxide tension	Pa_{CO_2}	35-45 mm Hg (average, 40)
Oxygen tension	Pa_{O_2}	80-100 mm Hg
Oxygen percent saturation	Sa_{O_2}	97
Hydrogen ion concentration	pH	7.35-7.45
Bicarbonate	HCO_3^-	22-26 mEq/L

TABLE 36-4 Acid-base Changes in Acidosis and Alkalosis

Acid-base Disturbance	pH	HCO_3^-	Pa_{CO_2}
Respiratory acidosis	↓	↑	↑
Respiratory alkalosis	↑	↓	↓
Metabolic acidosis	↓	↓	↓
Metabolic alkalosis	↑	↑	↑

TABLE 36-5 Changes in Ventilatory Function as a Result of Pulmonary Disease

Test	Obstructive Pattern	Restrictive Pattern
RV	↑	↓
FRC	↑	↓
TLC	N or ↑	↓
VC*	N or ↓	↓
FVC	N or ↓	↓
MBC	↓	N or ↓
FEV_1†	↓	N or ↓
FEV_1/FVC	↓ (<80%)	N or ↑ (>80%)
MMFR	↓	N or ↓
CV	↑ for age or > FRC	
Compliance	N or ↑ (slight)	↓
Pa_{O_2}	↓	N (↓↓ exercise)
Pa_{CO_2}	↑	N or ↓
pH	↓ (during exacerbations)	N or ↑

Modified from Crofton J, Douglas A: *Respiratory diseases,* ed 3, Oxford, 1981, Blackwell; and Cherniak RM: *Pulmonary function testing,* Philadelphia, 1977, Saunders.
N, Normal; ↓, decreased or tending to decrease; ↑, increased or tending to increase. See earlier text in chapter for test abbreviations.
*Useful test to monitor progress of restrictive lung disease.
†Most useful test to monitor progress of obstructive lung disease.

sented in Chapter 22. In this chapter the technique used for the collection of blood to measure the blood gases and some general guidelines for the interpretation of measurements are presented.

Usually a sample of arterial blood is used for the blood gas analysis. Fig. 36-7 demonstrates the correct technique for drawing a blood sample. The radial (or brachial) artery is often chosen because of its accessibility. The wrist is extended by positioning it over a rolled towel. After the skin has been sterilized, the artery is stabilized with two fingers of one hand while the arterial puncture is made with the other hand using a heparinized syringe. After 5 ml of blood has been drawn into the syringe, air is removed and the blood is placed on ice and taken immediately to the blood gas laboratory for analysis. Obtaining the blood sample is usually performed by the intensive care nurse. Table 36-3 lists the normal values for the arterial blood gases (ABGs).

The Pa_{CO_2} is the best index of $\dot{V}_A$. When the Pa_{CO_2} rises, the direct cause is always generalized *alveolar hypoventilation.* Hypoventilation causes *respiratory acidosis* and a fall in the pH of the blood. Alveolar hypoventilation may occur if the V_T is decreased (the deadspace effect), as occurs in rapid, shallow breathing. Hypoventilation may also occur if the respiratory rate is decreased, as occurs in narcotic or barbiturate drug overdose. The Pa_{CO_2} may also rise to compensate for a *metabolic alkalosis.* Consequently, to interpret the Pa_{CO_2} correctly, one must also consider the blood pH and bicarbonate levels to determine whether a change is caused by a primary respiratory condition or is compensating for a metabolic condition.

The direct cause of a lowered Pa_{CO_2} is always *alveolar*

hyperventilation. Hyperventilation causes *respiratory alkalosis* and a rise in the pH of the blood. Hyperventilation is common in asthma and pneumonia and represents an effort to raise the Pa_{O_2} at the expense of excreting excess CO_2 from the lungs. Hyperventilation may also be caused by brain injury or tumor, aspirin poisoning, or anxiety, or it may be a compensation for *metabolic acidosis*. Table 36-4 summarizes the acid-base changes in compensated acidosis and alkalosis. The thicker arrows indicate the primary disorder. The change in the bicarbonate level represents the kidneys' attempt to compensate for the respiratory acidosis or alkalosis, whereas the change in the $Paco_2$ in the metabolic disorders represents the lung's role in compensation. The purpose of the compensation is to return the blood pH to normal.

When the Pao_2 falls below the normal value, *hypoxemia* results. Pao_2 levels fall slightly with age, so it is normal for persons over age 60 years to have a Pao_2 as low as 70 mm Hg. In severe respiratory failure the Pao_2 may fall to 30 to 40 mm Hg. Hypoxemia resulting from respiratory disease is caused by one or more of the following mechanisms: (1) ventilation-perfusion imbalance (most

common cause), (2) alveolar hypoventilation, (3) impaired diffusion, or (4) intrapulmonary anatomic shunts. Hypoxemia resulting from the first three abnormalities can be corrected by administering O_2. However, the intrapulmonary anatomic shunt (arteriovenous shunt) cannot be corrected by O_2 therapy.

Changes in the ABGs are critical measurements in the diagnosis of respiratory or ventilatory failure, which may be insidious in onset. Respiratory insufficiency exists when the Pao_2 falls below the normal values, and respiratory failure exists when the Pao_2 falls to 50 mm Hg. The $Paco_2$ may be increased or decreased below the normal values in respiratory insufficiency or failure. Respiratory failure is discussed in greater detail in Chapter 41. Table 36-5 summarizes some of the common changes in ventilatory function and ABGs in restrictive and obstructive patterns of pulmonary disease.

QUESTIONS

▼ *Answer the following on a separate sheet of paper.*

1. List six radiologic methods frequently used to detect pulmonary disease.
2. List four distinct features that are depicted on a routine chest radiograph.

▼ *Circle the letter that correctly answers the question.*

3. Which of the following diagnostic methods is *not* used to detect pulmonary disease and adequacy of pulmonary function?
   a. Blood gas measurements
   b. Ventilatory function tests
   c. Intravenous pyelogram
   d. Fluoroscopy

▼ *Match each of the diagnostic tests in column A to its description in column B.*

Column A

4. _____ Bronchography
5. _____ Angiography of pulmonary vessels
6. _____ Fluoroscopy
7. _____ Perfusion lung scan
8. _____ Percutaneous needle biopsy of lung
9. _____ Bronchoscopy
10. _____ Sputum studies
11. _____ Computed tomography
12. _____ Mediastinoscopy

Column B

a. Most accurate method of diagnosing pulmonary embolism
b. Used to obtain information about how various zones of the lung behave during respiratory cycle

Column B—cont'd

c. Reveals the size and appearance of the tracheobronchial tree; useful in confirming the diagnosis of bronchiectasis
d. Closed technique to obtain lung biopsy specimen
e. Useful technique to obtain aspiration of secretions for cytologic examination or biopsy specimen under direct visualization
f. Radiologic technique providing detailed radiographs of "slices of the lung"
g. Technique used to assess spread of lung cancer to hilar lymph nodes
h. Involves injection into a peripheral vein of albumin microspheres tagged with an isotope
i. Specimen may be obtained by aspiration of gastric contents

▼ *Match each of the diagnostic procedures in column A with the potential hazards and precautions in column B. Letters in column B may be used more than once.*

Column A

13. _____ Fluoroscopy
14. _____ Bronchography
15. _____ Bronchoscopic biopsy
16. _____ Perfusion and ventilation scans
17. _____ Pulmonary angiography
18. _____ Lung biopsy by open and closed techniques

Column B

a. Food and fluids are withheld after this examination until the gag reflex returns.
b. The major risk during this procedure is development of cardiac dysrhythmia.
c. This is a safer procedure for the diagnosis of pulmonary embolism but less definitive.
d. Excess radiation is the chief hazard associated with this procedure.
e. Percussion and postural drainage should follow this procedure.
f. Pneumothorax and bleeding are possible complications.
g. Laryngospasm or edema is a possible complication after this procedure.

Continued.

QUESTIONS—cont'd

▼ *Answer the following on a separate sheet of paper.*

19. Describe the role of ventilatory function tests and blood gas analysis in the diagnosis and treatment of pulmonary disorders. Are any of these tests specifically diagnostic?

20. Explain why alveolar ventilation is a better index of effective ventilation than minute volume or tidal volume.

21. Describe the procedure for the measurement of compliance of the lungs and thoracic cage. How is compliance calculated from the measurements?

22. List three common causes of decreased lung compliance and three causes of decreased chest wall compliance.

23. Why does a patient with emphysema adopt a slow, deep pattern of respiration?

24. What breathing pattern might a patient with normal airway resistance but very stiff lungs (low compliance) adopt? Why?

25. Describe the correct technique for the collection of blood in the measurement of arterial blood gases.

26. List three causes of alveolar hyperventilation and hypoventilation.

27. List four causes of hypoxemia. Which one is *not* corrected by oxygen administration?

▼ *Circle T if the statement is true and F if it is false. Correct any false statements.*

28. T F Rapid, shallow breathing results in less effective ventilation because the respiratory rate is greater than the normal rate per minute.

29. T F The ratio of physiologic dead space to tidal volume does not normally exceed 30% to 40%.

30. T F Alveolar ventilation in a 120-pound woman with a tidal volume of 200 ml and a respiratory rate of 30 breaths/minute is about 6 L/minute.

31. T F The work of breathing refers to the form of energy expenditure required to move the chest bellows (the amount of oxygen consumed by the respiratory muscles).

32. T F Elastic properties of the lung are the result of the surface tension of fluid lining the alveoli and the elastic fibers throughout the lung.

33. T F The maximum breathing capacity test is a good test to measure pulmonary reserve.

34. T F Nonelastic resistances consist of the frictional resistance to flow in the airways.

▼ *Circle the letter preceding each item below that correctly completes the statement. More than one answer may be correct.*

35. The primary lung volume that measures the amount of air inhaled or exhaled with each breath is the:
    a. Tidal volume (V_T)
    b. Expiratory reserve volume (ERV)
    c. Inspiratory reserve volume (IRV)
    d. Residual volume (RV)

36. The lung capacity that measures the maximum volume of air that can be expired after a maximum inspiratory effort is the:
    a. Total lung capacity (TLC)
    b. Vital capacity (VC)
    c. Inspiratory capacity (IC)
    d. Functional residual capacity (FRC)

37. The spirometer directly measures the combination:
    a. V_T, TLC, RV, IC
    b. FRC, TLC, ERV, VC
    c. V_T, IRV, ERV, VC, IC

38. In healthy young persons the 1-second forced expiratory volume/forced vital capacity ratio is approximately:
    a. 30%   c. 80%
    b. 50%   d. 100%

39. The normal range for $Paco_2$ is:
    a. 22 to 30 mm Hg
    b. 35 to 45 mm Hg
    c. 50 to 62 mm Hg
    d. 85 to 100 mm Hg

40. Alveolar hypoventilation can be readily diagnosed by measuring the:
    a. Pao_2
    b. pH of arterial blood
    c. Respiratory rate
    d. $Paco_2$
    e. Tidal volume

41. Physiologic dead space can be increased by:
    a. Enlargement of the anatomic dead space
    b. High ventilation/perfusion ratios of pulmonary units
    c. Low ventilation/perfusion ratios of pulmonary units

42. Laboratory test results that indicate adequate compensation for a respiratory acidosis are:
    a. Increase in pH toward 7.4
    b. Decrease in serum bicarbonate
    c. Increase in serum bicarbonate

43. Which of the following pulmonary function tests is *most* sensitive in detecting early obstructive lung disease of the peripheral airways?
    a. MMFR
    b. R_{AW}
    c. FEV_1/FVC
    d. CV/VC

44. The single-breath nitrogen test can be used to measure:
    a. RV
    b. V_D
    c. Uneven distribution of alveolar ventilation
    d. CC/TLC
    e. All the above

▼ *Match each of the pulmonary functions in column A to its definition in column B.*

Column A		Column B
45. _____ FVC	a.	Carbon dioxide tension in arterial blood
46. _____ FEV_1	b.	Volume of air exchanged in the airway in 1 minute
47. _____ V_D/V_T	c.	Volume of air expired during first second of the FVC maneuver
48. _____ V_A	d.	Proportion of tidal volume that is physiologic dead space
49. _____ V_E	e.	Effective ventilation per minute
50. _____ $Paco_2$	f.	Expiration performed as rapidly and as forcefully as possible after a maximum inspiration
51. _____ MMFR	g.	Nonelastic resistance of the large airways
52. _____ R_{AW}	h.	Maximum flow rate during the middle two quarters of the FVC maneuver

QUESTIONS—cont'd

▼ *Complete the table as directed.*

53. Indicate the common changes in ventilatory function and blood gases in restrictive and obstructive patterns of pulmonary disease by filling in the blanks in the table. Use the following key: N = normal, ↓ = decreased, ↑ = increased.

Changes in Ventilatory Function as a Result of Pulmonary Disease

Test	Obstructive Pattern	Restrictive Pattern
Residual volume		
Functional residual capacity		
Total lung capacity		
Vital capacity		
Forced vital capacity		
Maximum breathing capacity		
FEV_1		
FEV_1/FVC		
Compliance		
Pao_2		
$Paco_2$		
pH		

CHAPTER 37

Cardinal Signs and Symptoms of Respiratory Disease

LORRAINE M. WILSON

Pulmonary diseases may give rise to both respiratory and general signs and symptoms. Respiratory signs and symptoms include cough, excessive or abnormal sputum, hemoptysis, dyspnea, and chest pain. General signs and symptoms include cyanosis, digital clubbing and hypertrophic osteoarthropathy, and other manifestations related to inadequate gas exchange. The reader is referred to other textbooks for a discussion of adventitious chest sounds and systematic assessment of the respiratory status.

COUGH

Coughing is a protective reflex caused by irritation of the tracheobronchial tree. The ability to cough is an important mechanism in clearing the lower airways, and many adults normally cough a few times on first arising to clear the trachea and pharynx of secretions that have accumulated during sleep. Coughing is also the most common symptom of respiratory disease. Any cough persisting for longer than 3 weeks should be investigated to determine the cause.

Stimuli that typically produce a cough are mechanical, chemical, and inflammatory. Inhalation of smoke, dust, and small foreign bodies is the most common cause of cough. Smokers often have a chronic cough as a result of inhaling foreign bodies (smoke) and chronic inflammation of the airways. Mechanical stimulation from tumors either extrinsic or intrinsic to the airways is another cause of cough (the most common tumor causing cough is bronchogenic carcinoma). Any inflammatory process of the airways, with or without exudate, may produce a cough. Chronic bronchitis, asthma, tuberculosis, and pneumonia typically have coughing as a prominent symptom. A cough may be productive, hacking and non-productive, brassy (as with pressure on the trachea), frequent, infrequent, or paroxysmal (intermittent coughing episodes).

SPUTUM

The normal adult produces about 100 ml of mucus in the respiratory tract per day. This mucus is transported to the pharynx by the normal cleansing actions of the cilia that line the airways. When excess mucus is formed, the normal process of removal may be ineffective and may result in the accumulation of mucus. When this occurs, the mucous membrane is stimulated, and the mucus is coughed up as sputum. Excess mucus production may be caused by physical, chemical, or infective insults to the mucous membrane.

Whenever a patient produces sputum, it is important to observe its source, color, volume, and consistency. Sputum produced by clearing the throat is most likely to have originated in the sinuses or nasal passages rather than in the lower respiratory tract. Profuse purulent sputum suggests the presence of a suppurative process such as lung abscess, whereas sputum production that gradually increases over a period of years suggests chronic bronchitis or bronchiectasis.

The color of sputum is also important. Yellow sputum indicates an infection. Green sputum is indicative of stagnant pus. The green color is produced by the presence of verdoperoxidase, which is liberated from polymorphonuclear neutrophils (PMNs) in the sputum. Green sputum is common in bronchiectasis because of the stagnation of sputum in dilated, infected bronchioles. Many patients with lower respiratory tract infection report having green sputum early in the morning, which becomes yellow as the day progresses. This phenomenon is probably caused by the accumulation of purulent sputum during the night, with the consequent release of verdoperoxidase.

The character and consistency of sputum also yield useful information. Pink, frothy sputum is characteristic of acute pulmonary edema. Sputum may be mucoid, sticky, and gray or white in chronic bronchitis. A foul odor to the sputum may indicate a lung abscess or bronchiectasis.

HEMOPTYSIS

Varying amounts of blood may be mixed with sputum, or blood may compose the entire expectoration. *Hemoptysis* is the term applied to the expectoration of both pure blood and blood-streaked sputum. Any process resulting in interruption of the continuity of the pulmonary blood vessels may result in bleeding. The expectoration of pure blood is a serious symptom and may be the first manifestation of active tuberculosis. Other common causes of hemoptysis are bronchogenic carcinoma, pulmonary infarction, bronchiectasis, and lung abscess. Blood-streaked sputum (which may be rust colored) is a common feature of pneumococcal pneumonia. Sputum may have the appearance of currant-jelly (brick red) in *Klebsiella* pneumonia. Table 37-1 summarizes some of the gross characteristics of sputum in some pulmonary disorders. When blood or blood-streaked sputum is expectorated, it is important to determine whether the source is actually the lower respiratory tract rather then the nasal passages or gastrointestinal (GI) tract. Blood originating in the GI tract *(hematemesis)* is usually dark, similar to coffee grounds, from partial digestion and is associated with nausea, vomiting, and anemia; blood originating in the lower airways (below the glottis) is usually bright red, frothy, and associated with a history of cough with or without anemia. Blood originating in the upper air passages (e.g., nosebleed or bleeding after a tonsillectomy) is often associated with frequent swallowing and may have the appearance of partially digested blood when vomited.

TABLE 37-1   Characteristics of Sputum Seen in Various Pulmonary Disorders

Appearance	Likely Cause
Mucoid, translucent, grayish white	Atypical pneumonia, asthma
Currant-jelly (brick red)	*Klebsiella pneumoniae*
Rusty (prune juice color)	Pneumococcal pneumonia
Pink, frothy	Pulmonary edema
Salmon colored or creamy yellow	Staphylococcal pneumonia
Mucopurulent sputum: yellow, greenish, or dirty gray	Bacterial pneumonia; acute or chronic bronchitis
Purulent and foul smelling	Oral anaerobes (aspiration), lung abscess, bronchiectasis

DYSPNEA

Dyspnea, or *breathlessness,* is the subjective sensation of difficulty in breathing and is a cardinal symptom of cardiopulmonary disease. A patient with dyspnea is likely to complain of shortness of breath or a sensation of suffocation. Dyspnea is by no means always an indication of disease; the normal person usually experiences this sensation after varying degrees of physical exertion.

It is important to distinguish dyspnea from other signs and symptoms that may have an entirely different clinical significance. *Tachypnea* refers to a rapid respiratory rate greater than the normal 12 to 20 breaths/minute that may be present with or without dyspnea. *Hyperventilation* refers to ventilation that is greater than the amount required to maintain normal carbon dioxide (CO_2) elimination; it is identified by observing an arterial CO_2 partial pressure, or tension ($Paco_2$), that is less than the normal 40 mm Hg. Dyspnea is a common complaint in the *hyperventilation syndrome* in otherwise healthy individuals who are emotionally stressed (see Chapter 22). Finally, the symptom of *exertional fatigue* must be distinguished from dyspnea. The normal person experiences exertional fatigue after varying degrees of physical exertion, and this symptom may also be experienced with cardiovascular, neuromuscular, and other nonpulmonary diseases.

In recent years there has been a surge of scientific interest in the measurement and neurophysiologic mechanisms of dyspnea (Mahler, 1990). However, no totally satisfactory explanation for dyspnea under all circumstances is yet available. The proposed sources of dyspnea include (1) the mechanical receptors in the respiratory muscles, lung, and chest wall; according to the *length-tension theory,* sensory elements, particularly muscle spindles, play a central role in comparing the tension in the muscles with the degree of stretch; dyspnea is experienced when the tension is inappropriately large for a

TABLE 37-2　American Thoracic Society Dyspnea Scale

Grade	Degree	Criteria
0	None	Is not troubled with breathlessness except with strenuous activity
1	Slight	Is troubled by shortness of breath when hurrying on the level or walking up a slight hill
2	Moderate	Walks slower than most people of the same age because of breathlessness or has to stop for breath when walking at own pace on the level
3	Severe	Stops for breath after walking 100 yards or after a few minutes walking on level ground
4	Very severe	Too breathless to leave the house or breathless when dressing/undressing

From Brooks SM, chairman: *ATS News* 8:12-16, 1982.

particular muscle length (volume of breath achieved); (2) chemoreceptors for CO_2 and oxygen tensions (P_{CO_2} and P_{O_2}) *(oxygen-debt theory);* (3) increased work of breathing with the consequent sensation of increased effort; and (4) an imbalance between respiratory work and the capacity to ventilate. The length-tension inappropriateness mechanism is the most widely accepted theory because it explains most of the cases of clinical dyspnea. The key factor that seems to determine whether dyspnea is experienced is whether the level of ventilation or effort is appropriate to the degree of activity. However, the stimuli, sensory receptors, and nerve pathways by which the appropriateness is recognized have not been established with certainty.

The amount of exertion sufficient to induce dyspnea varies with age, gender, altitude, state of physical fitness, and emotional involvement in the task. It is important to correlate dyspnea in a client with the minimum level of activity sufficient for its induction, that is, to determine whether dyspnea is experienced after strenuous or moderate activity or while at rest. Table 37-2 outlines a dyspnea scale developed by the American Thoracic Society that may be appropriate for the clinical assessment of chronic dyspnea. There are also some variations of the general symptom of dyspnea. *Orthopnea* is shortness of breath on assuming the recumbent position. It is usually quantified by describing the number of pillows or angle of elevation required to prevent the sensation. A common cause of orthopnea is congestive heart failure resulting from the increased blood volume in the central vasculature on assuming the recumbent position. Orthopnea is also a common symptom in many respiratory disorders. *Paroxysmal nocturnal dyspnea* refers to the onset of dyspnea during the night with the urgent need to sit up to breathe. It differs from orthopnea in that the onset usually occurs after several hours of recumbency. The cause is the same as in the orthopnea of congestive heart failure, and the delayed onset is related to the mobilization of peripheral edema fluid and its addition to the central intravascular volume.

Those patients who have dyspnea as a principal symptom usually have one of the following conditions: (1) cardiovascular disease, (2) pulmonary emboli, (3) interstitial or alveolar disease of the lung, (4) disorders of the chest wall or muscles, (5) obstructive disease of lung, (6) disorders of the chest wall or muscles, or (7) anxiety. Dyspnea is a prominent symptom of pulmonary edema, congestive heart failure, and valvular heart disease. Pulmonary embolism is characterized by the sudden onset of dyspnea. Dyspnea is a prevalent symptom in diseases that affect the tracheobronchial tree, lung parenchyma, and pleural space. It is frequently associated with restrictive diseases in which respiratory work is increased as a result of increased elastic resistance of the lung (pneumonia, atelectasis, congestion) or chest wall (obesity, kyphoscoliosis) or in obstructive airways disease with increased bronchial nonelastic resistance (emphysema, bronchitis, asthma). When the work of breathing is increased chronically, however, the patient may adapt to the new level and not experience dyspnea. Dyspnea may also be experienced if the respiratory muscles are weak (e.g., myasthenia gravis), paralyzed (e.g., poliomyelitis, Guillain-Barré syndrome), fatigued as a result of increased work of breathing, or less able to perform mechanical work (e.g., severe emphysema or obesity). Finally, persons with hyperventilation syndrome secondary to anxiety or emotional stress often complain of dyspnea. Their breathing pattern is frequently strange, with irregularities in both frequency and tidal volume. At other times the pattern is one of such sustained hyperventilation that the patient complains of tingling in the extremities and even a feeling of faintness (see respiratory alkalosis in Chapter 22). If the abnormal breathing pattern disappears during sleep, psychogenic causes should be suspected.

CHEST PAIN

Chest pain has many causes, but the most characteristic pain of lung disease is that resulting from inflammation of the pleura *(pleurisy).* Only the parietal layer of the pleura is a source of pain, since the visceral pleura and the lung parenchyma are regarded as insensitive organs.

Typically pleurisy usually is abrupt in onset but may develop gradually. The pain occurs at the site of inflammation and is usually well localized. It is cutting and sharp in character and is aggravated by coughing, sneezing, and deep breathing, so the patient often adopts a pattern of rapid, shallow breathing and avoids unnecessary movement. The pain may be somewhat relieved by applying pressure (splinting) over the involved area. The most common causes of pleuritic pain are pulmonary infection or infarction, although such conditions may be present without pain. Patients with pneumothorax or massive atelectasis may occasionally experience chest pain that is thought to be caused by traction on the parietal pleura by adhesions attached to the visceral pleura.

DIGITAL CLUBBING AND HYPERTROPHIC OSTEOARTHROPATHY

Digital clubbing is a peculiar change in the shape of the tips of the fingers and toes characterized by a bulbous appearance. It is a significant physical sign because it is associated with a number of serious conditions. Pulmonary disease (e.g., bronchogenic carcinoma, bronchiectasis, lung abscess, pulmonary tuberculosis) is the most common cause of digital clubbing (70% to 80% of cases). Cardiovascular disease (e.g., congenital intracardiac shunting, infective endocarditis) ranks second (10% to 15% of cases); and 5% to 10% of the cases of digital clubbing are associated with chronic diseases of the GI tract, including the liver. The pathogenesis of digital clubbing is not understood. A popular hypothesis ascribes it to hypoxia, but this does not explain its presence in many entities. Clubbing often develops early in bronchogenic carcinoma and is not associated with arterial desaturation. It is curious that the chronic hypoxia of emphysema rarely seems to be associated with digital clubbing, but the chronic hypoxia of tetralogy of Fallot is often associated with severe clubbing. The box at right

CONDITIONS ASSOCIATED WITH DIGITAL CLUBBING

A. Pulmonary disease
  1. Pulmonary neoplasms (5%-10%)
    a. Bronchogenic carcinoma
    b. Mesothelioma
    c. Hodgkin's disease
  2. Infections
    a. Lung abscess
    b. Bronchiectasis
    c. Cystic fibrosis
    d. Empyema
    e. Chronic obstructive pulmonary disease (COPD)
    f. Tuberculosis with cavitation
B. Cardiovascular disease
  1. Cyanotic congenital heart disease
  2. Infective endocarditis
  3. Infected vascular prosthesis
C. Gastrointestinal disease
  1. Cirrhosis of the liver
  2. Inflammatory bowel disease
    a. Ulcerative colitis
    b. Crohn's disease
  3. Sprue
  4. Familial polyposis
  5. Neoplasms of the esophagus, liver, or small and large bowels
D. Miscellaneous
  1. Primary hereditary finger clubbing
  2. Graves' disease

lists some conditions that are typically associated with digital clubbing.

It is important to detect clubbing as early as possible because of its diagnostic significance. The earliest sign is a loss of the angle between the nail and the dorsum of the terminal phalanx; this angle is normally 160 degrees. Fig. 37-1 illustrates the normal variations and early and advanced clubbing. In early clubbing the skin at the base of the nail may have a shiny appearance, and gentle pressure on the nail root reveals a spongy feeling (floating nail). Normally the nail plate rests firmly against the bone. Early clubbing must be differentiated from the normal curved nail that is common in African Americans. If one views the normal curved nail from the side, the base angle is still about 160 degrees. In early clubbing the base angle of the nail becomes greater than 160 degrees. As the condition progresses, the tissue at the root of the nail becomes heaped up and the curvature of the nail becomes pronounced, until the soft tissue of the digit tip becomes bulbous, producing the classic drumstick appearance.

A condition closely related to digital clubbing is *hypertrophic osteoarthropathy* (HOA). HOA is characterized by digital clubbing, periosteal new bone formation,

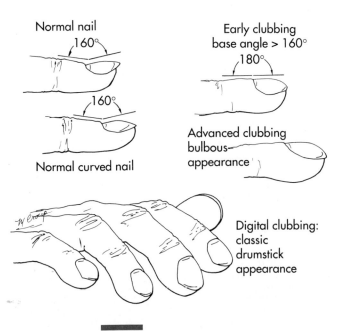

Normal nail
160°

160°

Normal curved nail

Early clubbing base angle > 160°
180°

Advanced clubbing bulbous appearance

Digital clubbing: classic drumstick appearance

FIG. 37-1   Digital clubbing.

and arthritis. HOA is seen most frequently in bronchogenic carcinoma and may be confused with arthritis. HOA may precede the radiographic appearance of lung cancer by many months. Patients may experience severe skeletal pain before the appearance of clubbing or HOA. It is unclear whether digital clubbing alone is a partial expression of HOA or is a separate entity (Gilliland, 1994). Other joints besides the digits may be affected by HOA.

SIGNS OF INADEQUATE GAS EXCHANGE

Cyanosis

Cyanosis is a bluish coloration of the skin and mucous membranes that develops as a result of an increase in the absolute amount of reduced hemoglobin (hemoglobin [Hb] not united with O_2). It may be a sign of respiratory insufficiency, although this is a highly unreliable indication. There are two types of cyanosis: central and peripheral. *Central cyanosis* resulting from insufficient oxygenation of Hb in the lungs is most easily observed on the face, lips, and earlobes and under the tongue. Cyanosis is generally not detected until the absolute amount of reduced Hb is 5 g/dl or more in a person with normal Hb concentration (oxygen saturation [Sao_2] less than 90%). The normal amount of reduced Hb in the capillary bed is 2.5 g/dl. In the person with a normal Hb concentration,

Sao_2 is about 75% and the arterial oxygen tension (Pao_2) is 50 mm Hg or less when cyanosis is first detected. Anemic patients (low Hb concentration) may never become cyanotic, even though they have severe tissue hypoxia, because the absolute amount of reduced Hg is not likely to reach 5 g/dl. On the other hand, a person with polycythemia (high Hb concentration) can easily have 5 g/dl of reduced Hb when there is only mild hypoxia. Other factors that make cyanosis difficult to recognize are variations in skin thickness, pigmentation, and lighting conditions.

In addition to cyanosis caused by respiratory insufficiency (central cyanosis), *peripheral cyanosis* occurs when severely reduced blood flow causes a great reduction in the venous saturation, thereby turning an area blue. Peripheral cyanosis may result from cardiac insufficiency, obstruction of blood flow, or vasoconstriction resulting from cold temperatures.

Cyanosis may also be produced by small amounts of circulating methemoglobin and by even smaller amounts of sulfhemoglobin, although these causes occur infrequently. These variations in cause and the difficulty in recognizing cyanosis make it an unreliable sign of respiratory insufficiency.

Hypoxemia and Hypoxia

The term *hypoxemia* refers to values of Pao_2 that are abnormally low and is frequently associated with *hypoxia,* or inadequate tissue oxygenation. Hypoxemia is not nec-

▶ TABLE 37-3   Indicators of Hypoxemia and Hypoxia

Blood Gases/System	Laboratory Findings/Clinical Signs

Arterial blood gases	Pao_2*: 80-100 mm Hg (normal)
	        60-80 mm Hg (mild hypoxemia)
	        40-60 mm Hg (moderate hypoxemia)
	        <40 mm Hg (severe hypoxemia)
	Sao_2: 95%-97% (normal)
	        <90% (may indicate hypoxemia)
	pH: 7.35-7.45 (normal)
	        <7.35 (acidemia)
	        >7.45 (alkalemia)
	$Paco_2$: 35-45 mm Hg (normal)
	        >45 mm Hg (hypoventilation)
	        <35 mm Hg (hyperventilation)

Respiratory system	Tachypnea, decreased tidal volume, dyspnea, yawning, use of accessory respiratory muscles, flared nostrils
Central nervous system	Headache (from cerebral vasodilation) Mental confusion, bizarre behavior, restlessness Agitation, anxious facial expression, sweating Drowsiness progressing to coma when hypoxia is severe
Cardiovascular system	Tachycardia early; bradycardia later when the heart muscle is not receiving adequate O_2 Rise in blood pressure followed by a drop when hypoxia remains uncorrected; dysrhythmias
Skin	Cyanosis of lips, oral mucosa, and nailbeds

*Pao_2 values are for a person less than 60 years of age breathing room air; subtract 1 mm Hg for each year person is over 60 years of age to obtain lower limits of normal.

essarily accompanied by tissue hypoxia. One can have normal tissue oxygenation with hypoxemia, just as one can have a normal PaO_2 with tissue hypoxia (because of the abnormalities of O_2 delivery and utilization by the cells, discussed in Chapter 35). A relationship exists, however, between the PaO_2 and tissue hypoxia, although the precise PaO_2 at which impairment of tissue use of O_2 occurs is variable. All things being equal, the more rapid the onset of hypoxemia, the more extensive are the tissue abnormalities. In general, PaO_2 values that are persistently less than 50 mm Hg are associated with tissue hypoxia and acidosis (caused by anaerobic metabolism). Because hypoxia may exist with both normal and low values of PaO_2, evaluation of blood gas measurements must always be correlated with clinical observation of the patient. Cyanosis is an unreliable sign of hypoxia because SaO_2 must be less than 75% in persons with normal Hb before it is detectable. Table 37-3 lists clinical signs and laboratory findings that indicate hypoxia.

Hypercapnia and Hypocapnia

Just as ventilation is considered adequate when O_2 supply is matched with O_2 demand, so must CO_2 elimination through the lungs be matched with CO_2 production for adequate ventilation. Because CO_2 is highly diffusible, the CO_2 tensions are equal in alveolar air and arterial blood; thus $PaCO_2$ is the direct and immediate reflection of the alveolar ventilation in relation to the metabolic rate. Adequate ventilation maintains the $PaCO_2$ at about 40 mm Hg. *Hypercapnia* is defined as a rise in the $PaCO_2$ above 45 Hg; *hypocapnia* occurs when the $PaCO_2$ is less than 35 mm Hg. The direct cause of CO_2 retention is alveolar hypoventilation (ventilation inadequate to cope with CO_2 production). Hypercapnia is always accompanied by some degree of hypoxia when the patient is breathing room air.

The major causes of hypercapnia are obstructive airways disease, respiratory depressant drugs, weakness or paralysis of the respiratory muscles, chest trauma or abdominal surgery causing shallow respirations, and loss of lung tissue. Clinical signs associated with hypercapnia are mental confusion progressing to coma, headache (as a result of cerebral vasodilation), asterixis or flapping tremor of the outstretched hands, and a pulse of large volume with warm, sweaty extremities (as a result of the peripheral vasodilation caused by the hypercapnia). In chronic hypercapnia resulting from chronic pulmonary disease, the patient may become abnormally tolerant to the high $PaCO_2$, so that the principal drive to respiration is hypoxia. Under these circumstances, if O_2 is administered at a high concentration, respiration is diminished and the hypercapnia is increased.

Excessive loss of CO_2 from the lungs (hypocapnia) occurs when there is hyperventilation (ventilation in excess of metabolic need to remove CO_2). Common causes of hyperventilation are listed in Chapter 36 and also include excessive mechanical ventilation, anxiety states, cerebral trauma, aspirin poisoning, and compensatory response to hypoxia. Signs and symptoms typically associated with hypocapnia include frequent sighing and yawning, dizziness, palpitations, tingling and numbness in the extremities, and muscular twitches. Severe hypocapnia ($PaCO_2$ less than 25 mm Hg) may cause convulsions.

QUESTIONS

▼ *Match the signs and symptoms in column B with the possible causative factors in column A. Each letter may be used only once.*

Column A

1. ____ Interruption in the continuity of the pulmonary blood vessels
2. ____ Inflammation of the pleura
3. ____ Increase in the absolute amount of reduced hemoglobin
4. ____ Physical, chemical, or infectious insults to the mucous membrane of the respiratory tract
5. ____ Protective reflex initiated by irritation of the tracheobronchial tree
6. ____ Pathogenesis unknown; associated with early stage of bronchogenic carcinoma and with certain chronic respiratory, cardiovascular, and gastrointestinal diseases
7. ____ Increased ventilatory work as correlated with the minimum level of activity sufficient for its induction

Column B

a. Cough
b. Excess sputum production
c. Hemoptysis
d. Dyspnea
e. Digital clubbing
f. Chest pain
g. Cyanosis

▼ *Circle T is the statement is true and F if it is false. Correct any false statements.*

8. T F Hypoxia refers to inadequate tissue oxygenation.
9. T F PaO_2 values that are persistently less than 85 mm Hg are associated with tissue hypoxia.
10. T F Cyanosis is a reliable sign of hypoxia.
11. T F Confusion, restlessness, and agitation are clinical signs that may indicate hypoxia.
12. T F Anemic patients frequently become cyanotic even with moderate degrees of hypoxemia.
13. T F The $PaCO_2$ is the best index of alveolar ventilation adequacy.
14. T F Hypercapnia refers to a rise in the $PaCO_2$ above 45 mm Hg.
15. T F The direct cause of hypocapnia is alveolar hypoventilation.
16. T F Symptoms of headache, drowsiness, and asterixis are associated with hypercapnia.

▼ *Answer the following questions on a separate sheet of paper.*

17. What is digital clubbing? Why is it important to detect?
18. How would you detect cyanosis in an African-American patient?

CHAPTER 38

Obstructive Patterns of Respiratory Disease

LORRAINE M. WILSON

PATTERNS OF RESPIRATORY DISEASE

Respiratory diseases have been classified on the basis of etiology, anatomic site, chronicity, and changes in structure and function. None of these classifications is entirely satisfactory. The etiologic agents are unknown in some cases, whereas in others the same causal agent may affect different anatomic sites and produce different pathophysiologic effects. In this chapter and Chapter 39, respiratory diseases are classified according to ventilatory dysfunction and are divided into two categories: diseases that produce primarily an *obstructive ventilatory disorder* and those that produce a *restrictive ventilatory disorder.* This classification was chosen because spirometric and other tests of ventilatory function are carried out almost routinely, and most respiratory diseases affect ventilation. There are two limitations to this approach. In some respiratory disorders the ventilatory abnormality may produce a mixed pattern (e.g., chronic emphysema with superimposed pneumonia), whereas in other disorders affecting respiration, ventilatory function may be normal (e.g., anemia or right-to-left shunt). The following pulmonary disorders, which do not readily fit into obstructive or restrictive patterns of disease, are discussed separately: cardiovascular diseases affecting the lung, respiratory insufficiency and failure, pulmonary neoplasms, and tubercu-

losis. Only those disorders most frequently encountered in hospital practice are considered.

CHRONIC OBSTRUCTIVE PULMONARY DISEASE

Chronic obstructive pulmonary disease (COPD) is a term often applied to a group of pulmonary diseases of long duration characterized by increased resistance to airflow as the main pathophysiologic feature. Chronic bronchitis, pulmonary emphysema, and bronchial asthma make up the entity known as COPD. There appears to be an etiologic and sequential relationship between chronic bronchitis and emphysema that does not seem to exist between these two diseases and asthma. This is particularly true in regard to etiology, pathogenesis, and treatment, as discussed later in this chapter.

Chronic bronchitis is a clinical disorder characterized by excessive production of mucus in the bronchi and is manifested by a chronic cough and production of sputum for a minimum of 3 months/year for at least 2 consecutive years. This definition assumes that diseases such as bronchiectasis and tuberculosis, which also cause chronic cough and sputum production, have been excluded. The sputum produced in chronic bronchitis may be mucoid or mucopurulent.

Pulmonary emphysema is an anatomic alteration of the lung parenchyma characterized by abnormal enlargement of the alveoli and alveolar ducts and destruction of the alveolar walls.

Asthma is a disease characterized by hypersensitivity of the tracheobronchial tree to various stimuli. It is manifested by periodic, reversible airway narrowing caused by bronchospasm.

Note the different bases of the definitions (American Thoracic Society, 1962) of the preceding diseases: chronic bronchitis is defined by clinical symptoms, pulmonary emphysema by pathologic anatomy, and asthma by clinical pathologic physiology. Although each disease may exist in its pure form, it is more usual for chronic

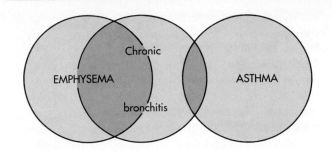

FIG. 38-1   Interrelationship between the disease entities making up COPD.

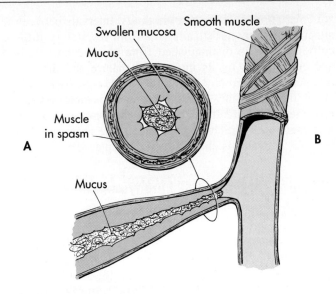

FIG. 38-2   Factors causing expiratory obstruction in bronchial asthma. **A**, Cross section of bronchiole occluded by muscle spasm, swollen mucosa, and mucus in lumen. **B**, Longitudinal section of bronchiole.

bronchitis and emphysema to exist together in the same patient. Asthma is more easily separated from chronic bronchitis and emphysema on the basis of a history of paroxysmal attacks of wheezing beginning in childhood and associated with allergies. Occasionally, however, patients with chronic bronchitis have asthmatic features to their disease. Fig. 38-1 illustrates the interrelationship of chronic bronchitis, asthma, and emphysema. The darkly shaded areas represent those persons with features of more than one disease; the lightly shaded areas represent each disease in the predominantly pure form. For purposes of clarity, asthma is considered separately from chronic bronchitis and emphysema because it is more easily separated from the other two diseases. A detailed discussion of asthma is included in Chapter 10.

Asthma

The term *asthma* comes from the Greek word for "panting" and means attacks of shortness of breath. Although in the past this term has been used for the clinical picture of shortness of breath resulting from any cause, today it is confined to a condition of abnormal responsiveness of the air passages to various stimuli, causing widespread airway narrowing.

The pathologic changes involved in airway obstruction are found in the medium-sized bronchi and in bronchioles as small as 1 mm in diameter. Airway narrowing is caused by bronchospasm, mucosal edema, and hypersecretion of viscous mucus (Fig. 38-2).

Asthma can be divided into three categories. *Extrinsic,* or *allergic, asthma,* found in a minority of adult patients, is clearly caused by a known allergen. This form generally begins in childhood in a member of a family with a history of atopic diseases, including hay fever, eczema, and dermatitis as well as asthma. Allergic asthma results from the sensitization of such a person to an allergen, usually a protein, in the form of an inhaled pollen, animal dander, mold spores, feathers, dust, lint, or, less often, to a food such as milk or chocolate. Exposure to the allergen, even in minute quantities, produces an asthmatic attack. *Intrinsic,* or *idiopathic, asthma,* on the other hand, is characterized by the absence of clearly defined precip-

itating factors. Nonspecific factors such as the common cold, exercise, or emotion may trigger the asthmatic attack. The intrinsic type of asthma is more apt to develop after age 40, with the onset of attacks after infections of the nasal sinuses or tracheobronchial tree. The attacks become more frequent over time, and the condition merges into chronic bronchitis and sometimes emphysema. Most patients develop *mixed asthma,* which is composed of components of both extrinsic and intrinsic asthmas. Often patients with intrinsic asthma later develop the mixed type; children who have the extrinsic type often have complete recovery at adolescence.

The pathogenesis of asthma is discussed in Chapter 10. The clinical manifestations are easy to recognize. After exposure to the causative allergen or precipitating factor, dyspnea may begin suddenly. Patients feel as if they are suffocating and must stand or sit up and devote all their energy to breathing. On the basis of the anatomic changes previously described, it is apparent that the major difficulty is with expiration. The tracheobronchial tree widens and lengthens during inspiration, but it is difficult to force air out of the constricted, edematous, mucus-filled bronchioles, which normally contract to a certain degree during expiration. Air is trapped distal to the obstruction, so there is progressive hyperinflation of the lungs. Prolonged wheezing expirations are thus characteristic as the patient struggles to force the air out. It is usual for an asthmatic attack to last from a few minutes to several hours, followed by a cough that is productive of considerable whitish sputum. Treatment consists of administration of bronchodilator drugs, specific long-term desensitization, avoidance of known allergens, and occasionally administration of corticosteroid drugs. Intervals between attacks are characteristically free from respiratory difficulty. Asthma is distinguished from chronic bronchitis and emphysema by its intermittent nature and the fact that destructive emphysema rarely occurs. An asthmatic attack that continues for days and is intractable to ordinary methods of treatment is called *status asthmaticus*. In these patients, ventilatory function may be so impaired as to result in cyanosis and death (see Chapter 10).

Chronic Bronchitis and Emphysema

Although chronic bronchitis and emphysema represent two distinct processes, they are often found in combination in patients with COPD. An estimated 13 million Americans have chronic bronchitis and/or emphysema, which was responsible for more than 90,000 deaths in 1991. The incidence of COPD has risen 450% since 1950, and it is now the fourth leading cause of death. COPD affects men twice as often as women, presumably because men have been heavier smokers; however, the incidence of COPD in women has increased 600% since 1950, presumably reflecting their smoking behavior (U.S. Public Health Service, 1993).

The main pathologic findings in chronic bronchitis are hypertrophy of the bronchial mucosal glands and an increase in the number and size of goblet cells, accompa-nied by inflammatory cell infiltration and edema of the bronchial mucosa. The resulting increased production of mucus leads to the characteristic symptoms of cough and expectoration. The chronic cough in the presence of increased bronchial secretions appears to affect the minute bronchioles to the point of destruction and dilation of their walls. The primary etiologic factors seem to be cigarette smoking and the forms of air pollution common to the industrial environment. Continued air pollution also predisposes to recurrent infections by slowing down ciliary and phagocytic activity, causing increased mucus accumulation at the same time that defense mechanisms are weakened.

Emphysema is classified according to the pattern of involvement of the acini. Although several morphologic patterns have been described, two types are most important in relation to COPD. *Centrilobular emphysema* (CLE) selectively affects the respiratory bronchioles and alveolar ducts. Fenestrations develop in the walls, enlarge, become confluent, and tend to form a single space as the walls disintegrate (Fig. 38-3). Initially, the more distal alveolar ducts and sacs and the alveoli are preserved. CLE usually affects the upper portions of the lung more severely, but it tends to be unevenly distributed. CLE is more prevalent in men than in women, is usually associated with chronic bronchitis, and is seldom found in nonsmokers.

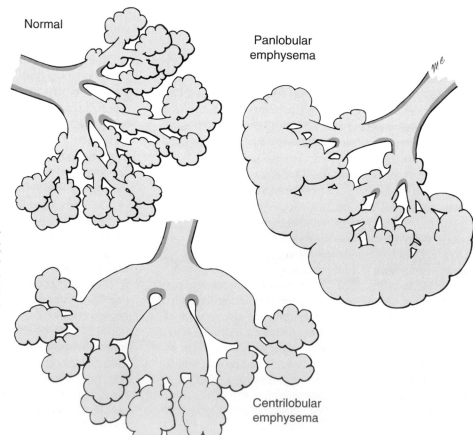

FIG. 38-3   Morphologic types of emphysema. Panlobular: entire pulmonary lobule involved; destruction and distention distal to the respiratory bronchioles. Centrilobular: destruction is central, primarily involving the respiratory bronchioles.

Panlobular emphysema (PLE), or *panacinar emphysema,* is a less common morphologic pattern in which there is nearly uniform enlargement and destruction of the alveoli distal to the terminal bronchiole; both the central and the peripheral portions of the acinus are involved (Fig. 38-3). As the disease progresses, there is gradual loss of all components of the acinus until only a few strands of tissue remain, which are usually blood vessels. PLE is characteristically uniform in distribution throughout the lung, although the basal sections tend to be more severely affected. PLE, but not CLE, is associated with a small group of patients with primary emphysema. This form of emphysema is characterized by the insidious development of increased airway resistance without evidence of chronic bronchitis. It has an early onset and usually produces symptoms between ages 30 and 40 years. In England, fewer than 6% of patients with COPD have *primary emphysema,* which affects women as often as men. The cause of this form of emphysema is unknown, but a familial type associated with a deficiency of the enzyme alpha$_1$-antiprotease has been described.

It has been hypothesized that *alpha$_1$-antiprotease* * is essential in protection of the lung against the naturally occurring proteases and that a deficiency of this antiprotease may play a role in the pathogenesis of emphysema (Cherniak, Cherniak, 1983). Proteases are produced by bacteria, polymorphonuclear neutrophils (PMNs), monocytes, and macrophages during the phagocytic process (see Chapter 4) and have the ability to break down the elastin and other macromolecules in lung tissue. In the healthy person, lung tissue damage is prevented by the action of antiproteases, which inhibit protease activity. This theory is based on the discovery of a small group of patients with an inherited deficiency of alpha$_1$-antiprotease. Genetic typing has revealed that most members of the normal population with normal levels of alpha$_1$-antiprotease have two M genes and are designated as type MM. Two of the most common genes associated with emphysema are the S and Z genes. Homozygous SS or ZZ individuals have serum levels of alpha$_1$-antiprotease that are near zero or very low and have a 70% to 80% chance of developing emphysema of the primary type (panlobular or emphysematous). Heterozygous MS or MZ individuals with one abnormal gene have intermediate levels of alpha$_1$-antiprotease and are believed to have an increased predisposition to develop emphysema, usually of the bronchitic type (centrilobular). In persons of the latter group, smoking can produce an inflammatory response with consequent release of proteolytic enzymes (proteases), while at the same time the oxidants in smoke inhibit alpha$_1$-antiprotease. The heterozygous state is common, with

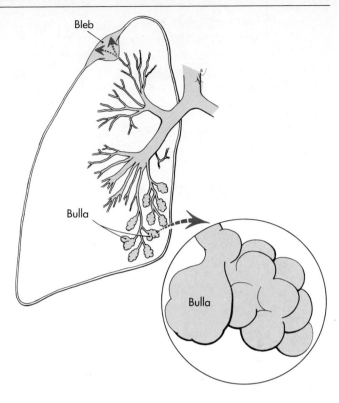

FIG. 38-4   Pulmonary blebs and bullae.

an estimated incidence of 5% to 14% of the general population affected.

PLE, although characteristic of primary emphysema, may also be associated with the emphysema of aging and with chronic bronchitis. It is believed that the deterioration of the elastic and reticular fibers of the lung, with the resultant loss of elastic recoil of the lung, leads to progressive generalized distention of the lung in the aging process. *Senile emphysema,* however, is not true emphysema because most of these elderly patients do not develop significant impairment of lung function. The PLE associated with chronic bronchitis is thought to be an end stage of progressive CLE because both morphologic patterns may exist in the same lung.

When the thorax of a patient who has emphysema is opened during surgery or at autopsy, the lungs are seen to be grossly enlarged; they remain filled with air and do not collapse. They are whiter than normal and feel downy or billowy. Subpleural air-filled spaces called *blebs* and parenchymal air-filled spaces greater than 1 cm in diameter called *bullae* are typically seen (Fig. 38-4). There is also generalized dilation of the air spaces. Bullae are common in both PLE and CLE but may exist in the absence of either. Bullae generally develop because of a check-valve bronchiolar obstruction (Fig. 38-5). During inspiration the bronchiolar lumen widens so that air is able to pass by the obstruction caused by thickening of the mucosa and excess mucus. During expiration, however, when the bronchiolar lumen normally becomes nar-

---

*Formerly known as alpha$_1$-antitrypsin; it is now known as alpha$_1$-antiprotease because it has been found to inhibit the action of other proteases as well as trypsin.

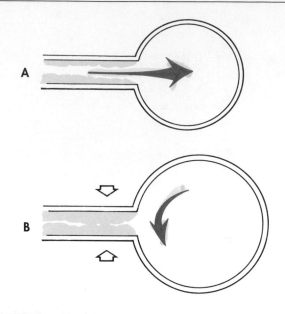

FIG. 38-5   Check-valve bronchiolar obstruction. **A,** During inspiration, lumen widens enough to allow air entry. **B,** During expiration, premature collapse and narrowed lumen prevent egress of air that becomes trapped in alveoli.

rowed, the obstruction may prevent the egress of air. A loss of elasticity of the bronchiolar walls in emphysema may also cause premature collapse. Air is thus trapped in the affected pulmonary segment, leading to overdistention and coalescence of several alveoli. This effect is caused by fragmentation of the interalveolar elastic tissue and subsequent rupture of the attenuated interalveolar septa, resulting in a bulla. In emphysema there may be a single bulla or many bullae, which may or may not communicate with each other. Blebs, which are formed by ruptured alveoli, may rupture into the pleural cavity and cause a spontaneous pneumothorax (collapse of the lung). Other changes frequently seen in the COPD lung are a reduction in the capillary bed and histologic evidence of chronic bronchiolitis (involvement of the minute bronchioles).

The flow diagram in Fig. 38-6 illustrates the pathogenesis of COPD and the morphologic types of emphysema that result. This diagram emphasizes that although a genetic predisposition may be a factor in the development of pulmonary emphysema and smoking and air pollution are the prime factors in the pathogenesis of the bronchitic type of emphysema, an interaction exists between the two. For example, persons with a genetic predisposition might develop emphysema if exposed to varying degrees of air pollution. Although senile dilation of the air spaces is not considered true emphysema, it is possible that normal loss of elasticity of the lung parenchyma associated with aging is a factor in the development of true emphysema.

The clinical course of patients with COPD ranges from

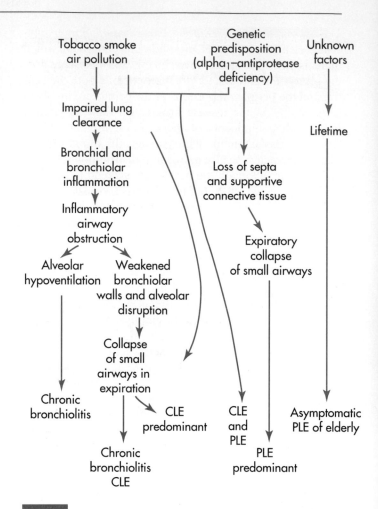

FIG. 38-6   Pathogenesis of COPD. *CLE,* Centrilobular emphysema; *PLE,* panlobular emphysema. (Modified from *Chronic obstructive pulmonary disease: a manual for physicians,* ed 3, New York, 1972, National Tuberculosis and Respiratory Disease Association.)

what is known as the pink puffers to the blue bloaters. The clinical hallmark of *pink puffers* (associated with primary PLE) is the development of dyspnea without significant cough and sputum production. Usually the dyspnea begins between ages 30 and 40 years and becomes increasingly severe. In advanced disease the patient may be too breathless to eat and characteristically has a thin, wasted appearance. Later in the course of the disease, the pink puffer may develop secondary chronic bronchitis. The chest of the patient is barrel shaped; the diaphragm is low and moves poorly. Polycythemia and cyanosis are rare (thus the term *pink*), and cor pulmonale (heart disease resulting from pulmonary hypertension and lung disease) rarely develops until the terminal stage. Minimal ventilation-perfusion imbalance occurs, so by hyperventilating, the pink puffer is usually able to keep blood gases within the normal range until late in the course of the disease. The lungs are usually greatly enlarged, and thus total lung capacity (TLC) and residual volume (RV) increase greatly.

TABLE 38-1   Differentiation of Clinical Types of COPD

Feature	Pink Puffer (Emphysematous)	Blue Bloater (Bronchitic)
Onset	30 to 40 years of age	20s and 30s: cigarette cough
Age at time of diagosis	60± years	50± years
Cause	Unknown factors	Unknown factors
	Genetic predisposition	Smoking
	Smoking	Air pollution
	Air pollution	Climate
Sputum	Minimal	Copious
Dypsnea	Relatively early	Relatively late
$\dot{V}/\dot{Q}$ ratio	Minimal $\dot{V}/\dot{Q}$ imbalance	Marked $\dot{V}/\dot{Q}$ imbalance
Body build	Thin, asthenic	Well nourished
Anteroposterior diameter of chest	Barrel chest common	Not increased
Pathologic lung anatomy	Panlobular emphysema	Centrilobular emphysema predominant
Respiratory pattern	Hyperventilation and marked dyspnea, which may occur at rest	Diminished respiratory drive
		Hypoventilation common, with resultant hypoxia and hypercapnia
Lung volume	Low FEV_1	Low FEV_1
	Increased TLC and RV	Normal TLC; moderate increase in RV
$Paco_2$	Normal or low (35-40 mm Hg)	Elevated (50-60 mm Hg)
Pao_2	65-75 mm Hg	45-60 mm Hg
Sao_2	Normal	Much desaturation because of $\dot{V}/\dot{Q}$ imbalance
Hematocrit	35%-45%	50%-55%
Polycythemia	Hemoglobin and hematocrit normal until late	Elevated hemoglobin and hematocrit common
Cyanosis	Rare	Common
Cor pulmonale	Rare, except terminally	Frequent, with many episodes

$\dot{V}/\dot{Q}$, Ventilation/perfusion; $Paco_2$, Pao_2, arterial carbon dioxide, oxygen tensions; Sao_2, oxygen saturation; FEV_1, forced expiratory volume in 1 second; TLC, total lung capacity; RV, residual volume.

At the other extreme of the COPD range are the *blue bloaters* (bronchitis with little evidence of obstructive emphysema). These patients usually have a productive cough and frequent respiratory infections that continue for years before there is noticeable functional impairment. Eventually, however, they develop dyspnea on exertion. These patients show a diminished respiratory drive; they hypoventilate and become hypoxic and hypercapnic. There is also an extremely distorted ventilation/perfusion ($\dot{V}/\dot{Q}$) ratio. The chronic hypoxia stimulates the kidney to produce erythropoietin, which in turn stimulates increased production of red blood cells, resulting in secondary polycythemia. Hemoglobin (Hb) levels may be 20 g/dl or higher, and cyanosis is more readily apparent because there may easily be 5 g/dl of reduced Hb when only a small proportion of the circulating blood Hb is in the reduced form (thus the name *blue bloater*). Because these patients are not dyspneic at rest, they appear to be comfortable. There is generally not a great weight loss, and body build is normal. The TLC may be normal, and the diaphragm is in the normal position. Death usually results from cor pulmonale (which develops early) or from respiratory failure. At autopsy, emphysema is often,

although not always, seen. The emphysema tends to be of the centrilobular type, although the panlobular type may also be present.

Table 38-1 contrasts the pure bronchitic (blue bloater) and emphysematous (pink puffer) types of COPD. Most patients with COPD lie somewhere between these two extremes.

The typical course of COPD is long, beginning in the patient's 20s and 30s with a "cigarette cough" or "morning cough" and the production of a small amount of mucoid sputum. Minor respiratory infections tend to persist longer than usual in these patients. Although exercise tolerance may decrease somewhat, it usually goes unnoticed as the patient becomes less energetic over time. Eventually episodes of acute bronchitis occur more regularly, particularly in the winter, and the patient's working capacity decreases, so that work may have to be given up sometime in the patient's 50s or 60s. In patients of the predominantly emphysematous type, the course appears to be less protracted, with no previous history of a productive cough; severe debilitating dyspnea may develop within a few years. When hypercapnia, hypoxemia, and cor pulmonale develop, the prognosis is poor and death usually comes within a few years after the onset. A combination of respiratory failure and heart failure precipitated by pneumonia is the usual cause of death.

Therapy for the patient with chronic bronchitis and obstructive emphysema requires measures to relieve obstruction of the small airways. Although airway collapse secondary to emphysema is irreversible, many patients have some degree of bronchospasm, retention of secretions, and mucosal edema, which may be relieved by the appropriate therapy. Of paramount importance is cessation of smoking and avoidance of other forms of air pollution or allergens that may aggravate symptoms. Often the cessation of smoking alone may bring about a marked relief of symptoms and improvement of ventilation. Infection should be treated promptly, and patients who are particularly susceptible to respiratory infection may be directed to use prophylactic antibiotics. The patient is instructed to seek this medication whenever dyspnea or the amount of sputum production increases. Tetracycline, ampicillin, and penicillin are usually the drugs of choice. All patients should receive influenza vaccine.

Additional measures to relieve airway obstruction include provision of adequate hydration to thin bronchial secretions, use of expectorants, and use of bronchodilator drugs to relieve smooth muscle spasm. Sympathomimetic drugs such as albuterol, terbutaline, and xanthines (e.g., aminophylline) are commonly administered. Ipratropium bromide (Atrovent), an anticholinergic agent in a metered-dose inhaler, is an effective bronchodilator in patients with chronic bronchitis. For patients with copious secretions, percussion and postural drainage are used to assist in removing obstructive secretions, which may also predispose to infection. Breathing exercises may also be helpful. The patient is taught to use slow, relaxed expiration against pursed lips. This exercise prevents collapse of small bronchioles and reduces the amount of trapped air. A graduated program of physical exercise during the administration of low-concentration oxygen may be helpful in improving the patient's sense of well-being. Oxygen, however, must be administered with caution in the later stages of the illness when the patient has hypercapnia and hypoxemia. Respiratory failure may be precipitated, since these patients depend on hypoxia to stimulate breathing. The treatment of cor pulmonale and respiratory failure complications are discussed in Chapters 40 and 41.

BRONCHIECTASIS

Bronchiectasis is a condition characterized by chronic dilation of the medium-sized bronchi and bronchioles (about fourth to ninth generations). Two anatomic types are usually described: saccular and cylindrical (Fig. 38-7). *Saccular bronchiectasis* consists of rounded cavity-like dilations, often found in dilated bronchi and typically in adults. Bronchiectasis develops when the bronchial walls are weakened by chronic inflammatory changes involving the mucosa and muscular coat. As seen in Fig. 38-7, purulent materials collect in these dilated areas and lead to persistent infection of the affected segment or lobe. Chronic infection causes further damage to the bronchial walls, and a vicious circle is set up. There is no single, specific cause of bronchiectasis, since it is a disease based on an abnormal anatomic condition. Most often, bronchiectasis begins in childhood after repeated lower respiratory tract infections, which develop as a complication of measles, whooping cough, or influenza. Bronchial obstruction resulting from a neoplasm or an aspirated foreign body (es-

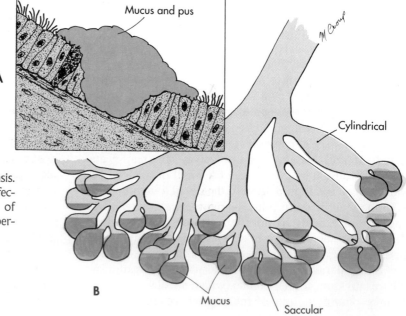

FIG. 38-7 Pathologic changes in bronchiectasis. **A,** Longitudinal section of bronchial wall: chronic infection causes damage to bronchial walls. **B,** Collection of purulent material in dilated bronchioles leading to persistent infection.

pecially if it is organic, such as a peanut) may also lead to bronchiectasis and secondary infection of the distal bronchial tree. Bronchiectasis of the upper lobes may be associated with tuberculosis, although it is frequently asymptomatic because bronchial drainage is achieved by gravity. Cystic fibrosis and Kartagener's syndrome (bronchiectasis associated with sinusitis and displacement of the heart to the right side of the thorax) are examples of congenital diseases associated with bronchiectasis.

The principal clinical feature of bronchiectasis is a chronic, loose cough productive of a large amount of mucopurulent, foul-smelling sputum. Coughing is most severe when the patient changes position. The amount of sputum varies with the stage of the disease but may be 200 ml daily in severe cases. Hemoptysis is common, usually consisting of blood streaks in the sputum. Characteristic features of advanced untreated disease are recurrent pneumonia, malnutrition, digital clubbing, cor pulmonale, and right ventricular failure.

The degree of functional disturbance depends on the extent of involvement of pulmonary tissue. Bronchiectasis localized to one or two segments of the lung may cause little impairment of pulmonary function, whereas diffuse bronchiectasis may be associated with anastomoses between the bronchial and pulmonary circulation, with resultant right-to-left shunting.

The most important feature of treatment is daily, vigorous bronchial hygiene with postural drainage, which generally must be continued for the rest of the patient's life. Antibiotic therapy for the control of infection is another important aspect of therapy. Before the advent of antibiotics, bronchiectasis was much more common and the prognosis was poor. Patients rarely lived beyond the age of 40 years. Bronchiectasis is much less common today and, except for the congenital forms of the disease, should be regarded as preventable. Timely vaccinations against childhood diseases frequently complicated by pneumonia, vigorous antibiotic and other appropriate treatment of pneumonia, and prompt removal of aspirated foreign bodies are all preventive measures.

CYSTIC FIBROSIS

Cystic fibrosis (CF), or *mucoviscidosis,* is a disease of genetic origin, occurring in about 1 in 2000 births among Caucasians but is rarely seen in African Americans or Asians. The name cystic fibrosis was formulated originally to describe the pathologic changes of the lungs and pancreas in afflicted individuals. Obstruction of exocrine ducts followed by cystic dilation and fibrosis is accompanied by pancreatic insufficiency and inability to clear pulmonary secretions, which lead to the clinical hallmarks of CF, recurrent respiratory infections and malabsorption.

CF is an autosomal recessive disease. The gene responsible for CF, located on the long arm of chromosome 7, was cloned in 1989; the CF gene protein product

known as the *cystic fibrosis transmembrane conductance regulator* (CFTR) was also identified (Harris, Argent, 1993). The CFTR protein is thought to be the chloride channel in epithelial cells, which explains the pathophysiologic basis of the disease: the primary abnormality is aberrant regulation of chloride transport across epithelial cells in the lungs, intestines, pancreas, and apocrine sweat glands. This defect impairs clearance of secretions in a variety of organs. The secretions of the exocrine glands that produce mucus and some other exocrine fluids produce abnormally viscid secretions. (Sweat and saliva are not particularly viscid but do contain abnormal amounts of salt.) The viscid secretions typically cause obstruction of the pancreatic and hepatic ducts and the bronchioles. The obstruction, in turn, can lead to fibrotic changes in the involved organs.

Most individuals with CF are diagnosed in the first few years of life, when recurrent respiratory infections, steatorrhea, and growth retardation prompt a *sweat chloride test.* Under standardized conditions for collection of sweat after pilocarpine administration (which stimulates sweating), more than 99% of CF patients have sweat chloride levels greater than 60 mEq/L (Denning et al., 1980). Normal chloride values range from 10 to 35 mEq/L.

The course of CF, largely determined by the degree of pulmonary involvement, varies from patient to patient. However, deterioration is inevitable, leading to debilitation and death. The prognosis has improved over the past few decades, mainly because of aggressive treatment before the onset of irreversible pulmonary changes. Median survival time has increased from less than 2 years in the 1940s to 26 years in the 1990s. The respiratory disease and complications that accompany CF account for more than 95% of the deaths. The sequence of events proceeds from recurrent pulmonary infections that gradually develop into bronchiectasis from retention of thick secretions to chronic pneumonia, fibrosis, ventilation-perfusion imbalance, chronic hypoxemia, cor pulmonale, and respiratory failure. Pulmonary function studies invariably show an obstruction pattern, although restrictive lung volumes may be present with advanced disease. Patients with advanced disease may produce up to 200 ml of sputum per day. Finger clubbing is common.

Because pulmonary dysfunction is the overriding factor in determining survival, the management of this aspect of the disease is crucial, with removal of the obstructing bronchial secretions as the most crucial aspect of treatment. Generally, aerosol therapy is used to liquefy secretions and is followed by percussion and postural drainage. A number of agents for increasing mucus clearance are being tested. The development of an aerosolized recombinant human deoxyribonuclease (DNase) that degrades thickened mucus and allows it to be cleared more easily appears promising. *Gelosin,* a protein that dismembers actin, may prove useful as a mucolytic agent. Prevention of respiratory infection and its prompt treatment with sputum-sensitive specific antibiotics is also a central aspect of treatment.

QUESTIONS

▼ *Answer the following on a separate sheet of paper.*

1. What is the ventilatory functional disorder associated with COPD?
2. Describe the interrelation of chronic bronchitis, pulmonary emphysema, and asthma.
3. Describe the symptoms of an asthmatic attack. How is it treated? What is *status asthmaticus*?
4. Contrast the two morphologic patterns of emphysema according to anatomic changes, distribution in lung, gender prevalence, type of associated COPD, and etiology.
5. What are the objectives of treatment for chronic bronchitis and emphysema?
6. What are the two criteria for establishing a diagnosis of chronic bronchitis? What is the time within which these symptoms must be manifested (months per year and consecutive years)?
7. Describe the pathologic anatomic changes in the lung parenchyma in pulmonary emphysema.
8. What are subpleural air-filled spaces called? What is their cause?
9. What are parenchymal air-filled spaces more than 1 cm in diameter called? What generally causes them?
10. How does the tracheobronchial tree of the asthmatic patient respond to various stimuli? How is this manifested?
11. What anatomic changes occur in bronchiectasis? What are some possible precipitating factors, and what features tend to cause persistence and progression of the disease?
12. What are the principal clinical features of bronchiectasis?
13. Identify the mode of treatment for bronchiectasis.
14. What is the most crucial aspect of treatment of cystic fibrosis?

▼ *Match each of the diseases in column A with its basis for definition in column B.*

Column A
15. _____ Chronic bronchitis
16. _____ Pulmonary emphysema
17. _____ Asthma

Column B
a. Pathologic anatomy
b. Clinical symptoms
c. Pathophysiology

▼ *Circle the letter preceding each item below that correctly completes the statement. More than one item may be correct.*

18. The pathologic changes associated with chronic bronchitis include:
    a. Hypertrophy of the bronchial mucosal glands
    b. Destruction of alveolar walls
    c. Increase in the number of goblet cells
    d. Edema, scarring, and increased thickness of bronchioles
    e. Decreased production of surfactant

19. In bronchial asthma:
    a. Bronchiolar smooth muscle is atrophic.
    b. Medium-sized and small bronchi are plugged with viscid mucus.
    c. The lungs are pale and emphysematous.
    d. The patient is usually free from symptoms between attacks.

20. Emphysema is an anatomic entity that:
    a. Has one basic morphologic pattern
    b. Causes serious respiratory insufficiency when it develops as a result of the aging process
    c. Is characterized by increased size of the air spaces distal to the terminal bronchioles with associated parenchymal destruction
    d. Is always related to chronic bronchitis

21. The major source of disability and death in pediatric patients with cystic fibrosis is:
    a. Malnutrition
    b. Recurrent pulmonary infection
    c. Hyponatremia resulting from the loss of salt in sweat and saliva
    d. Chronic pancreatitis

22. Centrilobular emphysema:
    a. Is more common than PLE
    b. Appears to be related to cigarette smoking
    c. Usually affects the upper lobes more severely
    d. Is associated with deficiency of alpha₁-antiprotease

23. The pathophysiology of asthma is characterized by:
    a. Bronchodilation
    b. Alveoli filled with exudate
    c. Loss of support of bronchiolar walls
    d. Bronchiolar narrowing

▼ *Circle T if the statement is true and F if it is false in regard to cystic fibrosis. Correct any false statements.*

24. T F Mucoviscidosis is another name for the disease.
25. T F It is a disease of genetic origin.
26. T F It is more common in African Americans than in Caucasians.
27. T F Up to 200 ml of mucopurulent, foul-smelling sputum may be produced daily.
28. T F The exocrine glands are affected by this disease.
29. T F Digital clubbing is a characteristic feature of advanced disease.
30. T F The prognosis of cystic fibrosis is generally good.

QUESTIONS—cont'd

▼ *Match the pink puffer and blue bloater types of COPD in column B with their associated features in column A.*

Column A
31. _____ PLE
32. _____ CLE predominant
33. _____ Genetic predisposition
34. _____ Late onset of dyspnea
35. _____ Minimal sputum
36. _____ Polycythemia common
37. _____ Early cor pulmonale
38. _____ Marked $\dot{V}/\dot{Q}$ imbalance
39. _____ Thin, wasted appearance
40. _____ Hypercapnia (early)

Column B
a. Pink puffer
b. Blue bloater

▼ *Match the type of asthmatic condition in column A with the appropriate descriptive features in column B. Each item in column B may be used more than once.*

Column A
41. _____ Extrinsic asthma
42. _____ Intrinsic asthma
43. _____ Mixed asthma

Column B
a. A clearly defined precipitating factor is absent.
b. The condition is clearly caused by a known allergen and usually develops in early childhood.
c. Attacks may be associated with infection of the tracheobronchial tree or of the nasal sinuses.
d. This type affects most asthmatic patients.
e. Exposure to the allergen precipitates an asthmatic attack.

▼ *Circle the letter preceding each item below that correctly completes the statement.*

44. Individuals with homozygous alpha₁-antiprotease deficiency (SS or ZZ phenotypes) have a _____ chance of developing primary emphysema:
   a. <20%
   b. 20%-40%
   c. 40%-60%
   d. >70%

45. The lung pathology associated with homozygous alpha₁-antiprotease deficiency (SS or ZZ phenotypes) is believed to result from:
   a. Unopposed effect of inhaled irritants
   b. Defective repair of microbial-induced damage
   c. Unopposed effect of host phagocytic proteolysis
   d. Unopposed effect of host trypsin liberation

46. The type and distribution of lung disease in homozygous alpha₁-antiprotease is usually:
   a. CLE predominant at the bases
   b. PLE predominant at the bases
   c. Generalized airway disease or chronic bronchitis

   d. Uniform bullous or cystic disease

47. Individuals who are heterozygous with respect to alpha₁-antiprotease (MS or MZ phenotypes) have an increased predisposition to developing emphysema of the _____ type, and the estimated incidence of these individuals is as high as _____ of the general population.
   a. Panlobular; 1%
   b. Panlobular; 14%
   c. Centrilobular; 1%
   d. Centrilobular; 14%

48. A 50-year-old heavy smoker has two episodes of "chest infection" after colds in one winter. On questioning, he states that he has had a morning cough productive of clear sputum on most days for the past 5 to 10 years. Tuberculosis and bronchiectasis were considered and ruled out at the time of the second recent infection. Which of the following diagnoses is most likely?
   a. Emphysema
   b. Chronic bronchitis
   c. Asthma
   d. Lung cancer

49. An 8-year-old boy presents with non-seasonal recurrent upper and lower respiratory infections. He has persistent cough and sputum production even between infections and recently has begun to be dyspneic on mild effort. He has no obvious gastrointestinal problems, but his mother states that he has bulky, foul-smelling stools. He has had measles but not pertussis or chickenpox. He is undersized and has finger clubbing and rales over both apices. Which of the following is his most likely problem?
   a. Post-measles bronchiectasis
   b. Cystic fibrosis
   c. Hypogammaglobulinemia
   d. Nontropical sprue (celiac disease)

50. The boy's condition in question 49 would be confirmed by which of the following test results?
   a. Stool fat determination shows higher than normal fat excretion.
   b. Sweat chloride test is 78 mEq/L (normal, 10 to 35 mEq/L).
   c. Sputum culture is positive for *Staphylococcus aureus.*
   d. Chest computed tomography scan shows areas of bronchiectasis.

CHAPTER 39

Restrictive Patterns of Respiratory Disease

LORRAINE M. WILSON

A restrictive ventilatory disorder is characterized by increased stiffness of the lungs or thorax or both, resulting from decreased compliance and a reduction in all lung volumes, including the vital capacity. The work of breathing increases to overcome the elastic forces of the respiratory apparatus, so a pattern of rapid, shallow breathing is adopted. The physiologic consequences of a restricted pattern of ventilation are alveolar hypoventilation and an inability to maintain normal blood gas tensions.

A number of diseases may contribute to pulmonary restriction through varying mechanisms. In this chapter, these diseases are divided into two classes: extrapulmonary disorders, including neurologic, neuromuscular, and thoracic cage disorders; and diseases of the pleura and lung parenchyma.

EXTRAPULMONARY DISEASE

Neurologic and Neuromuscular Disorders

In reference to extrapulmonary disorders, the term *extrapulmonary* implies that the lung tissue itself may be quite normal. The common pathophysiologic disturbance in these disorders is *alveolar hypoventilation,* although this is not entirely true in the case of kyphoscoliosis.

A number of disorders directly affecting the medullary respiratory center may cause alveolar hypoventilation. Carbon dioxide (CO_2) retention from a variety of causes may depress rather than stimulate respiration when the arterial CO_2 partial pressure, or tension (Pa_{CO_2}), exceeds about 70 mm Hg. A number of drugs are capable of depressing the respiratory center, thereby causing alveolar hypoventilation. For example, narcotic or barbiturate drug overdose is a common cause of death resulting from respiratory depression and failure. Acute "overdose" of ethanol also can cause death by depression of respiration. Anatomic damage to the respiratory center resulting from head trauma or cerebral lesions caused by a cerebrovascular accident (CVA, stroke) can also cause respiratory center depression and alveolar hypoventilation. Abnormalities of neural or neuromuscular transmission to the respiratory muscles may result in paresis or paralysis and alveolar hypoventilation. Amyotrophic lateral sclerosis, poliomyelitis, Guillain-Barré syndrome, and myasthenia gravis are neurologic disorders that may produce ventilatory insufficiency. The muscles themselves are diseased in progressive muscular dystrophy. The severity of the respiratory involvement in any of these diseases depends on the amount of anatomic involvement: vital capacity (VC) is reduced in proportion to the degree of paresis of the respiratory muscles. Although parenchymal lung disease is not primary, secondary infection is common because of ineffective coughing and limitation of respiratory excursions. Table 39-1 summarizes the extrapulmonary disorders causing alveolar hypoventilation and the mechanism responsible.

Thoracic Cage Disorders

Four major types of fixed chest wall deformities may restrict ventilation by interfering with the bellows mechanism: kyphoscoliosis, pectus excavatum, ankylosing spondylitis, and healed thoracoplasty.

Kyphosis is a term that refers to any posterior angulation of the spine (hunchback), and *scoliosis* refers to a lateral displacement of the spine. Kyphoscoliosis is therefore characterized by angulation of the spine both poste-

TABLE 39-1   Extrapulmonary Disorders Causing Alveolar Hypoventilation

System or Structure	Disease or Altered Condition	Altered Mechanism
Neurologic (central nervous system, CNS)	$Paco_2$ >70 mm Hg Narcotics and barbiturates	Depression of the respiratory center
	Head trauma, CNS lesions	Direct anatomic damage to the respiratory center
	Poliomyelitis	Interruption of nerve transmission to respiratory muscles because of lower motor neuron lesion
	Amyotrophic lateral sclerosis	Interruption of nerve transmission to respiratory muscles because of upper motor neuron lesion
Neurologic (peripheral nervous system)	Guillain-Barré syndrome	Interruption of nerve transmission to respiratory muscles as a result of inflammation involving ganglion cells and peripheral nerves
	Myasthenia gravis	Interruption of nerve transmission to respiratory muscles because of disease involving the neuromuscular junction
Muscular	Progressive muscular dystrophy	Paresis of the respiratory muscles because of diffuse disease of the skeletal muscles
Chest cage	Kyphoscoliosis	Deformity of the chest cage causing abnormal positioning and functioning of the respiratory muscles and compression of the chest cage contents
	Closed chest wall trauma	Voluntary restriction of ventilation as a result of pain or paradoxical movement of the chest wall and thoracic contents in flail chest injury
	Pickwickian syndrome (extreme obesity)	Limitation of thoracic movement by accumulated body fat

Paco₂, Arterial carbon dioxide tension.

riorly and laterally. About 80% of cases are idiopathic; the remaining 20% result from the aftereffects of poliomyelitis or tuberculosis of the spine (Pott's disease). Kyphoscoliosis is quite common, with about 1% of the American population affected, although the defect is severe enough to produce cardiopulmonary symptoms in only a small proportion of these persons. Severe kyphoscoliosis is associated with marked asymmetry of the chest and leads to abnormal functioning and positioning of the respiratory muscles and to compression of the lungs.

Fig. 39-1 shows the sequence of events that may lead to both respiratory and cardiac failure in kyphoscoliosis. In these persons, breathing entails a high work and energy cost, so a rapid, shallow pattern is adopted. This in turn leads to alveolar hypoventilation by preferential ventilation of the anatomic dead space at the expense of alveolar ventilation. In addition, compression of the lungs by the thoracic deformity causes a small lung volume and unequal distribution of ventilation and perfusion because both alveoli and pulmonary blood vessels are compressed. The consequent physiologic shunting leads to hypoxemia. When alveolar ventilation is also limited, the result is hypoxemia, hypercapnia, and respiratory acidosis. Compression of the pulmonary blood vessels and the acidosis also lead to pulmonary hypertension and cor pulmonale. The common cause of death from this chain of events is a combination of respiratory failure and heart failure.

Pectus excavatum (funnel chest) is a congenital deformity in which the lower end of the sternum is attached to the thoracic spine by fibromuscular bands, giving the lower sternal area a caved-in appearance. Compare this deformity with kyphoscoliosis in Fig. 39-2. Pectus excavatum, unlike severe kyphoscoliosis, rarely causes more than mild restriction of ventilation.

Thoracoplasty is a surgically induced depression of the thoracic cage that was once performed for the treatment of tuberculosis but is no longer common. Because this procedure is performed for an underlying lung disease, the subsequent pulmonary dysfunction is usually more closely related to the original disease than to the induced deformity.

Ankylosing spondylitis is a disease that causes symmetric reduction in mobility of the bony thorax as a result of the ossification of the vertebral joints and ligaments (see Chapter 75). Rib fixation and increased stiffness of the chest wall cause mild ventilatory restriction, which is not usually symptomatic.

Closed chest wall injury may also restrict ventilation. The most common chest wall injury is simple rib fracture. As a result of the pain and muscle splinting, there is ventilatory restriction of tidal volume (V_T), increase in respiratory frequency (f), and voluntary inhibition of the cough reflex. Healthy young persons tend to tolerate these changes well, but in elderly persons these changes may lead to impaired clearing of secretions, respiratory tract infection, blood gas abnormalities, and

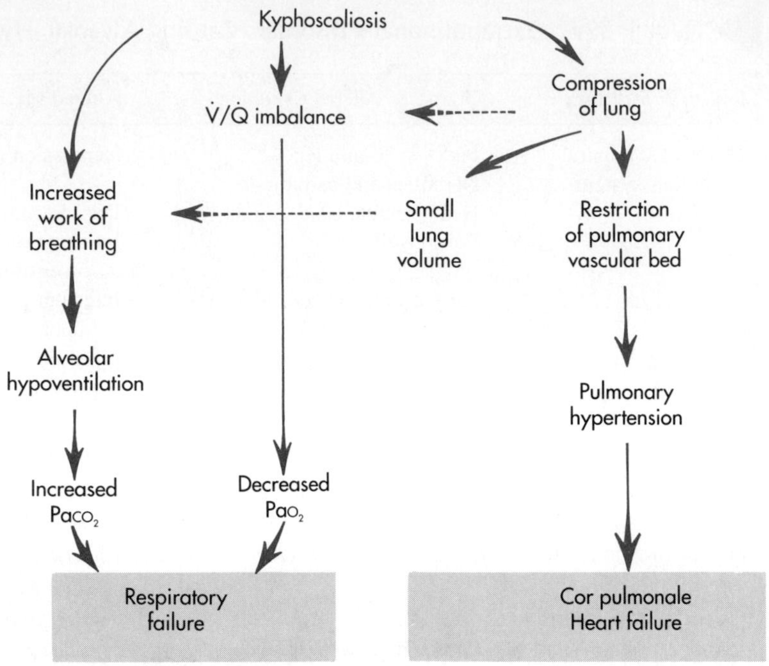

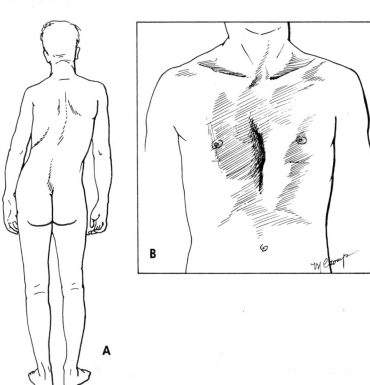

FIG. 39-1 Pathogenesis of respiratory failure and heart failure in kyphoscoliosis. $\dot{V}/\dot{Q}$, Ventilation/perfusion; $PaCO_2$, arterial carbon dioxide tension; PaO_2, arterial oxygen tension.

FIG. 39-2 Thoracic deformities restricting ventilation. **A,** Kyphoscoliosis. **B,** Pectus excavatum (funnel chest).

even respiratory failure. Flail chest is a major defect in chest wall continuity caused by a crushing chest injury (typically seen in steering wheel injuries in motor vehicle crashes) with multiple rib fractures. The resulting instability of the chest wall causes a paradoxical movement of the chest wall accompanied by pendulum movement of the mediastinal contents during the breathing cycle. This condition may cause interference with venous return to the heart and cause dead-space air to be shunted back and forth between the lungs *(pendelluft)*, as illustrated in Fig. 39-3. The treatment for flail chest is stabilization of the chest wall and mechanical ventilation with positive end-expiratory pressure (PEEP).

Pickwickian syndrome is the term used to describe a group of clinical features found in persons who are extremely obese. These features include chronic alveolar hypoventilation, somnolence, polycythemia, hypoxemia, and hypercapnia. (The syndrome was named after the

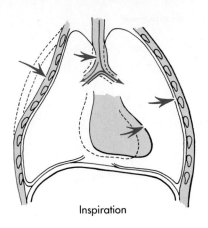
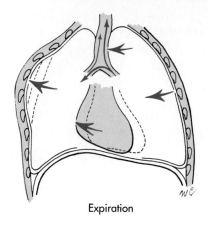

Inspiration   Expiration

FIG. 39-3   Altered cardiopulmonary dynamics in flail chest injury. Arrows indicate the direction of motion; arrows within the trachea and bronchi indicate air being shunted back and forth between lungs during respiratory cycle (pendelluft). Note paradoxical motion of the unstable portion of the chest wall on the right side. (From Burrows B, Knudson RJ, Kettle LJ: *Respiratory insufficiency*, Chicago, 1975, Mosby.)

sleepy fat boy in Dickens' *Pickwick Papers*.) The somnolence common to this syndrome can be related to the CO_2 retention that depresses the central nervous system (CNS); polycythemia is the compensatory response to chronic hypoxia. In persons with pickwickian syndrome, the accumulated body fat appears to limit thoracic movement and greatly increases the work of breathing. Respiratory impairment may progress to the point of cor pulmonale and respiratory failure. It is now known that pickwickian syndrome is only one subtype of a group of disorders called *sleep apnea syndromes*, in which elements of upper airway obstruction (which results in snoring) or central hypoventilation or both may be present (Phillipson, 1994). Nonobese persons may also be afflicted. It is important to note also that not all extremely obese persons develop alveolar hypoventilation and blood gas abnormalities. Weight reduction, if successful, seems to be the most effective treatment for pickwickian syndrome and may reverse the respiratory insufficiency.

DISEASES OF THE PLEURA AND LUNG PARENCHYMA

Pleural Disorders

The pleura and pleural space are the sites of a number of disorders that may restrict the expansion of the lungs or the alveoli or both. This reaction may result from compression of the lung as a result of the accumulation of air, fluid, blood, or purulent material in the pleural cavity. Pain resulting from inflammation or fibrosis of the pleura may also cause limitation of chest expansion.

Pleural effusion

The parietal and visceral pleura are opposed to each other and are separated by a thin layer of serous fluid. This thin layer of fluid represents a balance between transudation from the pleural capillaries and reabsorption by the visceral and parietal veins and lymphatics, as discussed in Chapter 35. *Pleural effusion* is the term applied

to a collection of fluid in the pleural cavity (Fig. 39-4, *A*). Pleural effusions may be transudates or exudates. A *transudate* occurs if there is a rise in pulmonary venous pressure, as in congestive heart failure. In these cases the balance of forces favors the passage of fluid out of the vessels. Transudation may also occur if there is hypoproteinemia, as in liver and renal disease. The accumulation of transudate in the pleural cavity is called *hydrothorax*. The pleural fluid tends to accumulate at the base of the lungs as a result of the force of gravity. The accumulation of an *exudate* is secondary to involvement of the pleura by inflammation or malignant growth and results from increased capillary permeability or impaired lymphatic absorption. An exudate is differentiated from a transudate by the protein content and specific gravity of the pleural fluid. Transudates have a specific gravity of less than 1.015 and a protein content of less than 3%; exudates have a higher specific gravity and protein content because of their cellular content.

When the pleural effusion contains pus, the condition is termed *empyema*. Empyema is the result of extension of infection from contiguous structures and may be a complication of pneumonia, lung abscess, or perforation of a carcinoma into the pleural cavity. Empyema that is not adequately treated by drainage may have disastrous effects on the thoracic cage. The inflammatory exudate becomes organized, and fibrous adhesions weld the parietal and visceral pleura together. This condition is termed *fibrothorax* (Fig. 39-4). If the fibrothorax is extensive, it may cause serious mechanical restriction of the underlying tissue. Surgical peeling, called *decortication*, is sometimes necessary to separate the pleural membranes.

The term *hemothorax* is used to designate frank bleeding into the pleural cavity and does not designate a hemorrhagic pleural effusion. Trauma is the most common cause of hemothorax. The trauma may be classified as *penetrating* (e.g., knife wound) or *nonpenetrating* (e.g., fractured rib, which in turn lacerates the lung or an intercostal blood vessel). The thoracic duct can also drain lymph into the pleural cavity as a result of trauma or malignant tumor, a condition termed *chylothorax*.

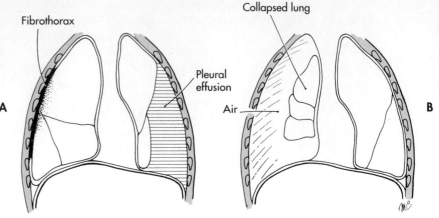

FIG. 39-4   Disorders of the pleura. **A,** Fibrothorax resulting from organization of inflammatory exudate and pleural effusion. **B,** Collapse of lung because of open pneumothorax.

Pneumothorax

The presence of air in the pleural cavity caused by a breach in the pleura is termed *pneumothorax.* A pneumothorax may be classified according to cause as traumatic or spontaneous. It may also be classified according to the sequence of events that follow the breach in the pleura as open, closed, or tension pneumothorax.

A penetrating wound to the chest is a common cause of *traumatic pneumothorax.* As the air enters the pleural space, which is normally subatmospheric in pressure, the lung collapses to a variable extent. If the communication is open, a massive collapse occurs until the pressure in the pleural cavity is equal to that of the atmosphere (*open pneumothorax,* Fig. 39-4, *B*). The mediastinum shifts in the direction of the collapsed lung and may shift to and fro during the respiratory cycle as air moves in and out of the pleural cavity. Emergency treatment of a penetrating chest wound consists of applying an airtight seal immediately over the wound. If the defect causing the communication between the pleural space and the atmosphere seals itself off, it is called a *closed pneumothorax.* On the other hand, if the defect remains open during inspiration and closes during expiration (check-valve effect), a large volume of air may collect in the pleural space so that pressure builds up above that of the atmosphere, causing complete collapse of the lung. This is termed *tension pneumothorax.* Tension pneumothorax is a serious emergency that must be treated immediately by aspiration of air from the pleural cavity.

Spontaneous pneumothorax is the term used to designate a sudden, unexpected pneumothorax, which may occur with or without underlying pulmonary disease. Common pulmonary diseases that may cause a spontaneous pneumothorax include emphysema (rupture of blebs or bullae), pneumonia, and neoplasms. A pneumothorax occurs when there is communication between a bronchus or alveolus and the pleural cavity so that air gains access to the pleural cavity through the defect, which may result in an open, closed, or tension pneumothorax. A spontaneous pneumothorax may occur in apparently healthy young persons, usually between ages 20 and 40 years, and is termed *idiopathic spontaneous pneumothorax.* The usual cause is rupture of a subpleural bleb at the surface of the lung or localized bullous disease (see Fig. 38-4). The cause of such a bleb or bulla in otherwise healthy persons is unknown, but a familial predisposition has sometimes been reported.

Both pleural effusion and pneumothorax limit function by restricting the expansion of the underlying lung. The degree of functional impairment and disability depends on the size and the rapidity of development. If fluid accumulates slowly, as is usually the case in pleural effusion, a large amount of fluid may be accommodated with little apparent distress. On the other hand, rapid decompression of a lung from a massive pneumothorax may be accompanied by rapid development of shock. Table 39-2

 TABLE 39-2   Signs and Symptoms of Pleural Effusion and Pneumothorax

Pleural Effusion	Pneumothorax
Dyspnea variable	Dyspnea (if large)
Pleuritic pain usually precedes effusion if secondary to pleuritic disease	Pleuritic pain severe
Trachea deviated away from the side of effusion	Trachea deviated away from the side of pneumothorax
Bulging of intercostal spaces (large effusion)	Tachycardia
	Cyanosis (if large)
Diminished and delayed chest movement on the involved side	Diminished and delayed chest movement on the involved side
Flat percussion note over the pleural effusion	Hyperresonant percussion note over pneumothorax
Egophony over compressed lung next to effusion	Flatness to percussion over collapsed lung
Decreased breath sounds over pleural effusion	Decreased or absent breath sounds on affected side
Decreased vocal and tactile fremitus	Decreased vocal and tactile fremitus

summarizes the signs and symptoms of pleural effusion and pneumothorax. The presence of both conditions is confirmed by radiography.

A first pneumothorax is treated by conservative observation if the collapse is 20% or less. The air is gradually absorbed through the pleural surfaces, which act as wet membranes, allowing oxygen (O_2) and CO_2 to diffuse through them. If the pneumothorax is large and dyspnea severe, a thoracotomy tube attached to water-sealed drainage will be necessary to aid reexpansion of the lung. If bloody effusion is associated with pneumothorax, it must be removed by drainage because clotting and organization lead to extensive pleural fibrosis. A pleural effusion is treated by needle aspiration *(thoracentesis)*. This treatment is particularly important if the effusion is an exudate, because fibrothorax may result. A small, noninflammatory effusion (transudate) may be resorbed into the capillaries once the cause of the effusion has been reversed.

Lung Parenchymal Disorders

A large number of diseases affecting the lung alveoli and/or interstitium lead either locally or diffusely to respiratory impairment of varying degrees. Damage to healthy lung tissue may result from invasion by bacteria, viruses, fungi, protozoa, or malignant cells and inhalation of irritating dust and fumes. Damage to the alveolar capillary endothelium from a variety of causes leads to interstitial, alveolar wall, and intraalveolar edema. Excess fibrotic tissue may be deposited as a sequela to a variety of diseases, usually inflammatory or allergenic in nature. The result is a reduction in lung compliance (stiff lungs) and interference with the gas diffusion pathway. A deficiency of surfactant, as in respiratory distress syndrome, may also produce the same results.

The physiologic abnormalities seen in patients with disease of the lung parenchyma vary widely and depend, to some degree, on the extent of the pathologic process. A restrictive defect with its concomitant decrease in lung volume and a rapid, shallow breathing pattern is common. Hypoxemia is the most important blood gas abnormality and is typically caused by a ventilation-perfusion imbalance, resulting in excess wasted ventilation or wasted perfusion caused by shunting. None of the physiologic abnormalities is specific, but pulmonary function tests are helpful in quantifying the degree of abnormality, guiding therapy, and assessing the results. Only selected, frequently encountered lung parenchymal diseases are discussed in this chapter.

Atelectasis

Atelectasis, although not a disease per se, is associated with disease of the lung parenchyma. *Atelectasis* is a term meaning "imperfect expansion," and it implies that the alveoli in the affected part of the lung have become airless and collapsed. Atelectasis should not be confused

with pneumothorax. Although alveolar collapse occurs in both conditions, the cause of the collapse is very different. Atelectasis occurs because alveoli become underinflated or uninflated, whereas pneumothorax occurs because air enters the pleural space. In most patients, pneumothorax is not preventable, but atelectasis is preventable with the proper nursing interventions. There are two major causes of collapse: absorption atelectasis secondary to bronchial or bronchiolar obstruction, and atelectasis caused by compression.

In *absorption atelectasis,* obstruction of the airway prevents air from entering the alveoli distal to the obstruction. The air already present in the alveoli is then absorbed gradually into the bloodstream, and the alveoli collapse. (It takes more air pressure and work to reinflate an alveolus from a completely collapsed position, just as one must blow harder at the beginning when blowing up a balloon.) Absorption atelectasis may result from intrinsic or extrinsic bronchial obstruction. Intrinsic bronchial obstruction is most frequently caused by retained secretions or exudate. Extrinsic pressure on a bronchus typically results from neoplasm, lymph node enlargement, aneurysm, or scar tissue. This discussion is concerned with intrinsic obstruction resulting from retained secretions, the more common and preventable cause.

The physiologic defense mechanisms that act to keep the lower respiratory tract sterile have already been discussed. Some of these mechanisms also act to prevent atelectasis by preventing obstruction. These mechanisms include the combined action of the "ciliary escalator," which may be assisted by cough to move noxious particles and bacteria to the posterior pharynx, where they are swallowed or expectorated. Another mechanism that prevents atelectasis is collateral ventilation. Recent experimental studies of collateral ventilation, a subject of debate for the past 50 years, leave no doubt that air can pass from one lung acinus to another by other than the normal airways. It is now well established that small pores, called the *pores of Kohn* after their discoverer in 1873, between the alveoli provide a path for collateral ventilation.

Fig. 39-5 illustrates how collateral ventilation prevents absorption atelectasis in the presence of bronchiolar obstruction by a mucus plug. Also illustrated is one of the causes of ineffective ventilation and its effect. Only deep inspiration is effective in opening up the pores of Kohn and providing collateral ventilation to an adjacent obstructed alveolus. Collapse caused by absorption of gases in the obstructed alveolus is thus prevented. (Normally gas absorption into the blood is favored because the total partial pressure of the blood gases is slightly less than atmospheric pressure because more O_2 is absorbed into the tissues than CO_2 is excreted.) During expiration the pores of Kohn close, and pressure builds up in the obstructed alveolus, which aids in the expulsion of the mucus plug. Even greater expiratory force may be built up if, after taking a deep breath, the glottis is closed and then suddenly opened as in the normal cough. In contrast, the

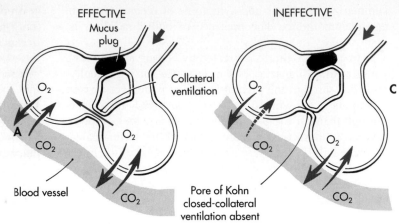

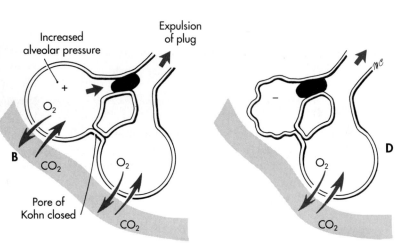

FIG. 39-5 Role of collateral alveolar ventilation in prevention of absorption atelectasis. Effective ventilation: **A,** during deep inspiration, pores of Kohn open and air enters adjacent obstructed alveolus; **B,** during expiration, pores of Kohn close; positive pressure builds up in obstructed alveolus and aids in expulsion of mucus plug. Ineffective ventilation: **C,** pores of Kohn do not open during shallow inspiration, so collateral ventilation is not provided to obstructed alveolus; **D,** obstructed alveolus collapses as alveolar gases are absorbed into bloodstream. (Modified from Kroeker EJ: *Hosp Med* 5:67-76, 1969.)

pores of Kohn remain closed with shallow inspiration, so that there is no collateral ventilation to the obstructed alveolus; pressure adequate to expel the mucus plug is thus not attained. Absorption of alveolar gases into the bloodstream continues, resulting in collapse of the alveolus. As the air leaves the alveolus, it is gradually replaced by edematous fluid.

This discussion emphasizes the importance of coughing and deep-breathing exercises and other physical activity to prevent atelectasis in predisposed persons. These measures are particularly important in postoperative, bedridden, or otherwise debilitated patients because atelectasis is the prevalent cause of morbidity in this population group. Atelectasis at the lung bases is especially common in patients whose respirations are shallow as a result of pain, weakness, or abdominal distention. Retained secretions may lead to pneumonia and more extensive atelectasis.

Prolonged atelectasis may lead to the replacement of the involved lung tissue with fibrous tissue. Adequate prevention also requires familiarity with factors that interfere with normal lung defense mechanisms. Some of these factors, discussed previously, are listed in Table 39-3 for added emphasis and consideration.

Compression atelectasis results from extrinsic pressure on all or part of the lung, driving the air out and causing collapse. Common causes are pleural effusion, pneumothorax, or abdominal distention that elevates the diaphragm. Compression atelectasis is much less common than absorption atelectasis.

Infections of the lung parenchyma: pneumonias

Acute inflammation of the lung parenchyma, which is usually infectious in origin, is called *pneumonia* or *pneumonitis.* The first term is preferable, since the second term has frequently been used to designate a nonspecific pulmonary inflammation of unknown cause. Pneumonia is a common malady and affects about 1% of the American population annually. Despite the development of antibiotics, pneumonia is still the sixth leading cause of death in the United States. The emergence of nosocomial (hospital-acquired) antibiotic-resistant organisms and newly discovered organisms (e.g., *Legionella*), the increased number of immunocompromised hosts, and diseases such as acquired immunodeficiency syndrome (AIDS) have expanded the range and severity of etiologic possibilities and explains why pneumonia remains a significant health care problem. The infant and young child are particularly susceptible because of poorly developed immune responses. Pneumonia is frequently the terminal event in elderly patients and those debilitated by chronic diseases. Alcoholic and postoperative patients

▶ TABLE 39-3   Lung Defense Mechanisms That Prevent Atelectasis

Protective Mechanism	Factors That Cause Interference With Mechanism
Mucus and ciliary action	General dehydration causes production of viscous mucus and scant volume. Inhalation of dry air increases viscosity of mucus so that crusting occurs. Excess mucus production (e.g., chronic bronchitis) overwhelms ciliary escalator. Cigarette smoke reduces or paralyzes ciliary action. Trauma (suctioning) reduces ciliary action. Anesthetics and atropine-like drugs reduce both mucus production and ciliary action.
Cough	Pain reduces expiratory force. Sedatives and narcotics inhibit cough initiation. Chronic obstructive pulmonary disease (COPD) reduces airflow rate.
Collateral ventilation	Shallow breathing is caused by pain or sedation. Pulmonary edema results from congestion or infection. Constant tidal volume respiration occurs in a patient on a mechanical respirator. Anesthetic gases and oxygen are rapidly absorbed, allowing less time for collateral ventilation.
Pharyngeal clearing	Unconsciousness; obtundation favors aspiration of gastric contents or upper respiratory tract secretions.

RISK FACTORS FOR PNEUMONIA

- Age >65 years
- Aspiration of oropharyngeal secretions
- Viral respiratory infection
- Chronic illness and debilitation (e.g., diabetes mellitus, uremia)
- Chronic respiratory disease (e.g., chronic obstructive pulmonary disease (COPD) asthma, cystic fibrosis)
- Cancer (especially lung cancer)
- Prolonged bedrest
- Tracheostomy or endotracheal tube
- Abdominal or thoracic surgery
- Rib fractures
- Immunosuppressive therapy
- AIDS
- Smoking history
- Alcoholism
- Malnutrition

and those with chronic respiratory disease or viral infections are particularly vulnerable. As many as 60% of critically ill patients in intensive care units may develop pneumonia, and half of these patients will die. *Pneumocystis carinii* pneumonia is currently the major terminal infection in patients with AIDS because of their immunodeficiency. The box at right summarizes the risk factors for pneumonia.

Microbial agents causing pneumonia have three primary modes of transmission: (1) aspiration of secretions that contain pathogenic microorganisms that have colonized the oropharynx, (2) inhalation of infectious aerosols, and (3) hematogenous spread from an extrapulmonary site. Aspiration and inhalation of infectious agents are the two most common modes of acquiring pneumonia respectively, whereas hematogenous spread occurs infrequently. Consequently, predisposing factors include any deficiency in the defense mechanisms of the respiratory system. Colonization of the oropharynx with gram-negative bacilli and subsequent aspiration as a pathogenic mechanism of acquiring many gram-negative

pneumonias have been the subjects of recent research (see later discussion).

The pathologic picture depends, to some extent, on the etiologic agent. *Bacterial pneumonia* is characterized by an intraalveolar suppurative exudate with consolidation. The infectious process may be classified anatomically. There is consolidation of an entire lobe in *lobar pneumonia,* whereas *lobular pneumonia,* or *bronchopneumonia,* refers to a patchy distribution of infectious areas about 3 to 4 cm in diameter surrounding and involving the bronchi. *Viral* or *Mycoplasma pneumoniae pneumonias* are characterized by an interstitial inflammation with accumulation of an infiltrate in the alveolar walls, although the alveolar spaces themselves are free of exudate and there is no consolidation. If the infecting agent is a *fungus* or *Mycobacterium tuberculosis,* the common pathologic pattern is a patchy distribution of granulomas, which may undergo caseous necrosis with the development of cavities. Fig. 39-6 illustrates the forms of pneumonia and the common causative agent.

It is also important to differentiate between community-acquired and hospital-acquired pneumonias. The relative frequencies with which individual agents cause pneumonia are quite different in these two locations (Table 39-4). Nosocomial infections are more likely to be caused by enteric gram-negative bacteria or *Staphylococcus aureus* and less likely to be caused by pneumococci or *Mycoplasma.*

The pattern of response also depends on the specific etiologic agent. *Streptococcus pneumoniae* (pneumococcus) is the most common cause of bacterial pneumonia, both in the community (accounting for as many as 75% of the cases) and in the hospital. Among the bacterial

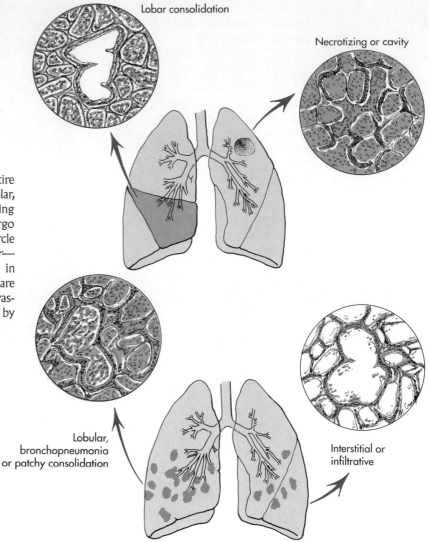

FIG. 39-6 Forms of pneumonia: *lobar*—entire lobe consolidated, exudate chiefly intraalveolar, *pneumococcus* and *Klebsiella* common infecting organisms; *necrotizing*—granuloma may undergo caseous necrosis and form cavity, fungi and tubercle bacillus infections are common causes; *lobular*—patchy distribution, fibrinous exudate chiefly in bronchioles, *Staphylococcus* and *Streptococcus* are common infecting organisms; *interstitial*—perivascular exudate and edema between alveoli, caused by virus or mycoplasmal infection.

▶ **TABLE 39-4**   Most Common Causes of Community-acquired and Nosocomial Pneumonias

Location of Acquisition	Causes
Community	*Streptococcus pneumoniae*
	Mycoplasma pneumoniae
	Haemophilus influenzae
	Legionella pneumophila
	Chlamydia pneumoniae
	Oral anaerobes (aspiration)
	Influenza A and B
	Adenovirus
Hospital	Enteric gram-negative bacilli (e.g., *Escherichia coli, Klebsiella pneumoniae*)
	Pseudomonas aeruginosa
	Staphylococcus aureus
	Oral anaerobes (aspiration)

pneumonias, the pathogenesis of pneumococcal pneumonia has been the most extensively studied. Pneumococci usually reach the alveoli in droplets of mucus or saliva. The lower lobes of the lung are frequently involved because of the effect of gravity. Once established in the alveolus, the pneumococcus elicits a typical response involving four successive stages*:

1. Engorgement (first 4 to 12 hours): serous exudate pours into alveoli from the dilated, leaking blood vessels.
2. Red hepatization (next 48 hours): lung assumes a red, granular appearance (*hepatization* means liverlike) as red blood cells, fibrin, and polymorphonuclear leukocytes fill the alveoli.
3. Gray hepatization (3 to 8 days): lung assumes a grayish appearance as the leukocytes and fibrin consolidate in the involved alveoli.

*These stages represent the temporal course in untreated pneumococcal pneumonia. With the use of antibiotics the course is now run in about 3 days.

4. Resolution (7 to 11 days): exudate is lysed and resorbed by macrophages, restoring the tissue to its original structure.

The onset of pneumococcal pneumonia is typically sudden, with chills, fever, pleuritic pain, cough, and rust-colored sputum. Rales and a friction rub may be heard over the involved tissue because of the exudate and fibrin that are in the alveoli and may be deposited on the pleural surface. There is almost always some degree of hypoxemia as a result of the shunting of blood through the non-ventilated, consolidated area of lung; the patient may have a dusky appearance. Chest radiograph, white blood cell count, and sputum examination—including gross appearance, microscopic examination, and culture—may all be helpful in making the diagnosis and following the course of the pneumonia.

The general treatment of patients with pneumonia consists of administering antibiotic drugs effective against the specific organism, providing O_2 therapy for hypoxemia, and treating complications. Likely complications and mortality are related to the specific infecting organism. Pneumococcal pneumonia generally runs an uncomplicated course, resulting in restoration of normal tissue structure. The most likely complication is a small pleural effusion. The treatment of choice is penicillin G. Before the era of antibiotics there was a 20% to 40% mortality rate for pneumococcal pneumonia, but this has now been reduced to 15% to 20% (Johnson, Finegold, 1994). Death is more likely to occur in elderly, chronically ill persons. The presence of bacteremia also affects the prognosis for pneumonia. The mortality in patients with bacteremia is about double that observed in the absence of bacteremia. Transient bacteremia may occur in all patients with pneumococcal pneumonia. Demonstrable bacteremia suggests ineffective localization of the pulmonary process, and not surprisingly, the mortality is higher in this group. The consequences of bacteremia may be metastatic lesions resulting in such conditions as meningitis, bacterial endocarditis, and peritonitis.

A vaccine for pneumococcal pneumonia is currently available and in adults is 80% to 90% effective against the most common pneumococcal serotypes. The vaccine is generally given to persons at high risk of fatal outcome, for example, those with sickle cell anemia, multiple myeloma, nephrotic syndrome, or diabetes mellitus.

Other less common causes of bacterial pneumonia in the adult include streptococci other than *Streptococcus pneumoniae* and *Haemophilus influenzae* (a gram-negative bacteria). These organisms are more apt to cause infection in children. Generally, nontypical strains of *H. influenzae* are responsible for pneumonia in adults and most often affect patients with preexisting chronic obstructive pulmonary disease (COPD).

Staphylococcus aureus (a gram-positive coccus) and gram-negative aerobic bacilli, including *Pseudomonas aeruginosa, Klebsiella pneumoniae,* and *Escherichia coli,* are responsible for most nosocomial pneumonias.

These pneumonias cause extensive damage to the lung parenchyma, and complications such as lung abscess and emphysema are common. Mortality figures for nosocomial pneumonias are as high as 33%.

Oropharyngeal and gastric colonization play a critical role in the pathogenesis of pneumonia in the hospitalized patient. The oropharynx becomes colonized by many species of gram-negative organisms within 48 hours of hospitalization. Aspiration of oropharyngeal secretions occurs during sleep and is enhanced by such factors as a nasogastric tube, altered consciousness, depressed gag reflex, or delayed gastric emptying. The role of gastric colonization has been recognized in recent years. Gastric bacterial counts rise in the presence of medications that raise the gastric pH, such as H_2 blockers (e.g., ranitidine) and antacids given to prevent stress ulceration. Sucralfate is a medication that heals ulcers without altering the gastric pH and should be used alone.

Some patients who survive *Klebsiella* (or Friedländer's) pneumonia develop a chronic pneumonia with severe progressive destruction of lung tissue that ultimately converts the patient into a respiratory cripple. A thick "red currant jelly" sputum is characteristic of this pneumonia. Most cases of *Klebsiella* pneumonia occur in middle-age or elderly males who are chronic alcoholics or who have some other chronic disease. Pneumonia caused by *Pseudomonas* organisms is most common in hospitalized patients who are terminally ill or who have marked suppression of immunologic body defenses (e.g., a patient with leukemia or a person who has had a renal transplant and is receiving large doses of immunosuppressive drugs). Other predisposing factors in gram-negative pneumonias include prior antimicrobial therapy, which alters the normal resident flora of the respiratory tract and allows overgrowth of certain microorganisms. Contaminated ventilatory equipment is a common source of *Pseudomonas* infection. *S. aureus* is commonly a secondary infection in hospitalized, debilitated patients and is most likely to cause a bronchopneumonia.

Viral infections typically occur in community epidemics, and are generally limited to the upper respiratory tract. Although viruses are the most common cause of pneumonia in children, viral pneumonias in adults account for only about 10% of cases. Persons with chronic diseases or elderly persons are more susceptible. Characteristic signs and symptoms include headache, fever, generalized aching of muscles, extreme fatigue, and a dry cough.

Most of these pneumonias are mild, do not require hospitalization, and leave no permanent lung damage. Types A and B influenza virus and adenovirus are common infecting agents. The treatment of viral pneumonia is symptomatic and palliative because antibiotics are not effective against viruses. Vaccination may give protection for a limited time but does not give protection against the many other types of viruses (some unidentified) that may cause respiratory infections. Viral pneumonia may set the stage for secondary invasion by bacteria, which has already been discussed. More rarely, a fatal patchy or diffuse pneumonitis may be attributed to the virus.

Pneumonia caused by *Mycoplasma pneumoniae* is generally discussed with viral pneumonias even though the infecting organism is a bacterium. Most mycoplasmal infections are restricted to pharyngitis or bronchitis, but about 10% of infected patients develop pneumonia. Mycoplasmal pneumonia typically affects young adults, especially college students and military recruits, and may be implicated in as many as 50% of all cases. The clinical picture of mycoplasmal pneumonia is similar to influenza virus pneumonia with evidence of interstitial pneumonitis. It is highly contagious and, unlike viral pneumonia, responds to erythromycin, tetracycline, or doxycycline. Mycoplasmal pneumonia is often referred to as primary atypical pneumonia or "walking pneumonia."

Legionella pneumophila, a gram-negative bacteria, was first recognized as an agent in pneumonia in the late 1970s after an outbreak of disease at a convention of the American Legion. *Legionella* infections (legionnaires' disease) account for up to 7% of community-acquired pneumonias and up to 10% of nosocomial pneumonias. Legionellae thrive in aquatic environments. Diverse natural reservoirs harbor these organisms, including mud, hot streams, and stagnant lakes. Transmission to humans occurs chiefly by aspiration of contaminated water. Hot water systems, shower heads, hot tubs, humidifiers, and air-conditioning systems with stagnant water may harbor legionellae and provide a source for human infection. Infection may occur sporadically or in outbreaks. It is most often seen in older adults, smokers, and others with impaired lung defenses. After an incubation period of 2 to 10 days, the illness usually begins gradually with malaise, dry cough, chills, fever, headache, confusion, diffuse myalgias, anorexia, and diarrhea. The diagnosis of *Legionella* infection may be made by culturing the organism or identifying its antigens. Chest radiographs show a patchy or lobar distribution pattern. The treatment of choice for legionnaires' disease is erythromycin. The overall mortality rate is 15% but is much higher in immunocompromised or untreated patients (Bernstein, Locksley, 1994).

Chlamydia pneumoniae is now recognized as a common cause of acute respiratory tract infection and pneumonia. Serologic studies have demonstrated that about 10% of community-acquired and hospital-acquired pneumonias are caused by this organism. *C. pneumoniae* is a member of the genus *Chlamydia* but distinct from the species *C. psittaci* and *C. trachomatis,* which cause psittacosis and genital infections, respectively. *C. pneumoniae* appears to be a pathogen spread by close personal contact. The pneumonia caused by this organisms is generally quite mild, with signs and symptoms resembling mycoplasmal pneumonia. As with mycoplasmal pneumonia, it generally responds to erythromycin or tetracycline therapy.

Pneumocystis carinii, a protozoan parasite, is the causal agent in *P. carinii* pneumonia (PCP). Recurrent PCP affects more than half of all AIDS patients and is a common cause of death in this population. PCP is an opportunistic infection and may also occur in other immunocompromised hosts such as patients receiving immunosuppressive therapy for cancer or organ transplantation. The three most common signs and symptoms of PCP are fever, shortness of breath, and a dry cough. The chest radiograph shows diffuse, patchy infiltrates. Trimethoprim-sulfamethoxazole or pentamidine is the treatment of choice for PCP.

Aspiration pneumonia refers to the pathologic consequences of the entry of oropharyngeal secretions, particulate matter, or gastric contents into the lower airway. Most people aspirate small amounts of oropharyngeal secretions during sleep, and the secretions are normally cleared without sequelae by the normal defense mechanisms. Three distinct aspiration syndromes may be distinguished because of the differing nature of the aspirate, signs and symptoms, and pathophysiology.

As noted previously, aspiration of pathogenic microorganisms colonizing the oropharynx is the most common mode of infecting the lower airways and causing bacterial pneumonia. *Anaerobic pneumonias* are caused by the aspiration of oropharyngeal secretions containing anaerobes such as the *Bacteroides, Fusobacterium, Peptococcus,* and *Peptostreptococcus* species common among patients with poor dental hygiene. Anaerobic pneumonia is most common in hospitalized patients and persons with chronic alcoholism with infected gums and a predisposition toward aspiration. Nearly all such pneumonias acquired in the hospital are caused by a mixture of both anaerobic and aerobic microorganisms (e.g., gram-negative bacilli, *S. aureus*). The onset of symptoms is usually gradual over 1 to 2 weeks, with fever, weight loss, anemia, leukocytosis, dyspnea, and cough productive of foul-smelling sputum. Lung abscesses form as the lung parenchyma is destroyed, and empyema may develop as the microbes make their way to the pleural surface. Most of the abscesses form in the right lung in the posterior and basilar bronchopulmonary gravity-dependent segments because of the more direct path of the right mainstem bronchus. Finger clubbing is common if the abscess is chronic. Treatment consists of prolonged antibiotic therapy, usually with clindamycin or a combination of penicillin and metronidazole (Flagyl), and drainage of empyema, if present.

A second type of aspiration syndrome called *Mendelson's syndrome* is related to the regurgitation and aspiration of the acidic stomach contents. In contrast to the slow onset of anaerobic pneumonia, the resulting *chemical pneumonitis* or *aspiration pneumonitis* may develop within hours and be extremely fulminant. Massive inhalation of gastric contents may lead to sudden death from obstruction, whereas aspiration of smaller quantities of gastric contents may lead to widespread edema, tachypnea, dyspnea, tachycardia, fever, leukocytosis, and respiratory failure. The severity of the inflammatory response depends on the pH of the aspirate more than any other factor. Aspiration pneumonitis always results when the pH of the aspirate is 2.5 or less. Aspiration pneumonitis follows three common patterns: (1) rapid recovery (usually when the quantity of aspirate is small or more alkaline), (2) rapid development of acute respiratory distress syndrome (see Chapter 41), or (3) bacterial superinfection. The bacterial pneumonia that develops is partly chemical as a result of the reaction to the gastric juice and partly from the bacterial superinfection that occurs over days from organisms that may inhabit the mouth or stomach. Abscesses, bronchiectasis, and gangrene are common complications of aspiration pneumonia. The mortality rates are very high and have been reported as 30% to 50%. Aspiration of gastric contents is most common during or after anesthesia (especially in obstetric patients and surgical emergencies because of the lack of surgical preparation), in infants, and in any obtunded patient with depressed gag and cough reflexes.

It is important to realize that vomiting is not a prerequisite to the entrance of gastric contents into the tracheobronchial tree, since silent regurgitation may occur in obtunded patients. Proper positioning to drain oropharyngeal secretions from the mouth is most important in the care of these patients.

A third type of aspiration syndrome is related to the aspiration of particulate matter (usually food) or nonacid fluids (e.g., near-drowning or tube feeding) causing *mechanical obstruction*. When fluid is aspirated, the trachea should be suctioned immediately to relieve the obstruction. When solid matter is aspirated, the presenting symptoms depend on the size of the object and where it is lodged in the airways. If the object is lodged high in the trachea, causing complete obstruction, apnea, aphonia, and rapid death may ensue. If the object cannot be dislodged by means of the finger sweep or the Heimlich maneuver, an emergency tracheotomy (cricothyrotomy) may be performed. If the object (e.g., a peanut) becomes lodged in the smaller airways, the presenting signs and symptoms may include a chronic cough and recurrent infection. Therapy consists of removing the object, usually by means of bronchoscopy.

Hypostatic pneumonia is a pneumonia that develops frequently at the lung bases and is caused by shallow breathing and constantly remaining in the same position. Gravity causes blood to become congested in the dependent part of the lung, and infection aids the development of true pneumonia.

Fungi may be the cause of pneumonia, although they are a much less common cause than bacteria. A few fungi are capable of producing a chronic granulomatous, suppurative lung disease that is often mistaken for tuberculosis. Many of these fungal infections are endemic to certain geographic regions. The most important fungal infections in the United States are *histoplasmosis* (Midwest

and East), *coccidioidomycosis* (Southwest), and *blastomycosis* (Southeast). Spores of these fungi are found in the soil and are inhaled. Spores carried into the smaller divisions of the lung are phagocytized and cause an allergic reaction. After allergy develops, the reaction becomes inflammatory, with tubercle formation, central caseation, scarring, calcification, and even cavity formation. All the pathologic changes resemble tuberculosis so closely that differentiation can be made only by identification and culture of the fungus from lung tissue. Serologic and delayed hypersensitivity skin tests are not positive until a few weeks after the initial infection and may even be negative with severe disease.

It is not unusual for fungal pneumonia to complicate the final stages of terminal diseases such as cancer or leukemia. *Candida albicans,* a yeast frequently found in the sputum of healthy persons, may invade the pulmonary tissue under these conditions. Infection with *Candida* is termed *candidiasis.* Prolonged use of antibiotics may also alter the natural body flora and permit invasion of *Candida.* Amphotericin B is the drug of choice for the pulmonary fungal infections.

Pulmonary fibrosis

Pulmonary fibrosis is not a disease entity but a pathologic term that denotes an excessive amount of connective tissue in the lung. Fibrosis results from a method of tissue repair that may follow any disease process of the lung, producing inflammation or necrosis. The most common type of pulmonary fibrosis is *localized fibrosis,* which follows localized damage to the lung parenchyma caused by such conditions as tuberculosis, pulmonary abscess, bronchiectasis, or unresolved pneumonia. Less often, pulmonary fibrosis may diffusely involve the lung parenchyma, particularly affecting the interalveolar septa. Unlike localized fibrosis, diffuse pulmonary fibrosis is a disabling and frequently fatal disorder. Diffuse pulmonary fibrosis represents end-stage lung disease from a host of known and unknown causes. A few of the more common causes of diffuse pulmonary fibrosis are listed in the box on p. 612.

The *pneumoconioses* are a group of diseases caused by the inhalation of certain inorganic and organic dusts. Some dusts, when inhaled in sufficient concentration into the lungs, produce a fibrous tissue reaction, whereas others are quite inert. The dust inhalation diseases are of particular interest because exposure is usually related to certain occupations, and these diseases are theoretically preventable by the institution of industrial safety standards. Only a few examples of noxious dusts or gases causing pulmonary fibrosis are listed in the box. Whether a particular dust causes disease depends on (1) the size of the particle—the most dangerous dust particle seems to be 1 to 5 μm because larger particles never reach the alveoli; (2) the concentration and length of exposure—high concentration is usually required to overcome the action of the ciliary escalator, and long exposure is usually re-

COMMON CAUSES OF DIFFUSE PULMONARY FIBROSIS

DISEASES OF KNOWN CAUSE

1. Pneumoconioses (occupational inhalation of dusts)
   a. Inorganic dusts
      Silica: silicosis
      Coal: "black lung"
      Iron: siderosis
      Asbestos: asbestosis
      Talc: talcosis
      Beryllium: berylliosis
   b. Organic dusts
      Cotton: byssinosis
      Sugar cane: bagassosis
      Moldy hay: "farmer's lung"
      Maple bark
2. Noxious gas inhalation of nitrogen oxides (silo filler), chlorine, sulfur oxides, or metal fumes
3. Drug sensitivity to diphenylhydantoin (phenytoin, Dilantin) or busulfan (Myleran)
4. Irradiation injury
5. Viral pneumonias
6. Chronic pulmonary edema

DISEASES OF UNKNOWN CAUSE

1. Hamman-Rich syndrome
2. Sarcoidosis
3. "Collagen diseases," progressive systemic sclerosis
4. Chronic interstitial pneumonia
5. Mucoviscidosis (cystic fibrosis)

---

quired (e.g., coal miner's pneumoconiosis, or black lung disease, usually requires 20 years of exposure before there is extensive pulmonary fibrosis); and (3) the nature of the dust—certain materials (particularly the organic dusts such as cotton fiber, which causes *byssinosis;* sugar cane [*bagassosis*]; and moldy hay [*farmer's lung*]) have an unusual antigenic effect and cause an allergic alveolitis. The chemical natue of inorganic dusts also influences their capacity to produce disease. Silica dust (frequently inhaled by grinders, sandblasters, and rock quarry workers), which causes *silicosis,* is particularly harmful. It is thought that these dust particles regularly destroy the macrophages by which they are phagocytized, resulting in the formation of fibrotic nodules. Widespread fibrosis is produced by the coalescence of the fibrotic nodules.

Asbestos is a compound of magnesium and iron silicate. Because of its unique physical characteristics (durability, heat resistance, flexibility), it is widely used in industry (e.g., shipbuilding, car brake and clutch lining, air filters, insulation materials, roofing). *Asbestosis* is an interstitial process that slowly develops into a diffuse, nonnodular pulmonary fibrosis involving the terminal airways, alveoli, and pleurae. The disease is usually recognized after 20 years of exposure and tends to progress after exposure has ended. The major complications of asbestosis are bronchogenic carcinoma, malignant mesothelioma, and pleural plaques. The risk of bronchogenic carcinoma is largely confined to cigarette smokers, in whom the risk is greater than in smokers without asbestosis (see Chapter 42). Asbestos exposure occurs not only from mining and the manufacture of asbestos products, but also from general community air pollution. Asbestos fibers have been found in the autopsied lungs of a high percentage of city dwellers. The potential health hazard of such low concentrations is not clear.

The inhalation of noxious gases may be associated with certain occupations. The result is a chemical pneumonitis. Of particular interest is *silo filler's disease,* which is not a pneumoconiosis but is caused by the inhalation of nitrogen oxides from fermentation of the vegetation in a freshly filled silo. The severity of reaction to noxious gases depends on the concentration of gas and length of exposure. Viral pneumonias, chronic pulmonary edema, irradiation involving the chest, and certain drugs that produce a hypersensitivity reaction (e.g., diphenylhydantoin [phenytoin], busulfan) are other known causes of diffuse pulmonary fibrosis.

Among diseases of unknown cause leading to diffuse pulmonary fibrosis is the *Hamman-Rich syndrome.* This syndrome is an unusual interstitial pneumonia that may have a rapidly fatal course or a more protracted one, both with the development of severe intraalveolar and interstitial fibrosis. Other chronic interstitial pneumonias also tend to result in progressive pulmonary fibrosis, as do certain systemic diseases such as sarcoidosis, collagen diseases (especially scleroderma), and mucoviscidosis.

The systemic symptoms in the group of diseases causing pulmonary fibrosis vary widely. In the early stages there may be no symptoms at all. The pulmonary symptoms, however, are strikingly similar. The primary symptom seems to be a progressive dyspnea on exertion. The common pathologic denominator is interstitial fibrosis, with the extent of fibrosis determining the effect on pulmonary function. When the fibrosis is extensive, there is a decrease in lung elasticity, total lung capacity (TLC), VC, and residual volume (RV), which all indicate restrictive lung disease. The dyspnea reflects the poor compliance and results in a concomitant increase in the work of breathing. With marked destruction of alveoli and pulmonary vessels, hypoxemia, pulmonary hypertension, cor pulmonale, and heart failure may result. In many patients, however, symptoms do not progress beyond mild exertional dyspnea.

QUESTIONS

▼ *Match each of the extrapulmonary disorders causing alveolar hypoventilation in column A with its appropriate altered mechanism in column B.*

Column A

1. _____ Kyphoscoliosis
2. _____ Progressive muscular dystrophy
3. _____ Pa_{CO_2} 70 mm Hg
4. _____ Myasthenia gravis
5. _____ CNS lesion
6. _____ Amyotrophic lateral sclerosis

Column B

a. Depression of the respiratory center
b. Interruption of nerve transmission to respiratory muscles from disease involving the neuromuscular junction
c. Interruption of nerve transmission to respiratory muscles because of upper motor neuron lesion
d. Direct anatomic damage to the respiratory center
e. Paresis of the respiratory muscles because of diffuse disease of the skeletal muscles
f. Deformity of the chest cage causing abnormal positioning and functioning of its respiratory muscles

▼ *Circle T if the statement is true and F if it is false. Correct any false statements.*

7. T F In kyphoscoliosis, compression of the lungs by the thoracic deformity causes a small lung volume and unequal distribution of ventilation and perfusion.

8. T F Pectus excavatum refers to a lateral displacement of the spine.

9. T F Flail chest injury is associated with paradoxical movement of dead-space air between the airways of the right and left lungs during the respiratory cycle.

10. T F Ankylosing spondylitis is a disease that causes asymmetric deformity of the chest cage.

▼ *Circle the letter preceding each item below that correctly completes the statement. Only one answer is correct.*

11. The pickwickian syndrome is characterized by all the following *except:*
    a. Hypoxemia
    b. Hypercapnia
    c. Increased arterial pH
    d. Polycythemia
    e. Cor pulmonale

12. Patients with kyphoscoliotic lung disease would be expected to exhibit all the following physiologic abnormalities *except:*
    a. Increased nonelastic work of breathing
    b. Increased elastic work of breathing
    c. Decreased lung compliance
    d. Decreased vital capacity

13. Alveolar hypoventilation results in all the following abnormalities of the blood gases *except:*
    a. Low Pa_{O_2} c. High Pa_{CO_2}
    b. Low PA_{O_2} d. Low PA_{CO_2}

14. Children with muscular dystrophy are most likely to exhibit the following abnormalities of pulmonary function:
    a. Obstructive ventilatory pattern
    b. Restrictive ventilatory pattern
    c. Pulmonary diffusion block
    d. Normal ventilatory function

▼ *Answer the following on a separate sheet of paper.*

15. What are two physiologic alterations that occur as a consequence of a restricted pattern of ventilation?

16. List possible causes of traumatic and spontaneous pneumothorax.

17. Describe the emergency treatment of a penetrating chest wound.

18. Why does a pneumothorax occur when there is a communication between a bronchus or alveolus and the pleural cavity?

19. Describe the treatment for a large pneumothorax and a large pleural effusion.

20. What is a collection of fluid in the pleural cavity called?

21. When a transudate occurs, there is a rise in pressure so that the balance of forces favors the passage of fluid out of the vessels. What is this pressure called?

22. What is formed in the pleural cavity as the result of increased capillary permeability or impaired lymphatic absorption?

23. What is pleural fluid called that has a specific gravity of less than 1.015 and a protein content of less than 3%?

24. List five general disorders that may cause damage to the lung alveoli and interstitium. State the specific damage to lung tissue that each disorder causes.

25. Contrast absorption and compression atelectasis with respect to the common cause of each and the mechanism involved.

26. Why are the pores of Kohn important in maintaining collateral ventilation? Illustrate how collateral ventilation prevents absorption atelectasis caused by bronchial obstruction by a mucus plug.

27. List in sequence the four stages describing the pathologic changes in the lung in untreated pneumococcal pneumonia (include name of stage, time period, and description of lung changes).

28. List three principles of treatment for patients with pneumonia.

29. List three criteria used to predict whether a particular dust will cause disease of the lung parenchyma. State the reason why each of these criteria is important.

30. List the three most important fungal infections in the United States causing lung disease.

31. What are two consequences of pulmonary fibrosis?

32. The manifestations of extensive diffuse pulmonary fibrosis are typical of what type of pattern of ventilatory dysfunction?

▼ *Complete the following statements by filling in the blanks.*

33. Pulmonary fibrosis is characterized pathologically by _____ fibrosis.

34. Pneumonia caused by gram-negative or staphylococcal organisms causes extensive damage to the lung _____. Common complications include _____ and _____. The prognosis is generally _____.

▼ *Circle T if the statement is true and F if it is false. Correct any false statements.*

35. T F Patients with Friedländer's pneumonia occasionally develop a chronic pneumonia after the original infection.

36. T F Gram-negative pneumonias often occur in hospitalized or debilitated patients.

37. T F Viral pneumonia typically has a poor prognosis.

Continued.

QUESTIONS—cont'd

38. T F Viral pneumonia is successfully treated with erythromycin.
39. T F The clinical picture of mycoplasmal pneumonia is similar to that of viral pneumonia.
40. T F Aspiration pneumonia develops at the lung bases and is caused by shallow breathing and constantly remaining in the same position.
41. T F Amphotericin B is the drug of choice for the treatment of candidiasis.
42. T F Fungal pulmonary lesions are often granulomatous and similar to lesions caused by *Mycobacterium tuberculosis.*

▼ *Match the type of pneumothorax in column A with the correct description in column B.*

Column A		Column B
43. _____	Open	a. Communication between pleural cavity and atmosphere is sealed off.
44. _____	Closed	
45. _____	Tension	b. Communication between pleural cavity and atmosphere open during inspiration and closed during expiration.
		c. Communication between pleural cavity and atmosphere does not seal off.

▼ *Match each of the anatomic patterns of pneumonia in column A with its pathologic description or common causative agent in column B. More than one letter may be used for each blank in column A.*

Column A		Column B
46. _____	Lobar consolidation	a. Fungi or *Mycobacterium tuberculosis*
47. _____	Lobular consolidation	b. Viral or *Mycoplasma* pneumonia
48. _____	Necrotizing or cavity formation	c. *Pneumococcus*
		d. *Staphylococcus* or *streptococcus*
49. _____	Interstitial	e. Perivascular exudate and edema between the alveoli
		f. May undergo caseous necrosis
		g. Exudate chiefly intraalveolar
		h. Fibrinous exudate chiefly in bronchioles
		i. Patchy distribution of infection
		j. Whole lung lobe infected

▼ *Match each of the protective mechanisms in column A with the factors that cause interference with it in column B. More than one letter may be used for each blank in column A.*

Column A		Column B	
50. _____	Cough	a.	Cigarette smoke
51. _____	Mucus and ciliary action	b.	General dehydration
52. _____	Collateral ventilation	c.	Pain
53. _____	Pharyngeal clearing	d.	Shallow breathing
		e.	Constant tidal volume breathing
		f.	Sedatives and narcotics
		g.	Atropine-like drugs
		h.	Unconsciousness
		i.	Reduction of airflow rate

▼ *Match each item in column A with its description or cause in column B. Items are associated with occupational diseases resulting in diffuse pulmonary fibrosis.*

Column A		Column B
54. _____	Organic dusts	a. Caused by inhalation of nitrogen oxides
55. _____	Silica dust	b. Caused by inhalation of cotton dust
56. _____	Farmer's lung	c. Mechanism of adverse reaction is allergic alveolitis.
57. _____	Silo filler's disease	d. Caused by moldy hay
58. _____	Byssinosis	e. Mechanism of adverse reaction is production of chemical pneumonitis.
59. _____	Black lung disease	f. Mechanism of adverse reaction is destruction of macrophages with formation of fibrotic nodules.
		g. Common occupational disease among rock quarry workers, grinders, and sandblasters
		h. Caused by inhalation of coal dust

▼ *Circle the letter preceding each item below that correctly answers the question. More than one answer may be correct.*

60. Which of the following are common causes of diffuse pulmonary fibrosis?
   a. Tuberculosis
   b. Inhalation of noxious gases
   c. Inhalation of silica dusts
   d. Sarcoidosis
   e. Diphenylhydantoin (Dilantin) therapy

61. Which of the following are *typical* signs, symptoms, and findings associated with pneumococcal pneumonia:
   a. "Red currant jelly" sputum
   b. "Rusty" sputum
   c. Dry, nonproductive cough
   d. Decreased white blood cell count
   e. Fever, chills, pleuritic pain
   f. Lobar consolidation evident on chest radiograph

62. What percentage of the American population is affected by pneumonia annually?
   a. 1%
   b. 5%
   c. 10%
   d. 15%

63. Which of the following abnormalities are frequently seen in patients with disease of the lung parenchyma?
   a. A restrictive pattern of pulmonary dysfunction
   b. An obstructive pattern of pulmonary dysfunction
   c. Rapid, shallow breathing pattern
   d. Slow, deep breathing pattern
   e. Decrease in lung volume
   f. Hypercapnia
   g. Hypoxemia

64. Inadequately treated empyema may result in which of the following conditions?
   a. Hydrothorax
   b. Chylothorax
   c. Hemothorax
   d. Fibrothorax

65. Which of the following statements is the best description of a pneumothorax?
   a. Air within the pleural cavity
   b. Cohesion and positive intrapleural pressure
   c. A pathologic lesion of the lung

QUESTIONS—cont'd

d. Accumulation of fluid in the pleural cavity

66. What is the most common cause of idiopathic spontaneous pneumothorax in healthy young adults?
    a. Bulging of the intercostal spaces
    b. Rupture of a subpleural bleb or localized bullous disease
    c. Lesions of the parietal pleura
    d. Diffuse emphysematous disease of the lungs

67. Which of the following signs and symptoms would best differentiate between a pleural effusion and a pneumothorax?
    a. Moderate dyspnea
    b. Diminished and delayed chest movement on the involved side
    c. Decreased vocal fremitus over the involved area
    d. Diminished or absent breath sounds on the affected side
    e. Egophony over lung above effusion (bleating sound heard by stethoscope when patient speaks)

68. A patient with pneumonia is having severe pain in the right lateral portion of the chest accompanying respiratory movements. Why is this?
    a. Inflamed lung is painful.
    b. Visceral pleura is inflamed and sensitive to pain.
    c. Parietal pleura is inflamed and sensitive to pain.
    d. Patient has an intercostal peripheral neuritis.

69. Nosocomial (arising from hospitalization) infections associated with respirators, resuscitation equipment, and humidifiers are especially likely to be caused by:
    a. *Klebsiella pneumoniae*
    b. *Staphylococcus aureus*
    c. Fungi
    d. *Pseudomonas* organisms

70. The normal respiratory tract is sterile:
    a. Below the oropharynx
    b. Below the larynx
    c. Below the mainstem bronchi
    d. Below the terminal bronchioles
    e. Nowhere

71. The usual course of pneumococcal lobar pneumonia terminates with:
    a. Diffuse pulmonary fibrosis

b. Organization of the inflammatory exudate
    c. Complete resolution of the pulmonary inflammation
    d. Abscess formation and empyema

72. Conditions that increase the risk for pneumonia include all the following *except:*
    a. Hyperventilation
    b. Smoking history
    c. Altered level of consciousness
    d. Viral respiratory infection
    e. Lung cancer

73. Which of the following pulmonary infections is considered to be opportunistic?
    a. *Pneumocystis carinii*
    b. *Pseudomonas aeruginosa*
    c. *Streptococcus pneumoniae*
    d. *Chlamydia pneumoniae*

74. All the following organisms are common etiologic agents in nosocomial pneumonias *except:*
    a. *Mycoplasma* pneumoniae
    b. Gram-negative bacilli *(Escherichia coli, Klebsiella)*
    c. *Staphylococcus aureus*
    d. *Pseudomonas aeruginosa*
    e. Oral anaerobes

75. The most common mode of infection in nosocomial bacterial pneumonia is:
    a. Aspiration of secretions containing pathogens colonizing the oropharynx
    b. Hematogenous spread from an extrapulmonary site of infection
    c. Inhalation of infectious aerosols
    d. Direct innoculation

76. To reduce the risk of colonization of the oropharynx with gram-negative organisms, stress ulcer prophylaxis in critically ill patients should consist of therapy with:
    a. Ranitidine (H_2-receptor antagonist)
    b. Antacids
    c. Sucralfate
    d. Only a and b
    e. All the above

77. *Pseudomonas aeruginosa* infection of the respiratory tract can be acquired:
    a. From mechanical ventilators
    b. From tracheostomy sites

c. In patients on corticosteroids
    d. All the above

78. The hallmark of anaerobic pulmonary infection is:
    a. No organisms seen in sputum or pus
    b. Failure to respond to first-line antibiotics
    c. Severe systemic reaction to the infection
    d. Foul-smelling, putrid sputum

79. The vast majority of anaerobic pleuropulmonary infections take the form of:
    a. Limited acute bronchitis
    b. Lung abscess
    c. Fulminating pneumonia and sepsis
    d. Empyema

80. The clinical course of anaerobic pulmonary infection is typically:
    a. Fulminant and fatal
    b. Chronic and indolent
    c. Benign
    d. Unpredictable
    e. Relapsing over the years

81. The antibiotic of choice to treat suspected anaerobic pulmonary infection is:
    a. Erythromycin
    b. Clindamycin
    c. Vancomycin
    d. Streptomycin

82. Which of the following are particularly associated with pulmonary aspiration?
    a. General anesthesia
    b. Drug addiction
    c. Neurologic disorders
    d. Childbirth
    e. All the above

83. Aspiration pneumonitis is:
    a. Also called Mendelson's syndrome
    b. Associated with a mild pneumonia when associated with bacterial superinfection
    c. Associated with a more severe reaction the lower the pH of the gastric aspirate
    d. Associated with a high mortality rate

84. The reduced lung compliance in kyphoscoliosis can be attributed to:
    a. Atelectasis
    b. Inability to inflate the lungs adequately
    c. Multiple pleural effusions
    d. Abnormal surfactant secretion

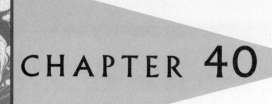

CHAPTER 40

Cardiovascular Disease and the Lung

LORRAINE M. WILSON

Chronic lung disease is an increasingly frequent cause of heart disease, and conversely, heart disease with decompensation or vascular disease may cause changes in the structure and function of the lung. This close interrelationship relates to the functional position of the lungs in the circulation (see Fig. 35-4). This chapter discusses pulmonary embolism, pulmonary edema, and cor pulmonale, all diseases demonstrating the close relationship between the heart and lungs.

PULMONARY EMBOLISM

Pulmonary embolism (PE) occurs when an embolus, usually a blood clot that breaks free from its attachment in a vein of the lower limbs, circulates through the blood vessels and the right side of the heart to become lodged in the main pulmonary artery or one of its branches. *Pulmonary infarction* is the term used to describe a local focus of necrosis resulting from the vascular obstruction (Fig. 40-1; see also Fig. 7-9).

The true incidence of PE cannot be determined because of the difficulty of the clinical diagnosis, but it is an important cause of morbidity and mortality in a hospital population and is said to account for more than 200,000 deaths in the United States annually. PE has been described in more than 50% of consecutive autopsies in some studies, suggesting that many cases are clinically undetected.

Three basic factors are related to the development of venous thrombosis and subsequent PE: (1) venous stasis or slowing of the blood flow, (2) injury to the vein wall, and (3) hypercoagulability (see box, on p. 617). Several diseases and activities seem to increase the risk of forming a thrombus, and patients in these states should be watched closely to detect any evidence of thrombus formation. The risk of thrombus formation is increased by pregnancy, the use of oral contraceptive drugs, obesity, heart failure, varicose veins, abdominal infection, cancer, sickle cell anemia, and any prolonged inactivity such as plane, train, or bus rides. Many of these conditions are common in hospitalized patients. Venous thrombosis and PE occur predominantly in bedridden patients. The single most important condition predisposing to venous thrombosis is congestive heart failure; the postoperative state is next in importance. The most common site for a blood clot to form is in the ileofemoral deep veins of the legs (90%), although clots may form in the pelvic veins and in the right side of the heart. Emboli of nonthrombotic origin occur infrequently (fewer than 10% of pulmonary emboli) but include obstruction caused by air, fat, malignant cells, amniotic fluid, parasites, vegetations, and foreign material.

The signs and symptoms of a PE are extremely variable, depending on the size of the clot or clots. The clinical picture may range from no signs to sudden and almost immediate death caused by a massive saddle embolus at the bifurcation of the main pulmonary artery, resulting in blockage of the entire outflow of the right ventricle. In a patient with the signs of thrombophlebitis in leg veins, the classic syndrome associated with a moderate-size PE consists of sudden onset of unexplained dyspnea, tachypnea, tachycardia, and restlessness. Pleuritic pain, friction rub, hemoptysis, and fever are not usually present unless infarction has occurred.

RISK FACTORS FOR PULMONARY EMBOLISMS

A. Conditions promoting venous stasis
  1. Prolonged bedrest/immobilization
  2. Postpartum status
  3. Orthopedic surgery/casts
  4. Obesity
  5. Older age
B. Injury to the vein wall
  1. Postsurgical, especially involving the thorax, abdomen, pelvis, or legs
  2. Pelvic or hip fractures
  3. Intravenous therapy
C. Conditions that increase blood coagulability
  1. Malignancy
  2. High-estrogen oral contraceptives
  3. Polycythemia
D. High-risk disorders
  1. Stage IV congestive heart failure
  2. Postoperative status
    a. Hip surgery
    b. Extensive abdominal or pelvic surgery for malignancy
  3. Postpartum status
  4. History of deep venous thromboses (DVT), pulmonary embolism (PE), varicosities
  5. Long-bone fractures
  6. Abdominal infection
  7. Diabetes mellitus
  8. Sickle cell anemia
  9. Chronic lung disease

Massive PE may result in a sudden shocklike state with tachycardia, hypotension, cyanosis, stupor, or syncope. Death usually follows within a few minutes. Frequently, however, the symptoms of PE are subtle, such as unexplained fever or worsening of a preexisting cardiac or cardiopulmonary condition. These subtle symptoms are apt to be associated with recurrent small, multiple pulmonary emboli. They may go unnoticed until right ventricular hypertrophy and failure direct attention to the pulmonary vascular disease.

The effect of PE is to produce an area of lung that is ventilated but underperfused, thus increasing physiologic dead-space ventilation. Reflex bronchoconstriction occurs in the affected area and is thought to result from the release of histamine or serotonin from the clot. Reflex bronchoconstriction is considered to be compensatory in the occluded area, since it reduces the unevenness of ventilation and perfusion. In adjacent areas, however, reflex bronchospasm may result in considerable hypoxemia. If the pulmonary vascular bed is sufficiently reduced by a large embolus or by recurrent multiple emboli, pulmonary hypertension may result. It is estimated that two thirds of the vascular bed must be obliterated before this happens.

A localized area of ischemic necrosis *(infarction)* is an uncommon complication of PE because of the lung's dual blood supply. Pulmonary infarction is usually associated with occlusion of a medium-size lobar or lobular artery and insufficient collateral flow from the bronchial circulation (Fig. 40-1). A pleural friction rub and a small pleural effusion are common signs.

Few diagnostic tests specifically distinguish a pulmonary infarction from a pulmonary infiltrate. Radioac-

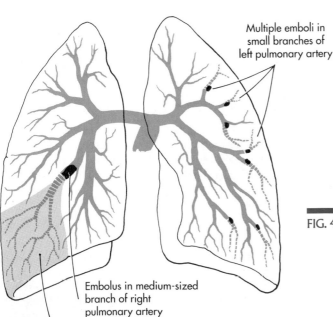

Multiple emboli in small branches of left pulmonary artery

Embolus in medium-sized branch of right pulmonary artery

Infarcted area

FIG. 40-1   Pulmonary embolism and infarction.

tive lung perfusion scans are abnormal in either case or in the presence of emphysema. The chest radiograph may be normal or a pleural effusion may be present in both cases. Physiologic tests and serum enzymes are likewise of little value in distinguishing an infarction from pneumonia. In addition, the signs and symptoms of pneumonia may be similar to those of PE. The most reliable method of diagnosis is pulmonary angiography.

Treatment of PE is directed toward prevention of initial or recurrent embolism, relief of symptoms resulting from the embolus, and surgical removal of a massive embolus. In high-risk patients the effectiveness of oral anticoagulants in preventing PE has been clearly shown. Low-dose heparin (3000 to 5000 units every 8 to 12 hours subcutaneously) has also been a valuable prophylactic agent. Another prophylactic measure frequently used for high-risk patients is external compression of the lower extremities with an intermittently inflating pneumatic device.

The early detection of patients with deep venous thrombosis (and therefore at high risk for PE) has been greatly improved by the use of three relatively new non-invasive diagnostic techniques: Doppler ultrasonic examination, impedance plethysmography, and iodine-125– (^{125}I-)labeled fibrinogen uptake (see Chapter 34). The combined approach of early detection of deep venous thrombosis by these improved techniques and the use of low-dose heparin in persons at high risk of having deep venous thrombosis offers promise for the reduction of PE.

Treatment of an acute PE includes general cadiopulmonary support with oxygen (O_2), digitalization, intensive care monitoring, elastic stockings, and the administration of aqueous heparin in full doses of 20,000 to 40,000 units/day by continuous infusion or divided doses. Surgical embolectomy is considered only when the embolus is massive because the mortality rate from this type of surgery is about 50%. Other surgical measures to prevent recurrent pulmonary emboli from the lower extremities include ligation of the inferior vena cava and the insertion of a filtering device or screen in the inferior vena cava (see Chapter 34).

PULMONARY EDEMA

Pulmonary edema is an excessive accumulation of serous or serosanguinous fluid in the interstitial spaces and alveoli of the lungs. If the edema is acute and extensive, death may rapidly ensue. Pulmonary edema may be precipitated by an increase of hydrostatic pressure within the pulmonary capillaries, a decrease in the colloid osmotic pressure as in nephritis, or damage to the capillary walls. Damage to the capillary walls may result from the inhalation of noxious gases, inflammation as in pneumonia, or local interference with oxygenation. The most common cause of pulmonary edema is left ventricular failure

resulting from arteriosclerotic heart disease or mitral stenosis (mitral valve obstruction). If the left side of the heart fails while the right side continues to pump blood, the pulmonary capillary pressure rises until pulmonary edema results. There are two stages in the formation of pulmonary edema: (1) interstitial edema characterized by engorgement of the perivascular and peribronchial spaces and increased lymphatic flow and (2) alveolar edema when fluid moves into the alveoli. Blood plasma is poured out into the alveoli faster than coughing or the lymphatics of the lung can clear it. This plasma interferes with diffusion of O_2, and the consequent tissue hypoxia further increases the tendency to edema. Asphyxia may result unless measures are taken to reverse the pulmonary edema. Emergency treatment for acute pulmonary edema includes measures to reduce pulmonary hydrostatic pressure, such as placing the patient in Fowler's position with the feet dependent; rotating tourniquets; or phlebotomy (removal of about a pint of blood). Other measures include the administration of diuretics, O_2, and digitalis to improve myocardial contractility.

In the presence of chronic passive congestion of the lungs, structural changes in the lung (i.e., pulmonary fibrosis) may result. These changes enable the lung to function for a time with the increased hydrostatic pressure without the development of pulmonary edema. The balance, however, is precarious, and the patient may have attacks of dyspnea at night (paroxysmal nocturnal dyspnea) because of the increase in pulmonary hydrostatic pressure that results from a horizontal position.

COR PULMONALE

Cor pulmonale is the condition in which hypertrophy and dilation of the right ventricle, with or without right ventricular failure, develop as a result of disease affecting the structure or function of the lung or its vasculature. By this definition, neither disease of the left side of the heart nor congenital heart disease is responsible for the pathogenesis. Cor pulmonale may be acute (e.g., massive pulmonary embolism) or chronic. The following discussion concerns the chronic condition.

The exact incidence of cor pulmonale is unknown, since it often goes unrecognized both clinically and at autopsy. The estimated incidence of cor pulmonale is 6% to 7% of all heart disease based on studies using the criterion of postmortem ventricular wall thickness (Fishman, 1994).

Normal Function of the Pulmonary Circulation

The pulmonary circulation is interposed between the right and left ventricles for the purpose of gas exchange. Normally, flow through the pulmonary vascular bed de-

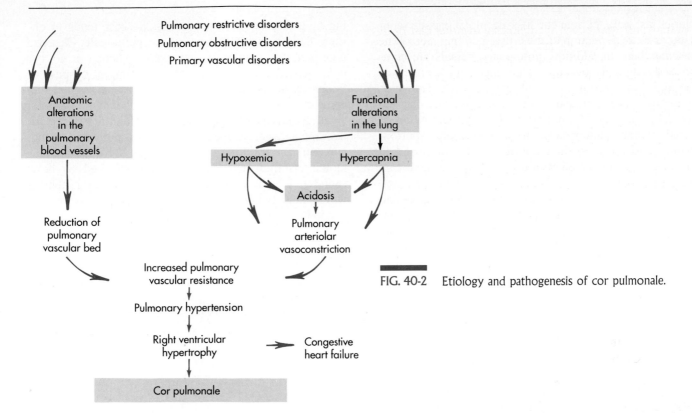

FIG. 40-2   Etiology and pathogenesis of cor pulmonale.

pends not only on the right ventricle, but also on the pumping action of breathing movements. Because the pulmonary circulation is a low-pressure, low-resistance circulation under normal circumstances, cardiac output can increase many times (as happens during exercise) without significant increase in pulmonary artery pressure. This condition occurs because of the enormous capacity of the pulmonary vascular bed, which is normally about 25% perfused at rest, and its ability to recruit more vessels during exercise.

Etiology and Pathogenesis

The etiology and pathogenesis of cor pulmonale are illustrated in Fig. 40-2. The diseases causing cor pulmonale are those in which the pulmonary vasculature is primarily involved, such as recurrent pulmonary emboli, and those in which the impediment to pulmonary blood flow is secondary to obstructive or restrictive respiratory diseases. Chronic obstructive pulmonary disease (COPD), especially the bronchitic type, is the most common cause of cor pulmonale. Restrictive respiratory diseases leading to cor pulmonale include "intrinsic" diseases, such as diffuse pulmonary fibrosis, and "extrinsic" disorders, such as extreme obesity, kyphoscoliosis, or severe neuromuscular dysfunction that affects the respiratory muscles. Finally, pulmonary vascular disease that causes obstruction to blood flow and cor pulmonale is quite rare and usually results from recurrent pulmonary emboli.

Regardless of the initiating disease, the common path-

way and prerequisite for cor pulmonale is the development of increased pulmonary vascular resistance and pulmonary hypertension. Pulmonary hypertension, in turn, increases the workload of the right ventricle, causing it to hypertrophy and eventually fail. The critical point in the sequence seems to be an increase in pulmonary vascular resistance through the small arteries and arterioles.

Two basic mechanisms produce an increase in pulmonary vascular resistance: (1) hypoxic vasoconstriction of pulmonary blood vessels and (2) obstruction and/or obliteration of the pulmonary vascular bed. The first of these two mechanisms seems to be the most critical in the pathogenesis of cor pulmonale. The hypoxemia, hypercapnia, and acidosis that characterize advanced bronchitic COPD provide an excellent example of how these mechanisms operate. The *alveolar (tissue) hypoxia,* rather than the hypoxemia, provides a potent stimulus to pulmonary vasoconstriction. In addition, chronic alveolar hypoxia promotes hypertrophy of smooth muscle in the pulmonary arterioles, which then respond more vigorously to acute hypoxia. The hypercapneic acidosis and hypoxemia act synergistically to augment the vasoconstriction. Increased blood viscosity arising from secondary polycythemia and increased cardiac output stimulated by chronic hypoxia and hypercapnia make an additional contribution to increased pulmonary artery pressure.

The second mechanism that makes a contribution to increased vascular resistance and pulmonary artery pressure is anatomic in origin. Emphysema is characterized by gradual destruction of the alveolar structure with formation of bullae and complete obliteration of nearby capillaries as well. Permanent loss of blood vessels contributes to the reduction of the cross-sectional area of the vascular bed. In addition, pulmonary vessels are compressed externally because of the mechanical effects of the high lung volumes in obstructive disease. However, anatomic obstruction and obliteration of the vascular bed are believed to be less important than hypoxic vasoconstriction in the pathogenesis of cor pulmonale. Approximately two thirds to three fourths of the vascular bed must become obstructed or destroyed before a significant rise in pulmonary artery pressure occurs. Chronic respiratory acidosis is present in a number of obstructive and respiratory diseases as a result of generalized alveolar hypoventilation or as a consequence of ventilation-perfusion abnormalities. It is evident from this discussion that any pulmonary disease that affects gas exchange, ventilatory mechanics, or the pulmonary vascular bed may result in cor pulmonale.

Clinical Manifestations

Diagnosis of cor pulmonale rests mainly on two criteria: (1) presence of a respiratory disease with associated pulmonary hypertension and (2) evidence of a hypertrophied right ventricle. Presence of persistent hypoxemia, hypercapnia, and acidosis or of right ventricular enlargement on radiographs should suggest the possibility of underlying lung disease. Presence of emphysema tends to obscure the diagnostic features of cor pulmonale. Dyspnea is present as a feature of emphysema whether or not cor pulmonale is present. A sudden worsening of dyspnea or fatigue, syncope on exertion, or substernal anginal discomfort should suggest cardiac involvement. Physical signs of pulmonary hypertension include a systolic lift over the parasternal area, a loud second pulmonic sound, and murmurs resulting from functional tricuspid and pulmonic insufficiency. Gallop rhythm (S_3 and S_4 heart sounds), jugular venous distention with prominent A waves, hepatomegaly, and peripheral edema may be seen in patients with right ventricular failure.

Treatment

Treatment of cor pulmonale is aimed at correcting the alveolar hypoxia (and consequent pulmonary vasoconstriction) by the judicious administration of low-concentration O_2. Continuous use of O_2 can decrease pulmonary hypertension, polycythemia, and tachypnea; improve well-being; and reduce mortality (Kersten, 1989). Bronchodilators and antibiotics help relieve airflow obstruction in patients with COPD. Fluid restriction and diuretics relieve signs attributed to right ventricular failure. Long-term anticoagulation therapy is necessary when recurrent pulmonary emboli are present.

QUESTIONS

▼ *Answer the following on a separate sheet of paper.*

1. List three factors that directly relate to the development of venous thrombosis.

2. What disease is the most common cause of cor pulmonale in the United States?

3. List four conditions that may precipitate pulmonary edema.

4. What is paroxysmal nocturnal dyspnea?

5. Define cor pulmonale.

6. What is the relationship between left-sided heart failure and pulmonary edema? Is this condition the most frequent cause of pulmonary edema?

7. List three objectives in the treatment of pulmonary embolism.

8. What are the two goals in treatment of cor pulmonale?

9. Describe two mechanisms that can lead to increased pulmonary vascular resistance.

▼ *Circle the letter preceding each item below that correctly answers the question. More than one answer may be correct.*

10. The classic signs and symptoms associated with a moderate-sized pulmonary embolism (PE) without infarction are:
    a. Dyspnea
    b. Rapid respiratory rate
    c. Tachycardia
    d. Unconsciousness and death within minutes
    e. Hemoptysis

11. Which of the following types of PE is more frequent?
    a. Massive occlusion at bifurcation of main pulmonary artery
    b. Moderate-sized occlusion of lobar or lobular pulmonary artery
    c. Occlusion of small pulmonary vessels as a result of recurrent multiple emboli

12. Which of the following are effects of PE?
    a. Pulmonary infarction
    b. Ventilation/perfusion ($\dot{V}/\dot{Q}$) imbalance resulting in increased dead space
    c. $\dot{V}/\dot{Q}$ imbalance resulting in increased shunting

    d. Reflex bronchoconstriction

13. The most reliable method of diagnosing a PE is:
    a. Chest radiograph
    b. Perfusion lung scan with albumin tagged with radioactive isotope
    c. Pulmonary angiography
    d. Physical examination

14. The usual treatment of an acute PE includes:
    a. Oral anticoagulants in low dosage
    b. Intensive care monitoring
    c. General cardiopulmonary support with O_2
    d. Elastic stockings
    e. Surgical embolectomy

15. What is the approximate mortality rate for surgical removal of a massive PE?
    a. 1%
    b. 10%
    c. 50%

16. Emergency treatment of acute pulmonary edema might include:
    a. Placing the patient in a high Fowler's position with the feet dependent
    b. Placing the patient in a horizontal position with the feet elevated
    c. Rotating tourniquets
    d. Rapid infusion of intravenous solutions

17. A PE usually occurs when a thrombus from a leg vein breaks off and:
    a. Circulates through the left ventricle and lodges in the main pulmonary artery or its branches
    b. Circulates through the right ventricle of the heart and lodges in the pulmonary vein
    c. Circulates through the right side of the heart and lodges in the main pulmonary artery or its branches

18. The most likely location for the formation of a blood clot causing a PE is:
    a. A deep vein in the legs
    b. The left ventricle
    c. An artery in the legs
    d. The right ventricle

19. Which of the following conditions is associated with an increased risk of PE?
    a. Carcinoma of the small bowel
    b. Postoperative bedridden status
    c. Thombophlebitis
    d. Congestive heart failure

20. The condition associated with the highest incidence of pulmonary embolism is:
    a. Congestive heart failure
    b. Postoperative bedridden status
    c. Postpartum status
    d. O_2
    e. Venous insufficiency

21. All the following have a place in the treatment of cor pulmonale. The single most important therapeutic modality is:
    a. Digitalis
    b. Diuretics
    c. Bronchodilators
    d. O_2
    e. Phlebotomy

22. Continuous low-concentration O_2 therapy in hypoxemic patients with chronic obstructive pulmonary disease (COPD) has the following effects:
    a. Improves pulmonary function
    b. Improves exercise tolerance
    c. Has no effect on red cell mass
    d. Reduces pulmonary artery hypertension

▼ *Circle T if the statement is true with respect to pulmonary infarction and F if it is false. Correct any false statement.*

23. T F It is a localized area of ischemic necrosis.

24. T F It is an infrequent complication of pulmonary embolism as a result of the lung's dual blood supply.

25. T F It is frequently associated with a small pleural effusion.

26. T F It is easily differentiated from pneumonia on chest radiographs.

▼ *Complete the following statements by filling in the blanks.*

27. A freely circulating blood clot that lodges in a blood vessel causing an obstruction is called a(n) _____.

28. A prerequisite for the development of cor pulmonale is increased pulmonary vascular resistance leading to _____ _____.

CHAPTER 41 ▷ Respiratory Failure

LORRAINE M. WILSON

Respiratory failure is a relatively common problem, which is usually, but not always, the end result of chronic disease affecting the respiratory system. Increasingly, this condition is encountered as a complication of acute trauma, septicemia, or shock.

Respiratory failure, as with the failure of any other organ system, may be characterized on the basis of clinical features or laboratory tests. One must remember, however, that the correlation between the clinical features and deviations of laboratory tests from the normal range is far from straightforward in respiratory failure.

Respiratory failure is said to exist when the lung cannot fulfill its primary functions of gas exchange, namely, oxygenation of the arterial blood and carbon dioxide elimination. There are various grades of respiratory failure, and the condition may be acute (and possibly remittent), or chronic. *Chronic respiratory insufficiency or failure* refers to long-term functional impairment that persists many days or months and represents a compromise between the pathologic processes leading to failure and the compensatory processes stabilizing the situation. Blood gases may be mildly abnormal or within normal limits at rest but markedly abnormal during situations of increased demand such as exercise. Increased work of breathing (and thus decreased respiratory reserve) and reduction of physical activity are the two broad coping mechanisms in chronic respiratory insufficiency.

ACUTE RESPIRATORY FAILURE

Acute respiratory failure is numerically defined as respiratory failure with an arterial oxygen partial pressure (or tension, Pao_2) of 50 to 60 mm Hg or less with or without an arterial carbon dioxide partial pressure (or tension, $Paco_2$) of 50 mm Hg or greater under resting conditions at sea level. This numeric definition based on arterial blood gases (ABGs) has been established because the line between chronic respiratory insufficiency and respiratory failure is subtle and clinical observations alone are unreliable. On the other hand, one must understand that the definition based on ABGs is not absolute; the significance of the numbers depends on the patient's past history. A previously healthy person who develops this degree of abnormality of ABGs after a near-drowning accident might be expected to be comatose, whereas many patients with chronic obstructive pulmonary disease (COPD) can function with some degree of physical activity at the same levels.

Two broad classifications of respiratory failure are based on ABG pathophysiology: (1) *hypoxemic,* or *normocapnic, respiratory failure* (hypoxemia with normal or low $Paco_2$) and (2) *hypercapnic,* or *ventilatory,* failure (hypoxemia and hypercapnia). This chapter discusses the clinical features, causes, pathogenetic mechanisms, and management of these two types of respiratory failure.

Pathogenesis and Etiology

The successful treatment of acute respiratory failure depends not only on its recognition at an early stage, but also on identification of the mechanisms at fault. Early recognition may be difficult when the onset is insidious because the clinical signs and symptoms are nonspecific.

CAUSES OF RESPIRATORY FAILURE

A. Disorders extrinsic to the lungs
 1. Respiratory center depression
  a. Drug overdose (sedatives, narcotics)
  b. Cerebral trauma or infarction
  c. Bulbar poliomyelitis
  d. Encephalitis
 2. Neuromuscular disorders
  a. Cervical cord injury
  b. Guillain-Barré syndrome
  c. Amyotrophic lateral sclerosis
  d. Myasthenia gravis
  e. Muscular dystrophy
 3. Pleural and chest wall disorders
  a. Chest injury (flail chest, rib fracture)
  b. Pneumothorax
  c. Pleural effusion
  d. Kyphoscoliosis
  e. Obesity: pickwickian syndrome
B. Disorders intrinsic to the lungs
 1. Diffuse obstructive disorders
  a. Emphysema, chronic bronchitis (COPD)
  b. Asthma, status asthmaticus
  c. Cystic fibrosis
 2. Diffuse restrictive disorders
  a. Interstitial fibrosis of various causes (e.g., silica, coal dust)
  b. Sarcoidosis
  c. Scleroderma
  d. Pulmonary edema
   (1) Cardiogenic
   (2) Noncardiogenic (ARDS)
  e. Atelectasis
  f. Consolidated pneumonia
 3. Pulmonary vascular disorders
  a. Pulmonary emboli
  b. Severe emphysema

PRECIPITATING FACTORS OF RESPIRATORY FAILURE IN CHRONIC LUNG DISEASE

Infection of tracheobronchial tree, pneumonia, fever
Change in tracheobronchial secretions (increased volume or viscosity)
Bronchospasm (inhalation of irritants or allergens)
Disturbance in ability to clear secretions
Sedatives, narcotics, anesthesia
Oxygen therapy (high FiO_2)
Trauma, including surgery
Cardiovascular disorders (heart failure, pulmonary embolism)
Pneumothorax

Although tissue hypoxia cannot be assessed directly, ABG measurements (one step in the long process that determines tissue oxygenation) can be helpful in drawing inferences about inadequate tissue oxygenation and the faulty mechanisms. Knowledge of the mechanisms at fault provides insight into the pathophysiology of a patient's lung disease, which leads in turn to appropriate treatment.

An important first step in the recognition of impending respiratory failure is awareness of the conditions and settings likely to lead to respiratory failure. The box above lists some of the common lung disorders causing respiratory failure, classified as extrinsic or intrinsic. Most of these conditions were discussed in previous chapters. *Extrinsic lung disorders* (with lungs that are normal or nearly normal) lead to ventilatory, or hypercapnic, respiratory failure through (1) depression of central respiratory drive or (2) interference with the ventilatory response. Narcotic overdose is one of the most common causes of respiratory center depression resulting in ventilatory failure. Interference with ventilatory response occurs when there is disease or injury of the neural pathways or ventilatory muscles or mechanical dysfunction of the thoracic bellows caused by injury, pain, or deformity. Some of the possible causes of a decreased ventilatory response are listed under neuromuscular and pleural and chest wall disorders.

Although extrapulmonary, or extrinsic, lung disorders are important causes of respiratory failure, the *pulmonary, or intrinsic, lung disorders* are even more important. Chronic obstruction of the airways results in ventilatory failure, with COPD the most common cause. Diffuse restrictive disorders of the lung parenchyma and vasculature generally cause mild hypoxemic respiratory failure; however, acute intrinsic abnormalities of the lung parenchyma such as massive pulmonary edema, atelectasis, extensive consolidated pneumonia, and adult respiratory distress syndrome (ARDS) may cause profound hypoxemia. ARDS accounts for a significant portion of the population of respiratory intensive care units and has a high mortality rate. This condition is discussed separately from the other causes of respiratory failure later in this chapter.

Finally, it is important to know that a number of precipitating factors can result in acute respiratory failure in persons with chronic lung disease (see box above). Retained secretions, infection, and bronchospasm are the most common precipitating factors in patients with COPD causing *acute-on-chronic respiratory failure.* Important iatrogenic factors include the injudicious administration of narcotics or high fractions of inspired oxygen (FiO_2). Cor pulmonale, pulmonary embolism (especially in patients with polycythemia), and pneumothorax from an emphysematous bleb are other less common precipi-

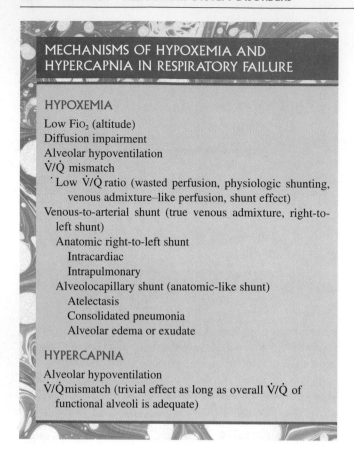

MECHANISMS OF HYPOXEMIA AND HYPERCAPNIA IN RESPIRATORY FAILURE

HYPOXEMIA

Low Fio_2 (altitude)
Diffusion impairment
Alveolar hypoventilation
$\dot{V}/\dot{Q}$ mismatch
  Low $\dot{V}/\dot{Q}$ ratio (wasted perfusion, physiologic shunting, venous admixture–like perfusion, shunt effect)
Venous-to-arterial shunt (true venous admixture, right-to-left shunt)
  Anatomic right-to-left shunt
    Intracardiac
    Intrapulmonary
  Alveolocapillary shunt (anatomic-like shunt)
    Atelectasis
    Consolidated pneumonia
    Alveolar edema or exudate

HYPERCAPNIA

Alveolar hypoventilation
$\dot{V}/\dot{Q}$ mismatch (trivial effect as long as overall $\dot{V}/\dot{Q}$ of functional alveoli is adequate)

tating causes of respiratory failure. Some of these precipitating factors cannot be eliminated, but many of them can; this has important implications for patient education and the management of chronic respiratory disease.

Mechanisms of hypoxemia and hypercapnia

By definition, hypoxemia is present in respiratory failure. *Hypoxemic respiratory failure* is characterized by hypoxemia and either normocapnia or hypocapnia, whereas *ventilatory failure* is characterized by hypoxemia and hypercapnia. The treatment implications of this distinction will become evident as this discussion proceeds.

The box above lists the pathogenetic mechanisms involved in hypoxemia and hypercapnia. Only the last three mechanisms shown in the box (alveolar hypoventilation, low ventilation/perfusion [$\dot{V}/\dot{Q}$] ratio, and shunting) are important causes of hypoxemia. The primary cause of hypercapnia is alveolar hypoventilation, but $\dot{V}/\dot{Q}$ inequality generally has a trivial effect on the $Paco_2$. It should be noted that alveolar hypoventilation causes both hypercapnia and hypoxemia, whereas $\dot{V}/\dot{Q}$ mismatch generally causes only hypoxemia.

The determination of the $Paco_2$ with respect to the lungs is relatively simple: the $Paco_2$ is directly related to CO_2 production and nearly inversely proportional to alveolar ventilation (West, 1995), as follows:

$$Paco_2 \propto \frac{\dot{V}co_2 \text{ (production of } CO_2)}{\dot{V}_A \text{ (alveolar ventilation)}}$$

Thus, if alveolar ventilation ($\dot{V}_A$) is halved, the $Paco_2$ will be doubled provided CO_2 production remains constant. Conversely, if $\dot{V}_A$ should double as in hyperventilation, the $Paco_2$ would be halved. Ventilatory failure with hypercapnia always involves the mechanism of alveolar hypoventilation. Pure hypoventilation, although relatively infrequent, is associated with the extrapulmonary conditions listed in the box on p. 623, in which the lungs are relatively normal (with the exception of kyphoscoliosis). Alveolar hypoventilation develops in these conditions because the minute ventilation falls, as in respiratory center depression from narcotic overdose, or there is a disproportionally high work of breathing or total body metabolism (increased CO_2 production) for a given $\dot{V}_A$, as in obesity or chest deformity (Cherniack, Cherniack, 1983). The hypoxemia associated with pure hypoventilation is generally mild (Pao_2 = 50 to 80 mm Hg) and is directly caused by the elevation of the alveolar Pco_2 ($PAco_2$). This fact can be explained by recalling that the partial pressure of all the alveolar or all the arterial blood gases must add up to the total (atmospheric) pressure. Thus, when $Paco_2$ increases, the Pao_2 must decrease, and vice versa, at a constant total atmospheric pressure. The relationship between the rise in Pco_2 and the fall in the Po_2 that occurs in hypoventilation can be predicted by the *alveolar gas equation* if we know the composition of the Fio_2 and the *respiratory exchange ratio* (R or RQ), as follows:

$$PAo_2 = Fio_2 (PB - PH_2O) - \frac{Paco_2}{R}$$

where PAo_2 is the partial pressure of O_2 in the alveolus; Fio_2 is the inspired O_2 fraction (0.21 when breathing air); PB is the barometric pressure (760 mm Hg at sea level); PH_2O is the partial pressure of water vapor in the trachea (47 mm Hg at normal body temperature); and $Paco_2$ is the partial pressure of CO_2 in the arterial blood and is assumed to be equal to that in the alveolus.* R or RQ is determined by body metabolism and is equal to the volume of CO_2 produced divided by the volume of O_2 consumed ($\dot{V}co_2/\dot{V}o_2$). R is 0.7 when pure fat is burned, 1.0 when pure carbohydrate is burned, and about 0.8 on a mixed diet. When a healthy person is breathing room air with a normal $Paco_2$ of 40 mm Hg and we assume that R = 0.8:

$$PAo_2 = 0.21(760 - 47) - \frac{40}{0.8}$$

$$PAo_2 \approx Pao_2 = 100 \text{ mm Hg}$$

---

*Equality of alveolar and arterial CO_2 gas tensions is assumed, as well as equality of alveolar and arterial O_2 gas tensions, although this is not strictly accurate. The Pao_2 is about 5 mm Hg lower than the PAo_2 because of a small $\dot{V}/\dot{Q}$ mismatch and shunt in the normal lung, but the effect on $PAco_2$ and $Paco_2$ differences is negligible.

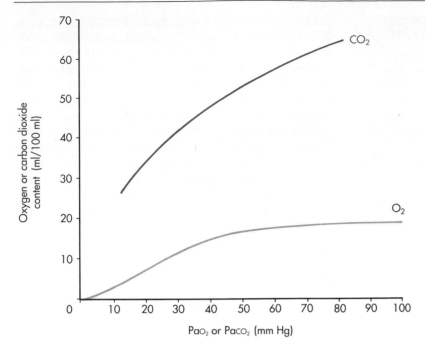

FIG. 41-I   Oxyhemoglobin and carbon dioxide dissociation curves plotted on the same scale. (Modified from Comroe JH Jr: *The lung*, ed 2, Chicago, 1962, Mosby.)

If a person should hypoventilate breathing room air and the normal $PaCO_2$ should rise from 40 to 70 mm Hg, the PAO_2 and PaO_2 would necessarily fall from 100 mm Hg to about 62 mm Hg:

$$PAO_2 = 0.21(760 - 47) - \frac{70}{0.8}$$

$$PAO_2 \approx PaO_2 = 62.23 \text{ mm Hg}$$

(NOTE: For each 10 mm Hg rise in $PaCO_2$ above normal, the PaO_2 will fall 12.5 mm Hg.)

It is apparent from an examination of the alveolar gas equation that the hypoxemia that develops from pure hypoventilation can easily be corrected by administering O_2 and raising the FiO_2. The equation also shows that if the drop in the PaO_2 is greater than expected, other mechanisms causing hypoxemia must be operating (shunting or $\dot{V}/\dot{Q}$ mismatch). Although the degree of hypoxemia that develops from pure hypoventilation in the example is not serious (because O_2 saturation is about 90% at a PaO_2 of 62 mm Hg), this degree of $PaCO_2$ will depress the respiratory center and cause a serious acidosis.

$\dot{V}/\dot{Q}$ inequality, or mismatch, is by far the most important mechanism causing hypoxemia in persons with chronic airway obstruction and plays a role in most other intrinsic lung disorders. $\dot{V}/\dot{Q}$ inequality refers to the *regional* imbalance of ventilation and blood flow in the pulmonary gas-exchanging units discussed in Chapter 35. Some pulmonary units have relatively high $\dot{V}/\dot{Q}$ ratios (wasted ventilation or dead-space-like units), whereas others have low $\dot{V}/\dot{Q}$ ratios (wasted perfusion, physiologic shunt, venous admixture). If some alveoli receive too little ventilation in proportion to perfusion (low $\dot{V}/\dot{Q}$),

there is a fall in PaO_2 and a rise in $PaCO_2$ in the blood leaving these alveoli. In effect, blood is shunted past the alveoli without adequate gas exchange taking place (venous admixture effect). Conversely, alveoli that receive too little perfusion in proportion to ventilation (high $\dot{V}/\dot{Q}$) produce high PaO_2 and low $PaCO_2$ in the blood flowing from them. Recall that the healthy lung has some $\dot{V}/\dot{Q}$ inequality because of the effects of gravity (see Chapter 35), but this is not significant enough to cause blood gas abnormalities. Low $\dot{V}/\dot{Q}$ ratios can cause significant hypoxemia in lung disease but generally have little effect on the $PaCO_2$. The relationship between the partial pressures and content of these two gases accounts for the difference.

Fig. 41-1 illustrates the oxyhemoglobin and CO_2 dissociation curves drawn on the same scale for comparative purposes. This figure makes the important point that the oxyhemoglobin curve has a flat portion, but the CO_2 curve does not. At a PaO_2 of about 60 (when the curve starts to flatten), the O_2 content of the blood has reached more than 80% of the maximum content of about 19.5 vol %. A large increase in the PaO_2 (e.g., from 60 to 100 mm Hg) causes only a small increase in O_2 content. In contrast, CO_2 transport in the blood is much more efficient. Because the CO_2 curve is steep in the physiologic range of the $PaCO_2$, a small change (e.g., from 40 to 50) causes a large change in CO_2 content. In terms of $\dot{V}/\dot{Q}$ imbalance, this means that alveoli with high $\dot{V}/\dot{Q}$ ratios cannot fully compensate for those with low $\dot{V}/\dot{Q}$ ratios with reference to O_2 transport. The hemoglobin (Hb) from the better ventilated units, when already nearly saturated (flat part of oxyhemoglobin dissociation curve), cannot carry the excess O_2 that would be needed to compensate for the deficit caused by poorly oxygenated blood from the low $\dot{V}/\dot{Q}$ units. Because the CO_2 dissociation curve is more nearly linear in the physiologic range, the hyperventilating units with a high $\dot{V}/\dot{Q}$ ratio can compensate for hypoventilating units with a low $\dot{V}/\dot{Q}$ ratio. The result is that the mixed blood leaving the high and low $\dot{V}/\dot{Q}$ units will have a normal $Paco_2$. However, progressive involvement of more and more of the lung by the disease process will result in more and more alveolocapillary units with low $\dot{V}/\dot{Q}$ ratios. Eventually a point is reached at which the remaining high $\dot{V}/\dot{Q}$ units cannot compensate for the low units, and hypercapnia ensues. Therefore those diseases characterized by $\dot{V}/\dot{Q}$ abnormalities (most of the intrinsic lung diseases and kyphoscoliosis) demonstrate progression through hypoxemic respiratory insufficiency and failure (which occurs first) to hypercapnic, or ventilatory, failure (which occurs later).

The important principles to remember from this discussion so far are that (1) the factors determining oxygenation and ventilation are different and must be analyzed separately; (2) the $Paco_2$ must be regarded as a function of the *overall* ventilation of the entire lung, without regard to local inequalities of distribution of ventilation and perfusion; (3) the Pao_2, on the other hand, depends not only on the amount of $\dot{V}_A$, but also on $\dot{V}/\dot{Q}$ matching; and (4) hypercapnia must be viewed as representing a problem not only with oxygenation, but also with ventilation.

The third important mechanism causing hypoxemia is venous-to-arterial, or right-to-left, shunting of blood, which bypasses the gas-exchanging units of the lung. A true anatomic right-to-left shunt may exist in congenital heart disease, as when an opening exists between the right and left chambers of the heart or, rarely, when an arteriovenous fistula exists within the lung (West, 1995). There is a small true shunt in normal lungs (see Fig. 35-12) amounting to about 2.5% of pulmonary blood flow. In addition to these rare anatomic vascular abnormalities and the small normal shunt, shunting may also occur when alveolar spaces are nonfunctional, as when the alveoli are collapsed (atelectasis) or filled with edema fluid or with exudate, as in pulmonary edema or pneumonia. This type of shunting may be regarded as an extreme type of $\dot{V}/\dot{Q}$ mismatch in which ventilation of the involved units is zero while perfusion continues. If a large number of gas-exchange units are involved in shunting, the resulting hypoxemia can be severe. However, the $Paco_2$ is generally normal or low because the subject can usually increase ventilation sufficiently in the remaining normal lung to blow off the CO_2 adequately. When overall hyperventilation occurs in response to severe hypoxemia, hypocapnia and respiratory alkalosis may result. Hypoxemic respiratory failure caused primarily by shunting is difficult to treat because the hypoxemia is not readily correctable by O_2 therapy.

Another type of extreme $\dot{V}/\dot{Q}$ imbalance is that exemplified by a pulmonary unit in which there is ventila-

tion but no perfusion (dead space). The classic example of alveolar dead-space disease is acute pulmonary embolus. Another common cause is acutely decreased pulmonary perfusion resulting from acutely decreased cardiac output or acute pulmonary hypertension with increased pulmonary vascular resistance (Shapiro, Peruzzi, Kozlowski-Templin, 1994). Destruction of the alveolar septal walls in emphysema, with replacement of several alveoli by large air spaces, results in reducing the surface area for gas exchange. The anatomic dead space can be greatly increased by a rapid, shallow breathing pattern, as illustrated in Table 36-2. The normal physiologic dead space is 30% of the tidal volume (V_D/V_T). If dead-space ventilation is increased significantly (wasted ventilation), overall ventilation must increase to maintain effective $\dot{V}_A$. In advanced disease the work of breathing may be so great as to cause hypercapnia and hypoxemia. When there is both high minute volume and high physiologic dead space, the condition is referred to as *high-output ventilatory failure*.

Hypoxemia caused by high altitude can generally be ignored in the treatment of respiratory failure because it is constant for a particular locale. At sea level, P_B is 760 mm Hg. With increasing altitude the total P_B and the Po_2 of inspired air decrease, although the percentage of O_2 in the air remains constant at 20.93%. For example, in Boston at sea level the P_B is 760 mm Hg and the inspired Po_2 is 159 mm Hg, whereas in Denver the P_B is 632.3 mm Hg and the inspired Po_2 is 132.3 mm Hg (Comroe, 1974).

Most authorities no longer consider diffusion impairment to be a significant factor in producing hypoxemia, although it may play a minor role when there is thickening of the alveolocapillary membrane, as in pulmonary fibrosis and sarcoidosis. The normal contact time between alveolar gas and pulmonary blood is 0.75 second under resting conditions, and equilibration is normally completed in 0.25 second. Thus there is ample diffusion time in reserve (Cherniack, Cherniack, 1983; Shapiro, Peruzzi, Kozlowski-Templin, 1994). When diffusion time is somewhat reduced during exercise, it is possible for diffusion limitation to make a greater contribution to hypoxemia.

In summary, when hypoxemic respiratory failure is present, the principal mechanisms involved are low $\dot{V}/\dot{Q}$ ratio or shunting, either alone or in combination. Diffusion impairment may possibly make a minor contribution to the hypoxemia, although this is controversial. Hypoxemic respiratory insufficiency or failure is usually associated with restrictive or vascular diseases of the lung. Even though the work of breathing is increased in these conditions (with consequently increased CO_2 production and O_2 consumption for ventilatory work), the subject has enough strength to increase ventilation sufficiently to maintain a normal $Paco_2$. Any slight rise in the $Paco_2$ will stimulate increased ventilation. When the Pao_2 falls to about 50 to 60 mm Hg, this also stimulates ventilation.

Consequently, hyperventilation may result, so that the $Paco_2$ is decreased below normal levels (respiratory alkalosis or hypocapnia). Hyperventilation while breathing room air is generally ineffectual in correcting hypoxemia because of the sigmoid shape of the oxyhemoglobin dissociation curve. O_2 therapy is quite effective in correcting hypoxemia caused by $\dot{V}/\dot{Q}$ imbalance or diffusion impairment but ineffective if the cause is shunting.

Hypercapnic, or ventilatory, failure may be caused by hypoventilation alone or in combination with any or all of the other hypoxemic mechanisms—$\dot{V}/\dot{Q}$ imbalance, shunting, or possibly diffusion impairment. Pure ventilatory failure occurs in extrapulmonary disorders involving failure of neural or muscular control of breathing. The classic example of hypercapnic respiratory failure occurs in COPD and involves $\dot{V}/\dot{Q}$ imbalance and hypoventilation. When respiratory failure is precipitated by retained secretions and pneumonia in such patients, considerable shunting may also occur. Although obstructive disorders of the airways generally result in hypercapnic respiratory failure, reversible airway disease, as in asthma, is an exception to the rule. An acute asthmatic attack is generally characterized by hypoxemia and hypocapnia because the subjects are usually able to hyperventilate. A rise of the $Paco_2$ even to normal levels in a sustained asthmatic attack may be a signal that the functional status is deteriorating (Cherniack, Cherniack, 1983). The primary focus in ventilatory failure is on measures to improve ventilation and at the same time prevent serious tissue hypoxia. Methods of differentiating between the mechanisms involved in hypoxemia and hypercapnia are discussed subsequently.

Clinical Features

The manifestations of acute respiratory failure represent a combination of the clinical features of the underlying disease, the precipitating factors, and the manifestations of hypoxemia and hypercapnia. Thus the clinical picture may be quite variable because various factors may precipitate it. The presence or absence of preceding chronic respiratory insufficiency is another factor that modifies the clinical picture.

The signs and symptoms of hypoxemia are a direct result of tissue hypoxia. (These were presented in Chapter 37 but are reviewed here.) The more frequently cited signs and symptoms do not develop until the Pao_2 is in the range of 40 to 50 mm Hg. Tissues highly sensitive to O_2 depletion are principally affected, including the brain, heart, and lungs. The most prominent signs and symptoms are neurologic: headache, mental confusion, impairment of judgment, slurring of speech, asterixis, impairment of motor function, agitation, and restlessness that may progress to delirium and unconsciousness. In some cases the neurologic signs and symptoms of hypoxic persons have been misinterpreted as alcoholic inebriation. The initial cardiovascular responses to hypoxemia are tachycardia and increased cardiac output and blood pressure. When the hypoxia persists, bradycardia, hypotension, decreased cardiac output, and dysrhythmias may occur. Hypoxemia causes vasoconstriction of the pulmonary blood vessels. The metabolic effect of tissue hypoxia is anaerobic metabolism resulting in metabolic acidosis. Although cyanosis is often regarded as a sign of hypoxia, it is unreliable (see Chapter 37). The classic symptom of dyspnea may also be absent, especially when respiratory center drive is decreased, as in the respiratory failure of narcotic overdose.

Hypercapnia while breathing room air is always accompanied by hypoxemia. Consequently the signs and symptoms of ventilatory failure represent the effects of both hypercapnia and hypoxemia. The major effect of increases in the $Paco_2$ is depression of the central nervous system (CNS). For this reason, severe hypercapnia is sometimes referred to as CO_2 narcosis. Hypercapnia results in cerebral vasodilation, increased cerebral blood flow, and increased intracranial pressure. The resultant headache, worse on awaking in the morning (since $Paco_2$ increases slightly during sleep) is characteristic. Other resultant signs and symptoms include papilledema, neuromuscular irritability (asterixis), fluctuations of mood, and increased drowsiness, which may progress to frank coma. Although an increased $Paco_2$ is normally the most powerful stimulus to respiration, it has a depressive effect on respiration at levels greater than 70 mm Hg. In addition, persons with COPD and chronic hypercapnia develop insensitivity to increased $Paco_2$ and depend on hypoxic drive. Hypercapnia causes constriction of the pulmonary blood vessels, thus aggravating any pulmonary artery hypertension that may be present. When CO_2 retention is severe, decreased myocardial contractility, systemic vasodilation, heart failure, and hypotension may ensue. Hypercapnia causes respiratory acidosis, which is often combined with metabolic acidosis when there is tissue hypoxia. This combination can cause a serious depression of the blood pH. The renal compensatory response to respiratory acidosis is reabsorption of bicarbonate to restore pH to normal. This response takes about 3 days, so respiratory acidosis is much more severe when the onset is rapid.

Diagnosis

A number of situations can occur during which anyone can recognize respiratory failure. Examples are cardiac arrest, complete obstruction of the upper airways by, for example, a piece of meat, head injury serious enough to stop the breathing mechanism, or labored breathing in a person who is cyanotic. However, in many patients the presence of respiratory failure may not be so obvious. The onset of respiratory failure is insidious in many persons with chronic respiratory insufficiency. Signs and symptoms may be nonspecific and correlate poorly with the degree of respiratory impairment until the situation is

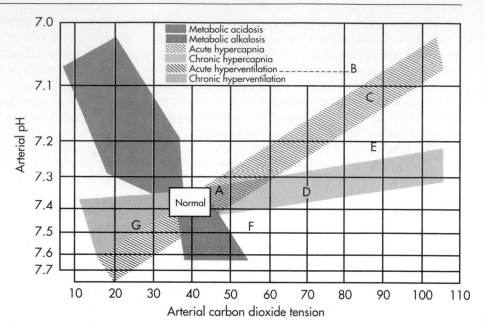

FIG. 41-2 Nomogram for acid-base disturbances. This graph displays the quantity and direction of changes in pH and Paco₂ in various types of acid-base disturbances. The shaded areas represent the range of variability in persons with pure acid-base disorders. In general, values outside the significant bands represent mixed acid-base disorders. See text for explanation of letter points. [Modified from Burrows B, Knudson RJ, Kettel LJ: *Respiratory insufficiency,* Chicago, 1975, Mosby.]

catastrophic. Great astuteness is needed to recognize every case of respiratory failure. Thus the clinician needs to have a high degree of suspicion and be ready to obtain measurements of ABGs when respiratory failure is suspected because this is the only way a definitive diagnosis can be made. In general, a Paco₂ of 50 mm Hg or more or a Pao₂ of 50 to 60 mm Hg or less at sea level is accepted as indicating respiratory failure.

Assessment of respiratory function

Measurement of respiratory function is indispensable in the provision of adequate respiratory care, not only for accurate diagnosis, but also for evaluation of response to treatment. Measurement of ABGs provides valuable information for establishing the degree and type of respiratory failure and for identifying the mechanisms involved. A number of bedside measurements of ventilatory function are also frequently used to assess ventilatory reserve and the need for mechanical ventilation. The ventilatory status and the acid-base status are assessed by examining the Paco₂, bicarbonate (HCO₃⁻), and pH.

A nomogram may be helpful in determining whether hypercapnic respiratory failure is acute or chronic or whether a mixed acid-base disorder is present. Fig. 41-2 shows the relation between the Paco₂ and pH and the alterations seen in respiratory and metabolic disorders of acid-base balance. Data that fall within a particular band usually represent the primary disorder, and data outside the band represent a mixed disorder. The following equivalences need to be emphasized: (1) respiratory acidosis = hypercapnia = alveolar hypoventilation, and (2) respiratory alkalosis = hypocapnia = alveolar hyperventilation. The lettered points on the nomogram represent common values in respiratory failure. Any sudden, severe decrease in ventilation resulting in the retention of

CO_2 in the blood will produce acute respiratory acidosis *(C)*. This acidosis is frequently aggravated by a coexisting metabolic acidosis from excess lactic acid produced by the tissue hypoxia that also results from decreased ventilation *(B)*. The renal compensation for a rise in the Paco₂ is retention of HCO₃⁻ to restore blood pH to normal. This process normally takes about 3 days. Thus point *D* represents chronic hypercapnia, frequently seen in patients with COPD. Point *E* could represent partially compensated acute hypercapnia or a mixture of acute and chronic hypercapnia, which might occur when a patient with COPD develops a respiratory infection. Point *F* represents a mixture of chronic hypercapnia and metabolic alkalosis, which might be caused by rapid correction of the hypercapnia by artificial ventilation. When the Paco₂ is lowered rapidly in a person with compensated respiratory acidosis (hypercapnia) and consequently with an increased HCO₃⁻, there is an excess of base bicarbonate (metabolic alkalosis) until the kidneys can excrete the excess. Point *G* represents chronic hyperventilation (respiratory alkalosis), which is common in hypoxemic respiratory failure. Point *A* represents a mild hypercapnia. The acute and the chronic forms cannot be distinguished unless the patient's usual Paco₂ is known.

Evaluation of oxygenation involves examination of several parameters, including Pao₂, the alveolar-arterial O₂ difference or gradient [the P(A − a)o₂ or (A − aD)o₂], cardiac output, and hemoglobin. The Pao₂ should be related to the Paco₂, pH, and HCO₃⁻ to determine the type of respiratory failure (hypoxemic versus hypercapnic) and the pathophysiologic mechanism. The Fio₂ must be taken into account when interpreting ABGs. Pure hypoventilation while breathing air (Fio₂ = 0.21) can be distinguished from the other mechanisms (V̇/Q̇ and/or shunt) by calculating the expected value of the Pao₂ for a given change in the $Paco_2$. This can be calculated using the alveolar gas equation (see pp. 624-625). If the change is greater than expected (e.g., $Pao_2 = 45$ mm Hg), $\dot{V}/\dot{Q}$ mismatch and/or shunting must also be involved.

The $P(A - a)o_2$ gradient is even more helpful in distinguishing between the pathophysiologic mechanisms. The normal $P(A - a)o_2$ gradient is about 10 mm Hg because of a small amount of normal shunting. Knowing that high concentrations of inspired O_2 correct hypoventilation and $\dot{V}/\dot{Q}$ imbalance (and diffusion impairment) but not absolute shunting allows one to distinguish between the mechanisms, using the $P(A - a)o_2$ gradient. The $P(A - a)o_2$ gradient is normal while breathing room air if the cause of the hypoxemia is pure hypoventilation caused by an extracardiopulmonary disorder. A $P(A - a)o_2$ gradient greater than 20 mm Hg (25 in older adults) when breathing room air is considered abnormal, and the cause is a cardiopulmonary disorder. Provided that a congenital heart defect or an intracardiac (anatomic) shunt has been ruled out, the cause of the hypoxemia is a disorder within the lung. The $P(A - a)o_2$ gradient can help determine how much the physiologic shunt is caused by $\dot{V}/\dot{Q}$ mismatch (venous admixture) rather than absolute intrapulmonary capillary shunting. Intrapulmonary shunting may be considered as an extreme case of low $\dot{V}/\dot{Q}$ ratio to distinguish it from venous admixture—so low that the administration of 100% O_2 no longer provides enough O_2 to the affected pulmonary capillaries to oxygenate the blood in them. The Pao_2 can be calculated by using a simplified version of the alveolar gas equation and then calculating the alveolar-arterial partial pressure difference ($Pao_2 - Pao_2$), as follows:

$$PAo_2 = Pio_2 - \frac{Paco_2}{R}$$

where:

$$Pio_2 = Fio_2 \times (PB - PH_2O)$$

Using the figures of 760 mm Hg for PB at sea level, 47 mm Hg for the partial pressure of H_2O at normal body temperature, and 20.93% O_2 for the Fio_2, the Pio_2 is seen to be 149.3 mm Hg ($0.2093 \times [760 - 47]$).

Making a concrete application of this formula, the following room air (PB = 750 mm Hg) ABG values were obtained on a 30-year-old man during an asthmatic attack: $Paco_2 = 60$ mm Hg and $Pao_2 = 40$ mm Hg. Thus $Pio_2 = 0.2093 \times (750 - 47) = 147$, and $P(A - a)o_2 = 147 - (60/0.8) - 40$ mm Hg $= 32$ mm Hg. Because $P(A - a)o_2$ is greater than 20, alveolar hypoventilation alone does not account for the hypoxemia, and there is either additional $\dot{V}/\dot{Q}$ mismatch or shunting.

$\dot{V}/\dot{Q}$ mismatch may be differentiated from true intrapulmonary shunting by determining the $P(A - a)o_2$ after having the patient breathe 100% O_2 for 15 minutes to wash out the nitrogen gas from the alveoli. Since $Fio_2 = 1.0$ when pure O_2 is breathed, the alveolar gas equation simplifies as follows:

$$PAo_2 = (PB - 47) - Paco_2$$

A healthy person breathing 100% O_2 at sea level would thus have a PAo_2 of 673 mm Hg ($760 - 47 - 40$). The normal Pao_2 is greater than 500 mm Hg and the $P(A - a)o_2$ gradient 30 to 50 mm Hg when 100% O_2 is breathed. $\dot{V}/\dot{Q}$ mismatch is largely corrected by administration of 100% O_2; a Pao_2 less than 500 mm Hg indicates significant shunting (Cherniack, Cherniack, 1983). The $P(A - a)o_2$ gradient is also increased.

The measurement of the $P(A - a)o_2$ gradient has serious limitations in estimating the magnitude of intrapulmonary shunting, since the values change with different cardiac outputs and Fio_2 concentrations. Using a high Fio_2 will improve shunting because of venous admixture but may aggravate intrapulmonary capillary shunting by causing absorption atelectasis. For these reasons, other indexes for estimating shunt have been developed and the classic $P(A - a)o_2$ shunt determination using 100% O_2 is no longer popular. One such index is the *arterial-alveolar oxygen tension ratio* ($P[a/A]o_2$), which is not affected by supplemental O_2. An example of a normal value is the following:

$$P(a/A)o_2 = \frac{Pao_2}{PAo_2} = \frac{80 \text{ mm Hg}}{100 \text{ mm Hg}} = 0.8$$

The PAo_2 is estimated using the alveolar gas equation. The normal $P(A/a)o_2$ value is about 0.8, and the value decreases with increased shunting.

The $\dot{Q}_S/\dot{Q}_T$ *physiologic shunt equation* is another method of measuring shunt. It measures the portion of the total cardiac output ($\dot{Q}_T$) that is not oxygenated during passage through the lungs ($\dot{Q}_S$). However, it is not always used because it requires a sample of blood from an indwelling pulmonary artery catheter. Shapiro, Peruzzi, and Kozlowski-Templin (1994) have introduced an *estimated shunt equation* that only requires measured values for Pao_2, mixed-venous O_2 tension ($P\overline{v}o_2$), O_2 saturation (Sao_2), and hemoglobin (Hb), as follows:

$$\frac{\dot{Q}_S}{\dot{Q}_T} = \frac{Cćo_2 - Cao_2}{3.5 + (Cćo_2 - Cao_2)}$$

$Cćo_2$ is the pulmonary capillary O_2 content; Cao_2 is the arterial O_2 content; and $C\overline{v}o_2$ is the mixed-venous O_2 content. These values are calculated by the following formulas:

$$Cao_2 = Hb \times 1.34 \times Sao_2 + (Pao_2 \times 0.0031)$$
$$C\overline{v}o_2 = Hb \times 1.34 \times S\overline{v}o_2 + (P\overline{v}o_2 \times 0.0031)$$
$$Cćo_2 = Hb \times 1.34 \times 1.0 + (PAo_2 \times 0.0031)$$

The first parts of the previous equations represent the portion of O_2 carried by Hb and the second parts the portion dissolved in the plasma. In estimating the pulmonary capillary O_2 content, it is assumed that all the available Hb is 100% saturated and that the pulmonary capillary O_2 content is equal to the PAo_2 (which is solved using the alveolar gas equation). The 3.5 constant in the equation rep-

TABLE 41-1 Measurements of Respiratory Function

Test	Significance	Normal Value	Critical Value
TESTS OF VENTILATORY FUNCTION			
Respiratory rate (frequency, f) per minute	Overall indicator of respiratory distress and work of breathing	12-20	>35 or <10
Tidal volume (V_T), ml	Volume of air exchanged during each breath at rest	500-700	<350
Minute ventilation ($\dot{V}_E$), L	Overall indicator of ventilation	5-10	>10
Forced vital capacity (FVC), ml/kg ideal body weight	Indicates ventilatory reserve; best indicator of need for ventilatory support	65-75	<15
Forced expiratory volume in 1 second (FEV_1), ml/kg	First-second expired volume of FVC; useful in assessing ventilatory reserve in patients with COPD as well as efficacy of measures to overcome airway obstruction	50-60	<10
Maximum inspiratory force (MIF), cm H_2O	Indicates reserve of ventilatory effort	75-100	<25
V_D/V_T	Dead space/tidal volume ratio; allows estimate of ventilation in excess of perfusion; requires collecting sample of expired air to measure P_{ECO_2} and Pa_{CO_2}; $V_D/V_T = Pa_{CO_2} - (P_{ECO_2}/Pa_{CO_2})$	0.25-0.40	>0.60
Pa_{CO_2}, mm Hg	Reflects ability of lung to eliminate CO_2; trend should be followed in patient with chronic hypercapnia along with pH of arterial blood; serious acidemia when pH 7.2 or less	35-45	>55
TESTS OF OXYGENATION STATUS			
Pa_{O_2} (breathing air), mm Hg	Adequacy of oxygen tension in arterial blood; expected Pa_{O_2} can be calculated from alveolar gas equation when patient breathing higher Fi_{O_2} than air (O_2 therapy)	80-100	<50-60
$P(A - a)_{O_2}$ or $(A - aD)_{O_2}$, mm Hg (breathing 100% O_2)	Alveolar-arterial oxygen tension difference; indicates oxygenation reserve	30-50	>÷50
$\dot{Q}_S/\dot{Q}_T$, %	Proportion of cardiac output shunted past alveoli	<5	>20
TESTS OF ACID-BASE STATUS			
Pa_{CO_2}, mm Hg		40 ± 5	
Arterial blood pH		7.35-7.45	
HCO_3^-, mEq/L		24 ± 3	

Values from Cherniack RM, Cherniack L: *Respiration in health and disease,* ed 6, Philadelphia, 1983, Saunders; and Bendixen HH et al: *Respiratory care,* St Louis, 1965, Mosby.

resents arteriovenous content difference, $C(a - \bar{v})_{O_2}$, normally 4.5 to 6.0 ml/dl in healthy adults, but assumed to be at the lower value of 3.5 in critically ill patients. The normal value for $\dot{Q}_S/\dot{Q}_T$ in a healthy person is 3% to 5%. High values indicate increased shunting.

Finally, clinicians may want to estimate the degree of shunt from the Pa_{O_2} alone. Normally the Pa_{O_2} should be approximately equal to $Fi_{O_2} \times 6$. For example, while breathing 40% O_2, the Pa_{O_2} should be about 240 mm Hg. When 100% O_2 is administered, the shunt is estimated by adding 5% to the shunt for every 100 mm Hg the Pa_{O_2} is less than 700 mm Hg. Thus a Pa_{O_2} of 300 mm Hg represents a 20% shunt, and a Pa_{O_2} of 100 mm Hg represents a 30% shunt. A shunt of 20% or more indicates a need for ventilatory support. A 50% shunt is compatible with life only if the patient is breathing 100% O_2.

Table 41-1 lists some of the common measurements used by intensive care physicians and nurses to assess ventilatory function and oxygenation for patients in respiratory failure. The critical values listed are used as criteria of the need for mechanical ventilation. It must be emphasized that these values are only guidelines. Good

clinical judgment is based on a thorough understanding of the pathophysiology of respiratory failure and involves the integration of qualitative observations with quantitative measurements.

Treatment

Priorities in the management of respiratory failure vary according to the etiology, but the primary aims of treatment are the same for all patients, that is, to treat the cause of the respiratory failure and at the same time ensure adequate ventilation and clear airways.

Because the most life-threatening feature of respiratory failure is the impairment of gas exchange, the first goal of therapy is to ensure that hypoxemia, acidemia, and hypercapnia do not reach hazardous levels. A Pa_{O_2} of 40 mm Hg or a pH of 7.2 or less is poorly tolerated by adults and can result in cerebral, kidney, and cardiac impairment and the development of cardiac dysrhythmias. A Pa_{CO_2} of 60 mm Hg that has developed slowly in a patient with COPD is usually well tolerated, but rapid development to this level is not. A Pa_{CO_2} of 70 mm Hg or

TABLE 41-2 Priorities and Principles in Treatment of Hypercapnic Respiratory Failure

Priority	Problem	Treatment
1	Retained secretions (ineffective cough)	Adequate hydration, expectorants, aerosols Supervised coughing Catheter aspiration (deep suction) Bronchoscopic suction Endotracheal tube aspiration Tracheostomy
2	Hypoxemia	Graduated O_2 therapy with frequent monitoring of ABGs to direct therapy
3	Hypercapnia	Respiratory stimulants (drug overdose) Avoidance of sedation Artificial ventilation via endotracheal tube or tracheostomy
4	Respiratory infection	Antibiotics
5	Bronchospasm	Bronchodilatory drugs (isoproterenol by inhalation therapy; intravenous, oral, or rectal aminophylline; corticosteroid drugs)
6	Cardiac failure	Diuretics Digoxin (with caution if given at all)

more is usually poorly tolerated in any patient and causes CNS depression and coma.

O_2 may be delivered at a concentration of 40% to 60% to a patient with hypoxemia and a normal or low $Paco_2$ (mask or catheter at 8 L/minute with adequate humidification) to achieve a rapid correction of the hypoxemia. However, this concentration should not be continued for more than a few hours, since it has a direct toxic effect on alveolar cells, causing decreased synthesis of surfactant and decreased pulmonary compliance. Prolonged administration of O_2 (more than 24 to 48 hours) at high concentrations (greater than 50%) also causes absorption atelectasis.

Hypoxemia with hypercapnia is always treated with low, graduated O_2 therapy, beginning with a mask that delivers 24% O_2. The concentration is increased to 28% O_2 if necessary to maintain a Pao_2 of 50 mm Hg or more. Careful monitoring of ABGs is used at all times to ensure that the O_2 therapy does not cause a deterioration in the patient's respiratory status: In the patient with COPD, attempts are made to achieve Pao_2 values that are normal for the patient (e.g., 50 to 70 mm Hg) and not those normal for the healthy adult (80 to 100 mm Hg). When it is not possible to achieve Pao_2 values of 50 mm Hg, artifi-

cial ventilation with a respirator may be required. See Table 41-1 for critical values indicating need for ventilatory support.

Table 41-2 lists the priorities and aims in the treatment of hypercapnic respiratory failure. The approach to the problem of retained lung secretions includes measures to liquefy and remove them. Liquefaction is best achieved by adequate hydration of the patient. Drugs such as potassium iodide taken orally or aerosol delivery of water may also help in the mobilization of sputum. Secretions are best removed by encouraging the patient to cough or assisting the patient's efforts by percussion, vibration, and postural drainage. When the patient is too depressed or weak to cough, secretions may be removed by aspiration via an endotracheal tube or bronchoscopy. If these methods fail, tracheostomy may be necessary.

If bronchospasm is present in respiratory failure, bronchodilatory or corticosteroid drugs may be used. Respiratory infection, which is a common cause of hypoxemic respiratory failure, is treated with the appropriate antibiotics.

Finally, a thorough search is made for other factors that may have induced the respiratory failure, such as pulmonary embolism or left ventricular failure.

A number of excellent books dealing with the management of respiratory failure are suggested in the bibliography at the end of Part Seven for those who want to know more about this subject.

ADULT RESPIRATORY DISTRESS SYNDROME

Adult respiratory distress syndrome (ARDS) is a distinct form of respiratory failure characterized by profound hypoxemia refractory to conventional treatment. It is preceded by a variety of serious illnesses, all of which result in a characteristic diffuse noncardiogenic pulmonary edema. The term was coined by Petty and Ashbaugh (1971) after observing acute life-threatening respiratory distress in patients with no previous lung disease. Although this syndrome has been called by a variety of other names (shock lung, wet lung, adult hyaline membrane disease, stiff lung syndrome), the term adult respiratory distress syndrome has been more widely accepted. It has been estimated that 250,000 persons have ARDS each year, and the mortality rate is 50% (Raffin, 1987).

Etiology and Pathogenesis

ARDS develops when the lung is injured directly or indirectly by various processes. Some of the most common conditions that lead to ARDS are listed in the box on p. 632.

The mechanism by which such a diversity of insults could produce a common clinical and pathophysiologic syndrome is not clear. The common denominator causing the characteristic alveolar edema seems to involve injury

CAUSES OF ADULT RESPIRATORY DISTRESS SYNDROME

Shock from various causes (especially hemorrhagic, hemorrhagic acute pancreatitis, gram-negative sepsis)

Sepsis without shock, with or without disseminated intravascular coagulation (DIC)

Overwhelming viral pneumonia

Critical trauma
 Head injury
 Direct chest injury
 Multiple organ trauma with hemorrhagic shock
 Multiple fractures
  Fat embolization (associated with fracture of long bones such as the femur)

Aspiration/inhalation injury
 Aspiration of gastric contents
 Near-drowning
 Smoke inhalation
 Irritant gas inhalation (e.g., chlorine, ammonia, sulfur dioxide)
 Prolonged exposure (>48 hours) to high concentration of inhaled oxygen (FiO_2 >50%)
 Narcotic overdose

Postperfusion cardiopulmonary bypass surgery

to the alveolocapillary membrane with the production of a capillary leak. Electron microscopy studies reveal that the air-blood barrier consists of type I pneumocytes (supporting cells) and type II pneumocytes (source of surfactant) along with basement membrane on the alveolar side; these are back to back with capillary basement membrane and endothelial cells. In addition, the alveolus has connective tissue cells that serve as support and regulate volume. The alveolocapillary membrane is normally quite impermeable to particles. However, with injury this permeability is altered, with an influx of fluid, red blood cells and white blood cells, and blood proteins. The fluid first accumulates in the interstitium; when the capacity of the interstitium is exceeded, the fluid accumulates in the alveolus, causing congestive atelectasis. The point of vulnerability seems to be the interdigitations (small spaces about 60 Å wide) between the capillary endothelial cells, which become widened, allowing the influx of small particles, which then cause a shift in oncotic pressure. Thus the formation of pulmonary edema depends on the disruption of the normal relations of the Starling forces: hydrostatic pressure, oncotic pressure, and tissue pressure. In addition, alterations in the surfactant system undoubtedly play a role in the diffuse microatelectasis. In fact, light microscopy reveals that the proteinaceous material may be organized into hyaline membranes lining the alveolus. The pathologic picture is similar to that of the respiratory distress syndrome occurring in the infant. The consequence of the diffuse edema

and atelectasis is marked intrapulmonary shunting, which may affect more than 40% of the cardiac output.

The poor prognosis of patients with ARDS has provided considerable impetus to elucidating the mechanisms that initiate pulmonary vascular injury. These seem to depend on the interaction of activated inflammatory cells, humoral mediators, and endothelial cells. A better understanding of these mechanisms will determine the development of effective pharmacologic interventions. Recent research (Demling, 1993; Fishman, 1992) has focused on the mechanisms leading to the activation of inflammatory cells (particularly the polymorphonuclear neutrophil leukocytes, PMNs), platelets, and other clotting factors, since it is becoming increasingly clear that ARDS is part of an inflammation-induced systemic state that can evolve into multiple organ failure.

Clinical Features

The primary features of ARDS include a marked degree of intrapulmonary shunting with hypoxemia, a progressive loss in lung compliance, and extreme dyspnea and tachypnea resulting from both the hypoxemia and the increased work of breathing secondary to the loss of lung compliance. The normal compliance of the lungs and thorax together is about 100 ml/cm H_2O. In ARDS, compliance may be as low as 15 to 20 ml/cm H_2O. Functional residual capacity is also reduced. These features are a consequence of the interstitial and alveolar edema. The result is a stiff lung that is difficult to ventilate. A hallmark of ARDS is that the hypoxemia cannot be relieved by O_2 administration during spontaneous breathing. The full-blown clinical state may become manifest 1 to 2 days after the initiating injury.

Establishing a correct diagnosis of ARDS largely depends on obtaining an accurate clinical history. The earliest laboratory finding is hypoxemia, so measuring ABGs in the appropriate clinical setting is important. The $PaCO_2$ is generally normal or low. Early chest radiographic findings may be normal despite the hypoxemia. Later, as the alveolar and interstitial fluid accumulates and the congestive atelectasis spreads, the chest radiograph shows a diffuse "whiteout" appearance. Thus another name for ARDS is *white lung*.

Treatment

The management of ARDS is aimed at correcting the accompanying shock, acidosis, and hypoxemia. Almost all patients require mechanical ventilation and high concentrations of O_2 to avoid serious tissue hypoxia. The use of positive end-expiratory pressure (PEEP) with the volume respirator is a major advance in the treatment of this condition. PEEP helps to correct the respiratory distress syndrome by reexpanding previously atelectatic areas and by reversing the flow of atelectatic edema fluid from capillaries. Another benefit of PEEP is that it allows administration of lower concentrations of FiO_2. This is important because on the one hand a high Fio_2 is generally needed to achieve a minimally acceptable Pao_2, and on the other hand high O_2 concentrations are toxic to the lung and cause ARDS. The net effect of PEEP is to improve Pao_2 and allow reduction in Fio_2. Potential hazards from the use of PEEP are pneumothorax and interference with cardiac output because of high pressures. Close monitoring and attention are directed toward achieving "best PEEP," that is, ventilation at the end-expiratory pressure that results in the best lung compliance and least reduction in the Pao_2 and cardiac output.

Because sequestration of fluid in the lung is a problem, restriction of fluids and diuretic therapy are other important measures in the treatment of ARDS. Appropriate antibiotics are given to treat infection. Although the use of corticosteroids is controversial, many centers use them in the treatment of ARDS even though their benefit has not been clearly established. Another potentially promising treatment is surfactant replacement therapy for adults with the syndrome. Surfactant therapy has already been applied to infants with respiratory distress syndrome with dramatic results in reducing morbidity and mortality. Its application to ARDS awaits the results of current research (Fishman, 1992).

QUESTIONS

▼ *Answer the following on a separate sheet of paper.*

1. What is the relationship between respiratory insufficiency and maintaining normal arterial blood gases (ABGs)?

2. What is the most common cause of chronic respiratory insufficiency?

3. List the two types of respiratory failure based on ABG changes.

4. Explain why high concentrations of O_2 must not be administered in hypercapnic respiratory failure.

5. What level of Pao_2 or $Paco_2$ would not be well tolerated in most adults?

6. List at least three measures used to treat the problem of retained secretions and pulmonary infection in hypercapnic respiratory failure.

7. What is the primary goal and first priority in the treatment of respiratory failure?

8. What are the three most common precipitating factors of acute-on-chronic respiratory failure in patients with COPD? Name two iatrogenic precipitating factors. Name as many other factors as you can remember.

9. Why is a patient breathing air with a $\dot{V}/\dot{Q}$ mismatch able to maintain a normal $Paco_2$ by increasing alveolar ventilation but is unable to achieve a normal Pao_2? (Explain with respect to the oxyhemoglobin and CO_2 dissociation curves.)

10. A 25-year-old male heroin addict was admitted to the hospital with severe hypoventilation because of drug overdose. The barometric pressure was 760 mm Hg. His body temperature was normal, so the partial pressure of water in his trachea was 47 mm Hg. On admission his Pao_2 was 50 mm Hg and $Paco_2$ 80 mm Hg while breathing air. Is this pure hypoventilation? Calculate the $P(A - a)o_2$ gradient to answer the question. He was given O_2 ($Fio_2 = 50\%$).

Measurement of ABGs then revealed $Pao_2 = 246$ mm Hg and $Paco_2 = 80$ mm Hg. What would you expect his Pao_2 to be when receiving 50% O_2? Do you now think that his hypoxemia was caused by pure hypoventilation? (Assume that his respiratory exchange ratio [R] is 0.8.)

11. A 60-year-old man with COPD was admitted to the hospital because of respiratory distress. He reported an increase in sputum production; the sputum was purulent, although his temperature was normal. Measurement of ABGs revealed Pao_2 of 35 mm Hg and $Paco_2$ of 55 mm Hg. Barometric pressure was 747 mm Hg. Assume $R = 0.8$. What was his $P(A - a)o_2$ gradient? Is his hypoxemia caused by either hypoventilation or $\dot{V}/\dot{Q}$ imbalance alone or by both these mechanisms? He was given 24% O_2. Two days later his ABGs were Pao_2 of 50 mm Hg and $Paco_2$ of 45 mm Hg. Is his condition better or worse? Calculate his $P(A - a)o_2$ to answer this question.

▼ *Circle T if the statement is true and F if it is false. Correct any false statements.*

12. T F The clinical signs of respiratory failure are most easily detected in a patient who has chronic respiratory insufficiency that has progressed to respiratory failure.

13. T F Cyanosis is the most reliable index of respiratory failure.

14. T F Acute respiratory failure may be manifested by cardiovascular and neurologic signs and symptoms.

15. T F Hypoxemia with a normal or low $Paco_2$ is associated with conditions affecting the alveolar wall and interstitium of the lung.

16. T F Hypoventilation may cause the $Paco_2$ to fall below normal because CO_2 excretion is directly related to ventilation.

17. T F Hyperventilation when breathing room air fails to correct hypoxemia.

18. T F Cerebral oxygenation may become impaired when significant hypocapnia is combined with hypoxemia.

19. T F Impaired cerebral oxygenation can be explained by the shift of the oxyhemoglobin dissociation curve to the left as a result of respiratory alkalosis.

20. T F When the $Paco_2$ rises to 70 mm Hg in pure hypoventilation, one expects a normal Pao_2 of 95 mm Hg to be decreased to about 45 mm Hg.

21. T F Hypoventilation or hyperventilation may be accurately identified at the bedside by observing the respiratory rate and depth.

22. T F A forced vital capacity (FVC) of 700 ml in a 70 kg man of average build indicates a need for ventilatory support.

23. T F A Pao_2 of 80 mm Hg with a $Paco_2$ of 24 mm Hg after breathing 100% O_2 for 15 minutes indicates a serious shunting problem. ($P_B = 747$ mm Hg.)

24. T F A person with viral pneumonia and a 50% shunt would be considered as being in good condition.

25. T F Absorption atelectasis is an expected complication with the prolonged administration of 60% O_2.

26. T F Hypercapnia causes decreased cerebral blood flow and decreased intracranial pressure.

Continued.

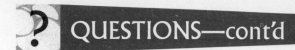

27. T F PEEP is the treatment of choice for ARDS.
28. T F Papilledema observed in some persons with acute ventilatory failure is indirectly caused by hypercapnia.
29. T F Pa_{CO_2} is inversely related to CO_2 production and directly related to $\dot{V}_A$.
30. T F Hypoxemic respiratory failure may progress to hypercapnic respiratory failure as the patient tires from the increased work of breathing.

▼ *Circle the letter preceding each item below that correctly answers the question or completes the statement. More than one answer may be correct.*

31. Ventilation failure is numerically defined as:
    a. $Pa_{O_2} = 80$ mm Hg, $Pa_{CO_2} = 60$ mm Hg
    b. $Pa_{O_2} = 70$ mm Hg, $Pa_{CO_2} = 35$ mm Hg
    c. $Pa_{O_2} \geq 60$ mm Hg, $Pa_{CO_2} \geq 40$ mm Hg
    d. $Pa_{O_2} \leq 50$ mm Hg, $Pa_{CO_2} \geq 50$ mm Hg

32. Which of the following best describes the primary causes of respiratory failure?
    a. Hypersensitivity of the tracheobronchial tree to various stimuli
    b. $\dot{V}/\dot{Q}$ imbalance that increases physiologic shunt or dead space
    c. Alveolar hypoventilation associated with obstructive or restrictive disease
    d. Impaired diffusion from alveolocapillary block

33. The major cause of hypoxemia with hypercapnia is:
    a. Alveolar hypoventilation
    b. Alveolar hyperventilation
    c. Neither a nor b
    d. Both a and b

34. Treatment of patients with hypoxemia with hypercapnia includes:
    a. O_2 delivered at a concentration of 40% to 60% to achieve a rapid correction of hypoxemia
    b. Low graduated O_2 therapy beginning with a mask that delivers 24% O_2 concentration
    c. Careful monitoring of ABGs
    d. Achievement of a Pa_{O_2} of 90 to 100 mm Hg for all these patients

35. Tissue hypoxia may occur even when the Pa_{O_2} is normal if:
    a. Severe anemia is present.
    b. Cardiac output is low.

c. The oxyhemoglobin curve is shifted to the left.
d. Local vasoconstriction is present.

36. Alveolar hypoventilation results in:
    a. Low PA_{CO_2}
    b. Low Pa_{CO_2}
    c. High PA_{CO_2}
    d. High Pa_{CO_2}

37. Which of the following mechanisms can contribute significantly to hypoxemia?
    a. Alveolar hypoventilation
    b. Perfusion of underventilated lung units
    c. Ventilation of underperfused lung units
    d. Diffusion impairment
    e. Left-to-right shunt

38. A low Pa_{O_2} can theoretically be the result of any of the following *except:*
    a. Shunting of arterial blood
    b. $\dot{V}/\dot{Q}$ abnormalities
    c. Alveolocapillary diffusion block
    d. Alveolar hypoventilation
    e. Anemia

39. The predominant cause of hypoxemia in asthma is:
    a. Hypoventilation
    b. Diffusion impairment
    c. Increased dead-space ventilation
    d. Areas of low $\dot{V}/\dot{Q}$ ratio
    e. True right-to-left shunts

40. Decreased pulmonary diffusing capacity plays a role in:
    a. Narcotic overdose
    b. Sarcoidosis
    c. Myasthenia gravis
    d. Asbestosis

41. Even when the Pa_{O_2} is normal, tissue hypoxia can occur if:
    a. Severe anemia is present.
    b. Cardiac output is low.
    c. P_{50} is low (oxyhemoglobin curve shifted to the left).
    d. Local vasoconstriction is present.

42. Hypoxemia can always be significantly improved by administration of O_2 *except* when caused by:
    a. Low $\dot{V}/\dot{Q}$ ratio
    b. High $\dot{V}/\dot{Q}$ ratio
    c. Alveolar hypoventilation
    d. True right-to-left shunt
    e. Diffusion defect

43. Which of the following findings is(are) compatible with diffusion limitation alone?
    a. Low Pa_{O_2}, high Pa_{CO_2} at rest
    b. Normal Pa_{O_2}, normal Pa_{CO_2} at rest
    c. Low Pa_{O_2}, normal Pa_{CO_2} during exercise
    d. Low Pa_{O_2}, normal Pa_{CO_2} during exercise

44. Which of the following findings is compatible with $\dot{V}/\dot{Q}$ mismatch alone?
    a. Low Pa_{O_2}, high Pa_{CO_2}
    b. Low Pa_{O_2}, low Pa_{CO_2}
    c. Low Pa_{O_2}, normal Pa_{CO_2}
    d. Normal Pa_{O_2}, normal Pa_{CO_2}

45. Which of the following findings is compatible with true shunting alone?
    a. Low Pa_{O_2}, high Pa_{CO_2}
    b. Low Pa_{O_2}, low Pa_{CO_2}
    c. Low Pa_{O_2}, normal Pa_{CO_2}
    d. Normal Pa_{O_2}, normal Pa_{CO_2}

46. Some major effects of hypoxemia causing significant tissue hypoxia are:
    a. Vasoconstriction of the pulmonary blood vessels
    b. Anaerobic metabolism and metabolic acidosis
    c. Impaired judgment
    d. Increased or decreased cardiac output
    e. Cardiac dysrhythmias

47. Place the following sequence of events in proper order to explain why a patient with COPD might complain of morning headaches.
    a. Normal hypoventilation during sleep
    b. Increased cerebral blood flow
    c. Chronic hypercapnia
    d. Increase in retained respiratory secretions
    e. Additional rise of Pa_{CO_2}
    f. Morning headache
    g. Increased intracranial pressure

48. Which of the following is the best definition of respiratory failure?
    a. Respiratory alkalosis or acidosis
    b. Any increase or decrease in $\dot{V}_A$
    c. CO_2 retention when O_2 is administered
    d. Inability to maintain normal ABG values
    e. Hypoxemia at rest

49. High-output ventilatory failure is characterized by:
    a. High effective $\dot{V}_A$ and low V_D
    b. High V_T and high urine output
    c. High $\dot{V}_E$ and high V_D
    d. High respiratory frequency and low $\dot{V}_E$
    e. High cardiac output and high effective $\dot{V}_A$

50. Impaired synthesis of surfactant occurs in:
    a. O_2 toxicity
    b. ARDS
    c. Infant respiratory distress syndrome
    d. Hypercapnia

51. Physiologic correlates of ARDS include:
    a. Severe hypoxemia, usually with hypocapnia

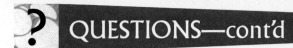

b. Increased intrapulmonary shunting
c. Increased V_D
d. Reduction of FRC
e. Increased $P(A - a)O_2$ gradient

52. Pathophysiologic changes in ARDS include:
   a. Low compliance
   b. Diffuse atelectasis
   c. Loss of pulmonary surfactant
   d. Interstitial and alveolar edema and hemorrhage

53. Which of the following test results indicate a need for mechanical ventilation?
   a. Respiratory rate >35/minute
   b. V_D/V_T >0.6
   c. $P(A - a)O_2$ >450 on 100% O_2
   d. FVC <15 ml/kg ideal body weight
   e. MIF <25 cm H_2O

54. Physiologic effects of PEEP when used to treat ARDS include:
   a. Reduction of $P(A - a)O_2$ gradient
   b. Increased cardiac output
   c. Increased FRC
   d. Improved compliance

55. Complications of PEEP for ARDS include:
   a. Pneumothorax
   b. Interference with cardiac output
   c. Infection
   d. None of the above

56. O_2 toxicity is associated with:
   a. FiO_2 >50% for >48 hours
   b. Loss of surfactant
   c. Alveolar collapse
   d. Reduced lung compliance

57. Satisfactory method(s) of reducing oxygen toxicity is(are):
   a. Frequent observation for signs of toxicity
   b. Hyperbaric O_2 treatment
   c. Limitation of O_2 administration to 48 hours
   d. Maintenance of the FiO_2 at 40% or less
   e. Intermittent O_2 administration

▼ Match each type of respiratory disorder in column B with the type of respiratory failure it is likely to be associated with in column A.

Column A

58. _____ Hypoxemic respiratory failure
59. _____ Hypercapnic respiratory failure

Column B

a. COPD
b. Respiratory center depression
c. Asthmatic attack
d. Bacterial pneumonia
e. ARDS
f. Myasthenia gravis
g. Silicosis

▼ Match the acid-base status in column B with the findings it fits best in column A. (Use the acid-base nomogram in Fig. 41-2 to check your answers.)

Column A

60. _____ Patient with cystic fibrosis and chronic hypercapnia
61. _____ Patient with head injury, $PaCO_2$ = 40 mm Hg, HCO_3^- = 24 mEq/L, pH = 7.41
62. _____ Patient with COPD and respiratory infection, $PaCO_2$ = 75 mm Hg, pH = 7.1
63. _____ COPD patient above after being on mechanical ventilator, $PaCO_2$ = 55 mm Hg, pH = 7.48, HCO_3^- = 39 mEq/L
64. _____ Patient with lobar pneumonia, $PaCO_2$ = 24 mm Hg, pH = 7.46, PaO_2 = 60 mm Hg
65. _____ Patient who aspirated vomitus during a cerebrovascular accident, 2 days later $PaCO_2$ = 20 mm Hg, pH = 7.32, PaO_2 = 35 mm Hg

Column B

a. Normal acid-base status
b. Chronic respiratory alkalosis
c. Mixed acute and chronic respiratory acidosis
d. Mixed respiratory alkalosis and metabolic acidosis
e. Mixed chronic respiratory acidosis and metabolic alkalosis
f. Chronic respiratory acidosis

▼ Answer the questions below related to the following case study.

A 25-year-old female was found in her apartment by neighbors in a semicomatose condition. Paramedics brought her to the emergency room, and the physician diagnosed her condition as acute narcotic overdose. The following ABG results were obtained (breathing room air) before admission to the ICU:

pH = 7.22 HCO_3 = 34 mEq/L
PaO_2 = 39 mm Hg SaO_2 = 62%
$PaCO_2$ = 84 mm Hg   Hb = 12 g/dl

66. The PaO_2 of 39 indicates severe _____.
67. The $PaCO_2$ of 84 indicates marked _____.
68. Calculate her $P(A - a)O_2$ using the alveolar gas equation: _____. Assume PB = 760 mm Hg, PH_2O = 47 mm Hg, and R = 0.8. Is it normal?
69. Calculate her arterial O_2 content in ml/dl: _____. Is it normal?
70. The patient's hypoxemia is a result of:
   a. A problem with gas exchange intrinsic to the lungs
   b. A problem with the respiratory pump (extrinsic to the lungs) secondary to depression of the respiratory center
   c. Hyperventilation causing a left shift of the oxyhemoglobin dissociation curve and reduced SaO_2
   d. Marked left-to-right intrapulmonary shunting
71. The patient's acid-base status is best characterized as:
   a. Marked hyperventilation and metabolic acidosis
   b. Partially compensated primary respiratory acidosis
   c. Chronic respiratory alkalosis
   d. Mixed respiratory alkalosis and metabolic acidosis
72. The greatly depressed PaO_2, elevated $PaCO_2$, and low pH are diagnostic of:
   a. Hypoxemic respiratory failure
   b. Hypercapnic respiratory failure
73. Acute ventilatory failure is associated with:
   a. Alveolar hypoventilation   c. Alveolar hyperventilation
   b. Severe hypoxemia   d. Severe hypocapnia

CHAPTER 42

Pulmonary Malignant Neoplasms

LORRAINE M. WILSON

More than 90% of primary lung tumors are malignant, and about 95% of these malignant tumors are bronchogenic carcinoma. Whenever lung cancer is mentioned, bronchogenic carcinoma is the tumor being referred to because most primary malignant tumors of the lower respiratory tract are epithelial in nature and arise from the mucosa of the bronchial tree.

Although once considered a rare form of malignant growth, the incidence of lung cancer in the industrialized countries has risen to epidemic proportions since 1930. Some of the alarming statistics were cited in the introduction to this part of the text. Cancer of the lung is now the leading cause of cancer death in both men and women. The peak incidence occurs between ages 55 and 65 years. This increase is believed to be related to increased cigarette smoking and therefore is largely preventable.

BRONCHOGENIC CARCINOMA

Etiology

Although the exact cause of bronchogenic carcinoma is unknown, three factors appear to account for the increase in incidence: smoking, industrial hazards, and air pollution. Of these factors, *smoking* appears to play the major role, accounting for 85% of the cases (Carr, Hoyle, 1994). Massive statistical evidence indicates that a relationship exists between heavy cigarette smoking and the development of lung cancer. Three prospective studies, one involving nearly 200,000 men ages 50 to 69, followed for 44 months, revealed that the death rate from cancer of the lung per 100,000 was 3.4 in the male nonsmoker, 59.3 in those who smoked 10 to 20 cigarettes daily, and 217.3 in those who smoked 40 or more cigarettes daily. Those who give up smoking permanently reduce their risk to that of a nonsmoker after an abstinence of 15 years.

Great interest has arisen about the relationship of *passive smoking,* or the inhalation of other persons' smoke in an enclosed area, to the risk of developing lung cancer. Some studies have shown that nonsmokers exposed to second-hand smoke double their risk of developing lung cancer. Mortality from lung cancer is related to atmospheric pollution, but its effect is small compared with that of cigarette smoking. The death rate from cancer of the lung is twice as high in cities as in rural areas. Statistical evidence also shows that the disease is more common in the lowest socioeconomic classes and decreases in higher classes. This may be partly explained by the fact that persons in the lowest social classes are more apt to live near their jobs, where the atmosphere may be more polluted. A *carcinogen* (cancer-producing material) that has been found in polluted air (and also in cigarette smoke) is 3,4-benzpyrene. The nicotine in cigarette smoke is not a carcinogen.

In certain instances, bronchogenic carcinoma appears to be an occupational disease. Of the various industrial hazards, the most important is undoubtedly *asbestos,* which is widely used in the construction industry. The risk of lung cancer in asbestos workers is about 10 times greater than that in the general population. Local benign or diffuse malignant mesotheliomas of the pleura are rare tumors that have been specifically associated with asbestos exposure. There is also increased risk in those who work with uranium, chromate, arsenic (insecticide used in agriculture), iron, and iron oxides. The risks of lung cancer from both asbestos and uranium exposure are greatly enhanced in those who also smoke cigarettes.

Two other factors that may play a role in the risk of developing lung cancer are *diet* and *familial tendency.* Several studies have shown that smokers who eat a diet low in vitamin A are at increased risk for developing lung cancer. Evidence also suggests that family members of lung cancer patients are at increased risk for developing the disease, although it is unknown whether this is truly hereditary or because of the shared family environment.

In many tissues, chronic inflammatory changes are known to precede cancer. Evidence supports the view that chronic inflammation of the bronchial mucosa from inhaled irritants may be of greater importance than the carcinogenic effect of any one substance. Another factor that has not received much attention is the close correspondence between the increase in the number of motor vehicles and the incidence of lung cancer.

These facts suggest that although smoking clearly plays a major part in the increasing incidence of lung cancer, it is by no means the only factor. Chronic infection; air pollution from motor vehicles and industry; occupational exposure to carcinogens; and dietary, familial, and perhaps other unknown factors may (either alone or in combination) predispose to cancer of the lung.

WORLD HEALTH ORGANIZATION (WHO) CLASSIFICATION OF PLEUROPULMONARY NEOPLASMS

BRONCHOGENIC CARCINOMAS

   I. Epidermoid (squamous) carcinomas
  II. Small cell carcinoma (includes oat cell)
 III. Adenocarcinomas (includes alveolar cell carcinoma)
  IV. Large cell carcinoma
   V. Combined epidermoid and adenocarcinoma

OTHERS

  VI. Carcinoid tumors (bronchial adenomas)
 VII. Bronchial gland tumors
VIII. Papillary tumors of the surface epithelium
  IX. Mixed tumors and carcinosarcomas
   X. Sarcomas
  XI. Unclassified
 XII. Mesotheliomas
XIII. Melanomas

From Kreyberg L, Liebow AA, Uehlinger EA: *Histological typing of lung tumors,* ed 2, Geneva, Switzerland, 1981, World Health Organization.

Pathology

Primary lung cancer is usually classified according to histologic type (see the box above), all of which have different natural histories and responses to treatment. Although more than a dozen types of primary lung cancer exist, bronchogenic cancer, which includes the first four cell types, makes up 95% of all lung cancer.

Bronchogenic carcinoma is usually divided into *small cell lung cancer* (SCLC) and *non–small cell lung cancer* (NSCLC) for the purposes of determining therapy. NSCLC includes the epidermoid, adenocarcinoma, large cell types, or mixtures of these. In general, SCLC is primarily managed with chemotherapy, with or without radiation therapy, whereas NSCLC, if localized at the time of diagnosis, is treated by surgical resection. The approximate frequency of the various histologic types are as follows: epidermoid (17%), adenocarcinoma (40%), large cell carcinoma (15%), and small cell carcinoma (25%). Ninety percent of the patients with bronchogenic carcinoma of all cell types are smokers, and the remaining 10% of nonsmokers who develop lung cancer usually have adenocarcinoma (Minna, 1994).

Squamous cell (epidermoid) carcinoma, a common histologic type of bronchogenic carcinoma, arises from the surface of the bronchial epithelium. Epithelial changes, including metaplasia or dysplasia from long-term smoking, typically precede the appearance of tumor. Squamous cell carcinoma is usually centrally located near the hilus and projects into the large bronchi. The tu-

mor is seldom more than a few centimeters in diameter and tends to spread by direct extension to the hilar lymph nodes, chest wall, and mediastinum. Squamous cell carcinoma often presents with manifestations of cough and hemoptysis as a result of irritation or ulceration, pneumonia, and abscess formation from the obstruction and secondary infection. Because this type of lung cancer generally metastasizes late, early treatment improves prognosis.

Adenocarcinomas, as the name implies, show a cellular organization resembling that of bronchial glands and may contain mucus. The majority of these tumors arise in the peripheral segmental bronchi and are sometimes associated with focal lung scars and chronic interstitial fibrosis. These lesions invade blood and lymph vessels early in their development and often give rise to distant metastases before the primary lesion causes symptoms.

Bronchial-alveolar cell carcinoma, a rare subtype of adenocarcinoma, arises from the epithelium of the alveoli or possibly the terminal bronchioles. The onset is generally insidious, with signs resembling pneumonia. In some cases this neoplasm grossly resembles the uniform consolidation of lobar pneumonia. Microscopically, groups of alveoli are lined with clear mucus-secreting cells, and there is abundant expectoration of mucoid sputum. The prognosis is poor unless surgical removal of the diseased lobe is performed early. Adenocarcinoma is the only histologic type of lung cancer that does not have a clear association with smoking.

Large cell carcinomas are those with large, poorly differentiated malignant cells with abundant cytoplasm and variably sized nuclei. They tend to develop in the peripheral lung tissue, grow rapidly, and spread to distant sites early and extensively.

Small cell carcinomas, as with the squamous cell type, are usually centrally located about the mainstem bronchi. Unlike other lung cancers, this type of tumor arises from Kulchitsky's cells, a normal component of the bronchial epithelium. Microscopically, the tumor may be made up of small cells (about twice the size of lymphocytes) with dense hyperchromatic nuclei and little cytoplasm. The cells often resemble oat seeds, thus the term *oat cell carcinoma.* Small cell carcinomas have the fastest doubling time and the worst prognosis of all the bronchogenic carcinomas. Early metastasis to the mediastinal and hilar lymph nodes, as well as hematogenous spread to distal organ sites, often occur. About 70% of patients have evidence of extensive disease (distal metastases) at the time of diagnosis, and the 5-year-survival is less than 5%.

OTHER FORMS OF LUNG CANCER

In addition to bronchogenic carcinoma, other forms of primary lung cancer include bronchial adenomas, sarcomas, and mesotheliomas (see box, p. 637). Despite their rarity, these tumors are important because they simulate bronchogenic carcinoma and are life-threatening.

Bronchial adenomas are a group of small, malignant neoplasms of low aggressiveness arising in the lower trachea or major bronchi, the most important being the bronchial carcinoid and the rarer cylindroma. *Bronchial carcinoids,* as with small cell carcinomas, are derived from Kulchitsky's cells of the bronchial mucosa. These tumors constitute about 4% of all bronchial tumors. They may become apparent during the teens to late middle age (average age of diagnosis, 45 years), with males and females affected equally. Signs and symptoms of bronchial obstruction such as chronic cough, hemoptysis, or pneumonitis are common. Bronchial carcinoids are similar to carcinoid tumors of the intestines.* Some of these tumors secrete serotonin, 5-hydroxytryptophan, and other biologically active substances that give rise to a symptom complex known as the *carcinoid syndrome.* Symptoms include flushing, bronchoconstriction and wheezing, and diarrhea. Carcinoid tumors follow a relatively benign course, and surgical resection is usually quite successful, resulting in a 5-year-survival rate of more than 90% with typical carcinoids.

Malignant mesothelioma is an uncommon tumor of the pleura associated in the great majority of patients with prior asbestos exposure. This exposure may have been brief, and the usual time between exposure and clinical onset is 25 years. Malignant mesotheliomas are highly malignant, with survival time averaging less than a year from the time of diagnosis.

Both *primary sarcoma of the lung* and *primary malignant melanoma of the lung* are very rare but highly malignant forms of lung cancer. It is more likely that either type of these lung cancers represents metastasis from an undiagnosed primary tumor rather than a primary tumor site.

Finally, one should remember that the lung is affected by metastatic cancer much more often than by a primary malignant neoplasm. The lung is a common site for secondary deposits of cancer cells originating in other organs because blood-borne microscopic tumor emboli are likely to become enmeshed in the pulmonary capillary bed. Lymph-borne tumors from the lower half of the body and abdominal cavity may also be arrested as they pass through the thoracic duct. The most common neoplasms giving rise to pulmonary metastasis in descending order of frequency are carcinomas of the breast, gastrointestinal tract, female genital tract, and kidneys; melanomas; and male genital cancer.

MANIFESTATIONS OF BRONCHOGENIC CARCINOMA

Bronchogenic carcinoma imitates a variety of other pulmonary diseases and has no typical mode of onset. It often masquerades as a pneumonitis that fails to resolve. Cough is a common symptom often ignored by the patient or attributed to smoking or bronchitis. When bronchial carcinoma develops in a patient with chronic bronchitis, cough often becomes more frequent or the volume of sputum may increase. Hemoptysis is another common sign. Initial symptoms of localized wheeze and mild dyspnea may result from varying degrees of bronchial obstruction. Chest pain may appear in various forms but is usually experienced as an ache or discomfort caused by neoplastic spread to the mediastinum. Pleuritic pain may occur when secondary involvement of the pleura occurs, resulting from neoplastic spread or pneumonia. Rapid development of digital clubbing is an important sign because it is often associated with bronchogenic carcinoma (30% of cases, usually NSCLC). General symptoms such as anorexia, fatigue, and weight loss are late symptoms.

Symptoms of intrathoracic or extrathoracic spread may also be present when the patient is first seen by the physician. Local extension of the tumor to the mediastinal structures may produce hoarseness as a result of involvement of the recurrent laryngeal nerve, dysphagia

---

*Carcinoid tumors are more common in the gastrointestinal tract than in the lungs. Although usually benign, they can be malignant.

from involvement of the esophagus, and paralysis of the hemidiaphragm from involvement of the phrenic nerve. Symptoms of extrathoracic spread depend on the site of metastasis. Structures typically involved are the scalene lymph nodes (especially in peripheral lung tumors), adrenals (50%), liver (30%), brain (20%), bone (20%), and kidneys (15%). Oat cell tumors are known to produce virtually any of the polypeptide hormones such as parathyroid hormone (PTH), adrenocorticotropic hormone (ACTH), or antidiuretic hormone (ADH), so the patient may exhibit features that resemble hyperparathyroidism, Cushing's syndrome, or fluid retention with hyponatremia.

DIAGNOSIS AND STAGING OF LUNG CANCER

The main tools in the diagnosis of lung cancer are radiology, bronchoscopy, and cytology. A solitary, circumscribed nodule, or *coin lesion,* on the chest radiograph is of particular importance and may be the earliest indication of bronchogenic carcinoma, although it may also occur in many other conditions. Computed tomography (CT) scan may be of further help in differentiating the suspected lesion. Bronchoscopy with biopsy is the most successful technique in the diagnosis of squamous cell

▶ TABLE 42-1   TNM Staging System for Lung Cancer: 1986 American Joint Committee on Cancer

TNM Designation		Definition
PRIMARY TUMOR (T)		
T0		No evidence of primary tumor
Tx		Occult cancer seen in bronchial washing cytologies but not on radiograph or bronchoscopy
TIS		Carcinoma in situ
T1		Tumor ≤3 cm in diameter surrounded by normal lung or visceral pleura
T2		Tumor >3 cm in diameter or any size that invades the visceral pleura or has associated atelectasis extending to hilum; must be >2 cm distal to carina
T3		Tumor of any size with direct extension into the chest wall, diaphragm, mediastinal pleura, or pericardium without involving heart, great vessels, trachea, esophagus, or vertebral bodies; or within 2 cm of carina without involving the carina
T4		Tumor of any size with invasion of the mediastinum or involving heart, great vessels, trachea, esophagus, vertebral bodies, or carina; or with the presence of malignant pleural effusion
REGIONAL LYMPH NODES (N)		
N0		No demonstrable metastasis to regional lymph nodes
N1		Metastasis to peribronchial and/or ipsilateral hilar nodes
N2		Metastasis to ipsilateral mediastinal or subcarinal lymph nodes
N3		Metastasis to contralateral mediastinal or hilar lymph nodes; ipsilateral or contralateral scalene or superclavicular lymph nodes
DISTANT METASTASIS (M)		
M0		No known distant metastasis
M1		Distant metastasis present with site specified (e.g., brain)
STAGE GROUPING		
Occult carcinoma	TxN0M0	Sputum contains malignant cells but no other evidence of primary tumor or metastasis
Stage 0	TISN0M0	Carcinoma in situ
Stage I	T1N0M0 T2N0M0	Tumor classified as T1 or T2 without evidence of metastasis to regional lymph nodes or distal site
Stage II	T1N1M0 T2N1M0	Tumor classified as T1 or T2 with only evidence of metastasis to ipsilateral peribronchial or hilar lymph nodes
Stage IIIa	T3N0M0 T3N1M0	Tumor classified as T3 with or without evidence of metastasis to ipsilateral peribronchial or hilar lymph nodes; no distal metastasis
Stage IIIb	Any T N3 M0 T4 any N M0	Any tumor classification with metastasis to contralateral hilar or mediastinal lymph nodes or to the scalene or supraclavicular lymph nodes; or any tumor classified as T4 with or without any regional lymph node metastasis; no distal metastasis
Stage IV	Any T any N M1	Any tumor with distant metastasis

From Mountain CF: *Chest* 89:225S-233S, 1986.

carcinoma, which is generally located centrally. Scalene node biopsy is most successful in the diagnosis of those cancers inaccessible to bronchoscopy. Cytologic examination of the sputum, bronchial brushings, and examination of the pleural fluid also play an important role in the diagnosis of lung cancer.

Both the histology and the stage of disease are important to determine the prognosis as well as the treatment plan. Distinguishing between SCLC and NSCLC is crucial. Lung cancer staging consists of two parts: (1) anatomic staging to determine the extent of the tumor and its resectability and (2) physiologic staging to determine the patient's ability to withstand various antitumor treatments.

The *TNM staging system* for lung cancer formulated by the American Joint Committee on Cancer is a widely accepted method of determining the extent of disease for NSCLC. The various T (tumor size), N (regional lymph node metastasis), and M (presence or absence of distal metastasis) factors are combined to form different stage groups (Table 42-1). Tumor size and histology are determined by radiology and examination of tissue specimen. In addition, mediastinoscopy is often useful to confirm the diagnosis and to separate operable from inoperable tumors. Tests to detect distal metastases include bone scan, brain scan, liver function studies, and gallium scan of liver, spleen, and bone.

When the TNM system was developed for bronchogenic carcinoma, the treatment of SCLC gave such poor results that it did not seem worthwhile to apply the TNM system to this variety of lung cancer. Thus a simple two-staging system is applied to SCLC. *Limited-stage disease* is defined as SCLC confined to one hemithorax and regional lymph nodes, and *extensive-stage disease* is defined as involvement more extensive than these parameters. In part, the limited-stage disease definition is related to whether the tumor can be encompassed within a tolerable radiation therapy port.

Patients with lung cancer often have cardiopulmonary and other medical conditions related to chronic obstructive pulmonary disease (COPD). Physiologic staging of these patients is necessary to predict their ability to tolerate a lobectomy or pneumonectomy. A preoperative forced expiratory volume in 1 second (FEV_1) less than 2 L may result in a FEV_1 of 0.8 L or less after pneumonectomy, a value generally considered to preclude surgery. Other major contraindications for surgery include history of recent myocardial infarction, uncontrolled major dysrhythmias, carbon dioxide (CO_2) retention, and severe pulmonary hypertension.

TREATMENT AND PROGNOSIS OF LUNG CANCER

After the histologic diagnosis and anatomic and physiologic staging procedures are completed, an overall treatment plan is formulated. The most common treatment regimens are combinations of surgery, radiation, and chemotherapy.

Surgery is the treatment of choice for patients in stages I, II, and selected stage IIIa NSCLC unless the tumor is nonresectable or other conditions (e.g., cardiac disease) rule out surgery. Surgery may include partial or total lung removal. Approximately 30% of patients with NSCLC are considered resectable for cure. The 5-year survival rate for this resectable group is about 30%. Thus most patients initially thought to have a curable resection die of metastatic disease (usually within 2 years). The prognosis for the remaining 70% of patients who have unresectable NSCLC is even worse. *Radiation therapy* is generally recommended for stages I and II lesions if surgery is contraindicated and for stage III lesions when the disease is confined to the involved hemithorax and ipsilateral supraclavicular lymph nodes. When NSCLC is disseminated, radiation therapy may be applied to local sites for palliative purposes (e.g., spinal cord compression from metastasis to vertebrae). *Combination chemotherapy* may be prescribed for some patients with NSCLC. The median survival time for unresectable patients with NSCLC is less than 1 year, even with radiation and/or chemotherapy. A small group (6%) will survive 5 years.

The cornerstone of therapy for patients with SCLC is chemotherapy, with or without radiation therapy. Chemotherapy and chest radiotherapy may be administered to patients with limited-stage disease if they are physiologically able to withstand the treatment. Patients with extensive-stage disease are treated with chemotherapy alone. Some frequently used combination chemotherapy regimens include cyclophosphamide, doxorubicin (Adriamycin), and vincristine (CAV) and cyclophosphamide, doxorubicin, vincristine, and etoposide (CAVE). Combination chemotherapy increases median survival from 6 to 17 weeks, untreated, to 40 to 70 weeks. Radiation therapy is also used as prophylaxis against cerebral metastases and for the palliative management of pain, recurrent hemoptysis, effusions, or obstruction of the airways or the superior vena cava (Carr, Hoyle, 1994; Minna, 1994).

The overall prognosis for patients with bronchogenic carcinoma is poor (14% 5-year survival; American Cancer Society, 1995) and has improved only slightly over the past few years, despite the introduction of multiple new chemotherapeutic agents. Thus the emphasis must be placed on prevention. Health care professionals should advise people not to smoke cigarettes or live in an environment polluted by industry. Protective measures must also be taken for those who work with asbestos, uranium, chromium, and other carcinogenic materials.

QUESTIONS

▼ *Answer the following on a separate sheet of paper.*

1. What is the carcinoid syndrome, and what type of tumor causes it?
2. What are some common signs and symptoms of bronchogenic carcinoma, and why is it difficult to diagnose on the basis of these signs and symptoms?
3. List three major diagnostic tools used for the detection of lung cancer, and describe the significant findings of each technique.

▼ *Match each histologic type of bronchogenic carcinoma in column A with its characteristics in column B.*

Column A		Column B
4. _____ Squamous cell		a. Located centrally within large bronchi
5. _____ Oat cell		b. Located in peripheral lung
6. _____ Adenocarcinoma		c. Most common type
7. _____ Large cell		d. Least common type
		e. Most aggressive type, poorest prognosis
		f. Relatively slow to metastasize
		g. No clear association with smoking
		h. SCLC histologic type
		i. NSCLC histologic type
		j. Often associated with abnormal hormone secretion

▼ *Circle T if the statement is true and F if it is false. Correct any false statements.*

8. T F Three factors that appear to account for the increase in lung cancer over recent decades are cigarette smoking, industrial hazards, and air pollution.

9. T F Statistical evidence indicates a negative relationship between heavy cigarette smoking and bronchogenic carcinoma.

10. T F Of the industrial hazards, the most common material responsible for increasing the risk of developing lung cancer is uranium.

11. T F Primary malignant neoplasms of the lung are more common than secondary metastasis to the lung from another primary site.

12. T F About 95% of primary malignant neoplasms of the lung are bronchogenic carcinoma.

13. T F About one third of malignant bronchogenic tumors are centrally located about the hilus and first few orders of bronchi.

▼ *Circle the letter preceding each item below that correctly answers the question or completes the statement. More than one choice may be correct.*

14. The lung is a common site for secondary metastasis because:
    a. Blood-borne tumor emboli are likely to become enmeshed in the capillary beds of the lungs.
    b. It is anatomically close to the abdominal organs.
    c. All the lymph of the body passes through the thoracic duct and may transport lymph-borne tumor cells to the lungs.

15. The overall 5-year survival rate for patients with primary lung cancer is about:
    a. 75%
    b. 50%
    c. 14%
    d. 1%

16. Methods of treatment of lung cancer include:
    a. Irradiation
    b. Lung scan
    c. Surgical resection
    d. Chemotherapy

17. Of the four patients with the following TNM stages of lung cancer, which would probably not be recommended for surgical resection?
    a. T1N1M0
    b. T2N1M0
    c. T2N2M1
    d. T1N0M0

18. Which of the following individuals would be at higher risk for the development of bronchogenic carcinoma than the general population?
    a. A 50-year-old man who has a history of asbestos exposure
    b. A 65-year-old woman with a 50-pack-per-year cigarette smoking history
    c. A uranium worker
    d. A chromate worker
    e. All the above

CHAPTER 43 ▶ Pulmonary Tuberculosis

SYLVIA A. PRICE

Tuberculosis (TB) is an infectious communicable disease caused by *Mycobacterium tuberculosis*. The aerobic, acid-fast rods include both pathogenic and saprophytic organisms. Several pathogenic mycobacteria exist, but only the bovine and human strains are pathogenic to humans. The tubercle bacillus is 0.3 × 2 to 4 μm, which is smaller than a red blood cell.

PATHOGENESIS

The portals of entry for the *M. tuberculosis* organism are the respiratory tract, the gastrointestinal (GI) tract, and an open wound in the skin. Most TB infections are contracted by the airborne route, through the inhalation of droplet nuclei containing organisms of the tubercle bacillus from an infected individual. The GI tract is the usual portal of entry for the bovine strain, which is spread by contaminated milk. However, in the United States, with widespread pasteurization of milk and detection of diseased cattle, bovine TB is rare.

TB is a disease controlled by a cell-mediated immunity response. The effector cell is the macrophage, and the lymphocyte (usually T cell) is the immunoresponsive cell. This type of immunity is basically local, involving macrophages activated at the infection site by lymphocytes and their lymphokines. This response is referred to as a cellular (delayed) *hypersensitivity reaction* (see Chapter 5).

The tubercle bacilli that reach the alveolar surfaces are usually inhaled in units of one to three bacilli; larger clumps of inhaled bacilli tend to impinge on the mucociliary surfaces of the nasal passages and bronchial tree and do not cause disease. Once in the alveolar space, usually in the lower part of the upper lobe or the upper part of the lower lobe, the tubercle bacillus evokes an inflammatory reaction. Polymorphonuclear leukocytes appear on the scene and phagocytize the bacteria but do not kill the organism. After the first few days, leukocytes are replaced by macrophages. The involved alveoli are consolidated, and acute pneumonia develops. This cellular pneumonia may resolve itself so that no residue remains, or the process may continue, with the bacteria continuing to be phagocytized or to multiply within the cells. Lymphatic drainage of the bacilli also occurs into the regional lymph nodes. The infiltrating macrophages elongate and partially fuse to form the epithelioid cell tubercle, surrounded by lymphocytes. This reaction usually takes 10 to 20 days.

Necrosis of the central portion of the lesion results in a relatively solid, cheesy appearance called *caseous necrosis*. The area of caseous necrosis and the surrounding granulation tissue of epithelioid cells and fibroblasts evoke different responses. The granulation tissue may become more fibrous, forming collagenous scar tissue, which results in a capsule surrounding the tubercle.

The primary lesion in the lung is called the *Ghon focus,* and the combination of regional lymph node involvement and the primary lesion is termed the *Ghon complex.* A calcified Ghon complex may be seen on a routine chest radiograph of healthy persons.

Another response that may occur at the site of the necrotic area is liquefaction, with the liquid material sloughing into a connecting bronchus and producing a cavity. The tubercular material sloughed from the walls of the cavity enters the tracheobronchial tree. The process may be repeated in other parts of the lung, or bacilli may be carried to the larynx, middle ear, or gut.

Even without therapy, small cavities close and leave a fibrous scar. As inflammation subsides, the bronchial lumen may be narrowed and closed by scarring near the junction of the cavity and the bronchus. The caseous material may thicken and be unable to flow through the communicating channel, so the cavity fills with this material and the lesion becomes similar to the unsloughed encapsulated lesion. It may remain in a quiescent stage for long periods or reestablish its bronchial communication and be the site of active inflammation.

The disease may spread through the lymphatics or blood vessels. The organisms that pass through the lymph nodes reach the bloodstream in small numbers and may initiate occasional lesions in various organs. This dispersal of the organisms, referred to as *lymphohematogenous dissemination,* is usually self-limited. *Hematogenous dissemination,* an acute phenomenon, usually gives rise to miliary TB; it occurs when a necrotic focus erodes a blood vessel, allowing large numbers of organisms to enter the vascular system and be disseminated to the various organs.

EPIDEMIOLOGY

The case incidence rate of and mortality from TB declined rapidly after the advent of chemotherapy. In recent years, however, the decline has reached a plateau, and the incidence is generally increasing. Factors associated with this trend include socioeconomic and health-related problems (e.g., alcoholism, homelessness, a rise in acquired immunodeficiency syndrome/human immunodeficiency virus [AIDS/HIV] infection), with the increased incidence noted particularly among minority group members and refugees who have entered the United States from areas where TB is endemic.

In 1993, 25,313 new cases of TB were reported to the Centers for Disease Control and Prevention (CDC). This is a case incidence rate of 10.4/100,000 U.S. population, an increase of 18% since 1985. In the United States it is estimated that 10% of the population, are currently infected with TB. An adult tuberculin reactor with an abnormal chest radiograph consistent with TB has a 5% to 10% chance of developing clinical evidence of TB in the next 2 years. More than 80% of the reported new cases of TB are in persons over 25 years of age, the majority of whom were infected in the past. In the United States only

about 5 of 100 of the newly infected population will contract (develop) pulmonary TB 1 or 2 years after infection. Of the remaining 95, another 5 will typically "break down" and develop clinical disease at some future point. Therefore about 10% of infected individuals will develop clinical TB during their lifetime, but the risk is higher for immunosuppressed individuals, especially those with HIV infection. Lymphocytes and monocytes, which are the primary defense cells against the TB infection, are destroyed by HIV. During 1990 to 1999 worldwide an estimated 88 million persons will develop TB, and 8 million of these cases will be attributed to HIV infection (Dolin, Raviglione, Kochi, 1994).

When considering a person's susceptibility to TB, two risk factors must be examined: the risk of acquiring the infection and the risk of developing clinically active disease after infection has occurred. The risks of acquiring the infection and of developing clinical disease depend on the infection's existence in the population, especially among persons infected with HIV; immigrants from areas of high prevalence of TB; high-risk racial and ethnic minority groups (e.g., African Americas, Native Americans, Alaskan natives, Asians, Pacific Islanders, and Hispanics); and those residing in high-risk environments for the transmission of TB, such as correctional facilities, homeless shelters, hospitals, and nursing homes.

DIAGNOSIS AND CLINICAL MANIFESTATIONS

The symptoms associated with pulmonary TB are a productive, prolonged cough (duration of more than 3 weeks), chest pain, and hemoptysis. Systemic symptoms include fever, chills, night sweats, fatigue, loss of appetite, and weight loss. Individuals suspected of having TB should be referred for a physical examination, a Mantoux tuberculin test, chest radiography, and bacteriologic or histologic examination. Tuberculin skin testing should be performed in all individuals suspected of having clinically active TB, but its value is limited by false-negative reactions, particularly in immunosuppressed individuals (e.g., those with HIV infection). Those individuals who have symptoms suggestive of TB, especially prolonged productive cough and hemoptysis, should receive a chest radiograph even though they have a negative reaction to the tuberculin skin test.

According to the CDC, a case of TB is verified by a positive bacteriologic culture for the *M. tuberculosis* organism. It is imperative to query individuals suspected of having TB regarding their history of exposure and previous TB or infection. Demographic factors (e.g., country of origin, age, ethnic or racial groups) and medical conditions (e.g., HIV infection) that may increase the individual's risk for exposure to TB must also be considered.

HYPERSENSITIVITY REACTION

The pathogenicity of the bacillus does not arise from any intrinsic toxicity but from its capacity to induce a hypersensitive reaction in the host. *Tuberculoproteins* derived from the bacillus appear to induce this reaction. The tissue responses of inflammation and necrosis are the results of a cellular (delayed) hypersensitivity response of the host to the tubercle bacillus. A TB hypersensitivity reaction usually develops 3 to 10 weeks from the onset of infection. Persons who have been exposed to the tubercle bacillus develop sensitized T lymphocytes. If *purified protein derivative* (PPD) of tuberculin is injected into the skin of a person whose lymphocytes are sensitized to tuberculoprotein, the sensitized lymphocytes interact with the extract and attract macrophages to the area.

Intradermal (Mantoux) Tuberculin Test

The standard technique (Mantoux test) is the intradermal injection of 0.1 ml of PPD tuberculin containing 5 tuberculin units (TU) into the upper third of the volar aspect or dorsal surface of the forearm after the skin has been cleansed with alcohol. A disposable tuberculin syringe with a 26- to 27-gauge needle is usually preferred. The short needle is held so that the bevel faces upward, and the tip of the needle is inserted beneath the surface of the skin. A wheal 6 to 10 mm in diameter and resembling a mosquito bite should be produced when the prescribed 0.1 ml amount is accurately injected (see Fig. 9-8).

The skin reaction requires 48 to 72 hours to reach its peak after the injection, and the reaction should be read during that period, in a good light, with the subject's forearm slightly flexed. The reaction must be recorded as the diameter of the induration in millimeters, measured transversely to the long axis of the forearm. Only induration (palpable swelling), not erythema alone, is significant. Induration may be determined by inspection and by palpation (stroking the area with a finger).

The interpretation of the skin test identifies various types of reactions (see box above). An indurated area measuring 5 mm or larger is considered a positive reaction in selected groups, reflecting sensitivity resulting from infection with the bacillus. An induration of 10 mm or larger is also classified as positive in certain groups, whereas an induration of 15 mm or greater is positive in all persons with no known risk factors for TB.

A positive reaction to the tuberculin test indicates the presence of infection but does not necessarily signify clinical disease. However, this test is an important diagnostic tool in the evaluation of an individual patient and is also useful in determining the prevalence of TB infection in a population.

CLASSIFICATION OF TUBERCULIN REACTIONS: INTRADERMAL MANTOUX TEST (WITH 5 TU PPD TUBERCULIN)

≥5 mm of induration is classified as positive in the following groups:
1. Persons known to have or suspected of having HIV infection
2. Persons who have had close contact with a person with infectious TB
3. Persons who have chest radiograph findings suggestive of previous TB and who have received inadequate or no treatment
4. Persons who inject drugs and whose HIV status is undetermined

≥10 mm of induration is classified as positive in persons who do not meet the above criteria but who have other risk factors for TB, including the following:
1. Persons with certain medical conditions (excluding HIV infection), such as substance abuse (especially drug injection), recent infection with *M. tuberculosis,* chest radiograph findings suggestive of previous TB (in a person who received inadequate or no treatment), diabetes mellitus, silicosis, prolonged corticosteroid therapy, endstage renal disease, chronic malabsorption syndromes, and low body weight (10% or more less than the ideal)
2. Medically underserved, low-income populations, including high-risk racial and ethnic groups (Asians and Pacific Islanders, African Americans, Hispanics, Native Americans)
3. Residents of long-term care facilities, such as correctional facilities and nursing homes
4. Children younger than 4 years of age
5. Other groups identified locally as having an increased prevalence of TB, such as migrant farm workers or homeless persons

≥15 mm is positive in the following:
All persons with no known risk factors for TB

Modified from Centers for Disease Control and Prevention: *Core curriculum on tuberculosis: what the clinician should know,* ed 4, Atlanta, 1994, CDC.

Anergy Testing

Anergy is the absence of tuberculin reactivity in infected individuals. For example, in immunosuppressed persons, a cellular delayed-type hypersensitivity response such as a tuberculin reaction may either decrease or disappear. The etiology of anergy may result from HIV infection, severe or febrile illness, measles or other viral infections, Hodgkin's disease, sarcoidosis, live-virus vaccination, and the administration of corticosteroids or immunosuppressive drugs. According to the CDC (1994), on the average, 10% to 25% of patients with TB disease have negative reactions when tested with the tuberculin skin test.

Approximately one third of HIV-infected persons and more than 60% of AIDS patients may have skin test reactions less than 5 mm although they are infected with *M. tuberculosis*. HIV infection may suppress the skin test response because of the CD4+ T lymphocyte count, which decreases to less than 200 cells/mm^3. Anergy can also occur with a relatively high CD4+ T lymphocyte count.

BCG Vaccination

Bacille Calmette-Guérin (BCG), an attenuated living strain of bovine tubercle bacilli, is the most widely used vaccine in many countries. In BCG vaccination these organisms are injected into the skin to produce a well-circumscribed, calcified, walled-off primary focus. BCG has retained its capacity to increase the immunologic resistance of animals and humans. Primary infection of BCG has the advantage over primary infection by virulent organisms because no danger exists of producing progressive disease in the host.

Vaccination with BCG usually leads to the development of tuberculin sensitivity. The degree of sensitivity is variable, depending on the strain of BCG used and the population vaccinated. There is no way of distinguishing tuberculin reactions caused by vaccination with BCG from those caused by natural mycobacterial infections.

Despite the worldwide acceptance of BCG, vaccination is not generally recommended against TB in the United States because of the low risk of infection and the variable effectiveness of the vaccine. BCG vaccination is only 50% effective against all forms of TB. According to the CDC (1988) recommendations, BCG should be given only to (1) infants and children with negative skin test results who cannot be given isoniazid preventive therapy but who will be continuously exposed to a person with infectious TB who is resistant to isoniazid and rifampin and (2) those who belong to groups in whom the rate of new infection exceed 1% per year and in whom the usual surveillance and treatment programs have not been successful.

RADIOLOGIC EXAMINATION

Radiologic examination often suggests the presence of TB, but it is almost impossible to make a diagnosis on this basis alone, since almost all the manifestations of TB can be mimicked by other diseases.

Pathologically, the earliest manifestation of TB involvement of the lung is usually a parenchymal lymph node complex. In adults the apical and posterior segments of the upper lobe or the superior segments of the lower lobe are the usual sites of lesions, which may appear dense and homogenous. There may also be evidence of cavity formation and scattered disease, which is often bilateral.

BACTERIOLOGIC STUDIES

Although catheterized urine, cerebrospinal fluid, and gastric contents may be microscopically examined, the most important bacteriologic study in the diagnosis of TB is examination of the sputum. The *Ziehl-Neelsen staining method* may be used. The slide is flooded with steaming carbolfuchsin and then decolorized with acid alcohol. It is then counterstained with methylene blue or brilliant green. The preferred method of staining is the auramine-rhodamine technique of fluorescent staining; the auramine-rhodamine solution, once attached to the mycobacteria, resists acid-alcohol decolorization. The clinician is provided with an estimate of the number of acid-fast bacilli (AFB) detected on the slide. A positive specimen gives the clinician a preliminary indication of the diagnosis, but a negative specimen does not rule out infection with the disease.

The most accurate diagnostic method is the *culture technique*. Culture examinations should be done on all specimens. The mycobacteria are slow growing and require a complex medium. Mature colonies are cream or buff colored and warty and cauliflower-like in appearance. As few as 10 bacteria/ml of digested, concentrated material can be detected on the culture medium. The mycobacterial growth observed on the culture medium should be quantified as to the number of colonies present. The microorganism takes 6 to 12 week at 36° to 37° C to grow when using conventional biochemical tests. However, when a liquid medium is inoculated for growth using the BACTEC radiometric system and rapid methods are used for species identification, culture results should be available within 10 to 14 days of specimen collection.

Tests are currently available that permit identification of most species of mycobacteria, and computerized programs have been developed that aid in the interpretation of data. For example, nucleic acid probes can identify the species in 2 to 8 hours. *High-performance liquid chromatography* (HPLC) detects differences in the spectrum of mycolic acids in the cell wall and is equally as rapid. *Polymerase chain reaction* (PCR) techniques are being developed that could be performed on sputum or other clinical specimens to diagnose TB disease more rapidly. This technique is in the experimental phase and is not available for routine diagnosis of TB.

TREATMENT

Tuberculosis is treated primarily by prolonged administration of antimicrobial drugs. These drugs can also be used to prevent an infected person from developing clinical disease.

The American Thoracic Society (ATS) (1994) emphasizes three principles on which treatment for TB are based: (1) regimens must include multiple drugs to which the organisms are susceptible; (2) the drugs must be taken regularly; and (3) drug therapy must continue for a sufficient time to provide the safest and most effective therapy in the shortest period. In 1994 the CDC and ATS published new guidelines for the treatment of TB disease and infection, including the following:

1. A 6-month drug regimen consisting of isoniazid (isonicotinic acid hydrazide, INH), rifampin, and pyrazinamide given for 2 months followed by INH and rifampin for 4 months is recommended for the initial therapy of TB for patients with fully susceptible organisms who adhere to treatment. Ethambutol (or streptomycin in children too young to be monitored for visual acuity) should be included in the initial regimen until the results of drug susceptibility studies are available, unless little possibility exists of drug resistance (e.g., less than 4% primary resistance to INH in the community; patient has had no previous treatment with antituberculosis medications, is not from a country with a high prevalence of drug resistance, and has no known exposure to a drug-resistant case). This four-drug, 6-month regimen is effective even when the infecting organism is resistant to INH. In the presence of HIV infections, it is important to assess clinical and bacteriologic responses. If a slow or suboptimal response occurs, therapy should be prolonged or judged on a case-by-case basis.

2. A 9-month regimen of INH and rifampin is acceptable for person who cannot or should not take pyrazinamide. Ethambutol (or streptomycin in children too young to be monitored for visual acuity) should be included in the initial regimen until the results of drug susceptibility studies are available, unless little possibility exists of drug resistance. If INH resistance is demonstrated, rifampin and ethambutol should be continued for a minimum of 12 months.

3. More widespread use of directly observed therapy (DOT) is recommended, treating all patients with DOT.

4. Multidrug-resistant TB (MDR TB) with resistance to INH and rifampin is difficult to treat. Treatment must be individualized and prolonged, based on medication history and susceptibility studies. Clinicians unfamiliar with treatment of MDR TB should seek expert consultation.

5. Children should be managed in the same ways as adults, using adjusted doses of the drugs.

6. A 4-month regimen of INH and rifampin, preferably with pyrazinamide for the first 2 months, is recommended for adults who have active TB and who are smear and culture negative, if little possibility exists of drug resistance.

The critical factor for the successful outcome of treatment is patient adherence to the drug regimen. DOT is a way to ensure that patients adhere to therapy. With DOT, a health care worker or designated individual observes the patient swallow each dose of TB medication. Measures such as DOT are designed to foster adherence and ensure that patients take the drugs as prescribed.

The response to antituberculosis chemotherapy for patients who have positive sputum cultures is evaluated by repeated examinations of the sputum. Specimens for culture should be obtained monthly until the culture converts to negative. Patients who have converted to negative sputum cultures *after* 2 months of treatment should have at least one more sputum smear and culture at the end of the drug therapy regimen. Patients with MDR TB should have monthly cultures for the entire course of therapy. A chest radiograph at completion of the therapy provides a baseline for comparison of future films. Patients with a negative sputum *before* treatment, however, should have a chest radiograph and the clinical evaluation. The intervals for the procedure depend on the clinical circumstances and differential diagnosis.

Routine follow-up after therapy is not necessary for patients who have had a satisfactory and prompt bacteriologic response to 6- or 9-month therapy with INH and rifampin. Patients whose organisms were susceptible to the drugs administered should report any symptoms of TB, such as prolonged cough, fever, or weight loss.

INH is also used prophylactically in a dosage of 300 mg/day for adults, usually for 12 months. Recent evidence indicates that 6 months of preventive therapy confers considerable protection. It is important to emphasize that persons with HIV infection should receive 12 months of therapy.

The following high-priority groups (persons with positive skin tests) should be considered for preventive therapy:

1. Persons known to have or suspected of having HIV infection, including those who inject drugs (HIV status unknown)
2. Close contacts of persons with infectious TB
3. Persons who have a chest radiograph suggestive of TB and who have received inadequate treatment
4. Persons who inject drugs and known to be HIV negative
5. Persons with certain medical conditions (e.g., diabetes mellitus, silicosis, cancer of the head and neck, end-stage renal disease)
6. Persons whose tuberculin skin test reaction converted from negative to positive within the past 2 years
7. Persons younger than 35 years of age with a reaction to the tuberculin test of greater than 10 mm
8. Foreign-born persons from areas where TB is common (e.g., Asia, Africa, and Latin America)
9. Medically underserved, low-income populations, including high-risk racial and ethnic groups (e.g., Asians and Pacific Islanders, African Americans, Hispanics, Native Americans)
10. Residents of long-term care facilities

TABLE 43-1   Drugs for Treatment of Tuberculosis in Adults (Dosage in mg/kg)

Drug	Daily	Twice Weekly	Thrice Weekly	Adverse Reactions	Monitoring Reactions	Remarks
FIRST-LINE DRUGS						
Isoniazid (INH)	5 (300 mg)	15 max (900 mg)	15 max (900 mg)	Hepatitis Peripheral neuropathy Mild central nervous system effects	Measure baseline levels of hepatic enzymes.	Pyridoxine can prevent peripheral neuropathy.
Rifampin	10 (600 mg)	10 (600 mg)	10 (600 mg)	GI upset Drug interactions Hepatitis Bleeding problems	Perform baseline complete blood count measurements.	Significant interactions occur with methadone, contraceptives, and other drugs. Rifampin colors body fluids orange.
Pyrazinamide (PZA)	15-30 (2 g)	50-70 (4 g)	50-70 (3 g)	Liver injury Hyperuricemia GI upset Rash	Measure baseline levels of uric acid and hepatic enzymes.	Treat hyperuricemia only if patient has symptoms.
Ethambutol	15-25	50	25-30	Optic neuritis	Perform baseline and monthly tests of visual acuity and color vision.	Other ocular effects and increased renal failure may occur.
Streptomycin	15 (1 g)	25-30 (1.5 g)	25-30 (1.5 g)	Ototoxicity Renal toxicity	Perform baseline and repeat tests as needed for hearing and kidney function.	Avoid or reduce dose in adults over 60 years old.
SECOND-LINE DRUGS						

Capreomycin	15-30 (1 g)	—	—	Toxicity:
				  Auditory
				  Vestibular
				  Renal
					Assess vestibular and hearing function.
					Perform BUN and creatinine tests.
						Use with caution in older adults.

Ethionamide	15-20 (1 g)	—	—	GI upset Hepatotoxicity Hypersensitivity	Measure hepatic enzymes.	Start with low dosage and increase as tolerated.
Cycloserine	15-20 (1 g)	—	—	Psychosis Convulsions Headaches Drug interactions	Assess mental status. Measure serum drug levels.	Start with low dosage increase as tolerated.

Kanamycin	15-30 (1 g)	—	—	Toxicity:
				  Auditory
				  Vestibular
				  Renal
					Assess vestibular and hearing function.
					Perform BUN and creatinine tests.
						Use with caution in older adults.

Para-aminosalicyclic acid (PAS)	150 (12 g)	—	—	GI upset Hepatotoxicity Hypersensitivity Sodium load	Measure hepatic enzymes. Assess volume load.	Start with low dosage and increase as tolerated. Monitor cardiac patients for sodium level.

Modified from American Thoracic Society: *Am J Respir Crit Care Med* 149(5):1359-1374, 1994.
GI, Gastrointestinal; *BUN*, blood urea nitrogen.

11. Children younger than 4 years
12. Other groups identified locally as having an increased prevalence of TB (e.g., migrant farm workers, homeless persons)

Table 43-1 describes the antimicrobial drugs used to treat TB.

PREVENTION AND CONTROL

Public health measures are designed for early detection and treatment of cases and sources of infection. By law, TB must be reported to the health department. Screening of high-risk groups is a significant function of state and local health departments. The purpose of early detection of persons with TB infection is to identify those individuals who would benefit from preventive therapy to stop development of clinically active TB. This preventive health measure benefits not only the infected individual, but the community as well. To this end, populations at risk for developing TB must be identified, and priorities for establishing drug treatment programs must take into account the risk of therapy versus the benefit to the individual.

The CDC recently revised the guidelines for preventing transmission of TB in health care facilities. These guidelines emphasize that severely immunosuppressed health care workers should receive anergy testing, counseling by employee health professionals, and the opportunity for job reassignment.

TB eradication involves a combination of effective chemotherapy, prompt case and contact identification and follow-up, management of persons exposed to patients with infectious MDR TB, and chemoprophylactic therapy of high-risk population groups.

QUESTIONS

▼ *Answer the following on a separate sheet of paper.*

1. What groups are the most likely to develop tuberculosis (TB) once they become infected?
2. Describe the two risk factors that must be examined when a person's susceptibility to TB is considered.
3. Explain the rationale for administering at least two drugs in the treatment of TB.
4. List the three principles on which treatment for TB is based.
5. Describe the preventive therapy regimen for HIV-infected persons with a positive tuberculin skin test reaction.
6. Evaluate the role of bacille Calmette-Guérin (BCG) in the control of TB in the United States.
7. What is the purpose of directly observed therapy (DOT) in the treatment of TB?
8. What are the factors most likely to be responsible for multidrug-resistant TB (MDR TB) in patients with no previous history of TB treatment?
9. What are the public health measures for prevention and control of TB in the United States?

▼ *Circle the letter preceding each item below that correctly completes the statement. More than one answer may be correct.*

10. *Mycobacterium tuberculosis* is described as a(n):
    a. Nonpathogenic organism
    b. Acid-fast rod
    c. Aerobic bacillus
    d. Exotoxin
11. Which of the following diagnostic test results confirm(s) that an individual has TB?
    a. Abnormal chest radiograph
    b. Culture positive for *M. tuberculosis*
    c. Reaction greater than 10 mm to a 5 TU PPD
    d. Positive AFB smear
12. The portal of entry into the body by the tubercle bacillus that is responsible for most TB infections in the United States is the (an):
    a. Respiratory tract
    b. Lymphoid tissue of the oropharynx
    c. Gut
    d. Open wound in the skin
13. The most common site of implantation of the tubercle bacillus is the alveolar surface of the lung parenchyma in the:
    a. Lower part of the upper lobe
    b. Upper part of the lower lobe
    c. Both a and b
    d. Neither a nor b
14. The tissue lesion or tubercle produced by the causative agent *M. tuberculosis* usually results in:
    a. Hyperplasia of epithelial tissue with many mature cells
    b. Dilation and erosion of a pulmonary artery
    c. Bacilli surrounded by lymphocytes and fibroblasts
    d. Erosion of the epithelial lining of the mainstem bronchus

15. The earliest reaction to the tubercle bacillus is:
    a. Cavity
    b. Fibrosis
    c. Calcification
    d. Caseous necrosis
16. The development of caseous necrosis in TB occurs as a result of:
    a. Immunity
    b. Hypersensitivity
17. The period from the onset of infection with tubercle bacilli to the development of a tuberculin hypersensitivity reaction is usually:
    a. 4 to 6 months
    b. 3 to 10 weeks
    c. 2 to 4 days
    d. 8 to 12 hours
18. A tuberculin skin test detects:
    a. A humoral sensitivity reaction to the tubercle bacillus
    b. TB infection with disease
    c. Cellular (delayed) immunologic sensitivity to the tubercle bacillus
    d. Caseous necrosis
19. A nonsignificant reaction to the tuberculin skin test usually indicates that a person:
    a. Is immune to TB
    b. Has been treated for TB with drugs
    c. Has not been exposed to *M. tuberculosis*
    d. Has not been exposed to the tubercle bacillus or, if recently exposed, has not developed a tuberculin hypersensitivity reaction
20. A significant reaction to the tuberculin

QUESTIONS—cont'd

test for persons known to have or suspected of having HIV infection is indicated by:
a. Formation of a vesicle followed by a pustule
b. A region of ≥10 mm of erythema
c. An area of ≥10 mm of induration

d. An area of ≥5 mm of induration with erythema
21. The signs and symptoms associated with pulmonary TB include:
a. Chest pain
b. Hemoptysis
c. Increase in sputum production and prolonged cough

d. Low-grade fever
22. In the treatment of adult pulmonary TB the usual daily dosage (in mg) of INH and rifampin is, respectively:
a. 100, 300
b. 200, 400
c. 300, 600
d. 500, 800

▼ *Match the drug in column A with the associated adverse reactions in column B. Reactions may be used more than once.*

Column A	Column B
23. _____ Rifampin	a. Optic neuritis
24. _____ Isoniazid (INH)	b. Hyperuricemia
25. _____ Para-aminosalicylic acid (PAS)	c. Bleeding problems
26. _____ Ethambutol	d. Hepatotoxicity
27. _____ Cycloserine	e. Immunosuppression
28. _____ Pyrazinamide	f. Psychoses
	g. GI upset
	h. Ototoxicity
	i. Nephrotoxicity
	j. Hypersensitivity
	k. Hepatitis
	l. Drug interactions
	m. Peripheral neuropathy

▼ *Circle T if the statement is true and F if it is false. Correct any false statements.*

29. T F For adults with a positive culture for pulmonary TB in areas where primary INH resistance is increased, a three-drug regimen consisting of INH, rifampin, and capreomycin is recommended.
30. T F On the average, 5% to 10% of patients with TB disease have negative reactions when tested with the tuberculin skin test.
31. T F The polymerase chain reaction (PCR) test is the preferred staining method for identifying most species of mycobacteria.
32. T F The etiology of anergy may result from HIV infection, severe or febrile illness, measles or other viral infections, Hodgkin's disease, sarcoidosis, live-virus vaccination, and the administration of corticosteroids or immunosuppressive drugs.
33. T F Short-course therapy for TB refers to treatment duration of 9 months with INH only.
34. T F It is estimated that 20% of infected persons will likely develop clinical TB during their lifetime.

BIBLIOGRAPHY ▼ PART VII

Aitken ML, Fiel SB: Cystic fibrosis, *Dis Mon* 39:1, 1993.

Aitken ML et al: Recombinant human DNAase inhalation in normal subjects and patients with cystic fibrosis, *JAMA* 267:1947, 1992.

American Cancer Society: Lung cancer, *CA* 43(4):201-225, 1993.

American Cancer Society: Cancer statistics 1995, *CA* 45(1):1-31, 1995.

American Thoracic Society: Chronic bronchitis, asthma, and pulmonary emphysema: a statement by the Committee on Diagnostic Standards for Nontuberculosis Respiratory Diseases, *Am Rev Respir Dis* 85:762-768, 1962.

American Thoracic Society: Diagnostic standards and classification of tuberculosis in the United States, *Am Rev Respir Dis* 142(3):725-735, 1990.

American Thoracic Society: Control of tuberculosis in the United States, *Am Rev Respir Dis* 146(6):1623-1633, 1992.

American Thoracic Society: Treatment of tuberculosis and tuberculosis infection in adults and children, *Am J Respir Crit Care Med* 149(5):1359-1374, 1994.

Bernstein MS, Locksley RM: *Legionella* infections. In Isselbacher KJ et al, editors: *Harrison's principles of internal medicine,* ed 13, New York, 1994, McGraw-Hill.

Bukowski DM, Peters JI: Acute respiratory failure, *Hosp Med* 30(12):52-59, 1994.

Burney LE: Smoking and lung cancer: a statement of the Public Health Service, *JAMA* 171:1829, 1957.

Carr DT, Hoyle PY: Bronchogenic carcinoma. In Murray JF, Nadel JA, editors: *Textbook of respiratory medicine,* vol II, Philadelphia, 1994, Saunders.

Continued.

BIBLIOGRAPHY ▼ PART VII

Centers for Disease Control and Prevention: Management of persons exposed to multidrug-resistant tuberculosis, *MMWR* 41(RR-11):1-8, 1992.

Centers for Disease Control and Prevention: Prevention and control of tuberculosis in migrant farm workers, *MMWR* 41(RR-10):1-11, 1992.

Centers for Disease Control and Prevention: Prevention and control of tuberculosis in U.S. communities with at-risk minority populations and prevention and control of tuberculosis among homeless persons, *MMWR* 41(RR-5):1-29, 1992.

Centers for Disease Control and Prevention: *Core curriculum on tuberculosis: what the clinician should know,* ed 4, Atlanta, 1994, CDC.

Centers for Disease Control and Prevention: Guideline for preventing the transmission of *Mycobacterium tuberculosis* in healthcare facilities, *MMWR* 43(RR-13):1-112, 1994.

Cherniack RM: *Pulmonary function testing,* Philadelphia, 1977, Saunders.

Cherniack RM, Cherniack L: *Respiration in health and disease,* ed 3, Philadelphia, 1983, Saunders.

Comroe JH Jr: *Physiology of respiration,* ed 2, Chicago, 1974, Mosby.

Demling RH: Acute respiratory distress syndrome: current concepts, *New Horiz* 1(3):388-401, 1993.

Denning CR et al: Cooperative study comparing three methods of sweat tests to diagnose cystic fibrosis, *Pediatrics* 66:752, 1980.

Dolin P, Raviglione M, Kochi A: *A review of epidemiological data and estimations of current and future incidence and mortality from tuberculosis,* Geneva, 1994, World Health Organization.

Fairbanks DNF: Snoring: not funny, not hopeless, *Hosp Med* 20(3):173-189, 1984.

Fishman AP: *Update: pulmonary disease and disorders,* New York, 1992, McGraw-Hill.

Fishman AP: *Pulmonary disease and disorders,* ed 2, New York, 1994, McGraw-Hill.

Fishman AP: Pulmonary hypertension and cor pulmonale. In Fishman AP, editor: *Pulmonary disease and disorders,* ed 2, New York, 1994, McGraw-Hill.

Gilliland BC: Relapsing polychondritis and miscellaneous arthritides. In Isselbacher KJ et al, editors: *Harrison's principles of internal medicine,* ed 13, New York, 1994, McGraw-Hill.

Griffith DE, Wallace RJ: Bacterial pneumonia in the adult: diagnosis and therapy, *Hosp Med* 24(1):188-203, 1988.

Harris A, Argent BE: The cystic fibrosis gene and its product CFTR, *Semin Cell Biol* 4:37, 1993.

Johnson CC, Finegold SM: Pyogenic bacterial pneumonia, lung abscess, and empyema. In Murray JF, Nadel JA, editors: *Textbook of respiratory medicine,* vol I, Philadelphia, 1994, Saunders.

Kersten LD: *Comprehensive respiratory nursing,* Philadelphia, 1989, Saunders.

Light RW: Postoperative pleural effusion: pathophysiology, clinical importance, and principles of management, *Respir Care* 29(5):540-549, 1984.

Light RW: Pneumothorax. In Murray JF, Nadel JA, editors: *Textbook of respiratory medicine,* vol II, Philadelphia, 1994, Saunders.

Loeb S, editor: *Springhouse's illustrated guide to diagnostic tests,* Springhouse, Pa, 1994, Springhouse.

Mahler DA: *Dyspnea,* Mount Kisco, NY, 1990, Futura.

Martin L: Acute respiratory failure, *Hosp Med* 25(1):54-69, 1989.

Minna JD: Neoplasms of the lung. In Isselbacher KJ et al, editors: *Harrison's principles of internal medicine,* ed 13, New York, 1994, McGraw-Hill.

Mitchell RS, Petty TL, Schwarz MI: *Synopsis of clinical pulmonary disease,* ed 4, St Louis, 1989, Mosby.

Morgan WKC, Seaton AS: *Occupational lung diseases,* ed 3, Philadelphia, 1995, Saunders.

Moser KM: Pulmonary thromboembolism. In Isselbacher KJ et al, editors: *Harrison's principles of internal medicine,* ed 13, New York, 1994, McGraw-Hill.

Mountain CF: Value of new TNM staging for lung cancer, *Chest* 96:475, 1989.

Murray JF: New presentations of bronchiectasis, *Hosp Pract* 26:55, 1991.

Murray JF, Nadel JA, editors: *Textbook of pulmonary medicine,* Philadelphia, 1988, Saunders.

Parkes WR: *Occupational lung diseases,* ed 2, London, 1982, Butterworth.

Petty TL, Ashbaugh RS: The adult respiratory distress syndrome, *Chest* 60:233-239, 1971.

Phillipson EA: Sleep disorders. In Murray JF, Nadel JA, editors: *Textbook of respiratory medicine,* vol II, Philadelphia, 1994, Saunders.

Raffin TA: ARDS: mechanisms and management, *Hosp Pract* 22:65, 1987.

Rubin EM: Lung abscess, *Hosp Med* 25(6):128-144, 1989.

Shapiro BA, Peruzzi WT, Kozlowski-Templin R: *Clinical application of blood gases,* ed 5, St Louis, 1994, Mosby.

Snider D et al: Multidrug-resistant tuberculosis, *Sci Am Sci Med* 1(2):16-25, 1994.

Snider GL, Faling LJ, Rennard SI: Chronic bronchitis and emphysema. In Murray JF, Nadel JA, editors: *Textbook of respiratory medicine,* vol I, Philadelphia, 1994, Saunders.

Stockley RA: Alpha1-antitrypsin and the pathogenesis of emphysema, *Lung* 169:S205, 1991.

US Department of Health and Human Services: *The health consequences of smoking: nicotine addiction. A report of the surgeon general,* Washington, DC, 1988, DHHS.

US Public Health Service/US Department of Health and Human Services: *Health, United States,* Washington, DC, 1993, PHS/DHHS.

Vasconcellos CA et al: Reduction in viscosity of cystic fibrosis sputum in vitro by gelosin, *Science* 263:969, 1994.

Victor LD: *Clinical pulmonary medicine,* Boston, 1992, Little, Brown.

Weinberger SE: *Principles of pulmonary medicine,* ed 2, Philadelphia, 1992, Saunders.

West JB: *Pulmonary pathophysiology,* ed 4, Boston, 1992, Williams & Wilkins.

West JB: *Respiratory physiology,* ed 5, Boston, 1995, Williams & Wilkins.

World Health Organization: *Histological typing of lung tumors,* ed 2, Geneva, 1982, WHO.

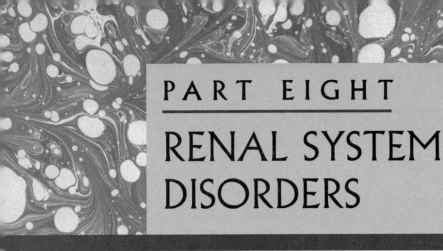

PART EIGHT

RENAL SYSTEM DISORDERS

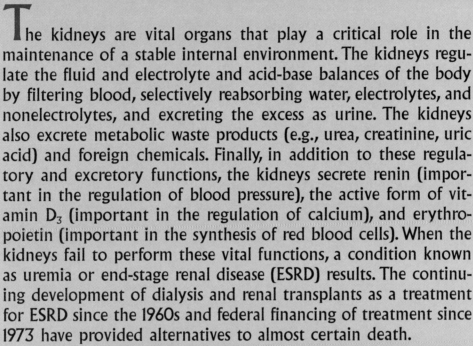

The kidneys are vital organs that play a critical role in the maintenance of a stable internal environment. The kidneys regulate the fluid and electrolyte and acid-base balances of the body by filtering blood, selectively reabsorbing water, electrolytes, and nonelectrolytes, and excreting the excess as urine. The kidneys also excrete metabolic waste products (e.g., urea, creatinine, uric acid) and foreign chemicals. Finally, in addition to these regulatory and excretory functions, the kidneys secrete renin (important in the regulation of blood pressure), the active form of vitamin D_3 (important in the regulation of calcium), and erythropoietin (important in the synthesis of red blood cells). When the kidneys fail to perform these vital functions, a condition known as uremia or end-stage renal disease (ESRD) results. The continuing development of dialysis and renal transplants as a treatment for ESRD since the 1960s and federal financing of treatment since 1973 have provided alternatives to almost certain death.

Part Eight focuses on acute and chronic renal failure. ESRD is a major cause of morbidity and mortality in the United States. Almost 1 person in 10,000 annually in the United States develops ESRD. The number of people living with ESRD has increased dramatically since the early 1970s. In 1989 it was estimated that 202,000 people had a diagnosis of ESRD in the United States (US Renal Data System, 1991), and the number is expected to rise to 240,000 by the year 2000 (Levinsky, Rettig, 1991). In 1990 ESRD costs totaled about $7.3 billion, of which the federal government paid about 72% through the Medicare ESRD program (US Renal Data System, 1993). Approximately 41,000 people receive a renal transplant annually, and the remainder receive some form of intermittent dialysis treatment. ESRD is the largest categoric chronic disease program in many states. Acute renal failure is a common clinical problem characterized by a relatively abrupt decline in renal function. Approximately 5% of all hospitalized patients develop acute renal failure, and the majority of cases are

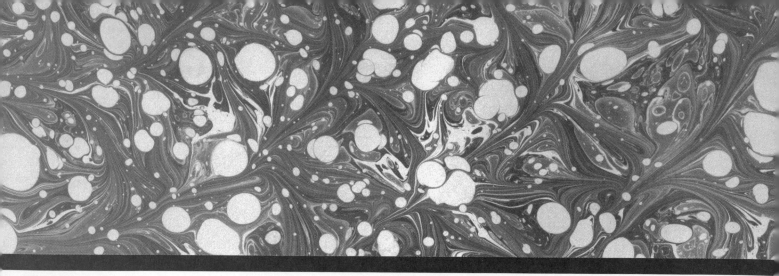

related to surgery or trauma. Mortality for acute renal failure varies between 30% and 60%, depending on the underlying medical condition.

An understanding of normal renal structure and function is essential for understanding renal failure, and this is the topic of discussion in Chapter 44. Chapter 45 discusses the means of detecting renal disease. The cause and pathophysiology, consequences, and treatment of chronic renal failure are discussed in Chapters 46, 47, and 48. Finally, acute renal failure is discussed in Chapter 49. Chronic renal failure is discussed before acute renal failure because once the pathophysiology and treatment of chronic renal failure are understood, the principles of acute renal failure become easy to grasp. Another reason for this sequence is because acute-on-chronic renal failure is fairly common, although acute renal failure rarely becomes chronic. ▼

CHAPTER 44

Anatomy and Physiology of the Kidneys and Urinary Tract

LORRAINE M. WILSON

ANATOMY OF THE KIDNEYS AND URINARY TRACT

The kidneys perform the vital function of regulating the volume and chemical composition of the blood (and the internal environment) by selectively excreting solutes and water. If both kidneys were to fail to perform this function for any reason, death would follow within 3 or 4 weeks. The kidney's vital function is accomplished by filtering the blood plasma through the glomerulus, followed by reabsorbing the appropriate amounts of solute and water along the renal tubules. Excess solutes and water are excreted in urine through the urinary collecting system to the outside of the body. This chapter reviews the gross and microscopic anatomy of the kidney and discusses its physiologic functions.

Urinary Tract

The urinary tract consists of the kidneys, which constantly manufacture urine, and the various tubes and reservoirs necessary to carry urine to the outside of the body (Fig. 44-1).

The kidneys are bean-shaped organs situated on either side of the vertebral column. The right kidney is slightly lower than the left because it is pushed down by the liver. Its upper pole lies on the level of the twelfth rib. The upper pole of the left kidney lies at about the level of the eleventh rib.

The two ureters are tubes about 10 to 12 inches (25 to 30 cm) long extending from the kidneys to the bladder. Their only function is to convey urine to the bladder.

The bladder is a collapsible muscular bag located behind the symphysis pubis. There are three openings in the bladder—two from the ureters and one into the urethra. The bladder has two functions: (1) it serves as a reservoir for urine before it leaves the body, and (2) aided by the urethra, it expels urine from the body.

The urethra is a small dilatable tube leading from the bladder to the outside of the body. It is about $1\frac{1}{2}$ inches (4 cm) long in females and about 8 inches (20 cm) long in males. The opening to the outside of the body is called the *urinary meatus*.

Anatomic Relations of the Kidney

The kidneys lie at the back of the upper abdomen behind the peritoneum, in front of the last two ribs and three major muscles—the transversus abdominis, quadratus lumborum, and psoas major (Fig. 44-2). They are kept in position by a heavy cushion of fat. The adrenal glands are situated over the upper pole of each kidney.

The kidneys are well protected from direct trauma—posteriorly by the ribs and overlying muscles and anteriorly by a thick cushion of intestines. When they are injured, it is almost always as a result of a force acting on the twelfth rib, which rotates inward and squeezes the kidney between it and the bodies of the lumbar vertebrae.

This excellent protection from direct injury also accounts for their difficult position for palpation and surgical access. The normal-size left kidney generally is not palpable on physical examination, because the upper two thirds of the anterior surface is overlaid by the spleen.

The lower pole of the normal-size right kidney, however, may be bimanually palpated in many persons. Gross enlargement or displacement of either kidney may be detected by palpation, although this is more easily accomplished on the right.

Gross Structure of the Kidney

In the adult, each kidney is about 12-13 cm ($4\frac{7}{10}$ to $5\frac{1}{10}$ inches) in length, 6 cm ($2\frac{2}{5}$ inches) wide, and 2.5 cm (1 inch) in thickness and weighs about 150 g. The size does not vary appreciably with body fluid. A difference of more than 1.5 cm ($\frac{3}{5}$ inch) in the pole-to-pole length of a particular kidney (compared with its mate) or a change in the shape is significant, since the majority of renal diseases are manifested by structural changes in the organ.

The anterior and posterior surfaces, upper and lower poles, and lateral margin of the kidney have a convex contour, whereas the medial margin is concave because of the presence of the hilus (Fig. 44-3, *A*). Several structures enter or leave the kidney through the hilus, including the renal artery, renal vein, nerves, lymphatics, and ureter. The kidney is encased in a thin, fibrous, glistening capsule, which is loosely adherent to the underlying tissue and can be easily stripped from the surface.

A longitudinal section of the kidney reveals two distinct regions—the outer cortex and inner medulla (Fig. 44-3, *B*). The medulla is divided into triangular wedges called *pyramids*. The pyramids are interspersed with cortical material called the *columns of Bertin*. Pyramids have a striated appearance because they are made up of seg-

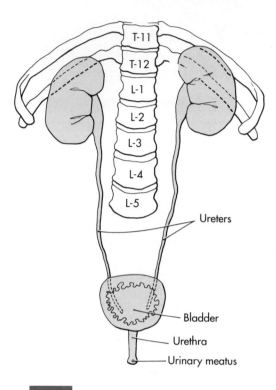

FIG. 44-1   Urinary tract, anatomic relations.

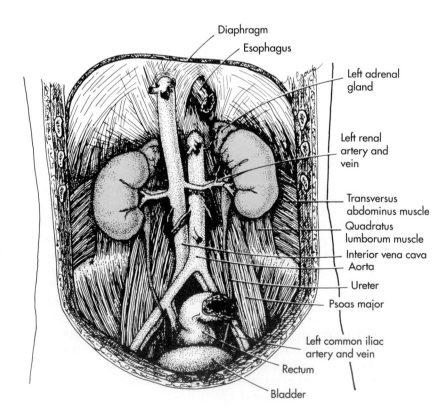

FIG. 44-2   Kidneys, anatomic relations.

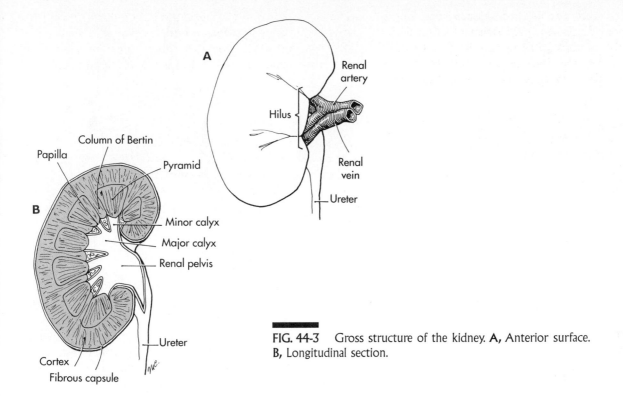

FIG. 44-3   Gross structure of the kidney. **A,** Anterior surface. **B,** Longitudinal section.

ments of the tubules and collecting ducts of the nephron. The *papilla* (apex) of each pyramid forms the papillary ducts of Bellini, which in turn are created by the terminal fusion of many collecting ducts. Each papillary duct is thrust into a cup-shaped terminal extension of the renal pelvis called a *minor calyx* (L. *calix,* cup). Several minor calyces unite to form major calyces, which in turn unite to form the pelvis of the kidney. The *renal pelvis* is the main reservoir for the renal collecting system. The ureter connects the renal pelvis to the urinary bladder.

Knowledge of renal anatomy is basic to understanding urine formation. Urine formation begins in the cortex and continues as the material flows through the tubules and collecting ducts. The formed urine then flows into the papillary ducts of Bellini, enters the minor calyces, major calyces, and renal pelvis, and finally exits the kidney via the ureter to the urinary bladder. The walls of the calyces, pelvis, and ureter contain smooth muscles, which contract rhythmically and help to propel urine along its course by peristalsis.

Gross Vascular Supply of the Kidney

The renal arteries arise from the abdominal aorta at approximately the level of the second lumbar vertebra. Because the aorta is to the left of the midline, the right renal artery is longer than the left (see Fig. 44-2). Each renal artery branches as it enters the hilus of each kidney.

The renal veins that drain each kidney empty into the inferior vena cava, which lies to the right of the midline. Consequently, the left renal vein is about twice as long as the right. Because of these anatomic features, the trans-

plant surgeon generally prefers the left kidney from the donor, which is rotated and placed in the right pelvis of the recipient. Few technical difficulties are encountered with a short renal artery that is anastomosed with the internal iliac (hypogastric) artery. The renal vein, however, must be longer, since it is implanted directly into the external iliac vein (see Fig. 48-8).

As the renal artery enters the hilus, it divides into the interlobar arteries, which pass between the pyramids to form the arcuate branches, which arch over the bases of the pyramids (Fig. 44-4).

The arcuate arteries give rise to the interlobular arterioles, which form a parallel array in the cortex. These interlobular arterioles give rise to afferent arterioles.

Each afferent arteriole supplies blood to a tuft of capillaries called the *glomerulus* (pl., glomeruli). The capillaries of the glomerulus converge into the *efferent arteriole,* which in turn subdivides into a portal network surrounding the tubules, sometimes called the *peritubular capillaries* (not shown). The blood passing through this portal network drains into a venous network to the interlobular, arcuate, interlobar, and renal veins to reach the inferior vena cava.

Special features of renal blood flow

The kidneys are perfused with blood, about 1200 ml/min—a volume equal to 20% to 25% of the cardiac output (5000 ml/min). This fact is quite remarkable when one considers that the combined weight of the kidneys is less than 1% of the total body weight.

More than 90% of the blood perfusing the kidney is distributed to the cortex, whereas the remainder is dis-

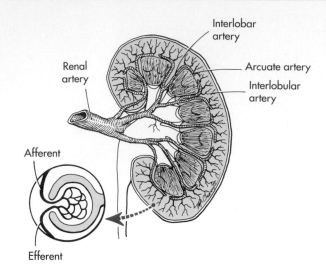

FIG. 44-4   Vascular supply to the kidney. Approximately 90% of the blood is distributed to the cortex and 10% to the medulla. *Inset* depicts the glomerular capillary tuft with afferent and efferent arterioles.

tributed to the medulla (the physiologic significance of this for urine concentration is discussed later).

Another special feature of renal blood flow is autoregulation of blood flow through the kidney. The afferent arterioles have an intrinsic capacity to vary their resistance in response to changes in arterial blood pressure, thus keeping renal blood flow and glomerular filtration constant. It is effective over an arterial pressure range of 80 to 180 mm Hg. The result is the prevention of large changes in solute and water excretion. Autoregulation, however, can be overpowered in certain circumstances, even in the autoregulatory range. The mechanisms involved in renal autoregulation are discussed later in this chapter. Renal nerves may cause vasoconstriction in states of emergency and shunt blood away from the kidneys to the heart, brain, or skeletal muscles at the expense of the kidney. Disturbances in autoregulation and the distribution of intrarenal blood flow may be important in the pathogenesis of acute oliguric renal failure (see Chapter 49).

Variations in renal vascular supply

Multiple arteries or veins can supply the kidneys (Fig. 44-5). Anomalies of the renal arteries are far more common than anomalies of the veins. In fact, about 25% or more of the population have more than one renal artery supplying a kidney. These additional arteries usually originate as small multiple branches from the aorta and supply the poles of the kidney. An arteriogram of the renal blood supply is essential in the donor before kidney transplantation is attempted because of the possibility of these variations, which may present technical difficulties for the surgeon.

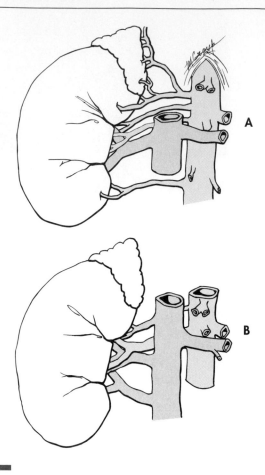

FIG. 44-5   Anomalies in renal vasculature. **A,** About 25% of the population have multiple renal arteries supplying a kidney. **B,** Multiple renal veins. (Modified from Netter FH: Kidneys, ureters, and urinary bladder. In *The Ciba collection of medical illustrations,* vol 6, West Caldwell, NJ, 1973, Ciba Medical Education Division.)

Microscopic Structure of the Kidney
Nephron

The functional work unit of the kidney is called the *nephron.* There are about 1 million nephrons in each kidney, basically similar in structure and function. Thus the work of the kidneys may be considered to be the sum total of the function of all the nephrons put together. Each nephron consists of the Bowman's capsule, which surrounds the glomerular capillary tuft, the proximal convoluted tubule, the loop of Henle, and the distal convoluted tubule, which empties into the *collecting ducts* (Fig. 44-6). A normal person can survive, albeit with difficulty, with less than 20,000 nephrons, or 1% of the total nephron mass. Thus it is possible to donate one kidney for transplantation without endangering life.

Renal corpuscle

The renal corpuscle consists of the Bowman's capsule and the glomerular capillary tuft. The term *glomerulus* is often used interchangeably with *renal corpuscle,* although it properly refers only to the capillary tuft.

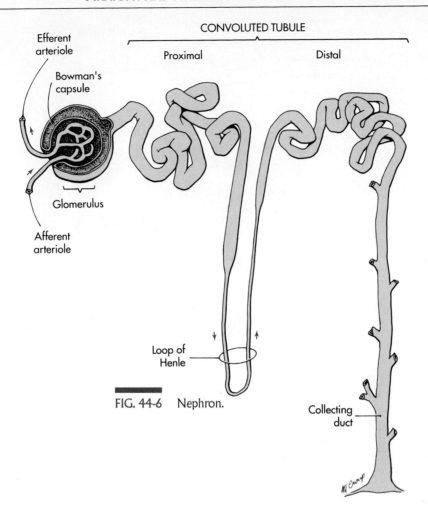

FIG. 44-6   Nephron.

Bowman's capsule is a specialized invagination of the proximal tubule (Fig. 44-7). A urine-containing space exists between the capillary tuft and Bowman's capsule called *Bowman's space,* or the *capsular space.*

Bowman's capsule is lined with epithelial cells. *Parietal epithelial cells* are flat and form the outermost part of the capsule; the much larger *visceral epithelial cells* form the innermost part of the capsule and line the outer side of the capillary tuft. Foot processes, or *podocytes,* form extensions of the visceral epithelial cells that come in contact with the basement membrane at intervals, leaving many areas free of epithelial cell contact. The area between the foot processes, usually referred to as the *slit pore,* has an average width of about 400 Å (angstrom units).

The *basement membrane* forms the middle layer of the capillary wall, sandwiched between the epithelial cells on one side and the endothelial cells on the other. The capillary basement membrane is continuous with that of the tubule. It is composed of a hydrated gel of intertwined collagenous fibers. No pores are visible in the basement membrane, although it behaves as if it had pores about 70 to 100 Å in diameter.

Endothelial cells form the innermost layer of the capillary tuft. Unlike the epithelial cells, the endothelial cells are in continuous contact with the basement membrane. However, there are numerous windowlike openings called *fenestrations,* which are about 600 Å in diameter. The endothelial cells are continuous with the endothelial lining of the afferent and efferent arterioles.

The endothelial cells, basement membrane, and visceral epithelial cells are the three layers that make up the glomerular filtration membrane. The glomerular filtration membrane allows ultrafiltration of the blood by separating the formed elements of the blood and the large protein molecules from the rest of the plasma and delivering the plasma as filtrate to the urinary space of Bowman's capsule. The discriminatory nature of glomerular ultrafiltration is a result of the unique structural arrangement and the chemical composition of the ultrafiltration barrier. The glomerular basement membrane appears to be the structure that limits the passage of solute into the urinary space on the basis of size. In addition, the filtration barrier has a negative charge owing to clusters of anion-rich macromolecules within the basement membrane and lining the epithelial and endothelial cell margins. This negative charge is why anionic albumin (which has a diameter slightly less than the smallest pore size) does not normally enter the urinary space. Larger protein molecules and blood cells do not normally appear in the filtrate and urine.

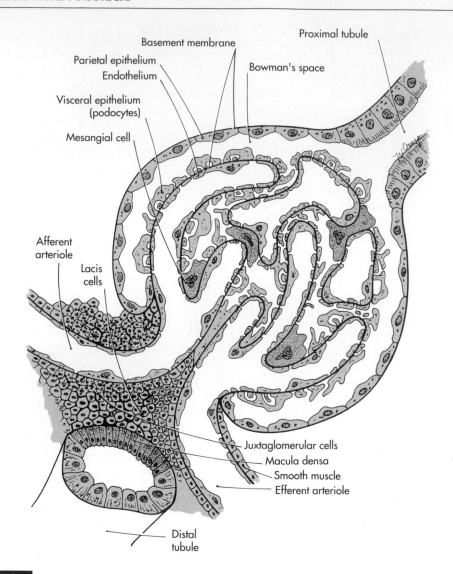

FIG. 44-7   Renal corpuscle. The glomerular capillary filter consists of three layers of cells: the endothelium, basement membrane, and visceral epithelium containing podocytes or foot processes. Mesangial cells (between the capillaries) form a supporting network for the glomerular tuft. The juxtaglomerular apparatus consists of a specialized group of cells (the macula densa and juxtaglomerular cells) near the vascular pole of the glomerulus and is important in the regulation of blood pressure. Extraglomerular mesangial cells located at the vascular pole are called *lacis cells.*

Another important component of the glomerulus is the *mesangium,* which consists of *mesangial cells* and *mesangial matrix.* Mesangial cells form a continuous network between the capillary loops of the glomerulus and are thought to function as a supporting framework. Mesangial cells are not part of the filtration membrane but do secrete the mesangial matrix. Mesangial cells have phagocytic activity and secrete prostaglandins. Because mesangial cells have contractile ability and are located adjacent to glomerular capillaries, they may have a role in influencing the glomerular filtration rate (GFR) (see above) by regulating flow through the capillaries. Mesangial cells that lie outside the glomerular tuft near the vas-

cular pole of the glomerulus (between the afferent and efferent arterioles) are called *lacis cells* (see Fig. 44-7).

Juxtaglomerular apparatus

The juxtaglomerular apparatus (JGA) consists of a specialized group of cells near the vascular pole of each glomerulus that has an important role in the regulation of renin release and the control of extracellular fluid (ECF) volume and blood pressure. The JGA consists of three types of cells: (1) the *juxtaglomerular (JG) cells* (which produce and store renin) in the wall of the afferent arteriole, (2) the *macula densa* of the distal tubule, and (3) the extraglomerular mesangial or *lacis cells.* The macula densa is a group of special-staining, distal tubular epithelial cells. These cells are contiguous with both the lacis cell compartment and the renin-secreting JG cells (see Fig. 44-7).

In general, renin secretion is controlled by both extrarenal and intrarenal factors. Two important mechanisms controlling renin release involve the JG cells and the macula densa. Either decreased wall tension in the afferent arteriole or decreased salt delivery to the macula densa in the distal tubule stimulates the JG cells to release renin from granules where it is stored within the cells. The JG cells, which are specialized myoepithelial cells cuffing the afferent arterioles, also act as miniature pressure transducers, sensing renal perfusion pressure. A decrease in the actual ECF volume or *effective circulating volume* (ECV)* results in decreased renal perfusion pressure, which is sensed as decreased stretch by the JG cells. Renin is then released into the circulation by the JG cells, which in turn activates the renin-angiotensin-aldosterone mechanism (discussed near the end of this chapter).

A second control mechanism for renin release centers in the macula densa cells, which may function as chemoreceptors, monitoring the chloride load presented to the distal tubule. Under conditions of volume contraction, less sodium chloride (NaCl) is delivered to the distal tubule (since more is absorbed in the proximal tubule); feedback from the macula densa cells to the JG cells then causes increased release of renin. The mechanism by which the chloride signal is translated into changes in renin secretion is not well understood. An increase in the ECF volume causing an increase in renal perfusion pressure and increased NaCl delivery to the distal tubule has the opposite effect of the example given of decreased ECF volume—it *suppresses* renin secretion.

Other factors influencing renin secretion include the renal sympathetic nerves, which stimulate renin release through beta$_1$-adrenergic receptors in the JGA, and angiotensin II, which inhibits renin release. Numerous other circulating factors may also alter renin secretion, including plasma electrolytes (calcium [Ca^{++}] and potassium [K^+]) and various hormones, including atrial natriuretic hormone, dopamine, ADH, ACTH, and prostaglandins. It is probable that the JGA is a site for the integration of these diverse inputs and that renin secretion reflects the interaction of all the factors.

---

*The effective circulating volume is not a measurable and distinct body fluid compartment; rather, it is related to the adequacy of tissue perfusion, that is, to the "fullness" and "pressure" within the vascular tree. ECV is made up of three components: absolute intravascular volume, cardiac output, and systemic vascular resistance. A change in any one of these three parameters without a compensatory change in the others will affect the fullness of the circulation and thus the ECV. Normally the actual ECF and the ECV parallel each other, but under some pathologic conditions (e.g., congestive heart failure) the ECV can be reduced yet the ECF volume may be increased above normal.

BASIC RENAL PHYSIOLOGY

The primary function of the kidney is to maintain the volume and composition of the extracellular fluid within normal limits. The composition and volume of the extracellular fluid are controlled by glomerular filtration and by tubular reabsorption and secretion, discussed in the following sections. The box below presents a list of renal functions that may be helpful to review at this point. These functions will be discussed again at the end of this chapter.

Glomerular Ultrafiltration

Urine formation begins with glomerular filtration of plasma. Renal blood flow (RBF) is equal to about 25% of the cardiac output, or 1200 ml/min. Assuming a normal hematocrit of 45%, renal plasma flow (RPF) is equal to 660 ml/min ($0.55 \times 1200 = 660$). Approximately one fifth of the plasma, or 125 ml/min, passes through the glomerulus into Bowman's capsule. This is called the *glomerular filtration rate* (GFR). Filtration at the glomerulus is termed *glomerular ultrafiltration,* because the pri-

MAJOR FUNCTIONS OF THE KIDNEY

EXCRETORY FUNCTIONS

Maintains plasma osmolality near 285 mOsm by varying the excretion of water

Maintains the extracellular fluid (ECF) volume and blood pressure by varying the excretion of sodium (Na^+)

Maintains the plasma concentration of each individual electrolyte within normal range

Maintains the plasma pH near 7.4 by eliminating excess hydrogen (H^+) and regenerating bicarbonate (HCO_3^-)

Excretes the nitrogenous end-products of protein metabolism, chiefly urea, uric acid, and creatinine

Serves as excretory route for most drugs

NONEXCRETORY FUNCTIONS

Synthesizes and activates hormones

  Renin: important in the regulation of blood pressure

  Erythropoietin: stimulates red blood cell production by bone marrow

  $1,25(OH_2)D_3$: final hydroxylation of vitamin D_3 to its most potent form

  Prostaglandins: most are vasodilators, act locally, and protect against renal ischemic damage

Degradation of polypeptide hormones

  Insulin, glucagon, parathormone, prolactin, growth hormone, antidiuretic hormone (ADH), and gastrointestinal (GI) hormones (gastrin, vasoactive intestinal polypeptide [VIP])

mary filtrate has the same composition as plasma with the exception of the absence of proteins. Blood cells and large protein molecules or negatively charged proteins, such as albumin, are effectively restrained by the size-selective and charge-selective characteristics of the glomerular filtration membrane barrier, whereas molecules of smaller size or with a neutral or positive charge, such as water and crystalloids, are readily filtered. Calculation reveals that 173 L of fluid is filtered through the glomerulus in 1 day—an astonishing amount in organs whose combined weight is about 10 oz. As the filtrate travels through the tubules, various substances are added to or subtracted from it so that eventually only about 1.5 L/day is excreted as urine.

The forces that account for this high GFR are entirely passive, and no metabolic energy is expended. The filtration force is a result of the pressure gradient between the glomerular capillary and Bowman's capsule. The hydrostatic pressure of the blood in the glomerular capillaries favors filtration, and this force is opposed by the hydrostatic pressure of the filtrate in Bowman's capsule and the oncotic pressure of the blood. The oncotic pressure in Bowman's capsule is essentially zero, since the filtrate is normally devoid of protein. Although never measured in humans, the glomerular capillary pressure was estimated by Pitts (1974) to be about 50 mm Hg and intracapsular pressure to be about 10 mm Hg. These estimates are based on measurements in rats. Oncotic pressure of the blood is about 30 mm Hg. Net glomerular filtration pressure is thus about 10 mm Hg. The glomerular filtration is influenced not only by these physical forces, but also by the permeability of the filtration membrane (K_f). K_f is a product of the intrinsic permeability of the glomerular capillary and the glomerular surface area for filtration. The filtration rate is much higher in the glomerular capillaries than in other body capillaries because K_f is approximately 100 times higher (173 L/day versus about 2 L/day). The balance of forces involved in glomerular ultrafiltration may be summarized as follows:

$$GFR = K_f \times \left(\begin{bmatrix} \text{Intracapillary} \\ \text{hydrostatic} \\ \text{pressure} \end{bmatrix} - \begin{bmatrix} \text{Intracapsular} & \text{Intracapillary} \\ \text{hydrostatic} & + \text{ oncotic} \\ \text{pressure} & \text{pressure} \end{bmatrix} \right)$$

$$\text{Net filtration pressure} = 50 - (10 + 30)$$
$$= 10 \text{ mm Hg}$$

The most accurate way to measure the GFR is to use a substance such as inulin, which is freely filtered at the glomerulus and is neither secreted or reabsorbed by the tubules. The clearance of a substance is the volume of plasma from which that substance is completely cleared by the kidneys per unit of time. The rate of clearance of inulin is exactly equal to the GFR. This is measured by the administration of inulin at a constant intravenous (IV) drip rate to ensure a constant plasma concentration level. Measurement of inulin concentration in plasma (P_{in}) in mg/dl, urine (U_{in}) in mg/dl, and the volume of urine (V) in ml/min permits calculation of inulin clearance (C_{in}) in

ml/min. The result must be corrected for body surface area, estimated with a nomogram that relates height and weight to body surface area. For example, if a person is passing urine at the rate of 4.2 ml/min, the inulin concentration in the urine specimen is 600 mg/dl and the plasma inulin concentration is constant at 25 mg/dl, then

$$GFR = C_{in} = \frac{(U_{in})\ 600 \text{ mg/dl} \times (V)\ 4.2 \text{ ml/min}}{(P_{in})\ 25 \text{ mg/dl}}$$
$$= 100 \text{ ml/min}$$

The calculated GFR of 100 ml/min would then be normalized by correcting it to the standard normal body surface area of 1.73 m². This correction makes it possible to compare function in persons of varying physical statures. The GFR of normal young men averages 125 ± 15 ml/min/1.73 m², and that of normal young women is 110 ± 15 ml/min/1.73 m².

Autoregulation of renal plasma flow and glomerular filtration rate

The rate of glomerular filtration is not totally dependent on the physical forces operating at the glomerular membrane. The kidney has the ability to maintain the RPF and the GFR at a relatively constant level in spite of the normal daily fluctuations in systemic blood pressure and renal perfusion pressure. This phenomenon, intrinsic to the kidneys, is termed *autoregulation.* The purpose of maintaining the GFR within a narrow range is to prevent inappropriate fluctuations in salt and water excretion. Autoregulation is effective over an arterial blood pressure range of about 80 to 180 mm Hg but may be overridden even in this range under certain pathologic conditions.

Two mechanisms are largely responsible for the autoregulation of RPF and the GFR: (1) myogenic stretch receptors in vascular smooth muscle of the afferent arteriole and (2) tubuloglomerular feedback (TGF). In addition, norepinephrine, angiotensin II, and other hormones can influence autoregulation. The glomerular capillaries differ from other capillary beds in being interposed between two (afferent and efferent) arterioles. As a result, the intracapillary hydrostatic pressure (P_{gc}) is determined by three factors: (1) the systemic blood pressure and (2) and (3) the resistances at the afferent and efferent arterioles. This arrangement allows rapid regulation of the GFR by altering the resistance in the afferent or efferent arterioles. For example, a rise in systemic blood pressure and renal perfusion pressure would be expected to increase the P_{gc} and thus the rate of RPF and the GFR. However, the increased renal perfusion pressure will be sensed by the myotonic stretch receptors in the afferent arteriole, resulting in constriction of the afferent arteriole. The efferent arterioles, however, do not directly respond to changes in stretch so do not contribute to the myotonic response. The result of afferent arteriolar vasoconstriction is a reduction of RPF, P_{gc}, and GFR, thus offsetting a large increase in GFR that would be expected with the increased renal perfusion pressure (Fig. 44-8, *A*).

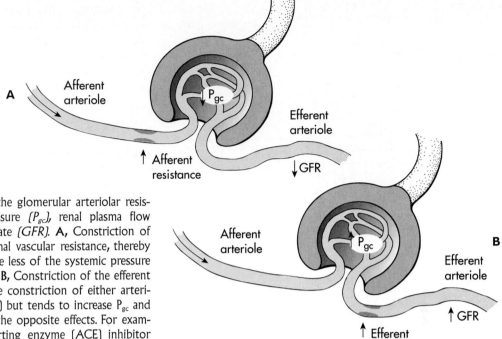

FIG. 44-8   Relationship among the glomerular arteriolar resistances, glomerular capillary pressure (P_{gc}), renal plasma flow (RPF), and glomerular filtration rate (GFR). **A,** Constriction of the afferent arteriole increases renal vascular resistance, thereby decreasing RPF, P_{gc}, and GFR (since less of the systemic pressure is transmitted to the glomerulus). **B,** Constriction of the efferent arteriole also decreases RPF (since constriction of either arteriole raises renal vascular resistance) but tends to increase P_{gc} and GFR. Arteriolar vasodilation has the opposite effects. For example, giving an angiotensin-converting enzyme (ACE) inhibitor drug, which reduces formation of angiotensin II, will reduce systemic blood pressure and P_{gc}.

On the other hand, when systemic hypotension is present, the renin-angiotensin system is activated with the generation of angiotensin II. Angiotensin II causes vasoconstriction of the efferent arteriole and vasoconstriction of the afferent arteriole, but to a lesser degree. The result is a reduction of renal perfusion pressure and RPF (because of increased afferent arteriolar resistance) and an increase in P_{gc} (because of increased efferent arteriolar resistance). The net result is that angiotensin II has counteracting effects on the regulation of GFR: the decrease in RPF will tend to reduce GFR, whereas the increase in P_{gc} will tend to increase GFR (see Fig. 44-8, *B*). Norepinephrine (released from the renal sympathetic nerves or from the adrenal cortex) enhances the vasoconstrictive effect of angiotensin II. Angiotensin II also stimulates the release of vasodilator prostaglandins (e.g., PGI_2, PGE_2) from the glomeruli, which minimizes the likelihood of renal ischemia under conditions of systemic hypotension.

The second mechanism responsible for GFR autoregulation, tubuloglomerular feedback (TGF), refers to alterations of GFR that can be induced by changes in the flow rate of fluid in the distal tubule. TGF is mediated by the macula densa cells in the distal tubule (contiguous with the glomerular pole), which are sensitive to the chloride composition of the tubular fluid. A high rate of sodium chloride in the distal tubules leads to constriction of the afferent arteriole and thus a reduction in the GFR of that nephron. According to this mechanism, the nephron itself is quite literally a feedback loop. An increase in GFR leads to increased sodium chloride delivery to the distal

nephron and hence to increased salt transfer across the macula densa cells. A reduction of the GFR follows. Conversely, if GFR is low, little salt is available for transport across the macula densa cells. The afferent arteriole dilates, and the GFR increases.

Tubular Reabsorption and Secretion

Three classes of substances are filtered at the glomerulus (Fig. 44-9): electrolytes, nonelectrolytes, and water. Some of the most important electrolytes are sodium (Na^+), potassium (K^+), calcium (Ca^{++}), magnesium (Mg^{++}), bicarbonate (HCO_3^-), chloride (Cl^-), and phosphate ($HPO_4^=$). Important nonelectrolytes are glucose, amino acids, and the metabolic end-products of protein metabolism: urea, uric acid, and creatinine.

The second step in urine formation after filtration is the selective reabsorption of filtered substances. Most of the substances filtered are reabsorbed through minute "pores" in the tubule, where they pass back into the peritubular capillaries that surround the tubule. In addition, some substances are secreted from the surrounding peritubular blood vessels into the tubule.

Reabsorption and secretion take place by active and passive transport mechanisms. A mechanism is active if it transports a substance against an electrochemical gradient (i.e., against a gradient of electrical potential, chemical potential, or both). Work is performed directly on the substance reabsorbed or secreted by the tubular cells, and energy is expended in the process. A transport mecha-

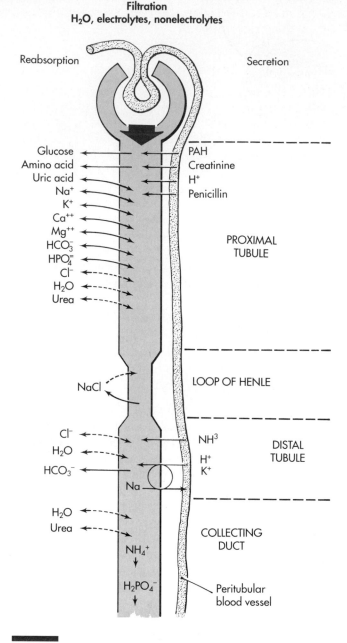

FIG. 44-9 Tubular reabsorption and secretion along the glomerular nephron. *Solid arrows* indicate active transport, and *broken arrows* indicate passive transport.

nism is passive if the substance being reabsorbed or secreted moves down an electrochemical gradient. No energy is expended in moving the substance.

Along the proximal tubule, glucose and amino acids are completely reabsorbed by active transport. Almost all the potassium and uric acid are actively reabsorbed, and both are secreted into the distal tubule. At least two thirds of the filtered sodium is actively reabsorbed in the proximal tubule. Reabsorption of sodium continues in the loop of Henle, distal tubule, and collecting ducts, so that less than 1% of the filtered load is excreted in the urine. Most

of the calcium and phosphate is reabsorbed in the proximal tubule by active transport. Water, chloride, and urea are reabsorbed in the proximal tubule by passive transport. As large numbers of positively charged sodium ions leave the tubular lumen, negatively charged chloride ions must follow for reasons of electrical neutrality. The exit of a large number of ions and nonelectrolytes from the proximal tubular fluids leaves it osmotically dilute, and as a result, water diffuses out of the tubule into the peritubular blood. Urea then diffuses passively down a concentration gradient established by the reabsorption of water. Hydrogen ion (H^+), organic acids such as para-amino-hippurate (PAH) and penicillin, and creatinine (an organic base) are all actively secreted in the proximal tubule. About 90% of the bicarbonate is reabsorbed in the proximal tubule indirectly by $Na^+ - H^+$ exchange. When H^+ is secreted into the tubular lumen (in exchange for Na^+), it combines with the HCO_3^- present in the glomerular filtrate to give carbonic acid (H_2CO_3). The H_2CO_3 dissociates to water and carbon dioxide (CO_2). Both CO_2 and H_2O diffuse out of the tubular lumen into the tubular cell. In the tubular cell, carbonic anhydrase catalyzes the reaction of CO_2 and H_2O to form H_2CO_3 once again. The dissociation of H_2CO_3 produces HCO_3^- and H^+. The H^+ is secreted, and the HCO_3^- passes into the peritubular blood along with Na^+.

In the loop of Henle, Cl^- is actively transported out of the ascending limb, followed passively by Na^+. NaCl then diffuses passively into the descending limb. This process is important for urine concentration and is discussed later in this chapter.

The selective process of secretion and reabsorption is completed in the distal tubule and collecting ducts. Two important functions of the distal tubule are the final regulation of water balance and acid-base balance. If the cells are to function normally, the pH of the extracellular fluid must be maintained within the narrow range of 7.35 to 7.45. Several biologic mechanisms working in coordination contribute toward maintaining the pH within normal limits. The principal blood buffer is the bicarbonate–carbonic acid system given by the equation:

$$CO_2 + H_2O \underset{}{\overset{\text{carbonic anhydrase}}{\rightleftharpoons}} H_2CO_3 \rightleftharpoons H^+ + HCO_3^-$$

The blood pH is given by the Henderson-Hasselbalch equation:

$$pH = pK + \log \frac{[HCO_3^-] \text{ (kidneys)}}{[H_2CO_3] \text{ (lungs)}}$$

where pK is the dissociation constant of carbonic acid. The lungs eliminate CO_2, which is produced when H^+ is buffered by HCO_3^- (left shift of the reaction above), and thus play an important role in stabilizing the pH. The role of the kidneys in maintaining acid-base balance is the reabsorption of most of the filtered HCO_3^-. When considering disturbances in acid-base balance, it should be remembered that the serum pH is largely a function of the

HCO_3^-/H_2CO_3 ratio and that the numerator is largely regulated by renal mechanisms, whereas pulmonary mechanisms regulate the denominator (through control of CO_2 elimination). A change in the numerator or denominator is followed by a unidirectional change in the other. This change, known as *compensation,* serves to protect the pH.

In addition to reabsorbing and conserving most of the HCO_3^-, the kidneys also eliminate excess H^+. About 80 mEq of acids other than H_2CO_3 is produced in the body each day. Because these acids cannot be eliminated by the lungs, they are called *fixed acids.* These acids are eliminated in the tubular fluid, so that it is possible for the urine to achieve a pH as low as 4.5 (a hydrogen ion gradient that is 800 times that in the plasma). All along the tubule, H^+ is secreted into the tubular fluid. The H^+ may then be excreted by combination with filtered dibasic phosphate ($HPO_4^=$) or with ammonia (NH_3). Thus H^+ is excreted as the titratable monobasic acid salt (NaH_2PO_4) or as ammonium ion (NH_4^+). NH_3 diffuses readily into the tubular lumen, but after combination with H^+ to form the charged particle NH_4^+, it is unable to diffuse back into the tubular cell. Because the minimum urine pH that can be achieved is 4.5, the amount of free H^+ that can be excreted is limited. Therefore the ammonium mechanism (and the phosphate mechanism) is important in eliminating an acid load, since NH_4^+ does not affect the urine pH. The buffering of H^+ by NH_3 or $HPO_4^=$ also has the effect of adding a new HCO_3^- to the plasma for every H^+ excreted into the urine. The H^+ that is secreted is derived from H_2CO_3 in the tubular cell, leaving HCO_3^- behind in equimolar amounts. In contrast, when HCO_3^- is reabsorbed from the tubular fluid by the mechanism previously described, HCO_3^- is merely conserved, since one H^+ is returned to the plasma for each one that is secreted into the tubular fluid. Therefore the regeneration of HCO_3^- (i.e., the de novo synthesis) by the buffering mechanism is very important in preventing acidosis.

Both uric acid and potassium are secreted into the distal tubule, as already mentioned. Normally about 5% of the filtered potassium load is excreted in the urine. Water reabsorption is also completed in the distal tubule and collecting ducts.

Several hormones regulate the tubular reabsorption and secretion of solutes and water. Water reabsorption depends on the presence of antidiuretic hormone (ADH). Aldosterone influences Na^+ reabsorption and K^+ secretion. Increased aldosterone causes increased Na^+ reabsorption and increased K^+ secretion. A decrease in aldosterone has the opposite effect. Parathyroid hormone (PTH) regulates Ca^{++} and $HPO_4^=$ reabsorption along the tubule. Increased PTH results in increased reabsorption of Ca^{++} and increased $HPO_4^=$ excretion. A decrease in PTH has the opposite effect.

Fig. 44-9 summarizes the major function of each part of the nephron. This selective reabsorption and secretion along the tubule enables the kidney to regulate the inter-nal body environment in a precise manner. The following discussion examines in greater detail the role of the kidney in water metabolism.

Regulation of Water Balance

The total solute concentration of body fluids is remarkably constant in the normal person despite wide fluctuation in water and solute intake and excretion. It is through the production of urine much more concentrated or dilute than the plasma from which it is derived that the concentration of the plasma and body fluids is maintained within narrow limits. When a large volume of fluids is ingested, causing dilution of body fluids, the urine becomes dilute and the excess water is rapidly excreted. Conversely, when water deprivation or excess solute intake causes the body fluids to become concentrated, the urine becomes highly concentrated so that solute is lost in excess of water. The water retained tends to return the body fluids to a normal solute concentration.

Before the processes involved in the regulation of body fluid balance can be understood, it is necessary to understand the concept of osmolality, a term used to express the concentration of body fluids.

Osmotic concentration

Osmotic concentration *(osmolality)* refers to the number of particles dissolved in a solution. When a solute is added to water, the effective concentration (activity) of water is lowered relative to that of pure water. Osmotic activity is influenced only by the relative number of solute and solvent particles and is ideally independent of the nature of the solute. Solute particles that differ in mass, shape, and charge have the same effect on the osmotic activity of the solvent, provided they are equal in number. Thus six sodium and chloride ions that are completely dissociated have the same effect on the osmotic activity as six glucose molecules in 1 kg of water even though they are quite different in mass, shape, and charge (Fig. 44-10).

Colligative properties of solutions. The addition of solute particles to a solvent lowers the vapor pressure and freezing point and raises the boiling point and osmotic pressure of the solvent. These phenomena are referred to as the *colligative properties* of solutions. All these properties depend on osmotic concentration.

Fig. 44-11 illustrates the four colligative properties of solutions. The first two colligative properties are vapor pressure lowering and boiling point elevation. When particles are added to water, it is more difficult for the water to escape from the surface, since the effective concentration of water is decreased. Consequently, pure water boils at 100° C, whereas a solution of glucose and water has a boiling point higher than 100° C.

When solute particles are added to water, the osmotic pressure is increased, which is a third colligative property of a solution. In Fig. 44-11, note that there are two glucose molecules in the left compartment and six in the right compartment separated by a semipermeable membrane. The pores in the membrane are too small to allow glucose to diffuse readily. Water, a smaller molecule, diffuses easily from the area of low osmotic concentration in the left-hand compartment to the area of higher osmotic concentration in the right-hand compartment. This process is called *osmosis*. Actually, water is moving from an area of higher water concentration (in the left compartment) to an area of lower water concentration (in the right compartment). Osmosis is thus only a special case of diffusion.

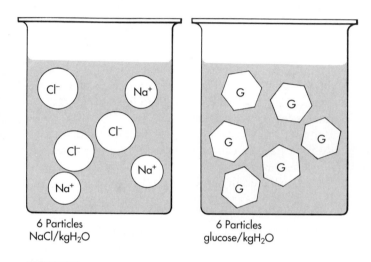

FIG. 44-10   Osmotic concentration equals the number of particles per kilogram of water. It does not depend on the mass, shape, or charge of the particles in an ideal solution.

The diffusion of water from the left to the right compartment continues until osmotic equilibrium is achieved, with the result that the fluid level is elevated in the right compartment. The force driving the water through the semipermeable membrane is called *osmotic pressure*. To prevent the water from diffusing into the right-hand compartment, it would be necessary to apply physical pressure over the solution in the right-hand compartment that would be equal to the higher potential of water in the left compartment. It is common usage to speak of the osmotic pressure of a solution, although it is virtually never measured. Several other properties of solutions vary in exact proportion to the osmotic pressure and are more easily measured (e.g., depression of the freezing point and vapor pressure lowering). In fact, even the use of the term "osmotic pressure" is rather loose, since it is commonly expressed in terms of concentration rather than pressure (see below).

The principle of osmosis is basic to the movement of water between compartments in the body. This principle is also applied in dialysis by putting high concentrations of glucose in the dialysis bath to facilitate the removal of excess fluid that accumulated while the kidneys were not functioning adequately.

The fourth colligative property of a solution is the freezing point depression. Particles added to water cause the solution to have a lower freezing point than that of pure water, which freezes at 0° C.

Measurement of osmotic concentration. Two common methods measure the osmotic concentration of body fluids. The freezing point depression as measured by the osmometer is a true measure of osmotic concentration, but

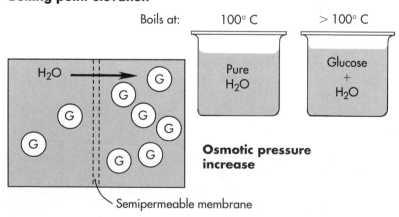

FIG. 44-11   Colligative properties of solutions. *G*, Glucose molecule.

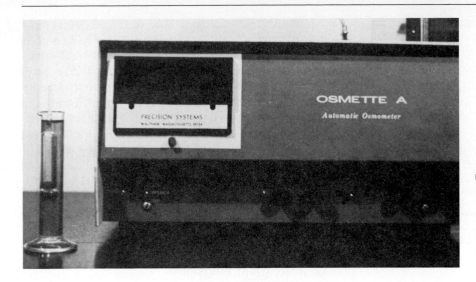

FIG. 44-12 Osmometer and urinometer. The osmometer measures the freezing point depression of a solution used to calculate osmolality. The urinometer *[left]* does not actually measure osmotic concentration but rather the density of a solution.

the measuring procedure is complex and must be carried out in a laboratory.* It is based on the principle that the freezing point of a solution consisting of 1 gram-molecular weight (mole or mol) of any nondissociated substance dissolved in 1 kg of water will be −1.86° C.† Such a solution is called an *osmolal solution,* and it contains 1 g-osmol of solute particles (i.e., the number of particles needed to lower the freezing point of water by 1.86° C). The change in temperature is called the *molal freezing point constant* (K_f) and is equal to 1 osmol.

In the absence of dissociation, each molecule of solute behaves as a single particle. Therefore, since molecular size has no effect on colligative properties, 1 g-mole of albumin (mol wt 70,000) affects the freezing point of water to the same degree as 1 g-mole of glucose (mol wt 180). If dissociation occurs, as with sodium chloride, for example, and two ions are formed, each molecule has the effect of two particles. In this case, then, 1 osmol is one-half the molecular weight.

To calculate the osmotic concentration (osmolality) of a solution, it is necessary only to measure the lowering of the freezing point below that of pure water (ΔT). This number is then divided by K_f, the molal freezing point constant:

$$\text{Osmolality} = \frac{\Delta T}{K_f}$$

For example, blood plasma freezes at −0.53° C. When this number is divided by −1.86 (K_f), the calculated concentration is 285 mOsm (1 milliosmol = 0.001 osmol):

$$\text{Plasma concentration} = \frac{-0.53° \text{ C}}{-1.86° \text{ C}} \times 1000$$

$$= 285 \text{ mOsm}$$

In the healthy person, plasma concentration is 285 ± 10 mOsm/kg H_2O.

The second method of estimating concentration of body fluids is to measure the specific gravity with the urinometer (see photographs of the urinometer and osmometer in Fig. 44-12). Specific gravity is not a true measure of concentration, but because of its simplicity, it is commonly used in the clinical unit. What is actually being measured is the density (which depends on the weight of the solute particles) and not the concentration (which depends on the number of solute particles). However, estimating the concentration of urine by measuring specific gravity is fairly accurate, provided the urine has normal constituents. The correlation between the osmolal and specific gravity measurements is discussed in Chapter 45.

Osmolality versus osmolarity. In the literature and in practice the term osmolarity is frequently used in place of or interchangeably with the term osmolality when speaking of the concentrations of IV solutions or body fluids. This interchange often causes confusion. *Osmolality* is an expression of concentration in terms of 1000 g of water. Accordingly, neither temperature nor space taken up by the solids present in the solution has any bearing on the osmolality figure, and a direct comparison can be made of various body fluids with different water or solids content. On the other hand, such a comparison is not possible when concentration is expressed in terms of 1 L of solution (i.e., *osmolarity*). The amount of water in 1 L of solution is a function both of its temperature and the space occupied by the solids in solution. Inasmuch as colligative properties are determined only by the ratio of solute to solvent particles, the osmolarity of various body fluids is not directly comparable. The difference between osmolality and osmolarity is apparent in the diagram in Fig.

---

*More recently a device to measure osmotic concentration on the basis of vapor pressure lowering has been used in some laboratories. This method is more rapid and less complicated than the osmometer method.

†One mole of any element or molecular compound contains the same number of particles (Avogadro's number: 6.02×10^{23} molecules/mol) as any other.

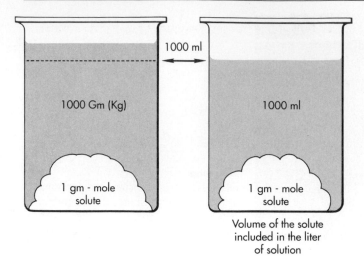

FIG. 44-13 Osmolality versus osmolarity. Osmolarity is an expression of concentration in terms of 1000 g of water. Osmolarity is concentration expressed in terms of 1000 ml of solution. Osmolality is approximately equal to osmolarity for dilute solutions when the volume occupied by the solute is small.

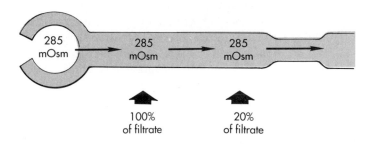

FIG. 44-14 Eighty percent isoosmotic reabsorption of the globular filtrate in the proximal tube.

44-13. To make up a 1-osmol solution, 1 g-mole of solute particles is added to a beaker with exactly 1000 g of water. The volume of the solution is thus greater than 1 L. The 1-osmolar solution is made by first adding 1 g-mole of solute particles to the beaker and then sufficient water to reach the 1-L mark. Thus the volume of the solute is included in the solution. It is obvious that the concentrations of the two solutions are not equal. The difference between osmolality and osmolarity is negligible in the range of concentration and temperature of body fluids. It is, however, important to use osmolal units of concentration in the accurate preparation of IV solutions.

It is the function of the kidneys to keep the concentration of the body fluids constant at 285 mOsm. How this is accomplished is explored in the following sections.

Isoosmotic reabsorption in the proximal tubule

When the glomerular filtrate first enters the proximal tubule, it has the same concentration as the plasma—285 mOsm. It is therefore called *isoosmotic*. Along the

proximal tubule as much as 80% of the filtrate is reabsorbed into the peritubular capillaries.* This reabsorption is isoosmotic, since both water and solutes are reabsorbed in the same proportion as they exist in the filtrate. So at the end of the proximal tubule the concentration of the filtrate is still 285 mOsm, and about 20% of the filtrate still remains (Fig. 44-14). Even though the flow has been significantly reduced (from 125 to about 25 ml/min), urine excretion directly out of the proximal tubule would be about 1500 ml/hr. At this rate of urine excretion, death would occur within a few hours from dehydration, since a loss of 12% to 14% of the body weight in water is fatal. The next step in the process of urine formation is to greatly reduce the volume of the filtrate before it is expelled as urine.

Countercurrent mechanism

In the kidney there are two types of nephrons—the cortical and the juxtamedullary (next to the medulla), illustrated in Fig. 44-15. The juxtamedullary nephron has a much longer hoop of Henle than the cortical nephron, and its peritubular blood supply is in the form of hairpin loops of vessels that dip down beside the loop of Henle. These blood vessels are called the *vasa recta*. These anatomic features of the juxtamedullary nephrons largely account for the concentration of urine. In fact, the longer the hairpin loop, the greater the concentrating ability of an animal. The kangaroo rat, a desert rodent, has unusually long loops and can excrete urine with an osmolality of about 6000 mOsm. In humans, about one of seven nephrons is juxtamedullary, with long loops, and the maximum concentration of urine is about 1400 mOsm.

The countercurrent mechanism, which is responsible for the conservation of water by the kidney, actually involves two basic processes: (1) the countercurrent multiplier of concentration in the loop of Henle and (2) the countercurrent exchanger in the vasa recta, which also takes the form of a hairpin loop. The loop of Henle makes the interstitial fluid in the medulla hyperosmotic and the tubular fluid that emerges from it into the distal tubule hypoosmotic; these changes permit the concentration of the final urine to be modified over a wide range. The vasa recta prevent the dissipation of the osmotic gradient in the medullary interstitial fluid that has been built up by the loop of Henle. Along the nephron, the fundamental processes involved in the production of a concentrated or dilute urine are the active reabsorption of chloride in the ascending limb of Henle and the variable permeability to the passive diffusion of water and urea along their concentration gradients.

First, let us examine the overall relationships during the production of a concentrated urine (Fig. 44-16). Beginning at the glomerulus, where filtration starts, the fil-

---

*Reported values of filtrate reabsorption in the proximal tubule vary from 66.6% to 87.5%, depending on the source (Pitts, 1974).

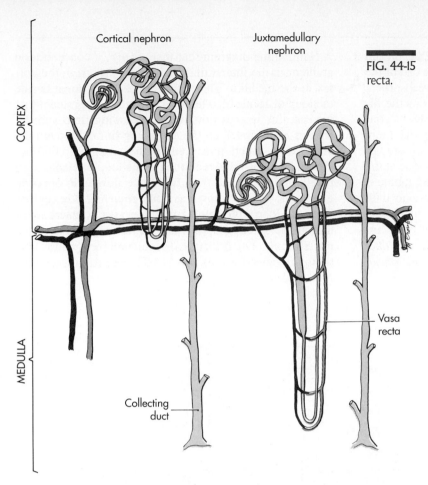

Cortical nephron   Juxtamedullary nephron

FIG. 44-15 Cortical and juxtaglomerular nephrons with vasa recta.

CORTEX

MEDULLA

Vasa recta

Collecting duct

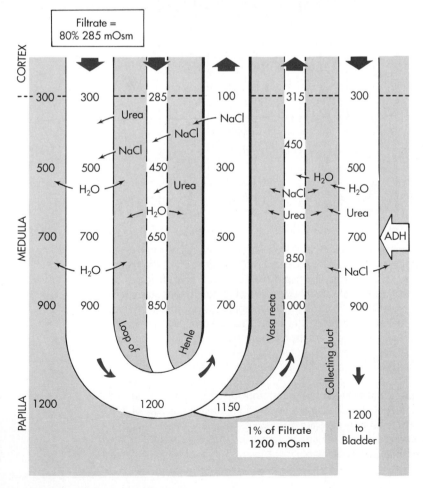

Filtrate = 80% 285 mOsm

CORTEX

MEDULLA

PAPILLA

300 — 300 — 285 — 100 — 315 — 300

Urea — NaCl
NaCl
NaCl

500 — 500 — 450 — 300 — 450 — 500

H₂O — Urea
H₂O — NaCl — H₂O
H₂O
Urea — Urea

700 — 700 — 650 — 500 — 500 — 700

H₂O
850
NaCl

900 — 900 — 850 — 700 — 1000 — 900

Loop of   Henle   Vasa recta   Collecting duct

ADH

1200 — 1200 — 1150 — 1200 to Bladder

1% of Filtrate 1200 mOsm

FIG. 44-16 Countercurrent mechanism. Summary of passive and active exchanges of water and ions in the nephron in the course of elaboration of hyperosmotic urine. Concentrations of tubular urine, peritubular fluid, and blood in vasa recta are in milliosmoles per liter. Boxed numbers represent proportion of glomerular filtrate within the tubule at each level. *ADH,* Antidiuretic hormone. [Modified from Netter FH: Kidneys, ureters, and urinary bladder. In *The Ciba collection of medical illustrations,* vol 6, West Caldwell, NJ, 1973, Ciba Medical Education Division.]

trate is isoosmotic with the plasma at 285 mOsm (rounded to 300 mOsm in the diagram). By the end of the proximal tubule, 80% of the filtrate has been reabsorbed, although the concentration is still 285 mOsm. As the filtrate moves down the descending limb of Henle, its concentration reaches a maximum at the tip of the loop. Then, as it moves up the ascending limb, the filtrate becomes more and more dilute until it is hypoosmotic at the top of the limb. As it proceeds along the distal tubule it becomes more concentrated, until it is isoosmotic with the blood plasma at the top of the collecting duct. As it moves down the collecting duct, it again becomes increasingly concentrated. At the end of the collecting duct about 99% of the water has been reabsorbed and about 1% of the filtrate is excreted as urine.

Note on the diagram that there is also a concentration gradient in the interstitial fluid, increasing from the cortex to the medulla. The vasa recta that dip down beside the loop of Henle also have a concentration gradient that increases as it goes down the descending limb and decreases as it moves up the ascending limb, although the decrease is much less than in the ascending limb of Henle. Note also that the limbs of the loop of Henle form parallel columns and that the filtrate flow is in opposite directions. This is known as *countercurrent flow* and allows the loop of Henle to function as a countercurrent multiplier, building up the concentration gradient in the interstitium. (The principle of countercurrent multiplication is reviewed in Fig. 44-17.) The entire process may now be described in greater detail.

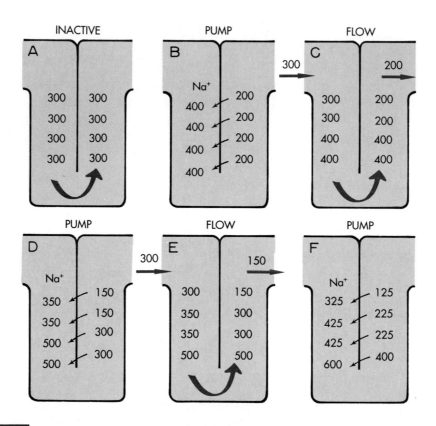

FIG. 44-17   Principle of countercurrent multiplication of concentration is based on the assumption that at any level along the loop of Henle, a gradient of 200 mOsm can be achieved between the limbs by active transport of chloride and passive diffusion of sodium ions. The changes in the concentration along the loop are illustrated in a series of discontinuous steps. *Step A:* multiplier not active, filtrate enters at 300 mOsm. *Step B:* flow stopped, ion pump activated, generating a horizontal gradient of 200 mOsm between the limbs. *Step C:* flow started, more filtrate enters at 300 mOsm, pushing some fluid around the tip from the descending to ascending limb; some fluid is ejected. *Step D:* flow stopped, ion pump activated, generating another gradient of 200 mOsm between the limbs. *Step E:* more filtrate enters at 300 mOsm, pushing filtrate around the tip from descending to ascending limb. *Step F:* flow stopped; ion pump activated, generating another gradient of 200 mOsm between the limbs; note that the concentration of the filtrate at the tip of the loop is now 600 mOsm, and there is a longitudinal gradient of 275 mOsm, whereas the ion pump was only able to generate a horizontal gradient of 200 mOsm. Continuation of this process further increases the longitudinal gradient. (Modified from Pitts RF: *Physiology of the kidney and body fluids,* ed 3, Chicago, 1974, Mosby.)

The operation of the countercurrent multiplier in the loop of Henle is initiated by the active transport of chloride out of the ascending limb. This causes sodium to passively follow down the potential gradient created by the active chloride transport. Water, however, cannot passively follow the sodium chloride transport, since the ascending limb is impermeable to water (indicated by the heavy lines in Fig. 44-16). Consequently, the filtrate becomes hypoosmotic as the top of the ascending limb is approached. The interstitial fluid becomes more concentrated, setting up an osmotic gradient between the interstitial fluid and the descending limb of Henle. Water flows out of the descending limb and sodium chloride passively enters, causing the filtrate to become increasingly concentrated. As this process continues, a concentration gradient increasing from cortex to medulla is established in the descending limb of Henle and the interstitium until a steady state is reached.

The vasa recta, which dip down beside the loop of Henle, act as a countercurrent exchanger by passive diffusion (active transport is not involved). The blood in the vasa recta is in osmotic equilibrium with the interstitial fluid. As blood flows through the descending limb of the vasa recta, sodium chloride passively moves in and water moves out, causing the blood to become increasingly concentrated as it approaches the tip of the loop. In the ascending limb of the vasa recta, opposite events occur. Sodium passively diffuses out into the interstitium while water is reabsorbed into the blood vessel and is returned to the general circulation. The fact that the blood flow through the vasa recta is sluggish allows it to act as an efficient exchanger (recall that the medulla receives only 10% of the blood supply to the kidney). If the blood flow were rapid, the sodium chloride that entered the descending limb would be washed away. Thus the vasa recta, acting as a countercurrent exchanger, prevent the dissipation of the concentration gradient in the interstitium built up by the loop of Henle, which acts as a countercurrent multiplier of concentration.

Along the distal tubule, sodium (chloride) is actively reabsorbed. Under conditions of antidiuresis, the hypoosmotic filtrate at the beginning of the distal tubule becomes isoosmotic by the time it reaches the top of the collecting duct. The final concentration of urine takes place in the distal tubule and collecting ducts under the control of antidiuretic hormone (ADH). The distal tubule and collecting ducts are permeable to water in the presence of ADH. Water diffuses out into the interstitium in response to the osmotic gradient in the medulla and then enters the ascending limb of the vasa recta and is returned to the general circulation. The final urine produced is low in volume and high in osmotic concentration.

In contrast, under conditions of diuresis and in the absence of ADH, the distal tubule and collecting ducts are virtually impermeable to water. Sodium (chloride) is actively reabsorbed from the distal tubule and collecting ducts, but water does not diffuse out to maintain osmotic equilibrium. Because sodium is reabsorbed and water is left behind, a large volume of dilute urine is produced.

Urea also diffuses out of the collecting ducts into the interstitial fluid, where it contributes to the high osmotic concentration in the medulla. Some of the urea also enters the descending limb of the loop of Henle and the vasa recta and is recirculated. The effect is to trap urea in the medullary interstitium. A person on a low-protein diet is unable to concentrate urine as well as a person on a normal diet or high-protein diet, since urea is the end-product of protein metabolism.

ADH mechanism for the regulation of plasma osmolality

The ADH mechanism helps maintain the volume and osmolality of the extracellular fluid (ECF) at a constant level by controlling the final volume and osmolality of the urine (see also Chapter 20). Deviations of the ECF volume or osmolality from normal values control the release of ADH. ADH is produced in the supraoptic nuclei of the hypothalamus and descends along nerve fibers to the posterior pituitary, where it is stored for subsequent release. ADH is controlled by a feedback mechanism with two pathways (Fig. 44-18).

ADH release is stimulated by an increase in the ECF osmolality (from the ideal 285 mOsm) or a decrease in ECF volume. Increased osmolality or decreased ECF volume, for example, may be caused by factors such as water deprivation; fluid loss from vomiting, diarrhea, burns, or sweating; or displacement of fluid as in ascites. The subjective feeling of thirst is also stimulated by a decrease in ECF volume or an increase in ECF osmolality. For example, increased thirst is a common symptom in a person who is hemorrhaging (decreased ECF volume) or in the person who has just eaten a candy bar (increased ECF osmolality because of more glucose particles in the blood).

Osmoreceptor cells located in the hypothalamus near the supraoptic nuclei sense as little as a 1% to 2% change in the osmolality of the blood in the internal carotid circulation. Neuronal signals from the osmoreceptor then stimulate the release of ADH from the pituitary gland and simultaneously stimulate thirst. The centers that mediate thirst are located in the hypothalamus. Actions of ADH in the kidney augment the key events that occur in the loop of Henle by two related mechanisms: (1) blood flow through the vasa recta of the medulla is diminished by the presence of ADH, thus minimizing solute depletion in the interstitium; and (2) ADH increases the permeability of the collecting ducts, so that more water diffuses out to equilibrate with the hyperosmotic interstitial fluid. The net effect of these two mechanisms is increased water reabsorption and excretion of a small volume of concentrated urine. Drinking water and conservation of water by the kidneys both aid in the restoration of the ECF osmolality to normal.

When the ECF volume is reduced by about 10%, wa-

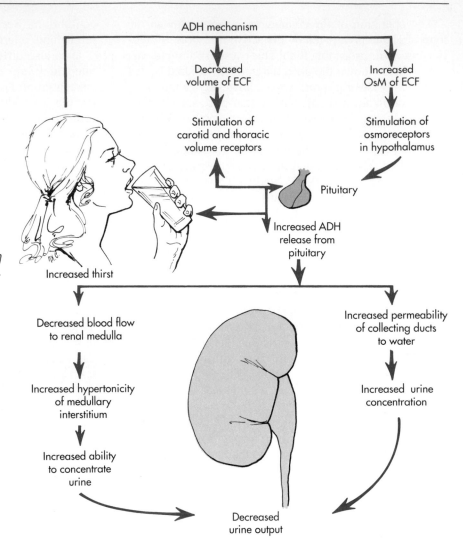

FIG. 44-18 Antidiuretic hormone *(ADH)* mechanism for the regulation of plasma osmolality. *ECF,* Extracellular fluid.

ter repletion is activated as a means of restoring ECF volume regardless of ECF osmolality. In this case, baroreceptors in the arterial and venous circulations stimulate ADH release through neuronal pathways. This nonosmotic stimulation of ADH occurs independently of osmoreceptor function. Thirst is also stimulated but is probably mediated through angiotensin II (see below). The ECF volume stimulus for ADH release can override the osmotic stimuli, so that significant ECF volume depletion is a cardinal cause of hyponatremia.

Conversely, low ECF osmolality or volume expansion from increased water intake activates mechanisms that counterregulate water conservation. Thirst is suppressed, and ADH release is inhibited. PGE_2, a prostaglandin produced in the kidney, inhibits the action of ADH on the collecting ducts. The net effect of these processes is decreased water intake and the excretion of a greater volume of dilute urine.

Even in extreme cases of a huge volume of fluid ingestion or of limited fluid intake, normal humans have amazing flexibility in maintaining the osmolality of the ECF at a constant 285 mOsm. To accomplish this, hu-

mans are able to excrete urine as dilute as 40 mOsm or as concentrated as 1200 to 1400 mOsm. As will be shown later, the patient with renal insufficiency loses this great flexibility.

Regulation of Body Sodium Content
Renin-angiotensin-aldosterone system

Regulation of the effective circulating volume or ECF volume is achieved primarily through the modification of urinary Na^+ excretion in contrast to the regulation of ECF osmolality, which is achieved through alterations of water balance. Na^+ handling is not directly involved in osmoregulation unless there are also concurrent changes in volume. Osmolality is determined by the ratio of solutes (mostly Na^+ and K^+ salts) to water, whereas the ECF volume is determined by the absolute amounts of Na^+ and water present. The renin-angiotensin-aldosterone mechanism plays a major role in regulation of body Na^+ content.

Renin is the first enzyme in the biochemical cascade of the renin-angiotensin-aldosterone system. The function

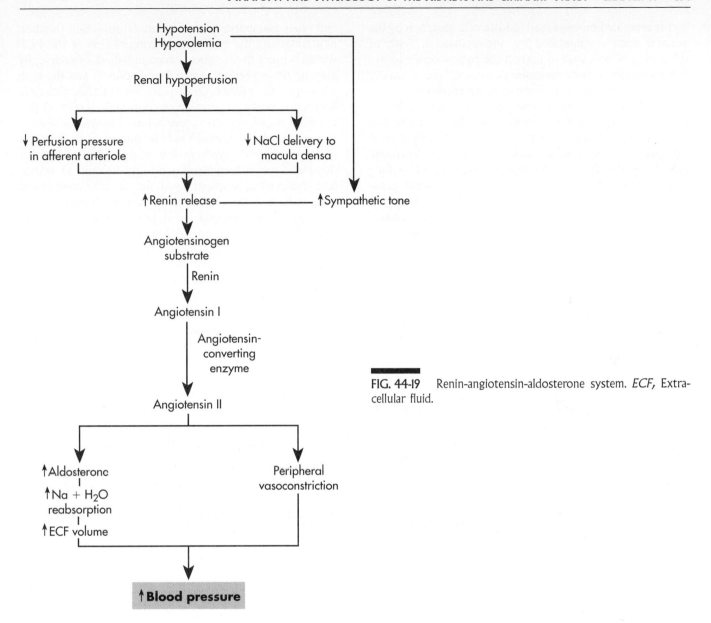

FIG. 44-19   Renin-angiotensin-aldosterone system. *ECF,* Extracellular fluid.

of this system is maintenance of ECF volume and tissue perfusion pressure by altering vascular resistance and renal Na^+ and water excretion. Renal hypoperfusion, produced by hypotension and volume depletion, and increased sympathetic activity are the major stimuli to renin secretion, as shown on the top of the diagram in Fig. 44-19. Input from the JGA of the nephron, which serves as an intrarenal baroreceptor and a chemoreceptor of distal tubular Na^+ delivery, was described previously. Input to the central nervous system (CNS) is provided by centrally located baroreceptors via the vagus and glossopharyngeal nerves, which in turn influence sympathetic outflow: baroreceptors located within the low-pressure cardiac atria and pulmonary vasculature respond primarily to the volume or fullness of the vascular tree. Increased intravascular volume distends the cardiac atria and leads to a decrease in renal sympathetic activity and the release of atrial natriuretic peptide (see below); these

both increase renal Na^+ excretion. Decreased intravascular volume has the opposite effect. Baroreceptors located within the high-pressure aortic arch and carotid sinus respond primarily to arterial blood pressure. A decline in blood pressure produces an increase in renal sympathetic activity, leading to Na^+ and water retention. An increase in intravascular pressure has the opposite effect.

The release of renin from the JG cells into the circulation initiates a sequence of events that begins with cleavage of the substrate angiotensinogen (a serum glycoprotein produced by the liver) into angiotensin I. Angiotensin I is then converted into angiotensin II by angiotensin-converting enzyme (ACE) found in high concentration in the lungs but also present in a variety of sites, including the kidney. Once generated, angiotensin II has two major systemic effects: arteriolar vasoconstriction and enhanced renal Na^+ and water reabsorption by the distal tubules and collecting ducts. The second effect is mediated by increased aldosterone secretion by the adrenal cortex, stimulated by angiotensin II. Both of these actions will tend to correct the hypovolemia or hypotension (thus restoring tissue perfusion) that is usually responsible for the stimulation of renin secretion.

The cardiac atria possess an additional mechanism for the control of renal Na^+ excretion and ECF volume that is counterregulatory to the renin-angiotensin-aldosterone mechanism. The cardiac atria synthesize a hormone called *atrial natriuretic hormone* (ANP), which is then stored in granules. ANP is released from the atrial granules in response to stretch (i.e., increased ECF volume). ANP induces Na^+ and water excretion by the kidneys. This diuretic effect is mediated by its vasodilatory properties resulting in enhanced renal blood flow and its suppressive action on aldosterone and ADH secretion.

Functions of the Kidney

The major functions of the kidneys are summarized in the box on p. 659, which emphasizes their regulatory role in the body. Vander (1991) summarized the function of the kidneys when he said, "This regulatory role is obviously quite different from the popular conception of the kidneys as glorified garbage-disposal units which rid the body of assorted wastes and poisons." The kidneys do excrete certain foreign chemicals (e.g., drugs), hormones,

and other metabolites, but their most important function is maintaining the volume and composition of the ECF within normal limits. This is accomplished, of course, by varying the excretion of water and solutes, and the high filtration rate allows great precision in this function. Renin and erythropoietin production and vitamin D metabolism are all important nonexcretory functions. Excessive renin secretion, which may be important in the cause of some forms of hypertension, is discussed in Chapter 46. Deficiency of erythropoietin and vitamin D activation, believed to be important in the cause of anemia and bone disease in uremia, are discussed in Chapter 47.

The kidneys also play an important role in degradation of insulin and production of a group of compounds of possible endocrine significance—the prostaglandins. About 20% of the insulin produced by the pancreas is degraded by the renal tubular cells. Consequently, diabetic patients with renal failure may require less insulin. Prostaglandins (PG) are unsaturated fatty acid hormones present in many tissues of the body. The renal medulla produces PGA_2 and PGE_2, which are potent vasodilators. Prostaglandins may play a role in the regulation of renal blood flow, renin release, and Na^+ reabsorption. It is also possible that prostaglandin deficiency may contribute to some forms of secondary renal hypertension, although there is insufficient evidence of this at present.

? QUESTIONS

▼ *Label the figures with the appropriate terms from each group.*

1. The urinary tract (Fig. 44-20).
   Urinary meatus
   Right kidney
   Left kidney
   Ureter
   Bladder
   Uretha

2. Posterior abdominal wall, vertebrae, and ribs (Fig. 44-21).
   Eleventh rib
   Twelfth rib
   Psoas major muscle
   Transversus abdominis muscle

3. Cross section of the kidney (Fig. 44-22).
   Pyramid
   Ureter
   Renal pelvis
   Papilla
   Cortex
   Minor calyces
   Major calyx
   Fibrous capsule
   Medulla
   Column of Bertin

4. The nephron (Fig. 44-23).
   Proximal convoluted tubule
   Distal convoluted tubule
   Collecting duct
   Loop of Henle
   Bowman's capsule
   Macula densa
   Juxtaglomerular cells
   Afferent arteriole
   Efferent arteriole
   Glomerular capillary tuft

5. On the diagram for question 2, draw the kidneys in their correct relation to the ribs and vertebrae.

6. Trace the formation and transit of urine from the renal cortex to the bladder by lettering the following structures in sequence.
   _____ Ureter
   _____ Renal pelvis
   _____ Collecting ducts
   _____ Bowman's capsule
   _____ Proximal convoluted tubule
   _____ Bladder
   _____ Minor calyces
   _____ Distal convoluted tubule

   _____ Major calyces
   _____ Papillary ducts of Bellini

7. This list contains the names of blood vessels supplying and draining the kidneys. Letter it in the correct sequence beginning with the blood vessels supplying the kidney.
   _____ Renal vein
   _____ Afferent arterioles
   _____ Abdominal aorta
   _____ Arcuate arteries
   _____ Inferior vena cava
   _____ Interlobar veins
   _____ Glomerular capillaries
   _____ Interlobular arterioles
   _____ Interlobar arteries
   _____ Arcuate veins
   _____ Renal artery
   _____ Peritubular capillaries (portal network)
   _____ Interlobular veins
   _____ Efferent arterioles

▼ *Answer the following on a separate sheet of paper.*

8. Why is it especially important to obtain

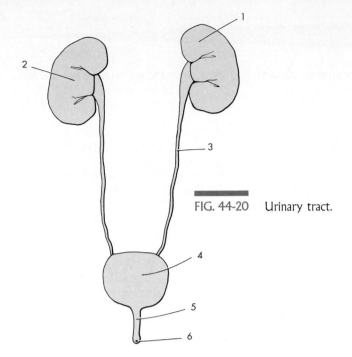

FIG. 44-20   Urinary tract.

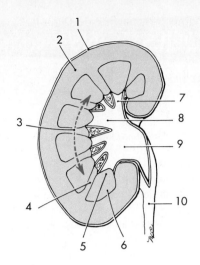

FIG. 44-22   Cross section of the kidney.

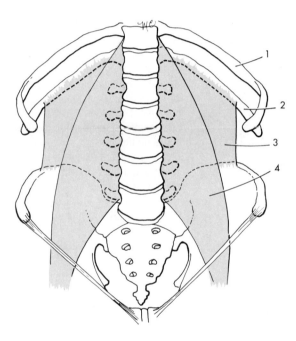

FIG. 44-21   Posterior abdominal wall, vertebrae, ribs.

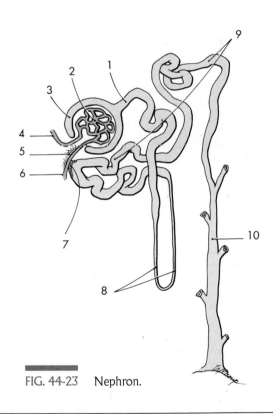

FIG. 44-23   Nephron.

a renal arteriogram in a healthy person who is supplying a donor kidney for transplantation?

9. Explain how the juxtaglomerular cells and macula densa cells help to control blood pressure.

10. Why is a heavy blow over the twelfth rib particularly dangerous to the kidney?

▼ *Match the type of renal corpuscular cell in column A with its proper description in column B by placing the correct letter in the blank.*

Column A

11. _____ Parietal epithelium
12. _____ Visceral epithelium
13. _____ Podocytes
14. _____ Endothelial cells
15. _____ Basement membrane
16. _____ Mesangial cells

Column B

a. Network between capillary loops of the glomerulus

b. Extensions of visceral cells in contact with basement membrane

c. Layer that separates epithelial from endothelial cells

d. Flat cells, outermost part of capsule

e. Innermost layer of capillary tuft containing fenestrations

f. Large cells that line the outside of the capillary tuft

Continued.

▼ *Circle the letter preceding each item below that correctly completes the statement. Only one answer is correct.*

17. The glomerular filtration membrane is composed of all the following cell layers except:
    a. Endothelial cells
    b. Basement membrane
    c. Visceral epithelium
    d. Mesangial cells

18. Factors that are important in preventing protein molecules from leaking through the glomerular filtration membrane include:
    a. Size of the smallest pores in the glomerular filtration barrier effectively restricts filtration of protein molecules
    b. Negative surface charge of the glomerular filtration barrier
    c. Negative surface charge of protein molecules
    d. All of the above
    e. Only a and b

19. Pole-to-pole length of the normal-sized kidney is about:
    a. 6-7 cm (2⅖ to 2⅘ inches)
    b. 9-10 cm (3½ to 4 inches)
    c. 12-13 cm (4⁷⁄₁₀ to 5¹⁄₁₀ inches)
    d. 16-19 cm (6³⁄₁₀ to 7½ inches)

20. The normal-sized kidney that is not generally palpable during physical examination is the:
    a. Right
    b. Left

21. The minimal number of nephrons needed to sustain life is about:
    a. 2 million   c. 200,000
    b. 1 million   d. 20,000

22. All of the following are components of the juxtaglomerular apparatus (JGA) *except:*
    a. Renin-producing granular cells
    b. Macula densa cells
    c. Angiotensin-producing cells
    d. Extraglomerular mesangial (lacis) cells

23. The proportion of the cardiac output normally delivered to the kidneys is:
    a. 90%   c. 25%
    b. 50%   d. 10%

24. The cortex/medulla ratio of blood distribution in the kidney is normally about:
    a. 9:1   c. 1:1
    b. 1:9   d. 1:3

▼ *Answer the following on a separate sheet of paper.*

25. Why is glomerular filtration called ultra-filtration?

26. How is net filtration pressure derived?

27. Define and give the normal numerical value of the GFR for men and women.

28. What kind of substance must be used to measure the GFR, and why?

29. During an inulin clearance test, the following values were obtained from a patient: concentration of inulin in plasma 25 mg/dl and in urine 500 mg/dl; urine volume 2 ml/min. Calculate this patient's GFR ignoring body surface area. Is it within normal range?

30. What are the two most important functions of the distal tubule and collecting ducts?

31. Explain how the kidneys and lungs work together in the regulation of acid-base balance in the body.

32. How do phosphate excretion and ammonia secretion contribute to the excretion of acid by the kidney?

33. List the major functions of the kidney.

34. How are the four colligative properties of a solution affected by the addition of particles to water?

35. What does the osmometer measure? the urinometer? Which is the most accurate in estimating concentration and why?

36. Write the formula to calculate plasma osmotic concentration from the freezing point. Given that plasma freezes at $-0.53°$ C, calculate the concentration of plasma in milliosmols.

37. Draw a cortical and juxtamedullary nephron, illustrating their position in relation to the cortex and medulla.

38. What are the vasa recta and what do they do?

39. What is the purpose of the countercurrent mechanism? What are the two basic processes involved?

▼ *Circle the letter preceding each item below that correctly completes the statement. Only one answer is correct, with exceptions noted.*

40. The forces that determine the glomerular filtrate are:
    a. Hydrostatic pressure of the blood in the glomerulus
    b. Plasma protein concentration
    c. Hydrostatic pressure of the fluid in Bowman's capsule
    d. All of the above

41. Tubular secretion involves the movement of substances:
    a. From the peritubular capillaries into the tubular lumen
    b. From the tubular lumen into the peritubular capillaries
    c. From the glomerular capillaries into the tubular lumen
    d. From the tubular lumen into the bladder

42. Normal renal plasma flow is about:
    a. 1200 ml/min   c. 125 ml/min
    b. 660 ml/min   d. 1 ml/min

43. The fraction of plasma filtered by the glomerulus (filtration fraction) is:
    a. 100%   c. 20%
    b. 50%   d. 1%

44. In humans, the most exact measurement of GFR is the:
    a. Endogenous creatinine clearance test
    b. Exogenous creatinine clearance test
    c. Inulin clearance test
    d. Urea clearance test
    e. Combined creatinine and urea clearance test

45. Autoregulation of renal circulation and GFR:
    a. Is localized almost entirely in the afferent arterioles
    b. Is dependent on blood hormones
    c. Is dependent on intrinsic nerves
    d. Resides wholly within the kidney
    e. Is effective over a blood pressure range of about 80 to 180 mm Hg

46. Mechanisms responsible for renal autoregulation include:
    a. Myogenic stretch receptors in vascular smooth muscle cells of the afferent arteriole
    b. Tubuloglomerular feedback responsive to flow rate of fluid in the distal tubule
    c. Osmoreceptors in the central nervous system
    d. Aldosterone secretion

47. According to the tubuloglomerular feedback theory, an increase in the flow of tubular fluid delivered to the macula densa will result in:
    a. A decrease in the GFR of the same nephron
    b. An increase in renal blood flow
    c. Activation of the renal sympathetic nerves
    d. An increase in solute and water reabsorption by the proximal tubule

48. Constriction of the afferent arteriole, induced by the myogenic mechanism in response to an increase in renal perfusion pressure, causes:
    a. Decreased renal plasma flow (RPF)
    b. Decreased glomerular capillary pressure (P_{gc})
    c. Decrease in GFR induced by myogenic mechanism
    d. Decrease in GFR induced by tubuloglomerular feedback

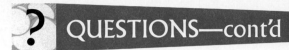

e. All of the above

49. The adaptive value of renal autoregulation is:
   a. Increase in the total renal blood flow in response to hypotensive shock
   b. Decrease in renal cortical blood flow in response to hypotensive shock
   c. Increase in renal medullary blood flow in cases of dehydration shock
   d. Increase in sodium and water retention in severe cases of hypertension
   e. Prevention of large changes in solute and water excretion in response to fluctuations in mean arterial pressure

50. Substances normally filtered by the glomerulus include all of the following except:
   a. Electrolytes   d. Blood cells
   b. Nonelectrolytes   e. Proteins
   c. Water

51. The type of transport involving the movement of a substance up a chemical or electrical gradient (requiring energy expenditure) is called:
   a. Osmosis
   b. Passive diffusion
   c. Active transport
   d. Hydrostatic transport

52. In humans, nitrogen is excreted in urine as:
   a. Urea   d. Ammonia
   b. Uric acid   e. All of the above
   c. Creatinine

53. The proximal tubule passively reabsorbs:
   a. Glucose   d. Water
   b. Sodium   e. Amino acids
   c. Chloride

54. Parathyroid hormone regulates the renal reabsorption and excretion of:
   a. Potassium   c. Phosphate
   b. Calcium   d. Bicarbonate

55. Increased aldosterone secretion causes:
   a. Increased renal Na^+ reabsorption (decreased excretion)
   b. Decreased renal Na^+ reabsorption (increased excretion)
   c. Increased renal K^+ reabsorption (decreased excretion)
   d. Decreased renal K^+ reabsorption (increased excretion)

56. Which factor has the most significant effect on Na^+ reabsorption in the proximal tubule?
   a. Aldosterone
   b. Acute change in the ECF volume
   c. Glomerular filtration rate
   d. Change of renal blood flow

57. If the serum Na^+ concentration increased by 25%, which of the following has occurred?

a. Total body water has decreased by 25%
b. Total body water has decreased by 50%
c. ECF water has decreased by 25%
d. ECF water has decreased by 50%

58. Which of the following statements related to renal regulation of acid-base balance is false?
   a. H^+ secretion in exchange for Na^+ in the proximal tubule results in the reclamation of nearly all of the HCO_3^- filtered at the glomerulus.
   b. The most important site for the excretion of fixed acids is the collecting ducts.
   c. Most of the 50 to 100 mEq of nonvolatile acids produced each day is excreted as nonbuffered H^+ in the distal tubule.
   d. Most of the daily nonvolatile acid load is excreted in buffered form, usually as phosphates ($H_2PO_4^-$) or ammonium (NH_4^+) in the collecting ducts.
   e. The buffering of H^+ by NH_3^+ or $HPO_4^=$ has the effect of adding a new HCO_3^- to the plasma for every H^+ excreted in the urine.

59. The ratio of juxtaglomerular nephrons to cortical nephrons in the human kidney is about:
   a. 1:1   c. 1:7
   b. 1:3   d. 1:15

60. The osmolality of a solution depends on:
   a. Density of the particles
   b. Size of the particles
   c. Electrical charge of the particles
   d. Number of the particles
   e. All of the above

61. Osmolality is solute concentration:
   a. Per 1000 ml of solution
   b. Per 1000 g (kg) of water

62. The normal serum osmolality is about:
   a. 50-100 mOsm
   b. 100-250 mOsm
   c. 280-290 mOsm
   d. 320-340 mOsm

63. Urine is elaborated by:
   a. Glomerular ultrafiltration, tubular reabsorption, and tubular secretion
   b. Glomerular filtration alone
   c. Tubular secretion alone
   d. Tubular reabsorption alone

64. The proportion of glomerular filtrate reabsorbed in the proximal tubule is about:
   a. 20%
   b. 25% to 50%
   c. 67% to 80%
   d. 99%

65. Reabsorption of solutes and water in the proximal tubule is:
   a. Isoosmotic
   b. Hypoosmotic
   c. Hyperosmotic
   d. Active for all ions and passive for water
   e. Complete

66. Production of a concentrated urine (1200 mOsm) requires:
   a. The presence of ADH
   b. Active chloride reabsorption in the ascending limb of Henle
   c. Medullary hyperosmolality of at least 1200 mOsm
   d. Collecting duct responsive to ADH
   e. All of the above

67. Urine concentration is increased under all of the following conditions except:
   a. Presence of a long loop of Henle
   b. Presence of ADH
   c. An increase in medullary blood flow
   d. Delivery of a relatively small volume of fluid from the proximal tubule into the loop of Henle

68. In water diuresis:
   a. The chloride pump continues to operate in the ascending limb of Henle
   b. The chloride pump does not operate in the ascending limb of Henle
   c. The distal tubule is highly permeable to water
   d. The collecting duct is highly permeable to water

69. The site of final concentration of urine is the:
   a. Ascending limb of the loop of Henle
   b. Collecting duct
   c. Distal tubule and ascending limb of loop of Henle
   d. Proximal and distal tubules

70. The countercurrent mechanism in the nephron is designed to accomplish which of the following functions?
   a. Retaining creatinine
   b. Eliminating H^+ ions
   c. Concentrating urine
   d. Increasing water loss

71. The ascending limb of the loop of Henle:
   a. Actively transports sodium
   b. Is permeable to water
   c. Is hyperosmotic
   d. Actively transports chloride
   e. Actively transports water

72. The medullary interstitial fluid in health is:
   a. Always hypoosmotic
   b. Always hyperosmotic
   c. Hyperosmotic during diuresis only
   d. Hyperosmotic during antidiuresis and hypoosmotic during diuresis

Continued.

73. Under conditions of severe water deprivation in humans, maximum urine osmolality is greater than plasma osmolality by a ratio of about:
    a. 10:1
    b. 5:1
    c. 3:1
    d. 2:1

74. Under conditions of excess water ingestion in humans, maximum renal diluting capacity results in the excretion of urine with an osmolality of about:
    a. 40 mOsm
    b. 100 mOsm
    c. 285 mOsm
    d. 1400 mOsm

75. Factors that determine the effective circulating volume include all of the following except:
    a. Intravascular volume
    b. Systemic vascular resistance
    c. Cardiac output
    d. Heart rate

76. ADH is synthesized:
    a. By the liver and released into the circulation
    b. By the juxtaglomerular cells and released into the renal circulation
    c. By hypothalamic nuclei and stored in the posterior pituitary
    d. By the macula densa cells and released into tubular fluid

77. ADH release is stimulated by:
    a. Decreased serum osmolality
    b. Increased serum osmolality
    c. Decreased ECF volume
    d. Increased ECF volume
    e. Increased urine sodium

78. Which of the following are effects of ADH?
    a. Stimulates thirst
    b. Decreases isoosmotic reabsorption in the proximal tubule
    c. Decreases blood flow in the renal medulla
    d. Decreases urine output
    e. Decreases permeability of collecting ducts to water.

79. The adaptive purpose of the ADH mechanism is to:
    a. Maintain the serum osmolality within the normal physiologic range by varying the excretion of water
    b. Maintain tissue perfusion and blood pressure by preserving ECF fluid volume by varying the excretion of sodium
    c. Maintain blood pH within the normal physiologic range
    d. All of the above

80. Renin is secreted by the:
    a. Glomerular endothelium
    b. Juxtaglomerular cells surrounding the afferent arteriole
    c. Proximal tubule cells
    d. Adrenal cortical cells
    e. Macula densa cells in the distal tubule

81. Which of the following statements about renin release from the JGA is false?
    a. A reduction in renal perfusion pressure is sensed by baroreceptors in the afferent arteriole and results in renin secretion.
    b. A decrease in the effective circulating volume increases renin release.
    c. Stimulation of renal sympathetic nerve fibers increases renin secretion.
    d. Increased delivery of NaCl to the macula densa cells increases renin secretion.
    e. Hypovolemia stimulates renin release.

82. Which of the following statements regarding angiotensin I is true?
    a. It is the most powerful vasoconstrictor known.

b. It is acted on in the lung by angiotensin-converting enzyme.
    c. It stimulates aldosterone release.
    d. An angiotensin-converting enzyme (ACE) inhibitor drug, such as enalapril (Vasotec), lowers blood pressure by blocking conversion of angiotensin I to angiotensin II.

83. All of the following are actions of angiotensin II except:
    a. Stimulates thirst
    b. Stimulates aldosterone secretion from the adrenal cortex
    c. Inhibits proximal tubular reabsorption of Na^+
    d. Causes vasoconstriction of the arterioles
    e. Stimulates release of vasodilator prostaglandins in kidney

84. Atrial natriuretic peptide:
    a. Release is stimulated by ECF volume excess
    b. Is released from cells in the cardiac atria
    c. Causes salt and water diuresis
    d. Has a suppressive action on aldosterone and ADH
    e. All of the above

▼ Match the regulating factors in column A with the correct response in column B to a sudden decrease in the effective circulating volume secondary to the loss of 800 ml of blood.

Column A		Column B
85. _____ Renin-angiotensin		a. Increase
86. _____ Aldosterone		b. Decrease
87. _____ Atrial natriuretic peptide		
88. _____ ADH		
89. _____ PGE_2		
90. _____ Sensation of thirst		

▼ Match the appropriate osmotic concentration in column B with each region of the nephron or interstitium in column A:

Column A		Column B
91. _____ Bowman's space		a. Hypoosmotic
92. _____ Ascending limb of Henle		b. Isoosmotic
93. _____ Descending limb of Henle		c. Hyperosmotic
94. _____ Proximal tubule		d. Isoosmotic or hypoosmotic
95. _____ Distal tubule		
96. _____ Collecting duct		
97. _____ Medullary interstitium		
98. _____ Cortical interstitium		

▼ Match the correct estimated pressures in column B with the proper glomerular filtration forces in column A.

Column A		Column B
99. _____ Glomerular hydrostatic pressure		a. 50 mm Hg
100. _____ Colloid osmotic pressure		b. 30 mm Hg
101. _____ Net filtration pressure		c. 10 mm Hg
102. _____ Hydrostatic pressure in Bowman's capsule		

CHAPTER 45

Diagnostic Procedures in Renal Disease

LORRAINE M. WILSON

BIOCHEMICAL METHODS

This chapter discusses some of the commonly performed diagnostic tests for the detection of renal disease and evaluation of renal function. These tests are divided into methods that are predominantly biochemical or predominantly morphologic. These diagnostic tests are especially important in the detection of renal disease, since many serious renal diseases do not produce symptoms until renal function is significantly impaired.

Chemical Examination of Urine

Chemical testing of the urine has been greatly simplified by the introduction of impregnated paper strips that detect substances such as glucose, acetone, bilirubin, protein, and blood. The pH of the urine can also be measured by a dipstick test. Of particular importance in renal disease are the detection of protein or blood in the urine, the measurement of osmolality or specific gravity, and microscopic examination of the urine (discussed later under "Morphologic Methods").

Proteinuria

Healthy adults normally excrete small amounts of protein in the urine—up to 150 mg per day—consisting mainly of albumin and Tamm-Horsfall protein. The latter is secreted by the distal tubule. Proteinuria in amounts greater than 150 mg/day is considered pathologic.

Because it is easy to use, the dipstick test (Albustix, Combistix) is the most commonly used test for proteinuria. The end of the stick is dipped in urine and removed immediately, and the urine is shaken off by tapping the stick on the side of the container. The result is compared with the color on the label. Grading is from 0 to 4+, indicating the amount of protein in the urine (see box on p. 678). Although the dipstick test is generally accurate, there are a number of pitfalls and difficulties in interpretation. Early morning samples are normally more concentrated and should preferably be tested for protein. A "trace" response found in an early morning specimen is probably within normal limits, less than 150 mg/day. On the other hand, if the urine specimen is collected later in the day and is more dilute (e.g., specific gravity 1.006), a trace response might indicate significant proteinuria. A common cause of a false-positive result in women is contamination of the urine with vaginal secretions. All routine urine examinations should include a simple test for protein for purposes of screening. More accurate quantitative tests for protein may be carried out in the laboratory on a 24-hour specimen.

Persistent proteinuria almost always indicates renal disease, especially involving the glomerulus. The direct cause of proteinuria is always an increase in glomerular permeability. Recall that the glomerulus is composed of three layers (endothelium, basement membrane, and epithelium), which have a series of pores of varying sizes. Normally, the glomerular membrane allows only proteins of low molecular weight to enter the filtrate (e.g., immunoglobulin light chains, amino acids) and restricts the filtration of macromolecules (e.g., albumin, IgG). The renal tubules then reabsorb most of these proteins, normally excreting a small amount that is undetectable on a screening test. Albuminuria is common in the various

SCREENING TEST FOR PROTEINURIA

DIPSTICK GRADE	PROTEIN CONCENTRATION (mg/dl)
0	0-5
Trace	5-20
1+	30
2+	100
3+	300
4+	1000

types of glomerulonephritis. *Heavy proteinuria* refers to the passage of 3.5 g/day or more and is the laboratory definition of the nephrotic syndrome (discussed later). Some patients with the nephrotic syndrome may pass as much as 20 or 30 g of protein per day. *Moderate proteinuria* is associated with a broad spectrum of renal diseases; *minimal proteinuria* (less than 1 g/day) is more apt to be associated with renal diseases such as chronic pyelonephritis, with less glomerular involvement.

Hematuria

The dipstick test for occult blood is an excellent screening test for hematuria. Whenever it is positive, the urine should be examined microscopically. Hematuria is a common finding in a number of renal diseases and pathologic processes in the lower urinary tract, including infections, stones, trauma, and neoplasms. Hematuria is a prominent feature of glomerulonephritis but not of pyelonephritis. The dipstick test is easy for patients to use as they check the course of hematuria during their treatment.

Hydrogen ion concentration

In the healthy adult, urine pH ranges widely from 4.5 to 8.0, but the average pooled specimen is quite acidic, at 6.0, because of acidic metabolites produced by the normal breakdown of body tissues and nutrients. The usual diurnal pattern consists of a rise of pH after a meal (alkaline tide) followed by a gradual fall until the next meal is ingested, whereas during normal sleeping hours, the pH reaches its minimum (nocturnal acid tide caused by hypoventilation during sleep). A diet high in animal protein tends to produce an acid urine, whereas a predominantly vegetable diet tends to produce an alkaline urine.

A persistently acidic urine may occur in respiratory or metabolic acidosis and in pyrexia (fever). A persistently alkaline urine is suggestive of urinary tract infection with urea-splitting organisms. For example, in *Proteus* infections, the urine pH is consistently at 8 or higher. Persistently alkaline urine also occurs in renal tubular acidosis (a renal disease in which there is inability to conserve bicarbonate), in potassium depletion, and in

Fanconi's syndrome (a renal disease in which ammonia excretion is defective).

Although random pH readings are of little diagnostic value, they are helpful in the management of certain clinical conditions in which the pH of the urine should be kept persistently high or low by diet or drugs. Alkaline urine is desirable in the treatment of patients with calculi that form in acid urine, and acid urine is desirable in patients with calculi that form in alkaline urine or who have urinary tract infections (Table 45-1).

Common stones formed in acid urine are composed of calcium oxalate, uric acid crystals, or cystine. About two thirds of all urinary calculi are of the calcium oxalate type. Idiopathic hypercalciuria is an important predisposing factor. Thiazide diuretics decrease calcium excretion and are quite effective in preventing recurrence (Coe, Favus, 1994). Cystine stones are rare and are related to a hereditary renal tubular transport disorder involving certain amino acids. Cystine, a metabolic product of dietary methionine, is the least soluble of the naturally occurring amino acids. The excess urinary excretion of cystine (cystinuria) in an acid urine results in cystine urolithiasis. Treatment of this disorder is directed toward a reversal of risk factors by forced hydration and administration of bicarbonate or acetazolamide (Diamox) to maintain the urine pH above 7.5 (Coe, Favus, 1994). Hyperuricemia leading to uric acid crystallization is a particular hazard in patients who are receiving cytotoxic drugs for cancer or leukemia. Uric acid is formed principally as an end-

▶ **TABLE 45-1   Factors Contributing to the Formation of Urinary Tract Calculi and Their Prevention**

Urinary Stone Content	Predisposing Factors	Preventive Therapy to Achieve Desired Urine pH*
	ACID URINE	ALKALINE URINE (pH >6)
Calcium oxalate	Hypercalciuria	Vegetables, milk, fruit (except plums, prunes, cranberries)
Uric acid crystals	Chemotherapy, gout	Sodium bicarbonate or citrate
Cystine	Aminoaciduria	
	ALKALINE URINE	ACID URINE
Triple phosphate	Urinary tract infection	Meat, breads, protein foods, cranberry juice, prunes, plums
Calcium phosphate	Hypercalciuria Prolonged immobility	Mandelamine

*High fluid intake is the most important preventive measure against all calculi.

product of nucleoprotein metabolism. With increasing proliferation and destruction of cells, a proportional increase in uric acid occurs because of degradation of cellular nucleoproteins. The physician may order the administration of sodium bicarbonate or citrate to alkalinize the urine. It is important to encourage a high fluid intake in these patients, especially before bedtime, when the urine normally becomes more acidic, to prevent crystallization of uric acid in the renal tubules and interstitium and consequent obstruction. Some foods that help alkalinize the urine are milk, vegetables, and fruits (except prunes, plums, and cranberries).

Common stones formed in alkaline urine are composed of calcium phosphate or magnesium ammonium phosphate (triple-phosphate or struvite stones). Calcium phosphate or oxalate is often present in triple-phosphate stones. Triple-phosphate stones are often associated with urinary tract infections, especially with urea-splitting organisms. These stones occasionally grow to occupy the entire pelvicalyceal system (see Fig. 3-11). Such a stone, referred to as a "staghorn" calculus because of its shape, must be removed surgically. Because 90% of all calculi contain calcium, hypercalciuria is an important predisposing cause. Hypercalciuria is associated with hyperparathyroidism, renal tubular acidosis, and prolonged immobilization. All are associated with mobilization of calcium salts from bone. Meat, bread, protein foods, cranberry juice, plums, and prunes tend to produce an acid urine and thus help prevent the formation of these

stones. The physician may order a drug such as methenamine mandelate (Mandelamine) to acidify the urine for persistent urinary tract infections. Probably the most important factor in the prevention of all stones regardless of composition is a high fluid intake sufficient to produce a urine output of 2.5 to 3 L/day.

The pH of the urine may be tested by using Squibb Nitrazine paper or a dipstick test. The following points should be kept in mind while performing this test: (1) only fresh urine should be used (when urine is allowed to stand, urea breaks down to ammonia and the pH becomes more alkaline); (2) the test strip should be removed promptly after being dipped in the urine to avoid washing out the test reagent; and (3) the color comparison with the standard should be made immediately in good light (daylight is preferable, and fluorescent light should be avoided).

Specific gravity

Specific gravity is commonly measured in the clinical unit to determine the concentration of urine. It is measured by the flotation of the hydrometer or urinometer in a cylinder of urine (Fig. 45-1). The proper procedure for measuring the specific gravity of urine is as follows:

1. Check the accuracy of the urinometer against distilled water to read 1.000 at its calibration temperature. Most urinometers are calibrated at a temperature of 16° C (60.8° F). This procedure is necessary, since the density of water changes with temperature.
2. Fill the cylinder about three fourths full of well-mixed urine. A uniform solution is necessary, since solute concentration is being measured.
3. Give the urinometer a gentle spin as it is plunged into the urine to avoid errors of surface tension at the stem and to prevent it from adhering to the sides of the cylinder.
4. Read from top to bottom. The urinometer is calibrated in units of 0.001, starting with 1.000 at the top and progressing downward to 1.060. The correct reading is at the level of the bottom of the meniscus, which should be read at eye level.
5. Correct the specific gravity reading if the temperature of the specimen deviates from the calibration temperature of the urinometer. Use a thermometer to determine the actual temperature of the urine. Add 0.001 to the reading for every 3° C (5.4° F) above the calibration temperature and subtract 0.001 for each 3° C below. For example, if a urinometer calibrated at 16° C is placed in a freshly voided urine specimen with a temperature of 31° C (88° F) and shows a reading of 1.015, 0.005 is added to the reading

$$31° C - 16° C = 15° C \times \frac{0.001}{3° C} = 0.005$$

The true specific gravity corrected for temperature is 1.020.

Although specific gravity measurement is simple and convenient, it is important to realize that density is being

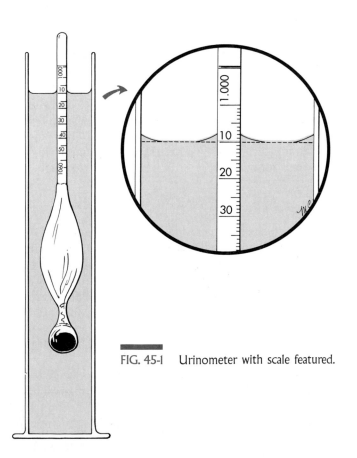

FIG. 45-1   Urinometer with scale featured.

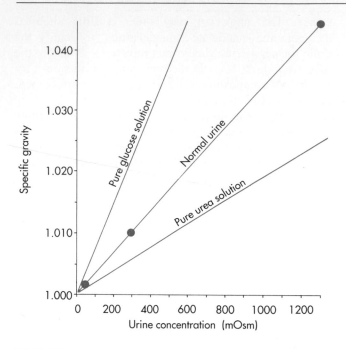

FIG. 45-2   Relationship between specific gravity and osmolality of the urine. (Modified from De Wardner HE: *The kidney,* ed 4, New York, 1973, Longman.)

measured. The density depends on the weight as well as on the number of solute particles in solution. The kidney's capacity to concentrate, however, is related to the concentration of particles in solution (i.e., osmolality) and not to their weight. True concentration, osmolality, is measured by freezing point depression or vapor pressure lowering, although this is more expensive and time consuming to measure.

Fortunately, when urine contains only normal constituents (mainly NaCl), the correlation between specific gravity and osmolality is sufficiently close to use specific gravity as a clinical guide to the osmolality of the urine. The relation between specific gravity and the osmolality of urine is shown in Fig. 45-2. When the urine contains normal constituents (middle line), a specific gravity of 1.010 corresponds to the osmolality of the blood at 285 mOsm. When given large amounts of water, the healthy person can excrete urine with a minimum specific gravity of 1.001 (about 40 mOsm). When deprived of fluid, maximum specific gravity is about 1.040 (1300 mOsm). If the urine should contain glucose or protein (dense particles), the specific gravity would be greater at a fixed osmolality than in normal urine (shifted toward the pure glucose curve); and conversely, if the urine contains much urea (a less dense molecule), the specific gravity will be lower. For example, at a concentration of 400 mOsm, the specific gravity of urine with normal constituents is about 1.013. At the same osmolality, if the urine contained a large amount of protein or glucose, the specific gravity would be about 1.030; if it contained a large amount of urea, the specific gravity would be about 1.007. These

factors must be considered when the specific gravity measurement is used to estimate the ability of the kidneys to concentrate urine.

In chronic renal disease, the kidney first loses the ability to concentrate urine. Later, the ability to dilute urine is lost as well, so that the specific gravity of urine becomes fixed near 1.010 (the specific gravity of the plasma). This generally occurs when 80% of the nephron mass has been destroyed.

Glomerular Filtration Rate

One of the most important indices of renal function is the glomerular filtration rate (GFR), which indicates the amount of functioning renal tissue. As noted in Chapter 44, the most accurate way to measure the GFR is by means of the inulin clearance test. However, this test is infrequently used in the clinical unit because it involves an intravenous infusion at a constant rate and timed collections of urine by catheterization. The endogenous creatinine clearance test is much simpler to carry out.

Creatinine clearance test

Creatinine is an end-product of muscle metabolism that is liberated from the muscles at a virtually constant rate and is excreted in the urine at the same rate. The plasma (serum) level is therefore nearly constant, ranging from 0.7 to 1.5 mg/dl (higher value in men than in women because of men's greater muscle mass). Creatinine is excreted in the urine by filtration at the glomerulus, but it is not reabsorbed by the tubules. A small amount, however, is secreted by the tubules, especially when serum creatinine levels are high. Despite the small amount secreted, the creatinine clearance test is a convenient test from which to estimate the GFR in the clinical unit. To perform the creatinine clearance test, it is only necessary to collect a 24-hour urine specimen and a blood specimen during the same 24-hour period (Fig. 45-3). Creatinine clearance (C_{cr}) is then calculated from the clearance formula:

$$C_{cr} = \frac{U_{cr}V}{P_{cr}}$$

Creatinine clearance is a fairly good index of the GFR, although it is not a true measurement, since creatinine is secreted by the tubules to some extent and the slight secretion of creatinine tends to cause overestimation of the GFR. Plasma creatinine also may be overestimated because of the difficulties inherent in the laboratory determination. Luckily, these two errors are of nearly the same magnitude and cancel each other out, so that creatinine clearance approximates the GFR.

In chronic renal disease and some forms of acute renal failure, the GFR is decreased below the normal value of 125 ml/min. GFR also decreases with advancing age: every year after the age of 30, it decreases at the rate of 1 ml/min.

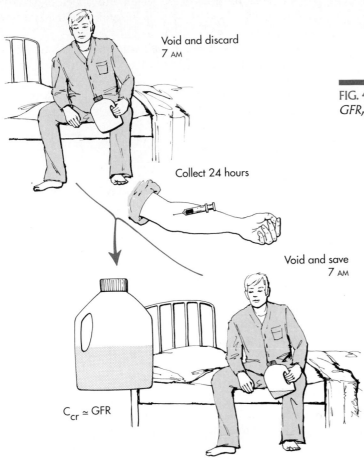

FIG. 45-3   Creatinine clearance test. C_{cr}, Creatinine clearance; *GFR,* glomerular filtration rate.

Void and discard
7 AM

Collect 24 hours

Void and save
7 AM

$C_{cr} \simeq GFR$

Plasma creatinine and blood urea nitrogen

The plasma creatinine and blood urea nitrogen (BUN) concentrations are also guides to the GFR. The normal BUN concentration is about 10 to 20 mg/dl, and plasma creatinine concentration is 0.7 to 1.5 mg/dl. Both of these substances are nitrogenous end-products of protein metabolism normally excreted in the urine. When the GFR decreases, as in renal insufficiency, the plasma levels of creatinine and BUN rise. This condition is called *azotemia* (nitrogenous substances in the blood). The level of plasma creatinine as an index of the GFR is more accurate than the BUN, since creatinine production is mainly a function of the size of the muscle mass, which changes very little. The BUN, however, is affected by the amount of protein in the diet and the catabolism of body protein. The relation of a rising plasma creatinine and BUN level to a decreasing GFR is discussed in Chapter 46.

Tubular Function Tests

A number of tests are carried out to evaluate the function and integrity of the renal tubules. The function of the tubules is selective reabsorption of the contents of the tubular fluid and secretion of substances into the tubular lumen, which are either circulating in the peritubular capillaries or are formed at the tubular cell. These processes are under the control of a wide variety of hormones, gas pressures, and plasma electrolyte concentrations. Common tests of proximal tubular function include the phenolsulfonphthalein (PSP) and para-aminohippurate (PAH) excretion tests. Distal tubular function tests include tests of concentration, dilution, acidification, and sodium conservation. The fractional excretion of sodium (FE_{Na}) is an important calculation in differentiating prerenal azotemia from acute tubular necrosis and is discussed in Chapter 49.

PSP excretion test

Phenolsulfonphthalein (PSP) is a nontoxic dye eliminated primarily by secretion into the proximal tubule. Binding of PSP to plasma proteins is so high that only about 4% is excreted by glomerular filtration. With the usual 6 mg dose, the plasma level of the dye is only about one fifth of the tubular capacity to excrete PSP. The excretion rate of PSP is therefore usually limited by the rate of delivery to the tubules via the renal plasma flow and, in severely impaired kidneys, by proximal tubular function. The 15-minute PSP test is most commonly performed (Fig. 45-4).

Thirty minutes before the PSP dye is given, the patient is asked to drink two or three glasses of water to ensure sufficient bladder urine for urination. Exactly 1 ml (6 mg) of PSP is injected intravenously, using a tuberculin syringe for accuracy. Exactly 15 minutes after the dye is given, the patient is asked to completely empty the bladder. All the urine is then placed in a 1-L volumetric flask; 5 ml of 10% sodium hydroxide (NaOH) is added, as well as enough water to bring the volume up to 1 L. A test tube of the pink, diluted specimen is then compared with the appropriate standards visually or by the use of a colorimeter. The person with normal renal function should excrete a minimum of 28% of the dye in 15 minutes.

The primary value of the PSP excretion test is in the detection of functional impairment early in the course of renal disease. Many physicians no longer perform this test and consider the creatinine clearance test alone to be an adequate assessment of renal function. The analysis of the PSP test is so simple that it can be performed without the aid of a clinical laboratory, so it might be useful in situations where such a facility is not available.

PAH excretion test

Para-aminohippurate is a substance that is filtered by the glomerulus and secreted by the proximal tubule. When given in low concentrations to humans, about 92% of it is cleared in one circulation through the kidneys. It is therefore a fairly accurate measure of renal plasma flow (RPF). In the adult, RPF is approximately 600 ml/min. If the plasma concentration is further increased until secretory capacity is exceeded, the secretory capacity of the proximal tubule can be calculated from the filtered load and urinary excretion. This test is most commonly used in research.

Concentration and dilution tests

The measurement of urine specific gravity after water restriction is a sensitive measure of the ability of the renal tubules to reabsorb water and produce a concentrated urine. Renal function is considered normal if an early morning urine specimen has a specific gravity of 1.025 or more. When concentrating ability is doubtful, a more elaborate concentration test, such as the Fishberg concentration test, may be carried out. To ensure accuracy of results, the patient must be on a normal diet (normal salt, protein, and fluid intake) and must not be taking diuretics before the administration of the test. The patient is instructed to eat a normal evening meal at 6 PM and not to take food or fluids until the test is completed the next morning. Urine specimens are collected the next morning at 6, 7, and 8 AM. At least one of these specimens should have a specific gravity of 1.025 (800 mOsm) or more (Fig. 45-5).

The urinary dilution test is performed by having the patient drink 1 L of water within 30 minutes. Urine specimens are then collected over the next 3 hours. At least one of these specimens should have a specific gravity of 1.003 (80 mOsm) or less (Fig. 45-5). The urinary dilution test is much less useful than the concentration test, since nonspecific factors, such as nausea or emotions, may in-

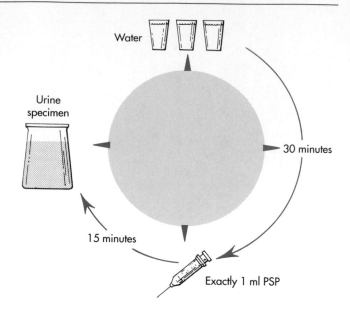

FIG. 45-4   Fifteen-minute phenolsulfonphthalein (PSP) excretion test; 28% or more of the dye normally is excreted in 15 minutes.

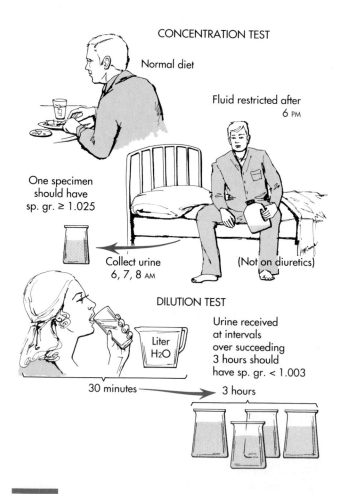

FIG. 45-5   Urine concentration and dilution tests. *sp. gr.,* Specific gravity.

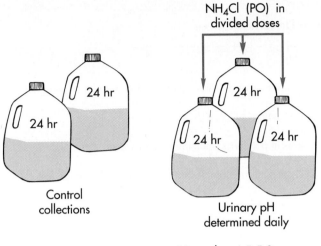

NH₄Cl (PO) in
divided doses

Control
collections

Urinary pH
determined daily

Normal = 4.5-5.3
Renal tubular acidosis >5.3

FIG. 45-6   Urine acidification test. *NH₄Cl,* Ammonium chloride; *PO,* by mouth.

terfere with water diuresis even in normal subjects. Diluting ability may be defective in adrenal insufficiency, hepatic disease, and cardiac failure. The ability to dilute urine is lost late in most renal diseases, whereas concentrating ability is lost early. Neither the concentration nor the dilution tests should be carried out on azotemic patients, since dehydration and water intoxication, respectively, could result.

Urine acidification test

The urine acidification test is designed to measure the maximum acid-excreting capacity of the kidney and is specific for the diagnosis of renal tubular acidosis.

In the 5-day test, control urine is collected for 2 days. The patient is then given ammonium chloride (about 12 g/day in the adult) for the next 3 days. The ammonium chloride is metabolized to urea and hydrogen chloride, producing acidosis in the patient. The urinary pH is determined daily, and on the fifth day ammonium and titratable acids are also measured. Normally the kidney excretes the acid load and the urine pH is 5.3 or less (Fig. 45-6). In renal tubular acidosis, a hydrogen ion gradient between the tubular lumen and the plasma cannot be maintained and a low urine pH is not achieved. Many patients with chronic renal failure can achieve a urine pH of 5.3, but excretion of ammonium and titratable acids is impaired.

Sodium conservation test

Healthy persons can produce urine that is virtually sodium free under conditions of dietary restriction of sodium. In renal disease, the ability to conserve sodium may be lost, and some patients suffer sodium depletion. If a person is losing more sodium than is ingested, the result is a contraction of the plasma volume, a decrease in

the GFR, and an accelerated course toward final renal failure. A salt-losing nephritis is more common in patients who have chronic pyelonephritis or polycystic disease. Both diseases involve primarily the renal tubules. Many patients in renal failure oscillate between states of sodium retention and depletion, so their daily intake of sodium must be defined within very narrow limits.

The sodium conservation test is sometimes used to determine how much sodium is needed in the diet of a patient with a salt-losing nephritis. The patient eats a low-sodium diet (10 mEq, or 500 mg). Sodium excretion in the urine normally falls to equal sodium intake within 1 week. In salt-losing nephritis, a large amount of sodium continues to be lost in the urine despite the restricted intake. Additional sodium may be added to the diet when the magnitude of the deficit is determined. For example, a patient who is excreting 50 mEq of sodium in urine on a 10-mEq sodium diet should be allowed an additional 40 mEq of sodium in the diet, or 50 mEq.

MORPHOLOGIC METHODS

Diagnostic methods in renal disease that are primarily morphologic include microscopic and bacteriologic examination of the urine, renal radiologic examination, and renal biopsy. These methods are discussed briefly.

Microscopic Examination of Urine

Microscopic examination of the urine is carried out on a freshly collected, centrifuged specimen, the deposit from which is suspended in 0.5 ml of urine. In health, the urine contains a small number of cells and other elements derived from the entire length of the genitourinary tract—casts, epithelial cells from the lining of the urinary tract and vagina (females), spermatozoa (males), mucus threads, and no more than one or two red blood cells (RBCs) and three or four white blood cells (WBCs) per high-power field.

The most common abnormal constituents of the urine are RBCs, WBCs, bacteria, and casts. All casts arise in the kidney and are thought to be "moldings" of renal tubules. Thus they indicate conditions exclusively within the kidneys and, for this reason, are of great diagnostic value. Casts consist of a mucoprotein matrix, the Tamm-Horsfall mucoprotein, in which cells or debris is embedded and in which a variety of serum and renal proteins may be absorbed. The Tamm-Horsfall protein is secreted by the distal tubule cells. As it passes down the tubule, it dehydrates and takes on the shape of the tubule. *Hyaline casts* consist of this protein and appear as clear cylinders. Cellular elements may be incorporated into hyaline casts (cellular casts) at the time of their formation. In this way, various types of casts are formed, depending on the cell type embedded in the cast (Fig. 45-7). Normally not

▶ TABLE 45-2   Common Normal and Abnormal Findings in Urinalysis

Characteristic	Normal	Abnormality and Possible Significance
Appearance	Clear	Cloudy: large numbers of RBCs or WBCs as in UTI or precipitation of urate or phosphate crystals
Color	Straw yellow	Red or brown: hematuria, hemoglobinuria Red: beets, pyridium Brown: bile in jaundice, porphyrins in porphyria; melanin in melanoma Orange: Pyridium
Odor	Slightly aromatic	Unpleasant odor common in UTI; acetone smell in diabetic ketoacidosis; ammonia smell usual in specimen after standing because of bacterial degradation of urea
Specific gravity	1.001-1.035	Relatively constant near 1.010 in renal failure
pH	5-6.5	>7.5 suggests UTI with urea-splitting organisms
Protein	0 to trace <150 mg/day	Most renal diseases are characterized by proteinuria; nephrotic syndrome: >3.5 g/day
Glucose	Negative	Diabetes mellitus
Ketones	Negative	Diabetes mellitus; starvation
RBCs	0-2/hpf	Larger number may be seen in UTI, glomerulonephritis, neoplasm, stone, papillary necrosis, coagulopathy
WBCs	0-4/hpf	Increased numbers seen in UTI and a variety of other conditions
Epithelial cells	0-5/hpf	Excessive number of renal epithelial cells suggests renal disease
Bacteria	0	Bacteria seen in fresh unspun urine signify UTI
Oval fat bodies	0	Seen in nephrotic syndrome
Casts	0-1/hpf (hyaline)	Coagulated protein formed in renal tubules and collecting ducts; excessive number or specific types are associated with renal disease (see text)
Crystals	Many types	Cystine: abnormal aminoaciduria

hpf, High power field; *UTI,* urinary tract infection; *RBCs,* red blood cells; *WBCs,* white blood cells.

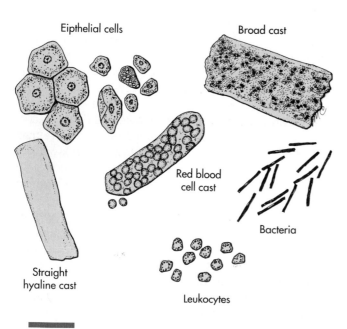

FIG. 45-7   Some formed elements in the urine sediment.

enough protein is present in the renal tubules to provide more than an occasional cast. *Cylindruria* (excessive excretion of casts in the urine) usually means increased proteinuria or renal excretion of cells, or both, and indicates renal disease.

Casts are classified according to shape or constituents.

Cellular casts may contain RBCs, WBCs, bacteria, or tubular epithelial cells or may be mixed. RBCs and *red cell casts* are seen in active glomerulonephritis. *White cell casts* are often seen in pyelonephritis. Oval fat bodies and *fatty casts* are common in the nephrotic syndrome. Oval fat bodies are the remains of degenerated fat-filled tubular cells. *Granular casts* or *waxy casts* represent stages in the degeneration of a cellular cast, and the progression is from coarse to fine and finally to waxy. Broad granular casts are a typical finding in end-stage kidney disease. They are granular because of dead cells and broad because they are formed in the collecting ducts, owing to decreased urinary flow. These broad granular casts are sometimes called *renal failure casts.* Table 45-2 summarizes some common normal and abnormal findings in routine urinalysis.

Bacteriologic Examination of Urine

Urine is normally sterile, and a significant number of bacteria may indicate the presence of urinary tract infection (UTI) (kidneys, bladder, or urethra) or prostatitis. Bacterial counts may be carried out by inoculating the surface of a nutrient agar plate, using a calibrated loop that delivers 0.001 ml of urine (Fig. 45-8). The agar plate is then incubated for 24 hours at 37° C, and colonies are counted. *Significant bacteriuria* is defined as more than 10^5 (100,000) colony-forming units of bacte-

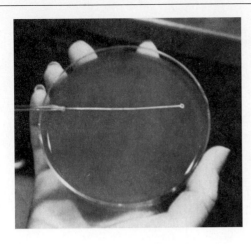

FIG. 45-8   Inoculation of the surface of a blood agar plate by means of a calibrated loop. The plate is incubated for 24 hours at 37° C. Significant bacteriuria is 10^5 (100,000) or more organisms per milliliter of urine.

ria per milliliter of urine (cfu/ml) from a midstream clean-catch specimen. This number is based on epidemiologic studies that show that an asymptomatic individual with a count of this magnitude has an 85% chance of having a UTI. If the individual has signs or symptoms of UTI (fever, dysuria, urinary frequency), a count lower than 10^5 cfu/ml may be significant. The bacteria may be subcultured for identification and for an antibiotic sensitivity test. This procedure is commonly referred to as a C & S, or *culture and sensitivity,* test. The results of this test are a useful guide in the choice of an antibiotic for the most effective treatment.

For a bacteriologic study of the urine to have validity, the specimen must be free of contaminating bacteria from the urethra, external genitalia, and perineum. Proper techniques and precautions are therefore important in the collection of urine specimens. Collection of the urine by catheterization into a sterile container is the best way to ensure that the specimen is uncontaminated. Catheterization, however, is avoided if possible, because of the danger of introducing bacteria into the urinary tract. A "sterile-voided" specimen is generally considered adequate for a bacteriologic study. Men, and particularly women, are instructed to wash the area around the urinary meatus with soap and water. A midstream specimen is then collected in a clean or sterile specimen container. The urine is examined within 30 minutes, or a preservative is added and it is refrigerated at 4° C. Refrigeration prevents the growth of bacteria, and the preservative prevents the deterioration of casts and cells.

Radiologic Examinations

A number of radiologic procedures are available to evaluate the urinary system. The excretory urogram, or intravenous pyelogram (IVP), is the most common and important radiologic examination of the kidneys and is usually performed first. Other imaging examinations include ultrasonography, radionuclide (isotopic) imaging, computed tomography (CT), magnetic resonance imaging (MRI), voiding cystourethrography, and renal angiography.

Intravenous pyelogram

The usual procedure for performing the IVP includes a flat plate (plain film) radiograph of the abdomen followed by IV injection of contrast medium. The contrast medium circulates via the bloodstream and heart to the kidneys, where it is excreted. After injection, a radiograph is taken every minute for the first 5 minutes to visualize the cortex of the kidney. The cortex is thinned in glomerulonephritis and has a moth-eaten appearance in pyelonephritis and ischemia. Adequacy of filling of the calyces is evaluated by examination of the 3- and 5-minute radiographs. At 15 minutes another radiograph is taken, at which time the calyces, pelvis, and ureters can be visualized. Cysts, lesions, and obstructions cause a distortion of these structures. A final radiograph is taken at 45 minutes, in which the bladder is visible. If the patient is severely azotemic (BUN >70 mg/dl), an IVP is not usually done, since this indicates that the GFR is very low. Consequently the dye will not be excreted and the pyelogram will be difficult to visualize.

Sometimes a *retrograde pyelogram* is done by passing a catheter up the ureter and injecting contrast medium directly into the kidney. The main indications for this procedure are urologic, for example, further investigation of a nonfunctioning kidney or when visualization of the IVP is not clear. This procedure is avoided if at all possible because it involves anesthesia and there is a real danger of infection.

The standard IVP serves many purposes. It can establish the presence and position of the kidneys and evaluate their size and shape. The effect of different disease states on the kidney's ability to concentrate and excrete the dye can also be evaluated. Fig. 45-9 shows some typical abnormalities revealed by the IVP. The small, atrophic kidney may be caused by unilateral renal ischemia or unilateral chronic pyelonephritis (Fig. 45-9, *A*). Bilaterally small kidneys are common findings in chronic nephrosclerosis, pyelonephritis, and glomerulonephritis. Distortion of the renal pelvis with clubbing of the calyces is a common finding in chronic pyelonephritis (Fig. 45-9, *B*). Note also the irregular shape and the greatly thinned cortex.

Renal ultrasonography

High-frequency sound waves (ultrasound) directed at the abdomen are reflected from tissue surfaces of varying density. The reflected waves, or echoes, are used to construct images (sonograms) representing sections of the kidney. Ultrasonography is particularly useful in distinguishing solid tumors from fluid-filled cysts. Because ul-

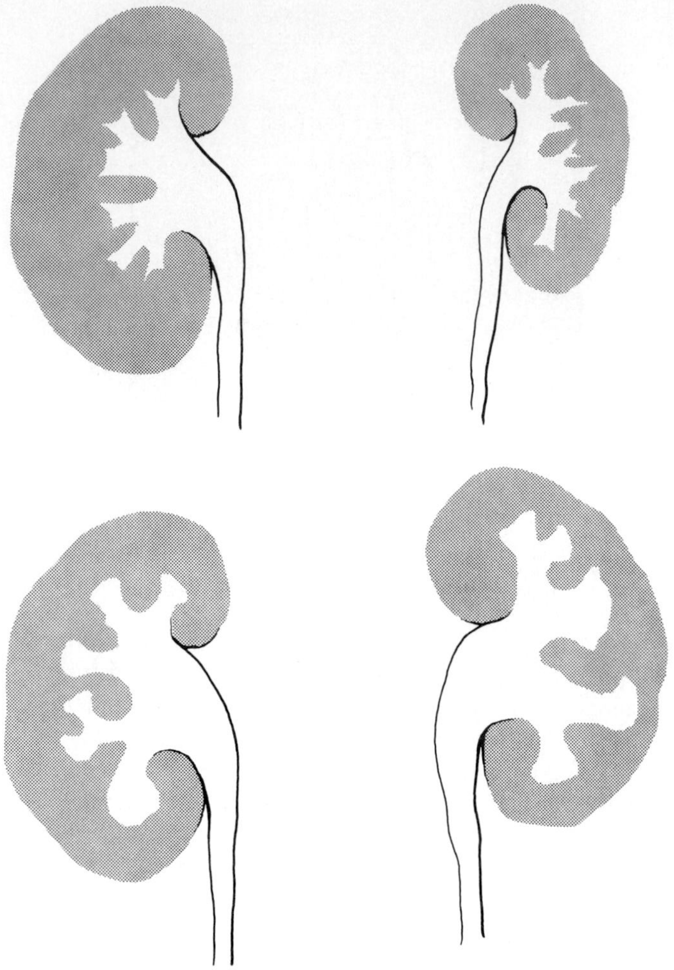

FIG. 45-9   Diagram of abnormalities viewed on the intravenous pyelogram (IVP). **A,** Small, atrophic kidney caused by unilateral renal ischemia. **B,** Clubbing of the calyces, irregularity of contour, and thinning of cortical substance may be found in chronic pyelonephritis.

trasound evaluation does not depend on renal function, it can be applied to patients in severe renal failure who have kidneys that cannot be visualized on the IVP. Kidney size can be determined accurately, and an obstruction can be identified. Other applications include evaluation of a unilateral nonvisualizing kidney (often caused by hydronephrosis), evaluation of renal transplants (perirenal abscess or hematoma, for example, can be differentiated from acute rejection), and renal localization for needle placement for percutaneous renal biopsy.

Renal radionuclide imaging

Radionuclide imaging involves the injection of a radioactive material that is subsequently detected externally by a scintillation (gamma) camera that picks up the radioactive emissions. Information is provided for the evaluation of both structure and function. The properties of a compound that bind the radioisotope determine how it is handled by the kidney—whether it is retained within the vasular system, filtered by the glomerulus, or secreted into the tubule. Three main procedures may be performed together or independently: *renal scintiangiography* uses serial imaging of the aorta and renal vasculature; *renal scintiscanning* uses imaging of the renal parenchyma using various ^{99m}Tc-labeled compounds; and *renography* is

the original technique of radionuclide evaluation of the kidneys using ^{131}I hippuran, which is excreted by tubular secretion. Radionuclide imaging is used for many purposes in renal evaluation but is particularly helpful in renal transplant evaluation. Renal function may be followed, impaired diffusion detected, and acute rejection differentiated from acute tubular necrosis.

Voiding cystourethrogram

The voiding cystourethrogram procedure involves filling the urinary bladder with contrast material via a urinary catheter. Films of the lower urinary tract are taken before, during, and after voiding. Its major diagnostic uses are to investigate abnormalities of the urethra (e.g., stenosis) and to determine whether there is vesicoureteral reflux.

Computed tomography

The application of CT to the abdomen has been a fairly recent development. The radiograph reveals the anatomy of series of "slices" of the body about 10 mm thick so that abnormalities may be identified. Because CT is more expensive than more conventional radiographic techniques, an important question is what it can show that other investigative methods cannot. One use-

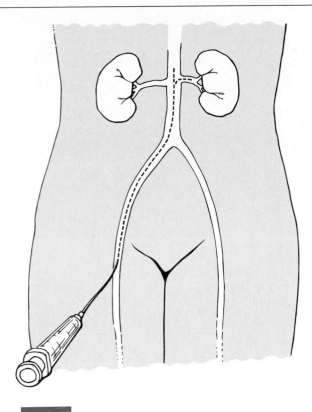

FIG. 45-10   Transfemoral approach in renal angiography.

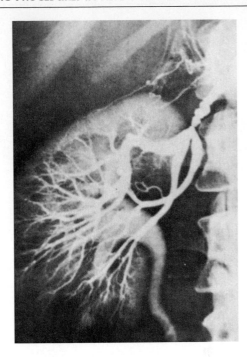

FIG. 45-11   Renal arteriogram showing stenosis of the right renal artery.

ful application of renal CT is the detection of retroperitoneal masses (e.g., tumor spread) that may be difficult to detect by angiography.

Magnetic resonance imaging

MRI is a noninvasive imaging technique that gives the same information as the renal CT scan, but it has the advantages of not requiring exposure to ionizing radiation nor the administration of contrast media. MRI is based on the principle that certain atoms, such as the hydrogen ion contained in the molecules and tissues of the body, act as tiny magnets. If the patient is placed in a strong magnetic field, some of the atomic nuclei align themselves in the same direction as the magnetic force. When a radiofrequency pulse is applied, some of the nuclei absorb the energy, causing them to wobble in and out of alignment (resonate) with the magnetic field. Signals emitted during the return of the magnetization vector to its equilibrium position can be analyzed to provide a detailed structural image. MRI has the disadvantages of high cost and relative unavailability except in large medical centers.

Renal arteriogram

The renal blood vessels may be visualized in an arteriogram. The usual procedure is to introduce a catheter via the femoral artery and abdominal aorta to the level of the renal artery. Contrast medium is injected at this level and then flows into the renal artery and its accessory branches. Additional information often can be obtained by selective renal angiography; the tip of the catheter is maneuvered into the renal artery and more contrast medium is injected (Fig. 45-10). This procedure may be used (1) to visualize renal artery stenosis, which may cause some cases of hypertension; (2) to visualize the blood vessels of a neoplasm; (3) to visualize the blood supply of the cortex, which, for example, may have a patchy appearance in chronic pyelonephritis; and (4) to ascertain the structure of the renal blood supply of a donor before renal transplantation. Fig. 45-11 is an arteriogram showing marked narrowing of the right renal artery.

Angiography is not done without discomfort and some hazard. The patient usually experiences an intense burning sensation for a few seconds as the solution enters the blood vessel. Before injection the patient is usually tested for iodide sensitivity to avoid an anaphylactic response. Other complications following arteriogram include thrombus or embolus formation and local inflammation or hematoma at the site of entry. Although these complications are rare, vital signs are checked every 15 minutes until stable and then every 4 hours for 24 hours. Peripheral pulses are also checked for diminished strength to detect occlusion of blood flow because of a thrombus.

Renal Biopsy

Renal biopsy is one of the most important diagnostic techniques developed during the past few decades. It has resulted in considerable advancement of knowledge of

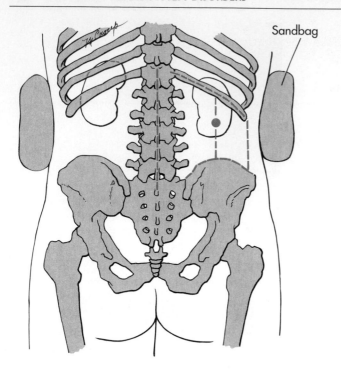

FIG. 45-12   Percutaneous renal biopsy. Site is located by radiographic reference; patient lies prone with sandbag under abdomen to fix kidney against back. Vital signs are monitored.

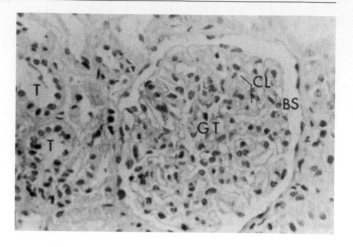

FIG. 45-13   Light microscopy of normal renal biopsy section. *BS,* Bowman's space; *GT,* glomerular tufts; *CL,* capillary lumen; *T,* tubule.

the natural history of renal disease. Renal biopsy is used chiefly for the diagnosis of diffuse renal disease and for following its progress.

Usually the percutaneous procedure is used for renal biopsy. The patient lies prone, with sandbags under the abdomen to fix the kidney against the back (Fig. 45-12). Local anesthesia is used. The usual site for the biopsy is over the right renal angle just below the twelfth rib. The site is located by radiographic reference. A biopsy needle is used to obtain a specimen of renal tissue. The tissue is examined, after appropriate preparation, by light microscopy, electron microscopy, and immunofluorescent microscopy. Fig. 45-13 illustrates the appearance of a normal renal biopsy by light microscopy.

Renal biopsy should be performed only by a skilled nephrologist. The procedure is dangerous in patients who are uncooperative or who have a coagulative disorder or a solitary kidney. The most common complications are intrarenal bleeding and perirenal bleeding. Serious bleeding with gross hematuria occurs in about 5% and death in about 0.17% of cases. Arteriovenous fistula is the second most common complication.

Immediately after the biopsy, pressure is applied over the biopsy site for 10 minutes with 4 × 4-inch sponges, and the patient is kept in a prone position for 30 minutes. A pressure dressing is then applied to the biopsy site. The dressing from above and the sandbag from below provide pressure on the kidney and aid in the prevention of extrarenal bleeding. Lying on the sandbag is usually uncomfortable for the patient, but it immobilizes the kidney in the anteroposterior plane and is a necessary measure to ensure hemostasis. The patient should be kept in bed and as quiet as possible for the next 24 hours and should be instructed not to cough or sneeze. During this period frequent observations of the vital signs, abdomen, and urine should be made. The patient is kept on bed rest as long as hematuria occurs.

? QUESTIONS

▼ *Answer the following on a separate sheet of paper.*

1. Contrast the amount of protein a healthy adult and a person with nephrotic syndrome might excrete in a day. Explain the significance.
2. What is always the direct cause of proteinuria, regardless of the underlying disease process?
3. Explain why only fresh urine should be used for measuring pH.
4. Hyperuricemia leading to uric acid crystallization in the renal tubules is a particular hazard for patients receiving cytotoxic drugs. Why?
5. What are the most common factors predisposing to formation of calculi in alkaline urine? Explain.
6. What is the most important preventive measure against all calculi?
7. What are the five important points that must be considered in obtaining an accurate specific gravity measurement with the urinometer?
8. What is creatinine, and what is its normal range of values in the plasma?
9. Why is the creatinine clearance test not a true measure of GFR?
10. What effect does increasing age have on the GFR?
11. What test most accurately measures effective renal plasma flow?
12. Which is the more accurate index of renal function, the BUN or the plasma creatinine level? Why? What is azotemia?
13. Give two examples of difficulties that may be encountered in the interpretation of the dipstick test for proteinuria.

▼ *Fill in the blanks with the correct words or numbers or circle the appropriate letter to complete the following sentences.*

14. Protein excreted in the urine of the healthy adult consists mainly of _____ and _____ protein.
15. The average pooled daily urine specimen has a pH of about _____.
16. After a meal, one expects a (a) rise or (b) fall in the urine pH. This is referred to as the _____ tide.
17. During normal sleeping hours the urine pH reaches its (a) maximum or (b) minimum because of (c) hypoventilation or (d) hyperventilation during sleep. This is referred to as the _____ tide.
18. When the urine contains normal constituents, a specific gravity of 1.010 corresponds to the normal osmolality of the blood at _____ mOsm.
19. When given large amounts of water, the healthy human being can dilute urine to a minimum specific gravity of about _____ (40 mOsm). Under conditions of water deprivation a normal person can excrete a concentrated urine with a maximum specific gravity of about _____ (1300 mOsm). What is the purpose of this great flexibility?
20. In the 15-minute PSP test the kidneys normally excrete _____% of the dye in the urine.
21. After about 14 hours of water deprivation, the urine of a person with normally functioning kidneys has a specific gravity of _____ or more. After a water load (1 L in 30 minutes) the specific gravity should be _____ or less within the next 3 hours.
22. The_____ _____ test is specific for the diagnosis of renal tubular acidosis (RTA). The urine pH should be _____ or less in the 5-day test.
23. The _____ _____ test is used to determine the proper dietary intake of sodium, especially in a patient with "salt-losing" nephritis. A negative sodium balance is most frequently found in patients with renal disorders primarily involving the (a) tubules or (b) glomerulus.

▼ *Circle the letter preceding each item that correctly completes the statement. Only one answer is correct, with exceptions noted.*

24. The normal pH range of the urine is:
   a. 7.0-14.0   c. 4.5-8.0
   b. 6.0-12.0   d. 3.0-6.0

25. The most clinically useful test for the measurement of the glomerular filtration rate is:
   a. Urea clearance
   b. Uric acid clearance
   c. Creatinine clearance
   d. PSP excretion

26. The following foods tend to produce an acidic urine (more than one answer may be correct):
   a. Meat
   b. Vegetables
   c. Cranberry juice, prunes
   d. Milk

27. The following data were obtained from a creatinine clearance test on a patient: 24-hour urine volume = 1440 ml; urine creatinine level = 50 mg/dl; plasma creatinine level = 2 mg/dl. The creatinine clearance (uncorrected for body surface area) is:
   a. 100 ml/min
   b. 1440 ml/min
   c. 25 ml/min
   d. 36,000 ml/min

28. At the usual rate of decrease with aging, the GFR in a 90-year-old man would be about:
   a. 25% of normal
   b. 50% of normal
   c. 75% of normal
   d. 100% of normal

▼ *Answer the following on a separate sheet of paper.*

29. Name the most common abnormal constituents of the urine sediment.
30. When is bacteriuria significant? List proper conditions of urine collection and significant bacterial count.
31. Differentiate between an intravenous pyelogram (IVP) and a retrograde pyelogram. State the purpose of each.
32. List four reasons for performing a renal arteriogram.
33. Why is it not worthwhile to perform an IVP on a patient who is severely azotemic (BUN level greater than 70 mg/dl)?
34. Outline a plan of care for a patient after a renal arteriogram.
35. Outline a plan of care for a patient during and after a renal biopsy. What observations should be made?

Continued.

QUESTIONS—cont'd

▼ *Fill in the blanks with the correct words.*

36. Four types of morphologic renal investigations are:
    a. _____ examination of the urine sediment
    b. _____ study of the urine
    c. Renal _____, a method that reveals the shape, size, and position of the kidneys
    d. Renal _____, a method that reveals the microscopic structure of the kidney

37. Hyaline casts are made up of coagulated _____ _____ protein secreted by the _____ tubule.

38. Excessive excretion of casts in the urine is called _____ and usually means that there is an increased glomerular permeability to _____.

39. A _____ and _____ test is sometimes done to determine the best choice of an antibiotic for treating a urinary tract infection.

40. An abnormality seen on the IVP that is diagnostic of chronic pyelonephritis is _____ of the calyces.

▼ *Circle the letter preceding each item that correctly answers each question or completes the statement. Only one answer is correct.*

41. Casts are classified according to:
    a. Number of particles
    b. Shape and constituents
    c. Number of bacteria

42. Long-standing renal ischemia usually results in which condition of the kidney?
    a. Atrophy
    b. Hypertrophy

43. Above what level of RBCs per high-power field would microscopic examination of urine sediment reveal significant hematuria?
    a. 100,000
    b. 5000-9000
    c. 1-2

44. Which of these statements with respect to renal biopsy is false?
    a. Death occurs in 1% of patients.
    b. The procedure is dangerous in patients who are uncooperative.
    c. Postbiopsy hematuria occurs in 5% of patients.
    d. During the procedure the patient lies in a prone position on a sandbag.

▼ *Match the renal disease in column B with the type of cast most frequently seen in the urine sediment in Column A.*

Column A	Column B
45. _____ Broad granular casts	a. Pyelonephritis
46. _____ Red blood cell casts	b. Nephrotic syndrome
47. _____ Leukocyte casts	c. Advanced renal disease
48. _____ Fatty casts and oval fat bodies	d. Active glomerulonephritis

▼ *Match the radiologic technique in column B with its description or application in column A.*

Column A	Column B
49. _____ Used to detect vesicoureteral reflux	a. Computed tomography
50. _____ No radiation hazard involved; fluid-filled cysts can be distinguished from solid tumors	b. Voiding cystourethrogram
	c. Ultrasonography
51. _____ Uses radioisotopes; useful for evaluation of renal transplant	d. Radionuclide imaging
52. _____ Image reveals serial "slices" of the body	

CHAPTER 46 ▶ Chronic Renal Failure

LORRAINE M. WILSON

This chapter gives an overview of the course of deteriorations in progressive renal failure, its general pathophysiology, and its causes.

Renal failure is usually divided into two broad categories—chronic and acute. Chronic renal failure is a progressive, slow development of renal failure, usually over a period of years, as contrasted with acute renal failure, which develops over a period of days or a few weeks. In both cases the kidneys lose their ability to maintain normal volume and composition of the body fluids under conditions of normal dietary intake. Although the terminal functional disability is similar in the two types of renal failure, acute renal failure has some unique features and is discussed separately in Chapter 49.

Chronic renal failure follows a great number of conditions that devastate the nephron mass of the kidney. Most of these conditions involve diffuse, bilateral disease of the renal parenchyma, although obstructive lesions of the urinary tract may also lead to chronic renal failure. In the beginning, some renal diseases involve primarily the glomerulus (glomerulonephritis), whereas others involve primarily the renal tubules (pyelonephritis or polycystic kidney disease) or may interfere with blood perfusion to the renal parenchyma (nephrosclerosis). In all cases, however, if the disease process is not halted, the entire nephron is progressively destroyed and replaced by scar tissue. The individual features of the various parenchymal renal diseases are discussed later in this chapter.

Despite the diversity of causes, the clinical features of chronic renal failure are remarkably similar, because progressive renal failure may be explained simply as a deficiency in the total number of functioning nephrons, and a fairly fixed combination of disturbances is inevitable.

OVERVIEW: CLINICAL COURSE OF CHRONIC RENAL FAILURE

An overview of the general course of chronic renal failure may be obtained by looking at the relation of the creatinine clearance and glomerular filtration rate (GFR), as a percentage of the normal, to the serum creatinine and blood urea nitrogen (BUN) levels as the nephron mass is progressively destroyed by chronic renal disease (Fig. 46-1).

The general course of progressive renal failure may be divided into three stages (designated as I, II, and III in Fig. 46-1). The first stage is called *decreased renal reserve.* During this stage, the serum creatinine and BUN levels are normal and the patient is asymptomatic. Impairment of renal function may be detected only by imposition of severe demands on the kidney, such as a prolonged urine concentration test, or by careful testing of the GFR.

The second stage in the progression is called *renal insufficiency,* when more than 75% of the functioning tissue has been destroyed (GFR is 25% of normal). At this point the BUN level is just beginning to rise above the normal range. The rise in BUN concentration is variable, depending on the dietary intake of protein (compare the BUN graphs for a low and normal protein intake). The serum creatinine level also begins to rise above normal during this stage. The azotemia is generally mild unless, for example, the patient is stressed by infection, heart failure, or dehydration. It is also during the stage of renal insufficiency that the symptoms of nocturia and polyuria (caused by impaired concentrating ability) begin to appear. These symptoms occur in response to stress and sudden changes in food or fluid intake. The patient usually takes little note of these symptoms, so they may be revealed only by careful questioning. *Nocturia* (urinating at night) is defined as persistent nocturnal output of 700 ml or having to get up more than once to void during the night. Nocturia is caused by loss of the normal diurnal pattern of concentrating urine to a greater degree at night. The ratio of day to night urine is normally 3 : 1 or 4 : 1. Of course, nocturia may occasionally occur in response to anxiety or to a high fluid intake, especially of tea, coffee, or beer taken just before retiring. *Polyuria* means a persistent increase in the volume of urine. Normal urine output is about 1500 ml/day and varies considerably with fluid intake. Polyuria of renal insufficiency is usually greater in diseases that affect primarily the tubules, although it is generally moderate and rarely exceeds 3 L/day.

The third and final stage of progressive renal failure is called *end-stage renal disease* (ESRD) or *uremia.* End-stage renal disease occurs when about 90% of the nephron mass has been destroyed, or only about 200,000 nephrons remain intact. The GFR is 10% of normal, and the creatinine clearance may be 5 to 10 ml/min or even less. At this point the serum creatinine and BUN levels rise sharply in response to small decrements in the GFR. During ESRD the patient begins to suffer severe symptoms as the kidneys are no longer able to maintain fluid and electrolyte homeostasis in the body. The urine becomes isoosmotic with the plasma at a fixed specific gravity of 1.010. The patient usually becomes oliguric (urine output less than 500 ml/day) because of glomerular failure, even though the renal tubules may have been initially affected by the disease process. The complex of biochemical changes and symptoms, called the *uremic syndrome,* affects every system in the body and is discussed in detail in Chapter 47. In ESRD, unless the patient receives dialysis or renal transplantation, death will surely follow.

Although the clinical course of chronic renal disease has been divided into three stages, in practice no sharp divisions exist between the stages. The hyperbolic shape of the graph of azotemia plotted against GFR reflects this continuous but slowly accelerating course.

General Pathophysiology of Chronic Renal Failure

Two theoretic approaches are generally offered to account for the impaired function of the kidneys in chronic renal failure. The traditional point of view is that all the nephron units are diseased to varying degrees and that specific parts of the nephron concerned with particular functions may be destroyed or their structure altered. For example, organic lesions of the medulla disrupting the anatomic arrangement of the loop of Henle and vasa recta or the chloride pump in the ascending limb would interfere with countercurrent multiplication and exchange. The second approach, known as the *Bricker hypothesis*

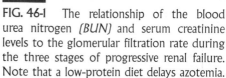

FIG. 46-1   The relationship of the blood urea nitrogen *[BUN]* and serum creatinine levels to the glomerular filtration rate during the three stages of progressive renal failure. Note that a low-protein diet delays azotemia.

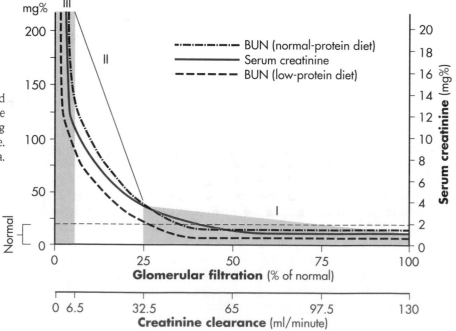

or *intact nephron hypothesis,* maintains that nephrons, when diseased, are totally destroyed. The remaining intact nephrons behave normally. Uremia results when the total number of nephrons is so reduced that fluid and electrolyte balance can no longer be maintained. The intact nephron hypothesis is most useful in explaining the orderly pattern of functional adaptation in progressive renal disease, that is, the ability to maintain a balance of body water and electrolytes despite a marked decrease in the GFR.

The sequence of events in the general pathophysiology of progressive renal failure may be outlined in terms of the intact nephron hypothesis. As chronic renal disease advances, the amount of solute that must be excreted by the kidney to maintain body homeostasis does not change, although there is a progressive reduction in the number of nephrons performing this function. Two important adaptations occur in the kidney in response to the threat of fluid and electrolyte imbalance. The remaining intact nephrons hypertrophy in an attempt to carry the entire work load of the kidneys (Fig. 46-2). There is an increase in filtration rate, solute load, and tubular reabsorption in each individual nephron, even though the GFR for the entire nephron mass of the kidneys is decreased below normal. This increased single-nephron GFR (SNGFR), (i.e., hyperfiltration) occurs by dilation of the glomerular afferent arterioles, resulting in enhanced single-nephron plasma flow. This adaptive mechanism is successful in maintaining body fluid and electrolyte balance down to low levels of renal function. Finally, when about 75% of the nephron mass is destroyed, the filtration rate and solute load per nephron are so high that glomerular-tubular balance (balance between increased filtration and increased tubular reabsorption) can no longer be maintained (note that six of the eight nephrons are destroyed in Fig. 46-2). A loss of flexibility occurs in both the excretion and conservation of individual solutes and water. Modest dietary changes may upset the precarious balance, because the lower the GFR (which means fewer nephrons), the greater must be the change in excretion rate per nephron. Loss of the ability to concentrate or dilute causes the specific gravity of urine to become fixed at 1.010, or 285 mOsm (the concentration of plasma), and accounts for the symptoms of polyuria and nocturia. For example, a person on a normal diet excretes about 600 mOsm of solute each day. If that person is incapable of concentrating urine from the normal plasma osmolality of 285 mOsm, there is an obligatory loss of 2 L of water with the 600-mOsm solute excretion (285 mOsm/L) regardless of water intake. In response to the same solute load and water deprivation, the normal person could concentrate urine to about four times the plasma concentration and thus excrete a small volume of concentrated urine. As the GFR progresses toward zero, it becomes increasingly important to regulate the intake of water and solutes precisely to accommodate the decreased flexibility in renal function.

The intact nephron hypothesis is supported by several

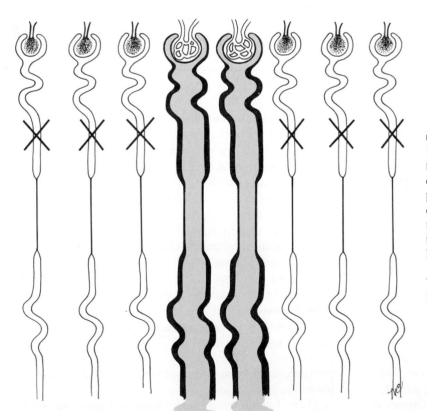

FIG. 46-2 Intact nephron hypothesis. As chronic renal disease advances and nephrons are progressively destroyed, the remaining intact nephrons hypertrophy in an attempt to carry on the entire work load of the kidney. Solute load per nephron is increased, resulting in osmotic diuresis, that is, rise in urine flow and reduction in concentration. (Modified from Netter FH: Kidneys, ureters, and urinary bladder. In *The Ciba collection of medical illustrations,* vol 6, West Caldwell, NJ, 1973, Ciba Medical Education Division.)

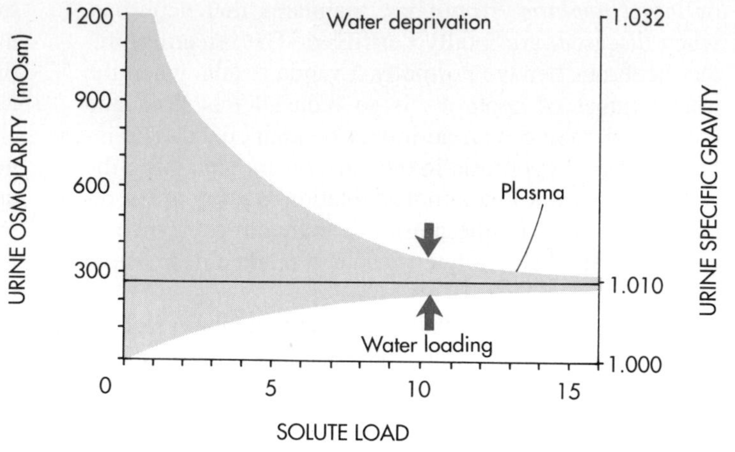

FIG. 46-3   The response of normal kidneys to an increasing solute load under conditions of water loading and deprivation. Ability to concentrate or dilute urine is progressively lost as the solute load increases. Urine specific gravity becomes fixed near 1.010 (285 mOsm). [Modified from Gordon A, Maxwell MH: *Hosp Med* 5[I]:6-18, 1969.]

experimental observations. Bricker and Fine (1969) have shown that in patients with naturally occurring pyelonephritis and in dogs with experimental destruction of the kidney, the surviving nephrons hypertrophy and become more active than normal. Also, when one kidney is removed in the healthy person, the remaining kidney undergoes hypertrophy and the capacity of this kidney approaches that formerly possessed by both.

Normal kidneys under conditions of increased solute load behave much like the kidney in progressive renal failure, giving further support to the intact nephron hypothesis. The experimental data in Fig. 46-3 illustrate the concept that with progressive increases in solute load, the ability to concentrate the urine under conditions of water deprivation (upper curve) or to dilute the urine under conditions of high water intake (lower curve) is progressively lost. Both curves approach the specific gravity of 1.010 until the urine is isoosmotic with the plasma at 285 mOsm, so that a fixed specific gravity exists.

The experimental conditions just described could be induced in a normal person by giving mannitol (an osmotic diuretic). The number 10 on the *x* axis is arbitrarily chosen to show that the kidneys are excreting 10 times the usual solute load. At this point each normal nephron is undergoing an osmotic diuresis with an obligatory loss of water. The kidney has lost its flexibility to either concentrate or dilute the urine from the plasma osmolality of 285 mOsm.

Similar events probably occur in the patient with progressive renal failure. The patient with 90% destruction of nephron mass is at the same point on the graph as the normal person with an induced solute load that is 10 times normal. The remaining 10% of the nephrons are forced to excrete 10 times the normal solute load and therefore lose their flexibility; they are unable to compensate properly by the usual changes in tubular reabsorption for excesses or deficiencies of sodium or water.

It has been noted for some time that chronic renal failure is often progressive even if the inciting cause of injury is removed. For example, children with chronic pyelonephritis caused by vesicoureteral reflux and recurrent urinary tract infections (UTIs) develop pyelonephritic scars involving the tubules and interstitium, but when the reflux is corrected surgically and renal infection halted with antibiotics, progressive renal failure continues. These observations have led to recent major research efforts to learn the reasons for the progression of renal disease and methods to halt or slow its progression.

The most popular current explanation for progressive renal failure in the absence of active primary renal disease is the *hyperfiltration hypothesis*. According to the hyperfiltration theory, the intact nephrons are eventually injured by the increased plasma flow and GFR and increased glomerular intracapillary hydrostatic pressure (P_{gc}). Even though the increased SNGFR is adaptive in the short run, in the long run it is maladaptive.

Most of the evidence for the hyperfiltration theory of secondary injury is derived from the *remnant kidney* model in the rat. When one kidney in the rat was removed and two thirds of the other kidney destroyed, it was noted that the animal developed end-stage renal failure within 6 months even though a primary renal disease was not present. The rat developed proteinuria, and renal biopsy of the remnant kidney revealed widespread glomerulosclerosis similar to lesions in many primary renal diseases. One explanation for renal lesions and progressive renal failure is based on the functional and structural changes that occur when the number of intact nephrons is reduced in an experimental animal.

Functional adaptations to a reduction of the nephron mass lead to systemic hypertension and increased SNGFR (hyperfiltration) in the remaining intact nephrons. Increased SNGFR is largely accomplished through dilation of the afferent arterioles. At the same time the efferent arteriole constricts because of the local release of angiotensin II. Consequently, renal plasma flow and P_{gc} increase, since most of the systemic pressure is transmitted to the glomerulus.

These functional compensations are associated with significant structural changes. The volume of the glo-

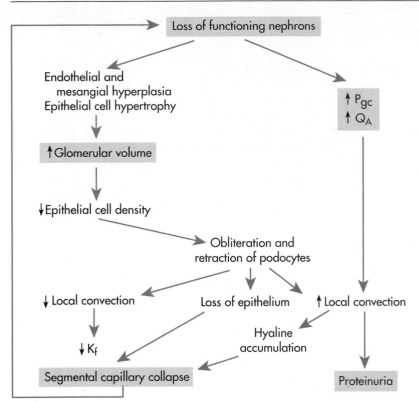

FIG. 46-4 Pathogenesis of focal glomerulosclerosis in the progression of chronic renal failure. P_{gc}, Glomerular intracapillary hydrostatic pressure; Q_A, single nephron plasma flow; K_f, ultrafiltration coefficient (a measure of the number of small pores allowing filtration of water and small solutes). (Redrawn from Brevis M, Epstein FH: *Kidney Int* 26:375, 1984.)

merular tuft increases without an increase in the number of visceral epithelial cells, resulting in a reduction of cell density within the enlarged glomerular tuft. It is believed that the combination of glomerular hypertension and hypertrophy is the significant change that causes secondary injury of the glomerular tuft and progressive destruction of nephrons. Decreased visceral epithelial density leads to fusion of the foot processes and a loss of the size-selective barrier so that increased protein is lost in the urine. The increase in permeability and intraglomerular hypertension also favors the accumulation of large proteins (e.g., fibrin, IgM, complement) in the subendothelial space. The accumulation of these subendothelial deposits along with proliferation of mesangial matrix eventually leads to a narrowing of the capillary lumen from the compression. Other secondary injuries include microaneurysm formation from intraglomerular hypertension and thrombus formation from endothelial cell dysfunction. The aggregate effect is collapse of the glomerular capillaries and glomerulosclerosis, manifested by proteinuria and progressive renal failure. In addition, this sequence leads to a positive feedback loop with acceleration of the destructive process as fewer and fewer nephrons remain intact. The structural and functional changes that lead to secondary injury of the glomerulus are summarized in Fig. 46-4 (Rose, Rennke, 1994).

Recent progress in understanding the mechanisms of progressive renal failure through the hyperfiltration hypothesis has caused clinicians to focus treatment on the prevention of secondary glomerular injury rather than to focus on the primary renal disease. Large clinical trials are now in progress with dietary protein restriction and antihypertensive therapy as a means of slowing the progress of chronic renal failure. This treatment is discussed in Chapter 48.

CAUSES OF CHRONIC RENAL FAILURE

Chronic renal failure is a clinical state of progressive, irreversible renal damage arising from many different causes. The rate of progression of these chronic renal diseases varies greatly. The course terminating in ESRD may vary from 2 to 3 months to 30 to 40 years. The most common causes of chronic renal failure may be divided into the eight classes listed in Table 46-1. No attempt is made to be all-inclusive, and only selected examples are listed under each class. These diseases are discussed in this chapter but not necessarily in the same order in which they appear in the table. It should be emphasized that although the early stages of renal disease may be quite variable, the end stages are remarkably similar and in many cases the original cause cannot be identified.

Currently, diabetes and hypertension are responsible for the largest proportion of ESRD, accounting for 34.2% and 29.4% of the total cases, respectively. Glomerulonephritis is the third most common cause of ESRD (14.4%). Infectious tubulointerstitial nephritis (chronic

TABLE 46-1   Classification of the Causes of Chronic Renal Failure

Disease Classifications	Disease
Infectious tubulointerstitial disease	Chronic pyelonephritis or reflux nephropathy
Inflammatory diseases	Glomerulonephritis
Hypertensive vascular disease	Benign nephrosclerosis
	Malignant nephrosclerosis
	Renal artery stenosis
Connective tissue disorders	Systemic lupus erythematosus
	Polyarteritis nodosa
	Progressive systemic sclerosis
Congenital and hereditary disorders	Polycystic kidney disease
	Renal tubular acidosis
Metabolic disorders	Diabetes mellitus
	Gout
	Hyperparathyroidism
	Amyloidosis
Toxic nephropathy	Analgesic abuse
	Lead nephropathy
Obstructive nephropathy	Upper urinary tract: calculi, neoplasms, retroperitoneal fibrosis
	Lower urinary tract: prostatic hypertrophy, urethral stricture, congenital anomalies of the bladder neck and urethra

pyelonephritis or reflux nephropathy) and polycystic kidney disease (PCKD) each account for 3.4% of ESRD (US Renal Data System, 1993). The remaining 14% of the causes of ESRD are relatively uncommon and include obstructive uropathy, systemic lupus erythematosus (SLE), and others to be discussed in the following pages. The current distribution of the primary causes of ESRD has changed greatly from its distribution in 1967, when chronic glomerulonephritis and chronic pyelonephritis (now called *reflux nephropathy*) accounted for two thirds of the cases of ESRD. This change reflects changing practices of patient acceptance into ESRD programs, with the inclusion of a greater proportion of minorities and older patients.

The four major risk factors for the development of ESRD are age, race, gender, and family history. The incidence of diabetic renal failure increases greatly with age. ESRD caused by hypertensive nephropathy is 6.2 times more common in African Americans than in whites. Overall, the incidence of ESRD is greater in males (56.3%) than in females (43.7%), although certain systemic diseases causing ESRD, such as type II diabetes mellitus and SLE, are more common in females. Finally, family history is a risk factor for the development of diabetes and hypertension. PCKD is transmitted by autosomal dominant heredity, and there are a variety of uncommon recessive or sex-linked renal diseases.

Urinary Tract Infection, Pyelonephritis, and Reflux Nephropathy

UTIs are common and affect people throughout the life span, especially women. UTI accounts for nearly 7 million visits to physicians' offices annually in the United States (Hooten, 1995). Microbiologically, UTI exists when significant bacteriuria is present (10^5 pathogenic microorganisms/ml are detected in the urine of a properly collected midstream "clean catch" sample). The only abnormality may be colonization of the urine (asymptomatic bacteriuria), or bacteriuria may be associated with symptomatic infection of any of the structures of the urinary tract. UTI is commonly divided into two general subcategories: lower urinary tract infection (urethritis, cystitis, prostatitis) and the upper urinary tract (acute pyelonephritis). *Acute cystitis* (infection of the bladder) and *acute pyelonephritis* (infection of the renal pelvis and interstitium) are the most significant in terms of morbidity, but they rarely result in progressive renal failure. *Chronic pyelonephritis* (PN) refers to progressive renal injury, associated with parenchymal scarring on intravenous pyelogram (IVP), induced by recurrent or persistent infection of the kidneys. Recent evidence indicates that chronic PN occurs in patients with UTI who also have a major anatomic abnormality of the urinary tract, such as vesicoureteral reflux (VUR), obstruction, calculi, or neurogenic bladder (Kunin, 1987; Rose, Rennke, 1994). It is thought that the renal damage in chronic PN, also called *reflux nephropathy,* results from the reflux of infected urine up the ureters and then into the renal parenchyma (intrarenal reflux). Chronic PN caused by VUR is a major cause of end-stage renal failure in children and is theoretically preventable by the control of UTIs and correction of the structural abnormalities of the urinary tract that cause obstruction. Unfortunately, VUR may not be discovered in childhood, and the progressive renal damage may be silent until the signs and symptoms of ESRF are discovered in the adult.

Etiology and pathogenesis

The most common infecting organism of the urinary tract is *Escherichia coli,* which accounts for more than 80% of the cases. *E. coli* is a normal inhabitant of the colon. Other infecting organisms often include *Proteus, Klebsiella, Pseudomonas, Enterococcus,* and *Staphylococcus* organisms. In most cases the organisms gain access to the bladder via the urethra. The infection, beginning as cystitis, may remain confined to the bladder or may ascend via the ureter to the kidney. Organisms may also reach the kidney via the bloodstream or lymphatics, but this is believed to be uncommon. The bladder and upper urethra are normally sterile, although bacteria are present in the lower urethra. The flushing action of urine flow enables the normal urinary tract to rid itself of bacteria before they have a chance to invade the mucosa. Other defense mechanisms include the antibacterial ef-

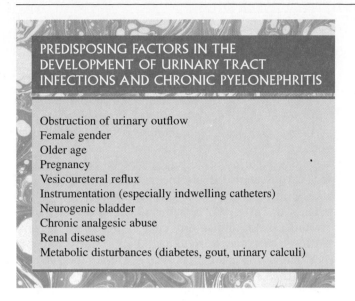

PREDISPOSING FACTORS IN THE DEVELOPMENT OF URINARY TRACT INFECTIONS AND CHRONIC PYELONEPHRITIS

Obstruction of urinary outflow
Female gender
Older age
Pregnancy
Vesicoureteral reflux
Instrumentation (especially indwelling catheters)
Neurogenic bladder
Chronic analgesic abuse
Renal disease
Metabolic disturbances (diabetes, gout, urinary calculi)

fect of the urethral mucosa, the bactericidal properties of prostatic fluid in men, and the phagocytic properties of the bladder epithelium. Despite these defenses, urinary infections may occur and they may be related to certain predisposing factors listed in the box above.

Obstruction of the urinary outflow proximal to the bladder can result in the accumulation of fluid under pressure in the renal pelvis and ureter. This alone is enough to cause severe atrophy of the renal parenchyma. It is a condition called *hydronephrosis*. In addition, obstruction below the level of the bladder is often associated with vesicoureteral reflux (see below) and infection of the kidney. Common causes of obstruction are renal or ureteral scarring, calculi, neoplasms, prostatic hypertrophy (common in men older than 60 years), congenital anomalies of the bladder neck and urethra, and urethral stricture.

Girls and women have a much higher incidence of UTIs and acute pyelonephritis than boys and men, presumably because of a shorter urethra and its proximity to the anus and consequent fecal contamination. Epidemiologic studies have shown that significant bacteriuria (10^5 organisms/ml of urine) exists in 1% to 4% of school-age girls, 5% to 10% of women of childbearing age, and about 25% of women older than 60 years (Papper, 1978). Only a few of these persons have clinical symptoms of UTI. Long-term follow-up studies in school-age girls reveal that girls with significant bacteriuria are more apt to have recurrent UTIs during adulthood, usually shortly after marriage or during the first pregnancy (Kunin, 1987). Although these UTIs are responsible for considerable morbidity, they rarely result in chronic pyelonephritis and ESRD except in those hidden cases with childhood damage from urologic abnormalities—mostly high grades of VUR. Infection in males is rare, and when it occurs, it is usually related to obstruction.

It has been known for some time that hydroureter and hydronephrosis, most marked on the right, always occur during pregnancy and persist for some time afterward. The dilation is attributed partly to muscular relaxation caused by the high progesterone levels and partly to obstruction of the ureters by the enlarged uterus. About 5% to 7% of the women so affected have asymptomatic bacteriuria (Whalley, 1967; Norden, Kass, 1968). In a controlled study, Kass (1960) found that 42% of a placebo-treated group of women ($n = 48$) who had asymptomatic bacteriuria during early pregnancy developed pyelonephritis later during the pregnancy or during the first few weeks postpartum, although none of the group treated with antibiotics for the bacteriuria ($n = 42$) developed symptomatic infection. Cystitis and pyelonephritis are not more common in women with toxemia than in other women. An increased incidence of infant prematurity and mortality occurs when women develop upper UTIs during pregnancy (Stamm, 1994).

When the renal pelvis becomes distended with newly formed urine, the smooth muscle contracts, propelling a bolus of urine into the ureter. Dilation of the ureter then initiates a peristaltic wave, which carries the urine into the bladder. Urinary flow is normally unidirectional, from the renal plevis to the bladder, and reverse flow (reflux) is prevented by the *ureterovesicular valve* (located where the ureter is implanted into the bladder). The action of this one-way valve is vitally important in preventing backflow during the act of micturition when intravesicular pressure rises, because transmission of this pressure can damage the kidney directly. *Vesicoureteral reflux* (VUR) is defined as retrograde flow of urine from the bladder into the ureter, especially during micturition. VUR is graded from I to V, with grade I indicating reflux only into the lower ureter and grade V indicating massive reflux into the renal pelvis and calyces. VUR may be detected by injecting contrast material into the bladder through a catheter until the bladder is distended to the point at which the patient has the urge to void. Serial radiographs are taken with the bladder distended and during and after the act of voiding. The entire procedure is known as *voiding cystourethrography*. VUR has been associated with congenital malformation of the intravesicular ureter, obstruction of the bladder outlet (bladder neck or urethra), and cystitis. VUR has been demonstrated in a high proportion of patients, especially children, with recurrent UTIs and appears to be the mechanism by which organisms ascend to the kidney. It is generally believed that the reflux of infected urine into the renal parenchyma is responsible for the prominent renal scarring in humans (reflux nephropathy). The net effect is that chronic pyelonephritis caused by VUR accounts for about 20% to 30% of end-stage renal failure in children (Rose, 1987).

Urethral and ureteric catheterization and cystoscopy commonly introduce infective organisms into the bladder or kidney. About 2% of simple, single bladder catheterizations result in infection. There is a 98% incidence of infection within 48 hours when an indwelling catheter is placed, unless meticulous attention is directed to keeping a closed drainage system. Even when the system is closed, the urine is sterile for only about 5 to 7 days. These facts indicate that catheterization is a procedure to avoid if possible.

The bladder is a distensible reservoir for urine from which the urine is evacuated at suitable intervals. The innervation of the bladder consists of a reflex arc at the S2 and S4 level of the spinal cord, whose function is modified by sensory and motor connections to the higher centers in the brain. The act of micturition (urination) involves the coordinated contraction of the detrusor muscle (smooth muscle of the bladder wall), abdominal wall, and muscles of the pelvic floor; fixation of the chest and diaphragm; and relaxation of the internal and external sphincter muscles. Accordingly, both autonomic and voluntary activities are involved. Contraction of the detrusor muscle is reflex (stimulated when the bladder contains about 300 ml of urine), and this reflex contraction may be both inhibited and facilitated by supraspinal portions of the nervous system under voluntary control. Interference with efferent or afferent limbs of the reflex arc or with efferent or afferent pathways connecting the sacral spinal cord to the central facilitory or inhibitory mechanisms can disrupt normal micturition; these conditions are referred to as *neurogenic bladder.*

Lapides (1976) identified five types of neurogenic bladder dysfunction, each associated with a particular neural lesion: (1) uninhibited neurogenic bladder, (2) reflex neurogenic bladder, (3) autonomous neurogenic bladder, (4) sensory paralytic neurogenic bladder, and (5) motor paralytic neurogenic bladder.

Uninhibited neurogenic bladder involves a defect of the corticoregulatory tract. This condition is common in patients who have lesions involving the cerebral cortex, as in cerebrovascular accidents, or those who have disseminated cord lesions involving the corticoregulatory tracts, as in multiple sclerosis. The uninhibited neurogenic bladder resembles that of an infant. The patient is aware of a sudden desire to urinate as the bladder fills but may be unable to inhibit the desire to void even though the situation may not be appropriate. Uninhibited neurogenic bladder dysfunction is the type most frequently encountered in clinical practice. In children the upper motor neuron dysfunction is manifested in persistent diurnal and nocturnal diuresis beyond the age of 2 to 3 years. Uninhibited neurogenic bladder dysfunction may be associated with recurrent UTI, especially in young girls. The patient may be able to suppress urination by voluntarily contracting the striated muscles around the urethra but is unable to control the uninhibited bladder contractions. The resultant rise in intravesicular pressure causes ischemia of the bladder wall and a lowering of local tissue immunity, with consequent infection.

Reflex neurogenic bladder results from disconnection of the sacral reflex arc from higher centers, as in cord injury or transection above the S2 level. All bladder sensation is lost, and emptying occurs reflexly whenever intravesicular pressure rises above a critical level. Emptying of the bladder is incomplete because of the lack of motor input from higher centers, and vesicoureteral reflux occurs because of the high intravesicular pressures. Both the VUR and residual urine predispose the patient with spinal cord injury to cystitis and pyelonephritis.

Autonomous neurogenic bladder results from destruction of both limbs of the bladder reflex arc, as by sacral or cauda equina lesions (e.g., gunshot wound, abdominal-perineal resection surgery, neoplasia, congenital anomalies such as spina bifida and myelomeningocele). Patients with this type of lesion can neither perceive bladder fullness nor initiate urination in the normal fashion. However, they may learn to pass their urine by voluntarily straining and manual pressure over the suprapubic region (Credé's maneuver).

Sensory paralytic neurogenic bladder results from lesions of the sensory limb of the bladder reflex arc, as in diabetic neuropathy or multiple sclerosis. There is a gradual loss of bladder sensation, infrequent urination, and overdistention. Overdistention causes the bladder muscle to lose its tone, so that emptying is incomplete and there is residual urine.

Motor paralytic neurogenic bladder involves interruption of the motor limb of the bladder reflex arc, commonly associated with poliomyelitis, tumor, or trauma. The sensation of bladder fullness is intact, but the patient has either partial or total inability to initiate urination. Painful overdistention may result, requiring catheterization and drainage.

The pathogenic mechanisms predisposing to UTI in neurogenic bladder dysfunction include ischemia of the bladder wall from overdistention, which lessens resistance to bacterial invasion; residual urine, which provides a medium for bacterial growth; and VUR associated with increased intravesicular pressures. The use of catheters and urinary drainage is an additional predisposing factor.

Chronic analgesic abuse alone may cause chronic interstitial nephritis (see p. 716), which may be difficult to distinguish from chronic pyelonephritis. In addition, recurrent UTI is common in analgesic nephropathy. Various underlying renal diseases increase susceptibility to infection and pyelonephritis. Finally, metabolic disturbances such as diabetes, gout, and renal stones are often complicated by renal infection.

Acute pyelonephritis

The clinical features of acute pyelonephritis are usually quite characteristic. In about 90% of the cases, the patient is a woman. There is an abrupt onset of fever, chills, malaise, back pain, tenderness to palpation over the costovertebral area, leukocytosis, pyuria, and bacteriuria. These signs and symptoms are often preceded by dysuria, urgency, and frequency, indicating that the infection began in the lower urinary tract. The finding of leukocyte casts indicates that the infection is in the kidney.

Fig. 46-5 illustrates the gross and microscopic appearance of the kidney in acute pyelonephritis. The kidney is swollen, with multiple small abscesses on the surface. On cross section, abscesses appear as yellowish gray streaks in the pyramids and cortex. Microscopically, numerous polymorphonuclear leukocytes (PMNs) are found within the tubules *(arrow)* and in the interstitium surrounding the tubules. Segments of the tubules are destroyed, and this leukocytic material is flushed out into the urine as casts.

E. coli is the most common infecting organism in acute, uncomplicated pyelonephritis. Of patients with this infection, 90% respond to antibiotic therapy and the remaining 10% may have acute recurrent infections or persistent asymptomatic bacteriuria. When acute pyelonephritis is complicated by obstruction, recurrent or persistent bacteriuria occurs in 50% to 80% of patients within 2 years. It is not known with certainty how many of these patients will develop significant renal damage or how long the process might take. Treatment is directed toward appropriate antibacterial therapy, correction of predisposing factors, and careful long-term follow-up, with urine cultures at intervals to ensure that the urine is sterile.

Chronic pyelonephritis

The identification and the causes of chronic pyelonephritis are controversial. A major problem in identification is that many other inflammatory and ischemic diseases of the kidney produce segmental focalized areas of disease indistinguishable from those produced by bacterial infection. For example, nonbacterial disorders such as arteriolar nephrosclerosis and toxic nephropathies caused by analgesic abuse, lead exposure, and certain drugs (see pp. 716-717) result in tubulointerstitial damage similar to chronic pyelonephritis. It is now apparent that only a small proportion of these lesions result from infection. In the past, the diagnosis of chronic pyelonephritis was almost universally applied when these tubulointerstitial abnormalities were found. The notion that a severe degree of VUR can produce the renal scarring, atrophy, and dilated calyces (reflux nephropathy) commonly diagnosed as chronic pyelonephritis is now well accepted. The mechanism causing the scarring is believed to be the combined effects of (1) VUR, (2) intrarenal reflux, and (3) infection (Kunin, 1987; Rubin et al., 1991; Rose, Rennke, 1994). The severity of the VUR is the single most important determinant of whether renal damage will occur. Most of the evidence suggests that the renal involvement in reflux nephropathy occurs early in childhood before the age of 5 to 6 years, because new scar formation rarely occurs after this age. The explanation for this observation is that intrarenal reflux ceases as the child grows older, probably because of renal growth even though VUR may continue.

In adults, VUR and reflux nephropathy may be associated with obstructive and neurologic conditions that cause

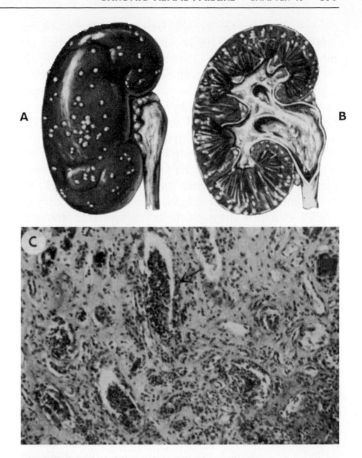

FIG. 46-5   Gross and microscopic appearance of the kidney in acute pyelonephritis. **A,** The kidney is swollen with multiple abscesses on the surface. **B,** Abscesses appear as yellowish gray streaks on the cross section. **C,** Histologically, many PMNs appear in the interstitium and within the tubules. (Illustration by Judy Simon, Department of Medical and Biological Illustrations, University of Michigan.)

obstruction of urinary drainage (as in renal calculi, or neurogenic bladder in diabetes or spinal cord injury). However, most adults with renal scarring of chronic pyelonephritis developed these lesions during early childhood. Evidence to support the reflux-infection mechanism comes from animal models and the following human observations: 85% to 100% of children and 50% of adults with renal scarring have VUR, and 50% of children and 5% to 23% of adults with recurrent UTIs have VUR (Rubin et al., 1991).

Despite the fact that the reflux neuropathy occurring in early childhood may explain the renal scarring and damage seen in many patients, the problem of how to explain progressive renal damage remains, since a sizable proportion of adults with end-stage chronic pyelonephritis do not have concurrent reflux or UTI. Some patients do not even recall a history of recurrent UTI. As discussed previously in this chapter, the most popular theory explaining progressive renal failure in the presence of corrected reflux and sterile urine is the *intrarenal hemo-*

dynamic theory or *hyperfiltration hypothesis* (Rose, 1987; Rose, Rennke, 1994). According to this theory, the initial infection-induced nephron loss leads to compensatory increases in glomerular capillary pressure and hyperperfusion in the remaining relatively normal nephrons. The intraglomerular hypertension then appears to produce glomerular injury and eventual sclerosis. The concept of hemodynamically mediated glomerular injury is supported by an increasing body of evidence from animal and human studies. Experimental evidence shows that the control of systemic hypertension, especially by the administration of angiotensin-converting enzyme (ACE)–inhibitor drugs such as captopril or enalapril maleate, slows the decline of GFR in many patients with chronic renal failure. These drugs lower glomerular capillary pressure by opposing the action of angiotensin II and dilating the efferent arteriole. Preferential lowering of glomerular pressure also occurs when dietary protein is restricted to 20 to 30 g/day, supplemented with amino acids and their keto analogues. Multiple protein-restriction studies have demonstrated marked slowing (75% to 90%) or even a cessation of the decline in GFR in many patients, although the mechanism by which protein intake affects GFR is uncertain. Moreover, this effect occurred in a wide variety of chronic renal diseases, including chronic pyelonephritis and chronic glomerulonephritis.

In contrast to acute pyelonephritis, the clinical features of chronic pyelonephritis are quite vague. The diagnosis is often made when a patient presents with symptoms of chronic renal insufficiency or hypertension, or proteinuria may be discovered in a routine examination. In some cases there is a documented history of UTIs dating from childhood. In other cases, careful questioning may reveal a history of vague symptoms of dysuria, frequency, and sometimes loin pain. Many patients are asymptomatic until the disease is advanced. Typical findings in chronic pyelonephritis include intermittent bacteriuria and WBCs or white cell casts in the urine. Proteinuria is usually minimal. Because chronic pyelonephritis is chiefly a medullary interstitial disease, the concentrating ability of the kidney is affected early in its course, before a significant decrease in the glomerular filtration rate occurs. Consequently, polyuria, nocturia, and urine with a low specific gravity are prominent early symptoms. Many patients also have a tendency to lose salt in the urine. About one half of the patients may develop hypertension. Azotemia is common in the course of chronic pyelonephritis, but advancement to renal failure usually progresses slowly.

The IVP reveals clubbing of the calyces, a thinned cortex, and small, irregular-shaped kidneys that are usually asymmetric (see Fig. 45-9, *B*). Fig. 46-6 illustrates the pathologic changes in chronic pyelonephritis. The surface of the kidney is coarsely granular, with U-shaped depressions (Fig. 46-6, *A*), subcapsular scars, and a dilated and fibrosed pelvis and calyces seen on the cross section (Fig. 46-6, *B*). Microscopic examination of tissue sections reveals characteristic parenchymal changes: many

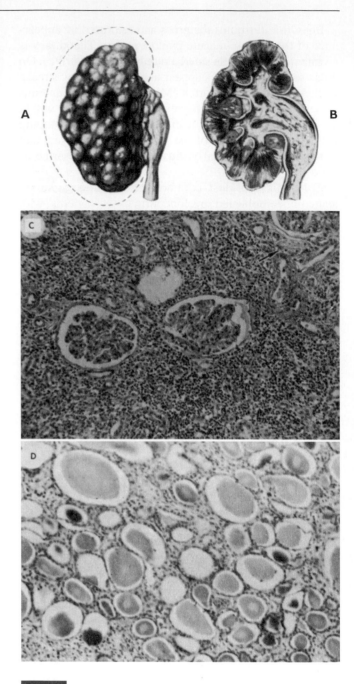

FIG. 46-6 Gross and microscopic appearance of the kidney in chronic pyelonephritis. **A,** Coarsely granular surface with U-shaped depressions. **B,** Thinning of the cortex, subcapsular scars; dilated, fibrosed pelvis; and calyces. **C,** Chronic inflammatory cells throughout interstitium; small, atrophied tubules; and an area of interstitial fibrosis *(arrows)*. **D,** Thyroid-gland appearance caused by dilated tubules containing glassy-looking casts. (Illustration by Judy Simon, Department of Medical and Biological Illustrations, University of Michigan.)

chronic inflammatory cells consisting of plasma cells and lymphocytes (dark-staining dots) are scattered throughout the interstitium. The three glomeruli are intact but surrounded by many tubules that are small and atrophied or dilated. There is an area of interstitial fibrosis near the glomerulus (*arrow,* Fig. 46-6, *C*). Large areas of thyroidization (having the appearance of thyroid gland tissue) are seen, consisting of dilated tubules lined with flattened epithelial cells and filled with glassy-appearing casts (Fig. 46-6, *D*).

Glomerulonephritis

Glomerulonephritis is a bilateral inflammatory disease of the kidneys that begins in the glomerulus and is manifested by proteinuria and/or hematuria. Although the lesions are primarily glomerular, entire nephrons may eventually be destroyed, leading to chronic renal failure. The original disease described by Richard Bright in 1827 *(Bright's disease)* is now known to be a collection of many diseases of different causes (most of which are unknown), although immune responses seem to be implicated in several forms of glomerulonephritis.

In recent years, knowledge of the pathologic changes in renal disease has been greatly expanded by renal biopsy studies using light, immunofluorescent, and electron microscopy. As knowledge has expanded, new categories have emerged based on a greater ability to define the nature of renal lesions. Numerous attempts have been made to separate and classify the various types of glomerulonephritis by relating histologic and clinical features. Unfortunately, the various categories are not exclusive. This overlap is understandable, since the kidney has only a limited number of morphologic and functional responses. To add to this confusion, many systemic and metabolic disorders may, when there is renal involvement, have changes in the glomeruli that are indistinguishable from primary glomerulonephritis.

Table 46-2 lists the various ways in which glomerulonephritis is described and classified. This table serves as a guide for the discussion in the remainder of this chapter and should be read before proceeding. The general term *glomerulonephritis* (GN) is commonly used to refer to a number of primary renal diseases predominantly affecting the glomeruli, but it is also used to refer to glomerular lesions that may or may not be the result of the primary renal disease. For example, the renal lesion in systemic lupus erythematosus may be referred to as proliferative glomerulonephritis. The following discussion focuses on primary renal diseases that cause glomerulonephritis, although references are made to systemic diseases that cause similar lesions in the kidney. Systemic diseases causing renal injury are considered in more detail later in this chapter.

Acute glomerulonephritis

The classic case of acute glomerulonephritis follows a streptococcal infection of the throat or sometimes of the skin after a latent period of 1 to 2 weeks. The responsible organism is usually a type 12 or 4, group A, beta-hemolytic streptococcus; rarely others. However, the streptococcus itself does not cause renal damage by infection. It is believed that antibodies are directed against a specific antigen that is a constituent of the specific streptococcal plasma membrane. An antigen-antibody complex is formed in the blood and circulates to the glomerulus, where it is mechanically trapped in the basement membrane. Complement is fixed, resulting in injury and inflammation, which attracts PMNs and platelets to the damaged site. Phagocytosis and release of lysosomal enzymes also damage the endothelium and glomerular basement membrane (GBM). As a response to injury there is proliferation of endothelial cells and then of mesangial cells, and later epithelial cells may increase as well. The resulting increased porosity of the glomerular capillary permits proteins and blood cells to escape into the forming urine, causing proteinuria and hematuria. It is presumably these antigen-antibody-complement complexes that appear as

► TABLE 46-2   Classifications of Glomerulonephritis

Classification	Description
DISTRIBUTION	
Diffuse	Involves all the glomeruli; most common form results in chronic renal failure
Focal	Only a portion of the glomeruli are abnormal
Local	Only a part of the glomerular tuft is abnormal, such as a single capillary loop
BROAD CLINICAL FORMS OF DIFFUSE GLOMERULONEPHRITIS	
Acute	Classic, benign disorder that is nearly always preceded by a streptococcal infection and associated with immune-complex deposition in the GBM and proliferative cellular changes
Subacute	Rapidly progressive form of glomerulonephritis characterized by intense cellular proliferative changes that destroy the glomeruli and result in death from uremia within a few months from the onset
Chronic	Slowly progressive glomerulonephritis leading to sclerosing and obliterative changes in the glomeruli; small, contracted kidneys; and death from uremia; entire course varies from 2-40 years

Continued.

▶ TABLE 46-2   Classifications of Glomerulonephritis—cont'd

Classification	Description

PATHOGENETIC IMMUNE MECHANISM AND IMMUNOFLUORESCENT PATTERN

Immune-complex, granular	Antibody (Ab) to either exogenous or endogenous nonglomerular antigens (Ag) is involved in the formation of circulating Ab-Ag complexes, which are passively trapped in the GBM. Complement fixation and the release of immunologic mediators result in glomerular injury; deposit is along epithelial surface and reveals a lumpy or granular pattern on immunofluorescent microscopy; associated with poststreptococcal GN, idiopathic membranous GN, and the GN of serum sickness, subacute bacterial endocarditis, malaria, and anaphylactoid purpura
Nephrotoxic (anti-GBM), linear	Antibodies form that react with the patient's own GBM as the antigen (anti-GBM or antikidney antibodies). True autoimmune disease in contrast to immune-complex GN, in which the GBM is like an innocent bystander; immune deposits are subendothelial and result in a ribbonlike linear pattern on immunofluorescence; associated with RPGN and Goodpasture's syndrome

HISTOLOGIC PATTERN

Minimal change	Also called lipoid nephrosis or foot-process disease; glomeruli appear normal or nearly normal on light microscopy, whereas electron microscopy reveals fusion of the foot processes; only major form of GN without evidence of immunopathology; commonly presents as the nephrotic syndrome in children 1-5 years of age; responds well to corticosteroid therapy; prognosis excellent
Proliferative change	Deposition of immunoglobulin, complement, and fibrin leads to proliferation of endothelial, mesangial, and epithelial cells; latter leads to crescent formation that may encircle and obliterate the glomerular tuft—ominous sign, common in RPGN and advanced CGN
Membranous change	Epimembranous deposit of immune material along GBM causing the GBM to thicken, but there is little or no inflammation or cellular proliferation, although the capillary lumen may eventually be obliterated; most common lesion in adults with the nephrotic syndrome; responds poorly to corticosteroid and immunosuppressive therapy; generally poor prognosis and slow progression to renal failure; membranous changes are also common in systemic nephritic diseases such as diabetes mellitus and SLE
Membranoproliferative change	Also called mesangiocapillary, lobular, or hypocomplementemic GN; immune-complex material deposited between the GBM and endothelium, causing GBM thickening and proliferation of the mesangial cells and giving the glomerulus a lobular or "wire-loop" appearance on light microscopy; characterized by low serum complement level, hematuria, and the nephrotic syndrome; responds poorly to therapy, generally progresses slowly to renal failure
Focal glomerulonephritis	Proliferative or sclerosing lesions that occur at random throughout the kidneys (focal as opposed to diffuse), often affecting only part of the glomerular tuft (local); occurs during at least part of the course of SBE, SLE, polyarteritis nodosa, Goodpasture's syndrome, and purpura; idiopathic focal GN sometimes appears in children; prognosis good

CLINICAL SYNDROMES

Acute nephritic syndrome	Acute nephritis of sudden onset, usually associated with poststreptococcal GN but can occur in many other renal diseases and as an acute exacerbation of CGN
Nephrotic syndrome	Clinical complex characterized by massive proteinuria (>3.5 g/day), hypoalbuminemia, edema, and hyperlipidemia. Occurs in many primary renal and systemic diseases; 50% of patients with CGN have it at least once
Persistent asymptomatic urine abnormalities	"Latent" stage in CGN, characterized by minimal proteinuria and/or hematuria but without symptoms; glomerular function relatively stable or may show slow progression ("silent azotemia")
Uremic syndrome	Symptomatic end-stage renal failure

AGN, Acute glomerulonephritis; *GBM*, glomerular basement membrane; *GN*, glomerulonephritis; *CRF*, chronic renal failure; *CGN*, chronic glomerulonephritis; *SLE*, systemic lupus erythematosus; *SBE*, subacute bacterial endocarditis; *RPGN*, rapidly progressive or subacute glomerulonephritis.

subepithelial nodules (or epimembranous humps) on electron microscopy and as a granular, "lumpy-bumpy" pattern on immunofluorescent microscopy; by light microscopy the glomeruli appear swollen and hypercellular, with invasion of PMNs (Fig. 46-7).

Acute poststreptococcal glomerulonephritis (APSGN) most frequently affects children between 3 and 7 years of age, although adolescents and young adults are also affected. The ratio of males to females is about 2:1.

The common presenting features of APSGN include hematuria, proteinuria, oliguria, edema, and hypertension. Common symptoms associated with the onset are fatigue, anorexia, and sometimes fever, headache, nausea, and vomiting. Elevation of the antistreptolysin O

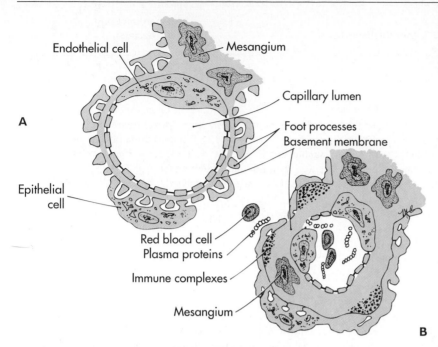

A

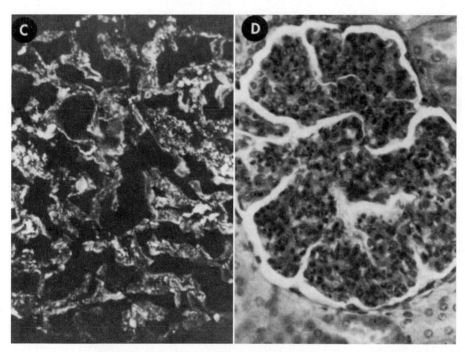

FIG. 46-7   Acute poststreptococcal glomeru-lonephritis. **A,** Diagram of electron microscopy appearance of a single capillary loop of the glomerular tuft. **B,** Diagram of electron microscopy appearance of subepithelial deposits of immune complex, thickened basement membrane, cellular proliferation, and damage to capillary. **C,** Photomicrograph of immunofluorescent preparation, showing lumpy pattern of immunoglobulin and complement deposits along glomerular capillary walls in circulating immune-complex disease. **D,** Light microscopy slide from kidney of a patient with acute poststreptococcal glomerulonephritis (APSGN), showing infiltration with polymorphonuclear leukocytes (PMNs) and hypercellularity that crowd the glomerulus filling Bowman's space. (Modified from Netter FH: Kidneys, ureter, and urinary bladder. In *The Ciba collection of medical illustrations,* vol 6, West Caldwell, NJ, 1973, Ciba Medical Education Division. Immunofluorescent micrograph courtesy of Michael J. Deegan, MD, University of Michigan Medical School.)

(ASO) titer may indicate the presence of antibodies to streptococcal organisms. Serum complement levels may be low, owing to depletion. This common finding gives further support to the hypothesis that the disease has an immune basis.

The major physiologic disturbances in APSGN are depicted on the diagram in Fig. 46-8. The GFR is usually depressed (although renal plasma flow is generally normal). Consequently the excretion of water, sodium, and nitrogenous substances may be decreased, resulting in edema and azotemia. Increased aldosterone may also play a role in sodium and water retention. Facial edema, particularly periorbital edema, is extremely common in the morning, although it may become more apparent in the lower extremities as the day progresses. The degree of edema usually depends on the severity of the glomerular inflammation, whether there is concomitant congestive heart failure, and how soon dietary salt is restricted.

Hypertension almost always occurs, although the rise in blood pressure may be only moderate. Whether the hypertension results from an expansion of the extracellular fluid (ECF) volume or from vasospasm is not clear.

Damage to the glomerular capillary tuft results in hematuria and albuminuria, as previously described. The urine may be grossly bloody or coffee colored. Microscopic examination of the sediment reveals cylindruria (many casts), red blood cells (RBCs), and red cell casts. The latter establish the glomerular origin of the bleeding.

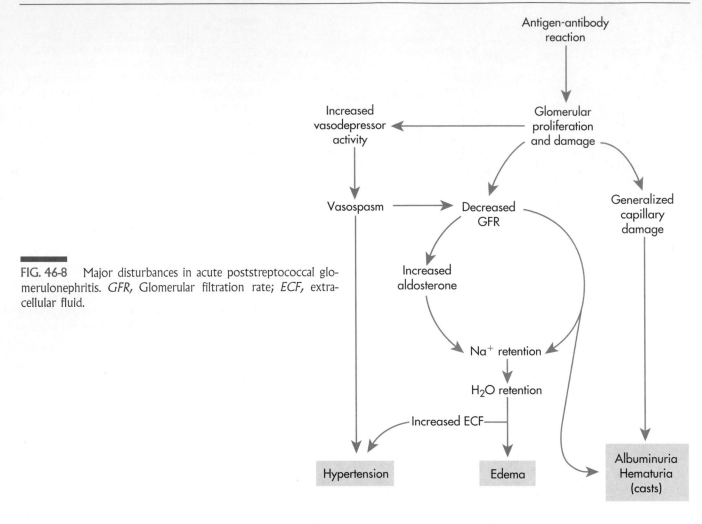

FIG. 46-8   Major disturbances in acute poststreptococcal glomerulonephritis. *GFR*, Glomerular filtration rate; *ECF*, extracellular fluid.

The loss of protein is usually not great enough to cause hypoalbuminemia, and the nephrotic syndrome rarely occurs in APSGN. The urine specific gravity is usually high despite azotemia, a combination rarely occurring in renal diseases other than APSGN. This finding is explained by the fact that tubular function has been affected very little by the acute disease.

The usual treatment of APSGN is penicillin to eradicate any residual streptococcal infection, bed rest during the acute phase, sodium restriction in the presence of edema or signs of heart failure, and antihypertensive drugs if indicated. Corticosteroid drugs have no known beneficial effect in APSGN. Symptoms usually subside within days, although microscopic hematuria and proteinuria may persist for months. It is estimated that more than 90% of children have a complete recovery. The prognosis is less favorable for adults (30% to 50%). Death occurs in 2% to 5% of all patients during the acute phase. In the remainder of patients, the disease may advance to a rapidly progressive glomerulonephritis (RPGN) or a more slowly progressive chronic glomerulonephritis (CGN). In RPGN, death from uremia usually occurs within a few months, whereas the entire course may vary from 2 to 40 years in CGN.

The natural history of the various forms of dif-

fuse glomerulonephritis is depicted in the diagram in Fig. 46-9. Contrary to popular belief, only a small percentage of the cases of RPGN and CGN have their origin in APSGN. The precipitating factors are usually unknown.

Although APSGN has been more clearly defined, it should be noted that an acute nephritic syndrome may be associated with many other diseases affecting the kidney (e.g., subacute bacterial endocarditis [SBE], malaria, anaphylactoid purpura, the collagen diseases). An acute nephritic syndrome may also occur during the course of CGN (Table 46-2).

Rapidly progressive glomerulonephritis

Rapidly progressive glomerulonephritis (formerly called *subacute*) is a term used to designate a fulminant renal disease with characteristic clinical and morphologic features. There is hematuria, proteinuria, and rapidly progressive azotemia resulting in death within 2 years. At autopsy, the salient features are widespread parietal epithelial crescent formation and diffuse glomerular involvement. Goodpasture's syndrome, a rare disease most common in young men, is a good example of this type of disease. The onset may be insidious or acute and is associated with lung hemorrhage and hemoptysis. There is

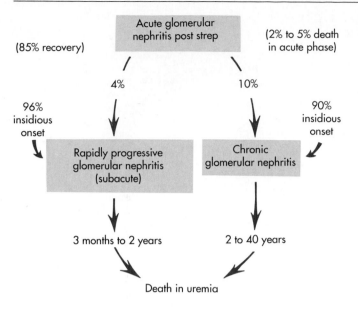

(85% recovery)

Acute glomerular
nephritis post strep

(2% to 5% death
in acute phase)

4%

10%

96%
insidious
onset

Rapidly progressive
glomerular nephritis
(subacute)

Chronic
glomerular nephritis

90%
insidious
onset

3 months to 2 years

2 to 40 years

Death in uremia

FIG. 46-9 Natural history of the various forms of diffuse glomerulonephritis.

usually no preceding illness to suggest the origin of the antibodies against the glomerular basement membrane that develop in the patient's blood. Subendothelial immune-complex material is seen with electron microscopy, and a linear pattern of immunofluorescence suggests that a nephrotoxic immune mechanism is involved in the pathogenesis (Fig. 46-10). Immunoglobulin deposits have also been found along the basement membrane in the lung alveoli. Patients who are treated aggressively early in the course of the disease with a combination of plasmapheresis (to remove anti-GBM antibodies), corticosteroids, and cytotoxic agents, such as cyclophosphamide or azathioprine, are more likely to recover. Approximately 20% of the patients regain normal renal

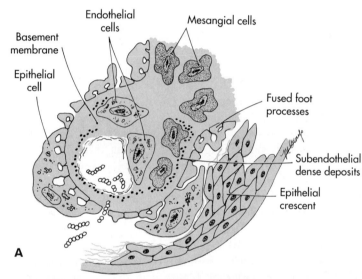

A

FIG. 46-10 Rapidly progressive glomerulonephritis. **A,** Cross section of a single capillary loop showing subendothelial dense deposits and glomerular damage. **B,** Photomicrograph of immunofluorescent preparation showing linear pattern of immune deposit typical of anti–glomerular basement membrane (GBM) disease. **C,** Light microscopy slide from a patient with rapidly progressive glomerulonephritis, showing large fibroepithelial crescent *(arrows)* crowding a lobulated glomerular tuft. (**A** modified from Netter FH: Kidneys, ureters, and urinary bladder. In *The Ciba collection of medical illustrations,* vol 6, West Caldwell, NJ, 1973, Ciba Medical Education Division. **B** from Fish AJ, Michael AF, Good RA: Pathogenesis of glomerulonephritis. In Strauss MB, Welt LG, editors: *Diseases of the kidney,* ed. 2, Boston, 1971, Little, Brown.)

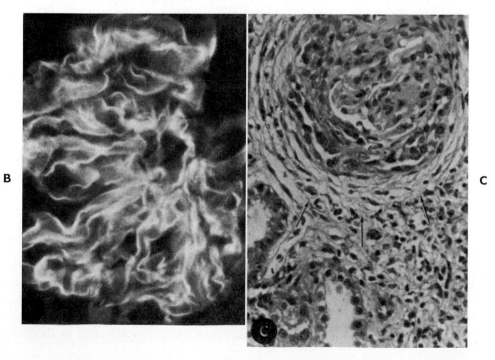

B

C

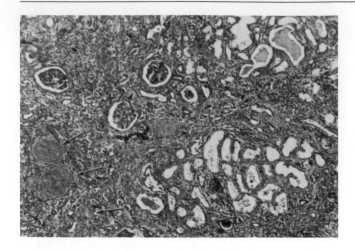

FIG. 46-11   End-stage kidney (light microscopy) from a patient with chronic pyelonephritis, showing marked distortion of the renal architecture. There is interstitial fibrosis, several glomeruli are completely hyalinized *(arrows)*, and three are spared. Marked tubular distortion and atrophy are present, and casts appear in several tubules.

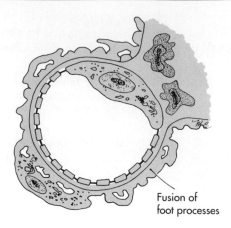

Fusion of foot processes

FIG. 46-12   Schema of glomerular loop showing fusion of foot processes in minimal change glomerulonephritis. (Modified from Netter FH: Kidneys, ureters, and urinary bladder. In *The Ciba collection of medical illustrations,* vol 6, West Caldwell, NJ, 1973, Ciba Medical Education Division.)

function. The greater the number of glomeruli that are involved, the less the chance of recovery. The exact mechanism of autoantibody elimination is not known. Dialysis support may be required for patients who develop progressive renal failure. Renal transplantation may be used after the anti-GBM antibodies have disappeared. Early diagnosis and vigorous treatment have increased survival of patients with this disease to more than 50% compared with 10% to 15% a decade ago (Brenner, Rector, 1991).

Chronic glomerulonephritis

Chronic glomerulonephritis (CGN) is characterized by slow, progressive destruction of the glomeruli from long-standing glomerulonephritis. In most instances, CGN has no known relationship to APSGN and RPGN but appears to represent de novo disease. The onset tends to be insidious, and it is usually discovered late in its course when symptoms of renal insufficiency appear. According to the stage of the disease, there may be polyuria or oliguria, proteinuria of varying degrees, hypertension, progressive azotemia, and death from uremia.

In advanced CGN the kidneys are grossly contracted, sometimes weighing as little as 50 g, and the surface is granular. These changes are caused by ischemia and the loss of nephrons. Microscopically, most of the glomeruli are altered. There may be a mixture of membranous and proliferative changes and epithelial crescent formation. Eventually there is atrophy of the tubules, interstitial fibrosis, and thickening of the arterial walls. When marked damage to all structures has occurred, the organ is called an *end-stage kidney,* and it may be difficult to determine whether the original lesion was glomerular, interstitial, or vascular (Fig. 46-11).

Nephrotic syndrome. Although many patients with CGN

have persistent, asymptomatic proteinuria throughout the course of the disease, about 50% develop the nephrotic syndrome. The nephrotic syndrome is a clinical state in which there is massive proteinuria (>3.5 g/day), hypoalbuminemia, edema, and hyperlipidemia. Usually the BUN level is normal.

The nephrotic syndrome is associated with several primary (idiopathic) glomerular diseases, or it may be associated with a large variety of systemic disorders in which the kidneys are secondarily involved. Examples of primary renal diseases associated with the nephrotic syndrome include minimal change glomerulonephritis, membranous glomerulonephritis, focal glomerulosclerosis, mesangial proliferative glomerulonephritis, and membranoproliferative glomerulonephritis (discussion follows). Examples of systemic diseases associated with the nephrotic syndrome include diabetes glomerulosclerosis; systemic lupus erythematosus (SLE); amyloidosis; Henoch-Schönlein purpura; drugs (e.g., gold, captopril, street heroin); other immune-complex diseases caused by chronic infection (e.g., hepatitis B, endocarditis, shunt infections); neoplasm; and acquired immunodeficiency syndrome (AIDS). Children and adults differ in the prevalence of the etiologies of the nephrotic syndrome. The cause of the nephrotic syndrome in children is predominantly primary glomerular disease, whereas it is most often associated with a systemic disorder in adults.

Minimal change glomerulonephritis (GN) is the typical lesion of the nephrotic syndrome in childhood (<15 years) accounting for about 70% to 80% of the cases. Older names for this disease include *lipoid nephrosis, nil disease,* or *foot-process disease.* The latter name is related to the observation that the normally discrete foot processes (podocytes) of the glomerular epithelial cells appear on electron microscopy to be fused together (Fig. 46-12). The cause is unknown although the disease is preceded by an upper respiratory infection in about one third of the cases. Minimal change GN is the only major form of glomerulonephritis in which immune pathogenic mechanisms do not appear to be involved. The onset of the nephrotic syndrome is usually sudden in children ages 2 to 6 years, with a male to female ratio of 2:1. This lesion is less common in adults and accounts for only 15% to 20% of the cases of idiopathic nephrotic syndrome.

Because the etiology and pathogenesis of minimal change GN are unknown, treatment is empiric and symptomatic. More than 95% of children respond to corticosteroid therapy with complete disappearance of the proteinuria within 8 weeks. The response to corticosteroids may take longer in adults with a less favorable outcome. In the minority of patients who do not respond to steroid therapy or who have relapses, immunosuppressive drugs such as cyclophosphamide (Cytoxan) or azathioprine (Imuran) may be helpful. The small proportion of patients who do not recover generally follow a long, remitting, relapsing course ending in uremia (Glassock, Brenner, 1994; Schrapner, Robson, 1993).

Focal glomerulosclerosis (FGS) accounts for 10% to 15% of the cases of idiopathic nephrotic syndrome in children and 10% to 20% of the cases in adults. The lesion is characterized by sclerosis and hyalinosis of some of the glomeruli (hence the term *focal*). Immunofluorescence reveals deposition of IgM and C3. The cause of the lesion is unknown. Some patients respond to corticosteroid therapy with a lasting remission, but about half of the patients with heavy proteinuria develop end-stage renal failure within 10 years. If the patient receives a renal transplant, the disease commonly recurs in the transplanted organ (Glassock, Brenner, 1994).

Membranous glomerulonephritis is the most common cause of idiopathic nephrotic syndrome in adults, accounting for 30% to 40% of the cases, but it is rare in children (<5%). The lesions are diffusely distributed and involve all the glomeruli. The predominant histologic change seen by light microscopy is thickening of the basement membrane. IgG and C3 are seen in a granular pattern along the glomerular basement membrane. Membranous change GN follows a slowly progressive course with intermittent remissions and exacerbations. About one third of the patients develop end-stage renal failure within 5 to 10 years. Corticosteroids, sometimes in combination with cyclophosphamide, are used in an attempt to obtain a remission but do not seem to greatly alter the course of the disease (Glassock, Brenner, 1994).

Mesangial proliferative glomerulonephritis is characterized by diffuse involvement of glomeruli and proliferation of the mesangial cells and endothelial cells. It represents a heterogeneous group of glomerular diseases. Immunofluorescence microscopy reveals a variety of patterns. A granular pattern of IgA and C3 deposits in the mesangium may predominate, in which case it is called *IgA nephropathy* or *Berger's disease*. In other cases there may be IgG or IgM deposits in the mesangium that may represent resolving poststreptococcal GN or other sys-

temic diseases such as systemic lupus erythematosus or Henoch-Schönlein purpura. This lesion is responsible for about 5% of idiopathic nephrotic syndrome in adults and 5% to 10% in children. It is more common in older children and young adults. Patients who have a remission of proteinuria after corticosteroid therapy tend to do well, with less inclination to develop progressive renal failure. Progressive renal failure develops in about 20% to 30% of the patients with steroid-unresponsive nephrotic syndrome (Glassock, Brenner, 1994). Since it was first identified in 1968, IgA nephropathy is becoming the most frequently identified primary glomerular disease in the world (although in most cases the proteinuria is mild). Diffuse mesangial IgA deposition is seen in 10% of renal biopsies performed for diagnostic purposes in North America, 20% to 25% in Europe and Australia, and as many as 30% to 40% in the Asian-Pacific region (D'Amico, 1987; Glassock et al., 1991).

Membranoproliferative glomerulonephritis (MPGN) is characterized both by thickening of the capillary loops and mesangial hypercellularity. It is also called *mesangiocapillary* or *lobular glomerulonephritis*. There are two main subgroups (types I and II), which have different histologies. Type I MPGN is characterized by subendothelial deposits of C3 in a granular pattern around the capillary loop. This type of pattern may also be seen in SLE. Type II MPGN is uncommon, where long segments of densely staining deposits occur within the basement membrane, causing thickening; the alternate name is *dense deposit disease*. The dense deposits may contain C3 and IgM.

MPGN is found in about 5% of cases of idiopathic nephrotic syndrome in children, especially between the ages of 8 and 16 years, and is somewhat less common in adults. The clinical presentation is quite varied. Type I accounts for about two thirds of the cases, affecting males and females equally. Some 50% to 75% present with the nephrotic syndrome. The remainder have proteinuria in the nonnephrotic range that is accompanied by hematuria. Circulating immune complexes are often present, and serum C3 levels are depressed. Type II may be associated with partial lipodystrophy with loss of subcutaneous fat in the face or other parts of the body. Low plasma C3 in type II MPGN is associated with the presence of C3-nephritic factor (C3NeF), an IgG antibody to C3-convertase, which has the effect of protecting C3-convertase from enzymatic degradation, with resultant low C3 levels.

The cause of MPGN is unknown, although in some cases there is a history of a preceding upper respiratory infection. Both types I and II MPGN are aggressive and progressive diseases with approximately half of the patients dying or developing ESRD within 10 years. The prognosis for type II lesions is worse than for type I.

The major physiologic disturbances leading to edema in the nephrotic syndrome are depicted in Fig. 46-13. The initial event in most cases is an antigen-antibody reaction at the glomerulus, resulting in increased GBM permeability, massive proteinuria, and hypoalbuminemia. Patients

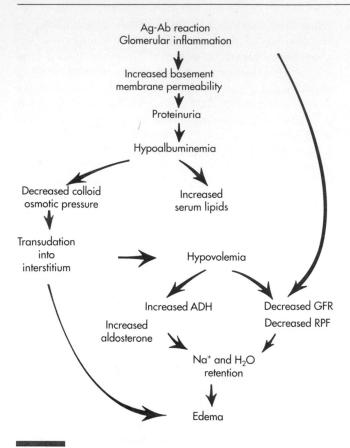

FIG. 46-13   Pathogenesis of nephrotic edema. (Modified from Schreiner FE: The nephrotic syndrome. In Strauss MB, Welt LG, editors: *Diseases of the kidney*, ed 2, Boston, 1971, Little, Brown.)

with the nephrotic syndrome commonly pass 5 to 15 g of protein every 24 hours. Hypoalbuminemia, by decreasing colloid osmotic pressure (COP), favors the transudation of fluid out of the vascular compartment into the interstitium. This is a fairly direct mechanism for the production of edema. In addition, the hypovolemia results in a decrease of renal plasma flow (RPF) and GFR, activating the renin-angiotensin mechanism. The hypovolemia also activates volume receptors in the left atrium. The result is increased aldosterone and ADH production. Salt and water are retained by the kidneys, further aggravating the edema. By repetition of this chain of events, massive edema (anasarca) may occur. The amount of protein lost, however, does not correlate precisely with the severity of the edema, since people vary in the rate of protein synthesis to replace that which is lost. The cause of the hyperlipidemia that often accompanies the nephrotic syndrome is obscure. Serum cholesterol, phospholipids, and triglycerides are all usually increased. Note that the mechanism of nephrotic edema differs from that of acute poststreptococcal glomerulonephritis (APSGN).

Complications of the nephrotic syndrome include hyperlipidemia and hypertension, which may predispose to atherosclerosis when prolonged. There is also an increased susceptibility to infection, which may be caused by loss of immunoglobulins in the urine. Thrombosis is a common complication in the nephrotic syndrome, leading to renal vein thrombosis, deep venous thrombosis in the legs, and pulmonary embolism.

The nephrotic syndrome is treated with corticosteroid and immunosuppressive drugs directed toward the nature of the lesion, a high-protein and salt-restricted diet, diuretics, sometimes intravenous infusion of albumin, and restricted activity during the acute phase. When diuretics are used, they must be used with caution since excessive diuresis will cause ECF volume depletion and increase the risk of thrombosis and renal hypoperfusion. It is also important to isolate patients from sources of infection. Patients with the nephrotic syndrome are highly susceptible to infection, and before antibiotic drugs were discovered, they often died of empyema, pneumonia, or peritonitis. Angiotensin-converting enzyme (ACE) inhibitors can reduce protein loss by reducing intraglomerular pressure and GFR. This reduction in protein loss, reduction in intraglomerular pressure, and inhibition of angiotensin II may also be helpful in reducing the fluid retention. ACE inhibitors are also the first-line drugs of choice to control systemic hypertension, which may be caused by the renal disease and may be a side effect from corticosteroid therapy. Long-term management is important, since many patients follow a course of repeated exacerbations and remissions over a period of years, but with advancing glomerular hyalinization, proteinuria usually diminishes as azotemia progresses.

Hypertensive Nephrosclerosis

Hypertension and chronic renal failure are closely related. Hypertension may be the primary disease and damage the kidneys, and conversely, severe chronic renal disease may cause hypertension or contribute to its maintenance through the mechanism of sodium and water retention, the vasopressor effects of the renin-angiotensin system, and possibly prostaglandin deficiency. Sometimes it is difficult for the nephrologist to determine which was the primary disease. Nephrosclerosis (hardening of the kidneys) refers to the pathologic changes in the renal blood vessels as a result of hypertension. It is one of the leading causes of chronic renal failure, particularly in the nonwhite population.

Essential hypertension and the kidneys

Hypertension is defined as a sustained elevation of blood pressure above the accepted normal values of 90 mm Hg diastolic or 140 mm Hg systolic. According to this definition, about 5% of the United States population have hypertension. However, as many as 25% of individuals may have this disorder by the age of 50 years. The cause of hypertension is unknown in about 90% of the cases and is termed *essential hypertension* (unknown etiology and pathogenesis). The onset of essential hypertension usually occurs between the ages of 20 and 50 years, and it is more frequent in African Americans. Essential hypertension is classified as benign or malignant. *Benign hypertension* is slowly progressive, whereas in *malignant hypertension* there is rapid acceleration in the course of the hypertensive disease, resulting in severe organ damage.

The rate of progression of benign essential hypertension is variable, but it generally runs a slowly progressive course over a period of 20 to 30 years. Longstanding hypertension produces structural changes in the arterioles throughout the body, characterized by fibrosis and hyalinization (sclerosis) of the blood vessel walls. The chief target organs of this condition are the heart, brain, kidneys, and eyes. The usual cause of death is myocardial infarction, congestive heart failure, or cerebrovascular accident. If essential hypertension remains benign, patients are not likely to suffer renal damage sufficient to die of uremia. Most of the cases of renal insufficiency attributed to benign nephrosclerosis have underlying renal disease (Nolan, Schrier, 1992). Proteinuria and mild azotemia may exist for years without symptoms, and most patients who die of uremia do so as a result of the hypertension entering the malignant phase. This occurs in less than 10% of the cases of essential hypertension.

Malignant hypertension implies severe hypertension with diastolic blood pressure greater than 120 to 130 mm Hg, grade IV retinopathy,* and renal excretory dysfunction, ranging from proteinuria to hematuria to azotemia. Malignant hypertension may occur at any time during the course of benign hypertension but usually occurs after many years. Occasionally it occurs de novo, especially in African American men in their third and fourth decades.

In the kidney, renal arteriosclerosis caused by longstanding hypertension results in *benign nephrosclerosis.* This disorder is the direct result of ischemia caused by the narrowed lumen of the intrarenal blood vessels. The kidney may be reduced in size, usually symmetrically, and has a granular, pitted surface. Histologically, the essential lesion is sclerosis of the small arteries and arterioles, which is most marked in the afferent arterioles. The closure of the arteries and arterioles leads to destruction of the glomeruli and atrophy of the tubules, so that entire nephrons are destroyed.

Malignant nephrosclerosis designates the structural renal changes often associated with the malignant phase of essential hypertension.† The kidneys may be of normal size, with minimal granularity and some petechiae from

---

*Grade IV retinopathy refers to the most severe changes in the retina caused by hypertension. These changes may be viewed with the ophthalmoscope and consist of vascular sclerosis, exudates, hemorrhages, and papilledema.

†Although these gross and microscopic renal lesions are characteristic of the malignant phase of essential hypertension, they are not specific and may be superimposed on a variety of diseases associated with hypertension (e.g., chronic pyelonephritis, chronic glomerulonephritis, polyarteritis nodosa).

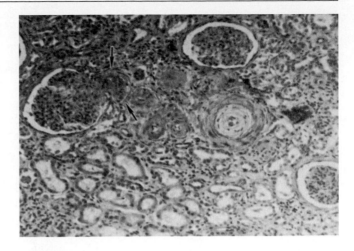

FIG. 46-14   Malignant nephrosclerosis. Light microscopy slide showing several hyalinized arterioles *(center field),* dilated tubules with atrophied lining cells *(lower center),* and an area of fibrinoid necrosis *(arrows).*

rupture of arterioles, or they may be shrunken and scarred. Histologically there are three types of lesions: (1) proliferative endarteritis, (2) fibrinoid necrosis of arteriolar walls, and (3) fibrinoid necrosis of glomerular tufts. At first there is marked thickening of the intima of the interlobular arteries caused by proliferation of the endothelial cells. These changes produce an appearance often referred to as "onion skin." The narrowed lumina produce ischemia of the afferent arterioles and the release of renin, and the blood pressure rises still further. Focal necrosis then occurs in the walls of the afferent arterioles, and because the necrosed areas contain fibrin, the change is called *fibrinoid necrosis.* Fibrinoid necrosis of the glomerular tufts is probably an extension of the fibrinoid necrosis of the feeding afferent arterioles. If the blood pressure remains elevated, these localized changes become widespread, with the formation of thrombi, glomerular hemorrhage, infarction of entire nephrons, and rapid death of all renal cells. Fig. 46-14 illustrates some of the above lesions. The treatment of hypertension is discussed in Chapters 31 and 48.

Renal artery stenosis

The renal artery may be occluded by atherosclerotic plaques or fibromuscular dysplasia, causing hypertension that is often of the rapidly progressive type. Atherosclerosis is found chiefly in older men and usually involves the proximal one third of the renal artery near the aorta. Fibromuscular dysplasia is characterized by excesses in fibrous connective tissue within the layers of the blood vessel and is most apt to occur in the middle and distal thirds of the renal artery, sometimes involving segmental branches. There are several histologic types of fibromuscular dysplasia, and the disorder is most common in women between the ages of 20 and 50 years.

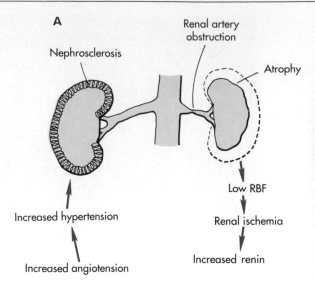

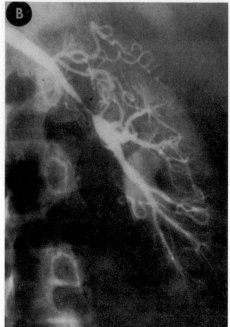

FIG. 46-15   **A,** Pathogenesis of nephrosclerosis in the contralateral kidney in renal artery stenosis. **B,** Renal arteriogram showing renal artery stenosis caused by fibromuscular dysplasia. *RBF,* Renal blood flow. (**B** from Stanley JC, Fry WF: *Arch Surg* 110:922, 1975. Copyright 1975, American Medical Association.)

Renal artery stenosis may be unilateral or bilateral. If the caliber of the artery is reduced by 70% or more, renal ischemia occurs. The renal ischemia activates the renin-angiotensin system, and hypertension follows. Although uncommon (about 0.5% of hypertension cases), renal artery stenosis is important because surgical correction may alleviate or markedly ameliorate the hypertensive state (Working Group on Renovascular Hypertension, 1987).

Unilateral renal artery stenosis not only causes ischemic atrophy of the involved kidney but also may eventually cause hypertensive nephrosclerosis of the contralateral kidney. The pathogenetic mechanism is depicted in Fig. 46-15. If the contralateral kidney has developed significant nephrosclerosis from the renin-induced hypertension, the function of the ischemic kidney may even be the better of the two, since the stenosed renal artery protects the occluded kidney from the full effects of the systemic hypertension.

Renal artery stenosis should be suspected when hypertension develops in persons younger than 30 years, when there is a truly abrupt-onset hypertension at any age, or when there is a definite worsening of previously well-controlled hypertension. Physical findings suggestive of renal artery stenosis include a continuous systolic and diastolic bruit heard over the epigastrium or the flank. Differences in carotid, brachial, or femoral pulses or blood pressure in the extremities, indicative of generalized atherosclerosis, are other nonspecific clues.

A captopril screening test is the procedure of choice for suspected renal artery stenosis, since this test has a specificity and sensitivity greater than 95% (Badr, Brenner,

1994). Rapid-sequence IVP is no longer used as a screening tool, since it has a false-positive rate of 12% in the hypertensive population. The captopril test measures the increase in plasma renin activity (PRA) in response to the administration of captopril, which is exaggerated in persons with renovascular hypertension compared with persons with essential hypertension. If the captopril test is positive, more invasive tests are administered. The most definitive diagnostic procedure is bilateral arteriography with repeated bilateral renal vein and systemic renin determinations. If the arteriogram shows unilateral renal artery stenosis and if renal vein renin measurements from the two kidneys differ by a ratio of 1.5:1 or more, the chance of curing the hypertension by surgical reconstruction is almost 90% (Badr, Brenner, 1994). A renin ratio below 1.5:1 does not exclude the diagnosis of renovascular hypertension, especially if bilateral disease is present.

The aim of treatment is to control systemic blood pressure and restore perfusion to the ischemic kidney. Surgical treatment consists of revascularization of the ischemic kidney, often by means of a saphenous vein bypass graft. Alternately, percutaneous transluminal angioplasty (PCTA) may be used to enlarge the vessel lumen. Success rates with surgery or PCTA in young persons with fibromuscular dysplasia are 50% cure and 30% improvement in blood pressure; renovascular hypertension is improved in about 50% of older persons so treated. Even if PCTA or surgery fails to normalize blood pressure, these procedures allow easier medical control of hypertension. ACE inhibitor drugs are particularly effective in treating patients with renovascular hypertension, but caution must be exercised in bilateral renal artery stenosis or stenosis of a solitary kidney, since acute renal failure may follow converting enzyme inhibition under these circumstances. This adverse effect is presumed to be the result of the loss of angiotensin II effects on the glomerular efferent arterioles, which serve to maintain the GFR in the setting of renal hypoperfusion (see Chapters 44 and 49). It should be emphasized that, although the risk of precipitating acute renal failure is greatest with ACE inhibitor drugs, any antihypertensive drug can lead to acute renal failure if the stenosis is severe (Conlin et al., 1992; Schrier, 1995).

Connective Tissue Disorders

The connective tissue disorders (collagen diseases) are systemic diseases whose manifestations are mainly attributable to the soft tissues of the body (see Part Twelve). They are of particular interest in nephrology because of the high incidence of renal involvement. About two thirds of patients with SLE and progressive systemic sclerosis (scleroderma) have clinical evidence of renal involvement. The incidence is about 80% for patients with polyarteritis nodosa. Renal involvement is relatively uncommon in rheumatoid arthritis. When it does occur, it is usually a complication of therapy (gold salts, D-penicillamine) or a manifestation of secondary amyloidosis (Glassock, 1992).

Systemic lupus erythematosus

SLE is a multisystem disease of unknown etiology characterized by circulating autoantibodies to deoxyribonucleic acid (DNA). The diagnosis of SLE is confirmed by positive tests for antinuclear antibodies (ANA) (a useful screening test) and the more specific test for anti-DNA antibodies. SLE predominantly affects young women between the ages of 20 and 40 years, who account for 90% of the cases. Renal involvement is a major cause of morbidity in patients with SLE. Although renal failure is becoming less common with modern treatment, about 25% of those with SLE eventually develop renal failure.

Lupus nephritis is caused by circulating immune complexes that become trapped in the glomerular basement membrane and cause damage. The mechanism is similar to that in APSGN except that the source of the antigen is the body's own DNA rather than the streptococcal plasma membrane. In SLE the body produces antibody against its own DNA. The clinical picture may be one of acute glomerulonephritis or of nephrotic syndrome. Although the basic cause is thought to be the same in both cases, focal, membranous, and proliferative changes in the glomeruli may all be seen. The earliest change often involves only part of the glomerular tuft (local), or only scattered glomeruli may be involved (focal). Focal glomerulonephritis and local glomerulonephritis respond quite well to corticosteroid drugs, and a complete remission may occur. The prognosis is poor for those who de-

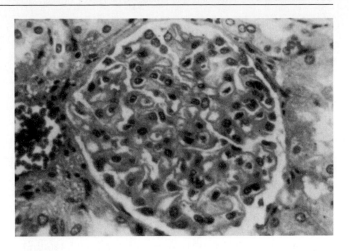

FIG. 46-16   Glomerulus from a patient with membranous lupus nephritis. Capillary walls (basement membrane) are uniformly thickened, but there is no increase in cellularity. Note the wire-loop appearance. Note the red blood cells in the lumen of the tubule *(left center)*.

velop diffuse membranous or proliferative changes, and these patients often develop ESRD within 10 years (Fig. 46-16). A combination of corticosteroid and cytotoxic drugs is often given to patients with active, proliferative lesions in an attempt to better preserve renal function. Patients with SLE tolerate dialysis quite well and, if transplanted, do not develop a recurrence of the renal lesions.

Polyarteritis nodosa

Polyarteritis nodosa (PAN) is an inflammatory and necrotizing disease involving the medium-size and small arteries throughout the body, with secondary ischemia of the tissues supplied by the affected vessels. Early signs and symptoms of PAN are nonspecific, including fever, malaise, weight loss, and abdominal pain. Intractable hypertension secondary to the arteritis is often present. Men are more commonly affected than women, and the mean age of onset is 48 years. Although the exact cause and pathogenesis are unknown, evidence suggests some form of hypersensitivity mechanism. In many cases the onset is associated with a sensitivity reaction to drugs.

Renal lesions are of two types. If the medium-size vessels within the kidney are affected, areas of renal infarction develop. If the disease is confined to the arterioles, the renal histology is that of severe focal, proliferative glomerulonephritis and fibrinoid necrotic changes with epithelial crescents.

The prognosis of untreated PAN is extremely poor, with a 5-year survival rate of 13%. Death commonly results from renal failure, bowel infarction, or cardiovascular or CNS complications. Recently, the prognosis of PAN has been greatly improved by a therapeutic regimen consisting of corticosteroids, cytotoxic agents (cyclophosphamide or azathioprine), and plasma exchange, resulting in a 90% remission rate. Early antihypertensive therapy can lessen the morbidity and mortality associated with the renal, cardiac, and CNS complications of PAN.

Progressive systemic sclerosis

Progressive systemic sclerosis, or *scleroderma,* is an uncommon systemic disease characterized by diffuse sclerosis of the skin and other organs. The disease affects the vasculature of several organs, including the kidneys. Women are affected more often than men. The onset is usually between the ages of 20 and 50 years. As in SLE, a variety of antibodies may be found in the serum, suggesting that immune mechanisms may be involved in the pathogenesis.

The interlobar arteries typically show changes resembling hypertensive nephrosclerosis. Progressive renal impairment may develop slowly over a period of years. In a few cases, hypertension and uremia may follow a malignant course, with the development of end-stage renal failure within weeks.

No effective therapy is available for scleroderma, but aggressive antihypertensive therapy with ACE inhibitors may significantly prolong life and forestall the development of renal failure. Dialysis may also prolong life, but most patients will eventually die from extrarenal disease, especially myocardial failure or pulmonary fibrosis.

Congenital and Hereditary Disorders

Renal tubular acidosis and polycystic disease of the kidneys are hereditary disorders affecting primarily the renal tubules and may terminate in renal failure, although this is more common in polycystic disease. Both diseases have an infantile and an adult form, whose manifestations may be quite distinct.

Polycystic kidney disease

Polycystic kidney disease (PCKD) is characterized by bilateral, multiple, expanding cysts that gradually encroach on and destroy the normal renal parenchyma by compression. The kidney may be enlarged (sometimes as large as a football) and filled with grapelike clusters of cysts (Fig. 46-17). The cysts are filled with clear or hemorrhagic fluid.

The rare infantile form of the disease appears to be inherited as an autosomal recessive trait. The cysts are closed, blind pouches into which the glomerular filtrate flows. The course of the disease is rapidly progressive, usually resulting in death before the age of 2 years.

In contrast, adult polycystic disease is much more common (about 1 per 500 population). It is an autosomal dominant trait, the cysts communicate with the tubules, and the course is slowly progressive, with symptoms of renal insufficiency usually occurring during the fourth decade. Flank pain, hematuria, polyuria, proteinuria, and palpably enlarged, "knobby" kidneys are often the presenting signs and symptoms. Hypertension and urinary tract infections are common complications.

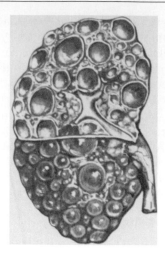

FIG. 46-17   Polycystic kidney. (Illustration by Judy Simon, Department of Medical and Biological Illustrations, University of Michigan.)

Treatment for patients with PCKD is aimed at preventing complications and preserving renal function. Patients and family members should be educated about the inheritance and manifestations of the disease. Therapy is directed toward the control of hypertension and the early treatment of UTI. Patients with PCKD have a tendency to be salt losers, so dehydration and inadequate salt intake should be avoided. The disease progresses to ESRD in about 25% of patients by the age of 50 years and in about 50% by the age of 70 years. Some patients may have a normal life span and die of nonrenal causes. ESRD is managed by dialysis or renal transplantation. Bilateral nephrectomy may be necessary before transplantation in patients with greatly enlarged kidneys.

Renal tubular acidosis

Renal tubular acidosis (RTA) refers to a group of disorders in which there is defective renal H^+ tubular excretion or loss of HCO_3^- in the urine despite preservation of an adequate GFR. The result is a sustained metabolic acidosis. RTA may be hereditary or acquired, and it is commonly divided into four subtypes:

- Type 1 RTA is characterized by defective H^+ secretion in the distal tubule.
- Type 2 RTA is characterized by defective HCO_3^- reabsorptive capacity in the proximal tubule.
- Type 3 RTA occurs in infants and is a rare form of a mixture of types 1 and 2, with both a urine acidification defect and excessive loss of HCO_3^- in the urine.
- Type 4 RTA is most commonly associated with the hyporeninemic hypoaldosteronism syndrome.

This discussion focuses on types 1 and 2 RTA.

Classic *type 1,* or *distal, RTA* is characterized by the inability to maximally acidify the urine to less than pH 5.3 even in the presence of acidemia. The patient is unable to excrete the daily metabolic acid load, resulting in a progressive systemic acidemia with a plasma HCO_3^- that may be less than 10 mEq/L.

Distal RTA may occur as a primary isolated defect or in association with other diseases and disorders. The primary disorder is the most common form in childhood and is transmitted by autosomal dominant inheritance with a variable degree of expression. Females are affected more than males. Autoimmune diseases, such as Sjögren's syndrome, are probably the major cause of this rare condition in adults. Although the exact nature of the defect responsible for the abnormalities of acidification in distal RTA is unclear, proposed mechanisms include (1) failure to transport H^+ against a steep pH gradient between the tubular lumen and peritubular fluid or (2) excessive back diffusion of H^+ from lumen to blood (Coe, Kathpalia, 1994).

The classic feature of distal RTA is the presence of a normal–anion gap hyperchloremic metabolic acidosis with a urine pH that is persistently above 5.3. Urine osmotic concentration and K^+ conservation are usually impaired, resulting in hypokalemia and polyuria. Bone disease, renal calculi, and nephrocalcinosis are other common manifestations of distal RTA caused by disturbed Ca^{++} metabolism. The chronic acidosis results in mobilization of Ca^{++} salts from the bone and hypercalciuria. Bone resorption is manifested as osteomalacia in adults and as rickets and stunted growth in children. Ca^{++} salts may precipitate diffusely in the renal parenchyma (nephrocalcinosis) or within the collecting system, causing calculi. Precipitation of $CaPO_4$ in the kidney is favored by low urinary citrate (which normally inhibits crystallization) and the elevated urine pH. Renal failure may be secondary to these complications.

The diagnosis of distal RTA is confirmed by the NH_4Cl loading test (see Chapter 45). NH_4Cl is metabolized in the liver to HCl. The excess H^+ normally excreted in urine causes the urine pH to fall below 5.3, but the urine pH remains above 5.3 in the person with distal RTA.

The acidemia in distal RTA may be corrected by the administration of sodium or potassium HCO_3^- or citrate (metabolized into HCO_3^- in the body). The usual dose is 1 to 3 mEq/kg/day. Infants and children respond well to this therapy, and the condition is usually completely reversed. In some adults the calcium deposits are reabsorbed after prolonged alkali therapy, whereas in others the nephrocalcinosis is permanent. The prognosis depends on the extent of renal damage before treatment is initiated.

Type 2, or *proximal, RTA* is characterized by an alkaline urine pH and bicarbonaturia at mildly or moderately reduced plasma HCO_3^- levels. In contrast to distal RTA, the urine pH can fall below 5.3 if the patient is sufficiently acidotic, indicating that distal acidification is intact. The basic mechanism causing proximal RTA is defective reabsorption of HCO_3^- in the proximal tubule. Normally about 85% of the filtered HCO_3^- is reabsorbed

in the proximal tubule at normal plasma concentrations. A large quantity of HCO_3^- is thus shunted to the distal tubule. Because the distal tubule has a limited capacity to reclaim HCO_3^-, an HCO_3^- diuresis occurs.

The loss of large quantities of HCO_3^- in the urine produces hyperchloremic metabolic acidosis. The severe progressive acidosis characteristic of distal RTA does not occur in proximal RTA, and the plasma HCO_3^- is usually stabilized at a moderate level between 13 and 20 mEq/L. The bicarbonaturia induces renal losses of Na^+ and K^+; therefore, ECF volume depletion and hypokalemia also occur. In contrast to distal RTA, nephrocalcinosis and nephrolithiasis do not usually occur.

As with distal RTA, proximal RTA may be inherited or acquired. When inherited, it is often associated with Fanconi's syndrome, a generalized tubular defect associated with inadequate absorption of glucose, phosphate, amino acids, and uric acid. Failure to thrive and stunting of growth, as in distal RTA, are regular features in growing children. Acquired proximal RTA in adults may be associated with multiple myeloma, Sjögren's syndrome, or amyloidosis.

Proximal RTA cannot be diagnosed by the NH_4Cl test, since these patients can acidify the urine when presented with an acid load. Rather, the diagnosis is made by the HCO_3^- infusion test. In this test, sufficient HCO_3^- is infused to raise the serum HCO_3^- level to just below the normal range (20 to 22 mEq/L) and then the urine pH and the fraction of the filtered HCO_3^- that is excreted are measured. In proximal RTA the urine pH rises above 7 and the fractional excretion of HCO_3^- exceeds 15% (since the reabsorptive threshold for HCO_3^- has been exceeded). However, in distal RTA, the urine pH remains unchanged and the fractional excretion of HCO_3^- is less than 3% (Coe, Kathpalia, 1994).

Treatment of proximal RTA may not be necessary in adults if the patient is asymptomatic and if the acidemia is mild. In children, treatment is always indicated, since even mild acidemia may retard growth. Proximal RTA is generally more difficult to treat than distal RTA. Larger dosages of alkali may be necessary (10 to 15 mEq/kg/day) to keep plasma HCO_3^- in the normal range, and a K^+ supplement is usually needed since therapy causes increased losses in the urine. Thus a combination of potassium and sodium citrate (Polycitra) is the drug of choice.

Metabolic Disorders

Metabolic disorders that may lead to chronic renal failure include diabetes mellitus, gout, primary hyperparathyroidism, and amyloidosis.

Diabetes mellitus

Diabetic nephropathy (renal disease in diabetics) is one of the most important causes of death in long-standing diabetes mellitus. Nearly one third of all new patients entering ESRD programs have diabetic renal failure. It

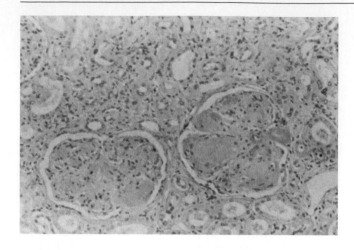

FIG. 46-18 Diabetic nephropathy (light microscopy) showing the typical nodular lesion in the two central glomeruli. Nodular appearance is caused by the deposit of mesangial matrix within the core of the peripheral capillary lobules. Initially the capillary lumina are patent, but they are gradually obliterated as the disease progresses. Note also the thickening of the basement membrane of the tubules in the lower central field.

has been estimated that about 50% of type I (insulin-dependent) diabetics develop chronic renal failure within 15 to 25 years after the onset of diabetes. Fewer individuals with type II diabetes (non–insulin-dependent) develop chronic renal failure (about 6%) with the exception of Pima Indians where the incidence is nearly 50%. Native Americans and African Americans have a particularly high risk of developing diabetic renal failure.

Diabetes mellitus affects the structure and function of the kidney in many ways. *Diabetic nephropathy* is a term that encompasses all of the lesions occurring in the kidney in diabetes mellitus. Glomerulosclerosis is the most characteristic lesion and may be diffuse or nodular. *Diffuse diabetic glomerulosclerosis,* the most common lesion, consists of diffuse thickening of the mesangial matrix* with eosinophilic material accompanied by thickening of the capillary basement membrane. *Nodular diabetic glomerulosclerosis* (also known as the *Kimmelstiel-Wilson lesion*) is less common but very specific for this disease; it consists of rounded, nodular accumulations of eosinophilic material that are usually located in the periphery of the glomerulus within the core of the capillary lobule (Fig. 46-18). Nonglomerular abnormalities in diabetic nephropathy include chronic tubulointerstitial nephritis, papillary necrosis, hyalinosis of the efferent and afferent arterioles, and ischemia. Diabetic glomerulosclerosis is nearly always preceded by diabetic retinopathy, characterized by microaneurysms around the macula.

---

*The mesangial matrix is a spongy network of basement membrane–like trabeculae at the center of the glomerular lobule surrounding the mesangial cells. It merges with the capillary basement membrane.

STAGES OF DIABETIC NEPHROPATHY

STAGE 1 (EARLY FUNCTIONAL CHANGES)

Renal hypertrophy
Increased glomerular capillary surface area
Increased glomerular filtration rate (GFR)

STAGE 2 (EARLY STRUCTURAL CHANGES)

Thickening of the glomerular capillary basement membrane
Normal or slightly elevated GFR

STAGE 3 (INCIPIENT NEPHROPATHY)

Microalbuminuria (30-300 mg/24 hr)
Elevated blood pressure

STAGE 4 (ESTABLISHED OR CLINICAL NEPHROPATHY)

Proteinuria (>300 mg/24 hr)
Decreased GFR

STAGE 5 (PROGRESSIVE RENAL INSUFFICIENCY OR FAILURE)

Rapidly declining GFR (−1 ml/month)
Kidney loses up to 3% of function every month

From Dunfee TP: *Hosp Med* 30(5):45, 1995, McGraw-Hill.

The natural history of diabetic nephropathy from onset to ESRD may be divided into five phases or stages (see box above). Recent research has demonstrated that some of the long-term complications of diabetes, such as diabetic retinopathy, neuropathy, and nephropathy, can be prevented or delayed by strict control of blood glucose and hypertension and dietary protein restriction (see Chapter 48).

Stage 1, or the phase of *early functional changes,* is characterized by renal hypertrophy and hyperfiltration. Stage 1 findings are present in virtually all patients at the diagnosis of insulin-dependent diabetes mellitus (IDDM) and develop at the onset of the disease. An elevation of the GFR commonly occurs, up to 40% above normal. This elevation is multifactorial in origin, with contributing factors including high blood glucose levels and abnormalities in glucagon, growth hormone, renin, angiotensin II, and prostaglandin effect. The kidneys exhibiting the increased GFR are larger than normal, and individual glomeruli are larger with increased surface area. It is believed, as discussed earlier in this chapter, that these changes may lead to focal glomerulosclerosis.

Stage 2, or the phase of *early structural changes,* is characterized by thickening of the glomerular capillary basement membrane and gradual accumulation of mesangial matrix material. This stage is present at approximately 5 years from the onset of IDDM and appears to develop in all patients with diabetes mellitus. The severity of mesangial thickening or expansion observed in stage 2 is positively correlated with the future development of proteinuria and decline in renal function. The accumulation of mesangial matrix may impinge on the glomerular capillary lumina, causing ischemia and decreased surface area for filtration, but the GFR is usually still in the high-normal range (reduced from the greatly elevated GFR during stage 1). Urinary albumin excretion is generally normal during stage 2, except for bouts of reversible microalbuminuria.

Persistent hyperglycemia seems to be the most important factor in the pathogenesis of the diabetic glomerulosclerosis and involves several mechanisms, including (1) vasodilation with increased permeability of the microcirculation allowing increased leakage of solutes into the vascular walls and surrounding tissues; (2) glucose disposal via the polyol pathway (independent of insulin), leading to accumulation of polyols and decreased levels of vital cellular components, including the glomeruli; and (3) glycosylation of glomerular structural proteins. In hyperglycemia, glucose reacts with circulating and structural proteins nonenzymatically (e.g., the glycosylation of hemoglobin produces hemoglobin A_{1c}). Glycosylation of basement membrane and mesangial proteins may be the major factor responsible for the increase in mesangial matrix and the alterations in membrane permeability leading to proteinuria.

Stage 3 diabetic nephropathy is referred to as the phase of *incipient nephropathy* and typically develops about 10 years after the onset of diabetes. The hallmark of this stage is persistent microalbuminuria (urinary albumin excretion between 30 and 300 mg/24 hr) detectable only by radioimmunoassay or other sensitive laboratory methods. Normal urinary albumin excretion is below 30 mg/24 hr, whereas albumin excretion above 300 mg/24 hr is referred to as "overt" proteinuria to distinguish it from microalbuminuria. Persistent microalbuminuria is documented with three or more separate urine collections over a 3- to 6-month period. Persistent microalbuminuria can be detected in 25% to 40% of patients, and the likelihood of progressing to stages 4 and 5 nephropathy is high in those who develop it and low in those who do not. Normal to high-normal levels of GFR and increasing blood pressure are also important features of stage 3 diabetic nephropathy.

Stage 4, or the phase of *established* or *clinical diabetic nephropathy,* is characterized by dipstick-positive proteinuria (>300 mg/24 hr) with a progressive decrease in the GFR. Diabetic retinopathy, as well as hypertension, is almost always present with stage 4 diabetic nephropathy. This stage is present approximately 15 years after the onset of IDDM and leads to ESRD in most cases. However, many patients never reach ESRD because of premature death from atherosclerotic heart disease or stroke.

Stage 5, or the phase of *progressive renal insufficiency or failure,* is characterized by azotemia (elevated BUN and serum creatinine) caused by a rapid decline in the GFR, leading to the eventual development of ESRD and the need for dialysis or renal transplanation. The average time required to reach stage 5 from the onset of IDDM is 20 years. The rate of decline in the GFR averages 1 ml/mo so ESRD occurs in approximately 5 to 10 years after the onset of proteinuria. The rate of progression may be retarded by appropriate interventions (see below). The advanced diabetic nephropathy of stage 5 is generally accompanied by retinopathy, peripheral neuropathy, and hypertension (Dunfee, 1995; Schrier, Gottschalk, 1995).

The results of a number of studies, including the 1993 Diabetes Control and Complications Trial with 1441 patients, have shown that precise regulation of blood glucose (achieved through meticulous attention to diet, exercise, self-monitoring of blood glucose, and multidose daily insulin) can slow the rate of nephropathy, retinopathy, and neuropathy significantly, especially if the therapy is begun during the third or microalbuminuria stage. Dietary protein restriction and lowering the blood pressure with ACE inhibitors decrease albumin excretion and slow progression of diabetic nephropathy. ACE inhibitors are effective in slowing progression to renal failure because they are the only antihypertensive drugs that act by dilating the efferent arterioles, thus lowering intraglomerular pressure. By contrast, calcium antagonists (e.g., verapamil) cause dilation of the afferent arterioles in the kidney, which may increase intraglomerular pressure rather than lowering it.

Renal replacement therapy should be introduced at a much earlier stage than with nondiabetics, since uremia is associated with acceleration of other diabetic complications (e.g., retinopathy). Continuous ambulatory peritoneal dialysis is the treatment of choice. Generally, mortality among diabetics on long-term dialysis is about three times higher than among nondiabetics of comparable age. Renal transplantation may be successful in younger diabetics.

Gout

Gout is a metabolic disease characterized by hyperuricemia (increased plasma uric acid concentrations). There are two forms of the disease. Primary gout is an hereditary disorder of deranged uric acid metabolism affecting males in 95% of cases. Secondary gout may arise either from increased uric acid production in conditions such as leukemia, polycythemia vera, or multiple myeloma or from decreased uric acid secretion, as in chronic renal failure. The source of the increased uric acid in the myeloproliferative disorders is the massive breakdown of cells (which contain nucleoproteins).

The major lesions of gout are principally caused by the deposition and crystallization of urates in the fluids and tissues of the body. The joints and kidneys are the prime targets. In chronic gout, deposit of urate crystals in the renal interstitium causes interstitial nephritis, nephrosclerosis, and slowly progressive renal failure. At present, chronic urate nephropathy is believed to be a rare cause of renal failure, unless marked hyperuricemia persists for several decades (serum uric acid >13 mg/dl in men and >10 mg/dl in women). There is some evidence that chronic lead intoxication (see p. 717) may play a role in some hyperuricemic patients with chronic renal failure, since lead interferes with uric acid excretion and produces progressive renal damage (Rose, 1987). Acute renal failure may develop secondary to complete obstruction of renal tubules by uric acid during cytotoxic drug therapy for malignant disease (see Chapters 45 and 49).

Hyperparathyroidism

Primary hyperparathyroidism, resulting in hypersecretion of parathyroid hormone, is a relatively rare disease that can result in nephrocalcinosis and subsequent renal failure. The usual cause is adenoma of the parathyroid glands. Secondary hyperparathyroidism is a common complication of chronic renal failure. Whether the disease is primary or secondary, the manifestations are similar. These are discussed in detail in Chapters 21 and 47.

Amyloidosis

Amyloidosis is a metabolic disease in which amyloid, an insoluble, waxy glycoprotein, is deposited in the various soft tissues of the body, where it can produce pressure and cause atrophy of the contiguous cells. The cause of amyloid production and its deposition in tissues is unknown. Immunologic derangements have been implicated—B cell activation, T cell suppression, macrophage involvement—but all such abnormalities have been nonspecific. At present, two major clinical forms are recognized, although differentiation is not always clearcut. In primary or congenital amyloidosis, amyloid is more often found in the tongue, heart, gastrointestinal tract, and peripheral nerves than in the kidneys. Secondary amyloidosis is frequently associated with chronic infectious disease, such as tuberculosis, chronic rheumatoid arthritis (25%), and multiple myeloma (10% to 20%), and with paraplegia (40%). The kidneys are frequently involved in secondary amyloidosis. The nephrotic syndrome and death from renal failure are common in this condition.

Toxic Nephropathy

The kidney is especially vulnerable to the toxic effects of drugs and chemicals for the following reasons: (1) it receives 25% of the cardiac output, so it may readily be exposed to large amounts of a chemical; (2) the hyperosmotic interstitium allows chemicals to be concentrated in a relatively hypovascular region; and (3) the kidney is an obligatory excretory route for most drugs, so renal insufficiency results in drug accumulation and increased concentration in the tubular fluid. The most frequently encountered nephrotoxins result in acute renal failure and

are discussed in Chapter 49. Chronic renal failure may result from analgesic abuse and exposure to lead.

Analgesic abuse

It is generally accepted that chronic abuse of analgesics can cause renal injury. Chronic renal failure associated with excessive consumption of analgesics is a relatively common problem and perhaps the most preventable form of renal disease. Its incidence varies, depending on regional differences in analgesic intake. Analgesic abuse accounts for about 1% to 2% of end-stage renal failure cases in the United States as a whole, as many as 10% in northwestern North Carolina, and 20% of the cases in Australia (Rose, 1987). The responsible ingredient causing nephropathy was first thought to be phenacetin, a common pain reliever. However, recent evidence indicates that it is the combination of aspirin and phenacetin that causes renal damage, since renal insufficiency is rarely a problem in patients taking aspirin, phenacetin, or acetaminophen (the major metabolite of phenacetin) alone. Clinically evident renal disease usually requires the ingestion of 2 to 3 kg each of aspirin and phenacetin (Murray, Goldberg, 1978). Most compound analgesics (which are now rarely available) contain 150 mg phenacetin. Therefore clinically evident renal disease would develop after taking six to eight tablets (about 1 g) every day for 5 to 8 years. Middle-aged women with a history of chronic headache or backache are the most frequent anaglesic abusers.

The mechanism by which these agents combine to produce renal damage is incompletely understood. One theory is that aspirin potentiates the toxic effect of phenacetin metabolites on the kidney in the following two ways (Cotran et al., 1986):

1. Aspirin causes medullary ischemia by inhibiting the local production of prostaglandin (a potent renal vasodilator hormone), thus enhancing the toxic effect of phenacetin metabolites and slowing down their removal.

2. Aspirin interferes with the hexose monophosphate shunt, thereby lowering the concentration of glutathione, which normally inactivates phenacetin metabolites.

The characteristic renal lesion is papillary necrosis and interstitial nephritis. The papillary tips may slough off completely and be excreted in the urine. Because the distal tubule bears the brunt of the disease, urine concentration and acidification tend to be severely impaired, and a salt-losing state may also develop. Common clinical features are hematuria (in cases of papillary necrosis), renal colic (flank pain), and urinary tract infection, including chronic pyelonephritis. Frequently the disease progresses insidiously, so the patient may have advanced chronic renal failure and hypertension at the time of diagnosis. Early diagnosis is particularly important in analgesic nephropathy, because progressive renal injury may be halted by cessation of analgesic intake.

Lead nephropathy

Exposure to lead occurs in a number of occupations, and lead may be ingested in illicitly distilled whiskey. Lead intoxication is still a problem in the United States, although not as great as when lead-based paints were used. Lead is incorporated chiefly into the bone and gradually released over a period of years; it is also incorporated into renal tubular cells. Patients with lead nephropathy typically have hyperuricemia. Acute gouty arthritis occurs in about one half of the patients with lead nephropathy, in contrast to other forms of renal failure in which gout is rare. Hypertension is also common. The basic renal lesion is interstitial nephritis, and there is slowly progressive renal failure.

QUESTIONS

▼ *Answer the following on a separate sheet of paper.*

1. What is the major difference between acute and chronic renal failure, and what happens to the function of the kidneys in both categories?

2. Name in order the three stages in the natural history of progressive renal failure. What percentage of nephrons are destroyed in each?

3. Indicate whether the laboratory values of BUN and plasma creatinine would be normal, rising just above normal, or rising sharply in each of the three stages of renal failure.

4. What happens to the creatinine clearance in progressive renal failure?

5. What is the difference between polyuria and oliguria? Define *nocturia*.

6. Explain why polyuria and oliguria occur as more and more functioning nephrons are destroyed in chronic renal failure. Explain how renal lesions could cause these symptoms.

7. Explain how the normal kidney responds to an increasing solute load, how this condition might be induced, and how the evidence supports the intact nephron hypothesis.

8. What happens to the remaining functioning nephrons in progressive renal failure (size, filtration rate, tubular reabsorption, solute load)?

9. Explain why the original cause of chronic renal failure may be difficult to identify in some cases.

10. Discuss several predisposing factors in the development of UTI and chronic pyelonephritis (PN).

11. What is the significance of asymptomatic bacteriuria in school-aged children?

12. Name the three mechanisms believed to be responsible for reflux nephropathy.

13. Explain the intrarenal hemodynamic theory of progressive renal failure. How well does this theory explain silent (asymptomatic) chronic PN in patients who may be unaware of any renal disease until symptomatic end-stage renal failure occurs? What are the treatment implications of this theory?

14. Name three types of glomerulonephritis, based on clinical classification. What is the prognosis of each type, generally speaking? Describe their natural history and relationship.

▼ *Circle the letter preceding each item below that correctly answers the question or completes the statement. More than one answer may be correct.*

15. Which of the following best describes nocturia?
    a. A decrease in the volume of urine
    b. Loss of the normal diurnal pattern of concentrating urine to a greater degree at night
    c. Both a and b
    d. Neither a nor b

16. The earliest signs or symptoms of chronic renal failure are:
    a. Secondary hyperparathyroidism and pruritus
    b. Oliguria and proteinuria
    c. Polyuria and nocturia
    d. Anemia and fatigue

17. The main cause of polyuria in early chronic renal failure is:
    a. Excessive water intake
    b. Solute diuresis in the remaining intact nephrons
    c. Failure of the renal tubules to respond to ADH
    d. Inadequate secretion of ADH

18. If a patient with chronic renal failure caused by polycystic kidney disease (with little ability to concentrate or dilute the glomerular filtrate) excretes 900 mOsm of solute per day, his urine volume will be about:
    a. 900 ml
    b. Equal to intake
    c. 3000 ml
    d. 450 ml
    e. 4500 ml

19. The salt-losing tendency in early chronic renal failure (especially in tubulointerstitial diseases) is caused by:
    a. Obligatory sodium wastage to preserve acid-base balance
    b. Defective sodium reabsorption
    c. An osmotic diuresis in each functioning nephron
    d. Decreased aldosterone production

20. Persistent azotemia (increased BUN and serum creatinine) and the uremic syndrome occur when renal compensatory mechanisms fail. This occurs when about what percentage of the nephrons have been destroyed by the renal disease?
    a. 10%-20%
    b. 75%-80%
    c. 90%-99%
    d. 100%

21. The progression of renal failure when the primary renal disease is no longer present (e.g., vesicoureteral reflux [VUR], pyelonephritis during childhood) is best explained by:
    a. Secondary glomerular injury for the long term from the compensatory mechanisms involved in maintaining renal function in remaining intact nephrons
    b. Decreased intraglomerular capillary pressure
    c. Loss of protein in the urine
    d. Excessive secretion of prostaglandins

22. Mechanisms that explain the pathogenesis of proteinuria and focal glomerulosclerosis in progressive renal failure are:
    a. Dilation of the afferent arteriole and constriction of the efferent arteriole leading to increased intraglomerular capillary pressure
    b. Enlargement of the glomerular tuft without an increase in the number of visceral epithelial cells leading to increased permeability of the filtration barrier and proteinuria

Continued.

c. Accumulation of large proteins in the subendothelial space and proliferation of mesangial matrix leading to compression of the glomerular capillary lumen

d. Intraglomerular hypertension leading to microaneurysm and thrombus formation

e. All of the above

23. Rank the leading causes of chronic renal failure and ESRD for the 1990s by placing a number (1 to 4) in front of each renal disease:
   a. ___ Polycystic kidney disease
   b. ___ Diabetic glomerulosclerosis
   c. ___ Hypertensive nephrosclerosis
   d. ___ Chronic glomerulonephritis

24. The most common infecting organism in UTI is:
   a. *Staphylococcus aureus*
   b. *Proteus vulgaris*
   c. *Klebsiella pneumoniae*
   d. *Escherichia coli*

25. Significant bacteriuria is defined as _____ microorganisms/ml urine.
   a. 10^2 c. 10^4
   b. 10^3 d. 10^5

26. In the male, UTI is less common than in the female because:
   a. The urethra is longer
   b. The distance between the urethra and anus is greater
   c. Prostatic fluid contains bacteriocidal substances
   d. All of the above

27. The bacterial population in the bladder is significantly increased by:
   a. Hydration
   b. Residual urine
   c. Frequent micturition
   d. Quantity of IgA in the urine

28. A simple, single bladder catheterization leads to UTI in approximately what percentage of cases?
   a. <1%   c. 5%
   b. 2%   d. 10%

29. Factors predisposing to UTI include:
   a. Urethral stricture
   b. Indwelling catheter drainage
   c. High progesterone levels in pregnancy
   d. Vesicoureteral reflux
   e. Prostatic hypertrophy

30. Pathogenic mechanisms predisposing to UTI in persons with neurogenic bladder include:
   a. Ischemia of the bladder wall from overdistention

b. Residual urine providing a medium for bacterial growth

c. Vesicoureteral reflux associated with increased intravesicular pressures

d. Frequent use of bladder catheters and urinary drainage

e. All of the above

31. Renal infection is usually caused by:
   a. Blood-borne infection
   b. Reflux of bladder urine into kidney
   c. Lymphatic spread
   d. Absence of vesicoureteral valve

32. All of the following are true of acute pyelonephritis except:
   a. Common in females
   b. Common in pregnancy
   c. Common with urinary obstruction
   d. Commonly progresses to chronic renal failure and ESRD

33. The most reliable evidence of acute renal parenchymal infection is:
   a. Leukocyte casts in the urine
   b. Bacteriuria >100,000/ml
   c. Numerous WBCs per high power field
   d. Renal biopsy

34. Mechanisms believed to be responsible for reflux nephropathy include:
   a. Vesicoureteral reflux
   b. Intrarenal reflux
   c. Renal infection secondary to reflux of infected bladder urine
   d. All of the above

35. The scars of chronic pyelonephritis (reflux hypertrophy) are characteristically:
   a. V shaped
   b. U shaped
   c. Located at a pole of the kidney
   d. Circular

36. The "thyroid" appearance of renal tubules is considered typical of:
   a. Chronic glomerulosclerosis
   b. Malignant hypertension
   c. Diabetic nephropathy
   d. Chronic reflux nephropathy (chronic pyelonephritis)

37. Glomerulonephritis is a broad term used to describe:
   a. Infection of the glomeruli
   b. Poststreptococcal renal damage
   c. An inflammatory process involving the entire nephron
   d. An inflammatory process involving the glomerulus

38. Glomerulonephritis can be classified as:
   a. Primary or secondary glomerular injury
   b. An acute self-limited condition

c. An asymptomatic form of acute renal failure

d. A systemic inflammatory disease

39. Glomerulonephritis is manifested by:
   a. Weight loss, anemia, arthralgias
   b. Proteinuria, hematuria, and/or edema
   c. Fever, chills, flank pain
   d. Anuria, hypotension, and/or vasculitis

40. Immunofluorescent technique used in microscopy identifies:
   a. Immunoglobulins (antibodies) in biopsied renal tissue
   b. Areas of sclerosis in the glomeruli
   c. Only diffuse renal disease
   d. The probability of curing the renal disease

41. Which of the following statements is false with respect to immune-complex glomerulonephritis?
   a. Ag-Ab complexes form in the blood and circulate to the glomerulus
   b. PMNs produce glomerular injury by the release of lysosomal enzymes
   c. Immunofluorescent studies show a pattern of granular deposits along the glomerular capillary
   d. The major injury is caused by streptococcal renal infection

42. Complement is implicated in glomerular diseases because of the potential for:
   a. Inflammation-mediated damage to innocent tissues
   b. Dampening the immune response
   c. Stimulating anti–glomerular basement membrane (GBM) antibodies
   d. Hypotension during complement activation

43. Acute glomerulonephritis may follow infection with:
   a. *E. coli* urinary tract sepsis
   b. Type 4 or 12 group A beta-hemolytic streptococci
   c. Group A staphylococci
   d. Type 12 group B streptococci

44. Streptococcal infection is followed by:
   a. Nephritis after a latent period of 3-4 weeks
   b. Nephritis after a latent period of 1-2 weeks
   c. Rheumatic fever after a latent period of 10 days
   d. Rheumatic fever and nephritis with a serologically similar organism

45. Which of the following is least characteristic of acute poststreptococcal glomerulonephritis (APSGN)?

QUESTIONS—cont'd

a. Most common in children ages 3-7 years
b. Low serum complement levels
c. Hypertension
d. Edema
e. Urine with low osmolality

46. Which of the following statements concerning APSGN is not true?
   a. Most cases of chronic glomerulonephritis evolve from APSGN
   b. RBC casts are characteristic urinary findings in APSGN
   c. Corticosteroid drugs have no known beneficial effect in APSGN
   d. Immunofluorescent microscopy shows a lumpy-bumpy pattern of immune deposits along the glomerular capillaries

47. Which of the following findings is uncommon in APSGN?
   a. Decreased serum complement
   b. Ability to produce concentrated urine
   c. RBC casts
   d. Massive proteinuria (nephrotic syndrome)

48. All of the following are characteristic of Goodpasture's syndrome except:
   a. The renal injury is caused by anti-GBM antibodies
   b. It results in a rapidly progressive glomerulonephritis
   c. It has been successfully treated with a combination of corticosteroids, cytotoxic agents, and plasmapheresis
   d. The prognosis is generally excellent
   e. Renal biopsy shows extensive extra-capillary proliferation or crescents in most patients

49. Which of the following statements is false concerning the histologic changes in the end-stage kidney of chronic glomerulonephritis?
   a. Only the glomeruli are involved in the pathologic destruction
   b. Destructive lesions involving the glomeruli, renal tubules, and vasculature are all present
   c. Some glomeruli are completely hyalinized
   d. Epithelial crescents are frequently seen

50. Nephrotic range proteinuria is defined as urinary protein losses of:
   a. 150 mg/24 hr   c. 1.0 g/24 hr
   b. 300 mg/24 hr   d. >3.5 g/24 hr

51. The nephrotic syndrome is characterized by:
   a. Hypoalbuminemia

b. Hyperlipidemia
c. Generalized edema
d. Proteinuria >3.5 g/day
e. All of the above

52. The initiating event that leads to the development of the symptoms associated with the nephrotic syndrome is:
   a. Thickening of the glomerular basement membrane
   b. Decreased GFR
   c. Increased permeability of the glomerular filtration barrier to proteins
   d. Acute tubular necrosis

53. The glomerular basement membrane normally:
   a. Acts as a barrier to protein molecules because of their size, shape, and electrical charge
   b. Allows no filtration of plasma proteins
   c. Acts as a mechanical barrier to plasma proteins
   d. Acts as a barrier to positively charged small ions

54. Most of the protein found in the urine of nephrotic patients is:
   a. Tamm-Horsfall protein
   b. Albumin
   c. Bence Jones protein
   d. Low–molecular weight proteins

55. The most common cause of the nephrotic syndrome in children is:
   a. Minimal change glomerulonephritis
   b. Focal glomerulosclerosis
   c. Diabetic glomerulosclerosis
   d. Focal glomerulosclerosis
   e. Renal amyloidosis

56. Which of the following statements regarding minimal glomerulonephritis (GN) change is false?
   a. More than 95% of children achieve a remission with corticosteroid therapy within a few weeks
   b. Adults with this lesion never develop progressive renal failure
   c. Immune mechanisms do not appear to be involved in this renal disease
   d. Electron microscopy shows fusion of the foot processes of the glomerular epithelial cells

57. Complications of idiopathic nephrotic syndrome include:
   a. Infection caused by loss of immunoglobulins in the urine
   b. Atherosclerosis from long-term hyperlipidemia
   c. Renal vein thrombosis and pulmonary embolism from altered coagulation

d. Progressive renal failure
e. All of the above

58. IgA nephropathy is characterized histologically by:
   a. Segmental accumulation of complement
   b. Proliferation of the glomerular visceral epithelial cells
   c. Granular deposits of IgA confined primarily to the mesangial matrix
   d. Focal glomerular sclerosis

59. What percentage of documented cases of IgA nephropathy progress to ESRD?
   a. 5%
   b. 10%
   c. 20%-30%
   d. 50%

60. The most significant lesion in uncomplicated membranous glomerulonephritis is located in the:
   a. Proximal convoluted tubules
   b. Distal convoluted tubules
   c. Tubular basement membrane
   d. Glomerular capillary basement membrane

61. Which of the following statements is false concerning membranoproliferative glomerulonephritis?
   a. Characterized both by thickening of the basement membrane and proliferation of the mesangial cells
   b. There are two types
   c. Frequently associated with the nephrotic syndrome
   d. May be associated with lupus nephritis
   e. Rarely progresses to ESRD

62. Hypertension is defined as:
   a. Systolic blood pressure ≥140; diastolic ≥90 consistently
   b. Systolic blood pressure ≥150; diastolic ≥90 consistently
   c. Systolic blood pressure ≥160; diastolic ≥90 consistently
   d. Systolic blood pressure ≥140; diastolic ≥90 on any single random measurement

63. The percentage of patients with hypertension-induced ESRD admitted to dialysis/transplant treatment programs in the 1990s is about:
   a. 5%   c. 15%
   b. 10%   d. 30%

64. The characteristic lesion of benign nephrosclerosis is:
   a. Hyalinized thickening of the arteriolar walls with narrowing of lumina

Continued.

QUESTIONS—cont'd

b. Fibrinoid necrosis, glomerular hemorrhage
c. Nodular glomerulosclerosis
d. Widespread infarction of entire nephrons

65. In malignant nephrosclerosis:
   a. Rapidly progressive renal failure develops
   b. Fibrinoid necrosis of the arteriolar walls and glomerular occurs
   c. Entire nephrons may be destroyed by infarction
   d. Prognosis is poor
   e. All of the above

66. Which of the following statements concerning unilateral renal artery stenosis is false?
   a. Most common type of surgically correctable hypertension
   b. Reveals delayed visualization of the affected kidney on IVP
   c. A frequent cause is fibromuscular dysplasia
   d. The affected kidney is longer by at least 1.5 cm
   e. Most frequently affects females between the ages of 20 and 50 years

67. Pathologic changes in the kidney produced by accelerated hypertension in unilateral renal artery stenosis are least marked:
   a. When hypertension is caused by chronic renal failure
   b. When hypertension is caused by adrenal adenoma
   c. When hypertension is caused by pheochromocytoma
   d. In the kidney with renal artery stenosis

68. Findings that should make the clinician suspicious of the presence of renal artery stenosis in a patient include:
   a. Bruit heard over the epigastrium
   b. History of hypertension with an abrupt onset
   c. Hypertension in a young female in her 30s
   d. Difference in blood pressure between the right and left lower extremities
   e. All of the above

69. The diagnosis of renal artery stenosis is confirmed by:
   a. An increase in the plasma renin activity when given captopril (Capoten)
   b. An IV pyelogram showing delayed visualization of one kidney
   c. Roentgenographic evidence of difference in the size of the two kidneys

d. Renal arteriographic evidence of luminal narrowing and/or a difference in renal vein renin from the two kidneys by a factor of 1.5:1

70. ACE inhibitors can cause acute renal failure in patients with bilateral renal artery stenosis or unilateral renal artery stenosis *because* they reduce arterial pressure combined with dilation of the efferent arterioles.
   a. Statement is correct, but reason is incorrect
   b. Statement is incorrect, but reason is correct
   c. Both statement and reason are correct
   d. Both statement and reason are incorrect

71. Which of the following antibodies is most significant in the pathogenesis of the glomerulonephritis of systemic lupus erythematosus (SLE)?
   a. Anti–glomerular basement membrane (GBM)
   b. Anti–RNA
   c. Anti–DNA
   d. Anti–platelet

72. All of the following statements are true with respect to SLE except:
   a. Renal lesions are present in about two thirds of the patients
   b. A combination of corticosteroid and cytotoxic drugs is often successful in effecting a remission
   c. The most common finding in lupus nephritis is proteinuria
   d. The prognosis is poor for those who develop diffuse membranous or proliferative renal lesions
   e. Hemodialysis for renal failure is never necessary for patients with lupus nephritis

73. Which of the following statements is false concerning polyarteritis nodosa (PAN)?
   a. Affects women more frequently than men
   b. Arterial lesions in the kidney are common
   c. Intractable hypertension secondary to the arteritis is common
   d. Corticosteroids, cytotoxic agents, and early antihypertensive therapy have greatly improved the prognosis

74. Which of the following statements are true concerning scleroderma?
   a. Renal lesions resemble those of hypertensive nephrosclerosis
   b. Incidence is higher in women than in men

c. Immune mechanisms may be involved in the pathogenesis
d. Onset between the ages of 20 to 50 years is most common
e. All of the above

75. Hereditary transmission in adult polycystic kidney disease (PCKD) is:
   a. Autosomal recessive
   b. Autosomal dominant
   c. Sex-linked recessive
   d. Autosomal dominant with poor penetrance

76. Adult PCKD:
   a. Results in rapidly progressive chronic renal failure
   b. Is characterized by multiple cysts that communicate with the tubules
   c. Is associated with small, contracted kidneys
   d. Is not usually associated with hypertension

77. "Salt-wasting" nephropathies:
   a. Are commonly associated with PCKD and chronic pyelonephritis
   b. Are characterized by polyuria and the loss of large amounts of sodium in the urine
   c. Are associated with renal diseases that damage the structure and function of the tubules more than the glomeruli
   d. Are commonly associated with tubulointerstitial diseases
   e. All of the above

78. The major clinical characteristics of type I (distal or classical) renal tubular acidosis (RTA) include:
   a. Persistently alkaline urine (pH >5.3) in the presence of normal–anion gap metabolic acidosis
   b. Polyuria and hypokalemia
   c. Nephrocalcinosis, rickets, and failure to thrive common in children with distal RTA
   d. Diagnosis confirmed by the ammonium chloride loading test
   e. Treatment involving the administration of potassium bicarbonate or citrate

79. The percentage of patients with insulin-dependent diabetes mellitus (IDDM) who develop ESRD within 15-25 years after the onset of diabetes is about:
   a. 25%   c. 50%
   b. 30%   d. 67%

80. Diffuse diabetic glomerulosclerosis, the most common lesion in diabetic nephropathy, is characterized by:
   a. Widening of the glomerular basement membrane together with gen-

QUESTIONS—cont'd

eralized expansion of the mesangial matrix
b. Nodular accumulations of eosinophilic material deposited in the periphery of glomerular tufts (Kimmelstiel-Wilson lesion)
c. Hyalinization of the efferent arteriole
d. Necrosis of the papillary ducts

81. A major contributing factor in the pathogenesis of diabetic nephropathy may be:
a. Glycosylation of glomerular structural proteins
b. Albuminuria
c. Hypokalemia
d. Hyperlipidemia

82. Early functional changes (stage I) in the natural history of diabetic nephropathy include:
a. Renal hypertrophy
b. Hyperfiltration with elevated GFR up to 40% above normal
c. Persistent microalbuminuria
d. Structural changes in the glomerulus

83. Factors that are predictive of the development of clinical diabetic nephropathy include all of the following except:
a. Increased GFR
b. Hypokalemia
c. Renal hypertrophy
d. Persistent microalbuminuria

84. Microalbuminuria is defined as the urinary albumin excretion of:
a. 30 mg/24 hr
b. >150 mg/24 hr
c. 30-300 mg/24 hr
d. 1.0 g/24 hr

85. Interventions that may slow the progression of diabetic nephropathy include all of the following except:
a. ACE inhibitors
b. Dietary protein restriction
c. Strict control of blood glucose
d. Weight reduction

86. ACE inhibitors lower intraglomerular pressure by:
a. Dilating the afferent arteriole
b. Dilating the efferent arteriole
c. Constricting the afferent arteriole
d. Stimulating renal vasodilator prostaglandins

87. Amyloidosis of the kidneys:
a. Is frequently associated with the nephrotic syndrome
b. Is associated with multiple myeloma
c. May be secondary to rheumatoid arthritis
d. Is associated with chronic infections such as tuberculosis

e. All of the above

88. Analgesic (NSAID)–induced nephropathy with papillary necrosis:
a. Is of historic interest only
b. Is associated with the use of aspirin alone
c. Is associated with long-term combined aspirin and phenacetin abuse
d. Is related to the total amount of drug ingested over time

89. Most, if not all, NSAID-induced renal disturbances are:
a. Due to their inhibiting effects on the production of renal vasodilator prostaglandins

b. Irreversible
c. Specific for a given NSAID class
d. More apt to occur in patients with hypertension

90. The kidney is vulnerable to the toxic effects of drugs because:
a. It is the obligatory excretory route for most drugs
b. The hyperosmolality of the medulla allows drugs to be concentrated in a relatively ischemic area
c. It receives 25% of the cardiac output so may be exposed to a large amount of the chemical
d. All of the above

▼ Match the descriptions in column B with the terms in column A that refer to the distribution of glomerular lesions.

Column A		Column B
91. _____	Diffuse	a. Only a portion of the glomeruli are involved
92. _____	Local	b. Part of the glomerulus is involved
93. _____	Focal	c. All the glomeruli are affected

▼ Match the descriptive characteristics in column B with the appropriate pathogenic immune mechanism in column A.

Column A		Column B
94. _____	Circulating immune complex	a. Associated with Goodpasture's syndrome
95. _____	Anti-GBM	b. Associated with acute poststreptococcal glomerulonephritis (APSGN) and SLE
		c. Immunoglobulin is deposited subepithelially
		d. Immunoglobulin is deposited subendothelially
		e. Autoimmune mechanism
		f. Linear or ribbonlike pattern of deposit on immunofluorescent biopsy slide
		g. Ag-Ab complexes are mechanically trapped in the filtration membrane
		h. Results in more serious injury to the glomerulus

▼ Match the appropriate description in column B with the histologic type of glomerulonephritis in column A. Letters may be used more than once.

Column A		Column B
96. _____	Minimal change GN	a. Primary change in the glomerulus is an increase in endothelial, mesangial, or epithelial cells
97. _____	Membranous GN	b. Predominant change is thickening of the basement membrane
98. _____	Proliferative GN	c. Only morphologic change is fusion of the foot processes
		d. Most common lesion in children associated with the nephrotic syndrome
		e. Nephrotic patients with these lesions often progress to renal failure

Continued.

QUESTIONS—cont'd

▼ *Match the descriptive phrases in column B with the terms in column A to which they apply. Letters may be used more than once.*

Column A
99. _____ Polycystic kidney disease (adult form)
100. _____ Polycystic kidney disease (infantile form)
101. _____ Distal RTA
102. _____ Proximal RTA
103. _____ Kimmelstiel-Wilson disease
104. _____ Gout
105. _____ Hyperparathyroidis
106. _____ Amyloidosis

Column B
a. Characteristic lesion of diabetic nephropathy
b. May be a hereditary disorder
c. Commonly presents as failure to thrive
d. Nephrocalcinosis is a common complication
e. Deposits in kidney common in rheumatoid arthritis, paraplegia, and multiple myeloma
f. Cysts communicate with tubules
g. Cysts are closed
h. Urate crystals may be deposited in the renal tubules or interstitium
i. Treated with sodium bicarbonate or sodium and potassium citrate
j. Urine acidification test may aid in diagnosis

▼ *Circle T if the statement is true and F if it is false. Correct any false statements.*

107. T F Surgical correction of renal artery stenosis or removal of the ischemic kidney always results in cure of the hypertension.
108. T F About one third of all patients with SLE, PN, and scleroderma have clinical evidence of renal disease.
109. T F SLE patients with focal and local glomerular lesions respond well to corticosteroid therapy, and the prognosis is good.
110. T F About 50% of type I (IDDM) diabetic patients develop ESRD after 20 years.
111. T F Hypoproteinemia is important in the pathogenesis of edema in APSGN.

112. T F In advanced chronic renal failure, the kidney is larger than normal, with multiple petechiae on the surface.
113. T F Polyuria and "salt wasting" are common clinical features of analgesic nephropathy.
114. T F Chronic renal failure may cause hypertension.
115. T F Widespread epithelial crescent formation signifies remission and a good prognosis in chronic renal failure.
116. T F Immunopathic mechanisms are probably involved in the pathogenesis of most of the connective tissue disorders.
117. T F Aspirin inhibits the synthesis of prostaglandins in renal cells, thus favoring medullary ischemia.
118. T F Renal tubular acidosis is a syndrome of abnormal renal acidification causing hyperchloremic (normal–anion gap) metabolic acidosis in which the overall renal function is relatively unimpaired.
119. T F The basic defect in type 2 (proximal) RTA is impaired reabsorption of filtered bicarbonate resulting in bicarbonaturia.
120. T F Diabetic retinopathy almost always precedes the development of ESRD in diabetic nephropathy.

▼ *Fill in the blanks with the correct words.*

121. In acute pyelonephritis, _____ (inflammatory cells) are usually found throughout the cortex and medulla and segments of the _____ are destroyed, whereas in chronic pyelonephritis, in the interstitium there are many _____ and _____ cells.

122. Label Fig. 46-19 by matching the letters with the renal histologic findings from the list below.
___ Normal tubule
___ Area of interstitial fibrosis
___ Hypertrophied tubule with atrophy of epithelial cells
___ Atrophied tubule containing cast
___ Inflammatory cells (PMNs)

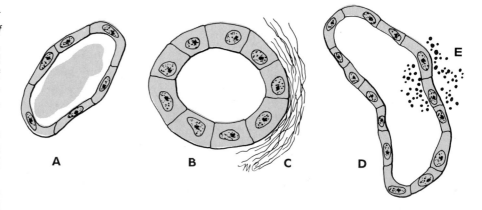

FIG. 46-19   Histologic findings in chronic pyelonephritis.

CHAPTER 47

End-Stage Renal Disease

THE UREMIC SYNDROME

LORRAINE M. WILSON

Each of the principal kidney diseases that lead to chronic progressive renal failure has unique features that relate to the cause, pathogenesis, and morphology. These differences were discussed in Chapter 46. It was also pointed out that these diseases produce many similar morphologic changes. This is particularly true when the terminal stage of chronic renal disease is reached, when it may be difficult to determine the cause of the chronic renal failure by examining the end-stage kidney.

As also explained in Chapter 46, from a functional point of view, regardless of cause, there is a common sequence of changes in renal function caused by the progressive destruction of nephrons. The rate of destruction can vary greatly, with quiescent periods and exacerbations, and the duration from beginning to end may vary from months to as long as 40 years. However, once the glomerular filtration rate (GFR) begins to fall and the blood urea nitrogen (BUN) and creatinine levels rise, there is a tendency toward rapid progression to end-stage renal failure. Because of these common functional patterns, it is possible to consider the events in the pathophysiology of chronic renal failure as a single phenomenon rather than discuss the changes in function on a disease-by-disease basis.

The common sequence of changes has this effect on the patient: when the GFR falls to 5% to 10% of normal and progresses toward zero, the patient develops what is called the *uremic syndrome.* The uremic syndrome is a symptom complex that results from or is associated with retention of nitrogenous metabolites because of renal failure. In advanced uremia, some functions of virtually every organ system in the body may become abnormal.

Two groups of clinical symptoms are present in the uremic syndrome. First, symptoms referrable to deranged regulatory and excretory functions are prominent: fluid volume and electrolyte abnormalities, acid-base imbalance, retention of nitrogenous and other metabolites, and anemia caused by renal secretory deficiency. A second group of clinical features includes a constellation of cardiovascular, neuromuscular, gastrointestinal, and other abnormalities. Surprisingly little is known about the basis of these multiple-system abnormalities, though diligent research is now being conducted to uncover these mysteries. Table 47-1 lists some of the common manifestations of the uremic syndrome discussed in this chapter.

> TABLE 47-1 Manifestations of the Uremic Syndrome

Body System	Manifestations	Body System	Manifestations
Biochemical	Metabolic acidosis (serum HCO_3^- 18-20 mEq/L	Gastrointestinal	Anorexia, nausea, vomiting, leading to weight loss
	Azotemia (decreased GFR, leading to increased BUN, creatinine)		Ammoniacal odor to breath
	Hyperkalemia		Metallic taste, dry mouth
	Sodium retention or wasting		Stomatitis, parotitis
	Hypermagnesemia		Gastritis, enteritis
	Hyperuricemia		GI bleeding
Genitourinary	Polyuria, progressing to oliguria, progressing to anuria		Diarrhea
		Intermediary metabolism	Protein—intolerance, abnormal synthesis
	Nocturia, reversal of diurnal rhythm		Carbohydrate—hyperglycemia, decreased insulin need
	Fixed urine sp gr 1.010		
	Proteinuria; casts		Fat—increased levels of triglycerides
	Loss of libido, amenorrhea, impotence, sterility		Easy fatigability
Cardiovascular	Hypertension	Neuromuscular	Muscle wasting, weakness
	Hypertensive retinopathy, encephalopathy		Central nervous system
	Circulatory overload		Decreased mental acuity
	Edema		Poor concentration
	Congestive heart failure		Apathy
	Pericarditis (friction rub)		Lethargy/restlessness, insomnia
	Dysrhythmias		Mental confusion
Respiratory	Kussmaul's breathing, dyspnea		Coma
	Pulmonary edema		Muscle twitching, asterixis, convulsions
	Pneumonitis		Peripheral neuropathy
Hematologic	Anemia leading to fatigue		Slowed nerve conduction, "restless leg" syndrome
	Hemolysis		
	Bleeding tendency		Sensory changes in the extremities—paresthesias
	Decreased resistance to infection (urinary tract infection, pneumonia, septicemia)		Motor changes—foot drop progressing to paraplegia
Cutaneous	Pallor, pigmentation	Calcium and skeletal disorders	Hyperphosphatemia, hypocalcemia
	Hair and nail changes (nails brittle, thin, ridged, alternating red and light bands associated with protein wasting)		Secondary hyperparathyroidism
			Renal osteodystrophy
			Pathologic fractures (demineralization of bones)
	Pruritus		
	Uremic "frost"		Calcium salts deposited in soft tissue (around joints, blood vessels, heart, lungs)
	Dry skin		
	Bruises		Conjunctivitis (uremic red eye)

HCO_3^-, Bicarbonate; *GFR,* glomerular filtration rate; *BUN,* blood urea nitrogen; *sp gr,* specific gravity; *GI,* gastrointestinal.

BIOCHEMICAL DISTURBANCES

Metabolic Acidosis

Renal failure is characterized by a wide variety of biochemical disturbances. One of the constant abnormalities exhibited by the uremic patient is metabolic acidosis. On a normal diet, the kidney has to excrete 40 to 60 mEq of hydrogen ion (H^+) daily to prevent acidosis. In renal failure, impaired ability of the kidney to excrete H^+ results in a systemic acidosis, with a decrease in the plasma pH and bicarbonate (HCO_3^-) concentration. The HCO_3^- level decreases because it is used up in buffering H^+. Ammonium ion (NH_4^+) excretion is the kidney's most important mechanism for the excretion of H^+ and the regeneration

of HCO_3^- (since it allows de novo addition of new HCO_3^- rather than just reabsorption of the filtered HCO_3^- to the extracellular fluid). Total NH_4^+ excretion is decreased in renal failure because of the diminished number of nephrons. Phosphate excretion provides another mechanism for the excretion of H^+ as titratable acid (i.e., phosphate-buffered H^+). The rate of phosphate excretion, however, is determined by the need to maintain phosphate balance rather than acid-base balance. Phosphate tends to be retained in renal failure because of the diminished nephron mass and factors related to calcium metabolism, which are discussed later. The retention of sulfate and other organic anions also contributes to the depletion of HCO_3^-.

The serum bicarbonate level usually stabilizes at about 18 to 20 mEq/L (moderate acidosis) and rarely drops below this level. The most likely explanation for this lack of progression in the presence of a positive hydrogen ion balance is that hydrogen ion is being buffered by calcium carbonate from the bone.

It is possible that the symptoms of anorexia, nausea, and lethargy common in the uremic patient may be partly because of the acidosis. One symptom that is undoubtedly caused by acidosis is Kussmaul's respiration, although this symptom may be less prominent in chronic acidosis. *Kussmaul's respiration* is the deep, sighing respiration that occurs because of the need to increase carbon dioxide excretion and thus reduce the severity of the acidosis.

Potassium Imbalance

Potassium (K$^+$) imbalance is one of the serious disturbances that may occur in renal failure, because only a narrow plasma concentration range is compatible with life (normal = 3.5 to 5.5 mEq/L). About 90% of the normal daily intake of 50 to 150 mEq is excreted in the urine. Hypokalemia may be associated with the polyuria of early chronic renal failure, particularly in tubular diseases such as chronic pyelonephritis. However, as the patient becomes oliguric in end-stage renal failure, hyperkalemia invariably develops.

The systemic acidosis also contributes to the hyperkalemia by causing K$^+$ to shift from the cells to the extracellular fluid. The major life-threatening effect of hyperkalemia is its influence on the electrical conduction of the heart. Fatal dysrhythmias or cardiac standstill may occur when serum K$^+$ levels reach 7 to 8 mEq/L.

Sodium Imbalance

The average American diet contains 2 to 10 g sodium (Na$^+$) (or 5 to 25 g sodium chloride [NaCl])/day. In most normal persons there is great flexibility in the kidney's ability to vary excretion of sodium in response to a variable intake. Salt excretion may vary from nearly zero to more than 20 g daily. Patients with chronic renal failure lose this great flexibility and may be "poised on a razor's edge" with respect to the ability to vary sodium output. In early renal insufficiency when polyuria is present, sodium wasting may occur because of the increased solute load of each intact nephron. The osmotic diuresis results in obligatory sodium losses. This sodium-losing tendency is more common in chronic pyelonephritis and polycystic kidneys, which primarily affect the tubules.

When oliguria supervenes in terminal renal failure, the patient is more likely to retain sodium. The retention of sodium and water may result in circulatory overload, edema, hypertension, and congestive heart failure. The development of congestive heart failure secondary to the hypertension and the increased aldosterone levels present in uremic patients may also play a major role in sodium retention.

Hypermagnesemia

Like potassium, magnesium (Mg^{++}) is chiefly an intracellular cation and is excreted chiefly by the kidneys. The normal serum level is 1.5 to 2.3 mEq/L. The ability to excrete magnesium is reduced in the uremic patient. However, hypermagnesemia is generally not a serious problem, since intake of magnesium is usually reduced because of anorexia, reduced protein intake, and decreased absorption from the gastrointestinal (GI) tract. A sudden load of magnesium from the ingestion of laxatives such as milk of magnesia or magnesium citrate may cause death by depressing neuromuscular activity.

Azotemia

As previously discussed, a sharp rise in the plasma urea and creatinine levels generally signals the onset of terminal renal failure and accompanies uremic symptoms. There is much evidence, however, that urea itself is not responsible for the symptoms and metabolic defects found in uremia. Some of the substances found in the blood of uremic patients that might act as toxins are the guanidines, phenols, amines, urate, creatinine, aromatic hydroxy acids, and indican. Some of these compounds act as potent enzyme inhibitors. It is likely that a combination of factors such as the acidosis and other electrolyte disturbances, hormonal disturbances, and retained toxins produce the metabolic defects and the multiple-system involvement. Present research postulates that the uremic toxins may lie in the middle molecular range in size (urea is a small molecule; albumin is a large molecule), and this has led to the *middle molecular hypothesis* and research into more efficient removal of these molecules. Hemodiafiltration and hemoperfusion are new, experimental types of dialysis now undergoing clinical trials to test the middle molecular hypothesis (see Chapter 48).

Hyperuricemia

The intimate association of gout and the kidney was alluded to in Chapter 46. A rise in serum uric acid concentration and the formation of obstructive crystals in the kidney can cause chronic or acute renal failure. On the other hand, the serum uric acid level generally rises early in the course of chronic renal failure because of excretory impairment of the kidneys. The kidneys normally account for about 75% of the excreted uric acid. A rise in serum uric acid concentration above the normal 4 to 6 mg/dl may or may not be associated with symptoms. It is not uncommon, however, for uremic patients to have attacks of gouty arthritis from the deposition of urate salts in the joints and soft tissues.

GENITOURINARY DISTURBANCES

Urinary symptoms in uremia are intimately associated with water metabolism; these findings have been discussed in previous chapters. Polyuria caused by osmotic diuresis gradually gives way to oliguria and even anuria as the nephron mass is gradually destroyed. Nocturia and a reversal of the normal diurnal pattern of urine excretion, resulting in a relatively constant rate of urine formation throughout the day and night, is another important symptom caused by the osmotic diuresis. A constant urine specific gravity near 1.010 in the uremic patient reflects loss of the ability to concentrate or dilute the urine from the plasma concentration. These changes make the uremic patient vulnerable to acute changes in water balance. Diarrhea or vomiting may quickly cause dehydration (with subsequent hypovolemia, decreased GFR, and further deterioration of renal function), and excess water intake may cause circulatory overload, edema, and congestive heart failure.

As the nephron mass and the GFR decrease, proteinuria, which may have been prominent earlier in the chronic renal disease, may become insignificant or may disappear altogether. Broad granular casts may occasionally be found in the urine sediment and are characteristic of advanced renal failure.

Young uremic women cease to menstruate, and the men are generally impotent and sterile when the GFR falls to 5 ml/min. Both genders experience a loss of libido as the uremia becomes more severe. Sexual and reproductive function may return after renal transplantation or a regular hemodialysis program. Most physicians, however, advise women not to become pregnant when advanced renal insufficiency is present.

CARDIOVASCULAR ABNORMALITIES

Hypertension and congestive heart failure often accompany the uremic syndrome. About 90% of the hypertension is volume dependent and related to sodium and water retention, whereas probably less than 10% is renin dependent. The combination of hypertension, anemia, and circulatory overload caused by sodium and water retention contributes to the increased propensity to congestive heart failure. Other side effects of severe hypertension include retinopathy and encephalopathy. The symptoms of these disorders are the same as in nonuremic patients.

Pericarditis, once a frequent complication of chronic renal failure, is now infrequent because of the early initiation of dialysis. Retained metabolic toxins are believed to be the cause of the pericarditis. The clinical presentation of patients with uremic pericarditis is similar to that of other etiologies. The patient may complain of pain on deep inspiration or when lying down, but about two thirds of the patients are asymptomatic. A to-and-fro friction rub may be heard over the precordium with auscultation. The chest radiograph may reveal an enlarged cardiac silhouette when a pericardial effusion is present. Occasionally the patient with uremic pericarditis may develop a massive hemorrhagic effusion and cardiac tamponade, especially when anticoagulants are used during hemodialysis. In the event of this emergency, prompt aspiration of the fluid by the physician may be lifesaving.

Finally, it must be remembered that cardiac dysrhythmias commonly associated with K^+ imbalance in renal failure are also affected by imbalances in Na^+, H^+, calcium (Ca^{++}), and Mg^{++}.

RESPIRATORY CHANGES

The deep, sighing (Kussmaul's) respiration of severe acidosis has already been mentioned. However, the patient with moderate acidosis of chronic renal insufficiency is more apt to complain of dyspnea on exertion, and the increased depth of breathing is overlooked except by an experienced observer.

Other respiratory complications of renal failure are the "uremic lung" and pneumonitis. Chest radiographs of the uremic lung reveal a bilateral butterfly-shaped infiltration of the lungs (Fig. 47-1). It is actually pulmonary edema and is inevitably associated with fluid overload caused by

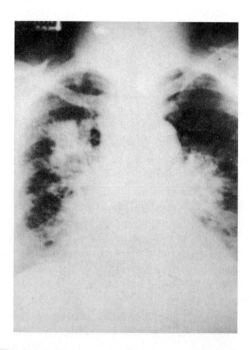

FIG. 47-1   Uremic lung, showing marked central distribution of pulmonary edema. (From Bailey GL: *Hemodialysis*, New York, 1972, Academic Press.)

sodium and water retention and/or left ventricular failure. The butterfly configuration of the pulmonary edema is the result of increased permeability of the alveolar capillary membrane around the hilus of the lung. Bilateral infection causing a pneumonitis may be superimposed on the chronically wet lung. Pulmonary congestion disappears with the reduction of body fluids by salt restriction and hemodialysis.

HEMATOLOGIC PROBLEMS

A characteristically normochromic, normocytic anemia is an inevitable feature of the uremic syndrome. Usually the hematocrit falls to the 20% to 30% range and parallels the degree of azotemia. The primary cause of the anemia is decreased red blood cell (RBC) formation. Decreased RBC formation is caused by deficient production of erythropoietin by the failing kidney. There is also some evidence that uremic toxins may inactivate erythropoietin or suppress the response of the bone marrow to its action. A second factor contributing to the anemia is that the life span of the RBC in a patient with renal failure is about half that in the normal person. The increased hemolysis of RBCs appears to be caused by the abnormal chemical environment in the plasma and not by a defect in the cells themselves. In addition to the deficient erythropoiesis and hemolytic tendency, blood loss in the GI tract may further aggravate the anemia. Other factors contributing to the anemia include iatrogenic blood loss and iron and folic acid deficiency. The blood loss caused by frequent sampling for laboratory tests and loss in the hemodialysis tubing may be considerable (average loss is 4.6 L/yr in one study). Iron deficiency may result from blood loss and from poor GI absorption (antacids taken for hyperphosphatemia also bind iron in the gut). Folic acid deficiency is associated with uremia, and if the patient is receiving hemodialysis treatment, water-soluble vitamins are lost through the dialysis membrane. The bleeding tendency of uremia is apparently caused by a qualitative defect in the platelets and consequently results in defective adhesion. Inhibition of certain coagulation factors may also play a role.

Pallor as a result of persistent anemia is characteristic of the uremic patient. The anemia undoubtedly contributes to the symptoms of fatigue. Dyspnea on exertion may be experienced when the hemoglobin is 8 g/dl or less. Bruising, nosebleeds, and GI bleeding may be manifestations of the coagulation defect.

Infection is a fairly common complication of patients with advanced renal insufficiency. The white blood cell (WBC) count is usually normal in end-stage renal disease (ESRD), but there is evidence of defective granulocyte, lymphocyte, and monocyte-macrophage function. Decreased chemotaxis causes impairment of the acute inflammatory response and decreased delayed hypersensi-

tivity. Uremic patients also tend to have less fever in response to an infection (Ruiz et al., 1990; Tolkoff-Rubin, Rubin, 1990). Poor nutrition, pulmonary edema, and the use of cannulas and indwelling catheters may be predisposing factors in the increased susceptibility to infection. The use of large doses of corticosteroid and other immunosuppressive drugs after renal transplant to suppress tissue rejection makes these patients unusually susceptible to severe infection that may result in death.

CUTANEOUS CHANGES

The accumulation of urinary pigments (principally urochrome) combined with anemia in advanced renal insufficiency gives the skin of the light-skinned person a peculiar waxy yellow cast. In the brown-skinned person this is observed as a yellowish brown coloration, and in the black-skinned person as an ashen gray color with yellow tones, particularly on the palmar and plantar surfaces. The skin may be dry and scaly, and the hair may be brittle and may change color. The nails may be thin, brittle, and ridged and show alternating light and reddish bands. These nail changes are characteristic of chronic protein wasting (Muehrcke lines). Pruritus is common in the uremic patient and is considered to be a manifestation of increased parathyroid gland function and deposition of calcium in the skin. When the BUN level is very high, fine white crystals of urea may appear on areas of the skin where there is heavy perspiration. This is called *uremic frost.* Multiple bruises caused by minor trauma are often seen on the skin of the uremic patient because of increased capillary fragility.

GASTROINTESTINAL SIGNS AND SYMPTOMS

The GI manifestations of uremia can cause the patient great distress. Anorexia, nausea, and vomiting are common in uremia and are often the first symptoms of disease. They are responsible in part for the extensive weight loss in chronic renal failure. The entire GI tract itself becomes affected in uremia. Patients often complain of a metallic taste in the mouth, and there may be an odor of ammonia to the breath. The mouth may become inflamed and ulcerated (stomatitis), and the tongue may be dry and coated. Occasionally parotitis (inflammataion of the parotid gland) occurs. The normal flora of the mouth contains organisms (tooth calculus bacteria) that can split urea in the saliva to produce ammonia. This accounts for the uriniferous odor to the breath and the altered sense of taste and predisposes the tissue to the inflammation and infection. Mucosal ulcerations may occur in the stomach and the small or large intestine and may result in profuse bleeding. The effect of GI hemorrhage is extremely serious, as the fall in blood pressure lowers the GFR even further and the digestion of the blood causes a precipitous rise in the BUN level. Diarrhea occurs at times and may cause serious dehydration.

INTERMEDIARY METABOLISM ABNORMALITIES

Abnormalities of intermediary metabolism are characteristic of the uremic syndrome, although the physiologic mechanisms are poorly understood.

Protein

Whatever other elements are responsible for uremic symptoms, the breakdown products of protein metabolism are of prime importance. The dietary restriction of protein generally relieves somewhat the symptoms of lassitude, nausea, and anorexia, and increasing evidence exists that it may retard the progression of renal deterioration (see Chapter 48). The patient tends to decrease protein intake voluntarily as azotemia progresses, since the appetite for protein foods generally is lost. Another reason for protein restriction in uremia is that H^+, K^+, and phosphates are derived chiefly from protein foods and must be restricted to prevent their accumulation in the blood. Abnormal protein synthesis in uremia is manifested by elevation or depression of selected amino acids. The significance of this phenomenon is not known.

Carbohydrates and Fats

Defective carbohydrate metabolism is commonly associated with uremia. Fasting blood sugar levels are elevated in more than 50% of uremic patients but not usually over 200 mg/dl. Insensitivity of the peripheral tissues to insulin is the possible cause. On the other hand, insulin-dependent diabetic patients who develop uremia may improve their carbohydrate metabolism and require a lower dosage of insulin, in apparent contradiction to the glucose intolerance of nondiabetic patients. A possible explanation is an elevated serum insulin level because of a prolonged half-life (the kidney normally inactivates about 20% of the insulin) in uremia. Carbohydrate metabolism generally becomes normal with regular hemodialysis.

Abnormal fat metabolism is manifested by high serum triglyceride levels in uremic patients, even in those who regularly undergo dialysis. Contributing factors in the elevated triglycerides may include the elevated glucose and insulin levels and the acetate used in the dialysate. The abnormal carbohydrate and fat metabolism undoubtedly contributes to the accelerated atherosclerosis in chronic dialysis patients.

NEUROMUSCULAR ABNORMALITIES

Involvement of the neuromuscular system is a nearly universal complication of uremia. Both the central and the peripheral nervous systems are involved, with diverse consequences. Muscles may be involved partly because of the peripheral neuropathy and partly because of muscle wasting.

Central Nervous System

The degree of cerebral disturbance roughly parallels the degree of azotemia. Early symptoms are decreased mental acuity and ability to concentrate, apathy, and lethargy. The patient complains of feeling weak and tired and may be unable to perform a normal day's work without frequent rest periods. Lethargy may alternate with periods of restlessness and insomnia. The untreated patient will eventually become confused and comatose. If convulsions occur, they are usually associated with hypertensive encephalopathy. Neuromuscular irritability is reflected by involuntary jerking and twitching of muscles. *Asterixis* (flapping tremor of the hands) may sometimes be present and is a manifestation of cerebral toxicity. The physical sign is induced by having the patient raise both arms with forearms fixed and fingers extended; this will result in alterations of flexion and extension at the wrist (flapping tremor).

Peripheral Neuropathy

Affliction of the peripheral nervous system follows a characteristic course. The earliest sign of peripheral neuropathy is the slowing of nerve conduction. This is generally tested on the peroneal nerve in the leg. A decreased velocity of nerve conduction may begin before the onset of clinical symptoms. The "restless leg syndrome" may sometimes be an early symptom. The patient may describe this symptom as a peculiar feeling that is relieved by walking or moving the legs. The second stage in the development of peripheral neuropathy is the advent of sensory changes in the extremities. The patient experiences burning pain, numbness, or tingling (paresthesias) of the toes and feet, which progress up the leg in a stockinglike fashion. Later, paresthesias may occur in the fingers and hands. Finally, motor nerves are involved. Motor involvement usually begins as a foot drop and may progress to paraplegia. Pathologically there is a patchy loss of myelin and damage to the peripheral nerves, possibly caused by uremic toxins and electrolyte imbalance.

Hemodialysis may halt the progress of peripheral neuropathy, but once these changes occur, they are poorly reversible (sensory) or are irreversible (motor). Therefore hemodialysis (or transplantation preparations) should be started before clinical signs and symptoms occur.

CALCIUM AND SKELETAL DISORDERS (RENAL OSTEODYSTROPHY)

If a patient with chronic renal failure survives long enough, calcium and phosphate imbalances with skeletal involvement are inevitable. The skeletal disorders called *renal osteodystrophy* comprise three lesions.

Osteomalacia is the most common bone disorder and is seen in about 60% of all patients with chronic renal failure. It consists of defective mineralization of bone. It is caused by a deficiency of 1,25-dihydroxycholecalciferol ($1,25[OH]_2D_3$), the most active form of vitamin D metabolized by the kidneys. The deficiency of the most active form of vitamin D leads to severely impaired absorption of calcium from the gut. In the bone, osteoblasts continue to manufacture osteoid tissue (the framework on which calcium salts are laid down to produce bone), but

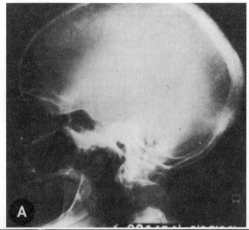

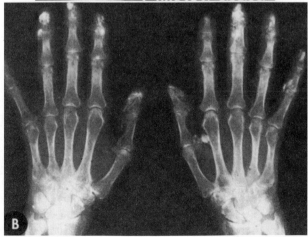

FIG. 47-2 Renal osteodystrophy. **A,** Skull radiograph shows spotty demineralization of bone, producing a "moth-eaten" appearance. **B,** Subperiosteal resorption is present in all the phalanges but is seen best on the middle phalanx of both the right and left hands, producing a jagged appearance. (Courtesy of DE Schteingart.)

the low serum calcium level and ineffective action of vitamin D on the bone do not allow mineralization. Osteoid tissue eventually replaces normal bone, producing osteomalacia in adults and rickets in children. Osteoid is structurally weak and may fracture or deform under stress. On radiographs, osteomalacia presents as a generalized decrease in bone density, especially of the hands, skull, ribs, and spine. In addition, recent evidence indicates that the accumulation of aluminum metabolites in bone results in a form of vitamin D–resistant osteomalacia. The sources are aluminum hydroxide antacids commonly used as dietary phosphate-binding agents. Aluminum is also common in the community water and may be transferred to the patient during dialysis.

Osteitis fibrosa, occurring in more than 30% of patients, is characterized by osteoclastic resorption of bone and replacement by fibrous tissue. The bone demineralization may be localized and may present as cystlike lesions (osteitis fibrosa cystica) or may appear on a radiograph as a generalized decrease in bone density. Osteitis fibrosa is caused by the increased levels of parathyroid hormone (PTH) (secondary hyperparathyroidism) in chronic renal failure. The classic radiographic appearance of osteitis fibrosa is often seen in the fingers as subperiosteal bone resorption and in the skull as a patchy loss of bone density (Fig. 47-2).

Osteosclerosis, the third, less common bone disorder, is often manifested as a banded or striped appearance of the vertebrae ("rugger jersey spine") on radiographs. It is caused by alternate bands of decreased and increased bone density.

Any of the lesions just described may occur alone, but a combination is more common. Hemodialysis alone does not prevent renal osteodystrophy. Only within the past few years has research uncovered some of the complex relationships in the pathogenesis of renal osteodystrophy so that effective treatment is possible. The principal factors are decreased renal function, secondary hyperparathyroidism, and vitamin D deficiency or resistance.

Pathogenesis of Renal Osteodystrophy

The sequence of events leading to secondary hyperparathyroidism and renal osteodystrophy is most easily followed in Fig. 47-3 (also see Chapter 21).

Normally the serum calcium and phosphate are in equilibrium with solid-phase calcium and phosphate in the bones. The absorption from the gut, excretion by the kidneys, and deposition and resorption from the bone of these minerals are primarily controlled by PTH and 1,25-dihydroxycholecalciferol ($1,25[OH_2]D_3$). Moreover, serum calcium and phosphate levels have a reciprocal relationship; that is, when serum calcium levels go up, serum phosphate levels go down and vice versa. This interrelation serves the purpose of keeping the serum calcium-phosphate cross product constant so that calcium phosphate is not precipitated in the vascular system. For

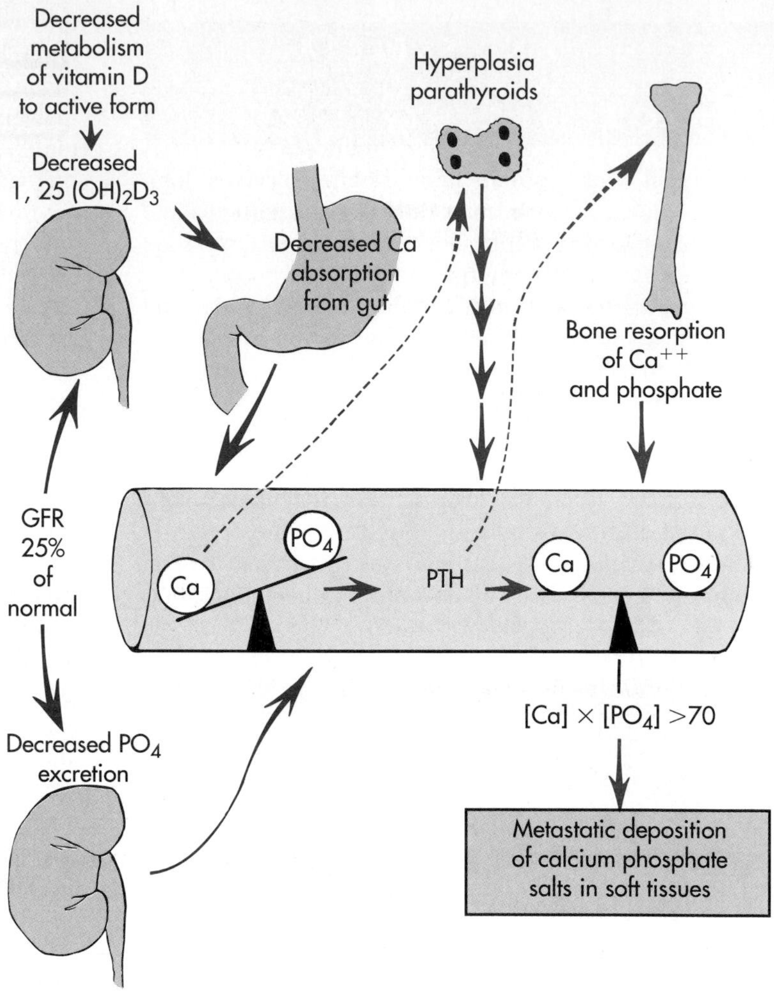

FIG. 47-3 Pathogenesis of renal osteodystrophy. *1,25[OH]₂D₃,* 1,25-Dihydroxycholecalciferol; *GFR,* glomerular filtration rate; *PTH,* parathyroid hormone; *Ca⁺⁺,* calcium.

example, the normal serum calcium level is 9.0 to 11.0 mg/dl, and the normal phosphate level is 3.0 to 4.5 mg/dl. The normal cross-product value in milligrams per deciliter of calcium and phosphate is thus 3 to 4.5 × 9 to 11 = 27.0 to 49.5. Precipitation of calcium phosphate salts in the soft tissues is believed to occur when their cross product exceeds 60 to 70 mg/dl.

As renal disease advances, calcium-phosphate interrelations become progressively disrupted. When the GFR falls to about 25% of normal, phosphate is retained by the kidneys. Phosphate retention causes the depression of serum calcium levels. The azotemic state also interferes with vitamin D₃ activation by the kidney, which is necessary for the absorption of calcium from the gut. Both these factors tend to cause hypocalcemia. Hypocalcemia stimulates the parathyroid glands to put out more PTH, which causes bone resorption of calcium and phosphate, increased excretion of phosphate, and activation of vitamin D₃ by the kidneys. Serum calcium and phosphate levels thus tend to be restored to normal. As the GFR continues to decrease, however, the low serum calcium and high phosphate levels increasingly stimulate parathyroid activity. The parathyroid glands may show hyperpla-

sia of the secretory cells, with apparent independence of physiologic controls. The result is increasing demineralization of the bony skeleton. A rise in the serum alkaline phosphatase level is evidence that this process is occurring. The calcium phosphate cross product may become exceedingly high, resulting in the precipitation of calcium phosphate salts in the soft tissues of the body.

Common sites for the deposition of calcium salts are in and around joints, resulting in painful arthritis; in the kidney (nephrocalcinosis), resulting in obstruction; in the blood vessels, which may have the appearance of an arteriogram on radiographs; in the heart and lung, leading to dysrhythmias, cardiomyopathy, and pulmonary fibrosis; and in the eyes. The deposition of calcium salts in the conjunctiva and cornea of the eye is called *band keratopathy.* Band keratopathy appears as grayish or whitish granular opacities in the form of a crescent on the nasal or temporal side of the limbus (where cornea and sclera meet at colored and white parts of the eye) (Fig. 47-4). Precipitation of calcium phosphate salts occurs on the surface of the eye because here the pH is high and favors precipitation. These deposits can be seen with the naked eye but are most easily outlined by slit lamp examination.

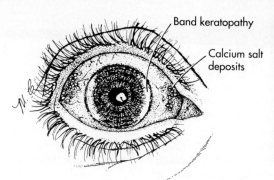
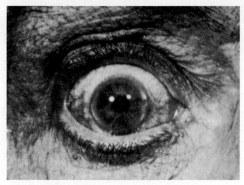

Band keratopathy

Calcium salt deposits

FIG. 47-4   Band keratopathy caused by deposit of calcium salts in the eye. Conjunctival deposits of calcium salts are also present. Diagram of abnormalities seen in photograph. (Photograph from Maxwell MH, Kleeman CR, editors: *Clinical disorders of fluid and electrolyte metabolism*, ed 2, New York, 1972, McGraw-Hill Book Co.)

The conjunctival deposits sometimes cause intense irritation with redness and watering of the eyes ("uremic red eye").

This completes the description of the syndrome called uremia. Not all components are present in every patient, and the dominant features may vary from one patient to another. The prevention and treatment of these complications are considered in Chapter 48.

QUESTIONS

▼ *Answer the following on a separate sheet of paper.*

1. What is meant by uremic syndrome?
2. What are the two groups of clinical symptoms present in the uremic syndrome? How does the middle molecular hypothesis account for some of these symptoms? What are the implications of this theory?
3. Explain why total NH_4^+ excretion is decreased in renal failure.
4. Why does the acidosis of chronic renal failure generally stabilize at a moderate level when there is a positive H^+ balance? What relation might the acidosis of renal failure have to the bone abnormality?
5. Why is salt wasting associated with polyuria in early renal insufficiency?
6. Name two common laxatives that, if administered to the uremic patient, might result in death.
7. Explain the meaning of a constant finding of urine specific gravity at 1.010.
8. How are sexual and reproductive functions affected in terminal renal failure? (Explain the effects in men and women.)
9. Name four factors that contribute to the development of infection in the uremic patient.
10. Describe skin color changes in uremic patients who are white skinned, brown skinned, and black skinned.
11. Illustrate the mechanisms by which gastrointestinal bleeding, vomiting, or diarrhea could cause the deterioration of renal function. (Draw flow diagrams.)
12. List several changes you might expect to observe in the mental, emotional, and neuromuscular status and rest pattern of a patient who is developing uremia.
13. List the stages in the development of peripheral neuropathy and the signs and symptoms you would expect to observe in the patient with renal failure.
14. Illustrate the radiographic appearance of the phalanges when there is subperiosteal bone resorption in renal osteodystrophy.
15. Draw a flow diagram of the pathogenesis of secondary hyperparathryoidism and list several examples of the consequences of this condition.
16. A uremic patient has a serum phosphate level of 8 mg/dl and a calcium level of 10 mg/dl. Would you expect metastatic calcification in the soft tissues of the body? Explain.
17. What is band keratopathy? Illustrate. What causes "uremic red eye"?

▼ *Circle the letter preceding each item below that correctly answers the question or completes the statement. Only one answer is correct, with exceptions noted.*

18. In renal failure there is an impaired ability to excrete H^+. This results in:
    a. Respiratory acidosis
    b. Metabolic acidosis
    c. Respiratory alkalosis
    d. Metabolic alkalosis
19. Which of the following describes the plasma pH and bicarbonate levels in the condition of renal failure?
    a. Increase in pH and decrease in HCO_3^-
    b. Decrease in pH and increase in HCO_3^-
    c. Decrease in both pH and HCO_3^-
    d. Increase in both pH and HCO_3^-
20. Which of the following mechanisms is most important for the excretion of H^+ by the kidney?
    a. Excretion of H^+ as NH_4 by combination with NH_3
    b. Excretion of H^+ as acid phosphate

Continued.

21. Hypokalemia associated with polyuria is most apt to be associated with:
    a. Acute renal failure
    b. Acute pyelonephritis
    c. Chronic pyelonephritis

22. As the patient becomes oliguric in end-stage renal failure, which of the following K^+ disturbances usually develops?
    a. Hypokalemia
    b. Hyperkalemia

23. Metabolic acidosis contributes to hyperkalemia by which of the following mechanisms?
    a. Shift of K^+ from the intracellular fluid (ICF) to the extracellular fluid (ECF)
    b. Shift of Mg^{++} from the ICF to the ECF
    c. Shift of K^+ from the ECF to the ICF
    d. Shift of Mg^{++} from the ECF to the ICF

24. Fatal dysrhythmias and cardiac arrest are most apt to occur when serum K^+ levels reach:
    a. 3.5-4.5 mEq/L
    b. 4.5-5.5 mEq/L
    c. 6.5-7.5 mEq/L

25. When oliguria occurs in terminal renal failure, the patient is likely to do which of the following? (More than one answer may be correct.)
    a. Increase sodium-losing tendency
    b. Retain sodium
    c. Increase circulatory overload
    d. Increase aldosterone secretion

26. Symptoms of gouty arthritis experienced by some uremic patients are most likely caused by serum elevations of:
    a. Urea
    b. Creatinine
    c. Uric acid
    d. Bicarbonate

27. Which of the following factors contribute to the development of congestive heart failure in uremic patients? (More than one answer may be correct.)
    a. Anemia
    b. Hypertension
    c. Excess sodium and water intake
    d. Circulatory overload

28. Which statements are true in relation to anemia in a uremic patient? (More than one answer may be correct.)

a. It is caused by excess hemolysis.
b. It is caused by iron deficiency.
c. It is normochromic, normocytic.
d. It is caused by excess production of erythropoietin.
e. When severe, it may cause symptoms of fatigue, dyspnea, and pallor.

29. What is the mechanism of the bleeding tendency in uremia? (More than one answer may be correct.)
    a. Defective platelet adhesion
    b. Severe thrombocytopenia
    c. Inhibition of some of the circulating coagulation factors

30. Symptoms of uremia generally begin when the GFR falls to which of the following ranges of normal?
    a. 80%-90%
    b. 50%-60%
    c. 30%-40%
    d. 4%-10%

31. A 40-year-old woman with ESRD has a hemoglobin (Hb) of 7.4 g/dl and a hematocrit (Hct) of 21. Her blood pressure is 172/94, and her heart rate is 103 bpm. What is the most likely explanation of her Hb and Hct values?
    a. The values are normal
    b. The values are abnormally low because of a reduced cardiac output
    c. The values are low because of a deficit of erythropoietin
    d. The values are elevated because of hemoconcentration

32. Which of the following statements does not apply to uremic neuropathy?
    a. Sensory changes are more marked than motor changes in the early stages
    b. Nerve conduction times may be depressed even when clinical neuropathy is absent
    c. Once motor neuropathy is present, it is poorly reversible by dialysis
    d. The earliest manifestations occur in the upper extremities

33. The half-life of insulin is prolonged in ESRD because:
    a. The kidney is the main site of insulin degradation
    b. Excretion of insulin is impaired
    c. Uremia impairs peripheral degradation of insulin

d. Peripheral antagonism of insulin action occurs

34. All of the following statements are true regarding renal osteodystrophy except:
    a. Intestinal absorption of calcium is usually impaired
    b. Parathormone levels are invariably high
    c. $1,25(OH_2)D_3$ levels are elevated
    d. Metastatic calcification occurs when the Ca-PO_4 cross product exceeds 60 to 70 mg/dl

35. The most important factor causing uremic bleeding is:
    a. Thrombocytopenia
    b. Hypoprothrombinemia
    c. Abnormal platelet function
    d. Abnormal plasma factor IX

▼ *Circle T if the statement is true and F if it is false. Correct any false statements.*

36. T F Anorexia, nausea, and lethargy are common symptoms in the uremic patient and may be partly the result of metabolic acidosis.

37. T F Kussmaul's respiration is the shallow respiration that occurs because of the need to decrease CO_2 excretion by the lungs.

38. T F The symptoms of anorexia, nausea, and lassitude are often relieved by the dietary restriction of protein.

39. T F Dietary protein restriction may retard the progression of chronic renal failure.

40. T F Dietary protein restriction helps reduce K^+, H^+, and phosphate intake.

41. T F There is no evidence of abnormal protein synthesis in uremia.

42. T F Hypoglycemia is the usual manifestation of abnormal carbohydrate metabolism in uremia.

43. T F Insulin-dependent diabetic persons who become uremic often require lower dosages of insulin.

44. T F Elevation of serum triglycerides in uremia is related to abnormal fat metabolism in uremia.

QUESTIONS—cont'd

▼ *Fill in the blanks with the correct words.*

45. Organisms normally in the mouth split _____, producing _____, which contributes to the uriniferous odor to the breath, inflammation and ulceration of the mucous membranes, predisposition to _____, and altered taste sensation common in the uremic patient.

46. Three types of bone lesions seen in renal osteodystrophy are (a) _____ caused by hyperparathyroidism; (b) _____ caused by vitamin D deficiency; and (c) _____, which gives a banded ("rugger jersey") appearance to the spine because of alternating areas of bone demineralization and sclerosis.

▼ *Match the abnormality found in uremia in column A with the most likely complication resulting from that abnormality in column B. More than one letter may be used for each condition in column A.*

Column A	Column B
47. _____ Pericarditis	a. Pneumonia
48. _____ Circulatory overload	b. Retinopathy
49. _____ Hypertension	c. Cardiac tamponade
	d. Pulmonary edema
	e. Encephalopathy

▼ *Match the following integumentary manifestations of the uremic syndrome in column B with the probable causative factor in column A.*

Column A	Column B
50. _____ Urochrome	a. Bruises
51. _____ Anemia	b. Yellow cast
52. _____ Urea	c. Pruritus
53. _____ Proteinuria	d. Fine, white crystal deposits in areas of increased perspiration
54. _____ Calcium deposits in skin	e. Brittle, ridged nails with alternating light and red bands
55. _____ Capillary fragility	f. Pallor

CHAPTER 48

Treatment of Chronic Renal Failure

LORRAINE M. WILSON

methods of retarding the progression of chronic renal failure caused by secondary glomerular injury from hyperfiltration in intact nephrons are currently under intensive investigation. Dietary protein restriction and antihypertensive therapy (especially with the use of angiotensin-converting enzyme [ACE] inhibitors) are the two major interventions being investigated (see p. 735).

The second stage of treatment begins when conservative measures are no longer effective in sustaining life. End-stage renal disease (ESRD) or terminal renal failure exists at this point (glomerular filtration rate [GFR] is usually <2 ml/min), and the only effective treatment is either intermittent dialysis or renal transplantation. However, before this point is reached, a number of physiologic alterations occur, many of which are detrimental. Therefore dialysis is usually begun before true ESRD is reached. The box on p. 735 summarizes the principles of management of chronic renal failure discussed in this chapter.

The treatment of chronic renal failure can be divided into two stages. The first stage consists of conservative measures designed to temper or delay the progressive deterioration of renal function. Conservative measures are begun when the patient becomes azotemic. The physician makes every effort to determine the primary cause of the renal failure and search out any reversible factors such as the following:

1. Extracellular fluid (ECF) volume depletion caused by the overzealous use of diuretics or a salt restriction that is too stringent
2. Urinary tract obstruction from calculi, prostatic enlargement, or retroperitoneal fibrosis
3. Infection, especially of the urinary tract
4. Severe or malignant hypertension

These factors are likely causes of a sudden deterioration of renal function in a patient with chronic renal failure (Schrier, 1992). Treatment of reversible factors may stabilize and prevent any further deterioration of renal function. In addition to the correction of reversible factors,

CONSERVATIVE MANAGEMENT

The basic principles of conservative management are quite simple and are based on an understanding of the range of excretion that can be achieved by the failing kidney. Dietary regulation of individual solutes and fluid is then adjusted to the limitations. In addition, therapy is directed toward prevention and treatment of complications as they occur.

Dietary Regulation of Protein

Dietary regulation is of primary importance in the treatment of chronic renal failure. It is customary to restrict the protein intake of the azotemic patient, although there is controversy about how severe this restriction should be. The restriction of protein not only reduces the blood urea nitrogen (BUN) level and perhaps other poorly defined toxic products of protein metabolism, but also reduces the intake of potassium, phosphate, and the hydrogen-ion production that stem from protein. Symptoms of nausea, vomiting, and fatigue may be ameliorated. More important, recent studies have demonstrated that abnormal intrarenal hemodynamics contribute to the progression of chronic renal failure in several modes of renal disease (see Chapter 46). Restriction of dietary protein intake has been demonstrated to normalize these aberrations and retard progression to renal failure. The probable mechanism is related to the fact that a low-protein intake reduces the ex-

MANAGEMENT OF CHRONIC RENAL FAILURE

CONSERVATIVE MANAGEMENT

Determination and treatment of the cause
Optimization and maintenance of salt and water balance
Correction of any urinary tract obstruction
Early detection and treatment of infection
Control of hypertension
Low-protein, high-calorie diet
Control of electrolyte balance
Prevention and treatment of renal bone disease
Modification of drug therapy with alterations in renal function
Detection and treatment of complications

RENAL REPLACEMENT THERAPY

Hemodialysis
Peritoneal dialysis
Renal transplantation

cretory load, thus reducing glomerular hyperfiltration, intraglomerular pressure, and secondary injury of the intact nephrons.

Recall from the discussion in Chapter 46 that once the kidneys have sustained a substantial degree of damage, progressive deterioration of renal function takes place because of the deleterious effects of glomerular hypertension within the intact nephrons. When renal failure is progressive, the GFR tends to decline in a linear fashion over time so that plotting serial measurements of GFR allows prediction of the time to ESRD when dialysis treatment will be necessary. However, the measurement of GFR at low levels is inaccurate. A common method of assessing the results of protein restriction in retarding the progression of chronic renal disease to ESRD is to plot the reciprocal of the plasma creatinine concentration ($1/P_{cr}$) versus time instead of the GFR. Recall that

$$GFR \approx \text{Creatinine clearance} = \frac{U_{cr}V}{P_{cr}}$$

where U_{cr} is the urine creatinine concentration, V is the urine flow rate, and P_{cr} is the plasma creatinine concentration. If body muscle mass is stable, production and excretion rates of creatinine per unit time ($U_{cr}V$) will be relatively constant so that

$$GFR \approx \frac{\text{Constant}}{P_{cr}} \propto \frac{1}{P_{cr}}$$

Thus the reciprocal of the plasma creatinine concentration ($1/P_{cr}$) can be used to track changes in the GFR. The approximate time until ESRD is reached can be predicted by extrapolation of the $1/P_{cr}$ versus time relationship. Changes in the slope of $1/P_{cr}$ plotted against time can be used to indicate the rate of progression of renal failure. A

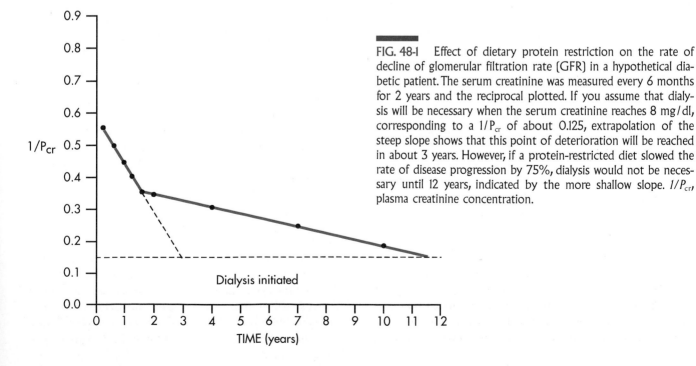

FIG. 48-1   Effect of dietary protein restriction on the rate of decline of glomerular filtration rate (GFR) in a hypothetical diabetic patient. The serum creatinine was measured every 6 months for 2 years and the reciprocal plotted. If you assume that dialysis will be necessary when the serum creatinine reaches 8 mg/dl, corresponding to a $1/P_{cr}$ of about 0.125, extrapolation of the steep slope shows that this point of deterioration will be reached in about 3 years. However, if a protein-restricted diet slowed the rate of disease progression by 75%, dialysis would not be necessary until 12 years, indicated by the more shallow slope. $1/P_{cr}$, plasma creatinine concentration.

decrease in slope would mean that progression to ESRD is slower than expected and is the expected result of effective therapy (Fig. 48-1).

Several studies have demonstrated the possibility of retarding the rate of progression of renal failure by reducing protein intake. Using a diet containing the minimum daily requirement (MDR) of protein (0.6 g/kg) versus an unrestricted protein diet (average protein intake in the United States is 1.2 to 1.6 g/kg), Oldrizzi et al. (1985) showed that the rate of increase in creatinine was 11 times lower in the protein-restricted group of patients with chronic glomerulonephritis and 19 times lower in the protein-restricted group of patients with chronic pyelonephritis than in the control groups. In another study in which protein intake was less than the MDR, Giordano (1981) noted that the average time to reach ESRD was 16 months in the noncompliant group but increased to 7.6 years in the protein-restricted group. Preliminary results of studies in patients with diabetic nephropathy showed that the rate of progression was reduced by 75% in protein-restricted groups (Diabetes Control and Complications Trial Research Group, 1993).

The long-term effects of severely restricted protein diets (i.e., <MDR) on nutritional status are of obvious concern. It is possible to maintain nitrogen balance on a 20-g protein diet, provided the protein is of highest biologic value (i.e., contains all the essential amino acids as do milk and eggs) and adequate calories are provided in the form of fats and carbohydrates to prevent the breakdown of body protein to satisfy caloric requirements. One approach to this problem is to supplement very low–protein diets by using either a mixture of essential amino acids (EAA) or combinations of EAAs and alpha-keto or alpha-hydroxy analogues of amino acids (KA). This approach allows more variety in the diet and therefore may be more acceptable to some patients. Carbohydrate supplements may be given to ensure adequate calories to prevent breakdown of body protein. Mitch (1991) found that this therapy minimizes uremic symptoms, secondary hyperparathyroidism, and metabolic acidosis. Vitamin B complex, pyridoxine, and ascorbic acid supplements should be given with such regimens.

Although preliminary evidence suggests that low-protein diets may slow the progression of renal failure, dietary treatment does not seem to have much effect once the GFR has fallen to 4 to 5 ml/min. The current clinical recommendation for stable, predialysis, chronic renal failure patients is 0.6 g/kg/day protein with 35 calories/kg (Mitch, Klahr, 1988). The protein allowance may be liberalized to 1.0 g/kg/day when the patient is receiving regular dialysis.

Dietary Regulation of Potassium

Hyperkalemia generally becomes a problem in advanced renal failure, and it becomes necessary also to restrict dietary intake of potassium. The typical dietary allowance is 40 to 80 mEq/day. Care must be taken not to adminis-

ter foods or drugs that are high in potassium. These include salt substitutes (which contain ammonium chloride and potassium chloride), expectorants, potassium citrate, and foods such as soups, dates, bananas, and pure fruit juices. Inadvertent administration of food or drugs high in potassium could cause a serious hyperkalemia.

Dietary Regulation of Sodium and Fluids

The dietary regulation of sodium is important in renal failure. The typical sodium allowance is 40 to 90 mEq/day (1 to 2 g of sodium), but the optimal sodium intake must be determined individually for each patient to maintain good hydration. An intake that is too liberal can lead to fluid retention, peripheral edema, pulmonary edema, hypertension, and congestive heart failure. Sodium retention is generally a problem in glomerular disease and in advanced renal failure. On the other hand, if sodium is restricted to the point of negative sodium balance, hypovolemia, decreased GFR, and a deterioration of renal function will ensue. Sodium depletion is more common in tubulointerstitial disease and may be precipitated by vomiting or diarrhea. It is therefore important to determine the optimum sodium intake for each patient. The sodium conservation test and a careful observation of the daily weight, signs of edema, and other complications may all be helpful.

In the sodium conservation test the patient eats a low-sodium diet for 5 days (e.g., 10 mEq/day). The normal person will conserve sodium and come into balance during this period. On the fifth day, 24-hour urine samples are collected and the sodium is measured. The sodium lost in the urine at this time represents an obligatory loss and thus the "sodium floor." For example, a patient on a 10 mEq sodium diet who loses 50 mEq in the urine on the fifth day has a negative sodium balance of 40 mEq (50 − 10 = 40); 40 mEq of sodium must be added to the diet. The "sodium ceiling" is determined by observing weight, blood pressure, and other signs of ECF excess. As stated previously, the range between sodium deficit and sodium excess can be very narrow.

The intake of fluids requires careful regulation in advanced renal failure, because the patient's thirst is an unreliable guide to the state of hydration. Daily weight is the critical parameter to follow, in addition to accurate intake and output records. An intake that is too liberal may result in circulatory overload, edema, and water intoxication, and less than optimal intake will result in dehydration, hypotension, and a deterioration in renal function. The general rule for fluid intake is urine output during past 24 hours + 500 ml, the 500 ml representing insensible loss. For example, if the patient's urine output during the past 24 hours was 400 ml, the total intake per day should be 500 + 400 ml = 900 ml. Anephric patients are allowed 800 ml/day, and patients in dialysis are given sufficient fluid to allow a 2- to 3-pound weight gain between treatments. Obviously, both sodium and fluid intake must be manipulated to achieve fluid balance.

Prevention and Treatment of Complications

The second category of conservative measures used in the treatment of renal failure comprises those directed toward the prevention and treatment of complications.

Hypertension

Renal function deteriorates more rapidly if severe hypertension develops. In addition, extrarenal complications such as retinopathy and encephalopathy may develop. Hypertension can usually be controlled effectively by sodium and fluid restriction and by ultrafiltration when the patient is on hemodialysis, since more than 90% of hypertension is volume dependent. In some cases an antihypertensive drug (with or without a diuretic) may be given to achieve blood pressure control. The most common antihypertensive drugs given are methyldopa (Aldomet), propranolol (Inderal), and clonidine (Catapres), and the most common diuretic is furosemide (Lasix). Recent evidence suggests that ACE inhibitor drugs (e.g., captopril) may be particularly beneficial. In addition to lowering systemic blood pressure, these drugs directly lower the intraglomerular pressure by selectively dilating the efferent arteriole (see Chapter 46). ACE inhibitor drugs also reduce proteinuria. Because ACE inhibitor drugs lower the intraglomerular pressure and slow the progression of chronic renal failure, treatment with these drugs has been advocated even for patients who are normotensive. When the patient is receiving hemodialysis, it is important to withhold the antihypertensive drug before treatment to prevent hypotension and shock that may result as intravascular fluid is removed through ultrafiltration if the normal vascular vasoconstrictive reaction is blocked by the drug. In a small number of cases (<10%) the hypertension may be renin dependent and refractory to sodium-volume control or control with a mild antihypertensive. A more potent antihypertensive drug such as minoxidil (Loniten) can usually bring the blood pressure under control. Bilateral nephrectomy may be considered as a last resort when all other methods have failed. Bilateral nephrectomy causes the anemia to become more severe, since even the end-stage kidney produces some erythropoietin (Rose, Black, 1988).

Great care is taken to lower the blood pressure gradually so that the patient does not become hypotensive, with consequent lowering of GFR and further deterioration of renal function. Hypertension in the majority of uremic patients is caused by fluid overload and is most effectively restored to normal by regulation of sodium and fluid intake and intermittent dialysis.

Hyperkalemia

One of the most serious complications in the uremic patient is the development of hyperkalemia. When serum potassium (K^+) reaches a level of about 7 mEq/L, serious dysrhythmias and cardiac arrest may occur (see Chapter 21). In addition, hypocalcemia, hyponatremia, and acidosis intensify the deleterious effects of hyperkalemia. For this reason the patient's heart may be monitored to detect the effect of the hyperkalemia (and the effects of all the other ions) on cardiac conduction.

Acute hyperkalemia may be treated by the administration of intravenous (IV) glucose and insulin, which drives K^+ into the cells, or by the careful (IV) administration of 10% calcium gluconate, with continuous electrocardiogram (ECG) monitoring if the patient is hypotensive with widening of the QRS complex. The effect of these measures is only temporary, and the hyperkalemia must subsequently be corrected by dialysis. When it is not possible to lower K^+ by dialysis, the cation exchange resin sodium polystyrene sulfonate (Kayexalate) may be used. Each gram of the resin binds 1 mEq of K^+. Kayexalate may be given by mouth or by rectal instillation. When given rectally, 50 to 100 g is mixed with 200 to 300 ml of water. To facilitate the K^+ exchange, 25 to 30 ml of 70% sorbitol (a poorly absorbed, osmotically active alcohol that has a laxative effect) is added. Obviously, orange juice (high K^+ content) should not be given to disguise the taste when Kayexalate is administered orally.

Anemia

Anemia is a nearly universal finding in patients with advanced renal disease, and hematocrits of 18% to 20% are common. The cause of the anemia is multifactorial, including deficiency of erythropoietin production; circulating factors that appear to inhibit erythropoietin; shortened RBC life span; increased gastrointestinal (GI) blood loss caused by platelet abnormalities; iron and folic acid deficiency; and blood losses from hemodialysis or from frequent samples for laboratory tests. Although all of the listed factors may contribute to the anemia of chronic renal failure, it appears that erythropoietin deficiency is the major cause of the anemia, since patients respond so well to replacement of this hormone. In 1985 the human erythropoietin gene was isolated and cloned (Jacobs et al., 1985; Lin et al., 1985), facilitating unlimited amounts of the hormone. The recent widespread availability of recombinant human erythropoietin (EPO) has revolutionized the management of the anemia of chronic renal failure (CRF). A 6% to 10% increase in the hematocrit and a reduction of the anemia-related symptoms of weakness and fatigue can be expected. EPO is commonly administered as a subcutaneous injection (25 to 125 U/kg of body weight) three times per week. The major complication of EPO therapy is hypertension, which occurs in about one half of the patients. The rise in blood pressure caused by EPO therapy has been attributed to an increase in blood viscosity and the reversal of the anemia-induced peripheral vasodilation. The risk of hypertension can be ameliorated by aiming for a subnormal hematocrit of 30% to 35%.

In addition to EPO therapy, other measures to alleviate anemia in CRF patients include minimizing blood losses and giving vitamins and blood transfusions. Iatrogenic blood loss can be reduced by taking the smallest blood sample possible for laboratory tests and by minimizing residual blood left in the tubing in hemodialysis treatment. A multivitamin and a folic acid preparation are usually given each day, since water-soluble vitamins are depleted by dialysis. Oral iron or dextran iron complex (Imferon) may be given parenterally, since iron deficiency may result from blood loss and binding by antacids. Until recently, blood transfusions of packed RBCs were commonly used to treat anemia in patients with CRF but are now generally restricted to patients with hematocrits less than 24%.

Acidosis

The mild chronic metabolic acidosis of the uremic patient usually stabilizes at a plasma bicarbonate level of 16 to 20 mEq/L. It does not usually progress beyond this point, since hydrogen ion (H^+) production is balanced by bone buffering. The renal acidosis is not usually treated unless the plasma bicarbonate (HCO_3^-) falls below 15 mEq/L, when symptoms of acidosis may appear. Severe acidosis may be precipitated by the superimposition of an acute acidosis on the mild chronic acidosis. This might occur, for example, in profuse diarrhea with its HCO_3^- loss. When severe acidosis is corrected by the parenteral administration of sodium bicarbonate ($NaHCO_3$), it is important to be aware of the hazard involved. Overcorrection of blood pH may precipitate tetany, convulsions, and death. It should be remembered that patients with chronic renal failure are usually hypocalcemic. A mild degree of induced alkalosis may reduce the ionized fraction of serum calcium (Ca^{++}) (usually in an acidic environment) to the point of severe hypocalcemia. The most logical mode of treatment, finally, is dialysis.

Renal osteodystrophy

One of the most crucial therapeutic measures used to prevent the development of secondary hyperparathyroidism and its consequences is a low-phosphate diet along with the administration of agents that bind phosphate in the bowel. The prevention and correction of hyperphosphatemia preclude the sequence of events leading to calcium and bone disorders discussed in Chapter 47. A low-protein diet is also low in phosphate. The treatment should begin early in the course of progressive renal failure, when the GFR is down to one third of normal. The phosphate-binding agent of choice is currently calcium carbonate or calcium acetate. In the past, most nephrologists prescribed aluminum antacid gels (Amphogel or Basojel) as phosphate binders. However, it is now known that this regimen creates a new problem of aluminum intoxication caused by the gradual accumulation of aluminum in tissues. The major manifestations of aluminum toxicity occur in bone and skeletal muscle, leading to vitamin D–resistant osteomalacia and muscle pain. Calcium carbonate (1 to 2 g) should be taken with each meal to ensure maximum effectiveness in binding dietary phosphate and thus preventing its absorption. The goal of therapy is to maintain the serum phosphate at about 4.5

mg/dl and the calcium at about 10 mg/dl. Studies in patients with CRF show that correction of hyperphosphatemia can at least partially correct the hypocalcemia, $1,25(OH)_2D_3$ deficiency, and excess parathyroid hormone (PTH) secretion.

Magnesium-containing antacids should never be substituted as phosphate binders, since patients with CRF have reduced ability to excrete this ion and could develop a serious hypermagnesemia. The major complication in patients taking calcium carbonate as a phosphate binder is the occasional development of hypercalcemia from increased intestinal absorption of calcium. One approach to preventing this complication is to lower the calcium in the dialysate from the standard 3.25 to 3.50 mEq/L to 2.5 mEq/L. Both serum calcium and phosphate levels should be monitored at least monthly to ensure that the calcium-phosphate cross product is in the normal range to avoid metastatic calcification.

If severe skeletal involvement occurs for lack of or despite preventive therapy with phosphate-binding agents, subtotal parathyroidectomy or vitamin D therapy may be indicated. Severe bone demineralization, hypercalcemia, or intractable pruritus is considered an indication for parathyroidectomy. When the predominant lesion is osteomalacia, the nephrologist must begin vitamin D therapy with great care. This treatment may be quite hazardous. Not only may calcium absorption be increased, but it may in fact lead to progressive soft tissue calcification when bone resorption and hyperphosphatemia continue unabated.

Hyperuricemia

Allopurinol is usually the drug of choice for treating the hyperuricemia of advanced renal disease. This drug reduces uric acid levels by blocking the biosynthesis of some part of the total uric acid produced by the body. Colchicine (antiinflammatory drug for gout) may be given for the relief of symptoms of gouty arthritis.

Peripheral neuropathy

Usually, symptomatic peripheral neuropathy does not occur until renal failure is far advanced. There is no known treatment for these changes except dialysis, which stops their progression. Therefore the development of sensory neuritis is a signal that dialysis should not be delayed any longer. Motor neuropathy may be irreversible. Nerve conduction velocity tests are commonly performed every 6 months to monitor the progress of peripheral neuropathy.

Prompt treatment of infection

Patients with chronic renal failure have an increased susceptibility to infection, particularly urinary tract infection. Because infection of any sort may accentuate the catabolic process and impair adequate nutrition and fluid and electrolyte balance, infections should be treated promptly to prevent further deterioration of renal function. However, the detection of infection in a patient with

ESRD requires a high degree of suspicion and attention to less specific indicators such as tachycardia, fatigue, or a slight rise in temperature. This is because hypothermia is one of the clinical features of the uremic syndrome and because many patients with ESRD do not exhibit the expected rise in body temperature or white blood cell (WBC) count when an infection is present (Lewis, 1992).

Cautious drug administration

Because many drugs are excreted by the kidney, they must be cautiously administered to the uremic patient. The half-life of drugs excreted by the kidney is greatly prolonged in uremia, so toxic serum levels may occur and the dosages of these drugs must therefore be reduced. The nephrologist chooses antibiotics (nonnephrotoxic) and their dosages with these facts in mind. Particular caution is necessary when digitalis drugs are ordered for the treatment of intrinsic cardiac disease in the uremic patient. In fact, cautious drug administration to the uremic patient should be the rule.

In progressive renal failure, conservative therapeutic measures finally become inadequate. Dialysis or renal transplantation is then the only means of preserving life. Continuation of many of the conservative measures may be necessary, particularly with dialysis.

DIALYSIS AND RENAL TRANSPLANTATION

The treatment of end-stage renal failure has been transformed by the development of techniques for dialysis and renal transplantation during the past 30 years. In the past, patients with renal failure were doomed to die when all conservative methods failed. Now their lives may be prolonged many years with maintenance dialysis or renal transplantation.

There is an intimate relation between these two techniques, and closely paralleled advances in both have been made. For example, the uremic patient may choose to undergo renal transplantation with a related or cadaver donor rather than be maintained on chronic intermittent dialysis. Nevertheless, dialysis will undoubtedly play an important role in the treatment. Dialysis may be used to maintain the patient in an optimum clinical state until the donor kidney is available. In the case of a cadaver renal transplant, the patient may have to wait many months. There are several choices of treatment, depending on the resources available. The initial treatment will be carried out in the medical center hemodialysis unit. The patient may then undergo home dialysis training to permit self-administration of the procedure at home until the donor kidney is available; or more commonly, treatment may be given in a satellite (out-of-hospital) or mobile hemodialysis unit near the patient's home. Dialysis may sustain the renal transplant patient through periods of postoperative oliguria, and it provides an alternative if the transplanted kidney should fail because of rejection or other complications. Renal transplantation and chronic maintenance dialysis offer about the same prognosis in regard to longevity. Each mode of treatment has its own unique problems. Renal transplantation, if successful, probably offers a better quality of life because it is less restrictive: there are usually no dietary restrictions, and it is not necessary to commit large blocks of time several times each week for dialysis.

Preparation of the Patient

It is important that the patient be prepared for the transition from conservative management to more definitive therapy long before the need arises for maintenance dialysis or renal transplantation. Not only does this give the patient hope, but it also allows time for indoctrination of the patient in preparation for the treatment and makes it possible for the treatment to start at the proper time.

Originally, extremely rigid criteria were used to select patients for either renal transplantation or maintenance dialysis, especially because of limited facilites and the high cost of treatment. The increase in facilites, financial support by the federal government, improvements in techniques, and success in treating some children, older individuals, diabetic persons, and patients with systemic lupus erythematosus are all factors that have helped to liberalize the criteria so that a greater number of patients can be helped.

When to Begin Treatment

There are no clear-cut guidelines in terms of measurable blood levels of creatinine or BUN to determine when definitive therapy should begin. Most nephrologists' decisions are based on the well-being of the patient, who is followed closely as an outpatient. Therapy is generally begun when the patient is no longer able to work full-time, develops peripheral neuropathy, or shows other signs of clinical deterioration. The serum creatinine level is generally above 6 mg/dl in males (4 mg/dl in females), and the GFR is below 4 ml/min. In no case should the patient be allowed to become bedridden or so sick that usual activities are impossible.

Sometimes, despite being carefully followed, the patient may deteriorate rapidly over a period of a few days, usually in response to an infectious disease. Sometimes one or two peritoneal dialyses will restablize the patient. If this is not successful, intermittent hemodialysis may be initiated. If a decision for a renal transplant has been made, transplantation may be done on an elective basis at a later date.

Dialysis

Dialysis is a process by which solutes and water are diffused through a passive, porous membrane from one fluid compartment to another. Hemodialysis and peritoneal

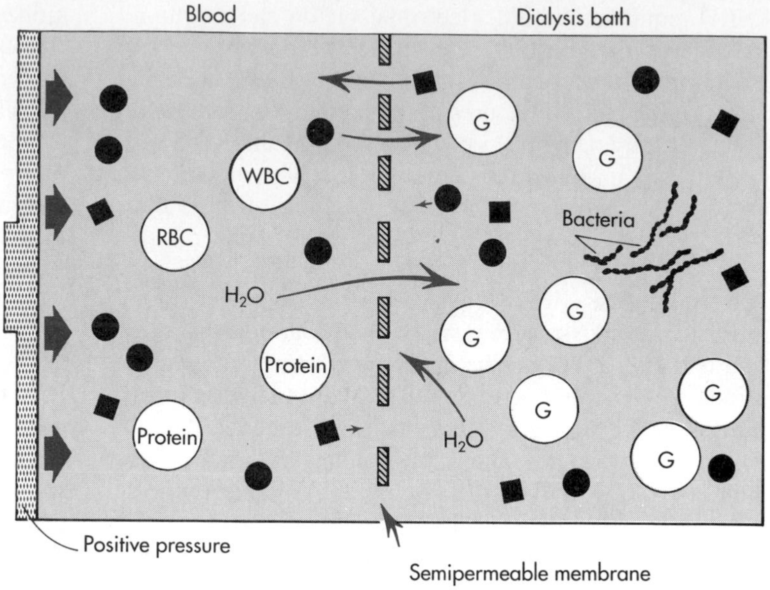

FIG. 48-2 Basic principles of diffusion and osmotic and hydrostatic pressures involved in dialysis. *RBC,* Red blood cell; *WBC,* white blood cell; *G,* glucose.

dialysis are the two major techniques used in dialysis, and the basic principles involved are the same for both—diffusion of solutes and water from the plasma to the dialysis solution in response to a concentration or pressure gradient.

Fig. 48-2 illustrates the basic principles of diffusion and osmotic and hydrostatic pressure gradients involved in dialysis. Given a semipermeable membrane with the patient's blood on one side and a solution of known composition on the other side (the *dialysate,* or dialysis bath), substances to which the membrane is permeable will move from where their concentration is high to where it is low. If the blood potassium level is high and the potassium level in the dialysis bath is low *(round dots),* the net movement of potassium will be out of the blood into the dialysis bath *(long arrows indicate direction of net diffusion).* The *black squares* represent solutes that are in higher concentration in the dialysate (e.g., bicarbonate), so that net diffusion is from the bath solution to the blood. Ultrafiltration (water removal) may be achieved by two methods: (1) creating a hydrostatic pressure gradient (e.g., by mechanically increasing the positive pressure in the blood compartment) and (2) creating an osmotic pressure gradient by increasing the concentration of glucose in the dialysis bath. The resulting osmotic and hydrostatic pressure gradients cause a net movement of water from the blood to the dialysis bath.* The positive pressure in the blood compartment also speeds up the diffusion of both solutes and water. Ultrafiltration in hemodialysis is achieved primarily by using the first method, whereas peritoneal dialysis uses the second method. Note that protein, blood cells, and bacteria are too large to pass through the pores in the dialysis membrane.

By using a dialysis solution that contains the important electrolytes in normal concentrations, the concentration of these electrolytes can be corrected in the blood of the patient with renal failure. The basic practical problem in dialysis is to bring enough blood into contact with enough dialysis solution across a semipermeable membrane of adequate area. This may be accomplished inside the patient's body, using the peritoneum as the semipermeable membrane (peritoneal dialysis), or outside the body, using an "artificial kidney" and Cuprophane or Polysulfone as the semipermeable membrane (hemodialysis).

Hemodialysis

An artificial kidney machine, or hemodialyzer, consists simply of a semipermeable membrane with blood on one side and dialysis fluid on the other. There are two principal types of dialyzers in use today. The *parallel plate dialyzer* consists of two Cuprophane sheets sandwiched between two rigid supports to form an envelope. Two or more envelopes are arranged in parallel. Blood flows between the membrane layers, and dialysis fluid may flow in the same direction as the blood or in the opposite direction (countercurrent), as shown in Fig. 48-3. The *hollow fiber* or *capillary dialyzer* consists of thousands of tiny capillary fibers arranged in parallel (Fig. 48-4). Each fiber has a wall thickness of 30 μm, an inside diameter of 200 μm, and a length of 21 cm. (For comparative purposes, a red blood cell has a diameter of 7 μm.) Blood flows down the center of these tiny tubes, and dialysis fluid bathes the outside. The flow of the dialysis fluid is opposite to that of the blood. This dialyzer is small and compact because of the large surface area provided by the many capillary tubes. Fig. 48-5 is a diagrammatic representation of a hemodialysis system using a hollow fiber dialyzer.

A dialysis system consists of two circuits—one for the blood and one for the dialysis fluid. When the system is

---

*Some glucose does diffuse from the dialysis bath into the blood, but since water diffuses much more rapidly than glucose, the major shift will be that of water from blood to bath.

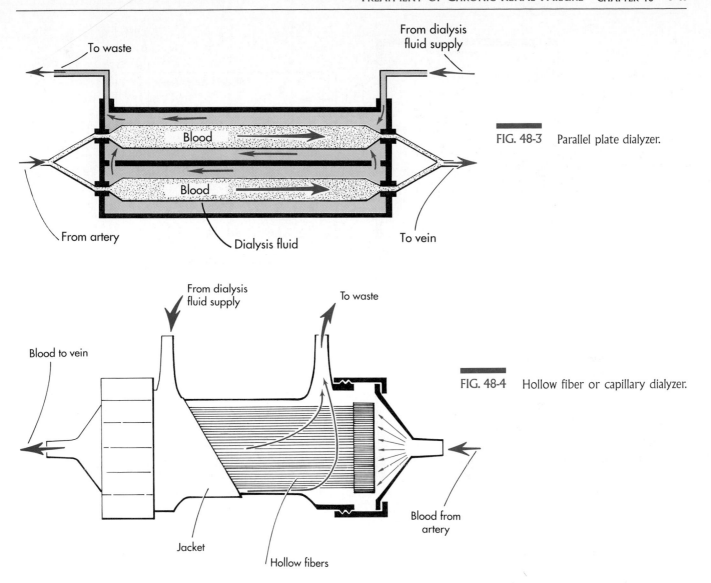

FIG. 48-3   Parallel plate dialyzer.

FIG. 48-4   Hollow fiber or capillary dialyzer.

in operation, blood flows from the patient through plastic tubing (arterial line), through the hollow fibers of the dialyzer, and back to the patient through the venous line. The dialysis fluid forms the second circuit. Tap water is filtered and heated to body temperature and is then mixed with a concentrate by a porportioning pump to make the dialysate, or bath. The bath is then delivered to the dialyzer, where it flows on the outside of the hollow fibers before exiting to a drain. Equilibrium between the blood and the dialysate takes place across the dialyzing membrane by the processes of diffusion, osmosis, and ultrafiltration described in Fig. 48-1.

The composition of the dialysis bath is designed to approximate the ionic composition of normal blood, modified slightly to correct the common fluid and electrolyte disorders that accompany renal failure (see box to right). The usual components are sodium (Na^+), K^+, Ca^{++}, magnesium (Mg^{++}), chloride (Cl^-), acetate, and glucose. Urea, creatinine, uric acid, and phosphate diffuse readily from the blood to the dialysis fluid, since they are not present in the dialysis fluid. Sodium acetate, which is in

DIALYSATE COMPOSITION	
COMPONENT	mEq/L
Sodium	138-145
Potassium	0-4.0
Chloride	100-107
Calcium	2.5-3.5
Magnesium	0.4-1.0
Acetate	30-37
Glucose*	100-250*

*Glucose concentration in milligrams per deciliter.

higher concentration in the dialysis bath, diffuses into the blood. The purpose of adding the acetate is to correct the uremic patient's acidosis. Acetate is metabolized into bicarbonate in the patient's body. The reason for using acetate rather than bicarbonate is to avoid the problem of

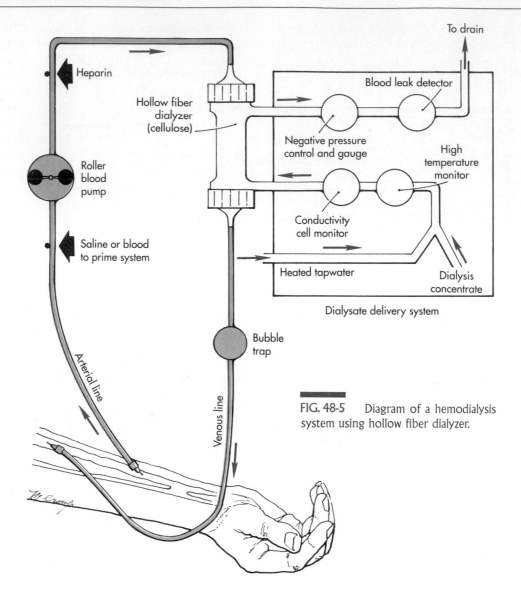

FIG. 48-5   Diagram of a hemodialysis system using hollow fiber dialyzer.

calcium bicarbonate precipitation when calcium and bicarbonate are added to the same dialysis fluid. Recently, machines have been developed that can use two separate dialysates—one with calcium and the other with bicarbonate, which avoids the problem of precipitation. A low concentration of glucose (200 mg/dl) is added to the dialysis bath to prevent glucose diffusion into the dialysis bath with the consequent loss of calories. In hemodialysis a high concentration of glucose is not necessary, because fluid removal may be achieved by effecting a hydrostatic pressure gradient between the blood and dialysis fluid. The hydrostatic pressure gradient is achieved by increasing the positive pressure within the dialyzer blood compartment by increasing resistance to venous outflow (not shown) or by exerting a vacuum effect in the dialysis fluid compartment by manipulating the negative pressure control. The hydrostatic pressure gradient across the dialyzing membrane also increases the diffusion rate of the solutes.

The blood circuit of the dialysis system is initially primed with saline or blood before connection to the circulation of the patient. The blood pressure of the patient may be adequate to propel the blood through the extracorporeal circuit, or a blood pump may be used to assist the flow (about 200 to 400 ml/min is a desirable flow rate). Heparin is continuously delivered to the arterial line by a slow infusion pump to prevent clotting. A clot and bubble trap in the venous line prevents air or blood clots from returning to the patient. To ensure patient safety, monitors with alarms for various parameters are included in modern hemodialyzers. A conductivity cell monitors the chemical composition of the dialysis fluid. Dialysis fluid at body temperature increases the rate of diffusion, but a temperature that is too high would cause hemolysis of red blood cells (RBCs), with possible death to the patient. Any tear in the dialysis membrane causing either a minor or a massive leak is detected by a photocell in the dialysate outflow.

Maintenance hemodialysis is usually performed three times per week, and the length of a single treatment

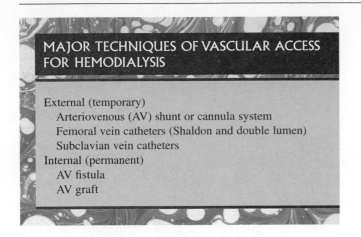

MAJOR TECHNIQUES OF VASCULAR ACCESS
FOR HEMODIALYSIS

External (temporary)
   Arteriovenous (AV) shunt or cannula system
   Femoral vein catheters (Shaldon and double lumen)
   Subclavian vein catheters
Internal (permanent)
   AV fistula
   AV graft

varies from 3 to 5 hours, depending on the type of dialysis system used and the condition of the patient.

Vascular access for hemodialysis

Long-term intermittent hemodialysis requires reliable access to the vascular system. Blood must exit and return to the patient at the rate of 200 to 400 ml/min. The box above lists the major vascular access techniques classified as external (usually temporary) and internal (permanent). Vascular access remains the most vulnerable aspect of hemodialysis because of the many complications and failures. Thus numerous methods of vascular access have been developed over the years. The common denominator in most of these vascular access techniques is access to the arterial circulation and return to the venous circulation.

External (temporary) vascular access. The *external arteriovenous (AV) shunt* or *cannula system* is created by placing Teflon cannula tips in an artery (usually the radial or posterior tibial) and a nearby vein (Fig. 48-6, *A*). The cannula tips are then connected by silicone rubber tubing and

a Teflon bridge to complete the shunt. At the time of dialysis, the external shunt tubing is separated, and connection is made to the dialyzer. Blood then flows from the arterial line, through the dialyzer, and then back to the vein. The cannula system was devised in 1960 (Quinton et al., 1960) and made chronic intermittent hemodialysis possible for the first time. The main problem with the external AV shunt is its short life span because of clotting and infection (average life 9 months). The external AV shunt has been largely supplanted by other means of angioaccess (see below) and is mainly of historic interest. Occasionally, however, it is used when dialytic therapy is required for short periods, as in dialysis for drug overdose or poisoning, acute renal failure, and the initial phase of dialytic treatment for chronic renal failure.

Femoral and subclavian vein catheters are used most often in cases of acute renal failure when temporary angioaccess is required or when other means of vascular access are temporarily nonfunctional in chronic dialysis patients. Both types of catheters may be inserted at the bedside by an experienced physician.

There are two types of femoral dialysis catheters. The Shaldon catheter is a single-lumen catheter that requires a second access. If two Shaldon catheters are used, they may be placed bilaterally or in the same vein with the outflow catheter placed distally to the inflow catheter. The newer type of femoral catheter has a double lumen— one for blood outflow to the dialyzer and one for blood return to the patient. Complications associated with femoral vein catheters include laceration of the femoral artery, hemorrhage, thrombosis, embolus, hematoma, and infection.

Subclavian vein catheters are gaining wide acceptance as a temporary means of angioaccess because insertion is easier and there are fewer complications than with femoral vein catheters (Raja et al., 1984). The subclavian

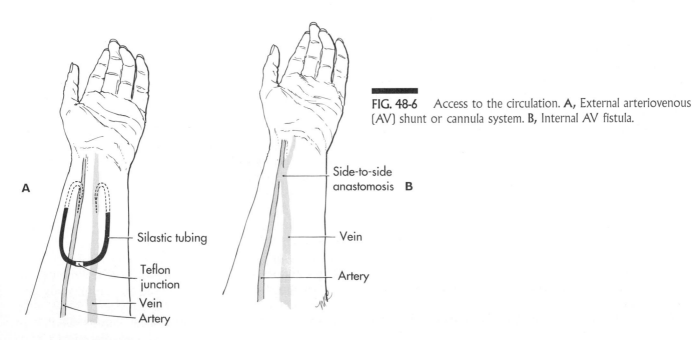

FIG. 48-6   Access to the circulation. **A,** External arteriovenous (AV) shunt or cannula system. **B,** Internal AV fistula.

vein catheter also has a double lumen with inflow and outflow lines. Subclavian catheters may be used for as long as 4 weeks, but femoral vein catheters are usually removed 1 to 2 days after insertion.

Catheters left in place between dialysis treatments are filled with a saline-heparin solution or irrigated periodically with a saline-heparin solution to prevent clotting. If catheters are removed at the end of dialysis, pressure must be applied to the entry site until complete clotting occurs and the site must be observed for several hours thereafter to detect any recurrent bleeding.

Complications associated with subclavian vein catheterization are similar to those with femoral vein catheterization, including pneumothorax, laceration of the subclavian artery, hemorrhage, thrombosis, embolus, hematoma, and infection.

Internal (permanent) vascular access. The *AV fistula* was developed by Cimino and Brescia (1962) in response to the many complications with the AV shunt. An AV fistula is constructed by anastomosing an artery directly to a vein (usually the radial artery and the cephalic vein at the wrist) in the nondominant arm (Fig. 48-6, *B*). Blood is shunted from the artery to the vein, causing the vein to enlarge ("ripening") after a few weeks. Venipuncture with large-bore needles becomes easy and gives access to blood flowing under arterial pressure. Connection with the dialysis system is made by placing one needle distally (arterial line) and the other needle proximally (venous line) in the arterialized vein. The average life of the AV fistula is 4 years, and there are far fewer complications than with the AV shunt. The main problems are painful venipuncture, formation of aneurysms, thrombosis, difficult postdialytic hemostasis, and ischemia of the hand *(steal syndrome).*

In some cases it is not possible to create a fistula from the patient's own blood vessels because of disease, damage from previous procedures, or small size. An *AV graft* may then be anastomosed between an artery and vein (usually in the arm), where it serves as a conduit for the flow of blood and the site for needle puncture during dialysis. The graft creates a raised area just under the skin and looks like a raised vein. An AV graft is a prosthetic tube device made out of biologic materials (bovine carotid artery, human umbilical cord artery) or a synthetic material (Gore-Tex, or polytetrafluoroethylene, a material similar to Teflon). A segment of Gore-Tex may also be used to patch AV fistulas that have stenosed or formed aneurysms. AV graft complications are similar to those of the AV fistula, including thrombosis, infection, aneurysm, and hand ischemia caused by the shunting of blood through the prosthesis and away from the distal circulation (steal syndrome).

Peritoneal dialysis

Peritoneal dialysis is an alternative to hemodialysis for the treatment of acute and chronic renal failure. Although peritoneal dialysis existed 20 years before hemodialysis, it was not commonly used for long-term treatment. How-

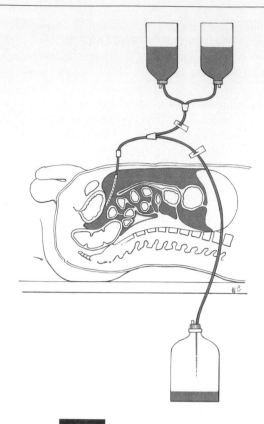

FIG. 48-7   Peritoneal dialysis.

ever, recent engineering and medical developments have led to peritoneal dialysis becoming an alternative to hemodialysis as a treatment for chronic renal failure. Approximately 9% of ESRD patients undergo some type of peritoneal dialysis (US Renal Data System, 1991).

Peritoneal dialysis is very similar to hemodialysis, except that the peritoneum functions as the semipermeable membrane. Access to the peritoneal cavity is achieved by paracentesis using either a straight, rigid trocar for acute peritoneal dialysis or the more permanent, soft Tenckhoff catheter for chronic peritoneal dialysis. Peritoneal dialysis is performed by infusing 1 to 2 L of dialysis solution into the abdomen through the catheter (Fig. 48-7). The dialysate stays in the abdomen for a variable period of time (dwell time) and then is drained off by gravity into a container placed below the patient. After the drainage is complete, new dialysate is infused and a new cycle begins. Solute removal is accomplished by diffusion, whereas ultrafiltration (water removal) is accomplished by osmosis rather than by hydrostatic pressure gradients as in hemodialysis. Glucose is added to the dialysate to make it slightly hyperosmotic. Ultrafiltration can be enhanced by raising the glucose concentration and therefore the osmolality of the dialysate (1.5%, 2.5%, and 4.5% glucose concentrations are available).

The following are four modes of peritoneal dialysis in current use, one for acute and three for chronic dialysis:
1. Manual intermittent peritoneal dialysis
2. Continuous ambulatory peritoneal dialysis (CAPD)
3. Continuous cycler-assisted peritoneal dialysis (CCPD)

4. Automated intermittent peritoneal dialysis (IPD)

Until 15 years ago, *manual intermittent peritoneal dialysis* was the most common method of performing peritoneal dialysis. A catheter is placed in the peritoneal cavity by paracentesis. In the adult, 2 L of sterile dialysis solution is allowed to run into the peritoneal cavity through the catheter for 10 to 20 minutes. Equilibrium between the dialysis fluid and the highly vascular peritoneal semipermeable membrane then takes place during the dwell time, usually 30 minutes. The fluid is then allowed to drain by gravity into a closed, sterile collecting system. The cycles (each lasting about 1 hour) are repeated over a period of 1 to 2 days. In acute renal failure, one or two such treatments each week usually provide acceptable control of fluid and electrolytes and azotemia.

The main advantages of the manual method of IPD are its simplicity (it does not require highly skilled personnel nor sophisticated equipment) and that it does not require access to the bloodstream. Disadvantages of this method include the large nursing time committment, confinement during the procedure, and the relatively high risk of peritonitis. It is less efficient than hemodialysis, requiring about six times as long to achieve the same results.

CAPD is a self-dialysis technique using 2-L exchanges of dialysate four times per day, with the last exchange performed at bedtime and allowed to dwell in the peritoneal cavity overnight. The empty bag and tubing are continually attached to the catheter and concealed beneath the clothing during the 4-hour dwell time. After the dwell time, the bag is lowered to the floor and allowed to fill by gravity. CAPD was devised in the late 1970s and is the most popular method of peritoneal dialysis used today for the treatment of chronic renal failure.

Advantages of CAPD include greater freedom for the ESRD patient because it can be performed anywhere; absence of peaks and valleys in blood chemistry levels characteristic of intermittent hemodialysis; simplicity; and ease of learning. The primary disadvantage of CAPD is the risk of peritonitis, which occurs on the average of once every 40 patient weeks. Various methods have been designed to reduce the risk of contamination. One such device is an ultraviolet light used to sterilize the catheter spike and outlet port of the dialysis bag. Other disadvantages of CAPD include catheter tunnel infection, moderate protein loss, hypercholesterolemia, hypertriglyceridemia, obesity (excess calories from absorption of the glucose), and inguinal and abdominal hernias. Lower cost is not an advantage of peritoneal dialysis as originally expected because of the cost of dialysate and of hospitalization related to peritonitis. The cost to each patient receiving dialysis (whether hemodialysis or peritoneal dialysis) is estimated to be about $35,000 per year. Finally, many patients are unwilling to make the continuous time commitment of 3 to 4 hours each day to perform the exchanges.

CCPD is a variation of CAPD in which an automatic cycler machine delivers multiple overnight exchanges and an additional exchange in the morning. The dialysate then remains in the abdomen during the day for one long cycle. Both CAPD and CCPD require the abdomen to be full on a continuous basis. CCPD may be more acceptable to some patients but must be performed either at home or at a dialysis center, whereas CAPD can be performed anywhere.

An alternate to CAPD and CCPD is automated *IPD*. which allows for "dry periods" when the abdomen is empty. IPD is typically performed nightly with the aid of automated (cycler-assisted) equipment, and the peritoneal cavity remains empty during the day.

New Approaches to Solute Removal

Many patients continue to manifest various disturbed metabolic functions despite vigorous hemodialysis that maintains the concentration of classic uremic metabolites (e.g., urea, creatine, phosphate) at near normal levels. These observations have led investigators to postulate that there is a series of uremic toxins intermediate in molecular weight between the classic small molecules such as urea ($<$500 daltons) and the plasma proteins ($>$50,000 daltons) that may partially account for the clinical abnormalities (middle molecular hypothesis).

Two new experimental techniques of removing solutes include *hemofiltration* (HF) (also called *hemodiafiltration*) and *absorbent therapy*. Both methods assume the presence and pathophysiologic significance of middle molecules. The HF technique is based on the principle of convection rather than diffusion, and is more analogous to the function of the human glomerulus than is hemodialysis. In HF the standard hemodialysis technique is modified by sequentially prediluting the blood with an electrolyte solution resembling plasma and subsequently ultrafiltering it under high hydraulic pressures. The principal advantage of this technique is more efficient removal of solutes in the middle molecular range that are inefficiently removed by hemodialysis; supposedly, this may partially explain why patients on HF feel clinically well and have less hemodynamic instability.

Additional approaches to solute removal include adjunctive techniques designed to be used with maintainance hemodialysis or in patients with significant residual renal function (GFR equals 5 to 10 ml/min). All involve the use of absorbents for solute removal. Absorbents may be used through direct action on the bloodstream (hemoperfusion), through regeneration of dialysate (REDY sorbent hemodialysis), or by means of introduction into the gut (oral ingestion of oxystarch or charcoal).

Hemoperfusion uses activated charcoal, encapsulated in membranes, as the absorbent. Charcoal hemoperfusion systems are efficient in removing middle molecules but do not effectively remove many of the significant uremic solutes, including urea, electrolytes, and water.

The *REDY sorbent dialysis system* uses an enzyme-sorbent disposable cartridge for reprocessing dialysate so that a small volume may be used. The sorbent consists of zirconium compounds and carbon. The REDY system is widely used to treat patients requiring special dialysis solutions; to dialyze in community hospitals lacking a dialysis facility; whenever moving a dialysis machine to the patient is preferable to moving the patient; and for home dialysis.

The oral *ingestion of absorbents* such as oxystarch or activated charcoal is a third absorbent method of solute removal. The technique of using the gastrointestinal (GI) tract for solute removal is in a primitive state of development, although the use of oral aluminum hydroxides and Kayexalate (orally or by enema) is conventional practice for the control of phosphates and K^+, respectively.

Renal Transplantation

A successful renal transplant is the preferred method of treatment for patients in end-stage renal failure, although some patients may elect self-dialysis in their own home after being taught the procedure by a home-training nurse.

The first successful renal transplant was performed on identical twins in 1954 by Murray, Merrill, and Harrison in Boston. In 1989, 40,812 or 25% of the patients with ESRD underwent transplantation. Renal transplantation costs about $40,000 to $50,000. However, after a successful transplantation, the cost of care falls to less than $10,000 per year, making renal transplantation the most cost-effective treatment for ESRD patients (US Renal Data System, 1991). Dialysis by comparison costs about $35,000 per year, and the quality of life is less than with successful transplantation. However, the demand for renal transplantation far exceeds the number of available living-related and cadaver kidneys, limiting transplantation as a treatment option.

The surgical technique involved in renal transplantation is relatively simple and is generally performed by a surgeon with a background in urologic, vascular, or general surgery. It is standard procedure to rotate the donor kidney and place it in the contralateral iliac fossa of the recipient. The ureter then lies anterior to the renal vessels and is more readily anastomosed or implanted into the recipient bladder. The renal artery is anastomosed end-to-end to the internal iliac artery, and the renal vein is anastomosed to the external or common iliac vein (Fig. 48-8).

Tissue typing and immunogenetics

An *autograft* (transfer of an individual's own tissue) from one part of the body to another (e.g., skin) is always accepted. A *syngenetic graft* is a transfer of tissue between genetically identical individuals (i.e., identical twins) and usually "takes" permanently. A *xenograft* is the transfer of tissue between different species (e.g., baboon to human) and is always rejected by an immunocompetent recipient. An *allograft* is a graft between genetically different members of the same species (from one human to another) and is the most common type of tissue transplantation. The major limiting factor in this procedure is the body's immunologic response that leads to rejection of the transplanted kidney. Rejection may be cell mediated or humoral. Cell-mediated rejection involves T lymphocytes produced in response to antigens in the donor kidney that are recognized as foreign cells. These lymphocytes invade the foreign donor kidney and contribute to its destruction. Humoral rejection involves the production of antibodies against antigens in the donor kidney, which the recipient's plasma cells recognize as foreign. Rejection can occur within hours or several years after transplantation.

Tissue typing or histocompatibility testing to ensure the closest possible tissue match between donor and re-

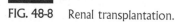

FIG. 48-8   Renal transplantation.

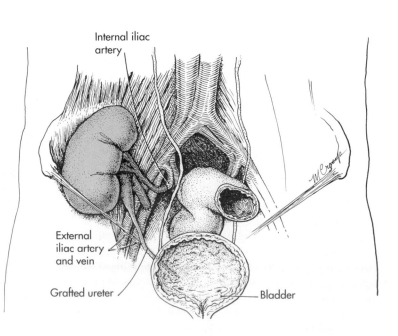

TABLE 48-1   The ABO Blood Group System

Type	Antigen	Distribution in Population		Potential Donor
A	A	W	40%	A, O
		B	27%	
		I	16%	
		O	28%	
B	B	W	11%	B, O
		B	20%	
		I	4%	
		O	27%	
AB	A and B	W	4%	AB, A, B, O
		B	4%	
		I	1%	
		O	5%	
O	None	W	45%	O
		B	49%	
		I	79%	
		O	40%	

From Ambrose MW, editor: *Illustrated guide to diagnostic tests,* Springhouse, Pa, 1994, Springhouse.
W, Caucasian; *B,* African American; *I,* American Indian; *O,* Oriental.

 TABLE 48-2   Potential HLA Antigens by Locus

	Class I Antigens			Class II Antigens
Locus	A	B	C	DR
	A1	B5	B49	CW1	
	A2	B7	BW50	CW2	DR1
	A3	B8	B51	CW3	DR2
	A9	B12	BW52	CW4	DR3
	A10	B13	BW53	CW5	DR4
	A11	B14	BW54	CW6	DR5
	AW19	B15	BW56	CW7	DRW6
	A23	B16	BW57	CW8	DR7
	A24	B17	BW58	CW9	DRW8
	A25	B18	BW59	CW10	DRW9
	A26	B21	BW60	CW11	DRW10
	A27	BW22	BW61		DRW11
	A29	B27	BW62		DRW12
	A30	B35	BW63		DRW13
	A31	B37	BW65		DRW14
	A32	B38	BW67		DRW15
	AW33	B39	BW70		DRW16
	AW34	B40	BW71		DRW17
	AW36	BW41	BW72		DRW18
	AW43	BW42	BW73		DRW52
	AW66	B44	BW75		DRW53
	AW68	B45	BW76		
	AW69	BW46	BW4		
	AW74	BW47	BW6		
		BW48			

From Roitt I, Brostoff J, Male D, editors: *Immunology,* ed 3, St Louis, 1993, Mosby.

cipient and suppressing the immune response with drugs are the two general approaches used to promote successful renal transplant and prevent rejection. Two major antigenic groups have been identified as important in determining histocompatibility: the ABO blood group system and human leukocyte antigens (HLA).

ABO blood group antigens. ABO antigens are present in most tissues of the body as well as on RBCs. The ABO antigens determine blood type and are identified serologically. Type A blood has the A antigen; type B blood has the B antigen; type AB blood has both the A and B antigens; and type O blood has neither. Naturally occurring antibodies are present in the blood serum when a particular antigen is lacking on the cells. Anti-A antibodies are found in persons who do not have the A antigen (blood types B and O), and anti-B antibodies are found in persons without the B antigen (blood types A and O). Individuals with type AB blood have neither antibody, since they have both antigens. The same general rules apply to renal transplants with respect to ABO compatibility as apply to blood transfusions (Table 48-1). An O kidney can be transplanted into any recipient, whereas an A kidney can be given only to an A or AB recipient. Unlike blood transfusions, the rhesus (Rh) factor is not a concern with organ transplantation, since Rh antigens are not found on vascular endothelial tissues (the principal target tissue in rejection). ABO typing is always performed before blood transfusions and organ transplantation. Transplantation between ABO-incompatible persons is not done, since it generally leads to immediate hyperacute rejection.

Human leukocyte antigen system. The second antigen system important in organ transplantation is the major histocompatibility complex (MHC) discussed in Chapter 5. This antigen system is called the human leukocyte antigen (HLA) system in humans, since the antigens were first discovered on WBCs. The genes that code for the HLA antigens are located on the short arm of chromosome 6. Four major HLA sites or loci important for transplantation, designated A, B, C, and DR, have been identified in this region. Each sublocus controls a series of antigenic factors, and more than 100 have been identified (Table 48-2). Three of these genes (HLA-A, HLA-B, and HLA-C) code for *class I antigens.* Class I antigens are found on the surface of all nucleated cells in the body and on RBCs and platelets. Class I antigens are recognized by CD8 lymphocytes, which are the cytotoxic or "killer" T cells. Class I antigens present the major target for T cell and antibody reactions to transplanted grafts. Three genes at the D sublocus code for *class II antigens* (HLA-DR, HLA-DQ, and HLA-DP), but only the HLA-DR (D-related) gene is important in transplanted organ rejection. Class II antigens have a more limited distribution in the body than class I antigens and are present on the surface

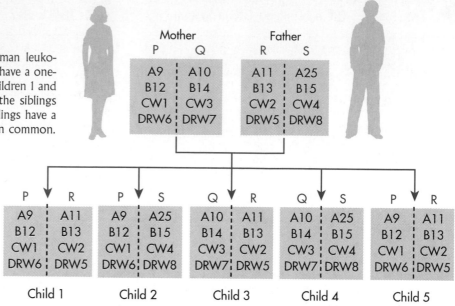

FIG. 48-9   Pattern of inheritance of human leuko-cyte antigen (HLA) antigens. All children have a one-haplotype mismatch with each parent. Children 1 and 5 are HLA-identical siblings; the rest of the siblings have a one-haplotype mismatch. Some siblings have a two-haplotype mismatch or no antigens in common.

of antigen-presenting cells (e.g., B cells, activated macrophages, some activated T cells, and vascular endothelial cells) (Hutchinson, 1993). CD4 cells (helper T cells) recognize class II antigens. Helper T cell activity depends on *both* the recognition of the foreign antigen on antigen presenting cells (APCs) and the presence on these cells of "self" class II HLA antigens. Note that T cells recognize antigens only when the antigens are presented on the surface of cells (in association with either class I or II HLA self antigens). B cells do not have this requirement and can recognize antigens in plasma with their surface monomer, IgM, acting as the antigen receptor.

In addition to the major antigens encoded by the HLA genes, an unknown number of *minor antigens* are encoded by genes at sites other than that of the HLA locus. These minor antigens can induce a weak immune response that can cause slow rejection of a graft. However, these antigens are not tested for, since laboratory tests do not exist for minor antigens.

Haplotype inheritance of the HLA antigens. The complex of the four histocompatibility genes (A, B, C, and DR) important in transplantation is known as a haplotype and is codominantly expressed. Because chromosomes are paired, an individual has a total of 8 HLA genes (two pairs on each of the two chromosomes). Each of the chromosome sets is called a haplotype and is inherited as a set. The genotype of an individual consists of two haplotypes. In other words, each individual inherits two half-sets (haplotypes)—one set from each parent. Within a single family, only four genotypes can be present. For example, if the HLA genotype of the mother is PQ and that of the father is RS, four possible combinations exist for the children: PR, PS, QR, and QS. By the laws of simple Mendelian inheritance, 25% of the children will be HLA-identical, 50% will have one haplotype in common, and 25% will have a two-haplotype mismatch (Fig. 48-9).

In general, the closer the genetic similarity between donor and recipient, the greater the chance of a successful transplant. When the donor and recipient are identical twins or HLA-identical siblings, some 95% of the renal transplants survive at the end of 1 year and the subsequent half-life is 25 years. A renal transplant of a one-HLA haplotype match from a family member has a 1-year graft rate of 85% with an 11- to 12-year half-life. With increasing numbers of mismatches for cadaver (unrelated) persons, 1-year kidney graft survival declines to about 70% and the half-life declines to about 7 years (Opelz, 1991).

Prevention of rejection by HLA matching. Obviously, the ideal donor for an organ transplant is a monozygotic (identical) twin, one who can provide a perfect genetic match for the recipient. Unfortunately, this cicumstance rarely occurs. One way to overcome rejection of transplanted tissue is by tissue matching for histocompatibility antigens. The antigens expressed by the cells vary with different tissues, and some cells do not have antigens that present antigens for processing. For example, corneas are easily grafted because they are avascular and the lymphatic supply of the eye prevents many antigens from triggering an immune response, so the proportion of successful corneal transplants is very high. Bone marrow has the greatest capability of inducing rejection, followed by the skin, heart, kidney, and liver. HLA matching is not used for the liver, which seems to tolerate HLA antigen differences quite well.

Tissue typing is a technique developed to predict the outcome of organ transplantation based on a particular match of antigens between donor and recipient. The overriding consideration for organ allograft rejection is whether the donor graft carries any antigens that are not present in the recipient—called the *host-versus-graft reaction principle*.* Three tests of the HLA system antigens are commonly performed before renal transplantations: (1) the Terasaki microcytotoxicity assay; (2) the mixed lymphocyte culture/mixed lymphocyte response; and (3) the white blood cell (WBC) cross match.

The *Terasaki microcytotoxicity assay* is used to type class I HLA antigens (A, B, and C loci). A blood serum (lymphocyte) sample is exposed to monospecific antiserums to the class I antigens and complement. If the serum "recognizes" its HLA antigen on the lymphocyte cell surface, the complement cascade is activated and the cell membrane is lysed, permitting a marker dye to enter the cell; they may then be detected by phase microscopy (Terasaki et al., 1978). This test, along with the test for class II antigens, is used to identify the haplotypes of donors being considered for transplant surgery and to determine how well they match the recipient.

Class II antigens (related to the D locus) were first demonstrated by the *mixed lymphocyte culture* (MLC) or *mixed lymphocyte response* (MLR). In the MLC test, lymphocytes from a potential donor and recipient are cultured together for 4 or 5 days. Ordinarily both sets of cells would undergo blast transformation in response to antigenic disparity between their cell membrane antigens. However, it is only the antigens present in the donor and lacking in the recipient that are of interest in renal transplantation, since they cause host-versus-graft rejection. Thus to test only the reactivity of the recipient cells, the donor cells are pretreated with irradiation or mitomycin C to inactivate them with respect to capacity to undergo blast transformation without destroying surface antigens. When the two cultures are mixed, only those of the potential transplant recipient undergo blast transformation. The degree of blast transformation is measured by titrated thymidine added to the culture. If the recipient's cells are stimulated by the donor cells, greater quantities of thymidine are taken up for the synthesis of nucleoprotein during blast transformation.

The genes that control the class I and class II antigens are closely linked to the MHC region. Hence among siblings, compatibility of class I and class II antigens is positively correlated (i.e., they are inherited as a haplotype) except in rare cases when a break has occurred during meiosis. In the latter case, a new haplotype appears in the child who may be identical for class I antigens but different for class II antigens. When there is strong stimulation of the MLC test, the majority of grafts are rejected even when the HLA-A and HLA-B antigens (class I antigens of major importance) are identical. Thus matching at the HLA-DR locus is the most important factor in predicting the success of a renal transplant.

Because the MLC test requires several days to complete, it is useful only for pretransplant matching of living, related donors with recipients and not for cadaver kidneys, which can be preserved only for 2 to 3 days before transplantation. Fortunately, a serologic test has been developed recently that can rapidly type HLA-DR antigens (24 to 36 hours) so it can be applied to HLA-DR typing of cadaver kidneys. This test is done on B lymphocytes (which express class II HLA antigens on their surface). Prior development of methods of separating the B and T lymphocytes in blood sera allowed the development of the rapid typing of HLA-DR antigens (Carpenter, Lazarus, 1994).

In addition to ABO blood typing and assessing class I and class II antigens, another test that is routinely performed before renal transplantation is the *WBC cross match* to determine if there are preformed antibodies to the lymphocytes of a potential donor. The sera of the potential donor and recipient are incubated, and a marker for cell death is added. Death of more than 10% of the potential donor cells is considered a positive cross match and precludes transplantation, since the likely outcome would be hyperacute rejection of the donor kidney. Table 48-3 summarizes the tests used to assess pretransplant compatibility.

Pretransplant blood transfusion

It was formerly believed that numerous blood transfusions in a patient awaiting renal transplantation would cause sensitization to a large number of HLA antigens in the general population and decrease the chances of a successful graft. Thus the policy of many transplantation units was to keep blood transfusions to a minimum and to use only packed, washed RBCs (minus WBCs and platelets). However, the overall experience with the nontransfused patients was the opposite of what was expected. Nontransfused patients had the highest risk of graft failure. This discovery was followed by a period during the 1980s in which some nephrologists employed donor-specific transfusions (e.g., from a parent) before transplantation. The result was a transplant success rate of 95% to 100%. Unfortunately, about 30% of the patients receiving donor-specific transfusion developed antidonor antibodies and could not receive the kidney as planned, for fear of hyperacute rejection (Salvatierra et al., 1980). The beneficial effect of pretransplant blood transfusions was also documented in patients receiving random transfusions, perhaps from chance exposure to antigens that happened to be on their transplant. In fact, the more transfusions that a potential recipient received, the greater the probability of graft survival (Opelz,

---

*The major exception to this principle is graft-versus-host disease, which can be a major complication of bone marrow transplantation. This reaction occurs because grafted immunocompetent T cells proliferate in the irradiated, immunocompromised host and "reject" cells with class II proteins, resulting in severe organ dysfunction, especially in the skin, liver, and GI tract.

► **TABLE 48-3   Tissues Typing for Renal Transplantation**

Test	Explanation
ABO compatibility	Test for RBC surface antigen compatibility also located on vascular endothelium, and on most tissues of body Compatibility is the same as for blood transfusion crossmatching: type O, universal donor; type AB, universal recipient ABO compatibility between donor and recipient is of critical importance; major blood group mismatch will result in an antibody-mediated hyperacute rejection
Histocompatibility (Terasaki microcytotoxicity assay)	Tests for class I HLA locus antigen match (HLA-A, HLA-B, and HLA-C antigens) between donor and recipient; present on all nucleated body cells T leukocytes in venous blood tested Important test for living, related donor transplantation (the chances of an identical match between siblings is 1:4)
Mixed lymphocyte culture (MLC)/ mixed lymphocyte response (MLR)	Assesses class II HLA-D locus antigens found mainly on the surface of B lymphocytes Lymphocytes of donor and recipient are grown together in a culture, only the response of the recipient to the donor cells is important; preferred donor is the one who provokes the lowest MLR in the recipient Test requires 4-5 days to complete so not suitable for selection of cadaver kidneys; used for living, related donors. 24-hour *HLA-DR typing* is now possible and allows rapid assessment of the D locus in cadaver kidneys
White-cell cross match	Performed to detect preexisting cytotoxic antibodies to donor antigens Positive cross match will result in hyperacute rejection and is a contraindication for transplantation

RBC, Red blood cell; *HLA,* human leukocyte antigen.

Terasaki, 1978). One proposed mechanism to explain the blood transfusion effect and active enhancement of graft survival is induction of anergy. Alternately, the mechanism might involve the production of enhancing antibodies specific for donor antigen, thus interfering with the graft rejection process by masking antigens in the graft and preventing their recognition by T cells (Hutchinson, 1993).

The success of treating rejection with cyclosporine has largely precluded the use of pretransplant transfusion to avoid the risk of presensitization and the transmission of HIV or hepatitis infection. Therefore current practice is to use as few blood transfusions as possible. The effectiveness of recombinant erythropoietin in maintaining RBC mass further reduces the need for blood transfusions.

Renal transplant rejection

The nature of the body's immunologic defense against entry of foreign proteins is such that almost all organ transplantation from another person (with the possible exception of an identical twin) is followed by an attempt on the part of the recipient to reject that organ. There are three types of rejection.

Hyperacute rejection occurs within minutes or hours after completion of the transplant and inevitably leads to organ loss. It is caused by ABO incompatibility or previous exposure to transfused WBCs or platelets from another person whose tissues contain the same antigens as the kidney donor. The recipient has preformed circulating antibodies, and such grafts undergo rejection via the humoral immune system, in which the B cell mechanism predominates. The antibodes are deposited along the kidney vascular endothelium, and complement is activated with consequent tissue damage. The end result is diffuse vascular thrombosis and cortical necrosis (Rose, Black, 1988). Hyperacute rejection can be prevented for the most part by appropriate ABO and lymphocyte cross matching before transplantation.

Acute rejection usually occurs within the first 12 weeks after transplantation. Acute rejection episodes may recur at any time after the initial one, but the incidence decreases with time. The greater the HLA antigenic disparity between donor and host (including an unrelated cadaver donor), the greater the likelihood of severe acute rejection episodes. Preformed antidonor antibodies are not present in acute rejection (as in the hyperacute case).

The overall scheme in the development of effector mechanisms in allograft rejection is illustrated in Fig. 48-10. In response to the allograft, cytotoxic (CD8) T cells recognize the class I HLA (A, B, C) antigens on the surface of the foreign cells. Helper (CD4) T cells recognize the foreign class II HLA-DR antigens on certain antigen presenting cells (APCs), such as the macrophage, in the graft. The activated T helper (CD4+) cell then releases cytokines, which are required as growth and differentiation factors for other cells involved in the rejection reac-

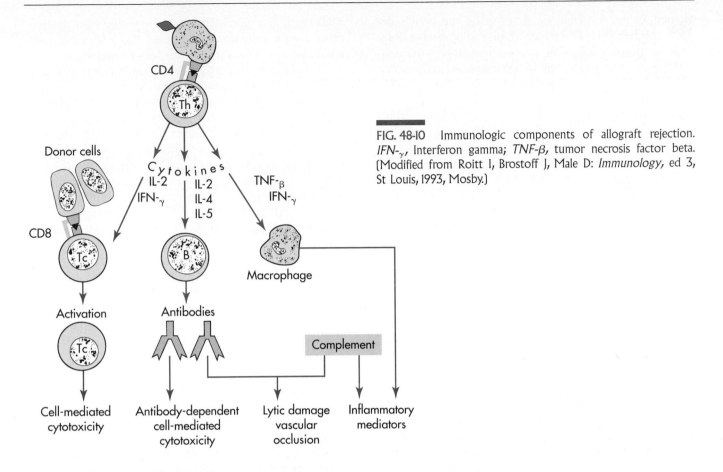

FIG. 48-10   Immunologic components of allograft rejection. *IFN-γ*, Interferon gamma; *TNF-β*, tumor necrosis factor beta. (Modified from Roitt I, Brostoff J, Male D: *Immunology,* ed 3, St Louis, 1993, Mosby.)

tion. Interleukin-2 (IL-2) and interferon-gamma (IFN γ) stimulate the cytotoxic T cells to form a clone of cells. These cytotoxic "killer" T cells then attack the cells in the allograft. IL-2, IL-4, and IL-5 are involved in B cell activation; lymphotoxin (tumor necrosis factor beta [TNF-β]) in concert with IFN γ causes activation of macrophages. In addition to direct killing of graft cells by cytotoxic T cells, the cells can be killed by a combination of antibody and phagocytic cells called *antibody-dependent cellular cytotoxicity* (ADCC). In this process, antibody bound to the surface of the foreign graft cell is recognized by phagocytic cells (e.g., macrophages or NK cells) and the cell is killed. B cell activation leading to the production of anti-graft IgG antibodies and complement activation can also cause damage to the vascular endothelium. The result is platelet aggregation within the vessel, thrombosis, hemorrhage, and damage to the parenchymal cells of the allograft, as well as the release of inflammatory mediators (Roitt et al., 1993; Carpenter, Lazarus, 1994). In summary, CD4+ T cells play a central role in initiating the rejection response by binding to class II HLA-DR antigens and subsequently enhancing the effector phase of the immune reaction by stimulating cytotoxic (CD8+) T cell, B cell, and macrophage mechanisms of allograft destruction.

Histologic evidence in the rejected kidney indicates that the critical targets for destruction are the vascular endothelium of the microvasculature and the renal tubules.

There is perivascular accumulation of monocytes and varying degrees of vascular injury and tubular necrosis. Immunofluorescent micrographs of the vascular epithelium show deposits of fibrin, complement, and IgG, indicating involvement of the humoral immune system in the organ rejection (Carpenter, Lazarus, 1994).

The first rejection episode commonly occurs about 2 weeks after transplantation and is characterized by renal insufficiency (rising BUN and serum creatinine), oliguria, and sometimes swelling of the graft and fever. A biopsy of the graft may be necessary to make the diagnosis and determine the extent of the lesion. Acute rejection is often reversible with appropriate drug therapy, which is aimed primarily at suppressing T cells (see below). Recovery usually takes 2 to 4 weeks, and during this time the patient requires dialysis.

Chronic rejection occurs months to years after the initial transplant and is characterized by hypertension, proteinuria, and slow loss of renal function. The cause is poorly understood but could be non-HLA minor antigens, a low-grade cell-mediated rejection, or the deposition of antigen-antibody complexes in the graft. Histologically, the primary changes are in the renal arteries and glomeruli and resemble a recurrence of the primary renal disease. Unlike acute rejection, this type of rejection responds poorly to drugs and has a poor prognosis (Rose, Black, 1988).

Immunosuppressive treatment. The survival of the transplanted kidney depends on minimizing the body's defense mechanisms. The major immunosuppressive drugs used to prevent rejection are azathioprine, corticosteroids, and cyclosporine, and in some centers, antilymphocyte globulin (ALG) or antithymocyte globulin (ATG), and monoclonal antibodies.

Azathioprine (Imuran [PO or IV]) and corticosteroids (prednisone [PO] or Solu-Medrol [IV]) are the standard drugs ordered. Azathioprine, an antimetabolite, is a derivative of 6-mercaptopurine. It inhibits the proliferation of lymphocytes by interfering with nucleic acid synthesis. Corticosteroids also suppress T cell proliferation by interfering with the release of interleukin-2 from monocytes. These drugs make the patient more susceptible to infection. Consequently, overwhelming infection is a major complication in a renal transplant recipient and the principal cause of death. To minimize the danger of both infection and rejection, the general approach is to increase the dosage of corticosteroids for a limited period of time during the initial transplant period and to treat rejection episodes while keeping the maintenance dose low at other times.

Cyclosporine is a potent fungal metabolite and a specific immunosuppressant that prevents the replication of T cells by inhibiting the production of interleukin-2. Since its approval by the US Food and Drug Administration (FDA) in 1983, it has revolutionized organ transplantation. In the United States, 1-year cadaver graft survival now rivals the 80% graft survival from HLA-identical related donors (Carpenter, Lazarus, 1994). Opelz (1991) reported the results of a large international collaborative transplant study involving cadaveric renal transplants between 1982 and 1989. Cyclosporin was given to virtually all of the 30,000 transplant recipients. This study showed that although the 1-year cadaver graft survival was high, long-term graft survival at 5 years after transplant was not improved. Five-year cadaver graft survival ranged between 45% and 65%, depending on the number of mismatches for HLA-A, -B, and -DR antigens.

Thus the major advantage of cyclosporine over azathioprine is during the first 1 or 2 years after cadaveric transplant and not in the rate of graft loss thereafter.

Cyclosporine may be given in combination with azathioprine and corticosteroids. The usefulness of this drug is limited by its adverse side effects, most notably its nephrotoxicity. Hypertension, hirsutism, gum hyperplasia, and increased susceptibility to infection are other side effects. The incidence of malignancy (especially lymphoma) is increased, especially when cyclosporine is used in combination with other immunosuppressants.

Antilymphocyte globulin (ALG) and antithymocyte globulin (ATG) are produced by injecting human lymphocytes (ALG) or thymocytes (ATG) into animals, which then make antibodies against them. These antibodies are then injected into the transplant patient to prevent or treat rejection. The major effect of ALG or ATG is to deplete T cells. Side effects include susceptibility to infection and to the foreign protein that can lead to fever, chills, and anaphylaxis.

Monoclonal OKT3 antibodies are administered intravenously and cause suppression of T cells. The drug acts by opsinizing the T3 molecule present in the cell membrane of all peripheral T cells, thus rendering them incapable of an immunologic response. OKT3 antibody is highly effective in the treatment of acute rejection (Rose, Black, 1988).

A final consideration is that there is limited choice in opting for renal transplantation as a treatment modality, since there are more than 21,000 newly diagnosed persons with end-stage renal failure each year and a limited supply of good-quality kidneys for transplantation even for ideal recipients. Consequently, the overwhelming majority of patients will receive dialysis as a chronic form of treatment. However, the recent significant advances in tissue typing and improved immunosuppression, especially with cyclosporine, offer hope for greater success in those patients receiving cadaver transplants (the commonest source of organs).

? QUESTIONS

▼ *Answer the following on a separate sheet of paper.*

1. When are conservative measures of treatment begun for the patient with chronic renal failure? What are the basic principles of conservative treatment? Name four causes of sudden deterioration of renal function in your answer.

2. When conservative therapeutic measures are no longer adequate in the treatment of the uremic patient, what are the alternatives?

3. Mr. Walker, who is oliguric and uremic,

has had a total urine output of 500 ml during the past 24 hours. What should his approximate fluid intake be for the next day?

4. What are the two modalities of treatment for the end-stage renal failure patient and how are they related?

5. Define dialysis.

6. Differentiate between an external and an internal shunt.

▼ *Circle the letter preceding each item below that correctly answers the question or completes the sentence. Only one*

answer is correct, with exceptions noted.

7. To slow the progression of end-stage renal failure, in some patients, a/an:
   a. Diet high in carbohydrates is prescribed
   b. Early dialysis is recommended
   c. Course of corticosteroids is recommended
   d. Low-protein diet and control of hypertension are recommended

8. Common treatments to ameliorate the anemia of end-stage renal failure are: (More than one answer may be correct.)

QUESTIONS—cont'd

a. Erythropoietin
b. Weekly blood transfusions
c. Iron and folic acid
d. Minimizing blood loss caused by hemodialysis and laboratory tests

9. The IV administration of sodium bicarbonate to correct the systemic acidosis in renal failure may result in which of the following complications?
a. Tetany and convulsions
b. Hypermagnesemia
c. Azotemia
d. Renal osteodystrophy

10. Phosphate binding agents for the uremic patient are properly administered:
a. One hour before meals
b. During meals
c. One hour after meals
d. Ad lib by patient for gastric distress

11. Which of the following findings in a patient with renal insufficiency would indicate that dialysis treatment should be initiated? (More than one answer may be correct.)
a. BUN 60 mg/dl
b. K+ 6.3 mEq/L
c. Unable to carry on usual job as telephone operator
d. Burning sensation on soles of feet

12. Peritoneal dialysis removes waste products from the blood because of all the following principles except:
a. Water moves across the semipermeable membrane by osmosis
b. The peritoneal surface acts as a semipermeable membrane
c. Red blood cells are removed by ultrafiltration
d. Na+ and K+ are removed by diffusion

13. The objectives of hemodialysis are all the following except:
a. Removal of excess extracellular and intracellular fluid
b. Diffusion of K+ out of the blood
c. Stimulation of urine production by the osmotic pressure gradient
d. Diffusion of urea out of the blood

14. The most compact of the basic types of hemodialyzer is the:
a. Coil dialyzer
b. Parallel plate dialyzer
c. Hollow fiber dialyzer

15. All the following substances may leave the blood and enter the dialyzing fluid except:
a. Albumin   c. Magnesium
b. Urea   d. Potassium

16. In hemodialysis, blood is pumped through a _____ tubing bathed in a dialysis fluid that is similar to plasma in composition.
a. Permeable   c. Osmotic
b. Semipermeable   d. Ultrafiltrate

17. The purpose of adding sodium acetate to the dialyzing fluid is to:
a. Correct the hyperuricemia
b. Decrease the incidence of peripheral neuropathy
c. Alleviate pruritus
d. Provide bicarbonate to the body to correct acidosis
e. Increase the osmolality of the dialysing solution to provide for ultrafiltration

18. The flow of blood through an artificially created internal AV fistula causes the vein to enlarge and is referred to as:
a. Fistulation
b. Ripening
c. Ultrafiltration
d. Cannulation

19. Which of the following drugs is used to prevent clotting of blood during extracorporeal circulation?
a. Protamine
b. Heparin
c. Warfarin sodium (Coumadin)
d. Fibrinogen

20. The purpose of histocompatibility testing is:
a. To rule out noncompatible donors
b. To demonstrate matching of MHC genes that control synthesis of certain proteins
c. To prevent posttransplant diuresis
d. None of the above

21. Body cells used in kidney donor and recipient matching include:
a. Endothelial cells of the glomerulus
b. Renal tubular cells
c. Red blood cells
d. White blood cells

22. The probability of HLA-identical siblings in a family is:
a. 10%
b. 25%
c. 50%
d. 75%

23. The most important antigens from the point of view of renal transplant are: (More than one answer may be correct.)
a. ABO blood group
b. Leukocytes
c. Hemoglobin
d. Thrombocytes

24. In general, a donor kidney from which of the following persons would be most likely to be successful?
a. Parent
b. Sister
c. Cadaver
d. Cousin

25. Transplantation should not be carried out with:
a. Cadaver donor with two-antigen HLA matching
b. Cadaver donor with two-antigen DR matching
c. Related donor with four-antigen matching and different blood group
d. Recipient with weak stimulation on the MLC test to related donor
e. Recipient with a history of multiple blood transfusions

26. Which of the following statements are true concerning the procedure for renal transplantation? (More than one answer may be correct.)
a. The left kidney of the donor is rotated and placed in the right iliac fossa of the recipient.
b. The left kidney of the donor is rotated and placed in the left iliac fossa of the recipient.
c. The left kidney of the donor is placed in the left upper abdominal cavity of the recipient, and the renal artery is anastomosed to the recipient's renal artery.
d. The renal vein is anastomosed to the common iliac vein.
e. The renal artery is anastomosed to the internal iliac artery.
f. The ureter of the transplanted kidney is implanted into the colon.

27. The immune response to transplantation in acute rejection is mediated by:
a. Humoral antibodies
b. T cells
c. Complement and humoral antibodies
d. Humoral antibodies acting synergistically with T cells

28. The most common cause of failure of a renal transplant is:
a. Obstruction of the ureterovesicular anastomosis
b. Infection of the transplanted kidney
c. Immunologic rejection of the transplanted kidney
d. Recurrence of the patient's original kidney disease

29. The most common cause of death in kidney transplant recipients is:
a. Surgical complications

Continued.

QUESTIONS—cont'd

b. Hypertension
c. Viral infections
d. Combined relentless rejection and overwhelming infection

30. The advantage of kidney transplant is:
   a. Generally eliminates the need for dialysis
   b. Side effects easily treated with corticosteroids
   c. No danger to the donor
   d. Minimal danger of postoperative infections

▼ *Match the uremic complications in column A with the common therapies for the prevention or treatment of the condition in column B. Conditions may have more than one treatment.*

Column A	Column B
31. _____ Hyperkalemia	a. Cardiac monitor
32. _____ Hyperparathyroidism	b. Kayexalate
33. _____ Hypertension	c. Colchicine
34. _____ Osteomalacia	d. IV glucose + insulin
35. _____ Hyperuricemia	e. ACE inhibitor drugs
36. _____ Peripheral neuropathy	f. Allopurinol
37. _____ Gouty arthritis	g. Calcium carbonate
	h. Vitamin D
	i. IV calcium gluconate
	j. Progress halted only by dialysis
	k. Sodium restriction

▼ *Match the histocompatibility test in column A with the antigens or antibodies it detects in column B.*

Column A	Column B
38. _____ RBC type and cross match	a. Class I antigens
39. _____ Microcytotoxicity assay	b. ABO antigens
40. _____ Mixed lymphocyte culture	c. Lymphocyte antibodies
41. _____ WBC cross match	d. Class II antigens
	e. HLA-DR antigens

▼ *Circle T if the statement is true and F if it is false. Correct any false statements.*

42. T F It is only the antigens present in the donor and lacking in the recipient that cause immunologic rejection in a transplanted kidney.

43. T F The presence of preformed antibodies against donor ABO antigens or lymphocytes causes hyperacute rejection in the kidney transplant recipient.

44. T F Hemodialysis is never needed after a successful renal transplantation.

45. T F An immunologic response does not occur when the kidney donor is an HLA-identical sibling.

46. T F If acute rejection episodes are untreated, the cells of the transplanted kidney are destroyed.

47. T F Most of the immunosuppressive drugs used to prevent or treat transplantation rejection act by depleting T cells.

▼ *Answer the following on a separate sheet of paper.*

48. Name two new developments that have potential for greatly increasing survival of cadaver kidney transplants.

49. Name several experimental approaches to the removal of uremic solutes. How are they related to the middle molecular hypothesis?

50. Which of the following statements regarding the major histocompatibility locus of genes (called HLA in humans) is least accurate?
   a. These genes code for class I and class II proteins, which play a major role in the rejection of allografts
   b. Class I proteins are expressed on virtually all body cells
   c. Class II proteins are found only on certain cells (e.g., B lymphocytes, macrophages)
   d. These genes may have different alleles at both class I and class II loci; thus the corresponding proteins on the surface of human cells are very polymorphic
   e. Matching of the class I proteins between donor and recipient is the strongest predictor of allograft success

51. A recipient of a two-haplotype HLA-matched kidney from a sibling still needs immunosuppression therapy to prevent graft rejection because:
   a. Graft-versus-host disease will be a problem
   b. Class II HLA antigens will not be matched
   c. Immunosuppression decreases the chance of infection at the surgical site
   d. Minor histocompatibility antigens will not be matched

52. Kidney grafts between monozygotic (identical) twins:
   a. Are not rejected, even without immunosuppression therapy
   b. Are subject to hyperacute rejection
   c. Are rejected slowly as a result of minor histocompatibility antigens
   d. Are rejected only if immunosuppression therapy is omitted

53. What is the role of class II HLA antigens in graft rejection?
   a. They are a recognition element for T helper cells, which then promote the response of cytotoxic T cells
   b. They are the recognition element for cytotoxic T cells
   c. They enhance the function of T suppressor cells
   d. They can induce the production of blocking antibodies that protect the graft

CHAPTER 49   Acute Renal Failure

LORRAINE M. WILSON

Acute renal failure is a clinical syndrome characterized by a rapid decline in renal function (usually within a few days) leading to rapidly progressive azotemia. The rapid decline in glomerular filtration rate (GFR) causes the serum creatinine to rise as much as 0.5 mg/dl/day and the blood urea nitrogen (BUN) as much as 10 mg/dl/day over several days. Acute renal failure (ARF) is usually associated with oliguria (urine output <400 ml/day). This criterion of oliguria is not arbitrary but is related to the fact that the average American diet contains about 600 mOsm of solute. If the maximum urine-concentrating ability is 1200 mOsm/L water, there is an obligatory loss of about 500 ml of water per day in the urine. Thus, when urine output falls below 400 ml/day, the solute load cannot be eliminated and the BUN and creatinine rise. However, oliguria is not a necessary feature of ARF. Recent evidence suggests that in one third to one half of ARF cases, urine output exceeds 400 ml/day and may be as high as 2 L/day. This form of ARF is called *nonoliguric*, or *high-output*, acute renal failure. ARF results in signs and symptoms similar to those of the uremic syndrome in chronic renal failure, reflecting failure of the kidney's regulatory, excretory, and endocrine functions. However, anemia and renal osteodystrophy are not usually features of ARF because of its acute onset.

ARF is a very common clinical syndrome, occurring in approximately 5% of hospitalized patients and as many as 30% of patients admitted to intensive care units. A wide variety of diseases, drugs, pregnancy-related complications, trauma, and surgical procedures may lead to ARF. In contrast to chronic renal failure, the majority of patients who develop ARF usually have prior normal renal function and the condition is generally reversible. In spite of these facts, mortality from ARF is very high (about 60%), even with the availability of dialysis treatment, perhaps reflecting the critical illnesses with which it is usually associated.

CAUSES OF ACUTE RENAL FAILURE

The causes of acute renal failure are generally considered under three diagnostic categories: prerenal azotemia, postrenal azotemia, and intrinsic acute renal failure (see box, p. 756). This classification stresses that only in the third category (renal) is renal parenchymal damage sufficient to cause functional failure in itself. If prolonged, prerenal and postrenal factors are likely to lead to intrinsic renal failure, but with proper diagnosis they are readily reversible. The most common intrinsic renal disease that leads to ARF is *acute tubular necrosis* (ATN), which describes a renal lesion in response to prolonged ischemia or exposure to a nephrotoxin. The diagnosis of ATN is made on the basis of excluding prerenal and postrenal causes of azotemia followed by exclusion of other causes of intrinsic renal failure (glomerular, vascular, and tubulointerstitial renal diseases).

Prerenal azotemia is the single most frequent cause of acute azotemia (>50% of cases), which may lead to ATN-type acute renal failure. The common denominator of the prerenal causes of ARF is *prolonged renal ischemia* from decreased renal perfusion. Renal hypoperfusion is associ-

COMMON CAUSES OF ACUTE RENAL FAILURE

PRERENAL AZOTEMIA (DECREASED RENAL PERFUSION)

1. Absolute extracellular fluid (ECF) volume depletion
   a. Hemorrhage: major surgery*; trauma, postpartum
   b. Excessive diuresis
   c. Severe gastrointestinal (GI) losses: vomiting, diarrhea
   d. Third space losses: burns*; peritonitis; pancreatitis
2. Decreased effective arterial circulating volume
   a. Reduced cardiac output: myocardial infarction; dysrhythmias; congestive heart failure; cardiac tamponade; pulmonary embolism
   b. Peripheral vasodilation: sepsis*; anaphylaxis; drugs: anesthesia, antihypertensives, nitrates
   c. Hypoalbuminemia: nephrotic syndrome; liver failure (cirrhosis)
3. Primary renal hemodynamic alterations
   a. Prostaglandin synthesis inhibitors: aspirin and other NSAIDs
   b. Vasodilation of efferent arteriole: angiotensin-converting enzyme (ACE) inhibitors (e.g., captopril)
   c. Vasoconstrictor drugs: alpha-adrenergic agents (e.g., norepinephrine); angiotensin II
   d. Hepatorenal syndrome
4. Bilateral renal vascular obstruction
   a. Renal artery stenosis, emboli, thrombosis
   b. Bilateral renal vein thrombosis

POSTRENAL AZOTEMIA (URINARY TRACT OBSTRUCTION)

1. Urethral obstruction: urethral valves; urethral stricture
2. Bladder outflow obstruction: prostatic hypertrophy*, carcinoma*
3. Bilateral ureteral obstruction (unilateral if one functional kidney)
   a. Intraureteral: calculi, blood clots, sloughed papillae
   b. Extraureteral (compression): retroperitoneal fibrosis; neoplasm of bladder, prostate, or cervix; accidental surgical ligation or injury
4. Neurogenic bladder

INTRINSIC ACUTE RENAL FAILURE

1. Acute tubular necrosis
   a. Postischemic
      (1) Shock, sepsis, open heart surgery, aortic surgery (all causes of severe prerenal azotemia)
   b. Nephrotoxic
      (1) Exogenous nephrotoxins
         (a) Antibiotics: aminoglycosides, amphotericin B
         (b) Iodinated contrast media (especially in diabetics)
         (c) Heavy metals: cisplatin, bichloride of mercury, arsenic
         (d) Solvents: carbon tetrachloride, ethylene glycol, methanol
      (2) Endogenous nephrotoxins
         (a) Intratubular pigments: hemoglobin; myoglobin
         (b) Intratubular proteins: multiple myeloma
         (c) Intratubular crystals: uric acid
2. Primary renal glomerular or vascular disease
   a. Acute poststreptococcal or rapidly progressive glomerulonephritis
   b. Malignant hypertension
   c. Acute-on-chronic renal failure related to salt or water depletion
3. Acute tubulointerstitial nephritis
   a. Allergic: beta-lactams (penicillins, cephalosporins); sulfonamides
   b. Infection: e.g., acute pyelonephritis

*Most common causes.

ated with a large variety of conditions resulting in intravascular volume depletion, decreased effective arterial circulating volume, or, rarely, renal vascular obstruction. Some of the most common prerenal conditions with increased risk of ARF are abdominal aortic surgery, open heart surgery, cardiogenic shock, extensive burns, and septic shock. Most of these conditions are associated with systemic hypotension with compensatory activation of the sympathetic nervous system and the renin-angiotensin-aldosterone system. Angiotensin causes vasoconstriction of the renal, cutaneous, and splanchnic vascular beds, and aldosterone causes salt and water retention. This response is designed to maintain the systemic mean arterial pressure and perfusion to the vital organs. At the same time, renal autoregulatory mechanisms are activated to maintain the GFR and protect the kidney against ischemia. Angiotensin II preferentially causes constriction of the glomerular efferent arteriole (thus increasing intraglomerular pressure and GFR) and at the same time stimulates the production of vasodilator renal prostaglandins. The renal protective effect of prostaglandins can be negated by the administration of nonsteroidal antiinflammatory drugs (NSAIDs), such as aspirin, which block the production of these hormones. Thus administration of NSAIDs in the presence of renal hypoperfusion states from prerenal causes has been increasingly recognized as a precipitating cause of ischemic damage of the kidney in ARF. Angiotensin-converting enzyme (ACE) inhibitor drugs (which inhibit angiotensin II) may also precipitate ARF under conditions of renal hypoperfusion or renal vascular obstruction and so should be used with caution. The early treatment of prerenal azotemia may prevent its progression to ARF.

Postrenal causes of azotemia that may lead to ARF are less common (5%) than prerenal causes and refer to obstruction to the flow of urine at any level of the urinary tract. Prostatic enlargement (caused by cancer or benign hypertrophy) is the most common cause of bladder outlet obstruction. Cervical cancer may also cause obstruction of the urinary tract. Obstruction above the bladder (commonly caused by calculi) must be bilateral to cause urinary outflow obstruction, unless there is only one functioning kidney. It is important to realize that prolonged obstruction of urinary outflow will lead to hydronephrosis, severe damage to the renal parenchyma, and ARF. Thus the early identification and correction of urinary tract obstruction are crucial.

Acute tubular necrosis (ATN) is the most common renal lesion causing ARF (75%). ATN arises from either prolonged renal ischemia (from prerenal conditions already identified) or from exposure to nephrotoxins. Unfortunately, the terms *ATN* and *ARF* are used interchangeably in the clinical arena although this is not correct. ATN refers to a type of lesion that is commonly but not invariably associated with ARF (see below). ARF may be present without ATN. Other intrinsic renal causes of ARF without tubular necrosis include primary renal glomerular or vascular diseases such as acute poststreptococcal glomerulonephritis or malignant hypertension, respectively. Acute-on-chronic renal failure can also result from stresses such as infection or fluid loss from vomiting and diarrhea in a person with chronic renal failure and little renal reserve. Acute tubulointerstitial nephritis caused by an allergic reaction to an antibiotic or an acute pyelonephritis may likewise result in ARF. These other non-ATN causes of ARF must be ruled out before a diagnosis of ATN is made.

Nephrotoxic causes of ATN include both exogenous and endogenous nephrotoxins commonly causing the nonoliguric type of ARF. Exogenous nephrotoxins are categorized into four major groups: antibiotics, contrast media, heavy metals, and solvents.

Aminoglycoside antibiotic therapy is complicated by ARF in about 10% of the courses (e.g., gentamicin, kanamycin, tobramycin).

A variety of heavy metals are potent nephrotoxins and produce ARF with ATN. Cisplatin (platinum salt), a drug used to treat certain solid neoplasms, is the most common agent in this category. ATN caused by mercury, arsenic, chromium, or uranium is usually the result of occupational exposure, or the substance is ingested in a suicide attempt.

Both cyclosporine (used to treat transplant rejection) and contrast media can contribute to ARF by causing intrarenal vasoconstriction. Diabetics are particularly vulnerable to nephropathy from the use of contrast media. Additional risk factors for contrast media nephropathy

include preexisting renal insufficiency, advanced age, volume depletion, multiple myeloma, and multiple exposures to contrast agents within a short period.

Nephrotoxic tubular injury can result from the ingestion of solvents such as ethylene glycol (antifreeze) or methanol (wood alcohol). The inhalation of fumes from carbon tetrachloride (CCl_4), a common ingredient in spot remover and other cleaning fluids, accompanied by the ingestion of ethyl alcohol (CH_3CH_2OH), is particularly dangerous because of a chemical reaction between these two compounds that forms a potent nephrotoxin. This set of circumstances (e.g., alcohol ingestion at a party and removing a clothing stain with spot remover) has resulted in ARF in a number of unsuspecting persons. For the same reasons, hobbyists using organic solvents and glues should work in well-ventilated rooms and refrain from drinking alcohol at the same time.

Endogenous nephrotoxins include hemoglobin, myoglobin, and Bence Jones protein (abnormal immunoglobulin produced in multiple myeloma). Hemolysis of red blood cells (RBCs) with the release of hemoglobin into the blood serum is usually caused by a mismatched blood transfusion. Large amounts of myoglobin are contained within muscles and may be released after a massive crush injury (rhabdomyolysis). When hemoglobin, myoglobin, or Bence Jones proteins are excreted in the urine, they have a direct toxic effect on the renal tubular cells and cause ARF. Finally, precipitation of uric acid crystals in the renal tubules, causing obstruction and ARF, may complicate certain "high turnover" malignancies (e.g., leukemia) or more commonly chemotherapy with cytotoxic agents. In both of these situations, massive cell lysis causes the release of large amounts of purine uric acid precursors. Uric acid crystallizes most readily in an acidic environment so precipitation can be prevented by administering allopurinol (inhibits uric acid synthesis) before chemotherapy or giving sodium bicarbonate to alkalinize the urine and forcing fluids.

PATHOLOGY OF ACUTE TUBULAR NECROSIS

The term *acute tubular necrosis* (ATN) is commonly applied to both nephrotoxic and ischemic renal injuries, although it does not reflect the nature and severity of the observed tubular changes. Two types of histologic lesions are commonly observed in ATN: (1) necrosis of the tubular epithelium leaving the basement membrane intact, commonly resulting from the ingestion of nephrotoxic chemicals; and (2) necrosis of both the tubular epithelium and the basement membrane, commonly associated with renal ischemia.

The severity of tubular damage in ATN caused by nephrotoxins is highly variable, and the prognosis varies accordingly. There may be necrosis of the proximal tubule epithelium with complete healing in 3 or 4 weeks. Bichloride of mercury and carbon tetrachloride commonly produce this type of lesion. The prognosis is generally good with conservative management or supportive dialysis. In contrast, other poisons such as glycols may produce irreversible renal failure with infarction of the entire nephron, termed *acute cortical necrosis*. The prognosis in this case is poor. Calcification commonly occurs in the area of cortical necrosis if the patient is fortunate enough to survive.

Tubular damage caused by renal ischemia is also highly variable. It depends on the extent and duration of the decreased renal blood flow and ischemia. There may be patchy or widespread destruction of the tubular epithelium and basement membrane or cortical necrosis. Many cases of acute cortical necrosis have followed complications of pregnancy, particularly premature separation of the placenta, postpartum hemorrhage, eclampsia, and septic abortion. When the basement membrane is disrupted, epithelial regeneration occurs in a random, haphazard manner, frequently leading to obstruction of the nephron at the site of necrosis. The prognosis depends on the extent of this type of change.

PATHOPHYSIOLOGY OF ACUTE RENAL FAILURE

Although there is now agreement concerning the pathology of the kidney damaged by ATN-type ARF, there is still considerable controversy over the pathogenesis of the suppression of renal function and the usually accompanying oliguria. Most modern concepts concerning possible causative factors are based on studies using animal experimental models in which nephrotoxic acute renal failure is produced by injections of mercuric chloride, uranyl nitrate, or chromate, whereas ischemic damage is produced by injecting glycerol or clamping the renal arteries. Several theories have been proposed to explain the moderate reduction in renal blood flow and reduction in GFR observed in both experimental animals and humans, including (1) tubular obstruction; (2) backleak of tubular fluid; (3) decreased glomerular permeability; (4) vasomotor dysfunction; and (5) tubuloglomerular feedback. None of the proposed mechanisms can account for all the variable aspects of ATN-type ARF. Schrier (1992) summarized the supporting and the contradictory evidence for each of the proposed mechanisms.

The tubular obstruction theory proposes that ATN leads to the desquamation of necrotic tubular cells and other proteinaceous materials, which then form casts and occlude the tubule lumina. Cellular swelling as a result of the initial ischemia may also contribute to the obstruction and perpetuate the ischemia. Intratubular pressure increases, so that net glomerular filtration pressure is reduced. Tubular obstruction may be an important factor in ARF caused by heavy metals, ethylene glycol, or prolonged ischemia.

The tubular backleak hypothesis proposes that glomerular filtration continues normally but that the tubular fluid "leaks" out of the lumina through the damaged tubular cells into the peritubular circulation. Disruption of the basement membrane may be seen with severe ATN, which provides an anatomic basis for this mechanism.

Although the syndrome of ATN implies an abnormality of the renal tubule, recent evidence suggests that in some circumstances the glomerular capillary endothelial cells and/or basement membrane cells undergo changes that reduce permeability or the surface area for filtration. The result is a reduction of glomerular ultrafiltration.

Total renal blood flow (RBF) may be reduced to as low as 30% of normal in oliguric ARF. This level of RBF could be compatible with a substantial GFR. In fact, RBF in chronic renal failure is often as low as or lower than that found in the acute form, yet reduced but adequate renal function persists. Furthermore, experimental evidence suggests that RBF must be less than 5% before renal parenchymal damage occurs (Merrill, 1971). Thus it appears that renal hypoperfusion alone cannot account for the degree of reduction in GFR and the tubular lesions found in ARF. However, there is evidence of marked changes in the intrarenal distribution of blood flow from the cortex to the medulla during acute and prolonged hypotension (Merrill, 1971). It will be recalled from Chapter 44 that in the normal kidney about 90% of the blood is distributed to the cortex (where the glomeruli are located) and 10% goes to the medulla. This allows the kidney to concentrate urine and perform its functions. In contrast, in ARF the ratio of renal cortical to medullary blood distribution may be reversed, so there is relative ischemia of the renal cortex. Constriction of the afferent arterioles provides a vascular basis for the marked reduction in GFR. Renal ischemia would then activate the renin-angiotensin system and perpetuate cortical ischemia after the initiating stimulus has disappeared. The highest concentration of renin is found in the outer cortex of the kidney (the site where ischemia is greatest) in animals and humans with acute renal failure (Schrier, 1992). Some authors have postulated a role for prostaglandins in the vasomotor dysfunction of ARF (Harter, Martin, 1982). Renal hypoxia normally stimulates the renal synthesis of prostaglandin E and prostaglandin A (PGE and PGA) (potent vasodilators), causing renal blood flow to be redistributed to the cortex with resulting diuresis. It is possible that acute severe or prolonged ischemia may block the synthesis of these renal prostaglandins. Prostaglandin inhibitors such as aspirin are known to reduce renal blood flow (RBF) in normal persons and potentiate ATN (Schrier, 1992).

Tubuloglomerular feedback (TGF) is a phenomenon in which the flow to the distal nephron is regulated by receptors in the macula densa of the distal tubule, which lies in proximity to the glomerular pole. If distal flow of tubular filtrate were inappropriately increased, the reab-

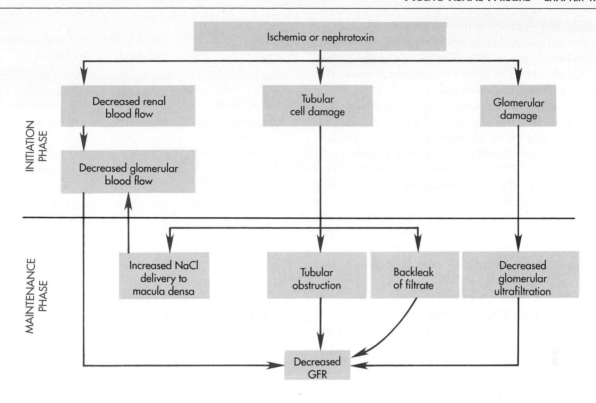

FIG. 49-1   Pathogenesis of acute renal failure. *NaCl,* Sodium chloride; *GFR,* glomerular filtration rate. (Redrawn from Harter HR, Martin KJ: *Postgrad Med* 72[6]:191, 1982).

sorptive capacity of the distal tubule and collecting ducts could be overwhelmed and lead to extracellular fluid (ECF) volume depletion. Thus TGF is a protective mechanism. In ATN, proximal tubular damage greatly reduces the absorptive capacity of the tubules. TGF is believed to be at least partly responsible for the decrease in GFR in the presence of ATN by causing constriction of the afferent arteriole and/or mesangial contraction, which lower intraglomerular capillary pressure (P_{gc}) and permeability, respectively. Thus a decrease in GFR caused by TGF could be considered an adaptive mechanism in ATN.

Fig. 49-1 illustrates a schema in which the various factors involved in the pathogenesis of ARF are combined. The initiating event is generally an ischemic insult or a nephrotoxin, which damages the tubules or glomeruli or reduces renal blood flow. Acute renal failure is then maintained through several possible mechanisms that may be present or absent and are a result of the initial injury. Each mechanism differs in the importance of its contributions to the pathogenesis according to the different theories cited. It is likely that the relative importance of these mechanisms varies with the situation and depends on the evolution of the disease process as well as the severity of the pathologic damage. The pathophysiology of ARF is far from settled, and much more research is needed to define the relative importance of the various factors.

CLINICAL COURSE OF ACUTE RENAL FAILURE

The clinical course of acute renal failure has been divided traditionally into three stages: oliguria, diuresis, and recovery. This tradition is followed in the discussion below while recognizing that acute renal failure and azotemia may be present with urine output of more than 400 ml/24 hr. The clinical courses of oliguric and nonoliguric acute renal failure are similar. However, abnormalities of blood chemistry are generally milder and the prognosis for recovery better in cases of nonoliguric acute renal failure.

Oliguric Stage

The clinical picture is often dominated by the surgical, medical, or obstetric calamity causing the acute renal failure. Oliguria is usually present within 24 to 48 hours after the initial injury, although this symptom may not occur until several days after exposure to nephrotoxic chemicals. Azotemia accompanies the oliguria.

It is critically important to recognize the onset of oliguria, determine the cause, and begin treatment of any reversible causes. Acute renal failure of the ATN type must be differentiated from prerenal (hypoperfusion) and postrenal (urinary tract obstruction) failure and other intrarenal disorders (e.g., acute poststreptococcal glomerulonephritis, acute pyelonephritis, acute-on-chronic renal failure). The diagnosis of acute renal failure is made only after the other causes are excluded.

Oliguria caused by acute-on-chronic renal failure is usually evident from the history. Because patients with chronic renal failure have a limited ability to adjust fluid and electrolyte balance, they may be easily thrown into acute renal failure by relatively minor upsets. Examples are the patient with chronic glomerulonephritis who has a gastrointestinal upset with vomiting or diarrhea or the patient with chronic pyelonephritis who gets a superimposed acute renal infection. Occasionally, a patient with undiagnosed chronic renal insufficiency may present in acute renal failure. A history of long-standing nocturia, hypertension, systemic diseases such as systemic lupus erythematosus or diabetes mellitus, radiographic evidence of small, contracted kidneys, and signs of long-standing renal disease such as renal osteodystrophy are suggestive of chronic renal insufficiency. The patient can usually be restored to the previous state of health by treatment of the infection, correction of the fluid and electrolyte imbalance, and treatment by peritoneal dialysis if necessary.

Postrenal obstruction must be ruled out, especially if the cause of the renal failure is not apparent. The presence of anuria or of periods of anuria alternating with periods of normal urine flow suggests obstruction. Urethral and bladder neck obstruction can be evaluated by catheterization and determining residual urine in the bladder after an attempt at complete voiding. If outlet obstruction is ruled out but bilateral obstruction proximal to the bladder is suspected, ultrasound or radioisotope renal scan and retrograde pyelography may be performed.

Ultrasonography reveals renal size and may show evidence of obstructing calculi in the renal pelves or ureters. Radioisotope scans may be used to evaluate the integrity of the major renal vessels and are useful when occlusion of the renal artery or vein by an embolus or thrombus is suspected. Retrograde pyelography is used in selected cases of obstructive uropathy and may be therapeutic as well as diagnostic. Potential causes of obstruction are listed in the box on p. 756. Prolonged obstruction will lead to intrinsic and often irreversible renal failure. Treatment involves immediate removal of the obstruction. Finally, prerenal oliguria is the most common antecedent situation leading to ARF and must be distinguished from ATN.

Prerenal Oliguria Versus Acute Tubular Necrosis

Prerenal oliguria and azotemia are physiologic and potentially reversible. They result from shock, decreased plasma volume, and consequent decrease in renal blood flow and GFR. Prerenal oliguria may result from any of

TABLE 49-1 Renal Indices in Prerenal Azotemia and Acute Renal Failure

Laboratory Test	Prerenal Azotemia	Acute Tubular Necrosis
Urinary Na^+ concentration	<20 mEq/L	>40 mEq/L
Urine/plasma creatinine ratio	>40:1	<20:1
Urine/plasma urea ratio	>8:1	<2:1
FE_{Na} (%)	<1	>1
BUN/creatinine ratio	>10:1	About 10:1
Urine osmolality	>500 mOsm	Near 287 mOsm (fixed)
Urine/plasma osmolality ratio	>2:1	<1.1:1
Urine specific gravity	>1.015	Near 1.010 (fixed)
Urinary sediment	Normal	Casts, cellular, debris

Na^+, Sodium; FE_{Na}, fractional excretion of sodium; *BUN,* blood urea nitrogen.

the prerenal causes of acute renal failure previously discussed. If left uncorrected, prerenal oliguria may progress to ATN. Serial determinations of the urine output, BUN level, creatinine level, and electrolytes should therefore be made after any major surgery, trauma, serious infection, or obstetric complication.

A few simple tests on the sediment and chemical constituents of the urine are helpful in distinguishing prerenal oliguria or azotemia from the true acute renal failure of the ATN type (Table 49-1).

In prerenal oliguria, when there is not yet any damage to the renal parenchyma, the response of the kidney to decreased perfusion is to conserve salt and water. In contrast, intrinsic renal tubular damage is associated with impaired ability to conserve sodium. Consequently, urine sodium concentration is low in prerenal oliguria (<20 mEq/L) and high in ATN (>40 mEq/L).

Water reabsorption by the kidney is assessed by the concentration of a nonreabsorbable solute, such as creatinine, usually expressed as the ratio of the concentration of creatinine in urine to that of plasma (U/P creatinine). A U/P creatinine ratio of 2.0 indicates that 50% of the filtered water is reabsorbed, whereas a U/P creatinine ratio of 100 indicates that 1% of the filtered water is reabsorbed. Thus in prerenal azotemia the U/P creatinine ratio is high (>40), whereas it is low in the presence of intrinsic tubular renal disease (<20).

The U/P urea ratio is more than 8 in prerenal oliguria and less than 2 in established ATN. The U/P urea ratio is somewhat lower than the creatinine ratio, since there is some back diffusion of urea but not of creatinine. Thus the U/P creatinine ratio is a truer estimate of water reabsorption across the nephron.

The normal ratio of BUN to creatinine is 10:1. In prerenal azotemia this ratio is greater than 10:1 and may be 20:1 or greater. The high ratio of BUN to serum creatinine indicates the disproportionate rise of the blood levels of urea. Blood urea levels rise faster than creatinine because of the greater back reabsorption (its molecule is smaller than that of creatinine) in the situation of reduced renal perfusion. The production of urea may also increase markedly and contribute to the disproportionate increase in the BUN, since a catabolic state is often present in the acute illness and trauma associated with the development of prerenal azotemia.

Urine osmolality, specific gravity, and U/P osmolality ratio are additional indices of water handling by the kidney. In prerenal oliguria, urine osmolality is more than 500 mOsm (specific gravity >1.015) but decreases to about 287 mOsm (specific gravity 1.010) in established ATN as ability to concentrate is lost (Rose, Rennke, 1994). The U/P osmolality progresses toward 1:1 in established ARF, indicating that the urine is isoosmotic with the plasma.

The urinary sodium concentration and U/P creatinine are the most reliable indices in distinguishing prerenal azotemia from ATN. When these indices are combined, the fractional excretion of sodium (FE_{Na}) can be calculated. The FE_{Na} is less than 1% in prerenal azotemia and is usually greater than this in established ATN. The FE_{Na} is a sensitive index in differentiating prerenal azotemia from established acute renal failure. Fractional excretion of sodium is calculated by the following formula (Harter, Martin, 1982):

$$FE_{Na} = \frac{U_{Na}}{P_{Na}} \times \frac{P_{Cr}}{U_{Cr}} \times 100\%$$

where

U_{Na} = urinary concentration of sodium in mEq/L
P_{Na} = plasma concentration of sodium in mEq/L
U_{Cr} = urinary concentration of creatinine in mg/dl
P_{Cr} = plasma concentration of creatinine in mg/dl

Misleading results are occasionally obtained when (1) residual urine that has remained in the bladder for several hours is used; (2) a diuretic has been administered; (3) there is preexisting chronic renal disease; or (4) there is intermittent urinary tract obstruction.

Examination of the urine sediment may also be helpful in the differential diagnosis of ARF. In prerenal azotemia, the urine sediment is essentially normal with a few hyaline casts; brown, granular casts and many epithelial cells are likely to be present in ATN. Prerenal azotemia is fairly easy to exclude on the basis of the clinical setting and the urine chemistry. However, urine chemistry may not be helpful in differentiating postrenal obstruction from ATN and other criteria must be used.

Prevention of ATN in patients at high risk or those with prerenal azotemia or oliguria is an important therapeutic consideration. Correction of circulatory insufficiency and the resulting renal hypoperfusion is important in preventing the progression of prerenal oliguria to ATN. Blood transfusion to replace any losses and hydration with intravenous fluids may be successful in restoring circulation and increased urine output. Mannitol and furosemide have sometimes been successful in inducing diuresis and reducing the risk of oliguric ATN.

Harter and Martin (1982) suggest the following approach. After careful assessment of ECF volume and cardiac function (to exclude ECF volume excess), give 500 ml of intravenous normal saline rapidly to exclude prerenal oliguria. If urine output is unchanged, mannitol, 25 g, is given slowly IV, followed by furosemide, 80 to 320 mg IV. If diuresis occurs (urine output >40 ml/hr), these doses may be repeated every 3 to 4 hours to maintain high urine flow rates. If this regimen is unsuccessful (urine output still <30 ml/hr), established ATN probably exists.

In established ATN the period of oliguria may last no longer than a day or it may last as long as 6 weeks. The average duration of the oliguria is from 7 to 10 days. During the oliguric phase, the usual rise in BUN level is 25 to 30 mg/dl daily and creatinine rises at the rate of about 2.5 mg/dl daily. The retention of fluids, electrolytes, and nitrogenous substances causes the rapid development of uremic symptoms.

Diuretic Stage

The diuretic stage of acute renal failure begins when the urine output increases to more than 400 ml/day. This stage generally lasts 2 to 3 weeks. Daily urine output rarely exceeds 4 L, provided the patient is not overhydrated. The high urine volume of the diuretic phase is caused partly by the osmotic diuresis produced by the high blood urea concentration and partly by the impaired ability of the recovering tubules to conserve filtered salts and water. During the diuretic phase, patients may develop deficits of potassium, sodium, and water. If the urinary losses are not replaced, death may end the diuresis. During the early diuretic stage, the BUN level may continue to rise, largely because urea clearance does not keep up with endogenous urea production. As the diuresis continues, however, the azotemia gradually disappears and there is great clinical improvement.

Recovery Stage

The recovery stage of acute renal failure lasts as long as a year, during which time the anemia and concentrating ability of the kidneys gradually improve. Some patients, however, are left with a permanent reduction in the GFR.

Even though damage to tubular epithelium is theoretically reversible, ATN is a dangerous condition with a serious prognosis. The mortality is still about 50% (down from a previous rate of about 90% three decades ago) despite the most careful management of fluid and electrolyte balance and the aid of dialysis. About two thirds of those with ATN die during the oliguric stage and about one third during the diuretic stage. Mortality is related to the causal background of the associated illnesses leading up to the acute episode. Mortality is about 60% in cases after surgery, crush injuries, and other major trauma, about 25% after incompatible blood transfusions and carbon tetrachloride poisoning, and 10% to 15% in obstetric cases. In general, patients with nonoliguric ARF have a better prognosis than those with oliguric ARF: only about 25% of the former die.

TREATMENT OF ESTABLISHED ACUTE TUBULAR NECROSIS

After the diagnosis of ATN is established, the primary consideration in management is the maintenance of fluid and electrolyte balance. The same principles of conservative management that were discussed in the treatment of chronic renal failure also apply to acute renal failure. The early use of hemodialysis to prevent severe fluid and electrolyte imbalance and uremic symptoms has undoubtedly reduced the mortality. Careful attention to fluid and electrolyte balance is necessary not only during the oliguric stage, but also during the diuretic stage, when severe sodium and potassium depletion may occur. The most frequent complication in acute renal failure resulting in death is infection. It is the contributing cause of death in about 70% of patients and the primary cause in about 30%. Not only is the uremic patient more susceptible to infection, but once it is established, it is more difficult to control. The presence of infection may go unrecognized because of the lack of the usual symptom of fever, since hypothermia is common in renal failure. Once infection is identified, it should be treated with non-nephrotoxic antibiotics.

QUESTIONS

▼ *Answer the following on a separate sheet of paper.*

1. Why is it particularly hazardous to use organic solvents (containing CCl_4) and drink an alcoholic beverage at the same time?

2. List the two major mechanisms of renal injury in acute intrinsic renal failure.

3. What is meant by acute-on-chronic renal failure? What are the precipitating causes?

4. What is the difference between the two types of histologic lesion commonly observed in ATN? What is the common cause?

5. What is acute cortical necrosis? List the common causes, complications, and prognosis.

6. What is the most common complication resulting in death in acute renal failure?

7. What is the advantage of considering the causes of acute renal failure under the prerenal, postrenal, and renal diagnostic categories?

8. List examples of common conditions causing obstructive uropathy at the level of the bladder outlet, ureters, and kidneys.

9. Name one penicillin and three aminoglycoside antibiotics that are frequently the cause of nephrotoxic acute renal failure. What are the characteristics of patients at high risk?

10. Name and briefly describe five factors suggested as contributing to the pathogenesis of acute renal failure.

11. What is the most sensitive laboratory test in differentiating prerenal azotemia from established acute renal failure? By what formula is it calculated? Name some circumstances that may cause misleading laboratory test results.

12. Name two drugs commonly given in an attempt to correct prerenal oliguria and prevent progression to establish acute renal failure.

▼ *Circle the letter preceding each item below that correctly answers the question or completes the statement. Only one answer is correct, with exceptions noted:*

13. Acute renal failure usually refers to the sudden cessation of renal function resulting in urine output of less than:
    a. 800 ml/day
    b. 1200 ml/day
    c. 400 ml/day

14. In ATN, proximal tubular epithelial damage associated with CCl_4 or $HgCl_2$ poisoning (mild exposure) usually results in:
    a. Irreversible renal failure with infarction of the entire nephron
    b. Complete healing of the lesion in 3 to 4 weeks

15. Acute tubular necrosis may result from:

(More than one answer may be correct.)
    a. Exposure to nephrotoxic chemicals
    b. Obstruction of the ureteropelvic junction
    c. Hyperkalemia
    d. Massive crush injuries
    e. Excessive sodium restriction
    f. Prolonged shock

16. Which of the following will not cause necrosis of the tubular epithelial cells?
    a. CCl_4
    b. Severe acute renal ischemia
    c. Transfusion reactions
    d. Mercuric ions
    e. Diodrast (x-ray contrast medium)

17. Which of the following statements is true concerning the treatment and differentiation of prerenal azotemia and established ATN? (More than one answer may be correct.)
    a. Oliguric urine is concentrated in established ATN.
    b. The urine/plasma osmolality ratio is greater than 2:1 in prerenal azotemia.
    c. The urine/plasma urea concentration is less than 1 in established ATN.
    d. The correction of circulatory insufficiency by blood and IV administration of fluids may prevent the progress of prerenal azotemia to ATN.
    e. The administration of IV mannitol will correct established ATN.

QUESTIONS—cont'd

18. The risk of radiographic contrast media–induced acute renal failure is increased by: (More than one answer may be correct.)
    a. Age >60 years
    b. Dehydration
    c. Diabetes mellitus
    d. Plasma creatinine >2.0 mg/dl
    e. Double dose of contrast medium
19. Sudden deterioration of renal function in a person with diabetes mellitus suggests:
    a. Renal calculi
    b. Acute poststreptococcal glomerulonephritis
    c. Chronic pyelonephritis
    d. Papillary necrosis
20. Which of the following conditions is suggested by complete anuria for more than 48 hours?
    a. Severe prerenal azotemia
    b. Acute-on-chronic renal failure
    c. Nephrotoxic antibiotic-induced renal failure
    d. Bilateral renal artery or renal vein occlusion
21. Which of the following statements is incorrect regarding nonoliguric acute renal failure?
    a. Urine volume is >400 ml/day
    b. Tubular damage is generally less severe than in oliguric ARF
    c. Azotemia is absent
    d. It is commonly induced by nephrotoxic antibiotics

22. Mortality is less in nonoliguric than in oliguric ARF but still about:
    a. 10%
    b. 25%
    c. 35%
    d. 50%
23. Which of the following findings is most consistent with ATN?
    a. Urinary Na, 50 mEq/L
    b. U/P creatinine ratio, 70
    c. Urinary sediment, a few hyaline casts
    d. Fe_{Na}, 0.8%
    e. U/P osmolality ratio, 2:1

▼ *Circle T if the statement is true and F if it is false. Give reasons for your answer.*

24. T F   Progressive azotemia is a defining characteristic of nonoliguric acute renal failure.
25. T F   In acute arterial hypotension, re-

nal cortical blood flow increases from about 10% to about 80% to 90% whereas renal medullary blood flow decreases by the same percentage.
26. T F   Nephrotoxic ARF induced by CCl_4 is potentiated by the ingestion of ethyl alcohol.
27. T F   Rhabdomyolysis results in the release of large amounts of Tamm-Horsfall protein into the urine, inducing ARF.
28. T F   Anuria alternating with episodes of polyuria suggests ARF from prerenal causes.
29. T F   During prerenal oliguria the BUN usually increases faster than serum creatinine because of greater back diffusion and catabolism of body protein.

▼ *Match the stage in the clinical course of acute renal failure in column B with the statement that best applies to it in column A.*

Column A	Column B
30. _____ Azotemia gradually subsides in this stage.	a. Oliguric stage
31. _____ Concentrating ability of the kidneys gradually improves during this stage (may last up to 1 year).	b. Diuretic stage
32. _____ BUN may rise 25 to 30 mg/dl daily during this stage.	c. Recovery stage
33. _____ Average duration is 7 to 10 days.	
34. _____ Most deaths occur during this stage.	
35. _____ Most common complications during this stage are hyperkalemia, pulmonary edema, and cardiac failure.	
36. _____ About one third of the deaths occur during this stage.	

BIBLIOGRAPHY ▼ PART VIII

Badr KF, Brenner BM: Vascular injury to the kidney. In Isselbacher KJ et al, editors: *Harrison's principles of internal medicine,* ed 13, New York, 1994, McGraw-Hill.

Ballerman BJ, Zeidel ML, Gunning ME, Brenner BM: Vasoactive peptides and the kidney. In Brenner BM, Rector FC, editors: *The kidney,* ed 4, Philadelphia, 1991, WB Saunders.

Bennet WM et al: Tubulointerstitial disease and toxic nephropathy. In Brenner BM, Rector FC, editors: *The kidney,* ed 4, Philadelphia, 1991, WB Saunders.

Bosch JP, Stein JH: *Contemporary issues in nephrology: hemodialysis: high efficiency treatments,* New York, 1993, Churchill Livingstone.

Brenner BM, Myer TW, Hostetter TH: Dietary protein intake and the progressive nature of kidney disease, *N Engl J Med* 307:652, 1982.

Brenner BM, Rector FC: *The kidney,* vols I and II, ed 4, Philadelphia, 1991, WB Saunders.

Bricker NS, Fine LG: On the meaning of the intact nephron hypothesis, *Am J Med* 46:1, 1969.

Carpenter CB, Lazarus JM: Dialysis and transplantation in the treatment of renal failure. In Isselbacher KJ et al, editors: *Harrison's principles of internal medicine,* ed 13, New York, 1994, McGraw-Hill.

Cimino JE, Brescia MJ: Simple venipuncture for hemodialysis, *N Engl J Med* 267:608, 1962.

Coe FL, Favus MJ: Nephrolithiasis. In Isselbacher KJ et al, editors: *Harrison's principles of internal medicine,* ed 13, New York, 1994, McGraw-Hill.

Coe FL, Kathpalia S: Hereditary tubular disorders. In Isselbacher KJ et al, editors: *Harrison's principles of internal medicine,* ed 13, New York, 1994, McGraw-Hill.

Continued.

BIBLIOGRAPHY ▼ PART VIII

Conlin PR, Dluhy RG, Williams GH: Disorders of the renin-angiotensin-aldosterone system. In Schrier RW, editor: *Renal and electrolyte disorders,* ed 4, Boston, 1992, Little, Brown.

Cotran RS, Rubin RH, Tolkoff-Rubin NE: Tubulointerstitial diseases. In Brenner BM, Rector FC, editors: *The kidney,* vol II, ed 3, Philadelphia, 1986, WB Saunders.

D'Amico G: The commonest glomerulonephritis in the world: IgA nephropathy, *Q J Med* 64:709-727, 1987.

Diabetes Control and Complications Trial Research Group: Effects of intensive treatment of diabetes on the development and progression of long-term complications in insulin-dependent diabetes mellitus, *N Engl J Med* 329:977, 1993.

Dunfee TP: The changing management of diabetic nephropathy, *Hosp Med* 30(5):45-55, 1995.

Dunn MJ, editor: *Renal endocrinology,* Baltimore, 1983, Williams & Wilkins.

Eschbach JW, Egrie JC, Downing MR: Correction of anemia of ESRD with recombinant human erythropoietin, *N Engl J Med* 316:73, 1987.

Fine LG: The uremic syndrome: adaptive mechanisms and therapy, *Hosp Pract* 22(9):63-73, 1987.

Fitzsimmons SC, Agodoa L, Striker L, et al: Kidney disease of diabetes mellitus, *Am J Kidney Dis* 13(1):7-10, 1989.

Friedman EA: *Strategy in renal failure,* New York, 1978, John Wiley & Sons.

Gault MH et al: Syndrome associated with the abuse of analgesics, *Ann Int Med* 68:906-925, 1968.

Giordano C: Early diet to slow the course of chronic renal failure. Presented at Eighth International Congress of Nephrology. In Zurukzoglu W, editor: *Advances in basic and clinical nephrology,* Basel, Switzerland, Sept 1981.

Glassock RJ: The pathophysiology of acute glomerulonephritis, *Hosp Pract* 23(2):163-178, 1987.

Glassock RJ: The glomerulopathies. In Schrier RW, editor: *Renal and electrolyte disorders,* ed 4, Boston, 1992, Little, Brown.

Glassock R, Adler S, Ward H, Cohen A: Primary glomerular diseases. In Brenner BM, Rector FC, editors: *The kidney,* ed 4, Philadelphia, 1991, WB Saunders.

Glassock RJ, Brenner BM: The major glomerulopathies. In Isselbacher KJ et al, editors: *Harrison's principles of internal medicine,* ed 13, New York, 1994, McGraw-Hill.

Gutch GF: *Review of hemodialysis for nurses and dialysis personnel,* ed 5, St Louis, 1993, Mosby.

Harter HR, Martin KJ: Acute renal failure, *Postgrad Med* 72(6):175-197, 1982.

Hooten TM: A simplified approach to urinary tract infection, *Hosp Pract* 30(2):23-30, 1995.

Hutchinson I: Transplantation and rejection. In Roitt I, Brostoff J, Male D: *Immunology,* ed 3, St Louis, 1993, Mosby.

Jacobs K, Shoemaker C, Rudersdorf R, et al: Isolation and characterization of genomic and cDNA clones of human erythropoietin, *Nature* 313:806-810, 1985.

Jacobson HR, Striker GE, Klahr S: *The principles and practice of nephrology,* ed 2, St Louis, 1995, Mosby.

Kass EH: Bacteriuria and pyelonephritis of pregnancy, *Arch Intern Med* 105:194, 1960.

Kunin CM: *Detection, prevention, and management of urinary tract infections,* ed 3, Philadelphia, 1987, Lea & Febiger.

Lapides J: *Fundamentals of urology,* Philadelphia, 1976, WB Saunders.

Levinsky NG, Rettig RA: Special report: the Medicare end stage renal disease program: a report from the Institute of Medicine, *N Engl J Med* 324:1143-1148, 1991.

Lewis SL: Fever: thermal regulation and alterations in end-stage renal disease patients. *ANNA J* 19(1):13-18, 1992.

Lin FK, Suggs S, Lin CH, et al: Cloning and expression of the human erythropoietin gene, *Proc Nat Acad Sci USA* 87:7580-7584, 1985.

Massry SG, Glassock RJ, editors: *Textbook of nephrology,* Baltimore, 1995, Williams & Wilkins.

Merrill JP: Acute renal failure. In Strauss MB, Welt LG, editors: *Diseases of the kidney,* ed 2, Boston, 1971, Little, Brown.

Mitch WE: Dietary protein restriction in patients with chronic renal failure, *Kidney Int* 40:326-341, 1991.

Mitch WE, Klahr S: *Nutrition and the kidney,* Boston, 1988, Little, Brown.

Murray TG, Goldberg M: Analgesic-associated nephropathy in the USA: epidemiologic, clinical, and pathogenetic features, *Kidney Int* 13:64, 1978.

Narins RG: *Maxwell & Kleeman's clinical disorders of fluid and electrolyte metabolism,* ed 5, New York, 1994, McGraw-Hill.

Netter FH: Kidneys, ureters, and urinary bladder. In *The Ciba collection of medical illustrations,* vol 6, West Caldwell, NJ, 1973, Ciba Medical Education Division.

Nolan CR, Schrier RW: The kidney in hypertension. In Schrier RW, editor: *Renal and electrolyte disorders,* ed 4, Boston, 1992, Little, Brown.

Nolan MT, Augustine SM: *Transplantation nursing: acute and long-term management,* Norwalk, Conn, 1995, Appleton & Lange.

Norden CW, Kass EH: Bacteriuria of pregnancy—a critical appraisal, *Ann Rev Med* 19:431-470, 1968.

Oldrizzi L, Rugiu C, Valvo E: The progression of renal failure in patients with renal disease of diverse etiology on protein-restricted diet, *Kidney Int* 27:553-557, 1985.

Opelz G: HLA matching should be utilized for improving kidney transplant success rates, *Transplant Proc* 23:46, 1991.

Opelz G, Terasaki PL: Improvement of kidney graft survival with increased number of blood transfusions, *N Engl J Med* 299:799, 1978.

Papper S: *Clinical nephrology,* ed 2, Boston, 1978, Little, Brown.

Pitts RF: *Physiology of the kidney and body fluids,* ed 3, Chicago, 1974, Mosby.

Quinton W, Dillard D, Scribner DH: Cannulation of blood vessels for prolonged hemodialysis, *Trans Am Soc Artific Intern Organs* 6:104-109, 1960.

Raja RM, Fernandes M, Kramer MS: Comparison of subclavian vein with femoral vein catheterization for hemodialysis, *Am J Kidney Dis* 2:474, 1984.

Roitt I, Brostoff J, Male D: *Immunology,* ed 3, St Louis, 1993, Mosby.

Rose BD: *The pathophysiology of renal failure,* ed 2, New York, 1987, McGraw-Hill.

Rose BD, Black RM: *Manual of clinical problems in nephrology,* Boston, 1988, Little, Brown.

BIBLIOGRAPHY ▼ PART VIII

Rose BD, Rennke HG: *Renal pathophysiology: the essentials,* Baltimore, 1994, Williams & Wilkins.

Rubin RH, Tolkoff-Rubin NE, Cotran RS: Urinary tract infection, pyelonephritis, and reflux nephropathy. In Brenner BM, Rector FC, editors: *The kidney,* vol II, ed 4, Philadelphia, 1991, WB Saunders.

Ruiz P et al: Impaired function of macrophage Fc-gamma receptors in end-stage renal disease, *N Engl J Med* 322(11):717-722, 1990.

Sandler DP et al: Analgesic abuse and chronic renal disease, *N Engl J Med* 320:1238, 1989.

Salvatierra O Jr, Vincent F, Amend W, et al: Deliberate donor-specific blood transfusions prior to living related renal transplantation, *Ann Surg* 192:543, 1980.

Schrapner HW, Robson AM: Nephrotic syndrome: minimal change disease, focal glomerulosclerosis, and related disorders. In Schrier RW, Gottschalk CW, editors: *Diseases of the kidney,* ed 5, Boston, 1993, Little, Brown.

Schrier RW, editor: *Renal and electrolyte disorders,* ed 4, Boston, 1992, Little, Brown.

Schrier RW: *Manual of nephrology,* ed 4, Boston, 1995, Little, Brown.

Schrier RW, Gottschalk CW, editors: *Diseases of the kidney,* ed 5, Boston, 1993, Little, Brown.

Stamm WE: Urinary tract infections and pyelonephritis. In Isselbacher KJ et al, editors: *Harrison's principles of internal medicine,* ed 13, New York, 1994, McGraw-Hill.

Terasaki PL, Bernoco D, Park MS, et al: Microdroplet testing for HLA-A, -B, -C, and -D antigens, *Am J Clin Pathol* 69:103, 1978.

Thompson C: The spectrum of renal cystic diseases, *Hosp Pract* 23(4):165-175, 1988.

Tolkoff-Rubin NE, Rubin RE: Uremia and host defense, *N Engl J Med* 322(11):770-772, 1990.

US Renal Data System: *USRDS 1991 annual data report,* Bethesda, Md, 1991, National Institutes of Health.

US Renal Data System: USRDS 1993 annual data report, Bethesda, Md, March 1993, The National Institutes of Health, National Institute of Diabetes and Digestive and Kidney Diseases.

Vander AJ: *Renal physiology,* ed 4, New York, 1991, McGraw-Hill.

Whalley P: Bacteriuria in pregnancy, *Am J Obstet Gynecol* 97:723-738, 1967.

Working Group in Renovascular Hypertension: Detection, evaluation, and treatment of renovascular hypertension: final report, *Arch Int Med* 147:820, 1987.

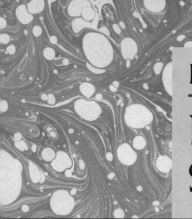

PART NINE

NEUROLOGIC SYSTEM DISORDERS

More than 200 clinical syndromes associated with dysfunction, disease, and injury of the nervous system are recognized. The clinical manifestations of disease involving the nervous system are perhaps the most complex and intriguing in all of medicine. Signs and symptoms of these diseases vary in type and range from relatively simple, objective, and easily elicited signs to complex and highly individualized signs.

Only a small number of neurologic disorders are presented in this part of the text. It begins with a concise overview of neuroanatomy, since accurate diagnosis and treatment usually depend on the localization of the disorder within the nervous system. For health care professionals to respond to the patient with a neurologic disorder in an intelligent, empathetic, and therapeutic manner, a working knowledge of neuroanatomy is essential. ▼

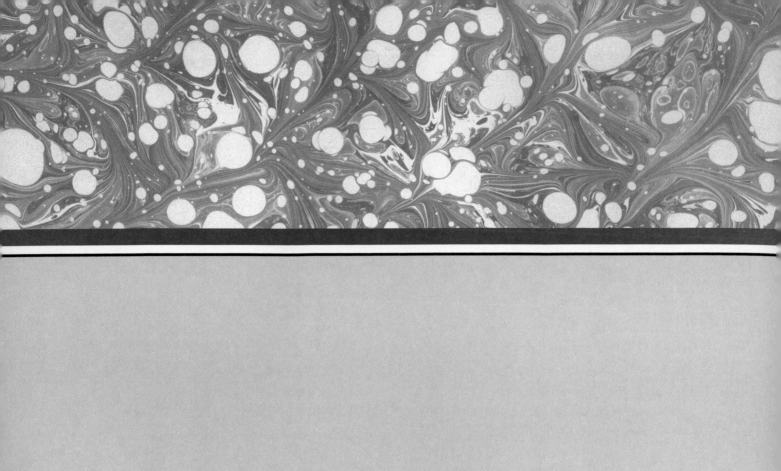

CHAPTER 50

Anatomy and Physiology of the Nervous System

LORRAINE M. WILSON
MARY S. HARTWIG

The human nervous system is a complex, highly specialized, interconnected network of neural tissue. It coordinates, interprets, and controls the interactions between the individual and the surrounding environment. This important body system also regulates the activities of most of the other body systems. The body is able to function as a harmonious unit because of the neural regulation of communications among the various systems. The phenomena of consciousness, thought, memory, language, sensation, and movement all originate within this system. Thus the ability to comprehend, learn, and respond to stimuli is a result of the integrated functioning of the nervous system, which culminates in the personality and behavior of the individual.

OVERVIEW OF THE HUMAN NERVOUS SYSTEM

This chapter provides a brief overview of selected anatomic and physiologic concepts concerning neural tissue. The constraints and the focus of this textbook do not permit an extensive coverage of this material. Readers are urged to seek the references given at the end of Part Nine to review and expand their knowledge of the nervous system.

The nervous system consists of nerve cells (neurons) and supporting cells (neuroglia and Schwann cells) so correlated and integrated that they function as a single unit. *Neurons* are the specialized excitable cells of the nervous system that receive the *sensory*, or *afferent*, input from specialized endings of the peripheral nerves or sensory receptor organs and transmit the *motor*, or *efferent*, output to muscles and glands, the effector organs. Certain neurons, called *interneurons*, have the sole function of receiving and transmitting neural data to other neurons. These interneurons, also called *association neurons*, are especially numerous in the gray matter of the spinal cord, where their interconnections are responsible for the many integrative functions of the spinal cord. *Neuroglia* provide support, protection, and nutrients for the neurons of the brain and spinal cord. *Schwann cells* protect and support the other neurons and neuronal processes outside the central nervous system.

The nervous system is divided into the central nervous system (CNS) and the peripheral nervous system (PNS). The brain and spinal cord constitute the CNS. The PNS is composed of the afferent and efferent neurons of the somatic nervous system and neurons of the autonomic (or visceral) nervous system.

The CNS is encased by the bones of the skull and vertebral column. It is further protected by suspension in cerebrospinal fluid (CSF), which is produced within the ventricles (cavities) of the brain. The CNS is also covered by three layers of tissue collectively referred to as the *meninges* (dura mater, arachnoid, and pia mater).

The brain is divided into the forebrain, midbrain, and hindbrain on the basis of embryologic development. These categories are further subdivided on the basis of anatomic organization of the mature brain (see box on p. 771). The midbrain, pons, and medulla oblongata together are called the *brain stem*.

The spinal cord is a single continuous structure that extends from the medulla oblongata through the foramen magnum of the skull and down the vertebral column to the lower level of the first lumbar vertebra (L1) in adults. The spinal cord is divided into 31 segments, from which originate the 31 pairs of spinal nerves. These segments are named after the vertebrae corresponding to the exit

site for the associated nerve roots, thus giving rise to the cervical, thoracic, lumbar, and sacral divisions of the spinal cord (Fig. 50-1).

The PNS is divided anatomically into 31 pairs of spinal nerves and 12 pairs of cranial nerves. A *peripheral nerve* may consist of neurons relaying afferent (sensory) neural messages toward the CNS and/or relaying efferent (motor) neural messages from the CNS. The spinal nerves carry both afferent and efferent neural messages and are thus called *mixed nerves*. The cranial nerves arise from the surface of the brain; five pairs are motor, three pairs are sensory, and four pairs are mixed nerves. Functionally, the PNS is divided into the somatic nervous system and the autonomic nervous system.

The *somatic nervous system* (SNS) is composed of mixed nerves. The afferents convey conscious and unconscious sensory information (e.g., pain, temperature, touch, conscious and unconscious proprioception, vision, taste, hearing, smell) from the head, body wall, and extremities. The efferents are involved primarily with the skeletal musculature of the body. The SNS is concerned with interaction and response to the external environment.

The *autonomic nervous system* (ANS) is a mixed ner-

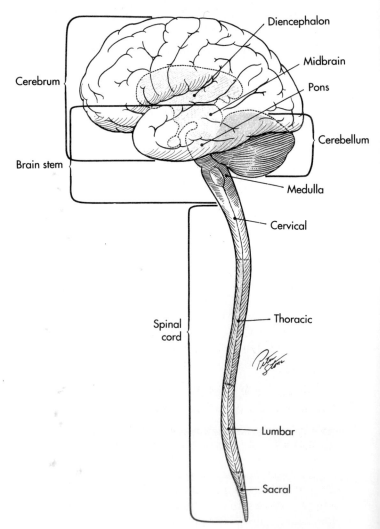

FIG. 50-1 Lateral view of the central nervous system. (From Langley LL, Telford JR, Christensen JB: *Dynamic anatomy and physiology,* ed 5, New York, 1980, McGraw-Hill.)

THE FIVE MAJOR SUBDIVISIONS OF THE BRAIN*

Telencephalon (endbrain)
  Cerebral hemispheres
    Cerebral cortex
    Rhinencephalon ("nosebrain"); limbic system
    Basal ganglia
      Caudate
      Lenticular (putamen, globus pallidus)
      Claustrum
      Amygdala
Diencephalon (interbrain)
  Epithalamus
  Thalamus
  Subthalamus
  Hypothalamus
Mesencephalon (midbrain)
  Corpus quadrigemina
    Superior colliculus
    Inferior colliculus
  Tegmentum
    Red nucleus
    Substantia nigra
  Cerebral peduncles
Metencephalon (afterbrain)
  Pons
  Cerebellum
Myelencephalon (marrow brain)
  Medulla oblongata

*The *prosencephalon* (forebrain) = telencephalon + diencephalon; the *rhombencephalon* = metencephalon + myelencephalon.

▶ TABLE 50-1   Autonomic Effects on Various Organs

Effector Organ	Effect of Sympathetic Stimulation	Effect of Parasympathetic Stimulation
Eye		
Pupil	Dilation (mydriasis)	Contraction (miosis)
Ciliary muscle	Relaxation (far vision)	Contraction (near vision)
Glands of head		
Lacrimal	Decreased secretion	Stimulation of secretion
Nasopharyngeal	Decreased secretion	Stimulation of secretion
Salivary	Scanty, viscous secretion	Profuse, watery secretion
Heart	Increased rate	Decreased rate
	Increased conduction velocity	Decreased conduction velocity
	Increased force of beat	Decreased force of beat
Blood vessels*		
Coronary	Vasodilation	Minimal
Skeletal muscle	Vasodilation	Minimal
Abdominal viscera	Vasoconstriction	Minimal
Cutaneous	Vasoconstriction	Minimal
Blood		
Coagulation	Increased	
Glucose	Increased	
Free fatty acids	Increased	
Lungs	Bronchodilation	Bronchoconstriction
Gut		
Lumen	Decreased peristalsis and tone	Increased peristalsis and tone
Sphincters	Increased tone (usually contraction)	Decreased tone (usually relaxation)
Secretions	Possible inhibition	Stimulation
Liver	Glycogenolysis	
Gallbladder and ducts	Inhibition of contraction	Stimulation of contraction
Adrenal medulla	Secretion of epinephrine and norepinephrine	
Bladder muscle	Relaxation (usually)	Contraction
Sex organs	Ejaculation	Erection
Sweat glands	Stimulation of certain sweat glands	
Pilomotor muscles	Contraction	
Adipose tissue	Lipolysis	

*Effects of sympathetic stimulation depend on whether alpha$_1$-adrenergic receptors (vasoconstriction) or beta$_2$-adrenergic receptors (vasodilation) are stimulated.

vous system. Its afferent fibers carry input from visceral organs (concerning the regulation of heart rate, blood vessel diameter, respiration, digestion, hunger, nausea, elimination, etc.). The motor efferents of the ANS innervate smooth muscle, cardiac muscle, and glands of the viscera. The ANS regulates primarily visceral functions and interactions with the internal environment.

The two divisions of the ANS are the parasympathetic autonomic nervous system (PANS) and the sympathetic autonomic nervous system (SANS). The *sympathetic division* leaves the CNS from the thoracic and lumbar (thoracolumbar) regions of the spinal cord; the *parasympathetic division* leaves from the brain (via components of cranial nerves) and the sacral portion (craniosacral) of the spinal cord. The SANS increases heart and respiratory rates and decreases activity of the gastrointestinal (GI) tract. Its primary focus is to prepare the body for stress, the so-called fight-or-flight responses. In contrast, the PANS decreases heart and respiratory rates and increases GI motility as needed for digestion and elimination; it aids in conservation and homeostasis of body functions. Table 50-1 lists some of the important functions of the sympathetic and parasympathetic divisions of the ANS.

NEURAL TISSUE

Neuroglia, Schwann Cells, and Myelin

Neuroglia are the supporting cells for the neurons of the CNS, whereas Schwann cells have this function in the PNS. The neuroglia compose about 40% of the volume of the brain and spinal cord. They outnumber the neurons approximately 10:1. Four distinct neuroglial cell types have been identified: microglia, ependymal cells, astroglia, and oligodendroglia (Fig. 50-2).

Microglia have phagocytic properties; when nervous tissue is damaged, these cells ingest and digest tissue debris. They are found throughout the CNS and also have a role in fighting infection. These cells have properties similar to those of histiocytes (macrophages) found in peripheral connective tissue.

Ependymal cells (or *ependymocytes*) are involved in the production of CSF. They are the neuroglia that line the ventricular system of the CNS. These cells provide the epithelial lining (ependyma) of the choroid plexus of the cerebral ventricles.

Astroglia (or *astrocytes*) provide essential nutrients to neurons and assist neurons in maintaining the proper bioelectrical potentials for impulse conduction and synaptic transmission. Astroglia have star-shaped cell bodies with multiple processes. Because many of the astrocyte processes terminate on blood vessels as perivascular "feet" or foot processes, they are thought to be involved

in a system of rapid transport of metabolites. The role of astrocytes in preventing certain substances from passing from the blood vessels to neural tissue, the *blood-brain barrier,* is yet to be determined. It was formerly believed that the foot processes surrounding the capillary wall functioned as the major blood-brain barrier. Most authorities presently believe that the tight junctions between the endothelial cells of the blood capillaries are primarily responsible for the blood-brain barrier (Fig. 50-3).

Another important barrier to passage of substances into the brain is the *blood–cerebrospinal fluid barrier,* which exists because of the secretory function of the choroid plexus. The blood-CSF barrier is formed by tight junctions between the cuboidal epithelial cells of the choroid plexus in the ventricles, which actively secrete CSF (Fig. 50-4), and not at the choroid capillaries, which are fenestrated. The ependymal lining of the ventricles and the pia-glial surface of the brain do not impede exchanges between CSF and brain. Thus the CSF may serve as a channel for intracerebral transport.

The primary role of the blood-brain and blood-CSF barriers is to provide control systems that regulate and maintain an optimal, stable chemical environment for the neurons of the CNS. In general, the barriers are highly permeable to water, oxygen (O_2), carbon dioxide (CO_2), glucose, and essential amino acids and are less permeable to electrolytes such as sodium (Na^+), chloride (Cl^-), and potassium (K^+) ions. The barriers are relatively impermeable to macromolecules such as proteins, hexoses

FIG. 50-2   Diagrammatic representation of the arrangement of different types of neuroglial cells. Note that there are two types of astrocyte. *Fibrous* astrocytes are found mainly in white matter, whereas *protoplasmic* astrocytes are found in gray matter. [From Snell RS: *Clinical neuroanatomy,* ed 3, Boston, 1992, Little, Brown.]

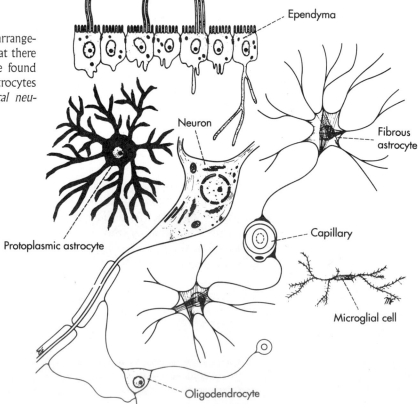

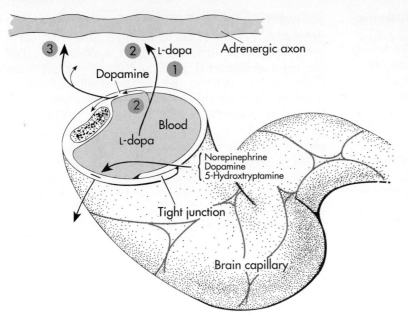

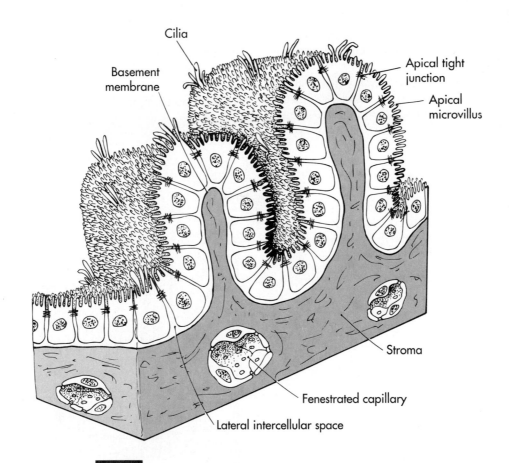

FIG. 50-3   Diagram of a brain capillary demonstrating a tight junction between endothelial cells that constitute the blood-brain barrier. The endothelial cells of brain capillaries contain enzymes that regulate the specific transport of brain biogenic amines (norepinephrine; dopamine; 5-hydroxytryptamine [5-HT], or serotonin; amino acids). Levodopa (L-dopa), an amino acid precursor of dopamine used in the treatment of Parkinson's disease, passes the blood-brain barrier *(1)*, is decarboxylated in the capillary endothelium *(2)*, and enters neural tissue *(3)*, where it is degraded by monoamine oxidase. Decarboxylation of L-dopa to dopamine *(2)* also takes place after its incorporation into axonal varicosities of aminergic neurons. (Redrawn from Carpenter MB: *Core text of neuroanatomy,* ed 4, Baltimore, 1991, Williams & Wilkins.)

FIG. 50-4   Blood–cerebrospinal fluid (CSF) barrier. Diagram of a choroid plexus villus covered by a single layer of cuboidal epithelium, with apical microvilli protruding into the CSF of the ventricles. The blood-CSF barrier is formed by the apical tight junctions between the epithelial cells. The choroid capillaries in the underlying connective tissue are fenestrated.
(Redrawn from Carpenter MB: *Core text of neuroanatomy,* ed 4, Baltimore, 1991, Williams & Wilkins.)

other than glucose, free fatty acids, many drugs, and toxic substances.

In newborns, when these barriers are not fully developed, toxic substances such as bilirubin can readily enter the CNS, causing a condition called *kernicterus* (see Chapter 27). Any injury to the brain, whether from trauma, inflammation, or toxins, causes a breakdown of the blood-brain barrier, allowing free diffusion of large molecules into the nervous tissue.

When neurons die as a result of injury, astrocytes proliferate and fill in the space formerly occupied by the nerve cell body and its processes, an activity known as *replacement gliosis* (see following comments on nerve cell damage). When extensive destruction of CNS tissue occurs, a cavity may be formed that becomes lined with astrocytes.

Oligodendroglia (or *oligondendrocytes*) are the glial cells responsible for myelin production within the CNS. Each oligodendroglion surrounds several neurons, and its plasma membrane wraps around the neuronal processes to form the myelin sheath. The Schwann cells form the myelin in the PNS.

Tumors of the neuroglia are referred to as *gliomas* and account for 40% to 50% of intracranial tumors (see Chapter 57).

Myelin is a white lipid-protein complex that insulates the nerve process. When present, it almost completely prevents the flow of Na$^+$ and K$^+$ ions across the neuronal membrane. Myelin is not continuous along the nerve processes, and the intervals where it is absent are called the *nodes of Ranvier* (Fig. 50-5). Nerve processes in the CNS and PNS may or may not be myelinated. Nerve fibers with myelin sheaths are called *myelinated fibers* and within the CNS are called *white matter.* Fibers that have no myelin are called *nonmyelinated fibers* and are present within the *gray matter* of the CNS. Transmission of nerve impulses along myelinated fibers is faster than along nonmyelinated fibers, since the impulses travel, or "jump," from node to node along the myelin sheath; this is known as *saltatory conduction.*

Schwann cells form the myelin and the neurilemma of peripheral nerves (Fig. 50-5). The plasma membrane of Schwann cells concentrically wraps around nerve processes of the neurons in the PNS to form the myelin sheath. Not all neurons of the PNS are myelinated. The *neurilemma* is a delicate cytoplasmic membrane formed by Schwann cells that wraps around all PNS neurons (myelinated and nonmyelinated). The neurilemma provides structural support and protection for the nerve processes.

When there is damage to a nerve cell process in the PNS, a potential exists for regeneration of the nerve fiber. A complex series of degenerative and regenerative changes occurs along the damaged area as long as the cell

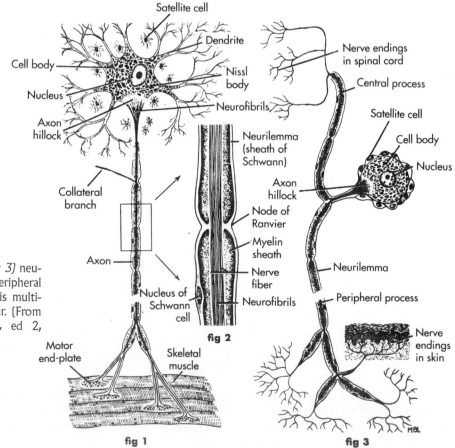

FIG. 50-5   Motor *[fig 1]* and sensory *[fig 3]* neurons. *Fig 2,* Structure of a myelinated peripheral nerve. The motor neuron illustrated here is multipolar, and the sensory neuron is unipolar. [From Crouch JE: *Functional human anatomy,* ed 2, Philadelphia, 1972, Lea & Febiger.]

body is still viable. When possible, the neurilemma regenerates along its original course, and a new process sprouts and grows within the neurilemma from the cell body of the damaged neuron.

No neurilemma exists in the CNS; and thus little or no regenerative potential exists for damaged central neuronal processes. The damaged areas of the CNS neurons are filled with glial cells (primarily astrocytes) through the process of replacement gliosis. A gliotic scar after brain injury may result in focal epilepsy (see Chapter 55).

Neurons

A *neuron* is a nerve cell and is the basic anatomic and functional unit of the nervous system (Fig. 50-5). Each neuron has a cell body that gives rise to one or more processes. *Dendrites* are processes that conduct information toward the cell body. The single long process that conducts information away from the cell body is called an *axon.* Dendrites and axons are often referred to, collectively, as *nerve fibers* or *nerve processes.* The ability to receive, convey, and transmit neural messages is a result of the specialized neuronal cell membrane properties of excitability and electrical-chemical conductivity. The human nervous system is composed of approximately 10^{11} neurons, as many (it is estimated) as there are stars in our galaxy. They vary in size, shape, and length of processes. A distinction is also made according to the direction of flow of neural impulses. Thus there are afferent (sensory) neurons, efferent (motor) neurons, and internuncial (associational) neurons.

Neurons are classified as unipolar, bipolar, or multipolar according to the number and pattern of processes arising from the cell body. *Unipolar neurons* have a single process that divides into two branches a short distance from the cell body. One branch is directed toward the periphery, and the other branch travels toward the CNS. An example of a unipolar neuron is the sensory neuron of a spinal nerve (Fig. 50-5). *Bipolar neurons* have two processes, one axon and one dendrite. Retinal rod and cone cells are bipolar neurons. *Multipolar neurons* have several dendrites and one axon, which may undergo extensive branching. Most neurons of the CNS are multipolar; for example, the motor neurons arising in the ventral horn of the spinal cord have axons that extend to skeletal muscle (Fig. 50-5).

Neurons are also classified by the length of their processes. *Golgi type I* neurons have a long axon that may extend more than a meter in length, for example, a motor neuron from the sacral spinal cord that extends to the tips of the toes. The long fiber tracts of the brain and spinal cord and the nerve fibers of the PNS are composed of axons of this type of neuron. *Golgi type II* neurons have short axons that terminate close to the cell body. The dendrites are also short and are clustered around the cell body. Golgi type II neurons are numerous in the brain and spinal cord and are much more common than type I neurons.

A neuron, or nerve cell, shares in the biochemical machinery of all other living cells. In addition to production of energy to maintain and repair themselves, the metabolically active nerve cells make and release chemicals called neurotransmitters. Neurons primarily use glucose as a metabolic fuel but are essentially restricted to oxidative metabolism.

Most neuronal intracellular organelles are present in the cell body cytoplasm, although some are present within the cell processes. Cellular organelles and inclusions include protein-synthesizing *Nissl substance,* composed of rough endoplasmic reticulum; protein-storing and protein-processing Golgi bodies; and energy-producing mitochondria, neurofibrils, microfilaments, and microtubules involved in intracellular transport. The cell body and dendritic cytoplasm are about equivalent in the types of organelles present, but the axons notably lack Nissl substance. The region of the axon known as the *axon terminal* (see following discussion) is metabolically active and contains a high concentration of intracellular organelles, especially mitochondria. The nucleus and the prominent nucleolus are located in the cell body. The centrosome may be seen in neurons prenatally and during the first few months of postnatal life, when mitosis is still possible. Centrosomes are generally absent from mature neurons, however, because these cells are incapable of dividing and increasing their numbers.

Dendrites may be long neuronal processes and branch only at their ends, or they may be short and have multiple branches. Dendrites usually transmit neural impulses toward the cell body and may be considered as extensions of the cell body to increase the receptive area for neural messages. Dendrites undergo terminal branching, and the terminal branches are called *dendritic spines.*

Each neuron has only one axon, which may be short, long, or of an intermediate length, depending on the function of the given neuron. Axons within the human nervous system can be less than 1 mm or more than 1 m in length. Axons usually arise from the cell body in an area called the *axon hillock.* The axon may give rise to a branch along its course called an *axon collateral.* Close to the site of termination, axons branch profusely. The terminal branches, called *telodendria,* are slightly enlarged at the distal ends. The enlargements are called *synaptic boutons* or *knobs.* The diameters of axons vary from neuron to neuron and are related to the function of the neuron: the larger the diameter, the faster the conduction of the impulse. The conduction of a neural impulse along an axon is also affected by whether myelin is present, since conduction along myelinated fibers is faster.

Neurotransmitters are chemicals synthesized in the neurons, stored in synaptic vesicles in the axon terminals, and released from the axon terminal by *exocytosis.* Some neurotransmitters are totally reabsorbed and recycled by the neuron that secreted them (e.g., norepinephrine). Other neurotransmitters are lysed by enzymes within the synaptic cleft, and part of the lysed molecule is reabsorbed and recycled. The best known example of the latter is the reabsorption of choline after acetylcholine is lysed by cholinesterase. Neurotransmitters are the method of communication between neurons. Each neuron releases one transmitter. These chemicals change the cell permeability of a neuron, making it more or less able to conduct an impulse, depending on the neuron and the transmitter. There are about 30 known or suspected neurotransmitters, including norepinephrine, acetylcholine, dopamine, serotonin, gamma-aminobutyric acid (GABA), and glycine.

Neurons conduct neural signals throughout the body. Neuronal impulses are electrical along the length of a neuron and chemical between neurons. Neurons are not anatomically continuous with one another. The areas where neurons come in contact with other neurons or effector organs are called *synapses*. The synapse is the only location where an impulse can pass from one neuron to another or to an effector. The space between one neuron and the next neuron (or effector organ) is called the *synaptic cleft*. The neuron bringing the nerve impulse toward the synapse is called the *presynaptic neuron;* the one leaving is the *postsynaptic neuron*. An estimated 10^{14} synapses exist in the human nervous system. Synapses can be between an axon and a dendrite *(axodendritic synapse)*, between an axon and a cell body *(axosomatic synapse)*, between axons *(axoaxonic synapse)*, and also between dendrites *(dendrodendritic synapse)*. One neuron can make synaptic contact with many neurons *(divergence)* and may receive synaptic contact from many neurons *(convergence)* (Fig. 50-6).

The electrical component of neural transmission deals with the transmission of the neural impulses along the length of the neuron. Neurons have cell membranes with a variable selective permeability to Na^+ and K^+ ions that is affected by chemical and electrical changes in the neuron, most notably neurotransmitters and receptor organ stimuli, respectively. In the resting state the cell membrane permeability creates a high intracellular K^+ concentration and a low intracellular Na^+ concentration even in the presence of a high extracellular Na^+ concentration. Electrical impulses are generated by the separation of charges caused by the intracellular and extracellular ion concentration differences across the cell membrane.

FIG. 50-6   **A,** Convergence of neural input. **B,** Divergence of neural input. Convergence and divergence are important neural mechanisms of processing and integrating information. (From Vander AJ, Sherman JH, Luciano DS: *Human physiology,* ed 3, New York, 1975, McGraw-Hill.)

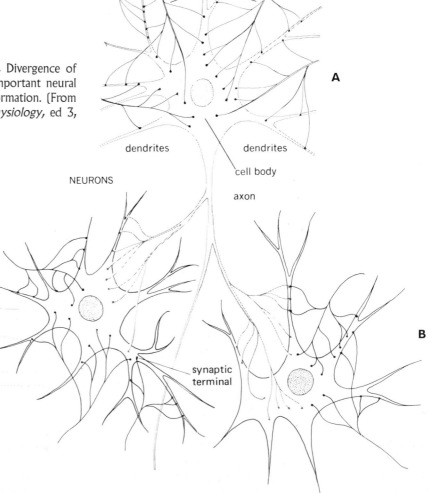

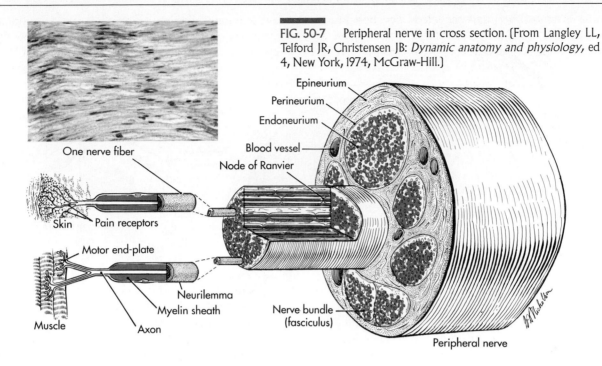

FIG. 50-7   Peripheral nerve in cross section. (From Langley LL, Telford JR, Christensen JB: *Dynamic anatomy and physiology,* ed 4, New York, 1974, McGraw-Hill.)

If the stimuli causing electrical changes in the neuronal cell membrane cause an increased permeability to K⁺ ions, the neuron becomes *hyperpolarized* and inhibited. Hyperpolarized neurons are unable to carry a nerve impulse. When the stimulus causing the electrical changes results in an increased permeability to Na⁺ ions, the neuron becomes excited or *depolarized.* If the membrane is depolarized to a critical level, called the *excitation threshold,* a change of membrane permeability occurs, with sudden influx of Na⁺, rapid depolarization, and generation of an action potential at the point of stimulation.

An *action potential* is transmitted along the axon as an all-or-none phenomenon rather than as a graded response. When the action potential reaches the axon terminal, it causes a release of the neurotransmitter from synaptic vesicles by exocytosis into the synaptic cleft. The transmitter attaches itself to a receptor site on the postsynaptic neuronal or effector membrane and may or may not initiate an action potential in the postsynaptic membrane. Each neuron is covered with many synapses. Whether an action potential will develop is determined by the balance of the excitatory and inhibitory impulses the neuron receives at that time from all its synaptic connections. This is another demonstration of the diversity and extensive intercommunication that exist in the nervous system.

Nerves

A *nerve* is a group or bundle of nerve cell fibers surrounded by a connective tissue sheath outside the CNS. (Nerves do not exist in the CNS. The proper term for a group of fibers conducting impulses within the CNS is *fiber tract.*) The peripheral nerves are the cranial and spinal nerves and their branches. Nerves of the autonomic branch of the PNS are associated with both cranial and spinal nerves.

A peripheral nerve is composed of a bundle of nerve fibers surrounded by connective tissue layers thought to be continuous with CNS meningeal layers (Fig. 50-7). *Endoneurium* surrounds the individual nerve fibers adjacent to the myelin (if present) and the neurilemma and is continuous with the pia. Bundles of nerve fibers (also called *fasciculi*) are wrapped in *perineurium,* which is continuous with the arachnoid. The *epineurium* contains blood vessels and fat cells, surrounds the various fasciculi of a peripheral nerve, and is continuous with the dura.

COVERINGS OF THE BRAIN AND SPINAL CORD

The gelatinous tissue of the brain and spinal cord is protected by bone (skull and vertebral column) and by three connective tissue layers: the pia mater, the arachnoid, and the dura mater. Each is a separate, continuous sheet; connections between the pia and arachnoid are called *trabeculae.* The dura is also called the *pachymeninx;* the pia mater and arachnoid are collectively referred to as the *leptomeninges* (Fig. 50-8).

The *pia mater* is directly continuous with brain and spinal tissue and follows the contour of their external structure. It is a vascular layer through which blood ves-

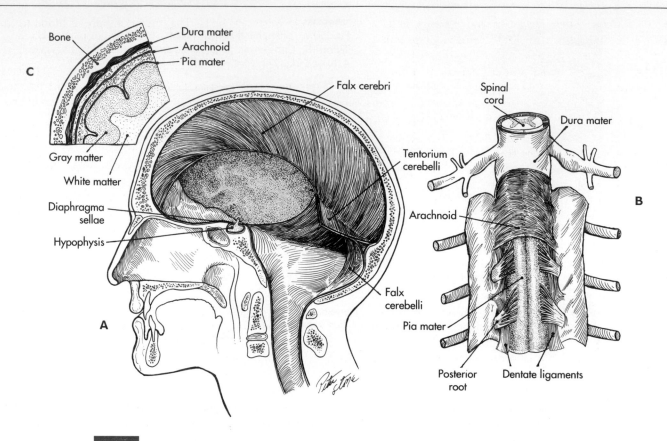

FIG. 50-8   Meninges. **A,** Extensions of the dura mater in the cranial cavity, sagittal view. **B,** Dura and arachnoid sheathe spinal nerves at their origin. The dentate ligament separates dorsal from ventral roots and adheres to the dura. **C,** A vertical section through a portion of the calvaria (cranium) and cortex. (From Langley LL, Telford JR, Christensen JB: *Dynamic anatomy and physiology,* ed 5, New York, 1980, McGraw-Hill.)

sels pass to the internal CNS structures to nourish the neural tissue. The pia extends below the spinal cord, which, as previously mentioned, ends at about the lower level of L1. The end of the spinal cord is cone shaped and is called the *conus medullaris.* A slender filament of pia called the *filum terminale* extends from the conus medullaris.

The *arachnoid* is a thin, fine, avascular, fibrous membrane. It hugs the brain and spinal cord but does not follow every contour as does the pia mater. The area between the arachnoid and pia mater is called the *subarachnoid space* and contains cerebral arteries, veins, arachnoid trabeculae, and the CSF that bathes the CNS. Enlargements in the subarachnoid space are called *cisterns.* One notable enlargement is the lumbar cistern in the lumbar region of the vertebral column. The lower lumbar region (usually between L3 and L4 or L4 and L5) is the area where spinal taps are performed to obtain CSF for examination.

The *dura mater* is a tough, inelastic, leatherlike tissue composed of two layers: the outer endosteal dura and the inner meningeal dura. The *endosteal* layer forms the inner periosteum of the skull and is continuous with the periosteal lining of the vertebral canal of the spinal cord.

The inner *meningeal* dura is a thick membrane that covers the brain and dips in between brain tissues to provide support and protection. The layer becomes continuous with the spinal dura mater. The spinal dura continues to the level of the second sacral vertebra (S2), where it fuses with the filum terminale and forms the coccygeal ligament. This extends to the coccyx, where it becomes continuous with the periosteum and anchors the spinal cord in the vertebral canal.

The spinal cord is stabilized along the length of the vertebral canal by a series of 20 to 22 paired longitudinal ligaments referred to as the *dentate* or *denticulate ligaments.* These ligaments, which are attached to the dura at intervals, are lateral extensions of collagenous pial tissue separating the dorsal and ventral roots.

Four major sheaths of the meningeal dura extend into the cranial cavity (Fig. 50-8, *A*). The *falx cerebelli* separate the two cerebellar hemispheres. The left and right cerebral hemispheres are separated along the longitudinal fissure of the *falx cerebri.* The *tentorium cerebelli* separates the cerebrum from the cerebellum. Finally, overlying the pituitary and penetrated by the hypothalamohypophyseal portal system is the *diaphragma sellae.*

The venous sinuses are located between the two layers

of dura mater where they separate. Venous sinuses are valveless channels for the drainage of cerebral blood and CSF. No vascular tissue exists in these sinuses; they are composed of dura mater with an endothelial lining.

When damage occurs to the vasculature of the brain, there may be bleeding into the *extradural* or *epidural space* (between the bone of the skull and the endosteal dura), the *subdural space* (between the meningeal dura and the arachnoid), the *subarachnoid space* (between the arachnoid and pia mater), or beneath the pia mater into the brain itself. The inner table of the skull contains grooves in which lie the anterior, middle, and posterior meningeal arteries. A fracture line running through any of these grooves may damage the contained artery and is the most common cause of *extradural* or *epidural hematoma.* A blow to the head over the parietotemporal region damaging the middle meningeal artery is the most frequent cause of extradural hematoma. *Subdural hematoma* is often caused by damage to the venous vasculature traversing the subdural space. A ruptured aneurysm of the arteries supplying the base of the brain results in *subarachnoid hemorrhage. Intracerebral hemorrhage* occurs when the vessels that penetrate brain tissue are involved so that blood enters the brain tissue itself.

The scalp is an additional structure that must be included in considering the coverings of the CNS. Overlying the skull, to which it is attached by the frontalis and occipitalis muscles, is a freely movable, dense fibrous tissue called the *galea aponeurotica* (Latin *galea,* meaning "helmet"). The galea helps absorb the force of external trauma, especially glancing blows; without the protection of the scalp, the skull would be much more readily fractured. Overlying the galea is a membranous layer containing large blood vessels, a fatty layer, skin, and the hair of the scalp. When severed, the blood vessels constrict poorly and may cause severe bleeding that, however, can be controlled by digital pressure. Between the galea and the outer table of the skull is a potential space called the *subaponeurotic space.* The *diploic* and *emissary veins* (see Figure 56-5) penetrate the skull from the dural sinuses into the subaponeurotic space and act as a safety feature (pressure valve) in case of increased intracranial pressure. These veins are also potential access sites for intracranial infection from a pyogenic focus in the scalp or sinuses or in cases of traumatic laceration of the galea. Thus meticulous removal of foreign particles, careful débridement, and flushing with normal saline and sometimes with a bactericidal agent are essential to reduce this hazard whenever the galea has been lacerated.

VASCULAR SUPPLY OF THE BRAIN AND SPINAL CORD

The CNS, as with all body tissue, depends on an adequate blood supply for its nutrients and for removal of meta-

bolic waste products. The arterial supply of blood to the brain is a branching network of vessels that is highly interconnected to ensure adequate blood supply to the cells. This blood supply is provided via two pairs of arteries, the vertebral arteries and the internal carotid arteries, branches of which anastomose to form the cerebral arterial circle of Willis (Figs. 50-9 and 50-10).

The venous brain drainage does not closely parallel the arterial supply; it leaves the brain through the large dural sinuses and returns to the general circulation via the internal jugular veins.

The spinal cord arterial and venous systems are quite close parallels of each other and also have extensive branching interconnections to adequately supply the tissue.

Carotid Arterial Supply

The *internal* and *external carotid arteries* branch from the common carotid arteries at about the level of the thyroid cartilage. The left common carotid artery stems directly from the aortic arch, but the right common carotid artery is derived from the innominate or brachiocephalic artery (a 1-inch remnant of the right aortic arch). The external carotid arteries supply the face, thyroid, tongue, and pharynx. A branch from the external carotid arteries, the *middle meningeal artery,* supplies the deep structures of the face and sends a large branch to the dura mater. A slight dilation in the internal carotid arteries just past the bifurcation is called the *carotid sinus.* Specialized nerve endings within the carotid sinuses respond to changes in arterial blood pressure to reflexly maintain blood supply to the brain and body.

The internal carotid arteries enter the skull and divide, at about the level of the optic chiasm, into the anterior cerebral arteries and the middle cerebral arteries. The middle cerebral arteries are direct continuations of the internal carotid arteries. Just after entering the subarachnoid space and before dividing, the internal carotid arteries give rise to the *ophthalmic arteries,* which enter the orbits and supply the eyes and other orbital contents, portions of the nose, and air sinuses. Occlusion of this branch of the internal carotids (e.g., during a stroke) can result in monocular blindness.

The *anterior cerebral arteries* provide blood supply to structures such as the caudate and putamen nuclei of the basal ganglia, portions of the internal capsule and corpus callosum, and portions (mainly medial) of the frontal and parietal lobes of the cerebrum, including the somesthetic and motor cortices. An occlusion in the main trunk of an anterior cerebral artery results in a contralateral hemiplegia that is greater in the leg than in the arm (lower extremity more involved than upper extremity). Bilateral paralysis and sensory impairment result when there is total occlusion of both anterior cerebral arteries, again more severe in the lower extremities than in the upper.

The *middle cerebral arteries* supply arterial blood to

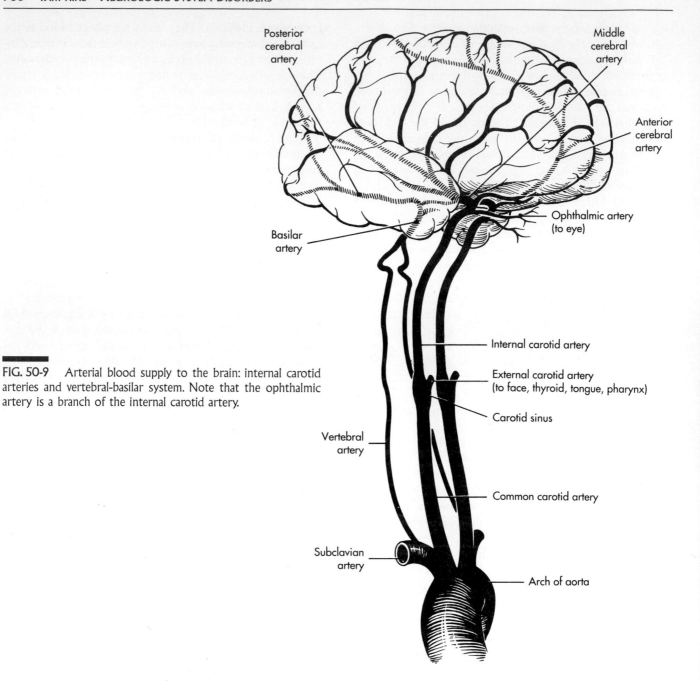

FIG. 50-9   Arterial blood supply to the brain: internal carotid arteries and vertebral-basilar system. Note that the ophthalmic artery is a branch of the internal carotid artery.

portions of the temporal, parietal, and frontal lobes of the cerebral cortex and form a fanlike distribution over the lateral surfaces. This artery represents the major supply of blood to the precentral and postcentral gyri. Auditory, somesthetic, motor, and premotor cortices are supplied by the artery, as are the association cortices concerned with higher integrated functions in these central lobes. Occlusion of the middle cerebral artery near the origin of the main cortical branches (in the main trunk of the artery) results in severe aphasia when the language-dominant cerebral hemisphere is involved, contralateral sensory loss of position sense and two-point tactile discrimination, and a severe contralateral hemiplegia predominantly in the upper extremities and the face.

Vertebral-Basilar Arterial Supply

The right and left *vertebral arteries* originate from the subclavian arteries of their respective sides. The right subclavian is a branch from the innominate artery, and the left subclavian comes directly off the aorta. The vertebral arteries enter the skull via the foramen magnum, and at the level of the medullary pontine junction of the brain stem (where the medulla oblongata and the pons meet), they fuse to form the basilar artery. The *basilar artery* continues to the level of the midbrain, where it bifurcates to form the paired posterior cerebral arteries. The medulla, pons, cerebellum, midbrain, and part of the diencephalon are supplied by branches from the vertebral-basilar artery system. The posterior cerebral arteries and

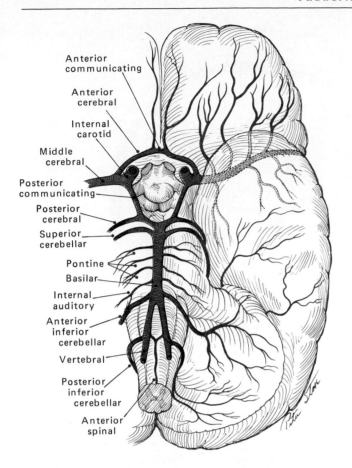

FIG. 50-10   Arteries of the brain. The circle of Willis *(center)* joins branches of the basilar and internal carotid arteries. (From Langley LL, Telford JR, Christensen JB: *Dynamic anatomy and physiology,* ed 5, New York, 1980, McGraw-Hill.)

their branches supply a portion of the diencephalon, parts of the occipital and temporal lobes, the cochlear apparatus, and the vestibular organs. In the occipital lobe the primary visual cortex is supplied by the calcarine artery, which is a branch of the posterior cerebral artery. Occlusion of a calcarine artery can result in a contralateral homonymous hemianopsia (see Chapter 57). However, macular sparing may result from anastomosis of posterior and middle cerebral arteries in the occipital lobe.

Arterial Circle of Willis

Although the internal carotid arteries and the vertebral-basilar arteries are two separate arterial systems delivering blood to the brain, they are united by anastomosing vessels to form the cerebral arterial *circle of Willis* (see Fig. 50-10). The *posterior cerebral arteries* are connected to the middle cerebral (and anterior cerebral arteries) by the posterior communicating arteries. The anterior cerebral arteries are connected by the *anterior communicating arteries* to complete the circle. There is usually only slight blood flow in the communicating arteries un-

der normal conditions; they are a safety feature in case of dramatic changes in arterial blood pressure. The branches of the internal carotid and the vertebral-basilar systems also have anastomosing vessels.

Conducting and Penetrating Arteries

In general, cerebral arteries are either conducting or penetrating. The *conducting arteries* (the internal carotid arteries; anterior, middle, and posterior cerebral arteries; vertebral-basilar arteries; and the main branches from these arteries) form an extensive vascular network over the surface of the brain. The *penetrating arteries* are nutrient vessels derived from branches of the conducting arteries. They enter the brain at right angles and provide blood to the deep cerebral structures, such as the diencephalon, basal ganglia, internal capsule, and parts of the midbrain. For example, the *lenticulostriate (striate) arteries* are penetrating branches of the middle cerebral artery supplying the internal capsule and parts of the basal ganglia (see Figs. 53-1 and 53-3). These small arteries are often implicated in the stroke syndrome. Occlusion or rupture of the striate arteries may interrupt the motor pathways of the internal capsule and result in paralysis.

Venous Drainage of the Brain

The venous drainage for the brain stem and cerebellum closely parallels the arterial vascular distribution in those areas. Most of the venous drainage from the cerebrum occurs via the deep veins draining into superficial venous plexuses and into dural sinuses. The sinuses eventually drain into the internal jugular veins at the base of the skull, which rejoin the general circulation. The dural sinuses include the superior and inferior sagittal and the transverse (lateral) sigmoid, straight, and cavernous venous sinuses (Fig. 50-11). When a skull fracture may be present, one must consider the possibility of trauma to the cerebral venous sinuses, which may result in a subdural hematoma.

Spinal Cord Vasculature

The spinal cord receives its supply of nourishing blood via the branches of the vertebral arteries (the anterior and posterior spinal arteries and their branches) and from segmented regional vessels arising from the thoracic and abdominal aorta (the radicular arteries and their branches). From where they branch off the vertebral arteries along the surface of the medulla, the anterior and posterior spinal arteries descend into the spinal cord. The segmental arteries enter the spinal portion of the CNS through intravertebral foramina and divide into anterior and posterior vessels; they encircle the cord, forming an extensive anastomosing vascular plexus on the surface of the cord that also interconnects with the vessels from the vertebral

FIG. 50-11   Venous (dural) sinuses of the head. Superficial veins of the face empty into the cavernous sinus. (From Langley LL, Telford JR, Christensen JB: *Dynamic anatomy and physiology,* ed 5, New York, 1980, McGraw-Hill.)

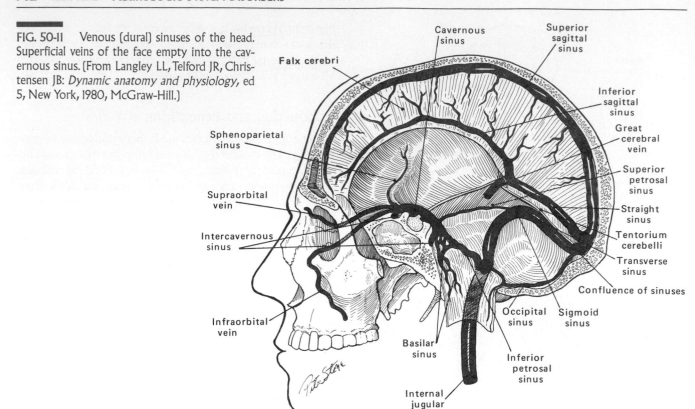

system. Branches from this superficial vascular plexus then penetrate the cord to supply the deep tissue.

The venous drainage primarily follows the arterial distribution. Some spinal cord veins have valves, in contrast to the valveless brain veins and venous sinuses. The vascular system of the spinal cord is directly continuous with the brain venous system. When the venous pressure is increased in the spinal cord, as in coughing or lifting heavy objects, an increase in central venous pressure may temporarily impede brain venous drainage.

VENTRICLES AND CEREBROSPINAL FLUID

The ventricles are a series of four interconnected cavities within the brain that are lined with ependymal cells (type of epithelial cell that abuts on all cavities of the brain and spinal cord) and contain CSF. There is one lateral ventricle in each cerebral hemisphere (Fig. 50-12). The third ventricle is in the diencephalon, whereas the fourth ventricle is in the pons and medulla. The lateral ventricle communicates with the third ventricle via the paired interventricular *foramina of Monro.* The third and fourth ventricles are connected via the narrow *aqueduct of Sylvius* in the midbrain. Three openings extend from the fourth ventricle: the paired lateral *foramina of Luschka* and the single medial *foramen of Magendie,* which are

continuous with the subarachnoid space of the brain and spinal cord.

Within each ventricle is a specialized secretory structure known as the *choroid plexus.* It is composed of a network of blood vessels of the pia mater in intimate contact with the ependymal lining. The choroid plexus secretes the clear, colorless CSF that provides a protective fluid cushion around the CNS. The CSF contains water, electrolytes, O_2 and CO_2 gases in solution, glucose, a few leukocytes (principally lymphocytes), and a slight amount of protein. This fluid differs from other extracellular fluids in that it has higher Na^+ and Cl^- ion concentrations and its glucose and K^+ ion concentrations are lower, indicating that it is a secretion rather than a simple filtrate.

Once in the subarachnoid space, the CSF circulates around the brain and spinal cord and then exits into the vascular system (no lymph system exists in the CNS). Most of the CSF is reabsorbed into the blood through special structures called *arachnoid villi,* or *arachnoid granulations,* which project from the subarachnoid spaces into the superior sagittal venous sinus of the brain. There is constant production and reabsorption of CSF in the CNS. The total volume of CSF in the entire cerebrospinal cavity is about 125 ml, and the rate of choroidal secretion is about 500 to 750 ml/day. The CSF pressure is a function of the rate of fluid formation and the resistance to reabsorption of the arachnoid villi. The CSF pressure is commonly measured during a lumbar punc-

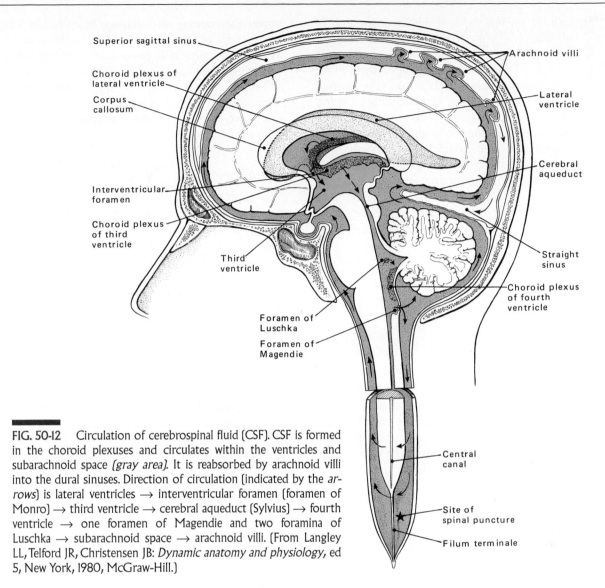

FIG. 50-12   Circulation of cerebrospinal fluid (CSF). CSF is formed in the choroid plexuses and circulates within the ventricles and subarachnoid space *(gray area).* It is reabsorbed by arachnoid villi into the dural sinuses. Direction of circulation (indicated by the *arrows*) is lateral ventricles → interventricular foramen (foramen of Monro) → third ventricle → cerebral aqueduct (Sylvius) → fourth ventricle → one foramen of Magendie and two foramina of Luschka → subarachnoid space → arachnoid villi. (From Langley LL, Telford JR, Christensen JB: *Dynamic anatomy and physiology,* ed 5, New York, 1980, McGraw-Hill.)

ture procedure and normally averages about 130 mm H_2O (13 mm Hg) in the recumbent position.

Hydrocephalus

Excessive CSF in the cerebrospinal cavity may elevate the pressure sufficiently to damage nervous tissue. This condition is called *hydrocephalus,* a term meaning "excess water in the cranial vault." Hydrocephalus may result from excess formation of fluid by the choroid plexuses, inadequate absorption, or obstruction to flow out of one or more of the ventricles. There are two types of hydrocephalus: noncommunicating, in which the flow of fluid from the ventricular system into the subarachnoid space is obstructed; and communicating, in which no such obstruction exists.

Noncommunicating hydrocephalus is the most common pediatric neurosurgical problem and usually has its onset in the immediate postnatal period. It is usually caused by a congenital narrowing of the aqueduct of Sylvius, so as fluid is formed by the choroid plexuses of

the two lateral and third ventricles, the volumes of these three ventricles increase greatly. This flattens the brain into a thin shell against the skull. The increased pressure also causes the whole head to swell in the newborn. Obstructive hydrocephalus is also frequently associated with *meningomyelocele,* a congenital condition in which fusion of the neural tube fails to occur and thus the spinal cord is open, with cord, nerves, dura, and the more superficial coverings of the cord completely disarranged. Most children with meningomyelocele develop hydrocephalus, especially after surgical repair of the meningomyelocele. In adults, obstructive hydrocephalus is most often caused by a posterior fossa tumor with deformity of the aqueduct of Sylvius or fourth ventricle.

Communicating hydrocephalus may be caused by overdevelopment of the choroid plexuses in the newborn, so much more fluid is formed than can be reabsorbed by the arachnoid villi. Fluid therefore collects inside the ventricles and on the outside of the brain, causing the head to swell tremendously and severely damaging the brain. Communicating hydrocephalus, however, is more frequently caused by interference with reabsorption of the CSF. This situation is usually secondary to meningitis or an irritant that occludes or scars the subarachnoid CSF spaces. This is by far the most common form in the adult. Because of the irritating effect of blood in the subarachnoid space, communicating hydrocephalus can follow subarachnoid hemorrhage by several weeks. A syndrome that often follows communicating hydrocephalus in the adult, especially after subarachnoid hemorrhage, is *low-pressure hydrocephalus* (or *normal-pressure hydrocephalus*). The presenting symptoms include difficulty with walking, followed rapidly by dementia, lassitude, and eventual urinary incontinence. It is important to recognize the syndrome of low-pressure hydrocephalus, since it is a treatable form of dementing disease.

All types of hydrocephalus can be treated by shunting the CSF to the extracranial venous system.

BRAIN

The brain accounts for approximately 2% of the total body weight of an adult (about 3 pounds). It receives approximately 20% of the cardiac output, demands 20% of the body's O_2 use, and requires about 400 kcal of energy daily. The brain is the most energy-consuming tissue in the entire body and is primarily sustained by the oxidative metabolism of glucose. The tissue is fragile, and the demand for O_2 and glucose via the blood supply is constant. Brain metabolism is steady and continuous, with no rest periods. Consciousness may be lost in as little as 10 seconds once blood flow has ceased, and a lapse of even a few minutes may cause irreversible damage. Sustained

hypoglycemia may also damage brain tissue. The ceaseless activity of the brain is related to its crucial function as an integration and coordination center between the sense organs and peripheral effector systems of the body, serving to organize incoming information, stored experiences, outgoing impulses, and behavior. The following discussion briefly considers the structure and function of selected parts of the brain.

Brain Stem

The brain stem is continuous with the spinal cord caudally and with higher brain centers rostrally. The parts of the brain stem from below upward are the medulla oblongata, pons, and midbrain (Fig. 50-13). Many ascending and descending tracts exist throughout the brain stem. It is an important relay and reflex center of the CNS.

Except for the olfactory and optic nerves, the nuclei of the cranial nerves are located in the brain stem. One or more of the cranial nerves are often involved in brain stem lesions, and location and expansion of such lesions can be detected by testing cranial nerve function. Cranial nerves I (olfactory) and II (optic) are actually *CNS tracts,* since they are the axons of the secondary sensory neurons carrying signals from primary sensory neurons in the nasal epithelium and the retina, respectively. As a CNS tract, the optic nerve is subject to CNS diseases (e.g., multiple sclerosis) and tumors.

The *medulla oblongata* is an important reflex center for cardiac, vasoconstrictor, respiratory, sneezing, coughing, swallowing, salivation, and vomiting reflexes. All the ascending and descending tracts of the cord are represented. On its anterior surface are two enlargements called the *pyramids,* which contain mainly voluntary mo-

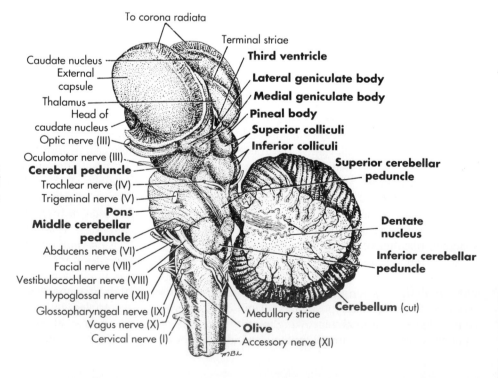

FIG. 50-13 Diencephalon and brain stem. (From Crouch JE: *Functional human anatomy,* ed 2, Philadelphia, 1972, Lea & Febiger.)

tor fibers. Posteriorly, the medulla also has two enlargements that are the fasciculi of the dorsal columns' ascending tracts, the *fasciculus gracilis* and *fasciculus cuneatus.* These tracts carry pressure, conscious muscle proprioception, vibratory sensations, and two-point tactile discrimination. The medulla contains nuclei of the last four cranial nerves, IX through XII.

The *pons* (Latin for "bridge") consists of a bridge of fibers that connects the halves of the cerebellum and joins the midbrain above with the medulla below. The pons forms an important connecting link in the corticocerebellar path by which the cerebral hemispheres and the cerebellum are united. The lower portion of the pons has a role in respiratory regulation. Nuclei of the trigeminal (cranial nerve V), abducens (VI), facial (VII), and vestibulocochlear or auditory (VIII) nerves are located here.

The *midbrain* is the short part of the brain stem that lies above the pons. It consists of (1) a posterior part, the *tectum,* containing the superior and inferior colliculi, and (2) an anterior part, the cerebral peduncles. The *superior colliculi* are involved in visual reflexes and in the coordination of visual tracking movements. Auditory reflexes, such as turning one's head toward a sound, are mediated through the *inferior colliculi.* The *cerebral peduncles* (or the basis pedunculi) are composed of bundles of descending motor fibers from the cerebrum. Two cranial nerves arise from the midbrain: the oculomotor (III) and the trochlear (IV). The trochlear nerves are the only ones of the 12 sets of cranial nerves that exit the brain stem on its posterior surface and cross to the opposite side. Therefore the superior oblique muscle is innervated by the contralateral trochlear nucleus. Because of its long intracranial course and its position just inferior to the free edge of the tentorium cerebelli, the trochlear nerve is at risk during surgical procedures of the midbrain. The substantia nigra and red nucleus, located in the midbrain, are part of the extrapyramidal or "involuntary" motor pathways. The *substantia nigra* has many connections, including those to the cerebral cortex, basal ganglia, red nucleus, and reticular formation. It is believed to have a complex inhibitory role in the areas to which it has interconnections. Lesions of the substantia nigra produce muscular rigidity, fine tremor at rest, slow and shuffling gait, and a masklike facies. Parkinson's disease involves the substantia nigra and its neurotransmitter, dopamine (see Chapter 54). The *red nucleus* has connections with the cerebellum, cerebral cortex, substantia nigra, basal ganglia, reticular formation, and subthalamic nucleus. It has a role in postural reflexes and righting reflexes dealing with the orientation of the head in space.

Cerebellum

The cerebellum lies in the posterior cranial fossa, covered by the tentlike roof of dura mater, the *tentorium,* which separates it from the posterior part of the cerebrum. It is composed of a middle portion, the *vermis,* and two lateral hemispheres. The cerebellum is connected to the brain stem by three bands of fibers called *peduncles.* The *superior cerebellar peduncle* establishes connections with the midbrain; the *middle cerebellar peduncle* connects the two cerebellar hemispheres; and the *inferior cerebellar peduncle* contains fibers of the dorsal spinocerebellar tracts and connects with the medulla. All activities of the cerebellum are below the level of consciousness. Its main function is that of a reflex center through which coordination and refinement of muscular movements are affected and changes in tone and strength of contraction are related to maintaining posture and equilibrium.

Diencephalon

Diencephalon is a term used to designate structures surrounding the third ventricle and forming the inner core of the cerebrum. The diencephalon is commonly divided into four areas: thalamus, hypothalamus, subthalamus, and epithalamus. The diencephalon processes sensory stimuli and helps initiate or modify the body's reaction to those stimuli.

The *thalamus* is composed of two large ovoid structures, each with a complex of nuclei that are interconnected with the ipsilateral cerebral cortex, cerebellum, and many subcortical nuclear complexes, such as those in the hypothalamus, brain stem reticular formation, basal ganglia, and possibly substantia nigra. It is an important relay station in the brain and an important subcortical integrator as well. All the main sensory pathways (except the olfactory system) form synapses with thalamic nuclei on their way to the cerebral cortex. Evidence indicates that the thalamus acts as a center of primitive, uncritical sensation through which the individual becomes vaguely conscious of pain, pressure, simple touch, vibratory sense, and extremes of temperature. For example, pain can be felt but it cannot be localized. The finer sensory discriminations require cortical resolution. Emotional responses to the sensory stimuli, however, are possible at the thalamic level of integration. In addition to its role as a primitive sensory center, the thalamus also plays a key role in the integration of motor expressions because of its functional relation to the major motor centers in the cerebral motor cortex, cerebellum, and basal ganglia.

The *hypothalamus* lies beneath the thalamus. It regulates peripheral autonomic nervous system discharges accompanying behavior and emotional expression. The hypothalamus also plays an important role in hormonal regulation. Antidiuretic hormone and oxytoxin are synthesized in nuclei located in the hypothalamus and transported via axons to the posterior pituitary, where they are stored and released. The release of anterior pituitary hormones is also regulated by hypothalamic releasing and inhibiting factors. Regulation of body water and electrolyte composition, body temperature, the endocrine functions of normal sexual and reproductive behavior, and the

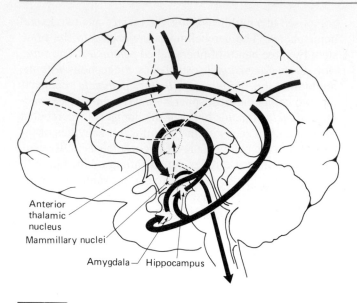

Anterior
thalamic
nucleus
Mammillary nuclei
Amygdala Hippocampus

FIG. 50-14 Diagram of the limbic system. The direction in which impulses flow is indicated by the arrows. Its principal function appears to be arousal of emotions. (From Stratton DB: *Neurophysiology,* New York, 1981, McGraw-Hill.)

expression of calm or rage, hunger, and thirst are among the many functions of the hypothalamus.

The *subthalamus* is an important extrapyramidal motor nucleus of the diencephalon. It has connections with the red nucleus, substantia nigra, and globus pallidus of the basal ganglia. Its function is not entirely understood, but a lesion here produces the dramatic dyskinesia known as *hemiballismus,* which is characterized by violent flinging movements of the limbs on one side of the body. The involuntary movement is usually more marked in the arm than in the leg.

The *epithalamus* is a narrow band of neural tissue that forms the roof portion of the diencephalon. The major structures of this area are the habenular nuclei and commissure, posterior commissure, striae medullaris, and pineal body. The epithalamus has connections with the limbic system and appears to play a role in some of the basic emotional drives and in the integration of olfactory information. The pineal body secretes melatonin and helps regulate the circadian rhythms of the body and inhibit gonadotropic hormones. In young boys, destruction of the pineal gland by a tumor may result in precocious puberty.

Limbic System

The term *limbic* means "border" or "fringe" and was introduced by Broca in 1878 to refer to two gyri forming a limbus or border around the diencephalon. The "limbic system" is a functional concept and has no universally accepted definition (Fig. 50-14). The principal cortical structures include the cingulate and hippocampal gyri and the hippocampus. Subcortical portions include the

amygdala, olfactory bulb and pathway, and septum. Some authors include the hypothalamus and part of the thalamus in the limbic system because of their close functional relationship. In the lower vertebrates the limbic system is involved primarily with the sense of smell; in humans its primary function is related to experiences and expressions of mood, feeling, and emotion, especially the reactions of fear, rage, and emotions related to sexual behavior. The limbic system is reciprocally connected to numerous central neural structures at several levels of integration, including the neocortex, hypothalamus, and the reticular activating system of the brain stem. It is influenced by input from all sensory systems, which integrates and expresses it as a behavioral pattern via the hypothalamus, which coordinates the autonomic, somatic, and endocrine responses. The limbic system is also believed to play a role in memory, since lesions of the hippocampus may result in the loss of recent memory. Psychomotor epilepsy begins with and may be confined to the limbic structures so involved in the processes of mood, feeling, and emotion. Perceptual distortions, especially memory recall, emotional crises, and alterations in relatedness to other persons and objects characteristic of psychomotor epilepsy, may be accounted for by involvement of limbic structures (see Chapter 55).

Cerebrum

The cerebrum is the largest and most prominent part of the brain. Nerve centers governing all sensory and motor activities as well as reason, memory, and intelligence are located here. The cerebrum is divided into right and left hemispheres by a deep groove or furrow called the great *longitudinal fissure.* The cerebral hemispheres have an outer covering of gray matter called the *cerebral cortex* spread over an inner core of white matter termed the *medullary center.* The two hemispheres are joined by a broad band of fibers called the *corpus callosum,* and gray masses called the *basal ganglia* are embedded in the white matter (see discussion of cerebral fiber tracts). Centers for sensory and motor activities are duplicated in each hemisphere and usually are associated with the opposite side of the body; that is, the right cerebral hemisphere controls the left side of the body and the left cerebral hemisphere controls the right side of the body. This functional concept is called *contralateral control.*

Cerebral cortex

The cerebral cortex, or gray mantle, of the cerebrum is thrown into numerous folds called *convolutions* or *gyri* (singular, gyrus). This arrangement enables a large surface area (estimated to be about 350 in²) to be contained within the narrow confines of the cranial vault. Furrows or grooves called *sulci* (singular, sulcus) created by the folds divide each hemisphere into distinct areas known as the frontal, parietal, temporal, and occipital lobes (Fig.

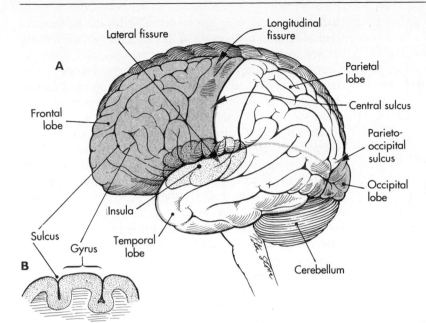

FIG. 50-15   A, Lateral view of the cerebrum. Note the line that demarcates the parietal and temporal lobes. B, Portion of the cortex in cross section. (From Langley LL, Telford JR, Christensen JB: *Dynamic anatomy and physiology,* ed 5, New York, 1980, McGraw-Hill.)

50-15). If the furrow is deep, it may be called a *fissure* rather than a sulcus. The *central sulcus* (fissure of Rolando) separates frontal and parietal lobes. The *lateral sulcus* (fissure of Sylvius) separates the temporal lobe below from the frontal and parietal lobes. The *parietooccipital sulcus* marks the boundaries of the occipital lobe. An additional subdivision of the cerebrum, the *insula,* lies within the lateral sulcus and is not visible on the surface.

Cerebral fiber tracts

The white matter of the cerebrum consists of neuron fiber tracts that may be grouped into three divisions: (1) association tracts, (2) commissural tracts, and (3) projection tracts.

The *association tracts* connect adjacent and distant cortical convolutions of the same hemisphere. The two hemispheres are linked by *commissural tracts,* the most prominent of which is a broad band of fibers called the *corpus callosum.* These tracts correlate the action of the two halves of the brain as, for example, in coordinating the actions of the two arms and hands in tossing and catching a ball. *Projection tracts* connect the cerebral cortex with other parts of the brain and spinal cord, for example, basal ganglia, diencephalon, and brain stem. The *internal capsule* is a large band of ascending and descending fibers (visible on coronal section as a white irregular mass) bounded by the thalamus and caudate on one side and lenticular nuclei on the other side. The internal capsule is the main pathway for sensory input and motor output between the cerebral cortex and the brain stem. The *corona radiata* is a mass of the fibers that leave the internal capsule in a fanlike radiation to go to various parts of the cerebral cortex.

Functional areas of cerebral cortex

Certain areas of the cerebral cortex are primarily concerned with specific functions. In 1909 Brodmann, a German neuropsychiatrist, mapped the cerebral cortex into 47 areas on the basis of cellular structure (*cytoarchitecture*). Many attempts have been made to ascribe specific functional importance to these areas. In many cases, however, specific functions may overlap several areas. Despite these limitations, the Brodmann map is a useful general guide for the discussion of cortical functions (Fig. 50-16).

The cerebral cortex can be viewed as having primary and association areas for certain functions. The primary area is that in which the perception or the movement occurs, but the association areas are necessary for integration and higher levels of behavior and intellect. The following discussion considers the highlights of frontal, parietal, temporal, and occipital cortical functions.

The frontal cortex contains the *primary motor area,* Brodmann area 4 (Fig. 50-17), which is responsible for voluntary movements. The primary motor area is located along the *precentral gyrus* (in front of the central sulcus) and is somatotopically organized. A lesion in area 4 results in a contralateral hemiplegia. The premotor cortex, area 6, is responsible for learned skilled movements such as writing, driving, or typing. A lesion in area 6 on the dominant side may result in loss of the ability to write, or *agraphia.*

Brodmann area 8 is called the *frontal eye field* and, in conjunction with area 6, is responsible for the voluntary scanning movements of the eyes and conjugate deviation of the eyes and the head. Voluntary eye movements have input from areas 4, 6, 8, 9, and 46.

Brodmann areas 44 and 45 are known as *Broca's mo-*

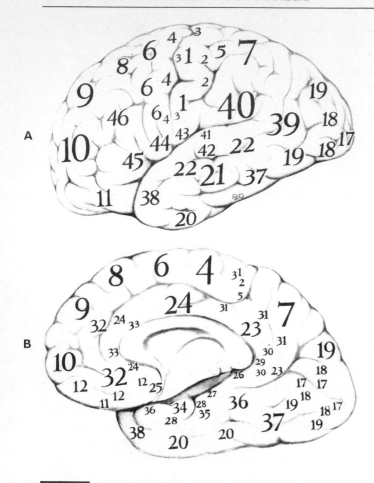

FIG. 50-16 Cytoarchitectural map of **A**, the lateral and **B**, the medial surface of the brain. Numbers represent the Brodmann areas. (From Noback CR, Demarest RJ: *The human nervous system*, ed 3, New York, 1981, McGraw-Hill.)

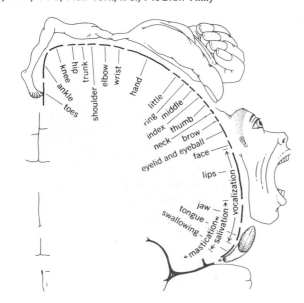

FIG. 50-17 Motor homunculus, showing the somatotopic organization of the motor cortex along the precentral gyrus. (From Vander AJ, Sherman JH, Luciano DS: *Human physiology*, ed 2, New York, 1975, McGraw-Hill.)

tor speech area; they are responsible for the motor execution of speech. Damage to this area results in difficulty in articulation (*motor,* or *expressive, aphasia*) when the lesion involves the dominant hemisphere. The dominant hemisphere controlling speech is the left in most adults, regardless of whether they are right-handed or left-handed.

The *prefrontal cortex,* areas 9 to 12, is associated with the personality of the individual. Complex intellectual activities, some memory functions, sense of responsibility for socially acceptable behavior, ideation, creative thought, judgments, and foresight are all primarily functions of the prefrontal cortex.

The parietal cortex has a major role in the higher level processing and integration of sensory information. The *primary somesthetic area* (areas 1 to 3) is located on the postcentral gyrus parallel to the motor cortex and posterior to the central sulcus. It is also somatotopically organized in a fashion resembling, but not identical to, the primary motor cortex. Sensations from all parts of the body are received in the primary sensory cortex, and it is here that they reach consciousness. These general sensations include pain, temperature, touch, pressure, and proprioception. The fine discrimination and more subtle aspects of sensory awareness are made possible by the primary sensory cortex. A lesion here produces contralateral sensory deficits.

The *somesthetic association area* (Brodmann areas 5 and 7) occupies the superior parietal lobe, extending to the medial surface of the hemisphere. It has many connections with other sensory areas of the cortex. The sensory association cortex receives and integrates different sensory modalities, for example, identifying a quarter placed in the hand without looking at it. The qualities of shape, form, texture, weight, and temperature are related to past sensory experiences so that the information may be interpreted and recognition can occur. Awareness of body image, of location of body parts and body posture, and of the self are also functions of this area. Language is a diffuse function that is located throughout many areas of the cortex. A lesion of the *angular gyrus* (area 39) in the dominant hemisphere results in *alexia* (inability to understand written language) and agraphia, although the individual may be able to speak normally. A lesion of the *supramarginal gyrus* (area 40) of the parietal cortex results in *astereognosis,* the inability to recognize objects by touch. A lesion in this area, such as may occur following a cerebrovascular accident (CVA, stroke), may also result in a defect in body awareness on the side contralateral to the lesion. For example, the affected person may be unaware of the arm on one side or fail to wash one half of the face.

The temporal lobe is the sensory receptive area for auditory impulses. The *primary auditory cortex* (areas 41 and 42) functions in the reception of sound, whereas the *auditory association cortex* (primarily area 22, although other parts of the temporal lobe are also included) is necessary for its comprehension. Brodmann area 22 is known as *Wernicke's area.* The temporal lobe (and the nearby hippocampus) also have a role in certain memory processes. The auditory association cortex is essential for the understanding of spoken language, and damage (especially on the dominant side) may result in a severe deficit in which language comprehension, naming objects, and repetition of things heard are severely impaired (*sensory,* or *Wernicke's, aphasia*). In Wernicke's aphasia, speech may be grammatically or phonetically correct, but the words chosen are inappropriate or consist of nonsensical syllables. This contrasts with *motor,* or *Broca's, aphasia,* in which comprehension may be unimpaired but expression is difficult. Both Wernicke's and Broca's areas (and many other areas of the brain) are necessary for normal speech communication, and these two areas are connected by a bundle of fiber tracts called the *arcuate fasciculus.*

The occipital lobe contains the *primary visual cortex,* area 17, where visual information is received and sense of colors becomes conscious. Damage to area 17 results in visual field defects (see Chapter 57). The primary visual cortex is surrounded by the visual association cortex (areas 18 and 19), where visual information becomes meaningful. This area also has a role in the reflex movement of the eyes when fixing on or following an object. Damage to areas 18 and 19 on the dominant side can result in a lack of recognition of objects and what they are used for even though faces may continue to be recognized. A lesion on the nondominant side may result in a failure to recognize faces (*prosopagnosia*) and to distinguish between forms of life (e.g., a cat versus a dog). The visual association cortex is adjacent to area 39 of the temporal lobe, and both are related to understanding the symbolism of language. Damage to this area results in *sensory alexia,* or inability to read with understanding.

Functional specialization of cerebral hemispheres

A characteristic of the brain with respect to sensation and motor control is that each half of the brain is concerned mainly with the opposite side of the body. Because the brain initially appears to be bilaterally symmetric, one might also assume that the two halves of the brain are functionally equivalent. However, this assumption is false. It has been known for some time that certain learned behaviors such as handedness, language perception, speech performance, and spatial relations are predominantly a function of one or the other hemisphere. About 90% of the population is right-handed, a trait controlled by the left side of the brain. It has been determined, from observations of patients with strokes and other brain lesions, that linguistic abilities (speech, reading, writing) are predominantly functions of the left side of the brain in about 96% of the population. Moreover, recent findings reveal anatomic asymmetry of the hemispheres. The Broca's and Wernicke's speech areas are generally larger in most persons. These observations led to the concept of *cerebral dominance,* with the left hemisphere considered dominant over the right.

In recent years the concept of cerebral dominance has been giving way to the newer concept of *cerebral specialization* and integration of thought processes, since it has become apparent that each hemisphere develops a specialization in many functions. The presence of massive fiber tracts connecting the two halves of the brain suggests that communication and integration of impulses into an overall pattern of action may be an important mode of brain functioning.

The evidence for cerebral specialization has been observed in patients who have undergone a cerebral *commissurotomy,* a surgical procedure in which the corpus callosum and other commissures joining the two hemispheres are severed for the relief of intractable epileptic seizures. Studies of such "split-brain persons" have provided increasingly detailed information on the separated hemispheres (Fig. 50-18). The behavior of such split-brain persons appears normal on casual observation. However, careful laboratory testing, in which it is possible to ensure that sensory information reaches only one hemisphere at a time and the motor response comes from only one hemisphere, reveals that the two hemispheres are almost completely independent with respect to perception, learning, memory, and ideation. The major hemisphere (usually the left) is specialized in language and mathematic calculation and is limited in spatial tasks. The minor hemisphere (usually the right) is specialized for grasping whole concepts and perceiving abstract visual patterns, music, and spatial locations, but it is unable to communicate through verbal language, although communication can take place through gestures and emotional activities. These observations of hemispheric specialization in split-brain persons have led to the notion of two modes of thought: the *rational-analytic* associated with the left side of the brain and the *gestalt-synthetic* associated with the right. The former mode of thought is believed to play an essential role in science, whereas the latter has an essential role in the creative arts, such as music, poetry, and imaginative expressions. Supposedly, some persons have left-hemisphere dominance and others are dominated by the right hemisphere. However, the specialization observed in the isolated hemispheres in split-brain experiments should not be overstated. Little is known about how the hemispheres interact in normal behavior, but the presence of the commissures suggests that there must be interaction.

Reticular formation

The reticular formation is a complex network of cell bodies and interlacing fibers that form the central core of the brain stem. It is continuous with the interneurons from the spinal cord below and extends upward into the diencephalon and telencephalon. The chief function of this diffuse reticular system is the integration of a large variety of cortical and subcortical processes, including determination of the state of consciousness and arousal, modulation of the transmission of sensory information to higher centers, modulation of motor activity, control of autonomic responses, and control of the sleep-wake cycle. This system is also the site of origin of most of the monoamines distributed throughout the CNS. The brain stem reticular formation is strategically located in the midst of ascending and descending neural pathways between the brain and spinal cord, enabling it to monitor traffic and participate in all brain stem–hemispheric transactions. It is diffusely receiving and diffusely projecting. The reticular formation receives input from the cerebral cortex, basal ganglia, hypothalamus and limbic system, cerebellum, spinal cord, and all sensory systems. The efferent fibers of the reticular formation are distributed to the spinal cord, cerebellum, hypothalamus and limbic system, and thalamus, which in turn project to the cerebral cortex and basal ganglia. In addition, an important group of monoamine fibers is distributed widely in ascending paths to subcortical and cortical structures and in descending paths to the spinal cord. Many synaptic endings also exist in the brain stem, so the reticular formation acts on itself. Thus the reticular formation influences and is influenced by all areas of the CNS.

One of the important functional components of the reticular formation is termed the *reticular activating system* (RAS). The RAS performs a general arousal function in which it activates the cerebral cortex to become receptive to stimuli from other parts of the body. The RAS is essential to maintain the waking state and the waking electroencephalogram (EEG). Damage to certain portions of the reticular formation may result in a coma from which the individual cannot be awakened. In addition to controlling the general state of arousal, the RAS performs a screening function with respect to stimuli so that arousal and attention are selective. The RAS also is believed to play a role in habituation, that is, decreased response to a monotonous stimulus, such as the background ticking of a clock. Certain stimuli that are significant to an individual may receive selective attention, whereas others are ignored. This could explain why restaurant signs attract our attention when we are driving on the highway and are hungry or why a mother may sleep through a loud thunderstorm yet awaken to the faintest

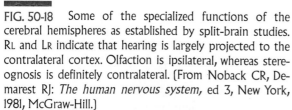

FIG. 50-18   Some of the specialized functions of the cerebral hemispheres as established by split-brain studies. Rᴸ and Lᴿ indicate that hearing is largely projected to the contralateral cortex. Olfaction is ipsilateral, whereas stereognosis is definitely contralateral. (From Noback CR, Demarest RJ: *The human nervous system*, ed 3, New York, 1981, McGraw-Hill.)

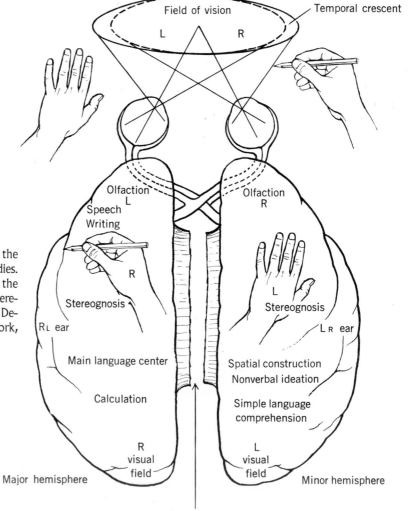

cry of her baby. Input from the cerebral cortex itself to the RAS, which in turn projects the impulses back to the cortex, may further increase cortical activity and arousal. This accounts for such states as a high degree of intellectual activity, worry, or anxiety possibly increasing cortical activity.

Several CNS monoamines, including dopamine, norepinephrine, and serotonin, play an important role in states of sleep and wakefulness. These monoamines are presumably produced in the cell bodies of neurons and distributed in vesicles via axoplasmic flow to nerve terminals. It has been demonstrated by histofluorescent staining techniques that the entire monoamine distribution system in the CNS originates in cell bodies located in the brain stem. Norepinephrine and serotonin pathways project upward to various parts of the brain and downward into the spinal cord, whereas dopamine pathways project only upward. The norepinephrine pathways as well as those of dopamine are believed to stimulate conscious wakefulness. Norepinephrine tracts are also responsible for rapid eye movement (REM) sleep. Destruction of the locus ceruleus (cell bodies that contain norepinephrine) in the brain stem can suppress REM sleep. Serotonin pathways arising from the raphe nuclei of the brain stem inhibit RAS arousal and promote both REM and non-REM sleep. Destruction of these nuclei produces insomnia. Certain pharmacologic agents that stimulate or inhibit the monoamines can alter sleep and arousal. For example, amphetamine, a drug that stimulates increased synthesis of norepinephrine, decreases total sleep time as well as REM sleep. The administration of *p*-chlorophenylalanine, a drug that blocks serotonin synthesis, results in insomnia, whereas the administration of 5-OH-tryptophan (a precursor of serotonin) restores normal sleep.

Another important function of the CNS monoamines is the regulation of emotional behavior through pathways that project to the hypothalamus and limbic system. The mechanisms effecting this control are poorly understood. The major tranquilizing drugs causing alteration in mood are believed to act on CNS monoamine neuronal systems.

CRANIAL NERVES

The cranial nerves arise directly from the brain and exit the skull via openings in the bone called *foramina* (sin-

 TABLE 50-2   Summary of Cranial Nerve (CN) Functions

Cranial Nerve	Nerve Component	Function
I Olfactory	Sensory	Smell
II Optic	Sensory	Vision
III Oculomotor	Motor	Elevation of upper lid Pupillary constriction Most extraocular movements
IV Trochlear	Motor	Downward inward movement of eye
VI Abducens	Motor	Lateral deviation of eye
V Trigeminal	Motor	Temporal and masseter muscles (jaw clenching, chewing); lateral movement of the jaw
	Sensory	Skin of face and anterior two thirds of scalp; mucosa of eyes; mucosa of nasal and oral cavities, tongue, and teeth Corneal or blink reflex: sensory limb carried in CN V, motor response in CN VII
VII Facial	Motor	Muscles of facial expression, including those of forehead and around eyes and mouth Lacrimation and salivation
	Sensory	Taste on anterior two thirds of tongue (sweet, sour, salty)
VIII Vestibulocochlear		
Vestibular branch	Sensory	Equilibrium
Cochlear branch	Sensory	Hearing
IX Glossopharyngeal	Motor	Pharynx: swallowing, gag reflex Parotid: salivation
	Sensory	Pharynx, posterior tongue, including taste (bitter)
X Vagus	Motor	Pharynx, larynx: swallowing, gag reflex, phonation; abdominal viscera
	Sensory	Pharynx, larynx: gag reflex; neck, thoracic, and abdominal viscera
XI Accessory	Motor	Sternocleidomastoid and upper portion of trapezius: head and shoulder movements
XII Hypoglossal	Motor	Tongue movements

gular, foramen). The 12 pairs of cranial nerves, designated by a name or Roman numeral, are olfactory (I), optic (II), oculomotor (III), trochlear (IV), trigeminal (V), abducens (VI), facial (VII), vestibulocochlear (VIII), glossopharyngeal (IX), vagus (X), accessory (XI), and hypoglossal (XII). Cranial nerves I, II, and VIII are purely sensory; III, IV, VI, XI, and XII are mainly motor but do carry proprioceptive fibers from the muscles they innervate; V, VII, IX, and X are mixed. Cranial nerves III, VII, and X also carry some nerve fibers of the parasympathetic branch of the ANS. The cranial nerves are discussed at length in Chapter 51. Table 50-2 is a summary of the major functions of the cranial nerves.

SPINAL NERVES

The spinal cord is composed of 31 segments of nervous tissue, each bearing a pair of spinal nerves that emerge from the vertebral canal through the intervertebral foramina (openings between the vertebral bones). The spinal nerves are named according to the intervertebral foramina through which they exit, except for the first cervical nerve pair, which exits between the occipital bone and the first cervical vertebra (C1). Thus there are 8 cervical nerve pairs (and only 7 cervical vertebrae), 12 thoracic nerve pairs, 5 lumbar nerve pairs, 5 sacral nerve pairs, and 1 coccygeal nerve pair (Fig. 50-19). When localizing a spinal lesion according to cord level rather than vertebral level, it is important to note that the two levels do not correspond. The disparity between the length of the spinal cord and that of the vertebral canal increases the distance between the attachment of the various nerve roots and the intervertebral foramina; therefore the nerve roots arising from the lumbar and sacral segments have to pass for some distance before making their exit.

The spinal nerve is attached to the lateral surface of the spinal cord by two roots: a *dorsal,* or *posterior (sensory), root;* and a *ventral,* or *anterior (motor), root* (Fig. 50-20). The dorsal root shows an enlargement, the *dorsal root ganglion,* composed of the cell bodies of afferent or sensory neurons. The cell bodies of all afferent neurons of the cord are in these ganglia. The dorsal root fibers are the processes of sensory neurons that bring impulses in from the periphery to the cord. The cell bodies of motor or ef-

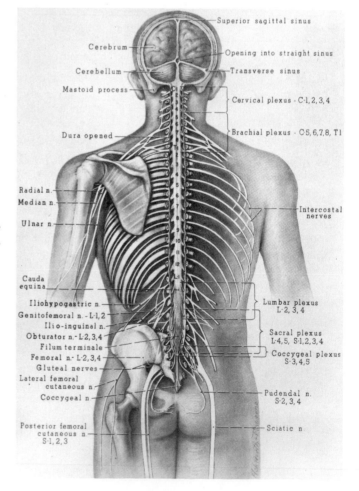

FIG. 50-19   Spinal nerves and plexuses. (From Jacob SW, Francone CA, Lossow WJ: *Structure and function in man,* ed 4, Philadelphia, 1978, Saunders.)

POSTERIOR

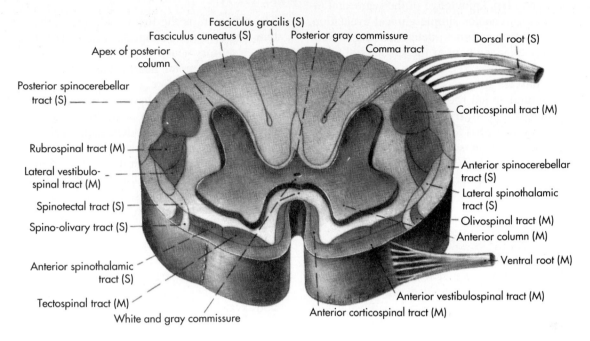

FIG. 50-20   Cross section of the spinal cord showing the major ascending sensory *(S)* and descending motor *(M)* tracts. (From Jacob SW, Francone CA, Lossow WJ: *Structure and function in man,* ed 4, Philadelphia, 1978, Saunders.)

ferent neurons are inside the cord in anterior and lateral columns of gray matter. Their axons form the ventral root fibers that pass to muscles and glands. The two roots emerge from the intervertebral foramen and join beyond it to form the spinal nerve, or nerve trunk. Thus all spinal nerves are mixed nerves; that is, they contain both sensory and motor fibers. After a short course the nerve trunk divides into dorsal and ventral divisions, or *rami* (singular, ramus). (There are also two more divisions: a meningeal branch, supplying the spinal cord meninges and ligaments; and a visceral branch, which has two portions, the white and gray rami, and belongs to the ANS.)

In general the *dorsal division* of the spinal nerves supplies the intrinsic muscles of the back and specific segments of the skin overlying them called dermatomes (see following discussion). The *ventral division* is large and forms the main part of the spinal nerve. The muscles and skin of neck, chest, abdomen, and extremities are supplied by the ventral division.

In all regions except the thoracic, the ventral divisions of the spinal nerves interlace to form networks of nerves called *plexuses.* The plexuses thus formed are the cervical, brachial, lumbar, sacral, and coccygeal. In each instance, branches are given off from the plexus to the parts supplied. These branches are the peripheral nerves and have specific names.

The first four cervical nerves (C1 to C4) form the *cervical plexus,* which innervates the neck and the back of

the head. One important branch is the phrenic nerve, which supplies the diaphragm.

The *brachial plexus* is formed from C5 through T1 or T2. This plexus supplies the upper extremity. Important branches are the radial, median, and ulnar nerves of the arm.

The thoracic nerves (T3 through T11) do not form a plexus but pass out in the intercostal spaces as the intercostal nerves. They supply intercostal muscles, upper abdominal muscles, and the skin areas of the chest and abdomen.

The *lumbar plexus* is derived from spinal segments T12 through L4, the *sacral plexus* from L4 through S4, and the *coccygeal plexus* from S4 through the coccygeal nerve. L4 and S4 contribute branches to both the lumbar and sacral plexuses. Nerves from the lumbar plexus innervate muscles and skin in the lower trunk and lower extremities. The major nerves from this plexus are the *femoral* and *obturator.* The major nerve from the sacral plexus is the *sciatic,* the largest nerve in the body. The sciatic nerve pierces the buttocks and runs down the back of the thigh. Its many branches supply the posterior thigh muscles, leg and foot muscles, and nearly all the skin of the leg. Nerves from the lower sacral levels and from the coccygeal plexus supply the perineum.

Each of the spinal nerves is distributed to specific segments of the body. The area of skin supplied by the dorsal root of each spinal nerve, and therefore a single segment of the spinal cord, is called a *dermatome.* Although the dermatomes overlap, knowledge of the segmental innervation of the skin enables simple clinical evaluation, using a pin or wisp of cotton to determine the sensory function of a particular segment of the spinal cord or peripheral nerve (see Chapter 51).

The skeletal muscles also receive a segmental innervation from the ventral spinal roots. The segmental innervation of the biceps brachii, triceps, brachioradialis, abdominal muscles, quadriceps femoris, gastrocnemius and soleus, and plantar flexor muscles should be memorized, since it is possible to test them by eliciting simple muscle reflexes using a reflex hammer (see Chapter 51).

SPINAL CORD

The spinal cord serves as a center for spinal reflexes and as a conducting pathway for impulses traveling to and from the brain. The spinal cord is composed of *white matter* (myelinated nerve fibers) with an internal core of *gray matter* (unmyelinated neuronal tissue). The white matter serves as a conducting pathway for afferent and efferent impulses traveling between various levels of the spinal cord and the brain. The gray matter is the integrative area for the cord reflexes.

When seen on cross section, the gray matter is in the form of the capital letter H. The two projections of the H that pass toward the front of the body are called *anterior,* or *ventral horns,* and the two projecting backward are the *posterior,* or *dorsal, horns* (see Fig. 50-20).

The ventral horn is composed primarily of cell bodies and dendrites of the multipolar motor efferent neurons of the ventral roots and spinal nerves. The *ventral horn cell,* or *lower motor neuron,* is commonly called the *final common pathway,* since any movement, whether initiated in the cerebral motor cortex, basal ganglia, or reflexly in the sensory receptor, must be translated into action via this structure.

The dorsal horn contains cell bodies and dendrites from which arise sensory fibers that go to other levels of the CNS after synapsing with sensory fibers from sensory nerves.

The gray matter also contains internuncial, or associational, neurons, ANS afferents and efferents, and axons originating at different levels of the CNS. Internuncial neurons transmit impulses from one neuron to another within the brain and spinal cord. In the spinal cord, internuncial neurons have many interconnections, and many of them directly innervate the ventral horn cells. Only a few incoming sensory impulses to the spinal cord or motor impulses from the brain terminate directly on the ventral horn cell or lower motor neuron. Instead, most of them are first transmitted through internuncial cells, where they are appropriately processed before stimulating the anterior horn cell. This arrangement allows highly organized patterns of muscle responses.

Reflex Arc

The reflex arc is the functional unit of the nervous system. Reduced to its simplest form, it consists of two neurons, a sensory neuron leading from a sensory receptor or ending and a motor neuron that conveys impulses to a muscle or gland. More generally the two neurons are not connected directly but have one or more internuncial neurons interposed between them. Such a mechanism is capable of response quite independent of the higher centers and is sufficient for the performance of such simple acts as withdrawing from painful stimuli. Reflexes may involve only one segmental level of the spinal cord or several levels. The impulses may spread upward or downward from the level at which they enter the cord by passing through internuncial neurons. Because of the multitude of interconnections of neurons within the cord, an almost infinite variety of responses is possible. Knowledge of the segmental levels of the reflexes and of the dermatomes is helpful in localizing lesions of the nervous system (see Chapter 51).

Pathways of Selected Spinal Cord Tracts

The white matter of the spinal cord conducts the long ascending and descending tracts by which afferent impulses from the spinal nerves reach the brain and those through which efferent impulses pass from motor centers in the brain to ventral horn cells of the cord and thus modify movement. The fibers that make up the white matter of the spinal cord are not scattered chaotically but are arranged in bundles that show a functional as well as an anatomic grouping.

Each lateral half of the spinal cord is divided into three longitudinal sections that run the length of the cord, called *dorsal, lateral,* and *ventral columns.* Within each of these divisions are distinct bands of fibers, called tracts, having quite difinite locations. A fiber tract is a bundle of fibers all having the same origin, termination, and function. The tracts may be ascending, descending, or associative.

Ascending tracts bring sensory information into the CNS and may travel to parts of the spinal cord and brain. The lateral spinothalamic tract is an important ascending tract that carries the fibers for the pain and temperature pathway. The fine touch, conscious proprioception, and vibratory pathways have fibers that compose the dorsal columns of the spinal cord white matter. Impulses from various parts of the brain to the motor neurons of the brain stem and spinal cord are called *descending tracts.* The lateral and ventral corticospinal tracts represent the voluntary motor pathway in the spinal cord (see Fig. 50-20 for the location of the tracts of these pathways). *Associative tracts* are short ascending or descending tracts; for example, they may travel between a few segments of the spinal cord and are thus called *intersegmental tracts.* Table 50-3 lists some of the most important ascending and descending tracts of the spinal cord.

TABLE 50-3   Major Ascending and Descending Tracts of the Spinal Cord

Tract	Function
ASCENDING	
Dorsal (posterior) columns	
Fasciculus cuneatus (T6 and above, upper body)	Fine touch capable of a high degree of localization of the stimulus, fine degree of discrimination of pressure and intensity (two-point discrimination, weight perception)
Fasciculus gracilis (T7 and below, lower body)	Conscious proprioception (position sense)
	Vibration (phasic sensations)
	Rapid transmission of sensory information
Spinothalamic	
Lateral spinothalamic	Pain
Ventral spinothalamic	Temperature, including warm and cold sensations
	Crude touch capable of much less localization of the stimulus and less discrimination of pressure and intensity
	Itching and tickling sensations
	Transmission of sensory information much slower than in dorsal columns
Spinocerebellar	
Dorsal spinocerebellar	Unconscious proprioception (muscle sense)
Ventral spinocerebellar	Coordination of posture and limb movement
	Sensory information transmitted originates almost entirely in the muscle spindles and Golgi tendon apparatus
	Large-tract fibers transmitting impulses faster than any other neurons in the body
DESCENDING	
Corticospinal	
Lateral corticospinal	Pyramidal tract carrying impulses for voluntary control of the muscles of the extremities
Ventral corticospinal	Pyramidal tract carrying impulses for voluntary control of the muscles of the trunk
Rubrospinal	Extrapyramidal tract concerned with unconscious integration and coordination of muscular movement adjusted to proprioceptive input
Tectospinal	Extrapyramidal tract concerned with reflex turning and scanning movements of the head and reflex movements of the arms in response to visual, auditory, or cutaneous sensation
Vestibulospinal	Extrapyramidal tract involved in equilibrium (maintaining balance) and coordination of head and eye movements

The spinal cord tracts are named to denote the origin and termination of their fibers. *Origin* means the location of the cell bodies of the tract, and *termination* refers to the point at which the axon forming the tract ends. Thus it is simple to determine whether a tract is an ascending sensory or descending motor tract by analyzing the name. For example, the rubrospinal tract is a descending motor tract with its cell bodies in the red nucleus of the midbrain and its axon termination in the spinal cord.

Ascending pathways

Sensory information from peripheral receptors is transmitted through the nervous system in a series of neurons organized into an ascending pathway system. The sensory chain consists of three neurons, each having a long axon. The *first-order neuron* has its cell body in a dorsal root ganglion and conducts the impulse from the receptor to the spinal cord. (If the receptors of the first-

order neuron lie in the regions supplied by cranial nerves, its axon enters the brain stem instead of the cord.) The cell body of the *second-order neuron* is located at variable levels of the gray matter of the spinal cord or brain stem and conveys the impulse within the white matter of the cord to the thalamus. The *third-order neuron* conducts impulses from the thalamus to the cerebral cortex, and its cell body lies in the thalamus. In general, the major sensory systems and their pathways are somatotopically organized and they are crossed pathways. This means that organization according to body surface area is present in the spinal cord and thalamus as well as the primary somesthetic cortex and that each side of the brain registers sensations from the opposite side of the body. It is usually the second-order neuron that crosses at some point on its way to the thalamus. Only two of the ascending pathways are discussed in detail here.

Pain and temperature pathway. The direct neural pathway

for the sensations of pain and temperature is the lateral spinothalamic pathway (see Fig. 51-7). The sensory nerve fibers carrying impulses from stimulated pain or temperature receptors enter the dorsal root of the spinal cord, and once in the white matter, they bifurcate and ascend or descend a few segments before synapsing with the second-order neuron in the gray matter of the dorsal horn. The axon of this second-order neuron crosses over to the contralateral side, where it joins the other fibers in the lateral spinothalamic tract. These fibers proceed to the thalamus, where they synapse with a third-order neuron that relays the impulses to the sensory cortex. In the thalamus, the pain and temperature sensations come into consciousness vaguely but are not localized. The full extent of these sensations is consciously perceived and localized as the impulses are received in the primary and secondary somesthetic cortex of the parietal lobe. (NOTE: There is also an indirect spinoreticular thalamic pathway for pain.)

Fine touch, conscious proprioception, and vibration pathway. The neural pathway for fine (discriminating) touch, conscious proprioception (awareness of body position and movement), and vibratory sense is called the *medial lemniscal system.* This system consists of the tracts that make up the dorsal white columns of the cord (the fasciculi cuneatus and gracilis) plus the medial lemniscus, a flat band of fibers extending through the brain stem.

General mechanoreceptors responsive to fine touch, vibration, body position, and movement conduct impulses into the cord through the dorsal root; they then ascend directly on the same side via the dorsal columns. The dorsal columns are somatotopically organized. First-order neurons in the dorsal cord transmit impulses from the lower part of the body (T7 and below) by fibers that form the tract known as the *fasciculus gracilis.* The fibers terminate in the *nucleus gracilis* of the medulla, where they synapse on the second-order neurons of the sensory pathway. Fibers transmitting impulses from the upper part of the body (T6 and above) occupy the more lateral dorsal column as the *fasciculus cuneatus,* which terminates in the *nucleus cuneatus,* also located in the medulla. The reason for this laminar organization is that the sacral and dorsal column fibers are pushed medially as fibers from higher segments are added. Thus the information for the feet is located in the midline of the cord, whereas information from the upper extremities is located on the most lateral side of the cord. (The laminar organization of the spinothalamic tract is opposite to that of the dorsal columns. Fibers from sacral and lumbar segments of the body are pushed laterally by fibers crossing the midline at successively higher levels. Thus the lamination is cervical to sacral segments represented from the medial to more lateral position. Because of this lamination, tumors arising outside the spinal cord first compress the spinothalamic fibers from sacral and lumbar areas, causing the early symptom of a loss of pain in the sacral area.)

Fibers from the second-order neurons cross to the opposite side of the medulla and ascend as a component of a tract called the *medial lemniscus.* The fibers of the medial lemniscus synapse with third-order neurons in the thalamus, which in turn sends fibers through the internal capsule to the somesthetic cortex of the parietal lobe. The sensory data reach the conscious level and become localized in the sensory cortex.

Descending pathways

There are two major systems of motor pathways, classified as pyramidal and extrapyramidal. *Pyramidal tracts* (lateral and ventral corticospinal) are those whose fibers come together in the medulla to form the pyramids, thus the name. Most of the descending motor pathways involve two principal neurons—the upper and lower motor neurons. The *upper motor neuron* has its cell body in the cerebral motor cortex or in subcortical areas of the brain and brain stem, and its fibers conduct impulses from the brain to the spinal cord (or from the cerebrum to the brain stem [corticobulbar tract]). The spinal motor neuron (or cranial motor neuron) that innervates the muscle is called the *lower motor neuron.* Thus the upper motor neuron is entirely within the CNS, whereas the lower motor neuron begins in the CNS (anterior horn of the spinal cord gray matter) and sends its fibers out to innervate muscles. The lower motor neuron is thus a part of the PNS.

Voluntary motor pathway. The lateral and ventral corticospinal tracts are the major voluntary motor tracts of the spinal cord. These tracts are concerned primarily with controlled skilled movements of the extremities. Another important function of the upper motor neuron is to influence reflex movement by sending down facilitating or inhibiting impulses to alpha and gamma motor neurons (see Fig. 51-4).

The upper motor neurons of the corticospinal tracts originate in area 4 of the primary motor cortex, area 6 of the premotor cortex, and various portions of the parietal lobe. From here, fibers descend through the internal capsule to synapse with internuncials at various levels of the spinal cord, which in turn synapse with neurons in the ventral horn gray matter. Some fibers, however, may synapse directly with lower motor neurons. It is also true that not all these fibers descend to spinal cord levels, since some may synapse with motor nuclei of cranial nerves (corticobulbar fibers) and in the reticular formation.

Approximately 85% of the descending fibers decussate (cross over) in the medulla and extend down the cord on the opposite side as part of the lateral corticospinal tract. The remaining 15% of the fibers remain uncrossed and descend on the same side of the cord as the ventral corticospinal tract. These fibers eventually cross the midline in the ventral gray column of the spinal cord segments (generally in the cervical and upper thoracic regions). Lesions of the corticospinal tracts produce Babinski's sign (see Fig. 51-6) and loss of performance of skilled voluntary movements, especially of the distal segments of the extremities.

EXTRAPYRAMIDAL SYSTEM AND BASAL GANGLIA

Precise delineation of the extrapyramidal system (all motor fibers not passing through the pyramids) is difficult anatomically. If the system is considered as an anatomic unit, it is composed of the (1) basal ganglia and their circuits, (2) cortical areas that project to the basal ganglia, (3) cerebellar areas that project to the basal ganglia, (4) parts of the reticular formation that have connections with the basal ganglia and cerebral cortex, and (5) thalamic nuclei that connect the basal ganglia and reticular formation.

The primary function of the extrapyramidal system is to provide coarse control for voluntary muscles. (Fine control is provided by the pyramidal or corticospinal system.) The whole system works as a unit providing for integration on three levels: cortical, striatal, and tegmental. The major effect is inhibition (Fig. 50-21).

The *basal ganglia*, or *basal nuclei*, are found in each cerebral hemisphere in paired groups and are formed from the central gray matter of the telencephalon. They

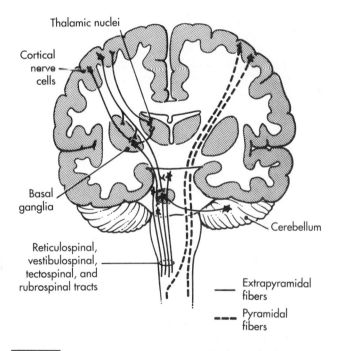

FIG. 50-21   Simplified diagram of pyramidal and extrapyramidal systems. Posture and performance of well-coordinated movements result from an integration of information received from both the cerebral cortex and the extrapyramidal systems. The cortex initiates movement, and the extrapyramidal system provides the facilitation or inhibition needed for production of purposeful, coordinated, controlled movements. Disruption of the extrapyramidal influence results in abnormal, uncontrolled movements. Components of the extrapyramidal system are the reticulospinal, vestibulospinal, tectospinal, and rubrospinal tracts. (Modified from *Medical notes on parkinsonism and pseudoparkinsonism*, 1972, Research Triangle Park, NC, Burroughs Wellcome.)

include the claustrum, putamen, globus pallidus, caudate, and amygdala (Fig. 50-22). The *caudate nucleus,* the most medial of the basal ganglia, is shaped like a comma with an extended tail. The *amygdaloid nucleus* lies as a knob of gray matter at the tip of the tail of the caudate. The putamen and globus pallidus together are called the *lenticular* (lens-shaped) *nucleus;* it extends from the head of the caudate. The *internal capsule* lies within borders formed by the thalamus, caudate nucleus, and lenticular nucleus. This crucial area is a passageway for all nerve fibers connecting the cerebrum with the rest of the CNS. The caudate and lenticular nucleus, along with the adjacent part of the internal capsule, are sometimes referred to as the *corpus striatum.*

Three nuclear masses located in the upper midbrain operate in close association with the basal ganglia and are considered to be part of the extrapyramidal system: the *red nucleus;* the *substantia nigra;* and the *subthalamic nucleus,* or *corpus Luysii.*

The basal ganglia have multiple connections with other portions of the CNS, including the cerebral cortex, cerebellum, thalamus, and reticular formation. They are important centers of coordination, especially in the control of automatic associated movements. The corpus striatum (caudate nucleus and putamen) is responsible for the initiation and inhibition of gross intentional body movements that are unconsciously performed in the normal person. They also provide muscle tone so that exact movements can be performed, such as fine handwork requiring the coordinated effort of the entire arm and trunk for the hand to be able to perform.

A feedback system seems to operate via circular pathways from the motor cortex to the basal ganglia, thalamus, and motor cortex. Motor signals from the cerebral cortex to the pons and cerebellum are also circuitous, with the return to the cortex being through the ventrolateral nucleus of the thalamus, through which signals from the basal ganglia also pass. Because of the proximity of these circuits, it is hypothesized that basal ganglia and cerebellum feedback signals could be integrated in this area.

Broadly speaking, the basal ganglia are involved in two general activities: control of the body's motor tone, and gross intentional movements. The general effect of basal ganglia excitation is of inhibitory signals to the bulboreticular facilitatory areas and of excitatory signals to the bulboreticular inhibitory areas. When the basal ganglia are not functioning adequately, the facilitatory areas become overactive and the inhibitory areas underactive. This results in rigidity throughout the body. The patient with an extrapyramidal disorder has great difficulty maintaining equilibrium while standing and posture while sitting, changing from a horizontal to a sitting position, rolling from a supine to a prone position, and walking. The righting reflex, the vestibular reflex, and proprioception are all disturbed. If the spinal cord is transected at the level of the mesencephalon, a *decerebrate rigidity* oc-

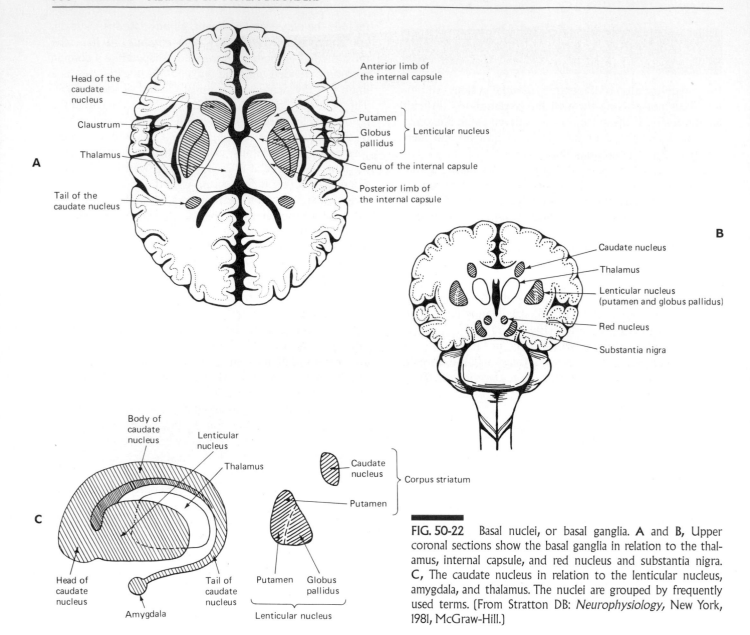

FIG. 50-22   Basal nuclei, or basal ganglia. **A** and **B,** Upper coronal sections show the basal ganglia in relation to the thalamus, internal capsule, and red nucleus and substantia nigra. **C,** The caudate nucleus in relation to the lenticular nucleus, amygdala, and thalamus. The nuclei are grouped by frequently used terms. (From Stratton DB: *Neurophysiology,* New York, 1981, McGraw-Hill.)

curs, indicating that the major effect of the basal ganglia is inhibition. The tremor (abnormal movements) observed in extrapyramidal disorders is a result of excess neural activity in one area of the brain from unopposed activity in another area. This characteristic is called the *release phenomenon* and occurs often with tissue destruction in the nervous system (a lesion in A removes the regulatory control that A exerted over B, and consequently B becomes overactive).

Both the corpus striatum and the motor cortex are instrumental in the control of gross intentional movements that are normally unconscious. The control is accomplished through two pathways: (1) the globus pallidus through the thalamus to the cortex and downward via corticospinal and extracorticospinal pathways into the spinal cord and (2) downward through the globus pallidus and substantia nigra to the reticular formation and reticulospinal tracts to the cord. The globus pallidus seems to provide the background muscle tone necessary for performing exacting movements, especially with the hands. Stimulation of the globus pallidus will stop the movement at any point and keep it locked at that point as long as the stimulation is continued.

Parkinson's syndrome and several extrapyramidal disorders of movement that involve the basal ganglia and extrapyramidal system are discussed in Chapter 54.

QUESTIONS

▼ *Circle T if the statement is true and F if it is false. Correct any false statements.*

1. T F The nervous system consists of two major cell types: (1) the neurons with their processes and (2) supporting connective tissue.

2. T F The nervous system is a communication system that directs and integrates all body activity.

3. T F Dendrites conduct impulses away from the neuron cell body.

4. T F The central nervous system (CNS) includes the brain, spinal cord, and cranial nerves.

5. T F All nerve cell bodies are located in the CNS.

6. T F Interneurons relay messages between other neurons in the CNS, and large numbers may be found in the gray matter of the spinal cord, forming intersegmental tracts.

7. T F Schwann cells form the myelin for neuronal processes within the CNS.

8. T F Spinal nerve trunks carry both afferent and efferent impulses to the CNS and are thus mixed nerves.

9. T F Nerves of the autonomic nervous system (ANS) are associated with both cranial and spinal nerves.

10. T F The parasympathetic branch of the ANS forms the thoracolumbar outflow from the spinal cord.

11. T F The ANS is primarily concerned with the regulation of visceral functions, such as heart rate, blood pressure, and intestinal motility.

12. T F Nerve cells are not mitotic; they do not reproduce.

13. T F The characteristic color of the white matter of the brain and spinal cord is the result of the presence of myelin-covered fiber tracts.

14. T F It is possible for a severed nerve fiber in the peripheral nervous system (PNS) to regenerate as long as the cell body is still viable.

15. T F Scar tissue in the CNS consists of astrocytes and may result in focal epilepsy.

16. T F Retinal rod and cone cells are examples of multipolar neurons.

17. T F Golgi type II neurons have extremely long axons.

18. T F The direction of a nerve impulse can be reversed.

19. T F Axons lack Nissl substance and thus cannot manufacture protein and must depend on the cell body for such production.

20. T F Convergence means that a single neuron receives input from two or more neurons, and the response is the summated effect of all the different types of information.

21. T F Convergence and divergence are important mechanisms enabling the nervous system to perform its integration and control functions.

22. T F The neurilemma is a thin membrane that envelops all nerve fibers.

23. T F A nerve fiber is the axon (or dendrite) of a nerve cell.

24. T F Bundles of nerve fibers found in the CNS are called cranial nerves.

25. T F The spinal cord terminates in the vertebral cavity at about L4.

26. T F Lesions of the brain stem affect cranial nerves I and II (olfactory and optic).

27. T F Tight junctions between epithelial cells of the choroid plexus provide the mechanism for the blood–cerebrospinal fluid (CSF) barrier.

▼ *Circle the letter preceding each item below that correctly answers the question or completes the statement. More than one answer may be correct.*

28. Which of the following structures is not included in the CNS?
    a. Glia cells
    b. Cerebellum
    c. Spinal cord
    d. Basal ganglia
    e. Ganglia of the sympathetic chain

29. Which of the following are characteristic of the ANS?
    a. Control of activities that are largely involuntary
    b. Atrophy of the muscle innervated if the nerve is destroyed
    c. Location outside the spinal cord

d. Invariable resultant excitation of the effector organ

30. The myelencephalon is composed of the:
    a. Medulla oblongata
    b. Cerebral hemispheres
    c. Pons
    d. Cerebellum

31. Subdivisions of the brain included in the prosencephalon (forebrain) include the:
    a. Myelencephalon   c. Diencephalon
    b. Metencephalon   d. Telencephalon

32. Regeneration of nerve fibers will occur if the cell body is intact and the fiber has:
    a. A myelin sheath   c. A dendrite
    b. An axon   d. A neurolemma

33. The processes of a neuron are:
    a. Cytoplasm
    b. Axon and one or more dendrites
    c. Cell body and one or more axons

34. The point at which the electrical activity from one neuron influences the excitability of another neuron is the:
    a. Sensory receptor   c. Synapse
    b. Effector   d. Cell

35. The nerve cell has a resting potential because its membrane is selectively permeable to different ions. The most important ions in the maintenance of resting membrane potential are:
    a. Calcium and phosphorus
    b. Magnesium and calcium
    c. Phosphorus and sodium
    d. Potassium and sodium

36. Which of the following statements is *false* concerning the meninges?
    a. The denticulate ligaments, located between the ventral and dorsal roots, are pial tissue that attaches to the dura at intervals.
    b. The pia mater is the innermost layer.
    c. The arachnoid is the outermost layer.
    d. The pia mater and arachnoid are collectively known as the leptomeninges.

37. The sheath of meningeal dura separating cerebrum from cerebellum is the:
    a. Falx cerebri
    b. Falx cerebelli
    c. Diaphragma sellae
    d. Tentorium cerebelli

38. An extradural hematoma is most often caused by:
    a. Rupture of the emissary veins

Continued.

QUESTIONS—cont'd

b. Damage to the cerebral venous sinuses
c. Laceration of the galea
d. Rupture of the middle meningeal artery
e. Rupture of the middle cerebral artery

39. The rupture of an aneurysm on the circle of Willis would likely cause bleeding into which of the following spaces?
   a. Epidural   c. Subarachnoid
   b. Subdural   d. Subaponeurotic

40. Head injury resulting in laceration of the galea is particularly hazardous and may lead to meningitis or brain abscess because:
   a. The emissary veins provide an access route for infection to enter the skull.
   b. The galea is part of the outer meningeal layer.
   c. The meningeal arteries form a direct connection between the scalp and dural sinuses through which infection can enter the skull.
   d. The source of infection is via the vertebral and internal carotids, since veins do not penetrate the skull.

41. The arterial supply to the brain is provided by the:
   a. External carotid arteries
   b. Internal carotid arteries
   c. Vertebral arteries
   d. Jugulars

42. Which of the following arteries is not included in the circle of Willis?
   a. Anterior communicating
   b. Posterior communicating
   c. Internal carotid
   d. Posterior cerebral
   e. Vertebral

43. The basilar artery is formed by the:
   a. Internal carotid arteries
   b. Anterior cerebral arteries
   c. Posterior cerebral arteries
   d. Vertebral arteries

44. A 65-year-old woman with hypertension reports episodes of blindness in the right eye and weakness in the left leg lasting 20 to 30 minutes. An arteriogram revealed atherosclerotic narrowing of an artery supplying the brain. Which artery accounted for the symptoms?
   a. Left internal carotid
   b. Right internal carotid
   c. Left posterior cerebral
   d. Vertebral-basilar

45. The major blood supply to the precen-

tral and postcentral gyrus is provided by the:
   a. Middle cerebral artery
   b. Anterior cerebral artery
   c. Posterior cerebral artery
   d. Anterior communicating artery

46. A compression fracture of the skull from a blow on the crown of the head would be most likely to damage which of the following dural sinuses?
   a. Straight sinus
   b. Superior sagittal sinus
   c. Cavernous venous sinus
   d. Sigmoid sinus

47. Which of the following statements is(are) *true* concerning the conducting and penetrating arteries of the brain?
   a. Conducting arteries form an array over the surface of the brain.
   b. Penetrating arteries branch off the conducting arteries at right angles to supply the internal capsule and other deep structures.
   c. Penetrating arteries from the middle cerebral artery are frequently implicated in a stroke syndrome.
   d. Occlusion of the penetrating blood vessels supplying the internal capsule results in paralysis.

48. Cerebrospinal fluid:
   a. Is formed at the rate of about 0.5 L/day
   b. Provides a protective cushion around the brain and spinal cord
   c. Is formed in the arachnoid granulations
   d. Flows out of the third ventricle into the fourth through the foramen of Magendie
   e. Has an average pressure of 130 mm H_2O when a patient is in the recumbent position during a spinal tap

49. Noncommunicating hydrocephalus:
   a. Is the most common form of hydrocephalus in the adult
   b. Is a form of low-pressure hydrocephalus
   c. Is frequently caused by a congenital narrowing of the aqueduct of Sylvius
   d. May be treated by shunting CSF to the jugular vein
   e. Does not usually cause swelling of the head

50. Which of the following does not apply to CSF?
   a. Clear, colorless
   b. Higher chloride and sodium content than blood plasma

c. Less glucose than plasma
   d. Absorbed into the arterial system
   e. Contains little protein

51. Which statement concerning the brain is *false?*
   a. Hypoglycemia can cause brain damage, since the brain is largely dependent on glucose for its energy supply.
   b. Brain tissue may be irreversibly damaged within a few minutes in the event of an untreated cardiac arrest.
   c. Brain metabolism decreases to an almost negligible level during sleep.
   d. The brain uses about 20% of the cardiac output.
   e. The brain is the most energy-consuming tissue in the entire body.

52. The brain stem includes:
   a. The medulla oblongata
   b. The pons
   c. The basal ganglia
   d. The midbrain

53. The following structures are located in the midbrain:
   a. Superior and inferior colliculi
   b. Hypothalamus
   c. Red nucleus
   d. Substantia nigra

54. The superior colliculi are concerned with:
   a. Auditory reflexes   c. Respiration
   b. Visual reflexes   d. Heart rate

55. An intact medulla is necessary for integration of reflexes involving:
   a. Swallowing
   b. Vomiting
   c. Cardiovascular control
   d. Respiration

56. The thalamus:
   a. Is an important sensory relay center
   b. Has many interconnections with the cerebral cortex
   c. Is a center of crude sensory awareness
   d. Relays impulses from the olfactory system
   e. Is the largest structure of the diencephalon

57. The hypothalamus:
   a. Contains nuclei that produce antidiuretic hormone
   b. Regulates hormone release by the anterior pituitary
   c. Is a control center of the ANS
   d. Contains a center for temperature control

58. Hemiballismus (violent flinging movements of the limbs on one side of the

? QUESTIONS—cont'd

body) may result from a lesion of the:
a. Pineal body
b. Primary motor cortex
c. Subthalamus
d. Hippocampus

59. The limbic system:
a. Is primarily involved with the expression of primitive emotions
b. Is involved in recent memory
c. Is believed to be involved in psychomotor epilepsy
d. Includes the corpus callosum

60. The two cerebral hemispheres are separated by the:
a. Central sulcus (fissure of Rolando)
b. Great longitudinal fissure
c. Fissure of Sylvius
d. Parietooccipital sulcus

61. Which of the following is not visible on the lateral surface of the brain?
a. Corpus callosum
b. Insula
c. Precentral gyrus
d. Occipital lobe

62. All the following structures are classified as projection tracts *except:*
a. Corona radiata
b. Internal capsule
c. Corpus callosum

63. Which sulcus separates the frontal lobe of the brain from the parietal lobe?
a. Parietooccipital   c. Central
b. Precentral   d. Postcentral

64. Projection fibers of the internal capsule are:
a. Afferent   c. Both
b. Efferent   d. Neither

65. The thin surface of the cerebrum is referred to as the:
a. Cortex   c. Corona radiata
b. Sulcus   d. Midbrain

66. Area 17 of the cerebral cortex is the principal visual cortex and is located in the:
a. Frontal lobe   c. Temporal lobe
b. Parietal lobe   d. Occipital lobe

67. The somesthetic area of the cortex:
a. Is located on the postcentral gyrus
b. Is located in the frontal lobe
c. Receives fibers from the thalamus
d. Is represented by areas 3, 1, and 2

68. Wernicke's area (area 22) is important for:
a. Voluntary scanning movements of the eyes
b. Comprehension of spoken language
c. Ability to recognize objects by touch
d. Ability to write
e. Comprehension of written language

69. The precentral gyrus is:
a. Somatotopically arranged with the facial areas in the most medial position
b. Areas 3, 1, and 2
c. The motor strip
d. Located in the frontal lobe
e. Area 4

70. The sensory association areas:
a. Are necessary for the interpretation and understanding of sensory input to the brain
b. Include areas 5 and 7 of the parietal lobe
c. Include areas 3, 1, and 2
d. Are involved with awareness of body image

71. A 70-year-old woman, on recovering from a cerebrovascular accident (stroke), was found to have difficulty in understanding written language (alexia) and inability to write (agraphia) but could understand spoken speech. Which area of the cortex was damaged by the stroke?
a. Broca's area
b. The angular gyrus (area 39)
c. Areas 5 and 7
d. Wernicke's area

72. A young college student was observed to have a marked change of behavior following a tobogganing accident in which he sustained a compression fracture of the skull. His dress became slovenly, and he failed to complete his assignments, contrary to his usual behavior. He was sent to the mental health clinic by a professor when he urinated in a wastebasket of the classroom. Which area of his brain was most likely injured and accounted for the behavior change?
a. Temporal lobe   c. Area 6
b. Prefrontal cortex   d. Area 40

73. Which of the following functional deficits would be most likely following a stroke involving the left middle cerebral artery?
a. Failure to recognize faces
b. Aphasia
c. Loss of topographic memory
d. Left-sided hemiplegia

74. The reticular substance extends through which of the following structures?
a. Thalamus
b. Midbrain
c. Pons
d. Medulla oblongata
e. Upper spinal cord

75. Some important functions of the reticular formation include:
a. Screening of sensory stimuli
b. Activation of the cerebral cortex to become sensitive to stimuli
c. Regulation of the sleep-wakefulness cycle
d. Modulation of motor activity

76. CNS monoamines produced in nuclei in the brain stem include:
a. Norepinephrine   c. Dopamine
b. Epinephrine   d. Serotonin

77. The CNS monoamines:
a. Are involved in the regulation of emotional behavior
b. Are affected by mood-altering drugs such as the tranquilizers
c. Are involved in the regulation of sleep and wakefulness

78. Cranial nerve V:
a. Is called the facial nerve
b. Is sensory to the face
c. Is motor to the muscles of mastication
d. Is a purely sensory nerve

79. The hypoglossal nerve:
a. Carries impulses for taste on the anterior two thirds of the tongue
b. Supplies the muscles of the tongue
c. Is a purely motor nerve
d. Is cranial nerve XI

80. The cranial nerve concerned with vision is the:
a. Optic   c. Trochlear
b. Oculomotor   d. Abducens

81. Which of the following statements is(are) *true* concerning the spinal nerves?
a. The dorsal root of a spinal nerve carries both sensory and motor fibers.
b. The motor fibers originate in the anterior horn of the spinal cord.
c. There are 31 pairs of spinal nerves.
d. Sensory components of the spinal nerves have their origin in the dorsal root ganglia.

82. Spinal nerve roots C5 through T1 or T2 give origin to the:
a. Brachial plexus
b. Femoral nerve
c. Radial nerve
d. Median nerve
e. Cervical plexus

83. The collection of nerve roots immediately below the spinal cord is called:
a. Fasciculus gracilis
b. Filum terminale
c. Cauda equina
d. Posterior columns

Continued.

QUESTIONS—cont'd

84. The simplest reflex arc involves how many neurons?
    a. One
    b. Two
    c. Three
    d. Four or more

85. All the following are ascending tracts in the spinal cord *except:*
    a. Fasciculus cuneatus
    b. Lateral spinothalamic
    c. Ventral spinocerebellar
    d. Ventral corticospinal

86. Which of the following sensations is(are) carried by the dorsal columns?
    a. Conscious proprioception
    b. Vibration sense
    c. Two-point discrimination
    d. Pain
    e. Temperature

87. The lateral spinothalamic tract:
    a. Carries the afferent impulses for fine touch
    b. Is the conscious pathway for pain and temperature
    c. Terminates in the fasciculus cuneatus and gracilis ·
    d. Is the motor pathway for voluntary muscle control

88. All the following statements concerning the conscious pathway for pain and temperature are true *except:*
    a. The cell body for the first-order neuron is located in the ipsilateral dorsal root ganglion.
    b. The cell body for the second-order neuron is located in the ipsilateral dorsal horn, but its axon crosses over to the opposite side of the spinal cord and courses up the lateral spinothalamic tract.

    c. The third-order neuron is located in the nucleus cuneatus.
    d. The axon of the third-order neuron terminates in the postcentral gyrus.

89. The lentiform nucleus includes the:
    a. Putamen
    b. Globus pallidus
    c. Amygdala
    d. Caudate

90. Which of the following fiber tract impulses are mediated through the ventral horn cell of the final common pathway (more than one answer may be correct)?
    a. Corticospinal
    b. Tectospinal
    c. Rubrospinal
    d. Vestibulospinal

91. The basal ganglia are (only one answer is correct):
    a. Masses of white matter embedded deep inside the cerebrum
    b. Paired structures found in each hemisphere
    c. Six distinct structures each independent of the others
    d. Cortical structures related to vegetative activities and having a steadying influence on muscle

92. All of the following diffuse across the blood-brain barrier *except:*
    a. Glucose
    b. Essential amino acids
    c. Free fatty acids
    d. Proteins

▼ *Match the numbers in column B with the appropriate item in column A.*

	Column A	Column B
93. _____	Pairs of cranial nerves	a. 7
94. _____	Pairs of spinal nerves	b. 3
95. _____	Number of cervical vertebrae	c. 8
96. _____	Pairs of cervical spinal nerves	d. 12
97. _____	Oculomotor nerve (cranial nerve number)	e. 31

▼ *Match the specialized functions in column B with the cerebral hemisphere they are more likely to be associated with in column A.*

	Column A	Column B
98. _____	Right hemisphere ·	a. Mathematical calculation
99. _____	Left hemisphere	b. Speech
		c. Spatial locations
		d. Grasping of whole concepts
		e. Music
		f. Right-handedness

▼ *Answer the following on a separate sheet of paper.*

100. Name and outline the components of the extrapyramidal system. What is its function? Name the basal ganglia.

CHAPTER 51

Evaluation of the Neurologic Patient

MARY CARTER LOMBARDO
MARY S. HARTWIG

clinical picture presented by most patients with a neurologic deficit. A complete and careful history and physical examination provides the final diagnosis in about 80% of patients. Despite the advances in diagnostic testing procedures, nothing has been found that can replace the history and physical examination.

For the neurologic examination to yield the necessary information, it is important, whenever possible, to gain the patient's cooperation. During the process of examination the patient is often requested to do something that may appear nonsensical or may sound ridiculous. Careful explanation before the neurologic examination should allay the patient's anxiety and clarify the importance of the examination to the diagnostic process. Explanation about the length of the examination, the procedure to be followed, and any pain that the patient can expect will help establish trust and confidence in the examiner. The patient should be requested to answer all questions as accurately as possible and follow all directions to the best of his or her ability. Time must be allotted for the patient's questions, both before and after the examination.

Neurology is a discipline that is concerned with diseases and disorders of the nervous system, a complex and vital network that allows the individual to cope and adapt to environmental stresses. Diseases of the nervous system may develop insidiously, with gradual loss of function (e.g., multiple sclerosis) or acutely, with sudden interference in normal functioning (e.g., ruptured aneurysm). Regardless of the cause, the professional health practitioner is dealing with a patient who must adapt to a new method of functioning, whether temporary or permanent.

Clinical examination of the patient with a neurologic disorder yields valuable information. Symptoms presented by patients seeking health care include the ones derived from the primary neurologic disorder and those arising from fear, depression, weakness, and other symptoms arising from the individual patient's method of adapting. A logical, systematic, thorough examination of the patient and the presenting complaints can assist the clinician in differentiating and analyzing the complex

NEUROLOGIC EXAMINATION

Evaluation of the patient with a neurologic disorder begins by systematically evaluating the patient and the complaints. The history, a summary of the patient's symptoms, and a discussion of similar or related complaints in family members will focus the clinician's thinking, direct the physical examination, and become the keystone for diagnosis of the problem. The close relationship between neurologic symptoms and symptoms of other medical disease states (e.g., diabetes mellitus, hypertension, thyroid disorders) necessitates a complete medical evaluation, even though the patient's symptoms suggest a neurologic problem. Explanations are especially important to help allay the patient's anxiety because the neurologic patient, more than any other patient, requires a clinician who sees beyond the symptoms and the disease process to the patient and family.

The neurologic history focuses on why the patient seeks medical attention. It is important that this information be elicited and recorded in the patient's own words, not in diagnostic terms. A detailed discussion of the neurologic examination is not included here because it can be found in many standard textbooks on neurology. A brief summary of the examination is included to help review some important points.

Important information includes past medical history, social history, family history, and onset of present symptoms. It is important to ask the patient what problems, if any, have been experienced with each major body system and part. The patient is asked specifically about dizziness, headaches, visual disturbances, bowel or bladder dysfunction, weakness, numbness, and pain. While eliciting this information, the clinician carefully observes the patient's behavior, attitudes, attention to personal appearance and grooming, ability to answer the questions appropriately, and ability to concentrate. Once this portion of the examination is completed, the clinician can substantiate suspicions and abnormal findings with further examinations and diagnostic tests. In some cases of neurologic disorder (e.g., migraine, trigeminal neuralgia), the diagnosis is made purely on the basis of the history because there are no significant physical findings.

Organization of the neurologic examination is very important. Following a particular order allows the clinician to evaluate the information and direct the later segments of the examination. The organization of the examination includes evaluation of (1) mental status and function, (2) level of consciousness, (3) cerebral functions, (4) language and speech, (5) cranial nerve function, (6) motor function (coordination and gait, muscle tone and strength), (7) reflexes, and (8) sensory function. Information from each segment of the examination is correlated with information previously gained, leading to a localization of the disease process.

Mental Status and Function

This portion of the examination evaluates the patient's ability to reason, abstract, plan ahead, and make judgments. Changes in behavior and personality may be associated with organic brain dysfunction; therefore these changes need to be elicited from the patient or the patient's family. In evaluating the patient's mental status, the examiner must be aware of socioeconomic, ethnic, and educational status. General knowledge and intellect may be evaluated by asking the patient to name five countries or five major rivers. The patient's ability to remember past events may be evaluated by asking the patient questions about his or her own past, but may be difficult to assess. Recent memory may be assessed by asking the patient to repeat at least six digits. Normal persons have the ability to remember and repeat seven digits forward and four backward. Important information is obtained by evaluating the patient's ability to produce abstract thoughts and generalizations from concrete statements. Asking the patient to interpret a common saying (e.g., "A rolling stone gathers no moss") is a frequently used method.

Level of Consciousness

Evaluating the patient's level of consciousness (LOC) is an essential component of the neurologic examination that should be performed thoughtfully, with meticulous attention to accuracy. Many tools are available today for categorizing LOC, using similar terms in different ways. (see Glasgow Coma Scale, Chapter 56). When using any tool, the most important criterion should be consistency, and a complete understanding of all terminology is essential. It is always better to describe the patient's behavior and responses exactly than to rely on such catch-all terms as *lethargic* or *stuporous*. Table 51-1 lists several terms used to describe LOC, with descriptions of behavior associated with these terms.

Cerebral Functions

Knowledge of the functions of the cerebral lobes and subsequently related symptoms associated with deficits of that particular area of the brain assist the clinician in pinpointing the neurologic deficit. Important observations about the patient's neurologic problems are made during the neurologic examination. Table 51-2 lists the cerebral lobes and some of their known functions.

Language and Speech

One of the most important functions of the dominant hemisphere is speech. The left hemisphere is dominant for speech in right-handed persons and in most left-handed persons. There are three speech disorders of neurologic origin: dysarthria, dysphonia, and aphasia.

Dysarthria is a defect in articulation, enumeration, and rhythm of speech related to a weakness in the muscles involved in speech. This abnormality is usually detected in ordinary conversation with the patient but may be confirmed by asking for repetition of a difficult word or phrase, such as "methodist episcopal." The causes for this weakness can be amyotrophic lateral sclerosis, pseudobulbar palsy, or myasthenia gravis.

Dysphonia is a disorder of vocalization giving a hoarse quality to the voice. The disorder can be confirmed by detecting hoarseness or a rough quality to the voice of a patient responding to a request to say "E" and by indirect laryngoscopy. This problem has many nonneurologic causes; among the neurologic causes are injury to the recurrent laryngeal nerve and tumors of the brain stem.

Aphasia is a general term meaning loss of the ability to comprehend, elaborate, or express speech concepts. *Motor aphasia* is loss of the ability to express thoughts in speech or writing, and *sensory aphasia* is loss of the abil-

TABLE 51-1   Levels of Consciousness

Term	Characteristics
Conscious	Freely aware of surroundings; oriented to person, place, and time Cooperative Can repeat several digits a few minutes after being told them
Automatism	Relatively normal behavior (e.g., capable of feeding self) Speaks in sentences but has difficulty with memory and judgment; no recollection of events before period of unconsciousness; may ask the same questions over and over Behaves automatically without immediate or late memory of behavior Obeys simple commands
Confusion	Performs purposeful activity (e.g., feeding) with clumsy movements Disoriented as to time, place, and/or person (acts as if in a daze) Memory impaired, unable to sustain thought or expression Generally difficult to arouse Becomes uncooperative
Delirium	Disoriented to time, place, and person Uncooperative Agitated, restless, resistive (may attempt to get out of bed; thrashes around in bed; pulls off dressings, IV, etc.) Difficult to arouse
Stupor	Quiet, may appear to be asleep Responds to loud verbal stimuli Annoyed by light Responds appropriately to painful stimuli
Deep stupor	Mute Very difficult to arouse (some arousal to painful stimuli) Responds to pain with automatic purposeless movements
Coma	Unconscious; body flaccid No response to verbal or painful stimuli Reflexes present; gag, knee jerk, corneal
Irreversible coma and death	Reflexes disappear Pupils become fixed and dilated Cessation of respirations and heartbeat

TABLE 51-2   Cerebral Functions and Deficits

Cerebral Lobe	Functions	Deficits
Frontal	Judgment Personality traits Complex mental skills (abstraction, conceptualizing, foresight)	Impaired judgment Impaired grooming and appearance Impaired affect Impaired thought process Impaired motor functions
Temporal	Auditory memory Recent memory Primary auditory area affecting awareness	Deficits in recent memory Psychomotor seizures Deafness
Parietal Dominant	Speech Calculation (mathematics) Topography of both sides of body	Aphasia Agraphia Acalculia Agnosia Sensory deficits (bilateral)
Nondominant	Sensory awareness Synthesis of complex memories	Disorientation Distortion of concept of space Loss of awareness of opposite side
Occipital	Visual memory Vision	Blindness and visual deficits

ity to comprehend spoken or written language. For evaluation, the patient may be directed to perform certain tasks by written or verbal orders, such as, "Fold this paper" and "Write your name." The most common cause of aphasia is a cerebrovascular disorder involving the middle cerebral artery, which supplies the speech and language center.

Cranial Nerve Function

Twelve pairs of cranial nerves arise from the undersurface of the brain through small foramina. They are numbered according to the order in which they emerge, from front to rear (Fig. 51-1).

The cranial nerves are composed of afferent or efferent fibers, and some, referred to as *mixed fibers,* are of both types. The cell bodies of the afferent fibers are located in ganglia outside the brain stem, whereas the cell bodies of the efferent fibers are located in various nuclei of the brain stem.

The cranial nerves are examined not in sequence but according to function. The method of examination of the cranial nerves and some pathophysiologic implications are discussed in the following sections.

Olfactory nerve (cranial nerve I)

The olfactory nerve conveys smells to the brain for appreciation. With the patient's eyes closed and one nostril occluded at a time, mildly aromatic substances, such as vanilla, cologne, and cloves, are offered for identification. The patient is requested to indicate the moment of first detection of the odor and, if possible, to identify the

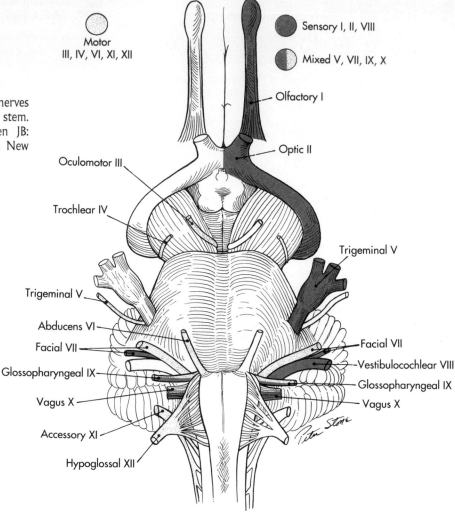

FIG. 51-1 Emergence of the cranial nerves from the ventral surface of the brain stem. (From Langley LL, Telford JR, Christensen JB: *Dynamic anatomy and physiology*, ed 5, New York, 1980, McGraw-Hill.)

substance. Perception of the odor is more important than correct identification of the substance.

Nasal disorders (e.g., sinusitis, allergies, upper respiratory infections) are the most common causes of loss of smell. A tumor in the olfactory groove (olfactory groove meningioma) is a neurologic cause for the loss of smell.

Anosmia may also occur after meningitis, subarachnoid hemorrhage, or head injury involving the nerve fibers as they pass through the cribriform plate.

Optic nerve (cranial nerve II)

The optic nerve transmits impulses from the retina to the thalamus via the optic chiasm. Higher-order visual pathways convey the information from the thalamus to the occipital cortex for recognition and interpretation. Examination of this nerve involves testing visual acuity either by using a Snellen test or, if this is not available, by asking the patient to read various sizes of newspaper print. Reduction of visual acuity is generally caused by diseases involving the eye, the optic nerve, or the optic chiasm. Visual field examinations provide information about the optic nerve and visual pathways from the eye to the occipital cortex. For general purposes as part of a

neurologic examination, visual fields are examined by confrontation by asking the patient to cover one eye. The examiner sits directly in front of the patient asking him or her to look straight ahead. A pencil or finger is brought into the field of vision from the four quadrants toward the uncovered eye. The patient is asked to identify when the pencil or finger first enters the visual field. This method provides a gross screening device. For a more thorough evaluation, a perimeter and tangent screen are used.

The optic disc is visualized by use of the ophthalmoscope. Neurologically the two most significant findings are papilledema and optic atrophy. Changes in the disc occur with tumors, infections, and trauma. Other changes visualized are exudates, hemorrhages, and arteriovenous abnormalities associated with diabetes and hypertension.

Oculomotor, trochlear, and abducens nerves (cranial nerves III, IV, and VI)

These three nerves are examined together, since they act conjugately to control the extraocular muscles (EOMs). In addition, the oculomotor nerve elevates the upper eyelid and innervates the constrictor muscle, which alters the pupil size. The innervation of the EOMs is ex-

PUPIL GAUGE (mm.)

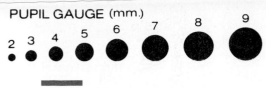

FIG. 51-2   Pupil size reference guide.

amined by asking the patient to follow a moving finger or pencil with eyes turning upward, downward, medially, and laterally. Weakness in muscles becomes evident when an eye cannot move in a certain direction. Pupils are examined in subdued light and should be round and approximately equal in size, although unequal pupils are found in approximately 20% to 25% of the population. However, the difference is rarely greater than 1 mm. Both pupils should react to light directly and consensually.

In recording the size of the pupils, it is essential to use millimeters (mm) to ensure accuracy in evaluating the patient's neurologic status. This practice is particularly important when the practitioner is evaluating a patient after a head injury. Fig. 51-2 provides a pupil size reference guide.

The nuclei of the oculomotor nerves and the trochlear nerve are located in the midbrain. The nuclei of the abducens nerve lies beneath the floor of the fourth ventricle in the lower pons and are close to fibers from the facial nerve nucleus.

Myasthenia gravis is an important cause of weakness of the EOMs, causing weakness in more than one muscle and ptosis (see Chapter 54). *Horner's syndrome* consists of ptosis of the lid, constriction of the pupil, and absence of sweating on the same side of the face. These symptoms can result from vascular lesions in the brain stem, cervical spinal cord injuries and tumors, or trauma affecting the sympathetic fibers in the neck or can be a temporary side effect of cerebral angiography.

Horizontal nystagmus (rapid lateral oscillations of the eye) is an important neurologic sign. It is seen normally on extreme lateral gaze. Nystagmus can occur in any direction of gaze and can be unilateral or bilateral. Neurologic causes include multiple sclerosis, lesions of one cerebellar hemisphere, and tumor of one side of the brain. Nonneurologic causes include the use of barbiturates and tranquilizers.

Trigeminal nerve (cranial nerve V)

The trigeminal nerve carries both motor and sensory fibers. It supplies innervation to the temporal and masseter muscles, which are the muscles of mastication. The motor division of this nerve is examined by asking the patient to clench the teeth and move the jaw from side to side while the examiner palpates the muscles and judges the strength of contraction.

The sensory fibers of the trigeminal nerve are divided into three main branches: ophthalmic, maxillary, and mandibular (Fig. 51-3). To evaluate areas of sensory loss, each area is tested by asking the patient to respond to a touch with a piece of cotton. The corneal reflex is tested in each eye: a wisp of cotton with a fine point is touched to the cornea, causing the patient to blink.

Tumors of the posterior fossa cause loss of corneal reflex and facial numbness as early signs. The most notable disorder affecting the trigeminal nerve is *trigeminal neuralgia,* or *tic douloureux,* causing brief, excruciating pain along the maxillary or mandibular divisions of the trigeminal nerve. Myasthenia gravis and amyotrophic lateral sclerosis cause weakness and fatigue of the muscles of mastication, making chewing difficult and at times impossible.

Facial nerve (cranial nerve VII)

The facial nerve has both sensory and motor function. It carries sensory fibers that mediate taste perception from the anterior tongue and motor fibers, which innervate all the muscles necessary for the varied facial expressions: smiling, frowning, grimacing, and so on.

The motor division of the facial nerve is evaluated by asking the patient to perform various facial movements and observing the patient speak. Weakness of the facial muscle may be evidenced by flattening of the nasolabial fold, drooping of one side of the mouth, and sagging of the lower eyelid. The sense of taste is evaluated by asking the patient to identify sweet, sour, and salty substances, which are applied to the tongue. The ninth cranial nerve, the glossopharyngeal, carries the sensation of bitterness. It is perceived only on the posterior segment of the tongue. This is an important point to remember when testing for the sensation of bitterness.

Because the nucleus of the facial nerve lies in the lateral portion of the lower pons, a lesion in the area of the brain stem will often cause facial nerve dysfunction. The facial nerve enters the temporal bone and is close to the middle ear, so it is subject to trauma from fractures of the base of the skull and the temporal bone, from surgical procedures, and from diseases of the ear. Other disorders that may result in facial nerve weakness include myasthenia gravis and Guillain-Barré syndrome. *Bell's palsy* is the most common type of nerve paralysis.

Vestibulocochlear nerve (cranial nerve VIII)

The vestibulocochlear nerve maintains balance and transmits impulses that allow a person to hear. Maintaining balance is the function of the vestibular division, whereas the cochlear division mediates hearing. The cochlear division can be tested by observing the patient's ability to hear a whisper from a distance of 2 feet. Another method of testing involves use of the tuning fork, which distinguishes between conductive hearing loss and sensorineural loss. People with normal hearing will hear a tuning fork placed in the midline of the head or forehead equally well in both ears. Also, they will hear the tuning fork better by air conduction than by bone conduction. Normally the tuning fork is heard twice as long

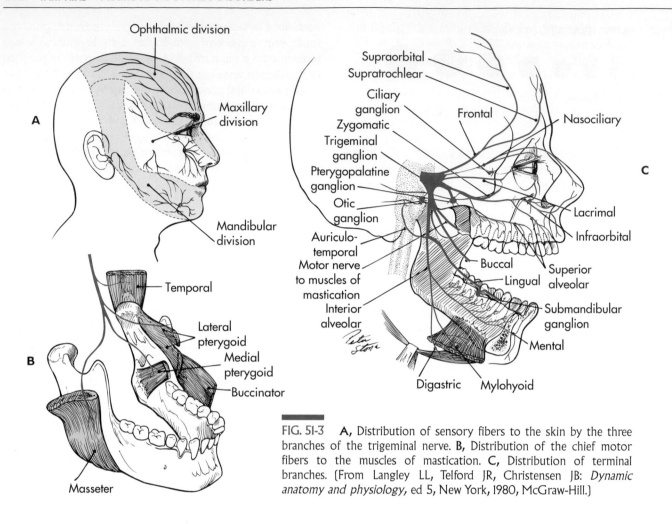

FIG. 51-3   **A,** Distribution of sensory fibers to the skin by the three branches of the trigeminal nerve. **B,** Distribution of the chief motor fibers to the muscles of mastication. **C,** Distribution of terminal branches. (From Langley LL, Telford JR, Christensen JB: *Dynamic anatomy and physiology,* ed 5, New York, 1980, McGraw-Hill.)

by air conduction. The two most common tuning fork–hearing tests are the Rinne and Weber tests. In the *Rinne test* a vibrating tuning fork is placed on the mastoid process; when the patient indicates that the vibration is no longer audible, the tuning fork is placed next to the ear. If the patient again hears the vibration, air conduction (AC) is better than bone conduction (BC). This is normal and is arbitrarily called a "positive" Rinne. A "negative" Rinne is indicative of middle ear disease causing conductive hearing loss. In the *Weber test* the vibrating tuning fork is placed on the top of the patient's head, in the middle of the forehead, or on the upper front teeth. The patient is asked where the sound is heard the loudest. Normally the sound is heard equally on both sides. If the sound lateralizes to one side, it may indicate a hearing loss. If the patient has conductive hearing loss, the sound will be heard better in the deafer ear, whereas with sensorineural loss it will be heard better in the healthy ear. If an abnormality is detected, a complete audiometer evaluation should be performed.

Acute dysfunction of the vestibular division of the vestibulocochlear nerve is manifested by vertigo, nausea, vomiting, and ataxia. The *cold caloric test* is used to screen for problems. It is performed with the patient up-

right. Ice water (5 ml) is injected into the ear. The normal response to this stimulus is nystagmus of both eyes, vertigo, nausea, and vomiting. Little or no reaction to this stimulus indicates an abnormality of the vestibular nerve. *Meniere's disease* involves a dilation of the endolymphatic channels in the cochlea, with eventual atrophy of the hearing mechanism resulting in vertigo, tinnitus, and hearing loss in the affected ear.

The vestibulocochlear nerve leaves the brain stem and travels along a path similar to that of the facial nerve. As with the facial nerve, it is subject to damage from fractures of the base of the skull and the temporal bone. Vascular occlusions and tumors of the brain stem are other causes of damage to this nerve.

Glossopharyngeal and vagus nerves (cranial nerves IX and X)

The glossopharyngeal and vagus nerves are closely related anatomically and functionally and are evaluated together. The glossopharyngeal nerve has a sensory division, which carries taste from the posterior portion of the tongue, innervates the carotid sinus and the carotid bodies, and supplies sensation to the pharynx. The motor division innervates the posterior wall of the pharynx. The vagus nerve innervates all the thoracic and abdominal viscera and conveys impulses from the walls of the intestines, the heart, and the lungs. It is not possible clinically to examine all these functions; therefore evaluation of the vagus nerve is directed toward evaluating the motor function of the palate, pharynx, and larynx.

The first step in evaluation of the glossopharyngeal and vagus nerves is inspection of the soft palate. The soft palate should be symmetric and should not deviate to either side. When the patient says "ah," the soft palate should rise symmetrically. To induce a *gag reflex,* the posterior wall of the pharynx is touched, causing elevation of the palate and constriction of the pharyngeal muscles. The patient's *swallowing reflex* is tested by observing the reaction to drinking a glass of water. Observations are made of difficulty in swallowing or regurgitation of fluid through the nose, which would indicate weakness of the soft palate and an inability to close off the nasopharynx when swallowing. *Indirect laryngoscopy* is performed when the patient's complaint is a voice disturbance or hoarseness. The vocal cords can be observed for paresis or lesions. Bilateral lesions may cause greater difficulty in swallowing and in the ability to mobilize secretions.

The glossopharyngeal and vagus nerves leave the skull through the jugular foramen with the internal jugular vein. Therefore trauma or a tumor close to this area would affect these structures. The recurrent laryngeal nerve, a branch of the vagus that supplies the larynx, is susceptible to injury during surgery of the neck because of its proximity to the thyroid gland. Amyotrophic lateral sclerosis and myasthenia gravis frequently cause weakness in the muscles innervated by the glossopharyngeal and the vagus nerves.

Accessory nerve (cranial nerve XI)

The accessory nerve is a motor nerve innervating the sternocleidomastoid muscle and the upper portion of the trapezius muscle. These two muscles flex the neck; also, the sternocleidomastoid muscle rotates the head from side to side, and the trapezius muscle rotates the scapula when the arm is raised.

The function of the accessory nerve is evaluated by observing the sternocleidomastoid and trapezius muscles for atrophy and assessing their strength. To test the sternocleidomastoid muscle, the patient is asked to turn the head toward one shoulder and to resist the examiner's attempts to move the head in the opposite direction. This test is repeated on the other side so that both the right and the left muscles are evaluated. The trapezius muscle is evaluated by asking the patient to shrug the shoulders while the examiner attempts to push downward. The patient is then asked to elevate both arms to a vertical position. A patient with weakness in the trapezius muscle will not be able to perform this action.

The accessory nerve lies close to the glossopharyngeal and vagus nerves. Tumors affecting these nerves frequently affect the accessory nerve. The cell bodies of the accessory nerve lie in the lower medulla and the upper part of the spinal cord at levels of the first through fifth cervical vertebrae and receive innervation from both cerebral hemispheres. Therefore a cerebral cortical lesion may cause little or no dysfunction in the two muscles innervated by this nerve. The most common cause for accessory nerve dysfunction is neck trauma, with direct damage to the cranial nerve cell body or axon.

Hypoglossal nerve (cranial nerve XII)

The hypoglossal nerve innervates the musculature of the tongue. Normal functioning of the tongue is essential for normal speech and swallowing. Slight bilateral weakness is characterized by difficulty in enunciating consonants and difficulty in swallowing. Severe bilateral weakness causes extreme difficulty with speech and swallowing.

The tongue is examined for asymmetry, deviation to one side, and the presence of fasciculations. This examination is first performed inside the mouth with the tongue at rest and then with the tongue protruded. Strength of the muscle is evaluated by asking the patient to push out a cheek with the tongue while the examiner opposes the effort with fingers on the patient's cheek.

The nuclei of the hypoglossal nerves lie within the medulla beneath the floor of the fourth ventricle and receive innervation from both cerebral hemispheres. Injuries to the neck may cause unilateral weakness of the tongue with atrophy and fasciculations. Tumors at the base of the posterior fossa near the foramen magnum may cause ipsilateral paralysis of the tongue. Bilateral weakness can result from amyotrophic lateral sclerosis and myasthenia gravis.

Motor Function

Motor performance depends on an intact muscle, a functioning neuromuscular junction, and intact cranial and spinal nerve tracts. To understand how the nervous system functions to coordinate muscle activity, it is important first to be able to distinguish between the upper and the lower motor neurons.

The *upper motor neuron* (UMN) originates in the cerebral cortex and projects downward, one part (the corticobulbar tract) ending in the brain stem and the other (the corticospinal tract) crossing in the lower medulla and descending into the spinal cord. The cranial nerve nuclei are the end point for the corticobulbar tracts. The corticospinal tracts terminate in the region of the anterior horn of the spinal cord from the cervical to the sacral areas. Those corticospinal fibers that travel through the medullary pyramids constitute the pyramidal tracts. Nerve fibers in the corticospinal tract mediate voluntary movement, particularly fine, discrete, conscious movement (Fig. 51-4).

The *lower motor neuron* (LMN) includes the motor

FIG. 51-4 Pyramidal motor pathways (corticospinal tracts). The tracts originate in pyramidal cells of the cortex. Fibers that cross at the medulla form the lateral corticospinal tracts, and the remaining fibers form the ventral corticospinal tracts. The basis pedunculi are part of the cerebral peduncles. (From Langley LL, Telford JR, Christensen JB: *Dynamic anatomy and physiology,* ed 5, New York, 1980, McGraw-Hill.)

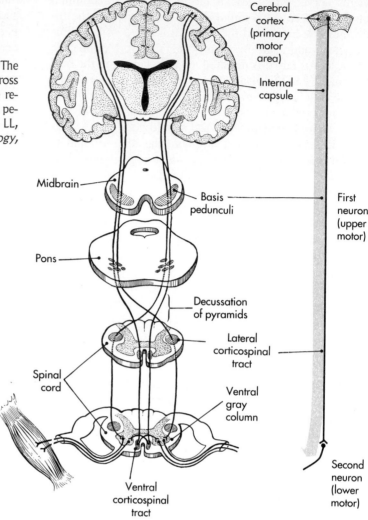

cells of the cranial nerve nuclei and their axons as well as the anterior horn cells of the spinal cord and their axons. The motor fibers leave through the anterior, or motor, root of the spinal column and innervate the muscles.

Lesions involving the UMN and the LMN produce characteristic changes in muscle response. Awareness of the differences in muscle weakness helps to locate the neurologic lesion. Table 51-3 summarizes this information.

Coordination and gait

Coordination is impaired by many disorders at any level of the motor system. Incoordination is a particularly relevant sign, generally indicating problems with cerebellar function and corticospinal tract interruption. Tests that reveal a lack of coordination include tandem walking (asking the patient to walk heel to toe), ability of the patient to follow through on simple rapid movements (placing the hand on the knee alternately using the palm and back of the hand), and ability of the patient to place the heel of one foot on the opposite knee and slide it down the front of the leg. Cerebellar disease causes these movements to be slow, nonrhythmic, and inaccurate.

Gait is usually observed by asking the patient to walk. Keeping in mind that most people tend to walk slowly and carefully when observed, the examiner looks for lack of arm swing or decreased arm swing, hemiplegia, rigidity, loss of coordinated movement, tremor, and/or apraxia (slow, shuffling steps and difficulty in lifting feet from the ground). Patients with cerebellar disease walk with a wide base of support and have a tendency to stagger laterally. Slow gait, small shuffling steps, and lack of arm swing are characteristics of Parkinson's disease.

Muscle tone and strength

Muscle tone, which is the resistance detected by the examiner when a joint is moved through passive range of motion, is frequently altered in nervous system disorders. UMN disorders increase muscle tone, whereas LMN disorders decrease muscle tone. Table 51-4 lists some of the alterations in muscle tone frequently seen in neurologic disorders.

Major muscle groups are observed for evidence of muscle wasting, fasciculations, or contractions. Muscle strength is tested by comparing the strength of the muscles on one side of the body with those on the other side

TABLE 51-3   Differentiation Between Upper and Lower Motor Neuron Weakness

Characteristic	Upper Motor Neuron*	Lower Motor Neuron†
Type and distribution of weakness	Lesions in brain: "pyramidal distribution," that is, distal, especially hand muscles; weaker extensors in arm and weaker flexors in legs. Lesions in cord: variable, depending on location	Depends on which lower motor neurons are involved, that is, which segments, roots, or nerves
Tone	Spasticity: greater in flexors in arms and extensors in legs	Flaccidity
Bulk	Slight atrophy of disuse only	Atrophy: may be marked
Reflexes	Accentuated, Babinski's sign present	Decreased or absent; no Babinski's sign
Fasciculations	No	Yes
Clonus	Frequently present	Absent

*Synonyms: pyramidal tract (referring to fibers in medullary pyramids), corticospinal tract, corticobulbar tract.
†Synonyms: anterior horn cell, ventral horn cell, somatic motor portions of cranial nerves, final common pathway.

as the patient resists the examiner's counterpressure. Age, gender, and physical condition must be considered when evaluating these tests. The patient is observed for any evidence of involuntary movements, including tremors, chorea, hemiballismus, and tic.

Reflexes

A *deep tendon reflex* is elicited by a brisk tap with a reflex hammer over a partially stretched tendon. The impulse then travels along afferent fibers to the spinal cord, where it synapses with a motor, or anterior horn, neuron. After it synapses, the impulse is transmittted down the motor neuron to the anterior nerve root through the spinal nerve and then the peripheral nerve. After it is transmitted across the neuromuscular junction, the muscle is stimulated to contract. In simplest form this is the reflex arc (Fig. 51-5).

The deep tendon reflexes, also known as *muscle stretch reflexes,* commonly tested are the biceps reflex, the triceps reflex, the brachioradialis reflex, the patellar reflex, and the Achilles reflex. The response to reflexes is graded on a scale of 0 to +4 (Table 51-5; see also Table 57-3). It

TABLE 51-4   Some Alterations in Motor Function Associated With Neurologic Disorders

Muscle Disorder	Clinical Findings	Neurologic Disorder
Dystonia	Persistent abnormal positions of body parts in which there is resistance to passive movement of the part	Extrapyramidal disease Wilson's disease Phenothiazine neuropathy Viral brain infection
Paratonia (gegenhalten)	Resistance to passive movement throughout the range of motion (somewhat proportional to the amount of force applied)	Frontal lobe disease
Decerebrate rigidity	Extension and pronation of the upper extremities and extension of the lower extremities	Severe brain injury above level of the pons
Hypotonia	Increased range of motion of joints (overextension and overflexion)	Cerebellar disease
Hemiballismus	Unilateral movements affecting side opposite the lesion and involving violent, flinging movements at the proximal joints	Cerebrovascular occlusions involving the subthalamic nucleus
Tremors	Involuntary rhythmic, tremulous movements Rest tremor: more pronounced at rest Intention tremor: worse when patient reaches for an object	Lesions of the cerebellar pathways

is important to compare sides when evaluating reflex responses.

Superficial reflexes are tested by stroking the skin with a firm object, such as the end of a reflex hammer or applicator, causing the muscles to contract. These reflexes include abdominal, cremasteric, plantar, and gluteal.

Assessment of reflexes gives the examiner information about the function of the reflex arc and specific spinal

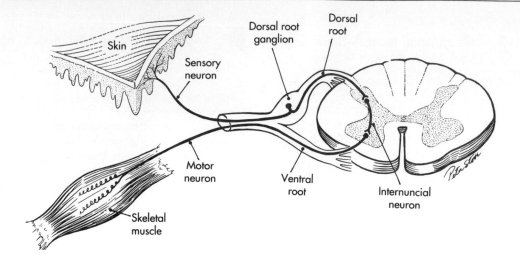

FIG. 51-5   Components of a simple reflex: a sensory, an internuncial, and a motor neuron. (From Langley LL, Telford JR, Christensen JB: *Dynamic anatomy and physiology,* ed 5, New York, 1980, McGraw-Hill.)

 TABLE 51-5   Grading of Reflexes

Grade	Significance
+4	Very brisk, suggestive of disease of the upper motor neuron, frequently associated with clonus (rhythmic oscillations between flexion and extension)
+3	Brisker than average but not necessarily indicative of disease
+2	Average/normal
+1	Somewhat diminished
0	No response

Modified from Bates B: *A guide to physical examination,* ed 4, Philadelphia, 1987, Lippincott.

cord segments. Reflexes are altered in disease states involving the UMNs and LMNs.

UMN paralysis is caused by an interruption of the descending motor tracts on one side of a segment of the spinal cord. Immediately after the lesion occurs, the deep tendon reflexes are temporarily depressed; this is known as *areflexia.* In addition, the paralyzed muscles are flaccid. Several weeks or months after the lesion occurs, the deep tendon reflexes become hyperactive; the superficial reflexes are lost, and Babinski's reflex is noted.

LMN paralysis is caused by destruction of the peripheral motor nerves and the anterior horn cells. When this occurs, the muscles become flaccid and hypotonic and the deep tendon reflexes are lost.

The plantar reflex is elicited by stroking the lateral aspect of the sole from the heel to the ball and curving medially across the ball of the foot. The normal response to this stimulus is flexion of the toes. An abnormal response, dorsiflexion of the great toe and fanning of other toes,

is known as *Babinski's reflex* and indicates UMN disease (Fig. 51-6). This reflex is seen (1) in children younger than 2 years; (2) during periods of deep sleep, general anesthesia, and postictal (after a seizure) depression; and (3) in persons who are drunk or in moderate to severe hypoglycemic shock.

Sensory Function

The sensory system plays a vital role in conveying to the central nervous system information about the environment. When examining the sensory system, the following four areas are investigated: (1) superficial tactile sensation, including pain, temperature, and touch; (2) proprioceptive sense, which is motion or position sense; (3) vibratory sense; and (4) cortical sensory functions. Patterns of sensory loss may lead to a diagnosis of lesions of the cerebral hemisphere, brain stem, spinal cord, nerve root, and single or multiple peripheral nerves.

Perceptions of pain and temperature are carried by nerve fibers to the dorsal root ganglia where the nuclei of these nerve fibers are located. After synapsing in the dorsal horn, they cross over the midline and enter the opposite lateral spinothalamic tract. This tract ascends through the entire length of the spinal cord, medulla, pons, and midbrain and terminates in the thalamus. The thalamus, acting as a relay station, transmits the impulse to the sensory cortex for interpretation. Simple touch sensation is transmitted by the ventral spinothalamic tract. A lesion involving the lateral spinothalamic tract will result in loss of pain and temperature sensation on the opposite side of the body below the level of the lesion. Lesions of the nerve roots and peripheral nerves impair the perception of touch (Fig. 51-7).

Fibers conducting sensations of position, vibration,

and touch requiring a high degree of localization, such as stereognosis, graphesthesia, and two-point discrimination, enter the spinal column and pass into the dorsal column system. Traveling upward to the lower medulla, where they synapse and cross over, the fibers ascend as the medial lemniscus, terminating in the thalamus. The fine distinction between and perception of these sensations are carried out in the parietal cortex.

The pattern of the dermatomes is shown in Fig. 51-8. Theoretically, a lesion in the dorsal root produces loss of sensation in the area supplied by the root. However, the nerve supply overlaps considerably, which frequently confuses the clinical picture.

Sensory testing is performed with the patient's eyes closed, using a wisp of cotton to test for touch, a safety pin to test for superficial pain, and test tubes filled with hot and cold water to test for temperature.

Proprioception, position, and motion sense are first evaluated in distal joints. If proprioception is normal in the distal joint, it is not necessary to test the proximal joint. A distal phalanx of one of the patient's fingers is grasped and slowly moved upward or downward, and the patient is asked to indicate the movement of the phalanx. The *Romberg test* evaluates the position sense for the legs and trunk; the normal person should be able to stand with feet together and eyes closed without swaying greatly or losing balance. Frequently, patients with abnormality in

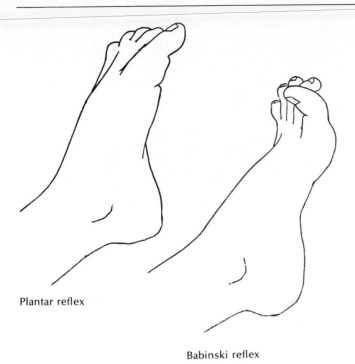

Plantar reflex

Babinski reflex

FIG. 51-6   Babinski's response. *Left,* Normal adult response to stimulation of the foot (flexion of all the toes). *Right,* Normal infant and abnormal adult response (dorsiflexion of the great toe and fanning of other toes).

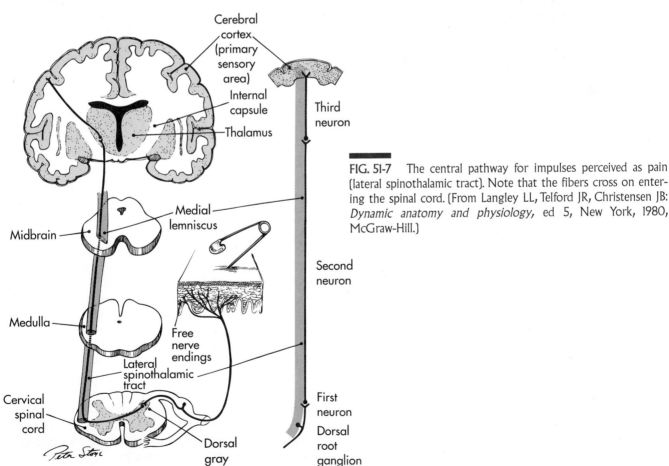

FIG. 51-7   The central pathway for impulses perceived as pain (lateral spinothalamic tract). Note that the fibers cross on entering the spinal cord. (From Langley LL, Telford JR, Christensen JB: *Dynamic anatomy and physiology,* ed 5, New York, 1980, McGraw-Hill.)

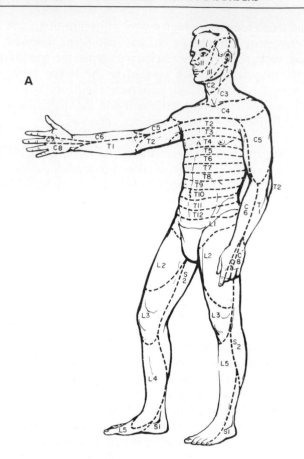
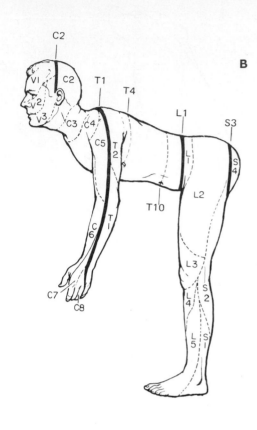

FIG. 51-8   Arrangement of the dermatomes. Each dorsal (sensory) spinal root innervates one dermatome. The first cervical nerve *(C1)* usually has no cutaneous distribution. The fifth cranial nerve *(C5)* supplies the sensory distribution to the face and anterior aspect of the head. The ophthalmic division is labeled I and VI, the maxillary division is II and V2, and the mandibular division is III and V3 in **A** and **B.** (**A** from Noback CR, Demarest RJ: *The human nervous system,* ed 3, New York, 1981, McGraw-Hill; **B** from Haymaker W: *Bing's local diagnosis in neurological diseases,* ed 15, St Louis, 1969, Mosby.)

the proprioceptive pathway can maintain their balance with eyes open because the visual orientation serves to keep them balanced. The patient with a cerebellar disorder, on the other hand, sways and loses balance with eyes open as well as closed.

DIAGNOSTIC TESTS

In addition to the clinical history and neurologic examination, the clinical practitioner can perform several diagnostic tests to help locate and define the neurologic problem. These tests help the examiner diagnose the problem but are not a substitute for a careful and thorough neurologic examination.

Invasive Procedures

Cerebral angiography is used to identify and locate cerebrovascular abnormalities. A contrast medium is injected into the carotid, femoral, or brachial artery, and a series of cerebrovascular radiographs is taken. The contrast media most commonly used contain iodinated compounds, which have the potential to provoke severe allergic reactions; therefore all patients are carefully screened for allergies to iodine and shellfish. Attendants should be alert for any signs of allergic reaction, such as itching, palpitations, dyspnea, dizziness, or gastrointestinal disturbances, during and immediately after the procedure. Vital signs and neurologic checks are an essential part of posttest care.

Digital subtraction angiography (DSA) is a type of angiography that combines radiography and a computerized subtraction technique to visualize vessels without the interference of surrounding bone and soft tissue. A computer subtracts the interfering structures for the radiographic image. This test is used in particular for visualizing cerebral blood flow and detecting aneurysms, tumors, and hematomas. The same precautions concerning allergy to iodine apply to this procedure.

Radioisotope brain scan is useful in the diagnosis of

► TABLE 51-6   Cerebrospinal Fluid Findings

Characteristics	Normal	Selected Abnormalities
Opening pressure	50 to 180 mm H_2O	Increased with intracranial mass from tumor, hemorrhage, or edema; decreased with spinal canal obstruction above LP site
Appearance	Clear, colorless	Xanthochromic (yellowish) appearance usually indicates presence of old blood or extreme elevation of protein in the CNS; cloudy appearance indicates infection (elevated WBC count, protein, microorganisms)
Cell count	0 to 5 WBCs/mm³	Increased with active disease: meningitis, acute infection, abscess, tumor, infarction, multiple sclerosis
	No RBCs	RBCs in subarachnoid hemorrhage or traumatic LP
Protein	20 to 45 mg/dl	Elevated in almost all serious pathologic CNS conditions
Glucose	40 to 70 mg/dl (normal = ²/₃ blood glucose)	Increased in systemic hyperglycemia; decreased in systemic hypoglycemia, bacterial meningitis
Microorganisms	None	Bacterial meningitis

LP, Lumbar puncture; *CNS,* central nervous system; *WBCs,* white blood cells; *RBCs,* red blood cells.

masses, vascular lesions, and ischemic or infarcted areas of the brain. After venous injection with a radionuclide, radiographs are taken as the radioisotope passes through the brain.

Electromyography is used to differentiate muscular disease from neurologic disorders. For this test, needles are placed in the muscles and electrical signals recorded during rest and contraction. This procedure can be painful for some patients, and an analgesic may be required during the posttest period.

Lumbar puncture (LP) is used to measure cerebrospinal fluid (CSF) pressure and to collect samples of the CSF for laboratory examination. Generally, an LP is contraindicated when there are signs of increased intracranial pressure, since the quick reduction of pressure from removal of CSF may cause herniation of the brain structures into the foramen magnum. The patient lies on one side and assumes a knee-chest position. The area of the third and fourth lumbar vertebrae is cleansed with a povidone-iodine solution and anesthetized with a lidocaine solution. A spinal needle is inserted and attached to a manometer to measure the pressure; specimens are collected in numbered test tubes from the manometer stopcock. After all specimens have been obtained, the needle is removed and the puncture covered with an adhesive plaster. Patients lie flat for several hours after the procedure and are encouraged to take fluids. Headaches are common after LP. Table 51-6 lists some common CSF normal and abnormal findings.

Noninvasive Tests

Brain stem auditory-evoked response is performed on comatose patients. It is a test of the cranial nerve VIII function, which remains intact even with severe brain stem destruction. An electrode is placed into the ear canal and stimulated. Responses are recorded on an electroencephalogram.

Computed tomography scan (CT scan) is useful in the diagnosis and monitoring of intracranial lesions or to evaluate and define the extent of a neurologic injury. Radiographs are taken by a computer in 1-degree intervals in a 180-degree arc. Enhanced studies are performed using contrast media injected into a vascular access. Whenever contrast media are used, allergy precautions must be taken. CT scans have replaced echoencephalography and have greatly enhanced diagnostic capabilities.

Magnetic resonance imaging (MRI) uses a strong magnetic field and a radiofrequency and, when combined with the radio frequencies released by the body's tissues, produces an image that is recorded. MRI is useful in the diagnosis of tumors, infarctions, and vascular abnormalities. This procedure does not expose the patient to radiation and is painless, although patients may complain of claustrophobia and distress from the clanking metallic sounds throughout the procedure.

Electroencephalogram (EEG) measures the electrical activity of the cerebral cortex's superficial layers via electrodes placed externally on the patient's skull. Wave patterns reflect the intensity and type of electrical potentials generated by neuronal activity within the brain. Normal wave patterns are labeled according to amplitude and frequency characteristics and are called *delta, theta, alpha,* and *beta.* The pattern of EEG waves are influenced by sleep state, drug use, disease, and aging.

Electronystagmogram (ENG) is an electrophysiologic test of vestibular function that may be used to diagnose disorders of the central nervous system. The test measures nystagmus (involuntary, rapid horizontal eye movements) induced by stimulation of the vestibular system. The test may cause some discomfort but is not dangerous to the patient. It consists of inserting air or water at different temperatures into the external ear canals, which stimulates the semicircular canals, and recording the resulting electrical activity generated by involuntary eye muscle movements.

QUESTIONS

▼ *Answer the following on a separate sheet of paper.*

1. What is the purpose of history taking during a neurologic examination?
2. List the six major areas of the neurologic examination.

▼ *Circle T for true and F for false. Correct any false statements.*

3. T F The highest integration and coordination center for perception and interpretation of sensory input is the frontal lobe.

4. T F The neurologic examination of mental status evaluates the patient's ability to reason, think abstractly, plan ahead, and make judgments.

5. T F The right hemisphere is dominant for speech in right-handed persons and in most left-handed persons.

6. T F Dysarthria is a defect in articulation, enunciation, and rhythm of speech related to a weakness in the muscles involved in speech.

▼ *Match the functions in column B with the location of their cerebral control in column A.*

Column A	Column B
7. _____ Medulla (brain stem)	a. Hearing
8. _____ Frontal lobe	b. Balance, coordination
9. _____ Precentral gyrus of frontal lobe (strip along central fissure in posterior part frontal lobe)	c. Relay center for sensory impulses
	d. Voluntary muscle movements
	e. Vital-organ functions: heartbeat, respiration
10. _____ Occipital lobe	f. Reception of fine sensory stimuli
11. _____ Temporal lobe	g. Sight
12. _____ Parietal lobe (strip along central fissure)	h. Intellect, memory, thought
13. _____ Cerebellum	
14. _____ Thalamus	

▼ *Circle the letter preceding each item below that correctly answers the question or completes the statement. More than one answer may be correct.*

15. During a cranial nerve examination, which of the following may be abnormal if there is damage to the medulla?
    a. Pupillary reflex
    b. Gag reflex
    c. Corneal reflex
    d. Patient's ability to shrug shoulders

16. During a cranial nerve examination, Mr. B. demonstrates the ability to smile without any apparent impairment but indicates that he is unable to chew. Where do you suspect the problem to be?
    a. Abducens (VI)
    b. Facial (VII)
    c. Trigeminal (V)
    d. Vestibulocochlear (VIII)
    e. Trochlear (IV)

17. Which of the following cranial nerves is responsible for vision?
    a. Olfactory (I)
    b. Optic (II)
    c. Oculomotor (III)
    d. Facial (VII)

18. Mrs. Jones presents with a dilated left pupil; left ptosis (drooping of the eyelid); and inability to look up, down, or medially with her left eye. These signs indicate a problem with:
    a. Right optic nerve
    b. Left optic nerve
    c. Left oculomotor nerve
    d. Left trochlear nerve
    e. Left abducens nerve

19. On neurologic examination, Babinski's reflex was demonstrated. Which of the following best describes this reflex?
    a. Extension of the leg when the patellar tendon is struck
    b. Tremor of the foot after brisk, forcible dorsiflexion
    c. Dorsiflexion of the great toe when the sole is stroked
    d. Flexion of the forearm when the biceps tendon is tapped

20. Mr. J. has an extensive tumor of the cerebellum. In view of the functions of this organ, which symptom would you expect to observe?
    a. Absence of the knee jerk and other reflexes
    b. Inability to execute smooth, precise movements

    c. Inability to respond to verbal commands
    d. All the above

21. Reflex activity of the central nervous system:
    a. Requires at least two nerve cells
    b. Is a simple process in higher mammals
    c. Requires more than three nerve cells to become activated
    d. Is a mechanical process

22. In the patellar reflex, efferent impulses originate from cell bodies located in the:
    a. White matter of the spinal cord
    b. Ventral gray column of the spinal cord
    c. Dorsal root spinal ganglion
    d. Ventral root spinal ganglion

23. A lesion in the corticospinal tract may cause:
    a. Problems with visual acuity
    b. Weakness with decreased reflexes
    c. Weakness with increased reflexes
    d. Problems with auditory reflexes

24. A lesion in the lateral spinothalamic tract may cause:
    a. Weakness with increased reflexes
    b. Problems with perception of pain and temperature
    c. Problems with perception of movement of joint
    d. Problems with integration of movement

25. Conductive hearing loss:
    a. Is associated with old age
    b. Is characterized by better hearing through bone conduction than through air conduction
    c. Is similar to nerve-type hearing loss
    d. Involves the inner ear

26. When Mrs. T. underwent a Weber test (a vibrating tuning fork placed at the midpoint of the top of the head), she stated that she heard the sound better in her right ear. Normally during a Weber test, the patient should hear the sound equally in both ears. Mrs. T.'s abnormal results could be caused by a:
    a. Sensorineural hearing loss in the left ear
    b. Sensorineural hearing loss in the right ear
    c. Conductive hearing loss in the right ear
    d. Mixed hearing loss in the right ear

27. A Rinne test is then performed on Mrs. T.'s right ear. She hears the tuning fork better when it is placed on her mastoid

QUESTIONS—cont'd

bone than when it is placed in front of her pinna. Which type of hearing loss does this suggest?
a. Conductive
b. Sensorineural

▼ Circle T if the statement is true and F if it is false. Correct any false statements.

28. T F Caloric tests are used in the diagnosis of disorders of the vestibular system.

▼ Match each testing procedure in column B with the correct cranial nerve in column A.

Column A	Column B
31. _____ Optic (II)	a. Occlude one nostril with digital compression; have patient indicate when odor is first detected and, if possible, identify substance.
32. _____ Trigeminal (V)	
33. _____ Facial (VII)	
34. _____ Vestibulocochlear (VIII)	b. Have patient say "ah" to note phonation and symmetry of the soft palate.
35. _____ Oculomotor (III)	
36. _____ Glossopharyngeal (IX)	c. Test positional sense.
37. _____ Vagus (X)	d. Cover one of the patient's eyes and bring finger into visual field.
38. _____ Accessory (XI)	
39. _____ Olfactory (I)	e. Test gag reflex
	f. Have patient raise eyebrows, frown, close eyes, and tightly close eyes; observe symmetry.
	g. Test for conductive versus sensorineural hearing loss.
	h. Ask patient to shrug shoulders and turn head with and without resistance.
	i. Have patient clench teeth; palpate masseters for tension.
	j. Check for ptosis of lids, and note quality of pupils.

▼ Match the cranial nerves in column A with responses indicating abnormality of the respective cranial nerves from column B.

Column A	Column B
40. _____ Trigeminal (V)	a. Dilation of the pupil, decreased reaction to light
41. _____ Glossopharyngeal, vagus (IX, X)	b. Loss of corneal reflex when cotton wisp is touched to cornea
42. _____ Oculomotor (III)	c. Absence of gag reflex when tongue blade is touched to posterior pharynx
43. _____ Accessory (XI)	d. Inability to shrug the shoulders
	e. Deviation of protruding tongue toward the weak side (muscle atrophy also present on paralyzed side)

29. T F A lesion of the lower motor neuron results in a spastic paralysis and hyperactive reflexes.

30. T F When reporting the evaluation of a patient's level of consciousness, one should describe behavior exactly rather than use terms such as coma or stupor.

▼ Answer the following on a separate sheet of paper.

44. List the four areas that are investigated when examining the sensory system.

▼ Fill in the blanks with the correct word or words.

45. Interruption of the proprioceptive fibers, as in tabes dorsalis (syphilitic infection of the brain and spinal cord), may cause inability to maintain balance when standing with the eyes closed. This is called a positive _____ sign.

46. A right-sided posterolateral herniated intervertebral disk compressing the _____ spinal cord roots might be expected to produce numbness over the lateral aspect of the right foot.

▼ Circle the letter preceding each item below that correctly answers the question or completes the statement. More than one answer may be correct.

47. The rationale for having the patient lie on the side in a knee-chest position during a lumbar puncture is to:
a. Prevent spinal cord injury
b. Gain easier access to the spinal canal
c. Prevent spinal headache
d. Prevent injury to the spinal nerves

48. A lumbar puncture is generally contraindicated in cases of increased intracranial pressure because:
a. Postprocedure headache is more likely.
b. Rapid reduction of pressure after cerebrospinal fluid withdrawal may cause brain herniation and sudden death.
c. The patient must lie flat for several days after the procedure.
d. There is greater risk of bleeding during and after the procedure.

49. The cerebrospinal fluid in a patient with bacterial meningitis usually:
a. Appears clear and colorless
b. Has a normal protein content
c. Has a normal cell count
d. None of the above

CHAPTER 52 Pain

MARY CARTER LOMBARDO
LORRAINE M. WILSON

Pain can be described as "an unpleasant sensory and emotional experience associated with actual or potential tissue damage, or described in terms of such damage" (International Association for Study of Pain, 1979). This description emphasizes that pain is *subjective* and is both a sensation and an emotion. For clinicians, pain is a perplexing problem. No test exists to measure or confirm the pain; instead, the clinician relies almost entirely on the patient's description of the pain and its severity. Pain is the most common reason given by patients when asked why they sought medical attention. The health care professional's commitment to manage and relieve the patient's pain is critical.

In most patients the sensation of pain is produced by an injury or by stimuli that are intense enough to be potentially injurious (noxious). In the case of injury or potential injury, pain serves a protective function, eliciting a stress response with withdrawal, escape, or immobilization of a body part (e.g., removal of a finger from a hot stove). Once this protective function has been completed, however, continuing unrelieved pain can compromise the individual, since it is often accompanied by a stress response with increased anxiety, heart rate, blood pressure, and respiratory rate. A prolonged stress response promotes the breakdown of body tissue, impairs immune functioning, and increases metabolic rate, blood clotting, and water retention, thus hindering rather than helping recovery. A painful experience leads to physical and behavioral reactions that, if not interrupted at an appropriate and early enough stage, will lead to a chronic pain syndrome. The longer these reactions and responses are allowed to occur unabated, the more likely that a self-perpetuating cycle of pain will develop, making it more difficult for the cycle to be interrupted.

Although pain is a subjective experience with unpleasant sensory and emotional components, some objective evidence of pain exists. Watching a patient's facial expression, listening to crying or moaning, and observing changes in vital signs (e.g, blood pressure, heart rate) may give the clinician a hint of the degree of pain the patient is experiencing. These observations are highly unreliable, however, putting patients at high risk for inadequate pain relief.

During the past 30 years, intense interest and research have focused on the nature of pain and its control, resulting in an expansion of knowledge related to this complex phenomenon. This chapter first discusses the physiology of pain generation and transmission, types of pain, and assessment and treatment of pain. This overview of pain is followed by a brief discussion of two common sites for pain: headache and back pain caused by intervertebral disk disease.

NEUROPHYSIOLOGY OF PAIN

Four distinct processes are involved between the stimulus of tissue injury and the subjective experience of pain: transduction, transmission, modulation, and perception. *Pain transduction* is the process by which noxious stimuli lead to electrical activity in the pain receptors. *Pain transmission* involves the process of transmitting pain impulses from the site of transduction over peripheral sensory nerves to their terminals in the spinal cord and the network of relay neurons that ascend from the spinal cord to the brain. *Pain modulation* involves neural activity via descending neural pathways from the brain that can influence pain transmission at the level of the spinal cord. Modulation also involves the chemical factors that produce or enhance activity in the primary afferent pain receptors. Finally, *pain perception* is the subjective experience of pain that is somehow produced by the neural activity of pain transmission.

Pain Receptors and Their Stimulation

The capacity of tissues to elicit pain when a noxious stimulus is applied to them depends on the presence of nociceptors. *Nociceptors* are primary afferent nerves for receiving and transmitting painful stimuli. The free nerve endings of nociceptors serve as receptors sensitive to painful mechanical, thermal, electrical, or chemical stim-

uli. The distribution of nociceptors varies throughout the body, with the largest number in the skin. Nociceptors are located in subcutaneous tissue, skeletal muscles, and joints. Pain receptors in the viscera are not located in the parenchyma of the internal organs themselves but rather are found in the peritoneal surfaces, pleural membranes, dura mater, and the walls of blood vessels.

A peripheral nerve consists of the axons of three different types of neurons: primary sensory or afferent neurons, motor neurons, and sympathetic postganglionic neurons. The cell bodies of the primary afferent neurons are located in the dorsal (posterior) root of the spinal nerve or in ganglia of the autonomic nervous system. Primary afferent fibers are classified according to their size, degree of myelination, and conduction velocity (Fig. 52-1). A-alpha (A-α) and A-beta (A-β) afferent fibers are largest in size and myelinated and have the fastest conduction velocity. These fibers respond to touch, pressure and kinesthetic sense. However, they do not respond to noxious stimuli and thus cannot be classified as nociceptors. In contrast, small-diameter, lightly myelinated *(A-delta (A-δ) primary afferent fibers* and unmyelinated *C primary afferent fibers* respond maximally only when noxious painful stimuli are applied to their receptive fields and thus are classified as nociceptors. Pain impulses are transmitted relatively slowly compared with sensory transmission in the large A-α and A-β fibers because of their small diameters and lack of myelin (C fibers).

A-δ and C primary afferents can be distinguished by the two types of pain they elicit, called fast pain and slow pain. *Fast pain* signals are transmitted to the spinal cord by the A-δ fibers and are felt within 0.1 second. Fast pain is generally well localized and has a prickling, sharp, or electrical quality. Fast pain is elicited in response to mechanical (e.g., cut, pinprick) or thermal stimuli on the skin surface but is not felt in most deeper tissues of the body. *Slow pain* is transmitted by the C afferent fibers and is felt 1 second after a noxious stimulus. Slow pain is less

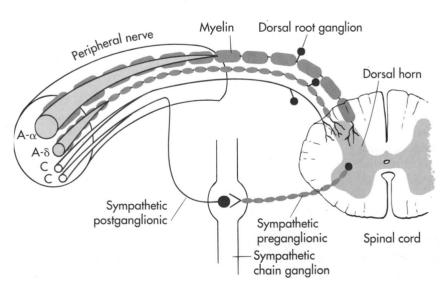

FIG. 52-1   Components of a typical cutaneous nerve. Two distinct functional categories of afferent neurons have cell bodies either in the dorsal root ganglion (somatic nerves) or in the sympathetic ganglion (autonomic nerves). Primary afferents include (1) the large, myelinated A-alpha *(A-α)* fibers and A-beta (A-β) fibers *(not shown)* carrying impulses mediating touch, pressure, and proprioception and (2) the small, myelinated A-delta *(A-δ)* and unmyelinated C fibers carrying impulses mediating pain. All sympathetic postganglionic fibers are unmyelinated C fibers. All these primary afferents converge on the spinal cord dorsal horn cells. (Modified from Fields HL: *Pain,* New York, 1987, McGraw-Hill.)

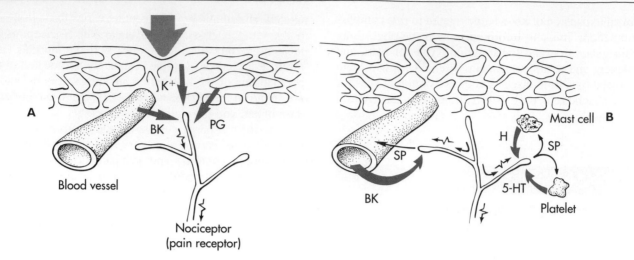

FIG. 52-2   Mechanisms of nociceptor activation and sensitization in an area of tissue injury. **A,** Direct activation by intense pressure and consequent cell damage. Cell damage leads to the release of intracellular potassium *(K+)* and to synthesis of prostaglandins *(PG)* and bradykinin *(BK)*. Prostaglandins increase the sensitivity of the pain receptor to bradykinin, the most potent pain-producing chemical. **B,** Secondary activation. Impulses generated in the pain receptor are transmitted not only to the spinal cord but also into other terminal branches, where they include the release of substance P *(SP)* and other peptides. Substance P causes vasodilation and neurogenic edema with further release of bradykinin; it also causes release of histamine *(H)* from mast cells and serotonin *(5-HT)* from platelets. (Redrawn from Fields HL: *Pain,* New York, 1987, McGraw-Hill.)

well localized and has a burning, throbbing, or aching quality. Slow pain may be elicited by mechanical, thermal, or chemical stimuli in the skin or most deep tissues or organs and is usually associated with tissue damage. Because of this double system of pain innervation, tissue injury often gives rise to two distinct pain sensations: an early sharp pain (transmitted by A-δ pain fibers) followed by a dull, burning, somewhat prolonged pain (transmitted by C pain fibers).

Transduction is the process by which a noxious stimulus depolarizes a nociceptor and initiates a pain stimulus. One possible mechanism of transduction is the activation of nociceptors by pain-producing chemicals released in an area of tissue injury (Fig. 52-2). In contrast to most other sensory receptors in the body, pain receptors adapt very little or not at all. In fact, with prolonged noxious stimulation, tissue damage, or inflammation, pain receptors become increasingly sensitized, called *hyperalgesia,* with a lowering of the pain threshold. Chemical substances found in an area of injury and believed to activate or sensitize nociceptors include potassium ions (K+) and histamine released from damaged tissue cells, serotonin (5-hydroxytryptamine, 5-HT) released from platelets, and bradykinin, one of the most potent pain-producing substances. Another class of substances synthesized in the area of damage includes the metabolic products of arachidonic acid, prostaglandins and leukotrienes.

In addition to substances released from damaged cells or synthesized in the area of injury, the nociceptors themselves release chemicals that enhance nociception, including substance P. *Substance P* is a neuropeptide that causes vasodilation, increased blood flow, edema with further release of bradykinin, release of serotonin from platelets, and release of histamine from mast cells.

Nociceptor activity produces several effects by this complex chain of events, including prolongation of the pain long after the stimulus has ceased and the gradual spread of hyperalgesia and tenderness (Fields, 1987). Pain may be reduced by drugs that block these chemicals, such as corticosteroids or nonsteroidal antiinflammatory drugs (NSAIDS, e.g., aspirin), which reduce inflammation and block the synthesis of prostaglandins.

Pain Pathways in Central Nervous System
Ascending pathways

The afferent A-δ and C nerve fibers transmitting pain impulses enter the spinal cord at the dorsal nerve root (Fig. 52-3). The fibers separate as they enter the cord and then reform in the dorsal (posterior) horn of the spinal cord. This area receives, transmits, and processes sensory impulses. The dorsal horn of the spinal cord is divided into cell layers called *laminae.* Two of these layers (laminae II and III), called the *substantia gelatinosa,* are particularly important in pain transmission and modulation. The substantia gelatinosa is hypothesized to be the site of the gating mechanism described in the gate control theory (see later discussion).

From the dorsal horn the pain impulses are conveyed to neurons that transmit information to the opposite side of the spinal cord in the anterior commissure and then converge on the *anterolateral spinothalamic tract* (formerly called lateral tract), which ascends to the thalamus and other brain structures. Just as two types of pain are transmitted by nociceptors (fast pain and slow pain), two parallel spinothalamic pathways transmit these impulses to the brain: the neospinothalamic tract and the paleospinothalamic tract.

The *neospinothalamic tract* is a *direct system* that carries sensory discriminative information about acute or fast pain from A-δ nociceptors to the thalamic areas. This system primarily terminates in an orderly fashion within the ventral posterolateral nucleus of the thalamus. Pain is called a *thalamic sense* because it is probably brought to consciousness in the thalamus. A neuron in the thalamus then projects its axon through the posterior limb of the internal capsule to carry the pain impulses to the primary somatosensory cortex of the postcentral gyrus. It is postulated that this organized pattern is important for the sensory-discriminative aspects of the acute pain experience, that is, its location, nature, and intensity.

The *paleospinothalamic tract,* which transmits impulses initiated in the slow-chronic type C nociceptors, is a multisynaptic, diffuse pathway that carries impulses to

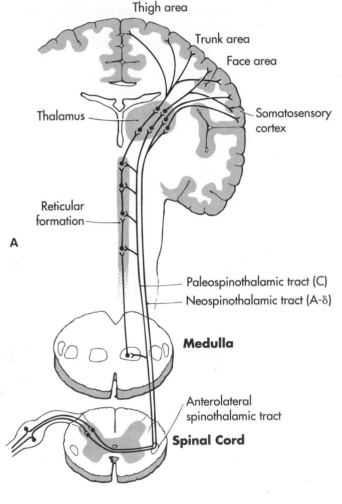

A

FIG. 52-3   Ascending pain pathways. **A,** The small A-δ and C pain fibers carrying acute-sharp and slow-chronic pain impulses, respectively, synapse in the substantia gelatinosa of the dorsal horn, cross the spinal cord, and ascend to the brain in either the neospinothalamic branch or the paleospinothalamic branch of the anterolateral spinothalamic tract. The neospinothalamic tract, principally activated by A-δ peripheral afferents, synapses in the ventroposterolateral nucleus (VPN) of the thalamus and proceeds directly to the somatosensory cortex of the postcentral gyrus, where pain is perceived as sharp and well localized. The paleospinothalamic branch, principally activated by C peripheral afferents, is a diffuse pathway that sends collaterals to the brain stem reticular formation and other structures, from which further fibers project to the thalamus. These fibers influence the hypothalamus and limbic system as well as the cerebral cortex. **B,** Afferent C pain fibers synapse primarily in the substantia gelatinosa (laminae II and III) of the dorsal horn, whereas A-δ pain fibers synapse primarily in laminae I and V.

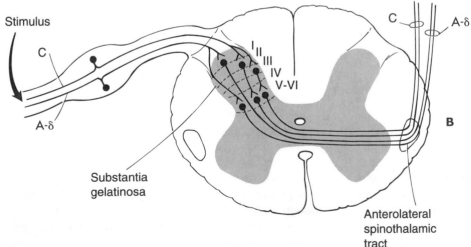

B

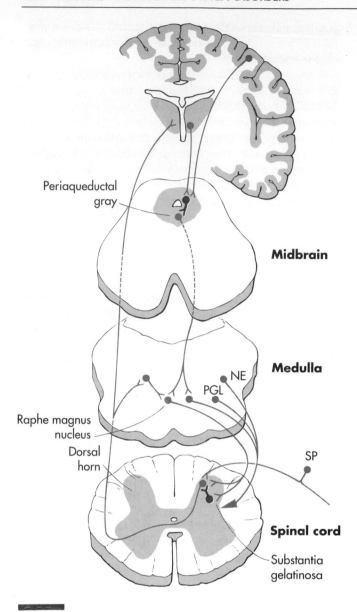

Periaqueductal gray

Midbrain

NE
PGL

Medulla

Raphe magnus nucleus

Dorsal horn

SP

Spinal cord

Substantia gelatinosa

FIG. 52-4 Descending pain-modulating pathways can inhibit incoming pain signals at the spinal cord level. Endorphin-containing neurons in the periaqueductal gray and substantia gelatinosa play an active role in pain modulation. *PGL*, Nucleus reticularis paragigantocellaris; *NE*, norepinephrine cells; *SP*, substance P. (Redrawn from Fields H, Bausbaum A: Endogenous pain control mechanisms. In Wall PD, Melzack R, editors: *Textbook of pain*, New York, 1984, Churchill Livingstone.)

the brain stem reticular formation before terminating in the parafascicular and other intralaminar nuclei of the thalamus, hypothalamus, limbic system nuclei, and forebrain cortex. Since pain impulses are transmitted more slowly than in the neospinothalamic tract, pain is associated with burning, aching, and poorly localized sensations. This system influences the expression of pain in terms of tolerance, behavior, and sympathetic autonomic responses. It is likely that visceral sensations are conveyed by this system. It is most important in chronic pain, mediating the associated autonomic responses, emotional behavior, and lowered thresholds that often occur. Thus

the paleospinothalamic pathway is referred to as an *affectational and motivational nociceptor system.*

It is important to note that neither of these tracts carries pain impulses exclusively; for example, the neospinothalamic tract also conveys crude touch and pressure sensations.

Descending pathways

Specific areas in the brain itself control or influence pain perception: the hypothalamus and limbic structures serve as the emotional center of pain perception, and the frontal cortex provides the rational interpretation and responses to pain. However, great variation exists in the way individuals perceive painful stimuli. One reason for this variation is because the central nervous system (CNS) has a variety of mechanisms for modulating or suppressing nociceptive stimuli.

Descending pathways of efferent fibers that extend from the cerebral cortex down the spinal cord can inhibit or modify incoming pain stimuli via a feedback mechanism involving the substantia gelatinosa and other layers of the dorsal horn. Consequently, descending pathways can influence pain impulses at the spinal level. One descending pathway that has been identified as important in the pain-modulating, or analgesic, system involves the following three components (Fig. 52-4; Fields, 1987; Guyton, Hall, 1996):

1. The first area is the *periaqueductal gray* (PAG) matter and *periventricular gray* (PVG) matter of the mesencephalon and upper pons surrounding the aqueduct of Sylvius.
2. Neurons from area 1 send impulses to the *raphe magnus nucleus* (NRM) located in the lower pons and upper medulla and the *nucleus reticularis paragigantocellularis* (PGL) in the lateral medulla.
3. Impulses are transmitted from the nuclei in 2 down the dorsolateral columns of the spinal cord to a pain inhibitory complex located in the *dorsal horns of the spinal cord.*

In animal studies, electrical stimulation of the PAG area or raphe nucleus areas can almost completely suppress strong pain signals entering via the dorsal spinal roots. A similar system may exist in humans, since stimulation of the nearby PVG area of the hypothalamus is reported to relieve clinical pain. In addition to the brain stem–to–spinal cord network, neural connections also exist from the hypothalamus and neocortex to the PAG, allowing for pain modulation by an individual's thoughts and feelings from the higher brain centers.

Sensory input to the spinal cord may also be influenced by chemical substances termed *neuroregulators.* These neuroregulators are known as either neurotransmitters or neuromodulators. *Neurotransmitters* are neurochemicals that inhibit or stimulate activity at postsynaptic membranes. Substance P, a neuropeptide, is a pain-specific neurotransmitter present in the dorsal horn of the spinal cord (at the gate in the gate control theory), among other sites. Other CNS neurotransmitters involved in pain transmission include acetylcholine, norepinephrine, epinephrine, dopamine, and serotonin.

Two neurotransmitters, serotonin and norepinephrine, are known to be involved in the downward inhibition of incoming pain signals. The rostroventral medulla (RVM) contains a high percentage of serotonergic neurons that project to the spinal dorsal horn. Serotonin inhibits dorsal horn nociceptor neurons, thus modulating pain transmission. Tricyclic antidepressant drugs, such as amitriptyline (Elavil), produce analgesia by enhancing the inhibitory action of serotonin on the spinal transmission neurons. This analgesic effect can be blocked by serotonergic antagonists. A significant number of neurons in the dorsolateral pons contain norepinephrine and have spinal projections, some of which terminate in the dorsal horn. Norepinephrine inhibition of nociceptive transmission is mediated by alpha$_2$-adrenergic receptors, which are highly concentrated in the superficial layers of the dorsal horn. When clonidine, an alpha$_2$-agonist, is administered spinally, pain is inhibited. Antagonist drugs to the alpha$_2$-adrenergic receptors can partially block the antinociceptive action of brain activation (Fields, 1987).

In addition to these serotonin and norepinephrine descending pain-modulating pathways, endogenous opioid peptides are present in all the regions thus far implicated in pain modulation. Moreover, connections from serotonin neurons to opioid-containing cells exist in the substantia gelatinosa. Opioid peptides, known as neuromodulators (pain reducing), are naturally occurring compounds that have morphine-like qualities. These are discussed in more detail later.

PAIN THEORIES

A number of theories have been proposed to explain the neurologic mechanisms that underlie the sensation of pain, including (1) the specificity theory, (2) the pattern theory, and more recently (3) the gate control theory and (4) the endorphin/enkephalin theory.

Specificity Theory

The specificity theory of pain, which dates back about 200 years to Descartes, proposes that pain travels from specific pain receptors over a specific neuroanatomic pathway to a pain center in the brain and that the relationship between the pain stimulus and response is direct and invariable. Although this theory is clearly an oversimplification in the light of present knowledge, two of its principles are still valid: (1) somatosensory receptors are specialized to respond optimally to one or more specific types of stimuli, and (2) the central destination of primary afferent neurons and ascending pathways is a critical factor in distinguishing the nature of the peripheral stimulus.

Pattern, or Summation, Theory

The pattern, or summation, theory of pain was first introduced by Goldscheider in 1898. He proposed that the summation of the skin sensory input at the dorsal horn cells produce the particular patterns of nerve impulses that evoke pain. Pain is produced by intense stimulation from nonspecific receptors, and it is the summation of the impulses that are perceived as pain. Goldscheider also identified a rapidly conducting pain fiber and a slower one. In 1943 Livingstone introduced the concept of *central summation*. One of the key concepts of the central summation theory is that nerve fiber circuits can become established in groups of spinal interneurons (a reverberating circuit) after an injury, causing ongoing pain without stimulation. This mechanism could explain such phenomena as phantom limb pain. However, such procedures as a cordotomy, which would sever the reverberat-

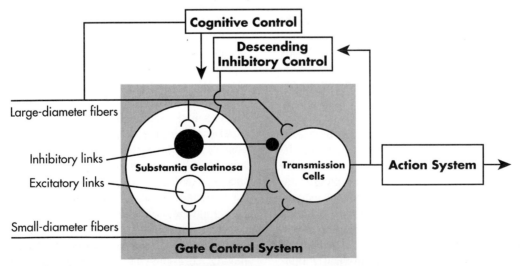

FIG. 52-5   The gate control theory of pain: Mark II. (From Melzack R, Wall PD: *The challenge of pain,* New York, 1983, Basic Books.)

ing circuit, usually do not relieve pain permanently (Melzack, 1973).

Gate Control Theory

Recent pain-related research has demonstrated that no single theory fully explains how pain is transmitted or perceived and that none reflects the complexity of the neuroanatomic pathways of pain transmission and modulation. The gate control theory was first developed in 1965 by Melzack and Wall to compensate for the deficiencies of the specificity and pattern theories of pain. Although some of its original assumptions have been disproved, this theory provides the most comprehensive and practical model for conceptualizing pain. The discovery of endogenous opioids in the early 1970s added another dimension to the understanding of pain modulation, but no single integrated theory yet exists.

The gate control theory of pain attempts to explain the variation in pain perception of identical stimulation. Melzack and Wall combined the available facts from the clinical literature and from neurophysiology to support their theory and used a schematic model to illustrate their ideas. This theory has been the focus of intense research over the past 30 years, and the model has been modified and updated (Fig. 52-5).

The basic tenets of the gate control theory are as follows (Melzack, Wall, 1983; Wall, Melzack, 1994):

1. Both the large, myelinated sensory fibers (L) carrying information about touch and proprioception from the periphery (A-α and A-β fibers) and the small fibers (S) carrying information about pain (A-δ and C fibers) converge on the dorsal horn of the spinal cord.
2. The transmission of nerve impulses from afferent fibers to spinal cord transmission (T) cells in the dorsal horn is modulated by a gating mechanism in the substantia gelatinosa cells. If the gate is closed, the pain impulses cannot proceed. If the gate is open or partially open, pain impulses stimulate the T cells in the dorsal horn and then ascend the spinal cord to the brain, where they are perceived as pain.
3. The spinal gating mechanism is influenced by the relative amount of activity in the large-diameter (L) and small-diameter (S) primary afferent fibers. Activity in large afferents tends to inhibit pain transmission (closes the gate), whereas small-fiber activity tends to facilitate pain transmission (opens the gate). The large-diameter afferents excite the inhibitory substantia gelatinosa neurons, thereby reducing input to the T cells and consequently inhibiting pain. In contrast, activity in the small-diameter fibers inhibits the inhibitory substantia gelatinosa cells, resulting in enhancement of transmission from primary afferents to the T cells and consequently increasing pain intensity. The inhibitions and facilitations are thought to occur by both presynaptic and postsynaptic mechanisms.
4. The spinal gating mechanism is influenced by nerve impulses that descend from the brain. This aspect of the mechanism is based on the enormous variety of psychologic factors known to influence pain and on the spinal cord dorsal horn being influenced by several pathways descending from the brain. These descending pain-modulating systems involving brain stem nuclei and serotonergic and noradrenergic neurons projecting to the substantia gelatinosa in the dorsal horn have already been discussed.
5. When the output of the spinal cord T cells exceeds a critical level, the "action system" for pain experience and response is activated. When this occurs, sensory input is being filtered, and continuing sensory and affective activity occurs at a series of CNS levels; for example, interaction occurs between the gate control system and the action system, or the brain may influence resetting of the gate as it analyzes and acts on the sensory input it receives.

In summary, the setting of the gate and therefore the ease with which information leading to pain generation passes through the gate depend on the balance of activity in large and small afferent fibers and in fibers descending from the higher centers.

The gate control theory of pain explains why rubbing or massaging a sore spot after an injury may relieve pain, since activity in large fibers is stimulated by this activity, closing the gate to small-diameter (pain) fiber activity. The use of transcutaneous electrical nerve stimulation (TENS or TNS) or effleurage to relieve pain are examples of clinical application of the theory. TENS therapy is reported to be effective in reducing self-reported pain and to reduce analgesic use after abdominal surgery, orthopedic surgery, thoracic surgery, and cesarean birth (Hargreaves, Lander, 1989).

Endorphin / Enkephalin Theory

The most important advance in the understanding of pain mechanisms has been the discovery of opiate receptor sites on synaptic membranes. Opiate receptor sites are especially concentrated in the PAG area, medial raphe nuclei, and dorsal horn of the spinal cord. Exogenous narcotic agents (e.g., morphine) and narcotic antagonists (e.g., naloxone) bind to these neuronal receptor sites. Opiates and opioids block pain (Fig. 52-6). Naloxone blocks inhibition and therefore increases pain. The presence of opiate receptor sites led to the search for endogenous *opioids,* substances with morphine-like properties that bind with the opiate receptors. In 1975 Hughes and his colleagues discovered enkephalin, the distribution of which appears to parallel opiate-binding sites.

There are three major families of endogenous opioid peptides, each derived from a different precursor and having a somewhat different anatomic distribution: the enkephalins, beta-endorphin, and dynorphin. *Met-enkephalin* and *leu-enkephalin* are peptide fragments de-

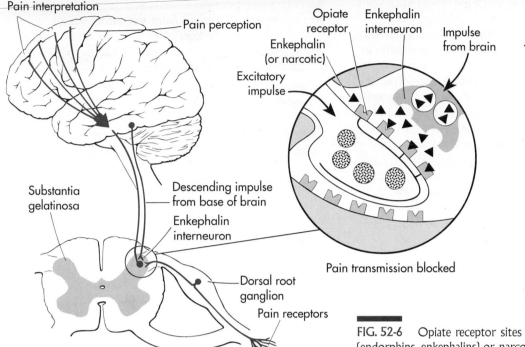

FIG. 52-6   Opiate receptor sites bind with endogenous opioids (endorphins, enkephalins) or narcotics and block transmission of pain impulses.

rived from pro-enkephalin and have the most extensive distribution in the CNS. Enkephalins are found in the hypothalamus, limbic system, PAG, RVM, (which contains a high proportion of serotonergic neurons), and dorsal horn of the spinal cord. Outside the CNS, enkephalins are also found in the gastrointestinal (GI) tract and adrenal glands. Electrical stimulation of the PAG and other parts of the brain can lead to analgesia. The analgesic effect can be reversed by naloxone, a morphine antagonist, demonstrating that endogenous opioids are involved. It is believed that enkephalin in some way may inhibit the release of substance P in the dorsal horn of the spinal cord. Enkephalins have a weaker analgesic effect than the other endorphins but are more potent and longer lasting than morphine.

Beta-endorphin is a peptide fragment derived from proopiomelanocortin (POMC), in the pituitary gland. Melanocyte-stimulating hormone (MSH) and adrenocorticotropic hormone (ACTH) are also derived from POMC. A significant amount of beta-endorphin exists in the hypothalamus and PAG and much less in the medulla and spinal cord. Beta-endorphin is a much more potent analgesic than enkephalin.

Dynorphin, the most recently discovered endorphin, is derived from prodynorphin, which is produced by the posterior pituitary gland. Its distribution roughly parallels that of the enkephalins. Dynorphin has the most potent analgesic effect—about 50 times more potent than beta-endorphin.

All the endogenous opiates act by combining with opiate receptor sites, with analgesic effects similar to those produced by exogenous opiate drugs. Thus opiate recep-

tors and endogenous opiates compose an intrinsic "pain suppression system." Experimental evidence suggests that such pain-reducing measures as placebo, acupuncture, and TENS may work because they stimulate release of endogenous opioids (Price, 1988). Epidural and intrathecal administration of opiates for the management of acute pain is a recent clinical application of knowledge about opiate receptors in the CNS. The epidural space is outside the dura mater of the spinal cord or brain, whereas the intrathecal space is inside the dura mater and contains the cerebrospinal fluid (CSF). Relatively small doses of opiate drugs (e.g., morphine) provide excellent and long-lasting analgesia and few systemic effects. The opiates bind with opiate receptors in the dorsal horn, providing pain relief without also causing sympathetic and motor nerve block (Dubner, Bennett 1989). Opiates can be injected intermittently or continuously through a small catheter placed in the intrathecal or epidural space by a procedure similar to lumbar puncture.

PAIN THRESHOLD AND TOLERANCE

The point at which a stimulus is perceived as painful is called the *pain threshold*. This varies minimally from individual to individual. One factor affecting pain threshold is perceptual dominance. This explains the clinical situation in which the pain felt in one area of the body diminishes or obliterates the pain felt in another area of the body. Not until the most severe pain is diminished does the patient perceive or acknowledge the other pain (Acute Pain Management Guideline Panel, 1992).

Pain tolerance refers to the length of time or intensity of pain that the patient endures before outwardly acknowledging it and seeking relief. In contrast to pain threshold, pain tolerance is more likely to vary from one individual to another. The patient's behavioral response to pain is influenced by a variety of factors, including personality type, psychologic state at the onset of pain, past experiences, sociocultural background, and meaning of the pain. Factors that decrease pain tolerance include repeated exposure to pain, fatigue, sleep deprivation, anxiety, and apprehension. Warmth, cold, distraction, alcohol consumption, hypnosis, and strong religious beliefs or faith act to increase pain tolerance (McCaffrey, Beebe 1989).

TYPES OF PAIN

To effectively assess and treat clients experiencing pain, it is important for clinicians to know that there are many different types of pain. Pain may be classified as acute or chronic according to duration. The character of pain may vary according to the location or source, such as whether it involves superficial somatic (cutaneous) structures, deep somatic structures, viscera, or damage to the CNS or peripheral nervous system (PNS). Pain may also vary according to the mode of transmission, giving rise to the phenomenon of referred pain.

Acute Pain Versus Chronic Pain

Acute pain and chronic pain are two types of pain, that differ in significant ways (Table 52-1). That is, chronic pain is not merely an extension of acute pain. Pain that resolves after successful intervention or healing is referred to as *acute pain*. Its onset is usually sudden and related to a specific problem that stimulates the person to act promptly to relieve the pain. The pain is short-lived (less than 6 months) and disappears when the internal or external factors that stimulated the pain receptors are eliminated. The duration of acute pain is correlated with the causative factor (acute injury or illness) and is generally quite predictable. The patient and the clinician expect the pain to diminish once the treatment begins.

The patient in acute pain displays a predictable neurologic response caused by sympathetic stimulation referred to as *autonomic hyperactivity*. These changes include tachycardia, tachypnea, increased peripheral blood flow, increased blood pressure (both systolic and diastolic), and the release of catecholamines (France, 1989). The intensity of the sympathetic response is generally proportional to the degree of stimulation of the pain receptors.

The prototype for acute pain is postoperative pain. The

▶ **TABLE 52-1   Characteristics of Acute and Chronic Pain**

Characteristic	Acute Pain	Chronic Pain*
Onset and duration	Abrupt onset; duration short, less than 6 months	Gradual onset; persistent, greater than 6 months
Intensity	Moderate to severe	Moderate to severe
Cause	Specific; biologically identifiable	Cause may or may not be well defined
Physiologic response	Predictable autonomic hyperactivity: increased blood pressure, pulse, and respiratory rate; dilated pupils; pallor; perspiration; nausea and/or vomiting	Normal autonomic activity
Emotional/behavioral response	Anxious; unable to concentrate; restless; distressed but optimistic about relief from pain	Depression and fatigue; immobility or physical inactivity; social withdrawal; sees no relief in sight, expects long-term pain
Response to analgesics	Effective pain relief	Often ineffective pain relief

*Chronic malignant, chronic nonmalignant, and chronic intermittent pain.

quality, intensity, and duration of the pain are related to the nature of the surgical procedure. Any trauma, including surgical trauma, results in tissue damage. Pain-producing substances released into the injured tissue lower the pain threshold. Incisions in the upper abdomen generally cause greater postoperative pain because of respiratory movements. Muscle spasm around the area of injury may contribute to the pain. Incisional pain is generally sharp and well localized because the skin and subcutaneous tissues are well supplied with nociceptors. When deeper structures with fewer pain receptors are injured, the pain tends to be dull and poorly localized or may be referred when visceral structures are involved (see following discussion). Fear and anxiety are often part of the affective-motivational aspects of acute pain and tend to reinforce each other. Thus measures to relieve the pain also reduce the anxiety, which tends to lessen the pain. Acute postoperative pain usually disappears with healing.

When pain continues despite treatment or apparent healing and serves no biologic purpose, the pain is called chronic. *Chronic pain* may be continuous, resulting from malignant or nonmalignant causes, or may be intermittent, as in recurrent migraine headaches. Pain that persists for 6 months or longer is generally classified as chronic. Chronic pain represents a major health care problem in U.S. society. It has been estimated that 25% of the population suffers from a chronic illness and chronic pain.

Patients with chronic pain have little or no autonomic hyperactivity but instead exhibit symptoms of irritability, lack of energy, and interference with the ability to concentrate. Chronic pain often encompasses every aspect of the person's life, creating emotional turmoil and distress, and interferes with physical and social functioning. Many factors are involved in the development of chronic pain, including organic, psychologic, social, and environmental factors (France, 1989).

Chronic pain syndromes usually have organic causes, but the patient's personality and psychologic status influence its development. Conditions associated with chronic pain with an organic origin vary widely and include headaches, back pain, arthritis, carcinoma, and neuropathologies (e.g., trigeminal neuralgia, phantom limb pain). Chronic pain syndromes are often accompanied by symptoms of anxiety, insomnia, and depression, with depression the most common. Chronic pain is a complex syndrome requiring a multidisciplinary approach for its management.

Superficial Somatic (Cutaneous) Pain

Cutaneous pain arises in the superficial structures of the skin and subcutaneous tissues. The effective stimulus for pain in the skin may be mechanical, thermal, chemical, or electrical. If the skin alone is involved, the pain is often described as tingling, sharp, cutting, or burning, but if blood vessels are contributing to the pain, it becomes throbbing in nature. The skin has many sensory nerves, and therefore damage to it is located more accurately and with greater precision than elsewhere. The area of pain may be localized along a distinct dermatome (skin segment) innervated by one dorsal (sensory) root (see Fig. 51-8). However, the dermatomes are not distinct and separate segments. Considerable overlap exists between any two adjacent dermatomes, and more so with pain and thermal senses than with tactile sensations. As a consequence, if one spinal nerve were completely nonfunctional, no area of complete anesthesia on the skin would be found, since the nerves from the two adjacent dermatomes would pick up the sensory stimuli. On the other hand, if a dorsal root of one spinal nerve were irritated, as in herpes zoster (shingles, a viral infection of a spinal ganglion), the noxious stimuli would be felt subjectively from the entire dermatome, including the overlap.

Deep Somatic Pain

Deep somatic pain refers to pain arising from muscles, tendons, ligaments, bones, joints, and arteries. These structures have fewer pain receptors, so the pain is often poorly localized. Pain is experienced as more diffuse than cutaneous pain and tends to radiate to adjacent areas. Pain from various deep structures differs. Pain from an acute injury of a joint is well localized and usually described as sharp or burning or as throbbing. In chronic inflammation of a joint (arthritis), dull aching pains are experienced on which movement superimposes sharp, stabbing pain. Bone pain arises from stimulation of pain receptors in the periosteum and is less well localized. It is often described as a dull aching or soreness. Skeletal muscle pain is also poorly localized and is described as a dull ache or cramp. Skeletal muscle pain is particularly severe during contraction under conditions of ischemia.

Visceral Pain

Visceral pain refers to pain arising from the body organs. Visceral pain receptors are sparse compared with somatic pain receptors and are located in the smooth muscle walls of hollow organs (stomach, gallbladder, bile ducts, ureter, urinary bladder) and in the capsules of solid organs (liver, pancreas, kidney). The visceral parenchyma is relatively insensitive to cutting, heat, or pinching. The main mechanisms that generate visceral pain are abnormal stretching or distention of the wall or capsule of the organ, ischemia, and inflammation. The gut is a source of either a gnawing or a cramping pain or the intermittent pain known as *colic* when irritated by the chemical substances produced by inflammation or when distended. Other distensible structures, such as the gallbladder, bile ducts, or ureters, can cause colicky pain, often from smooth muscle spasm. Obstruction of outflow and overdistention also cause ischemia and the release of chemicals that stimulate pain receptors.

The viscera are innervated by two routes: through nerves that supply autonomic functions (the true visceral pathway), such as the splanchnics, and through spinal nerves that supply somatic structures (the parietal pathway). The parietal pleura, peritoneum, and lower part of the pericardium are sensitive to pain but are supplied by spinal nerves instead of nerves of the autonomic nervous system (ANS). Pain transmitted via the true visceral pathway is poorly localized and is often referred to a *body surface area* (dermatome) distant from its origin. On the other hand, pain transmitted via the parietal pathway is felt directly over the painful area. All neurons stimulated by visceral afferent input have also been shown to receive somatic inputs. This dual innervation may be one reason for the poor localization of visceral stimuli and for the phenomenon of referred pain.

Visceral pain is transmitted through the sympathetic and parasympathetic fibers of the ANS. Visceral afferents are usually type C fibers, and the pain sensations generated usually have a dull or aching quality. Pain impulses from the thoracic and abdominal viscera are almost exclusively conducted through the sympathetic nervous system; they travel with the sympathetic nerve through the sympathetic ganglia without synapsing, and then

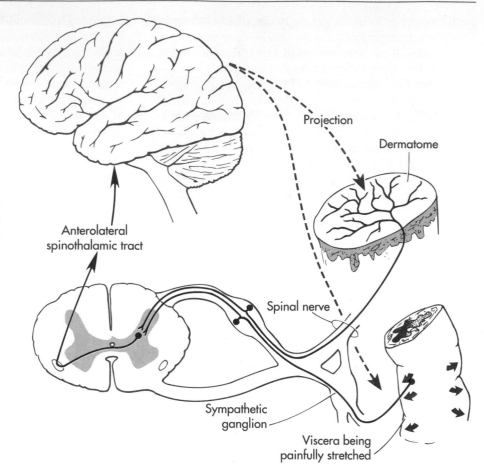

FIG. 52-7 The convergence-projection theory of referred pain. Afferent fibers from the viscus converge on the same pain projection neurons in the spinal cord as do afferent fibers from somatic structures (e.g., the skin). Thus visceral pain may be perceived as somatic pain.

reach the spinal nerves through the white ramus communicans and thence to the dorsal root ganglion. However, pain impulses from the pharynx, trachea, and esophagus are mediated by vagal afferents, and pain from the deep pelvic structures is transmitted in the sacral parasympathetic nerves. In the central pathways, visceral pain impulses, as well as other visceral sensations, travel the same route as impulses from somatic structures. This is an important factor in the frequent somatic referral of visceral pain.

Visceral pain is particularly unpleasant not only because of the affective component, which it shares with all pain, but also because so many visceral afferents excited by the same process that causes the pain have reflex connections that initiate nausea, vomiting, sweating, blood pressure changes, and other autonomic effects.

Visceral pain, as with deep somatic pain, initiates reflex contraction of nearby skeletal muscle. This reflex spasm is usually in the abdominal wall and is most marked when visceral inflammatory processes involve the peritoneum. The anatomic details of the reflex pathways by which impulses from diseased viscera initiate skeletal muscle spasm are unclear. The spasm protects the underlying inflamed structures from inadvertent trauma. This reflex spasm is sometimes referred to as muscle "guarding."

Referred Pain

Referred pain is defined as pain originating from one site in the body that is perceived as being localized in a different site. Visceral pain is often referred to dermatomes (skin areas) innervated by the same segments of the spinal cord as the painful viscus. When visceral pain is referred to the surface of the body, it is generally localized to the dermatomal segment from which the visceral organ originated in the embryo, not necessarily where the organ is located in the adult.

Presently, the most widely accepted explanation of referred pain is the *convergence-projection theory* (Fields, 1987). According to this theory, two types of afferents entering the spinal segment (one from the skin and another from the viscera or deep muscular structures) converge onto the same sensory projection cells (e.g., spinothalamic projection cells). Because the brain has no way of knowing the actual source of the input, it mistakenly "projects" the pain sensation to the somatic site (dermatome) (Fig. 52-7). For example, myocardial ischemia results in the patient experiencing severe pain over the middle of the sternum, often radiating down the medial side of the left arm, the root of the neck, and even the jaw. The pain is assumed to be caused by the accumulation of metabolites and oxygen deficiency, which stimulate the sensory nerve endings in the myocardium. The afferent

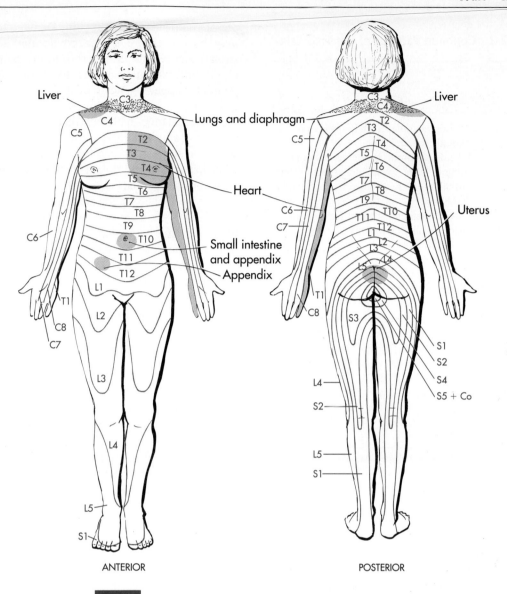

Liver
C3
C4
C5
Lungs and diaphragm
T2
T3
T4
T5
T6
T7
T8
T9
T10
T11
T12
C6
Heart
Small intestine and appendix
Appendix
L1
L2
C8
C7
T1
L3
L4
L5
S1

ANTERIOR

C3
C4
Liver
T2
T3
T4
T5
T6
T7
T8
T9
T10
T11
T12
L1
L2
L3
L4
L5
C5
C6
C7
Uterus
S3
S1
S2
S4
S5 + Co
T1
C8
L4
S2
L5
S1

POSTERIOR

FIG. 52-8   Common sites of referred pain originating in visceral organs. *C,* Cervical; *T,* thoracic; *L,* lumbar; *S,* sacral spinal nerves. *Co,* Coccyx.

nerve fibers ascend to the CNS through the cardiac branches of the sympathetic trunk and enter the spinal cord through the dorsal roots of the upper five thoracic nerves (T1 to T5). The cardiac pain is not felt in the heart but is referred to the skin areas (dermatomes) supplied by the corresponding spinal (somatic) nerves. The skin areas supplied by the upper five intercostal nerves and by the intercostal brachial nerve (T2) are therefore affected. A certain amount of spread of the pain impulses must occur within the CNS, since the pain is sometimes felt in the neck and jaw.

Another common example of referred pain is found in the early stages of acute appendicitis. Initially, visceral pain in the appendix is produced by distention of its lumen or spasm of its muscle. The visceral afferent pain fibers enter the spinal cord at the tenth thoracic (T10)

level, having ascended through the superior mesenteric plexus and the lesser splanchnic nerve. A vague aching or crampy pain is felt in the area of the umbilicus, which is innervated by the tenth (somatic) intercostal nerve. Later the pain shifts to the lower right quadrant of the abdomen, where the inflamed appendix irritates the parietal peritoneum, which is innervated by the twelfth thoracic and first lumbar spinal nerves (T12 to L1). Here the pain is sharp and precisely localized over the irritated peritoneum, since the impulses are transmitted directly via the spinal nerves (somatic or parietal pathway).

An understanding of the typical patterns of referred pain from visceral structures is helpful in diagnosing illness (Fig. 52-8). Table 52-2 identifies some of the dermatomes to which pain from damaged visceral structures are referred.

TABLE 52-2 Common Patterns of Referred Pain

Site of Visceral Pathology or Noxious Stimuli	Surface Areas of Referred Pain
Diaphragm	C3-C5 dermatomes: pain in ipsilateral shoulder or neck area
Heart	C3-T5 dermatomes: substernal pain radiating to back, down inner aspect of arm (usually left), and sometimes neck and jaw
Liver/gallbladder	T5-T9 dermatomes: pain in right costal margin radiating to back or right shoulder
Stomach	T7-T9 dermatomes: epigastric pain
Appendix/small intestine	T9-T11 dermatomes: periumbilical pain
Prostate	T10-T12 dermatomes: periumbilical and groin pain, sometimes radiating to scrotum and penis
Ovaries	T10 dermatome: periumbilical pain
Ureters	L1-L2 dermatomes: pain in groin and inner surface of thighs
Uterus	S1-S2 dermatomes: pain over sacrum
Rectum	S2-S4 dermatomes: low back pain radiating down posterior aspect of thigh and calf

C, Cervical; T, thoracic; L, lumbar; S, sacral spinal nerves.

Neuropathic Pain

The nervous system normally transmits noxious stimuli from the PNS to the CNS that result in pain. Thus lesions of the PNS or CNS can result in impairment or loss of pain sensation called *hypalgesia* and *analgesia,* respectively. Paradoxically, damage or dysfunction of the CNS or peripheral nerves can cause pain. This type of pain is called neuropathic pain, or *deafferentation.* Neuropathic pain arises from the peripheral nerves along their course or from the CNS because of abnormal functioning, without involving the excitation of specific pain receptors (nociceptors).

Neuropathic pain often has a burning, tingling, or electric shock–like quality. People with neuropathic pain suffer from instability of the ANS, and thus the pain is often made worse by emotional or physical (cold, fatigue) stress and relieved by relaxation, so they may fall asleep normally despite their pain. The most characteristic feature of neuropathic pain, which is never seen in tissue damage pain, is allodynia. *Allodynia* is pain triggered by stimuli that would ordinarily be innocuous, such as a light touch or even a puff of wind. A sensory defect is typically present in the area of the pain. Neuropathic pain is often severe and refractory to treatment with opiates.

Neuropathic pain may result from lesions of the CNS (*central pain)* or damage to the peripheral nerves (*peripheral pain).* The *thalamic pain syndrome* is an exam-

ple of central neuropathic pain. Damage to the thalamus may be caused by a cerebrovascular accident (CVA, stroke) and results in severe burning pain in the hemiplegic side, especially in the distal limb. One theory explaining the pathogenesis of thalamic pain is the loss of central inhibition. According to this theory, damage to the neospinothalamic pathway that spares the paleospinothalamic pathway releases the latter from inhibition, resulting in summation and hyperalgesia. This is similar to what happens when dorsal horn nociceptors excited by unmyelinated primary afferents are released from the inhibitory influence of the large, myelinated afferents, as described in the gate control theory. Activity of sympathetic efferents may also play a role in the pathogenesis of central neuropathic pain, since peripheral sympathetic blockade can sometimes relieve the pain (Fields, 1987).

Peripheral neuropathic pain occurs as a result of damage to peripheral nerves. Damage that is peripheral in origin leads not only to spontaneous firing of the affected peripheral nerve fibers, but also to spontaneous firing of the dorsal root ganglion cells of the damaged nerves. Examples of syndromes that may be present include postherpetic neuralgia, painful diabetic neuropathy, trigeminal neuralgia, causalgia, and phantom limb pain.

Postherpetic neuralgia is a dermatomal deafferentation pain that occurs as a sequela to herpes zoster (shingles). Herpes zoster is characterized by a painful vesicular rash, most often on the chest dermatomes (T3 to L3), caused by reactivation of the varicella-zoster virus (VZV). It is presumed that the virus infects the dorsal root ganglion during chickenpox and lies dormant until reactivated. Herpes zoster is most common in persons over age 50 years and in immunocompromised patients, such as those with Hodgkin's disease and non-Hodgkin's lymphoma. Persistent intractable pain occurs in the involved dermatomes months after the cutaneous lesions have healed in about 50% of older patients (postherpetic neuralgia). The exact cause is unknown, but scarring and degenerative changes in the spinal cord, ganglia, and nerve trunks may be important factors.

Diabetic neuropathy is a common complication of diabetes, especially after longstanding hyperglycemia. It may affect every part of the nervous system, with the possible exception of the brain. The most common clinical picture is that of bilateral peripheral polyneuropathy that is primarily sensory. In diabetic sensory neuropathy predominantly the small nerve fibers are affected, and these neuropathies are characteristically painful (Fields, 1987). Symptoms include numbness, paresthesias, severe hyperalgesias, and pain that is sometimes lancinating or "lightning" in type.

Trigeminal neuralgia (tic douloureux) is a severe neuralgia of the trigeminal nerve associated with pain in one of its divisions on the face, usually the maxillary or mandibular. It is characterized by paroxysmal, intense, stabbing facial pain that may be triggered by innocuous stimuli such as eating, talking, or drafts of cold air. The cause of this condition is believed to be patchy loss of myelin. Ectopic impulses may arise from a short patch of demyelination on a primary afferent nerve (Fields, 1987).

Causalgia is a term used to describe the intense burning pain in an extremity that may follow partial damage to a nerve trunk, typically the median nerve above the elbow or sciatic nerve above the knee. The pain usually begins soon after the injury and in time becomes associated with autonomic changes and trophic changes in the extremity. Causalgia is one subtype of a group of disorders known as *reflex sympathetic dystrophies,* and all give rise to allodynia, or pain triggered by innocuous stimuli. All tissues in the extremity waste, including bones, and there is evidence of sympathetic hyperactivity, including vasomotor changes and abnormal sweating. Pain relief follows sympathetic blockage. Other mechanisms of pain generation may include loss of afferent inhibition by the large, myelinated fibers and ectopic impulse generation at the site of injury. The causes of reflex sympathetic dystrophies include nerve damage, amputations, fractures of the small bones of the hand or foot, sprains, or thrombophlebitis.

Phantom limb pain is experienced by a patient as tingling, "pins and needles" sensation (paresthesias), or less often as a burning, crushing pain in a limb that the individual no longer possesses (because it has been amputated). This is possibly because some of the pain fibers have been pinched in the scar tissue of the limb stump, causing the generation of ectopic impulses. It is immaterial that the portion of the fiber attached to the receptor is missing, since a region still exists in the cerebral cortex for that portion of the extremity. All that is required is that an impulse reach the cortex for that area.

CLINICAL ASSESSMENT OF PAIN

The relief and management of pain require careful assessment to attempt to understand the patient's pain experience and identify the cause so that it can be removed, if possible. The clinician must first take a careful history, which should include the data about the pain listed in Table 52-3.

The patient can indicate the *location* of the pain by pointing to the body part or indicating the site on a drawing of a human figure. It is important to find out whether the pain is *superficial* or *deep*. Pain from a superficial lesion usually poses no problem because the cause and effect are obvious. However, exact location becomes especially important with deep pain that is referred to a dermatome when deep somatic structures or viscera are involved.

The *mode of onset* is an important factor in assessing pain. A pain that has a sudden onset and reaches a peak of intensity almost immediately suggests a rupture of tissue.

TABLE 52-3   Essential Data to Collect for Assessment of Pain

Characteristic of Pain	Questions for Patient
Location	Where does it hurt? Does the pain radiate? Is the pain superficial or deep?
Mode of onset	When did the pain start? Did it begin suddenly or gradually? Was there any particular event that appeared to produce the pain when it began?
Pattern (timing, frequency, duration)	What time of the day does the pain occur? How often does it appear? Is it constant or intermittent? How long does the pain last?
Aggravating and relieving factors	What seems to trigger the pain? What seems to make the pain worse (e.g., movement or changes in posture, coughing or straining, eating or drinking)? What seems to make the pain better (e.g., rest; sleep; changes in posture such as standing, sitting, lying down, or bending; food or antacids)?
Quality	What does the pain feel like (e.g., throbbing, dull, aching, sharp, stabbing, prickling, burning)?
Intensity	How strong is your pain? (Have patient rate the pain using a verbal or visual analog scale both before and after treatment.)
Associated symptoms	Are there any problems caused by your pain (e.g., anorexia, nausea, vomiting, insomnia)?
Effects on life-style	Does your pain interfere with your activities at home, work, or normal social interactions? Has the pain affected your life-style in any way (e.g., eating, sleeping, sexual activity, driving)?
Methods of pain relief	What has helped control your pain in the past? What has not worked in relieving your pain?

The pain of myocardial infarction or a ruptured peptic ulcer may develop in this manner.

The *pattern* of the pain, or the time and frequency of occurrence and duration, provides important information. Postural aches come after prolonged activity (usually late in the day) and disappear with rest, whereas arthritic pains are most severe during the first movements after prolonged inactivity (usually in the morning on awakening). Painful lesions of the bone, such as metastatic cancer, are likely to be most disturbing at night. Not all pain

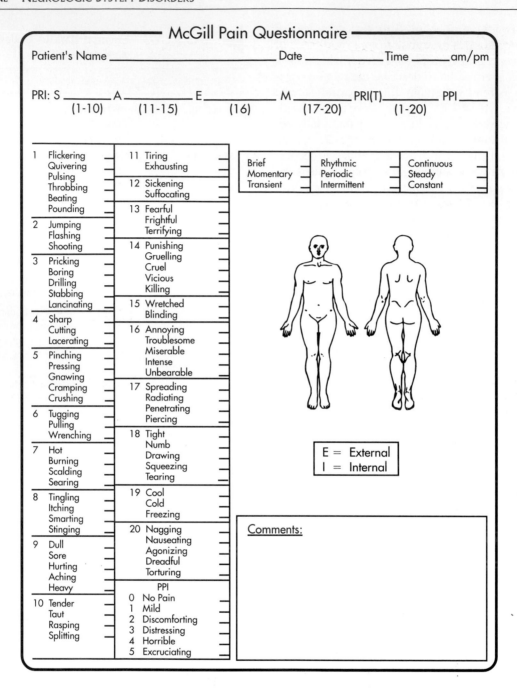

FIG. 52-9 McGill Pain Questionnaire. The pain rating index *(PRI)* is the sum of ranked values for the 20 words: *S,* subjective, 1 to 10; *A,* affective, 11 to 15; *E,* evaluative, 16; *M,* miscellaneous, 17 to 20 *PRI (T),* total PRI, (1-20); *PPI,* present pain index, a rating of pain intensity. The site of the pain is marked on the figure with an E (external) or I (internal), and the boxes above the figures are checked to describe the pattern of the pain. Comments include response to analgesics. (From Melzack R, Katz J, editors: Pain measurement in persons in pain. In Wall PD, Melzack R, editors: *Textbook of pain,* ed 3, New York, 1994, Churchill Livingstone.)

is constant. Intermittent pain that occurs several times a day can be equally disturbing. Attacks can last seconds, hours, or days and can affect the individual's ability to function normally (e.g., trigeminal neuralgia, migraine headache). Substernal pain lasting less than 15 minutes that is relieved by rest or nitroglycerin is characteristic of angina pectoris, but when the pain persists longer than 15 minutes, it may indicate myocardial infarction.

The *aggravating and relieving factors* of pain are more important than the quality of the pain in providing data concerning its mechanism. Pain related to breathing, swallowing, or defecation focuses attention on the respiratory system, esophagus, and lower bowel, respectively. Pain that is brought on by activity and relieved after a few minutes of rest suggests ischemia (e.g., angina pectoris, intermittent claudication). Pain occurring several hours

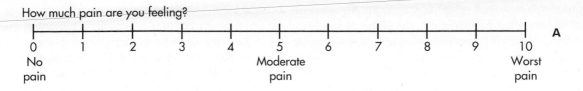

FIG. 52-10   Visual analog scales to assess intensity of pain. **A,** Numeric rating scale. **B,** Wong-Baker FACES Pain Rating Scale. Face 0 is smiling because it has no pain. Faces 1 to 5 have increasing amounts of pain (a little to the greatest imaginable) with increasingly sad expressions. [From Wong D, Baker C: *Pediatr Nurs* 14(1):9-17, 1988.]

after meals that is relieved by food or antacid ingestion is characteristic of duodenal ulcer. Pain that is increased or altered by cutaneous stimuli may be caused by disease or injury to the sensory tracts in the PNS or CNS (e.g., causalgia, thalamic syndrome).

The *quality* of the pain may be assessed by simply asking patients to describe the pain in their own words (e.g., dull, throbbing, burning). This can also be approached using a more formal assessment, such as the *McGill Pain Questionnaire* (Fig. 52-9), which is one of the most frequently used tools for assessing pain. It has been validated in several languages and can be used in both acute and chronic settings, as well as for research. The questionnaire measures the physiologic and psychologic dimensions of pain and is divided into four parts. In the first part the patient indicates the location of the pain on a drawing of a human body. In the second part the patient chooses 20 words that describe the sensory, affective, evaluative, and other qualities of the pain. In the third part the patient chooses words such as *brief, rhythmic,* or *steady* to describe the pattern of the pain. In the fourth part the patient rates the intensity of the pain on a scale of 0 to 5.

The tool most often used to assess the *intensity* or *severity* of the patient's pain is some form of a *visual analog scale* (VAS), which consists of a horizontal line evenly divided into 10 segments numbered 0 to 10 (Fig. 52-10, *A*). Patients are instructed that 0 represents "no pain at all" and 10 represents the "the most severe pain they can imagine." They are then asked to mark the number that best describes the level of pain they are experiencing at some given point in time. A modified VAS for use with children (or with cognitively impaired adults) substitutes a continuum of smiling or crying faces for numbers (Fig. 52-10, *B*).

It is important to ask the patient about *symptoms asso-* *ciated* with the pain. Autonomic responses such as nausea and vomiting are common with severe, acute pain. Auras often precede migraine headaches. The examiner should provide ample opportunity to discuss what the pain means to the patient by asking about its *impact on life-style.* Finally, it is important to document *methods of treatment for pain* that have been used by the patient in the past and their effectiveness.

In addition to collecting subjective data about pain, direct observation of *nonverbal and verbal behavior* may provide additional clues about the patient's pain experience. Nonverbal behaviors such as facial grimacing, tearing, abnormal gait or posture, muscle tension, and guarding of parts are common indicators of pain. Verbal and emotional signals indicating pain may include crying, moaning, irritability, expressions of anger or sadness, and changes in voice pitch or fluency. Gender and cultural differences exist in the types of displays used. As described previously, acute pain often activates a *sympathetic response,* resulting in increased heart and respiratory rates and blood pressure, pallor, flushing, sweating, and pupil dilation. Very brief and intense pain may also be followed by a rebound parasympathetic response.

Finally, the clinician should *inspect and palpate the painful area* to test range of motion of involved joints, determine if there is muscle guarding, and identify trigger points of pain and areas of decreased sensation or increased sensitivity.

MANAGEMENT OF PAIN

The overall goal in the treatment of pain is to provide the greatest relief from pain with the least possible side effects. There are two general methods for the treatment of pain: pharmacologic and nonpharmacologic. To achieve the goal of pain relief in the patient, the clinician needs to (1) use knowledge of the neuropathophysiology of pain as a basis for various interventions; (2) assess pain routinely using appropriate instruments, both before and after treatment; (3) use a variety of pharmacologic and nonpharmacologic pain-relieving methods; and (4) document the effectiveness of pain-relieving interventions. Planning is needed in consultation with the patient, and the clinician should create a relationship of warmth, empathy, and respect.

Pharmacologic Approaches

Medications are the most common form of pain control. There are three groups of pain medications: (1) nonopioid analgesics, (2) opioid analgesics, and (3) opioid antagonists and agonist-antagonists. A fourth group of medications is called *adjuvants* or *coanalgesics*. Pharmacologic management with analgesic drugs should be implemented using a stepwise approach.

Nonopioid analgesia: nonsteroidal antiinflammatory drugs (NSAIDs)

The first step, often effective for mild to moderate pain management, uses nonopioid analgesics, specifically acetaminophen (Tylenol) and the NSAIDs. A wide variety of NSAIDs are available with varying degrees of antipyretic, analgesic, and (except for acetaminophen) antiinflammatory actions. They also differ to some extent in their cost, duration of action, and side effects. Acetylsalicylic acid (aspirin) and ibuprofen (Motrin, Advil) are probably the most frequently used NSAIDs. NSAIDs are particularly effective in treating low-grade acute pain, chronic inflammatory conditions such as arthritis, and mild cancer-related pain.

NSAIDs produce analgesia by acting peripherally at the site of tissue injury by blocking the synthesis of prostaglandins from their arachidonic acid precursors. Prostaglandins, (mainly PGE_1, PGE_2, and PGI_2) sensitize nociceptors and work synergistically with other inflammatory products at the site of injury, such as bradykinin and histamine, to produce hyperalgesia. Thus NSAIDs interfere with the mechanism of transduction in primary afferent nociceptors by blocking prostaglandin synthesis.

In contrast to opioids, NSAIDs do not produce physical dependence or tolerance. All share a *ceiling effect;* that is, increasing the dose above a certain level does not increase the analgesic effect. However, the ceiling dose may be higher than the recommended starting dose, so a higher dose may be warranted. The most common complications associated with NSAIDs are GI upset, increased bleeding time (aspirin), blurring of vision, minor changes in liver function tests, and reduction in renal function.

Second only to aspirin, acetaminophen (Tylenol) is the next most frequently used analgesic agent (Taylor, Curran, 1985). Acetaminophen provides an analgesic and antipyretic effect similar to aspirin, but unlike the NSAIDs, it does not inhibit peripheral prostaglandin synthesis and thus does not have an antiinflammatory effect. On the other hand, acetaminophen does inhibit prostaglandin synthesis in the brain, which may account for its antipyretic and analgesic action (Flower, Moncada, Vane, 1990). If acetaminophen or aspirin is not effective alone in relieving pain, they may be combined with a weak narcotic such as oxycodone or codeine (which act centrally) for more effective pain relief.

Opioid analgesia

Opioids are currently the most potent analgesics available and are used in the management of moderately severe to severe pain. These drugs are the cornerstone in the treatment of postoperative and cancer-related pain. Morphine (from Morpheus, the Greek god of dreams) is an alkaloid derived from the dried juice of the opium poppy plant, and it has been used for centuries for its analgesic, sedative, and euphoric effects. Morphine is one of the most widely used drugs for the treatment of severe pain and remains the standard with which other analgesic drugs are compared.

In contrast to the NSAIDs, which act peripherally, morphine exerts its analgesic effect centrally. The actual mechanism of opioid action has become more clear since the discovery of endogenous opioid receptors in the limbic system, thalamus, PAG, substantia gelatinosa of the dorsal horn, and gut. Exogenous opioids such as morphine exert their effect by binding to opioid receptors in a manner similar to that of endogenous opioids (endorphins/enkephalins); that is, they have agonist action (enhance the receptor's action). By binding to opioid receptors in the brain stem pain-modulating nuclei, morphine exerts its effects on the descending pain-inhibiting systems. Morphine can also block the transmission of incoming nociceptor impulses at the level of the spinal cord dorsal horn by binding with opioid receptors in the substantia gelatinosa.

The action of opioids can depend on the type of receptor with which they interact. Three types of opioid receptors have been reasonably well defined: mu-, kappa-, and delta-receptors. The most important receptor type for clinical analgesia is called "mu" because of its affinity for morphine. Numerous drugs in the morphine class are mu-agonists, although they differ in potency (Jaffe, Martin, 1990). Table 52-4 lists some frequently used opioids with doses equivalent to 10 mg of morphine (*equianalgesic dose*). Knowledge of the equianalgesic doses of opioid drugs is essential when changing medications or routes of administration.

Opioid drugs have a very similar pattern of side effects, including respiratory depression, nausea and vomiting, sedation, and constipation. In addition, opioids all have the potential to produce tolerance, dependence, and addiction. *Tolerance* is the physiologic need for higher

▶ TABLE 52-4   Frequently Used Opioids and
Their Equianalgesic Drug Doses*

Opioid	Intramuscular Route	Oral Route	Comments
Morphine	10 mg	60 mg	Standard narcotic with which other analgesics are compared
Codeine	130 mg	200 mg	Often combined with acetaminophen (Tylenol #2, #3, or #4) or with aspirin (Empirin #2, #3, or #4)
Oxycodone	NA	30 mg	Often combined with acetaminophen (Percodan) or aspirin (Percocet)
Meperidine (Demerol)	75 mg	300 mg	
Hydromorphone (Dilaudid)	1.5 mg	8 mg	
Methadone (Dolophine)	10 mg	20 mg	
Levorphanol (Levo-Dromoran)	2 mg	4 mg	
Fentanyl (Sublimaze)	0.05 mg	NA	May be given transdermally as a patch or epidurally

NA, Not applicable.
*Compared with 10 mg of intramuscular morphine.

doses to maintain the analgesic effects of the drug. Tolerance to a particular opioid develops when it is administered chronically, as for cancer-related pain. Although considerable cross-tolerance occurs between the opioid drugs, it is not complete. This provides the theoretic basis for substituting another opioid drug when a particular one becomes ineffective. *Physical dependence* is also a physiologic process marked by the occurrence of a withdrawal syndrome after abrupt discontinuation of an opioid drug or after administration of an antagonist. The withdrawal syndrome is believed to result from rebound noradrenergic activity in the CNS that is depressed by chronic opioid use (Gossop, 1988). *Addiction,* or *psychologic dependence,* refers to a behavioral syndrome in which there is overriding concern with the use and acquisition of the drug, resulting in drug hoarding and unapproved escalation in the dose. It is important to understand the difference between tolerance, dependence, and addiction, since evidence indicates that patients are routinely undermedicated for pain because of an exaggerated fear (by both staff and patients) of the patient becoming addicted. This fear is unfounded because addiction is extremely rare when opioids are used to treat patients in pain (Porter, Jick, 1980). It is important to remember that patients vary in their analgesic dose requirements and that dosage must be individually titrated. In recent years, tremendous progress has been made in methods of opioid administration that help to provide greater relief from unnecessary pain.

One such advance in the method of opioid administration is "around-the-clock dosing" rather than PRN ("as-needed dosing," requiring the patient to request medication from the nurse). Around-the-clock dosing has the advantage of maintaining constant blood levels of analgesic and preventing the development of severe pain, which is more difficult to alleviate after it occurs. Because the best way to treat pain is to prevent it, *patient-controlled analgesia* (PCA) systems were developed. As the name implies, the PCA apparatus delivers a preset dose of morphine (or other opioid) through an indwelling intravenous (IV) line when the patient pushes a button. The device is loaded with enough drug to cover the patient's needs for 12 to 24 hours and is usually programmed so a minimal interval of 15 to 30 minutes elapses between doses. PCA devices are most often used to control postoperative and cancer-related pain. Some of the advantages of PCA include superior pain relief with less medication, less sedation, and a decrease in the delay between request for analgesia and relief. Epidural and intrathecal administration of morphine (preservative free) at the level of the spinal cord is a recent innovation requiring special expertise. The advantage of direct spinal administration of morphine is that it may provide analgesia with less side effects by activation of opioid receptors at the spinal level rather than at supraspinal levels. Successful analgesia can also be achieved with much lower doses (Lieb, Hurtig, 1985).

Opioid antagonists and agonist-antagonists

Opioid antagonists are drugs that counteract the effect of opioid drugs by binding to opioid receptors and blocking their activation. Naloxone, a pure opioid antagonist, reverses both the analgesia and the side effects of opioids. Naloxone is used to counteract the effects of a narcotic overdose, the most serious of which are respiratory depression and sedation.

Other opioid drugs are combinations of agonists and antagonists, such as pentazocine (Talwin) and butorphanol (Stadol). When these drugs are given to a patient dependent on narcotics, they can precipitate withdrawal symptoms. Opioid agonist-antagonists are effective analgesics when given alone and are less likely to produce undesirable side effects (e.g., respiratory depression) than pure agonist opioids.

Adjuvants or coanalgesics

Adjuvant or coanalgesic medications are agents originally developed for purposes other than pain relief but have been found to have analgesic properties or a complementary role in the management of patients with pain. Some of these drugs are particularly effective in the control of neuropathic pain that may not respond to opioids.

Anticonvulsants, such as carbamazepine (Tegretol) or phenytoin (Dilantin), have been found to be effective for the treatment of lancinating pains associated with nerve damage. Lancinating pains (brief flashing, stabbing, or shooting) are characteristic of trigeminal neuralgia, diabetic neuropathy, and postherpetic neuralgia and often occur after laminectomy and limb amputation. Animal studies suggest that anticonvulsants are effective for neuropathic pain because they suppress ectopic sites of impulse generation in damaged peripheral nerves (Fields, 1987). Anticonvulsants are not known to help other types of pain.

Tricyclic antidepressants, such as amitriptyline (Elavil) or imipramine (Tofranil), are very effective analgesics for neuropathic pain as well as a broad range of other painful conditions. Some specific applications include postherpetic neuralgia, invasion of neural structures by carcinoma, postsurgical pain, and rheumatoid arthritis. In the treatment of pain, tricyclics appear to have an analgesic effect independent of their antidepressant activity. It is believed that tricyclic antidepressants relieve pain by blocking reuptake of biogenic amines in the CNS. As mentioned previously, serotonergic and adrenergic neurons in the brain stem project to and inhibit pain transmission cells in the spinal cord dorsal horn and are part of the descending pain-modulating system. Tricyclics supposedly enhance the inhibitory action of serotonin and norepinephrine on these neurons for spinal pain transmission.

Other adjuvant medications useful in the treatment of pain include hydroxyzine (Vistaril), which has analgesic effects over a range of painful conditions and an additive effect when given with morphine; muscle relaxants such as diazepam (Valium), which are used to treat muscle spasm associated with pain; and steroids such as dexamethasone (Decadron), which have been used to control the symptoms associated with spinal cord compression or bone metastasis in cancer patients.

Nonpharmacologic Approaches

Despite the convenience of analgesic drugs, many patients and clinicians are dissatisfied with their long-term use for nonmalignant-related pain. This situation has led to the development of a number of nonpharmacologic methods of pain management. Nonpharmacologic methods of pain control can be divided into two groups: physical therapies and modalities and cognitive-behavioral strategies. Some of these modalities can be useful alone or used as adjuncts in the management of pain.

Physical therapies and modalities

Physical therapies for pain relief include various forms of cutaneous stimulation (massage, transcutaneous electrical nerve stimulation, acupuncture, heat/cold applications, exercise). The rationale for cutaneous stimulation is derived from the gate control theory of pain transmission. Cutaneous stimulation stimulates the large-diameter non-nociceptive fibers to "close the gate" to pain-conducting small-diameter fibers and thus relieves pain. It has been hypothesized that cutaneous stimulation may also cause the body to secrete endorphins and other pain-inhibiting neurotransmitters.

One of the oldest and most common strategies of cutaneous stimulation is rubbing or massage. *Massage* can be accomplished using varying amounts of pressure and stimulation of various myofascial trigger points throughout the body. An oil or lotion is used to reduce friction. Massage relaxes muscle tension and increases local circulation. Back massage is particularly relaxing and, if performed by a caring person, provides an additional dimension of emotional support.

Transcutaneous electrical nerve stimulation (TENS, or TNS) consists of a battery-operated device that sends weak electrical impulses via electrodes placed on the body. The electrodes are generally placed on or near the painful site. TENS units are used for the management of both acute and chronic pain: postoperative pain, low back pain, phantom limb pain, peripheral neuralgias, and rheumatoid arthritis. TENS is based on the gate control theory.

Acupuncture is an ancient Chinese technique involving the insertion of thin needles into various "acupuncture (trigger) points" throughout the body to relieve pain. An alternate, noninvasive method of stimulating the trigger points is to apply pressure with the thumbs, a technique called *acupressure.* Acupuncture is widely used in China and has even been used to perform major surgery without the use of an additional anesthetic. The use of acupuncture or acupressure techniques requires special training and has gained some popularity in the West. The gate control theory and the theory that acupuncture stimulates the release of endogenous opioids are possible explanations for its efficacy.

Range-of-motion (ROM) exercises (passive, assisted, or active) may be used to relax muscles, improve circulation, and prevent pain related to stiffness and immobility.

Heat application is a simple measure that has long been recognized as an effective method of reducing muscle spasm or pain. Heat can be delivered by conduction (hot-water bottles, electrical heating pads, lamps, hot wet compresses), convection (whirlpool, sitz bath, hot soaks), or conversion (ultrasound, diathermy). Pain from bruises, muscle spasms, and arthritis responds well to heat. Because heat dilates blood vessels and increases local blood flow, it should *not* be used after traumatic injuries when edema and inflammation are present. Because heat increases blood flow, it may relieve pain by removing the products of inflammation, such as bradykinin, histamine, and prostaglandins, that produce pain locally. It may also stimulate nerve fibers that close the gate, thus preventing the transmission of pain impulses up the spinal cord to the brain.

In contrast to heat therapy, which is effective for chronic pain, *cold application* is more effective for acute pain (e.g., trauma from burns, cuts, or sprains). Cold may be applied in the form of cold soaks or compresses, ice bags, Aquamatic K pads, and ice massage. Cold applications reduce blood flow to an area and reduce bleeding and edema. It is believed that cold therapy produces an analgesic effect by slowing the conduction velocity of nerves so that fewer pain impulses reach the brain. Another possible mechanism is that the perception of cold predominates and reduces the perception of pain.

Cognitive-behavioral strategies

Cognitive-behavioral strategies are useful in changing the patient's perception of pain, altering pain behavior, and giving the patient a greater sense of control over the pain. These strategies include relaxation, imagery, hypnosis, and biofeedback. Although most cognitive-behavioral methods emphasize either relaxation or distraction, in practice the two are almost inseparable.

With methods that emphasize *muscle relaxation,* the facilitator instructs the patient to focus on different muscle groups and voluntarily contract and relax them in sequence. Other means to induce relaxation include deep-breathing exercises, meditation, and listening to soothing music. Relaxation techniques reduce anxiety, muscle tension, and emotional stress and thus interrupt the pain-stress-pain cycle, in which pain and stress reinforce each other.

Distraction techniques reduce pain by focusing the patient's attention on another stimulus and away from the pain. Watching television, reading a book, listening to music, and engaging in a conversation are common examples of distraction. *Guided imagery* is a form of distraction in which the facilitator encourages the patient to visualize or think about a pleasant scene or desirable sensation to divert attention away from the pain. This technique is often combined with relaxation. *Hypnosis* is a cognitive method that depends on focusing the patient's attention away from the pain. It depends on the therapist's ability to guide the patient's attention to those images that are most constructive. Distraction interventions are most effective against acute pain but can also be effective against chronic pain. The ability of distraction interventions to relieve pain is based on the theory that when two separate stimuli are presented, focusing on one will negate the other. However, the more intense the pain, the more complex the distraction stimuli must be.

Biofeedback is a technique that depends on providing measurements of certain physiologic parameters to patients so that they may learn to control them, including skin temperature, muscle tension, heart rate, blood pressure, and brain waves. The biofeedback device transforms the physiologic parameters into visual signals viewed by the patient. The patient is first alerted to stress-related responses such as increased muscle tension, heart rate, or blood pressure and then taught how to regulate these responses through visual images, deep-breathing, or relaxation exercises. Several sessions are usually required before patients learn to control their responses. Although biofeedback has been used to manage a variety of chronic pain problems, its most common use has been to treat headaches. It is not clear how biofeedback reduces pain. Possible factors that produce the beneficial effects include muscle relaxation, reduced anxiety, distraction, and a feeling of increased control over the symptoms.

Ablative Procedures on Nociceptive Pathways

A treatment of last resort for the control of chronic pain is the interruption of nociceptive pathways by surgical or chemical means. These procedures may involve (1) interruption at the level of the peripheral nerve root, such as neurectomy, rhizotomy, or sympathectomy; (2) interruption at the level of the spinal cord, such as cordotomy; and (3) interruption at the level of the brain, such as thalamotomy. These procedures were performed more frequently in the past but are rarely done today except in terminal cancer patients when other means of pain control are not effective. An important exception is trigeminal neuralgia, which is often cured by surgical ablation of the trigeminal nerve.

MAJOR PAIN PROBLEMS

In 1985 Bristol-Meyers commissioned a large study of the prevalence and severity of pain using a cross section of 1254 individuals older than 18 years. Findings indicated that pain cost $55 billion and accounted for 4 billion workdays, making it a major health and economic problem (Sternbach, 1986). According to the findings, published as the Nuprin Pain Report, the two most common types of pain experienced by the subjects during the past year were headache (73%) and backache (56%). Fortunately, organic disease is an infrequent cause of headaches. The average headache is so common and its treatment with an analgesic so simple that most people do not seek medical help. Nevertheless, a severe headache can be very disabling and interfere with work performance and activities of daily living. Low back pain is one of the most prevalent medical problems in Western countries and the most prevalent cause of disability in those 18 years and older. Bonica (1982) estimated that 14% of employed American men and 21% of women ages 18 to 64 years suffered from low back pain. More than 10 million people are estimated as having mild to moderate functional limitations, and 3 million have severe limitations. Among them, more than 4 million cannot perform their work. The remainder of this chapter discusses these two major pain problems.

Headache (Cephalgia)

Headache is a common symptom that nearly all people experience, at least episodically, during their life span. Headache may be part of a sequela related to increased intracranial pressure (ICP), head injury, brain tumor, eyestrain, sinusitis, changes in atmosphere, food allergies, and so on. The list of possible causes is inexhaustible. Three basic types of headache are discussed here: (1) vascular (migraine and cluster headache), (2) muscular contraction (also called psychogenic or tension headache), and (3) traction inflammatory headache (usually secondary to an organic disease process).

General Considerations

Pain-sensitive cranial structures that are involved in headache include all the extracranial tissues, including skin, scalp, muscles, arteries, and periosteum of the skull; cranial sinuses; intracranial venous sinuses and their tributary veins; parts of the dura at the base of the brain and the arteries within the dura; and the trigeminal, facial, vagus, and glossopharyngeal cranial nerves and the cervical nerves (C2 and C3). The brain parenchyma, much of the meningeal tissue, and the skull (except for the periosteum) are insensitive to pain. Periosteal stretch may cause local pain.

The tentorium is a sheet of dura that serves as a line of demarcation and point of reference within the cranium. It separates the posterior fossa (brain stem and cerebellum) from the anterior cerebrum (see Fig. 50-8). The posterior area (about one third of the cranial cavity) is referred to as *infratentorial,* and the anterior area (two thirds of the cranial cavity) is referred to as *supratentorial.*

When head pain involves structures in the infratentorial area, it is referred to the occipital area of the head and neck by the upper cervical nerve roots. Supratentorial pain occurs in the anterior portion of the head (frontal, temporal, and parietal areas) and is mediated largely by the trigeminal nerve.

Some general mechanisms that seem to be responsible for evoking headache include the following (Lance, 1993):
- Distention or displacement of blood vessels: intracranial or extracranial
- Traction of blood vessels
- Contraction of head and neck muscles (muscular overaction)
- Stretching of periosteum (local pain)
- Degeneration of the upper cervical spine with compression of cervical nerve roots (e.g., arthritis of the cervical vertebrae)
- Deficiency of enkephalins (opiate-like brain peptides, active ingredient of endorphins)

The sympathetic nervous system (SNS) is basically responsible for neural control of the cranial and extracranial blood vessels.

ESSENTIAL DATA TO OBTAIN IN ASSESSING HEADACHE

- What, if anything, brings on the headache (precipitating factors)?
- When was the onset (number of years, medical conditions, past head injury)?
- Are there any early warnings (prodromal symptoms)?
- Does the headache occur alone or with associated features (nausea, vomiting, dizziness, photophobia, blurred vision)?
- How would you describe the headache (location, frequency, time of day, duration, quality, precipitating factors, relieving factors)?
- Does anyong else in your family have headaches or similar symptoms?

Assessment of the patient with headache

As with most conditions, competent history taking is essential to establish the correct diagnosis when the patient's complaint is headache. This is particularly so with headache, since positive neurologic findings are only occasionally found on physical examination. The box above presents some of the points that should be included in the history.

Patients must be rapidly assessed to rule out serious intracranial disease as a cause for the headache. Patients presenting with a "this is the worst headache of my life" scenario accompanied by vomiting, neck stiffness, photophobia, or neurologic deficits are at highest risk for serious neurologic disease. Worsening of the severity of the pain with defecating, coughing, stooping, or other maneuvers that are expected to increase ICP also deserve special attention.

New-onset headache in older persons should always be taken seriously. It may reflect depression or other emotional events, but since subdural hematoma and intracranial masses are more common in older persons, these more serious causes of the headache must be ruled out.

Details regarding the speed of onset, frequency, duration, and associated symptoms are important to establish. A headache that recurs regularly over years is most likely a tension or vascular headache, whereas a severe headache with a rapid onset would suggest meningitis, intracranial hemorrhage, or infarction.

Headache location can be valuable in determining etiology. Approximately two thirds of migraine headache are unilateral, but they may vary from one side to the other with different attacks. If recurring throbbing headaches are always located on the same side, an intracranial mass or vascular malformation should be considered. Cluster headaches, trigeminal neuralgia, and focal disease of the pain-sensitive structures of the head are exceptions to this rule of thumb. Tension headaches are usually bilateral or circumferential or may be localized, depending on the muscles involved.

The clinician must listen carefully to the patient's description of the pain. A headache described as pulselike or throbbing is generally vascular in origin. Patients with cluster headaches almost always complain of extremely intense, deep, boring pain that lasts 20 to 30 minutes.

Associated symptoms reported by the patient may also help in differentiating the cause of the headache. Although nausea and vomiting frequently accompany migraine headache, they may also be seen in any disease that elevates the ICP. The distinctive ANS findings (flushing of the forehead, injection and lacrimation of the conjunctiva, nasal congestion) are helpful in diagnosing cluster headache.

Patients should be queried about factors that precipitate or aggravate the headache. Headaches that worsen with head movement, coughing, sneezing, or walking are likely to be either vascular or inflammatory. Exposure to certain foods or other triggers (e.g., changes in barometric pressure) may precede the migraine headache.

Once the history of the headache is obtained, the clinician should evaluate the patient with a careful and deliberate physical examination, looking for the physical findings of life-threatening conditions sometimes associated with headaches.

Vascular headache

Vascular headaches include migraine, cluster, toxic vascular, and hypertensive varieties. Pulsation of the carotid artery can be demonstrated in some patients. Migraine headaches affect between 1% and 10% of men and 3% and 20% of women in the United States. They are most common in women younger than 40 years. Cluster headaches, on the other hand, are more common in men, who account for 90% of the cases. Seventy percent of patients with vascular headaches have a positive family history. Attacks are more likely to occur when the patient becomes overtired and fatigued. Many women experience attacks at a time related to menstruation (just before, during, or at the end). During pregnancy, most patients are without headache by the third month. A small number experience their initial attack during pregnancy. Oral contraceptives usually increase the problem, as does hormonal therapy in the postmenopausal patient.

Nearly every patient who suffers from migraine headaches has a *trigger.* These are individual and may include such factors as red wine, chocolate cake, the smell of perfume, flickering lights, alcohol, caffeine, nicotine, and food high in refined sugar. One particular trigger that is beginning to receive much attention is emotional stress. Emotional stress may be a significant contributor to migraines.

Migraine headache is the prototype, a throbbing vascular headache involving vasodilation and localized inflammation, which sensitizes the arteries to pain. Cere-

bral blood flow is decreased before the onset and increased during the actual headache.

The pathophysiology of migraine is not fully understood, but the most widely held theory postulates that the early vasoconstriction and subsequent vasodilation are induced by a release of biogenic amines such as serotonin, norepinephrine, and epinephrine in persons with a genetic predisposition to vascular hypersensitivity. Excretion of the degradation products of these amines increases during a migraine headache in some patients. A corresponding decrease in the blood serotonin levels has also been found. Because these amines are powerful vasoconstrictors, they may be responsible for the prodromal vasoconstriction. After their release, degradation, and depletion, a reactive hyperemia could account for the vasodilation during the migraine attack. This hypothesis is supported by the following: (1) the administration of reserpine, a drug that depletes serotonin levels in brain tissue and platelets, may induce a migraine attack; (2) the injection of serotonin may relieve migraine headache; and (3) the administration of methysergide, a serotonin antagonist, may prevent migraine in many instances.

Another vasoactive substance that has been implicated in migraine is *neurokinin,* a polypeptide similar to bradykinin. Neurokinin has been found in the fluid that collects around the involved cranial artery during a migraine attack and may be responsible for the inflammatory response.

There are two types of migraine headache. The *classic migraine* (migraine with aura) has a prodromal or preheadache phase lasting approximately 15 minutes and is associated with a disturbance of neurologic function. Symptoms may include bright flashing lights (*scintillation scotomata*) or other visual disturbances caused by cerebral vasoconstriction and ischemia. Other neurologic symptoms include paresthesias or paresis on one side of the body or a slight speech disturbance. These neurologic symptoms abate with the onset of the headache, which is frequently accompanied by nausea and vomiting. Unlike the classic migraine, the *common migraine* (migraine without aura) headache does *not* have a prodromal phase but rather is characterized by the immediate onset of the throbbing headache.

Most patients experience a unilateral headache that is initially a dull ache and finally a throbbing or pulsating pain, which may become bilateral. The frontal and temporal areas are the most frequently involved sites. However, the pain may occur behind the eye and in other regions of the face and neck. Two to four attacks per month, usually lasting 1 or 2 days, are most common.

The classic manifestations that frequently accompany migraine syndrome include photophobia, increased sensitivity to noise, vascular changes (cold hands and feet, pale skin), nausea and vomiting, and hyperesthesia of the scalp.

Medical management of migraine headache includes the use of vasoconstrictor substances, specifically ergot alkaloids (ergotamine tartrate) and Cafergot (a combination of caffeine and ergotamine taken at the onset of the headache to promote vasoconstriction). Beta-blocking agents, such as propranolol or calcium channel blockers (e.g., verapamil), are taken prophylactically to reduce the frequency of the headaches by interfering with the vasodilation of the cranial arteries. Cyproheptadine (Periactin), a serotonin and histamine antagonist, is used to reduce the pain and frequency of headaches. Once the headache is established, symptomatic treatment includes analgesics (including narcotics), sedatives, and anxiolytics. Because sleep tends to relieve the symptoms, hypnotics are often prescribed; chloral hydrate is a popular drug used for this approach. The newest drug available as a first-line treatment of migraine headaches is sumatriptan succinate (Imitrex). This drug inhibits neuronal transmission and blocks the release of vasoactive neuropeptides. Specifically, sumatriptan interacts with a particular subpopulation of serotonin receptors, especially with 1D receptors concentrated in the dorsal raphe. The final effect of sumatriptan is constriction of the dural arteries, which may account for its remarkable effectiveness in alleviating migraine headache (Ferrari et al., 1993). Nonpharmacologic therapy includes biofeedback, progressive muscle relaxation, and stress reduction, although these may have varying degrees of success.

The Physician's Health Study, conducted between 1982 and 1988 in the United States, studied male physicians 40 to 84 years of age with no prior history of cancer or cardiovascular disease (Buring et al., 1995). Although not the primary purpose of the study, anecdotal results demonstrated a correlation between the incidence of CVA and a history of migraine headache. Although in its preliminary stage, these research findings suggest that vascular events associated with migraine may also have causative importance in stroke in males. Further research to study this association is needed.

The other important vascular headache, although much less common than migraine, is the *cluster headache*. (Other synonyms include migrainous headache, histamine headache, Horton's headache, and paroxysmal nocturnal neuralgia.) It is so named because it tends to occur nightly for a few weeks or months (clusters) and then remains absent for years.

Cluster headaches occur much more frequently in men than in women. The characteristic pain is constant, severe, nonthrobbing, and unilateral and is often localized to the eye or side of the face. The onset is characteristically 2 or 3 hours after falling asleep and is apparently associated with rapid eye movement (REM) sleep. It lasts from minutes to hours and is associated with conjunctival injection, lacrimation, blocked nostril, and sometimes flushing of the cheek on the affected side. Alcohol is often mentioned as a precipitating factor if drinking occurs during a headache-prone period. Other assorted factors include stress, changes in the climate, and attacks of hay fever. The ophthalmic and extracranial arteries and the facial and scalp capillaries are usually dilated, and the internal carotid artery is narrowed.

At the peak of the headache, the pain is intolerable and incapacitating. In contrast to the person with migraine, the individual with cluster headache paces the floor restlessly and is unable to lie down or sit still. Many persons have even contemplated suicide. Drugs useful in the treatment of cluster headaches include the vasoconstricting agent ergotamine tartrate, the serotonin antagonist methysergide, the beta-blocking agent propranolol, and the phenothiazine agent chlorpromazine. Inhalation of 100% oxygen has also proved effective in some patients, probably resulting from the reduction of cerebral blood flow caused by the high oxygen concentration.

Muscular contraction headache (tension headache)

Muscular contraction, or tension, headache produces pain by a sustained contraction of the scalp, forehead, and neck muscles that is accompanied by extracranial vasoconstriction. The pain is characterized by a bandlike tightness around the head and tenderness of the occipito-cervical area. This type of headache is very common. The acute form is associated with conditions of temporary stress, anxiety, or fatigue generally lasting 1 or 2 days. The chronic tension headache is more common in women and is typically bilateral, unremitting (occurring during both day and night and lasting from months to years), dull, nonpulsating, and often associated with anxiety, depression, and repressed feelings.

Ideally, nonaddictive drugs should be prescribed for the person with chronic tension headache. Aspirin and acetaminophen are practical choices. Narcotic analgesics may be abused and may lead to tolerance (renal failure occurs in some persons who abuse phenacetin; see Chapter 46). Tranquilizers are probably not beneficial and may actually increase the depression. In patients who are tense and anxious, diazepam (Valium), 5 mg three times a day for 1 month, may be effective. If the patient is also depressed, the tricyclic antidepressant drug amitriptyline (Elavil), 25 mg three times a day, is added. In some headache treatment centers, tricyclic antidepressants are being used alone and are effective in increasing cerebral norepinephrine. Biofeedback, relaxation, self-hypnosis, and other conditioning techniques have been beneficial to some patients with headache and play an increasing role in therapy, since a real danger of overmedication exists in the patient with muscular tension headache.

Traction inflammatory headache

Traction inflammatory headache is usually secondary to organic disease. Masses of any origin (e.g., tumor, blood clot, abscess) may cause traction on and displacement of pain-sensitive structures. Headache is the outstanding symptom of a brain tumor (primary or metastatic), and as the tumor grows, the pain becomes more frequent and severe. By the time most patients with intracranial tumors present with headache, they have other significant diagnostic findings that suggest a tumor. Headache, vertigo, and other localizing neurologic signs are the usual manifestations of chronic subdural hematoma. A rapidly expanding intracranial mass causing increased ICP may displace cerebral structures, resulting in headache.

Headache is a symptom associated with many inflammatory processes. Meningitis, encephalitis, and infection of the sinuses, teeth, nose, or eyes frequently occur with the symptom of headache. Traction on the attached parts of the brain, especially the trigeminal and hypoglossal nerves, is likely to cause headache. Headache is also a symptom in particular immunologic disorders, especially periarteritis nodosa and giant cell arteritis.

Post–lumbar puncture headache

Headache after lumbar puncture (LP) occurs in one of four patients, usually within hours of the procedure. The headache is dramatically positional: it begins when the patient sits or stands upright and is diminished or eliminated by lying down. It is worsened by head shaking. The pain is usually in the frontal area and has the quality of a dull ache but may be throbbing. The symptoms usually resolve over a few days but may persist for weeks.

Although the exact mechanism of spinal headache is unknown, it is postulated that leakage of CSF through a tear in the dura caused by the LP results in a loss of the brain's supportive cushion. Thus, when the patient sits upright, there is dilation and tension on the brain's anchoring structures, the pain-sensitive dural sinuses, resulting in pain. Factors associated with spinal headache include use of a large-bore needle, withdrawal of a large volume of CSF, and repeat LPs. A small number of patients have a sterile meningitis.

To reduce the risk of spinal headache, the patient should remain flat in bed for at least 3 hours after an LP. Once a headache begins, treatment consists of bedrest in a quiet, dark room and analgesics of increasing strength. An epidural blood patch, accomplished by injecting about 15 ml of the patient's own blood into the epidural space at the site of the LP, is usually an effective treatment for those who are not helped by analgesics. The blood acts as a fibrin patch to seal the hole in the dura and prevent further leakage of CSF. In some persistent cases, a short course (10 days) of steroid therapy may be helpful (Kovanen et al., 1986).

Back Pain

Back pain, especially of the lower back, is a very common problem in the adult population. The numerous causes of back pain include arthritis of the spine, herniated intervertebral disk disease, and various soft tissue problems resulting from sprains, strains, and other trauma. Physiologic origins of low back pain are usually mechanical or biochemical irritations to nociceptive endings or to nerves and nerve roots in the lumbar spine. It is essential to rule out acute disk problems in any patient with a complaint of back pain, since failure to do so may result in permanent neurologic deficits.

Herniated intervertebral disk disease

One of the most common causes of back pain in the adult is herniated nucleus pulposus (herniated disk). Although more common in adults, disk disease can also occur in children and teenagers.

The vertebral column consists of a series of joints between the bodies of the adjacent vertebrae, the joints of the vertebral arches, the costovertebral joints, and the sacroiliac joints. Longitudinal ligaments and the intervertebral disks join the bodies of adjacent vertebrae. The *anterior longitudinal ligament,* a broad, thick band, runs longitudinally on the front of the vertebral bodies and intervertebral disks and fuses with the periosteum and annulus fibrosus. Lying within the vertebral canal on the posterior aspects of the vertebral bodies and intervertebral disks is the *posterior longitudinal ligament.*

Between the vertebral bodies, from the second cervical vertebra (C2) down to the sacral vertebrae, are the *intervertebral disks.* These disks form a resilient fibrocartilaginous joint between the vertebral bodies. The intervertebral disk consists of two basic parts: the nucleus pulposus at the center and the annulus fibrosus surrounding it. The disk is separated from the bone above and below it by two thin hyaline cartilage plates (Fig. 52-11).

The *nucleus pulposus* is the semigelatinous central portion of the disk. It contains bundles of collagenous fibers, connective tissue cells, and cartilage cells. This material functions as a shock absorber between adjacent vertebral bodies. It also plays an important role in the exchange of fluid between the disk and the capillaries.

The *annulus fibrosus* consists of concentric fibrous rings, which surround the nucleus pulposus. The functions of the annulus fibrosus are to permit motion between the vertebral bodies (because of the spiral structure of the fibers), to retain the nucleus pulposus, and to function as a shock absorber. Thus the annulus functions similar to the hoops around a water barrel or as a coiled spring, pulling the vertebral bodies together against the elastic resistance of the nucleus pulposus, whereas the nucleus pulposus acts as a ball bearing between the vertebral bodies (Fig. 52-12).

Intervertebral disks account for approximately one fourth of the length of the vertebral column. The thinnest disks are in the thoracic region, and the thickest ones are in the lumbar region. With increasing age the water content of the disks is reduced, and they become thinner (Schwartz, 1994).

Pathophysiology. The lumbar region is the most common area for herniation of the nucleus pulposus. The water content of the disk decreases with increasing age (from 90% in infancy to 70% in old age; Schwartz, 1994). In addition, the fibers become coarsened and hyalinized, which contributes to the changes that lead to herniation of the nucleus pulposus through the annulus with compres-

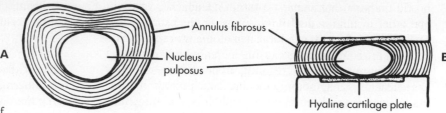

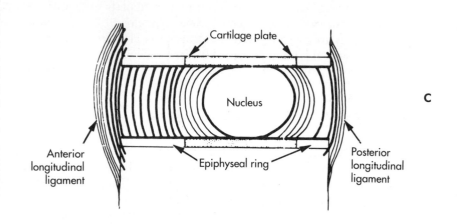

FIG. 52-11   A, Annulus fibrosus is composed of concentric fibrous rings that surround the nucleus pulposus. **B,** Nucleus pulposus abuts on the hyaline cartilage plate. **C,** Annulus fibers form three groups, with innermost fibers passing from one cartilage plate to the next, middle fibers passing between the epiphyseal rings of the vertebral bodies, and outermost fibers attaching between the vertebral bodies and the undersurface of the epiphyseal ring. Anterior fibers are more numerous and are supported by the powerful anterior longitudinal ligament, whereas the posterior longitudinal ligament gives only weak reinforcement to the less numerous posterior fibers. (From MacNab I: *Backache,* Baltimore, 1977, Williams & Wilkins.)

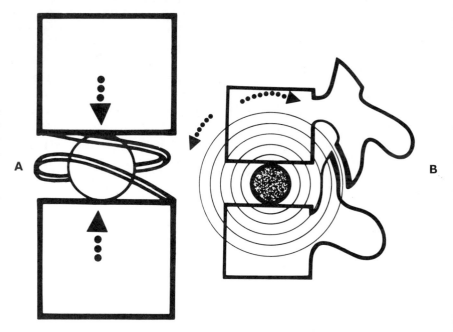

FIG. 52-12   A, Annulus acts as a coiled spring, pulling the vertebral bodies together against the elastic resistance of the nucleus pulposus. **B,** Nucleus pulposus acts as a ball bearing, with the vertebral bodies rolling over the incompressible gel in flexion and extension while the posterior vertebral joints guide and steady the movement. (From MacNab I: *Backache,* Baltimore, 1977, Williams & Wilkins.)

sion of the spinal nerve roots (Fig. 52-13). As a general rule, herniation is most likely to occur in regions of the vertebral column where a transition occurs from a more mobile segment to a less mobile one (lumbosacral and cervicothoracic junctions).

The vast majority of disk herniations occur in the lumbar area at the fourth to fifth lumbar (L4 to L5) or fifth lumbar to first sacral (L5 to S1) interspace. The most common direction of herniation of the nuclear material is posterolateral. Because the nerve roots at the lumbar area slant downward as they exit through the neural foramina, a disk herniation between L5 and S1 affects the S1 nerve root rather than L5 as might be expected. A herniation of the disk between L4 and L5 compresses the L5 nerve root (Fig. 52-14).

Cervical disk herniations, although less common than lumbar disk herniations, usually involve one of the three lower cervical roots. A cervical disk herniation is potentially serious, and spinal cord compression is possible, depending on the direction of protrusion. A lateral herniation of a cervical disk generally compresses the root below the disk level. Thus a C5 to C6 disk compresses the C6 nerve root, and a C6 to C7 disk involves the C7 root (Schwartz, 1994).

The patient generally gives a history of transient episodes of pain and gradual loss of spinal mobility. Although the patient tends to associate the problem with a particular incident of lifting or bending, herniation is a gradual process marked by periods of nerve root compression (causing many symptoms and periods of anatomic readjustment).

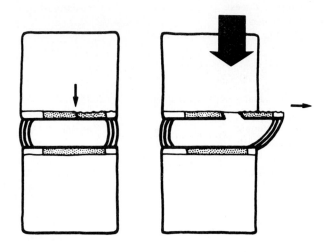

FIG. 52-13 The first morphologic change to occur in a disk rupture is a separation of the cartilage plate from the adjacent vertebral body. When a vertical compression force is then applied, the detached portion of the cartilage plate is displaced posteriorly, and the nucleus pulposus exudes through the torn fibers of the annulus. (From MacNab I: *Backache,* Baltimore, 1977, Williams & Wilkins.)

Clinical symptoms depend on the location of the herniation and variation in the individual anatomy. Table 52-5 provides a summary of the most common signs and symptoms.

The diagnosis of herniated intervertebral disk is often made from the history alone and can be confirmed during physical examination. Evaluating maneuvers such as leg raising and walking on the toes or heels is also helpful in making the diagnosis. Radiographs may be normal or may show evidence of distorted spinal alignment (generally caused by muscle spasm). They are also helpful to rule out other causes of back pain, such as spondylolisthesis (forward slippage of the anterior portion of a vertebral segment over a lower segment, usually at L4 or L5), spinal cord tumors, or bony spurs. However, it is impossible to diagnose a herniated disk by radiography alone. Myelograms, electromyography, and nerve conduction studies are used for final verification of the diagnosis and are particularly helpful in diagnosing the rare thoracic herniation.

Most patients respond to conservative treatment: 1 to 2 weeks of bedrest on a firm mattress, application of moist heat, and analgesics. Traction is useful in the care of patients with cervical herniations. Once the pain has subsided, the patient begins a program of graded exercise to strengthen the back and abdominal muscles. It is important that the patient limit lifting and use the proper body mechanics. Proper technique involves keeping the spine straight, bending the knees, and keeping the weight close to the body in order to use the powerful leg muscles and avoid using the back muscles. Surgery is generally reserved for patients who experience persistent in-

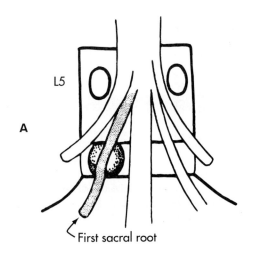

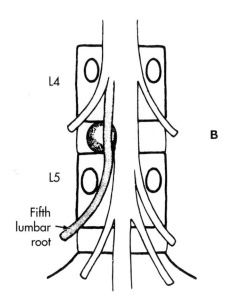

FIG. 52-14 **A,** Posterolateral herniation of the L5 to S1 disk generally compresses the S1 nerve root. **B,** Herniation of the L4 to L5 disk compresses the L5 root. (From MacNab I: *Backache,* Baltimore, 1977, Williams & Wilkins.)

▶ TABLE 52-5   Signs and Symptoms of Herniated Disk Disease

Location of Herniation	Nerve Root Involved	Pain	Weakness	Paresthesias	Atrophy	Reflexes
L4 to L5	L5	Over sacroiliac joint, hip, lateral aspect of thigh and calf, medial aspect of foot (pain that radiates down hip and leg is called *sciatica*)	May produce foot-drop, difficulty in dorsiflexion of foot and/or great toe; difficulty walking on heels	Lateral leg, distal portion of foot, between great and second toes (see dermatome map, Fig. 52-8)	Unremarkable	Usually unremarkable; knee or ankle reflexes may be diminished.
L5 to S1	S1	Over sacroiliac joint, posterior portion of entire leg to heel, lateral aspect of foot	May produce weakness of plantar flexion, abduction of toes and hamstring muscles; difficulty walking on toes	Midcalf and lateral aspect of foot, including fourth and fifth toes (see dermatome map, Fig. 52-8)	Gastrocnemius	Ankle reflex may be absent or diminished.
C5 to C6	C6	Neck pain radiating to shoulder, arm, and forearm	Biceps	Radial aspect of forearm, thumb, and index finger	Unremarkable	Biceps reflex is diminished or absent.

L, Lumbar; *S*, sacral; *C*, cervical

tractable pain or frequent attacks of pain, symptoms involving both sides, or the presence of a major neurologic deficit such as bowel and bladder incontinence or foot-drop. Surgery relieves the symptoms of nerve root compression but may not relieve the back pain.

Chemonucleolysis is gaining favor in the United States for the treatment of herniated disk disease. This treatment has been popular in Canada and Europe for 25 years. The treatment, which was approved by the U.S. Food and Drug Administration in late 1982, consists of injecting 2000 to 4000 units of chymopapain (an enzyme from the papaya tree) into the herniated disk. Chymopapain causes the hydrolysis of the proteins, decreasing their water-binding capacity in the nucleus pulposus. The enzyme attacks only the nucleus pulposus and not the annulus fibrosus. This treatment relieves the pressure on the nerve root, effectively relieving pain, and provides patients with an alternative to laminectomy.

 QUESTIONS

▼ *Circle the letter preceding each item below that correctly answers the question or completes the statement. More than one answer may be correct.*

1. Which of the following statements about pain is *false*?
   a. Pain has both a sensory and an emotional component.
   b. Objective signs of pain observed by the clinician are the most reliable signs that a patient is in pain.
   c. Pain is one of the most common complaints for which patients seek professional health care.
   d. Pain is an entirely subjective experience and exists when the patient says it exists.

2. The term *nociceptor* refers to:
   a. CNS receptors for endorphins
   b. Pain receptors in the somatosensory cortex
   c. Primary afferent nerve fibers for receiving and transmitting noxious stimuli
   d. Primary efferent nerve fibers

3. The term *transduction* refers to:
   a. The process by which noxious stimuli generate pain impulses in nociceptors
   b. The process of transmitting pain impulses over peripheral sensory nerves to the spinal cord
   c. Descending neural activity that can influence the transmission of pain impulses at the level of the spinal cord

   d. The translation of pain impulses into a subjective experience of pain or discomfort in the cerebral cortex

4. The cell bodies of primary afferent neurons for the transmission of pain impulses are located in the:
   a. Ventral (anterior) root ganglia of spinal nerves
   b. Dorsal (posterior) root ganglia of spinal nerves
   c. Sympathetic chain ganglia
   d. Substantia gelatinosa of the dorsal horn

5. Chemical substances responsible for sensitizing nociceptors in an area of injury include all the following *except*:
   a. Potassium

QUESTIONS—cont'd

b. Serotonin
c. Bradykinin and histamine
d. Prostaglandins
e. Endorphins

6. Primary afferent nerve fibers that carry noxious impulses resulting in pain perception include:
   a. A-alpha fibers
   b. A-beta fibers
   c. A-delta fibers
   d. C fibers

7. Noxious stimulation of primary afferent C fibers causes:
   a. Inhibition of pain
   b. Release of endogenous endorphins
   c. Release of substance P from pain receptors
   d. A reflex parasympathetic response

8. Structural and functional characteristics of A-delta fibers include:
   a. Lightly myelinated
   b. Unmyelinated
   c. Transmit rapid, sharp, or prickling pain sensations
   d. Transmit slow, diffuse, dull, or burning pain sensations

9. The paleospinothalamic tract:
   a. Carries messages relevant to the localization and intensity of pain
   b. Has connections to the reticular activating system and the limbic system, which underlies the arousal and emotional components of pain
   c. Transmits impulses initiated in the slow-chronic type C neural fibers
   d. Is the multisynaptic, diffuse pain pathway

10. The brain structure involved in the precise localization of cutaneous pain is the:
    a. Thalamus
    b. Hypothalamus
    c. Postcentral gyrus of the parietal lobe
    d. Precentral gyrus of the frontal lobe

11. Important components of the descending pain-inhibiting pathway include all the following *except:*
    a. Somatosensory parietal cortex
    b. Periaqueductal gray area
    c. Raphe magnus nucleus
    d. Substantia gelatinosa

12. The CNS structure responsible for initial consciousness of pain is the:
    a. Dorsal horn cells
    b. Thalamus
    c. Limbic system
    d. Somatosensory cerebral cortex

13. A nurse who states, "This patient requires too much pain medication for someone who is 3 days postop," is reflecting assumptions of:
    a. A specificity theory of pain
    b. A pattern-summation theory of pain
    c. The gate control theory of pain
    d. The endorphin/enkephalin theory of pain

14. In their gate control theory of pain, Melzack and Wall proposed that the location of the "gate" was in the:
    a. Thalamus
    b. Somatosensory cortex
    c. Serotonergic descending tract
    d. Dorsal horn substantia gelatinosa cells

15. According to the gate control theory of pain, stimulation of large, myelinated, A-alpha or A-beta fibers results in:
    a. Opening of the gate and increased pain
    b. Closure of the gate and increased pain
    c. Opening of the gate and decreased pain
    d. Closure of the gate and decreased pain

16. According to the gate control theory of pain, massaging or rubbing the skin may:
    a. Stimulate small-diameter A-alpha and C primary afferent nerve fibers
    b. Open the gate to pain relief
    c. Close the gate to pain transmission
    d. Allow more impulses to pass to transmission (T) cells

17. Opioids produce analgesia by:
    a. Inducing sleep
    b. Blocking pain impulses by binding with opioid receptors in the CNS
    c. Decreasing the pain threshold
    d. Enhancing the release of substance P in the spinal dorsal horn

18. The endogenous opioid with the most potent analgesic effect is:
    a. Met-enkephalin   c. Beta-endorphin
    b. Dynorphin   d. Leu-enkephalin

19. The point at which the intensity of a noxious stimulus causes a person to perceive pain is called:
    a. Pain threshold   c. Pain perception
    b. Pain tolerance   d. Pain modulation

20. Pain tolerance:
    a. Varies minimally from one individual to another
    b. Is decreased by anxiety, fatigue, and sleep deprivation
    c. Is increased by distraction
    d. Is affected by psychosocial factors, such as past experience, mood, and sociocultural background

21. In chronic pain:
    a. The successful relief of pain by placebos proves that the pain was psychologic.
    b. Strong pain medications are needed because the pain threshold is lower.
    c. Emotional depression is a factor in most chronic intractable pain states.
    d. Enkephalins are inhibitory to pain transmission to the cortex and are elevated by the belief that a placebo will be effective.

22. Which of the following statements is (are) *true* about visceral pain?
    a. It is well localized to the site of underlying disease.
    b. It is generally described as sharp and steady.
    c. It is usually diffuse and intermittent.
    d. It is often accompanied by nausea and vomiting.
    e. It is mediated by autonomic nerve fibers.

23. Which of the following statements is (are) *false* about parietal pain?
    a. It originates in the parenchyma of abdominal and thoracic organs.
    b. It is mediated via spinal nerve fibers from parietal structures in the thoracic and abdominal cavities.
    c. It is caused by inflammation of parietal structures.
    d. The patient describes it as steady and aching.
    e. It is aggravated by coughing and changes in peritoneal tension.

24. Referred pain is:
    a. Diffuse and poorly localized
    b. Described by patients as cramping and burning
    c. Always accompanied by tachycardia and restlessness
    d. Perceived at a site distant from the primary affected organ

25. The most widely accepted explanation for referred pain is:
    a. The specificity theory
    b. The pattern-summation theory
    c. The gate control theory
    d. The convergence-projection theory

26. Which of the following statements explain(s) why pain in acute appendicitis is experienced initially in the periumbilical area, then later becomes localized in the lower right quadrant with muscle guarding?
    a. Visceral pain impulses from the appendix enter the spinal cord at the T10 segmental level and are then

Continued.

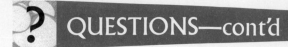

perceived as arising from the T10 dermatome (periumbilical area).

b. Inflammation of the parietal peritoneum over the appendix generates pain impulses that are transmitted directly over spinal nerves at the T12 segmental level (lower right quadrant of abdomen).

c. Pain is sharply localized when transmitted via parietal pathways.

d. Reflex muscle guarding commonly occurs over irritated peritoneum.

e. All the above are correct.

27. Neuropathic pain:
a. Often has a burning or electric shock–like quality
b. Is often triggered by innocuous stimuli (allodynia)
c. Results from CNS or peripheral nerve lesions damaging pain transmission pathways
d. Is often difficult to treat
e. All the above

28. In causalgia the:
a. Condition follows a partial injury to peripheral nerves, especially the median or sciatic.
b. Pain is almost continuous and is usually burning in nature.
c. Involved extremity shows signs of sympathetic hyperactivity.
d. Pain is not affected by tactile contact.

29. A 70-year-old woman presents with brief, intermittent episodes of excruciating, lancinating pain in the cheek, lips, and gums. These intense spasms of pain may be initiated by touching the lips or chewing movements. Results of physical examination and magnetic resonance imaging (MRI) of the head are normal. The most likely cause of this patient's pain is:
a. Neuroma of the acoustic nerve
b. Trigeminal neuralgia
c. Facial nerve palsy
d. Meningioma

30. Peripheral nerve damage caused by diabetes may result in:
a. Bilateral distal sensory neuropathy
b. Paresthesias
c. Incontinence
d. Hyperalgesia
e. All the above

31. Postherpetic neuralgia:
a. Follows the healing stage of shingles
b. Is most common in young individuals
c. Is believed to be caused by viral damage to the dorsal root ganglia
d. Almost invariably resolves in 1 to 2 days
e. Most frequently causes lancinating pain in the chest dermatomes

32. Pain assessment scales:
a. Rate pain objectively
b. Are only used for baseline assessment
c. Always use numeric ratings
d. Can be used to assess the effectiveness of an analgesic

33. Which of the following statements about the management of chronic pain is (are) true?
a. NSAIDs are effective for managing mild pain.
b. PRN drug administration is preferred.
c. Treatment begins with opioid drugs.
d. Parenteral drugs are preferred.

34. The analgesic effect of NSAIDs result from which of the following mechanisms?
a. Bind with mu–opioid receptors in dorsal horn substantia gelatinosa
b. Inhibit prostaglandin synthesis at the site of injury or inflammation
c. Inhibit prostaglandin synthesis in the brain
d. Relieve muscle spasm

35. The major narcotic antagonist agent is:
a. Morphine
b. Serotonin
c. Naloxone

d. Pentazocine (Talwin)

36. The dose of meperidine (Demerol) that is equianalgesic to 10 mg of morphine is:
a. 25 mg
b. 50 mg
c. 75 mg
d. 100 mg

37. Tricyclic antidepressants such as amitriptyline (Elavil) are effective against neuropathic pain because they:
a. Relieve the emotional depression associated with chronic pain
b. Relieve anxiety, which lowers the pain threshold
c. Enhance the inhibitory action of serotonin by blocking its reuptake in descending pain-modulating pathways
d. Stimulate the uptake of endogenous endorphins

38. PCA and TENS units both:
a. Produce numerous adverse reactions
b. Are invasive measures to reduce pain
c. Give the patient a sense of pain control
d. Reduce the opioid dosage needed to achieve analgesia

▼ Match each pain characteristic in column A with the type of pain (acute or chronic) in column B.

Column A	Column B
39. _____ Duration: 6 months or more	a. Acute pain
40. _____ Cause: may not be well defined	b. Chronic pain
41. _____ Onset: abrupt	
42. _____ Benefit: warns of danger	
43. _____ Autonomic response: sympathetic stress response	
44. _____ Emotional response: depression	
45. _____ Response to analgesics: often unresponsive	

▼ Match the source of the pain in column A with its description in column B.

Column A
46. _____ Superficial somatic pain
47. _____ Deep somatic pain
48. _____ Visceral pain

Column B
a. Poorly localized, diffuse, dull, aching; referred to dermatomes
b. Poorly localized, dull, aching, burning; radiates to adjacent areas
c. Well localized and defined, sharp, piercing or pricking

▼ Distinguish between narcotic physical dependence, tolerance, and addiction by placing the correct letters from column B in column A.

Column A
49. _____ Higher doses required to achieve pain relief
50. _____ A common fear of patients and some health care professionals
51. _____ Drug needed for normal function
52. _____ Abrupt discontinuation of the drug causes withdrawal symptoms
53. _____ Psychologic dependence on the drug

Column B
a. Physical dependence
b. Tolerance
c. Addiction

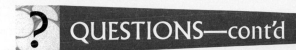

▼ Match the following classes of drugs in column A with their effects in column B.

Column A	Column B
54. _____ Opioid antagonists	a. Less likely to cause respiratory depression
55. _____ Opioid agonists	b. Only effective in treating lancinating pain associated with nerve damage
56. _____ Opioid agonist-antagonists	c. Relieve pain by blocking reuptake of serotonin and norepinephrine in CNS
57. _____ Tricyclic antidepressants	d. Bind to opioid receptors and block their activation
58. _____ Anticonvulsants	e. Reverse the effects of morphine

▼ Match the following modalities for coping with pain in column A with the most appropriate description in column B.

Column A	Column B
59. _____ Biofeedback	a. A form of distraction
60. _____ Guided imagery	b. Depends on monitoring physiologic responses
61. _____ Music therapy	c. Works best for acute pain such as a burn
62. _____ Cold applications	d. Reduces muscle tension and stress
63. _____ Progressive muscle relaxation	

▼ Circle T if the statement is true and F if it is false. Correct any false statements.

64. T F Addiction is extremely rare when opioids are used to treat patients in pain.

65. T F Evidence shows that patients are routinely undermedicated for pain because of an exaggerated fear of addiction by both patients and staff.

66. T F Pain from the diaphragm is usually referred to the epigastric area.

67. T F The convergence-projection theory posits that pain is perceived as arising from a particular cutaneous site because visceral and somatic afferents converge on the same spinal segment.

▼ Answer the following on a separate sheet of paper.

68. List nine categories of subjective data relevant to pain assessment.

69. List reactive and behavioral data relevant to pain assessment.

70. What is the physiologic function of the pain sensory system? What would be the advantages and disadvantages of having a congenital insensitivity to pain?

▼ Circle the letter preceding each item below that correctly completes each statement. More than one answer may be correct.

71. The most common type(s) of headache is (are):

a. Classic migraine
b. Cluster headache
c. Tension headache
d. Inflammatory headache

72. All the following are postulated mechanisms of headache except:

a. Dysfunction of the extracranial arteries
b. Traction of intracranial blood vessels
c. Compression of the cervical nerve roots
d. Pressure on the cranial nerves
e. Pressure on the brain parenchyma

73. Pain-sensitive structures of the head include:

a. All extracranial tissues, especially the arteries
b. Intracranial venous sinuses and their tributary veins
c. Cranial nerves V, VII, IX, and X plus the upper cervical nerves
d. Brain parenchyma
e. Some basal dural and basal arteries

74. Migraine headache:

a. Is more common in men
b. May be induced by reserpine, a drug that depletes serotonin
c. May be heralded by visual disturbances
d. May be continuous, lasting for weeks
e. May be aggravated by oral contraceptives

75. In migraine:

a. There is increased excretion of the metabolites of the biogenic amines.
b. Reserpine may cause a drop in the level of serum serotonin.
c. Neurokinin may be found in the

fluid surrounding the involved blood vessel.
d. Intense vasoconstriction occurs during the attack.
e. Methysergide, a serotonin antagonist, may prevent attacks.

76. In cluster headache:

a. The onset typically occurs at night during REM sleep.
b. The attacks last 1 to 2 days, then promptly subside.
c. The facial skin becomes pale.
d. The pain is unilateral and non-throbbing.
e. There may be conjunctival injection and tearing of the eye on the involved side.

77. In headache presumed to be caused by muscle contraction:

a. The patient often complains of a bandlike tightness around the head.
b. The headache may last for years.
c. The headache is often thought to have psychogenic causes.
d. There is commonly tenderness to palpation.
e. Tricyclic antidepressants may sometimes be used successfully.

▼ Circle T if the statement is true and F if it is false. Correct any false statements.

78. T F The common migraine headache is characterized by a vasoconstrictive prodromal phase associated with neurologic disturbances.

79. T F Post–lumbar puncture headache can often be avoided by using a small needle.

80. T F Horton's headache is a synonym for cluster headache.

81. T F Alcohol may induce attacks of cluster headache.

82. T F The pain in tension headache is often described as dull and non-pulsating.

83. T F Headache associated with an expanding intracranial mass such as a tumor generally becomes more severe as the mass enlarges.

▼ Answer the following on a separate sheet of paper.

84. List several questions you would ask a patient with a complaint of chronic headache during history taking.

Continued.

QUESTIONS—cont'd

▼ *Fill in the blanks with the appropriate word or words.*

85. Headache involving supratentorial structures is referred to the _____ two thirds of the head, and the pain pathway involves the _____ nerve.

86. Headache involving infratentorial structures is referred to the _____ area and is conveyed by the _____ nerves.

▼ *Match the headache characteristics in column B with the three categories of headache in column A. Letters may be used more than once.*

Column A	Column B
87. _____ Classic migraine headache	a. Flushed skin
88. _____ Cluster headache	b. Pale skin
89. _____ Tension headache	c. Generally unilateral
	d. Generally bilateral
	e. Throbbing quality
	f. Dull ache, constant day and night
	g. Precipitated by stress, fatigue
	h. Precipitated by alcohol
	i. Genetic predisposition
	j. Vasodilation during headache
	k. Mechanism involves sustained contraction of head and neck muscles

▼ *Circle the letter preceding each item below that correctly answers the question or completes the statement. Only one answer is correct.*

90. A herniated intervertebral disk:
   a. Is most common between L3 and L4
   b. Usually involves the nerve root of the interspace below the site of herniation in the lumbar area
   c. Involving S1 root compression may cause numbness of the web of the great toe
   d. Can easily be diagnosed by radiography alone

91. A herniated nucleus pulposus involving the L4 to L5 interspace may cause:
   a. Compression of the L5 nerve root
   b. Weakness of the dorsiflexors of the ankle
   c. Loss of sensation in the medial aspect of the foot
   d. Sciatica
   e. All the above

92. Herniated cervical disks may cause:
   a. Symptoms in the lower extremities
   b. Pain in the neck that radiates down the arms
   c. Weakness of the arm muscles and diminished biceps or triceps reflexes
   d. All the above

93. Which of the following statements is *true* of suspected herniated lumbar disks?
   a. Immediate surgery is advisable to prevent complications.
   b. Most patients recover completely without surgery.
   c. The pain may last for years.
   d. All the above are correct.

▼ *Fill in the blanks with the correct word or words.*

94. The semigelatinous central portion of the intervertebral disk that acts as a ball bearing and shock absorber is called the _____.

95. The _____ functions in a manner similar to a barrel hoop in the intervertebral disk.

96. The direction of herniation of the nucleus pulposus is frequently posterolateral because the _____ fibers are fewer in this area and the _____ ligament offers weak reinforcement.

CHAPTER 53

Cerebrovascular Disease

MARY CARTER LOMBARDO

Cerebral vascular (cerebrovascular) disease is a common neurologic condition. The manifestations of significant physiologic dysfunction caused by the disruption of cerebral blood flow have been known as early as the time of Hippocrates (460 to 370 BC). However, it was not until the advent of angiography that clinicians have been able to do more than take a "wait and see" approach to the care of patients experiencing a cerebrovascular accident, or stroke.

PATHOPHYSIOLOGY

The cerebrovascular system supplies the brain with a rich flow containing the nutrients critical for normal brain function. Interruption in cerebral blood flow (CBF) for 6 to 10 seconds results in unconsciousness and cerebral ischemia. Oxygen (O_2) deprivation of the neurons leads to loss of function. Excessive and sometimes irreversible changes in cellular homeostasis occur within minutes.

Normal CBF is 40 to 60 ml/100 g of brain tissue/minute. In a resting state the brain receives one sixth of the cardiac output; it uses 20% of the body's O_2. When CBF drops below 15 to 18 ml/100 g brain tissue/minute, several physiologic changes occur. The brain loses electrical activity and becomes electrically "silent," although neuronal membrane integrity and function remain intact. Clinically, these areas of the brain manifest a neurologic deficit, even though the brain cells are not dead. CBF less than 10 ml/100 g brain tissue causes cell membrane failure with subsequent alterations in extracellular fluid (ECF) potassium (K^+), rapid increases in intracellular fluid (ICF) calcium (Ca^{++}), rapid depletion of adenosine triphosphate (ATP), and profound ICF acidosis (Dobkin, 1989).

As energy stores become depleted in the brain, ion-exchange pumps fail, causing the ECF K^+ to rise and ICF sodium (Na^+) and Ca^{++} to rise. The brain cells respond to the ICF increase in Ca^{++} by using energy to contain the Ca^{++} within the mitochondria, which causes the uncoupling of oxidative phosphorylation. These changes are part of a chain of biochemical events that cause glial swelling and cerebral ischemia. Irreversible cellular damage occurs if ischemia is maintained. Even CBF levels of 10 to 18 ml/100 g brain tissue will lead to irreversible damage.

Glucose is the primary energy substrate of the brain, and it depends on a continuous supply to maintain its function. In contrast to other tissues of the body, the brain cannot use circulating free fatty acids (FFAs) as an energy source. A deficit of glucose supply to the brain, as with that of O_2, produces deranged function, tissue damage, or even death of brain cells if the deficit is prolonged.

Within 5 minutes of ischemia, brain ATP levels are depleted, and lactate levels begin to rise. Some research studies indicate that a relationship exists between elevated glucose levels and patient outcomes when the brain is ischemic. The reason for this is not fully understood. It is believed that high levels of glucose provide additional fuel for anaerobic metabolism in ischemic states, permitting the continued production of lactic acid, which worsens the ICF acidosis.

Other cellular metabolites may play a causative role in brain dysfunction secondary to stroke. During periods of anoxia, phospholipids are broken down into arachidonic acid, which is the precursor of vasospastic and thrombogenic compounds. Intracellular FFAs and their metabolites also increase, causing further ischemic damage.

When a cerebral vessel is occluded, the collateral circulation helps maintain some CBF to the ischemic area. The areas of the brain in which small amounts of CBF are maintained by collateral circulation are called *ischemic penumbra*. These are of intense interest to researchers, who are attempting to find ways to restore CBF to these areas and therefore reduce the permanent brain damage. In experimental animals, restoring CBF to ischemic areas in less than 2 hours is associated with reversible neurologic deficits, whereas occlusions lasting 6 hours are irreversible.

CEREBRAL CIRCULATION

As described in Chapter 50, the arterial blood to the brain is supplied by the two internal carotid arteries (anteriorly) and the two vertebral arteries (posteriorly). They arise from the aortic arch. On the right the brachiocephalic trunk (innominate) artery divides into the right common carotid artery, which supplies the head, and the right subclavian artery, which supplies the arm. On the left side the common carotid and left subclavian arteries each arise directly from the aortic arch.

In general the cerebral arteries are either conducting or penetrating. The *conducting arteries* (carotid; middle and anterior cerebral and vertebral; basilar; posterior cerebral) and their branches form an extensive network over the surface of the brain. The *penetrating arteries* are nutrient vessels derived from the conducting arteries. These vessels enter the brain at right angles and provide blood to structures below the cortical level (internal capsule, basal ganglia, etc.) (Fig. 53-1).

Circulation to the two hemispheres is generally symmetric, with each side retaining its own separate blood supply. However, anomalies of the classic distribution are common and generally insignificant. When a problem arises, these anomalies can cause confusion when an attempt is made to correlate clinical findings with pathophysiologic phenomena.

Collateral circulation may gradually develop when normal flow to a part is decreased. Most cerebral collateral circulation between major arteries is via the circle of Willis. It is estimated that anomalies in the circle of Willis occur in almost half the population. The brain also has collateral circulation sites, such as that between external and internal carotid arteries via the ophthalmic artery (see Fig. 50-9), that function only when other routes are impaired. Theoretically, these communicating channels are capable of providing an adequate blood supply to all areas of the brain. Practically, this is often not the case. A major vessel occlusion in one person will produce either no symptoms or a transient neurologic deficit; in another, the same occlusion site may cause a major

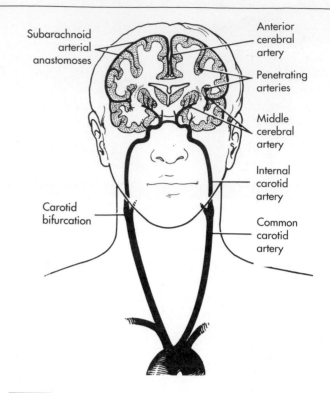

FIG. 53-1 Course of the internal carotid artery from the carotid bifurcation to its continuation as the middle cerebral artery. The penetrating lenticulostriate arteries arise from the first portion of the middle cerebral artery to supply the basal ganglia and internal capsule. These arteries are frequently implicated in a stroke syndrome. The middle cerebral artery continues to course over the cerebral hemisphere, sending short and deep penetrating arteries into the brain. The subarachnoid arterial anastomoses, which supply collateral circulation, are shown between the middle and anterior cerebral arteries. (Modified from *Essentials of stroke and diagnostic management,* rev ed, St Louis, 1973, Smith, Kline & French.)

loss of function. These differences would seem to be related to the state of the individual's collateral circulation.

The normal brain has the ability to regulate its own blood supply. "Normal" must be emphasized here because pathologic states are capable of altering or even abolishing this autoregulatory mechanism. Exactly how this mechanism functions is not entirely clear. McHenry (1976) has arbitrarily divided factors that control cerebral circulation into extrinsic, or extracranial, and intrinsic, or intracranial, as follows:

Extrinsic (Extracranial) Factors	Intrinsic (Intracranial) Factors
Systemic blood pressure	Cerebral autoregulatory mechanisms related to cerebral perfusion pressure
Cardiovascular function	Cerebral blood vessels
Blood viscosity	Intracranial or cerebrospinal fluid pressure

The extrinsic factors regulating CBF are related primarily to the cardiovascular system.

If systemic mean blood pressure (BP) drops below 60 mm Hg, the brain's autoregulatory mechanism becomes less effectual. The brain will initially attempt to compensate by extracting more O_2 from the available blood, but if the BP continues to drop until CBF is decreased to 30 ml/100 g of brain tissue/minute, signs of cerebral ischemia will appear.

Cardiac dysrhythmias can change cardiac output. If cardiac output is decreased by more than one third, there is often a fall in CBF.

The significance of blood viscosity is demonstrated by the fact that CBF may increase with anemia; in polycythemia it may decrease by 50%.

As noted previously, three intrinsic factors exist. First, McHenry (1976) calls the *cerebral perfusion pressure* the "driving force in cerebral circulation." It is the pressure difference between the cerebral arteries and veins. The CBF will remain constant (750 ml/minute) because of autoregulation even when systemic BP fluctuates. The range within which this mechanism can be effective is 150 to 60 mm Hg for the systemic BP. When systemic BP falls, a compensatory decrease occurs in cerebrovascular resistance (CVR). An elevation of BP results in an increase in CVR. The cerebral blood vessels are considered the most important factor relating to CVR.

Second, recent microcirculatory studies have identified a *myogenic response,* suggesting that the parenchymal tissue of arterioles releases a vasodilating metabolite in response to their O_2 needs and thereby exerts control on arterial smooth muscle tone:

Decreased perfusion pressure $\rightarrow$ Decreased CBF $\rightarrow$ Increased accumulation of metabolites $\rightarrow$ Vasodilation with restoration of CBF toward normal

The third intrinsic factor regulating CBF is *intracranial pressure* (ICP). An increase in ICP will increase CVR. CBF does not decrease until ICP has increased to 450 mm H_2O (normal range, 60 to 180 mm H_2O).

Three important metabolic factors (Guyton, Hall, 1996) follow:
1. *Carbon dioxide (CO_2) concentration.* High CO_2 tension (Pco_2) is a potent vasodilator, possibly because of accumulation of CO_2 in vasomotor centers. In normal subjects, CO_2 inhalations have produced up to 75% increase in CBF (raising Pco_2 by 9 mm Hg will raise CBF by 75%).
2. *Hydrogen ion (H^+) concentration.* An increase in H^+ yields an increase in CBF.
3. *Oxygen (O_2) concentration.* Low O_2 tension (Po_2) is a powerful vasodilator; high O_2 concentration is a moderate vasoconstrictor.

The brain is highly sensitive to changes in any of these factors. The brain's ability to adapt and compensate is poorly understood but basic in determining the extent of damage sustained from circulatory disruption. The brain copes most effectively when changes are gradual.

CEREBROVASCULAR ACCIDENTS

Cerebrovascular disease or accident (CVA, stroke) is, in general terms, a disturbance in cerebral circulation. A focal neurologic disorder, CVA may be secondary to a pathologic process within a cerebral blood vessel, such as thrombosis, embolus, rupture of a vessel wall, or basic vascular disease (e.g., atherosclerosis, arteritis, trauma, aneurysm, developmental malformations).

Stroke is responsible for 200,000 deaths in the United States each year and is the third most frequent cause of death. One-half million Americans each year have a new, acute CVA. An estimated 2 million people in the United States have a neurologic deficit that is a result of stroke. About 50% of all adult neurologic hospital admissions are the result of vascular disease.

The major causes of CVA, in order of importance, are atherosclerosis (thrombosis), embolism, hypertensive intracerebral hemorrhage, and ruptured saccular (berry) aneurysm. Stroke is generally accompanied by one or more associated medical problems, such as hypertension, cardiac disease, elevated blood lipids, diabetes mellitus, or peripheral vascular disease.

The severity of the CVA process is variable. Some infarcts are found on autopsy after death from unrelated causes. (Of all adults examined postmortem, 80% to 90% have significant atheromatous disease.) In others the stroke is sudden and dramatic, with the patient literally being "struck down." In this latter form, hemiplegia and unconsciousness both may be evident.

CVAs may be categorized according to cause or on the basis of their course. According to course, or *temporal profile,* which is defined as the chronologic pattern of clinical progression and regression of signs and symptoms, strokes may be divided into three types:
1. *Transient ischemic attacks (TIAs).* These are focal neurologic deficits that develop suddenly and disappear within a few minutes to hours.
2. *Progressive (CVA in evolution).* Evolution of stroke is gradual but acute.
3. *Completed CVA.* Deficits are maximal at onset, with little improvement.

Major clinical features associated with arterial insufficiency to the brain (points of bifurcation or angulation are most vulnerable) may be focal and temporary, or the dysfunction may be permanent, with actual tissue death and neurologic deficit. It is difficult to establish a close correlation between symptoms associated with a particular vessel and actual clinical manifestations in a particular patient because of the following:
1. There is individual variation of collateral circulation with regard to the circle of Willis (Fig. 53-2). Total occlusion of a carotid artery may produce no symptoms if the left anterior cerebral and left middle cerebral arteries receive adequate blood from the anterior com-

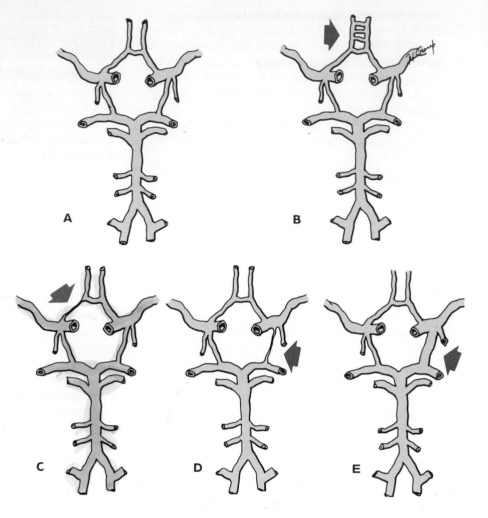

FIG. 53-2   The circle of Willis and some common anatomic variations. The anomalies are indicated by arrows. **A,** Normal circle of Willis. **B,** Reduplication of the anterior communicating artery. **C,** Stringlike anterior cerebral artery. **D,** Stringlike posterior communicating artery. **E,** Embryonic derivation of posterior cerebral artery from internal carotid artery. (Modified from Alpers BJ et al: *Arch Neurol Psychiatry* 81:409, 1959.)

municating artery. If this blood supply is not adequate, symptoms may include confusion, contralateral monoparesis or hemiparesis, and incontinence.

2. Leptomeningeal anastomoses are significant over the cerebral cortex between the anterior, middle, and posterior cerebral arteries. Anastomoses also exist between the anterior cerebral arteries of the two hemispheres across the corpus callosum.

3. Each of the cerebral arteries has a central area to supply with blood and a peripheral supply area, or border area, which it may share with another artery. Anastomoses exist between external and internal carotid arteries, as around the orbit, with blood from external carotid vessels going to the ophthalmic artery.

4. Various systemic and metabolic factors are significant in determining the symptoms that a particular pathologic process will produce. A stenosed vessel may produce no symptoms as long as systemic BP is 190/110 mm Hg, but if it is reduced to 120/70 mm Hg, variable symptoms may result, depending on the location of the stenotic area. Hyponatremia and hyperthermia are metabolic factors that facilitate development of neurologic deficits in the presence of stenotic blood vessels. Major clinical features associated with arterial insuffi-

ciency to the brain may be associated with the following signs and symptoms:

1. Vertebral-basilar (posterior circulation: manifestations usually bilateral)
   a. Weakness in one to four extremities
   b. Increased tendon reflexes
   c. Ataxia
   d. Bilateral Babinski's sign
   e. Cerebellar signs
   f. Dysphagia
   g. Dysarthria
   h. Syncope, stupor, coma, dizziness, memory disturbances
   i. Visual disturbances (diplopia, nystagmus, ptosis, paralysis of single eye movements)
   j. Numbness of face

2. Internal carotid artery (anterior circulation: symptoms usually unilateral). Most common location of lesion is the bifurcation of the common carotid into the internal and external carotids. Branches of the internal carotid are the ophthalmic, posterior communicating, anterior choroidal, anterior cerebral, and middle cerebral. Variable syndromes may develop. The pattern depends on the amount of collateral circulation.

a. Monocular blindness, episodic and called *amaurosis fugax,* on the side of the involved carotid. It is caused by retinal artery insufficiency. Sensory and motor symptoms involve contralateral extremities because of middle cerebral artery insufficiency.

b. Lesion in the area between the anterior and middle cerebral arteries or the middle cerebral artery. Symptoms initially develop in upper extremities (e.g., weak, numb hand) and may involve the face (supranuclear-type weakness). If the lesion is in the dominant hemisphere, expressive aphasia occurs because of involvement of Broca's motor-speech area.

3. Anterior cerebral artery (confusion is primary symptom)
   a. Contralateral weakness greater in leg; proximal arm also possibly involved; voluntary movement of that leg impaired
   b. Contralateral sensory deficits
   c. Dementia, grasp, pathologic reflexes (frontal lobe dysfunction)

4. Posterior cerebral artery (in lobe of midbrain or thalamus)
   a. Coma
   b. Contralateral hemiparesis
   c. Visual aphasia or word blindness (alexia)
   d. Third cranial nerve palsy: hemianopsia, choreoathetosis

5. Middle cerebral artery
   a. Contralateral monoparesis or hemiparesis (usually affecting arm)
   b. Occasional contralateral hemianopsia (blindness)
   c. Global aphasia (if dominant hemisphere is involved): disturbance of all functions involving speech and communication
   d. Dysphasia

Etiology

Cerebral thrombosis

Thrombosis (thromboocclusive disease) is the most common cause of CVA, accounting for about 40% of all strokes verified by pathologists. It is usually associated with local damage to the blood vessel wall caused by atherosclerosis.

The atherosclerotic process is characterized by fatty plaques that involve the intima of large arteries. The intima of the cerebral artery becomes thin and fibrous, with loss of muscle cells. The internal elastic lamina is split and frayed, and sclerotic material partly fills the lumen of the vessel.

The plaques show a tendency to form at branchings and curves. Thrombi are also associated with these specific sites. The blood vessels at risk, in decreasing order, are the internal carotid, upper vertebral, and lower basilar. The connective tissue is exposed from loss of the intima. Platelets adhere to this exposed, roughened surface.

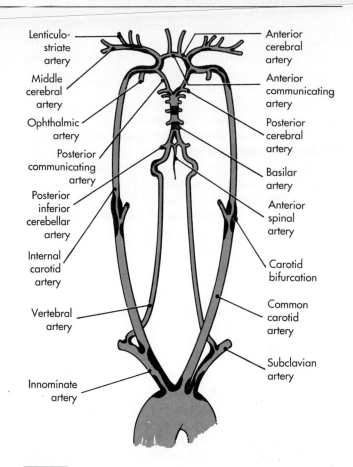

FIG. 53-3   Extracranial and intracranial arteries supplying blood to the brain. The circle of Willis and its principal branches are also shown. The sites of atherosclerosis of the cerebral blood vessels are designated *(dark areas),* the main locations being the carotid bifurcation and the takeoff of the branches from the aorta, innominate, and subclavian arteries. These are the sites that are amenable to surgery.

They release a chemical, adenosine diphosphate (ADP), which initiates the coagulation mechanism. This fibrinoplatelet plug may break off and embolize, or it may remain in place and eventually cause complete occlusion of the artery (Fig. 53-3).

Cerebral thrombosis is a disease of older age-groups; the peak age of occurrence is 60 to 69 years. In addition to atherosclerosis, hypertension appears to be an important underlying factor.

The onset of progression of symptoms tends to occur during sleep or soon after arising. Maximum intensity is generally realized within 48 hours. Progression is generally stepwise (a series of sudden changes) rather than smooth. Postural hypotension is more common in patients with cerebrovascular disease than in normal control subjects, possibly because of interference with the baroreceptor reflex. The pressor response to Valsalva's maneuver is often absent in older patients with atherosclerosis. Recumbency even for a night's rest can decrease sympathetic activity and lower BP in older persons. The surge in the amount of catecholamines (epinephrine, norepinephrine) released by the sympathetic nervous system in the early morning can play a role in the timing of CVAs. Additional factors, such as sedation or prolonged rest, can seriously compromise their precarious position.

TIAs are episodes of neurologic dysfunction that are usually of short duration (a few minutes) but may persist for 24 hours. TIAs involving the carotid arterial system last on the average about 14 minutes. Those involving the basilar-vertebral system last for about 7 minutes. TIAs are reversible, and the symptom pattern is the same with each attack because the same vessel is involved. This observation is important in terms of differential diagnosis, since small emboli from diseased heart valves might give similar symptoms, but no consistent patterns would exist, because different blood vessels might be involved each time. Other problems, besides cardiac emboli, that may initially be misdiagnosed as TIA include small strokes, seizures, migraine syndromes, postural hypotension, and Stokes-Adams syndrome.

Some TIAs seem to be related to vascular stenosis caused by atherosclerosis of the large arteries of the neck and less often of the intracranial arteries. TIAs are more frequent in men than in women (2:1). They occur less often in African Americans than in whites (although completed CVAs are more common in African Americans).

Additional research is necessary to establish the relationship between TIAs and CVAs. In the recent past this relationship seemed to be clear-cut, with 30% to 70% of patients reporting a history of TIAs before stroke. The validity of these data is now being questioned, and opinions vary concerning the risk of CVA when the patient has a history of TIAs.

Anoxic encephalopathy may occur with cerebral thrombosis. Symptoms and the clinical picture depend on location. The brain distal to the clot becomes swollen. Discoloration may occur, with a muddy-looking appearance. There is a loss of demarcation between the gray and white matter. As time passes, nerve cells disintegrate and are replaced by glia.

Pathologically, these infarcts may be classified as bland or ischemic because the infarct is arterial and does not have blood flowing into it (see Fig. 3-6).

Cerebral embolism

Cerebral embolism, the second morst common cause of CVA, affects younger persons more frequently than stroke caused by thrombosis. Most cerebral emboli originate from a thrombus in the heart, so this problem is essentially a manifestation of heart disease. Less frequently the embolus originates from an atheromatous plaque in the carotid sinus or internal carotid artery. Any area of the brain may be involved, but the embolus will lodge at a narrow point in a blood vessel. The middle cerebral artery, especially the upper division, is the most frequent site of cerebral emboli.

Symptoms may occur at any time and are rapidly pro-gressive. Symptoms of small emboli differ from those of TIAs in that the latter tend to occur with the same clinical picture each time (same vessel or vessels involved). With numerous small emboli, as from a chronic atrial fibrillation, the pattern varies with each episode, depending on the vessels involved.

In general, more tissue death occurs with emboli than with more gradually occurring situations because anastomotic vessels do not have time to dilate and thus compensate.

Cerebral hemorrhage

Cerebral hemorrhage is the third most frequent cause of CVA, accounting for one tenth of all cases. Ruptured cerebral arteries are the usual source of intracranial bleeding. Persons who have recently used cocaine are at risk for intracerebral hemorrhage because of the severe hypertension caused by this drug. Extravasation of blood occurs in the brain and/or subarachnoid space. Adjacent tissue may be displaced and compressed. Blood is particularly irritating to brain tissue, causing vasospasm in arteries adjacent to the bleeding site. This spasm may spread to the entire hemisphere and circle of Willis. The clot, which is originally soft and resembles red currant jelly, eventually resolves and decreases in size. Histologically, the brain adjacent to the clot may be swollen and necrotic. Through enzymatic action, liquefaction occurs and a cavity forms. Over several months all necrotic tissue is replaced. Astrocytes and new capillaries form a weavelike pattern in the cavity. Eventually, astroglial fibers proliferate and fill in the cavity.

Subarachnoid hemorrhage is often associated with a rupture of an aneurysm. Most aneurysms involve a vessel in the circle of Willis. Hypertension or a bleeding disorder may contribute to the occurrence of rupture. Often, more than one aneurysm are present.

Neurologic findings depend on the site and severity of the hemorrhage. The vessel involved is usually a penetrating artery such as one of the lenticulostriate branches of the middle cerebral artery that supply some of the basal ganglia and most of the internal capsule. The onset is abrupt and evolution rapid and steady, lasting minutes, hours, and occasionally days.

Frequently the clinical features include severe headache, nuchal rigidity, vomiting, stupor, coma, and convulsions. Cerebrospinal fluid (CSF) is bloody in 90% of patients (when hemorrhage is small and away from the ventricles, it may be clear). Of these patients, 70% to 75% die in 1 to 30 days, generally from hemorrhage extending into the ventricular system, temporal lobe herniation and midbrain compression, or seepage into vital centers.

Patients with cerebrovascular hemorrhage may do well if a vital center is not involved. An area in the cerebral hemisphere may tolerate a relatively large accumulation of blood (100 ml) with no significant clinical manifestations, whereas a 5 ml clot in the brain stem may be lethal (see Fig. 7-3).

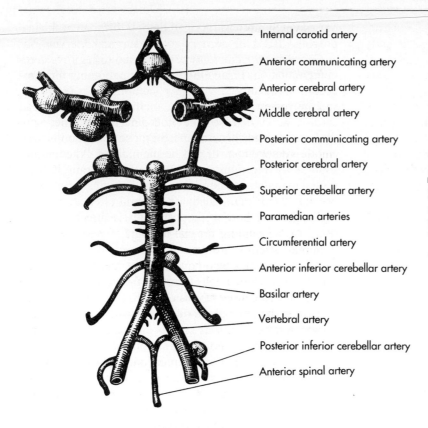

Internal carotid artery

Anterior communicating artery

Anterior cerebral artery

Middle cerebral artery

Posterior communicating artery

Posterior cerebral artery

Superior cerebellar artery

Paramedian arteries

Circumferential artery

Anterior inferior cerebellar artery

Basilar artery

Vertebral artery

Posterior inferior cerebellar artery

Anterior spinal artery

FIG. 53-4   The common sites of saccular (berry) aneurysms. Each is drawn in direct proportion to the frequency at that site. (From Beeson PB, McDermott W, Wyngaarden JB, editors: *Cecil textbook of medicine,* ed 15, Philadelphia, 1979, Saunders.)

When cerebral hemorrhage occurs because of a ruptured aneurysm, the patients are generally young and 20% have more than one aneurysm. As noted earlier, most cerebral aneurysms are located in the circle of Willis.

Saccular (or *berry*) *aneurysms* can be smaller than a pinhead or 2 to 3 cm in diameter. They are frequently the size of a pea and arise at or close to points of divisions of an artery. These aneurysms are thin-walled (covered only by intima) blisters protruding from the artery at a point where a local weakness exists. They gradually enlarge, and rupture can occur. Often they are asymptomatic until they rupture, which generally occurs during activity. The usual clinical pictures include sudden violent headache, "like something snapped in my head"; collapse; brief unconsciousness and confusion; no warning symptoms; and few, if any, lateralizing signs. An outstanding feature of aneurysms is their tendency to rebleed (Fig. 53-4).

Diagnosis

The differential diagnosis of stroke syndromes includes a variety of structural and metabolic causes. A thorough history and physical examination are done on all patients with suspected cerebrovascular disease. Generally, in any patient with a suspected CVA, the presence or absence of cerebral hemorrhage must be ruled out. This can be determined quickly and accurately with a routine, non-contrast-enhanced computed tomography (CT) scan. Brain scans may be helpful if the lesion has damaged the blood-brain barrier, which would allow the isotope to localize in the affected area. Electroencephalograms

(EEGs), if used, may demonstrate delta waves that are slower over the affected area.

Many disease states mimic the symptomatology of CVA, and these must be ruled out. Epidural and subdural hemotoma can cause altered mental status, focal neurologic deficits, and even coma. Older patients who are considered at high risk for stroke are also at high risk for recurrent falls that may lead to chronic subdural hematoma (see Chapter 56). Brain tumors and brain abscesses can cause the same focal deficits seen in CVA. Metabolic abnormalities, including hypoglycemia and Wernicke's encephalopathy, can mimic stroke. CVA can be confused not only with other severe diseases, but also with milder disorders such as labyrinthitis, migraine, or even dementia.

Treatment

In the acute care situation the critical factors to be considered are as follows:
1. Stabilization of vital signs
   a. Maintaining a patent airway: frequent and deep suctioning, O_2, tracheotomy, and respiratory assistance if brain stem is involved
   b. Blood pressure control on an individualized basis, which entails correcting hypotension as well as hypertension
2. Detection and correction of cardiac dysrhythmias
3. Bladder care: when feasible, indwelling catheters are avoided; they have been replaced by in-out catheterizations every 4 to 6 hours.
4. Proper positioning is stressed immediately.

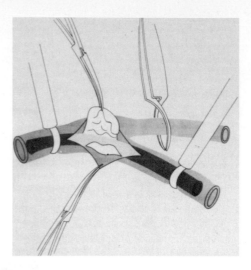

FIG. 53-5 Diagram of a carotid endarterectomy. A bypass tube is used during the removal of an atherosclerotic lesion at the carotid bifurcation. (From *Essentials of stroke and diagnostic management,* rev ed, St Louis, 1973, Smith, Kline & French.)

a. The patient should be turned every hour and passive range of motion (ROM) exercises instituted every 2 hours.

b. Within a few days, full ROM to a total of 50 times per day is recommended; this is necessary to avoid pressure areas and contractures, especially at the shoulder, elbow, and ankle.

No single method of treatment is consistently useful. Several modes of therapy seem useful, but mortality rates have not improved.

Conservative treatment

Vasodilators have increased CBF experimentally but have not proved beneficial in persons with CVA. Effective dilators of vessels in other areas of the body have little or no effect on cerebral vessels, especially when used orally (e.g., nicotinic acid, tolazoline, papaverine). On the basis of a few clinical trials, the following have been suggested as useful: histamine, aminophylline, acetazolamide, and intraarterial papaverine.

The use of vasodilators may also exert an adverse effect on CBF by lowering systemic BP and thereby decreasing intracerebral anastomotic flow.

Platelet antiaggregants such as aspirin are used to inhibit the platelet aggregation-release reaction that occurs after ulceration of an atheroma. Many patients and people at risk for developing clots are currently taking 650 mg (10 grains) of aspirin once or twice a day (in some cases once every other day) for prophylaxis against platelet aggregation.

Surgical therapy

Several surgical procedures are now used in patients with CVA. The proper selection of the individual who will most benefit from surgery remains a difficult task. Improving CBF is the primary goal of surgical intervention.

Carotid endarterectomy is performed to improve cerebral circulation (Fig. 53-5). Patients undergoing this procedure frequently have other complicating problems, such as hypertension, diabetes mellitus, and widespread cardiovascular disease. The procedure is performed with the patient under general anesthesia so that good airway and ventilatory control can be maintained. A temporary shunt is used to minimize ischemia to the brain. It is essential to maintain a normal or slightly high arterial blood pressure to maintain adequate cerebral circulation, since regional blood flow in these patients is directly proportional to the systemic arterial pressure.

In the 1960s, with the use of stereoscopic microscopes and microsuturing techniques, patent anastomoses were successfully performed through the revascularization procedure. *Revascularization procedures* are performed to increase regional blood flow to areas where circulation is compromised. Various vessels can be used; usually the superficial temporal artery is anastomosed to a superficial cortical artery. In another procedure (the subclavian–external carotid bypass graft), a segment of the saphenous vein is anastomosed to the subclavian artery and the proximal end of the external carotid artery. Revascularization is primarily a prophylactic procedure and is most likely to benefit patients with TIAs or those who are at an early stage in the course of a thrombosis-in-evolution. Patients manifesting fixed neurologic deficits can expect no benefit from these procedures and are not considered appropriate candidates.

Evacuation of blood clots is seldom beneficial in the acute stage of CVA. Exceptions are surface lesions when the patient is conscious and some cerebellar hemorrhages when surgical evacuation of the clot has led to improvement.

Surgical intervention in the case of aneurysms is directed toward prevention of a recurrence of the hemorrhage. Ligation of the common carotid artery in the neck is the most conservative treatment of aneurysm.

Intracranial procedures, such as clipping or ligating the neck of the aneurysm, necessitate major neurosurgical intervention. Aneurysms can also be painted with a physiologic glue, which provides an elastic cap and keeps them from rupturing. Before surgery can be undertaken, arteriograms are necessary. Arteriograms are a serious threat to the patient because (1) the dye, as with the original free blood, can cause vasospasm because of irritation; and (2) the pressure necessary to insert the dye may cause rebleeding in the newly ruptured area. The patient must be stabilized before surgery. The vasospasm must be resolved or minimal. Toward this end, the patient is placed on an aneurysm protocol, which may include the following precautions adapted to the individual patient:

1. Darkened room. No rectal temperatures are taken, since this may stimulate the vagus nerve and elevate blood pressure.

2. Phenobarbital, 30 mg intravenously (IV) every 6 hours to decrease possibility of seizures.
3. Dexamethasone (Decadron), 20 mg IV every 6 hours for its diuretic effect. Dexamethasone seems to protect the brain by stabilizing cerebral membranes and decreasing cerebral edema.
4. Cimetidine (Tagamet), 300 mg IV every 6 hours to prevent the gastrointestinal irritation that may be a side effect of dexamethasone administration.
5. Aminocaproic acid (Amicar), 2 g IV every 6 hours to prevent lysis of the clot. Amicar levels, streptokinase levels, and clot lysis times are monitored daily.
6. Hydralazine hydrochloride (Apresoline), 5 mg every 3 hours if blood pressure greater than 140 mm Hg systolic.
7. Fluid restriction based on serum osmolality; may be as severe as 800 to 1200 ml/24 hours.

Various shunt procedures may be performed (ventriculoatrial shunt) if obstructive hydrocephalus is an overriding concern. Free blood in the subarachnoid space may obstruct CSF circulation and cause acute hydrocephalus. Shunts are used more frequently than in the past and generally have replaced the decompression craniotomies formerly done to reduce the symptoms of increased ICP. Current research is focused on therapy that may save vital brain tissue that is compromised during the ischemic or hemorrhagic event. These therapies include calcium channel blockers, platelet inhibitors, thrombolytic agents, free-radical scavengers, and hemodilution.

One of the most promising research studies in treating CVA involves the use of *tissue plasminogen activator* (tPA), a thrombolytic agent approved for use in patients with acute myocardial infarction and pulmonary embolism. Research into the use of thrombolytics (streptokinase and tPA) to treat acute CVA caused by arterial occlusion is ongoing. This type of CVA accounts for approximately 80% of acute ischemic strokes. In the National Institute of Neurological Disorders and Stroke recombinant tPA (rtPA) CVA trial conducted between 1991 and 1994, significant benefits were found in a select group of patients treated with rtPA. These patients were 30 times more likely to demonstrate minimal or no neurologic deficit 3 months after the stroke than were pa-

tients not treated with rtPA. The key factors in this trial were (1) time to treatment (the target was 90 minutes and not later than 3 hours from onset of symptoms); (2) a smaller dose of rtPA (0.9 mg/kg, maximum dose 90 mg); (3) strict control of hypertension before, during, and after treatment with rtPA; and (4) identification of any patient with an intracranial hemorrhage (using a CT scan) (Marler, 1995). With the ongoing research into treatments for CVAs to minimize the death and dependency often associated with this devastating illness, breakthroughs can be expected.

Preventive measures

In a 24-year follow-up study by the American Heart Association involving 5184 men and women (ages 30 to 62 years at entry into the study), 345 had suffered CVAs; 60% of these had suffered thrombosis (called *atherothrombotic brain infarction, ABI*). Unlike other manifestations of atherosclerosis, ABI occurs equally among men and women. The most important risk factor identified was hypertension, which was even more dangerous when coupled with other factors such as diabetes, left ventricular hypertrophy identified by electrocardiography, elevated blood cholesterol level, cigarette smoking, and cardiac impairments. This study cites the control of blood pressure as the key to ABI prevention (American Heart Association, 1977).

Several other general preventive measures can be identified, as follows:
1. Decrease in salt intake, beginning early in life with salt-free or low-salt baby food
2. Especially with older persons, extreme care to maintain blood pressure during surgical procedures and avoidance of oversedation and prolonged bedrest
3. Increased activity: daily walking as part of a fitness program
4. Decrease in weight if overweight
5. Discontinuation of cigarette smoking
6. Discontinuation of oral contraceptive use by women who smoke, since the risk of cerebrovascular problems in a woman who smokes and takes an oral contraceptive is increased 16 times over that of a woman who does neither

QUESTIONS

▼ *Circle the letter preceding each item below that correctly answers the question or completes the statement. More than one answer may be correct.*

1. Which of the following is the most frequently occurring neurologic disease?
   a. Tumors of the nervous system
   b. Vascular disorders of the nervous system
   c. Spinal cord diseases
   d. Epilepsy

2. Two substances that must be supplied continuously to the brain to avoid irreversible brain cell damage are:
   a. Free fatty acids
   b. Glucose
   c. Oxygen
   d. Lactic acid

3. Death of brain cells from a lack of oxygen occurs in approximately:
   a. 15 minutes
   b. 10 minutes
   c. 4 minutes
   d. 1 minute

4. The major arterial blood vessels that supply blood to the circle of Willis are the:
   a. External carotid
   b. Internal carotid
   c. Ophthalmic
   d. Basilar-vertebral system

▼ *Answer the following on a separate sheet of paper.*

5. Describe the arterial blood supply to the brain.

6. Briefly describe the three extrinsic (extracranial) factors and the three intrinsic (intracranial) factors that are thought to be responsible for cerebral circulatory control.

7. Cerebrovascular accident (CVA, stroke) is responsible for how many deaths in the United States each year? Approximately how many people in the United States have a neurologic deficit that is a result of a stroke?

8. List and describe the three types of CVA according to the chronologic pattern of clinical progression and regression of signs and symptoms.

▼ *Circle the letter preceding each item below that correctly answers the question or completes the statement. More than one answer may be correct.*

9. Which of the following cerebral arteries are most likely to form fatty plaques, in order of occurrence?
   a. Ophthalmic
   b. Basilar
   c. Carotids
   d. Vertebral

10. Cerebral emboli can be composed of:
    a. Blood clot (especially with underlying heart or vascular disease)
    b. Fatty tissue
    c. Tumor cells
    d. Bacterial clumps (often from heart disease)

11. Major sites of origin of cerebral emboli causing a CVA include all the following *except:*
    a. Mural thrombi in the left atrium associated with atrial fibrillation
    b. Mural thrombi overlying ventricular infarcts
    c. Thrombi formed in rheumatic valve disease
    d. Thrombi formed on arteriosclerotic plaques in the aortic arch and carotid arteries
    e. Thrombi formed in the deep leg veins

▼ *Circle T if the statement is true and F if it is false. Correct any false statements.*

12. T F Cerebral thrombosis usually has a gradual onset, whereas cerebral embolism usually has a sudden onset.

13. T F In cerebrovascular disorders the signs and symptoms the patient experiences depend on which vessel is involved and the amount of collateral circulation in the affected area.

14. T F For a cerebrovascular disorder to be referred to as a transient ischemic attack (TIA), there must be evidence of cerebral tissue necrosis.

15. T F Cerebral thrombosis is a disease of the older age groups.

▼ *Circle the letter preceding each item below that correctly answers the question or completes the statement. More than one answer may be correct.*

16. Mr. B., a 60-year-old man, was admitted to the general hospital. On admission his vital signs were as follows: temperature 99.8°F, pulse 90 beats/minute, respirations 20 breaths/minute, and blood pressure 250/140 mm Hg. Lumbar puncture disclosed that the spinal fluid contained red blood cells and was under increased pressure. Shortly after admission, Mr. B. became comatose. He was diagnosed as having a cerebral hemorrhage. Which of the following symptoms would probably indicate a hemorrhage in the area of the brain involving the posterior cerebral artery and the thalamus?
    a. Contralateral hemiplegia or hemiparesis
    b. Ipsilateral numbness and sensory loss on the face
    c. Dementia
    d. Tremor

17. The predisposing factors that probably contributed to Mr. B.'s intracerebral hemorrhage include all the following *except:*
    a. History of preexisting hypertension
    b. Weakness of the vascular wall
    c. Sudden rise in blood pressure
    d. History of episodic hypotension

18. Miss K., a 32-year-old woman with a history of rheumatic heart disease complicated by mitral stenosis and atrial fibrillation, was admitted to the hospital with a high fever, changing heart murmurs, large tender spleen, and abrupt onset of a right hemiplegia and aphasia, which persisted for 48 hours. The *most likely* type of neurologic deficit is:
    a. Embolism
    b. TIAs
    c. Thrombosis
    d. None of the above

19. Mr. G., age 67, was referred to the neurologist by the public health nurse after he had experienced several TIAs. Symptoms experienced during these attacks included falling because of weakness of extremities, dizziness, and loss of equilibrium; double vision; and difficulty with speech. The most likely site of arterial occlusion is:
    a. Internal carotid artery

QUESTIONS—cont'd

b. Basilar-vertebral arteries
c. Radial artery
d. Anterior cerebral artery

20. Mr. K., a 75-year-old man with a history of mild diabetes mellitus and a previous myocardial infarction, was admitted to the hospital with a mild left hemiparesis, which evolved slowly over several hours with no other neurologic deficit. This deficit improved slightly after several days in the hospital but did not entirely clear. The most likely diagnosis is:
    a. Subarachnoid hemorrhage
    b. Wallenberg's syndrome (lateral medullary syndrome) on the right side of the medulla
    c. TIA involving the right middle cerebral artery
    d. Cerebral thrombosis involving the right middle cerebral artery

21. A subarachnoid hemorrhage is most frequently associated with:
    a. Mycotic aneurysms
    b. Severe hypertension
    c. Berry aneurysms
    d. Atherosclerotic aneurysms

22. Characteristics of TIAs include which *one* of the following?
    a. Lasting damage to the brain after an attack
    b. Similarity to epileptic attacks in the duration of neurologic dysfunction
    c. Return to "normal" after an attack
    d. Hemiparesis

23. Mr. O., a 50-year-old man, was admitted to a local general hospital convulsing and unconscious. His temperature was 99°F rectally, pulse rate 98 beats/minute, respirations 20 breaths/minute, and blood pressure 240/140 mm Hg. Twenty-four hours after admission,

Mr. O. regained consciousness. His right arm and right leg were paralyzed, and he was unable to speak. The hemorrhage responsible for his symptoms probably occurred from rupture of a branch of the:
    a. Anterior cerebellar artery
    b. Posterior cerebral artery
    c. Middle cerebral artery
    d. Vertebral artery

24. Berry aneurysms:
    a. Occur most often at the bifurcation of arteries
    b. Typically occur on or near the circle of Willis
    c. Are usually not discovered until they bleed
    d. Cause subdural hemorrhage when they rupture

25. A cerebral infarction in the distribution of the middle cerebral artery would be likely to cause all the following symptoms *except:*
    a. Contralateral hemiplegia
    b. Aphasia
    c. Cerebellar signs
    d. Homonymous hemianopsia (loss of vision in half the visual field)

26. A patient is admitted to the hospital with a diagnosis of mild CVA. The patient demonstrated left-sided weakness of upper and lower extremities. The patient probably has a lesion located in the:
    a. Left cerebral hemisphere
    b. Right cerebral hemisphere
    c. Brain stem
    d. Medulla

27. Which neurologic test would be most helpful in establishing the diagnosis in an individual with suspected CVA?

a. Electroencephalogram
b. CT scan of the head
c. Testing intactness of cranial nerves
d. Cold-water caloric test

28. Which of the following statements is(are) true with respect to the use of tissue plasminogen activator (tPA) for the treatment of acute stroke?
    a. Cerebral hemorrhage must be ruled out with a CT scan or MRI.
    b. Treatment must begin within 3 hours of the acute insult.
    c. Neurologic deficits are greatly reduced.
    d. Thrombotic CVA is an indication for this treatment.
    e. Cerebral hemorrhage is a possible complication.

▼ *Answer the following on a separate sheet of paper.*

29. For the acute period of a CVA, describe four critical factors in the patient's treatment.

30. Describe the effectiveness of vasodilators and platelet antiaggregants in the treatment of CVA.

31. State the primary goal of surgical intervention for stroke patients.

32. Describe a surgical procedure used to increase collateral blood flow to the brain.

33. What is the major purpose of clipping the neck of a berry aneurysm located on the anterior communicating artery of the brain?

34. What are the principles of prevention and therapy after neurologic deficit?

CHAPTER 54

Neurologic Disorders With Generalized Symptomatology

MARY S. HARTWIG

Diseases of the nervous system with a progressively downhill course traditionally have been referred to as *degenerative.* Pathologic processes of the nervous system are generally classified by their effects on a person's functioning rather than their causes, since for many the cause is under investigation or as yet undiscovered. The effects of a degenerative neurologic disease tend to be progressive, long lasting, or permanent, requiring the patient to learn new methods of adapting to increasing or changing disabilities. Families also are affected by the long-term nature of these neurologic disorders.

Many of the degenerative diseases affecting the nervous system present as distinct clinical syndromes, the recognition of which can assist in their identification. For example, Alzheimer's disease is characterized by progressive dementia with the absence of other neurologic deficits until the terminal stage. Amyotrophic lateral sclerosis is largely a motor neuron disease characterized by muscular weakness but without sensory changes. Distinct and gradually developing abnormalities of posture and movement characterize Parkinson's disease and Huntington's chorea. Multiple sclerosis, a demyelinating disease, is characterized by recurrent attacks of focal or multifocal neurologic deficits.

Other neurologic disorders discussed in this chapter include infections of the central nervous system and myasthenia gravis, a disease manifested by weakness and fatigability of the skeletal muscles caused by a deficiency of acetylcholine receptors at the neuromuscular junction.

DEMENTIAS

Primary Dementia: Alzheimer's Disease

Alzheimer's disease is a devastating, disabling disease that primarily affects persons older than 65 years. Current estimates are that approximately 10% of persons in this age-group have the disease. With the rapid expansion of the older population, it is estimated that 14 million persons will have Alzheimer's disease by 2050. These individuals not only will have a significant impact on the health care delivery system (demand for nursing homes, adult day-care centers, acute care facilities, research dollars), but also will cause significant stress in family members who must care for them.

Pathologically, the patient with Alzheimer's disease experiences a severe loss of hippocampal and cortical neurons with no loss of brain parenchyma. In addition, there are diffuse neurofibrillary tangles and senile plaques (the larger the number of senile plaques, the worse the symptoms). These last two pathologic changes are not unique to Alzheimer's disease—they are also found in patients with lead encephalopathy and Down's syndrome. The latest research findings indicate that problems with neurotransmitters and the enzymes associated with their metabolism are involved. It appears that choline acetyltransferase (the enzyme that synthesizes acetylcholine) is decreased. On autopsy the brain of patients with Alzheimer's disease shows significant reduction in the neurotransmitter acetylcholine; some brains contain as little as 10% of the normal amount. The amount of dementia is directly related to the reduction in brain acetylcholine. Its decrease is particularly remarkable in the cerebral cortex, the hippocampus, and the amygdala. Another area under investigation by researchers is peptide neurotransmitters, since somatostatin is decreased in the brain of those with Alzheimer's disease. An additional factor under investigation is aluminum neurotoxicity. Crapper, Quittkat, DeBon (1979) have suggested that the membrane transport system fails in patients with Alzheimer's disease, allowing an interaction between aluminum and chromatin that causes the pathologic changes in protein synthesis and neurofibrillary changes.

No one cause has been identified at present, but three major theories exist: (1) slow viruses, (2) an autoimmune process, and (3) aluminum toxicity. Currently the most popular theory (although still unproved) involves *slow viruses*. These viruses have an incubation period of 2 to 30 years; therefore transmission is difficult to prove. Certain varieties of viral encephalopathy (kuru, Creutzfeldt-Jakob disease) are characterized by pathologic changes that resemble the senile plaques seen in Alzheimer's disease.

The *autoimmune theory* is based on the presence of increased levels of brain-reactive antibodies in Alzheimer's disease. There are two types of amyloid (a protein complex with starchlike characteristics that is produced and deposited in certain pathologic states): one composed of immunoglobulin G (IgG) chains and the other of unknown composition. The theory suggests that the antigen-antibody complexes are catabolized by phagocytes and the immunoglobulin fragments degraded in lysosomes, leading to extracellular amyloid deposits.

The *aluminum toxicity theory* suggests that because aluminum is neurotoxic, it can induce neurofibrillary changes in the brain. Aluminum deposits have been identified in some patients with Alzheimer's disease, but some pathologic changes associated with the disease are different from those seen in aluminum toxicity. Most researchers believe that aluminum exposure is not the only answer, especially because aluminum is the most abundant metal in the Earth's crust and the human intestinal system does not absorb it well.

Genetic predisposition also plays a role in Alzheimer's disease. An estimated 10% to 30% of Alzheimer's patients develop the inherited type of the disease, referred to as *familial Alzheimer's disease* (FAD). Current research implicates a defect of chromosome 21. This theory is supported by the fact that persons with Down's syndrome, which involves the presence of an extra 21st

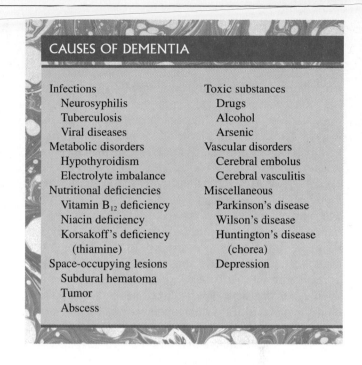

CAUSES OF DEMENTIA

Infections	Toxic substances
Neurosyphilis	Drugs
Tuberculosis	Alcohol
Viral diseases	Arsenic
Metabolic disorders	Vascular disorders
Hypothyroidism	Cerebral embolus
Electrolyte imbalance	Cerebral vasculitis
Nutritional deficiencies	Miscellaneous
Vitamin B_{12} deficiency	Parkinson's disease
Niacin deficiency	Wilson's disease
Korsakoff's deficiency	Huntington's disease
(thiamine)	(chorea)
Space-occupying lesions	Depression
Subdural hematoma	
Tumor	
Abscess	

chromosome, commonly develop Alzheimer's disease during the fourth decade of life.

Researchers have identified a gene encoding *amyloid precursor protein* (APP), a segment of which is present at the core of neural plaques. This 695–amino acid molecule protrudes through the outer membrane of the cell body and is broken off by other proteins and later broken down by proteases. The protein found in the plaques is an abnormal 42–amino acid piece of the APP that for unknown reasons has not broken down but instead accumulates in large concentrations in the brains of patients with Alzheimer's disease.

Diagnosis of Alzheimer's disease is complicated by the absence of a definitive test. Thus diagnosis is based on a collection of supportive data, clinical observations, and the family's description of the patient's behavior. Patients with the symptoms of dementia should be tested to detect potentially reversible nutritional, endocrine, and infectious causes for their symptoms. In addition to a complete physical and an extensive neurologic examination, diagnostic tests frequently ordered include complete blood count (CBC) and blood studies for syphilis, serum electrolytes, vitamin B_{12}, and thyroid function tests. A computed tomography (CT) scan may show ventricular widening and cortical atrophy and confirms the absence of brain tumor, brain abscess, or chronic subdural hematoma, which are treatable. Other treatable causes of dementia must also be ruled out. The box above lists causes of dementia other than Alzheimer's disease.

During the early stages of Alzheimer's disease, the patient remains somewhat independent but experiences diminished problem-solving capacity, diminished ability to cope with complex situations and think abstractly, emotional lability, forgetfulness, apathy, and loss of recent memory. As the disease progresses, the patient's behavior becomes more erratic and bizarre, with a tendency toward wandering and violent outbursts. Family members must remain constantly vigilant to protect the person from harm. Deterioration is predictable and occurs over a 3- to 10-year period. During the later stages of the disease, patients become incontinent and are unable to attend to any of their basic needs or to recognize family members. Death is usually the result of malnutrition or infection.

Management of the patient with Alzheimer's disease involves both the patient and the family. Tranquilizers and antidepressants may be useful in managing the patient's behavior. Experimental drugs are being used in some medical centers in an attempt to slow brain deterioration, but no approved drug therapy has been developed. Family support groups are essential to help families cope. Adult day-care centers, home health aides, and extended care facilities become indispensable to the family as the patient's condition deteriorates and total care is necessary. The challenge in the future will be to meet the needs of increasing numbers of these patients.

Secondary Dementias: Nutritional Degenerative Disease

Lack or deficiency of particular nutrients is known to have a deleterious effect on the brain. Several vitamins in particular are known to be essential for normal brain metabolism. Deficiencies of the B vitamins B_1, B_6, B_{12}, niacin, and pantothenic acid are associated with various neurologic disorders. Despite continued research, much remains unknown about the role of nutrition on the development of the nervous system and its healthy maintenance.

Alcoholism is a major problem in the United States. The alcoholic person is frequently the victim of severe nutritional deficiencies caused by decreased appetite; abusive drinking; and the presence of chronic illnesses, untreated infections, and anemia.

Wernicke-Korsakoff syndrome is associated with extensive alcohol abuse and nutritional deprivation (as in gastric carcinoma, thyrotoxicosis, and hyperemesis gravidarum). The term *cerebral beriberi* is used in reference to this disease. Pathologic changes involve necrosis of nerve cells and myelinated structures. Symptoms are related to the involved brain structures. Paralysis of gaze, nystagmus, and ataxia are caused by lesions in the midbrain, the cerebellar vermis, and the floor of the fourth ventricle. The psychologic symptoms, dull mentation, impairment of recent memory, and amnesia are generally caused by lesions of the thalamic nuclei and the hypothalamus. In addition, these patients have postural hypotension, dyspnea, tachycardia, cirrhosis of the liver, and anemia.

Thiamine is the therapy of choice for patients with Wernicke-Korsakoff syndrome. Improvement of symptoms varies; the disorders of mentation (apathy, inattentiveness, and listlessness) improve rapidly, whereas ataxia and nystagmus demonstrate slow but gradual improvement. Unfortunately, amnesia does not improve significantly.

CENTRAL MOTOR SYSTEM DISORDERS

Degenerative Diseases
Huntington's disease

Huntington's disease (chorea) is an uncommon inherited disease linked to a defect of chromosome 4. It is transmitted as an autosomal dominant trait with complete penetrance. The average age of onset of symptoms is 38 years. Patients experience a long (10 to 25 years), progressively debilitating course, eventually becoming completely bedridden, totally dependent for basic needs, and exhibiting socially problematic behaviors.

Pathologically, the disease is caused by a structural degeneration of neurons with cell loss in the basal ganglia (especially the caudate nucleus and putamen) and the cerebral cortex. The chorea-like movements may be related to a deficiency in gamma-aminobutyric acid (GABA) caused by a deficiency in glutamic acid decarboxylase and choline in the basal ganglia seen in patients with Huntington's disease.

The onset of Huntington's disease is insidious and generally begins with some chorea-like movements, emotional lability, intellectual deterioration, lack of attention to appearance, and forgetfulness. As the disease progresses, the symptoms become more debilitating and obvious to family and friends. Gradually the patient is unable to concentrate or attend to the activities of daily living and is subject to violent outbursts and combativeness.

No known definitive treatment or cure exists for Huntington's disease. Symptomatic treatment consists of administering haloperidol and chlorpromazine to minimize the chorea-like movements. As the disease progresses, family members can no longer cope with the constant attention required by these patients and confinement to an institution is necessary. Families require much emotional support to cope with the long-term and debilitating nature of the disease. It is also appropriate to offer genetic counseling and a thorough explanation of the disease because of its hereditary transmittal.

Amyotrophic lateral sclerosis

Amyotrophic lateral sclerosis (ALS), or Lou Gehrig's disease, is a progressive neurologic disease that affects persons in the fourth through seventh decades of life. The precise cause is yet unknown, although current research has provided several clues. The disease may be a result of (1) genetic predisposition, (2) a slow latent viral infection (e.g., mutated poliovirus), or (3) an autoimmune disorder.

Pathologic changes involve the anterior horn cells of the spinal cord and the lower brain stem and the motor neurons of the cerebral cortex that give rise to the corticospinal tract. Deterioration of these neurons cause neurogenic atrophy of the musculature they innervate. Sensory neurons are unaffected. This neuronal deterioration causes loss of fine motor control and muscle atrophy—the first symptoms noted by the patient. Atrophic weakness usually follows a proximal to distal pattern, which progresses to involve the neck, tongue, pharyngeal and laryngeal muscles and later the trunk and lower extremities. However, many patients have weaknesses beginning in the legs. Intellectual capacity remains unaffected, and patients generally remain in control of bowel and bladder functions. The average patient survives about 3 years after diagnosis, although some patients live 10 years or longer. Death is generally caused by respiratory failure, although long-term ventilatory therapy can prolong life. Treatment is supportive and symptomatic, and attention must be given to family members who are caring for a chronically ill, progressively deteriorating loved one.

Extrapyramidal Syndromes

Extrapyramidal syndromes are disorders concerned with movement that result from lesions involving those parts of the brain other than the corticospinal pathways, principally the basal ganglia (see Chapter 50). More data are available about the clinical aspects of extrapyramidal dysfunction than about its pathophysiologic basis. Neurochemical changes seem to be involved in some cases.

Tremor

Tremor is an involuntary movement that results from an excess of neuronal activity in one area as a result of unopposed activity in another area. The tremor is most marked peripherally. It may be suppressed by will or with vigorous activity. In general, there are alternating contractions of the flexor and extensor muscle groups, so movement is at right angles to the axis of the limb. The tremor of parkinsonism occurs at rest and temporarily disappears during voluntary activity. In contrast, a tremor caused by cerebellar deficiency is an *intention tremor* and is increased with purposeful activity.

Rigidity

Rigidity is characteristic of Parkinson's disease and classically shows a relatively constant resistance to muscle stretching. Rigidity must be differentiated from *spasticity,* which occurs with pyramidal tract disorders (upper motor neuron lesions). In spasticity, resistance at first increases as the stretching or pulling force increases because more motor units are brought into play. Additional force will finally cause a sudden loss of resistance ("clasp knife" effect). In contrast, rigidity produces a smooth, constant resistance to forceful stretching because, although the stretching causes some motor units to fire, motor units fall out as readily as others are recruited by the external force.

Chorea

Chorea refers to movements that are sudden, random, and involuntary. Fragments of purposeful movement are apparent, but normal progression is lacking and the movements are disorganized. Chorea may be generalized, as in Huntington's disease, or lateralized.

A *lateralized chorea* is seen with lesions in the ventrolateral thalamus or subthalamic nucleus. Occlusion of a penetrating branch of the posterior cerebral artery results in an infarct of the thalamic area and is often the basis of the hemichorea.

Chorea may involve proximal or distal extremities, face, head, and trunk. In some patients, speech and mastication are affected. The involuntary movements in the limbs may make walking and purposeful movement of the hands difficult. Choreiform movements tend to be aggravated by physical activity and environmental stimuli but may disappear during sleep.

The pathology in chorea involves extensive areas of the nervous system, most notably degeneration of the corpus striatum and the cerebral cortex. The pathophysiology in chorea may be related to an increased (or altered) response of striatal dopamine receptors. This hypersensitivity hypothesis is supported by biochemical and pharmacologic data. Levodopa (L-dopa) can cause an increase or exacerbation of chorea; neuroleptic drugs can decrease or ameliorate the abnormal movements, supposedly by competing with dopamine at the receptor sites.

Athetosis

Athetosis is marked by involuntary movements combined with instability of posture. It is evidenced by slow, rhythmic, writhing, wormlike movements that usually occur in the peripheral parts of the upper extremities, especially the fingers and hands. The face, neck, tongue, lips, and lower extremities may be affected. Attempts to perform a voluntary activity and emotional stimuli cause an exaggeration of the abnormal movements. Coordinated activity is not possible in the affected muscle groups.

The globus pallidus, putamen, and possibly the corpus striatum are involved in the pathology of athetosis. Hypoxia at birth is a causative factor in some cases; others are related to kernicterus, in which the unconjugated bilirubin is taken up by lipid-rich brain tissue (especially the basal ganglia, thalamus, cerebellum, and cerebral gray matter) and causes damage (see Chapter 27). Four types of *cerebral palsy* (a popular term referring to a motor dysfunction that is congenital or acquired during infancy) are identified: cerebral spastic diplegia (legs affected more than arms), the hemiplegic variety, double athetosis *(choreoathetosis),* and ataxic. Clinical manifestations often overlap. Cerebral palsy may be, but is not always, associated with mental retardation, disorders of perception and higher sensory function, and seizure disorders.

Dystonia

Dystonia is closely related to athetosis, differing only in that the larger axial muscles rather than the appendicular muscles are involved. Bizarre or grotesque postures of the limbs or trunk from excessive muscle tone are noted. Voluntary movement is seriously impaired, and sometimes the entire musculature of the body may be thrown into spasm by an effort to move an arm or leg or to speak. The pathology seems to involve the putamen and thalamus. Surgical lesions made in the ventrolateral thalamus may produce improvement.

Hemiballismus

Hemiballismus is the involuntary, violent movement of a large body area (entire leg, shoulder, pelvic girdle). It usually involves only one side of the body. Attempting a normal activity may invoke a ballistic movement instead. This syndrome is believed to be caused by extensive lesions of the subthalamic nuclei, usually secondary to hemorrhage or, less often, an infarct or a tumor. Death occurs in 4 to 6 weeks in 60% of patients and is generally the result of exhaustion, pneumonia, or congestive heart failure. The recent use of neuroleptics (dopamine antagonists), such as haloperidol and chlorpromazine, has improved the survival rate.

Parkinsonism

Parkinsonism is a syndrome characterized by rhythmic tremors, bradykinesia, rigidity of muscles, and loss of postural reflexes. The movement disorder results primarily from a defect in the dopaminergic (dopamine-producing) pathway that connects the substantia nigra to the corpus striatum (caudate and lenticular nuclei). (See basal ganglia in Figure 50-22.) The basal ganglia are part of the extrapyramidal system; influence the initiation, modulation, and completion of movement; and regulate automatic movements.

Parkinsonism is the most common disorder involving the extrapyramidal system, and several causes exist. The vast majority of cases are considered to be of unknown cause or idiopathic. *Idiopathic parkinsonism* is referred to as *Parkinson's disease* or *paralysis agitans.* Parkinson's disease affects more than one-half million Americans and is a leading cause of disability. It is a slowly progressive disease of middle or late life, with onset typically during the fifth and sixth decades. There is no apparent genetic cause and no known cure.

Parkinsonian symptoms, to a greater or lesser degree, accompany several other conditions that structurally damage the nigrostriatal pathway or interfere with the action of dopamine within the basal ganglia. *Postencephalic parkinsonism* was a common sequelae of an encephalitis (von Economo's disease) that occurred between 1918 and 1925; studies indicate that an influenza A virus may

have been responsible. *Drug-induced parkinsonism* may be a side effect of certain antipsychotic drugs, such as phenothiazines and butyrophenones (postsynaptic dopamine receptor blockers). Another type of dopamine receptor blocker, metoclopramide (useful for gastrointestinal disturbances), can also precipitate parkinsonism. Reserpine (an antihypertensive drug) is a presynaptic dopamine depleter that occasionally induces parkinsonism. Drug-induced parkinsonism is usually reversible when the drugs are discontinued, although some patients remain symptomatic for weeks to years. The use of an illicit designer drug, 1-methyl-4-phenyl-1,2,3,6-tetrahydropine (MPTP) induces parkinsonism by selectively destroying dopaminergic neurons of the substantia nigra. Parkinsonism is also associated with poisoning by heavy metals (lead, manganese, mercury) and carbon monoxide.

Major pathologic changes in Parkinson's disease involve the loss of dopamine-containing neurons in the substantia nigra and other pigmented nuclei. Many of the remaining neurons contain Lewy bodies (eosinophilic cytoplasmic inclusions). The loss of dopamine-containing neurons in the substantia nigra leads to a severe reduction of dopamine in nerve terminals of the nigrostriatal tract. The reduction of dopamine in the corpus striatum upsets the normal balance between dopamine (inhibitory) and acetylcholine (excitatory) neurotransmitters and underlies most of the symptoms in Parkinson's disease.

Although these pathologic changes are well known, the basic question concerning what triggers the nigrostriatal pathologic changes and concomitant neurochemical alterations remains unanswered. No convincing evidence supports a viral pathogenesis. The finding that MPTP, a meperidine derivative, produces parkinsonism that is clinically indistinguishable from idiopathic Parkinson's disease has generated renewed interest in exogenous toxins. Possible toxic agents in well water and agricultural pesticides have been proposed but not yet confirmed.

Clinical manifestations. The cardinal signs of parkinsonism are rigidity, tremor (especially at rest), akinesia or bradykinesia, and loss of postural reflexes. The dysfunction is chronic and progressive but with wide variation of symptoms among patients.

Rigidity may be isolated to one muscle group and primarily unilateral or may be widespread and bilateral. It decreases muscle strength and speed and is a major factor in the deformities associated with the syndrome. Passive movement of the involved limbs or trunk meets with a taffylike resistance that is relatively constant throughout the range of motion. It has been compared with bending a lead pipe and is sometimes called *lead-pipe rigidity.* "Catches" often occur during passive movement, giving a cogwheel or rachetlike character to the rigidity called *cogwheel rigidity.* Both flexor and extensor muscles are tightly contracted *(increased tonus),* indicating impaired control of opposing muscle groups.

When the rigidity involves the trunk, it is largely responsible for the gait and postural problems associated with parkinsonism. Patients stoop when they stand so that the chin is farther forward than the toes. They walk in shuffling, hasty, accelerating steps, as if stumbling forward and trying to hurry the feet back under them (*festinating gait*).

The tremor associated with parkinsonism occurs at rest and is called a *rest tremor*. When muscles are tensed to perform a purposeful act, the tremor usually stops. (About one third of patients have intention tremor along with rest tremor, but, as noted, intention tremors are generally associated with cerebellar dysfunction.) Tremors involving the hands are described as *pill rolling* and are the result of rhythmic movement of the thumb and first two fingers. Tremors are the result of regular alternating contractions (4 to 6 cycles/second) in antagonistic muscles. Tremors are likely to be worse when the patient is tired, under emotional stress, or focusing attention on the tremor. The basis for the tremor is not clear. Degeneration of the basal ganglia results in loss of inhibitory influence, and the increased feedback in various circuits may result in oscillation. Not every patient has an obvious tremor. If the patient incidentally has a cerebrovascular accident (CVA, stroke) and hemiplegia occurs, the tremor disappears on the paralyzed side.

Patients may experience either akinesia or bradykinesia. *Akinesia* is characterized by a decrease in spontaneous movement and difficulty in initiating spontaneous or new movements. *Bradykinesia* is characterized by an abnormal slowness in deliberate movement. Either symptom is very disabling and obvious when the patient attempts any voluntary activity such as walking, talking, or writing. Loss of associated movement is noted, for example, when the patient does not swing the arms while walking. The face is expressionless, and the voice is low and monotonous. Writing becomes progressively cramped and may reflect the tremor. *Micrographia* is the small handwriting that eventually trails off and cannot be deciphered. When automatic movement (normally unconscious) is performed consciously, much more work and energy are necessary. Thus patients with parkinsonism frequently complain of fatigue and muscle pain.

Secondary signs include gait disturbances, postural problems, and autonomic nervous system (ANS) disorders. Gait disturbances are characterized by increasing impairment of postural and righting reflexes. The patient cannot stop and turn quickly but turns *en bloc* rather than sequentially as a healthy person would. Because balance is poor, patients hurry along, trying to keep up with the center of gravity. They have difficulty in making adjustments to changes in position and tend to fall. Wheeled walkers may help prevent falls in some patients, although the conventional ones tend to roll away. A special autostop walker is currently available and is proving useful.

Autonomic manifestations of parkinsonism include sweating, oily skin accompanied frequently by seborrheic dermatitis, drooling, swallowing difficulties that lead to

TABLE 54-1	Major Neurologic Findings in Parkinson's Disease
Neurologic Finding	**Comment**
Rest tremor	Pill-rolling movement of fingers characteristic; tremor decreased with voluntary movement and during sleep
Masklike facies	Wide-eyed, unblinking, staring expression; blinks two or three times/minute (normal blinking, 12 to 20 times/minute)
Cogwheel rigidity	Motion interrupted by "catches"; resistance relatively constant throughout range of motion
Postural and gait abnormalities	Stooped, shuffling, festinating gait; unable to turn quickly, turns en bloc
Micrographia	Small handwriting that trails off; tremor may be obvious when drawing concentric circles
Monotone	Expressionless speech
Hyperactive glabellar (blink) reflex	Exaggerated sensitivity to finger tapping over glabella (between eyebrows) causes the patient to blink with each tap (it takes effort for a normal person to blink); early sign of Parkinson's disease

choking and gradually interfere with the ability to tolerate any oral feedings, constipation, and bladder problems, which are aggravated by anticholinergic drugs and prostatic hypertrophy.

Additional features of parkinsonism include the following:

- Oculomotor disorders: blurring convergence resulting from inability to sustain contraction of the ocular muscles
- Oculogyric crisis: spasms of the conjugate eye muscles, in which the eyes are fixed, usually in an upward gaze, for minutes to hours; associated with parkinsonism of exogenous etiology, such as drug induced or postencephalitic
- Extreme fatigue and muscle pain from muscles exhausted by rigidity
- Postural hypotension related to medication side effects as well as interference with blood pressure control mediated by the ANS
- Impaired respiratory function related to hypoventilation, inactivity, aspiration of food or saliva, and reduced airway clearance

Diagnosis. Diagnosis of parkinsonism is based on clinical findings. The key to making a diagnosis of true Parkinson's disease is a therapeutic response to levodopa (L-dopa). Other forms of parkinsonism involve degeneration of the neurons that formerly received the dopaminergic input and thus do not respond to L-dopa. Table 54-1 lists major neurologic features of the disease.

Treatment. Dopaminergic drugs are used to try to restore the balance between dopamine and acetylcholine. Dopamine does not cross the blood-brain barrier, but L-dopa, a metabolic precursor of dopamine, does cross it (see Fig. 50-3). However, L-dopa is largely decarboxylated in the periphery (stomach, liver, heart, kidneys), and only a small amount reaches the basal ganglia. Large doses are necessary to achieve results. To improve the efficiency of L-dopa, the drug was combined with a decarboxylase inhibitor that will not cross the blood-brain barrier. There is less breakdown of the drug in the peripheral tissues, so more is available to the brain and side effects are reduced. Sinemet (carbidopa and levodopa), approved in 1974, is available in the ratio of 1 part carbidopa to 10 parts levodopa. Therapy with these drugs is begun with small doses, which are gradually increased until symptoms disappear or side effects appear.

All patients on these drugs experience some side effects, including gastrointestinal (GI) effects such as nausea and vomiting (80% to 90% of patients lose weight). Administering the drug to patients after they have just eaten can reduce this side effect. Cardiac dysrhythmias, postural hypotension, and central nervous system (CNS) symptoms (nightmares, confusion, insomnia, hallucinations, depression) may also occur. Abnormal involuntary movements (dyskinesias) are bothersome and increase with long-term use of these drugs. These effects are dosage related, but decreasing the dosage often results in the return of the parkinsonism symptoms.

Despite progression of the disease, these drugs have maintained improvement in most patients for 5 to 10 years. Before these drugs were discovered, the average patient was totally disabled in about 9 years. After about 5 to 10 years, patients begin to experience an on-off phenomenon (sudden variation in response to drugs), which is believed to be related to a decrease of dopamine production that is outstripping the drug's replacement capacity.

Other drugs used in the treatment of parkinsonism include anticholinergics, antihistamines (which also have an anticholinergic action), and amantadine (a synthetic antiviral compound with dopaminergic effects used in the treatment of Asian influenza). These drugs are often used in combination with Sinemet (carbidopa and levodopa). The belladonna alkaloids atropine and scopolamine were the first centrally active anticholinergics used to treat parkinsonism but have been largely replaced by synthetic anticholinergics such as trihexyphenidyl (Artane) and benztropine (Cogentin). These drugs are used to block acetylcholine-stimulated nerve impulses, which lead to tremors, bradykinesia, and rigidity. Adverse effects include dry mouth, constipation, and urinary retention. The use of diphenhydramine (Benadryl) and other antihistamines is based on their central cholinergic blocking action. Dopamine agonists, such as bromocriptine (Parlodel), stimulate dopamine receptors left inactive when dopamine is in short supply. This drug works best early in treatment. Side effects include nausea, vomiting, headache, fatigue, lightheadedness, confusion, vertigo, and hypotension. The monamine oxidase B (MAO-B) inhibitor, selegiline (Eldepryl), is thought to block the activity of the brain enzyme MAO-B, which terminates the action of dopamine at synapses in the brain. In clinical trials this drug was found to prolong the effectiveness of L-dopa therapy in some patients; when given to patients with early symptoms, it appears to delay the onset of more disabling symptoms. Vitamin E therapy is also under investigation. Some evidence suggests that it may slow the biochemical oxidative activity that is toxic to brain cells in Parkinson's disease.

Surgical lesions (using stereotaxic techniques) made in the globus pallidus or ventrolateral thalamus may be a successful treatment in selected patients with parkinsonism. Rigidity may decrease, but there is no effect on the akinesia. Many patients do not benefit from surgery; this treatment is best reserved for those who do not respond to drug treatment, who have unilateral involvement and normal blood pressure, and who are relatively young. Experimental fetal tissue implantation shows promise, but the technique and the research are plagued by ethical considerations.

These therapies, along with physical and occupational therapy, help maintain function for a longer period than was previously possible. One must remember, however, that parkinsonism is a chronic, progressive disease that gradually causes severe disability.

Demyelinating Diseases

A large number of neurologic diseases are termed *demyelinating diseases* because their common pathologic feature is focal areas of destruction involving the myelin sheath of nerve fibers in the CNS. The axon often is damaged as well, but destruction of myelin is the primary change. Multiple sclerosis is the primary demyelinating disease and is the focus of this discussion.

Acute disseminated encephalomyelitis

Acute disseminated encephalomyelitis (postvaccinial or postinfectious), although rare, is a demyelinating disorder that deserves mention because it is essentially preventable. This is an acute encephalitic or myelitic process of variable course characterized by symptoms that indicate damage to the white matter of the brain or spinal cord. The pathologic findings consist of numerous circumscribed areas of perivascular demyelinization. About 1 week after measles and 10 days to 2 weeks after vaccination for rabies or smallpox, neurologic symptoms develop rapidly. These symptoms consist of headache, drowsiness, stupor, ocular palsies, and often a flaccid paralysis of all four limbs caused by a transverse cord lesion. Variations in severity are common.

Postvaccination encephalomyelitis may occur after rabies vaccination, presumably from sensitization to vaccine containing brain tissue. This type is essentially an allergic encephalitis and does not occur with the use of the newer duck embryo vaccines, which are free of nerve tissue. Encephalomyelitis may also follow smallpox vaccination, especially the primary vaccination, but the source of the material used for the vaccination seems to have little bearing on its occurrence. The incidence is estimated to be 1 in 5000 vaccinations. The recent decision not to include smallpox vaccination as part of the routine pediatric immunization program in the United States should decrease the incidence of this complication.

Postinfectious encephalomyelitis that develops after a viral infection, especially measles, occurs in about 1 in 1000 cases. The mortality rate is 10% to 20%, and about 50% of those who survive are left with some neurologic damage. The use of measles vaccine in the United States has greatly reduced the occurrence of encephalomyelitis. Some evidence indicates that the measles virus may play a role in the etiology of multiple sclerosis.

Multiple sclerosis

Multiple sclerosis (MS) is one of the most common neurologic disorders affecting young people. It is slightly more common in women. The mean age of occurrence is 30 years, with a range between 18 and 40 in most patients. It is characterized by the widespread occurrence of patches of myelin destruction followed by gliosis in the white matter of the CNS. The hard yellow plaques found on autopsy are responsible for its being so named. The characteristic course of MS is a series of isolated attacks that affect different parts of the CNS. Each attack subsequently shows some degree of remission, but the overall picture is one of deterioration.

Etiology and pathology. The fundamental nature of the disturbance that leads to MS is unknown and is consequently the subject of much speculation. The illness is more common in temperate climates (northern Europe, northern United States), with an incidence of 10 per 100,000 population, and it is rare in the tropics; in Japan, however, MS occurs infrequently at any latitude. There is also a slightly higher familial incidence of the disease: it is about eight times more common in close relatives of a person with MS than in the general population. Whether this increased familial occurrence is caused by a genetic predisposition (a hereditary pattern does not exist) or whether there is common exposure to an infectious agent (probably viral) during childhood, which in some way may lead to MS during early adulthood, is unknown. Migration studies reveal that if adults move from a high-risk to a low-risk area, they retain the high risk for developing MS. However, a person who emigrates before the age of 15 years acquires the low risk of the second residence. These data are consistent with a possible viral cause with a long latency period between initial exposure and clinical onset of disease. The mechanism of action may be that of an autoimmune reaction attacking myelin.

A number of viruses have been proposed as possible causative agents in MS. The measles (rubeola) virus is suspected by some investigators. Various measles antibodies have been found in the serum and cerebrospinal fluid (CSF) of patients with MS, and evidence suggests that these antibodies are produced in the brain. If the measles virus is involved, it probably invades the subject in early life, lies dormant for a number of years, and then stimulates an autoimmune response. Another theory suggests that certain genetic factors render some people more susceptible to CNS invasion by various "slow" viruses. Slow viruses have long incubation periods and possibly develop only in conjunction with an abnormal or deficient immune status. Certain histocompatibility antigens (HLA-A3, HLA-A7) have been found to be more common in MS patients than in control subjects. The presence of these antigens may be related to a deficient immunologic defense against viral infection. Other researchers are attempting to find a relationship between MS in humans and distemper in dogs and cats. In one dramatic case, a family dog with the neurologic disease distemper recovered, but later three family members began to exhibit symptoms of MS. Many view such supposed precipitating situations as having occurred by pure chance.

Several events are generally considered to be precipitating factors, among them pregnancy, infection (especially with fever), emotional stress, and injury. Complete recovery is usual after the first attack. Remission usually occurs within 1 to 3 months with successive attacks. Eventually, however, recovery is not complete, and patients are left with additional permanent damage after each bout.

The lesions of MS occur only in the white matter of the CNS. Autopsy examination shows that the lesions are most prominent in the pyramidal tracts and posterior columns of the cord, around the ventricles of the brain, in the optic nerve and tract, in the brain stem and cerebellar peduncles, and around large veins. In the acute phase the involved area is edematous, inflamed, and pinkish in color. The size may vary from a few millimeters to several centimeters in diameter. Macrophages remove the areas of degenerating myelin, and as the acute phase subsides, a reactive gliosis develops. The end result is a shrunken area of demyelination called a *plaque.* The axon cylinders and cell bodies are not destroyed, although the scar is capable of damaging the underlying axon fiber so that nerve fiber conduction is disrupted. The symptoms of MS caused by the demyelinization become irreversible as the condition progresses.

Clinical features. The location of the lesions determines the clinical manifestations of MS. Any combination of the following signs and symptoms may coexist:

1. *Sensory disorders.* Paresthesias (numbness, tingling, "dead" feeling, "pins and needles") may vary in degree from one day to the next. If there is a lesion of the posterior columns of the cervical cord, flexion of the neck causes shocklike sensations to run down the cord (Lhermitte's sign). Proprioceptive disorders often give rise to sensory ataxia and incoordination of the arms.

Vibration sense is often diminished. Because sensory disorders cannot be demonstrated objectively, these symptoms may be thought to be hysterical.

2. *Visual complaints.* Many patients experience visual problems as an initial symptom. Diplopia (double vision) is often reported, as well as blurred vision and abnormal visual fields with blind spots (scotomas) in one or both eyes. Vision may be totally lost in one eye for several hours to days. An optic neuritis is the basis for these visual disturbances. Diplopia from brain stem lesions affecting the nuclei or fiber tracts of the extraocular muscles and nystagmus are other common complaints.

3. *Spastic weakness of the limbs.* Weakness of a limb on one side of the body or an asymmetric distribution in all four limbs is a common complaint. The patient may complain of tiredness and heaviness in one leg and noticeably drags that foot and has poor control. The patient may complain that the leg jumps spontaneously, especially when in bed. More profound spasticity is accompanied by painful spasm of the muscles. The tendon reflexes may be hyperactive and abdominal reflexes absent; the plantar responses are extensor (Babinski's sign). These signs indicate involvement of the corticospinal pathways.

4. *Cerebellar signs.* Nystagmus (rapid oscillation of the eyeball horizontally or vertically) and cerebellar ataxia are other common symptoms and indicate involvement of the cerebellar and corticospinal tracts. Cerebellar ataxia is manifested by uncoordinated voluntary movements, intention tremors, balance disturbances, and dysarthria (scanning speech with words broken into syllables and pauses between syllables).

5. *Bladder dysfunction.* Lesions in the corticospinal tracts often cause disorders of sphincter control; hesitancy, urgency, and frequency are common and indicate a reduced-capacity spastic bladder. Acute retention and incontinence also occur.

6. *Disorders of mood.* Many patients develop euphoria—an unrealistic feeling of well-being. This feeling is believed to be caused by involvement of the white matter of the frontal lobes. Other signs of cerebral impairment may include loss of memory and dementia.

Diagnosis, prognosis, and treatment. Diagnosis of MS is usually made on the basis of a history of neurologic episodes that cannot be related to a single lesion of the CNS and are characterized by relapses and remissions. Plaques may sometimes be visualized by magnetic resonance imaging (MRI), and this finding, along with the history, can establish the diagnosis. The gamma-globulin level in the CSF is elevated in about 60% of patients with established MS, but this is not helpful in establishing an early diagnosis. One test helpful in determining the presence of acute demyelinization is the basic protein assay (BPA) of the CSF. The BPA level drops rapidly after acute exacerbation subsides (Antel, Arnason, 1991).

Progression of MS is extremely variable. The classic picture is one of intermittent relapses followed by more or less complete remission. Remission is less complete with each ensuing exacerbation, and thus within 10 to 20 years the patient is significantly disabled. Severe disability occurs within a few years in a rare, malignant form of the disease.

Treatment of MS is symptomatic. During an acute relapse the patient rests, although complete bedrest is avoided. Adrenocorticotropic hormone (ACTH) or glucocorticoids are used during the acute phase to hasten remission. The benefits of drug therapy are difficult to evaluate because of the episodic nature of the disease and are probably nonspecific or based on their antiinflammatory action. Immunosuppressive agents and plasmapheresis have been reported to be helpful in stabilizing patients and slowing deterioration. Patients experience alterations in all functions: vision, mobility and coordination, nutrition, elimination, and communication. Care of the patient with MS requires a total health care team approach.

MOTOR SYSTEM DISORDERS WITH PREDOMINANT LOWER MOTOR NEURON SIGNS

Myasthenia Gravis

The name *myasthenia gravis* means "grave muscle weakness." It is the only neuromuscular disease that incorporates both rapid fatigue of voluntary muscle and prolonged recovery time (recovery may actually take 10 to 20 times longer than normal). Mortality rates in the past have been as high as 90%. The death rate has been reduced drastically since medications and respiratory care units have become available.

The clinical syndrome was first described in 1600. In the late 1800s myasthenia gravis was distinguished from muscle weakness caused by true bulbar palsy. In the 1920s a physician with myasthenia gravis noticed an improvement after taking ephedrine for menstrual cramps. Finally, in 1934, another physician from England (Mary Walker) noted the similarity of symptoms in myasthenia gravis and curare poisoning. She used the curare antagonist physostigmine for myasthenia gravis and observed marked improvement.

The incidence of myasthenia gravis in the United States is cited as 4 in 10,000 population. The peak age of onset is 20 years, with the ratio of women/men being 3:1. A second peak, although lower than the first, occurs in older men in their 50s and 60s.

Mortality generally results from respiratory insufficiency, although with improvements in respiratory intensive care, this complication is becoming more manageable. Spontaneous remission may occur in 10% to 20% of patients and can be induced in selected patients by elective thymectomy. Young women who are in the early stages of the disease (first 5 years after onset) and do not respond well to drug therapy benefit most from this procedure.

Pathophysiology

Skeletal or striated muscles are innervated by large myelinated nerves that originate in the anterior horn cells of the spinal cord and the brain stem. They send their axons out in the spinal or cranial nerves to the periphery. Individual nerves branch many times and are capable of stimulating up to 2000 skeletal muscle fibers. The combination of the motor nerve and the muscle fibers it innervates is called a *motor unit.* Although each motor neuron innervates many muscle fibers, each muscle fiber is innervated by a single motor neuron.

The area of specialized contact between the motor nerve and the muscle fiber is called the *neuromuscular synapse* or *junction* (Fig. 54-1). The neuromuscular junction is a chemical synapse between a nerve and muscle consisting of three basic components: a presynaptic element, a postsynaptic element, and a synaptic cleft about 200 Å wide between two elements. The presynaptic element consists of the axon terminal, which contains synaptic vesicles filled with the neurotransmitter acetylcholine. Acetylcholine is synthesized and stored in the axon terminal (bouton). The plasma membrane of the axon terminal is called the *presynaptic membrane.* The postsynaptic element consists of the *postsynaptic membrane* (postjunctional membrane), or *motor end-plate,* of the muscle fiber. The postsynaptic membrane is formed by an invagination, called the *synaptic gutter* or *trough,* of the muscle membrane or sarcolemma into which the axon terminal protrudes. It has many folds (subneural clefts), which greatly increase the surface area. The postsynaptic membrane contains acetylcholine receptors and is capable of generating an end-plate potential, which in turn can generate a muscle action potential. Acetylcholinesterase, an enzyme that destroys acetylcholine, is also located in the postsynaptic membrane. The *synaptic cleft* refers to the space between the presynaptic and postsynaptic membranes. The space is filled with a gelatinous material through which extracellular fluid may diffuse.

When a nerve impulse reaches the neuromuscular junction, the presynaptic axon terminal membrane is depolarized, causing the release of acetylcholine into the synaptic cleft. The acetylcholine diffuses across the synaptic gap and unites with the acetycholine receptor sites in the postsynaptic membrane. This combination causes a change in permeability to both sodium and potassium in the postsynaptic membrane. The sudden influx of sodium ions and efflux of potassium ions lead to depolarization of the end-plate known as the *end-plate potential* (EPP). When the EPP reaches threshold, it generates an action potential in the nonjunctional muscle membrane, which is propagated along the sarcolemma. This action potential sets off a series of reactions, resulting in the contraction of the muscle fiber. Once transmission across the neuromuscular junction has occurred, acetylcholine is destroyed by the enzyme acetylcholinesterase. In normal persons the amount of acetylcholine released is more than sufficient to result in an action potential.

In myasthenia gravis, neuromuscular conduction is impaired. The number of normal acetylcholine receptors is

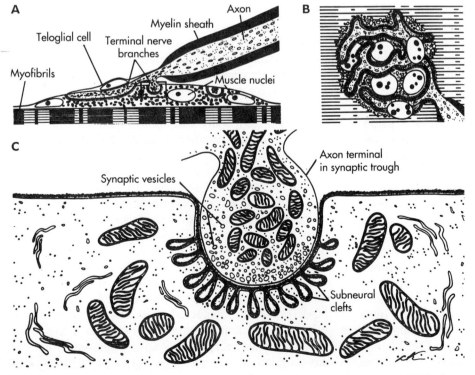

FIG. 54-1   Muscle and neuromuscular junction. Schematic representation of the motor end-plate as seen by light and electron microscopy. **A,** End-plate as seen in histologic sections in the long axis of the muscle fiber; **B,** as seen in surface view with the light microscope; **C,** as seen in an electron micrograph of an area such as that in the rectangle in **A.** (From Curtis B, Jacobson S, Marcus E: *An introduction to the neurosciences,* Philadelphia, 1972, Saunders.)

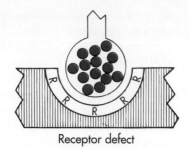
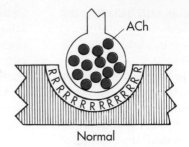

Normal   Receptor defect

FIG. 54-2   Defect in myasthenia gravis. Schematic representation of normal neuromuscular junction and one with a receptor deficit seen in myasthenia gravis. *ACh,* Acetylcholine; *R,* acetylcholine receptors. Circles indicate ACh-containing vesicles within nerve endings.

reduced, which is thought to be the result of an autoimmune injury. Antibodies to the acetylcholine receptor protein have been found in the serum of many myasthenia gravis patients. Determining whether this is a primary or secondary consequence of receptor damage caused by an unknown primary agent will be of great value in determining the exact pathogenesis of myasthenia gravis. Fig. 54-2 illustrates the probable defect in myasthenia gravis (Drachman, 1994).

In patients with myasthenia gravis the muscles appear normal macroscopically, although disuse atrophy may be present. Atrophy present results from disuse. Microscopically, in some patients lymphocytic infiltrates may be found within the muscle and other organs but no consistent abnormality is found in the skeletal muscle.

Clinical manifestations

As mentioned previously, it is currently hypothesized that myasthenia gravis is an autoimmune disorder that impairs acetylcholine receptor functioning and decreases the efficiency of the neuromuscular junction. It most frequently presents as an insidious, progressive disease characterized by muscle weakness and fatigability. However, it may remain localized to a specific group of muscles. Because the course is so variable from one patient to another, it is difficult to determine the prognosis. The box at right presents the hallmarks of the disease.

In 90% of patients, the initial symptoms involve the ocular muscles, causing ptosis and diplopia. The diagnosis can be established by attention to the levator palpebrae muscles of the eyelids. If the disease remains confined to the eye muscles, the course is very mild and is not associated with increased mortality.

The facial, laryngeal, and pharyngeal muscles are also frequently involved in myasthenia gravis. This involvement may result in regurgitation through the nose when swallowing is attempted (palatal muscles); abnormal, nasal speech; and failure of the mouth to close, which is termed the *hanging jaw sign.* With facial muscle involvement, a snarl-like appearance may be present when the individual attempts to smile.

Respiratory muscle involvement is evidenced by a weak cough, eventual attacks of dyspnea, and inability to clear mucus from the tracheobronchial tree. The shoulder and pelvic girdles may become involved in advanced

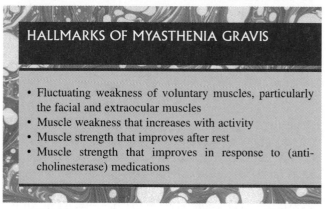

HALLMARKS OF MYASTHENIA GRAVIS

- Fluctuating weakness of voluntary muscles, particularly the facial and extraocular muscles
- Muscle weakness that increases with activity
- Muscle strength that improves after rest
- Muscle strength that improves in response to (anticholinesterase) medications

From National Nurses Advisory Board, National Myasthenia Gravis Foundation: *Myasthenia gravis: manual for the nurse,* Chicago, Ill, 1990, Author.

cases; generalized weakness of any skeletal muscles may occur. Standing, walking, or even holding the arms above the head as to comb the hair may become difficult.

Generally, symptoms of myasthenia gravis are relieved by rest and anticholinesterase agents. Symptoms are aggravated or exacerbated by (1) alterations in hormonal balance, as during pregnancy, fluctuations in the menstrual cycle, or disturbances in thyroid function; (2) concurrent illness, especially upper respiratory tract infections and those associated with diarrhea and fever; (3) emotional upsets—most patients experience more muscular weakness when they are upset; and (4) alcohol (especially with tonic water, which contains quinine, a drug promoting muscle weakness) and other drugs.

Diagnosis

A diagnosis can be made on the basis of the patient's history and the physical examination. One must acknowledge the reality of myasthenia gravis. Many patients have been bluntly told to see a psychiatrist because their symptoms have a psychologic basis only. Asking the subject to perform a repetitive action until tiredness is evident can help establish a diagnosis. Electromyography (EMG) reveals a characteristic falling off in the amplitude of motor unit potential with continued use. Measurement of antireceptor antibodies in plasma or in muscle biopsies also helps in making the diagnosis. The diagnosis is confirmed by the *Tensilon test.* Edrophonium chloride (Tensilon), a cholinesterase inhibitor drug, is given intravenously. In myasthenia patients, there is a marked improvement of muscle strength within 30 seconds. When a positive result is obtained, it is important to make a differential diagnosis between true myasthenia gravis and myasthenic syndrome. Patients with *myasthenia syndrome* have the same symptoms as those with true myasthenia gravis, but the cause is related to other pathologic processes, such as diabetes, thyroid abnormalities, and widespread malignancy. The age of onset of the two conditions is an important distinguishing factor. Patients with true myasthenia gravis are usually young, whereas those with myasthenic syndrome tend to be older. Symptoms in the myasthenic syndrome usually disappear if the basic disease can be controlled.

Abnormalities of the thymus gland occur in myasthenia gravis. Even when too small to be radiologically observable, the thymus glands of most patients are histologically abnormal. The tendency is for younger women to have thymic hyperplasia, whereas older men have thymic neoplasms.

Treatment

If the patient survives for 10 years, the disease usually remains benign, and death from myasthenia gravis itself would be rare. These patients must learn to live within the limits prescribed by their disease. They need 10 hours of sleep at night to awaken refreshed, and they need to alternate work and rest periods. They must avoid precipitating factors and must take their medications on time.

Medical treatment with *anticholinesterase drugs* is the treatment of choice. Neostigmine inactivates or destroys cholinesterase, so the acetylcholine is not destroyed immediately. The effect is restoration to almost normal muscular activity, at least 80% to 90% of former strength and endurance. Besides neostigmine (Prostigmin), pyridostigmine (Mestinon), and ambenonium (Mytelase), other synthetic analogs of the originally used drug, physostigmine (Eserine), are used. Disagreeable side effects in the GI tract (cramping, diarrhea) are called *muscarinic side effects.* It is important for the patient to realize that these symptoms can indicate too much medication has been taken on a particular day and that the next dose must be decreased accordingly to avoid a cholinergic crisis. Because neostigmine is the most apt to cause muscarinic effects, it may be prescribed initially so that the patient is made aware of exactly what this side effect is like.

Pyridostigmine is available in a time span form and is often used at bedtime so that the patient can sleep through the night without having to awaken to take medication. Corticosteroid therapy is associated with clinical improvement in many patients, although many serious side effects are associated with long-term use. Some patients respond well to a combined regimen of corticosteroids and pyridostigmine. Azathioprine, an immunosuppressive drug, is being used with good results; side effects are minor when compared with those associated with corticosteroids and consist mainly of GI upset, liver enzyme elevation, and leukopenia. Plasma exchange may be effective in myasthenic crisis because of its ability to remove antibodies to the acetylcholine receptors, but it is not useful in the chronic management of the disease.

Crisis in myasthenia gravis

When unable to swallow, clear secretions, or breathe adequately without artificial assistance, the myasthenic patient is in crisis. The two types of crises are (1) *myasthenic crisis,* a condition in which the patient needs more anticholinesterase drugs and (2) *cholinergic crisis,* a condition caused by an excess of anticholinesterase drugs. In either situation, ventilation and an adequate airway must be maintained. Tensilon (2 to 5 mg) is given intravenously as a test to differentiate between the types of crises. The drug produces a temporary improvement in myasthenic crisis and no improvement or worsening of symptoms in cholinergic crisis.

If in myasthenic crisis, the patient is maintained on the respirator. Anticholinesterase drugs are withheld because they increase respiratory secretions and may precipitate a cholinergic crisis. Medicines are restarted gradually, and often the dose can be lowered after a crisis.

In a cholinergic crisis, the patient may have taken an excess of medication by mistake or the dosage may have been excessive because of a spontaneous remission. Many who develop this type of crisis are called *brittle myasthenics.* They are difficult to control with medication and have a narrowed therapeutic range between underdose and overdose. Their response to drugs is often only partial. In cholinergic crisis, the patient is maintained on artificial ventilation, anticholinergic drugs are withheld, and 1 mg of atropine may be given intravenously and repeated if necessary. When atropine is administered, the patient must be carefully observed because respiratory secretions can thicken, making suctioning difficult, or a mucus plug can occlude a bronchus, causing atelectasis.

Guillain-Barré Syndrome

Guillain-Barré syndrome *(acute demyelinating polyneuropathy)* is an acute, primarily ascending motor paralysis with variable disturbances of sensory function. It is a lower motor neuron disorder in that the peripheral nerve, the final common pathway for motor movement, is involved. The syndrome, which is seen throughout the world, occurs in all seasons, similar to an endemic disease, and affects both genders and all age-groups. The incidence is approximately 3500 cases per year in the United States and Canada (Asbury, 1994). Attempts to isolate a causative infectious agent have been unsuccessful, and its cause remains unknown. The syndrome became well publicized in the United States in 1976 when an outbreak of more than 500 cases occurred during the national vaccination campaign against the swine influenza virus. Although there may be no known precipitating event, a careful patient history often reveals an unremarkable viral illness that occurred 1 to 3 weeks before the onset of motor weakness. Other typical preceding events are a mild respiratory or GI infection, surgery, immunizations, Hodgkin's disease or other lymphomas, and lupus erythematosus.

The neuropathies of Guillain-Barré syndrome result from an apparent autoimmune cellular reaction that specifically attacks the myelin sheath of peripheral nerves. The result is mild to severe demyelinating injury that interferes with impulse conduction in the affected peripheral nerves. (In contrast, the demyelination in MS is confined to the CNS.) Pathologic changes follow a consistent pattern: lymphocytic infiltrations occur in the perivascular spaces adjacent to the nerve and become the foci of myelin degeneration. In some cases the nerve axons themselves show evidence of wallerian degeneration, indicating a more proximal axonal lesion that has led to degeneration of the axon and myelin distal to it. The anterior horn cells of the spinal cord and the motor nuclei of the cranial nerves may become affected as the inflammation extends proximally from the peripheral nerve axons. If the nerve cell body is not destroyed, peripheral nerve regeneration may take place, with recovery of motor function. However, if the cell body of the lower motor neuron dies because of an aggressive inflammatory response, nerve regeneration cannot take place, affected muscles atrophy, and recovery is less complete. More than 80% of patients make a full or nearly complete recovery, which can take from a few weeks to several months, depending on the extent of myelin and axonal degeneration (Asbury, 1994).

Demyelination of peripheral nerve axons causes both positive and negative symptoms. The positive symptoms are pain and paresthesias arising from either abnormal impulse activity in sensory fibers or electrical "crosstalk" between damaged, abnormal axons. The negative symptoms are muscle weakness or paralysis, loss of tendon reflexes, and decreased sensation. The first two negative symptoms are caused by *motor* axon damage; the last results from *sensory* fiber damage. Three basic pathologic mechanisms are believed to underlie the negative symptoms: conduction block, slowed conduction, and impaired ability to conduct impulses at higher frequencies (Kandel, Schwartz, 1985).

In Guillain-Barré syndrome, sensory symptoms tend to be mild and may consist of pain, tingling, and numbness, as well as abnormalities in vibratory and position sense. However, the polyneuropathy is predominantly motor, and clinical findings may vary from mild muscular weakness to paralysis of the respiratory muscles requiring ventilatory management. Skeletal muscle weakness is often so acute that atrophy is not present, but loss of muscle tone and areflexia are readily detectable. Tenderness is usually elicited by deep pressure or squeezing of muscles. The arms may be spared, or their muscles may be less weakened than the leg muscles. Autonomic symptoms include postural hypotension, sinus tachycardia, and lack of ability to sweat. If cranial nerves are involved, paralysis of affected facial, ocular, and oropharyngeal muscles usually follows arm involvement. Cranial nerve symptoms include facial palsy and speech difficulties, visual disturbances, and swallowing difficulties. The term *bulbar palsy* is sometimes used to refer specifically to paralysis of the jaw, pharynx, and tongue musculature caused by damage to cranial nerves IX, X, and XI, which arise from the medulla oblongata, originally called the *bulb*.

Patient history and clinical findings of paralysis and paresthesias are especially important in diagnosing Guillain-Barré syndrome. Principal diagnostic tests are EMG, nerve conduction velocity, and lumbar puncture to examine the CSF. The CSF is under normal pressure and is acellular, although later in the course of the disease, high protein levels may be found. Body temperature is usually normal, and spleen and lymph node enlargement are not typical of this disease. Initial therapeutic management is supportive, with focus on support of ventilation, blood pressure, and cardiac function. Early plasmapheresis has been found to decrease the severity of symptoms. Intravenous administration of a high-dose immunoglobulin has also been beneficial, but glucocorticoid therapy has fallen into disuse because of lack of evidence of its efficacy. As soon as voluntary movement returns to skeletal muscles, intensive physiotherapy is initiated to prevent muscle and joint contractures.

Postpolio Syndrome

Postpolio syndrome, or *postpoliomyelitis neuromuscular atrophy,* is a progressive muscle weakness usually beginning 20 to 30 years after recovery from a viral poliovirus infection that attacked the anterior horn cells of the spinal cord, as well as cranial nerve nuclei. Symptoms are typical of a lower motor neuron paresis or paralysis: muscle pain, fasciculations, and muscle weakness that may reach a plateau or progress to muscle atrophy. The limbs are affected most often. However, the respiratory muscles may be involved, as well as head and neck muscles innervated by cranial nerves IX, X, and XI (bulbar paralysis). The result may be respiratory failure, severe sleep apnea, difficulty swallowing, episodes of choking, or aspiration. The cause of the long latent postpolio syndrome is controversial but usually is believed to involve an abnormality of surviving lower motor neurons, accompanied by a progressive, slow disintegration of peripheral nerve axons. Some evidence suggests that there is reactivation of latent or persistent poliovirus in the CNS (Ray, 1994). Treatment is supportive and directed toward maintaining respiratory function, alleviating symptoms, and preventing complications.

INFECTIOUS AND INFLAMMATORY DISORDERS

Infections of the central nervous system (CNS) constitute a serious medical problem requiring immediate recognition and treatment to minimize serious neurologic sequelae and ensure patient survival.

CNS infection by viruses occurs relatively infrequently but can be serious. Generally, viruses invade the CNS via the blood, although certain infections such as rabies and varicella-zoster invade the CNS via the peripheral nerves.

Signs and symptoms of viral CNS infections vary greatly according to the susceptibility of the different CNS cells to the virus. Infections limited to the meninges produce symptoms suggestive of meningitis (nuchal rigidity, headache, fever), whereas if the brain parenchyma is involved, the patient shows a decreased level of consciousness, seizures, focal neurologic deficits, and increased intracranial prcessure (ICP).

Viral Meningitis and Encephalitis

Viral meningitis is an infection involving the meninges; it tends to be benign and self-limiting. *Viral encephalitis* involves the brain parenchyma and is more serious. Various viruses are known to cause meningitis and encephalitis (see the box at right).

Viruses generally replicate themselves at the original site of infection (e.g., nasopharyngeal or GI systems), and then spread to the CNS via the vascular system. Contrary to previous thinking, the blood-brain barrier does not provide complete protection against the invasion of viruses. Encephalitis involves an inflammatory reaction of the brain parenchyma, causing degeneration and phagocytosis of neural cells.

Patients with viral meningitis present with abrupt onset of headache, fever, and nuchal rigidity; they may also experience malaise, sore throat, nausea, vomiting, and abdominal pain. In addition, viral meningitis caused by the enteroviruses is associated with rashes; mumps meningitis is associated with parotitis as well as oophoritis and pancreatitis. Type 2 herpes simplex meningitis may coincide with eruption of genital herpes lesions.

In addition to the meningeal signs, viral encephalitis presents with decreasing levels of consciousness, seizures, and focal symptoms, depending on the area of brain involved. Patients with herpes simplex encephalitis may show bizarre behavior and hallucinations.

In evaluating the patient with the signs and symptoms of viral meningitis and encephalitis, it is important to differentiate these diseases from other more treatable infections, such as subacute bacterial endocarditis or brain abscess. CSF pressure may be normal or elevated and may contain protein in small or large quantities; the electroencephalogram (EEG) may show changes, especially in en-

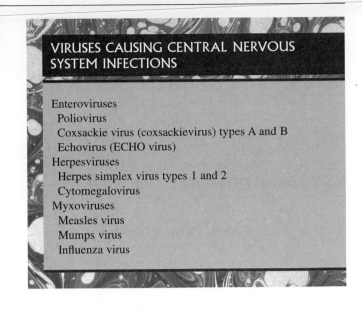

VIRUSES CAUSING CENTRAL NERVOUS SYSTEM INFECTIONS

Enteroviruses
  Poliovirus
  Coxsackie virus (coxsackievirus) types A and B
  Echovirus (ECHO virus)
Herpesviruses
  Herpes simplex virus types 1 and 2
  Cytomegalovirus
Myxoviruses
  Measles virus
  Mumps virus
  Influenza virus

cephalitis. Virologic studies can specifically identify the virus; this identification has become more important because herpes simplex encephalitis is currently treated with adenine arabinoside.

Other specific antiviral agents are not currently used, and patients are treated supportively. The prognosis is good for patients with meningitis but poorer for patients with encephalitis. Mortality rates vary from 50% in herpes simplex encephalitis to less than 1% in specific types of arbovirus encephalitis. Sequelae such as seizures, hydrocephalus, and other neurologic deficits are common.

Reye's Syndrome

Reye's syndrome is a rare, acute encephalitis and liver dysfunction seen in children and young adolescents after common viral infections. The children have a history of previous infection with influenza, varicella, adenovirus, coxsackievirus, echovirus, or parainfluenza virus, with apparent recovery from the original viral infection. It is now well accepted that a strong association exists between Reye's syndrome and the use of salicylates (aspirin) in children or adolescents with viral infections. The asymptomatic or recovery period in postviral infections varies from hours to days. Vomiting and convulsions followed by delirium and coma ensue after this apparent recovery.

Pathologically, the brain swells with injury to the neuronal mitochondria. Fatty infiltration of the liver occurs, spreading rapidly through the parenchyma. Fat deposits can also be found in the myocardium and renal tubules. The relationship between the viral infection and the encephalopathy and liver damage is unknown.

Coma and decerebrate posturing from increased intracranial pressure (ICP) are often seen. Electrolyte imbalances, especially hyponatremia, hypokalemia, and high serum ammonia levels, are serious problems. Treatment is nonspecific and is directed toward reducing ICP and correcting metabolic and electrolyte abnormalities.

Measures to control or reduce cerebral edema include hyperventilation and corticosteroids. Elevation of the head of the bed to approximately 30 degrees, hypothermia, and administration of intravenous mannitol are other means of reducing cerebral edema.

Hypertonic glucose solutions are used for hydration to maintain a blood sugar of 200 to 300 mg/dL, because low blood sugar leads to increased production of ammonia and fatty acids. Peritoneal dialysis has been used in some patients to reduce elevated blood ammonia levels.

Some children who recover have residual neurologic deficits, including impaired mental capacity, seizures, and hemiplegia. Mortality rates ranges from 25% to 50%, depending on factors such as age, severity of symptoms, and time of diagnosis and treatment.

Bacterial Infections

Bacterial infections of the CNS present a challenging problem. A variety of bacteria infect the meninges and brain parenchyma. The most common infecting bacteria are *Staphylococcus aureus*, *Streptococcus pneumoniae*, and *Haemophilus influenzae*. Isolation of the specific agent involved is essential in the treatment of bacterial CNS infections.

Bacteria enter the CNS by several different routes. The ears, sinus, mastoid, and face are the most common sites of the original infection. Bacteria are able to travel from the site of origin to the CNS because of the high vascularity of the face and neck and the anatomic structuring of the venous sinuses within the brain. Early and conscientious treatment of these primary infections significantly reduces the incidence of secondary CNS infections.

Brain abscess

Brain abscess is an infective process involving the brain parenchyma. It is caused primarily by the spread of an infection from adjacent foci or through the vascular system. A previous history of otitis media; mastoiditis; suppurative sinusitis; or infection of the face, scalp, or skull is common. Bronchiectasis, lung abscess, empyema, and bacterial endocarditis are also known to lead to brain abscess.

Infection may invade the brain several different ways. In otitis media the infection may extend through the tympanic cavity or through the mastoid and meninges to reach the brain tissue. The infection extends via the veins

TABLE 54-2 Focal Symptoms Seen in Brain Abscess

Lobe	Symptoms
Frontal	Drowsiness, inattentiveness, disturbed judgment, impaired intelligence, occasionally convulsions
Temporal	Inability to name objects; inability to read, write, or understand spoken words; hemianopia
Parietal	Impaired position sense and stereognostic perception, focal seizures, homonymous hemianopia, dysphasia, acalculia, agraphia
Cerebellar	Suboccipital headache, stiff neck, impaired coordination, nystagmus, impaired gait, intention tremor

of the inner ear, causing the veins to thrombose. This thrombosis impairs cerebral circulation, leading to ischemia and infarction, which facilitate the development of a local infection. Any tear in the dura caused by trauma is a potential source of infection of the brain.

Generally, abscesses are localized near the original site of infection. However, those resulting from retrograde venous propagation are located at some distance from the primary site in the distribution of the nearest venous sinus. Metastatic abscesses are generally located along the middle cerebral artery. Early in the course of the disease, the infected tissue is edematous and infiltrated with leukocytes. Gradually the outer portion becomes thickened because of the presence of collagen in the abscess wall. In the center of the abscess, liquefaction necrosis occurs. Abscess cavities can spread through the white matter, penetrating the walls of the ventricles or into the meninges.

Brain abscess most frequently occurs between the ages of 20 and 50 but has been found in all age-groups. The patient presents with headache and focal neurologic signs that vary with the location of the abscess (Table 54-2). Signs of increased ICP (especially nausea, vomiting, and decreasing level of consciousness) are the most common findings.

Generally a CT scan identifies and localizes the major abscess and surrounding smaller abscesses. Because of the danger of brain herniation, lumbar puncture is usually avoided when the presence of a large mass is suspected. Early diagnosis and prompt antibiotic therapy are essential if the patient is to survive. Residual neurologic deficits, especially convulsions, are common.

QUESTIONS

▼ *Answer the following on a separate sheet of paper.*

1. Name the sites in the brain that are affected in Parkinson's disease. How are these areas of the brain affected? Where are these areas located in the brain?

2. Name the type of fiber tract involved in Parkinson's disease. What is the general function of this fiber tract?

3. Define Parkinson's syndrome and name three types.

4. Discuss the role of dopamine in parkinsonism.

5. Name and briefly describe five movement disorders of the extrapyramidal motor tracts.

6. Name two drugs known to cause extrapyramidal dysfunction and parkinsonian signs and symptoms.

7. Name several neurologic findings (include one reflex) common in patients with Parkinson's disease.

8. What serious demyelinating disorder may follow measles or vaccination for rabies? How can this be prevented?

9. Describe the pathology in multiple sclerosis (MS). What are the most likely symptoms that would cause you to suspect MS in a patient?

10. List the major theories of the causes of Alzheimer's disease.

▼ *Circle the letter preceding each item below that correctly answers the question or completes the statement. Only one answer is correct, with exceptions noted.*

11. Which of the following is(are) a degenerative disease(s) of the nervous system?
    a. Brain abscess
    b. MS
    c. Amyotrophic lateral sclerosis
    d. Viral meningitis
    e. Wernicke-Korsakoff syndrome

12. The chief symptom complex of Parkinson's disease is:
    a. Rigidity, aphasia, and oculogyric crisis
    b. Hemiplegia, drooling, and tremor
    c. Tremor, rigidity, and weakness
    d. All the above

13. The preferred treatment for Parkinson's disease is:
    a. Medical treatment with L-dopa
    b. Surgical treatment of the older patient with bilateral disease
    c. Anticholinergic drugs
    d. Medical treatment with dopamine

14. Symptoms of Parkinson's disease include (more than one answer may be correct):
    a. Masklike face
    b. Intention tremor
    c. Bradykinesia
    d. Choreiform movements

15. The probable site of abnormality in athetosis is the:
    a. Neuromuscular junction
    b. Fifth cranial nerve
    c. Globus pallidus
    d. Motor cortex

16. In MS:
    a. Convulsions occur in about half the patients.
    b. Visual loss is generally unilateral.
    c. Headaches and aphasia are not unusual.
    d. Euphoria is an infrequent disturbance.

17. A patient who receives L-dopa should avoid taking large doses of:
    a. Thiamine (B_1)
    b. Pyridoxine (B_6)
    c. Cyanocobalamin (B_{12})
    d. Any of the B vitamins

18. MS is:
    a. Usually inherited
    b. Most common in tropical areas
    c. Often a familial disease
    d. Most common in the 20- to 40-year-old age group

19. Which of the following statements is *true* about myasthenia gravis?
    a. Ptosis of the eyelids is an infrequent symptom.
    b. By nature it is an acute disease common in cold climates.
    c. It is characterized by acetylcholine receptor deficiency at the junction of a motor nerve and skeletal muscle.
    d. Experimental evidence indicates that the parathyroid glands are involved in some way.

20. The only manifestations of myasthenia gravis are:
    a. Rigidity and tremor
    b. Flaccid and/or spastic paralysis of voluntary muscle
    c. Rapid fatigue of skeletal muscle and prolonged time for recovery of power
    d. Rapid fatigue of smooth muscle and prolonged time for recovery of power

21. Myasthenia gravis is often associated with disorders of the:
    a. Heart
    b. Thyroid
    c. Thymus
    d. Liver

22. Your patient has demonstrated a positive Tensilon test. Which of the following symptoms would indicate this result?
    a. Muscarinic effect on smooth muscle
    b. Immediate decrease in muscle strength
    c. Difficulty in keeping eyes open (ptosis)
    d. Immediate increase in muscle strength

23. Anticholinesterase drugs are used to treat myasthenia gravis. The most common side effects of these medications involve the:
    a. CNS
    b. Skeletal muscle
    c. GI tract
    d. Respiratory system

24. Which of the following is *not* used in the treatment of myasthenia gravis?
    a. Neostigmine
    b. Pyridostigmine
    c. Ambenonium
    d. Edrophonium

25. When a patient with myasthenia gravis is in crisis, the first consideration is to:
    a. Identify the type of crisis (cholinergic versus myasthenic)
    b. Control the hemorrage
    c. Establish an adequate airway
    d. Restore electrolyte balance

26. Signs and symptoms of Wernicke-Korsakoff syndrome include (more than one answer may be correct):
    a. Impairment of recent memory
    b. Postural hypotension
    c. Amnesia
    d. Anemia

27. Signs and symptoms of Alzheimer's disease include (more than one answer may be correct):
    a. Forgetfulness
    b. Cognitive rigidity
    c. Inability to cope with complex situations
    d. Bradykinesia
    e. Emotional lability

28. Which of the following are routes of entry of bacteria into the CNS?
    a. Ears
    b. Eyes

Continued.

QUESTIONS—cont'd

c. Nasal sinuses
d. Vascular system
e. All the above
29. Which of the following is(are) common in the previous history of patients with a brain abscess?
a. Otitis media
b. Face or scalp infection
c. Mastoiditis
d. Suppurative sinusitis
e. All the above
30. All the following are true statements concerning Guillain-Barré syndrome *except:*
a. It is an example of an upper motor neuron disease.
b. It involves demyelinization of peripheral nerves.
c. It is characterized by an ascending motor paralysis.
d. It may be helped by plasmapheresis early in the disease.
31. Which of the following statements about postpolio syndrome is *false?*
a. It involves an acute primary infection of the anterior horn cells of the spinal cord by the poliomyelitis virus.

b. It is characterized by progressive muscular paresis or paralysis 20 to 30 years after acute poliomyelitis.
c. It most often affects the limbs.
d. It may be caused by reactivation of the poliovirus in the CNS.

▼ *Circle T if the statement is true and F if it is false. Correct any false statements.*

32. T F Alzheimer's disease affects approximately 10% of the population over age 65.
33. T F Neurofibrillary tangles and senile plaques are unique to Alzheimer's disease.
34. T F Management of Alzheimer's disease involves the patient's family as well as the patient.
35. T F Metastatic brain abscesses are generally located along the middle cerebral artery.
36. T F Amyotrophic lateral sclerosis has been conclusively linked to arsenic toxicity.

37. T F Deficiencies of the B vitamins B_1, B_6, B_{12}, niacin, and pantothenic acid are associated with various neurologic disorders.
38. T F Niacin is accepted as the therapy of choice for patients with Wernicke-Korsakoff syndrome.
39. T F Viral meningitis is a viral infection involving the meninges; it tends to be benign and self-limiting.
40. T F Viral encephalitis involves the brain parenchyma and is potentially not a serious condition.
41. T F The blood-brain barrier provides complete protection against invasion by viruses.
42. T F Reye's syndrome is a rare acute encephalitis and liver dysfunction seen in children and young adolescents after common viral infections.
43. T F Fatty infiltration involves the liver, myocardium, and renal tubules in Reye's syndrome.

CHAPTER 55 Seizure Disorders

MARY CARTER LOMBARDO

Seizure disorders are relatively common neurologic problems and are the result of excessive paroxysmal discharge from a hyperexcitable population of neurons (the *epileptogenic focus*). They can also arise from normal brain tissue under certain pathologic conditions. The seizure itself is rarely damaging, but it can be a manifestation of a threatening underlying disorder such as metabolic derangement, intracranial infections, drug withdrawal, drug intoxication, or hypertensive encephalopathy. Depending on the location of these hyperexcitable neurons, the seizure is manifested as any combination of altered level of consciousness and disturbances in motor, sensory, or autonomic functions. The term *seizure* is generic, and other specific descriptions are applicable according to the characteristics observed. Seizures may be isolated or repetitive. Seizures spontaneously recurring over a span of years are termed *epilepsy*. Generalized motor seizures, involving loss of consciousness and some combination of tonic-clonic muscle contractions, are often called *convulsions*. Convulsive seizures typically produce severe, involuntary, skeletal muscle activity that may progress from one body part to the entire body or may occur suddenly, with total body involvement. *Status epilepticus* is a prolonged, continuous seizure or a series of repetitive seizures without interictal consciousness.

Data on seizure incidence are somewhat difficult to uncover. A frequently cited figure for epilepsy is 0.5% to 2% of the population. This figure, considered too conservative by many in the field, is estimated to be closer to 5% of the population. A greater percentage of persons have a seizure at least once in their lives; therefore higher rates are reported when isolated, nonrecurrent, and febrile seizures are included in the incidence. Gender-specific reports indicate slightly higher rates for males than females. Age-specific incidence shows a consistent pattern of the highest rate in the first year of life, a rapid decline toward adolescence, and a gradual leveling off during the remainder of life. More than 75% of patients with epilepsy have their first seizure before age 20; when the first seizure occurs after age 20, epilepsy is usually secondary. Epilepsy may be classified as idiopathic or symptomatic. In the *idiopathic,* or *essential, epilepsy,* no known cerebral lesion can be demonstrated. In *symptomatic,* or *secondary, epilepsy,* a cerebral abnormality promotes the seizure response. Among the many conditions that may be responsible for secondary epilepsy are head injuries (including those before and after birth), metabolic and nutritional disorders (hypoglycemia, phenylketonuria, vitamin B_6 deficiency), toxic factors (alcohol intoxication, narcotic withdrawal, uremia), encephalitis, hypoxia, circulatory disturbances, and neoplasms.

PATHOPHYSIOLOGY

Seizures result from excessive paroxysmal discharge either from an epileptogenic focus or from normal tissue under assault from a pathologic condition. The seizure activity depends partly on the location of the excessive discharge. Lesions in the midbrain, thalamus, and cerebral cortex are most likely to be epileptogenic, whereas lesions in the cerebellum and brain stem do not generally evoke seizures.

At the cell membrane level, certain biochemical phenomena characterize the epileptogenic focus, including the following:

- Instability of the nerve cell membrane, allowing the cell to be more susceptible to activation.

- Hypersensitive neurons with lowered thresholds for firing and firing excessively.
- Polarization abnormalities (excessive polarization, hypopolarization, or lapses in repolarization) caused by an excess of acetycholine or a deficiency of gamma-aminobutyric acid (GABA).
- Ionic imbalances that alter the chemical environment of the neuron. During a seizure the electrolyte balance at the neuronal level is altered. The imbalance causes the neuronal membrane to depolarize.

The metabolic changes that occur during and immediately after a seizure are caused in part by increased energy needs from the neuronal hyperactivity. Metabolic needs are drastically increased during convulsions; the electrical discharges of motor nerve cells may be increased to 1000/second. Cerebral blood flow is increased, as is tissue respiration and glycolysis. Acetycholine appears in cerebrospinal fluid (CSF) during and after seizures. Glutamic acid may be depleted during seizure activity.

Generally, no gross change is found at autopsy. Histopathologic evidence supports the hypothesis that the lesion is neurochemical rather than structural. No consistent pathologic factor has been identified. Focal abnormalities in the metabolism of potassium and acetylcholine are found to be present between seizures. Seizure foci seem especially sensitive to acetylcholine, a facilitatory transmitter; they are slow to bind and remove the acetylcholine.

TYPES OF SEIZURES

Each major clinical center for epilepsy uses the classification that works best for its purposes. Table 55-1 shows the classification (modified) adopted by the International League Against Epilepsy. Electroencephalographic study, clinical assessment, and history are used to identify the type of seizure.

The two major classes of epilepsy are *partial,* or *focal, seizures,* which begin in a specific area of the brain, usually the cerebral cortex, and the more common *generalized seizures,* presumably involving the entire cerebral cortex and diencephalon.

Partial seizures may present with elementary or complex symptoms. Partial seizures with elementary symptoms are focal attacks that involve motor or sensory symptoms. Jacksonian epilepsy is the most common form of this type of epilepsy, and generally the focus is located in the sensory or motor cortex. Psychomotor, or temporal lobe, epilepsy is an example of partial seizures with complex symptoms. Complex partial seizures involve disturbances in higher-level cerebral functions, such as memory and thought processes, as well as complex motor behavior, which is automatic. The epileptic focus for this type of epilepsy is often the temporal lobe. Both types of

partial seizure may spread and become generalized (major motor) seizures.

Jacksonian motor seizures are characterized by a focal onset thought to be caused by a lesion in the contralateral cortex. The seizure generally starts with either a tonic spasm or a clonic rhythmic twitching (e.g., of the fingers of one hand, face on one side). This disorder then spreads progressively, for example, from face to neck, hand, forearm, arm, trunk, and leg, all on one side of the body. Some patients experience progression to the opposite hemisphere with a loss of consciousness. It is extremely important to observe where the seizure begins, since this may offer a clue to location of the lesion.

Jacksonian seizures may also be sensory. The patient complains of transient abnormal sensations (e.g., numbness, crawling sensation, "pins and needles") that begin as focal phenomena and progressively spread to involve one side of the body. Usually some clonic movements are associated with the sensory seizure, since some motor representation exists in the sensory cortex.

Psychomotor (temporal lobe) seizures are characterized by transient mental disturbances and automatic, purposeless movements (e.g., clapping hands, smacking lips, chewing motions). Patients may have a clouded, "dreamy" feeling of unreality.

The patient is usually conscious during the attack but generally does not recall what has happened. Other behaviors associated with these seizures include sudden recollection of past events, hallucinations (visual or olfactory are common), forgetfulness, word-finding difficulty, personality change, antisocial behavior, and inappropriate moodiness. In the postictal (postseizure) period the patient may enter a fugue state in which complex and organized activities may be performed but not remembered (amnesia).

These attacks may be precipitated by music, blinking lights, and other stimuli. They may occur at any age but primarily occur in adults. Psychomotor seizures are often associated with small focal lesions in the anterior temporal lobe, especially in the hippocampal (uncinate) gyrus. They may also involve lesions outside the temporal lobe (in the insula, orbital cortex, anterior olfactory centers, and diencephalon). The involvement of these structures accounts for the fact that when an *aura* (warning symptoms of an impending seizure) occurs in psychomotor epilepsy, it often takes the form of a perceptual illusion, such as an unpleasant taste or smell.

Generalized seizures are characterized by the onset of bilateral, symmetric epileptic activity (not local). They include absences, or petit mal seizures, and the tonic-clonic, or grand mal, seizure.

Absence, or *petit mal, epilepsy* is characterized by short lapses of consciousness, rarely lasting more than a few seconds. For example, there may be a brief pause in conversation, a vacant look, or a rapid blinking of the eyes. The patient may experience one or two seizures a month or several a day. Absence seizures occur almost

▶ **TABLE 55-I   International Classsification of Epileptic Seizures**

International Classification	Traditional Name	Characteristics
1. Partial seizures		Consciousness not generally impaired.
a. Elementary symptoms (motor, sensory, or autonomic)	Jacksonian, or focal, epilepsy	Focal onset: usually unilateral spasm or twitching of the fingers or face, which may spread in a progressive march to involve the entire side Similar patterns when the symptoms are sensory
b. Complex symptoms	Psychomotor, or temporal lobe, epilepsy	Patient usually conscious during attack but does not recall what happened Transient mental disturbances, automatic purposeless movements (clapping hands, smacking lips) Sudden recollection of past events, visual or auditory hallucinations, personality changes, antisocial behavior, inappropriate moodiness Precipitated by music, blinking lights, and other stimuli
2. Generalized seizures		Bilateral, symmetric, and without local onset
a. Absence	Petit mal	Short lapses of consciousness lasting a few seconds indicated by a brief pause in conversation, a vacant stare, or rapid blinking of the eyes Almost exclusively in children; may disappear at puberty or be replaced by tonic-clonic epilepsy
b. Tonic-clonic	Grand mal	Classic seizure of epilepsy Generally preceded by an aura Loss of consciousness Generalized tonic and clonic spasms of the muscles Tongue may be bitten Bladder and/or bowel incontinence Mental confusion and amnesia for seizure event
3. Unilateral seizures		
4. Unclassified seizures		

Modified from Gastaut H: *Epilepsia* 11:102-113, 1970.

exclusively in children; onset is rare after 20 years of age. It may disappear after puberty or be replaced by other seizures, especially tonic-clonic.

Tonic-clonic, or *grand mal,* is the classic seizure of epilepsy. It may be characterized by an aura followed by a loss of consciousness and tonic-clonic spasms. The aura is a sensory indication of an impending seizure; it may consist of a momentary visual, auditory, or olfactory sensation.

The seizure starts with a rapid loss of consciousness. A cry may be uttered, from the forced expiration caused by thoracic or abnormal spasms. The patient experiences loss of upright position, tonic then clonic movements, and bladder and/or bowel incontinence, along with other autonomic dysfunctions. In the tonic phase, muscles contract and body position may be distorted. This phase lasts for a few seconds. The clonic phase involves opposing muscle groups contracting and relaxing, giving a jerking movement. The contractions gradually decrease in number but not in strength. The tongue may be bitten; this occurs in approximately half the patients (spasms of the jaw and tongue). The entire seizure lasts from 3 to 5 minutes and is followed by a period of unconsciousness that may

last from a few minutes to as long as a half hour. The patient regaining consciousness may appear confused, stuporous, or dull. This stage is referred to as the *postictal period.* Generally the patient has no recollection of the seizure.

Severe tonic-clonic seizures may cause systemic hypoxia with acidosis caused by respiratory spasm, excessive muscular activity, and cessation of breathing. Respiratory and cardiac arrest can result from prolonged seizure activity.

Febrile tonic-clonic seizures, frequently referred to as *fever convulsions,* are most common in children under 5 years of age. It is theorized that these seizures are caused by a rapid onset of hyperthermia related to a viral or bacterial infection. These seizures are generally of short duration, and there may a familial predisposition. In some instances, the seizures may continue beyond early childhood and the child may experience nonfebrile seizures later in life.

In addition to these common types of generalized seizures, some may be considered secondary. *Head injuries* continue to be the most common cause of acquired seizures. The incidence varies depending on the type and severity of the initial injury. Regardless of the mechanism, dura penetration is a significant risk factor for seizure development. With regard to epileptogenic pathophysiology, two major factors are considered. The primary injury results from traumatic mechanical forces that shear dendrite processes, destroy capillaries, and disrupt the extracellular environment. The secondary injury is produced by cerebral edema. Accumulation of toxic metabolic products and ischemia from systemic hypotension, hypoxia, and hypercarbia contribute to the cerebral edema. The pathophysiologic mechanisms for the occurrence of seizures after head trauma include ischemia resulting from an altered vascular supply, the mechanical effects of scarring, the destruction of dendrite inhibitory controls, defects in the blood-brain barrier, and changes in the extracellular ionic buffering systems.

Seizures may result from the acute phase or a sequela of a *central nervous system* (CNS) *infection* involving bacterial, viral, and parasitic organisms. It is noteworthy that seizures are typically the first clinical sign of a cerebral abscess. Infection accounts for about 3% of cases of acquired epilepsy.

Metabolic abnormalities, as an underlying cause of seizures, include hyponatremia, hypernatremia, hypoglycemia, hyperosmolar states, hypocalcemia, hypomagnesemia, hypoxia, and uremia. The neurologic symptoms of serum sodium alterations result from an increase or decrease in neuronal intracellular fluid volume and correlate with absolute levels of less than 125 mEq/L or greater than 150 mEq/L but, more important, correlate with the rapidity of the change. Advances in cardiopulmonary resuscitation (CPR) have contributed to an increased incidence of survival for patients experiencing cerebral hypoxia and its sequela, anoxic encephalopathy, causing it to become a more common cause of acquired seizure disorder.

Brain tumors are an additional cause of acquired seizures, particularly in patients 35 to 55 years of age. Whether a cerebral neoplasm produces seizures depends on its type, rate of growth, and location. Tumors that are supratentorial and involve the cortex are most likely to be associated with a seizure. The highest incidence occurs with tumors along the central sulcus with involvement of the motor strip. The farther the tumor is from this area, the less likely it is to cause seizures.

Arteriosclerotic cerebrovascular insufficiency and *cerebral infarctions* are the predominant causes of seizures in patients with vascular disorders, and these appear to be increasing as the older population increases. Large infarctions and deep infarctions extending to deep subcortical structures are more likely to cause recurrent seizures.

Numerous *toxic substances and drugs* are associated with seizures. With some therapeutic medications, seizures are manifested as a toxic effect. Drugs with this potential include aminophylline, antidiabetic medications, lidocaine, phenothiazines, physostigmine, and tricyclics.

Abuse of substances such as alcohol and cocaine may also lead to seizures.

STATUS EPILEPTICUS

Status epilepticus refers to a state in which a succession of seizures occurs with no recovery between them. Two types are possible: (1) *major motor status epilepticus,* in which one tonic-clonic seizure follows another; and (2) *absence-continuing status epilepticus,* involving a series of absence seizures. Status epilepticus is not a common phenomenon.

Major motor status epilepticus is an emergency and may be fatal if unrelieved. Several medications may be given to relieve this condition. Phenytoin (Dilantin) may be given intravenously (IV) and has the advantage of not altering neurologic signs and not depressing the patient. If this treatment is not successful in stopping the seizures, phenobarbital or diazepam (Valium) may be given IV. These drugs are more apt to cause cardiac or respiratory depression.

Status epilepticus often causes elevation of blood pressure and temperature, respiratory difficulty, and other systemic changes. Proper ventilation is crucial, and cardiopulmonary support systems may be warranted. Care must be taken to avoid aspiration of vomitus and saliva.

Fluid and electrolyte balance must be maintained. Exhaustion and acidosis may cause death. Once the patient is under control, causes of the episode should be explored. Abruptly stopping antiepileptic medications may be a precipitating factor, as may alcohol withdrawal.

ELECTROENCEPHALOGRAM

The electrical activity of the cortex is of extremely low voltage. It is amplified and recorded by an electroencephalograph. The record is called an *electroencephalogram* (ECG).

Brain waves are individualized and vary with activity (e.g., intense mental activity = low amplitude, high frequency; slow-wave sleep = low frequency, amplitude increased). Spikes indicate an irritative focus. Brain waves are slowed with hypoxia, anesthesia, sedatives, low carbon dioxide (CO_2), deep sleep, and relaxation; they are accelerated with increased CO_2 levels, sensory stimulation, light anesthesia, and drugs such as methylprednisolone (Medrol).

The superficial layers of cortex are responsible for the electrical activity recorded on EEGs. Masses of dendrites forming a dense network are thought to be the source. The cerebellum has a similar network, and a similar pattern can be recorded from that area.

EEGs should be used in conjunction with careful clinical evaluations. The EEG is a physiologic recording and does not distinguish one entity from another; for example, a tumor cannot be distinguished from a thrombosis by EEG. Ten percent of patients with seizures have normal EEGs. Also, an abnormal record does not mean a person has epilepsy. In fact, even in patients with diagnosed epilepsy, most seizure activity is non-clinical.

The EEG is only one test, not a conclusive diagnostic determination. Caution should be used in the interpretation of EEG tracings. For example, scalp electrodes frequently may not perceive the electrical activity from the inferior aspect of the frontal and temporal and occipital lobes.

Certain activating techniques such as hyperventilation, sleep, and visual stimulation are used to initiate abnormal electrical patterns in some patients.

In tonic-clonic seizures, EEG abnormalities depend on the frequency and duration of the seizures. EEG abnormalities are more common in patients with frequent seizures than in those with infrequent seizures. A normal EEG, however, is common in children with tonic-clonic seizures.

In some centers (e.g., Neuropsychiatric Institute at the University of California at Los Angeles), patients can be monitored on a 24-hour basis with radiotelemetry. Electrodes are implanted and attached to a telemetry pack that is secured to the patient's head. The EEG recordings along with a video camera are used to identify specific areas of the brain involved in abnormal discharges.

TREATMENT

The primary management mode for the seizure patient is drug therapy to prevent the occurrence of seizures or to reduce their frequency so that the patient can lead an essentially normal life. Approximately 70% to 80% of patients benefit from anticonvulsant drug therapy. The drug selected is determined by the type of seizure, and the doses are individualized. Table 55-2 lists some of the common drugs used for epilepsy and their side effects.

Historically, a combination of drugs was used on the premise that lower doses could be prescribed, thereby reducing the incidence of side effects. Today, many physicians use a monopharmacologic approach, preferring to minimize the number of drugs used.

Whichever approach is used, careful clinical assessment and frequent monitoring of drug levels are critical in patient management. Assessing drug levels allows individualization of drug dose to the patient's need. Patients metabolize drugs at varying rates. Factors such as serum protein levels and ability of the liver enzymes to biodegrade drugs influence the dose requirements and serum drug levels.

In the past, diet and surgery were also treatments for seizures, and these methods are still used occasionally today. A ketogenic diet was popular in the 1920s. A variation of the ketogenic diet, the *medium-chain triglyceride diet,* was introduced in the early 1970s. This high-fat, low-carbohydrate diet altered body chemistry by producing ketones. The resulting acidotic state seems to have an anticonvulsant effect on some children with myoclonic seizures.

Acetazolamide (Diamox), used in conjunction with anticonvulsant agents, produces a relative acidosis similar to a ketogenic diet. This state seems to create a climate less likely to produce seizure activity. Dehydration states also seem to decrease seizure activity, as does physical activity (possibly related to the production of lactic acid).

Surgical excision of cortical scars is a controversial treatment. It is restricted to focal epilepsy located in an area of the brain that is considered nonessential. Surgery is considered only after drug therapy has proved ineffective and certain criteria have been met, including the following:
- Focal lesion identified by EEG and compatible with clinical manifestations
- Accessible and nonessential area
- Patient a good candidate for rehabilitation (normal IQ, motivated)

Approximately 20% to 30% of patients with complex partial seizures of the temporal lobe are refractory to medical therapy. For some of these patients, *temporal lobe lobectomy* is an alternative to progressive deterioration caused by the seizures. The younger the patient at the time of surgery, the better is the outcome. Approximately 70% to 80% of patients are seizure free or have rare seizures after surgery. Rehabilitation after surgery is long term and ongoing. Often, patients are left with permanent deficits, but when this situation is weighed against continuing frequent uncontrolled seizures, patients often believe that the trade was well worth it.

Maintaining a patent airway and preventing injury are the two critical objectives in the care of the person experiencing a seizure. Maintaining the patient in a side-lying position reduces the risk of aspirating stomach contents and saliva and prevents the tongue from obstructing the airway. Preventing injury can be accomplished by protecting the head during the seizure and removing any objects that may cause harm.

The importance of the holistic approach in managing the person with a seizure disorder cannot be overstated. Patients and family need to understand the medication regimen and dosage and side effects, appropriate care for a person experiencing a seizure, the psychologic problems associated with seizures, and the public's attitude toward persons with seizures.

TABLE 55-2 Anticonvulsant Agents in the Treatment of Seizures

Drug	Therapeutic Uses (Type of Seizure)	Dose Blood Level	Adverse Effects
BARBITURATES			
Phenobarbital	Tonic-clonic seizures (often with hydantoins) Status epilepticus	15 to 40 μg/ml	Drowsiness (usually dosage related) Gastric distress Hyperactivity (especially in children, not dosage related)
Primidone (Mysoline)	Partial seizures (especially complex partial)	5 to 12 μg/ml	Drowsiness, vertigo, diplopia, ataxia Metabolized to phenobarbital and phenylethyl-malonamide
HYDANTOINS			
Phenytoin (Dilantin)	Tonic-clonic seizures (especially in adults) Partial seizures Complex seizures	10 to 20 μg/ml	May increase frequency of absence seizures Hirsutism, hypertrophic gums, gastric distress, diplopia, nystagmus, blurred vision, vertigo, hyperglycemia, macrocytic anemia, especially with long-term use because of blocking of folic acid synthesis Serum levels greater than 40 μg/ml associated with phenytoin encephalopathy
Mephenytoin (Mesantoin)	Partial seizures Tonic-clonic seizures	Adult: 200 to 800 mg/day Child: 100 to 400 mg/day	Slurred speech, confusion, insomnia Pancytopenia
IMINOSTILBENES			
Carbamazepine (Tegretol)	Complex partial seizures May be used in children	6 to 12 μg/ml	Bone marrow depression, gastric distress, drowsiness, blurred vision, constipation, skin rash
BENZODIAZEPINES			
Diazepam (Valium)	Status epilepticus only (IV)	Adult: 5 to 10 mg, up to 30 mg IV Child: 1 mg every 2 to 5 minutes, up to 10 mg	Sedation, cardiac and respiratory depression
Clonazepam (Klonopin)	Absence, myoclonic seizures	Adult: 1.5 to 20 mg/day Child: 0.1 to 0.2 mg/kg/day	Drowsiness, confusion, vertigo, syncope, headache
SUCCINIMIDES			
Ethosuximide (Zarontin)	Absence seizures	Adult: 20 to 40 mg/kg/day Child: 20 mg/kg/day; 40 to 90 μg/ml	Nausea, vomiting, weight loss, constipation, diarrhea, sleep disturbances, blood dyscrasias
Methsuximide (Celontin)	Absence seizures	Adult/child: 600 to 1200 mg/day	Drowsiness, ataxia, anorexia, aplastic anemia
VALPROIC ACID			
Valproic acid (Depakene)	Absence seizures	50 to 100 μg/ml	Nausea, hepatotoxicity

? QUESTIONS

▼ *Answer the following on a separate sheet of paper.*

1. Define epilepsy.
2. What is the incidence of epilepsy in the general population of the United States? For the offspring of epileptic persons?
3. What conditions may cause seizures?
4. List the areas of the brain associated with lesions that are likely to be epileptogenic.
5. Describe the factors that play an instrumental role in precipitating seizures.
6. Describe the metabolic changes that can occur during and immediately after a seizure.
7. Define status epilepticus.

▼ *Circle the letter preceding each item below that correctly answers the question or completes the statement. More than one answer may be correct.*

8. Which of the following statements about epilepsy is(are) *true?*
   a. The single most important factor in diagnosing epilepsy is careful observation and reporting of a seizure.
   b. Most patients can be brought under reasonable control.
   c. There are characteristic disease inheritance patterns.
   d. Epileptic persons may have difficulty in obtaining employment.
9. Complex partial seizures are usually characterized by:
   a. Inappropriate behavior
   b. A disturbance in the temporal lobe
   c. Most common occurrence in children
   d. Temporary loss of consciousness

10. Uncontrollable tonic, then clonic, muscular spasms with loss of consciousness are characteristic of the following type(s) of seizure:
    a. Elementary partial
    b. Absence
    c. Tonic-clonic
    d. Complex partial
11. A seizure involving a momentary loss of consciousness and often characterized by a blank stare and a facial twitch is referred to as:
    a. Elementary partial
    b. Tonic-clonic
    c. Complex partial
    d. Absence
12. Which of the following interventions are of primary importance when one encounters a patient having a seizure?
    a. Insertion of a tongue blade

b. Observation of the seizure to determine progression of muscular involvement
c. Restraint of the patient to limit outward movement of the arms and legs
d. Establishment of an open airway by maintaining the patient in a side-lying position

13. Which of the following are likely indications for the surgical treatment of an epileptic patient?
    a. Focal lesion identified by EEG and compatible with clinical manifestations
    b. Area accessible and nonessential
    c. Drug therapy not effective
    d. High motivation for a rehabilitation program

▼ *Match the type of drug in column A with the associated therapeutic uses and side effects in column B.*

Column A

14. _____ Phenytoin
15. _____ Ethosuximide
16. _____ Valproic acid
17. _____ Carbamazepine
18. _____ Diazepam
19. _____ Primidone

Column B

a. Hepatic damage, nausea
b. Drug of choice for tonic-clonic, complex, and partial seizures
c. Primary drug for absence seizures
d. Sedation, vertigo, ataxia, diplopia, nystagmus (drug metabolized to phenobarbital)
e. Drug of choice for complex partial seizures
f. Given IV to treat status epilepticus

CHAPTER 56

Central Nervous System Injury

MARY CARTER LOMBARDO
MARY S. HARTWIG

INCREASED INTRACRANIAL PRESSURE

Increased intracranial pressure (ICP) is defined as an increase in the pressure exerted within the cranial cavity. Normally the cranial cavity is occupied by brain tissue, blood, and cerebrospinal fluid (CSF). Each portion occupies a specific volume, giving a normal ICP of 50 to 200 mm H_2O or 4 to 15 mm Hg. ICP is normally influenced by everyday activities and rises temporarily to levels much higher than normal. A few of these activities are deep abdominal breathing, coughing, and straining. Temporary increases in ICP present no difficulty, but sustained increased pressure has a detrimental effect on living brain tissue.

The cranial cavity is a rigid compartment filled to capacity with incompressible substances: the brain (1400 g), CSF (approximately 75 ml), and blood (approximately 75 ml). An increase in the volume of any of these three major substances results in encroachment of the space occupied by the others and increased ICP. The *Monro-Kellie hypothesis* provides a conceptual model for understanding increased ICP. It states that because the bony skull cannot expand, if one of the three intracranial compartments expands, the other two must compensate by decreasing in volume, if the ICP is to remain constant. These compensatory mechanisms within the cranium are limited, but interruption of neural function can be severe when they fail. Compensation consists of increased drainage of CSF into the spinal canal and adaptation of the brain to increased pressure without increasing ICP. Compensatory mechanisms with potentially lethal consequences are reduction of blood flow to the brain and displacement of the brain downward or horizontally (herniation) when ICP becomes increasingly elevated. These last two compensatory mechanisms can have dire consequences for neural function. When the increase in ICP is serious and sustained, compensatory mechanisms are ineffective, and the pressure elevation can cause neuronal death (Fig. 56-1).

Brain tumors, brain injury, cerebral edema, and obstruction in CSF flow all contribute to increased ICP. Cerebral edema, perhaps the most common cause of increased ICP, itself has many causes. These include an increase in intracellular fluid, hypoxia, fluid and electrolyte imbalances, cerebral ischemia, meningitis, and injury. Regardless of the cause, the effects are basically the same.

ICP generally increases gradually. After head injury, edema formation may take 36 to 48 hours to reach its maximum. A rise in ICP to 33 mm Hg (450 mm H_2O) significantly reduces cerebral blood flow (CBF). The resulting ischemia stimulates the vasomotor centers, and the systemic blood pressure rises. Stimulation of the cardioinhibitory center produces bradycardia, and respiration is slowed. This compensatory mechanism, known as *Cushing's reflex*, helps to maintain CBF. (The decreasing respiration, however, leads to carbon dioxide [CO_2] retention and resultant cerebral vasodilation, which contribute to increasing ICP.) Systemic blood pressure will continue to rise proportionately to the increasing ICP, although eventually a point is reached when the ICP exceeds the arterial pressure and cerebral circulation ceases, with resultant brain death. Generally, this event is heralded by a rapidly decreasing arterial blood pressure.

The cycle of progressive neurologic deficit associated with cerebral contusion and edema (or any expanding intracranial mass lesion) is illustrated in Fig. 56-2. Brain trauma causes tissue fragmentation and contusion, resulting in a breakdown of the blood-brain barrier (BBB), with vasodilation and exudation of fluid, causing edema. Edema leads to an increase in tissue pressure and an

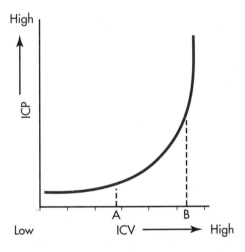

FIG. 56-1   The relationship of intracranial volume *(ICV)* to intracranial pressure *(ICP)*. Compensatory mechanisms are effective up to point *A* with expanding ICV, and ICP does not increase above the normal range. However, as the ICV continues to increase, a critical point *B* is reached where a small increase in ICV causes a large increase in ICP.

eventual increase in ICP, which in turn leads to decreased CBF, ischemia, hypoxia, acidosis (decreased pH and increased arterial carbon dioxide tension [$PaCO_2$]), and further breakdown of the BBB. This cycle continues so that cell death and edema formation increase progressively unless intervention occurs.

Clinical Manifestations and Assessment

Clinical manifestations of increased ICP are numerous and varied and may be subtle. Alteration of the patient's level of consciousness (LOC) is the most sensitive indicator of all the signs of intracranial hypertension. The clinical triad of symptoms is headache, caused by stretching of the dura and blood vessels; papilledema, caused by pressure and swelling of the optic disc; and vomiting, which is frequently projectile. The presence of widened pulse pressure and decreased pulse and respiratory rates signals brain decompensation and impending death. Other signs of increased ICP include hyperthermia, motor and sensory changes, altered speech, and seizures.

Decerebrate posturing is a condition that develops when a brain lesion or the consequences of increased ICP interrupt signals from higher structures to the pons and medulla and to the lower structures. The result is blockage of strong excitatory input from the cerebral cortex, red nuclei, and basal ganglia to the medullary inhibitor system. The pontine excitatory system becomes dominant, leading to generalized rigidity of upper and lower extremities (total extensor rigidity of the antigravity muscles of the neck, trunk, and legs, as shown in Fig. 56-3, *A*). This type of abnormal posturing is spastic as well as rigid, since the pontine antigravity signals preferentially excite the gamma motor neurons in the spinal cord, tightening muscle spindles and activating

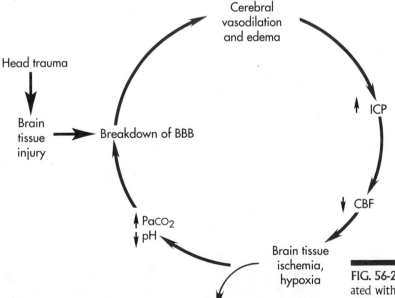

FIG. 56-2   The cycle of progressive neurologic deficit associated with an expanding intracranial mass lesion. *BBB,* Blood-brain barrier; *ICP,* intracranial pressure; *CBF,* cerebral blood flow; *PaCO₂,* arterial carbon dioxide tension.

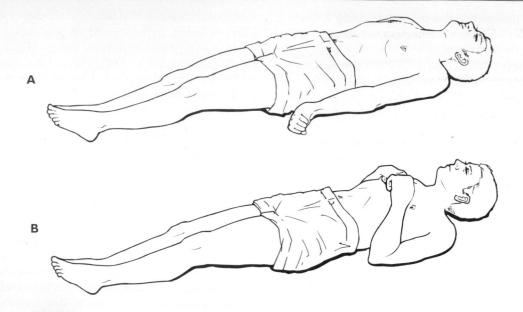

FIG. 56-3   Abnormal posturing. **A,** *Decerebrate posture* results from damage to the brain and brain stem. The jaws are clenched and the neck extended. The arms are adducted and stiffly extended at the elbows, with forearms pronated and wrists and fingers flexed. The legs are stiffly extended at the knees, with plantar flexion of the feet. **B,** *Decorticate posture* results from damage to one or both corticospinal tracts within or very near the cerebral hemispheres. In this posture the upper arms are held tightly to the sides, with elbows, wrists, and fingers flexed. The legs are stiffly extended and internally rotated, with plantar flexion of the feet.

stretch reflexes. The brain lesion may be bilateral or unilateral, with muscular rigidity on the side opposite the brain lesion. Decerebrate posturing has a particularly serious prognosis because it indicates severe damage to the cerebral hemisphere and imminent brain stem involvement, leading to interference with respiratory and cardiac centers in the medulla.

Decorticate posturing is another form of abnormal motor response with brain injury. It suggests a higher cortical lesion, with less severe damage to the cerebral hemisphere(s). Typically, the arm, wrist, and fingers are flexed and the upper extremity is adducted and internally rotated. In contrast, the lower extremity is either in extensor rigidity or unresponsive (Fig. 56-3, *B*).

The *Glasgow Coma Scale* (GCS) is the most widely used scale to assess the patient's arousability and reaction to a stimulus. This scale grades the patient's best response in three categories: eye opening, verbal responses, and motor responses. A deteriorating score indicates a worsening of the patient's neurologic status (Table 56-1).

Two general types of pathologic processes lead to coma with severely increased ICP: those that cause global ischemia of the cerebral hemispheres and those that depress or destroy brain stem–activating mechanisms. Coma occurs only when both cerebral hemispheres or brain stem divisions are dysfunctional. The major catastrophe of coma is death from brain herniation. The two main paths of herniation are through the tentorial notch and through the foramen magnum. *Uncal herni-*

ation involves displacement of the median aspect of the temporal lobe (uncus) through the tentorial notch, thus compressing the upper brain stem, the third cranial nerve (CN III), and the posterior cerebral artery (Fig. 56-4). *Central herniation* involves downward displacement of the diencephalon through the tentorial opening in the midline, which compresses the midbrain. In both cases there is a progression of rostral-to-caudal compression of first the midbrain, then the pons, and finally the medulla, leading to the appearance of neurologic signs and progressively diminished LOC.

Although the GCS scores the best response, it does not consider localized signs. The brain stem contains several intrinsic reflexes that are convenient to examine. When brain stem reflexes are normal, the cause of coma is generally diffuse cerebral dysfunction.

Normal pupillary symmetry, size, shape, and reaction to light indicate intact functioning of the midbrain and CN III. Equal, round, and reactive pupils (2.5 to 5 mm) (see Fig. 51-2) usually exclude midbrain damage as a cause of coma. An enlarged (greater than 5 mm) and poorly reactive pupil can result from transtentorial herniation and compression of the midbrain and CN III. Bilaterally dilated and unreactive pupils indicate severe midbrain damage. Oval-shaped pupils are often associated with early midbrain–CN III compression.

Evaluation of brain stem functioning includes spontaneous motion of each eye and the oculocephalic and oculovestibular tests. The resting position of eyes may be

► TABLE 56-1   Glasgow Coma Scale

Parameter/Response	Score	Parameter/Response	Score
EYE OPENING (E)		**BEST MOTOR RESPONSE (M)**	
Spontaneous: eyes open to approach	4	Obeys commands: for example, "raise your arm; hold up two fingers"	6
To speech: eyes open to name or command	3	Localizes pain: does not obey but locates and tries to remove painful stimulus	5
To pain: eyes open to digital pressure over proximal nailbed	2	Flexion withdrawal: flexes arm in response to pain with no purposeful attempt to stop stimulus and without abnormal flexion posture	4
None: does not open eyes to any stimulus	1		
BEST VERBAL RESPONSE (V)		Abnormal flexion to pain: flexes arms at elbow and pronates, making a fist (decorticate posturing)	3
Oriented: converses; knows who and where he or she is and month and year	5	Abnormal extension to pain: extends arms at elbow, usually adducts and internally rotates arm at shoulder (decerebrate posturing)	2
Confused: converses but disoriented in one or more spheres	4	None: no response to pain; flaccid	1
Inappropriate words: no sustained conversation; words disorganized or inappropriate	3		
Incomprehensible: makes sounds (e.g., moans) but no recognizable words	2		
None: no sounds even with painful stimuli	1		

Modified from Ropper AH: In Isselbacher KJ, editor: *Harrison's principles of internal medicine,* ed 13, New York, 1994, McGraw-Hill.

Coma score = E + V + M: 15 = fully alert; <8 = comatose. After head injury a score >11 indicates an 85% chance of a good recovery or moderate disability, whereas a score of 3 or 4 indicates an 85% chance of dying or remaining vegetative. Intermediate scores correlate with proportional chances of recovery.

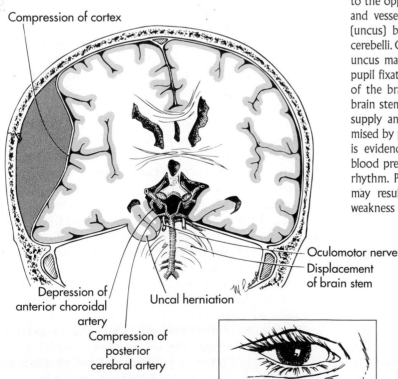

Compression of cortex

Depression of anterior choroidal artery

Compression of posterior cerebral artery

Uncal herniation

Oculomotor nerve
Displacement of brain stem

FIG. 56-4   Mechanisms of signs and symptoms of an expanding intracranial hematoma over the parietotemporal region. The expanding hematoma compresses the cortex, pushing the brain to the opposite side and displacing the brain stem, cranial nerves, and vessels. The extreme medial portion of the temporal lobe (uncus) becomes herniated under the edge of the tentorium cerebelli. Compression of the oculomotor nerve by the herniated uncus may lead to ipsilateral pupil dilation, ptosis, and eventual pupil fixation. Compression of the cerebral cortex and distortion of the brain stem result in depression of consciousness. In the brain stem the reticular activating system is involved. The arterial supply and venous return to the brain stem may be compromised by pressure. Interference with the cardiorespiratory centers is evidenced by irregularity or slowing of pulse; elevation of blood pressure; and abnormalities of respiratory rate, depth, and rhythm. Pressure on the corticospinal and associated pathways may result in a contralateral Babinski's sign and contralateral weakness or paralysis.

conjugate (both eyes in the same position), disconjugate (eyes in different positions), or skewed (vertical disconjugate position). An adducted eye at rest indicates paresis of the lateral rectus muscle resulting from a CN VI lesion, whereas abduction indicates paresis of the medial rectus muscle from a CN III lesion. A skewed deviation results from a lesion of the pons.

The *oculocephalic reflex* is tested by briskly turning the head from side to side while holding the eyes open. With an intact brain stem the eyes deviate conjugately in the direction opposite to the head turning (*doll's eyes present*). With a brain stem lesion, the eyes move in the same direction as the head is turned (*doll's eyes absent*). CN III (nuclei in midbrain) and CN VI (nuclei in pons) are responsible for eye movements, so this procedure is a good test to evaluate brain stem function. The *oculovestibular reflex* is tested by slowly injecting ice water into the external auditory canal until eye deviation or nystagmus occurs. This test, called the *ice-water caloric test,* is more powerful in eliciting eye reflexes, is used as an adjunct to testing the oculocephalic reflex, and has the same significance in the evaluation of brain stem pathways. The response of a comatose person with an intact brain stem is slow conjugate deviation of the eyes toward the irrigated ear, where they remain for 30 to 120 seconds. An extremely abnormal movement, such as skewing or jerky movements, usually indicates a brain stem lesion.

The *corneal reflex* is tested by touching a wisp of cotton to the cornea. The normal response is bilateral lid closure, which depends on the integrity of pontine pathways involving CN V and CN VII.

Finally, medullary function may be assessed by testing the *gag reflex* by touching a tongue blade to both sides of the posterior pharynx. The nuclei of CN IX and CN X mediating pharyngeal responses are located in the medulla.

The outcome of many neurologic conditions can be altered by the early recognition and treatment of increased ICP. ICP may be monitored directly by the use of epidural, subarachnoid, or intraventricular sensors. ICP monitoring is most often indicated after head injuries or brain surgery. A detailed discussion of ICP monitoring techniques, assessment, and treatment may be found in neurologic intensive care nursing textbooks.

HEAD INJURY

Anatomy

The brain is protected from injury by the hair, skin, and bones that surround it. Without this protection the delicate brain, which makes us what we are, would be extremely susceptible to injury and destruction. Moreover, a neuron once destroyed does not regenerate. Head injury can have catastrophic implications. Some problems are caused directly by the injury; many others are secondary to the injury. The medical team must work to prevent and detect the early effects of brain injury to avoid the sequence of events that leads to mental and physical deficit and even death.

Just above the skull lies the *galea aponeurotica,* a freely moveable, dense, fibrous tissue that aids in absorbing the force from external trauma. Between the galea and the skin is a fatty layer and a deep membranous layer that contains large vessels. When severed, these vessels constrict poorly and may cause significant blood loss in a patient with a scalp laceration. Directly beneath the galea is the subaponeurotic space, which contain the *emissary* and *diploic veins.* These vessels may carry infection from the scalp to deep within the skull, which underscores the extreme importance of thorough cleansing and débridement of the scalp whenever the galea has been torn (Schwartz, 1994).

In the adult the skull is a rigid compartment that does not allow for expansion of intracranial contents. The bone is actually composed of two walls or tables separated by cancellous bone. The outer wall is called the *outer table,* and the inner wall is called the *inner table.* This structure provides for greater strength and insulation with less weight. The inner table contains grooves in which lie the anterior, middle, and posterior meningeal arteries. When fracture of the skull involves tearing of one of these arteries, the resultant arterial bleeding, which accumulates in the epidural space, may lead to a fatal outcome unless it is detected and treated immediately. This constitutes one of the true neurosurgical emergencies, demanding immediate surgical intervention.

Covering the brain and providing added protection are the meninges. The three layers of the meninges are the dura mater, the arachnoid, and the pia mater. Each has a separate function and differs from the other two in structure (Fig. 56-5) (see Chapter 50).

The *dura* is the tough, semitranslucent, inelastic outer membrane that (1) protects the brain, (2) encloses the venous sinuses (which are composed of dura mater and endothelial lining only—no vascular tissue), and (3) forms the periosteum of the inner table. It is closely attached to the interior surface of the skull. Because of the problems that arise when a tear in the dura is not completely repaired and made airtight, its most important function may be protection. The fracture may expand instead of healing, and chronic leakage of CSF may occur, which may lead to the development of meningocerebral cicatrix, causing focal epilepsy. In some instances, however, the dura is purposely left open. These situations include cerebral edema (to allow for decompression of the bulging brain), drainage of CSF, or after exploratory trepanning (to allow for inspection and evacuation of clots).

The dura has a rich blood supply. The middle and posterior areas are supplied by the middle meningeal artery, which branches off the internal carotid and vertebral arteries. The anterior and ethmoid vessels are also branches of the internal carotid and supply the anterior fossa. A

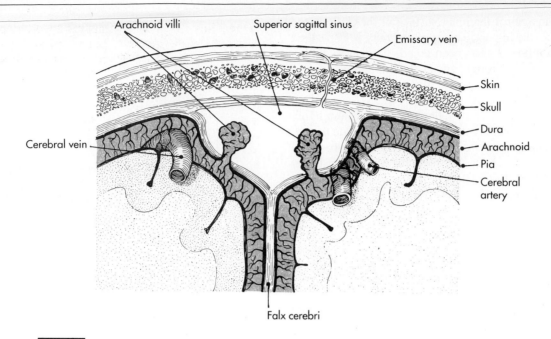

FIG. 56-5   Meninges in greater detail. Coronal section through the superior sagittal sinus. Emissary vein shown connecting scalp with superior sagittal sinus. The subarachnoid space is filled with cerebrospinal fluid. It enters the sinus through the arachnoid villi. (From Langley LL, Telford JR, Christensen JB: *Dynamic anatomy and physiology,* ed 5, New York, 1980, McGraw-Hill.)

branch of the occipital artery, the posterior meningeal, supplies blood to the posterior fossa.

Lying close to the dura but not attached to it is the fine, fibrous, elastic membrane known as the *arachnoid*. This membrane is not attached to the dura mater. However, the space between the two membranes—the subdural space—is a potential space. Bleeding between the dura and the arachnoid spreads freely, limited only by the barriers of the falx cerebri and tentorium. The cerebral veins passing through this space have little support except that provided by the dura and the arachnoid and therefore are susceptible to injury and rupture in head (cerebral) trauma.

Between the arachnoid and the pia mater (which lies directly beneath the arachnoid) is the *subarachnoid space*. This space widens and deepens in places and allows for circulation of CSF. In the superior sagittal and transverse sinuses, the arachnoid forms villous projections (pacchionian bodies), which serve as a pathway for the emptying of CSF into the venous system.

The *pia mater* is a delicate membrane that is richly supplied with minute blood vessels. It is the only meningeal layer that dips into all the sulci and blankets the ridges of the gyri; the other two layers bridge the sulci. In some of the fissures and sulci on the medial side of the hemispheres, the pia forms a barrier between the ventricles of the brain and the sulcus or fissure. This barrier provides a structural support for the choroid plexus of each of the ventricles.

The brain damage seen in head trauma can be caused in two different ways: (1) by the immediate effects of the trauma on the functioning brain and (2) by the later effects of the brain cells' response to the trauma.

Immediate neurologic damage is caused by the penetration and laceration of brain tissue by an object or piece of bone, by the effects of force or energy transmitted to the brain, and by the effects of acceleration-deceleration on the brain, which is confined in a rigid compartment.

The degree of damage caused by these problems can depend on the force applied: the greater the force, the greater the damage. Two kinds of force are applied in two ways, causing two different effects. First, local injury is caused by a sharp object with low velocity and little force. Disruption of neurologic functioning occurs in a localized area and is caused by penetration of the dura at the point of impact by the object or fragments of bone. Second, generalized injury occurs, which is more often seen in blunt trauma to the head and after motor vehicle crashes. The damage occurs as the energy or force is transmitted to the brain. Much of the energy or force is absorbed by the protective layers of hair, scalp, and skull; with violent trauma, however, these structures cannot protect the brain. The remaining energy is transmitted to the brain, causing damage and disruption along the way as delicate tissues are subjected to the force. If the head is moving and is suddenly and violently stopped, as in a motor vehicle crash, damage is caused not only by local injury to tissue, but also by acceleration and deceleration. The force of acceleration and deceleration causes the contents within the rigid skull to move, thereby forcing the brain against the inner surface of the skull on the side opposite the impact. This type of injury is also called *contrecoup injury*. As has been noted, some areas within the cranial vault are rough, and as the brain moves across them (e.g., the sphenoid ridge), they tear and lacerate the tissues. The damage is intensified when trauma also causes rotation of the skull. The areas of the brain likely to receive the greatest amount of damage include the anterior portion of the frontal and temporal lobes, the posterior sections of the occipital lobes, and the upper portion of the midbrain (Becker, 1992; Ropper, 1994).

The secondary effects of the trauma, which causes severe neurologic alterations, result from the tissue response to the injury. Whenever tissue is injured, it responds predictably by alteration in intracellular and extracellular fluid content, extravasation of blood, increased blood supply to the area, and mobilization of cells to repair damage and remove cellular debris.

The neurons, the functional cells within the brain, depend from minute to minute on a constant supply of nutrients in the form of glucose and oxygen and are very susceptible to metabolic injury when supplies are cut off. As a result of injury, the cerebral circulation may lose its ability to regulate the available circulating blood volume, causing ischemia of certain areas within the brain.

Epidural Hematoma

Epidural hematoma is a serious sequela to head injury and carries a mortality rate of approximately 50%. Epidural hematoma occurs most frequently in the parietotemporal area from a tear in the middle meningeal artery (Fig. 56-6, *B*). In the frontal and occipital areas, hematomas are frequently not suspected and produce poorly localizing signs. When epidural hematoma is not associated with additional brain injuries, early treatment is generally followed by recovery with little or no neurologic deficit.

The typical patient with epidural hematoma gives a history of head injury followed by a short period of unconsciousness. This is followed by a lucid period. It is important to note, however, that this lucid interval is not reliably diagnostic of epidural hematoma. First, the lucid interval may go unobserved, especially if it does not last long. Second, the patient with additional serious brain injury may remain stuporous (Becker, 1992).

An expanding hematoma in the temporal area causes the temporal lobe to be forced downward and inward. This pressure causes the medial portion of the lobe (the uncus and part of the hippocampal gyrus) to herniate under the edge of the tentorium, causing the neurologic signs observed by the medical team (see Fig. 56-4).

The pressure of the herniation of the uncus on the arterial circulation to the reticular formation of the medulla causes unconsciousness. Also located in this area are the nuclei to CN III (oculomotor). Compression of this nerve produces dilation of the pupil and ptosis of the eyelid.

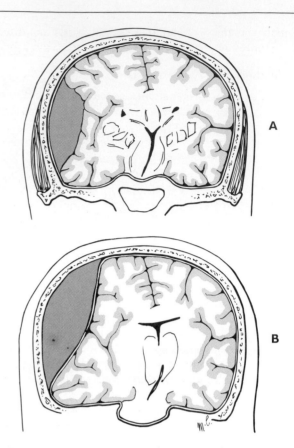

FIG. 56-6   **A,** Subdural hematoma, usually a result of laceration of the subdural vein. **B,** Epidural hematoma in the temporal fossa, usually a result of laceration of the middle meningeal artery.

Compression of the corticospinal pathways ascending in this area causes weakness in motor responses contralaterally (i.e., side opposite the hematoma), brisk or hyperactive reflexes, and Babinski's sign.

As the developing hematoma enlarges, it pushes the entire brain toward the opposite side, causing severe ICP. Late signs of increased ICP develop, including decerebrate rigidity and disturbances in vital signs and respiratory functioning.

Epidural hemorrhage is diagnosed from clinical signs and symptoms as well as by carotid arteriogram, echoencephalogram, and computed tomography (CT) scan. Treatment is by surgical evacuation of the hematoma and control of the bleeding from the lacerated middle meningeal artery. Surgical intervention must take place early, before serious compression of brain tissue causes brain damage. Mortality remains high even when the condition is diagnosed and treated early because of the associated severe brain trauma and sequelae.

Subdural Hematoma

Whereas an epidural hematoma is generally arterial in origin, a subdural hematoma is venous (Fig. 56-6, *A*). It is caused by rupture of the veins in the subdural space.

Subdural hematomas are divided into types that differ in symptoms and prognosis: acute, subacute, and chronic.

Acute subdural hematoma

Acute subdural hematomas cause serious and significant neurologic symptoms within 24 to 48 hours after injury. Frequently associated with serious brain trauma, these hematomas are also associated with a high mortality rate (Schwartz, 1994).

Progressive neurologic deficit results from compression of brain tissue with herniation of the brain stem into the foramen magnum, leading to compression of the brain stem. This quickly leads to cessation of respiration and loss of control of pulse and blood pressure.

Diagnosis is made by carotid arteriogram and echoencephalogram or CT scan. Acute subdural hematoma should always be considered in patients who have suffered severe neurologic trauma and show signs of deteriorating neurologic status. Because more than half of these hematomas are bilateral, it is extremely important to consider the type of injury incurred and to use appropriate diagnostic measures (e.g., bilateral arteriograms) to rule out the possibility of bilateral hematomas (Schwartz, 1994).

Treatment consists mainly of removal of the hematoma, decompression by removal of areas of skull and portions of the frontal or temporal lobes if necessary, and relaxation of the compressing dura. Even with prompt diagnosis and surgical intervention, mortality rates are about 60%, with most related to the severe brain trauma and major organ failure that accompanies severe trauma.

Subacute subdural hematoma

Subacute subdural hematoma causes significant neurologic deficit more than 48 hours but less than 2 weeks after injury (Schwartz, 1994). As with acute subdural hematoma, it is caused by venous bleeding into the subdural space.

The typical clinical history of a patient with a subacute subdural hematoma shows head trauma causing unconsciousness with subsequent gradual improvement in neurologic status. Over time the patient demonstrates signs of deteriorating neurologic status. The LOC begins to decrease gradually over a period of hours. As the ICP increases from the accumulating hematoma, the patient may become difficult to arouse and nonresponsive to verbal and painful stimuli. As with acute subdural hematoma, the shift of intracranial contents and the increasing ICP caused by the accumulation of blood leads to uncal or central herniation and gives rise to neurologic signs of brain stem compression.

Treatment, as in the treatment for acute subdural hematoma, is the early and prompt removal of the clot. This can be accomplished by various means, according to the patient's clinical condition. Because many of these clots are bilateral, both subdural spaces should be evaluated and, if indicated, surgically explored (Schwartz, 1994).

> **TABLE 56-2   Stages in the Natural History of Nonlethal Subdural Hematoma**

Stage	Description
Stage I	Dark blood spreads widely over the brain surface beneath the dura.
Stage II	Blood congeals and becomes darker, thicker, and gelatinous (2 to 4 days).
Stage III	Clot breaks down and after about 2 weeks has color and consistency of crankcase oil.
Stage IV	Organization begins with formation of encasing membranes: an outer thick, tough membrane derived from dura and a thin inner one from arachnoid. The contained fluid becomes xanthochromic.
Stage V	Organization is completed. Clot may become calcified or even ossified (or may resorb).

Modified from Jackson FE: *CIBA Clin Symp* 18(3):67-93, 1966.

Chronic subdural hematoma

Chronic subdural hematoma presents an interesting clinical history. The cerebral trauma responsible for it may be trivial or even nonexistent or forgotten. The onset of symptoms is usually delayed for weeks, months, and possibly years after the initial injury.

The initial trauma ruptures one of the veins transversing the subdural space. Slow bleeding thus occurs into the subdural space. Within 7 to 10 days after bleeding has occurred, the blood is surrounded by a fibrous membrane. As breakdown of blood cells within the hematoma occurs, an osmotic pressure gradient is built up, pulling fluid into the hematoma. This increase in the size of the hematoma may cause further bleeding by tearing the surrounding membrane or vessels, increasing the size and pressure of the hematoma. If allowed to follow its natural course, the contents of the subdural hematoma undergo characteristic changes (Table 56-2).

Chronic subdural hematoma has frequently been nicknamed "the imitator" because the signs and symptoms are generally nonspecific and nonlocalizing and could be caused by many different disease processes. Some patients complain of a headache. The most typical signs and symptoms include progressive alteration in LOC, including apathy, lethargy, and decreased attention span, and decreased ability to use higher cognitive skills. Hemianopsia, hemiparesis, and pupillary abnormalities are observed in less than 50% of patients. The CSF is rarely helpful in confirming a diagnosis and may be nonspecifically abnormal, with increased protein content and xanthochromia, or may contain a few red blood cells; the pressure is generally normal. When aphasia is present, it is usually an *anomic* type, which is characterized by well-articulated speech and normal grammar that conveys little or no information. The ability to understand the spoken word (comprehension) and the ability to repeat sentences and phrases remain unchanged.

Diagnosis is best made by arteriography. CT scan may demonstrate a hematoma, thereby avoiding the necessity of an arteriogram, but a negative CT scan does not necessarily rule out a diagnosis of subdural hematoma.

Small hematomas resolve spontaneously if allowed to follow their natural course. In patients with small hematomas with no neurologic signs, the best medical course is probably close monitoring. For the patient with progressive neurologic deficit and debilitating symptoms, however, the best course is surgical removal because the greatest danger in chronic subdural hematoma is that it may cause herniation of the temporal uncus and death (Schwartz, 1994).

SPINAL CORD INJURY

Approximately 10,000 new spinal cord injuries occur in the United States each year, primarily to young, single men. The cost of these injuries in terms of disability and rehabilitation is tremendous. The cause of such injuries is primarily automobile crashes, followed by falls and sports injuries. Contact sports and diving accidents are the primary sports causes of quadriplegia.

Mechanisms of Injury

The vertebral column is constructed with a circumferential bony ring that provides ideal protection for low-velocity penetrating injuries and contusions, but the intervertebral articulations are weak points for flexion, extension, or rotational stress. According to Schwartz (1994), dislocations and fractures that do not break the vertebral ring allow the vertebrae above and below the area of injury to act as fulcrums for other vertebrae and their attached soft tissue to undergo concussion, stretching, and contusion and thus disrupt the spinal cord.

The stresses of flexion, extension, and rotation, along with the relative weakness of the articulations of the vertebrae, cause fractures and dislocations to occur most often at points where a relatively mobile portion of the vertebral column meets a relatively fixed segment, that is, between the lower cervical area and the upper thoracic segment, between the lower thoracic and upper lumbar segments, and between the lower lumbar segment and the sacrum (Schwartz, 1994).

Most of the damage in spinal cord injury occurs at the time of injury. Secondary cord injury occurs from movement of the unstable vertebral column; the injury that occurs is a movement of the spinal cord against sharp fragments of bone projecting into the canal and continued compression of the spinal cord.

The primary changes that occur after spinal cord injury include small hemorrhages in the gray matter that occur as spinal cord blood flow decreases and hypoxia ensues, followed by edema. Hypoxia of the gray matter stimulates the release of catecholamines, which contribute to the hemorrhage and necrosis and cause further spinal cord dysfunction. This mechanism is still under investigation but has stimulated researchers to suggest cooling of the injured segment, norepinephrine blocking agents, and steroids as possible therapeutic measures to prevent additional damage.

When the spinal cord is completely severed, two functional disasters are immediately observed: (1) all voluntary activity in the body parts innervated by the spinal segments is permanently lost; and (2) all sensation, which depends on the integrity of the ascending spinal pathways, is lost. A third occurrence is immediate spinal areflexia, frequently called *spinal shock.*

Spinal Shock

Spinal shock is a temporary physiologic disorganization of spinal cord function that occurs immediately after the injury and may last from hours to months. This phenomenon is characterized by complete or nearly complete loss of reflex activity below the level of the cord injury. Flaccid paralysis, loss of deep tendon reflexes, loss of temperature control and vasomotor tone, and bowel and bladder paralysis that result in urinary retention and paralytic ileus are all frequently seen in these patients. Because spinal shock is associated with an instability in blood pressure and pulse, patients must be monitored closely.

Under normal conditions, axons descending from the supraspinal portions of the nervous system deliver low-frequency impulses to the neurons to maintain the neuron in a state of excitability or readiness. When the "background tone" (Mountcastle, 1980) is removed by the injury, the resting excitability of the spinal cord is greatly reduced.

Spinal shock may occur in partial transection of the cord. Mountcastle (1980) has demonstrated that the reticulospinal and vestibulospinal tracts, when severed, produce the phenomenon of spinal shock.

Transection of the spinal cord produces widespread alterations in visceral functions. Immediately after transection of the spinal cord, there is complete atony of the smooth muscle of the bladder wall. At the same time, constrictor tone of the sphincter muscle increases, probably because of loss of an inhibitory influence. With recovery of somatic reflexes, which may occur in 25 to 30 days after cord section, tone returns to the bladder muscles and reflex emptying of the bladder occurs. This is produced by simultaneous contraction of the smooth muscle walls and, to a certain extent, relaxation of the tone of the sphincter. After reflex emptying of the bladder, a considerable residual volume is left. Cutaneous stimulation to the abdomen, perineum, or lower extremities greatly facilitates reflex emptying.

In the intestinal tract it appears as if digestion and absorption proceed normally. Great difficulty is encountered in the evacuation of feces from the lower bowel and rectum. Normally the presence of fecal matter in the lower bowel and rectum passively stretching the walls produces active contraction and peristalsis; this, combined with relaxation of the sphincter, causes defecation. This mechanism is depressed during spinal shock. The sphincter ani muscles relax only slightly in response to passive dilation; therefore retention of fecal material occurs. With the recovery of reflex excitability, reflex evacuation of the bowel occurs, which is facilitated by tactile stimulus of the skin areas of the sacral segments and by manual dilation of the sphincter ani muscle.

Reflex actions on the peripheral vessels and organs innervated by the autonomic nervous system are profoundly affected by spinal shock. Transection of the spinal cord causes an immediate and profound fall in arterial pressure. This is the result of elimination of the bulbar vasoconstrictor mechanism; when spinal nerves are separated from the medullary centers, the important coordination between the state of the blood vessels and subsidiary centers in the spinal cord is lacking. In the person with an intact spinal cord, the spinal centers are regarded as subordinated to the higher vasoconstrictor center in the medulla. The hypotension persists for some time after transection. Spinal neurons innervating peripheral effectors concerned with body temperature control are permanently severed from the descending influences of the thermoregulatory center.

The duration of spinal shock varies greatly from one patient to another. In general the reappearance of any reflex that has been completely abolished by cord injury is a sign of recovery from spinal shock and of cord activity (Mountcastle, 1980).

Cervical Spinal Cord Injury

Until recently, high cervical spinal cord injuries were inevitably fatal, but advances in trauma management and stabilization have improved the survivability of this serious injury. To better classify these patients, Stauffer and Bell (1978) divide them into two categories: respiratory pentaplegia and respiratory quadriplegia.

The person with a first cervical vertabra (C1) functional level (i.e., the C1 level is the last neurologic level to function normally) is classified as a *respiratory pentaplegic*. This patient has little or no sensation or motor control of the head and therefore is totally ventilator dependent.

A C2- or C3-injured patient has some neck control, which allows the patient to develop tolerance for the upright position. Because innervation to the respiratory accessory muscles (sternocleidomastoid and scalenus muscles) are partially preserved, the patient is ventilator dependent but may be able to spend some time off the ventilator. These patients are termed *respiratory quadriplegics.*

The spinal respiratory center is located primarily at the C4 level. The phrenic nerve root must be intact if the patient is to develop any voluntary control of ventilation. Ventilatory capacity will not be normal in these patients, but depending on other factors, they may progress to a life without a ventilator that offers some measure of control and freedom.

Patients with a C5 injury retain control of their head, neck, shoulders, and diaphragm and may have partial control of the elbow. Partial control of the wrist is preserved after a C6 injury; in C7 injury the patient has full elbow extension, wrist flexion, and some finger control; in C8 to first thoracic vertebra (T1) injury the patient has reasonably good finger control, allowing independence with respect to many of the activities of daily living.

Autonomic Dysreflexia

Autonomic dysreflexia *(hyperreflexia)* is a potentially life-threatening reaction that can occur any time after the individual with complete or partial cord transection recovers from spinal shock. Dysreflexia is characterized by a generalized, undampened cardiovascular response to discharge from the sympathetic nervous system, which emerges from the thoracic and lumbar sections of the spinal cord. The abnormal mass reflex occurs because normal spinothalamic pathways carrying impulses to the brain from sensory receptors below the cord lesion are interrupted by the spinal cord lesion. The result is reflex sympathetic outflow from the thoracolumbar section of the spinal cord below the lesion. In turn, the autonomic motor pathways carrying efferent impulses back to the peripheral blood vessels and viscera are interrupted by the lesion. Thus the higher the lesion (sixth thoracic vertebra or above), the more likely an individual will develop autonomic dysreflexia.

The response is usually initiated by one or more noxious sensory impulses, such as a distended bladder, full rectum, shearing force against partially denervated skin, or exposed decubitus ulcer. Interruption of the ascending impulses triggers sympathetic outflow, causing intense arteriolar spasm and blood pressure elevation. The hypertension is sensed in the aortic and carotid sinus receptors and transmitted to the medulla oblongata via CN IX and the carotid sinus nerve. Parasympathetic stimulation causes the heart rate to decrease compensatorily, but the blood pressure remains elevated and even continues to climb because the descending autonomic responses that normally would provide negative feedback to the sympathetic outflow from the cord are interrupted by the cord lesion. Signs of autonomic hyperreflexia are sudden hypertension to levels greater than 200 mm Hg systolic; bradycardia as low as 30 to 40 beats/minute; severe, pounding headache; flushed skin and sweating above the level of the lesion; and pallor and "goose bumps" from pilomotor spasm below the level of the lesion. The patient may also complain of nausea and nasal congestion.

Because of the severe hypertension, immediate action must be taken to prevent a cerebrovascular accident (CVA, stroke). Elevating the head of the bed will often lower the blood pressure because of the venous pooling that occurs with high spinal cord injury. The source of the noxious stimulus must be removed; emptying a full bladder or bowel will produce relief. Similarly, careful attention to bowel and bladder regimens will dramatically reduce the incidence of dysreflexia. Anesthetic cream applied to the anus often prevents triggering dysreflexia when enemas or suppositories are administered. Intravenous antihypertensive medications such as trimethaphan camsylate (Arfonad), a ganglionic blocker, may be necessary if the hypertension is not relieved effectively by conservative measures.

Thoracic-Lumbar-Sacral Spinal Cord Injury

Patients with injuries of the thoracic (T), lumbar (L), and sacral (S) spine are considered paraplegic. The mechanism of injury in this area is typically a flexion injury caused by a fall onto the buttocks or a hyperextension injury, both of which cause compression fractures. A heavy direct blow is needed to fracture the midthoracic vertebral bodies unless they have been previously softened by osteoporosis or neoplasm.

The paraplegic patient is capable of achieving an independent life-style with respect to the activities of daily living. Patients with a T2 to T12 injury retain full upper extremity control and a limited amount of trunk control. In an L1 to L5 injury the patient may have full trunk control and, depending on the level of injury, hip, knee, ankle, and some foot control, which allows these patients to walk with braces. In a S1 to S5 injury the patient has some foot control but experiences bowel and bladder dysfunction.

Treatment of Spinal Cord Injuries

The early handling and treatment of patients with spinal cord injuries are critical for the prevention of further neurologic damage. Prehospital management should assume that trauma victims are spinal cord injured. This approach, combined with technical advances, has preserved remaining function in many patients. The types of trauma most likely to result in spinal cord injury include motor vehicle crashes (including all-terrain vehicles and motorcycles), gunshot wounds, diving accidents, and falls.

Patients with an injury at the C4 level or higher cannot breathe spontaneously. The jaw thrust maneuver is designed to minimize movement of the neck during resuscitation. Establishing an effective airway is the initial priority. Hypotension may occur because of disruption to the autonomic nervous system, causing loss of blood vessel tone and leading to pooling of blood in the extremities and abdomen. Fluid resuscitation does not correct this problem and, in fact, contributes to further complications; therefore it is critical to differentiate the cause of the hypotension (Table 56-3). Patients with injuries above the T6 level are at greater risk for circulatory complications caused by sympathetic nervous system disruption. As a consequence, on rare occasions, deep suctioning will stimulate a vasovagal response, leading to cardiac standstill.

TABLE 56-3   Neurogenic Versus Hypovolemic Shock

Parameter	Neurogenic	Hypovolemic
Blood pressure	Low	Low
Pulse	Bradycardia: slow, bounding	Tachycardia: rapid, weak, thready
Skin	Warm, dry	Cold, clammy

Once the patient has established effective ventilation, either breathing unassisted or with mechanical support, and the cardiovascular system is stable, the spinal cord injury can be assessed. Stabilization of the spinal cord is essential to reduce the risk of additional damage from body movements. The first 72 hours are critical in terms of preventing further deterioration of spinal cord function.

Spinal cord edema, one contributor to neurologic deterioration, is treated with methylprednisolone to protect the cells near the injury site (Ropper, 1994). The sooner corticosteroid therapy is initiated, the better the results. Another experimental technique to reduce spinal edema is intrathecal cooling with normal saline.

The primary treatment for cervical injury is reduction and stabilization of the fracture, most effectively achieved by skeletal traction with tongs or wires inserted in the skull to achieve and maintain reduction. Stabilization is achieved by anatomic reduction and by tension of the spinal ligaments and soft tissue of the cervical area. Slight extension of the neck creates tension in the anterior spinal ligament.

Reduction of fracture dislocations of the thoracic and lumbar spines is no longer recommended. At present, treatment consists of bedrest until pain subsides. Single compression fractures of the body of a vertebra, with flexion angulation of the spine without spinal cord deficit, may be treated by positioning on a specially designed frame (e.g., Stryker, Bradford, Foster), using extension to stretch the anterior spinal ligament and expand the vertebral body.

A controversial therapy is decompression of the spinal cord. There are two schools of thought on early surgical decompression. Some neurosurgeons believe (1) that severe injury to the cord can rarely be reversed, (2) that the damage that occurs in spinal cord injury occurs early in the injury, during which surgical intervention would seriously jeopardize the patient's life with little or no chance of improving postoperative functioning; and (3) that because function returns gradually over a period of up to 2 years, the risk of surgery is not warranted. Others believe that the postinjury edema and swelling of the spinal cord increase the neurologic deficit; therefore laminectomy with decompression always has some potential value. All surgeons agree that patients showing progressive deficit in neurologic function and those with open fractures benefit from surgical decompression.

QUESTIONS

▼ *Answer the following on a separate sheet of paper.*

1. What is normal intracranial pressure (ICP), in mm Hg? What causes increased ICP, and why is it dangerous?

2. Explain the mechanisms that account for the following signs and symptoms of intracranial hematoma: hemiparesis, seizures, mental dysfunction, depression of consciousness, changes in vital signs (increased systolic blood pressure, bradycardia), decerebrate rigidity, and dilated ipsilateral pupil.

3. What two general mechanisms account for brain damage in head trauma?

4. What is a contrecoup injury? What areas of the brain are most likely to be injured in a deceleration automobile accident?

5. List the three most common sites of spinal cord injury.

6. What is the foremost rule in the treatment of spinal cord injury?

7. Contrast the mechanisms for posttraumatic epidural and subdural hematomas.

▼ *Circle the letter preceding each item below that correctly answers the question or completes the statement. Only one answer is correct, with exceptions noted.*

8. Infection from a scalp wound may be transmitted to the brain tissue via the:
   a. Emissary and diploic veins
   b. Middle meningeal artery
   c. Cerebral veins of the subdural space
   d. Carotid artery

9. Brain injury can cause (more than one answer may be correct):
   a. Increased ICP
   b. Hypoxia
   c. Hypercarbia
   d. Hyperthermia

10. Billy, a 10-year-old boy, was hit by a baseball over the temporal area while playing sandlot baseball in the afternoon. Because of a short period of "dizziness," Billy sat on the bench for the next inning and then resumed playing the game. After dinner, Billy vomited, complained of a headache, lay down on the sofa, and appeared to be slightly confused. His mother took him to the emergency room of the local hospital. Which of the following types of brain hemorrhage might one suspect?
    a. Subdural
    b. Subarachnoid
    c. Subperiosteal
    d. Epidural

11. If the diagnosis suspected in question 10 is correct, which other of the following neurologic signs and symptoms would Billy be expected to develop if his case is untreated (more than one answer may be correct)?
    a. Ptosis of the contralateral eyelid
    b. Dilation of the ipsilateral pupil
    c. Positive Babinski's sign
    d. Ipsilateral hemiparesis
    e. Decrease in blood pressure

12. If the suspected diagnosis in question 10 is correct, therapy should consist of:
    a. Conservative observation for the next 24 hours before craniotomy
    b. A spinal tap with the removal of cerebrospinal fluid (CSF) to relieve the increased ICP
    c. Immediate surgical removal of the hematoma and interruption of the arterial bleeding
    d. Administration of a stimulant to improve mental alertness
    e. Administration of hypertonic urea to relieve cerebral edema, with craniotomy planned within the next 3 days

13. Which of the following changes in the neurologic status of a patient who was involved in a motorcycle accident would be most significant in indicating damage involving the central nervous system (CNS)?
    a. Localization of headaches
    b. Change from alertness to increasing lethargy
    c. Pain and edema located near the eye
    d. Increase in pulse and respiratory rate

14. Which of the following statements are *true* concerning chronic subdural hematoma (more than one answer may be correct)?
    a. Usually a result of trivial injury
    b. Develops very slowly
    c. Can be diagnosed by arteriogram
    d. Develops very rapidly

15. Which of the following mechanisms best explains the sign of ipsilateral pupil dilation in intracranial hematoma (more than one answer may be correct)?
    a. Hemorrhage from the anterior cerebral artery
    b. Herniation of the uncus into the tentorial ring, compressing the third cranial nerve.

    c. Hemorrhage from the middle cerebral artery
    d. Traction of the oculomotor nerve against the posterior cerebral artery

16. A young man with a head injury shows a rise in temperature together with a slowing of the pulse and respirations. Which of the following would probably be responsible for his symptoms?
    a. Injury to the cortical motor speech area
    b. Organization of the clot
    c. Injury to the vital centers within the medulla
    d. Lesion in the occipital lobe

17. A subdural hematoma that causes the development of significant signs and symptoms within 24 to 48 hours is classified as:
    a. Acute
    b. Subacute
    c. Chronic

18. An injury causing unilateral transection of the spinal cord causes which of the following changes below the level of the injury?
    a. Contralateral loss of vibration sense and ipsilateral loss of tactile sensation
    b. Contralateral loss of vibration sense and tactile discrimination and a contralateral increase in touch threshold
    c. An ipsilateral loss of the vibration sense and tactile discrimination and a contralateral increase in the touch threshold
    d. An ipsilateral loss of the vibration sense and tactile discrimination and an ipsilateral increase in the touch threshold

19. Which of the following changes is expected immediately after transection of the spinal cord (more than one answer may be correct)?
    a. A general increase in skeletal muscle tone
    b. A period of spinal shock lasting approximately 2 days
    c. Retention of urine and feces
    d. Hypotension

Continued.

QUESTIONS—cont'd

▼ Match each meningeal structure in column A with the appropriate statements from column B.

Column A

20. _____ Dura mater
21. _____ Arachnoid
22. _____ Pia mater

Column B

a. Fine, fibrous middle layer of the meninges
b. Inner meningeal layer closely applied to the brain and spinal cord
c. Encloses the venous sinuses and separates the brain into compartments
d. Circulation of CSF in a space directly under this layer
e. Middle and posterior portions supplied by the middle meningeal artery

---

▼ Circle T if the statement is true and F if it is false. Correct any false statements.

23. T F An epidural hematoma is a hemorrhage between the dura and the arachnoid.

24. T F Paraplegia may be caused by a bilateral lesion at C5.

25. T F A bilateral lesion in the middle or lower thoracic cord causes paraplegia.

26. T F Patients with cervical spinal cord injuries above the level of C3 are generally ventilator dependent.

27. T F A quadriplegic with a C6 injury might be expected to have partial function of the shoulder, elbow, and wrist.

28. T F The initial treatment of all serious spinal cord injuries consists of laminectomy with decompression.

29. T F An ipsilateral lesion of the spinal cord at C5 would cause hemiplegia.

30. T F Spinal shock is a temporary condition of decreased excitability of neurons above the level of the cord transection and may last for months.

▼ Circle the letter preceding each item below that correctly answers the question or completes the statement. Only one answer is correct.

31. The basic mechanism of a decreased level of consciousness (LOC) with an intracranial mass lesion is interference between the cerebrum and the:
   a. Autonomic nervous system
   b. Pons

c. Medulla
   d. Reticular activating system

32. A score of 6 on the Glasgow Coma Scale indicates:
   a. Full alertness
   b. Coma
   c. Brain death
   d. Damage to cranial nerve I

33. The oculocephalic (doll's eyes) reflex is:
   a. An indication of optic nerve function
   b. An abnormal reflex when present
   c. Absent in lesions of the brain stem at the pontine level
   d. Movement of the eyes in the direction the head is turned

34. The ice-water caloric test:
   a. Is called the oculocephalic test
   b. Is abnormal if nystagmus is elicited
   c. Assesses the hunger and satiety centers in the hypothalamus
   d. Assesses vestibular nerve function (CN VIII) in the pons

35. A good initial assessment of LOC is the patient's ability to:
   a. Solve an abstract problem
   b. Open the eyes when addressed
   c. Name objects correctly
   d. Squeeze your fingers tightly

36. A 52-year-old semiconscious man was admitted to the hospital after an automobile accident in which he sustained a head injury. A CT scan revealed diffuse cerebral edema but not a hematoma. The initial neurologic examination by the nurse revealed that he opened his eyes to his name. His speech was not understandable, although he did seem to make an effort to respond to questions. He also followed commands to move his arms or legs some of the time. His arm and leg strength was less

on the right than on the left. Compute a Glasgow Coma Scale score on the basis of these findings.
   a. 3
   b. 6
   c. 9
   d. 11

37. Signs present in autonomic dysreflexia include:
   a. Tachycardia and hypotension
   b. Bradycardia and hypertension
   c. Hyperthermia and hypertension
   d. Tachycardia and hypertension

38. The cause of autonomic dysreflexia is:
   a. Massive sympathetic outflow from interruption of spinothalamic pathways
   b. Injury to a peripheral nerve
   c. Increased ICP
   d. Injury to reflex centers in the brain stem

39. Stimuli that may trigger autonomic dysreflexia include:
   a. Full bladder
   b. Full bowel
   c. Shearing forces against partially denervated skin
   d. Débridement of a decubitus ulcer
   e. All the above

40. A serious manifestation of autonomic dysreflexia in a patient with spinal cord injury requiring urgent intervention is:
   a. Severe hypertension
   b. Severe hypotention
   c. Severe flushing and sweating above the level of the lesion
   d. Severe throbbing headache

41. Treatment of autonomic dysreflexia includes all the following *except:*
   a. Elevating the head of the bed
   b. Lowering the head of the bed to a flat position
   c. Intravenous antihypertensive drug (e.g., Arfonad)
   d. Emptying the bladder

42. Decerebrate posturing is characterized by:
   a. Abnormal flexion response
   b. Abnormal extension response
   c. Absent motor response
   d. Hyperflexion of the lower extremities

CHAPTER 57

Central Nervous System Tumors

MARY CARTER LOMBARDO

BRAIN TUMORS

Intracranial tumors include space-occupying lesions, both benign and malignant, that develop in the brain, meninges, and skull. Brain tumors derive from neuronal tissue, supportive brain tissue, the reticuloendothelial system (RES), brain coverings, and residual developmental tissues, or they metastasize from systemic carcinomas. Tumors metastasize to the brain most often from the lung, followed by breast, skin, kidney, gastrointestinal (GI) tract, prostate, and thyroid. Brain tumors can occur at any age; they may occur in children under age 10 but are most frequently found in adults during the fifth and sixth decades of life.

There are many classifications of brain tumors. Perhaps the one easiest to understand is the *Kernahan and Sayre classification,* in which the tumor is named for the cells present in the adult nervous system, in vascular tissue, and in developmental defects and the degree of malignancy is graded I to IV (IV being the most malignant) (Table 57-1).

Because patients with brain tumors have diverse and confusing symptoms, diagnosis may be difficult. Symptomatology of brain tumor depends on size, location, and invasiveness of the tumor.

Certain tumors occur more frequently in a particular age-group. During infancy and childhood, posterior fossa tumors are much more common than supratentorial lesions (middle or anterior fossa), which are more common in adults. The brain tumor of a child is likely to be a malignant astrocytoma of the cerebellum of grade I or II. In the middle-aged or older person the most common brain tumor is a glioblastoma multiforme, the most malignant glioma, characterized by a rapid growth rate.

Gliomas

Gliomas account for approximately 40% to 50% of brain tumors. Gliomas are classified on the basis of embryologic origin. In the adult the neuroglia of the central nervous system (CNS) provide for the repair, support, and protection of the delicate nerve cells. Gliomas consist of connective tissue and supporting cells. The neuroglia possess the potential to continue to divide throughout life. Glial cells congregate to form dense cicatricial scars in regions of brain where neurons disappear because of injury or disease (Snell, 1992).

There are three types of glial cell: microglia, oligodendroglia, and astrocytes. The *microglia* are of mesodermal embryologic origin and therefore are generally not classified as true glial cells. The microglia enter the CNS through the vascular system and function as phagocytes, clearing away the debris and combating infection.

The oligodendroglia and the astrocytes are true neuroglia and, as with neurons, arise from the ectoderm. *Oligodendroglia* are involved in myelin formation. The

TABLE 57-1   Brain Tumors

Tumor	Percent of All Brain Tumors
Gliomas	40-50
Astrocytoma grade I	5-10
Astrocytoma grade II	2-5
Astrocytoma grades III and IV (glioblastoma multiforme)	20-30
Medulloblastoma	3-5
Oligodendroglioma	1-4
Ependymoma grades I to IV	1-3
Meningioma	12-20
Pituitary tumors	5-15
Neurilemmomas (mainly cranial nerve VIII)	3-10
Metastatic tumors	5-10
Blood vessel tumors	
Arteriovenous malformations, hemangioblastomas, endotheliomas	0.5-1
Tumors of developmental defects	2-3
Dermoids, epidermoids, teratomas, chordomas, paraphyseal cysts	
Craniopharyngiomas	3-8
Pinealomas	0.5-0.8
Miscellaneous	
Sarcomas, papillomas of the choroid plexus, lipomas, unclassified, etc.	1-3

From Schwartz SI, editor *Principles of surgery,* ed 6, New York, 1994, McGraw-Hill.

function of astrocytes is still under investigation; evidence shows that they may play some role in impulse conduction and synaptic transmission of neurons and may serve as conduits between blood vessels and neurons (Mountcastle, 1980).

Astrocytomas infiltrate the brain and are frequently associated with cysts of various sizes. Although they infiltrate the brain tissue, the effect on brain functioning is minimal early in the illness. Generally, astrocytomas are nonmalignant, although they may undergo a malignant change to a glioblastoma, a highly malignant astrocytoma. These tumors are generally slow growing; therefore the patient frequently does not seek medical attention for several years, until debilitating symptoms occur, such as seizures or headaches. Complete surgical excision is generally not possible because of the invasive nature of the tumor, but it is sensitive to radiation.

The *glioblastoma multiforme* is the most malignant of the gliomas. This tumor has a rapid growth rate, and complete surgical excision is impossible. Life expectancy is usually about 12 months. The tumor may occur anywhere but most often involves the cerebral hemisphere and often spreads to the opposite side via the corpus callosum.

The *oligodendroglioma* is a slow-growing lesion similar to the astrocytoma but is composed of oligoden-

droglial cells. It is relatively avascular and is prone to calcification. It is usually found in the cerebral hemisphere of young people. Surgical excision and radiation are used to prolong life but are rarely curative.

Ependymoma is a malignant tumor arising from within the walls of the ventricle. In children the most common site is the fourth ventricle. This tumor invades the surrounding tissue and obstructs the ventricles. The tumor can be completely resected, although metastasis is possible during excision. Radiation treatment is used when complete resection is not possible.

Meningeal Tumors

The *meningioma* is the most important tumor arising from the meninges, the mesothelial lining cells, and the connective tissue cells of the arachnoid and the dura. Most meningeal tumors are benign and encapsulated and do not infiltrate adjacent tissue but rather compress the underlying structures. These tumors are often quite vascular and therefore take up radioactive isotopes during a brain scan. Complete surgical excision is possible, especially if the tumor is not in a critical area and diagnosis is made early. Meningiomas of the area around the brain stem and the base of the skull are often not accessible for complete excision. Because of the slow growth of this tumor, symptoms may be overlooked and the diagnosis missed completely. Symptoms include idiopathic epilepsy, hemiparesis, and aphasia.

Pituitary Tumors

Pituitary tumors arise from the chromophobe, eosinophil, or basophil cells of the anterior pituitary. These tumors cause headache, bitemporal hemianopsia (from pressure on the optic chiasm), and signs of abnormal secretion of hormones from the anterior pituitary. Fig. 57-1 illustrates the various visual field defects that typically occur when lesions involve the optic tract.

Chromophobe tumors are nonsecretory tumors that compress the pituitary gland, the optic chiasm, and the hypothalamus. Symptoms of this brain tumor include depression of sexual function, secondary hypothyroidism, and adrenal hypofunction (amenorrhea, impotence, loss of hair, weakness, hypotension, low basal metabolism, hypoglycemia, and electrolyte disturbances).

Eosinophilic adenomas are generally smaller and slower-growing tumors than chromophobe tumors. The symptoms include acromegaly in adults and gigantism in children, headache, sweating disturbance, paresthesias, muscular pain, and loss of libido. Disturbances in visual fields (bitemporal hemianopsia) are rare.

Basophil adenomas are generally small. These tumors are associated with the symptoms of Cushing's syndrome (obesity, muscle wasting, skin atrophy, osteoporosis, plethora, hypertension, salt and water retention, hypertrichosis, diabetes mellitus).

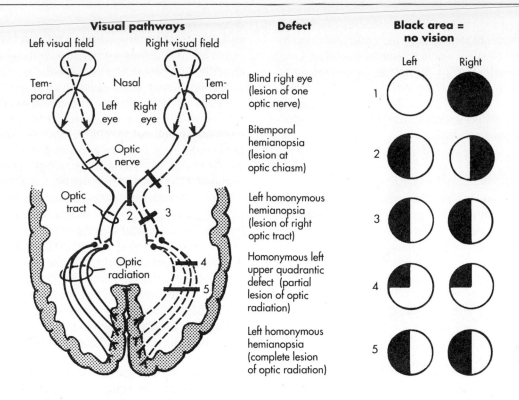

Visual pathways

Left visual field   Right visual field

Tem-poral   Nasal   Tem-poral

Left eye   Right eye

Optic nerve

Optic tract

Optic radiation

Defect

Blind right eye (lesion of one optic nerve)

Bitemporal hemianopsia (lesion at optic chiasm)

Left homonymous hemianopsia (lesion of right optic tract)

Homonymous left upper quadrantic defect (partial lesion of optic radiation)

Left homonymous hemianopsia (complete lesion of optic radiation)

Black area = no vision

Left   Right

FIG. 57-1   Visual field defects produced by selected lesions in the visual pathways. [Modified from *Programmed practice in anatomy and physiology of the nervous system,* Englewood Cliffs, NJ, 1972, Prentice-Hall.]

Neurilemmomas (Auditory Nerve Tumors)

Auditory nerve tumors constitute 3% to 10% of intracranial tumors. They probably arise from the Schwann cells of the nerve sheath. The nerve fibers in the eighth cranial nerve (CN VIII) are eventually destroyed. Bilateral auditory neurilemmoma may occur in von Recklinghausen's disease. Generally benign, these tumors occasionally undergo malignant change.

Symptoms of auditory neurilemmoma include first deafness, tinnitus, loss of caloric vestibular reactivity, and vertigo, followed by suboccipital discomfort, staggering gait, involvement of adjacent cranial nerves, and signs of increased intracranial pressure (ICP). Nystagmus, especially horizontal, is usually present. Treatment consists of complete removal of the tumor, if possible, because incomplete removal is generally accompanied by recurrence of the tumor. Surgery leaves the patient with facial paralysis and deafness.

Metastatic Tumors

Metastatic lesions, which account for approximately 5% to 10% of brain tumors, may originate from any primary site. The most common primary tumors are those of the lung and breast, but neoplasms from the genitourinary tract, GI tract, bone, and thyroid may also metastasize to the brain. The metastatic lesion may be single or multiple and may be a late stage in the metastatic process or the

first sign of a previously unrecognized primary tumor. Single lesions may be surgically excised to extend life or to reduce symptoms. The edema surrounding these lesions is responsive to corticosteroid therapy.

Blood Vessel Tumors

These tumors include the angiomas, hemangioblastomas, and endotheliomas and make up a small percentage of brain tumors. *Angiomas* are congenital arteriovenous (AV) malformations, present from birth, which slowly enlarge. They may compress surrounding brain tissue and bleed intracerebrally or into the subarachnoid space. *Hemangioblastomas* are neoplasms composed of embryologic vascular elements most often found in the cerebellum. The von Hippel-Lindau syndrome is a combination of cerebellar hemangioblastoma, angiomatosis of the retina, and cysts of the kidney and pancreas.

Tumors of Developmental Defects (Congenital)

Rare congenital tumors include *chordomas,* which are composed of cells derived from the embryonic notochord remnants and are found at the base of the skull. They grow slowly but are highly invasive, making complete surgical removal impossible. *Dermoids* and *teratomas* may occur anywhere in the CNS. *Teratomas* frequently occur in the ventricular system and obstruct the third ventricle, the aqueduct, or the fourth ventricle. *Craniopharyngiomas* arise from remnants of the embryonic craniopharyngeal duct (Rathke's pouch) and are usually located posterior to the sella turcica. Symptoms of congenital tumors generally manifest themselves early in a child's life but may be silent for many years. The symptoms include defects in visual fields, generally irregular, and hypothalamic and pituitary dysfunctions.

Pinealomas (Adnexal Tumors)

Pinealomas account for a small number of intracranial lesions and include tumors that originate within the pineal body *(pinealoma),* as well as those from the surrounding choroid plexus *(choroid papilloma).* Pinealomas compress the aqueduct, causing obstructive hydrocephalus, and the hypothalamus, giving rise to precocious puberty and diabetes insipidus. Choroid papilloma causes intraventricular bleeding and also obstructs the ventricular system.

Pathophysiology of Brain Tumors

Brain tumors give rise to progressive neurologic deficit. The symptoms occur on a continuum. This underscores the importance of the history when examining the patient. Symptoms should be discussed within a time perspective. When did the symptom develop? Was it associated with anything? How long have you had this?

The neurologic deficit in brain tumors is generally thought to be caused by two factors: the focal disturbances caused by the tumor and the increased ICP.

Focal disturbances occur when there is compression of brain tissue and infiltration or direct invasion of brain parenchyma with destruction of neural tissue. Dysfunction is greatest with the fastest-growing infiltrating tumors (e.g., glioblastoma multiforme).

Alteration in blood supply because of compression from the growing tumor causes necrosis of brain tissue. Interference with arterial blood supply is usually manifested by an acute loss of function and may be confused with primary cerebrovascular disorders.

Seizures as a manifestation of altered neuronal excitability are related to the compression, invasion, and alteration in the blood supply to the brain tissue. Some tumors form cysts, which also compress the surrounding brain parenchyma, increasing the focal neurologic deficit.

The increased intracranial pressure may result from several factors: an increase in the mass within the skull, edema formation around the tumor, and alteration in cerebrospinal fluid (CSF) circulation. The tumor's growth causes an increase in mass because it occupies space within the relatively fixed volume of the rigid compartment of the skull. Malignant tumors produce edema in the surrounding brain tissue. The mechanism is not completely understood, but it is thought that an osmotic gradient causes absorption of fluid by the tumor. Some tu-

mors may cause hemorrhage. Venous obstruction and edema caused by breakdown of the blood-brain barrier cause an increase in intracranial volume and ICP. Obstruction of CSF circulation from the lateral ventricles to the subarachnoid space causes hydrocephalus.

Increased ICP becomes life-threatening when any of the previously discussed causes develops rapidly. Compensatory mechanisms require days or months to be effective and therefore are not useful when increased ICP develops rapidly. These mechanisms include decreased intracranial blood volume, decreased CSF volume, decreased intracellular fluid contents, and decreased parenchymal cell numbers. Untreated increased ICP causes herniation of the uncus or the cerebellum. Uncal herniation is caused when the medial gyrus of the temporal lobe is displaced inferiorly through the tentorial notch by a mass in the cerebral hemisphere. This compresses the midbrain, causing loss of consciousness and compression of CN III. The cerebellar tonsils are displaced downward through the foramen magnum by a posterior mass in cerebellar herniation. Compression of the medulla and respiratory arrest rapidly ensue. Other physiologic changes that occur with rapidly developing increased ICP include progressive bradycardia, systemic hypertension with a widening pulse pressure, and respiratory failure (see Chapter 56).

Clinical Manifestations

The classic triad of symptoms in brain tumor consists of headache, vomiting, and papilledema. However, there is great variety in symptoms, depending on the site of the lesion and the rapidity of growth.

Headache

Headache is perhaps the most common symptom found in patients with brain tumors. The pain may be described as deep, aching, steady, dull, and sometimes agonizingly severe. It is most severe in the morning and is aggravated by activities that normally increase ICP, such as stooping, coughing, or straining at stool. The headache is somewhat relieved by aspirin and application of cold packs to the site.

The headache associated with brain tumor is caused by traction and displacement of pain-sensitive structures within the intracranial cavity. These pain-sensitive structures include the arteries, veins, venous sinuses, and cranial nerves.

The headache has a localizing value in that one third of headaches overlie the tumor site and the other two thirds are near or above the tumor. Occipital headache is the first symptom in tumors of the posterior fossa. Approximately one third of supratentorial lesions give rise to a frontal headache. A complaint of a generalized headache has little localizing value and usually indicates extensive displacement of intracranial contents with increased ICP.

Nausea and vomiting

Nausea and vomiting occur as a result of stimulation of the emetic center in the medulla. Vomiting is most frequent in children and in association with increased ICP with brain stem displacement. Vomiting may occur without preceding nausea and may be projectile.

Papilledema

Papilledema is caused by venous stasis, which leads to engorgement and swelling of the optic disc. When seen by funduscopy, it suggests increased ICP. It is often difficult to use this sign as diagnostic of brain tumor because the fundi in some persons may not show papilledema, even with very high ICP.

In association with the papilledema, some disturbances in vision may occur. These include enlargement of the blind spot and *amaurosis fugax* (fleeting moments of dimmed vision).

Localizing symptoms

Other signs and symptoms of brain tumor tend to have a greater localizing value. Tumors of the frontal lobe give symptoms of mental changes, hemiparesis, ataxia, and disturbances of speech. Mental changes are manifested by subtle changes in personality. Some patients experience periods of depression, confusion, or bizarre behavior. The most common changes involve higher level reasoning and judgment skills. Hemiparesis is caused by pressure on the neighboring motor areas and pathways. If the motor area is involved, jacksonian seizures and obvious motor weakness may occur. Tumors involving the lower end of the precentral cortex cause weakness of the face, tongue, and thumb, whereas tumors of the paracentral lobule produce weakness in the foot and lower extremity. Tumors of the frontal lobe may cause unsteadiness in the gait, often imitating cerebellar ataxia. When the left or dominant frontal lobe is affected, aphasia and apraxia may be evident.

Tumors of the occipital lobe may give rise to convulsive seizures preceded by an aura. With involvement of the occipital cortex, contralateral homonymous hemianopsia occurs (see Fig. 57-1). There may be visual agnosia, difficulty in judging distances, and a tendency to become lost in familiar surroundings.

Temporal lobe tumors cause tinnitus and auditory hallucinations, probably from irritation of the temporal auditory receptive or adjacent cortex. Varying degrees of sensory aphasia appear, beginning with difficulty in naming objects, when the temporal lobe of the dominant hemisphere becomes involved. Mental symptoms similar to those that develop with frontal lobe tumors may occur. Pressure from a growing tumor on the frontal cortex may result in facial weaknesses. Lesions of the anterior temporal pole cause a superior quadrantanopsia, which may progress to a complete hemianopsia.

Tumors in the parietal sensory cortex cause loss of cor-

TABLE 57-2 Disorders of Movement Seen in Cerebellar Tumors

Disorder	Description
Intention tremor	Oscillating tremor most marked at the end of fine movements
Asynergia	Lack of cooperation between muscles, for example, failure of the wrist extensors during flexion of the fingers, allowing the wrist to flex
Decomposition of movement	Performance of actions in successive parts rather than as a whole, for example, touching the nose by first flexing the forearm, then the arm, and lastly adjusting the wrist and forearm
Dysmetria	Errors in the range of movement, for example, in touching a point, stopping the action before reaching the point or moving past it
Deviation from line of movement	Example: carrying food to the ear instead of the mouth
Adiadochokinesia	Inability to perform alternating movements, for example, tapping quickly and smoothly
Nystagmus	Rapid oscillation of the eyes while fixing the gaze on region and object

tical sensory function and impairment of sensory localization, two-point discrimination, graphesthesia, position sense, and stereognosis. Visual defects from parietal or parietooccipital tumors usually involve inferior homonymous quadrants.

Cerebellar tumors cause early papilledema and frequently produce nuchal headache. Cerebellar lesions also cause disorders of movement, varying according to the size and specific location of the tumor within the cerebellum. Table 57-2 lists the most common of these disorders. Less conspicuous but equally characteristic of cerebellar tumor is *hypotonia* (absence of normal resistance to stretch or to displacement of a limb from a given posture) and hyperextensibility of joints. In speech the patient tends to decompose words into separate syllables pronounced in a staccato rhythm called *scanning speech*.

Tumors of the ventricles and hypothalamus produce varied deficits. Invasive lesions of the third ventricle and the hypothalamus produce somnolence, diabetes insipidus, obesity, and disturbances of temperature regulation. A small tumor in the third ventricle, on the other hand, causes steady headache and papilledema with few localizing signs. Tumors involving the fourth ventricle give rise to rapid development of increased ICP with papilledema and cerebellar symptoms.

Diagnosis

Any patient suspected of having an intracranial lesion should undergo a complete medical evaluation with special attention to the neurologic examination. Specific diagnostic studies are undertaken after the neurologic examination and proceed from the noninvasive procedures that cause the least risk to those that use more dangerous, invasive techniques.

Skull radiographs give valuable information about bone structure, thickening, and calcifications; the position of the calcified pineal gland; and the position of the sella turcica. The electroencephalogram (EEG) gives information about the altered excitability of the neurons. A shift of intracerebral contents can be seen on the echoencephalogram. A radioactive brain scan will show areas of abnormal accumulation of radioactive substances. Brain tumors and vascular occlusion, infection, and trauma cause breakdown of the blood-brain barrier, causing an abnormal accumulation of the radioactive substance.

Pneumoencephalography and cerebral angiography are two invasive procedures that aid in the final diagnosis and help the physician decide appropriate treatment.

Diagnosis of brain tumors has been aided considerably by the use of magnetic resonance imaging (MRI) and computed tomography (CT) scans. These procedures are now widely available and have become the diagnostic procedures of choice, replacing invasive techniques.

SPINAL CORD TUMORS

Spinal tumors develop in the spine or its contents and generally produce symptoms by involvement of the spinal cord or nerve roots. Primary cord tumors are about one-sixth as common as brain tumors and have a better prognosis because about 60% are benign. The spinal cord undergoes not only actual tumor growth, but also compression caused by an encroaching tumor. Spinal tumors occur in all age-groups but are rarely encountered before the age of 10 years.

Spinal tumors are classified according to the location of the tumor in relation to the dura and the spinal cord. The major classification divides tumors into extradural and intradural. Intradural tumors are then subdivided into extramedullary and intramedullary.

Extradural tumors generally arise from the bone of the spinal column or within the extradural space. Ninety percent of extradural tumors are malignant. The most common tumor affecting the spinal vertebral column is a metastatic carcinoma. Extradural neoplasms within the extradural space are typically metastatic carcinomas and lymphomas.

Intradural extramedullary tumors lie between the dura mater and the spinal cord (Fig. 57-2). The most common tumors in this area are benign neurofibromas and meningiomas. These tumors compress the spinal cord and can be surgically removed.

Intradural intramedullary tumors arise from within the spinal cord itself. The same tumors that affect the brain also affect the spinal cord. Ependymomas are the most common, followed by astrocytomas, glioblastomas, and oligodendrogliomas.

The spinal cord accommodates to compression that occurs slowly, as seen in meningiomas and neurofibromas, producing few signs and symptoms, especially in the early stages. Acute compression of the cord, such as that

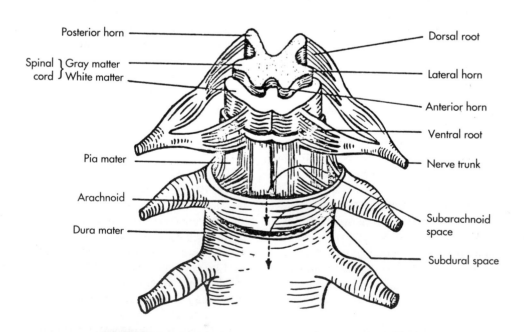

FIG. 57-2   Structure of the spinal cord. (From *Programmed practice in anatomy and physiology of the nervous system,* Englewood Cliffs, NJ, 1972, Prentice-Hall.)

► TABLE 57-3   **Symptoms and Signs of Common Vertebral Root Lesions**

Root	Location of Pain	Sensory Loss	Reflex Loss	Weakness and Atrophy
C5	Lower neck, tip of shoulder, arm	Deltoid area (inconsistent)	Biceps	Shoulder abductors, biceps
C6	Lower neck, medial scapula, arm, radial side of forearm	Radial side of hand, thumb, index finger	Biceps	Biceps
C7	Lower neck, medial scapula, precordium, arm, forearm	Index finger, middle finger	Triceps	Triceps
C8	Lower neck; medial arm and forearm, ulnar side of hand; fourth and fifth fingers	Ulnar side of hand, fourth and fifth fingers		Intrinsic hand muscles
L4	Low back, anterior and medial thigh	Anterior thigh	Quadriceps	Quadriceps
L5	Low back, lateral thigh, lateral leg, dorsum of foot, great toe	Great toe, medial side of dorsum of foot, lateral leg and thigh		Toe extensors, ankle dorsiflexors and evertors
S1	Low back, posterior thigh, posterior leg, lateral side of foot, heel	Lateral foot, heel, posterior leg	Achilles	Ankle dorsiflexion, plantar flexion

From Simpson J, Magee K: *Clinical evaluation of the nervous system,* Boston, 1973, Little, Brown.
C, Cervical; *L,* lumbar; *S,* sacral vertebrae.

occurring with metastatic lesions, causes rapid, progressive neurologic deficit. Resulting symptoms depend largely on the area affected as well as the location of the lesion within the spinal column.

Because of the anatomic organization within the cord, compression from lesions outside the cord generally produces symptoms well below the site of the lesion, with the level of sensory impairment gradually ascending as the compression increases and affects areas deeper within the cord. Lesions located deep within the cord may spare superficially arranged fibers and give rise to sensory dissociation, with loss of pain and temperature senses and preservation of the sense of touch. By disturbing position sense, cord compression may also result in ataxia.

Spinal Cord Compression at Different Levels
Tumors of the foramen magnum

Tumors of the foramen magnum are most often meningiomas. Symptoms of spinal cord compression at this level are caused by compression of the spinal cord, nerve roots, and intracranial contents. Suboccipital pain is perhaps the earliest symptom. This pain is aggravated by nodding. Nerve root compression causes sensory and motor weakness in the occipital region (second cervical [C2] dermatome) and the neck (C3 dermatome). Extension of the tumor into the intracranial cavity causes increased ICP, cerebellar dysfunction, nystagmus, and compression of cranial nerve nuclei, with trigeminal sensory loss and atrophy of the tongue.

Tumors of the cervical region

Cervical lesions produce radicular-like motor and sensory signs that involve the shoulders and arms and may involve the hands. Involvement of the hands from an upper cervical lesion (i.e., above C4) is thought to result

from compression of the descending blood supply to the anterior horns via the anterior spinal artery. The patient generally has weakness and atrophy involving the shoulder girdle and arms. Lower cervical tumors (C5, C6, C7) may cause the loss of upper extremity tendon reflexes (biceps, brachioradialis, triceps). Sensory loss extends along the radial border of the forearm and thumb in a C6 compression and involves the middle and index fingers in lesions at C7; C7 lesions cause sensory loss of the index and middle fingers (Table 57-3).

Tumors of the thoracic region

Patients with lesions of the thoracic area often present with insidious spastic weakness in the lower extremities and later paresthesias. Patients may complain of pain and a tight, binding feeling across the chest and abdomen, which may be confused with pain from intrathoracic and intraabdominal disorders. Patients with lower thoracic lesions may have loss of lower abdominal reflexes and Beevor's sign (the umbilicus elevates when the patient, in the supine position, raises the head against resistance).

Tumors of the lumbar-sacral region

A complex diagnostic situation exists in the case of a tumor involving the lumbar and sacral regions because of the proximity of the lower lumbar and sacral segments and the descending nerve roots from higher levels of the cord. Upper lumbar cord compression spares the abdominal reflexes, abolishes the cremasteric reflexes, and may produce weakness of hip flexion and spasticity of the lower legs. Patients have loss of the knee jerk reflex with brisk ankle reflexes and bilateral Babinski's signs. Pain is usually referred to the groin. Lesions involving the lower lumbar and upper sacral segments cause weakness and atrophy of perineal, calf, and foot muscles and loss of the ankle jerk reflex. Loss of sensation in the perianal and genital area with impairment of bowel and bladder control are characteristic signs of lesions involving the lower sacral area.

Tumors of the cauda equina

Lesions of the cauda equina cause early sphincteric symptoms and impotence. Other characteristic signs include dull, aching pain in the sacrum or perineum, sometimes radiating to the legs. Flaccid paralysis corresponds to the nerve roots involved and is sometimes asymmetric.

Symptoms are produced not only by the anatomic location of the spinal cord, but also by its position within the spinal canal. The pathology of extradural and intradural tumors is discussed next.

Extradural Tumors

Extradural tumors are primarily metastases from a primary lesion in the breast, prostate, thyroid, lungs, kidney, or stomach. Pain is generally the first symptom. It is described as being dull, constant, and localized over the area of the tumor, followed by pain radiating along the dermatome pattern. The localized pain is most severe at night and is aggravated by movements of the spine and bedrest. The radicular pain is intensified by coughing and straining. Pain may be present for weeks or months before spinal cord involvement.

The common clinical course of extradural tumors is rapid compression of the spinal cord from encroachment of the tumor on the cord, collapse of the vertebral column, or hemorrhage from within the metastasis. Once symptoms of spinal cord compression develop, they rapidly cause total loss of spinal cord function. Spastic weakness and loss of vibration and joint position senses below the level of the lesion are the first signs of cord compression. Without prompt surgical decompression, paresthesias and sensory loss progress quickly to irreversible paraplegia.

Extradural spinal cord tumors can be diagnosed by radiography of the spine. Most patients with tumors demonstrate osteoporosis or obvious bone destruction of the vertebral body and pedicles. A myelogram definitively localizes the tumor, although high-resolution CT scans are proving equal to myelograms in diagnostic accuracy. The CSF shows elevated protein and normal glucose levels.

Surgical decompression with laminectomy is the treatment of choice when symptoms of cord compression are present. Hormones, radiation, and chemotherapy are used as adjunctive measures.

Intradural Tumors

Intradural tumors, in contrast to extradural tumors, are generally benign. The clinical course is much slower and may extend over months to years. Intradural tumors are divided into two types: extramedullary and intramedullary.

Extramedullary tumors

Approximately 65% of all intradural tumors are extramedullary. They may be either neurofibromas or meningiomas.

Neurofibromas arise from the dorsal nerve roots. They sometimes form a dumbbell-like or hourglasslike growth extending into the extradural space. A small percentage of neurofibromas undergo sarcomatous changes and become invasive or metastasize.

Meningiomas are usually loosely attached to the dura, arising probably from the arachnoid membrane, and approximately 90% are found in the thoracic region. These tumors are more frequent in middle-age females. The posterolateral aspect of the cord is the most common site for these tumors.

Extramedullary cord lesions cause compression of the spinal cord and the nerve roots at the affected segment. The *Brown-Séquard syndrome* may result from lateral compression of the cord. This syndrome, caused by damage to one half of the cord, is characterized by ipsilateral signs of dysfunction of the corticospinal tract and the posterior column below the level of the lesion and contralateral reduction in pain and temperature perception below the level of the lesion. The patient complains of pain, first in the back and then along the spinal roots. As with extradural tumors, pain is aggravated by movement, coughing, sneezing, or straining and is most severe at night. The nocturnal aggravation of pain is caused by traction on the diseased nerve roots when the spine elongates with removal of the shortening effect of gravity. The sensory loss is at first vague and located below the level of the lesion (because of dermatome overlap). It gradually rises to below the segmented spinal cord level. Tumors of the posterior aspect may be manifested by paresthesias and later by proprioceptive sensory loss, adding ataxia to the weakness. Anteriorly situated tumors may cause little sensory loss but may cause severe motor disability.

With extramedullary tumors, CSF protein is almost always elevated. Spinal radiographs may show enlargement of a foramen and thinning of the adjacent pedicle. As with extradural tumors, myelograms, CT scans, and MRI are essential for precise localization. Early surgical removal is essential for a complete recovery.

Intramedullary tumors

The histologic structure of intramedullary tumors is essentially the same as that of intracranial tumors. More than 95% of these tumors are gliomas. In contrast to intracranial tumors, they tend to be more benign histologically and have a more benign course. Approximately 50% of intramedullary tumors are ependymomas, 45% are astrocytomas, and the rest are oligodendrogliomas and hemangioblastomas.

Ependymomas arise at all levels of the spinal cord but are found most often in the conus medullaris of the cauda equina. All other intramedullary tumors occur equally frequently in all areas of the spinal cord.

Intramedullary tumors grow into the central part of the spinal cord and destroy crossing fibers and neurons of the gray matter. The destruction of crossing fibers results in bilateral sensory loss of pain and temperature sense extending throughout the segments involved in the lesion, leading to damage to peripheral skin areas. The senses of touch, motion, position, and vibration are usually preserved unless the lesion is large. The loss of pain and temperature sensation with preservation of the other senses is known as *dissociated sensory loss*. Alteration in the function of muscle stretch reflexes results from damage to the anterior horn cells. Weakness, with atrophy and fasciculations, is caused by involvement of the lower motor neurons.

Intramedullary tumors may extend through several segments of the spinal cord. As the lesion progresses, involvement of the corticospinal and spinothalamic tracts causes loss of pain and temperature sense, and upper motor neuron signs extend below the level of the lesion. Table 51-3 lists some differentiating features between upper and lower motor neuron lesions.

Other signs and symptoms include dull, aching pain localized to the level of the lesion, impotence in males, and sphincter disturbances in both genders.

Radiography reveals visible widening of the spinal canal and erosion of the pedicles. On myelogram, CT scan, or MRI the spinal cord appears enlarged.

Surgical removal is sometimes possible with intramedullary tumors, especially ependymomas and hemangioblastomas, but recurrences are not uncommon. Again, early diagnosis is imperative to ensure a good prognosis.

QUESTIONS

▼ *Match the type of glioma in column A with its characteristic in column B.*

Column A
1. _____ Glioblastoma multiforme
2. _____ Medulloblastoma
3. _____ Oligodendroglioma
4. _____ Ependymoma

Column B
a. Often contains calcium
b. Most malignant
c. Typically arises in the fourth ventricle in children
d. Radiosensitive posterior fossa tumor of childhood

▼ *Match the brain tumors in column A with the statements in column B.*

Column A
5. _____ Chromophobe adenoma
6. _____ Basophilic adenoma
7. _____ Eosinophilic adenoma
8. _____ Craniopharyngioma
9. _____ Neurilemmoma
10. _____ Hemangioblastoma
11. _____ Pinealoma

Column B
a. Arises from remnants of Rathke's pouch; predominantly a tumor of childhood
b. Associated with acromegaly; does not cause chiasmal compression
c. Symptoms include tinnitus, deafness, vertigo, and caloric vestibular reactivity
d. Associated with Cushing's syndrome
e. Symptoms include hypopituitarism, hypothyroidism, hypoadrenalism, and often visual field defects
f. Often compresses the aqueduct, causing obstructive hydrocephalus, and the hypothalamus, causing precocious puberty and diabetes insipidus
g. Often bleeds intracerebrally or into the subarachnoid space; most common in cerebellum

▼ *Match the localizing symptoms of brain tumors in column A with their probable location in column B.*

Column A
12. _____ Homonymous hemianopsia
13. _____ Impairment of sensory localization, two-point discrimination
14. _____ Superior quadrantanopsia progressing to hemianopsia
15. _____ Disturbances of judgment; jacksonian seizures; ataxia and tremor
16. _____ Obesity and disturbance of temperature regulation

Column B
a. Frontal lobe
b. Temporal lobe
c. Occipital lobe
d. Parietal lobe
e. Hypothalamus

▼ *Answer the following questions on a separate sheet of paper.*

17. What makes the diagnosis of a brain tumor so difficult? What are the most common general signs and symptoms?

▼ *Circle the letter preceding each item below that correctly answers the question or completes the statement. Only one answer is correct, with exceptions noted.*

18. All the following statements concerning brain tumors are true *except:*
   a. A glioblastoma is the most malignant form of brain tumor.
   b. Brain tumors in children occur most often in the posterior fossa.
   c. Astrocytomas are generally nonmalignant.
   d. Glioblastomas are generally cured by surgical excision.
   e. Meningiomas are benign tumors of perineural tissue.

19. The two most common sources of metastasis to the brain are the:
   a. Lung and colon
   b. Colon and rectum
   c. Lung and breast
   d. Uterus in women and prostate in men

20. Which of the following statements concerning chordomas is *true*?
   a. They are highly invasive, making complete surgical excision impossible.
   b. They arise at the base of the skull.
   c. They grow slowly.
   d. All the above are correct.

Continued.

QUESTIONS—cont'd

21. Compensatory mechanisms for increased intracranial pressure (ICP) include all the following *except:*
    a. A decrease in the systemic blood pressure
    b. A decrease in intracerebral blood volume
    c. A decrease in the volume of cerebrospinal fluid (CSF)
    d. A decrease in the number of parenchymal cells

22. Noninvasive techniques helpful in the diagnosis of brain tumors include (more than one answer may be correct):
    a. History and neurologic examination
    b. Pneumoencephalogram
    c. CT scan
    d. Arteriogram
    e. MRI

23. The most common cause of extradural extramedullary cord compression is:
    a. Metastatic disease
    b. Glioma
    c. Astrocytoma
    d. Ependymoma

24. The most common types of intradural extramedullary spinal lesions are:
    a. Gliomas and angiomas
    b. Meningiomas and neurofibromas
    c. Sarcomas and lymphomas
    d. Gliomas and herniated nucleus pulposus

25. A spinal cord tumor that caused weakness and atrophy of the intrinsic hand muscles, sensory loss in the ulnar side of the hand, and Horner's syndrome, together with a "claw hand," would most likely be:
    a. Intramedullary at C6
    b. Extramedullary at C6
    c. Extramedullary at C7
    d. Intramedullary at C8

26. One of the most important tests in the diagnosis of spinal cord compression is:
    a. Ultrasound
    b. Myelography
    c. Spinal radiography

27. All the following are characteristics of lower motor neuron lesions *except:*
    a. Fasciculations
    b. Depressed reflexes below level of lesion
    c. Spastic paralysis below level of lesion
    d. Marked atrophy of muscle innervated below level of lesion

▼ *Match the disorders of movement seen in cerebellar tumors in column A with the proper descriptive statement in column B.*

Column A		Column B
28. _____	Nystagmus	a. Error in range of movement: carrying food to ear instead of mouth
29. _____	Dysmetria	b. Inability to perform tapping movement smoothly and quickly
30. _____	Asynergia	c. Quick oscillation of eyes while fixing gaze on an object
31. _____	Intention tremor	d. Lack of cooperation between muscles (e.g., failure of wrist extensors during flexion of the finger, allowing the wrist to flex)
32. _____	Deviation from line of movement	e. Oscillation tremor most marked at the end of fine movements
33. _____	Adiadochokinesia	f. Inability to arrest a movement at a given point and difficulty in performing successive movements

▼ *Circle T if the statement is true and F if it is false. Correct any false statements.*

34. T F An osmotic gradient causing absorption of fluid into a malignant brain tumor is the most likely mechanism of cerebral edema.
35. T F Hypotonia is an absence of normal resistance to stretch and is seen in cerebellar tumors.
36. T F Astrocytes function as cerebral phagocytes.
37. T F Oligodendroglia are involved in myelin formation.
38. T F Ependymoma is the most common type of intradural intramedullary spinal cord tumor.
39. T F Meningiomas of the spinal cord tend to be located in the cauda equina.
40. T F Papilledema is enlargement of the blind spot in the eye.

▼ *Match the site of spinal cord pathology in column A with the signs and symptoms in column B. Letters may be used more than once.*

Column A		Column B
41. _____	Pain increased by coughing or sneezing	a. Posterior (dorsal) root
42. _____	Loss of vibratory and position sense	b. Posterior column (major ascending tract)
43. _____	Babinski's sign	c. Corticospinal tract (major descending tract)
44. _____	Fasciculations	d. Anterior horn cells
45. _____	Spasticity	
46. _____	Ataxia	

BIBLIOGRAPHY ▼ PART IX

Acute Pain Management Guideline Panel: *Acute pain management: operative or medical procedures and trauma,* AHCPR Pub No 92-0032, Rockville, Md, 1992, Agency for Health Care Policy and Research, US Public Health Service, US Department of Health and Human Services.

Adams RD, Victor M: *Principles of neurology,* ed 5, New York, 1993, McGraw-Hill.

American Heart Association: *Stroke,* vol 8, no 1, Dallas, 1977, AHA.

American Heart Association: *Heart and stroke: 1994 statistics supplement,* Dallas, 1994, AHA.

Antel JP, Arnason BGW: Demyelinating diseases. In Wilson JD, editor: *Harrison's principles of internal medicine,* ed 12, New York, 1991, McGraw-Hill.

Appenzellar O: Pathogenesis of migraine, *Med Clin North Am* 75(3):763-789, 1991.

Asbury AK: Diseases of the peripheral nervous system. In Isselbacher KJ, editor: *Harrison's principles of internal medicine,* ed 13, New York, 1994, McGraw-Hill.

Basbaum AI, Field HL: Endogenous pain control mechanisms: review and hypothesis, *Ann Neurol* 4:451-462, 1978.

Becker DP: Injury to the head and spine. In Wyngaarden JB, editor: *Cecil textbook of medicine,* ed 19, Philadelphia, 1992, Saunders.

Bonica J: The nature of the problem. In Carron H, McLaughlin RE, editors: *Management of low back pain,* Littleton, Mass, 1982, Wright-PSG.

Bonica J, editor: *The management of pain,* vol I, Philadelphia, 1990, Lea & Febiger.

Buring J et al: Migraine and subsequent risk of stroke in the physician's health study, *Arch Neurol* 52:129-134, 1995.

Caplan LR: Stroke, *CIBA Clin Symp* 40(4):1-32, 1988.

Carpenter MB: *Core text of neuroanatomy,* ed 4, Baltimore, 1991, Williams & Wilkins.

Corbett A, Bennett MA, Kos S: Cognitive dysfunction following subcortical infarction, *Arch Neurol* 51:999-1007, 1994.

Cotran RS, Kumar V, Robbins SL: *Pathological basis of disease,* ed 5, Philadelphia, 1994, Saunders.

Crapper DR, Quittkat S, DeBon U: Altered chromatin formation in Alzheimer's disease, *Brain* 102:483-494, 1979.

Daake DR, Guelder SH: Imagery instruction and the control of postsurgical pain, *Appl Nurs Res* 2:114-129, 1989.

Diamond S: *Migraine headache prevention and management,* New York, 1990, Dekker.

Dobkin BH: The clinical problem of ischemic brain damage, *Ann Intern Med* 110:992-1000, 1989.

Drachman DB: Myasthenia gravis. In Isselbacher KJ, editor: *Harrison's principles of internal medicine,* ed 13, New York, 1994, McGraw-Hill.

Dubner R, Bennett GJ: Spinal and trigeminal mechanisms of nociception, *Annu Rev Neurosci* 6:381, 1989.

Ferrari M et al: Cerebral blood flow during migraine attacks without aura and effect of sumatriptan, *Arch Neurol* 52:135-139, 1995.

Fields HL: *Pain,* New York, 1987, McGraw-Hill.

Fields HL, editor: *Pain syndromes in neurology,* Boston, 1990, Butterworth.

Fields HL, Dubner R, Cervero F, editors: *Advances in pain research and theory,* New York, 1985, Raven.

Fields HL et al: Neurotransmitters in nociceptive modulatory circuits, *Annu Rev Neurosci* 14:219-245, 1991.

Flower RJ, Moncada S, Vane JR: Analgesic-antipyretics and the anti-inflammatory agents. In Gilman AG et al, editors: *Goodman and Gilman's the pharmacological basis of therapeutics,* ed 8, New York, 1990, Macmillan.

France R: Psychiatric aspects of pain, *Clin J Pain* 5:S30-S42, 1989.

Fromm G: First seizure management reconsidered: response I, *Arch Neurol* 44:1189, 1987.

Gossop M: Clonidine and the treatment of opiate withdrawal syndrome, *Drug Alcohol Depend* 21:253-259, 1988.

Gujol MC: A survey of pain assessment and management practices among critical care nurses, *Am J Crit Care* 3:123, 1994.

Guyton AC, Hall JE: *Textbook of medical physiology,* ed 9, Philadelphia, 1996, Saunders.

Haerer AF: *De Jong's the neurological examination,* Philadelphia, 1994, Lippincott.

Hardman JG et al, editors: *Goodman and Gilman's the pharmacological basis of therapeutics,* ed 9, New York, 1996, Macmillan.

Hargreaves A, Lander J: Use of transcutaneous electrical nerve stimulation for postoperative pain, *Nurs Res* 38(3):159-161, 1989.

Hauser SL: Multiple sclerosis and other demyelinating diseases. In Isselbacher KJ, editor: *Harrison's principles of internal medicine,* ed 13, New York, 1994, McGraw-Hill.

Hester NO, Foster RL: Cues nurses and parents use in making judgments about children's pain, *Pain* 5:S31, 1990.

Hoff JT, Boland MF: Neurosurgery. In Schwartz SI, editor: *Principles of surgery,* ed 6, New York, 1994, McGraw-Hill.

Hughes J et al: Identification of two related pentapeptides from the brain with potent opiate agonist activity, *Nature* 258:577-579, 1975.

International Association for the Study of Pain: Pain terms: a list with definitions and notes on usage, *Pain* 6:249, 1979.

Jaffe JH, Martin WR: Opioid analgesics and antagonists. In Gilman AG et al, editors: *Goodman and Gilman's the pharmacological basis of therapeutics,* ed 8, New York, 1990, Macmillan.

Kandel ER, Schwartz JH: *Principles of neural science,* ed 2, New York, 1985, Elsevier.

Kaplan R: Febrile seizures: when is treatment justified? *Postgrad Med* 82:63, 1987.

Kohr J: Measuring your patient's pain, *RN* 58:39-40, April 1995.

Kovanen J et al: Duration of postural headache after lumbar puncture: effect of needle size, *Headache* 26:224, 1986.

Lance JW: *Mechanism and management of headache,* ed 5, Boston, 1993, Butterworth.

Lieb RA, Hurtig JB: Epidural and intrathecal narcotics for pain management, *Heart Lung* 14:164, 1985.

Light AR: *The initial processing of pain and its descending control: spinal and trigeminal systems,* Farmington, Conn, 1992, Karger.

Marler J, project officer, The National Institute of Neurological Disorders and Stroke, rtPA Stroke Study Group: Tissue plasminogen activator for acute ischemic stroke, *N Engl J Med* 333:1581-1593, Dec 14, 1995.

Continued.

BIBLIOGRAPHY ▼ PART IX

McCaffrey M: *Nursing management of the patient with pain,* Philadelphia, 1979, Lippincott.

McCaffrey M, Beebe A: *Pain: a clinical manual for nursing practice,* St Louis, 1989, Mosby.

McCaffrey M, Ritchey K: Techniques of pain assessment, *Nurse Week* 5:16, 1992.

McHenry LC: Cerebral blood flow measurement and regulation in man. Part II. Current concepts in cerebrovascular disease, *Stroke* 11:5-8, 1976.

Melzack R: *The puzzle of pain,* New York, 1973, Basic.

Melzack R: The McGill pain questionnaire: major properties and scoring methods, *Pain* 22:1, 1975.

Melzack R: *Pain measurement and assessment,* New York, 1983, Raven.

Melzack R: The tragedy of needless pain, *Sci Am* 262(2):2-8, 1990.

Melzack R, Wall PD: *The challenge of pain,* New York, 1983, Basic Books.

Mountcastle VB: *Medical physiology,* ed 14, St Louis, 1980, Mosby.

Payan DG: Substance P: a modulator of neuroendocrine-immune function, *Hosp Pract* 24(2A):67-80, 1989.

Porter J, Jick H: Addiction rare in patients treated with narcotics, *N Engl J Med* 302:123, 1980.

Price DD: *Psychological and neural mechanisms of pain,* New York, 1988, Raven.

Raichle ME: The pathophysiology of ischemic brain damage, *Ann Neurol* 13(1):2-10, 1983.

Ray CG: Enteroviruses and reoviruses. In Isselbacher KJ, editor: *Harrison's principles of internal medicine,* ed 13, New York, 1994, McGraw-Hill.

Ropper AH: Trauma of the head and spine. In Isselbacher KJ, editor: *Harrison's principles of internal medicine,* ed 13, New York, 1994, McGraw-Hill.

Rowland LP: *Merritt's textbook of neurology,* ed 9, Baltimore, 1995, Williams & Wilkins.

Schwartz GR, editor: *Principles and practice of emergency medicine,* ed 3, Philadelphia, 1992, Lea & Febiger.

Schwartz SI, editor: *Principles of surgery,* ed 6, New York, 1994, McGraw-Hill.

Siedel HM et al: *Mosby's guide to physical examination,* ed 2, St Louis, 1991, Mosby.

Snell RS: *Clinical neuroanatomy,* ed 3, Boston, 1992, Little, Brown.

So EL: Update on epilepsy, *Med Clin North Am* 77:203, 1993.

Soloman S: Migraine: current approaches to diagnosis and management, *Hosp Pract* 26(4A):141-160, 1991.

Stauffer ES, Bell DG: Traumatic respiratory quadriplegia and pentaplegia, *Orthop Clin North Am* 9(4):1084-1089, 1978.

Sternbach RA: A survey of pain in the United States: the Nuprin Pain Report, *Clin J Pain* 2:49-53, 1986.

Sternbach RA: *Mastering pain,* New York, 1987, Putnam.

Taylor H, Curran NM: *The Nuprin Pain Report,* New York, 1985, Harris.

Wall PD, Melzack R: *The challenge of pain,* ed 3, New York, 1994, Churchill Livingstone.

White BC, Weigenstein JG, Winegar CD: Brain ischemia and anoxia, *JAMA* 251:1586-1590, 1984.

Wong D, Baker C: Pain in children: comparison of assessment scales, *Pediatr Nurs* 14(1):9-17, 1988.

Zejdlik CP: *Management of spinal cord injury,* Monterey, Calif, 1983, Wadsworth.

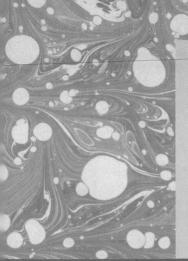

PART TEN

ENDOCRINE SYSTEM AND METABOLIC DISORDERS

This part discusses basic concepts in endocrinology and metabolism. These concepts should help the reader acquire an understanding of clinical problems associated with endocrine diseases. This part examines general physiologic concepts, including structure and mechanism of action of hormones, principles of neurohypothalamic control of pituitary function, circadian rhythms, feedback control of endocrine function, and mechanisms that control blood glucose.

The following clinical entities have been selected for discussion: Cushing's syndrome, Addison's disease, primary and secondary aldosteronism, hirsutism, pan-hypopituitarism, acromegaly, diabetes mellitus, hyperthyroidism, hypothyroidism, goiter, carcinoma of the thyroid, and pheochromocytoma. ▼

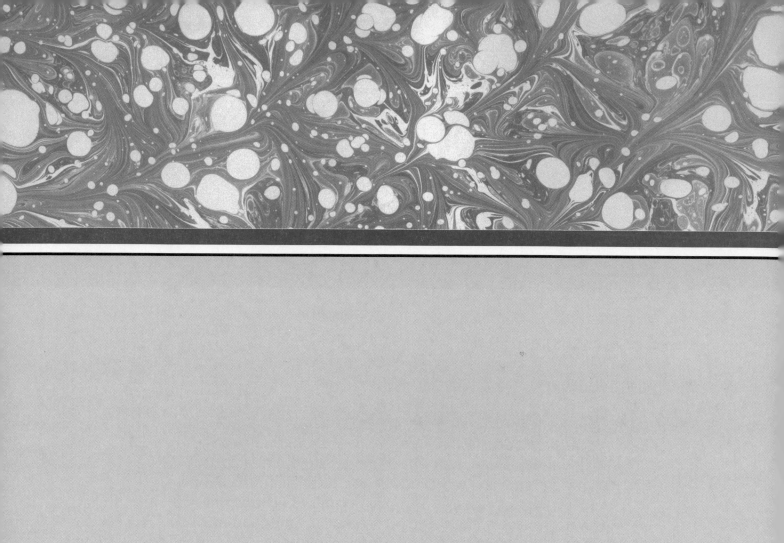

CHAPTER 58

Principles of Endocrine and Metabolic Control Mechanisms

DAVID E. SCHTEINGART

As living organisms develop complex structure and function, integration of their various components becomes essential to their survival. This integration is effected by two systems: (1) the central nervous system (CNS) and (2) the endocrine system. These two systems are related from the embryologic, anatomic, and functional standpoints. For example, many of the endocrine glands originate from the neuroectoderm, an embryonic layer that also gives origin to the CNS. In addition, there are anatomic connections between the developed CNS and the endocrine system, primarily through the hypothalamus. As a consequence, stimuli that disturb the CNS frequently also alter the function of the endocrine system. Conversely, a change in the function of the endocrine system may affect the function of the CNS. The integrated operation of the nervous and endocrine systems helps maximize the response of the organism to stressful stimuli.

FUNCTIONS OF THE ENDOCRINE SYSTEM

The endocrine system is made up of hormone-secreting glands that help maintain and regulate vital functions such as (1) response to stress and injury, (2) growth and development, (3) reproduction, (4) ionic homeostasis, and (5) energy metabolism.

When injury or stress occurs, the endocrine system triggers a series of responses aimed at maintaining blood pressure and preserving life. The hypothalamic-pituitary-adrenal axis is chiefly involved in this response.

Without the endocrine system there is failure to grow and reach maturity; infertility also occurs. The hypothalamic-pituitary-gonadal axis is chiefly involved in this function.

The endocrine system is important in maintenance of ionic homeostasis. Mammalian organisms live in an external environment that changes constantly. However, tissues and cells live in an internal environment that must remain constant. The endocrine system participates in the regulation of this internal environment through maintenance of sodium, potassium, water, and acid-base balance. Aldosterone and antidiuretic hormone (ADH) are responsible for this function. The calcium concentration is also controlled by endocrine function. Calcium is required for regulation of many biochemical reactions in living cells and for normal neural activation of muscle cell function. The parathyroid glands regulate calcium homeostasis.

Finally, the endocrine system acts as a regulator of energy metabolism. The basal metabolic rate is increased by thyroid hormone, and energy is made available to cells through the integrated action of gastrointestinal and pancreatic hormones.

HORMONES

The endocrine system is made up of glands that synthesize and secrete substances called *hormones*. Hormones cause the physiologic and biochemical changes that mediate the types of regulation described earlier. Once they are released into the bloodstream, hormones are transported to target tissues where they exert their effects. These effects frequently involve the regulation of ongoing enzymatic reactions. Hormones are generally secreted in very low concentrations. For instance, hormones are present in blood at a concentration of 10^{-6} to

10^{-12} molar. In contrast, another blood component, sodium, is usually present at a concentration of 10^{-1} molar. Despite these low concentrations, hormones exert marked metabolic and biochemical effects on their target tissues.

Hormones fall into two main classes: (1) steroids and thyronines, which are lipid soluble, and (2) polypeptides and catecholamines, which are water soluble. In addition, some hormones are in the category of glycoprotein, a combination of a sugar portion and a protein. The main characteristic of steroid hormones is the presence of a multicyclic structure, the cycloperhydrophenanthrene nucleus (Fig. 58-1). Examples of steroid hormones are the adrenocortical hormones and the hormones produced by the gonads. Polypeptides hormones are made up of chains of specific amino acids that vary in length, molecular weight, and constituent amino acids. Some polypeptide hormones, such as insulin, have a more complex structure with two amino acid chains linked together by disulfide linkages. The molecular structure of insulin is illustrated in Fig. 58-2. Other polypeptide hormones are parathormone or parathyroid hormone (PTH), the tropic

hormones of the pituitary gland (with the exception of thyroid-stimulating hormone [TSH], or thyrotropin, and gonadotropins), vasopressin, and glucagon. Examples of glycoprotein hormones are TSH and gonadotropins. Most hormones are synthesized as higher-molecular-weight precursors and are designated in their initial stages as pre-prohormones, prohormones, or higher-molecular-weight precursors. For example, insulin is synthesized as proinsulin, a continuous peptide, which—after losing a portion of the molecule, the C peptid—becomes a two-chain structure. Adrenocorticotropic hormone (ACTH) is derived from proopiomelanocortin (POMC), a 31,000-molecular-weight glycoprotein, which by sequential enzyme catalyzed cleavages generates a series of peptides, including opiates and the 39-amino-acid peptide ACTH.

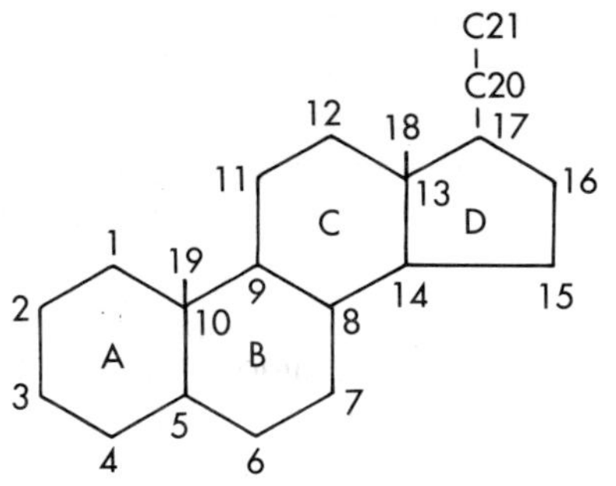

In addition to the classic hormones, which are produced by specific endocrine glands and act on specific target organs, a number of substances generated by hormone action act directly on cells and promote growth. Some of these substances have insulin-like activity, whereas others mediate the action of hormones, such as growth hormone. Somatomedin C is a well-recognized growth factor, generated in tissues under the effect of growth hormone, which is capable of promoting tissue growth. There are also compounds that are hormone-like in their mechanism of action but are produced in the blood itself. An example is angiotensin II, a polypeptide hormone that stimulates the adrenal cortex to secrete aldosterone. Angiotensin I is synthesized in the blood from renin substrate (a hepatic protein) under the catalytic effect of renin, an enzyme secreted by renal cells.

Although most hormones are synthesized by distinct endocrine glands, organs not classically considered endocrine glands contain groups of cells capable of synthesizing hormones. Many of these cells are derived from the neural crest and have the capacity to take up amine precursors and decarboxylate them for synthesis of hormones. These cells have been described as being part of the APUD (amine precursor uptake and decarboxylation)

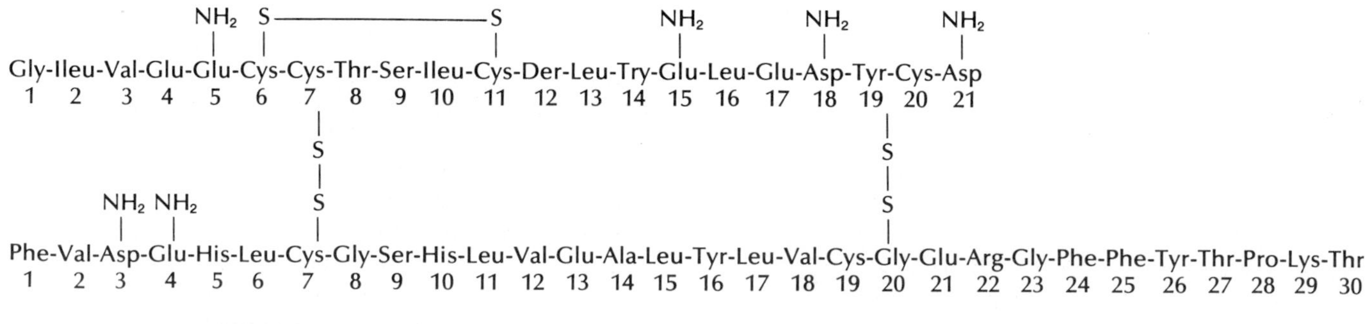

FIG. 58-1   A steroid nucleus. It has four rings: A, B, C, and D. The numbers designate the carbons within the molecule. Groups attached to different carbons are recognized by the respective numbers. For example, 17-hydroxy steroids have a hydroxyl group attached to the carbon in the 17 position.

FIG. 58-2   Molecular structure of insulin, a polypeptide hormone. The hormone has two chains, A and B. The A chain has 21 amino acids, and the B chain has 30 amino acids. The two chains are linked to each other by disulfide linkages.

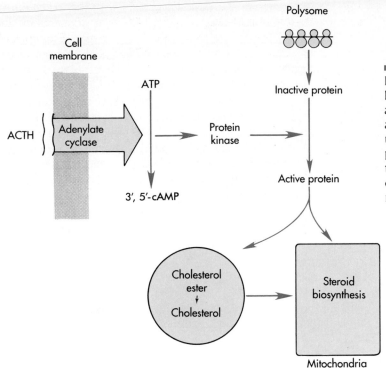

FIG. 58-3   Mechanism of action of adrenocorticotropic hormone [ACTH], a protein hormone. ACTH activates adenylate cyclase, increasing the synthesis of 3',5'-cyclic adenosine monophosphate [cAMP]. In turn, cAMP stimulates a protein kinase, which activates a rapid turnover protein. This protein causes increased release of cholesterol for use in steroid biosynthesis and stimulation of conversion of cholesterol to pregnenolone in the cell mitochondria. *ATP,* Adenosine triphosphate.

system. Tumors derived from these cells may acquire the capacity to secrete hormones that, because of their origin in cells outside the classic endocrine glands, are called *ectopic hormones.*

Much is known about the way hormones work on their target tissues or cells. Hormones influence cellular metabolic processes either directly or indirectly by first interacting with specific cell receptors. The combination of the hormone with its receptor may bring about changes within the cell by one of two mechanisms: (1) generation of a second messenger within the cell or (2) translocation of the hormone-receptor complex into the nucleus, where the complex induces new protein synthesis by the cell.

Polypeptide hormones and catecholamines appear to act via a second messenger mechanism, whereas steroid hormones are freely permeable to the cell membrane and exert their effects directly on the cell nucleus. More specifically, polypeptide hormones act by first interacting with a specific cell membrane receptor, and as a result of this interaction, a membrane-bound enzyme, adenylate cyclase, is activated and adenosine triphosphate (ATP) is converted to adenosine 3',5'-monophosphate (cyclic AMP). The latter then binds to the regulatory subunit of a protein kinase, thereby liberating a catalytic subunit of this enzyme. This in turn initiates the phosphorylation of certain key enzymes that specifically either activate or inactivate the biologic potency of these enzymes (Fig. 58-3).

Different polypeptide hormones activate different spe-

cific enzyme mechanisms, which mediate hormone action. For example, glucagon activates the enzyme phosphorylase by the process described, which brings about the enzymatic cleavage of glycogen to glucose-1-phosphate. ACTH increases steroidogenesis by activating one or several enzymes of the steroidogenic pathway. Insulin binds to the alpha subunit of the insulin receptor, a heterotetrameric glycoprotein in the cell membrane, and stimulates tyrosine phosphorylation of the beta subunit. A phosphorylation cascade then initiates a signal for the transport of glucose and the flux of certain ions across the cell membrane. In contrast to the way peptide hormones exert their effects, steroid hormones work directly inside the cell by entering the cell across the cell membrane and binding to cytosol receptor proteins. The steroid-receptor complex then is translocated to the nucleus of the cell, where it binds specifically to its locus on the deoxyribonucleic acid (DNA) and alters transcription, leading to the synthesis of one or several specific messenger ribonucleic acids (mRNAs). These products leave the nucleus and travel to the ribosome, where they direct the synthesis of proteins. By changing mRNA, steroids can modify the way protein is synthesized (Fig. 58-4).

In summary, hormonal action involves the combination of the hormone with its specific receptors in cells that are the targets of hormone action. The physiologic action of the hormone and the specificity of such action are intimately linked to the interaction of the hormone with its specific receptor.

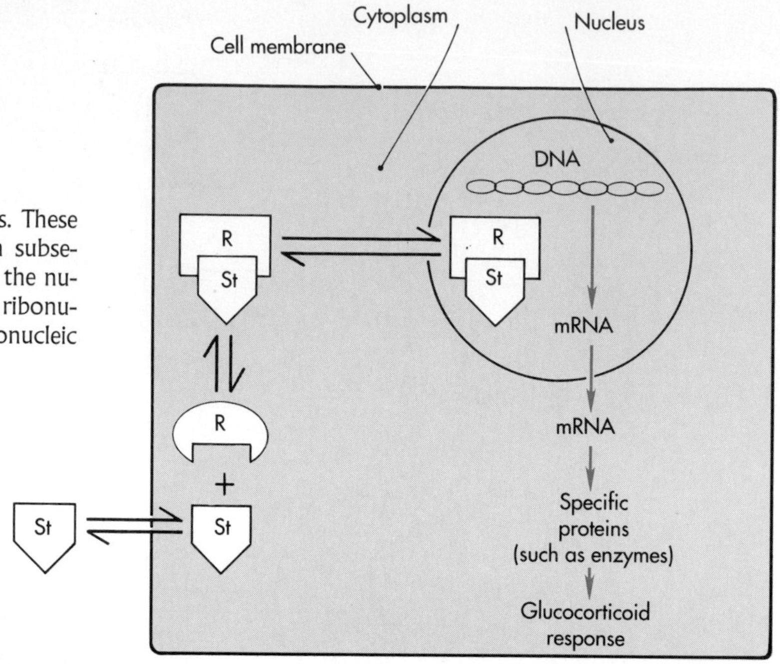

FIG. 58-4   Mechanism of action of steroid hormones. These hormones bind to intracellular receptor proteins, which subsequently carry the steroid molecule to the cell nucleus. In the nucleus the steroid modifies the formation of messenger ribonucleic acid (mRNA) and protein synthesis. DNA, Deoxyribonucleic acid; St, steroid hormone; R, receptor protein.

PHYSIOLOGY OF THE ENDOCRINE SYSTEM

The CNS is connected to the pituitary through the hypothalamus; this is the most clearly established link between the CNS and the endocrine system. The two systems are interrelated by both neural and vascular connections.

As demonstrated in Fig. 58-5, the pituitary is divided into an anterior, a posterior, and an intermediate lobe. Blood vessels link the hypothalamus with the cells of the anterior pituitary gland. These blood vessels end in capillaries at both ends and, for this reason, are known as a *portal system*. In this particular case the system connects the hypothalamus with the pituitary gland (hypophysis) and is called the *hypothalamic-hypophyseal* portal system. The portal system is an important vascular channel because it allows for the movement of releasing hormones from the hypothalamus to the pituitary gland, enabling the hypothalamus to modulate pituitary function. Stimuli originating in the brain activate neurons in the hypothalamic nuclei, which synthesize and secrete low-molecular-weight proteins. These proteins, or neurohormones, are known as *releasing hormones*. They are discharged into the blood vessels of the portal system, through which they reach cells in the pituitary gland. The pituitary gland responds to these releasing hormones by discharging pituitary tropic hormones. In this chain of events the hormones released by the pituitary gland travel with the blood and stimulate other glands, causing the release of target gland hormones. The target gland hormones, in turn, act on the neuromechanism or the pituitary cells and modify hormone secretion.

Fig. 58-6 illustrates a modality of feedback control in which the hormonal product of the target gland inhibits the release of the corresponding pituitary tropic hormone. This type of regulation of hormone secretion is known as a *negative-feedback control system*. In the hypothalamic-pituitary-adrenal system (Fig. 58-6, *A*), corticotropin-releasing hormone (CRH) causes the pituitary to release ACTH. Then ACTH stimulates the adrenal cortex to secrete cortisol. Cortisol, in turn, feeds back on the hypothalamic-pituitary axis and inhibits the production of CRH-ACTH. The system fluctuates, varying with the physiologic requirements for cortisol. If the system produces too much ACTH and therefore too much cortisol, the cortisol feeds back and inhibits the production of ACTH. This is a sensitive system, since an excessive production of cortisol or the administration of cortisol or other synthetic glucocorticoids can quickly inhibit the hypothalamic-pituitary axis and shut off the production of ACTH. The concept of feedback control has practical implications in patients receiving chronic corticosteroid therapy. These patients have suppressed ACTH release. If steroids are suddenly withdrawn, patients may develop adrenal insufficiency.

Another example of feedback control (Fig. 58-6, *B*) is the action of gonadotropin-releasing hormone (GnRH), which stimulates the pituitary to secrete follicle-stimulating hormone (FSH) and luteinizing hormone (LH). In women, estrogens are initially produced by the ovary in small amounts; the estrogens feed back on the hypothalamus, stimulating the secretion of GnRH. This in turn triggers FSH and LH release, ovulation, and secretion of estrogen and progesterone. The action of estrogens is an example of *positive feedback control*. A third example (Fig. 58-6, *C*) of feedback control is release of TSH-releasing hormone (TRH), which is se-

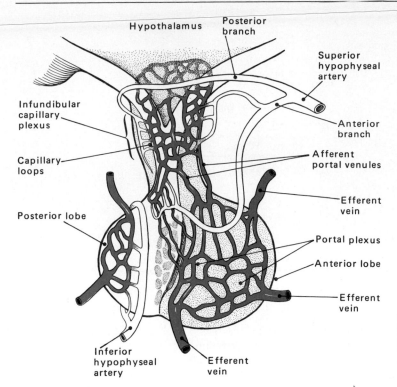

FIG. 58-5   Hypothalamic-hypophyseal portal system. (From Langley LL, Telford JR, Christensen JB: *Dynamic anatomy and physiology,* ed 4, New York, 1980, McGraw-Hill.)

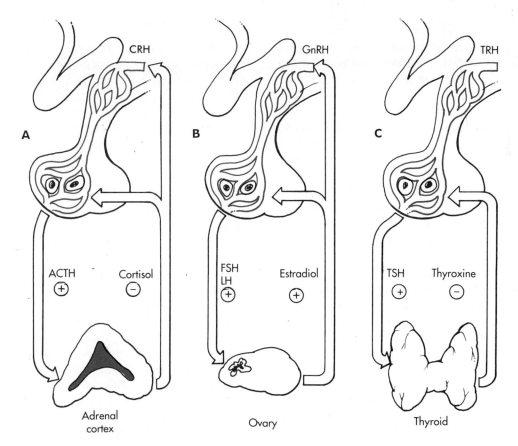

FIG. 58-6   Feedback-regulating systems where the target gland hormone feeds back to the hypothalamus. Pituitary release of the tropic hormone follows. **A,** Corticotropin-releasing hormone [CRH]. **B,** Gonadotropin-releasing hormone [GnRH]. **C,** TSH-releasing hormone [TRH]. ACTH, Adrenocorticotropic hormone; FSH, follicle-stimulating hormone; LH, luteinizing hormone; TSH, thyroid-stimulating hormone (thyrotropin).

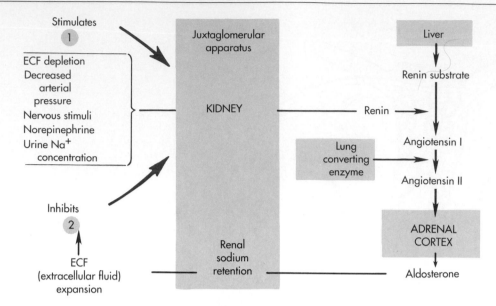

FIG. 58-7   Regulation of aldosterone secretion by the renin-angiotensin system. *1,* Extracellular fluid space *(ECF)* depletion, decreased arterial pressure, nervous stimuli, norepinephrine, and increased urinary sodium stimulate renin release. *2,* ECF expansion, by counteracting these factors, inhibits renin release.

creted by the hypothalamus and causes the pituitary to secrete TSH. In turn, TSH stimulates the thyroid to secrete thyroxine. Thyroxine then feeds back on the pituitary and inhibits production of TSH.

Although the interaction between pituitary hormones and the target gland hormones occurs through systemic circulation (the *long-loop system*), other interactions occur between pituitary hormones and their releasing factors (the *short-loop system*).

Other systems regulate hormone production independently of the hypothalamic-pituitary axis. One example is the *renin-angiotensin-aldosterone system.* As illustrated in Fig. 58-7, the kidney has juxtaglomerular (JG) cells, which are located in the wall of the afferent arteriole of the glomerulus. These cells secrete the enzyme *renin.* The production of renin is influenced by the perfusion pressure in the renal arteriole. Changes in the pressure of blood flowing through the afferent arteriole into the glomerulus are sensed by stretch receptors near the JG cells. This causes changes in the secretion of renin, which in turn activates angiotensin II. Angiotensin II stimulates the production of aldosterone by the adrenal cortex. Aldosterone promotes renal tubular reabsorption of sodium. As sodium is reabsorbed, volume is expanded, the pressure rises in the afferent arteriole, and renin production is shut off. Thus renin, angiotensin, and aldosterone release are determined by volume and pressure changes affecting the JG cells.

Fig. 58-8 illustrates another modality of feedback control, in which the metabolic substance controlled by the hormone acts directly on its release. In Fig. 58-8, *A*, insulin and glucose are depicted. Insulin responds to changes in the level of glucose in blood. When glucose levels increase, insulin is secreted. When glucose levels decrease, insulin is shut off. Although some of the pituitary hormones may indirectly influence insulin release, no clear evidence indicates that the pituitary gland directly and specifically controls insulin secretion.

PTH and calcium constitute another unique control system (Fig. 58-8, *B*). A drop in calcium level stimulates PTH secretion. Conversely, an increase in calcium shuts off PTH production.

Another physiologic characteristic of the hypothalamic-pituitary axis is the presence of rhythms. *Rhythms* are a common feature of the production of many hormones, and they originate in brain structures. ACTH provides an excellent example of rhythmic, or cyclic, hormone release. When ACTH and cortisol levels are measured on an hourly basis for 24 hours, the levels are seen to rise early in the day, decline later, and rise again during the night to reach a peak by the next morning (Fig. 58-9). This type of rhythm is referred to as a *diurnal,* or *circadian, rhythm.* Because hormonal release by the pituitary gland occurs in short spurts, it is also said that there is episodic hormonal release.

Gonadotropins, the tropic hormones of the pituitary gland that controls gonadal function, are involved in a different kind of cycle or rhythm. In women the release of gonadotropins is cyclic and occurs on a monthly basis rather than on a diurnal basis (Fig. 58-10). The presence

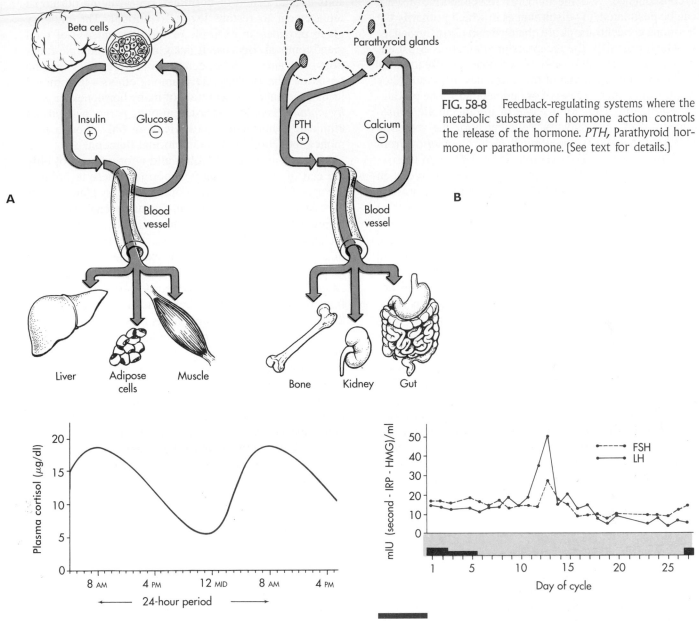

FIG. 58-8 Feedback-regulating systems where the metabolic substrate of hormone action controls the release of the hormone. *PTH,* Parathyroid hormone, or parathormone. (See text for details.)

FIG. 58-9 Circadian rhythm of cortisol secretion.

FIG. 58-10 Monthly cyclic release of gonadotropins in normal menstruating women. Depicted is the midcycle surge of follicle-stimulating hormone *(FSH)* and luteinizing hormone *(LH).*

of the normal cyclic release of gonadotropins is specific and characteristic of female reproductive endocrine function. In men, on the other hand, the release of the same gonadotropins does not have this cyclic nature, and it occurs at a constant rate. If the cyclic release of gonadotropins in a woman is abolished, cessation of normal menstrual cycles, disappearance of ovulation, and infertility occur.

Other hormones are not released with a spontaneous rhythm but are released in response to a stimulus. For example, insulin and growth hormone are released in response to food intake.

DISEASES OF THE ENDOCRINE SYSTEM

Hormones do not act directly on cells or tissues—they must first bind to specific receptors in the cell membrane or in the cytosol of the cell. For a metabolic event to occur, the metabolic steps distal to the interaction of the hormone and the receptor must all be intact. It thus appears that not only is the hormone concentration important for the final strength of the signal that turns on the cellular machinery, but the number and affinity of the receptors for the hormone are also critically important. As a consequence, two mechanisms for endocrine disease can be postulated: (1) disturbances in which primarily the hormone concentrations are changed and (2) disturbances in which primarily the receptors are defective. Most endocrine diseases can be understood conceptually in terms of the metabolic actions of the hormones involved. They result from either excessive or deficient hormone production or action. Thus knowledge of the metabolic consequence of the excessive or deficient hormone secretion will help to identify the clinical picture emerging from these disturbances. For example, if production of thyroxine, the thyroid hormone, is excessive, one can predict an increase in the basal metabolic rate and in heat production. In effect, patients with hyperthyroidism demonstrate a high metabolic rate, increased heat sensitivity, and weight loss. Conversely, lack of thyroxine results in the opposite metabolic effects, such as low basal metabolic rate and increased sensitivity to cold temperature. Primary disturbances at the receptor level have been described in patients with familial homozygous hypercholesterolemia. In this disorder, patients lack the low-density lipoprotein (LDL) receptor, which results in an inability of cells throughout the body to take up cholesterol, a lipid normally circulating in plasma and associated with the LDL lipoprotein fraction. A second type of disorder with a disturbance at the receptor level is Graves' disease, in which an autoimmune process forms antibodies against the TSH receptor, resulting in stimulation of thyroid function. Some forms of diabetes mellitus, such as the non-insulin-dependent type, are a consequence of a decreased sensitivity of peripheral tissues to the action of insulin, probably as a result of a decrease in the number or affinity of insulin receptors.

Treatment of Endocrine Diseases

The treatment of endocrine diseases is based on the change in hormone production underlying the specific disease. In simple terms, patients who have a disease caused by a *deficit* of hormone secretion are treated by replacement of these hormones. Consider the example of a diabetic patient whose body is not making enough insulin. Treatment for the metabolic consequence of insulin insufficiency is the administration of insulin. Similarly, a patient whose body is not making enough thyroid hormone and becomes hypothyroid is treated with replacement amounts of thyroxine.

The treatment of diseases of hormone *excess* is more complex, since several therapeutic alternatives are usually available. Removal of the whole gland or part of the gland that produces the hormone in excess is one such alternative. The removal of the entire gland, however, re-

sults in total deficit of hormone, necessitating hormonal replacement to restore levels to normal. The pituitary gland provides an example of the consequence of total gland removal. Because it is a gland with multiple functions—the anterior lobe secretes tropic hormones, and the posterior lobe secretes ADH, among others—its removal leads to cessation of secretion of many hormones, or *panhypopituitarism*. In contrast, removing part of a gland can eliminate a hormone excess, leaving only enough hormone production to maintain normal function.

Modern surgical techniques allow for removal of only the part of the gland that is abnormal. These techniques are used when a small tumor of the pituitary gland causes excessive hormone production. The tumor can be resected by microsurgical techniques without removal of the rest of the pituitary gland. In other cases, removal of only a part of a gland is not possible. For example, if the adrenal glands are removed, both the adrenal cortex and the adrenal medulla must be removed. Although the body can function well without the adrenal medulla, the capacity of the body to secrete catecholamines may be impaired.

Another alternative for dealing with hormone excess is the administration of drugs that interfere with hormone production by either blocking or destroying the tissue that makes the hormone. For example, a patient who has an overactive thyroid can be given radioactive iodine in large concentrations. The radioactive iodine concentrates in the thyroid gland and destroys the cells that make thyroxine, causing remission of the disease. Another example is adrenal hyperfunction, in which the glands can be blocked by drugs that interfere with the biosynthesis of adrenocortical hormones.

Suppression of hormone production is also illustrated by oral contraceptives. Estrogens and progestogens are given to inhibit pituitary release of gonadotropins; this in turn suppresses normal ovarian function and ovulation.

Another method of controlling excessive hormone effects is by *hormone antagonism*. An excess production of female hormone can be counteracted by administration of male hormone, or vice versa. Thus the metabolic effects of a hormone are opposed by the metabolic effects of an opposite hormone, causing cancellation of the effects of the first one. A hormone can also antagonize the effect of another hormone by blocking binding of the latter to its receptors in its target cells.

In summary, endocrine diseases are those of either hormone deficit or hormone excess. The deficit state is treated by replacing the deficient hormone. The excessive state can be treated either by surgically removing the whole gland or part of the gland that is working excessively or by giving drugs that block or destroy the tissues making the hormone.

? QUESTIONS

▼ *Answer the following on a separate sheet of paper.*

1. Cite two mechanisms by which hormones can work on their target cells.
2. In the table below list the two types of hormones that are differentiated by their chemical structure. State two examples of each type and identify the location of production for each example.

Type of hormone	Examples	Location of production	
a	1	1	
	2	2	
b	1	1	
	2	2	

3. Write a brief description of the way angiotensin II is synthesized in the blood and stimulates a peripheral gland.
4. Identify the role played by the hypothalamus in the hypothalamic-pituitary system.
5. What is the function of the hypothalamic-hypophyseal portal system?
6. Give an example of the way the feedback control mechanism operates to regulate endocrine hormone secretion.
7. Define circadian rhythm by identifying the hormonal levels (high or low) of adrenocorticotropic hormone (ACTH) and the time of day each level occurs.
8. Cite the two postulated mechanisms for endocrine disturbances.
9. State the rationale for providing hormone replacement or suppression as treatment for endocrine diseases caused by hormonal deficit or excess.

▼ *Circle the letter preceding each item below that correctly answers the question or completes the statement. More than one answer may be correct.*

10. The functions of the endocrine system include which of the following?
    a. Response to nutritional imbalance
    b. Regulation of growth and development
    c. Regulation of energy metabolism
    d. Response to stress and injury
11. The anterior lobe of the pituitary gland secretes:
    a. Antidiuretic hormone
    b. Tropic hormones
    c. Both a and b
    d. Neither a nor b
12. An overproduction of thyroxine may cause a condition referred to as:
    a. Panhypopituitarism
    b. Adrenal hyperfunction
    c. Hyperthyroidism
    d. Hypercalcemia

13. Thyrotropin-releasing hormone (TRH) secreted by the hypothalamus causes release of:
    a. Thyrotropic hormone (TSH)
    b. Gonadotropin-releasing hormone (GnRH)
    c. Follicle-stimulating hormone (FSH)
    d. Luteinizing hormone (LH)

▼ *Circle T if the statement is true and F if it is false. Correct any false statements.*

14. T F The system that connects the hypothalamus with the pituitary gland is described as a portal system.
15. T F Receptors for polypeptide hormone action are located in the membrane of the cell.
16. T F Receptors for hormone action are usually not specific for a particular hormone.

CHAPTER 59

Pituitary Gland Disorders

DAVID E. SCHTEINGART

GENERAL CONCEPTS

The pituitary gland is a complex structure at the base of the brain lying within a bony wall cavity, the *sella turcica,* in the sphenoid bone at the base of the skull. It is formed early in embryonic development from the fusion of two ectodermal hollow processes. An invagination from the roof of the primitive oral region, Rathke's pouch, extends upward toward the base of the brain and is met by an outpouching of the floor of the third ventricle, destined to become the neurohypophysis. The developed pituitary gland is thus formed by a posterior lobe, or *neurohypophysis,* in continuity with the hypothalamus and an anterior lobe, or *adenohypophysis,* connected to the hypothalamus through the pituitary stalk. A vascular structure, the hypothalamic-hypophyseal portal system, also connects the hypothalamus with the anterior pituitary gland. It is through this system that releasing hormones from the hypothalamus reach the cells of the pituitary gland to promote hormone release.

The anterior pituitary gland has multiple functions, and because of its ability to regulate the function of other endocrine glands, it is also known as the *master gland.* The anterior pituitary cells are specialized to secrete specific hormones. Seven such hormones have been well identi-

fied and their physiologic metabolic roles defined. These are adrenocorticotropic hormone (ACTH), melanocyte-stimulating hormone (MSH), thyroid-stimulating hormone (thyrotropin, TSH), follicle-stimulating hormone (FSH), luteinizing hormone (LH), growth hormone (GH), and prolactin (PRL). Some of these hormones (ACTH, MSH, GH, prolactin) are *polypeptides,* whereas others (TSH, FSH, LH) are *glycoproteins.* Morphologic studies indicate that each hormone is synthesized by a specific cell type. In a sense the anterior pituitary gland is a conglomeration of independent glands, all of which are under hypothalamic control.

The posterior lobe of the pituitary gland, or neurohypophysis, is concerned mainly with the regulation of fluid balance. Antidiuretic hormone (ADH) is synthesized primarily in the supraoptic and paraventricular nuclei of the hypothalamus and stored in the neurohypophysis.

PHYSIOLOGIC AND METABOLIC ROLES OF ANTERIOR PITUITARY HORMONES

GH, prolactin, and MSH have direct metabolic effects on target tissues. In contrast, ACTH, TSH, FSH, and LH exert their main effects through the regulation of secretion of other endocrine glands and are therefore known as *tropic hormones* (Table 59-1).

GH, or somatotropin, has major metabolic effects in children and adults. In children, GH hormone is required for somatic growth. In adults, GH may preserve normal adult organ size, and it participates in the regulation of protein synthesis and nutrient disposal. GH produces somatomedin, or insulin-like growth factor-1 (IGF-1), which appears to mediate the growth-promoting effect. It is likely that without somatomedin, GH cannot promote growth. Secretion of GH is regulated by a growth hormone–releasing hormone (GHRH) from the hypothalamus and by somatostatin, an in-

► TABLE 59-1   Anterior Lobe Pituitary Hormones and Function

Hormone	Releasing Hormone	Target	Function (Stimulates)
ACTH	CRH	Adrenal cortex	Steroidogenesis
MSH	CRH	Melanocytes	Pigmentation
TSH	TRH	Thyroid follicles	T_4, T_3
LH (men)	GnRH	Leydig cells	Testosterone
FSH (men)	GnRH	Seminiferous tubules	Spermatogenesis
LH (women)	GnRH	Corpus luteum	Progesterone
FSH (women)	GnRH	Follicular cells	Estrogens
Prolactin	TRH (+)	Mammary gland	Lactation
	Dopamine (−)		
GH	GHRH (+)	Systemic	Growth
	Somatostatin (−)		

See text for abbreviations.

hibiting hormone. The release of GH is stimulated by hypoglycemia and by amino acids such as arginine. It is also modified by stress and by exercise.

MSH is a constituent of proopiomelanocortin. It increases skin pigmentation by stimulating the dispersion of melanin granules in melanocytes. Its secretion is regulated by corticotropin-releasing hormone (CRH), and it is inhibited by a rise in cortisol. Deficient secretion of cortisol can stimulate MSH release, and high cortisol levels suppress its secretion.

Prolactin has a similar molecular structure to GH and some overlap with its biologic properties. Prolactin is one of a group of hormones necessary for breast development and milk secretion. The release of prolactin is under tonic inhibition by the hypothalamus through dopamine, secreted by the tuberohypophyseal dopaminergic neuron system. In its absence, increased prolactin secretion and lactation may occur. Thyrotropin-releasing hormone (TRH) stimulates prolactin secretion.

ACTH regulates the growth and function of the adrenal cortex and is especially important in the control of the production and release of cortisol. By itself, ACTH does not appear to have significant extraadrenal effects. CRH and arginine vasopressin (AVP) act synergistically to stimulate ACTH secretion.

TSH stimulates the growth and function of the thyroid gland. TSH causes thyroxine (T_4) and triiodothyronine (T_3) release, and these in turn regulate the secretion of TSH. TRH stimulates TSH secretion.

FSH and LH are also known as gonadotropins. In men, FSH maintains and stimulates spermatogenesis, and LH stimulates the secretion of testosterone by the Leydig, or interstitial, cells of the testes. FSH and LH are secreted in men in a continuous or tonic fashion. In contrast, in women, FSH stimulates follicular development and the secretion of estrogens by the follicular cells. LH induces ovulation and maintains and stimulates the secretion of progesterone by the corpus luteum, which develops from the follicle after ovulation has occurred. The release of FSH and LH in women follows a cyclic pattern so that the

levels of these two hormones rise at midcycle and slowly decline toward the end of the cycle, when menstruation occurs. FSH and LH secretion is modulated by the pattern of secretion of gonadotropin-releasing hormone (GnRH).

The clinical consequences of deficiencies in ACTH and TSH release are adrenal insufficiency and hypothyroidism, respectively. Absence of gonadotropin release leads to hypogonadism. Conversely, excessive secretion of ACTH leads to adrenocortical hyperfunction, or Cushing's syndrome. Syndromes of excessive TSH or gonadotropin release are more rare.

A clinical diagnosis of a pituitary disorder requires biochemical confirmation by specific tests that reveal the abnormality of pituitary function characteristic of the suspected condition. The pituitary hormones described, ACTH, MSH, TSH, FSH, LH, GH, and prolactin, can all be measured by radioimmunoassay in serum or plasma.

CLINICAL DISORDERS OF THE PITUITARY GLAND

Clinical syndromes associated with abnormal function of the pituitary gland include disorders of hormone deficit and hormone excess.

Hypopituitarism

Pituitary insufficiency typically affects all the hormones normally secreted by the anterior pituitary gland. The clinical manifestations of *panhypopituitarism* are therefore a composite of the metabolic effects caused by the deficient secretion of each one of the pituitary hormones.

Several pathologic processes may result in pituitary insufficiency: (1) pituitary tumor that destroys normal pituitary cells, (2) vascular thrombosis leading to necrosis of the normal pituitary gland, (3) infiltrative granulomatous diseases that destroy the pituitary, and (4) idiopathic or possible autoimmune destruction of pituitary cells.

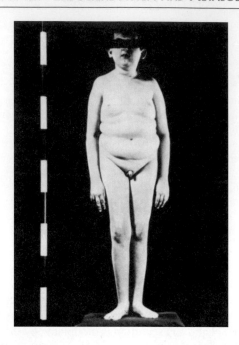

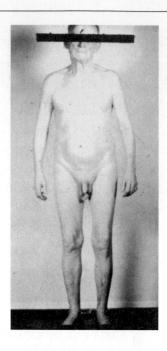

FIG. 59-1   Short stature and absence of secondary sexual characteristics in a patient with panhypopituitarism developing during childhood.

FIG. 59-2   Panhypopituitarism in the adult. There is pallor and a loss of body hair growth.

The clinical syndrome resulting from panhypopituitarism differs in children and in adults. In children, interference with somatic growth is caused by deficiency of GH release. *Pituitary dwarfism* develops as a consequence of this deficiency. As the child reaches adolescence, secondary sexual characteristics and the external genitalia fail to develop (Fig. 59-1). In addition, patients may present with various degrees of adrenal insufficiency and hypothyroidism. They may have difficulty in school and exhibit slow intellectual development. Their skin is usually pale because of the absence of MSH.

When hypopituitarism develops in adults, loss of pituitary function frequently has the following chronology: loss of GH, hypogonadism, hypothyroidism, and adrenal insufficiency. Because the adult has already completed somatic growth, adult patients with hypopituitarism are of normal height. Manifestations of GH deficiency may be expressed by unusual sensitivity to insulin and by fasting hypoglycemia. With the development of *hypogonadism*, men exhibit a decrease in libido, impotence, and a progressive decrease in body hair growth, beard, and muscular development (Fig. 59-2). In women, cessation of menstrual periods, or *amenorrhea,* is one of the early manifestations of pituitary failure. This is accompanied by atrophy of the breasts and the external genitalia. Both men and women show various degrees of hypothyroidism (see Chapter 60) and adrenal insufficiency (see Chapter 62). Deficiency of MSH causes a sallow or pale appearance in these patients.

Occasionally, patients exhibit isolated pituitary hormone failure. Under these circumstances the cause of the

deficiency is likely to be in the hypothalamus and involve the corresponding releasing factor.

In patients with panhypopituitarism, the baseline level of these hormones is low, as is the level of hormones produced by the target glands controlled by these hormones.

Patients with hypopituitarism have, in addition to low basal hormone levels, a blunted or absent response to the administration of hormone secretagogues. Combined pituitary function tests can be performed on these patients by injecting (1) insulin to produce hypoglycemia, (2) TRH, and (3) GnRH. Hypoglycemia, with a serum glucose level of less than 40 mg/dl, normally causes the release of GH, ACTH, and cortisol; TRH stimulates TSH and prolactin release; and GnRH stimulates the release of FSH and LH. Patients with panhypopituitarism fail to respond to any of these three secretagogues. In addition to the biochemical studies, radiographic examination of the pituitary gland is mandatory in patients with suspected pituitary disease, since pituitary tumors are a common cause of these disorders.

The treatment of hypopituitarism is simple. It consists of replacement of the deficient hormones. Human GH, the only one effective in humans, is produced by recombinant deoxyribonucleic acid (DNA) techniques and is available to physician specialists for the treatment of patients with GH deficiency. When administered to patients with pituitary dwarfism, it may cause significant increase in height. Pituitary hormones can be administered only by injection. Thus, for long-term daily replacement therapy, the hormones of the target glands affected by the pi-

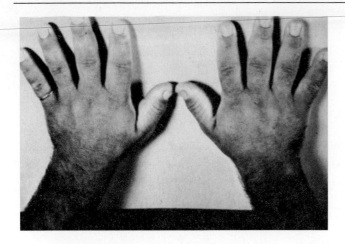

FIG. 59-3   Hands of a patient with acromegaly.

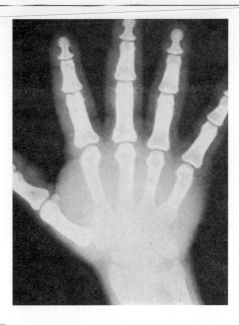

FIG. 59-5   Radiographic appearance of the hand of an acromegalic patient. There are increases in the soft tissues and in the density of the bones, squaring off the phalanges, and increased tufting of the terminal phalanges.

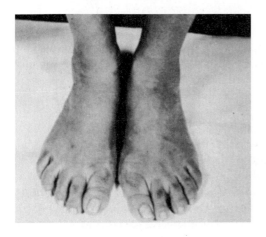

FIG. 59-4   Feet of a patient with acromegaly.

tuitary deficiency are administered instead. For example, adrenal insufficiency caused by deficiency of ACTH secretion is treated by giving hydrocortisone orally. Hypothyroidism caused by TSH deficiency is treated by giving thyroxine orally. Gonadotropin deficiency can be treated by administering androgens and estrogens. However, induction of ovulation necessitates the administration of gonadotropins.

Giantism and Acromegaly

Giantism and acromegaly are caused by excessive secretion of GH. This can result from a pituitary tumor that secretes GH or from a hypothalamic abnormality that leads to increased GH release. Some patients develop acromegaly in response to extrapituitary neoplasia that secretes GHRH ectopically. These patients have hyperplasia of pituitary somatotropes and hypersecretion of GH.

When GH excess occurs during childhood and adolescence, the patient experiences rapid longitudinal growth and becomes a giant. After somatic growth is completed,

GH hypersecretion will cause not giantism but thickening of bones and soft tissue. This condition is termed *acromegaly,* and patients with acromegaly exhibit enlargement of hands and feet. Hands become not only larger, but also more square (spadelike), and the fingers become more round and stubby (Fig. 59-3). Patients may relate the need for a larger size of glove. The feet also become larger and wider, and patients describe changes in shoe size (Fig. 59-4). The enlargement is usually caused by growth and thickening of bones and by increased growth of soft tissue (Fig. 59-5).

In addition, changes in facial features help diagnose the condition on simple observation. Facial features become coarse, and there is enlargement of the paranasal and frontal sinuses. Frontal bossing, prominence of the supraorbital ridges, and deformity of the mandible with development of prognathism and underbite (Fig. 59-6) also occur. Enlargement of the mandible causes the teeth to spread apart. Enlargement of the tongue occurs, which causes difficulty with speech (Fig. 59-7). The voice becomes deeper as a result of thickening of the vocal chords.

Deformities of the spine, caused by overgrowth of bone, lead to back pain and changes in the physiologic curvature of the spine. The radiographic examination of the skull in acromegaly shows typical changes, including enlargement of paranasal sinuses, thickening of the calvaria, deformity of the mandible (which resembles a boomerang), and most important, enlargement and destruction of the sella turcica suggesting a pituitary tumor (Fig. 59-8).

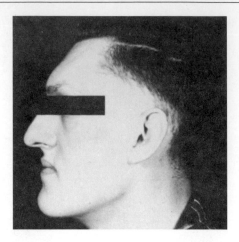

FIG. 59-6   Profile of a patient with acromegaly. There is prominence of the supraorbital ridges and of the nose (prognathism) and coarsening of facial features.

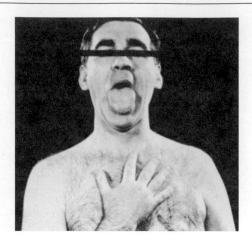

FIG. 59-7   Enlargement of the tongue in a patient with acromegaly. Note also acromegalic hand.

When acromegaly is associated with a pituitary tumor, the patients may exhibit bitemporal headaches and visual disturbance with bitemporal hemianopsia resulting from suprasellar extension of the tumor and compression of the optic chiasma.

Patients with acromegaly exhibit high basal GH levels and can be tested further by the administration of oral glucose. In normal subjects the induction of hyperglycemia by oral glucose suppresses GH levels. In contrast, patients with acromegaly or giantism fail to suppress GH levels.

Computed tomography (CT) scanning and magnetic resonance imaging (MRI) of the sella turcica demonstrate pituitary microadenomas as well as macroadenomas with extrasellar extension involving the suprasellar cistern, the parasellar regions, or the sphenoid sinus (Fig. 59-9).

Treatment of acromegaly or giantism is rather complex. Pituitary irradiation, surgery to the pituitary gland to resect a pituitary tumor, or combinations of these procedures may result in amelioration or remission of the disease. Medical treatment using a somatostatin analog is also available. This somatostatin analog can induce sustained suppression of GH and somatomedin C levels, decrease in tumor size, and marked clinical improvements.

Prolactin-Secreting Pituitary Tumors

The combination of persistent milk discharge and absent menses—*galactorrhea-amenorrhea*—is a relatively common endocrine syndrome in women. It is associated with increased prolactin secretion.

The presence of galactorrhea is usually demonstrated by manual expression of the nipple, although it may occur spontaneously and range from mild to severe. The associated amenorrhea is probably caused by the elevated prolactin levels. Prolactin is believed to inhibit the secretion of gonadotropic hormones by interfering with the

hypothalamic secretion of GnRH. In addition, prolactin may block the effect of gonadotropins on the gonad.

Approximately 20% of patients with galactorrhea exhibit a prolactin-secreting pituitary adenoma. In many instances, the adenoma is small and barely detectable by radiographic visualization of the sella turcica. In other instances, larger pituitary adenomas have been described. Normal prolactin levels range from 2 to 25 ng/ml. In patients with prolactin-secreting pituitary adenomas, levels may range from 100 ng/ml for small tumors to greater than 1000 ng/ml for large pituitary tumors.

Other patients may have galactorrhea and elevated prolactin levels without detectable pituitary adenomas. They may have undergone interruption of the normal tonic inhibition of prolactin release by the hypothalamus. Galactorrhea can be observed with (1) hypothalamic lesions that interrupt the release of dopamine, (2) drugs with effects on the central nervous system (phenothiazines, antidepressants, haloperidol, alpha-methyldopa), (3) oral contraceptives and estrogens, (4) endocrine disorders such as hypothyroidism and hyperthyroidism, (5) local neurogenic factors, (6) breast stimulation, (7) chest wall injury, and (8) spinal cord lesions.

In the presence of the galactorrhea-amenorrhea syndrome, it is necessary to obtain a basal serum prolactin level. If the prolactin level is elevated above normal, radiographic examination of the sella turcica should be performed, including CT with coronal cuts and MRI of the pituitary gland. These studies may demonstrate the presence of abnormalities suggestive of a pituitary microadenoma.

When the diagnosis of a prolactin-secreting pituitary tumor is confirmed, two forms of treatment are usually available: (1) transsphenoidal resection of the prolactin-secreting pituitary tumor and (2) suppression of prolactin secretion by the administration of bromocriptine, an ergot alkaloid derivative that acts as a dopamine agonist. Treat-

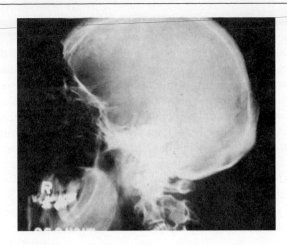

FIG. 59-8   Radiographic appearance of the skull of a patient with acromegaly. There is marked enlargement and destruction of the sella turcica and suggestion of intrasellar calcification. The calvaria is thick, and there is marked prominence of the frontal and paranasal sinuses. The angle of the mandible is rounded. There is also evidence of underbite.

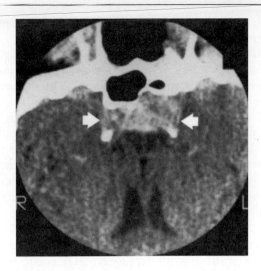

FIG. 59-9   Coronal cut of the sella turcica as shown on this computed tomography (CT) scan of a patient with a large prolactin-secreting macroadenoma. The enhancing intrasellar mass extends superiorly and laterally beyond the confines of the sella turcica. Also, there is destruction of the floor of the sella, which, instead of a straight horizontal contour, has an irregular appearance.

ment of hyperprolactinemia by the methods described frequently leads to disappearance of galactorrhea and restoration of normal menstrual cycles and fertility.

Prolactin-secreting pituitary tumors also occur in men, in whom the hyperprolactinemia is associated with hypogonadism and oligospermia. These tumors are frequently large and extend beyond the confines of the sella turcica. The management of prolactin-secreting pituitary microadenomas in men is similar to that described for women. In patients with large prolactin-secreting macroadenomas, bromocriptine may result in rapid and dramatic decrease in tumor size, without the need for surgical resection.

Disorders of Vasopressin Secretion

Arginine vasopressin (AVP) is an ADH synthesized in the supraoptic and paraventricular nuclei of the hypothalamus together with its binding protein, *neurophysin II*. AVP is then transported from the neuronal bodies, where it is produced, along the axons to nerve terminals in the posterior pituitary gland, where it is stored. AVP and its inactive neurophysin are then secreted in response to specific stimuli. The secretion of AVP is regulated by stimuli that arise in osmotic and volume receptors. An increase in extracellular fluid osmolality or a decrease in intravascular volume stimulate AVP secretion. AVP then increases the permeability of the renal collecting duct epithelium to water through a mechanism involving activation of *adenylate cyclase* and increased generation of cyclic adenosine monophosphate (cAMP). As a result, urine concentration increases and serum osmolality decreases to normal. Serum osmolality is usually kept constant within narrow limits between 290 and

296 mOsm/kg H_2O. With normal renal function, maximal renal concentration is associated with a urine osmolality of 1000 mOsm/kg H_2O.

Disturbances of AVP secretion include *diabetes insipidus* (DI) and the *syndrome of inappropriate ADH secretion* (SIADH) (also see Chapter 21). In patients with diabetes insipidus, the disorder may be secondary to a destruction of the hypothalamic nuclei where vasopressin is synthesized (*central* DI) or the result of unresponsiveness of the renal tubules to vasopressin (*nephrogenic* DI).

Several conditions may result in DI, including tumors of the hypothalamus, large pituitary tumors that extend above the sella turcica and destroy the hypothalamic nuclei, head trauma, surgical injury of the hypothalamus, intracerebral vascular occlusions, and granulomatous diseases. In many cases a lesion is not detectable by available imaging techniques. Nephrogenic DI results from a variety of renal diseases as well as systemic diseases that involve the kidney, including multiple myeloma, sickle cell anemia, hypercalcemia, hypokalemia, and lithium therapy.

Patients with central DI have *polydipsia* and *polyuria* with urine volumes between 5 and 10 L/day. These large renal losses of water are compensated for by increased water intake. Eventually, patients become dehydrated, experience weight loss, and have dry skin and mucous membranes. Because of the ingestion of large quantities of water required to maintain hydration, these patients also complain of epigastric fullness and anorexia. The thirst and urination usually continue during the night, and patients have interrupted sleep with frequent nocturia. Patients usually prefer the ingestion of ice cold water. Serum osmolality is increased with values frequently greater than 300 mOsm/kg H$_2$O. Concomitantly, urine osmolality is low, between 100 and 200 mOsm/kg H$_2$O. Because patients are dehydrated, renal function may be impaired and blood urea nitrogen (BUN) and serum creatinine may be increased. When patients with suspected DI are asked to withhold fluids for 18 hours, their urine specific gravity fails to increase and urine osmolality remains low. When patients adhere strictly to water deprivation during this test, thirst may become intense and they may develop orthostatic hypotension and experience significant weight loss. The subcutaneous administration of aqueous Pitressin is associated with a positive response. Urine volume decreases and the specific gravity increases immediately after the administration of Pitressin. Patients with nephrogenic DI fail to respond to AVP.

Central DI is treated with AVP. The most frequently used preparation is DDAVP (1-desamino-8 D-arginine vasopressin), which is administered intranasally and has a duration of action of 12 to 24 hours. If DDAVP cannot be given intranasally, an alternative form is available for parenteral administration. AVP is not effective in patients with nephrogenic diabetes insipidus.

SIADH is usually observed in association with diseases that affect the hypothalamus or the lungs or subsequent to drug administration. Patients develop a *hypoosmolar syndrome* with excessive and inappropriate water retention. Symptoms result from severe *hyponatremia* and involve the central nervous system with irritability, mental confusion, seizures, and coma, especially when the serum sodium decreases below 120 mEq/L. Serum osmolality is low, and urine osmolality is high and elevated above serum osmolality. In these patients, BUN and serum creatinine levels are low and urine sodium is greater than 20 mEq/L.

Treatment of SIADH is based on water restriction to less than 1000 ml/day and the administration of 3% to 5% sodium chloride solutions together with furosemide. The diuretic induces the loss of water and sodium chloride, which is restored in a hypertonic form. Demeclocycline, a drug that directly inhibits the effect of AVP at the renal tubule level, can be used effectively to reverse the hypoosmolality associated with SIADH.

QUESTIONS

▼ *Match the statements in column A with the structures of the pituitary gland in column B.*

Column A
1. _____ Derived from neural cells of the developing third ventricle
2. _____ Derived from Rathke's pouch
3. _____ Connected to the hypothalamus by the hypothalamic-hypophyseal portal system
4. _____ Confined within the sella turcica of the sphenoid bone

Column B
a. Adenohypophysis
b. Neurohypophysis
c. Both the above

▼ *Match the hormones in column A with one of the functions in column B.*

Column A
5. _____ Adrenocorticotropic hormone (ACTH)
6. _____ Growth hormone (GH)
7. _____ Luteinizing hormone (LH)
8. _____ Follicle-stimulating hormone (FSH)
9. _____ Prolactin
10. _____ Thyrotropin
11. _____ Melanocyte-stimulating hormone (MSH)
12. _____ Antidiuretic hormone (ADH)

Column B
a. Stimulates spermatogenesis in men
b. Stimulates the formation and release of thyroid hormones
c. Initiates milk secretion after parturition
d. Stimulates the secretory activity of the adrenal cortex
e. Stimulates somatomedin
f. Decreases free water clearance
g. Stimulates the corpus luteum to secrete progesterone in women
h. Increases pigmentation of the skin

▼ *Circle the letter preceding each item below that correctly answers the question or completes the statement. More than one answer may be correct.*

13. The hypothalamus secretes neurohormones that:
    a. Facilitate the formation of a corpus luteum in the ovary
    b. Inhibit the release of prolactin from the pituitary
    c. Increase the synthesis of hydrocortisone by the adrenal cortex
    d. Facilitate thyroid growth
    e. Increase the release of parathormone by the parathyroid glands

14. ADH is:
    a. Synthesized in the neurohypophysis
    b. Secreted by the adenohypophysis
    c. Synthesized in the supraoptic and paraventricular nuclei in the hypothalamus
    d. Stored and released from the neurohypophysis

15. MSH secretion is:
    a. Inhibited by high serum levels of cortisol
    b. Depressed in Cushing's disease caused by pituitary ACTH excess
    c. Greatly increased in Addison's disease.
    d. Controlled by a releasing hormone

16. Which of the following statements about GH is *false?*
    a. It is released in response to hypoglycemia.
    b. Its release is controlled by a hypothalamic releasing factor and somatostatin.
    c. Its release is inhibited by administration of arginine.
    d. Its anabolic effect is mediated through somatomedin.

17. Prepubertal panhypopituitarism may be manifested by:
    a. Acromegaly
    b. Retardation of growth

QUESTIONS—cont'd

c. Pale, dry skin
d. Precocious sexual development
e. Slow intellectual development

18. A 35-year-old multiparous woman seeks medical help because of vague symptoms of lethargy, lack of energy, and intolerance to cold. The history reveals that her menstrual periods ceased 1 year earlier, following the birth of her last child, which was complicated by postpartum hemorrhage. She is concerned that she is losing her sexual attractiveness. Physical examination reveals an asthenic female with thin hair, atrophied breasts, and thin pubic hair. Blood pressure is 94/60 mm Hg, temperature 97° F, pulse rate 54 beats/minute, and respirations 16 breaths/minute. Laboratory findings include low levels of TSH, normal serum cholesterol, depressed serum levels of ACTH, depressed urinary levels of 17-ketosteroids and 17-hydroxysteroids, and low serum level of FSH. The above data are suggestive of:
   a. Primary hypothyroidism
   b. Premature menopause in an otherwise healthy woman
   c. Galactorrhea-amenorrhea
   d. Primary adrenal insufficiency
   e. Panhypopituitarism

19. A possible explanation for this patient's condition is:
   a. A congenital disorder
   b. Postpartum necrosis of the pituitary
   c. Adrenal carcinoma
   d. A prolactin-secreting pituitary adenoma

20. Acromegaly results from:
   a. Hypersecretion of GH in a child
   b. Extrapituitary neoplasia that causes secretion of GHRH ectopically
   c. Hypersecretion of GH in an adult
   d. Parathormone hypersecretion
   e. Pituitary insufficiency

21. Physical signs of acromegaly include:
   a. Frontal bossing
   b. Prominence of the supraorbital ridges
   c. Broad, greatly enlarged, spade-shaped hands
   d. Prognathism

22. Patients with acromegaly often experience:
   a. Slurred speech
   b. Weight loss
   c. Hypoglycemia
   d. Headaches

23. Common radiologic signs in acromegaly include:
   a. Thickened calvaria
   b. Enlargement of the paranasal and frontal sinuses
   c. Increased length and thickness of the mandible
   d. Enlargement of the sella turcica

24. Signs and symptoms associated with central diabetes insipidus include:
   a. Polydipsia
   b. Dry skin and mucus membranes
   c. Hyperprolactinemia
   d. Polyuria

25. Human GH is used to treat:
   a. Pituitary dwarfism
   b. Adrenal insufficiency
   c. Hypopituitarism
   d. Hypothyroidism

26. The cause of vasopressin secretion associated with the syndrome of inappropriate ADH secretion (SIADH) includes:
   a. Destruction of hypothalamic nuclei
   b. Unresponsiveness of the renal tubules to vasopressin
   c. Both a and b
   d. Neither a nor b

▼ *Circle T if the statement is true and F if it is false. Correct any false statements.*

27. T F Gonadotropin deficiency in hypopituitarism may be treated by the administration of androgens and estrogens.

28. T F GH for treatment of hypopituitary dwarfs is obtained by extraction of the hormone from the pituitary glands of cattle and swine.

29. T F Giantism and acromegaly are caused by excessive secretion of somatotropin.

30. T F Patients with suspected pituitary disease require only biochemical confirmation by specific tests that reveal abnormality of pituitary function characteristic of the suspected condition.

31. T F Computed tomography (CT) scanning and magnetic resonance imaging (MRI) of the sella turcica demonstrate pituitary microadenomas and macroadenomas with extrasellar extension involving the suprasellar cistern, the parasellar regions, or the sphenoid sinus.

▼ *Answer the following on a separate sheet of paper.*

32. Explain the medical treatment currently being tested for treatment of acromegaly or giantism.

33. How is human GH produced?

34. List four pathologic processes that may result in pituitary insufficiency.

35. What are the likely complications when patients with suspected diabetes insipidus are requested to withhold fluids for 18 hours? Explain the rationale for the administration of aqueous Pitressin.

36. What is the rationale for the treatment of SIADH?

CHAPTER 60

Thyroid Gland Disorders

DAVID E. SCHTEINGART

GENERAL CONSIDERATIONS

The thyroid gland has two lobes joined by a thin isthmus and is located below the cricoid cartilage in the neck. Embryologically, the thyroid gland originates from an evagination of the pharyngeal epithelium, which carries with it cells from the lateral pharyngeal pouches. This evagination descends from the base of the tongue into the neck until it reaches its final anatomic location. Some thyroid tissue occasionally may be left along this track, giving rise to thyroglossal cysts, nodules, or a pyramidal thyroid lobe. The thyroid gland normally weighs between 10 and 20 g in adults. Histologically, the gland is made up of nodules composed of tiny follicles separated from each other by connective tissue (Fig. 60-1). The thyroid follicles are lined with cuboidal epithelium, and their lumen is filled with colloid. The follicular epithelial cells initiate the synthesis of thyroid hormones and activate their release into the circulation. The colloidal material, *thyroglobulin,* is where thyroid hormones are synthesized and eventually stored. The two principal hormones produced by the follicles are *thyroxine* and *triiodothyronine.* Another hormone-secreting cell within the thyroid gland is the *parafollicular cell,* or *C cell,* found in the basal portion of the follicle in contact with the follicular membrane. These cells originate in the embryologic ultimobranchial body. They secrete *calcitonin,* a hormone that lowers serum calcium levels, and thus contribute to the regulation of calcium homeostasis. The follicular thyroid hormones are derived from the iodination of tyrosyl residues in thyroglobulin. Thyroxine contains four iodine atoms (T_4), and triiodothyronine contains three iodine atoms (T_3) (Fig. 60-2). Thyroxine is secreted in larger quantities than triiodothyronine, but when compared on a milligram-per-milligram basis, triiodothyronine is the more active of the two hormones.

Biosynthesis and Metabolism of Thyroid Hormones

The biosynthesis of thyroid hormones involves a sequence of steps regulated by specific enzymes. These steps are (1) trapping of iodide, (2) oxidation of iodide to iodine, (3) organification of iodine into monoiodotyrosine and diiodotyrosine, (4) coupling of iodinated precursors, (5) storage, and (6) hormone release (Fig. 60-3). The trapping of iodide by the thyroid follicular cells is an active, energy-requiring process. This energy is derived from oxidative metabolism within the gland. Iodide is available to the thyroid from ingested food or fluids or that released by deiodination of thyroid hormones or iodinated agents. The thyroid takes up and concentrates 20 to 30 times the amount of iodide present in plasma. Iodide is converted to iodine, catalyzed by an iodide peroxidase enzyme. Iodine is then incorporated into a tyrosine molecule, a process described as *organification of iodine.* This process takes place at the cell-colloid interphase. The resulting compounds, monoiodotyrosine and diiodotyrosine, are then coupled as follows: two molecules of diiodotyrosine make T_4, and one molecule of diiodotyrosine and one molecule of monoiodotyrosine make T_3. The coupling of these compounds and the storage of the resulting hormones take place within thy-

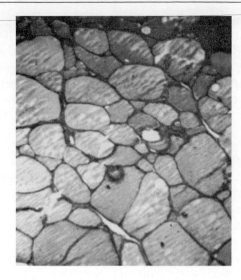

FIG. 60-1   Histology of the thyroid gland. Note colloid of filled follicles.

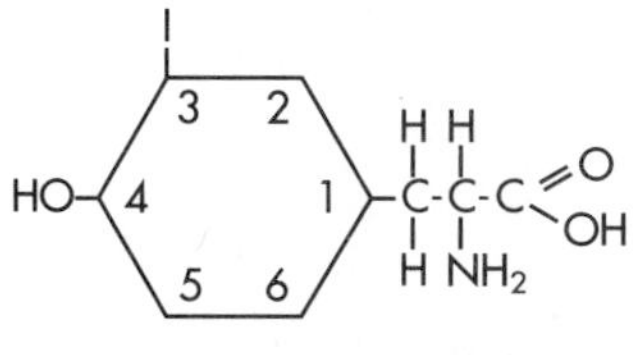

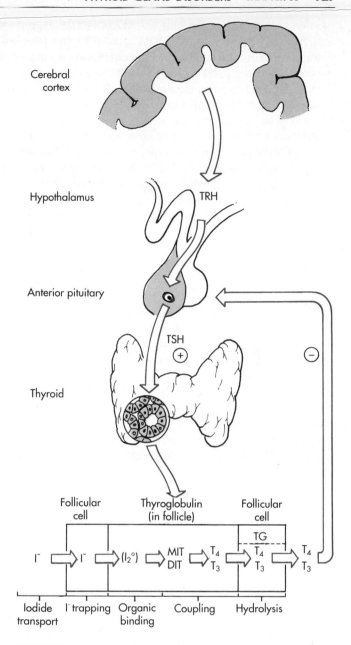

FIG. 60-3   Synthesis and secretion of thyroid hormones. The box indicates steps that occur within the thyroid gland. Thyroid function is regulated by the hypothalamic-pituitary axis. *TRH,* Thyrotropin-releasing hormone; *TSH,* thyroid-stimulating hormone (thyrotropin); *MIT,* monoiodotyrosine; *DIT,* diiodotyrosine; *TG,* thyroglobulin; T_3, triiodothyronine; T_4, thyroxine; I_2^0, iodine; I^-, iodide. [Modified from Ezrin C et al, editors: *Systematic endocrinology,* New York, 1973, Harper & Row.]

3 - MONOIODOTYROSINE

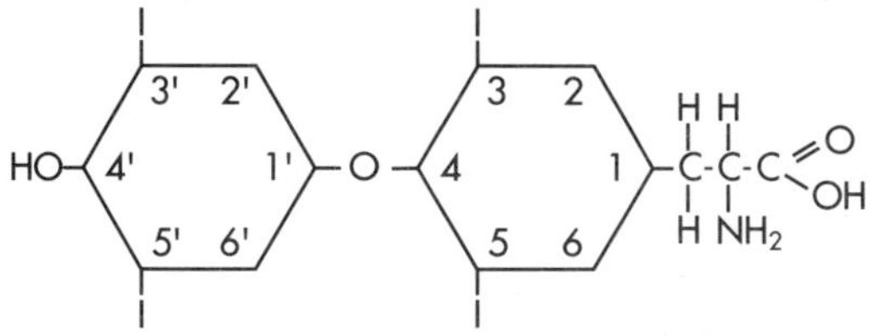

3,5,3',5'- TETRAIODOTHYRONINE (thyroxine; T_4)

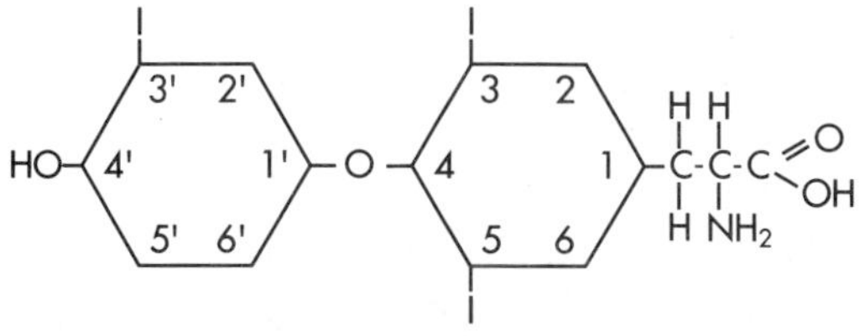

3, 5, 3'- TRIIODOTHYRONINE (T_3)

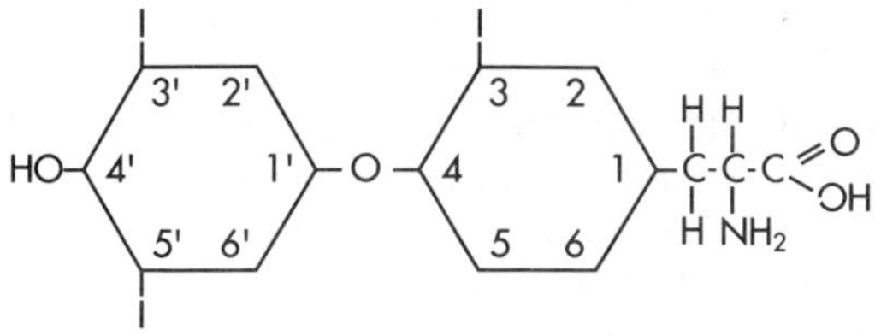

3, 3', 5'- TRIIODOTHYRONINE (reverse T_3; RT_3)

FIG. 60-2   Chemical structures of thyroid hormones.

roglobulin. Hormones are released from storage by incorporation of colloid droplets into the follicular cells by a process called *pinocytosis.* Within these cells, thyroglobulin is hydrolyzed and the hormones are released into the circulation. The various steps described are stimulated by thyrotropin (thyroid-stimulating hormone, TSH).

Thyroid hormones circulate in plasma bound to plasma

proteins: (1) thyroxine-binding globulin (TBG), (2) thyroxine-binding prealbumin (TBPA), and (3) thyroxine-binding albumin (TBA). Most of the circulating hormone is bound to these proteins, and a small proportion (less than 0.05%) is free. The bound and free hormones are in a state of reversible equilibrium. The free hormone is the fraction that is metabolically active, and the larger, protein-bound fraction is not readily accessible to target tissues. Of the three binding proteins, TBG binds thyroxine most specifically. In addition, thyroxine has greater affinity than triiodothyronine for these binding proteins. As a consequence, triiodothyronine is transferred more readily to its target tissues, a factor that accounts for its greater metabolic activity.

Thyroid hormones are chemically altered before excretion. An important alteration is *deiodination,* which accounts for the disposal of 70% of the secreted hormone. Another 30% is lost in the stool through biliary excretion as glucuronide or sulfate conjugates. As a result of deiodination, 80% of T_4 may be converted into 3,5,3'-triiodothyronine, and the remaining 20% is converted to reverse 3,3',5'-triiodothyronine (RT_3), a metabolically inactive hormone.

Thyroid function is controlled by the pituitary glycoprotein hormone TSH, which in turn is regulated by thyrotropin-releasing hormone (TRH), a hypothalamic neurohormone. Thyroxine exerts negative feedback regulation of TSH secretion by acting directly on the pituitary thyrotropes.

Several drugs and conditions can alter the synthesis, release, and metabolism of thyroid hormones. Drugs such as perchlorate and thiocyanate are capable of inhibiting thyroxine synthesis. As a result, they cause a decrease in thyroxine levels and, through negative feedback stimulation, an increase in release of TSH by the pituitary gland. This condition leads to enlargement of the thyroid gland and the development of a goiter. These drugs are therefore called *goitrogens.* Other drugs, such as thiourea derivatives and mercaptoimidazoles, can be used as antithyroid drugs because they inhibit the initial oxidation of iodide, the conversion of monoiodotyrosine to diiodotyrosine, or the coupling of iodotyrosine to produce iodothyronine. These drugs are useful in the treatment of conditions caused by excessive thyroid hormone secretion. Iodine, when given acutely and in large doses, is capable of blocking the organic binding and coupling reactions. The continued administration of large doses of iodine may lead to goiter development and a hyperthyroid state. Finally, drugs such as lithium carbonate and glucocorticoids inhibit thyroid hormone release.

Changes in the concentration of TBG can also cause changes in the level of total circulating thyroxine. Increases in TBG, as seen in pregnancy and with birth control pills, may lead to increased levels of protein-bound thyroxine. Conversely, decreases in TBG, as seen with chronic liver disease, severe systemic illness, nephrotic syndrome, and large doses of glucocorticoids, will cause a decrease in circulating protein-bound thyroxine.

Nutritional changes, such as observed during fasting or carbohydrate- and protein-deprived diets, can decrease the proportion of thyroxine deiodinated to T_3 and increase the less metabolically active RT_3. This alteration in the deiodination of thyroxine appears to be a mechanism for fuel conservation in states of food deprivation.

Action of Thyroid Hormones

The physiologic effects of thyroid hormones involve increased transcription of messenger ribonucleic acid (mRNA) and protein synthesis. This step appears to be necessary for the subsequent stimulation of cell respiration. Specifically, both thyroxine and triiodothyronine stimulate energy-producing electron transfer processes in the respiratory enzyme system of the cell mitochondria. The stimulation by thyroid hormones of oxidative processes leads to stimulation of thermogenesis. In addition to these thermogenic effects, thyroxine and triiodothyronine potentiate the action of epinephrine by increasing the sensitivity of beta-receptors to catecholamines. Thyroid hormones also stimulate somatic growth and are involved in the normal development of the central nervous system. In their absence, mental retardation and delayed neurologic maturation may be present at birth and in infancy.

Tests of Thyroid Function

The functional status of the thyroid gland can be ascertained by means of thyroid function tests. The following tests are presently used in diagnosis of thyroid disease:
1. Serum thyroxine and triiodothyronine
2. T_3 resin uptake
3. Free thyroxine
4. Serum TSH levels
5. Radioisotope thyroid uptake

The *serum thyroxine and triiodothyronine levels* can be measured by radioligand assays. Normal levels for thyroxine are 4 to 11 µg/dl; for triiodothyronine they are 80 to 160 ng/dl. The *T_3 resin uptake test* measures the saturation of thyroxine-binding protein by thyroxine and, together with the total thyroxine level, helps estimate the level of free thyroxine. When this test is performed, the patient's plasma is placed in a test tube with radioactive T_3 and a resin. The radioactive T_3 binds to both the plasma and the resin. Normally, 25% to 35% of the added T_3 is taken up by the resin. This result can also be expressed as a percent of normal values. A normal T_3 resin uptake ranges between 86% and 110% of normal. When the plasma level of thyroxine is high and the protein is completely saturated by thyroid hormone, more of the T_3 will be bound by the resin and less by the protein; the T_3 resin uptake will be high. Conversely, when the thyroxine level is low and the binding proteins are at a low level of saturation, more of the T_3 will bind to the protein and less to the resin; the T_3 resin uptake will be low. By combining the values of the serum thyroxine level and T_3

TABLE 60-1 Thyroid Function Tests

Test	Hyperthyroidism	Hypothyroidism
RAI uptake	Increased	Decreased
Serum thyroxine	Increased	Decreased
T_3 resin uptake	Increased	Decreased
Free thyroxine	Increased	Decreased
Serum TSH	Decreased	Increased

resin uptake, it is possible to estimate the level of metabolically active, circulating free thyroxine. The *free thyroxine index* (FTI) is an expression of this value and results from multiplying serum T_4 by T_3 resin uptake. The free thyroxine level can also be measured directly.

Plasma TSH levels can be measured by a radioimmunometric assay; normal values, by the third-generation assay, range from 0.02 to 5.0 µU/ml. The plasma TSH level measures the state of homeostatic control of thyroid function by the pituitary gland. Values are high in patients with primary hypothyroidism, in whom the low thyroxine levels are associated with a feedback increase in pituitary TSH release. Conversely, values are below normal in patients with autonomous increase in thyroid function (Graves' disease, hyperfunctioning thyroid nodules) or in those receiving suppressive doses of exogenous thyroid hormone. With the availability of highly sensitive TSH radioimmunometric assays, this test alone can be used in the initial evaluation of patients with suspected thyroid disease.

Some tests can measure the metabolic response to circulating thyroid hormone levels. These tests include the basal metabolic rate (BMR), which measures the oxygen consumption in the resting state; the serum cholesterol level; and the characteristics of response of the Achilles tendon reflex. In patients with hypothyroidism, the BMR is decreased and the serum cholesterol level is high. The Achilles tendon reflex shows slow relaxation. Opposite findings are seen in patients with hyperthyroidism.

The radioactive iodine (^123I) uptake test measures the ability of the thyroid gland to trap and organify iodide. The patient receives a tracer dose of ^{123}I, which the thyroid traps and concentrates over a 24-hour period. The radioactivity present over the thyroid is then calculated. Normally, the uptake ranges from 10% to 35% of the administered dose. Values are high in hyperthyroidism and low when the thyroid gland has been suppressed.

Hyperthyroidism and hypothyroidism are the two major functional abnormalities for which one needs reliable laboratory tools. Few supportive laboratory investigations may be required in severe cases. However, additional tests may be necessary in the diagnosis of mild cases of thyroid dysfunction. Table 60-1 summarizes the changes in thyroid function tests observed in patients with hypothyroidism and hyperthyroidism.

DISEASES OF THE THYROID GLAND

As with other endocrine diseases, those of the thyroid gland may involve the following:
1. Excessive thyroid hormone production (hyperthyroidism)
2. Deficient hormone production (hypothyroidism)
3. Thyroid enlargement (goiter) without evidence of abnormal thyroid hormone production

In addition, patients with severe systemic illnesses may develop changes in thyroxine metabolism and in thyroid function. These findings are known as euthyroid sick syndrome.

Hyperthyroidism

Also known as *thyrotoxicosis,* hyperthyroidism may be defined as the response of body tissues to the metabolic effects of excessive amounts of thyroid hormone. The condition may develop spontaneously or may result from the intake of excessive amounts of thyroid hormones. Occasionally, the therapeutic misuse of thyroid hormone leads to clinical manifestations of hyperthyroidism. Some patients with psychiatric illness may take large amounts of thyroxine or triiodothyronine and become thyrotoxic. These patients frequently deny taking thyroid hormones and pose a real challenge to the medical personnel attempting to establish the proper diagnosis. This form of thyrotoxicosis is called *thyrotoxicosis factitia.* Characteristic of it is the presence of high thyroxine levels and T_3 resin uptake with low radioactive iodine (RAI) uptake and TSH levels.

There are two types of spontaneous hyperthyroidism: (1) Graves' disease and (2) toxic nodular goiter. Graves' disease is the more common.

Graves' disease usually occurs in the third and fourth decades of life and more frequently in women than men. There is a familial predisposition to Graves' disease and frequent association with other forms of autoimmune endocrinopathy. In Graves' disease, the two major groups of features are thyroidal and extrathyroidal, either of which may be absent. The thyroidal features include a goiter, caused by hyperplasia of the thyroid gland, and hyperthyroidism, which results from excessive thyroid hormone secretion. Symptoms of hyperthyroidism include manifestations of hypermetabolism and of sympathetic overactivity. Patients complain of fatigue; tremor; heat intolerance; increased sweating with warm, moist skin; weight loss, often with increased appetite; palpitations and tachycardia; diarrhea; and muscle weakness and atrophy. The extrathyroidal manifestations include ophthalmopathy and localized skin infiltrations, usually confined to the lower legs. The ophthalmopathy, present in 50% to 80% of these patients, is characterized by stare, widening of the palpebral fissures, decreased blinking, lid lag, and failure of convergence. The lid lag is manifested by a

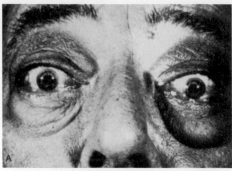
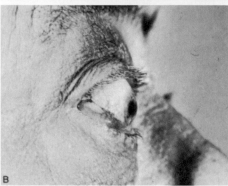

FIG. 60-4   Exophthalmos with periorbital edema in a patient with Graves' ophthalmopathy. **A,** Frontal view. **B,** Lateral view. (Courtesy of James C. Sisson, MD, Department of Internal Medicine, University of Michigan.)

slower movement of the eyelid relative to the eyeball when patients are asked to slowly lower their gaze. Infiltration of the orbital tissues and ocular muscles with lymphocytes, mast cells, and plasma cells leads to exophthalmos (proptosis of the eyeballs), congestive oculopathy, and weakness of extraocular movements (Fig. 60-4, *A* and *B*). The ophthalmopathy can be quite severe, and in extreme cases, vision may be threatened. Graves' disease appears to develop as a manifestation of an autoimmune disorder. An immunoglobulin (IgG) antibody is present in the serum of these patients. This antibody appears to react with the TSH receptor or the thyroid plasma membrane. As a result of this interaction, the antibody is capable of stimulating thyroid function independently of pituitary TSH, leading to hyperthyroidism. This thyroid-stimulating immunoglobulin (TSI) may result from an inherited abnormality of immune surveillance that permits a particular clone of lymphocytes to survive, proliferate, and secrete stimulatory immunoglobulins in response to some precipitating factor. A similar immune response appears to be responsible for the ophthalmopathy observed in these patients.

Toxic nodular goiter develops most frequently in older patients as a complication of chronic nodular goiter. The onset of hyperthyroidism in these patients is insidious, and the clinical manifestations of hyperthyroidism are less severe than in Graves' disease. Patients may present with dysrhythmias and heart failure resistant to digitalis

therapy. Patients may also show evidence of weight loss, weakness, and muscle wasting. The multinodular goiter usually present in these patients contrasts with the diffuse thyroid enlargement seen in patients with Graves' disease. Patients with toxic nodular goiter may show eye signs (stare, widening of palpebral fissure, decreased blinking) resulting from sympathetic overactivity. However, they lack the more dramatic manifestations of infiltrative ophthalmopathy seen in Graves' disease.

Patients with severe manifestations of hyperthyroidism may develop thyroid crisis or storm. In these cases, there is a general worsening of the clinical manifestations described earlier, to the point where they become life-threatening. Fever is almost always present and may be an important clue to the onset of serious complications. Crisis can be precipitated by minor trauma and stress, such as an infectious illness, surgery, or anesthesia.

In the presence of clinical manifestations of hyperthyroidism, laboratory tests show a high serum thyroxine and T_3 resin uptake. RAI uptake by the thyroid is increased, and serum TSH levels are low. In addition, TSH fails to respond to stimulation by TRH, the hypothalamic thyroid-releasing hormone.

Management of hyperthyroidism includes one or several of the following procedures:
1. Prolonged treatment with antithyroid drugs such as propylthiouracil or methimazole, given for at least 1 year; these drugs block thyroxine synthesis and release
2. Surgical subtotal thyroidectomy after preoperative drug therapy with propylthiouracil
3. Treatment with radioactive iodine

Treatment with radioactive iodine is used in most adult patients with Graves' disease. It is usually contraindicated in children and pregnant women. In patients with toxic nodular goiter, antithyroid drugs and ablative therapy with radioactive iodine can also be used. However, if the goiter is large and there are no contraindications for surgery, surgical resection of the goiter should be considered. Treatment of the ophthalmopathy of Graves' disease involves correction of hyperthyroidism and prevention of hypothyroidism that may develop after surgical or radiation ablative therapy. In many patients, the ophthalmopathy follows a self-limiting course and no further treatment is necessary. However, in severe cases in which vision is threatened, treatment with large doses of glucocorticoids and orbital decompression procedures may be necessary to salvage the eye. Hypothyroidism may develop in patients with hyperthyroidism receiving surgical or radioactive iodine therapy. Of patients treated with radioactive iodine, 40% to 70% may go on to develop hypothyroidism over the following 10 years.

Hypothyroidism

There are several types of hypothyroidism. Depending on the location of the initiating problem, the disease can be

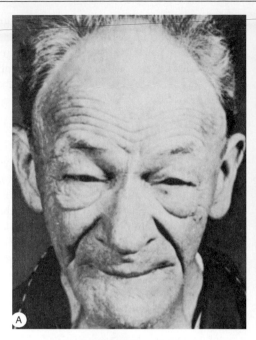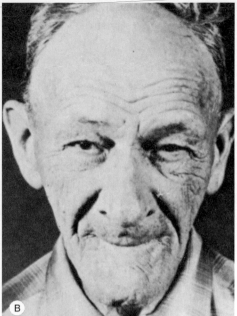

FIG. 60-5   Facial appearance of patient with myxedema. **A,** At the time of initial diagnosis. **B,** After replacement therapy with thyroxine. (Courtesy of James C. Sisson, MD, Department of Internal Medicine, University of Michigan.)

classified as (1) *primary,* resulting from a pathologic process that destroys the thyroid gland, or (2) *secondary,* caused by deficiency of pituitary TSH secretion. Depending on the age of onset of the hypothyroid state, the disease can be classified as (1) adult hypothyroidism, or *myxedema,* (2) juvenile hypothyroidism (onset after age 1 to 2 years), or (3) congenital hypothyroidism, or *cretinism* caused by lack of thyroid hormone before or shortly after birth.

Some patients with hypothyroidism have an atrophic or absent thyroid gland as a result of surgical or radioisotopic ablation of the gland or because of its destruction by circulating autoimmune antibodies. Developmental defects may also account for the absence of a thyroid gland in a patient with congenital hypothyroidism. Goiters are often observed in hypothyroid patients with hereditary defects in thyroid hormone biosynthesis; the concomitant increase in TSH release causes thyroid enlargement. Goiters may also be seen in patients with *Hashimoto's thyroiditis,* an autoimmune disease in which lymphocytic infiltration and destruction of the thyroid gland supervene in association with antithyroglobulin or antithyroid cell microsomal antibodies. Patients with secondary hypothyroidism may have pituitary tumors and be deficient in other pituitary tropic hormones.

The clinical manifestations of hypothyroidism in the adult and juvenile forms include fatigue; hoarseness; cold intolerance, decreased sweating; cool, dry skin; facial puffiness; and slow movements (Fig. 60-5). There is slowing of intellectual and motor activity and slow relaxation of deep tendon reflexes. Women with hypothyroidism frequently complain of hypermenorrhea.

Congenital hypothyroidism, or cretinism, may be present at birth or become evident within the first several months of life. Early manifestations of cretinism include persistent physiologic jaundice, hoarse cry, constipation, somnolence, and feeding problems. Subsequently, the child shows delay in reaching the normal milestones of development. The child with congenital hypothyroidism exhibits short stature; coarse features; a protruding tongue; broad, flat nose; widely set eyes; sparse hair; dry skin; a protuberant abdomen; and umbilical hernia.

Radiographic examination of the skeleton shows retarded bone age, epiphyseal dysgenesis, and delayed dental development. A major complication of unrecognized and untreated congenital and juvenile hypothyroidism is mental retardation, which is preventable by early correction of hypothyroidism. Health care personnel attending newborn and small infants must be alert for this condition.

Laboratory test results that confirm the presence of hypothyroidism include low serum thyroxine and triiodothyronine levels, low BMR, and elevated serum cholesterol. Serum TSH levels may be high or low, depending on the type of hypothyroidism. In primary hypothyroidism, serum TSH levels are high, together with low thyroxine. In contrast, both measurements are low in patients with secondary hypothyroidism.

Treatment of hypothyroidism includes the administration of thyroxine, which is usually begun at low dosage levels of 50 μg/day and gradually increased over days and weeks to a full maintenance dosage of 150 μg/day. The measurement of serum thyroxine levels and T_3 resin uptake as well as TSH levels in patients with primary hypothyroidism may be used to determine the adequacy of the replacement therapy. These levels should be maintained within the normal range.

Nontoxic Goiters

Nontoxic, diffuse, colloid goiters and colloid nodular goiters are common disorders that affect 16% of women and 4% of men age 20 to 60, as demonstrated in a survey of Tecumseh, a community in Michigan. Patients usually have no symptoms other than the cosmetic appearance, but occasional complications may occur. The thyroid may be diffusely enlarged and/or contain nodules.

The causes of nontoxic goiter include iodine deficiency or an intrathyroidal chemical defect caused by a variety of factors. As a result of this defect, the thyroid gland has an impaired capacity to secrete thyroxine, leading to increased TSH levels and hyperplasia and hypertrophy of the thyroid follicles. The enlarged thyroid gland frequently undergoes exacerbations and remissions, with hypervolution and involution of areas of the thyroid gland. Fibrosis may alternate with hyperplasia, and nodules containing thyroid follicles may develop.

Clinically, patients may demonstrate a protuberance in the lower third of the neck. With large goiters, mechanical compression problems may develop, including displacement of the trachea and esophagus and symptoms of obstruction.

If the impairment of thyroid function is severe, the goiter may be accompanied by hypothyroidism. To ascertain the functional status of the goiter, measurements of serum free T_4 and TSH levels may be necessary. In addition, radioactive iodine or technetium pertechnetate scintiscans show whether the nodules are "cold" or "hot." Cold nodules may represent carcinoma, and hot nodules are nearly always benign. Ultrasound scanning of the thyroid gland may be used to detect cystic changes in thyroid nodules. Cystic nodules are rarely cancerous.

Treatment of goiter involves suppression of TSH with thyroxine, which can eventually result in suppression of pituitary TSH and inhibition of thyroid function with atrophy of the thyroid gland. Surgery may be indicated for large goiters, to remove the mechanical and cosmetic problems they cause. In communities where goiters develop as a consequence of iodide deficiency, the use of iodized table salt should be encouraged.

Thyroid Neoplasms

Thyroid neoplasms usually present as discrete enlargements of the thyroid gland. At times, they may resemble a benign nodular goiter. Thyroid nodules are clinically palpable in approximately 5% to 10% of adults in the United States. The majority of these nodules are benign, but some nodular goiters are carcinomatous. To determine whether a thyroid nodule is benign or malignant, known risk factors and the clinical characteristics of the mass should be assessed and certain laboratory studies performed.

Risk factors

The risk of a carcinoma in a thyroid nodule is high, approximately 50%, in a child under 14 years of age. In contrast, the risk is less than 10% in adults. Men have a higher incidence of carcinomatous thyroid nodules than women. The recent appearance of a nodule or rapid enlargement of a preexisting nodule should raise a suspicion that the nodule is malignant. Previous exposure to therapeutic radiation of the head and neck regions may also increase the risk of developing thyroid carcinoma in the future. The incidence of radiation exposure during childhood in patients under 15 years of age with thyroid carcinomas has been reported to be as high as 50%; for patients under 30 years of age, 20%. Certain types of thyroid cancer, such as medullary thyroid carcinoma, may occur with familial incidence. The discovery of a goiter in a patient with a positive family history for this type of carcinoma is therefore significant for the diagnosis of a thyroid malignancy.

Clinical characteristics

A thyroid carcinoma should be suspected on clinical grounds if the nodule is single, hard on palpation, fixed to overlying tissue, and associated with satellite lymphadenopathy.

It is generally agreed that thyroid cancer can be subdivided clinically into a large group of well-differentiated neoplasms of slow growth and high curability and a smaller group of highly anaplastic tumors with a uniformly fatal outlook. There are four main types of thyroid cancer according to morphology and biologic behavior: (1) papillary, (2) follicular, (3) medullary, and (4) anaplastic.

Papillary carcinoma is the most common type of thyroid cancer and accounts for 80% of malignant thyroid tumors in children and in adults less than 40 years of age. It is approximately twice as common in females as in males. These neoplasms grow slowly and spread via lymphatics to regional nodes in approximately 50% of the cases. Treatment is surgical excision of the affected lobe with removal of regional lymph nodes if they are suspected of being involved.

Follicular carcinoma composes approximately 20% of all thyroid cancers. The gender and age distributions are similar to those of papillary cancer, although the incidence is somewhat higher later in life. In its most indolent form, the tumor closely resembles normal thyroid tissue, although at times it may be rapidly progressive, spreading rapidly to distant sites. These tumors not only resemble thyroid follicles histologically, but are also capable of taking up radioactive iodine. The mode of metastasis is via the bloodstream to distant sites, such as the lungs and bones. As with papillary tumors, the growth of this type of cancer is slow, with the disease evolving over many years. The treatment is total or nearly total thyroidectomy and removal of the involved lymph nodes. If metastases are present and capable of taking up radioactive iodine, ablation of the metastases with large doses of radioactive iodine can be carried out. After total thyroidectomy (by surgery or radioactive iodine), serum thyroglobulin should be undetectable. It is elevated in patients with metastatic disease, and a rise is indicative of recurring disease.

Medullary thyroid carcinoma is rather uncommon, comprising 5% to 10% of all cases. The cell of origin of this neoplasm is the parafollicular, or C, cell. Similar to its precursor cell, the tumor is capable of secreting calcitonin. Medullary thyroid carcinoma has been described in members of families with multiple endocrine neoplasia. Its progression and clinical course can frequently be followed by measurements of serum calcitonin levels. Although the tumor apparently grows slowly, it tends to metastasize to local lymph nodes at an early stage. Later, it spreads by the bloodstream to the lungs, liver, bones, and other organs. Because of the tendency for early metastases, these types of cancer are treated with total thyroidectomy.

Anaplastic carcinomas of the thyroid are histologically undifferentiated and extremely malignant and often prove fatal in weeks or months. They show evidence of early local invasion of structures surrounding the thyroid and of metastases, via both the lymphatics and the bloodstream. At present, this type of carcinoma is uniformly fatal regardless of the mode of treatment. Surgical resection should be attempted, followed by radiation therapy and chemotherapy.

Patients who have had resection of either papillary or follicular thyroid carcinomas should be followed for many years for evidence of recurrence or metastases. After thyroidectomy for papillary or follicular carcinoma, patients are placed on suppressive doses of levothyroxine. Periodically, patients are taken off thyroid replacement and stimulated with TSH. A large dose of radioactive iodine is administered, and the neck and the rest of the body are scanned for areas of radioactive uptake. If metastases are detected in this manner, large ablative doses of radioactive iodine can be administered.

Laboratory studies

Patients with a thyroid nodule suspected of being carcinomatous should be evaluated with a thyroid scan. The preferred scanning technique is the technetium-99m camera scan, which determines whether a nodule is solitary or part of a multinodular goiter. It can also determine whether the nodule is functioning. Solitary, nonfunctioning nodules have a 5% chance of being carcinomatous. Then an echographic study of the nodule can be performed. In this test, echoes produced by an ultrasonic beam directed into the thyroid nodule are analyzed to make an accurate differentiation between cystic and solid masses. Thyroid carcinomas are generally solid, and cystic masses usually represent benign cysts. In patients with a nonfunctioning solid nodule, a fine-needle aspiration biopsy of the nodule should be performed. If cytology shows or suggests papillary, medullary, or anaplastic carcinoma, the nodule should be surgically removed.

Euthyroid Sick Syndrome

Changes in thyroid function resembling hypothyroidism have been described in many hospitalized patients with severe systemic illness. In most of these patients the level of free thyroxine is normal, and these patients are not truly hypothyroid but have euthyroid sick syndrome. They have low levels of T_3 and increased levels of RT_3; occasionally, serum T_4 levels also decrease. TSH levels are usually normal or only slightly above normal. These findings are explained by changes in T_4 conversion to T_3 and decreased binding of T_4 to binding proteins. The biochemical change that leads to these changes in thyroid function is a decrease in $5'$ deiodination, which affects the conversion of T_4 to T_3 and the subsequent clearing of RT_3 to reverse T_2. A decrease in the total serum T_4 level is usually caused by a decrease in binding of T_4 to thyroxine-binding proteins. Patients with the most severe depression of serum thyroxine level have the least favorable prognosis.

QUESTIONS

▼ Circle the letter preceding each item below that correctly answers the question or completes the statement. More than one answer may be correct.

1. Which of the following are characteristics of triiodothyronine (T$_3$) as compared with thyroxine (T$_4$)?
   a. Has a lesser affinity for binding proteins, which results in a more potent effect on body tissues in regulating general metabolic rate
   b. Configuration consists of two molecules of diiodotyrosine
   c. Both a and b
   d. Neither a nor b

2. Which of the following levels of thyrotropin (TSH) indicate primary hypothyroidism (hypothyroidism of thyroidal origin)?
   a. Above-normal serum TSH levels
   b. Normal TSH levels
   c. Undetectable TSH levels

3. Parafollicular, or C, cells within the thyroid gland secrete:
   a. Thyroxine
   b. Triiodothyronine
   c. Calcitonin
   d. Renin

4. Which of the following are characteristic signs and symptoms of Graves' disease?
   a. Weight gain
   b. Diffuse hyperplasia of the thyroid gland
   c. Muscle fatigue
   d. Bradycardia

5. Mr. B., 40 years of age, was found to have Graves' disease. Which of the following treatment programs may be prescribed?
   a. Long-term administration of propylthiouracil
   b. Subtotal thyroidectomy following short-term administration of antithyroid drugs and ^{131}I treatment
   c. Total thyroidectomy
   d. Administration of 50 μg/day of thyroxine

6. A nurse in the newborn nursery observes a newborn baby boy who is very lethargic and has an umbilical hernia and dry skin. His respirations are noisy, and he has an abnormally hoarse cry. These signs suggest:
   a. Hyperthyroidism
   b. Cretinism

   c. Colloid goiter
   d. Euthyroidism

7. Which of the following signs and symptoms is characteristic of hypothyroidism?
   a. Weight loss
   b. Mental, physical slowness
   c. Cold intolerance
   d. Moist skin

8. Which of the following is characteristic of nontoxic goiters?
   a. Increase in TSH levels
   b. Hyperplasia and hypertrophy of the thyroid follicles
   c. Anti-TSH receptor IgG autoantibodies present in the serum

9. Which of the following is (are) not characteristic of a malignant thyroid nodule?
   a. It usually presents as a hot nodule.
   b. It usually appears as a single, firm, fixed nodule.
   c. It is functioning.
   d. Prognosis following early detection and treatment is excellent.

10. The most likely mechanism by which goitrogens inhibit thyroxine synthesis is to:
   a. Decrease thyroxine levels
   b. Increase release of TSH by the pituitary gland
   c. Convert monoiodotyrosine to diiodotyrosine
   d. Inhibit the initial oxidation of iodide

11. Ms. G., 40 years of age, was hospitalized with a diagnosis of acute monocytic leukemia. Her T$_3$ resin uptake test level was 100% of normal. She had low levels of T$_3$ and increased levels of reverse T$_3$. Serum T$_4$ levels were decreased. Her likely condition is:
   a. Hyperthyroidism
   b. Euthyroid sick syndrome
   c. Euthyroidism
   d. Graves' disease

12. The T$_3$ resin uptake test measures:
   a. Saturation of thyroxine-binding protein by thyroxine

   b. Radioactivity present over the thyroid
   c. Together with the total thyroxine level, the level of free thyroxine
   d. All the above

▼ Circle T if the statement is true and F if it is false. Correct any false statements.

13. T F The T$_3$ resin test measures the saturation of thyroxine-binding protein and indirectly the level of free thyroid hormone.

14. T F The most common form of hypothyroidism is caused by a lesion in the pituitary gland.

15. T F Hypothyroidism of all forms is best treated with thyroxine.

16. T F The process referred to as deiodination converts 80% of T$_4$ into 3,5,3'-T$_3$, and the remaining 20% is converted to RT$_3$.

17. T F Thyroid function is controlled by the hypothalamic glycoprotein hormone TSH and is regulated by thyrotropin-releasing hormone (TRH), a pituitary neurohormone.

18. T F Iodine is an essential element for the production of thyroxine.

▼ Answer the following on a separate sheet of paper.

19. Describe the location and function of the follicular epithelial cells in the thyroid gland.

20. List the steps and describe the process of biosynthesis of thyroid hormones.

21. List the tests that are presently used in the diagnosis of thyroid disease.

22. After a total thyroidectomy, what is the significance of elevated serum thyroglobulin in patients with metastatic disease?

23. Explain the radioactive (^{123}I) uptake test.

▼ Fill in the blanks with the appropriate word or number.

24. The thyroid takes up and concentrates _____ to _____ times the amount of iodide present in the plasma.

25. Solitary, nonfunctioning thyroid nodules have a _____ % chance of being carcinomatous.

26. Normal levels of thyroxine are _____ μg/dl; for triiodothyronine, _____ ng/dl.

27. Two types of spontaneous hyperthyroidism are _____ and _____.

CHAPTER 61

Adrenal Hypersecretion Disorders

DAVID E. SCHTEINGART

This chapter focuses on three selected adrenocortical clinical entities: Cushing's syndrome, aldosteronism, and androgen excess. In addition, pheochromocytoma, a rare catecholamine-secreting tumor of the adrenal medulla, is discussed. The first discussion concentrates on situations in which the plasma concentration of cortisol increases above normal physiologic levels and results in Cushing's syndrome. Causes of spontaneously abnormal elevations of plasma cortisol are considered. The second discussion focuses on another hormone of the adrenal cortex, aldosterone, and the condition known as aldosteronism. The third discussion deals with the pathophysiology and clinical manifestations of androgen excess. The chapter includes some aspects of the pharmacology of synthetic corticosteroids and the metabolic side effects that result from their chronic administration. Finally, the discussion of pheochromocytoma is important, since it is a cause of hypertension that is usually correctable if diagnosed and treated properly.

The adrenal cortex synthesizes and secretes four types of adrenocortical hormones: (1) glucocorticoids, (2) mineralocorticoids, (3) androgens, and (4) estrogens. The glucocorticoid hormone is cortisol; the mineralocorticoid hormone is aldosterone. There are other compounds, either naturally occurring or synthetic, with glucocorticoid or mineralocorticoid activity.

Cushing's syndrome results from the combined metabolic effects of persistently elevated blood levels of glucocorticoids. These high levels may occur spontaneously or as a result of the administration of pharmacologic doses of glucocorticoid compounds. To better understand the clinical manifestations of Cushing's syndrome, it is useful to begin with a review of the metabolic consequences of glucocorticoid excess.

METABOLIC EFFECTS OF GLUCOCORTICOIDS

Glucocorticoid excess causes alteration in the following:
1. Protein and carbohydrate metabolism
2. Distribution of adipose tissue
3. Electrolytes
4. The immune system
5. Gastric secretion
6. Brain function
7. Erythropoiesis

In addition, glucocorticoid excess also suppresses inflammation.

Glucocorticoids have catabolic and antianabolic effects on protein, causing a decrease in the ability of protein-forming cells to synthesize protein. As a consequence, there is loss of protein from tissues such as skin,

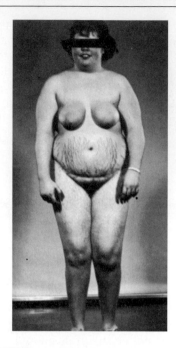

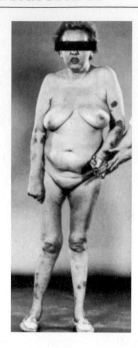

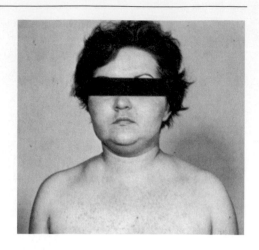

FIG. 61-3 Typical cushingoid facies with roundness of the face, double chin, prominent upper lip, and fullness of the supraclavicular fossae.

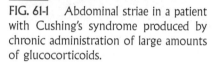

FIG. 61-1 Abdominal striae in a patient with Cushing's syndrome produced by chronic administration of large amounts of glucocorticoids.

FIG. 61-2 Marked protein catabolism in a patient with Cushing's syndrome. Muscles are markedly atrophic, and multiple ecchymoses are seen on the upper and lower extremities.

muscles, blood vessels, and bone. Clinically, the skin atrophies and breaks down easily; wounds heal slowly. Rupture of elastic fibers in the skin causes purple stretch marks, or *striae* (Fig. 61-1). Muscles also atrophy and become weak. Thinning of blood vessel walls and weakening of perivascular supporting tissue result in easy bruising (Fig. 61-2). This condition can be severe enough for petechiae or even large areas of ecchymosis to appear under the cuff when the patient's blood pressure is taken. Bone is also affected. The protein matrix of bone becomes weak, causing a condition known as *osteoporosis*. This may be a serious complication of glucocorticoid excess, since it causes the bone to become brittle and develop pathologic fractures. Osteoporosis occurs most frequently in the spine, causing vertebral collapse and resultant back pain and loss of height.

Carbohydate metabolism is also affected by abnormally high levels of glucocorticoids. Glucocorticoids stimulate gluconeogenesis and interfere with the action of insulin in peripheral cells. As a consequence, patients may develop hyperglycemia. In a person with an adequate insulin-secreting capacity, the effect of glucocorticoids is countered by increasing insulin secretion and subsequently normalizing glucose tolerance. In contrast, patients with diminished insulin-secreting capacity are unable to compensate, and they develop abnormal responses to glucose tolerance tests, fasting hyperglycemia, and clinical manifestations of diabetes mellitus.

Excessive glucocorticoid levels also affect the distrib-

ution of adipose tissue, which accumulates in the central areas of the body, causing development of truncal obesity, round face (moon face), supraclavicular fossa fullness, and cervicodorsal hump (buffalo hump) (Fig. 61-3). The truncal obesity and thinning of the upper and lower extremities as a result of muscle atrophy give patients the classic cushingoid appearance (Fig. 61-4).

Glucocorticoids have minimal effects on serum electrolyte levels. However, when given or produced in large concentrations, they may cause sodium retention and potassium waste, leading to edema, hypokalemia, and metabolic alkalosis.

Glucocorticoids can inhibit the immune response. Immune responses are of two major types: one results in production of humoral antibodies by plasma cells and B lymphocytes following antigenic stimulation; the other depends on sensitized T lymphocyte–mediated reactions. Glucocorticoids impair humoral antibody production and inhibit proliferation of germinal centers of spleen and lymphoid tissue in the primary response to antigen. Impairment of the immunologic response can occur at each of the stages of this response: (1) initial processing of antigens by cells of the monocyte-macrophage system, (2) induction and proliferation of immunocompetent lymphocytes and release of cytokines, (3) antibody production, and (4) the inflammatory reaction. Glucocorticoids also suppress delayed hypersensitivity reactions. For example, they may convert the skin test for tuberculosis from positive to negative. In addition, the glucocorticoid-mediated

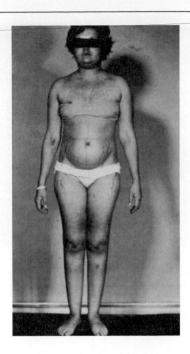

FIG. 61-4 Patient with Cushing's syndrome with acne over the chest, striae over the abdomen and upper thighs, and relatively thin upper and lower extremities. She also has pretibial edema.

inhibition of cellular immunity is probably important in suppressing transplant rejection.

Gastric secretory activity is increased by glucocorticoids. Hydrochloric acid and pepsin secretion may be increased in certain individuals taking glucocorticoids. It has also been suggested that mucosal protective factors are altered by steroids and that this may contribute to ulcer formation.

Psychologic changes are commonly seen with glucocorticoid excess. They are characterized by emotional lability, euphoria, insomnia, and episodes of transient depression. The neuropsychiatric manifestations of glucocorticoid excess occur in patients with spontaneous Cushing's syndrome and in those receiving pharmacologic doses of glucocorticoids. These changes are reversed when the patient's cortisol levels return to normal.

Glucocorticoids cause involution of lymphoid tissue, stimulation of neutrophil release, and enhancement of erythropoiesis.

The most important and clinically useful pharmacologic effect of glucocorticoids is their ability to suppress the inflammatory response. In this regard, glucocorticoids can inhibit hyperemia, extravasation of cells, cellular migration, and capillary permeability. They also inhibit the release of vasoactive kinins and suppress phagocytosis. By their effects on mast cells, glucocorticoids inhibit histamine synthesis and suppress the acute anaphylactic reaction based on antibody-mediated hypersensitivity. The antiinflammatory properties of glucocorticoids have placed them in the forefront of therapeutic agents available for the treatment of a variety of disor-

ders, such as collagen vascular diseases, in which suppression of inflammation is desirable. However, there are clinical conditions in which the immune suppression and antiinflammatory effect of glucocorticoids may be a disadvantage. With acute infection, the body may be unable to defend itself appropriately while receiving pharmacologic dosages of glucocorticoids.

Suppression of the Hypothalamic-Pituitary-Adrenal Axis

The administration of glucocorticoids in dosages that surpass physiologic concentrations can significantly suppress the ability of the hypothalamic-pituitary axis to release adrenocorticotropic (ACTH). Therefore the administration of corticoids on a long-term basis may result in adrenal insufficiency (1) when steroids are withdrawn and (2) in response to stress.

CUSHING'S SYNDROME

Cushing's syndrome may result from long-term administration of pharmacologic dosages of glucocorticoids (iatrogenic) or from excessive cortisol secretion caused by a disturbance in the hypothalamic-pituitary-adrenal axis (spontaneous).

Iatrogenic Cushing's syndrome is seen in patients with conditions such as rheumatoid arthritis, asthma, lymphoma, and generalized skin disorders who receive synthetic glucocorticoids as antiinflammatory agents. In *spontaneous Cushing's syndrome,* adrenocortical hyperfunction develops either as a result of excessive stimulation by ACTH or as a consequence of adrenal pathology leading to abnormal production of cortisol.

Cushing's syndrome can be divided into two types: (1) ACTH dependent and (2) ACTH independent (Fig. 61-5). Among the ACTH-dependent types, adrenocortical hyperfunction may result from abnormal and excessive secretion of ACTH by the pituitary gland. Because this is the type originally described by Harvey Cushing in 1932, it is also designated as Cushing's disease. Eighty percent of these patients have an ACTH-secreting pituitary adenoma. The remaining 20% have histologic evidence of pituitary corticotrope hyperplasia. It is not clear if either the microadenoma or the hyperplasia arises from a disturbed release of corticotropin-releasing hormone (CRH) by the neurohypothalamus. In either case there is excessive secretion of ACTH, loss of normal circadian rhythm of ACTH, and diminished sensitivity of the feedback control system to levels of circulating cortisol. ACTH may be secreted excessively in patients who have neoplasms with the capacity to synthesize and release peptides resembling ACTH both chemically and physiologically. The excessive amount of ACTH produced under these circumstances leads to excessive stimulation of cor-

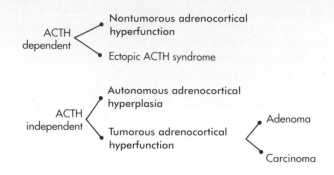

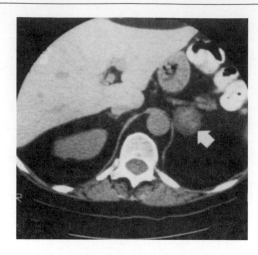

FIG. 61-5   Classification of Cushing's syndrome. *ACTH,* Adreno-corticotropic hormone.

FIG. 61-7   Computed tomography (CT) scan of the upper abdomen, demonstrating a left adrenal mass in a patient with Cushing's syndrome secondary to an adrenocortical adenoma.

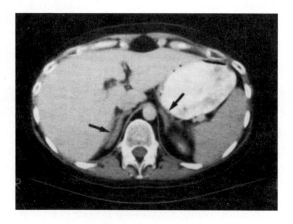

FIG. 61-6   Computed tomography (CT) scan of the upper abdomen, demonstrating bilateral adrenal enlargement in a patient with ACTH-dependent Cushing's syndrome.

tisol secretion by the adrenal cortex and, secondarily, to suppression of pituitary ACTH release. Thus the high ACTH levels in such a patient come from the neoplasm and not from the patient's own pituitary gland. A large number of neoplasms can cause the ectopic secretion of ACTH. These neoplasms are usually derived from tissues originating in the neuroectodermal layer during embryonic development. Oat cell carcinoma of the lung, bronchial carcinoids, thymomas, and islet cell tumors of the pancreas are among the most common. Some of these tumors are capable of ectopic CRH secretion. In that instance, ectopic CRH stimulates pituitary ACTH secretion, which causes excessive cortisol secretion by the adrenal cortex.

Adrenocortical hyperfunction can occur independently of ACTH control, such as when a tumor or bilateral, nodular adrenocortical hyperplasia with a capacity to secrete cortisol in an autonomous fashion develops in the adrenal cortex. Adrenocortical tumors leading to Cushing's syndrome may be benign (adenomas) (Fig. 61-6) or malignant (carcinomas) (Fig. 61-7).

The presence of Cushing's syndrome can be determined on the basis of the medical history and the physical findings already described. The diagnosis is usually confirmed by the measurement of abnormally high levels of cortisol in plasma and urine. Specific tests can determine the presence or absence of a normal circadian rhythm of cortisol release and a sensitive feedback control mechanism. Absence of circadian rhythm and diminished or absent sensitivity of the feedback control system are characteristics of Cushing's syndrome.

The types of Cushing's syndrome associated with excessive ACTH secretion—pituitary or ectopic—are frequently associated with hyperpigmentation. This hyperpigmentation is caused by the secretion of peptides related to ACTH and by breakdown fragments of ACTH that have melanotropic activity. The pigmentation is recognized in both skin and mucous membranes.

Adrenocortical adenomas may lead to severe Cushing's syndrome, but they usually develop slowly, and symptoms may be present for several years before the diagnosis is finally made (see Fig. 61-6). In contrast, adrenocortical carcinomas develop rapidly and may lead to metastasis and early death (see Fig. 61-7).

Several diagnostic procedures can be used to establish the nature of the underlying pathology in Cushing's syndrome and to localize a lesion amenable to surgical management.

Physiologic testing can help distinguish pituitary from ectopic or primary adrenocortical forms of Cushing's syndrome. In the ectopic and adrenocortical forms of Cushing's syndrome, the abnormal secretion of ACTH and/or cortisol is not likely to be altered by stimulating or suppressive maneuvers that test the presence or absence of a normal negative feedback control mechanism. For example, the administration of metyrapone, a drug

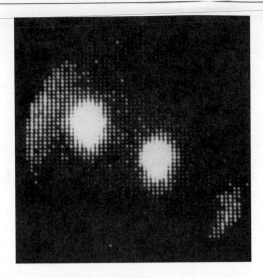

FIG. 61-8   [131]I 6-beta-iodomethyl-19-norcholesterol nuclear scan of the adrenal glands in a patient with ACTH-dependent Cushing's syndrome. There is bilateral increased uptake of radioactivity consistent with adrenocortical hyperfunction.

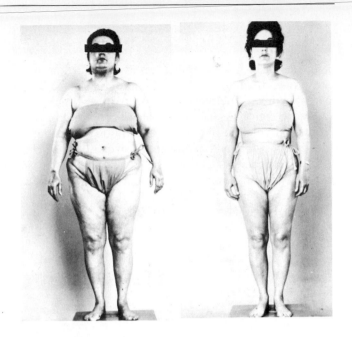

FIG. 61-9   Response to treatment of Cushing's syndrome with milotane, an adrenal inhibitor.

that blocks 11-beta-hydroxylation at the adrenocortical level and thus causes a decrease in plasma cortisol, is unable to stimulate ACTH release in patients with ectopic ACTH syndrome; in contrast, patients with pituitary ACTH-dependent Cushing's syndrome usually respond with an increase in ACTH release. Patients with either ectopic ACTH syndrome or primary adrenocortical disease do not suppress ACTH and/or cortisol levels with high doses of dexamethasone and do not stimulate these levels with the administration of ovine CRH; these features are characteristic of most patients with pituitary ACTH-dependent Cushing's syndrome.

Identification of the nature and localization of the lesion responsible for Cushing's syndrome is based on the radiographic visualization of pituitary and adrenal lesions and on nuclear scanning of the adrenal glands.

High-resolution computed tomography (CT) scanning of the pituitary gland can demonstrate areas of decreased density or enhancement consistent with a microadenoma in about 30% of these patients. Magnetic resonance imaging (MRI) with gadolinium contrast gives a positive finding in the majority of these patients. CT scanning of the adrenal glands usually shows adrenal enlargement in patients with ACTH-dependent Cushing's syndrome and adrenal masses in patients with adrenal adenoma or carcinoma.

Nuclear scanning of the adrenal glands involves the intravenous administration of radioactive cholesterol. Cholesterol labeled with ^{131}I is taken up and concentrated by the adrenal cortex. Images of the adrenal glands can be obtained by scanning techniques within 3 to 7 days after injection of the tracer (Fig. 61-8). Patterns suggestive of normal adrenal glands, adrenal hyperplasia, or adrenal adenoma or carcinoma can be obtained with adrenal photoscanning.

Treatment

Treatment of ACTH-dependent Cushing's syndrome differs, depending on whether the source of ACTH is pituitary or ectopic. Several approaches to therapy can be used in patients with pituitary hypersecretion of ACTH. If a pituitary tumor is recognized, a transsphenoidal resection of the tumor should be attempted. If there is evidence of pituitary hyperfunction but a tumor is not clearly detected, cobalt irradiation of the pituitary gland can be used instead. This treatment modality is particularly effective in young people with Cushing's syndrome. Cortisol excess can also be controlled by a total adrenalectomy and subsequent administration of physiologic dosage of cortisol or by chemical agents capable of blocking or destroying cortisol-secreting adrenocortical cells. When the treatment of Cushing's syndrome is successful, remission of the clinical manifestations occurs 6 to 12 months after institution of therapy (Fig. 61-9).

When adrenal neoplasms are the cause of cortisol excess, removal of the neoplasms followed by chemotherapy in patients with carcinoma is the preferred mode of treatment.

Treatment of ectopic ACTH syndrome is based on (1) resection of the neoplasm secreting ACTH or (2) adrenalectomy or chemical suppression of adrenal function, as prescribed for the patients with the pituitary ACTH-dependent type of Cushing's syndrome.

ALDOSTERONISM

Aldosteronism results from excessive production of aldosterone, the mineralocorticoid steroid hormone of the adrenal cortex. The metabolic effects of aldosterone relate to electrolyte and fluid balance. Aldosterone enhances proximal renal tubule reabsorption of sodium and causes potassium and hydrogen ion excretion. The clinical consequences of aldosterone excess are sodium and water retention, expansion of the extracellular fluid volume, and hypertension. In addition, hypernatremia, hypokalemia, and metabolic alkalosis occur.

There are two types of aldosteronism: (1) primary and (2) secondary. In *primary aldosteronism* the excessive production of aldosterone occurs as a result of a tumor (Fig. 61-10) or hyperplasia of the adrenal cortex. Most aldosterone-secreting tumors are benign and small—0.5 to 2 cm. Primary aldosteronism is a form of endocrine hypertension and probably affects 1% to 2% of patients with hypertension. Recognition of this condition can enable the cure of hypertension.

Secondary aldosteronism occurs in conditions in which afferent arteriolar pressure in the renal glomerulus decreases, leading to stimulation of the renin-angiotensin system. Angiotensin stimulates aldosterone production. Secondary aldosteronism is seen in congestive heart failure, cirrhosis of the liver, and nephrotic syndrome, conditions in which edema is a prominent clinical feature. Congestive heart failure exemplifies the way secondary aldosteronism may develop. Patients in congestive heart failure cannot pump blood normally and develop a fall in cardiac output. Perfusion pressure to the afferent arteriole of the renal glomerulus decreases. The fall in pressure is sensed by stretch receptors in the juxtaglomerular apparatus, and renin is secreted in increased amounts. Renin activates angiotensin production, which in turn stimulates aldosterone secretion by an otherwise normal adrenal

cortex. The increased production of aldosterone will, in turn, promote sodium and water reabsorption, expansion of the extracellular fluid compartment, and possibly an increase in afferent arteriolar pressure.

Secondary aldosteronism can also develop in conditions in which a partial occlusion of the renal artery occurs, leading to renal vascular hypertension.

The diagnosis of aldosteronism is based on the measurement of increased levels of aldosterone in plasma and urine and measurements of plasma renin. Plasma renin is low in primary aldosteronism and high in secondary aldosteronism.

CT scanning and nuclear photoscanning can also help detect and localize an adrenal lesion in patients with primary aldosteronism. In addition, samples of adrenal venous blood may be obtained by selective catheterization of the right and left adrenal veins. A significantly higher concentration of aldosterone on the side suspected of harboring a tumor helps confirm the presence of the lesion.

Treatment of primary aldosteronism includes partial adrenalectomy, with resection of an aldosterone-secreting adenoma. Patients with adrenal hyperplasia are treated by the administration of aldosterone antagonists such as spironolactone.

PHARMACOLOGY AND USE OF SYNTHETIC CORTICOSTEROIDS

Synthetic analogs of cortisol with glucocorticoid and antiinflammatory activity are frequently used either topically or systemically to treat many medical conditions. For example, steroids are used topically to treat skin disorders and systemically to treat conditions such as rheumatoid arthritis, asthma, and acute allergic reactions. Although therapeutically effective, steroids also have side effects. These side effects are related to the metabolic activity and action on various organ systems, as described earlier.

Altering the basic chemical structure of cortisol, the naturally occurring glucocorticoid, makes it possible to alter the pharmacologic characteristics of this compound (Fig. 61-11). For example, if a double bond is introduced between carbons 1 and 2 in the cortisol molecule, prednisolone is produced, which has, on a milligram-per-milligram basis, less sodium-retaining and more antiinflammatory activity than the parent compound, cortisol. That is, 1 mg prednisolone is a much more potent antiinflammatory and immunosuppressive agent than 1 mg cortisol. Another possible structural alteration is the introduction of a fluorine atom in an alpha position on carbon 9 of the steroid nucleus. The resulting compound, 9alpha-fluorocortisol, has strong sodium-retaining properties similar to aldosterone, a naturally occurring mineralocorticoid. By this substitution, a compound with pre-

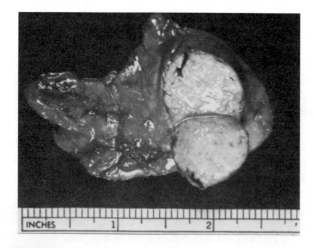

FIG. 61-10   Aldosterone-secreting adrenocortical adenoma.

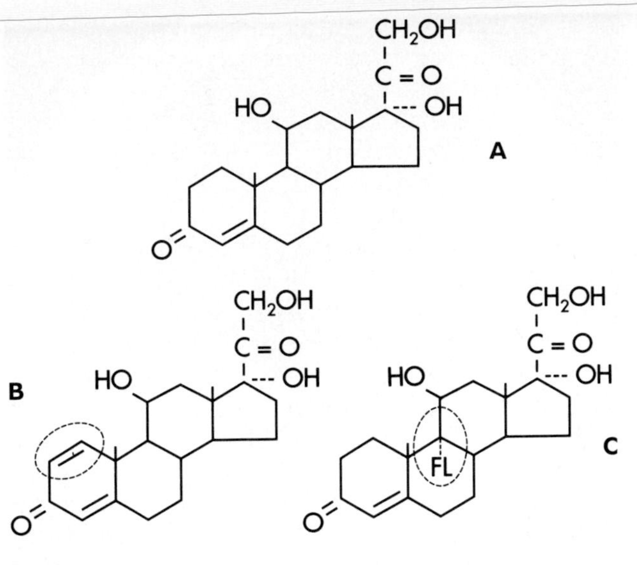

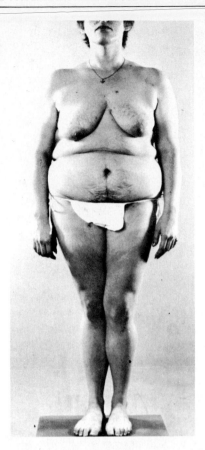

FIG. 61-11   Changes in the basic chemical structure of cortisol, leading to compounds with different pharmacologic characteristics from the parent compound. **A,** Cortisol. **B,** Prednisolone. **C,** 9 Alpha-fluorocortisol.

dominantly glucocorticoid activity becomes a mineralocorticoid.

Dozens of synthetic compounds have been created in the manner just described. In most cases the objective has been the development of steroid compounds with strong antiinflammatory activity and minimal adverse metabolic effects. Although this objective has been reached to some extent, therapy with any of the currently available synthetic corticosteroid preparations, if given long enough and in sufficiently high doses, results in Cushing's syndrome and persistent suppression of endogenous hypothalamic-pituitary-adrenal function. In many instances, steroids are the only effective treatment for serious systemic diseases. Under those circumstances the development of Cushing's syndrome may be a necessary trade-off in the control of a serious and crippling disease. The adverse effects of corticosteroid therapy can be minimized by administering a double dose of the drug on an alternate-day schedule instead of giving it daily and in divided doses. For example, if a patient needs prednisolone, 20 mg daily, instead of taking it in doses of 5 mg every 6 hours, the patient receives a 40 mg dose every other morning.

SYNDROMES OF ANDROGEN EXCESS

One of the most common problems seen by the endocrinologist among young women is hirsutism. It is the simplest and earliest clinical expression of androgen excess.

It is well documented that a complex relationship exists between the growth of hair in men and women and sex hormones. For example, the growth of beard; hair in the ears, nasal tip, and upper pubic triangle; and coarse hair over the trunk and limbs depend on adult male levels of circulating androgens. The growth of hair at the axilla, lower pubic region, and, in part at least, the limbs is initiated by pubertal events in both sexes and is mediated by weaker adrenal androgens. Androgen-type hair is coarse and dark. Certain hair growth appears to be independent of sex hormones. This hair is fine and light in color and includes lanugal hair, eyebrows, and eyelashes.

Hirsutism is defined as excessive growth of body hair in the female in a characteristic masculine distribution over the facial, periareolar, abdominal, and sacral areas (Fig. 61-12). It may be associated with baldness (Fig. 61-13) or temporal recession of the hairline (Fig. 61-14). It may be present by itself or be part of a virilizing syndrome, which is the clinical picture observed in girls and women of all ages with signs and symptoms of defeminization and masculinization. The characteristic findings in defeminization include amenorrhea, decrease in libido, atrophy of the breasts, and loss of feminine body contour. Masculization includes hirsutism, seborrhea, acne, deepening of the voice, increased muscular development, and enlargement of the clitoris (Fig. 61-15).

FIG. 61-12   Hirsutism in the female. Excess of body hair over the breasts, abdomen, and extremities.

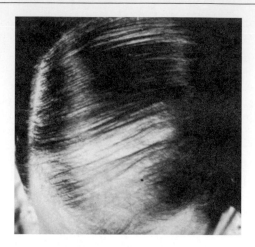

FIG. 61-13   Baldness in a woman with androgen excess.

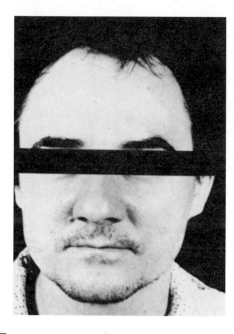

FIG. 61-14   Recession of the hairline in a woman with androgen excess. Note the excessive facial hair growth over the upper lip, chin, and sideburn areas.

True virilism is currently recognized as a rare condition, almost always associated with adrenal or ovarian tumors or with the syndrome of congenital adrenal hyperplasia. In contrast, hirsutism, often without any other signs of virilism but frequently accompanied by irregular or absent menstrual periods and acne, is a common clinical entity. Although it is often thought that simple hirsutism is a mild form of virilism because it has a similar cause, no specific hormonal abnormality or etiologic mechanism has been found as the sole cause of these types of hirsutism. Ethnic and genetic factors play important roles in the development of hair growth patterns. However, there is evidence that androgen excess is present in most cases of hirsutism.

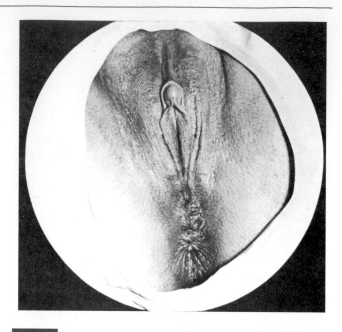

FIG. 61-15   Clitoral enlargement in a woman with androgen excess.

Androgen Physiology

Various androgens are normally secreted by both men and women. The three major types are (1) dehydroepiandrosterone, (2) delta 4-androstenedione, and (3) testosterone (Fig. 61-16).

Dehydroepiandrosterone (DHEA) and its metabolites, DHEA sulfate and androstenediol, are generally considered to be weak androgens. The adrenal gland is the main source of this type of androgen, although the ovary also contributes to the level of androstenediol. These androgens can be measured in the urine as 17-ketosteroids, of which DHEA makes up 60% of the total.

Delta 4-androstenedione is a stronger androgen product than DHEA but weaker than testosterone, of which it is a precursor. As with DHEA, delta 4-androstenedione is also produced by the adrenal cortex and the ovary.

Testosterone is the most potent of the three androgen compounds. There are several sources of testosterone, including the adrenal cortex, the ovary, the testes, and peripheral tissues. Testosterone is metabolized to a potent androgen, dihydrotestosterone (DHT); finally, both testosterone and DHT may be converted to androstenediol in peripheral tissues and excreted as such in the urine.

Testosterone can be produced in several endocrine and peripheral tissues from precursors. It circulates in the plasma partially bound to a carrier protein (sex hormone–binding globulin [SHBG]), and it is removed through metabolic degradation in the liver and other peripheral tissues (Fig. 61-17). Testosterone levels are therefore a balance between production and metabolic clearance. Although a large portion of circulating androgens is bound to SHBG, a small fraction is present in a free state. The biologic effects of circulating androgens are related to the levels of free androgens in plasma. Women with hirsutism usually have abnormalities in testosterone secretion and metabolism. For example, in normal women, testosterone is extracted and metabolized almost completely by the liver; in contrast, in virilized women, 32% of secreted testosterone is extracted and metabolized by extrahepatic peripheral tissues. These tissues are then subject to greater androgenic activity than that found in normal women. Similarly, hirsute women have less testosterone binding, higher free testosterone levels, and more active metabolic clearance tests than women without hirsutism.

Differential Diagnosis of Androgen Excess

Four major categories of conditions are associated with androgen excess: (1) adrenocortical, (2) ovarian, (3) simple or idiopathic hirsutism, and (4) miscellaneous states (see box on p. 946).

Among the adrenocortical states associated with androgen excess is Cushing's syndrome. In Cushing's syndrome, manifestations of androgen excess are superimposed on signs and symptoms of cortisol excess. Clinically, patients demonstrate coarse, dark hair growth; balding; deepening of the voice; and occasional clitoral enlargement. Biochemically, they demonstrate high levels of urinary 17-ketosteroids, DHEA, and androstenediol. Androgen excess is found most often among the ACTH-dependent type of Cushing's syndrome and in patients with adrenal carcinoma.

Some adrenocortical disorders are associated with androgen excess only, and the secretion of cortisol remains normal. Prenatally, such a disorder is found in patients with *congenital adrenal hyperplasia*. In this condition there is an inborn defect in one of the enzymes involved in cortisol biosynthesis. The most common type is a defect in 21-hydroxylase (Fig. 61-18). As a consequence of 21-hydroxylase deficiency, the adrenal cortex has an impaired capacity to secrete cortisol. The decrease in cortisol production causes an increase in ACTH secretion in

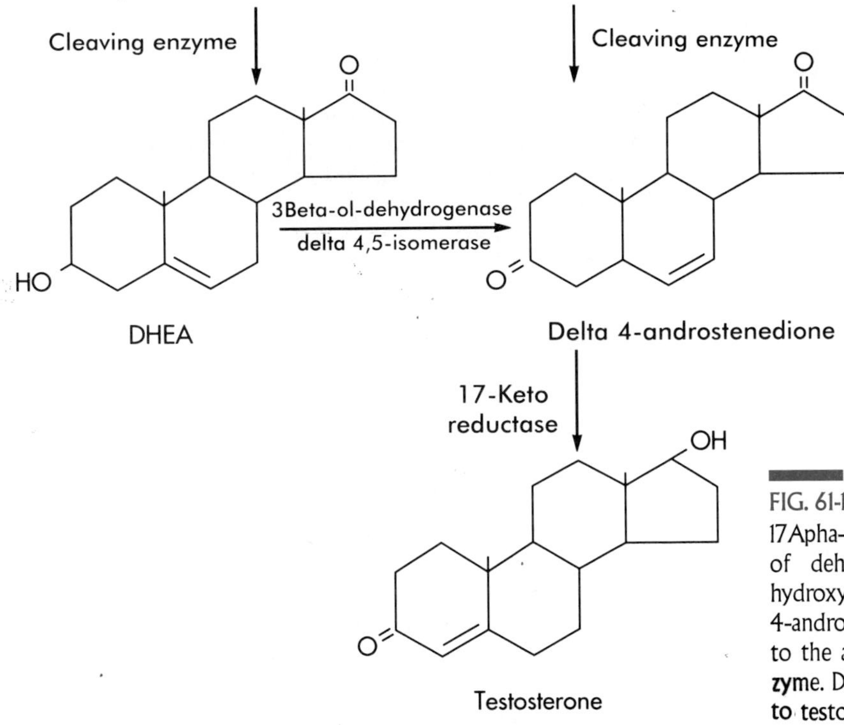

FIG. 61-16   Three major types of androgens in the female. 17Apha-hydroxypregnenolone is the immediate precursor of dehydroepiandrosterone (DHEA), whereas 17alpha-hydroxyprogesterone is the immediate precursor of delta 4-androstenedione. The transformation of the precursor to the androgen hormones is catalyzed by a cleaving enzyme. Delta 4-androstenedione can, in turn, be converted to testosterone by a step catalyzed by 17-ketoreductase.

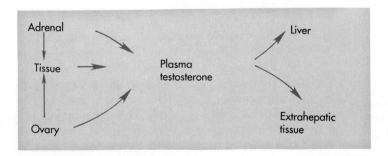

FIG. 61-17   Metabolism of plasma testosterone. The plasma level of testosterone results from a balance between the production of testosterone by adrenal, ovarian, and peripheral tissues and clearance by the liver and extrahepatic tissues.

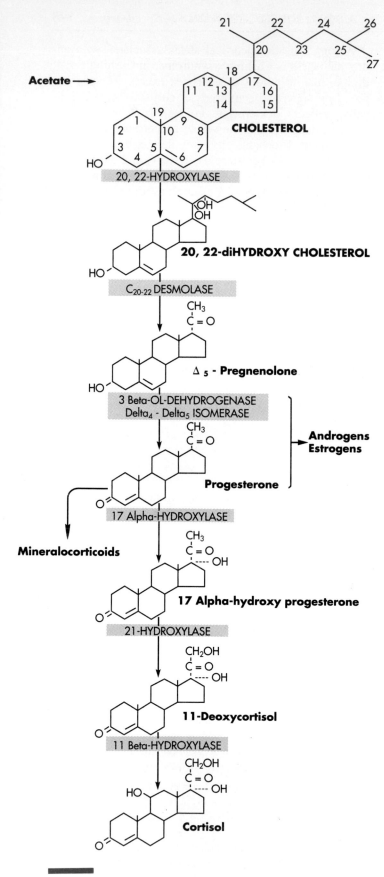

21 22 24 26
20 23 25 27

Acetate ⟶

CHOLESTEROL

20, 22-HYDROXYLASE

20, 22-diHYDROXY CHOLESTEROL

C$_{20-22}$ DESMOLASE

Δ$_5$ - Pregnenolone

3 Beta-OL-DEHYDROGENASE
Delta$_4$ - Delta$_5$ ISOMERASE

Progesterone

Androgens
Estrogens

17 Alpha-HYDROXYLASE

Mineralocorticoids

17 Alpha-hydroxy progesterone

21-HYDROXYLASE

11-Deoxycortisol

11 Beta-HYDROXYLASE

Cortisol

FIG. 61-18   Pathway of cortisol biosynthesis. Pregnenolone and progesterone are precursors of androgens and estrogens. Progesterone is also a precursor of mineralocorticoids. The biosynthesis of cortisol takes place in the adrenal cortex. Each step is controlled by specific enzymes. A defect in 21-hydroxylase is the cause of the most common type of congenital adrenal hyperplasia.

ANDROGEN EXCESS: DIFFERENTIAL DIAGNOSIS

I. Androgen excess of adrenocortical origin
  A. Cortisol excess: Cushing's syndrome
  B. Androgen excess only
    1. Prenatal: congenital adrenal hyperplasia (CAH)
    2. Postnatal: prepubertal
      a. Late manifestations of CAH
      b. Carcinoma
    3. Pubertal or postpubertal
      a. Hyperplasia, with or without polycystic ovaries
      b. Carcinoma
II. Androgen excess of ovarian origin
  A. Neoplasms: arrhenoblastoma, adrenal rest cell neoplasms, hilus cell neoplasms, luteoma
  B. Hilus cell or Leydig cell hyperplasia
  C. Polycystic ovary syndrome
III. Simple or idiopathic hirsutism
IV. Miscellaneous causes
  A. Endocrine
    1. Acromegaly
    2. Pregnancy
    3. Hypothyroidism
    4. Menopause
    5. Androgen therapy
    6. Inanition
  B. Nonendocrine
    1. Immobilization
    2. Body cast
    3. Porphyria
    4. Congenital ectodermal dysplasia

response to the negative feedback activation of pituitary function. ACTH stimulates the adrenal cortex, causing the precursors of cortisol biosynthesis to be shunted to the biosynthesis of androgens (Fig. 61-19). When the fetus is exposed to increased amounts of androgen, it undergoes changes in the development of the external genitalia. For example, a female fetus with this defect develops an enlargement of the clitoris and fusion of the labia majora. The genitalia then resemble male external genitalia. At the time of birth, this ambiguity in sexual development may create difficulties in sexual identification of the newborn. The syndrome of a masculinized genetically female fetus caused by androgen excess in utero is called *female pseudohermaphroditism* (Fig. 61-20).

Manifestations of androgen excess of adrenal origin can also develop postnatally and before puberty. Such a condition may be a late manifestation of congenital adrenal hyperplasia, as just described, or it may be caused by an androgen-secreting adrenal carcinoma. Finally, the clinical picture of androgen excess may develop at puberty or after puberty. About 4% to 12% of women with this condition may have a mild form of con-

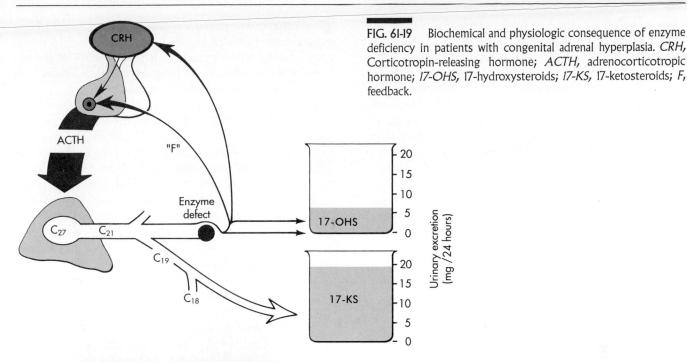

FIG. 61-19   Biochemical and physiologic consequence of enzyme deficiency in patients with congenital adrenal hyperplasia. *CRH*, Corticotropin-releasing hormone; *ACTH*, adrenocorticotropic hormone; *17-OHS*, 17-hydroxysteroids; *17-KS*, 17-ketosteroids; *F*, feedback.

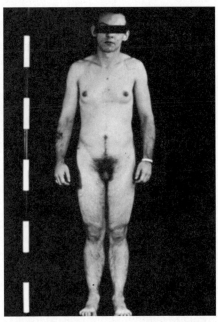

FIG. 61-20   Female pseudohermaphroditism in a patient with congenital adrenal hyperplasia caused by 21-hydroxylase deficiency. This patient had a male phenotype but was genetically a female. Note the masculine muscle development and body hair growth pattern. On casual examination the patient appeared to have a developed penis. On closer examination, however, this penis was seen to be an enlarged clitoris. The patient also had developed gynecomastia as a result of increased estrogen production accompanying the androgen excess.

genital adrenal hyperplasia (nonclassic form), with partial defects in 21-hydroxylase, 11-beta-hydroxylase, or 3-beta-ol-dehydrogenase delta 4,5-isomerase. In other patients the androgen excess may be part of the syndrome of polycystic ovaries or may be secondary to an adrenal carcinoma.

Several ovarian conditions can cause androgen excess. Tumors of the ovary, such as arrhenoblastomas and hilus cell neoplasms, are capable of secreting large amounts of testosterone. Other types of androgens are seen in patients with these tumors, depending on the cell type involved. Manifestations of androgen excess can also be seen in patients with Leydig cell hyperplasia. These patients usually have high plasma testosterone levels. Occasionally, masculinization in association with Leydig cell hyperplasia and Leydig cell tumors is seen in patients with gonadal dysgenesis, which is a sex chromosome abnormality leading to abnormal development of the ovaries.

In *polycystic ovary syndrome*, hirsutism is frequently associated with infertility, amenorrhea, obesity, and enlarged ovaries. In these patients, testosterone production rates are clearly increased and are responsible for the manifestations of androgen excess. The increased production of androgens in the polycystic ovary syndrome may be secondary to the hyperinsulinemia that develops in association with obesity or may result from abnormalities in the cyclic release of gonadotropins. Patients with polycystic ovary syndrome often have sustained elevations of serum luteinizing hormone. These changes in gonadotropin secretion may lead to anatomic changes in the ovary and stimulation of ovarian androgen production.

Many women have hirsutism without any other clinical manifestations of androgen excess. The problem usually begins after puberty and progresses slowly over years. Patients may or may not have menstrual irregularities and may or may not have polycystic ovaries. The urinary 17-ketosteroid level is frequently slightly or moderately elevated, and the testosterone production rate is increased. The free testosterone level is also elevated. The specific biochemical defect and the pathophysiology of this type of androgen excess are not well understood.

There are a number of miscellaneous causes of hirsutism. Some of them are of endocrine origin and include the hirsutism associated with acromegaly, pregnancy, hypothyroidism, menopause, androgen therapy, and inanition. Increased hair growth may occur without hormonal stimulation. It is seen in disorders such as porphyria and congenital ectodermal dysplasia or in areas of the body that have been either immobilized or placed in a body cast.

Clinical and Laboratory Evaluation of Hirsute Women

If a patient presents with complaints of excessive hair growth, it is necessary to determine whether the hirsutism is present by itself or accompanied by manifestations of virilization, as described earlier. It is also important to determine whether the symptoms are those of androgen excess alone or are accompanied by symptoms of cortisol excess. A history of recent onset and rapid progression of excessive hair growth frequently suggests a malignancy as the source of excessive androgen production. In that case, one should suspect either an adrenal or ovarian tumor and perform such procedures as a pelvic examination, laparoscopy, adrenal venography, and adrenal photoscanning to confirm or rule out this diagnosis. In patients with simple idiopathic hirsutism, measurements of androgens in the urine and plasma help confirm the presence of excessive androgen production.

Treatment

The treatment of androgen excess relates to the underlying pathology. If androgen excess is part of Cushing's syndrome, correction of Cushing's syndrome in the manner previously described will result in remission of the manifestations of androgen excess. Congenital adrenal hyperplasia can be effectively suppressed by chronic suppressive therapy with glucocorticoid analogs. Patients with adrenal or ovarian tumors should undergo resection of these tumors. Patients with simple or idiopathic hirsutism can be treated by androgen suppression with (1) oral contraceptives, (2) synthetic corticosteroids, (3) spironolactone, or (4) antiandrogens.

PHEOCHROMOCYTOMA

Pheochromocytoma, a rare cause of secondary hypertension, is an adrenal medullary or sympathetic chain (para-

ganglioma) tumor that releases excessive amounts of catecholamines (epinephrine and norepinephrine) in a sustained or intermittent manner. It affects 0.1% of the hypertensive population and may have a fatal outcome if undiagnosed or untreated. It occurs equally in men and women and has a peak incidence between ages 30 and 50. About 90% of these tumors are derived from adrenal medullary chromaffin cells, and 10% are extraadrenal, located in the retroperitoneal area (organs of Zuckerkandl), celiac and mesenteric ganglia, and urinary bladder. In patients with multiple endocrine neoplasia (MEN) II, an increased secretion of catecholamines with the clinical manifestations of a pheochromocytoma may result from bilateral adrenal medullary hyperplasia. Pheochromocytomas are usually benign (95% of cases), but they may be malignant and present with distant metastases.

The clinical manifestations of these tumors are related to the release of catecholamines. The most prominent feature is hypertension that may be paroxysmal (45% of cases) or sustained. Patients with paroxysmal symptoms develop acute episodes of severe hypertension (250/140 mm Hg) lasting minutes to hours. The episodes may be triggered by exercise, ingestion of tyrosine-containing foods (red wine, aged cheese, yogurt), caffeine-containing foods, abdominal palpation, or induction of anesthesia. Patients remain normotensive between episodes. Together with the hypertension, patients complain of pounding headaches on the top of their head, palpitations, pallor, diaphoresis, and dysrhythmias. Patients with sustained hypertension may also show variability in their high–blood pressure readings and complain of headaches and irregular heartbeat.

In patients suspected of a pheochromocytoma, the biochemical evaluation should be directed to the measurement of plasma epinephrine and norepinephrine levels and the quantitation of urinary catecholamine excretion rates. Because normal adrenal secretion of epinephrine and norepinephrine may vary greatly, distinction between physiologic and pathologic hypersecretory states may be difficult with a single determination of catecholamine levels. Circulating norepinephrine is derived from sympathetic neurons, whereas epinephrine is derived chiefly from the adrenal medulla. Norepinephrine can increase with a change from the recumbent to the upright position. Catecholamines are also increased with an acute myocardial infarction, volume depletion, hypothyroidism, and other physical or emotional stress. Peripheral vasodilators, cocaine, phenoxybenzamine, phentolamine, prazosin, and theophylline can increase catecholamine release. Insulin-induced hypoglycemia can evoke major increases in epinephrine and small increases in norepinephrine. Drugs such as clonidine, reserpine, guanethidine, haloperidol, thorazine, and alpha-methyldopa decrease plasma norepinephrine levels.

Basal plasma catecholamine levels should be obtained with the patient resting in the supine position for at least

30 minutes. Normal levels for epinephrine range from 0 to 100 pg/ml; for norepinephrine, 0 to 500 pg/ml; and for dopamine, 0 to 100 pg/ml. Markedly increased levels (epinephrine more than 500 pg/ml and norepinephrine greater than 1500 pg/ml) are virtually diagnostic of pheochromocytoma.

Basal urinary catecholamines should be collected for 12 hours during the night. Normal levels for epinephrine are 0 to 20 μg/day; for norepinephrine, 0 to 100 μg/day; for metanephrines, 0 to 300 μg/day; for normetanephrines, 50 to 800 μg/day; and for vanillyl mandelic acid (VMA), 0 to 7 mg/day. Patients with pheochromocytoma have high urinary catecholamine levels.

In borderline cases a clonidine suppression test may help differentiate normal subjects from patients with a pheochromocytoma. Clonidine, 0.3 mg, is administered orally after two baseline blood samples for epinephrine and norepinephrine are obtained; plasma epinephrine and norepinephrine samples are repeated 3 hours after clonidine administration. Patients with a pheochromocytoma fail to suppress catecholamine secretion, whereas clonidine will restore normal levels of catecholamines in other hyperadrenergic states.

Treatment consists of surgical resection of the pheochromocytoma and exploration of the retroperitoneal space for paraganglia-derived tumors. Patients' blood pressure should be stabilized preoperatively by alpha-adrenergic blocking agents, such as phenoxybenzamine, and beta-blockers, such as propranolol, when needed. Phenoxybenzamine is also used as medical treatment to block catecholamine effects in patients with malignant, unresectable pheochromocytomas.

QUESTIONS

▼ Circle the letter preceding each item below that correctly answers the question or completes the statement. More than one answer may be correct.

1. Glucocorticoids affect the following when present in excess:
   a. Adipose tissue distribution
   b. The immune system
   c. Protein metabolism
   d. Carbohydrate metabolism

2. When synthetic glucocorticoids are administered orally over a long time, which of the following events is likely to occur?
   a. The adrenal gland continues to function normally.
   b. The hypothalamic-pituitary axis is suppressed.
   c. Corticotropin-releasing hormone (CRH) and adrenocorticotropic hormone (ACTH) levels are increased.
   d. Endogenous cortisol secretion is stimulated.

3. Abrupt interruption of corticosteroid therapy may result in:
   a. Hyperglycemia
   b. Severe salt depletion
   c. Nausea, vomiting, hypotension
   d. Marked hyperpigmentation

4. Which of the following pathologic conditions may cause Cushing's syndrome?
   a. Pituitary adenoma
   b. Adrenal adenoma
   c. Ectopic hormone production by a neoplasm
   d. Atrophy of the adrenal glands

5. Which of the following diagnostic tests can be used to determine whether Cushing's syndrome is caused by an adrenal neoplasm or by an ACTH-secreting pituitary microadenoma?
   a. Adrenal computed tomography
   b. Adrenal biopsy
   c. Adrenal photoscanning
   d. Myelography

6. Mrs. A., 35 years of age, has the typical signs and symptoms of Cushing's syndrome. All the following signs and symptoms are characteristic of this condition except:
   a. Moon face (full, round face)
   b. Hypotension
   c. Purple abdominal striae
   d. Truncal obesity
   e. Osteoporosis

7. Which of the following are characteristic metabolic effects of aldosterone?
   a. Decreased potassium excretion
   b. Sodium retention
   c. Regulation of blood glucose
   d. Suppression of ACTH release

8. Primary aldosteronism occurs when the overproduction of aldosterone results from a tumor or enlargement of the:
   a. Pituitary gland
   b. Adrenal cortex
   c. Adrenal medulla
   d. Hypothalamus

9. Which of the following findings are characteristic of primary aldosteronism?
   a. Hypokalemia
   b. Hyponatremia
   c. Hypertension
   d. Nephrotic syndrome

10. The direct effect of stress is an increased secretion of corticotropin by the anterior pituitary. Corticotropin acts on the adrenal cortex to increase secretion, primarily, of:
    a. Glucocorticoids
    b. Mineralocorticoids
    c. Epinephrine

11. Cushing's syndrome may develop when which of the following secretes abnormal amounts of the stated hormone?
    a. Adrenal cortex, aldosterone
    b. Anterior pituitary, aldosterone
    c. Adrenal cortex, ACTH
    d. Anterior pituitary, ACTH

12. In physiologic testing for forms of Cushing's syndrome, patients who respond to metyrapone administration with an increase in ACTH release usually have which form of the disease?
    a. Ectopic
    b. Iatrogenic
    c. Primal adrenal
    d. Pituitary

13. A woman with hirsutism may present with which of the following signs and symptoms?
    a. Amenorrhea or irregular menstrual periods
    b. Increased breast size
    c. Hair growth under the chin
    d. Increased fertility

14. Androstenedione, a steroid precursor of testosterone, is:
    a. Produced in the ovary and adrenal cortex of women
    b. Produced only in male testes
    c. A 17-ketosteroid
    d. Present in higher concentration in the plasma of hirsute and virilized women

Continued.

QUESTIONS—cont'd

e. A less potent androgen than dehydroepiandrosterone

15. Congenital adrenal hyperplasia, of the 21-hydroxylase variety, is characterized by:
    a. A masculinized genetically female fetus
    b. A feminized genetically male fetus
    c. High ACTH levels
    d. Low serum cortisol levels
    e. Increased urinary 17-ketosteroid level

16. Which of the following conditions may result in excessive androgen production?
    a. Polycystic ovary syndrome
    b. Arrhenoblastoma
    c. Adrenal carcinoma
    d. Hilus cell tumor of the ovary

17. Manifestations of virilism include all the following *except:*
    a. Acne
    b. Receding hairline, balding
    c. Decreased body hair growth
    d. Clitoral enlargement
    e. Deepening of voice

18. Pheochromocytoma is:
    a. Found only in the adrenal medulla
    b. Manifested by hypotension
    c. A catecholamine-producing tumor
    d. Most often malignant

19. Signs and symptoms of pheochromocytoma include paroxysmal episodes of:

a. Severe hypertension
b. Flushing and profuse diaphoresis
c. Severe headache
d. Tachycardia and dysrhythmias

20. The urinary excretion of high levels of which of the following is important in establishing the diagnosis of pheochromocytoma?
    a. Free cortisol
    b. Potassium
    c. Catecholamines and their metabolites
    d. Aldosterone

21. The usual treatment of pheochromocytoma consists of:
    a. Surgical excision of the tumor
    b. Presurgical treatment with an alpha-adrenergic blocker such as phenoxybenzamine
    c. Radiation therapy
    d. Chemotherapy

▼ *Answer the following on a separate sheet of paper.*

22. Explain the statement that glucocorticoids have a catabolic effect on protein metabolism.

23. What effects do abnormally high levels of glucocorticoids have on glucose metabolism?

24. The hypothalamic-pituitary axis may be activated under stress. Explain the process by which it occurs.

25. How do the basic chemical structures of 9alpha-fluorocortisol and prednisolone differ? In relation to pharmacologic effects, what is achieved by altering the basic chemical structure of cortisol?

26. List three types of treatment for pituitary ACTH-dependent Cushing's syndrome. What is the purpose of the treatment modalities?

27. What is the preferred treatment for Cushing's syndrome that is secondary to an adrenal tumor?

28. Explain the way secondary aldosteronism develops in response to congestive heart failure.

▼ *Circle T if the statement is true and F if it is false. Correct any false statements.*

29. T   F   CRH is secreted by the hypothalamus.

30. T   F   CRH stimulates the release of ACTH from the anterior pituitary.

31. T   F   High plasma cortisol levels exert a negative feedback effect on CRH release in the normal state.

32. T   F   CRH directly initiates the secretion of cortisol.

33. T   F   A deficiency of 21-hydroxylase causes an increase in cortisol production and a decrease in ACTH secretion.

CHAPTER 62

Adrenal Hyposecretion Disorders

DAVID E. SCHTEINGART

Adrenocortical hormone secretion may be insufficient to maintain normal life because of (1) primary disease or insufficiency of the adrenal cortex or (2) deficient secretion of adrenocorticotropic hormone (ACTH). When the cause of adrenocortical insufficiency is a pathologic process of the adrenal cortex, the condition is known as *Addison's disease*. With pituitary ACTH insufficiency, secondary failure of the adrenal cortex occurs. Patients with Addison's disease have involvement of all zones of the cortex, resulting in deficiency of all the adrenocortical secretions: glucocorticoids, mineralocorticoids, and androgens. Occasionally, patients present with partial deficiencies of adrenocortical hormone secretion. This is seen in cases of hypoaldosteronism, which involves the zona glomerulosa only and its secretion of aldosterone, or in the adrenogenital syndrome, in which a partial enzyme defect blocks the secretion of cortisol.

Addison's disease has an incidence of 4 per 100,000 population. In the past, tuberculosis was the main cause of Addison's disease. Presently, with better chemotherapy for tuberculosis, fewer than 50% of patients with this condition develop adrenal insufficiency. Destruction of the adrenal cortex occurs as a manifestation of an autoimmune process in more than 50% of patients with Addison's disease. Adrenal antibodies are found in high titers in some patients with Addison's disease. These antibodies react with antigens in the adrenocortical tissue and cause an inflammatory reaction that eventually destroys the adrenal gland. Usually, more than 80% of both glands must be destroyed before signs and symptoms of insufficiency develop. Addison's disease may occur concurrently with other endocrine diseases in which autoimmunity plays a role. Among these are Hashimoto's thyroiditis, certain cases of insulin-dependent diabetes mellitus, and hypoparathyroidism. There also appears to be a familial predisposition for autoimmune endocrine disease, which is probably related to abnormal reactivity of the patient's immune system. Less common causes of Addison's disease are the chronic use of anticoagulants, granulomatous diseases, cytomegalovirus (CMV) infection in patients with acquired immunodeficiency syndrome (AIDS), and metastatic neoplasms that involve both adrenal glands.

METABOLIC CONSEQUENCES OF CORTISOL, ALDOSTERONE, AND ANDROGEN DEFICIENCIES

The clinical picture of Addison's disease results from the lack of cortisol, aldosterone, and androgens. *Cortisol insufficiency* causes diminished gluconeogenesis, decreased liver glycogen, and increased sensitivity of peripheral tissues to insulin. The combination of these changes in carbohydrate metabolism may cause inability to maintain normal blood glucose levels, leading to hypoglycemia in the fasting state. Because of the low glycogen storage, patients with adrenal insufficiency are unable to withstand food deprivation for a long time. Sensitivity to insulin observed in the presence of cortisol insufficiency may be a problem for patients with insulin-dependent diabetes mellitus who also develop Addison's disease. These patients may notice that the insulin dosage that kept them under control in the past now causes hypoglycemia.

Another consequence of cortisol insufficiency is an increase in the secretion of proopiomelanocortin (POMC)–derived peptides, including ACTH, and alpha–and beta–melanocyte-stimulating hormone (MSH). This occurs as a result of diminished feedback inhibition of the hypothalamic-pituitary axis. The clinical consequence of this hormonal response is hyperpigmentation.

Because cortisol is required for a normal stress response, patients with cortisol insufficiency are unable to withstand surgical stress, trauma, infection, and similar stresses. Under these circumstances a patient may become acutely adrenal insufficient and develop evidence of vascular collapse.

Aldosterone deficiency is manifested by increased renal sodium loss and enhanced potassium reabsorption. Salt depletion is associated with water and volume depletion. The decrease in circulating plasma volume leads to hypotension. This change is most strikingly evident when the patient changes from the recumbent to the upright position. Patients with Addison's disease may demonstrate a normal blood pressure when they are lying down but marked hypotension and tachycardia when they stand up for several minutes. By definition, postural hypotension occurs when systolic and diastolic blood pressures drop by more than 20 mm Hg when the patient assumes the upright position. Postural tachycardia exists when the pulse rate increases by more than 20 beats per minute (bpm) under these circumstances. The decrease in blood pressure and the increase in pulse rate usually persist for more than 3 minutes after the change in position. Thus a person with Addison's disease may have a blood pressure of 120/80 mm Hg when recumbent, but blood pressure may drop to 60/40 mm Hg after the patient assumes the upright position. Likewise, the pulse rate may rise from 80 to 140 bpm with a change in position.

The plasma renin activity is also affected in Addison's disease. The decreases in plasma volume and in arteriolar pressure cause stimulation of renin release and increased production of angiotensin II. The problem in Addison's disease is that since the adrenal cortex is destroyed, angiotensin II is not able to stimulate aldosterone production and bring the serum level back to its initial physiologic range. Therefore high renin levels and low aldosterone secretion are characteristic of aldosterone deficiency.

Androgen deficiency may affect growth of axillary and pubic hair. This effect is masked in men, in whom testicular androgens exert the major androgenic metabolic effects. In women, androgen insufficiency causes loss of axillary and pubic hair and decreased hair over the extremities.

Pigmentation in Addison's Disease

Hyperpigmentation is an important characteristic of primary adrenocortical insufficiency. It is found in the distal portion of the extremities and sun-exposed areas. It is also present in areas not normally exposed to the sun. These areas include the nipples, extensor surfaces of the extremities, genitalia, buccal mucosa, tongue, palmar creases, and knuckles. The assessment of pigmentation may be more difficult in an African American than in a white person. In African Americans the history of color change as ascertained by the patients or their relatives may be the only way of assessing the development of hyperpigmentation. Treatment of Addison's disease reverses the hyperpigmentation.

Diagnosis and Treatment

The diagnosis of Addison's disease is based on the recognition of cortisol, aldosterone, and androgen deficiency. In addition, laboratory tests can indicate primary adrenocortical insufficiency. Patients have decreased excretion of the degradation products or metabolites of cortisol, the urinary 17-hydroxycorticoids. Plasma cortisol levels are low, and plasma ACTH levels are elevated. If patients

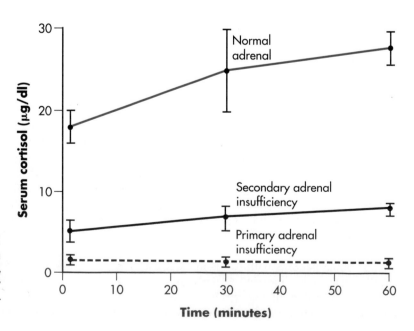

FIG. 62-1 Cortisol response to synthetic ACTH stimulation in normal subjects and in patients with adrenal insufficiency. In secondary adrenal insufficiency, baseline control levels are low but they respond slowly to ACTH. In primary adrenal insufficiency, this response is absent.

with Addison's disease receive an intravenous infusion with ACTH, the plasma cortisol levels do not rise in response to ACTH (Fig. 62-1). Serum electrolyte levels are abnormal in patients with Addison's disease, who demonstrate hyponatremia, hyperkalemia, and metabolic acidosis. Patients with adrenal insufficiency secondary to ACTH deficiency also have low levels of cortisol and its urinary metabolites. However, aldosterone levels are normal and plasma ACTH levels are low. When an intravenous infusion with ACTH is given to these patients, plasma cortisol levels rise, but in a subnormal manner. Adrenal imaging by computed tomography (CT) or magnetic resonance imaging (MRI) can also give information about the possible etiology of adrenal insufficiency. Patients with ACTH deficiency or autoimmune destruction

usually exhibit adrenal atrophy. In contrast, adrenal masses are found in patients with granulomatous disease, adrenal hematomas, or metastases.

Treatment of Addison's disease is based on replacement with cortisol, usually 20 to 30 mg/day in divided doses, and an aldosterone analog, 9alpha-fluorocortisol. When both cortisol and 9alpha-fluorocortisol are employed, patients may return to a normal metabolic state and be able to live a normal life. The dose of cortisol and 9alpha-fluorocortisol needs to be increased under conditions of stress (e.g., febrile illness, surgery, trauma).

In the past, Addison's disease was always fatal; however, patients with this condition, if properly treated, are now able to live a normal life and reach normal life expectancy.

QUESTIONS

▼ *Circle the letter preceding each item below that correctly answers the question or completes the statement. More than one answer may be correct.*

1. In Addison's disease:
   a. Levels of aldosterone increase.
   b. Both glucocorticoid and mineralocorticoid deficiencies develop simultaneously.
   c. Serum potassium levels decrease.
   d. Sodium reabsorption by the kidney increases.

2. Autoimmune destruction of the adrenal gland is caused by:
   a. Tuberculosis or other granulomatous diseases
   b. Malignant neoplasm of the lung that metastasizes to the adrenal gland
   c. Adrenal tissues becoming antigenic, causing the production of antibodies

3. Factors contributing to hypoglycemia in Addison's disease are:
   a. Decreased gluconeogenesis in the liver
   b. Increased glycogen storage in the liver
   c. Increased sensitivity of the peripheral tissues to insulin
   d. Increased insulin secretion by the pancreas

4. Which of the following sequences best explains the postural hypotension and tachycardia associated with Addison's disease?
   a. Aldosterone deficiency → increased sodium and water excretion → hypovolemia → fall in systolic and diastolic blood pressure on standing →

   compensatory increase in heart rate to maintain cardiac output
   b. Cortisol deficiency → decreased protein synthesis → hypoproteinemia → decreased osmotic pressure → edema → decreased intravascular plasma volume → fall in systolic and diastolic blood pressure on standing → compensatory increase in heart rate to maintain cardiac output
   c. Antidiuretic hormone deficiency → inability of kidney to conserve water → hypovolemia → fall in systolic and diastolic blood pressure on standing → compensatory increase in heart rate to maintain cardiac output

5. Adrenocortical insufficiency is associated with:
   a. Increased plasma renin activity and decreased plasma aldosterone
   b. Decreased plasma renin activity and increased plasma aldosterone
   c. Hyperkalemia and hyponatremia
   d. Hypokalemia and hypernatremia

6. The pigmentary changes observed in patients with Addison's disease are a result of:
   a. Decreased production of adrenocorticotropic hormone (ACTH) by the pituitary gland and associated increased production of melanocyte-stimulating hormone (MSH)
   b. Decreased production of cortisol, causing an increase in ACTH and MSH secretion
   c. Increased production of cortisol by the adrenal cortex, causing increased production of MSH

7. The diagnosis of primary adrenocortical insufficiency can be made with certainty when:
   a. Plasma cortisol levels are low.
   b. Hyperkalemia, hyponatremia, and hypertension are present.
   c. Urinary 17-hydroxycorticosteroid levels are less than 2 mg in 24 hours (normal, 2 to 8/24 hours) and fail to rise after ACTH infusion.
   d. Urinary 17-ketosteroid levels are less than 10 mg in 24 hours in an adult male (normal, 10 to 22 mg/24 hours).

8. Treatment of Addison's disease usually includes the administration of:
   a. ACTH
   b. Cortisol
   c. Pitressin
   d. 9Alpha-fluorocortisol
   e. Pituitary extract

9. Loss of pubic and axillary hair:
   a. May be a manifestation of adrenal androgen insufficiency in women but not in men
   b. Typically occurs in men with Addison's disease
   c. Occurs infrequently in men with Addison's disease, since serum testosterone levels are generally normal

10. In more than 50% of patients with Addison's disease, the destruction of the adrenal cortex results from:
    a. Tuberculosis
    b. Chronic use of anticoagulants
    c. Manifestation of an autoimmune process
    d. Granulomatous diseases

CHAPTER 63

Pancreas

GLUCOSE METABOLISM AND DIABETES MELLITUS

DAVID E. SCHTEINGART

ROLE OF THE PANCREAS IN REGULATING GLUCOSE METABOLISM

Carbohydrates are present in various forms, including simple sugars, or monosaccharides, and complex chemical units, such as disaccharides and polysaccharides. After ingestion, carbohydrates are broken down into monosaccharides and are absorbed, primarily in the duodenum and proximal jejunum. After absorption, the blood glucose level rises temporarily and eventually returns to baseline. The physiologic regulation of the blood glucose level largely depends on the liver (1) extracting glucose, (2) synthesizing glycogen, and (3) performing glycogenolysis. To a lesser extent peripheral tissues—muscles and adipocytes—extract glucose for their energy needs, thus contributing to the maintenance of normal blood glucose levels.

The liver's uptake and output of glucose and the use of glucose by peripheral tissues depend on the physiologic balance of several hormones that (1) lower blood glucose levels or (2) raise blood glucose levels. Insulin, the blood glucose–lowering hormone, is produced by the beta cells of the islets of Langerhans of the pancreas. Hormones that raise blood glucose levels include (1) glucagon, secreted by the alpha cells of the islets of Langerhans; (2) epinephrine, secreted by the adrenal medulla and other chromaffin tissues; (3) glucocorticoids, secreted by the adrenal cortex; and (4) growth hormone, secreted by the anterior pituitary gland. Glucagon, epinephrine, glucocorticoids, and growth hormone constitute a counterregulatory mechanism that prevents hypoglycemia under the effect of insulin (Fig. 63-1).

Tests of Carbohydrate Tolerance

A normal fasting plasma glucose level (Autoanalyzer technique) is 80 to 115 mg/dl. *Hyperglycemia* is defined as a fasting plasma glucose level more than 115 mg/dl and *hypoglycemia* as a level less than 80 mg/dl. Glucose is filtered by the renal glomerulus and is almost totally reabsorbed by the renal tubule as long as the plasma glucose concentration does not exceed 160 to 180 mg/dl. When the plasma glucose concentration rises above this level, glucose appears in the urine, a condition called *glycosuria*.

An individual's ability to regulate plasma glucose levels within the normal range may be determined by testing (1) the fasting plasma glucose level and (2) the plasma glucose response to a glucose load.

In the fasting state when food is not being absorbed, maintenance of normal fasting glucose levels depends on a well-integrated interaction among the liver, peripheral tissues, and hormones that lower and raise plasma glucose levels. If an individual is unable to regulate plasma glucose normally, this inability is reflected by either an increase or a decrease in the fasting plasma glucose level. For example, a patient with an insulin-producing tumor will develop hypoglycemia. On the other hand, a patient with insulin deficiency will be unable to maintain glucose levels at a normal range and will become hyperglycemic. Thus measuring the fasting plasma glucose level can help evaluate the integrity of the mechanism regulating plasma glucose.

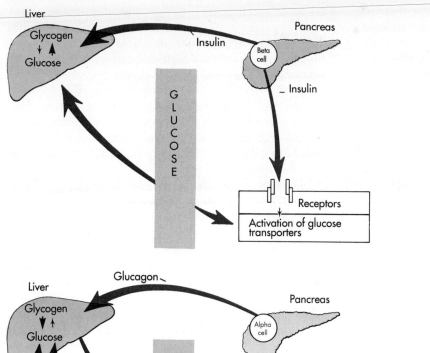

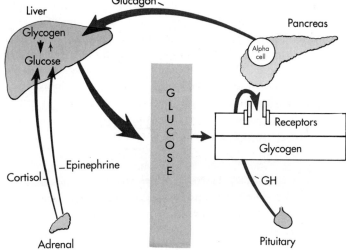

FIG. 63-1   Outline of regulation of blood glucose. *GH,* Growth hormone.

In a patient with diabetes mellitus (a condition of relative or absolute insulin deficiency), the fasting plasma glucose level becomes abnormal only in the late stage of the disease. Therefore its measurement does not provide information about early abnormalities in glucose metabolism.

A more sensitive method for uncovering abnormalities in glucose metabolism is the measurement of the plasma glucose level after a glucose load. A nondiabetic individual who ingests a glucose load absorbs this glucose and exhibits a temporary rise in plasma glucose levels. Mechanisms for glucose disposal are then brought into action, and the plasma glucose level returns to normal. The mechanism that mediates this response is insulin, and the main stimulus to insulin release is glucose. The tests used to make the pertinent measurements after a glucose load are (1) the 2-hour postprandial plasma glucose and (2) the oral glucose tolerance.

The *2-hour postprandial glucose test* is a simple screening test for an individual's ability to dispose of a glucose load. The test consists of measuring the patient's plasma glucose level 2 hours after the ingestion of a meal containing 100 g of carbohydrate or the administration of 75 g of glucose orally. If the plasma glucose level is equal to or less than 140 mg/dl 2 hours after the ingestion of the glucose load, it can be concluded that the plasma glucose level must have returned to baseline after an initial rise, indicating that the subject has a normal mechanism for glucose disposal. In contrast, if the patient's plasma glucose level is more than 140 mg/dl after 2 hours, it can be concluded that there is a disturbance in the mechanism regulating glucose levels.

If a 2-hour postprandial plasma glucose level is abnormal, an *oral glucose tolerance test* (OGTT) can provide more complete information about the presence of a disturbance in carbohydrate metabolism. For an OGTT, the fasting plasma glucose level is measured, and then the patient ingests 75 g of glucose within 5 minutes. The plasma glucose levels are measured at ½-hour intervals for 2 hours after the glucose load. In healthy, ambulatory people with normal glucose tolerance, the fasting plasma glucose level is 80 to 115 mg/dl. After the ingestion of glucose, the plasma glucose level rises initially but returns to baseline within 2 hours. Normal values for the OGTT have been defined as plasma glucose less than 200 mg/dl at ½, 1, and 1½ hours and less than 140 mg/dl at 2 hours (National Diabetes Data Group criteria). Criteria differing slightly from these values have been proposed by other investigators and health organizations.

DIABETES MELLITUS

Diabetes mellitus is a genetically and clinically heterogeneous group of disorders of metabolism manifested ultimately by loss of carbohydrate tolerance. In its fully developed clinical expression, diabetes mellitus is characterized by fasting hyperglycemia, atherosclerotic and microangiopathic vascular disease, and neuropathy. The clinical manifestations of hyperglycemia usually precede by many years the clinical recognition of vascular disease. Occasionally, however, patients with only a mild abnormality of glucose tolerance experience the severe clinical consequences of vascular disease.

Etiology

Evidence indicates that diabetes mellitus has diverse causes. Although different types of lesions may ultimately lead to insulin insufficiency, genetic determinants are usually critical in most patients with diabetes mellitus. *Insulin-dependent diabetes mellitus* (IDDM) is a genetically determined autoimmune disease with symptoms that develop at the end of a gradual process of immune destruction of insulin-producing cells. Genetically susceptible individuals appear to respond to a triggering event, probably a viral infection, by producing autoantibodies against the beta cells, which leads to a decline of glucose-stimulated insulin secretion. Clinical manifestations of diabetes mellitus occur when more than 90% of the beta cells have been destroyed. In the more severe forms of diabetes mellitus, beta cells are completely destroyed, resulting in insulinopenia and all of the associated metabolic abnormalities caused by insulin deficiency. Evidence for the genetic determination of IDDM is its association with specific histocompatibity (HLA) types. The type of histocompatibility genes associated with IDDM (DW3 and DW4) are the ones that code for proteins that play a critical role in monocyte-lymphocyte interactions. These proteins modulate T cell responses that are part of the normal immune response. When a defect occurs, the disordered T lymphocyte function plays an important role in the pathogenesis of islet cell destruction. There is also evidence of increased anti–islet cell antibodies that are directed to specific antigenic components of the beta cell. The triggering event that determines the autoimmune process in genetically susceptible individuals may be an infection with coxsackie B4 or mumps viruses. Outbreaks of new-onset IDDM have been observed at certain times of the year in members of the same social groups. Certain drugs known to trigger other autoimmune diseases may also initiate the autoimmune process in patients with IDDM. Anti–islet cell antibodies are present in a high percentage of patients with new-onset IDDM and provide strong evidence of an autoimmune mechanism in the pathogenesis of the disease. Immunologic screening and assessment of insulin secretion in persons at high risk for developing IDDM may allow early treatment with immunosuppressive therapy that could delay the onset of the clinical manifestations of insulin deficiency.

In patients with *non-insulin-dependent diabetes mellitus* (NIDDM), the disease has a strong familial pattern of occurrence. The concordance rate for NIDDM in monozygotic twins is almost 100%. The risk of developing diabetes is nearly 40% for siblings of patients with NIDDM and 33% for their offspring. The genetic transmission is strongest in *maturity-onset diabetes of the young* (MODY), a subtype of NIDDM in which the disease is transmitted in an autosomal dominant pattern. There is a 1:1 ratio of diabetic-to-nondiabetic children when one parent has NIDDM and about 90% of obligate carriers have NIDDM. NIDDM is characterized by defects in insulin secretion as well as in insulin action. The initial event appears to be the development of resistance to insulin in target cells of insulin action. Insulin initially binds itself to specific cell surface receptors, then starts a cascade of intracellular reactions that lead to increased glucose transport across the cell membrane. In patients with NIDDM, a defect exists in insulin receptor binding. This may be caused by a decreased number of receptor sites in the cell membrane of insulin-responsive cells or by abnormalities of the insulin receptor. As a consequence, abnormal coupling occurs between insulin receptor complexes and the glucose transport system. Normal glucose levels are maintained for a long time through an increase in insulin secretion, but eventually hyperglycemia occurs when insulin secretion declines and the amount of circulating insulin is no longer sufficient to maintain euglycemia. About 80% of patients with NIDDM are obese. Because obesity is associated with insulin resistance, it is likely that impairment of glucose tolerance and diabetes mellitus eventually develop in NIDDM patients as a consequence of their obesity. Weight reduction is frequently associated with improvement in insulin sensitivity and recovery of glucose tolerance.

Classification and Glucose Intolerance

Several classifications of diabetes mellitus have been proposed, based on the modalities of clinical presentation, age of onset, and natural history of the disease. The box on p. 957 describes a classification proposed by the National Diabetes Data Group of the National Institutes of Health, based on contemporary knowledge of the diabetic syndrome and disorders of glucose tolerance. Three clinical classes of disorders of glucose tolerance are de-

CLASSIFICATION OF DIABETES MELLITUS

CLINICAL CLASSES

1. Diabetes mellitus (DM)
    a. Insulin-dependent type (IDDM), type I
    b. Non-insulin-dependent type (NIDDM), type II
        (1) Nonobese NIDDM
        (2) Obese NIDDM
        (3) Maturity-onset diabetes of the young (MODY)
    c. Secondary diabetes
2. Impaired glucose tolerance (IGT)
3. Gestational diabetes (GDM)

STATISTICAL RISK CLASSES

1. Previous abnormality of glucose tolerance (Prev AGT)
2. Potential abnormality of glucose tolerance (Pot AGT)

Modified from National Diabetes Data Group: *Diabetes* 28(12): 1039-1057, 1979.

scribed: (1) diabetes mellitus (DM), (2) impaired glucose tolerance (IGT), and (3) gestational diabetes (GDM). Among individuals with diabetes mellitus, two types are recognized. Patients with IDDM, or type I, are ketosis prone. This has been termed juvenile-onset type in the past; however, it can occur at any age. NIDDM, or type II, patients are not prone to ketosis. Obesity is frequently associated with this type. MODY has strong familial prevalence and manifests itself before age 14 years. Patients are not ketosis prone and are frequently obese. *Secondary diabetes* develops in association with other conditions and syndromes, such as underlying pancreatic disease, Cushing's syndrome, and acromegaly. Some patients have primary insulin-receptor abnormalities such as those seen with acanthosis nigricans and the insulin-resistant syndrome.

In nonpregnant adults the diagnosis of diabetes mellitus is based on the findings of (1) classic symptoms of diabetes and unequivocal hyperglycemia, (2) fasting plasma glucose levels equal to or greater than 140 mg/dl on more than one occasion, and (3) if the fasting plasma glucose level is less than 140 mg/dl, glucose levels obtained during an OGTT equal to or greater than 200 mg/dl at 2 hours and at least at one other time between 0 and 2 hours after ingestion of glucose.

The diagnosis of diabetes mellitus in children is also based on the finding of classic symptoms of diabetes and a random plasma glucose greater than 200 mg/dl.

Patients with *impaired glucose tolerance* (IGT) do not meet the criteria described for diagnosis of diabetes mellitus. However, their OGTTs show abnormal values. These patients are asymptomatic. Biochemically, they exhibit fasting plasma glucose levels less than 140 mg/dl and values during an OGTT equal to or greater than 200

mg/dl at ½, 1, or 1½ hours and 140 to 200 mg/dl at 2 hours. Some patients with IGT may have underlying conditions that may be responsible for secondary types of diabetes. In other individuals, IGT may be the expression of an early stage in the development of diabetes. These individuals are not considered to have diabetes but are recognized as being at higher risk than the general population for the development of diabetes. Some of these patients may remain in this class for many years. Many return to normal glucose tolerance spontaneously, but 1% to 5% of persons with IGT proceed to overt clinical diabetes annually. Although clinically significant renal and retinal microangiopathic complications of diabetes are absent in patients with IGT, many studies of such groups have shown an increased prevalence of arterial disease, electrocardiographic abnormalities, and cardiac death or increased susceptibility to atherosclerotic disease. Appropriate intervention, including caloric restriction or weight loss in obese persons with IGT, may lead to improvement in glucose tolerance and a possible change in the occurrence of these complications.

Gestational diabetes mellitus (GDM) is the glucose intolerance that has its onset or recognition during pregnancy. Because of the increased secretion of various hormones with metabolic effects on glucose tolerance, pregnancy is a diabetogenic condition. Patients with a genetic predisposition for diabetes may show glucose intolerance or clinical manifestations of diabetes with pregnancy. The recommended criteria for the biochemical diagnosis of gestational diabetes are those proposed by O'Sullivan and Mahan (1973). According to these criteria, GDM is present when two or more of the following values are met or exceeded after a 100 g oral glucose challenge: fasting, 105 mg/dl; 1 hour, 190 mg/dl; 2 hours, 165 mg/dl; and 3 hours, 145 mg/dl. Recognition of GDM is important because these patients are at increased risk for perinatal morbidity and mortality and have increased frequency of viable fetal loss.

Two statistical risk classes of patients are included in the classification of diabetes. These are (1) *previous abnormality of glucose tolerance* (Prev AGT) and (2) *potential abnormality of glucose tolerance* (Pot AGT). Prev AGT applies only to individuals who at the time of their examination have a normal glucose tolerance but have previously demonstrated diabetic hyperglycemia or IGT that appeared spontaneously or in response to an identifiable stimulus. Included in this class are patients with GDM who have recovered glucose tolerance postpartum and patients with IGT or NIDDM who have normalized their glucose tolerance after weight reduction.

Persons with Pot AGT include those who have never exhibited abnormal glucose tolerance but who are at substantially increased risk for the development of diabetes, including persons with islet cell antibodies; monozygotic twins of individuals with IDDM; siblings of individuals with IDDM, especially those with identical HLA haplotypes; and offspring of individuals with IDDM. Individuals who are at an increased risk for NIDDM include monozygotic twins of individuals with NIDDM, first-degree relatives of individuals with NIDDM, mothers of neonates weighing more than 9 pounds, obese individuals, and members of racial or ethnic groups with a high incidence of diabetes. Patients with Pot AGT were formerly classified as prediabetic. However, this diagnosis can be established only retrospectively once individuals have developed diabetes and therefore cannot be used in individuals who may be at risk but who have normal glucose tolerance.

Epidemiology

The prevalence rate of diabetes mellitus is high. Estimates are that there are 10 million individuals with diabetes in the United States and that 600,000 new cases are diagnosed every year. Diabetes is the third leading cause of death by disease in the United States and the leading cause of blindness, through the development of diabetic retinopathy. The incidence of heart attack in individuals with diabetes is at least $2\frac{1}{2}$ times that of nondiabetic individuals of a comparable age.

Seventy-five percent of diabetic patients eventually die of vascular disease. Heart attacks, kidney failure, cerebrovascular accidents (CVAs, strokes), and gangrene are the major complications. In addition, there is an increased rate of intrauterine fetal death in infants of diabetic mothers.

The economic impact of diabetes is substantial as a result of medical expenses and lost wages in addition to the financial consequence of many of the complications such as blindness and vascular disease.

Clinical Manifestations

The clinical manifestations of diabetes mellitus are related to the metabolic consequence of insulin deficiency. Patients with insulin deficiency are unable to maintain normal fasting plasma glucose levels or glucose tolerance after ingesting carbohydrates. If the hyperglycemia is severe and exceeds the renal threshold for this substance, glycosuria supervenes. Glycosuria leads to osmotic diuresis, which causes increased urine output (polyuria) and thirst (polydipsia). Because of the loss of glucose through the urine, patients develop negative caloric balance and weight loss. Increased hunger (polyphagia) may also develop as the result of calorie loss. Patients complain of fatigue and sleepiness.

Patients with IDDM frequently exhibit an explosive onset of symptoms with polydipsia, polyuria, weight loss, polyphagia, fatigue, and somnolence occurring within a few days or weeks. They may become extremely ill and develop ketoacidosis, and they may die if treatment is not instituted promptly. They usually require insulin therapy for metabolic control and are generally sensitive to insulin. In contrast, patients with NIDDM may be com-

pletely asymptomatic, and the diagnosis may be made only after a laboratory examination of their blood and performance of OGTTs. With more severe degrees of hyperglycemia, these patients may develop polydipsia, polyuria, fatigue, and somnolence. They usually do not develop ketoacidosis. If the hyperglycemia is severe and patients do not respond to diet therapy, insulin therapy may be required to normalize glucose levels. These patients usually exhibit diminished peripheral sensitivity to insulin. Their own insulin levels may be diminished, normal, or high but inadequate to maintain normal blood glucose levels. They are also resistant to exogenous insulin. Because many of these patients are obese, it is postulated that high carbohydrate intake, large adipose cells, and impairment in intracellular glucose metabolism are responsible for their decreased sensitivity to insulin.

Management

The management of diabetes mellitus is based on (1) diet, (2) hypoglycemic agents, and (3) controlled physical activity.

In people without diabetes, an intact capacity to secrete insulin compensates for varying amounts of food intake and exercise. Individuals with diabetes are unable to secrete insulin normally, and so this ability is lost. The bodies of normal individuals adjust to hour-to-hour changes in food intake and exercise by varying their insulin secretion, but individuals with IDDM are unable to do so unless they concomitantly adjust their insulin dosage to prevent wide fluctuations in blood glucose levels.

The diet of diabetic patients is aimed at controlling the number of calories and the amount of carbohydrates ingested daily. The recommended number of calories varies, depending on the need for maintaining, reducing, or increasing body weight. For example, if the patient is obese, a calorie-restricted diet should be prescribed until the patient's weight has dropped into the ideal range for that person. In contrast, young patients with IDDM may lose weight during the state of decompensation. They should receive sufficient calories to restore their weight and for growth.

To prevent excessive postprandial hyperglycemia and glycosuria, diabetic patients should avoid excessive intake of carbohydrates. Usually, carbohydrates make up 50% of the total daily calorie allowance. This carbohydrate allowance must be distributed in such a way that the intake matches the patients' requirements throughout the day. For example, larger amounts are given at times of greater physical activity. Fat intake should be limited to 30% of the total daily caloric allowance, and at least half should be of the polyunsaturated type. A food exchange system has been developed to help patients manage their diet. This system groups together foods with similar amounts of carbohydrate, protein, and fat, and therefore calories. This allows patients to "trade" the food on each exchange list for any other food on the same list.

▶ TABLE 63-1   Oral Hypoglycemic Agents

Agent	Half-Life (Hours)	Timing Dose	Initial Dose	Maintenance Dose	Toxicity	Tablet Size
Glipizide (Glucotrol)	2 to 4	Four times or twice a day	5 mg	5 to 30 mg	Gastrointestinal Skin Hematologic	5 mg
Glyburide (Micronase, DiaBeta)	10	Four times or twice a day	5 mg	1.25 to 20 mg	Skin Gastrointestinal Hematologic	1.25 to 5 mg
Metformin (Glucophage)	1.3 to 4.5	Three times a day	1000 mg	1500 mg	Lactic acidosis	500 mg

Data from Hardman JG et al, editors: *Goodman & Gilman's the pharmacological basis of therapeutics,* ed 9, New York, 1996, McGraw-Hill.

▶ TABLE 63-2   Insulins

Type	Description	Effect on Blood Glucose (Hours after Administration)		
		Onset	Peak	Termination
SHORT ACTING				
Regular (crystalline zinc)	Clear	Immediate	2 to 4	6 to 8
Semilente (SL)*	Cloudy: amorphous insulin zinc suspension, no protamine	1	4 to 6	12 to 16
INTERMEDIATE ACTING				
NPH†	Cloudy: crystalline zinc insulin suspension, 50% saturated with protamine	2 to 3	8 to 12	18 to 24
Lente	Cloudy: mixture 30% SL + 70% UL, no protamine	2 to 3	8 to 12	18 to 24
LONG ACTING				
PZI†	Cloudy: excess protamine	6	14 to 20	24 to 36
Ultralente (UL)*	Cloudy: crystalline insulin suspension, high zinc content, no protamine	6	16 to 18	30 to 36

*Lente insulins (semi and ultra) do not contain protamine and are prepared in sodium acetate buffer. Their time of action depends on their variable zinc content and crystal size.
†Delayed action of NPH and PZI is controlled by their protamine content; they are prepared in sodium phosphate buffer.

Patients with mild symptoms of diabetes mellitus may be able to maintain normal blood glucose levels by means of a diet alone. However, diabetic patients with some remaining islet cell function (those with NIDDM) are good candidates for the use of *oral hypoglycemic agents,* such as the *sulfonylureas.* These drugs stimulate beta cell function and increase the secretion of insulin. Patients with IDDM have lost their islet cell function, and the oral hypoglycemics would be ineffective for them. Another type of oral hypoglycemic agent is *metformin.* It reduces blood glucose by decreasing hepatic glucose production and increasing peripheral glucose utilization. It is used alone or in combination with sulfonylureas.

There are potential adverse effects from the use of oral hypoglycemic agents (Table 63-1). However, the second-generation sulfonylureas have little or no antidiuretic effect, a potential problem with some of the first-generation agents.

Patients with severe insulin insufficiency, however, require injections of insulin in addition to dietary restrictions. Several preparations of insulin are available (Table 63-2). This insulin is identical to human insulin and is prepared by recombinant deoxyribonucleic acid (DNA) techniques. They are classified as short acting, intermediate acting, or long acting, according to the time required for the maximal plasma glucose–lowering effect to take place after their injection. *Short-acting insulins* produce their maximal effect within 2 to 6 hours after injection and are used to treat acute diabetic decompensation and to help manage patients with diabetic ketoacidosis. They also may be used to supplement longer-acting insulins. *Intermediate-acting insulins* have their peak within 8 to 12 hours after administration and are usually used for the day-to-day control of the diabetic patient. *Long-acting insulins* have a peak effect within 14 to 20 hours after administration and are rarely used in the routine management of diabetic patients.

Blood glucose control for insulin-requiring diabetic patients is often achieved by the use of intermediate-acting insulin administered before breakfast or as a split dose, with the larger portion given before breakfast and the smaller dose before supper. Short-acting insulin is frequently combined with intermediate-acting insulin for physiologic regulation of glucose during postprandial periods, particularly in patients with IDDM. More intense insulin therapy has been achieved using more frequent insulin injections or continuous subcutaneous insulin infusion systems. When frequent insulin injections are given, short-acting regular insulin is given before each meal, and intermediate-acting NPH or Lente insulin is given at bedtime. The dose of regular insulin is adjusted according to a preestablished algorithm that takes into account the prevailing glucose level and size of the meal. Several lightweight, portable insulin infusion pumps are available that deliver a continuous basal infusion, as well as preprandial boluses given 30 minutes before each meal. Patients on intensified insulin therapy must monitor their glucose level before each insulin dose. This is accomplished by finger stick, which produces a drop of capillary blood. The blood is applied to a test strip and read off a glucose meter. The meter can store the glucose values in its memory, and this information can be unloaded by the health care professional for further advice on the insulin program. Intensified insulin therapy frequently results in improved glucose control.

Physical exercise or labor also influences the control of blood glucose levels in patients with diabetes. Exercise appears to facilitate the transport of glucose into cells and to increase sensitivity to insulin. In nondiabetic individuals, insulin release decreases during exercise and hypoglycemia is avoided. However, patients who take insulin injections are unable to exert this control, and the increased glucose uptake during exercise can lead to hypoglycemia. This is particularly important when a patient engages in physical exercise when the insulin dose has reached its maximal or peak effect time. By appropriate timing of their physical exertion, patients may be able to improve the control of their glucose levels. For example, if patients exercise when their blood glucose level is high, they may be able to lower this level with exercise alone. Conversely, if patients need to exercise when the blood glucose level is low, they must receive additional carbohydrate to prevent hypoglycemia.

Patients with diabetes mellitus can lead a relatively normal life if they are well informed about their disease and its management. They can learn to administer their own insulin, monitor their blood glucose level, and use this information to regulate their insulin dosage and plan their diet and exercise to minimize hyperglycemia and hypoglycemia. For patients with NIDDM who are obese, are asymptomatic, and have moderately elevated glucose levels, the treatment of choice is dietary restriction and weight reduction. However, the success rate in weight reduction among these patients is low, and they may eventually require therapy with hypoglycemic agents.

A method for determining glucose control in all types of diabetes is the measurement of *glycated hemoglobin*. Hemoglobin does not normally contain glucose when it is first released from the bone marrow. During its 120-day life span in the red blood cell, hemoglobin normally incorporates glucose. If the ambient glucose level rises above normal, the amount of glycated hemoglobin will rise accordingly. Because of the slow hemoglobin turnover, a high value indicates that blood glucose levels have been high for 4 to 8 weeks. Table 63-3 summarizes the range of glycated hemoglobin observed in patients with diabetes.

Complications

Complications of diabetes mellitus can be divided into two major categories: (1) acute metabolic complications and (2) long-term vascular complications.

Acute metabolic complications

The metabolic complications of diabetes result from relatively acute changes in plasma glucose concentration. The most serious metabolic complication of IDDM is *diabetic ketoacidosis* (DKA). With severe insulin insufficiency, patients develop severe hyperglycemia and glycosuria, decreased lipogenesis, increased lipolysis, and increased oxidation of free fatty acids with production of ketone bodies (acetoacetate, hydroxybutyrate, and acetone). The increase in ketones in plasma causes ketosis. The increased production of ketones causes an increased hydrogen ion load and metabolic acidosis. Marked glycosuria and ketonuria also lead to osmotic diuresis and resultant dehydration and loss of electrolytes. Patients may become hypotensive and develop a state of shock. Eventually, because of decreased cerebral oxygen use, patients may become comatose and die. Coma and death from DKA are rare today, since patients and health care personnel are aware of the potential dangers of this complication and treatment of DKA can be instituted early.

DKA is treated by (1) reversing the metabolic derangement caused by the lack of insulin, (2) restoring water and electrolyte balance, and (3) treating conditions that may have precipitated ketoacidosis. Treatment with short-acting (regular) insulin—administered as a continuous intravenous infusion or as frequent intramuscular injections—and glucose in water or saline infusions increases glucose use, decreases lipolysis and ketone body production, and restores acid-base balance. In addition, patients may need potassium replacement. Because intercurrent infections can increase insulin requirements in patients with diabetes, it is not unusual for infection to

▶ TABLE 63-3   Glycated Hemoglobin Levels
in Diabetes

Normal/Glucose Control	Glycated Hemoglobin (%)
Normal value	2.2 to 4.8
Good glucose control	2.5 to 6.0
Fair glucose control	6.1 to 8.0
Poor glucose control	Greater than 8.0

precipitate acute diabetic decompensation and DKA. Thus treatment with antibiotics may be necessary in the management of patients with this condition.

Hyperglycemic, hyperosmolar, nonketotic coma (HHNK) is another acute metabolic complication that occurs most often in older individuals with NIDDM. Because of relative but not absolute insulin deficiency, hyperglycemia develops without ketosis. Hyperglycemia is severe, with serum glucose levels greater than 600 mg/dl. This causes hyperosmolality, osmotic diuresis, and profound dehydration. The patient may lose consciousness, and the mortality rate may be as high as 50%. The treatment of HHNK consists of rehydration, electrolyte replacement, and regular insulin. The major difference between HHNK and DKA is the lack of ketosis with HHNK. Because the patient has some residual ability to secrete insulin in NIDDM, the mobilization of fats for energy is avoided.

Another frequent metabolic complication of diabetes is *hypoglycemia* (insulin reaction, insulin shock), which is mainly a complication of insulin therapy. Insulin-dependent diabetic patients may, at times, receive insulin in amounts larger than needed to maintain normal glucose levels; hypoglycemia results. Symptoms of hypoglycemia are caused by epinephrine release (sweating, shakiness, headache, palpitations) and by lack of glucose in the brain (bizarre behavior, dullness of sensorium, coma). *It must be emphasized that hypoglycemic attacks are dangerous and, if frequent or prolonged, may cause permanent brain damage or even death.* Management of hypoglycemia requires the prompt administration of carbohydrate, either orally or intravenously. Occasionally, glucagon, a glycogenolytic hormone, is administered intramuscularly to raise blood glucose levels. Insulin-induced hypoglycemia in a diabetic patient can trigger the release of counterregulatory hormones (glucagon, epinephrine, cortisol, growth hormone), which results in a rise in glucose levels to a hyperglycemic range *(Somogyi effect)*. The lows and highs in glucose levels lead to poor diabetic control. Prevention of hypoglycemia by reducing the insulin dose also minimizes the rebound hyperglycemia.

Chronic long-term complications

The long-term vascular complications of diabetes involve small vessels—microangiopathy—and middle- and large-size vessels—macroangiopathy. *Microangiop-*

athy is a specific lesion of diabetes that affects capillaries and arterioles of the retina *(diabetic retinopathy)*, renal glomeruli *(diabetic nephropathy)*, peripheral nerves *(diabetic neuropathy)*, and muscles and skin. Histochemically, this thickening is accompanied by increased accumulation of glycoprotein. In addition, since the chemical components of the basement membrane can be derived from glucose, hyperglycemia causes an increased rate of formation of basement membrane cells. These cells do not require insulin for glucose use.

Histologic evidence of microangiopathy is already apparent in patients with IGT. However, clinical manifestations of vascular disease, retinopathy, or nephropathy usually appear 15 to 20 years after the onset of diabetes.

A strong relationship exists between hyperglycemia and the incidence and progression of retinopathy. An early manifestation of retinopathy is the presence of microaneurysms (tiny saccular dilations) of the retinal arterioles. Subsequently, hemorrhages, neovascularization, and retinal scars may lead to blindness (Fig. 63-2). The most successful treatment of retinopathy is panretinal photocoagulation. A laser beam is focused on the retina, producing a chorioretinal scar. Over the course of several sessions, an average of 1800 scars are placed throughout the posterior pole of the retina. This treatment approach appears to suppress neovascularization and subsequent hemorrhage.

Early manifestations of nephropathy are proteinuria and hypertension. As the loss of functioning nephrons progresses, patients develop renal insufficiency and uremia. At this stage, patients may require dialysis or renal transplantation. The pathogenesis of diabetic nephropathy and current research on interventions to slow its progression are discussed in Chapters 46 and 48.

Neuropathy and cataracts result from disturbances in the polyol pathway (glucose → sorbitol → fructose) caused by lack of insulin. In the lens, there is increased accumulation of sorbitol, leading to the formation of cataracts and blindness. In nerve tissue, there is an increased accumulation of sorbitol and fructose and a decreased concentration of myoinositol, leading to neuropathy. The biochemical alteration in nerve tissue interferes with metabolic activity of the Schwann cells and causes axonal loss. Motor conduction velocity decreases early in the course of neuropathy. Subsequently, the patient has pain, paresthesias, decreased vibratory and proprioceptive sensations, and motor impairment with loss of deep tendon reflexes, muscle weakness, and atrophy. Neuropathy may involve peripheral nerves (mononeuropathy and polyneuropathy) (Color plate 29), cranial nerves, or the autonomic nervous system. Involvement of the autonomic nervous system may be accompanied by nocturnal diarrhea, delayed gastric emptying with gastroparesis, postural hypotension, and erectile dysfunction.

Diabetic *macroangiopathy* has the histopathologic characteristics of atherosclerosis. A combination of biochemical disturbances caused by insulin insufficiency probably leads to this type of vascular disease. The dis-

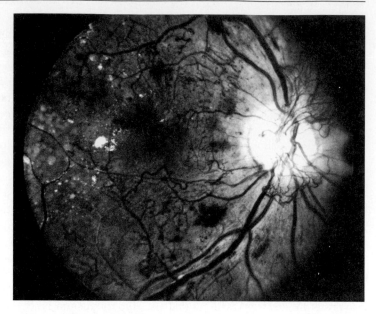

FIG. 63-2   Diabetic retinopathy. Note the hemorrhages, exudates, neovascularization, and dilation of the veins in the fundus of a patient with diabetes mellitus. (Reproduced with permission from the Ophthalmology Department, University Hospital, University of Michigan.)

turbances include (1) accumulation of sorbitol in the vascular intima, (2) hyperlipoproteinemia, and (3) abnormality in blood coagulation. Diabetic macroangiopathy eventually leads to vascular occlusion. When it involves peripheral arteries, it may result in *peripheral vascular insufficiency* with intermittent claudication and *gangrene of the extremities*. When it involves the aorta and coronary arteries, it may lead to angina and myocardial infarction.

Diabetes also interferes with pregnancy. Women with diabetes who become pregnant are prone to spontaneous abortions, intrauterine fetal death, large fetal size, and premature infants with a high incidence of respiratory distress syndrome and fetal malformations. The outcome of pregnancy in diabetic mothers has improved with tighter blood glucose control during pregnancy, early delivery, and advances in the field of neonatology and in the management of complications in the newborn. In general, a change in hormonal levels during pregnancy causes a progressive increase in insulin requirement, which reaches a peak in the third trimester, with a sharp drop in insulin requirements at delivery.

Present clinical and experimental evidence suggests that long-term diabetic complications develop because of the chronic abnormality in metabolism caused by insufficient insulin secretion. Diabetic complications can be minimized or prevented if the treatment of diabetes is effective enough to bring glucose levels, as indicated by glycated hemoglobin, to within the normal range. The importance of glucose control in ameliorating or preventing the complications of diabetes has been highlighted by the results of the Diabetes Control and Complications Trial (DCCT), conducted as a multicenter study over a 10-year period. Patients with IDDM who received intensified insulin therapy and decreased their glycated hemoglobin levels to within the normal range experienced a 50% to 75% reduction in the major microangiopathic complications, including retinopathy, nephropathy, and neuropathy.

The ultimate objective in the treatment of diabetes is *prevention*. The recognition of individuals at risk for developing IDDM may lead to early detection of the autoimmune process causing the destruction of beta cells and treatment with specific immunosuppressive agents. Once the disease has developed, pancreatic transplantation may restore the insulin-secreting capacity. In patients with NIDDM, a better understanding of the molecular mechanism of insulin resistance may lead to development of pharmacologic agents that could specifically enhance insulin action. Research in these areas is in progress.

QUESTIONS

▼ *Circle the letter preceding each item below that correctly answers the question or completes the statement. More than one answer may be correct.*

1. Glucose is removed from the bloodstream by:
   a. Conversion to glycogen by the liver
   b. Peripheral glucose use by muscle or adipose tissue

2. Fasting hypoglycemia will usually occur when there is:
   a. Pancreatic islet cell tumor
   b. Cirrhosis of the liver when the patient is unable to synthesize glycogen
   c. Excessive production of cortisol
   d. Excessive production of growth hormone

3. Which of the following tests is the most sensitive in the diagnosis of diabetes mellitus?
   a. Fasting plasma glucose
   b. 2-hour postprandial plasma glucose
   c. Standard oral glucose tolerance

4. The purpose of the 2-hour postprandial plasma glucose test is to:
   a. Assess the ability of an individual to dispose of a glucose load
   b. Test the insulin-secreting capacity of the islets of Langerhans under stress
   c. Determine insulin requirements
   d. Detect gestational diabetes

5. The major defect in diabetes mellitus is a disorder in the secretion of:
   a. Epinephrine
   b. Cortisol
   c. Insulin
   d. Growth hormone

6. Current theories of the pathogenesis of diabetes mellitus include:
   a. Autoimmune destruction of beta cells
   b. Viral destruction of beta cells
   c. Genetically determined defects in insulin release
   d. Decreased growth hormone production

7. The prevalence rate of diabetes mellitus is calculated at a minimum of how many million cases in the United States?
   a. 1
   b. 3
   c. 6
   d. 10

8. Robert M., a 30-year-old man, is being treated in an outpatient clinic. His history reveals that he has a bilateral family history of diabetes mellitus. His 2-hour postprandial blood glucose test shows levels of 115 mg/dl. Robert would most probably be classified as having:
   a. Insulin-dependent diabetes (IDDM)
   b. Potential diabetes
   c. Non-insulin-dependent diabetes (NIDDM)
   d. Impaired glucose tolerance

9. Which of the following are the usual characteristics of an NIDDM patient?
   a. Relative insensitivity to insulin
   b. Obesity
   c. Very low islet cell reserve
   d. Proneness to diabetic ketoacidosis

10. The individual with IDDM usually has all the following *except:*
    a. Weight gain
    b. Polydipsia
    c. Polyuria
    d. Fatigue
    e. Polyphagia

11. Jane S., 10 years old, is admitted to the hospital and diagnosed as having IDDM. The medical management that would most likely be prescribed for Jane is:
    a. A fixed amount of carbohydrate, fat, and protein distributed throughout the day plus an oral hypoglycemic agent
    b. A fixed amount of calories and carbohydrate, protein, and fat plus insulin therapy
    c. Education about diabetes and oral hypoglycemic agents

12. If a patient with diabetes is given an excessive dose of Lente insulin at 7 AM, when would one expect to see a hypoglycemic reaction (if such a reaction occurs)?
    a. Within ½ hour
    b. 11 AM
    c. 4 PM
    d. Midnight

13. The most common metabolic complication of insulin therapy is:
    a. Hypoglycemia
    b. Hyperglycemia
    c. Ketoacidosis
    d. Diabetic coma

14. Complications of diabetes mellitus include which of the following?
    a. Peripheral vascular insufficiency
    b. Diabetic nephropathy
    c. Ketoacidosis
    d. Retinopathy

15. IDDM is characterized by which of the following?
    a. Genetically determined autoimmune disease
    b. Anti–islet cell antibodies present in the initial stage of the disease
    c. Strong familial pattern of occurrence
    d. Defect in secretion as well as in insulin action

▼ *Answer the following questions on a separate sheet of paper.*

16. What is the purpose of measuring the fasting blood glucose level?

17. Administration of a glucose load to a nondiabetic individual causes a rise in blood glucose. Which mechanism brings glucose back to baseline levels?

18. What is the purpose of the food exchange system?

19. What are the advantages of the second-generation oral sulfonylureas?

20. Why is it important to identify individuals who are at risk for developing diabetes mellitus?

▼ *Match the glucose level in column B with the appropriate term in column A.*

Column A	Column B
21. _____ Hypoglycemia	a. 160 to 180 mg/dl
22. _____ Normal plasma glucose	b. 210 mg/dl
23. _____ Renal threshold for glucose	c. 40 mg/dl
24. _____ Hyperglycemia	d. 80 to 115 mg/dl

Continued.

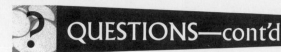

▼ *Circle T if the statement is true and F if it is false. Correct any false statements.*

25. T F Heart attacks occur at least 2½ times as often in patients with diabetes as in normal individuals of comparable age.

26. T F Twenty-five percent of all patients with diabetes eventually die of vascular disease, heart attacks, kidney failure, strokes, or gangrene.

27. T F Exercise tends to increase blood sugar by blocking transport of glucose into the tissues.

28. T F Obesity is a frequent finding in patients with NIDDM.

▼ *Match each statement in column A with the appropriate condition in column B.*

Column A

29. _____ Most likely to occur in an elderly person with NIDDM
30. _____ More likely to occur in a person with IDDM
31. _____ Often caused by inadequate food or missed meals
32. _____ Kussmaul's respirations are characteristic
33. _____ Hyperglycemia usually more severe
34. _____ Reversed by administration of glucose or glucagon
35. _____ Confusion, restlessness, and diaphoresis
36. _____ Rehydration and insulin used in treatment

Column B

a. Diabetic ketoacidosis (DKA)
b. Hyperglycemic, hyperosmolar, non-ketotic coma (HHNK)
c. Hypoglycemia

▼ *Circle the letter preceding each item below that correctly answers each question or completes the statement. More than one answer may be correct.*

37. Glucagon can best be described as a hormone that is:
   a. Secreted by the pancreatic alpha cells
   b. Effective in raising blood glucose levels
   c. Important in preventing hypoglycemia during the fasting state
   d. Important in preventing glycosuria
   e. Synergistic in its actions with insulin

38. Glucagon is used primarily to treat the patient with:
   a. DKA
   b. HHNK
   c. Insulin-induced hypoglycemia
   d. Hypokalemia

39. The diagnosis of hypoglycemic coma in an unconscious patient is *best* established by which of the following?
   a. Cerebrospinal fluid glucose of 45 mg/dl or less
   b. Blood glucose of 45 mg/dl or less and serum insulin of 100 μU/ml
   c. Blood glucose of 45 mg/dl or less with reversal of coma after rapid intravenous glucose administration
   d. An electroencephalogram showing slow delta waves

40. It is important to treat hypoglycemia *promptly* in a diabetic patient to prevent:
   a. Depletion of liver glycogen
   b. Permanent brain damage
   c. Peripheral neuropathy
   d. Retinopathy
   e. Weight loss

41. Central nervous system manifestations related to inadequate glucose for metabolism by the brain include:
   a. Bizarre behavior
   b. Seizures
   c. Coma
   d. Hypothermia

42. The clinical situation of large fluctuations in blood glucose in a patient with hyperglycemia is called:
   a. Somogyi effect
   b. Pancreatic instability
   c. Addison's response
   d. Cushing effect

43. Untreated hyperglycemia in a patient with IDDM results in:
   a. Metabolic alkalosis
   b. Metabolic acidosis
   c. Increasing lethargy → coma
   d. Respiratory acidosis
   e. Osmotic diuresis and dehydration

44. The primary difference between DKA and HHNK is:
   a. The level of hyperosmolality
   b. The level of hyperglycemia
   c. The amount of extracellular fluid volume depletion
   d. The amount of ketones produced

45. The chronic effect of diabetes on the nervous system is mainly a result of:
   a. Collapse of the vertebrae
   b. Increased incidence of seizures
   c. Peripheral neuropathy
   d. Degeneration of the anterior horn cells

46. Which of the following statements concerning intensive insulin therapy for diabetes (use of an external insulin pump or multidose insulin injections guided by frequent blood glucose monitoring) is *correct?*
   a. The DCCT study definitely showed that intensive insulin therapy reduced the likelihood of retinopathy, nephropathy, and neuropathy in patients with IDDM compared with standard therapy.
   b. Intensive insulin therapy failed to reduce the level of glycated hemoglobin.
   c. All patients with diabetes mellitus should receive such therapy.
   d. Hypoglycemia is a more frequent complication than the standard therapy.

47. A level of glycated hemoglobin indicating good control of hyperglycemia in a diabetic patient would be:
   a. 10% or more
   b. 8%
   c. 6% to 8%
   d. Less than 6%

BIBLIOGRAPHY ▼ PART X

Abboud CF: Laboratory diagnosis of hypopituitarism, *Mayo Clin Proc* 61:35-48, 1986.

Bischoff LG et al: Acute and chronic effects of hypoglycemia on cognitive and psychomotor performance, *Nebr Med J* 77(9):253-263, 1992.

Brink SJ, Stewart C: Insulin pump treatment in insulin-dependent diabetes mellitus children, adolescents, and young adults, *JAMA* 255:617, 1986.

DeGroot LJ, editor: *Endocrinology,* ed 2, Philadelphia, 1989, Saunders.

Diabetes Control and Complications Trial Research Group: Effects of intensive treatment of diabetes on the development and progression of long-term complications in insulin-dependent diabetes mellitus, *N Engl J Med* 329:977-986, 1993.

Eisenbarth GS: Genes, generator of diversity, glycoconjugates, and autoimmune B-cell insufficiency in type I diabetes, *Diabetes* 36:365, 1987.

Eisenbarth GS: Type I diabetes: clinical implications of autoimmunity, *Hosp Prac* 22(9):167-177, 1987.

Givens JR, Goodman RC: Hirsutism and polycystic ovary syndrome, *Hosp Prac* 21:10A, 81-104, 1986.

Greenspan FS, Baxter JD: *Basic and clinical endocrinology,* ed 4, East Norwalk, Conn, 1994, Appleton & Lange.

Henry RR: Glucose control and insulin resistance in non–insulin dependent diabetes mellitus, *Ann Intern Med* 124(1 pt 2):97-103, 1996.

Hurst JW, editor: *Medicine for the practicing physician,* ed 3, Boston, 1992, Butterworth-Hinemann, pp 515-518, 529-533.

Isselbacher KJ et al, editors: *Harrison's principles of internal medicine,* ed 13, New York, 1994, McGraw-Hill.

Kahn CR, White MF: The insulin receptor and the molecular mechanism of insulin action. *J Clin Invest* 82:1151-1156, 1988.

Kelley WN et al, editors: *Textbook of internal medicine,* ed 2, Philadelphia, 1992, Lippincott.

National Diabetes Data Group: Classification and diagnosis of diabetes mellitus and other categories of glucose intolerance, *Diabetes* 28(12):1039-1057, 1979.

O'Sullivan JB et al: Gestational diabetes and perinatal mortality rate, *Am J Obstet Gynecol* 116(7):901-904, 1973.

Rakel RE, editor: *The endocrine system,* Philadelphia, 1989, Saunders.

Schteingart DE: Cushing syndrome in medical therapy of endocrine tumors, *Endocrinol Metab Clin North Am* 18:311, 1989.

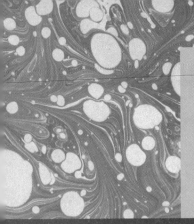

PART ELEVEN
REPRODUCTIVE SYSTEM DISORDERS

The male and female reproductive systems consist of gonads and tubular structures. The gonads produce gametes, ova, and spermatozoa, which are specialized cells that unite, male and female, to produce a new individual. The systems of both genders provide means for deposition of spermatozoa from the male reproductive system to the female reproductive system where the gametes unite and the resultant zygote is nurtured, grows, and develops until birth. Hormones direct and regulate the development and maintenance of the structures and sexual functions.

Dysfunctions of the reproductive system can be categorized broadly into developmental, endocrinologic, infectious processes, and neoplasms. Chapter 64 discusses disorders of the female system, such as menstrual problems, endocrine malfunctions, infections, and benign and malignant conditions of the reproductive organs and breasts. Chapter 65 discusses disorders of the male system, such as hypogonadism, functional alterations, infections, and benign and malignant neoplastic changes of the reproductive organs. Chapter 66 discusses sexually transmitted diseases, such as the classic venereal diseases of syphilis and gonorrhea, as well as other epidemiologically important infections transmitted sexually. ▼

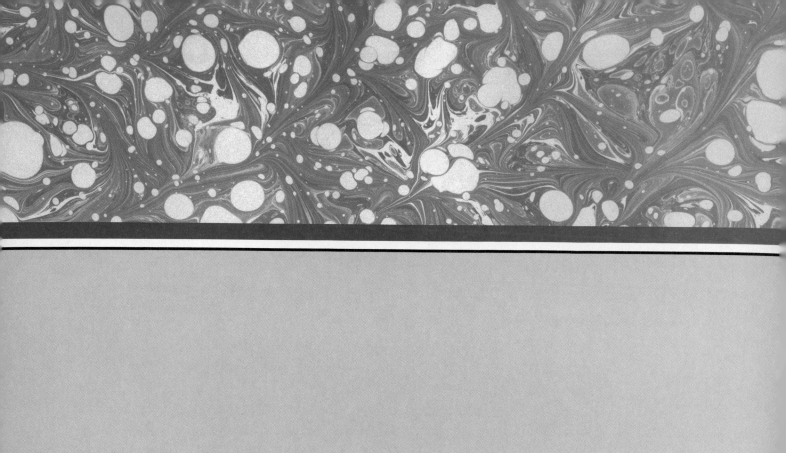

CHAPTER 64

Female Reproductive System Disorders

EVELYN J. PIEHL

ANATOMY AND PHYSIOLOGY

The internal organs of the female reproductive system are two ovaries, two fallopian tubes or oviducts, the uterus, and the vagina (Fig. 64-1). The external genitalia collectively are called the *vulva* and comprise the structures visible externally from the pubis to the perineum: the mons pubis, the labia majora, the labia minora, the clitoris, and the vestibule, an almond-shaped area inside the labia minora. The urethral meatus, the vaginal opening or introitus, and two sets of glands, Skene's glands and Bartholin's glands, open onto the vestibule (Fig. 64-2).

In the mature female the ovaries develop and release ova (oogenesis) and produce steroid hormones: the estrogens—estrone (E_1), estradiol (E_2), and estriol (E_3)—and androgens and progesterone. Small amounts of estrogens and androgens are also secreted by the adrenal cortex. The androgens are converted to estrogens peripherally in adipose tissue. Estradiol is the most potent estrogen and is secreted in the largest amounts by the ovaries.

The fallopian tubes extend from the ovaries to the uterus and open into the uterine cavity, providing a direct communication from the peritoneal cavity to the uterine cavity.

The uterus lies centrally in the pelvis and is divided structurally into the body or corpus and the cervix. The inner layer, the *endometrium,* consists of surface epithelium, glands, and connective tissue (stroma). The endometrium is shed during menstruation. At the lowest portion of the corpus is the *internal os* of the cervix. The *external os* is at the lower end of the cervix. The canal of the cervix provides a direct communication from the cavity of the uterine body, through the internal os and the external os, to the vagina.

The vagina extends from the cervix of the uterus to the *introitus* on the vestibule, the border between the internal and external genital structures. Thus there is continuous communication from outside the body to the peritoneal cavity through reproductive system structures. The internal pelvic organs can be palpated through the thin walls of the upper vagina, and there is ready access surgically through the vaginal wall behind the cervix to the peritoneal cavity.

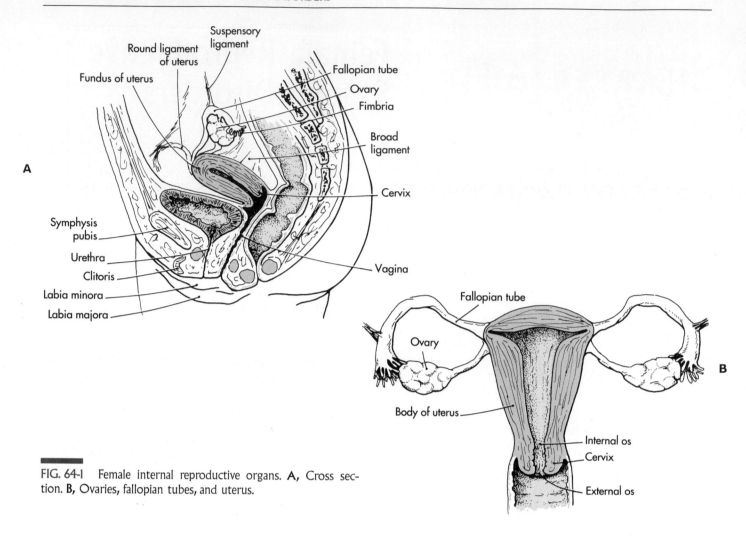

FIG. 64-1   Female internal reproductive organs. A, Cross section. B, Ovaries, fallopian tubes, and uterus.

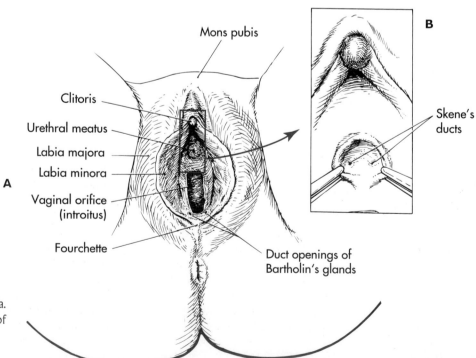

FIG. 64-2   Female external genitalia. A, Vulva. B, Paraurethral opening of Skene's glands.

The mons pubis lies over the anterior surface of the symphysis pubis and extends downward and is continuous with the labia majora. Medial to the labia majora are the labia minora. The labia minora converge and fuse inferiorly to form the fourchette and superiorly to form the prepuce of the clitoris. The *clitoris* is a small body of erectile tissue above the labia minora.

FUNCTIONS OF THE FEMALE REPRODUCTIVE SYSTEM

The female reproductive system functions by means of complex hormonal interactions to produce a mature ovum cyclically and to prepare and maintain an environment for conception and gestation (Fig. 64-3).

Hormonal Functions

Cyclic hormonal changes initiate and regulate ovarian function and endometrial changes. The regular, monthly occurrence of a menstrual cycle depends on a series of cyclic, well-coordinated steps, which involve hormone secretion at various levels of this integrated system. The center of hormonal control of the reproductive system is the hypothalamus. The two hypothalamic gonadotropic hormone–releasing hormones (GnRH), called follicle-stimulating hormone–releasing hormone (FSHRH) and luteinizing hormone–releasing hormone (LHRH), stimulate the anterior pituitary to secrete follicle-stimulating hormone (FSH) and luteinizing hormone (LH), respectively. The series of events initiated by the secretion of FSH and LH involves production of estrogens and progesterone from the ovary that result in physiologic changes in the uterus. Estrogen and progesterone in turn influence the production of the specific gonadotropic-releasing hormones in a feedback system that regulates gonadotropic hormone levels. These steps have been carefully studied through daily measurements of the levels of FSH and LH in the blood and levels of estradiol and progesterone in the blood and urine. The ovarian cycle, the endometrial cycle, and the changes in the levels of the hormones during a menstrual cycle are illustrated in Fig. 64-4.

Normal Menstrual Cycle

Menarche, the onset of menstruation, usually occurs between 12 and 13 years of age, with a range of 10 to 16 years. Menarche is normally preceded by a period of maturation that may span 2 years. During this interval, an orderly sequence of events occurs, which includes breast development, growth of pubic and axillary hair, and a spurt in somatic linear growth. Generally, the cycle interval ranges from 15 to 45 days, with the average being 28 days. Duration of flow varies with a range of 2 to 8 days,

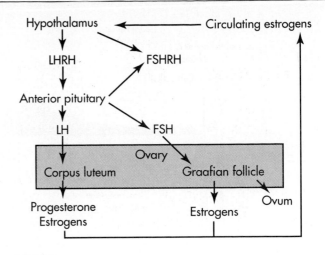

FIG. 64-3 Hypothalamic-pituitary ovarian hormone axis. *LHRH,* Luteinizing hormone–releasing hormone; *FSHRH,* follicle-stimulating hormone–releasing hormone.

with the average being 4 to 6 days. Menstrual blood does not clot. The amount lost each cycle ranges from 60 ml to 80 ml.

Ovarian cycle

Follicular phase. The cycle begins with the first day of menstrual flow, or sloughing of the endometrium. FSH induces the growth of several primordial follicles in the ovaries. Generally only one continues to grow and becomes the graafian follicle and the others degenerate. The follicle consists of an ovum and its two surrounding cell layers. The inner layer of granulosa cells synthesizes progesterone, which is secreted into the follicular fluid during the first half of the menstrual cycle and serves as a precursor for estrogen synthesis by the surrounding layer of theca interna cells. Estrogen is synthesized in the luteinized cells of the theca interna. The pathway of estrogen biosynthesis proceeds from progesterone and pregnenolone via 17-hydroxylated derivatives to androstenedione, testosterone, and estradiol. A high content of aromatizing enzyme in these cells facilitates the conversion of androgens to estrogens. In the follicle the primary oocyte begins to mature. At the same time the growing follicle secretes increasing amounts of estrogen into the system. Rising estrogen levels cause LHRH to be released by a positive feedback system.

Luteal phase. LH induces ovulation of the maturing oocyte. Just before the ovulation the primary oocyte completes its first meiotic division. High levels of estrogen now inhibit the production of FSH. Next estrogen levels begin to drop. After expulsion of the oocyte from the graafian follicle, the granulosa layer becomes vascularized and intensely luteinized, forming the yellow corpus luteum of the ovary. The corpus luteum continues to secrete small amounts of estrogen and increasing amounts of progesterone.

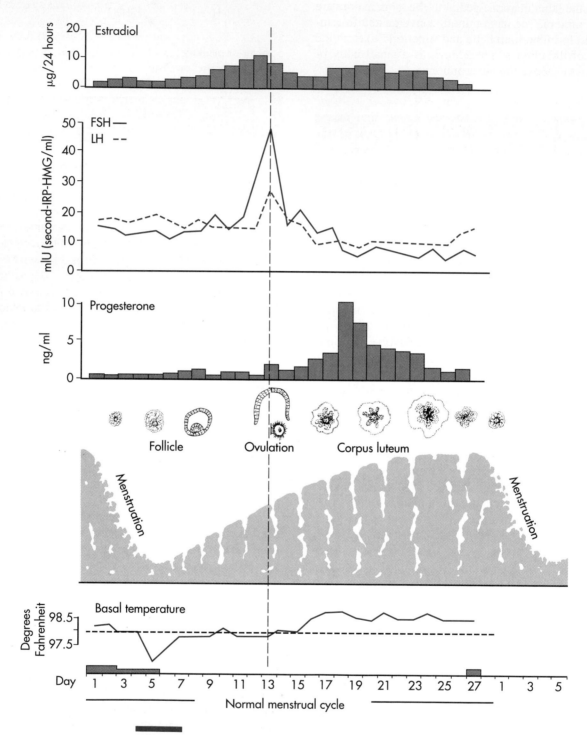

FIG. 64-4 Normal menstrual cycle. The horizontal bars on the time scale indicate the occurrence of menses. The interrupted vertical line at midcycle depicts the time of ovulation. Basal body temperature rises during the luteal phase of the cycle, coinciding with the onset of progesterone secretion. *FSH*, Follicle-stimulating hormone; *LH*, luteinizing hormone.

Endometrial cycle

Proliferative phase. Immediately after menstruation the endometrium is thin and in a resting state. This stage lasts about 5 days. Increasing levels of estrogen from the growing follicle stimulate the endometrial stroma to begin to grow and thicken, the glands to undergo hypertrophy and proliferation, and the blood vessels to become prominent. The glands and stroma grow at about an equal pace. As the glands become longer, they maintain their straight, tubular form. The glandular epithelium is columnar with uniform eosinophilic cytoplasm and central nuclei. The stroma is fairly compact in the basal layer but looser toward the surface. Vessels follow a slightly spiraling course and are smaller. The length of the proliferative phase varies widely among individuals, ending at ovulation.

Secretory phase. After ovulation, under the influence of increasing levels of progesterone and continuing estrogen from the corpus luteum, the endometrium becomes thick and velvetlike. There is greater and more elaborate convolution of glands and infolding of the glandular epithelium, giving a "sawtooth" appearance. The nuclei of the cells move downward, and the surface of the epithelium acquires a frayed appearance. The stroma becomes edematous. Heavy infiltration with leukocytes occurs, and the blood vessels become more and more tightly coiled and dilated. The length of the secretory phase among all women is constant at 14 ± 2 days.

Menstrual phase. The corpus luteum functions until about the twenty-third or twenty-fourth day of a 28-day cycle and then begins to regress. The resulting sharp drop in progesterone and estrogen removes the stimulation to the endometrium. Ischemic changes occur in the arterioles, and menstrual flow occurs.

CLIMACTERIC AND THE MENOPAUSE

The climacteric is the physiologic phase when regression of ovarian function takes place. Menopause, which is the cessation of regular cycle uterine bleeding, is just one event in the climacteric. Menopause usually occurs between the ages of 45 and 52 years. During the climacteric, estradiol levels decrease and the ovaries decrease in size and are virtually devoid of follicles. Microscopic examination reveals cortical thinning and a relative thickening of the medulla from increased fibrous connective tissue. Blood vessels at the hilus and medulla become progressively sclerotic. Anatomic involution of the ovaries is accompanied by a decrease in their ovulatory and endocrine functions. The decrease in circulating estradiol levels increases pituitary gonadotropin secretion by negative feedback. This increased production of FSH and LH continues for many years after the onset of menopause. Signs, symptoms, and physiologic changes associated with menopause result from decreasing circulating estrogen. Menopausal symptoms may begin before changes in the menstrual cycle occur. Regular menstrual bleeding may occur until the menopause, with cycles becoming shorter because of shorter follicular phases, or cycles may be variable and more widely spaced, with some being ovulatory and some being anovulatory. Any bleeding after 6 months of amenorrhea is abnormal, and the cause must be investigated to rule out carcinoma.

Common symptoms of menopause include hot flushes, palpitations, headache, cold hands and feet, irritability, vertigo, anxiety, nervousness, depression, insomnia, night sweats, forgetfulness, inability to concentrate, fatigue, and weight gain. The most common problem is vasomotor instability manifested by hot flushes. The typical sign of the hot flush is reddened and warm skin, principally of the head and neck, which lasts anywhere from a few seconds to 2 minutes. This is followed by cold chills. Other associated physiologic changes are increased heart rate, peripheral vasodilation, a rise in skin temperature, and concomitant pulsatile LH release. Bilateral oophorectomy at any age after menarche results in the same symptoms.

The skin of the genitalia and the lining of the vagina and urethra become thinner and dryer, resulting in a greater potential for irritation, infection, and dyspareunia. The labia, clitoris, uterus, and ovaries decrease in size. Skin elasticity decreases. An increase in facial or body hair growth may occur as a result of the decrease in estrogen levels and the unopposed effect of circulating androgens.

Osteoporosis occurs in about 25% of postmenopausal women within 15 to 20 years after menopause. Men of the same age can also be affected with the same type of osteoporosis as a part of the aging process, but the incidence and the extent of bone loss are greater in women. Vertebral fractures, Colles' fractures, and hip fractures are the major complications. Hip fractures are responsible for a mortality as high as 15% in women older than 60 years.

Symptomatic Therapeutic Measures

Any therapy chosen during the perimenopausal and postmenopausal years must be individualized. Estrogen replacement therapy decreases the incidence of osteoporotic fractures, prevents or reverses atrophic genital and urethral lining changes, diminishes hot flushes, and may decrease the incidence of atherosclerotic coronary disease. Estrogen replacement therapy is absolutely contraindicated in women with, or with a history of, estrogen-dependent tumors of the breast, uterus, or kidney; genital bleeding of unknown cause; deep vein thrombosis; cerebrovascular disease; or liver disease. Estrogens are relatively contraindicated in women with hypertension, diabetes mellitus, cholecystitis and cholelithiasis, pancreatitis, congestive heart disease, past endometriosis, or retinopathy.

Estrogen and a progestin are administered in a cyclic fashion to mimic the endometrial cycle and prevent hyperplasia of the endometrium. Several different regimens can be used. Uterine bleeding (menstrual periods) will occur in about 50% of women on replacement therapy. Estrogen alone may be administered continuously to women who have undergone a hysterectomy/salpingo-oophorectomy, although some clinicians prescribe cyclic therapy with estrogen and progestin in these women.

A thorough history and complete physical examination, including a mammogram, are mandatory before prescribing estrogen replacement therapy. Periodic Papanicolaou (Pap) smears of the cervix (or of the vaginal cuff in a woman who has had a hysterectomy), yearly mammograms, and endometrial biopsy every 1 to 2 years or if there is breakthrough bleeding should be performed to monitor for and rule out any malignant changes of the cervix, breast, or endometrium.

MENSTRUAL DISORDERS

Amenorrhea

Primary amenorrhea is the absence of menarche by the age of 17 years, regardless of the presence or absence of secondary sexual development; secondary amenorrhea is the absence of menses for 3 months or longer after having established menstrual cycles. Amenorrhea is physiologic in the prepubertal girl, the pregnant woman, and the postmenopausal woman; otherwise, amenorrhea is an indication of dysfunction or abnormality somewhere in the reproductive system. Amenorrhea is a symptom and not a disease entity. The cause of amenorrhea can be physiologic, endocrinologic, organic, or developmental (Table 64-1).

Girls with no evidence of onset of puberty by age 13 years or who do not develop menses by 5 years after onset of puberty should be evaluated. Mature women who are amenorrheic for 3 months should also be evaluated. A thorough history and physical examination, with attention to the influence of altered hormonal states, are essential first steps to clinical evaluation. Essential information involves dietary and exercise habits, evidence for psychologic disturbances, life-style, environmental stresses, family history of genetic disorders, abnormal growth and development, and signs of androgen excess. The physical examination includes inspection of the genitalia and palpation of the pelvic organs and evaluation of body dimensions, body habitus, the extent and distribution of body hair, and breast development and secretions. The normal arm span is about equal to body height; in hypogonadism, arm span is more than 2 inches greater than body height. Breast development and pubic hair are evaluated according to the Tanner developmental scale.

TABLE 64-1   Causes of Amenorrhea

Developmental Stage	Pathology
PRIMARY AMENORRHEA	
Absent or arrested secondary sexual development	Hypothalamic dysfunction Pituitary dysfunction Ovarian failure or dysgenesis
Normal secondary sexual development	Hypothalamic dysfunction Pituitary dysfunction Incomplete development of müllerian system
Abnormal secondary sexual development	Hypothalamic dysfunction Pituitary dysfunction Ovarian failure or dysgenesis Nonphysiologic sex hormone production Androgen insensitivity
SECONDARY AMENORRHEA	
Postmenarche	Endometrial dysfunction Ovarian dysfunction Hypothalamic dysfunction Pituitary dysfunction

Pelvic examination and palpation of the internal organs can usually rule out anomalies of müllerian duct derivatives, such as imperforate hymen, vaginal or uterine aplasia, or vaginal septum.

Laboratory assessment of amenorrhea

The first step is to determine whether hormonal failure is caused by a hypothalamic-pituitary problem or by a gonadal disorder. This determination is made by measuring serum FSH. If the serum FSH is repeatedly elevated, the woman most likely has a primary ovarian failure. If the serum FSH is normal or low, the problem most likely lies in the hypothalamus or the pituitary gland. In this case, evaluation of thyroid and adrenal function may determine if the patient has isolated gonadotropin deficiency or panhypopituitarism. In the presence of galactorrhea, a serum prolactin level should be obtained. A radiograph of the pituitary fossa and computed axial tomography (CT) of the pituitary gland may help determine if the patient has a pituitary tumor with or without suprasellar extension. In patients in whom amenorrhea is associated with hirsutism, measurement of 17-ketosteroids and serum testosterone and DHEA should be carried out. Levels are usually elevated in patients with excessive androgen secretion. More specific tests to determine the source of the excessive secretion of androgens include a pelvic examination, laparoscopy, adrenal scintiscan, and abdominal CT scan. Selective catheterization and sampling of blood from the adrenal and gonadal veins may help localize the source of androgen hypersecretion. Conditions related to androgen excess are discussed in Chapter 61.

Treatment of the amenorrheic patient

Treatment of amenorrhea is often based on the specific underlying pathologic condition. Women with prolactin-secreting pituitary adenomas should be treated with either transsphenoidal resection of the pituitary tumor or suppression of prolactin secretion with bromocriptine. Women with excessive androgen secretion should receive suppressive therapy with corticosteroids or oral contraceptives. Both of these preparations suppress the excessive secretion of androgens, probably by inhibiting gonadotropin release.

Women with hypothalamic-pituitary or ovarian deficiency should receive replacement therapy with estrogens and progesterone administered cyclically. Combined treatment with estrogens and progesterone helps to maintain secondary sexual characteristics and prevent vaginal and breast atrophy and osteopenia. Therapy can be continued through the expected time of menopause at age 45 to 52 years.

Women with primary gonadal disorders remain infertile. However, ovulation can be induced and fertility restored in some women with isolated gonadotropin deficiency, polycystic ovarian disease (PCOD), or excessive weight loss if weight is regained. Ovulation and fertility can be obtained with clomiphene citrate, a nonsteroidal compound that has both estrogenic and antiestrogenic properties, depending on the site of action. In responsive women, ovulation occurs 4 to 8 days and menstruation 14 to 21 days after clomiphene has been stopped. Several courses of treatment may be necessary before ovulation and fertility or normal menstrual cycles are established. An otherwise intact pituitary gland is required for a positive response to therapy.

In women with hypopituitarism or pituitary tumors, fertility can be restored by treatment with human FSH and human chorionic gonadotropin (hCG), which acts like LH. This therapy is expensive and requires careful control of dosage and estradiol response to avoid multiple pregnancies or the development of ovarian cysts.

Premenstrual Syndrome

Premenstrual syndrome (PMS) or premenstrual tension (PMT) is a constellation of physical and psychologic symptoms that occur during the luteal phase of the menstrual cycle and diminish with the onset of menses. They may be severe enough to interfere with some aspect of the person's (and her family's) life. In about 10% of women, premenstrual symptoms are severe enough that medical attention is sought. Although no specific definition of PMS is universally accepted, most experienced clinicians require three findings to make the diagnosis: (1) the symptom complex is consistent with PMS, (2) the symptoms occur exclusively during the luteal phase of ovulatory menstrual cycles, and (3) the symptoms are severe enough to disrupt the person's life. The symptoms

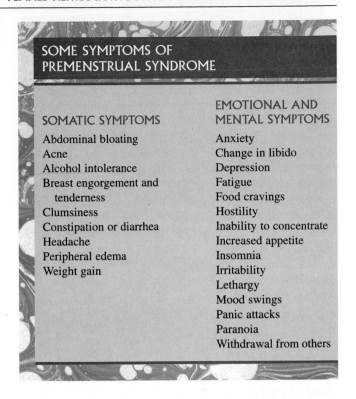

SOME SYMPTOMS OF PREMENSTRUAL SYNDROME

SOMATIC SYMPTOMS	EMOTIONAL AND MENTAL SYMPTOMS
Abdominal bloating	Anxiety
Acne	Change in libido
Alcohol intolerance	Depression
Breast engorgement and tenderness	Fatigue
Clumsiness	Food cravings
Constipation or diarrhea	Hostility
Headache	Inability to concentrate
Peripheral edema	Increased appetite
Weight gain	Insomnia
	Irritability
	Lethargy
	Mood swings
	Panic attacks
	Paranoia
	Withdrawal from others

associated with PMS are diverse, but each patient describes a unique set of multiple symptoms, all occurring during the characteristic time in the cycle. Psychologic disorders, including depression and anxiety, frequently are confused with PMS and must be ruled out before initiating therapy. At least 150 symptoms have been reported with this syndrome. Some are listed in the box above. Estimates of the incidence of PMS symptoms range from 25% to 100% of menstruating women. For many, the symptoms are only annoying and do not significantly interfere with their activities; for others, perhaps 5% to 10% of women with PMS, there are serious difficulties. The diagnosis of PMS is best made after the woman keeps a menstrual calendar with a daily symptom diary for 2 to 3 months. Fewer than 50% of these women are found to have a definite diagnosis of PMS when their records are evaluated for the cyclicity of symptomatology present with true PMS.

Symptoms may begin to occur at menarche and worsen with time; most women report that symptoms begin after childbirth and worsen after each pregnancy. Secondary psychologic difficulties such as marital discord, withdrawal from social activities, and difficulties maintaining relationships, including with their children, are often seen in women with long-standing PMS.

The cause of PMS is unknown. Theories include derangements in the amounts of estrogen and progesterone production, changes in other ovarian hormone production, altered central nervous system (CNS) effects of ovarian steroids, and changes in serotonin synthesis during the luteal phase.

The symptoms are so variable that no single therapy is effective for all women. The major goal of treatment is to provide as much relief as possible for the most significant symptoms. Simple interventions, such as exercise, alteration of diet, and avoidance of salt, alcohol, and caffeine, may result in dramatic improvement and should be given an adequate trial. Changes in life-style to reduce stress may also provide relief. For women in whom symptoms of anxiety predominate, a trial of anxiolytic agents administered during the luteal phase can be tried. However, the mainstay of treatment for PMS is use of agents that suppress ovarian function. Oral contraceptive pills may provide a simple and inexpensive solution. Alternatives to use for relief of symptoms for some women include GnRH agonists such as medroxyprogesterone acetate to suppress ovulation. Abnormal uterine bleeding and progestin-related adverse effects associated with this drug may limit its usefulness. Emotional support, education, and counseling for the woman and her family are also beneficial.

Dysmenorrhea

Dysmenorrhea is pain during menstruation caused by uterine muscle cramping. Primary dysmenorrhea occurs in the absence of any underlying physical disturbance and only during ovulatory cycles. The cause is the presence of excessive amounts of prostaglandin $F_{2\alpha}$ in menstrual blood, which stimulates uterine hyperactivity. The major symptom is pain that begins with the onset of menses. The pain may be sharp, dull, cyclic, or steady; it lasts for a few hours to 1 day. Occasionally symptoms last longer but rarely more than 72 hours. Associated systemic symptoms are nausea, diarrhea, headache, and emotional changes.

Treatment is use of nonsteroidal antiinflammatory agents, which block prostaglandin synthesis through inhibition of the enzyme cyclooxygenase. Therapy is most successful when begun before the onset of menstruation and continued until the symptoms have abated. Progesterone will also inhibit endometrial prostaglandin synthesis. Therefore treatment with oral contraceptives is also effective. These drugs reduce the amount of menstrual fluid and thus the prostaglandin concentration.

Secondary dysmenorrhea occurs because of an underlying physical problem such as endometriosis, uterine polyps, leiomyoma, cervical stenosis, or pelvic inflammatory disease (PID). In the case of an abnormal pelvic examination, further evaluation is necessary to establish the diagnosis. Dysmenorrhea may occur in women with increasing menometrorrhagia. A careful evaluation should be done to look for abnormalities within the uterine cavity or pelvis that may be precipitating both signs. Hysteroscopy, hysterosalpingogram (HSG), transvaginal sonogram (TVS), and laparoscopy are all procedures that may be used for evaluation. Treatment is aimed at correcting the underlying condition.

Dysfunctional Uterine Bleeding

Dysfunctional uterine bleeding is bleeding that occurs when no demonstrable organic cause is present. Most patients with dysfunctional bleeding are having anovulatory cycles. Anovulation occurs secondary to failure of any developing ovarian follicles to mature to the point of ovulation with subsequent formation of the corpus luteum. The exact cause of anovulation is not completely understood but probably results from dysfunction of the hypothalamic-pituitary-ovarian axis. This results in continued production of estrogen by the follicles and, without a corpus luteum, no production of progesterone. This altered hormone state results in alternating periods of anovulatory bleeding, which is usually very heavy, with amenorrhea. This situation is caused by the variation in the degree of estrogen stimulation to the endometrium, as well as to the degree of estrogen withdrawal. The frequency of the periodic bleeding episodes depends on variations in the number of functioning follicles. Several can be active at one time, producing high levels of estrogen. Under the influence of high estrogen levels and no progesterone, the endometrium can proliferate for weeks or months. In time, estrogen withdrawal will occur, caused either by the eventual degeneration of some follicles, causing levels to drop, or by the needs of the enlarging endometrial tissue becoming greater than the amount of estrogen produced can support. Both conditions result in estrogen breakthrough bleeding, which can vary in timing, duration, and amount.

In adolescents, irregular, prolonged, or excessive bleeding is commonly associated with the establishment of regular menstrual cycles secondary to immaturity of the hypothalamic-pituitary-ovarian axis and results in anovulatory cycles in 20% of cases. In the first 2 years after menarche, the incidence of anovulatory cycles is 75% or more and nearly 50% in the next 2 years. Forty percent of cases occur in women over 40 years of age. In this situation, premenopausal changes of the hypothalamic-pituitary-ovarian axis are occurring and result in anovulatory cycles. However, in older women, care is given to exclude pathologic causes because of the possibility of endometrial cancer. If bleeding is particularly heavy, an acute condition can develop that requires prompt intervention because hypovolemia and anemia may develop secondary to blood loss.

The diagnosis is made by history, absence of ovulatory cycle body temperature changes, and low serum progesterone levels. Diagnostic procedures are usually not necessary in young perimenarchal patients, but pelvic examination must be performed to exclude pregnancy or pathologic conditions. In the older perimenopausal woman, endometrial aspiration, curettage, or both should be done for tissue examination to clearly establish that anovulatory or dyssynchronous cycles are the cause and to rule out malignant changes.

Treatment initially is aimed at interrupting the process

TABLE 64-2   Abnormal Bleeding Patterns

Terminology	Pattern
Menorrhagia	Heavy or prolonged menstrual flow
Hypomenorrhea	Unusually light menstrual flow; spotting
Metrorrhagia	Bleeding at any time between periods
Polymenorrhea	Frequent menstrual periods
Menometrorrhagia	Bleeding at irregular intervals; amount and duration vary
Oligomenorrhea	Menstrual bleeding at more than 35-day intervals; decreased amount
Contact bleeding	Bleeding after coitus; caused by erosion, cervical polyps, vaginitis, or cervicitis

with use of hormonal therapy. Numerous regimens are available, including estrogens followed by progesterone, progesterone alone, or combination oral contraceptive pills. High-dose conjugated estrogens are prescribed daily until bleeding is controlled—usually 2 to 3 days; then a lower dose is prescribed daily during the remainder of the cycle. Medroxyprogesterone acetate daily is added from day 15 to day 25 of the cycle to stimulate the luteal phase. The hormones are discontinued on day 25. Menses should then occur within 3 to 4 days. Oral contraceptive pills alone at three or four times the usual dose can be effective and more simple than the sequential hormones. The dose is lowered when bleeding diminishes. Medroxyprogesterone acetate daily for 10 days can be used if biopsy examination shows proliferative endometrium. Therapy is continued for three to six cycles and then discontinued. Further evaluation is required if anovulatory cycles continue.

Abnormal Uterine Bleeding

Abnormal uterine bleeding includes bleeding caused by pregnancy, systemic disease, or cancer, as well as abnormal menstrual bleeding. Patterns of the bleeding have been defined and placed into seven categories, six of which are associated with the menstrual cycle (Table 64-2).

Evaluation of abnormal uterine bleeding requires a careful history and physical examination. Diagnostic and screening procedures include cytologic examination, endometrial biopsy, histologic examination, hysteroscopy, and dilation and curettage. Other procedures used are assay of the beta-subunit of human chorionic gonadotropin (hCG) for complications of pregnancy and trophoblastic disease, pelvic ultrasonography, and laparoscopy.

Management of these abnormal conditions depends on the specific diagnosis, realizing that more than one condition can be involved. If pathologic causes are excluded, if there is no significant risk of cancer developing, and if no acute life-threatening hemorrhage is occurring, many women with abnormal menstrual bleeding can be treated with hormone therapy.

REPRODUCTIVE ORGAN INFECTIOUS PROCESSES

Infections can occur in any of the reproductive organs and structures. The anatomy of the female reproductive system allows ascent of organisms from the lower tract to the upper tract and potentially the peritoneal cavity, as well as descent from the upper tract when there is hematogenous spread of the organism from a primary site elsewhere in the body.

Infections of the cervix, endometrium, and salpinx frequently occur concurrently, and they share overlapping microbial etiologies. Histopathologic studies show that 40% of women with mucopurulent cervicitis and 80% of women with acute salpingitis also have endometritis. Cervicitis and salpingitis are common infections of sexually active women during the reproductive years. These infections are a major public health concern because of the profound impact that salpingitis has on the reproductive health of women. Damage to the fallopian tubes that results from salpingitis is the major cause of tubal infertility and ectopic pregnancy.

Lower Genital Tract Infections
Vaginitis (vulvovaginitis)

Vaginal infections are the most common gynecologic complaint. Because the vulva is usually involved, the term *vulvovaginitis* is more correct. More than 90% of cases of vulvovaginitis are caused by bacteria of the *Candida* species or the bacterium *Trichomonas vaginalis*. The remaining 10% of cases are caused by a variety of etiologic agents.

Bacterial vaginosis. Bacterial vaginosis is a nonspecific vaginitis caused by a disturbance of the normal vaginal microbial ecosystem. No single bacterial species is responsible for the condition, but instead there is an overgrowth of a mixed flora that includes *Peptostreptococcus* and *Bacteroides* species, *Gardnerella vaginalis*, *Mobiluncus* species, and genital mycoplasmas. These overgrowths are associated with a loss of the normally dominant *Lactobacillus* species and rarely result in disease. Women who use an intrauterine contraceptive device, a cervical diaphragm, or spermicidal cream are more likely to have bacterial vaginosis. Prevalence is higher among sexually active young women than among their sexually inexperienced contemporaries. Sexual intercourse may be an inoculating event, but the role of sexual transmission is unknown.

With bacterial overgrowth, microbial decarboxylases facilitate the production of amines by anaerobes. Amines become volatile with high vaginal pH values, producing a fishy odor characteristic of vaginal secretions in bacterial vaginosis. Although 50% of women with bacterial vaginosis are asymptomatic, the cardinal symptom is the fishy vaginal malodor. Organisms associated with bacterial vaginosis have been isolated from amniotic fluid and with chorioamnionitis, postpartum endometritis, and bacteremia. Bacterial vaginosis in pregnancy may be associated with preterm premature rupture of membranes. In nonpregnant women, asymptomatic bacterial vaginosis may predispose to multiple-organism upper genital tract infections such as endometritis and salpingitis.

Diagnosis is made if at least three of the following four criteria are present: (1) adherent, white vaginal discharge, (2) a positive amine test (fishy odor noted when 10% potassium hydroxide (KOH) is added to vaginal secretions), (3) vaginal pH of 4.5 or higher, and (4) the presence of clue cells in vaginal secretions.

Treatment with metronidazole for 7 days results in immediate clearing of bacterial vaginosis; single-dose therapy results in immediate response also, but recurrence is more frequent. Clindamycin used as a cream or suppository for 7 days is also effective. In the past, women with asymptomatic bacterial vaginosis were not routinely treated. However, because it is known that there is a risk for development of upper tract disease, especially during pregnancy, treatment should be considered. During pregnancy, metronidazole is contraindicated in the first trimester.

Cervicitis

Cervicitis is an inflammatory condition of the cervix associated with pathologic organisms or puerperal infection. It is divided into two distinct syndromes. *Endocervicitis* is inflammation of the mucous membranes of the cervical canal and is most frequently caused by *Chlamydia trachomatis* and *Neisseria gonorrhoeae;* occasionally herpes simplex virus or *Haemophilus influenzae* causes endocervicitis. *Ectocervicitis* is inflammation of the stratified squamous epithelium of the cervix and is most often caused by *Trichomonas vaginalis, Candida albicans,* and herpes simplex virus. Cervicitis can be difficult to diagnose by clinical examination. Inflammation of the cervix may be visually evident at the time of examination; it may be apparent only with colposcopy or histopathologic examination; or there may be no inflammation even though organisms may be present. Cervical ectopy, the presence of endocervical columnar epithelium on the exposed visible exocervix (Fig. 64-5), also can cause an inflamed-looking cervix with mucus discharge. Women who are young, nulliparous, taking oral contraceptives, or pregnant tend to have a larger area of cervical ectopy. These populations may be at higher risk of developing cervicitis than other women.

Cervicitis caused by *Candida* species or associated with bacterial vaginosis may occur after overgrowth of these organisms in the vagina because of a change in vaginal flora and pH. The natural history of infection by

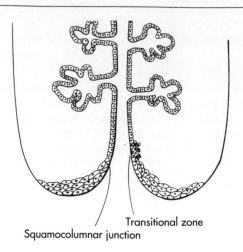

Transitional zone
Squamocolumnar junction

FIG. 64-5 Squamocolumnar junction of the uterine cervix.

these organisms has not been well studied. They can persist for extended periods if diagnosis and appropriate treatment are not done. The presence of abnormal organisms regardless of signs or symptoms should dictate whether therapy is necessary. Drug therapy should be instituted according to the etiology of the condition.

Upper Genital Tract Infections
Salpingitis (pelvic inflammatory disease)

Pelvic inflammatory disease (PID) is a general term used for a condition that more precisely is salpingitis or, if the ovaries are also involved, salpingo-oophoritis. Salpingitis is almost always a bacterial infection and occurs when microorganisms that are ordinarily confined to the cervix and vagina ascend through the cervix and, by means of the endometrium, through the uterus to the fallopian tubes. The ascent of the causative organism occurs most readily during menses. Salpingitis is most often caused by the sexually transmitted gonorrheal or chlamydial organisms and is more prevalent in women with multiple sexual partners. Some evidence exists that there can be spread to the salpinx by organisms that "piggyback" on motile sperm. About 17% of women become infertile from tubal occlusion, and 6% have an ectopic pregnancy after one episode of salpingitis.

The presence of an intrauterine device (IUD) is an independent risk factor for developing salpingitis, especially nongonococcal, nonchlamydial infections. The time of greatest risk for infection is soon after insertion of an IUD. More than half of infections with an IUD in place occur within 4 to 6 months of insertion. The administration of doxycycline at the time of insertion of an IUD is recommended because it reduces the risk of developing salpingitis.

Signs and symptoms with salpingitis vary widely. Half of women with acute salpingitis have more subtle manifestations, making a clear-cut diagnosis difficult to make based on symptoms. Typically, shortly after menstruation, there may be an abrupt onset of low abdominal pain with guarding, low-grade fever, and mucopurulent cervical discharge. With pelvic examination there is abdominal tenderness, cervical and uterine motion tenderness, adnexal tenderness, and perhaps an adnexal mass. Signs of more severe disease include temperature of at least 38° C or higher, purulent material from culdocentesis, and pelvic abscess. Abnormal laboratory tests include an elevated white blood cell count and gram-negative diplococci in cervical secretions. When salpingitis is suspected, the woman should have a serum pregnancy test done to rule out ectopic pregnancy as a cause of the signs and symptoms.

Treatment includes antibiotic therapy specific for any identified organism; optimal therapy includes treatment for gonorrhea and chlamydia. Severe manifestations such as peritonitis, nausea and vomiting, or high fever require hospitalization for intravenous (IV) antibiotic therapy. If an IUD is in place, it should be removed within 24 to 48 hours after initiating treatment. Healing frequently results in scarring of fallopian tube tissues and pelvic adhesions, which can occlude the tubes, causing infertility. Antimicrobial treatment may not prevent postinfection infertility because of irreversible tubal damage before treatment is begun (rate of 10% to 30%).

Oophoritis

Oophoritis occurs as a result of purulent material that drains from an infected fallopian tube. An abscess can form that involves the fimbriated end of the tube and ovary. Purulent material may also drain into the peritoneal cavity, causing peritonitis.

Primary oophoritis without accompanying salpingitis may occur by hematologic transmission from mumps, septicemia, or generalized systemic illness. The symptom of abdominal pain is usually mild and of short duration. Occasionally an abscess may form, but usually the infection subsides without severe symptoms or further problems.

SYSTEMIC INFECTION

Toxic Shock Syndrome

Toxic shock syndrome is an acute systemic illness caused by the toxin-producing *Staphylococcus aureus*. About 6% of women carry *S. aureus* vaginally, but only 2% have the types that are capable of producing the toxin. The toxin produces systemic effects by directly damaging cell membranes in peripheral tissues. The syndrome is highly associated with menstruation, particularly with tampon use, but is also associated with childbirth and major abdominal surgery.

Characteristic features are abrupt onset of high fever, myalgias, profuse nausea, vomiting, watery diarrhea, a diffuse sunburnlike rash, and skin desquamation that occurs 1 to 2 weeks after onset. Hypotension and frank shock develop, often with concomitant adult respiratory distress syndrome (ARDS). Abnormalities occur in all organ systems. Possible problems are acute renal failure with elevated blood urea nitrogen (BUN) or creatinine levels, altered state of mentation with coma, hepatic cell abnormalities, elevated muscle enzymes, thrombocytopenia, low serum calcium, and diffuse capillary leak syndrome with associated hypoalbuminemia.

Treatment requires hospitalization with fluid replacement and maintenance; antibiotics; and life-support measures as needed, including intubation and ventilation, vasopressor administration, and dialysis.

BENIGN LESIONS OF THE UTERUS AND OVARIES

Endometrial Hyperplasia and Polyps

Endometrial hyperplasia, an overgrowth of the endometrium, and *endometrial polyps,* soft pedunculated tumors, are caused by abnormal hormone production. The most common cause is anovulatory cycles, with prolonged production of estrogen and absence of progesterone. This condition is highly associated with dysfunctional uterine bleeding.

Diagnosis is made by examination of tissue after dilation and curettage (D and C) of the uterus. The diagnostic D and C often corrects the problem. In postmenopausal women, if hyperplasia progresses, hysterectomy may be indicated.

Leiomyomas

A *leiomyoma* is a benign, well-circumscribed uterine tumor. Other names for this tumor include fibroid, myoma, fibroma, and fibromyoma. Approximately 20% to 25% of women over the age of 35 years have a uterine leiomyoma. They are composed mostly of smooth muscle and some fibrous material.

Leiomyomas are classified according to their location. An *intramural* tumor is located in the muscle wall of the uterus and may distort the cavity as well as protrude from the external surface. A *subserous* tumor is just beneath the serosa and projects from the external surface of the uterus. This tumor may become pedunculated and extend into the pelvic or abdominal cavity. A *submucous* tumor is just beneath the endometrium. These tumors also may become pedunculated and may protrude into the uterine cavity, through the cervical os, into the vagina, or out the vaginal opening. In this last event, infection is a complication.

The size of leiomyomas varies greatly and can be large enough to fill the pelvic and abdominal cavities. They are subject to degeneration with alteration in blood supply caused by growth, pregnancy, or uterine atrophy in menopause. Torsion or twisting of a pedunculated leiomyoma may occur.

Leiomyomas can sometimes be palpated abdominally; most often they are diagnosed when masses are felt on bimanual pelvic examination. Most leiomyomas do not produce symptoms, and thus treatment is not necessary. Problems that may occur, however, include frequently excessive abnormal uterine bleeding and resultant anemia; pressure on the bladder that causes urinary frequency, urgency, and potential for cystitis; pressure on the rectum that causes constipation; and pain if the tumor degenerates or if there is torsion of a pedunculated leiomyoma.

No intervention is necessary for women who are asymptomatic or near menopause or who have small tumors. Regular examination should be performed to monitor changes. During the childbearing years, myomectomy may be performed if significant symptoms are present or if infertility occurs secondary to the leiomyoma. In some cases, hysterectomy may be performed if, for example, there is intractable abnormal uterine bleeding, particularly in the perimenopausal woman.

MALIGNANT CONDITIONS OF THE REPRODUCTIVE ORGANS

The five major sites for genital cancer in the female are the vulva, vagina, cervix, endometrium, and ovary. More rarely, cancer may occur in the fallopian tubes.

Carcinoma of the Vulva

Carcinoma of the vulva comprises 3% to 4% of all primary genital cancers in women. Ninety percent of the vulvar carcinomas are squamous cell cancer, and the remaining 10% are malignant melanoma, basal cell carcinoma, and adenocarcinoma of Bartholin's and Skene's glands. The classification of vulvar cancer ranges from carcinoma in situ to microinvasive carcinoma to invasive vulvar carcinoma. The median age for women with carcinoma in situ is 44 years; for microinvasive carcinoma, 58 years; and for frankly invasive carcinoma, 61 years. Sexually transmitted diseases are associated with vulvar carcinoma. These include granulomatous venereal disease, syphilis, herpes hominis type II, condylomata acuminata, and infection from human papillomavirus. The most common sites of primary vulvar carcinoma are the labia, occurring three times more frequently on the labia majora than the labia minora, and the clitoris. Metastasis is spread by direct invasion of the surrounding organs to the inguinal lymph nodes and then to the pelvic nodes. Malignant melanoma is the only vulvar carcinoma that is spread by the bloodstream.

The gross appearance of the lesions of cancer of the vulva is flat or raised and maculopapular or verrucous. They can be hyperpigmented (brown), red, or white. The various lesion patterns are referred to as Bowen's disease, erythroplasia of Queyrat, carcinoma simplex, and Paget's disease.

The initial signs and symptoms most frequently reported by the patient are a growth or mass on the vulva and pruritus. However, it is important to note that approximately 20% of women are asymptomatic and small lesions are often undetected or ignored. This may result in delayed diagnosis and treatment, and the tumor may spread to secondary sites. Health care professionals must be suspicious about any lesion and obtain a biopsy for diagnosis. Any evaluation for metastasis is necessary whenever invasive carcinoma is evident on biopsy. This evaluation includes careful inspection of the vagina and cervix, a Pap smear of the cervix, a bimanual examination, cystoscopy, proctoscopy, chest x-ray examination, CT scan, and biochemical profile. A barium enema examination of the rectum and descending colon may also be necessary.

Radical vulvectomy and inguinal node and pelvic node dissection were considered the most effective treatment. However, over the past 5 years less destructive procedures are being used that are contingent on the stage of disease. The depth of local invasion rather than the tumor size is related to the degree of spread. For example, carcinoma in situ of the vulva is treated with wide local excision of the tumor. Frequent follow-up examinations are necessary to check for recurrences. Tumors less than 2 cm in diameter with any degree of local invasion except the anus, vagina, or urethra may have lymph node metastasis. If the nodes are positive, radical vulvectomy and bilateral complete groin dissections are necessary; if negative, wide local excision of the lesion is done. With an invasion of 5 cm or more, a modified radical vulvectomy or hemivulvectomy with inguinofemoral lymphadenectomy is done. The treatment for more advanced stages involves radical vulvectomy, bilateral inguinal lymphadenectomy, and removal of a portion of the distal urethra or vagina and/or a portion of the rectum with postoperative pelvic irradiation. Tumors of the bladder or upper urethra require radical vulvectomy, inguinal node dissections, and possibly anterior exenteration. If the lesion involves the rectum, posterior exenteration may be done. If the tumor is fixed to bone or there are distant metastases, treatment is usually palliative and consists of irradiation and chemotherapy.

Treatment of other vulvar tumors such as malignant melanoma, basal cell carcinoma, and verrucous carcinoma of Bartholin's gland is managed by local excision; for deep melanomas, ipsilateral lymph node dissection may be done. Bartholin's gland carcinoma is usually treated by radical vulvectomy and bilateral inguinal node dissection.

Carcinoma of the Vagina

Primary vaginal carcinomas not involving the cervix or vulva are usually squamous cell cancers. Squamous cell carcinoma may appear as ulcerations, endophytic tumors, or exophytic tumors that may be manifested as dysplasia, carcinoma in situ, and invasion. This is not a common lesion and accounts for only 1% to 2% of all gynecologic cancers. The median age for carcinoma in situ is early in the fifth decade, whereas the median age for invasive carcinoma is in the middle of the sixth decade. Vaginal tumors that are secondary to tumors of other genital areas occur by direct extension or metastasis, especially from the cervix or rectum.

Significant risk factors for primary carcinoma of the vagina include (1) history of human papillomavirus infection, (2) hysterectomy before menopause, (3) history of an abnormal Pap smear, and (4) prior radiation for other carcinomas. The time between radiation therapy and development of vaginal carcinoma has been reported to be from 7 to 20 years. One percent to three percent of women with squamous cell carcinoma of the cervix also develop squamous cell carcinoma of the vagina. Carcinoma in situ of the vagina has been reported to occur from less than 2 years to 17 years after carcinoma in situ of the cervix.

In 1971 an increase was noted in the incidence of clear cell carcinoma of the vagina in young women who were exposed to diethystilbestrol (DES) in utero. Between 1946 and 1971, 2 to 3 million women took DES between the eighth and sixteenth weeks of pregnancy to prevent threatened spontaneous abortion. Women in their mid twenties whose mothers took DES are known to have sequelae that correspond with the time of fetal development during which the drug was used. DES causes development defects of the genital tract and adenoma of the vagina that may undergo malignant changes. The youngest DES-exposed daughter known to develop vaginal clear cell adenocarcinoma was 7 years old at diagnosis; the oldest at diagnosis was 33 years of age. Incidence rises sharply at 14 years, with the peak at 19 years. Clear cell adenocarcinoma in these women occurs most frequently in the upper third of the anterior vaginal wall. The risk that a DES-exposed woman will develop carcinoma is slight—the incidence is 0.4 to 1.4 per 1000 women, or less than 0.1%. The incidence stopped rising in the mid 1970s and continues to decline each year. Whether these women are at risk for development of other genital cancers as they become older is not known at this time. Therefore careful observation with regular examinations and cytologic and colposcopic studies is recommended for these women at risk.

Other malignant lesions that may occur in the vagina are malignant melanoma, which is the second most common primary cancer of the vagina (2% to 3% incidence), verrucous carcinoma, small cell carcinoma, and sarcomas (2% incidence, usually in the fifth and sixth decades). Sarcoma botryoides is rare but is the most common tumor of the genital tract in female children between 2 and 3 years old.

Carcinomas of the vagina can spread by direct extension to paracolpial, parametrial, and pararectal tissues and to the pelvic sidewalls or by the lymphatics to regional lymph nodes. Clear cell carcinoma frequently spreads to supraclavicular nodes or lungs.

Preinvasive lesions of the vagina are asymptomatic, and lesions can be undetected. Therefore careful inspection during routine physical examination is important for early detection of these lesions. Examination of the vagina by colposcopy is recommended for all women with abnormal cervical cytology. Vaginal discharge, and abnormal postmenopausal, postcoital, or intermenstrual vaginal bleeding are the most common signs. Pain or bladder and rectum problems usually occur with advanced disease. Diagnosis of invasive vaginal carcinoma is made by inspection, palpation, and biopsy. In addition, chest x-ray examination, biochemical profile, CT scan of the abdomen and pelvis, barium enema, cystoscopy, and proctoscopy are necessary for the diagnostic workup.

The primary treatment for vaginal squamous cell carcinoma is radiation therapy. Surgical excision is difficult because of the closeness of the bladder and rectum to the vagina. The thickness of the vesicovaginal and rectovaginal septa is usually only millimeters, making exenterative procedures necessary to allow adequate surgical margins around the tumor or tumors. Early lesions in clear cell carcinoma can be treated with surgery or radiation therapy; more advanced invasive lesions should be treated with surgery. Surgical procedures for any stage of the disease include radical hysterectomy, vaginectomy, and radical lymph node dissection.

Carcinoma of the Cervix

Carcinoma of the cervix is the second most frequent genital cancer in women. The majority of these cervical cancers are squamous cell carcinomas. Other types include adenocarcinoma, adenosquamous cell carcinoma, clear cell carcinoma, malignant melanoma, sarcoma, malignant lymphoma, and Hodgkin's disease.

Precancerous changes that are less than full thickness of the cervical epithelium are referred to as dysplasia; full-thickness changes of epithelium are carcinoma in situ of the cervix. Dysplasia and cancer in situ are classified as mild, moderate, or severe. Dysplasia and carcinoma in situ are termed *cervical intraepithelial neoplasia* (CIN) and are defined in grades from CIN 1 (mild dysplasia) to CIN 2 (moderate dysplasia) and CIN 3 (severe dysplasia and carcinoma in situ) (see Chapter 8).

Cervical cancer is routinely screened by the Pap smear test. This test has significantly reduced the mortality from cervical cancer. Current recommendation from the American College of Obstetricians and Gynecologists and the American Cancer Society is to perform a pelvic examination and screen annually all women who are or have been sexually active or have reached the age of 18 years. After three or more consecutive satisfactory normal annual examinations, the Pap test may be done less frequently at the discretion of the physician. The peak incidence of carcinoma in situ is 25 to 40 years of age, whereas the peak incidence of invasive cervical cancer is 48 to 55 years.

There are risk factors for development of cervical cancer that are suggestive of a sexually transmitted disease. The characteristics, known since the 1880s, that predispose a woman to cervical cancer include sexual activity at a young age, pregnancy at a young age, having several male sexual partners, having male partners who have a large number of sexual partners, being a prostitute, being married, and being multiparous. Other factors associated with a greater incidence of cervical carcinoma are low socioeconomic status and cigarette smoking.

Over the past 100 years, an association of cervical cancer with specific sexually transmitted diseases has been sought. Findings of a worldwide study (1995) report that human papillomavirus (HPV) deoxyribonucleic acid (DNA) is present in 93% of cervical tumors. These viruses are common in sexually transmitted disease, but only a small percentage of women infected with HPV develop cancer. More than 20 different types of human papillomavirus were involved with cervical cancer. Although the human papillomavirus that causes genital warts is a separate type from the types that cause cancer, an association does exist in that women who have genital warts were also infected with a virus type that causes cervical cancer.

Squamous cell carcinoma usually occurs at the junction of the squamous epithelium and the columnar mucous epithelium of the endocervix. It is preceded by cervical dysplasia and carcinoma in situ. Preinvasive carcinoma is not evident during a routine pelvic examination. The Pap smear is used as a screening test for detection of neoplastic changes. An abnormal smear is followed up with biopsy to obtain tissue for cytologic examination. Because the cervix has a normal appearance, colposcopy is used to define the abnormal area or areas for taking tissue samples. Punch biopsy of discrete areas or cone biopsy (the removal of a cone-shaped portion of tissue from the cervix that includes most or all of the transformation zone) of the whole squamocolumnar junction is performed.

Early forms of CIN may be removed completely by cone biopsy or eradicated by laser, cautery, or cryosurgery. Regular, frequent follow-up for recurrence of the lesion is important after these treatments.

Invasive carcinoma of the cervix occurs when the tumor invades the epithelium into the stroma of the cervix. Cervical cancer spreads by direct extension into the paracervical tissue. Continued growth results in a visible lesion that involves progressively more of the cervical tissue. Invasion may occur in several sites simultaneously as long strands of tumor cells extend deeply into the connective tissue and eventually invade lymph vessels and venules. Invasive cervical carcinoma may further invade or extend to the vaginal wall, the cardinal ligaments, and the endometrial cavity; invasion of lymph nodes and blood vessels results in metastases to distant parts of the body.

No signs or symptoms are specific for cancer of the cervix. Preinvasive cervical carcinoma produces no symptoms, but early invasive carcinoma can cause a vaginal discharge or vaginal bleeding. Although bleeding is the only significant sign, it does not necessarily occur early, so cancers can be far advanced before they are discovered. The most common type of vaginal bleeding is postcoital or intermenstrual spotting. Any discharge will be serosanguineous or purulent. As the tumor grows, late symptoms include low back or leg pain resulting from compression of lumbosacral nerves, urinary frequency, urgency, hematuria, or rectal bleeding.

Evaluation for cervical carcinoma includes examination by inspection or palpation, a biochemical profile (liver and renal functions), a chest x-ray film, cystoscopy, proctosigmoidoscopy, and a CT scan. Use of the CT scan is increasing because evaluation of findings in several studies is correlated with surgical-pathologic findings that are 97% specific in patients with advanced disease. Treatment of invasive carcinoma of the cervix is determined by clinical and surgical evaluation. Treatment modalities include surgical excision, irradiation therapy, chemotherapy, or combinations of these modalities.

Carcinoma of the Endometrium

Endometrial carcinoma is the most common female genital cancer and accounts for nearly half of all new genital cancer cases. The mortality from endometrial cancer makes up 23% of gynecologic cancer deaths. It occurs commonly after menopause between the ages of 55 and 60 years. The incidence is greater in women who are obese or nulliparous; who have late menopause, polycystic ovarian disease, or estrogen-secreting tumors of the ovary; or who take exogenous estrogen. Medical disorders associated with endometrial carcinoma are diabetes, hypertension, arthritis, and hypothyroidism. Most endometrial carcinomas are adenocarcinomas. Uncommon carcinomas are clear cell carcinoma, secretory carcinoma, and squamous cell carcinoma. Uterine sarcomas (carcinosarcoma, leiomyosarcoma, endometrial stromal sarcoma, müllerian adenosarcoma) cause about 1% to 6% of uterine body cancers. Surgery is the treatment of choice for these tumors.

Hyperplasia of the endometrium is associated with endometrial carcinoma. Adenomatous hyperplasia of the endometrium is usually physiologic if it occurs in an anovulatory hormonal environment before menopause. It can also represent a more active or advanced phase of endometrial hyperplasia, especially in postmenopausal women. Atypical adenomatous hyperplasia is a cause of concern in any woman regardless of menstrual status. The most severe form is a preinvasive cancer (which may be called carcinoma in situ of the endometrium) that occurs at 45 to 50 years, or about 10 years sooner than carcinoma of the endometrium.

Adenocarcinoma of the endometrium develops from a precancerous hyperplasia as a discrete lesion, such as a polyp, or in several different areas, usually the fundus and posterior wall of the uterus. It spreads to the surrounding endometrium and, if untreated, to the myometrium. In advanced stages the regional lymph nodes are involved and the ovary is the major site of metastasis. Further advancement involves the cervix, which is conducive to new routes for further spread. Hematogenous spread to the lungs or liver occurs late. Spontaneous perforation of the uterus causes seeding of tumor cells in the pelvic and abdominal cavities. Bleeding is the major sign of endometrial carcinoma and indicates ulceration. Women often note a serous discharge before frank bleeding. Pain is a late symptom and indicates widespread disease.

Malignant endometrial cells may occasionally be found in a Pap smear of asymptomatic women with endometrial carcinoma. The Pap smear findings must be followed up, but this is not a reliable screening or diagnostic modality to detect the disease. Diagnosis is made by examination of tissue from biopsy curettage of the endometrial cavity. The diagnostic workup includes a comprehensive history; physical examination, including a pelvic examination, chest x-ray, and CT scan; and barium enema, cystoscopy, and proctosigmoidoscopy, depending on the individual's situation.

Treatment involves total abdominal hysterectomy, bilateral salpingo-oophorectomy, and node dissection, depending on the stage of the disease. Radiation therapy is used in high-risk early-stage disease, in advanced disease, or for those patients who are medically unsuitable for hysterectomy. Prognosis depends on the age of the patient and the stage of the disease at the time of treatment.

Carcinoma of the Fallopian Tubes

Primary cancer of the fallopian tubes is rare. It accounts for the smallest number of primary malignant tumors of the female genital tract, namely, 0.5% to 1% of all gynecologic malignancies. Most malignant tumors that occur in the fallopian tubes are extensions from uterine or ovarian cancers. Therefore criteria exist to define any tumor as being a primary cancer of the fallopian tube. It must be located within the tube, and the uterus and ovary must not contain carcinoma; if either does contain cancer, the tumor in the fallopian tube clearly must be histologically different.

The most common primary malignant tumors of the fallopian tube are adenocarcinoma. Other tumors can be sarcomas such as leiomyosarcomas, chondrosarcomas, mixed mesodermal tumors, lymphomas, and choriocarcinomas. All of these types of malignancies in fallopian tubes are quite rare. Malignant tumors of the fallopian tubes metastasize by lymph vessels to regional nodes and spread by migration into the pelvic or abdominal cavities, or they may penetrate the serosa and shed cells directly into the pelvic or abdominal cavities. Signs and symptoms, if present at all, include vaginal discharge, abnormal vaginal bleeding or discharge, menstrual irregularities, and pain. Diagnosis of fallopian tube malignancy is usually made with exploratory laparotomy. Indication of a problem is made by noting an adnexal mass during pelvic examination. Pain is probably caused by tubal distention and therefore is similar to that caused by a tubal pregnancy. It may be intermittent and colicky or dull and aching. Prognosis depends on the depth of invasion of the carcinoma in the tube and whether the tumor has spread beyond the tube. Bilateral involvement has a poorer prognosis than unilateral disease.

Treatment is total abdominal hysterectomy, bilateral salpingoooophorectomy, and resection of as much gross disease as possible. Multiple biopsies of the peritoneum diaphragm, and pelvic and paraaortic nodes are done. It is important to evaluate the lymph nodes. Postoperative adjuvant therapy with radiation, chemotherapy, or both has been shown to improve prognosis.

Carcinoma of the Ovary

A definitive etiology of carcinoma of the ovary is unknown but is multifactorial. The risk of developing ovarian cancer is related to environmental, endocrine, and genetic factors. Environmental factors that are related to epithelial ovarian cancer are the subject of continuing debate and study. The highest incidence is in industrialized Western countries. Dietary habits, coffee and tobacco use, presence of asbestos in the environment, and use of talc have all been considered as possible cancer causes. No link between these factors and development of ovarian cancer has been found. Endocrine factors that relate to risk of ovarian cancer include women who are nulliparous, have early menarche, have late menopause, have their first pregnancy late, and have never breast-fed. Women with breast cancer have a two-fold greater risk for developing ovarian cancer. Use of oral contraceptives or other exogenous estrogen does not increase the risk and may be protective. Genetic factors have been shown to play a role in some families. Hereditary ovarian cancer that is autosomal dominant with variable penetrance has been documented in familial ovarian cancer registries. If two or more first-degree relatives have ovarian cancer, a woman has a 50% chance of developing it. Some physicians recommend a prophylactic oophorectomy at age 35 for women in this high-risk group.

More than 30 types of neoplasms have been identified to occur in the ovary. Ovarian tumors are grouped into three broad categories: (1) epithelial tumors, (2) gonadal stromal tumors, and (3) germ cell tumors.

Epithelial tumors make up 60% of all ovarian neoplasms and are classified as benign, borderline malignant, and malignant. Malignant forms of epithelial neoplasms make up 90% of all ovarian cancers. The most common epithelial malignancy is the serous adenocarcinoma.

Most neoplasms of epithelial origin develop from the surface epithelium, or serosa, of the ovary. In the embryo the gonadal ridge (ovaries) and the müllerian ducts (fallopian tubes, uterus, and vagina) have a common mesodermal origin. Therefore epithelial neoplasms of the ovary reflect cell types of müllerian differentiations: that is, serous, resembling fallopian tube, 46%; mucinous, resembling endocervix, 36%; endometroid, resembling endometrium, 8%; and clear cell, resembling endometrial glands in pregnancy, 3%. Other tumors are of urothelial cell type, mixed carcinomas, and undifferentiated carcinomas.

Ovarian cancer metastasizes by direct invasion of adjacent structures of the abdomen and pelvis and by cells seeding the abdominal and pelvic cavities. These cells follow the natural circulation of peritoneal fluid so that implantation and subsequent malignant growth can occur on all intraperitoneal surfaces. The lymphatics that drain the ovary are also a route for spread of malignant cells. All nodes of the pelvis and abdominal cavities will eventually be affected. Initial spread of ovarian cancer by the intraperitoneal and lymphatic routes occurs without specific signs or symptoms. Vague symptoms that will develop with time are feelings of pelvic heaviness, urinary frequency and dysuria, and changes in gastrointestinal functioning such as sensations of fullness, nausea, indigestion, early satiety, and constipation. Some women may have abnormal vaginal bleeding secondary to endometrial hyperplasia if the tumor is estrogen producing; some tumors produce testosterone and cause virilization. Symptoms of an acute condition in the abdomen can occur suddenly if there is hemorrhage into the tumor, rupture, or ovarian torsion. However, ovarian tumors are most often detected during routine pelvic examination.

In premenopausal women, most palpable adnexal masses are not malignant but are follicular or corpus luteum cysts. These functional cysts resolve in one to three menstrual cycles. If on pelvic examination the mass is felt to be less than 8 cm in size in a premenopausal woman, waiting and watching constitute an appropriate approach. The pelvic examination should be repeated in 1 to 2 months to reevaluate mass size and changes. However, in women who are premenarchal or postmenopausal, with any size mass, further immediate evaluation and perhaps surgical exploration are indicated. Because of a long asymptomatic period, diagnosis in 75% to 85% of women with epithelial ovarian cancer is not made until the tumor is well established throughout the peritoneal cavity.

The surgical intervention for ovarian cancer is a total abdominal hysterectomy, bilateral salpingo-oophorectomy with omentectomy, a complete abdominal exploration, and multiple biopsies of peritoneum, aortic nodes, and pelvic nodes. The 5-year survival rate is about 30% but varies with tumor involvement in other structures and the amount of disease that could not be removed by surgery. Other therapeutic measures include chemotherapy, radiation therapy, or a combination of these.

Prophylactic oophorectomy may be done for some women in families with documented transmission of familial ovarian cancer, but this procedure is not protective for all these high-risk women. Disseminated intraabdominal carcinomas that are histopathologically the same as ovarian carcinoma have occurred in some of these women after oophorectomy. The tissues at risk for carcinoma include those that develop from the same type of tissue from which the ovaries develop in the embryo.

Five percent of all ovarian neoplasms are gonadal stromal tumors; 2% of these account for 2% of ovarian malignancies. They are classified by the World Health Organization (WHO) into five types with multiple subtypes.

There are three major categories of germ cell tumors: (1) benign tumors (dermoid cysts), (2) malignant tumors (constituents of dermoid cysts), and (3) primitive malignant germ cell tumors (embryonic and extraembryonic cells) that are classified by WHO into seven types with multiple subtypes. Dermoid cysts make up 25% to 33% of all ovarian neoplasms; 1% of ovarian cancers develop from constituents of dermoid cysts. Two to three percent of ovarian cancers are primitive malignant germ cell tumors.

Accurate diagnosis of tumor type is important. Surgical excision is the primary treatment for all these ovarian tumors, with appropriate follow-up of any tumor determined to be malignant.

BREAST

Anatomy and Physiology

The mammary gland is developmentally and structurally related to the integument. Its sole function is to secrete milk for nourishment of the infant. This function is directed and mediated by the same hormones that regulate the functions of the reproductive system. Therefore the mammary gland is considered an accessory of the reproductive system. The mammary gland reaches its full potential with menarche in women; in the infant and child and in men, it is present only in rudimentary form (Fig. 64-6).

The breasts are composed of glandular, fibrous, and adipose tissue. They are separated from the chest wall muscles, the pectoral and anterior serratus, by connective tissue. Just a little below center of each mature breast is the nipple (mammary papilla), a pigmented projection

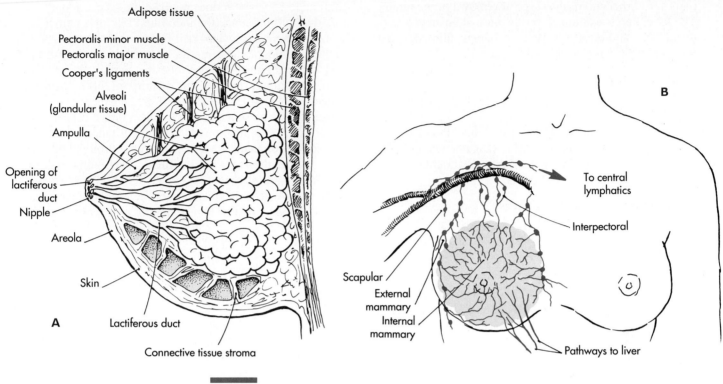

FIG. 64-6   Mature breast. **A,** Anatomy. **B,** Lymphatic drainage.

surrounded by the areola. It is perforated at the tip by several minute openings, the apertures of the lactiferous ducts. Montgomery's tubercles are sebaceous glands on the surface of the areola.

The glandular tissue forms 15 to 25 lobes arranged radially about the nipple and is separated by variable amounts of adipose tissue that surrounds the connective tissue (stroma) between the lobes. Each lobe is distinct so that disease that affects one lobe does not necessarily affect another. The lobes drain into the lactiferous sinuses, which then open into collecting ducts that open onto the nipple. The connective stroma in many places is concentrated into fibrous bands that course vertically through the substance of the breast, attaching the deep layer of the subcutaneous fascia to the dermis. These bands, *Cooper's ligaments,* are suspensory ligaments of the breast.

Changes During the Life Cycle

At puberty the breasts enlarge principally because of an increase in glandular tissue and a deposit of adipose tissue. With each menstrual cycle, there are typical changes of vascular engorgement, enlargement of the glands in the premenstrual phase followed by glandular regression in the postmenstrual phase. During late pregnancy and after parturition, the breasts secrete colostrum, a thin, yellowish fluid, until about 3 to 4 days postpartum, when secretion of milk begins in response to the stimulation of the infant's suckling. After weaning, the gland gradually regresses by loss of glandular tissue. At menopause the adipose tissue regresses more slowly then glandular tis-

sue but eventually disappears, leaving the breasts pendulous and small.

Benign Conditions
Infections

Bacterial infections commonly occur postpartum during early lactation when organisms gain access to breast tissue by fissures in the nipple. The organisms most commonly involved are *Staphylococcus aureus* or streptococci. The breast becomes reddened, hot to touch, swollen, and tender. Symptoms are high fever, chills, and malaise. The treatment is local heat, antipyretics and mild analgesics, periodic emptying of the breast by continued breast feeding and/or pumping, and oral antibiotic therapy. If an abscess occurs, hospitalization for administering IV antibiotics, aspiration, or incision and drainage may be necessary. Any aspirated material is sent for histologic evaluation to rule out malignancy.

Trauma

The most common injury to the breast is contusion. These injuries heal spontaneously but sometimes result in a fat necrosis, which is a mass that feels firm and irregular and occasionally causes skin retraction. For these reasons it is necessary to rule out carcinoma when this lesion occurs.

Fibroadenoma

Fibroadenomas are benign tumors and are well circumscribed with a firm, rubbery consistency. The treatment for fibroadenomas is surgical removal of the tumor. The specimen is examined to rule out malignancy. A cystosarcoma phyllodes is a type of benign fibroadenoma that can recur if not completely removed.

Intraductal papilloma

Papillomas that occur in the nipple ducts usually are too small to palpate but often cause a serosanguineous or bloody nipple discharge. The cause of any kind of abnormal nipple discharge, especially if sanguineous, must be determined and malignancy ruled out. Treatment is surgical excision of the involved ducts.

Fibrocystic disease of the breast

A number of changes of breast tissue are associated with fibrocystic disease. Included is cyst formation, ductal epithelial proliferation, diffuse papillomatosis, and ductal adenosis with formation of fibrous tissue. Clinically these changes can result in palpable nodules, masses, and nipple discharge. Fibrocystic breast disease occurs during the childbearing years; the cause is most likely caused by a relative excess of estrogen and a deficiency of progesterone during the luteal phase of the menstrual cycle. Approximately 50% of women have fibrocystic breast disease. The condition is usually bilateral.

Symptoms include swelling and tenderness of the breasts just before menstrual periods. Signs are palpable masses that move freely in the breast, a feeling of granularity of the breast tissue, and occasionally nonbloody nipple discharge. Many women are asymptomatic and seek medical care when they feel a palpable mass.

Treatment for symptomatic relief of tenderness is by use of mild analgesics and local heat. Improvement may result by avoiding coffee, tea, colas, and chocolate (with methylxanthines); cheese, wine, nuts, mushrooms, and bananas (with tyramines); and tobacco (with nicotine). About 30% of women with biopsy-proven fibrocystic disease have proliferative hyperplasia, which increases their risk for breast cancer by three times the general risk. The major problem for clinicians is distinguishing masses caused by fibrocystic disease and malignancy.

Carcinoma of the Breast

Breast cancer is the second most frequently occurring cancer (27%) in women after nonmelanoma skin cancers; it is the second leading cause of cancer deaths (20%) in women in the United States after lung cancer. Breast cancer is a slow-growing tumor in most cases. Initially there is hyperplasia of the cells with development of atypical cells. These cells progress to carcinoma in situ and then to stromal invasion. A cancer takes about 7 years to grow from a single cell to a mass large enough to palpate (about 1 cm in diameter). At that size about 25% of breast cancers have already metastasized.

A woman's lifetime risk of developing breast cancer is 1 in 9. This figure is general for all women based on a lifetime to 85 years; it does not take into account the factors that will influence the individual risk of a particular woman. There are several risk factors to consider. These include demographics, marital status, parity, menstruation history, family history, obesity, benign breast disease, radiation exposure, and history of prior primary cancer (Table 64-3). About 5% of breast cancer cases are caused by the presence of mutations in breast cancer susceptibility genes in families. The inheritance pattern is autosomal dominant; it can be inherited through both the paternal and the maternal families. The lifetime risk of developing breast cancer is greater than 80% for women in families with an autosomal dominant inheritance pattern. Often over half of female members of these families have breast or ovarian cancer. Research of cancer susceptibility genes is ongoing. Women who have a family history of multiple family members with breast or ovarian cancer should be counseled about their probable risk and monitored carefully to detect early the onset of malignant changes.

Breast cancers develop from mammary epithelial tissues. The causes of breast malignancy are multifactorial. Advances in molecular biology and current research in the biology of breast cancer (i.e., the genetic, molecular, and biochemical events involved in mammary epithelial cell changes in development of cancer) may result in important information about causes, pathophysiology, and prognosis and influence new modalities of earlier detection and treatment.

Breast carcinomas are classified as either ductal or lobular. Carcinoma in situ (i.e., ductal carcinoma in situ [DCIS] or lobular carcinoma in situ [LCIS]) is within the lumen of the ducts or lobules. Invasive or infiltrating carcinomas have spread into the stroma of the breast. Infiltrating ductal carcinoma is stony hard to palpation. Distant metastasis sites are bone, lung, liver, or brain. Infiltrating lobular carcinoma is characterized by an area of ill-defined thickening felt with palpation of the breast. Distant metastasis is usually to meningeal and serosal surfaces.

Paget's disease is an outward-growing malignancy along the nipple ducts from a deeper ductal or invasive ductal cancer with itching, burning, oozing, bleeding, or a combination of these, of the nipple. The underlying carcinoma is palpable in only 50% to 60% of patients. The malignant cells (Paget's cells) from the deeper tumor invade the epidermis of the nipple, causing a crusting, eczematoid appearance.

Inflammatory carcinoma is a rapidly growing tumor that is widespread dermal lymphatic invasion of carcinoma. The symptoms resemble an acute breast infection. The skin becomes reddened, hot, edematous, indurated, and painful. This type of cancer occurs in about 1% to 2% of women with breast cancer. Because the initial appearance is the same as in infection, diagnosis of cancer may be delayed. The prognosis of patients with inflammatory breast cancer is poor even with early diagnosis.

TABLE 64-3   Risk Factors and Incidence for Breast Cancer

Risk Factor	High Incidence	Low Incidence
Age	30-50 yr of age Rises sharply	Levels off at menopause Rises at ⅙ the earlier rate
Geographic location	Western Europe and North America: more than 6-10 times	Japan, most of Asia, Africa
Race	American-born, black women before 40 yr of age	White women before 40 yr of age
Socioeconomic status	Upper socioeconomic group	Lower socioeconomic group
Marital status	Single women 50% more likely to develop breast cancer	Married women
Parity	Nulliparous First birth after 35 yr of age Spontaneous abortions before first birth	Parous (decreases with each birth) High parity (four or more births) First birth before 20 yr of age
Menstrual history	Early age at menarche Late menopause: after 50 yr of age	Risk decreases 20% for each year delayed Natural onset of menopause before 45 yr of age Oophorectomy before 35 yr of age
Family history	First-degree female relatives (maternal or paternal families) of women with breast cancer: 2-3 times more likely to develop breast cancer Mother and sister, or 2 sisters have breast cancer: 5 times more likely to develop breast cancer	
Body habitus	Obesity (per 10-kg increment): 80% more likely to develop breast cancer	
Other breast disease	Ductal and lobular hyperplasia with atypia: 8 times more likely to develop breast cancer	
Radiation exposure	Increasing risk for each rad in young women and children; manifested after 30 yr of age; minimum latency period: 10-15 yr	
Second primary cancer	With primary ovarian cancer, risk of breast cancer 3-4 times greater With primary endometrial cancer, risk of breast cancer 2 times greater With colorectal cancer, risk of breast cancer 2 times greater	

The spread of cancer through the breast occurs by direct invasion of the breast parenchyma, along mammary ducts, in overlying skin, and through the extensive breast lymphatic network. Regional lymph node involvement includes the axillary, internal mammary, and supraclavicular nodes. Lymph node involvement must be determined histologically rather than by clinical examination.

Physical examination of the breasts by an experienced health professional and mammography are the main methods for early detection of breast cancer. The screening mammogram is used in an asymptomatic woman to detect any abnormality in a preclinical stage before invasion or axillary lymph node involvement when the rate of cure is high. The survival rate is directly related to tumor size and axillary lymph node status, making early diagnosis of prime importance. However, breast cancers are frequently first found by the woman herself during

 TABLE 64-4   Recommendations for Mammogram

Age	Mammogram
35-40 yr	Baseline
40-49 yr	Every 1-2 yr
50 yr and older	Annual

self–breast examination after the mass is palpable (about 1 cm). Current recommendations for mammography from the American Cancer Society guidelines are listed in Table 64-4.

Detection and diagnosis of breast cancer (see box on p. 988) begin with obtaining a thorough family and per-

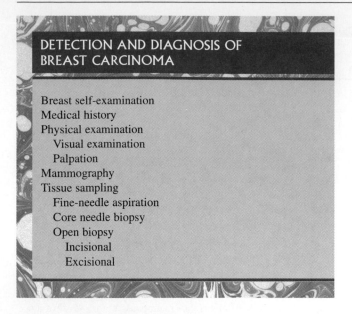

DETECTION AND DIAGNOSIS OF
BREAST CARCINOMA

Breast self-examination
Medical history
Physical examination
   Visual examination
   Palpation
Mammography
Tissue sampling
   Fine-needle aspiration
   Core needle biopsy
   Open biopsy
      Incisional
      Excisional

▶ TABLE 64-5   Treatment for Breast Cancer

Treatment	Description
SURGICAL	
Partial mastectomy	Ranges from tylectomy (lumpectomy) to segmental removal (wide tissue removal with overlying skin) to quadrantectomy (removal of one quadrant of the breast); removal or sample of axillary lymph nodes for staging
Total mastectomy with low axillary dissection	Excision of entire breast, all lymph nodes lateral to pectoralis minor muscle
Modified radical mastectomy	Excision of entire breast, all or most of axillary tissue
Radical mastectomy	Excision of entire breast, underlying pectoralis major and minor muscles; entire axillary contents
Extended radical mastectomy	Same as radical mastectomy with the addition of the internal mammary lymph nodes
NONSURGICAL	
Irradiation	To breast and other chest areas as local adjuvant after surgical procedure; to breast and regional lymph nodes for unresectable advanced cancers; to bony metastases; to axillary lymph node metastases; to local or regional recurrence of tumor after prior treatment
Chemotherapy	Systemic adjuvant after surgery; palliation for advanced disease
Endocrine and hormone therapy	Disseminated cancer-using estrogens, androgens, progesterones, antiestrogens, oophorectomy, adrenalectomy, hypophysectomy

sonal history of pertinent facts related to breast pathophysiology and a physical examination of the breasts. Mammography, which is a soft tissue radiograph, is an important adjunct to the physical examination. It can provide information during a diagnostic workup for an abnormality, as well as screen asymptomatic healthy women. It can detect masses too small to be felt and in many instances reveal the probable nature of a palpable mass. Tissue-sampling procedures done to obtain specimens for microscopic examination for diagnostic purposes include fine-needle aspiration, core needle biopsy, and open biopsy—either excisional (entire mass is removed) or incisional (some part of the mass is removed). If the specimen is malignant, further evaluation is necessary.

The type of treatment chosen for breast cancer depends on the extent of the tumor and presence of metastases. Pathologic staging (i.e., the amount and location of malignant disease) is determined from histologic examination of the removed tissue. The presence of malignancy in the lymph nodes and the number and location of nodes involved determine the prognosis and the need and kind of intervention. The treatment modalities for breast cancer are listed in Table 64-5.

Tamoxifen is a nonsteroidal agent with estrogen antagonist properties. Its major role in therapy of breast cancer appears to be as postsurgical adjuvant treatment of early breast cancer. It prolongs the disease-free interval with a low incidence of adverse effects. There is a 20% reduction in 5-year mortality with its use; the greatest benefit is in women over 50 years of age although it is also beneficial to premenopausal women and postmenopausal women who have advanced breast cancer. Research continues in use of this drug in prevention of primary disease in high-risk women.

QUESTIONS

▼ *Answer the following on a separate sheet of paper.*

1. What are the functions of the ovary in the adult female?
2. What hormonal and ovarian changes occur during the climacteric and menopause?
3. Describe the rationale for the treatment of the amenorrheic patient.
4. Describe the changes that occur in the ovaries and uterus during the menstrual cycle.
5. Explain how the position of the internal reproductive organs of the female is associated with the infectious process.
6. Describe the high-risk factors and prophylactic treatment associated with developing ovarian cancer.
7. Describe the breast tissue changes and cause of fibrocystic disease of the breast.
8. Explain the pathologic changes associated with the development of carcinoma of the breast.
9. Describe the process for the detection and diagnosis of breast cancer.

▼ *Circle the letter preceding each item below that correctly answers the question or completes the statement. More than one answer may be correct.*

10. Which of the following structures are part of the female reproductive system?
    a. Oviducts
    b. Epididymis
    c. Seminal vesicles
    d. Uterus
11. The fallopian tubes provide a direct communication from:
    a. Outside of the body to the peritoneal cavity
    b. Peritoneal cavity to the uterine cavity
    c. Cavity of the uterine body to the vagina
    d. Uterine cavity to the cervix
12. The cyclic events associated with a normal menstrual cycle are regulated by the:
    a. Cerebral cortex and the adrenal gland
    b. Parathyroid glands
    c. Hypothalamus and the anterior pituitary gland
    d. Cerebellum

13. The earliest hormonal event responsible for initiating a new cycle at the end of the luteal phase is a (an):
    a. Decrease in follicle-stimulating hormone
    b. Increase in serum estradiol levels
    c. Increase in luteinizing hormone
    d. Increase in follicle-stimulating hormone
14. Which of the following are characteristic signs and symptoms of the female climacteric?
    a. Menopause
    b. Regular cyclic uterine bleeding
    c. Enlargement of the ovaries
    d. Decrease in estradiol
15. The most common cause of secondary amenorrhea is:
    a. Use of oral contraceptives
    b. Pregnancy
    c. Endometrial dysfunction
    d. Pituitary tumors
16. A 25-year-old obese woman presents with secondary amenorrhea. A pregnancy test is negative. Physical examination reveals underdeveloped breasts and scanty pubic hair. Laboratory tests show an elevated FSH level and normal thyroid and adrenal function. These data are suggestive of:
    a. Gonadal dysgenesis
    b. Panhypopituitarism
    c. Primary ovarian failure
    d. Atrophic vaginitis
17. In postmenopausal women, the most common signs and symptoms associated with atrophy of the urogenital tissue include:
    a. Decreased vaginal secretions
    b. Increased acidity of vaginal secretions
    c. Dyspareunia
    d. Atrophic vaginitis
18. A 50-year-old woman with an intact uterus presents with erratic, episodic menstrual bleeding for the past 18 months. Initial treatment includes progestin on the last 7 days of each estrogen cycle. The *primary* rationale for this regimen is to:
    a. Reduce vasomotor flushes
    b. Prevent osteoporosis
    c. Prevent atrophic or reverse genital and urethral lining changes
    d. Enhance the spontaneous removal of the proliferated endometrium

19. Which of the following theories best describes the pathophysiology of women with premenstrual syndrome (PMS)?
    a. Progesterone levels are abnormally low and require pharmacologic treatment with progesterone.
    b. Elevated prolactin levels are responsible for the salt and water retention, and bromocriptine has been found to be an effective treatment.
    c. Chronic PMS is associated with secondary psychologic difficulties such as marital discord and withdrawal from social activities.
    d. The cause is unknown.
20. The cause of dysmenorrhea is usually associated with:
    a. Excessive amounts of prostaglandin F2 alpha in menstrual blood, which stimulates uterine hyperactivity
    b. Occurs secondary to failure of any developing ovarian follicles to mature to the point of ovulation and subsequent formation of the corpus luteum
    c. Presence of pathologic organisms or puerperal infection
    d. Purulent material draining from an infected fallopian tube
21. Anovulatory cycles with prolonged estrogen production and absence of progesterone production is associated with which of the following conditions:
    a. Endometrial hyperplasia
    b. Leiomyomas
    c. Cancer of the vulva
    d. Cervical carcinoma
22. Metastases by direct invasion of adjacent structures of the abdomen and pelvis and by peritoneal seeding of the abdominal and pelvic cavities is indicative of which of the following types of cancer?
    a. Uterine
    b. Ovarian
    c. Cervical
    d. Endometrial
23. The most common type of carcinoma affecting the female reproductive system is:
    a. Vaginal   c. Breast
    b. Cervical   d. Ovarian
24. The lifetime risk of developing breast cancer for women in families with an autosomal dominant inheritance pattern is greater than:
    a. 20%
    b. 40%

Continued.

QUESTIONS—cont'd

c. 60%
d. 80%

25. The causative organism responsible for toxic shock syndrome is:
    a. *Gonococcus*
    b. *Trichomonas*
    c. *Staphylococcus aureus*
    d. *Streptococcus*

▼ *Circle T if the statement is true and F if it is false. Correct any false statements.*

26. T F Climacteric is the physiologic phase when regression of ovarian function takes place.

27. T F Primary amenorrhea is the failure to begin spontaneous menstruation by 19 years of age.

28. T F Any vaginal bleeding in the postmenopausal patient must be investigated promptly to rule out endometrial cancer.

29. T F In menopausal women osteoporosis accelerates significantly because of the decrease in endogeneous estrogen production.

30. T F Salpingitis is frequently caused by gonorrheal or chlamydial infections of the cervix and is more prevalent in women with multiple sexual partners.

31. T F A leiomyoma is a malignant uterine tumor.

32. T F Invasive carcinoma of the vulva in the more advanced stages is usually treated by application of intravaginal radium plus external radiation.

33. T F Early forms of cervical intraepithelial neoplasia (CIN) can be removed completely by cone biopsy or eradicated by laser, cautery, or cryosurgery.

CHAPTER 65

Male Reproductive System Disorders

EVEYLN J. PIEHL

ANATOMY AND PHYSIOLOGY

The male reproductive structures are the penis; the testis (plural, testes) in the scrotal sac; the duct system, which includes the epididymis (plural, epididymides), the vas deferens (plural, vasa deferens), the ejaculatory ducts, and the urethra; and the accessory glands, which include the seminal vesicles, the prostate, and the bulbourethral glands (Fig. 65-1).

The testes are divided internally into lobules that contain the seminiferous tubules, Sertoli's cells, and Leydig's cells (Fig. 65-2). Sperm production, or spermatogenesis, takes place in the seminiferous tubules. Leydig's cells secrete testosterone. On the posterior portion of each testis is a coiled duct called the *epididymis*. The head is connected with the seminiferous tubule (outflowing duct) of the testis, and the tail is continuous with the vas deferens. The *vas deferens* is the excretory duct of the testis. It extends to the duct of the seminal vesicle, which it joins to form the ejaculatory duct. The ejaculatory duct joins the urethra, which is the common passageway to outside the body for both sperm and urine. The accessory glands communicate with the duct system. The prostate surrounds the neck of the bladder and the upper urethra. Its glandular ducts open into the urethra. The bulbourethral glands (Cowper's glands) are located near the urethral meatus. The penis is composed of three elongated cylindric masses of erectile tissue, which makes up the shaft of the penis. An inner mass is the *corpus spongiosum*, which contains the urethra, and two outer parallel masses, the *corpus cavernosa*. The distal end of the penis, known as the glans, is covered by the *prepuce* (foreskin). The prepuce may be removed surgically (circumcision).

FUNCTIONS OF THE MALE REPRODUCTIVE SYSTEM

The primary functions of the male reproductive system are to produce mature spermatozoa and deposit sperm in the female reproductive tract with coitus. The testes serve the exocrine function of spermatogenesis and the en-

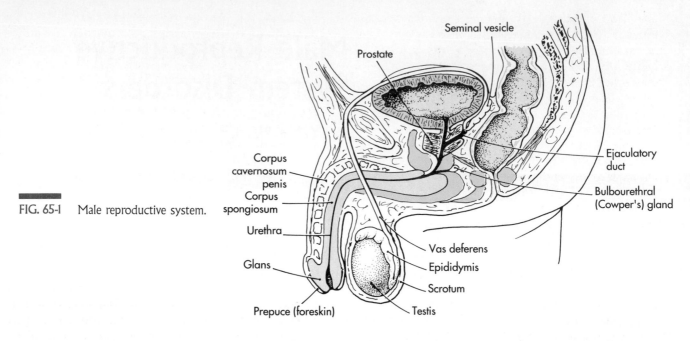

FIG. 65-1   Male reproductive system.

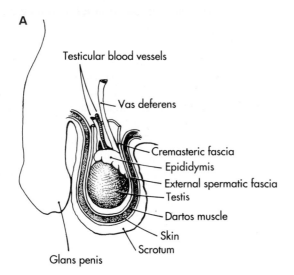

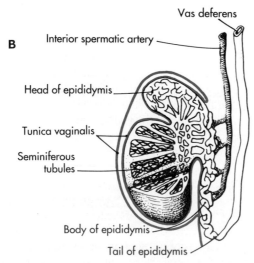

FIG. 65-2   The testes. **A**, External view. **B**, Sagittal section.

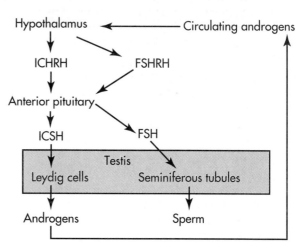

FIG. 65-3   Hypothalamic-pituitary-testicular hormone axis. *ICHRH,* Interstitial cell-hormone–releasing hormone; *FSHRH,* follicle-stimulating hormone–releasing hormone; *ICSH,* interstitial cell–stimulating hormone; *FSH,* follicle-stimulating hormone.

docrine function of secretion of sex hormones that control sexual development and function. All of the functions of the male reproductive system are regulated by means of complex hormonal interactions.

Hormonal Functions

The center of hormonal control of the reproductive system is the hypothalamic-pituitary axis (Fig. 65-3). Under the influence of various elements such as heredity, environment, psychogenic stimuli, and circulating hormone levels, the hypothalamus produces gonadotropic hormone–releasing hormones (GnRH). These hormones are follicle-stimulating hormone–releasing hormone (FSHRH) and luteinizing hormone–releasing hormone (LHRH). They are carried to the anterior pituitary to stimulate secretion of follicle-stimulating hormone (FSH), and luteinizing hormone (LH), more commonly called interstitial cell–stimulating hormone (ICSH) in men. Gonadotropins are secreted at a steady rate in men.

Testosterone directs and regulates characteristics of the masculine body; that is, development of the testes and male genitalia, descent of testes from the abdominal cavity to the scrotum during the fetal period, development of primary and secondary sexual characteristics, and spermatogenesis.

Testosterone production by the interstitial Leydig's cells in males increases greatly at the start of puberty. Puberty onset is marked by increasing ICSH levels, which is produced at first during sleep. The high levels early in puberty result in high levels of testosterone production by the testes. Estrone and estradiol are also produced and are derived from conversion of testosterone produced by the adrenals and testes and from androstenedione. Sex hormone–binding globulin levels fall during puberty, resulting in more free testosterone in the circulation. A growth spurt occurs in every organ system in the body except the central nervous system and the lymphatic system. Alterations in height, weight, and secondary sexual characteristics are the most prominent changes. The peak of the growth spurt occurs at about 14 years of age. The usual rate of growth at the 50th percentile is 5 inches from 12 to 14.5 years plus another 3 inches by 16 years; weight gain peaks at 14 years with about a 50% increase between the ages of 12 and 16 years, mostly as new muscle.

The earliest secondary sexual characteristic to appear is an increase in size of first the testes and scrotum and then the penis. Growth of the testes is caused by growth and development of the seminiferous tubules and the number of Leydig's and Sertoli's cells. Development of the genitalia to adult size and shape takes about 5 to 6 years. The primary sexual characteristics are then structurally at a level of full reproductive maturity. To achieve this, however, the male must produce viable sperm.

Spermatogenesis

Spermatogenesis begins with puberty, at about 13 years of age, and continues throughout life. In the seminiferous tubules, primary germ cells, the spermatogonia, begin to proliferate (mitosis). Some of the daughter cells remain spermatogonia, and others move to the lumen of the seminiferous tubule and enlarge into primary spermatocytes. The primary spermatocytes undergo meiotic division to form two secondary spermatocytes. Each secondary spermatocyte undergoes a second meiotic division, which results in two spermatids. Thus one spermatogonia produces four sperm. No further division occurs, and each spermatid undergoes a maturation and differentiation process to develop the head, neck, body, and tail of the

mature sperm. Spermatogenesis takes place continuously throughout life after puberty. Sperm are stored in the epididymides and vasa deferens and retain their fertility for as long as 42 days. In the absence of emission or ejaculation, spermatozoa are thought to be absorbed by the body. During sexual intercourse, sperm are deposited in the female vagina. After ejaculation the maximum life span of sperm at body temperature is 24 to 72 hours. At lowered temperatures semen may be stored for years.

Testicular Function

In the embryo, H-Y antigen produced by the Y chromosome induces differentiation of Sertoli's cells. These cells then direct the distribution of germ cells in the developing embryo/fetus and secrete müllerian-inhibiting substance (MIS). MIS causes regression of the müllerian duct system (which normally gives rise to female reproductive structures). Fetal Leydig's cells mature under the influence of the Y chromosome and, stimulated by ICSH, secrete testosterone. Testosterone causes differentiation of the vasa deferens and seminal vesicles; its metabolite, dihydrotestosterone (DHT), causes differentiation of the prostate and external genitalia.

During the first 6 months of life, Leydig's cells continue to produce low levels of testosterone but then regress until puberty. At puberty, FSH causes tubular and testicular growth and the testes begin the functions of the mature individual. ICSH stimulates Leydig's cells to produce testosterone, DHT, and estradiol; FSH binds to Sertoli's cells and influences sperm production. Simultaneous presence of a small amount of FSH potentiates the effect of ICSH. Testosterone must also be present in sufficient amount to complete the process of spermatogenesis. Thus both FSH and ICSH must be secreted by the anterior pituitary for spermatogenesis to occur. Testosterone, DHT, estradiol, and a tubular secretion—inhibin—in turn inhibit the secretion of ICSH and FSH by the anterior pituitary, thereby regulating circulating blood levels of testosterone by a negative feedback system.

CHANGES WITH AGING

The male climacteric is the term applied to that time when physiologic reproductive function declines related to increased chronologic age. It is difficult to separate the decline of reproductive function from the decline in physical fitness that occurs with advancing age, and it is possible that the decline in physical fitness is responsible for the decline in reproductive function. The decline is more gradual in men than in women; thus the male reproductive system retains enough of its function to allow for continued reproduction late in life. The seminiferous tubules of the testes continue to produce sperm, although in fewer numbers with advancing age. Ten percent of the seminiferous tubules have stopped producing sperm by 40 years of age, 50% by 50 years, and 90% by 80 years. Testosterone levels decrease gradually. The number of Leydig's cells may decrease, as well as the ability of the remaining cells to produce testosterone.

Failure to attain or maintain erection of the penis (impotence) is more common in aging men. Causes of this condition are not always identifiable; however, psychologic factors are thought to be involved in some cases. Physiologically, the veins and arteries that supply the erectile tissue of the penis are subject to the same sclerosis caused by aging as other blood vessels in the body, which may contribute to impotence.

DISORDERS OF THE MALE REPRODUCTIVE SYSTEM

Hypogonadism

Hypogonadism may be either primary, caused by dysfunction of Leydig's cells, or secondary, caused by dysfunction of the hypothalamic-pituitary unit. Secondary hypogonadism may be further divided into hypothalamic dysfunction and pituitary dysfunction. Hypothalamic or pituitary dysfunction will then result in Leydig's cell hypofunction.

Hypogonadism in the male is a condition characterized by an abnormal decrease in functional activity of the testes. It is the most common disorder of testicular function encountered in clinical practice. The androgens, testosterone and DHT, are essential for male development beginning with embryogenesis and for continuing male development at puberty and reproductive system functioning throughout life. Interruption of the complex hormonal interactions at any level is the cause of a great many syndromes and disorders that have common consequences including infertility, impotence, or complete lack of maleness (male pseudohermaphroditism) (Table 65-1). The specific outcome of male hypogonadism varies with (1) the time of onset of testosterone deficiency (i.e., during embryogenesis, before puberty, or after puberty), (2) the focus of the problem (i.e., a testicular defect or a hypothalamic-pituitary defect), and (3) the functioning status of the testes (i.e., low testosterone production followed by impairment of spermatogenesis, or normal testosterone production with isolated impairment of spermatogenesis). In some cases hypogonadism can be treated, but in other cases the condition is irreversible.

Hypogonadism may be caused by congenital or developmental disorders, acquired disorders, or systemic disorders. Lack of testosterone that causes primary hypogonadism results in increased production of GnRH and gonadotropins to stimulate testicular production of androgens. This type is called *hypergonadotropic hypogonadism.* Included in this category are Klinefelter's syndrome, Reifenstein's syndrome, male Turner's syndrome,

Sertoli-cell–only syndrome, anorchism, orchitis, and sequelae of irradiation. Lack of testosterone in secondary hypogonadism results from decreased levels of GnRH from the hypothalamus or decreased levels of gonadotropins from the pituitary. This type is called *hypogonadotropic hypogonadism.* Included in this category are hypopituitarism, isolated FSH deficiency, Kallmann's syndrome, and Prader-Willi syndrome.

Clinical presentation

Absence or decrease of testosterone in the developing XY chromosome complement embryo/fetus will result in development of female external genitalia or ambiguous external genitalia. In the late fetal period, the testes descend from the abdomen to the scrotum under the influence of testosterone. Without adequate levels of testosterone the testes fail to descend. This condition, *cryptorchidism,* is associated with potential morbidity later in life. Abnormalities of the levels of testosterone in the prepubertal and pubertal periods result in delayed closure of epiphyses and eunuchoidal skeletal proportions of arm span 2 inches or more greater than height, and heel-to-pubic-bone length 2 inches or more greater than pubic-bone-to-crown length. In addition, other changes under the influence of testosterone such as deepening of voice; growth of pubic and axillary hair; growth of beard; testes, penis, and prostate size; and development of male body habitus will not occur. Hypogonadism before puberty results in *eunuchoidism.* Absence or impairment of testicular functions after puberty results in loss of libido, lessening volume of semen ejaculate, possible hot flushes, and some regression of coarse sexual hair. In the adult mature male, testosterone is responsible for maintenance of male sexual characteristics, but loss of testosterone is usually not apparent clinically. However, inadequate testosterone during this period of life results in poor sexual functioning (i.e., impotence and loss of libido) and low sperm quality and quantity (i.e., infertility). Loss of libido and impotence are caused by hypogonadism in approximately 15% to 20% of men with that diagnosis. The normal sperm count in a healthy young man ranges from 20 million to 200 million/ml. About 6% of men in the reproductive age group are infertile, as defined by a sperm count less than 20 million/ml. In 90% of cases sperm count is reduced as the result of hypogonadism, 80% to 90% of which are idiopathic oligospermia with normal testosterone levels.

Assessment of hypogonadism

A thorough history and physical examination, with attention to altered hormonal states, are essential first steps in the clinical evaluation. Laboratory evaluation of hypogonadism includes obtaining serum testosterone levels, serum gonadotropin levels, and karyotype and performing a clomiphene stimulation test, GnRH stimulation test, hCG stimulation test, and semen analysis for sperm quantity and quality.

▶ TABLE 65-1   Causes of Male Hypogonadism

	Primary	Secondary	Androgen Resistance Syndromes
DEFICIENCY OF SPERM AND ANDROGEN PRODUCTION			
Congenital or developmental disorders	Klinefelter's syndrome and variants Functional prepubertal castrate syndrome Noonan's syndrome Myotonic dystrophy Polyglandular autoimmune disease Complex genetic disorders ? Normal aging	Hypogonadotropic eunuchoidism (Kallmann's syndrome) Hemochromatosis Complex genetic syndromes	Reifenstein's syndrome Idiopathic oligospermia or azoospermia
Acquired disorders	Orchitis (mumps, Hansen's disease) Surgical or traumatic castration Drugs (spironolactone, ketoconazole, alcohol, digitalis, cytotoxics) Irradiation	Hypopituitarism Hyperprolactinemia Estrogen excess Progestins Opiate-like drugs	
Systemic disorders	Chronic liver disease Chronic renal disease Sickle cell disease Paraplegia	Glucocorticoid excess (Cushing's syndrome) Acute stress or illness Nutritional deficiency Chronic illness Massive obesity	
ISOLATED DEFICIENCY OF SPERM PRODUCTION			

Congenital or developmental disorders	Germinal cell aplasia
	Cryptorchidism
	Varicocele
	Immotile cilia syndrome
	Myotonic dystrophy
		Androgen excess
		   Congenital adrenal hyperplasia
		   Androgenic anabolic steroids
		   Androgen-secreting tumors
		Hyperprolactemia
		Isolated FSH deficiency	

Acquired disorders	Orchitis Thermal trauma Irradiation Cytotoxic drugs Environmental toxins		
Systemic disorders	Acute febrile illness Paraplegia		
Idiopathic	Oligospermia or azoospermia		

FSH, Follicle-stimulating hormone.

The normal range of serum testosterone levels is wide (3 to 10 ng/ml). Elevated serum gonadotropin levels indicate testicular disease; elevated FSH indicates severe, irreversible tubular disease.

Clomiphene is a nonsteroidal weak estrogen agonist that stimulates the release of gonadotropins. A clomiphene stimulation or GnRH stimulation test should be performed if gonadotropin level is low in association with low serum testosterone level. In men with low levels of testosterone and gonadotropins, clomiphene should cause a 50% increase in ICSH. If ICSH does not increase, the clomiphene stimulation test indicates a hypothalamic-pituitary insufficiency. This test requires 100 mg clomiphene daily for 7 days.

Administering 100 μg of GnRH should cause a peak level three times the control of LH in 20 minutes. With hypothalamic dysfunction, a response may not occur until several injections are given over several days. An exaggerated response indicates a reduced feedback response secondary to low levels of testosterone and estradiol.

If there is no ambiguity of the male genitalia, a buccal smear is obtained to investigate for the presence of a Barr body, which would be diagnostic for Klinefelter's syndrome. Rarely a karyotype may be necessary.

Human chorionic gonadotropin (hCG) stimulates production of testosterone. An hCG stimulation test may be performed to determine Leydig's cell response of changes in production of testosterone. A 50% increase in serum testosterone in 1 to 3 days indicates normal functioning.

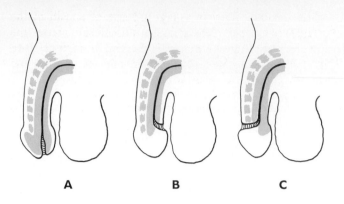

FIG. 65-4   **A,** Normal male urethral opening. **B,** Hypospadias and, **C,** epispadias developmental malformations.

Treatment of hypogonadism

Therapy undertaken for hypogonadism completely depends on the cause, diagnosis, underlying pathologic condition, and patient age. Testosterone deficiency from hypogonadism is treated with androgen replacement therapy. The goal of any therapy is to achieve normal physiologic effects of testosterone for that individual. Gonadotropin and LHRH therapy are used to stimulate spermatogenesis and establish or restore fertility. Once established, spermatogenesis can be maintained with use of hCG.

Cryptorchidism

At about 32 weeks gestation, the testes descend from the abdomen into the scrotum under the influence of testosterone. Cryptorchidism is the arrest of one testis or both testes in the normal path of descent. Unilateral cryptorchidism is the most common type, occurring in 30% of preterm infants, 3% to 4% of term infants, and 0.3% to 0.4% of 1-year-old boys. Spontaneous descent may occur by 1 year of age but is rare after 1 year. Most cases result from hypogonadism or mechanical obstruction. An ectopic testis fails to follow the normal path of descent and becomes lodged in an abnormal place. The common sites for an ectopic testis are the inguinal canal, the perineum, the thigh, the femoral area, or the base of the penis.

The undescended testis is usually smaller than normal, does not produce sperm well, and is susceptible to malignant change at some time in the individual's life. In some cases of a nonpalpable testis, there is testicular agenesis.

An undescended testis in the newborn may descend spontaneously by 1 year of age under the influence of endogenous testosterone secreted by the neonatal testes. Possible therapy after 1 year of age is administration of hCG to stimulate testosterone production. If there is no descent with hCG, the testis is surgically brought down into the scrotum through the inguinal canal and attached to the scrotum (orchiopexy). Intervention, whether medical or surgical, is carried out at about 1 to 2 years of age.

Diethylstilbestrol Exposure

Between 1946 and 1971, 2 to 3 million women took diethylstilbestrol (DES) between the eighth and sixteenth weeks of pregnancy as treatment to prevent threatened spontaneous abortion. Men (the youngest of whom are now in their mid-twenties) whose mothers took DES have sequelae that correspond with the time of embryologic development during which the drug was used. Abnormalities noted in boys and men whose mothers took DES during pregnancy are urethral meatal stenosis, hypospadias, epididymal cysts, varicoceles, increased incidence of cryptorchidism, and decreased fertility. The incidence of reproductive carcinoma in men as a result of DES exposure in utero or whether they are at risk for development of problems as they grow older is unknown.

Hypospadias

Hypospadias occurs in 1 in 300 male births and is the most common anomaly of the penis. Urethral development begins in utero at approximately 8 weeks and is complete by 15 weeks. The urethra is formed by the fusion of the urethral folds along the ventral surface of the penis. The glandular urethra is formed by canalization of an ectodermal cord that has grown through the glans to communicate with the fused urethral folds. Hypospadias results when midline fusion of the urethral folds is incomplete so that the urethral meatus opens on the ventral side of the penis (Fig. 65-4). There can be a spectrum of severity described as glandular (displacement of the meatus on the glans), coronal (at the coronal sulcus), penile (anywhere along the shaft of the penis), penoscrotal (at the ventral junction of the penis and scrotum), and perineal (on the perineum). The prepuce is absent on the ventral side and resembles a hood over the dorsal side of the glans. A band of fibrous tissue, called *chordee,* on the ventral side causes ventral curvature of the penis.

No physical problems are related to hypospadias in newborns or young children. However, in adults chordee will prevent sexual intercourse; infertility can occur in perineal or penoscrotal hypospadias; meatal stenosis may be present, causing difficulty in directing the urinary stream; and cryptorchidism is more common.

Treatment of hypospadias with chordee involves releasing the chordee and surgically restructuring the meatal opening. Repair should be done before the age of learning to stand to void, which is usually about 2 years. The foreskin is used in the reconstructive process; therefore an infant with hypospadias should not be circumcised. Chordee can occur without hypospadias and is treated by releasing the fibrous tissue to improve the function and appearance of the penis.

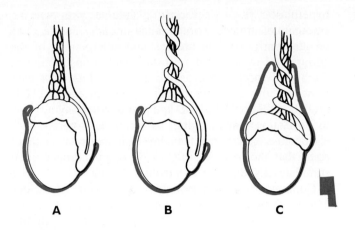

FIG. 65-5   Testicular torsion. **A,** Normal tunica vaginalis insertion. **B,** Extravaginal torsion. **C,** Intravaginal torsion with abnormally high vaginal insertion.

Epispadias

Epispadias is a congenital anomaly in which the urethral meatus is located on the dorsal surface of the penis (Fig. 65-4). The incidence of complete epispadias is approximately 1 in 120,000 males. This condition does not usually occur independently but rather with other urinary tract anomalies. Epispadias is classified according to the placement of the urinary meatus along the penile shaft: glandular (on the dorsal glans), penile (between the pubic symphysis and the coronal sulcus), and penopubic (at the junction of the penis and pubis). The urethral meatus is broad, and a dorsal groove extends from the meatus placement down through the glans. The prepuce hangs from the ventral side of the penis. The penis is flattened and small and may be curved dorsally because of chordee. Urinary incontinence occurs with penopubic (95%) and penile (75%) epispadias because of maldevelopment of urinary sphincters. Surgical repair is undertaken to correct the incontinence, remove the chordee, and extend the urethra to the glans. The foreskin is used in the reconstructive process; therefore an infant with epispadias should not be circumcised.

Testicular Torsion

A testis can twist within the scrotal sac (torsion) as a result of abnormal development of the tunica vaginalis and spermatic cord in the fetal period. An abnormally high insertion of the tunica vaginalis on the cord structures exists, which allows the testis mobility similar to a bell clapper within a bell and results in lack of the normal attachment of the testis to the visceral tunica vaginalis. The testis easily rotates and twists the spermatic cord. This type of torsion is called *intravaginal spermatic cord torsion* (Fig. 65-5). The incidence is higher in adolescents and young adults. Trauma may be a precipitating factor; in about 50% of patients the occurrence of torsion is

while the individual is asleep because of spasm of the cremaster muscle. Contraction of this muscle causes the left testis to rotate counterclockwise and the right testis to rotate clockwise. Blood supply is cut off, and edema forms; both events result in ischemia of the testis.

Symptoms are sudden onset of severe scrotal pain, low abdominal pain, nausea, and vomiting. Physical findings on examination are scrotal edema, erythema, tenderness, fever, new hydrocele, and loss of cremasteric reflex.

The epididymis will be palpated in an abnormal position if the examination is done before severe edema develops. Color Doppler sonography can show arterial flow rate. In torsion, blood flow is absent and the twisted testis is avascular.

This condition requires prompt surgical intervention because ischemia and necrosis with permanent damage to the testis occur in a short time. Testicular salvage is more likely when surgery is performed within 6 hours from onset of torsion. The salvage rate is about 70% during the 6 to 12 hours after torsion and drops to 20% at 12 hours after the event. In surgery detorsion of the testis is done and orchidopexy is performed on both testes as a prophylactic measure. Orchidectomy is not performed unless the testis is completely destroyed.

Torsion of the spermatic cord and testis can also occur in the fetus or neonate in utero or during birth. Twisting occurs in the inguinal portion of the cord above the insertion of the tunica vaginalis and is called extravaginal spermatic cord torsion (Fig. 65-5). Extravaginal torsion occurs only in neonates. It is generally asymptomatic and is most often found during the initial newborn physical examination as a firm, scrotal mass accompanied by a blue-colored area in the scrotal skin covering the mass (blue dot sign). Often the testis is completely necrotic. Orchidectomy is performed on the necrotic testis, and orchidopexy is performed on the contralateral testis.

Hydrocele

A hydrocele is a collection of fluid in the potential space between the two membrane layers of the tunica vaginalis. Congenital hydrocele occurs because of a patent processus vaginalis (a communication between the scrotal sac and the peritoneal cavity) so that peritoneal fluids can collect in the scrotum. An inguinal hernia is also often present. Because the fluid will reabsorb and the patency will close, no intervention is required. If an inguinal hernia is diagnosed and bowel is present in the sac, surgical repair is performed to avoid strangulation of the bowel.

In adults a hydrocele is noncommunicating with the peritoneal cavity; an acute onset of fluid collection is seen in response to infection, tumor, or trauma caused by either overproduction of fluid by the testis or obstruction of lymphatic or venous drainage in the spermatic cord. Chronic hydrocele usually occurs in men over 40 years of age. Fluid collects, and the resultant mass may be soft, cystic, or tense. The signs and symptoms are scrotal enlargement and a feeling of heaviness; a hydrocele is usually painless unless it is caused by an acute epididymal infection or testicular torsion. Diagnosis is aided by transillumination (a tumor does not transilluminate) and an ultrasound of the scrotum to visualize the testis and determine whether a tumor is present.

Active therapy is not always necessary. In an adult a tense hydrocele that impedes blood circulation or causes pain needs to be treated. The hydrocele in a neonate will usually resolve spontaneously. The processus vaginalis closes, and the fluid resorbs. When necessary, in a communicating hydrocele in a child, the processus vaginalis is ligated and the fluid drained. For a noncommunicating hydrocele, surgical drainage is done along with any indicated therapy for underlying causes.

Varicocele

A varicocele is an abnormal dilation (varicosity) of the pampiniform plexus of veins that drain each testis. It is more common on the left side. A varicocele on the right side may be a sign of obstruction caused by a tumor. A varicocele is palpable in 10% of men in the general population and 30% of men with infertility. Sperm concentration and motility are significantly decreased in 65% to 75% of men who have a varicocele. The mechanism for the relationship to infertility is unknown but may relate to testicular temperature increase because one of the functions of the pampiniform plexus is to keep the testes 1° to 2° F cooler than body temperature for optimal conditions for sperm production.

Usually no symptoms are associated with the presence of a varicocele, although some men describe a feeling of heaviness on the involved side and tenderness when it is palpated with examination. On physical examination a mass that feels like a "bag of worms" is palpable when the patient is in the upright position; when the patient is recumbent, the mass drains and cannot be felt. The sudden development of a varicocele in an older man is sometimes a late sign of renal tumor. Pressure from metastasized tumor mass in the renal vein will interfere with blood flow in the spermatic vein on the right side. Testicular atrophy may occur because of reduced blood flow. Surgical repair of the varicosities by ligation of the internal spermatic veins at the internal inguinal ring has been reported to improve sperm quality. Chronic pain can be helped with scrotal support.

Hyperplasia of the Prostate

Benign prostatic hyperplasia (BPH) is a disease of advancing age. Clinical evidence of BPH usually occurs in more than 50% of men over the age of 50 years. Prostatic hyperplasia is growth of multiple fibroadenomatous nodules in the prostate. It begins in the periurethral region as a localized proliferation and progresses to compress the remaining normal gland. The hyperplastic tissue is mostly glandular, with varying amounts of fibrous stroma and smooth muscle. The prostate surrounds the urethra, and enlargement of the periurethral region of the prostate causes obstruction of the bladder neck and prostatic urethra, which decreases urine outflow from the bladder. The cause of BPH is probably related to aging and the accompanying hormone changes. With aging, as serum testosterone levels decline, serum estrogen levels increase. It is theorized that the resulting higher estrogen/androgen ratio stimulates hyperplasia of prostate tissues.

Common signs and symptoms that occur in various combinations and severity are urinary frequency, nocturia, urgency, urgency incontinence, hesitancy, diminished force of the urinary stream, a feeling of incomplete emptying, overflow incontinence, and postvoid dribbling. A distended bladder may be felt on abdominal examination, and suprapubic pressure on a distended bladder causes a sense of urgency. The prostate is palpated during rectal examination to assess the size of the gland.

Diagnostic tests include an abdominal ultrasound to look for hydronephrosis or renal masses and to measure volume of postvoid residual urine and prostatic size. Cystoscopy is done to rule out bladder diverticula, stones, and tumors. Measurement of urinary flow rate and a retrograde urethrogram may also be done.

Obstruction of the bladder neck causing decreased or absent outflow of urine requires intervention to reestablish a patent outlet for urine. Possible procedures include partial prostatectomy, either transurethral resection of the prostate (TUR) or open incision prostatectomy, to remove the hyperplastic periurethral tissue; transurethral incision through muscle fibers of the bladder neck to enlarge the opening; balloon dilation of the prostate to enlarge the urethral lumen; and antiandrogen therapy to cause prostatic atrophy. Indwelling urethral stents placed in the prostatic urethra are a recently developed nonsurgical method of treatment.

REPRODUCTIVE ORGAN INFECTIOUS PROCESSES

Infections of the genital organs occur in men from venereal transmission, as a manifestation of systemic disease, or as a result of instrumentation (catheterization, surgery). Men seek medical care because of a variety of symptoms such as urethral discharge, dysuria, frequency, scrotal tenderness or pain, genital skin eruptions, dyspareunia, and low back and perineal pain.

Balanitis

Balanitis is an inflammation of the glans; *balanoposthitis* is inflammation of the glans and prepuce in the uncircumcised male. The inflammation can be caused by gonorrhea, trichomoniasis, syphilis, *Candida albicans,* tinea, or coliform organisms; as a complication of a dermatitis such as psoriasis; or by a contact dermatitis caused by clothing, use of condoms, or contraceptive jellies.

Balanoposthitis is also associated with a tight prepuce or poor hygiene. Normal secretions from under the foreskin become infected with anaerobic bacteria, causing inflammation and necrosis. Symptoms and signs are irritation, soreness, and a foul-smelling discharge; edema may cause phimosis. Ulceration can occur, causing enlargement and tenderness of the inguinal lymph nodes.

Culture of any discharge should be performed for identification of causative organisms or of secondary bacterial infection. Treatment includes saline irrigation several times daily and antibiotics. Circumcision may need to be considered if phimosis is present after the infection subsides.

Urethritis

Urethritis is inflammation of the urethra from any cause and is a common syndrome in males. Infectious urethritis is classified as either gonococcal or nongonococcal (NGU), depending on the causative organism. The most common organisms are *Neisseria gonorrhoeae, Chlamydia trachomatis, Ureaplasma urealyticum, Trichomonas vaginalis,* herpes simplex viruses (both HSV types 1 and 2), and human papillomavirus. These organisms are commonly transmitted by sexual activities. The classic signs and symptoms are a urethral discharge; inflammation of the meatus; and burning, itching sensation, frequency, and urgency with urination.

Acute urethritis is the most common finding in men with gonorrhea although some men with gonorrhea never develop overt signs or symptoms of urethritis. The discharge is a purulent, profuse discharge with a malodor with voiding. The incubation period for gonorrhea is 2 to 6 days.

The two most common organisms that cause NGU are *C. trachomatis* (30% to 50%) and *U. urealyticum* (25% to 35%). NGU may cause signs and symptoms similar to gonococcal urethritis, including urethral discharge, dysuria, and itching, but these are not as severe as with gonococcal infection. The usual incubation period for NGU is 1 to 5 weeks. *T. vaginalis* usually does not cause symptomatic disease in men and is often self-limiting. This organism is probably killed rapidly by components of prostatic secretions. Herpesvirus genital infections are sexually transmitted during periods of both symptomatic and asymptomatic viral shedding by the partner. An outbreak of lesions can cause meatal inflammation and dysuria. Vesicles may be present on urethral mucosa. Some human papillomavirus genotypes have been found to increase risk for malignancy. Intraurethral warts can cause urethral discharge, dysuria, bloody discharge, or hematuria. Intraurethral spread of warts can involve the bladder and ureters. Urethritis is not the presenting complaint in patients with herpes simplex virus or human papillomavirus infections but occurs after the infection is evident and the characteristic lesions are present.

Prostatitis

Prostatitis is inflammation of the prostate. It can be acute or chronic, and the cause can be either bacterial or nonbacterial. About 50% of men experience symptoms of prostatic inflammation during adult life, and only about 5% of these cases are caused by bacterial infection. Most bacterial infections of the prostate are caused by gram-negative organisms; the most common organism is *Escherichia coli*. Other causative organisms are enterococci, staphylococci, streptococci, *Chlamydia trachomatis, Ureaplasma urealyticum,* and *Neisseria gonorrhoeae*. Bacterial prostatic infections can be the result of a previous or concurrent urethral infection with direct ascent of bacteria from the urethra through the prostatic ducts into the prostate, reflux of urine from an infected bladder, or direct lymphatic or hematogenous spread.

Acute bacterial prostatitis occurs most often in men between the ages of 20 and 40 years. It causes fever as high as 39° to 40° C, chills, malaise, low back pain, perineal pain, dysuria, urethral spasm, and marked suprapubic tenderness. With rectal examination the prostate is found to be tender, swollen, warm, and firm. Palpation of the prostate should be done very carefully. Vigorous massage, in addition to being very painful for the patient, can cause secondary epididymitis or septicemia because of a shower of bacteria being released systemically. Because there is usually also a cystitis, a urinalysis and a urine culture will often identify the organism.

Treatment of bacterial prostatitis is with antibacterial agents specific for the causative organism. Supportive therapy includes bed rest, hydration, analgesics, antipyretics, and stool softeners.

Chronic bacterial prostatitis is a major cause of recurrent urinary tract infections (UTIs) in men. Symptoms are dysuria, urgency, frequency, and nocturia. Pain may occur in the back, perineal area, penis, scrotum, and suprapubic area. Palpation of the prostate gland by rectal examination may be negative. Often the individual is asymptomatic until a significant bacteriuria develops. Frequently there is recurrent symptomatic cystitis. When treated with antibiotics, these symptoms resolve and the urine culture becomes negative. However, the organism persists in the prostate and the individual may continue to have recurrent infections once antibiotics have been discontinued. Suppressive antimicrobial therapy usually results in complete symptomatic relief and reduces the risk of serious illness. Nonbacterial prostatitis causes the same symptoms as chronic prostatitis, but there is no UTI and no organism can be found. Occasionally the individual will notice mucous filaments in the urine. There is no specific treatment or cure.

Epididymitis

Epididymitis is an inflammatory response of the epididymis from infection or trauma. Infection spreads from an established urethritis or prostatitis, and it may be unilateral or bilateral. Chronic or recurring bacterial epididymitis is secondary to chronic infection in these sites or to the presence of a continuous indwelling urethral catheter. Abscess formation may also occur. Hematogenous spread from other sites is not common but does occur. Organisms from the pharynx and tuberculosis infection of the lungs are transmitted through the bloodstream.

The most common sign of epididymitis is scrotal pain and swelling with erythema; a hydrocele may form. A urethral discharge, dysuria, frequency, and urgency are usual symptoms. The onset may occur acutely over 1 to 2 days or develop more gradually. Laboratory tests done to identify the organism are a urethral smear, urinalysis, urine culture, blood culture, and cultures for sexually transmitted diseases.

Epididymitis is classified as nonspecific bacterial epididymitis and sexually transmitted epididymitis. Nonspecific bacterial epididymitis is caused by *E. coli,* streptococci, and staphylococci and is associated with an underlying urologic pathologic condition. Sexually transmitted epididymitis is caused by gonorrhea, *Chlamydia, Treponema pallidum,* and *T. vaginalis.* Identification of organisms and antibacterial treatment should begin immediately because sterility or infertility as a result of mechanical obstruction from scarring is a threat. Treatment is with antibiotic therapy, depending on the sensitivity of organisms identified. Supportive symptomatic therapy is bed rest, scrotal support, ice packs, and analgesics. In the case of chronic inflammation secondary to urethritis, prostatitis, or an indwelling catheter, vasectomy can be considered to avoid continuing spread of the organisms through the vas deferens.

Orchitis

Orchitis is inflammation of the testis; in combination with epididymitis it is called epididymoorchitis and is a serious complication of epididymitis. Orchitis differs from other infections of the genital tract in two ways: the major route of infection is hematogenous, and viruses are the most common organism to cause orchitis. It is classified as viral orchitis, pyogenic bacterial orchitis, or granulomatous orchitis.

Viruses cause the most cases of orchitis. Mumps orchitis is the most common viral infection seen although immunization against mumps in childhood has decreased the incidence. Twenty percent to thirty percent of mumps cases in adults are complicated by orchitis. It is bilateral in about 15% of men with mumps orchitis. In the pubertal or adult male, there usually is seminiferous tubule damage with risk for infertility and, in some cases, damage to Leydig's cells with resultant testosterone deficiency hypogonadism. Mumps orchitis rarely occurs in prepubertal males, but when it does, complete recovery can be expected without subsequent testicular dysfunction.

Signs and symptoms range from mild testicular discomfort and edema to severe testicular pain and marked edema in about 4 to 6 days after onset of the disease with high fever, nausea, and vomiting. Epididymitis and funiculitis (infection of the vas deferens) are possible complications.

Treatment for mumps orchitis is bed rest and scrotal support and elevation. Mild cases resolve in 4 to 5 days; severe cases resolve in 3 to 4 weeks.

Other viruses that can cause orchitis and present the same clinical picture are Coxsackie B virus, varicella, and mononucleosis.

Pyogenic bacterial orchitis is caused by bacteria (*Escherichia coli, Klebsiella pneumoniae, Pseudomonas aeruginosa*) and occasionally rickettsial or parasitic infections (malaria, filariasis, schistosomiasis, amebiasis) by spread from an epididymitis. Systemic diseases such as diphtheria, typhoid fever, paratyphoid fever, and scarlet fever may be transmitted by the bloodstream. The individual with pyogenic orchitis is acutely ill with high fever, edema, acute inflammatory hydrocele, and marked scrotal pain that radiates to the inguinal canal. Complications include testicular infarction, abscess, and pyocele of the scrotum.

Granulomatous orchitis is caused by syphilis, mycobacterial diseases, actinomycosis, fungal diseases, *Mycobacterium tuberculosis,* and *Mycobacterium leprae.* Genital tuberculosis that spreads hematogenously usually starts unilaterally in the lower pole of an epididymis. Infection may spread through the spermatic cord to the testis. Further spread involves the contralateral epididymis and testis, the bladder, and the kidneys.

Urine and blood cultures are done, as well as direct cultures of the infected testis to identify the causative organism. Treatment for these infections is with antibiotics specific for the organism causing the infection. Comfort measures are bed rest, scrotal support, ice packs, and analgesics.

MALIGNANT TUMORS OF THE MALE GENITAL TRACT

Carcinoma of the Prostate

Cancer of the prostate is the second most common malignancy in men in the United States and the third most common cause of cancer deaths in men over 55 years of age, after lung and colorectal cancer. Adenocarcinoma accounts for 95% of all prostate cancers; the remainder of neoplasms are transitional cell carcinomas, squamous cell carcinomas, and sarcomas. Adenocarcinoma of the prostate commonly develops in the periphery of the organ or in the periurethral tissue where benign prostatic hypertrophy occurs. No relationship exists between benign prostatic hyperplasia and the development of malignancy in the prostate.

As the tumor develops and progresses, there is direct extension to the urethra, bladder neck, and seminal vesicles. Prostatic cancer also spreads by lymphatic or hematogenous routes. The most common sites of metastases are to the pelvic lymph nodes and skeleton. Skeletal metastases are to bones of the pelvis, lumbar spine, femur, thoracic spine, and ribs, in that order. Organ metastases occur later and are commonly to liver and lung. Prostatic cancer is unpredictable in the course it will take. It can progress very slowly in some men; in others it grows and metastasizes rapidly and causes death early in the course of the disease. Therefore most clinicians treat patients with prostate cancer aggressively.

Symptoms are not present or are nonspecific early in the course of the disease, and men with advanced disease can also be asymptomatic. Common symptoms are dysuria, difficulty in voiding, urinary frequency, urinary retention, back pain, and hematuria; with increasing obstruction the patient may develop uremia. Signs of a pathologic condition are most often discovered during routine digital rectal examination.

On rectal examination of the prostate, the tumor feels harder than the normal or hyperplastic prostate as a firm mass within the substance of the gland. The diagnosis of prostate cancer is confirmed by either a transperineal or transrectal needle biopsy of the prostate or a transrectal fine-needle aspiration for a cytologic diagnosis. Also, transrectal ultrasound (TRUS) and measurement of serum prostate specific antigen (PSA) are done as part of the diagnostic workup. The TRUS can provide some information regarding location and size of any mass, and PSA is elevated in the presence of prostate malignancy.

The treatment of prostatic carcinoma depends on the size (volume) of the tumor or tumors and the absence or the extent of metastases (stage). Four major stages of prostate cancer are used. The first stage refers to tumors found incidentally in prostatic tissue removed for benign prostatic hypertrophy. These tumors are small and confined to the gland. The second stage refers to tumors that are palpable on rectal examination and are confined to the gland. The third stage refers to tumors that extend beyond the boundaries of the gland but are contained within the pelvis. The fourth stage refers to tumors that are metastatic. Evaluation of stage includes measurement of serum acid phosphatase, which is elevated with metastatic disease; a bone scan to look for bony metastases; and a pelvic lymphadenectomy to determine node metastases. Removal of lymph nodes has no bearing on the course of prostate carcinoma, but presence of metastases in lymph nodes can spare the patient from a radical prostatectomy.

Treatment in the first stage of disease is variable and depends on the age and medical condition of the patient.

Although the malignancy was probably removed in the first surgery, about 16% of these men will develop metastatic disease within 10 years. Therefore most physicians carry out aggressive therapy and close follow-up is done, especially in men under the age of 65 years. The second stage of disease is treated with either radical prostatectomy (removal of entire prostate and the seminal vesicles) or radiation therapy (external beam radiation or implanted interstitial radioactive seeds). Radical prostatectomy has an excellent cure rate of 15-year survival when the disease is localized in the gland. Serious complications are refractory incontinence and impotence. Radiation therapy is done less often but may be appropriate for men who do not want to undergo surgery or whose age or medical condition makes them unsuitable surgery candidates. Major complications of radiation therapy are proctitis and urethritis with possible stenosis.

The third stage of prostatic cancer is treated with radiation therapy as just described. The extent of the tumor in this stage and beyond is not curable surgically.

The fourth stage of prostatic cancer is treated with hormonal therapy. The object is to deprive the tumor of circulating androgens and thus achieve regression of the tumors, both prostatic and metastatic, to provide palliation. This can be accomplished surgically with castration or pharmacologically with use of estrogens (diethylstilbestrol), antiandrogens (flutamide), or luteinizing hormone–releasing analogs (leuprolide acetate). Survival after hormone therapy is variable; 10% survive less than 6 months, and 50% survive less than 3 years.

Carcinoma of the Testes

Testicular tumors compose about 1% of all cancers in men. The peak patient age for testicular cancer is 15 to 35 years, and it is the most common solid malignancy affecting men of these ages. Ninety-five percent of testicular tumors are malignant and derive from the germ cells. They are classified in order of increasing malignancy as seminoma, teratoma, embryonal carcinoma, teratocarcinoma, and choriocarcinoma. A testicular mass in a man over 50 years of age is most often a lymphoma.

Carcinoma in situ of the testes is found in subfertile males, those with varying degrees of cryptorchidism, and those with XY gonadal dysgenesis, making these conditions risk factors for subsequent development of invasive testicular carcinoma. About 25% of males with germ cell tumors have a history of infertility; a major risk for testicular malignancy is a history of cryptorchidism, even though the undescended testis had been brought down surgically. The contralateral testis is also at greater risk for developing malignant changes. Other risk factors for testicular cancer that have been mentioned include history of mumps orchitis after puberty, intrauterine exposure to estrogens, testicular atrophy, torsion, trauma, and elevated intrascrotal temperature.

The usual first sign of carcinoma is a painless scrotal

mass, which will cause pain as it increases in size. Early misdiagnosis or a delay in diagnosis because of patient fear or embarrassment results in advanced disease at diagnosis and a reduced survival rate. The origin of scrotal masses must be determined because most masses growing in or from the testes are malignant, and extratesticular masses are usually benign. Ultrasound can differentiate between extratesticular and testicular masses. The principal diagnostic measure is surgical exploration and microscopic identification of the tumor cells. Hormonal abnormalities or metastases cause late signs and symptoms that include gynecomastia, weight loss, abdominal mass with pain, nausea, vomiting, hemoptysis, shortness of breath, and back pain.

Germ cell tumors can spread by local extension or by lymphatic or hematogenous routes. The three stages are defined as testicular involvement only, retroperitoneal lymph node metastases, and visceral metastases.

Treatment is by radical inguinal orchidectomy. Retroperineal lymph node dissection is also usually performed if the tumor is a teratoma, teratocarcinoma, or embryonal carcinoma; this treatment is followed by multiple drug chemotherapy. Seminoma is treated by orchidectomy followed by irradiation to abdominal, mediastinal, and supraclavicular lymphatics. Chemotherapy is also used for control of metastatic tumor.

The 5-year survival prognosis ranges from nearly zero for the highly malignant choriocarcinoma to 80% with seminomas localized to the testis.

Non–germ cell tumors develop from Leydig's or Sertoli's cells. Most are benign, but 10% can be malignant and metastasize via the lymphatic system. They may secrete steroid hormones, causing feminization or virilization, depending on the hormone secreted. Gynecomastia occurs in about 30% of men with non–germ cell tumors.

Carcinoma of the Scrotum

Carcinoma of the scrotum is rare; the most common carcinoma involving the scrotum is squamous cell carcinoma. Other lesions include liposarcoma, leiomyosarcoma, basal cell carcinoma, extramammary Paget's disease, malignant melanoma, and metastatic lesions. In the 1940s the incidence of squamous cell carcinoma was thought to be related to the type of work the individual does, with laborers being at higher risk than white collar workers. Laborers were thought to be more exposed to industrial environmental irritants, mechanical irritation, and trauma. Carcinoma of the scrotum occurs more often in white men than black men and in urban populations than rural populations. Squamous cell carcinoma of the scrotum occurs most often in men 50 to 70 years of age. It begins as a solitary, slowly growing nodule that often goes undetected or ignored. Ulceration occurs after about 6 months of growth. Delay in medical assistance means that nearly 50% of men have palpable inguinal adenopathy with an advanced tumor stage when first seen by a

physician and the diagnosis is made. Excision of the lesion is done for evaluation by histologic examination for determining the depth of invasion. Palpable inguinal lymph nodes potentially can be caused by inflammation, so frequently a 6-week course of antibiotic therapy is prescribed. Enlarged pelvic or periaortic lymph nodes are aspirated for biopsy and a computed tomography (CT) scan of the abdomen and pelvis is done for staging. Wide local excision of the tumor with at least 2-cm margins and excision of the skin and underlying dartos muscle are done as treatment of early stage disease. Alternatively, laser therapy and Moh's micrographic surgery are used. Radiation therapy and chemotherapy are not effective. If inguinal lymph nodes are not palpable, biopsy is done to determine whether metastasis has occurred. If the inguinal lymph nodes are palpable after antibiotic therapy or the biopsy specimen is positive for malignancy, bilateral ilioinguinal lymphadenectomy is done.

The long-term survival rate is 70% if diagnosed and treated before metastases to the inguinal lymph nodes. Survival rates are significantly lower after metastases occur and with worsening stage of disease.

Basal cell carcinoma, extramammary Paget's disease, and sarcomas are all treated with wide excision of local disease with appropriate follow-up and further treatment for advanced disease, the same as for squamous cell carcinoma. Metastatic lesions to the scrotum are usually adenocarcinomas from primary tumors of the rectum, colon, and stomach.

Carcinoma of the Penis

Carcinoma of the penis occurs most commonly in men from 60 to 80 years of age but also is seen in men from 40 to 60 years of age. The incidence has been linked to the hygienic standards and differences in cultural and religious practices. It is more common in uncircumcised than in circumcised males. Neonatal circumcision has been said to eliminate the occurrence of penile carcinoma. Cervical carcinoma in sexual partners increases the risk of men developing penile cancer; and deoxyribonucleic acid (DNA) sequences of the sexually transmitted human papillomavirus have been identified in cases of penile cancer. Most malignancies of the penis are low-grade squamous cell carcinoma. Extent of metastasis to nodes indicates prognosis.

Carcinoma of the penis begins with a small lesion that begins beneath the prepuce or in the coronal region and gradually extends to involve the entire glans, prepuce, corona, and shaft. Carcinoma in situ (intraepithelial neoplasia) is also known as Bowen's disease of the penis or erythroplasia of Queyrat. This noninvasive form progresses to invasive carcinoma. It extends locally and first spreads through the lymphatic system to the inguinal lymph nodes. Metastatic enlargement of the regional inguinal lymph nodes eventually leads to skin necrosis, chronic infection, or hemorrhage from erosion into the femoral vessels. If penile carcinoma is untreated, death occurs within 2 years. Biopsies are necessary to determine extent of the tumor so that treatment can be planned. Small and noninvasive lesions are removed by wedge excision, or Moh's micrographic surgery may be used for excision; if the prepuce is involved, circumcision is done. Radiation therapy has also been successful for noninvasive lesions, as has topical application of 5-fluorouracil. CO_2 laser therapy and cryosurgery are other treatment options. Invasive tumors are treated by partial penectomy with a 2-cm margin around the tumor or by total penectomy with perineal urethrostomy. With advanced tumors more extensive surgery such as hemipelvectomy may be necessary. Chemotherapy may be used in combination with surgery.

BREAST

Benign Conditions of the Breast

Gynecomastia is hypertrophy of the breast and may be unilateral or bilateral. In boys during puberty, it is usually bilateral, but in men over 50 years of age, it is usually unilateral. It is a discoid enlargement beneath the areola. Often it is physiologic and will resolve spontaneously in 6 to 12 months. Other causes include conditions resulting in increased estrogen levels such as testicular tumors, pituitary tumors, some hypogonadism syndromes, cirrhosis of the liver, therapeutic use of estrogens for prostatic carcinoma, and use of steroidal preparations. Occasionally resection of extra breast tissue is performed for psychologic reasons, or biopsy is performed to rule out malignancy.

Malignant Conditions of the Breast

The incidence of cancer of the breast in men is about 1% of that in women, but clinically both are similar. The primary cause is thought to be excess estrogen synthesis, and many tumors are estrogen-receptor positive. Treatment is surgical excision of the mass, surrounding breast tissue, and lymph nodes as necessary. Surgical castration is carried out if there are metastases. Palliative procedures include adrenalectomy, hypophysectomy, and antiestrogen therapy.

QUESTIONS

▼ *Answer the following on a separate sheet of paper.*

1. What are the primary functions of the male reproductive system?
2. Explain the process of spermatogenesis.
3. In the assessment of hypogonadism, explain the rationale for performing the clomiphene or GnRH stimulation test.
4. What hormonal and physiologic changes of the reproductive organs are associated with aging in the male?
5. Explain the causative factors responsible for genital tract infections of the male reproductive system.
6. Trace the pathway of metastasis of adenocarcinoma of the prostate.

▼ *Circle the letter preceding each item below that correctly answers the question or completes the statement. More than one answer may be correct.*

7. Leydig's cells secrete:
   a. Gonadotropic releasing hormone (GnRH)
   b. Follicle-stimulating hormone (FSH)
   c. Interstitial cell–stimulating hormone (ICSH)
   d. Testosterone
8. The excretory duct of the testis is the:
   a. Seminal vesicle
   b. Ejaculatory duct
   c. Vas deferens
   d. Seminiferous tubules
9. The prostate glandular ducts open into the:
   a. Urethra
   b. Ureter
   c. Glans
   d. Epididymis
10. The center of hormonal control of the reproductive system is the:
    a. Adrenal gland
    b. Hypothalamic-pituitary axis
    c. Both a and b
    d. Neither a nor b
11. In the embryo, H-Y antigen produced by the Y chromosome induces:
    a. Regression of the müllerian duct system
    b. Differentiation of Sertoli's cells
    c. Secretion of follicle-stimulating hormone (FSH)
    d. Reabsorption of spermatozoa by the body
12. The most common disorder of testicular function is:
    a. Hypospadias
    b. Hypogonadism
    c. Cryptorchidism
    d. Epispadias
13. The normal sperm count in a healthy young man ranges from _____ to _____ million/ml.
    a. 5 to 75
    b. 10 to 150
    c. 15 to 175
    d. 20 to 200
14. Elevated serum gonadotropins indicate which of the following?
    a. Testicular disease
    b. Inflammation of the genital organs
    c. Adenocarcinoma of the prostate
    d. Gynecomastia
15. In benign prostatic hyperplasia, enlargement of the periurethral region of the prostate causes:
    a. Obstruction of the bladder neck and prostatic urethra
    b. Torsion of the spermatic cord and testis
    c. Inflammation of the testis
    d. Decrease in urine outflow from the bladder
16. A major cause of recurrent urinary tract infection in males is:
    a. Epididymitis
    b. Balanitis
    c. Chronic bacterial prostatitis
    d. Orchitis
17. The usual treatment for a diffuse, poorly differentiated carcinoma of the prostate is:
    a. Megavolt radiation
    b. Radical prostatectomy

Continued.

QUESTIONS—cont'd

c. Observation

d. Hormonal therapy

18. A scrotal mass in a young male that has increased in size with occasional pain may indicate which of the following:
    a. Testicular malignant tumor
    b. Prostatic carcinoma
    c. Cancer of the penis
    d. Carcinoma of the bladder

19. Which of the following organisms can cause epididymitis?
    a. Streptococci
    b. Gonorrhea
    c. *Chlamydia*
    d. Mumps virus

20. The rationale for the treatment of testosterone deficiency from hypogonadism with gonadotropin and luteinizing hormone–releasing factor (LHRF) is to:
    a. Stimulate spermatogenesis
    b. Establish or restore fertility
    c. Both a and b
    d. Neither a nor b

▼ Match the pathologic process in column B with the appropriate item in column A.

Column A

21. _____ Hypospadias
22. _____ Testicular torsion
23. _____ Benign prostatic hyperplasia
24. _____ Varicocele
25. _____ Hydrocele

Column B

a. Abnormally high insertion of the tunica vaginalis on the spermatic cord

b. Collection of fluid in the potential space between the membrane layers of the tunica vaginalis

c. Urethral meatus opening on the ventral side of the penis

d. Abnormal dilation of the pampiniform plexus of veins that drain the testes

e. Growth of multiple fibroadenomatous nodules in the prostate

CHAPTER 66

Sexually Transmitted Diseases

EVELYN J. PIEHL

Venereal or sexually transmitted diseases (STDs) are infections caused by dissimilar infecting organisms that are primarily transmitted by sexual contact (see box on p. 1006). In some cases, sexual transmission is the only mode of transmission; in other cases, sexual transmission is only one mode of transmission and nonsexual transmission is as epidemiologically important. Sexual contact (genital, oral-genital, oral-anal, and genital-anal) includes all heterosexual and homosexual behaviors. The variation of the incidence of venereal diseases is related to cultural and societal mores and attitudes, sexual behaviors, and life-styles of vulnerable individuals. The number and type of sexual partners and health-risk behaviors influence risk rather than sexual activity itself.

Historically, the incidence of venereal disease has been compiled by the U.S. Army since 1820. In the period of the Mexican, Civil, and Spanish Wars, the rates in peacetime were between 50 and 75 per 1000 and the rates doubled or tripled at time of war. In 1874 it was estimated that 1 in 20 members of the U.S. population was infected with syphilis. Gonorrhea was also recognized as a serious cause of chronic morbidity. In 1872 about 90% of sterile women were married to men who had contracted gonorrhea either before or during their marriages. All nations involved in World War I attempted to control venereal diseases among their troops. In the American Expeditionary Force in France, 246 venereal disease control officers were employed. After an initial rise in diseases, the incidence fell to below peacetime figures. The venereal disease corps was disbanded after the war, but the incidence continued to decline until 1940. In the 1920s Congress cut funding for venereal disease services and for state diagnosis and treatment clinics. With the onset of the depression in the 1930s, funding dropped even more. The chief of the Venereal Disease Division of the Public Health Service estimated in the late 1930s that 1 million mothers had syphilis and that 60,000 babies were born each year with congenital syphilis. The prescribed treatment at that time was arsenic or bismuth. In World War II, 300,000 draftees were diagnosed with syphilis and were treated with arsphenamine. After 1943 penicillin was found to be an effective treatment for syphilis. Rapid treatment centers in each state were established. In the 10 years after World War II, federal funding for venereal disease was again cut enormously because it was thought that penicillin would eradicate the problem. Throughout the 1950s the incidence of STDs was low, but public attitudes about established moral views on sexuality began to change during the 1950s and 1960s. Oral contraceptives were widely available by 1965. STDs increased in the 1960s among young persons, especially women. By 1970 the prevalence of syphilis and gonorrhea was at epidemic levels again.

In 1990, 50,223 cases of primary and secondary syphilis were reported—a 9% increase from 1989. This epidemic is linked to use of illegal drugs, especially crack cocaine. In the early 1990s, the incidence again declined,

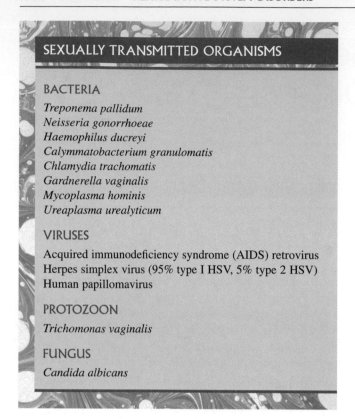

SEXUALLY TRANSMITTED ORGANISMS

BACTERIA

Treponema pallidum
Neisseria gonorrhoeae
Haemophilus ducreyi
Calymmatobacterium granulomatis
Chlamydia trachomatis
Gardnerella vaginalis
Mycoplasma hominis
Ureaplasma urealyticum

VIRUSES

Acquired immunodeficiency syndrome (AIDS) retrovirus
Herpes simplex virus (95% type I HSV, 5% type 2 HSV)
Human papillomavirus

PROTOZOON

Trichomonas vaginalis

FUNGUS

Candida albicans

with just 28,000 new cases in 1992 as compared with 50,000 annually between 1985 and 1990.

The annual age-specific incidence of gonorrhea tripled between 1963 and 1976; the incidence decreased each year for the next decade but then again began to rise. In 1991 in the United States, 1,300,000 cases were treated. The highest incidence occurs between the ages of 20 and 24 years in men and 15 and 19 years in women. In addition, more than 4 million cases of sexually transmitted *Chlamydia* infections occur annually in the United States. The direct and indirect costs of both acute symptomatic and asymptomatic *Chlamydia* illness exceed $2.4 billion annually.

Many STDs have a known serious impact on the health of the individual, some with long-term sequelae, including sterility, genital tract carcinoma, and possibly death. In addition, a variety of perinatal infections may be transmitted to the fetus or neonate. Sexually transmitted diseases are most common in young persons (about two thirds of cases occur in those 16 to 24 years of age), those with multiple sexual contacts, prostitutes, homosexual and bisexual men, and persons with infected partners.

Control of STDs requires facilities for evaluation, diagnosis, treatment, and follow-up observation after treatment to monitor effectiveness of treatment; partner tracing and treatment; patient and partner counseling about responsible sexual behavior; professional and lay education; and continued research to look for methods to produce immunity against infections.

DISEASES AND INFECTIONS

Syphilis

Syphilis is a chronic contagious infection caused by a spiral-shaped bacterium (spirochete), *Treponema pallidum.* There are three active phases: primary, secondary, and tertiary, or late phase, with a latent phase between the secondary and tertiary phases. The latent phase is divided into early and late. Transmission occurs most commonly by sexual intercourse with direct contact with a moist infectious lesion. Persons with untreated syphilis are highly infectious during the primary and secondary phases, and one third of exposed persons having sexual contact with untreated individuals become infected. Syphilis is characterized by a large variety of clinical manifestations. The incubation period averages 3 weeks and ranges from 10 to 90 days.

Primary syphilis

Typically the first clinical manifestation is a papule that develops at the site of contact. This papule progresses over one to several weeks (average 21 days) to form an ulcer called a *chancre* (Fig. 66-1 and Color plate 30). The chancre varies in size from a few millimeters to more than 2 cm. A typical chancre is a solitary painless lesion with a clean base and rounded borders. In heterosexual men the most common site is the penis, namely, the coronal sulcus, the shaft, the frenulum, and the urinary meatus, in that order. Nearly 50% of chancres in homosexual men are anal or perianal. In women chancres are found on the vulva, labia, or cervix. Chancres can be extragenital and are found on the tongue, lips, fingers, nipples, and pharynx. About half of people with primary syphilis will develop nonsuppurative, bilateral regional adenopathy. The chancre heals spontaneously in 4 to 6 weeks.

Dark-field microscopy is the most important diagnostic test and must be performed by an experienced examiner. The Venereal Disease Research Laboratory (VDRL) serologic test is positive in only 50% of cases when a chancre initially appears, whereas the fluorescent treponemal antibody absorption (FTA-ABS) test is positive in 90% of cases. In the diagnosis of primary syphilis, the chancre must be differentiated from herpes progenitalis, chancroid, granuloma inguinale, and drug eruptions. A characteristic indurated ulcer and positive dark-field examination, along with a positive FTA-ABS test, confirm the diagnosis of primary syphilis.

Secondary syphilis

Approximately 6 weeks to 6 months after exposure, individuals with untreated primary syphilis develop clinical manifestations of disseminated disease.

Early signs of secondary syphilis, which may begin before the primary chancre heals, frequently include a prodrome of malaise, low-grade fever, stiff neck, runny nose,

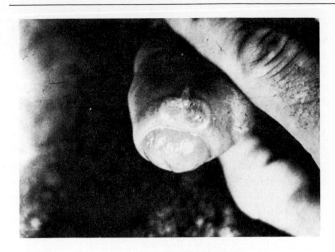

FIG. 66-1   Painless, hard ulcer of primary syphilitic chancre on the penis. (Courtesy of Marek A. Stawiski, MD, Associate Clinical Professor of Internal Medicine, Michigan State University.)

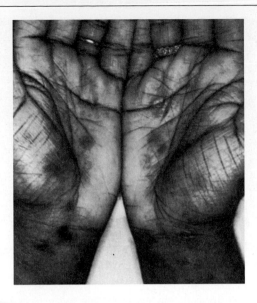

FIG. 66-2   Brownish macules over the palms in secondary syphilis.

lacrimation, anorexia, weight loss, and arthralgias. Secondary syphilis can affect every organ system in the body. The systems most commonly involved are skin, lymphatics, gastrointestinal (GI) tract, bones, kidneys, eyes, and central nervous system (CNS). Cutaneous lesions called *syphilids* occur in more than 80% of cases and are macular, maculopapular, papular, papulosquamous, and pustular. Macular and maculopapular lesions predominate, and pruritic eruptions may also occur. The lesions are usually symmetric and widespread; they may evolve from macular to papular or papulosquamous, or different forms may be present simultaneously. Many persons have lesions over the palms and soles (Fig. 66-2). Syphilids can resemble pityriasis rosea, psoriasis, or lichen planus. Other manifestations are patchy alopecia, thinning of eyebrows and beard, erythema of tonsils and pharynx, and superficial ulcers of oral and genital mucosa (mucous patches); moist, flat, wartlike condylomata lata can appear on the genitalia. All lesions of secondary syphilis are contagious. Lymphadenopathy is present in many patients and may take the form of lymphadenitis; abdominal pain, vomiting, and weight loss occur with gastric syphilis; GI involvement includes proctitis and colitis; elevated alkaline phosphatase occurs with syphilitic granulomatous hepatitis; destructive bony lesions involve skull, clavicle, tibia, and humerus, and bone pain occurs with osteitis or periostitis; renal involvement causes glomerulonephritis, hemorrhagic nephritis, or nephrotic syndrome; uveitis, acute pupillitis, and retinitis can occur and result in blindness. Syphilitic meningitis will usually occur within the first year of infection (during the secondary stage) and is characterized by headache, stiff neck, nausea, and vomiting. Very rarely, more severe neurologic disorders such as basilar meningitis, hydrocephalus, optic neuritis, or cerebrovascular syndromes develop. Cranial nerves III, VI, VII, and VIII are the most commonly involved. This manifestation is not the same entity as neurosyphilis seen in the tertiary stage.

The lesions of the secondary stage of syphilis heal spontaneously within 2 to 6 weeks, and a period of latency begins.

Latent syphilis

Latent syphilis is the stage in which the person is asymptomatic, there are no clinical signs of syphilis, and the cerebrospinal fluid (CSF) laboratory tests are normal. The Centers for Disease Control and Prevention (CDC) use 1 year after infection to demarcate early latent stage from late latent stage syphilis. During the early latent period, infectious relapses of secondary syphilis can occur. These relapses may continue to occur as long as 5 years after infection in 25% of patients. Eighty-five percent of relapses involve the appearance of mucocutaneous lesions.

Tertiary syphilis

Years to decades after the initial infection, three forms of tertiary syphilis can appear: late benign (gummatous) syphilis, cardiovascular syphilis, and neurosyphilis. About 30% of individuals with untreated primary and secondary syphilis will develop tertiary syphilis. The other 70% of individuals have no signs of disease.

Benign tertiary syphilis is a destructive inflammatory process that involves bone, skin, or mucous membranes. It occasionally may involve viscera, CNS, or eyes. Multiple episodes occur in about one third of individuals with this form of the disease. Lesions of tertiary syphilis of the skin vary from small nodules to deep ulcers. The characteristic lesion is the gumma (Fig. 66-3). Usually there is simultaneous active inflammation, formation of new lesions, and formation of scars in one or more areas.

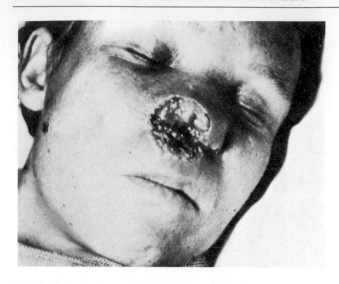

FIG. 66-3 Cutaneous gumma presenting as an ulcer over the nose. (Courtesy of Marek A. Stawiski, MD, Associate Clinical Professor of Internal Medicine, Michigan State University.)

Bone gummas begin as exquisitely tender points of periosteal inflammation, usually in long bones, clavicles, and skull. They progress to destructive and disfiguring lesions or draining sinuses. Hepatic gummas are the most common form of visceral involvement. Gummas in the heart or CNS can be so destructive or space occupying that they are fatal.

Asymptomatic syphilitic aortitis commonly occurs in cardiovascular syphilis. Widening of the aorta or linear calcification can be seen on chest x-ray film. Approximately 10% of these individuals develop symptomatic cardiovascular complications of aortic insufficiency and aortic aneurysm.

Three major forms of symptomatic cardiovascular syphilis, all of which are usually fatal, are aortic insufficiency with dilation of the aortic root, coronary vessel stenosis evidenced by angina, and aortic aneurysm.

Neurosyphilis is fundamentally a chronic meningitis. It is divided into asymptomatic, meningeal, meningovascular, and parenchymatous syndromes.

Asymptomatic neurosyphilis is without neurologic signs or symptoms but with abnormal CSF laboratory tests. It will either resolve spontaneously or (in 20% of cases) progress to symptomatic disease.

Meningeal neurosyphilis is the infection of the CSF early (in first year of infection) during secondary syphilis, and the person remains asymptomatic. CSF laboratory abnormalities may resolve spontaneously. If abnormalities persist 2 or more years after infection, there is a high probability of subsequent development of symptomatic neurosyphilis during the tertiary stage.

Meningovascular syphilis usually occurs 4 to 7 years after infection. Ischemia or infarction of the CNS occurs, resulting in signs and symptoms that mimic atherosclerotic cerebrovascular disease or a subacute encephalitic syndrome with superimposed cerebrovascular events. Symptoms include headache, loss of memory, personality changes, dizziness, and insomnia; seizures may also occur. These manifestations can involve any portion of the CNS.

Parenchymatous neurosyphilis syndromes are tabes dorsalis and general paresis. Demyelination of posterior columns of the spinal cord, dorsal roots, and dorsal root ganglions is the cause of tabes dorsalis. Paresthesias, diminished deep tendon reflexes, and poor pupillary response to light develop early. Severe visceral pain, loss of position and temperature sensations, impotence, bladder incontinence, and truncal ataxia develop over time, and optic atrophy may cause blindness. Charcot's joints, traumatic ulceration of the lower extremities, and a wide-spaced gait with foot slapping develop. An insidious dementia can develop with gradual onset of psychiatric symptoms, although onset can occur suddenly. Most common neurologic changes are pupillary abnormalities; lack of facial expression; tremors of lips, tongue, and facial muscles; and impaired handwriting and speech. Other manifestations include seizures, dramatic and bizarre changes in personality, and intellectual deterioration.

Congenital syphilis

Treponema pallidum can cross the placenta from the mother to the fetus, and congenital syphilis is acquired by the fetus in utero. Many infants with congenital syphilis have no obvious evidence of infection and are diagnosed based on maternal history and by serologic testing. Because they are infected in utero, symptomatic congenital syphilis in infants is analogous in many respects to the secondary stage of acquired infection. Serologic tests can be nonreactive among infants infected late during their mother's pregnancy. Clinical manifestations that appear in the first 2 years of life are designated early, and those appearing after 2 years of age are designated late. Fifteen to sixty percent of infants will have mucocutaneous lesions. Neonates will have cutaneous rashes such as bullae (pemphigus syphiliticus), vesicles, and maculopapules; mucous patches and condylomata lata may appear at 2 to 3 months of age. Bony lesions of early congenital syphilis are seen on x-ray examination. When the infection is severe, visceral involvement occurs such as hepatosplenomegaly, pancreatitis, pneumonia, and nephrosis. Hematologic abnormalities are also common in severe infection. CNS invasion may occur in as many as 60% of neonates, but effects may not be evident for months or years. Neonatal death can occur from liver failure, respiratory failure, or secondary bacterial infection.

Manifestations of late congenital syphilis include interstitial keratitis, dental anomalies (mulberry molars), eighth nerve deafness, osteitis, bilateral effusions of the knees, anterior bowing of the shins (saber shins), gummas, facial deformities, and neurosyphilis.

Diagnostic testing

Diagnosis with dark-field microscopy is the most rapid and direct means of identifying treponemes in specimen material from chancres of primary syphilis and mucocutaneous lesions of secondary syphilis. However, serologic tests for syphilis are the most frequently performed diagnostic tests. Available assays measure two distinctly different kinds of antibodies.

The nontreponemal tests, that is, the VDRL, the rapid plasma reagin (RPR), and the reagin screen test (RST), measure immunoglobulin G (IgG) and immunoglobulin M (IgM) flocculating antibodies to a defined mixture of cardiolipin, cholesterol, and lecithin. Treponemal tests detect *T. pallidum*–specific antibodies. These are the fluorescent treponemal antibody absorption test (FTA-ABS), the microhemagglutination assay for antibodies to *T. pallidum* (MHA-TP), and the hemagglutination treponemal test for syphilis (HATTS). Nontreponemal test antibody titers usually correlate with disease activity, and results are reported quantitatively. A fourfold change in titer, equivalent to a change of two dilutions (e.g., from 1:16 to 1:4 or from 1:8 to 1:32), is necessary to demonstrate a substantial difference between two nontreponemal test results that were obtained using the same serologic test.

Nontreponemal tests are used as the primary screening tests in cases of suspected syphilis and for serial measurement of nontreponemal antibody titers to assess disease activity after therapy. These tests are nonreactive in 25% to 33% of patients with primary, late latent, and tertiary disease. They are reactive in nearly 100% of cases of secondary disease. Temporarily false-positive nontreponemal tests are associated with several other diseases, such as *Mycoplasma pneumoniae* infections, Epstein-Barr virus infections, and malaria. Chronically false-positive tests, usually with low titers, are seen with systemic lupus erythematosus, leprosy, and addiction to narcotics.

Treponemal tests are done to confirm that reactive nontreponemal serologies are the result of treponemal infection. Falsely reactive treponemal tests occur in about 1% of the general population. A person who has a reactive treponemal test usually will have a reactive test for a lifetime, regardless of treatment or disease activity. Treponemal test antibody correlates poorly with disease activity and should not be used to assess response to treatment. No single test can be used to diagnose neurosyphilis among all persons. The diagnosis of neurosyphilis can be made based on various combinations of reactive serologic test results, abnormalities of CSF cell count or protein, or a reactive CSF VDRL or CSF FTA-ABS.

Treatment

Evaluation of infants for congenital syphilis should include those born to seropositive women who (1) have untreated syphilis; (2) were treated during pregnancy with erythromycin; (3) were treated for syphilis less than 1 month before delivery; (4) were treated for syphilis during pregnancy with the appropriate penicillin regimen but did not have a fourfold or greater decrease in nontreponemal antibody titers; (5) do not have a well-documented history of treatment for syphilis; or (6) were treated appropriately before pregnancy but had insufficient serologic follow-up to ensure an appropriate response to treatment.

Parenteral penicillin G is the drug of choice for therapy of all stages of syphilis. The susceptibility of *T. pallidum* to penicillin has not diminished since it was introduced for treatment in 1943. The dosage and the length of treatment depend on the stage and clinical manifestations of disease. Penicillin G is the only therapy considered adequate and with documented efficacy for neurosyphilis or for syphilis during pregnancy. Persons in these two situations who report penicillin allergy should almost always undergo desensitization, if necessary, and be treated with penicillin. During therapy the Jarisch-Herxheimer reaction may occur, and the patient should be informed about it before therapy. It is an acute febrile reaction accompanied by headache, myalgia, chills, tachycardia, and flushing that may occur within the first 24 hours after any therapy for syphilis.

Gonorrhea

Gonorrhea is a sexually transmitted infection of columnar and transitional epithelium caused by the bacterial organism *Neisseria gonorrhoeae*. Concomitant trichomoniasis or chlamydial infection is present in about 50% of persons with gonorrhea. The mode of transmission is almost exclusively sexual contact. Not everyone exposed to gonorrhea acquires the disease, and the risk of transmission from male to female is higher than the risk of female to male transmission. *N. gonorrhoeae* infects the urethra, endocervix, anal canal, conjunctiva, and pharynx directly. Infection can extend and involve the prostate, vas deferens, seminal vesicles, epididymis, and testes in men and Skene's glands, Bartholin's glands, endometrium, fallopian tubes, and ovaries in women. In homosexual men, gonococcal infection commonly involves the urethra, anal canal, and pharynx. Gonococcal infection in heterosexual men usually involves only the urethra; pharyngeal gonococcal infection occurs in 5% of those exposed by oral-genital contact. Systemic complications are dermatitis, arthritis, endocarditis, myopericarditis, meningitis, and hepatitis.

Signs and symptoms of urethritis develop from 2 to 30 days after inoculation. The first sign is a purulent yellow or green-yellow urethral discharge, dysuria, frequency, and malaise. Men who are uncircumcised may also develop balanoposthitis, resulting in a discharge from under the prepuce. A complication of balanoposthitis is phimosis from inflammation and edema of the glans. Most symptomatic men seek treatment, so the disease is halted without further problems. Those who develop no or minimal symptoms or ignore symptoms become a main source of spread of infection and also are at risk for developing systemic complications. If untreated, by about 10 to 14 days, infection ascends from the anterior urethra to the posterior urethra so that dysuria becomes more intense and malaise, headache, and regional lymphadenopathy develop. Continuing infection causes prostatitis, epididymitis, and cystitis in about 8% to 10% of men.

The incubation period in women is at least 2 weeks. The primary site of infection is the endocervix, with urethral infection in 70% to 90% of cases. Primary urethritis without cervical involvement is rare in women except in those who have undergone a total hysterectomy. More than half of women infected with gonorrhea have no symptoms or only mild symptoms that are frequently ignored, including vaginal discharge, dysuria, frequency, backache, abdominal pain, and pelvic pain. On examination the cervix is friable and edematous, often with a purulent or mucopurulent drainage. Bartholin's glands are likely to become infected with possible abscess formation. Infection ascending to the fallopian tubes, ovaries, and peritoneum occurs in about 20% of women. Gonococcal pelvic inflammatory disease (PID) symptoms are lower abdominal pain and general malaise. Possible sequelae of PID are chronic pelvic pain, dyspareunia, ectopic pregnancy, and sterility caused by adhesion formation and tissue scarring, even though treatment was successful.

Rectal mucosa can become infected in both men and women as a result of autoinoculation or anal intercourse. Infection of the pharynx is caused by oral-genital sexual contact. Direct contamination of the eye by fingers or towels causes gonococcal conjunctivitis. Neonates acquire gonococcal conjunctivitis by direct contact with the organism during birth through an infected birth canal.

Disseminated gonococcal infection is quite rare and occurs most often in women after menstruation when the organism has ready access to the upper genital tract. Signs and symptoms are skin rashes (macules, papules, pustules, or vesicles) (Fig. 66-4), arthritis, and arthralgias. Natural immunity after an infection by N. gonorrhoeae does not occur, so infection can be acquired more than once. Diagnosis is made by culture of discharge material from infected sites.

Gonorrhea was treated with penicillin beginning in the 1940s, but there have been major changes in antimicrobial resistance to treatment of gonorrhea. Resistance is increasing dramatically, worldwide, to penicillin G, sulfonamides, and tetracycline as each of these agents become commonly used for treatment. Currently, treatment for uncomplicated gonorrhea recommended by the CDC is ceftriaxone IM in a single dose or cefixime, ciprofloxacin, or ofloxacin orally in a single dose. Treatment of possible coinfection with *Chlamydia trachomatis* with a concomitant regimen for 1 week of doxycycline orally is recommended.

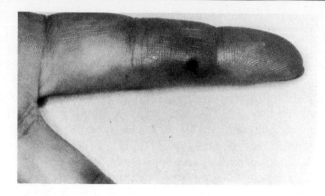

FIG. 66-4 Necrotic pustules over the palms are characteristic of disseminated gonorrhea. (Courtesy of Marek A. Stawiski, MD, Associate Clinical Professor of Internal Medicine, Michigan State University.)

Chlamydial Infection

The most common bacterial sexually transmitted disease worldwide is infection with *C. trachomatis*. Three species of *Chlamydia* are *trachomatis*, *pneumoniae*, and *psittaci*. Two serovars of *C. trachomatis* that cause disease in humans are lymphogranuloma (LGV) and trachoma. Strains of LGV serovar infect inguinal lymphatics and lymph nodes. Strains of trachoma serovar infect conjunctiva, causing the disease commonly called *ocular trachoma;* other strains infect urogenital columnar epithelial cells, causing a genital tract infection in adults, which is the disease commonly called chlamydia, and causing conjunctivitis and occasionally pneumonia in infants exposed at birth.

C. trachomatis infection of the genital tract is most common in sexually active adolescents and young adults in the United States. It is insidious, and symptoms are absent or minor among most infected women and many men. This large group of asymptomatic and infectious persons sustains transmission.

Chlamydial infection is transmitted by sexual intercourse, and in women the cervix is the primary site. The major signs and symptoms are a mucopurulent vaginal discharge with cervical ectopy and edema caused by cervicitis; dysuria is present when concomitant chlamydial urethritis is present. The urethra is not commonly a primary site for chlamydial infection in women. About 60% of women will not have symptoms, and untreated infections often persist for months. During this period many of these women transmit their infection to sexual partners and newborn infants and are also at high risk for developing upper urogenital tract infection and subsequent infertility. Endometritis and salpingitis occur as the organism ascends from the lower to the upper tract. Ascending infection usually causes mild to moderate abdominal pain. Progression of the infection causes PID in as many as 50% of women, resulting in scarring, adhesions, and occlusion of the fallopian tubes. Acute right upper abdominal pain indicates advancement of infection to perihepatic peritonitis, which can simulate acute cholelithiasis. Seventeen percent of women treated for PID will become infertile; an equal number will experience chronic pelvic pain; and of those who do conceive, 10% will have an ectopic pregnancy.

In men, urethritis is the most common site of infection caused by *C. trachomatis*. The infection usually remains localized to the urethra but may ascend the urogenital tract to cause epididymis or prostatitis. There is no associated inguinal lymphadenopathy or tenderness. The most common complaint of men with urethral infection is dysuria and discharge that ranges from clear to grossly purulent. It typically begins 7 to 10 days after sexual contact with an infected partner. More than half of men with chlamydial infection remain asymptomatic or have only mild symptoms.

C. trachomatis is the cause of 30% to 50% of cases of nongonococcal urethritis (NGU) and is found to coexist in about 20% of men with gonococcal urethritis. *C. trachomatis* is recovered from 60% to 70% of women partners of men with chlamydial NGU. Epididymitis occurs in about 5% of men, mostly under 35 years of age, with untreated chlamydial urethritis. Progression of the infection causes scarring and tissue damage of the duct system in men, which can lead to infertility. Untreated infection and/or asymptomatic infection is a source for spread of the organism to sexual partners.

An infant born to a woman with chlamydial infection of the endocervix has about a 70% chance of being infected. About 30% of infants born to infected women develop neonatal inclusion conjunctivitis, and 15% develop pneumonia; some have both diseases.

Chlamydia can be diagnosed by culture of secretions obtained from suspected infected sites. Other available diagnostic tests include direct fluorescent antibody (DFA) tests, enzyme-linked immunosorbent assay (ELISA), and DNA probe of secretions.

The recommended treatment regimens for uncomplicated urethral, endocervical, or rectal chlamydial infections in men and nonpregnant women are doxycycline or azithromycin given orally. Erythromycin is the treatment of choice for pregnant women and neonates.

Herpes Simplex Virus

Herpes simplex virus (HSV-1 and HSV-2) cause skin and mucosal disease. HSV-1 typically infects the oropharyngeal area, although it is the cause of primary genital infections in the United States. HSV-2 is the usual cause of genital herpes infection. Humans are the only natural reservoir of HSV, and because the organism is physically unstable and skin and mucous membranes are the major portals of entry to the body, HSV is spread only by close personal contact with infectious secretions from lesions. The primary mode of transmission of HSV-2 is sexual contact. Infection most often is introduced on mucous membranes or through injured or broken skin. HSV is characterized by a primary infection with recurrences. The course of each episode is self-limiting. There is no cure.

Primary infection typically begins 2 to 7 days after a sexual contact (range 1 to 45 days, mean 5.8 days). Type 1 and type 2 HSV genital infections are identical clinically. Individuals with a history of type 1 HSV oropharyngeal lesions and antibodies are likely to have a mild primary infection with type 2 HSV and may have few or no lesions or symptoms. Most of the source contacts have a history of genital herpes, but genital herpes may be acquired from persons who were not aware that they have a genital infection with HSV. Also they may be asymptomatic at the time of the sexual contact and not aware of the potential for transmission.

Signs and symptoms of primary infection include fever, malaise, and headache in about two thirds of women and one third of men. More than three fourths of persons develop tender inguinal adenopathy. Localized genital symptoms and severe pain occur in nearly everyone with primary infection. Most women also note vaginal discharge and dysuria, and some urinary retention may occur secondary to dysuria. About half of men have dysuria, and 25% have urethral discharge.

There are usually multiple bilateral genital lesions that begin as papules or vesicles and ulcerate within 3 to 6 days. The most common sites are the labia and mons in women, and in men the penile glans and shaft (Fig. 66-5). Contiguous skin sites can be involved, particularly on the buttocks or perianal area. Occasionally, these are the only sites involved. Autoinoculation may result in involvement of remote areas, such as the fingers. Herpetic pharyngitis may be present in up to 20% of cases of primary genital herpes. Perianal vesicles are common and may occur without prior rectal intercourse. True herpetic proctitis is most common in homosexual men or heterosexual women who have engaged in rectal intercourse. It may be present without other genital lesions and is second only to gonorrhea as an infectious cause of proctitis. Erosive cervicitis occurs in most women, and viral culture results of the cervix are positive in 90% of cases; vaginal mucosal lesions occur in less than 10% of cases. Cervical or vaginal lesions may be the only evidence of primary disease. Painful, ulcerative genital lesions persist for several days. In severe cases, lesions may be present for more than 2 weeks before healing.

After primary infection, HSV becomes latent in the dorsal root ganglia of the nerves supplying the infected areas. Recurrence of genital herpes is said to be related to menses, sexual activity, and stress. With reactivation, infectious virus is transported from the nerve root ganglia to the body surface along sensory nerves to skin sites, where development of characteristic lesions occurs. If HSV-1 is the cause of symptomatic primary genital infection, 40% to 55% of persons have a recurrence within

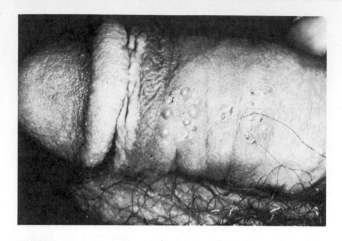

FIG. 66-5   Grouped, painful vesicles in herpes progenitalis. (Courtesy of Marek A. Stawiski, MD, Associate Clinical Professor of Internal Medicine, Michigan State University.)

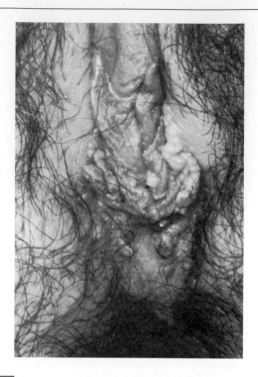

FIG. 66-6   Verrucous, moist nodules of condyloma acuminatum of the vulva. (Courtesy of Marek A. Stawiski, MD, Associate Clinical Professor of Internal Medicine, Michigan State University.)

1 year; with HSV-2, the recurrence rate is about 80%. Rates of recurrence vary widely among affected persons and from episode to episode in the same person. Typically, five to eight episodes occur per year for most persons, but some have recurrences monthly or more frequently; some will have symptoms with primary infection and then never again.

Recurrent herpes episodes tend to be milder than the primary infection. Half of persons experience a prodrome of burning or itching at the site of developing lesions. Systemic symptoms are usually absent, and lesions, which tend to occur unilaterally and always in the same areas, are fewer and smaller. Dysuria occurs with recurrent infection in 25% of women and 10% of men. Recurrent episodes usually last about 5 to 10 days, with pain lasting about 4 days. The recurrent vesicles and ulcers are infectious to sexual partners until the ulcers heal completely. Viral shedding during recurrences is short-lived, and titers are low. Transmission to others usually occurs when there are active, symptomatic lesions, but the virus can be shed and transmitted in the absence of active lesions as well. No signs or symptoms are present to alert an individual to this state. It is a common belief that recurrences diminish over time, but no reliable data substantiate this.

Herpes simplex virus infection can be diagnosed from culture of specimens obtained from vesicles (found in 90% of cultures), from ulcers (found in 70% of cultures), and from dry or crusted lesions (found in 30% of cultures).

Systemic acyclovir therapy provides partial control of the symptoms for herpes episodes when used during primary infections or for recurrent episodes when used as suppressive therapy after primary infection. When treatment with oral acyclovir for recurrent episodes is begun during the prodrome or within 2 days of onset of lesions, there is only limited benefit. Acyclovir does not eradicate

latent virus or affect subsequent risk, frequency, or severity of recurrences after the drug is discontinued. During an outbreak, topical therapy with acyclovir is substantially less effective in reducing symptoms than the oral drug, and its use is discouraged.

Immunocompromised persons may have prolonged episodes with extensive disease, and use of oral acyclovir for primary genital herpes and herpes proctitis is the recommended therapy. Hospitalization for IV acyclovir therapy may be necessary for severe disease or complications in some individuals. Therapy in persons not immunocompromised is not generally recommended.

Papillomavirus Infection

Human papillomaviruses (HPVs) are pathogens that commonly induce a variety of benign tumors called *warts;* they are also associated with several premalignant and malignant lesions. Exophytic genital and anal warts called *condylomata acuminata* are benign growths most commonly caused by HPV type 6 or 11. Other HPV types that may cause infection in the anogenital region (e.g., types 16, 18, 31, 33, and 35) have been strongly associated with dysplasia and carcinoma of the cervix. These types are usually associated with subclinical infection but are also found in exophytic warts and usually are present with type 6 or 11 (Fig. 66-6).

Condyloma acuminatum is the most common sexually transmitted viral disease in the United States. Transmission is by direct contact with an HPV-induced lesion. The incubation period can be weeks to months. Condyloma acuminatum occurs most often in young, sexually active adults. No generalized viral infection signs or symptoms are present with HPV infection. HPV-induced lesions of the respiratory tract (recurrent respiratory papillomatosis) can occur in infants and young children after exposure of the fetus or neonate to HPV during pregnancy or birth. The route of transmission, whether transplacental, via the birth canal, or postnatal, is unknown.

Condylomata acuminata are soft, fleshy, cauliflower-like exophytic lesions that may be tan, pink, or white on the skin of the genitalia, perineum, and perianal regions. They can spread from the point of inoculation, and single warts may multiply into cauliflower-like growths several centimeters in diameter. HPV infection manifestations may range from only mild involvement without symptoms to large growths with local irritation, pruritus, burning, ulceration, and secondary bacterial infection in both men and women. Evaluation for the presence of internal lesions in the vagina, cervix, urethra, anus, and rectum is important. Men who are sexual contacts of women with HPV-induced cervical lesions can develop small lesions on the shaft and glans of the penis. The warts are benign growths, but the association of the virus with eventual genital tract malignancies is significant. HPV DNA sequences have been found in 93% of cervical carcinomas and in some vulvar and penile carcinomas.

Condylomata acuminata can usually be identified clinically by their appearance. However, they must be distinguished from condylomata lata (the flat, whitish lesions of secondary syphilis) and molluscum contagiosum. Atypical lesions should be biopsied and examined histologically. Detection of HPV DNA sequences is an accurate way to diagnose HPV.

No therapy has been found to eradicate HPV. The goal of treatment is removal of exophytic warts for mechanical or cosmetic reasons and the amelioration of signs and symptoms. Removal of external genital warts is not likely to change the risk for the development of cervical cancer. In clinical trials it is reported that currently available therapeutic methods range from 22% to 94% effective in clearing external exophytic genital warts and that recurrence rates are at least 25% within 3 months regardless of treatment modality. In placebo-controlled studies, genital warts have cleared spontaneously without treatment in 20% to 30% of cases within 3 months. For external genital and perianal warts, recommended therapy is (1) cryotherapy with liquid nitrogen or cryoprobe, (2) topical Podofin 25% solution for self-treatment, or (3) topical podophyllin in 10% to 25% for application by a physician. Before treatment of cervical lesions, dysplasia must first be excluded. Vaginal, urethral meatus, or anal warts can all be ablated by cryotherapy with liquid nitrogen. During pregnancy the lesions have a tendency to proliferate and become friable. Topical podofilox and podophyllin are contradicted during pregnancy. Removal of visible warts is recommended during pregnancy, using cryotherapy, because of possible mechanical obstruction of the birth canal and bleeding during delivery of the baby.

Lymphogranuloma Venereum, Chancroid, and Donovanosis Infections

Lymphogranuloma venereum (LGV) is caused by serovars of *C. trachomatis.* It is also known as *Durand-Nicolas-Favre disease, tropical bubo,* and *lymphogranuloma inguinale.* LGV occurs in most areas of the world, but most cases are concentrated in tropical and subtropical areas. Local epidemics and sporadic cases number between 200 and 400 annually in the United States. The primary lesion is a small, painless herpetiform vesicle or ulcer, usually on the posterior vaginal wall in women and the coronal sulcus of the penis in men. It is present only a few days, heals without scarring, and causes no symptoms. The organisms are carried from the site of entry through the lymphatics to the regional lymph nodes. The nodes swell and form exquisitely tender masses. Abscesses develop that may erode through the skin to form sinus tracts. Local complications such as genital elephantiasis, strictures, and fistulas of the penis, urethra, and rectum may occur. The most common clinical manifestation of LGV among heterosexuals is tender inguinal lymphadenopathy that is most commonly unilateral. Secondary to anal intercourse, women and homosexual men may have proctocolitis or inflammatory involvement of perirectal or perianal lymphatic tissues resulting in fistulas and strictures.

Diagnosis of LGV is made serologically and by exclusion of other causes of inguinal lymphadenopathy or genital ulcers. Doxycycline is the preferred treatment.

Chancroid (soft chancre) is a sexually transmitted disease caused by the bacillus *Haemophilus ducreyi* that is endemic in many developing countries where it is the most common cause of genital ulcer disease. It also occurs in isolated, limited epidemics in industrialized societies where it occurs among and is spread by people who have traveled to endemic areas. The initial lesion is a papule that quickly ulcerates. The classic chancroidal ulcer begins as a tender papule that ulcerates within 24 hours. In men, chancroidal ulcers are common in six sites: 50% of lesions occur on the prepuce in uncircumcised males, then the coronal sulcus, then the skin of the penile shaft, followed by the glans, urethral meatus, and the scrotum. In women, the most common sites for ulcers are the labia majora, fourchette, labia minora, perineum, medial aspects of the thighs, clitoris, and perianal area. Cervical ulcers occur in 10% to 20% of cases. Many women will have few symptoms and continue to be sexually active. Definitive diagnosis can be made by identifying the organism *H. ducreyi* on a special culture medium not readily available to most laboratories. Diagnosis can also be made from clinical manifestations of chancroid ulcers plus no evidence of *T. pallidum* by serology and dark-field examination of ulcer exudate and no evidence of culture of HSV. However, as many as 10% of persons with chancroid may also be infected with *T. pallidum* or HSV. The recommended therapeutic agents are azithromycin or erythromycin orally or ceftriaxone intramuscularly.

Donovanosis is a sexually transmitted mucocutaneous ulcerative disease of the genital, inguinal, or perianal regions with low infectivity and morbidity. The causative organism is *Calymmatobacterium granulomatis*. The incidence is low in developed countries but is seen in the southeastern United States. It begins as one or more indurated papules at the site of contact, which, over several days to weeks, will ulcerate. The ulcers are bright, beefy-red, painless, and without inflammation or systemic manifestations. In women, the labia near the fourchette are the most common sites for lesions; in men, the foreskin and glans penis are the most common sites for lesions. The diagnosis is made by identifying Donovan bodies (the bacillus found in mononuclear cells) in smears or biopsies. No standardized serologic tests are available for diagnosis. Treatment regimens include use of chloramphenicol, streptomycin, cotrimoxazole, and the tetracyclines.

Trichomonas Infection

The causative organism of trichomoniasis, *Trichomonas vaginalis,* is a protozoan parasite. In women, the organism can infect the vagina, urethra, bladder, Skene's glands, and Bartholin's glands. In men, it can infect the urethra, prostate, seminal vesicles, and epididymides. Diagnosis is made when the organism can be identified by the clinician with microscopic examination of vaginal, cervical, or urethral discharge. The primary presenting symptom in women is vulvovaginitis and in men urethritis. Fifty percent of women with proven gonorrhea also have trichomoniasis; candidiasis and trichomoniasis also often coexist. Because *T. vaginalis* grows best at a pH of 5.5 to 5.8, conditions that raise vaginal pH, such as pregnancy, use of oral contraceptives, frequent douching, or cervical lesions, predispose to trichomoniasis. The organism is transmitted by coitus.

Signs and symptoms of trichomonas vaginitis are a profuse, malodorous, frothy vaginal discharge; dysuria with pruritus; edema of the vulva; and small, surface hemorrhages in the cervix (strawberry cervix). Associated problems can be dyspareunia and tenderness. However, more than 50% of women with trichomoniasis are asymptomatic. If untreated, symptoms may resolve but infection persists subclinically and may be associated with an abnormal Papanicolaou smear.

Most male sexual partners of women with the *Trichomonas* organism carry the organism in the urethra and prostate. The symptoms in men are mild to severe urethritis with dysuria and frequency, but many men may be asymptomatic or experience only transient symptoms, despite the presence of persistent subclinical infection. There is no evidence of severe complications or long-term sequelae from untreated *Trichomonas* infections.

Trichomonas infections are treated with an oral drug that can eradicate the organism from all the possible sites in which it can be harbored. Sexual contacts should also be treated. The organism is sensitive to the drug metronidazole, an imidazole compound. Short-term use in nonpregnant women is thought to be justified at this time, but pregnant women should be treated with clotrimazole.

Candida Infection

Candidiasis is not, strictly speaking, a venereal disease. However, vaginitis, vulvovaginitis, balanitis, or balanoposthitis caused by this organism have been identified after sexual contact.

Several *Candida* species are normally present in the mouth, throat, and large intestine of men and women and in the vagina of asymptomatic women. The common causative organism of genital candidiasis is *Candida albicans*. An overgrowth of this organism, which occurs when there is a change in host resistance or local bacterial flora, causes symptomatic vaginitis.

Predisposing factors for vaginal overgrowth of *Candida* are broad-spectrum antibiotic therapy, diabetes, pregnancy, menstruation, immunosuppressive drugs, and constrictive synthetic fiber underclothing. Use of oral contraceptives is associated with an increase in the presence of vaginal *Candida* organisms, but not with symptomatic candidal infection.

The most prominent symptom of yeast vaginitis in women is intense vulvar and vaginal pruritus and irritation. Vulvar edema, erythema, and fissures may occur, with dysuria secondary to inflamed tissue (external dysuria). A curdlike, cottage cheese–like vaginal discharge is often present. Examination reveals a dry, bright red vagina with adherent white plaques. Men are often asymptomatic. The most common signs are an erythematous "glazed skin" appearance on the penis and vesicles or erosions of the glans or inner surface of the prepuce. Symptoms include varying degrees of itching, burning, or irritation of the penis or glans. As infection progresses, the lesions appear crusted, adherent white cheesy patches may appear on the glans, and occasionally the scrotal skin has scaling pruritic lesions. Phimosis is a complication of candidal balanoposthitis. Most commonly, women become infected secondary to one of the predisposing factors that causes organism overgrowth. Men most commonly acquire infection from sexual contact with women who have vaginal candidiasis.

Genital candidiasis is treated with topical antifungal cream and suppository preparations. One of the imidazole compounds is the most effective agent. A cream is applied to the lesions of the penis or the vulva; a cream or suppository is used intravaginally for vaginal lesions.

Before applying topical preparations, the vulva or glans penis and prepuce should be washed with soap and water and dried well. Absorption of oral antifungal preparations from the GI tract is poor and is not considered effective for primary therapy.

Bacterial Vaginosis (Nonspecific Vaginitis)

Vaginitis that results from an overgrowth of both anaerobic bacteria and *Gardnerella vaginalis* (formerly *Haemophilus vaginalis*) is called bacterial vaginosis. *G. vaginalis* and anaerobes are part of the normal vaginal flora, but overgrowth can cause a vaginal discharge. The cause or causes of overgrowth are unknown.

Symptoms are the presence of a thin, yellow-gray, fishy-odor discharge that adheres to the vaginal walls and introitus. The vaginal epithelium is normal appearing. Addition of 10% potassium hydroxide to a slide preparation of the discharge accentuates the fishy odor and is diagnostic for this condition. Usually *G. vaginalis* also can be recovered from the urethra of 90% of male sexual contacts of infected women. The organism can be identified on the glans and under the prepuce. Signs and symptoms of infection in men are increased mucoid discharge from under the prepuce, fishy odor, and mild inflammation of the glans penis and prepuce.

Metronidazole is the most effective drug to eradicate this infection. Oral ampicillin is also an effective drug for treatment. Sexual contacts should also be treated.

Genital *Mycoplasma* Infection

Mycoplasma hominis, Ureaplasma urealyticum, and *Mycoplasma genitalium* are three *Mycoplasma* organisms frequently found in the genital tract, which are not highly virulent but have been associated with several different pathogenic conditions. The frequency of colonization with mycoplasma organisms increases with sexual contact. They have been recovered from the fallopian tubes of 5% to 15% of women with salpingitis and from the blood of 10% to 15% of women with postpartum fever. The presence of the organism in pregnant women has been associated with chorioamnionitis and low birth weight in the infant. The organisms have been recovered from mid-trimester abortuses, suggesting a relationship between the organisms and spontaneous abortion. The association of mycoplasma organisms and NGU in men is unknown. Balanitis may accompany *Mycoplasma* urethritis. *Mycoplasma* organisms are sensitive to tetracycline, aminoglycosides, and chloramphenicol.

QUESTIONS

▼ *Answer the following on a separate sheet of paper.*

1. Define the term venereal or sexually transmitted disease (STD).
2. What is the impact of sexually transmitted diseases on the health of individuals, and the economic consequences of STDs in the United States?
3. What is the causative organism in syphilis?
4. Describe the treatments for primary, secondary, early latent, and tertiary syphilis.
5. When the diagnosis of gonorrhea is confirmed by culture, what is the usual treatment?
6. What problems are associated with genital herpes infection?
7. What are the potential sequelae of condylomata acuminata infection?
8. Describe the treatment for chlamydial infections.

▼ *Circle the letter preceding each item below that correctly answers the question or completes the statement. More than one answer may be correct.*

9. One sign of primary syphilis that develops at the site of infection about 3 weeks after initial contact is:
   a. Skin rash
   b. Painless chancre
   c. Painful ulcers
   d. Pruritus
10. The principal test to positively confirm early primary syphilis is the:
    a. Fluorescent treponemal antibody absorption (FTA-ABS)
    b. Dark-field microscopy
    c. VDRL test
    d. KOH preparation
11. Which of the following statements are true of secondary syphilis?
    a. It develops several weeks to months after exposure.
    b. All lesions are contagious.
    c. Untreated, it almost always leads to cardiovascular syphilis.
    d. Chancre heals spontaneously.
12. Which of the following should always be included in a differential diagnosis of syphilis?
    a. Tinea versicolor
    b. Acne
    c. Pityriasis rosea
    d. Seborrheic keratosis

13. Which of the following are signs and symptoms of tertiary syphilis?
    a. Gummas on the skin, bones, or liver
    b. Ataxia, paresis, strokes, or personality changes
    c. Aortic aneurysms
    d. Malignant tumors as a result of GI involvement
14. Gonorrhea infections are increasing because:
    a. The majority of women with the disease are asymptomatic
    b. The incubation period for the causative organism in women is at least 2 weeks
    c. The gonococcus organism is usually resistant to penicillin
    d. Males can be asymptomatic carriers of the disease
15. Which of the following conditions is a sexually transmitted chlamydial disease?
    a. Lymphogranuloma venereum
    b. Chancroid
    c. Granuloma inguinale
    d. Trichomoniasis
16. The primary presenting symptom of women with a *Trichomonas* infection is:

Continued.

QUESTIONS—cont'd

a. Intense vulvar and vaginal pruritus
b. Presence of a thin, yellow-gray, fishy-odor discharge
c. Vulvovaginitis
d. Vulvar edema

17. The treatment for condylomata acuminata (external warts in the genital area) is:
    a. Caustic podophyllin resin 25% in tincture of benzoin
    b. Laser

c. Surgical excision
d. Clotrimazole

▼ *Circle T if the statement is true and F if it is false. Correct any false statements.*

18. T F It is estimated that nearly 20 million individuals are infected with genital herpes.
19. T F The human papillomavirus (HPV) responsible for condylomata acuminata is the same papovavirus that causes common warts.
20. T F The cervix is the primary site of chlamydial infection in women.
21. T F Candidiasis is classified as a venereal disease.
22. T F The presence of *Mycoplasma* organisms in pregnant women has been associated with chorioamnionitis and low infant birth weight.

BIBLIOGRAPHY ▼ PART XI

Arno JN, Jones RB: Venereal chlamydial infections. In Hoeprich PD, Jordan MC, Ronald AR, editors: *Infectious diseases,* ed 5, Philadelphia, 1994, Lippincott.

Cassell GH, Waites KB: Genital mycoplasma infections. In Hoeprich PD, Jordan MC, Ronald AR, editors: *Infectious diseases,* ed 5, Philadelphia, 1994, Lippincott.

Centers for Disease Control: Primary and secondary syphilis—United States, 1981-1990, *MMWR* 40:19, 1991.

Centers for Disease Control and Prevention: Recommendations for prevention and management of *Chlamydia trachomatis* infections, 1993, *MMWR* 42:RR12, 1993.

Centers for Disease Control and Prevention: Sexually transmitted disease treatment guidelines, *MMWR* 42:RR14, 1993.

Centers for Disease Control: Deaths from breast cancer—United States, 1991, *MMWR* 43:15, 1994.

Centers for Disease Control and Prevention: Results from the national breast and cervical early detection program, October 31, 1991–September 30, 1993, *MMWR* 43:29, 1994.

Centers for Disease Control and Prevention: Trends in sexual risk behaviors among high school students—United States, 1990, 1991, 1993, *MMWR* 44:7, 1995.

Council on Scientific Affairs: Estrogen replacement in the menopause, *JAMA* 249(3):359-361, 1983.

Danforth DN et al: *Obstetrics and gynecology,* Philadelphia, 1990, Lippincott.

Fife KH: Papillomaviruses and human warts. In Hoeprich PD, Jordan MC, Ronald AR, editors: *Infectious diseases,* ed 5, Philadelphia, 1994, Lippincott.

Fishman JR, deVereWhite RW: Prostate cancer screening, diagnosis, and staging. In Krane RJ, Siroky MB, Fitzpatrick JM, editors: *Clinical urology,* Philadelphia, 1994, Lippincott.

Gillenwater JY et al: *Adult and pediatric urology,* Chicago, 1987, Mosby.

Gleave ME, vonEschenbach AC: Testicular tumors. In Krane RJ, Siroky MB, Fitzpatrick JM, editors: *Clinical urology,* Philadelphia, 1994, Lippincott.

Goodman JL: Infections caused by herpes simplex viruses. In Hoeprich PD, Jordan MC, Ronald AR, editors: *Infectious diseases,* ed 5, Philadelphia, 1994, Lippincott.

Gusberg SB, Shingleton HM, Deppe G: *Female genital cancer,* New York, 1988, Churchill Livingstone.

Hacker NF et al: Vulva. In Hoskins WJ, Perez CA, Young RC, editors: *Principles and practice of gynecologic oncology,* Philadelphia, 1992, Lippincott.

Hanks GE, Myers CE, Scardino PT: Cancer of the prostate. In DeVita VT, Hellman S, Rosenberg A, editors: *Cancer: principles and practice of oncology,* ed 4, Philadelphia, 1993, Lippincott.

Hare MH, editor: *Genital tract infection in women,* Edinburgh, 1988, Churchill Livingstone.

Harris JR, Morrow M, Bonadonna G: Cancer of the breast. In DeVita VT, Hellman S, Rosenberg A, editors: *Cancer: principles and practice of oncology,* ed 4, Philadelphia, 1993, Lippincott.

Holmes KK et al, editors: *Sexually transmitted diseases,* ed 2, New York, 1990, McGraw-Hill.

Hoskins WJ, Perez CA, Young RC: Gynecologic tumors. In DeVita VT, Hellman S, Rosenberg A, editors: *Cancer: principles and practice of oncology,* ed 4, Philadelphia, 1993, Lippincott.

Hoskins KF et al: Assessment and counseling for women with a family history of breast cancer, *JAMA* 273(7):577-585, 1995.

Krieger JN: Infections of the genital tract. In Krane RJ, Siroky MB, Fitzpatrick JM, editors: *Clinical urology,* Philadelphia, 1994, Lippincott.

Krieger JN: Prostatitis, epididymitis, and orchitis. In Mandell GL, Bennett JE, Dolin R, editors: *Principles and practice of infectious diseases,* ed 4, New York, 1995, Churchill Livingstone.

Ledger WJ: *Infection in the female,* Philadelphia, 1986, Lea & Febiger.

Lichter AS et al: Breast cancer. In Hoskins WJ, Perez CA, Young RC, editors: *Principles and practice of gynecologic oncology,* Philadelphia, 1992, Lippincott.

Lippman ME, Lichter AS, Danforth DN: *Diagnosis and management of breast cancer,* Philadelphia, 1988, Saunders.

Lowrey G. *Growth and development of children,* Chicago, 1986, Mosby.

Markman M, Zaino R, et al: Carcinoma of the fallopian tube. In Hoskins WJ, Perez CA, Young RC, editors: *Principles and practice of gynecologic oncology,* Philadelphia, 1992, Lippincott.

McCormack WM, Rein MF: Urethritis. In Mandell GL, Bennett

BIBLIOGRAPHY ▼ PART XI

JE, Dolin R, editors: *Principles and practice of infectious diseases,* ed 4, New York, 1995, Churchill Livingstone.

Mead PB: Infections of the female pelvis. In Mandell GL, Bennett JE, Dolin R, editors: *Principles and practice of infectious diseases,* ed 4, New York, 1995, Churchill Livingstone.

Meares EM: Bacterial prostatitis. In Hoeprich PD, Jordan MC, Ronald AR, editors: *Infectious diseases,* ed 5, Philadelphia, 1994, Lippincott.

Morrissey JP, Cameron DW: Donovanosis. In Hoeprich PD, Jordan MC, Ronald AR, editors: *Infectious diseases,* ed 5, Philadelphia, 1994, Lippincott.

Morse SA, Holmes KK: Gonococcal infections. In Hoeprich PD, Jordan MC, Ronald AR, editors: *Infectious diseases,* ed 5, Philadelphia, 1994, Lippincott.

Perez CA, Kurman RJ, et al: Uterine cervix. In Hoskins WJ, Perez CA, Young RC, editors: *Principles and practice of gynecologic oncology,* Philadelphia, 1992, Lippincott.

Perez CA et al: Vagina. In Hoskins WJ, Perez CA, Young RC, editors: *Principles and practice of gynecologic oncology,* Philadelphia, 1992, Lippincott.

Perine PL: Lymphogranuloma venereum. In Hoeprich PD, Jordan MC, Ronald AR, editors: *Infectious diseases,* ed 5, Philadelphia, 1994, Lippincott.

Potosky AL et al: The role of increasing detection in the rising incidence of prostate cancer, *JAMA* 273(7):548-552, 1995.

Rallison M: *Growth disorders in infants, children, and adolescents,* New York, 1986, John Wiley and Sons.

Rein MF: Genital skin and mucous membrane lesions. In Mandell GL, Bennett JE, Dolin R, editors: *Principles and practice of infectious diseases,* ed 4, New York, 1995, Churchill Livingstone.

Rein MF: Vulvovaginitis and cervicitis. In Mandell GL, Bennett JE, Dolin R, editors: *Principles and practice of infectious diseases,* ed 4, New York, 1995, Churchill Livingstone.

Robey EL, Schellhammer PF: Scrotal cancer. In Krane RJ, Siroky MB, Fitzpatrick JM, editors: *Clinical urology,* Philadelphia, 1994, Lippincott.

Ronald AR: Chancroid. In Hoeprich PD, Jordan MC, Ronald AR, editors: *Infectious diseases,* ed 5, Philadelphia, 1994, Lippincott.

Sarosdy MF: Prostate adenocarcinoma: the management of pelvic confined disease. In Krane RJ, Siroky MB, Fitzpatrick JM, editors: *Clinical urology,* Philadelphia, 1994, Lippincott.

Schellhammer PF: Penile cancer. In Krane RJ, Siroky MB, Fitzpatrick JM, editors: *Clinical urology,* Philadelphia, 1994, Lippincott.

Schultz MJ, Crawford DE: Prostate adenocarcinoma: the management of metastatic disease. In Krane RJ, Siroky MB, Fitzpatrick JM, editors: *Clinical urology,* Philadelphia, 1994, Lippincott.

Skiner DG, Lieskovsky G: *Diagnosis and management of genitourinary cancer,* Philadelphia, 1988, Saunders.

Tanagho EA, McAninch JW: *Smith's general urology,* ed 14, Norwalk, Conn, 1995, Appleton & Lange.

Warshaw JB, editor: *The biological basis of reproductive and developmental medicine,* Amsterdam, 1983, Elsevier Biomedical.

Waugh MA: History of clinical developments in sexually transmitted diseases. In Holmes KK et al, editors: *Sexually transmitted diseases,* ed 2, New York, 1990, McGraw-Hill Information Services Co.

Wright DJM, editor: *Immunology of sexually transmitted diseases,* Boston, 1988, Kluwer Academic Publishers.

Estrogen stimulates the osteoblasts. Loss of estrogen after menopause lessens osteoblastic activity, resulting in a decrease in the organic matrix of bone. Generally, bone calcification is not affected in osteoporosis in women under the age of 65; instead, osteoporosis is caused by a loss of the organic matrix.

Osteoblastic function is also suppressed when large doses of *glucocorticoids* are administered. This can lead to osteoporosis from the failure of the osteoblasts to form new bone matrix.

JOINTS

Joints are the areas where two or more bones meet. These bones are held together by various means, such as joint capsules, fibrous bands, ligaments, tendons, fasciae, or muscles. The three types of joints are as follows:
1. Fibrous (synarthrodial) joints, which allow no movement
2. Cartilaginous (amphiarthrodial) joints, which have only minimal movement
3. Synovial (diarthrodial) joints, which are freely movable

Fibrous Joints

Fibrous joints do not have a cartilaginous lining, and the bones are joined by fibrous connective tissue. There are two types of fibrous joints: (1) the sutures between the bones in the cranium and (2) a *syndesmosis,* which consists of a interosseous membrane or a ligament between the bones. These fibers permit a slight "give" but no real movement. The attachment in the distal tibiofibular joint is an example of this type of fibrous joint.

Cartilaginous Joints

Cartilaginous joints are those in which the ends of the bones are covered by hyaline cartilage, supported by ligaments, and have only slight movement. There are two types of cartilaginous joints. *Synchondroses* are those in which the entire joint is covered by hyaline cartilage. The costochondral joints are an example of synchondroses. *Symphyses* are joints that have a fibrocartilage connection between the bones and a thin layer of hyaline cartilage covering articular surfaces. The pubic symphysis and the joints between the bodies of the vertebrae are examples of symphyses.

Synovial Joints

Synovial joints are the movable joints in the body. They have a joint cavity and hyaline cartilage over the articular surfaces of the bones (Fig. 67-3).

The *joint capsule* is made up of a dense fibrous outer covering, an inner layer of highly vascularized connec-

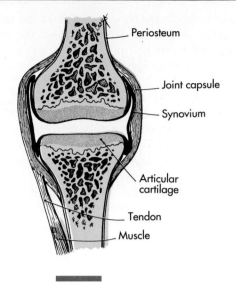

FIG. 67-3   Normal joint.

tive tissue, and synovium, which forms a sac that lines the entire joint and covers the tendons that pass through the joint. The *synovium* does not extend across to the articular surface of the joint. It is folded to allow full joint motion. The linings of the bursae throughout the body resemble synovium. The periosteum does not extend into the joint capsule.

The synovium produces a highly viscous liquid that lubricates the joint surfaces. Normal *synovial fluid* is clear, nonclotting, and either colorless or straw colored. Relatively small amounts (1 to 3 ml) are found in normal joints. The white blood cell count of the fluid is normally less than 200 cells/ml and is primarily of mononuclear cells. Hyaluronic acid is responsible for the viscosity of synovial fluid and is synthesized by synovial lining cells. The liquid component of the synovial fluid is thought to be a transudate from plasma. Synovial fluid also serves as a source of nutrition for the articular cartilage.

Hyaline cartilage covers the load-bearing portions of the bones in synovial joints. This cartilage serves an important role in distributing weight loads. Articular cartilage is made up of few cells and a large amount of ground substance. This ground substance consists of type II collagen and proteoglycans produced by the cartilage cells. The proteoglycans found in articular cartilage are very hydrophilic, which enables them to resist wear with heavy joint use.

Articular cartilage in the adult does not have any blood supply, lymphatic channels, or nerves. Oxygen and other necessary products for metabolism are carried by the synovial fluid that bathes the cartilage. Alterations may occur in collagen and proteoglycan synthesis after injury or with increasing age. Some of the new collagen produced at this time begins to resemble type I collagen and is much more fibrous. The proteoglycans can lose some of their hydrophilic abilities. These changes mean that the cartilage can lose its ability to resist wear with heavy usage.

The joint is lubricated by synovial fluid and by hydrostatic changes in the interstitial fluid of the cartilage. Pressure on the cartilage causes fluid to move from the cartilage to an area of less pressure. As the joint glides forward, this weeping fluid moves ahead of the load. The fluid moves back into the portions of the cartilage from which the pressure is relieved. The articular cartilage and the bones of the joint are normally held apart during action by the film of fluid. The articular cartilage cannot be worn out by excessive use as long as an adequate film of fluid is present.

The blood supply to the joint is richest in the synovium. The vessels arise from the subchondral bone at the level of the margin of the capsule. The capillary network is particularly thick in the portions of the synovium immediately adjacent to the joint space. This allows products from the plasma to diffuse easily into the joint space. The inflammatory process can be especially pronounced in the synovium, since there is such a rich supply of blood vessels as well as the presence of a large number of mast cells and other cells and chemicals that dynamically interact to stimulate and amplify the inflammatory response.

Autonomic and sensory nerves are widely distributed in the ligaments, joint capsule, and synovium. These nerves account for the sensitivity of these structures to position and movement. Nerve endings in the capsule, ligaments, and adventitia of blood vessels are particularly sensitive to stretching or twisting. Pain that arises from the joint capsule or synovium tends to be diffuse rather than localized. Joints are innervated by peripheral nerves that cross the articulation. This means that pain from one joint may be reported as coming from another; for example, pain arising in the hip may be felt as knee pain.

CONNECTIVE TISSUE

The tissues found in the joints and adjoining areas are primarily connective tissues composed of cells and ground substance. The two types of cells found in connective tissue include cells that permanently remain in or do not develop in connective tissue, such as mast cells, plasma cells, lymphocytes, monocytes, and polymorphonuclear leukocytes. These cells play an important role in the inflammatory and immune reactions seen in the rheumatic disorders. The second type of cells found in connective tissue includes those permanently located there, such as fibroblasts, chondrocytes, and osteoblasts. These cells synthesize the various fibers and proteoglycans of the ground substance and give each type of connective tissue its unique properties.

The fibers found in the ground substance include collagen and elastin. At least 14 forms of collagen can be classified by their molecular chain structure, location, and function. *Collagen* can be broken down by the action of collagenases. These proteolytic enzymes cleave the stable molecule so that it becomes unstable at physiologic temperatures and is hydrolyzed by other proteases. Alterations in the synthesis of cartilage collagen are seen with increasing age. Increased collagenase activity is seen in immune-mediated forms of rheumatic disorders such as rheumatoid arthritis.

Elastin fibers have a unique cross-linking property that provides important elastic properties. These fibers are found in the ligaments, the walls of the larger blood vessels, and the skin. Elastin is broken down by enzymes called *elastases*. Elastases may be important in the development of arteriosclerosis and emphysema. Some evidence suggests that changes in the cardiovascular system because of aging may result from increased breakdown of elastin fibers.

Proteoglycans are the other important product found in the ground substance along with the fibers. Proteoglycans are large molecules made up of long polysaccharide chains attached to polypeptide cores. Proteoglycans in articular cartilage cushion the joints to withstand great physical forces. The relationship of the proteoglycans to the inflammatory and immunologic processes is complex. Lymphokines can induce connective tissue cells to produce new proteoglycans, inhibit their production, or increase their breakdown. Proteoglycans can become the focus of autoimmune action in disorders such as rheumatoid arthritis. Increasing age changes the proteoglycans in cartilage; they become less able to aggregate with each other and interact with collagen. The major structural and functional changes that are a part of the normal aging process result from changes in the biochemistry of the connective tissues and occur primarily in the fibers and proteoglycans.

EVALUATION OF SYNOVIAL FLUID

The synovial fluid may be affected differently by each of the rheumatic disorders. Table 67-1 compares normal synovial fluid with the changes seen in some of the more common disorders. The *mucin clot test* is performed by adding acetic acid to the synovial fluid. This forms a precipitate by interaction with hyaluronic acid. The mucin clot has poor results with the more inflammatory fluids, since the hyaluronic acid has been broken down by the lysosomal enzymes and therefore is not available to precipitate when the fluid is treated with acetic acid. The clarity of normal synovial fluid is diminished by an increase in the cells and protein, as seen in some pathologic conditions.

▶ TABLE 67-1   Synovial Fluid

	Normal	Degenerative Joint Disease	Systemic Lupus Erythematosus (SLE)*	Gout†	Rheumatoid Arthritis	Reiter's Syndrome	Infectious Arthritis‡
Color and clarity	Straw colored; clear	Straw colored; clear	Straw colored; clear	Straw colored or white; cloudy	Straw colored or light yellow; cloudy	Opaque	Gray, purulent; cloudy
Mucin clot	Good	Usually good	Fair to good	Poor	Poor	Poor	Poor
White blood cell count (average)	200/mm³	1000/mm³	5000/mm³	10,000 to 20,000/mm³	15,000 to 20,000/mm³	20,000/mm³	50,000 to 75,000/mm³

*LE cells may be present.
†Uric acid crystals are present.
‡Bacteria can be cultured.

 QUESTIONS

▼ *Answer the following on a separate sheet of paper.*

1. List the structures of the musculoskeletal system.
2. What are the characteristics of woven bone as compared with lamellar bone?
3. List the various means by which joints are held together.
4. Explain the process by which a joint is lubricated.
5. What is the role of osteoclasts in the process of bone resorption?
6. What is the relationship of osteoid (organic matrix of bone) to the formation of new bone?
7. Why is it significant that some joints are innervated by peripheral nerves that cross the articulation?

▼ *Circle the letter preceding each item below that correctly answers the question or completes the statement. More than one answer may be correct.*

8. The major component of the musculoskeletal system consists of:
   a. Specialized tissues that connect bone structures
   b. Connective tissue
   c. Joints
   d. Bones
9. Which of the following are characteristics of bone?
   a. Provides the supporting and protective framework for the body's skeletal system
   b. Major tissue components are collagen and proteoglycans
   c. Composed of supportive, rigid connective tissue referred to as apatite
   d. Is uniform in nature

10. Which of the following *best* describes the periosteum?
    a. It is a region of longitudinal growth in children
    b. It is a heavy, fibrous band attached to the flared end of bone
    c. It is mainly composed of cortical tissue
    d. It contains proliferating cells that contribute to transverse growth of bone
11. In young children, epiphyseal fractures involving the area of provisional calcification most likely will result in:
    a. Retardation of longitudinal bone growth
    b. Hypertrophy of collagen fibers in the diaphysis
    c. Obliterated nerve supply to the diaphysis
    d. Progressive deformity of the involved limb
12. Which of the following cells are responsible for building bone by forming type I collagen and proteoglycans?
    a. Osteoblasts
    b. Osteocytes
    c. Osteoclasts
13. Which of the following is an example of a truly movable joint?
    a. Diarthrodial (synovial)
    b. Synarthrodial (fibrous)
    c. Cartilaginous
14. An example of a synarthrodial (fibrous) joint is:
    a. A skull suture
    b. The synovium
    c. The symphysis pubis
    d. An intervertebral disk

15. The function of ligaments is to:
    a. Attach muscle to bone
    b. Cover the surface of bones
    c. Hold bones together at joints
    d. Cover tendons that pass through joints
16. The load-bearing portions of the bones in synovial joints are covered with:
    a. Synovial fluid
    b. Hyaline cartilage
    c. Fibrocartilage
    d. Fascia
17. Which of the following contains the richest blood supply to the joint?
    a. Articular cartilage
    b. Synovium
    c. Hyaline cartilage
    d. Serous membrane
18. The cells that develop and remain in connective tissue are:
    a. Mast cells
    b. Plasma cells
    c. Fibroblasts
    d. Osteoblasts
19. The fibers in the connective tissue ground substance that are found in ligaments, walls of larger blood vessels, and skin are referred to as:
    a. Elastin
    b. Collagen
    c. Both the above
    d. Neither of the above
20. Which of the following is responsible for the synthesis of collagen fibers?
    a. Fibroblasts
    b. Proteolytic enzymes
    c. Polysaccharides
    d. Elastin
21. The function of proteoglycans in articular cartilage is to:

Continued.

QUESTIONS—cont'd

a. Allow full joint motion
b. Distribute weight loads
c. Lubricate the cartilage

▼ *Circle T if the statement is true and F if it is false. Correct any false statements.*

22. T F Pain from the synovium tends to be localized.

23. T F Autonomic and sensory nerves in the ligaments, joint capsule, and synovium account for the sensitivity of these structures to position and motion.

24. T F The mucin clot test is most effective with the more inflammatory fluids.

25. T F Type I collagen is primarily responsible for the deposition of calcium and phosphate in the bone matrix.

26. T F Articular cartilage in the adult has a blood supply, lymphatic channels, and nerves.

▼ *Match the conditions in column A with the synovial fluid white cell counts in column B.*

Column A	Column B
27. _____ Normal joint	a. 15,000 to 20,000/mm³
28. _____ Rheumatoid arthritis	b. 5000/mm³
29. _____ Infectious arthritis	c. 200/mm³
30. _____ Systemic lupus erythematosus	d. 50,000 to 75,000/mm³

31. Label the parts of the long bone in the accompanying diagram.

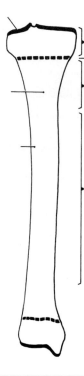

CHAPTER 68

Fractures and Dislocations

MICHAEL A. CARTER

FRACTURES

Classification of Fractures

A fracture is a break in a bone, usually caused by trauma or physical forces. The strength and angle of the force, the underlying condition of the bone, and surrounding soft tissue determine whether the fracture is complete or incomplete. Complete fractures result when a break extends completely through the bone, whereas incomplete fractures do not extend through the entire thickness of the bone. Several terms are used to describe fractures.

Angle of break

Transverse fractures proceed directly across the bone. When the broken segments of such a transversely fractured bone are repositioned, or reduced, back to their original location, they are stable and usually easy to control with casts (Fig. 68-1, *A*). *Oblique fractures* proceed at an angle across the bone. They are unstable and difficult to control (Fig. 68-1, *B*). *Spiral fractures* are the result of torsion of a limb. Of interest, these low-energy fractures are associated with little soft tissue damage, and such fractures tend to heal readily with external immobilization (Fig. 68-1, *C*).

Multiple fractures in one bone

Segmental fractures are two adjacent fractures that isolate a central segment from its blood supply. These fractures are difficult to treat. The fracture at one end of the avascular segment often fails to heal, and this situation may require surgical treatment (Fig. 68-2, *A*). *Comminuted fractures* are splinters or disruptions in continuity of tissue in which there are more than two fracture fragments.

Impaction fractures

Compression fractures occur when two bones crush (by impaction) a third bone between them, such as a vertebra between two other vertebrae. These fractures of the vertebal bodies are diagnosed by their radiographic appearance. Lateral views of the spine show a decrease in vertical height and a mild angulation at one or a few vertebrae. In young people a compression fracture may be associated with considerable retroperitoneal hemorrhage. As in pelvic fractures, the patient may rapidly develop hypovolemic shock and die if repeated accurate assessments of the pulse, blood pressure, and respiration are not obtained during the first 24 to 48 postinjury hours. Ileus and urinary retention may also result from these injuries (Fig. 68-2, *B*).

Pathologic fractures

Pathologic fractures occur through regions of bone that have been weakened by a tumor or some other pathologic process. The adjacent bone often shows decreased bone density. The most frequent cause of such fractures is a primary or metastatic tumor (Fig. 68-2, *C*).

Other stress (fatigue) fractures

Stress, or fatigue, fractures occur in individuals who have recently increased their activity level, such as recruits in the army in basic training or persons who have recently taken up jogging. With the onset of symptoms, the radiographs may not demonstrate the fracture. However, usually after 2 weeks, linear radiopaque lines appear perpendicular to the long axis of the bone. Such fractures heal well if the bone is immobilized for a few

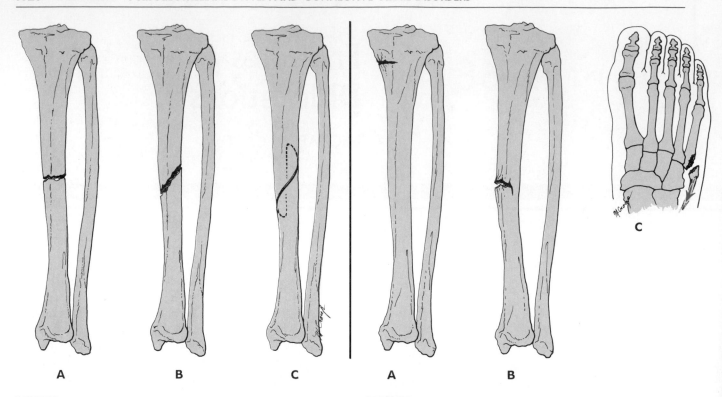

FIG. 68-1   Classification of fractures. **A,** Transverse. **B,** Oblique. **C,** Spiral.

FIG. 68-3   Other fractures. **A,** Stress (fatigue). **B,** Greenstick. **C,** Avulsion.

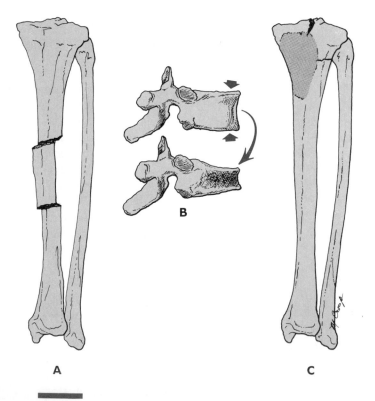

FIG. 68-2   Types of fractures. **A,** Segmental. **B,** Compression. **C,** Pathologic.

weeks. However, if the fractures are not diagnosed, the bones can become displaced and fail to heal properly. Thus any patient with severe extremity pain after a recent increase in activity may have such a lesion and should be protected by the use of crutches or an appropriate cast. After 2 weeks, radiographs should be obtained (Fig. 68-3, *A*).

Greenstick fractures

Greenstick fractures are incomplete fractures and are frequently seen in children. The cortex is partially intact, as is the periosteum. They will heal readily and rapidly remodel back to a normal shape and function (Fig. 68-3, *B*).

Avulsion fractures

Avulsion fractures separate a fragment of bone at a site of tendon or ligament insertion. Usually no specific treatment is required. However, if joint instability or another cause of disability is expected to result from such a fracture, the displaced fragment may be surgically excised or realigned in most cases (Fig. 68-3, *C*).

Joint fractures

Specific note should be made of fractures that involve joints, particularly if the joint geometry is significantly disturbed by displacement of these fragments. Unless adequately treated, this type of injury may lead to a progressive posttraumatic osteoarthritis of the injured joint (Fig. 68-4).

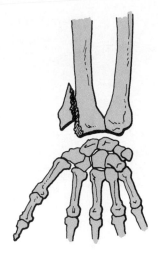

FIG. 68-4   Fracture of the distal radius with extension into the wrist joint.

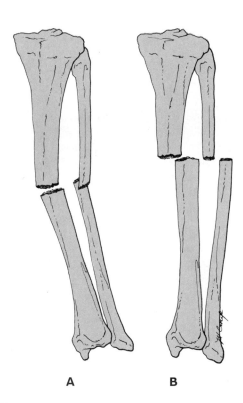

A   B

FIG. 68-5   Description of fractures. A, Angulation. B, Opposition.

Description of Fractures

Angulation and opposition are two terms frequently used in the description of long-bone fractures. The degree and direction of *angulation* from the normal position of a long bone may indicate the degree of fracture severity and the type of treatment program. Angulation is described by estimating the degrees of deviation of the distal fragment from the normal longitudinal axis, indicating the direction of the apex of the angle (Fig. 68-5, *A*). *Opposition* refers to the extent of displacement of the fracture surfaces and is used to describe what proportion of the fractured portion of one fragment touches its mate (Fig. 68-5, *B*).

Exposure to environment

Closed (simple) and open (compound) are terms commonly used in fracture description. A *closed,* or *simple, fracture* is one in which the skin is not perforated, so the fracture site is not exposed to the environment.

Technically, an *open,* or *compound, fracture* is one in which the skin on the involved limb has been penetrated. The important concept is whether the contaminated outside environment has come into contact with the fracture site. A fracture fragment may perforate the skin at the time of injury, become contaminated, and then return to near its normal position. Under these conditions, operative irrigation, débridement, and administration of intravenous antibiotics may be necessary to prevent osteomyelitis. In general, open fractures should have operative irrigation and débridement within 6 hours of the time of injury for the best chance of preventing infection.

Fracture Healing

When a bone is fractured, the adjacent soft tissues are damaged, the periosteum is separated from the bone, and considerable bleeding takes place. A blood clot develops in the area. The clot forms granulation tissue, within which the primitive bone-forming (osteogenic) cells differentiate into chondroblasts and osteoblasts. The chondroblasts secrete phosphate, which stimulates the deposition of calcium. A thickened band (callus) forms around the fracture site. The band continues to thicken and expand across the fracture site and converges with the band from the opposite fragment and fuses with it. Fusion of the two fragments (fracture healing) progresses as osteoblasts form trabeculae, which adhere to the bone and extend across the fracture site. This provisional bony union undergoes metaplastic transformation to become stronger and more organized. The bone callus remodels to assume the shape of intact bone as osteoblasts form new bone and osteoclasts remove the damaged and temporary bone (Fig. 68-6).

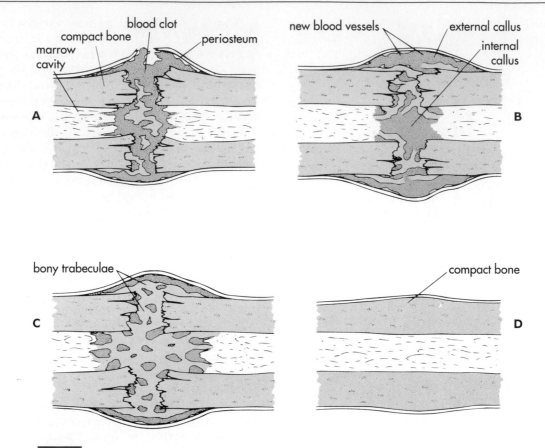

FIG. 68-6   **A,** In a fracture, usually the periosteum is torn, blood vessels are damaged, and bone fragments are separated. **B,** Rapid division of bone-forming and cartilage-forming cells in the region of the break forms a thickened band composed of an internal callus and an external callus. **C,** Osteoblasts form trabeculae, which adhere to existing bone and extend across the break. **D,** The break is bridged by compact bone, and the contour of the new, intact bone is remodeled. (From Luciano DF, Vander AJ, Sherman JA: *Human anatomy and physiology*, ed 2, New York, 1983, McGraw-Hill.)

HEALING POTENTIAL OF CHILDREN'S FRACTURES

Children's fractures usually heal rapidly and well. The active periosteal sleeve around the tubular bones in children is strong. Because this area is rarely completely ruptured, fracture fragments tend to be maintained in an acceptable position after fracture. Children's bones have great potential for corrective remodeling. Thus a considerable postreduction angular deformity may be accepted with confidence that the mature bone will be straight without evidence of injury. In addition, the injured limb tends to grow faster than the normal one. *Bayonet apposition* is often preferable to an end-on-end reduction to achieve equal adult limb lengths (Fig. 68-7). Although angular deformities do rapidly correct, there is no similar tendency for rotational deformities to resolve spontaneously. Normal rotational position during healing should be maintained.

Most fractures in children are appropriately treated by

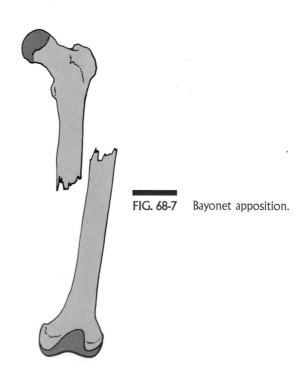

FIG. 68-7   Bayonet apposition.

closed reduction and external immobilization with casts or traction. Only a few children's fractures are optimally treated surgically. An example is a fracture of the lateral condyle of the humerus that extends into the joint and may also involve an injury to the epiphyseal growth plate. Failure to accurately reduce the fragment back to its normal anatomic position may lead to a reduction of elbow function and growth arrest of the limb, which may result in gross deformity developing with increasing maturity. Fractures of the head of the radius and of the hip in children also frequently demand surgical treatment. In general, fractures that extend into joints or that pass across or through growth plates are the ones most likely to require surgery.

DISLOCATION AND SUBLUXATION

The articular cartilage-bearing surfaces of normal joints fit one another with considerable accuracy (Fig. 68-8). *Subluxation* refers to any deviation from the normal relationship where the articular cartilage is still touching any portion of its mating cartilage. If no portion of its articular cartilage touches the usual mate, the joint is said to be *dislocated*. Early recognition and reduction of all dislocations are essential for a satisfactory end result.

Shoulder dislocations are most common in young people and usually result from a traumatic exaggerated abduction, extension, and external rotation position of the upper extremity (Fig. 68-9). The cocked position for throwing a ball is an example of the position that most frequently, if exaggerated, may cause dislocation. The humeral head is generally displaced anteriorly and inferiorly through a traumatic rent in the shoulder capsule. Characteristically the patient is seen sitting bent over, supporting the injured limb in a flexed position away from the chest or the side. The humeral head may be easily palpated in the anterior axilla. There is a palpable depression beneath the central origin of the deltoid at the acromion.

During the initial evaluation the neurovascular status of the limb is examined by testing the sensation in the area of the insertion of the deltoid on the humerus. This area is uniquely served by the sensory fibers of the axillary nerve. Local circumscribed anesthesia indicates the likelihood of an axillary nerve injury. Similarly, the patient's ability to minimally tense the deltoid in a voluntary attempt to initiate abduction also allows an estimate of the function of the axillary nerve. Axillary nerve function is necessary for shoulder abduction so that the patient may functionally position the arm. This nerve is frequently injured by the trauma of dislocation.

Ulnar nerve deficit occurs with nearly the same frequency as axillary nerve injury in shoulder dislocations.

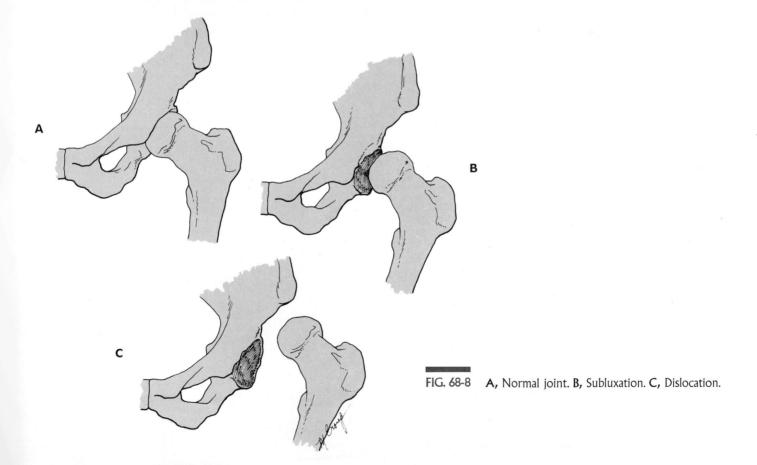

FIG. 68-8   A, Normal joint. B, Subluxation. C, Dislocation.

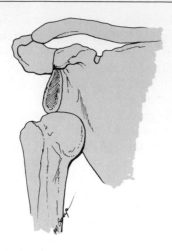

FIG. 68-9   Shoulder dislocation.

Ulnar nerve palsy has a severe effect on hand function.

Sustained anterior traction is the safest and most dependable method of reducing a dislocated shoulder. With this type of traction, the patient is given an analgesic, generally a narcotic, and is put in a prone position on an examination table or cart with the affected limb hanging over the side. Slow, gentle, sustained traction toward the floor is applied. Most patients can feel the reduction as a "clunk." This method of reduction is extremely successful and virtually without complications. A postreduction radiograph should demonstrate normal anatomy.

Dislocation of the hip is one of the few orthopedic emergencies. If a dislocated hip is not reduced within a few hours of the injury, the probability of the patient's developing aseptic necrosis is extremely great. Hip dislocation is recognized usually by gluteal, groin, and thigh pain in association with a rigid position of the limb in adduction, internal rotation, and flexion.

OSTEOMYELITIS

Osteomyelitis is infection of bone tissue and may be acute or chronic. The acute form is characterized by rapid onset of fever with systemic as well as local manifestations. In children, infections of bone develop as a complication of infection from other sites, such as the pharynx (pharyngitis), ear (otitis media), and skin (impetigo). The bacteria *(Staphylococcus aureus, Streptococcus, Haemophilus influenzae)* travel via the bloodstream to the metaphysis near the growth plates, where the blood flows into sinusoids. With bacterial proliferation and tissue necrosis, the localized area of inflammation is tender and painful.

Osteomyelitis, especially in children, must be diagnosed early so that appropriate antibiotic and surgical treatment can be administered to prevent the local spread of infection and crippling destruction of the entire bone. In adults, osteomyelitis may also be initiated by bloodborne bacteria but usually is the result of tissue contamination at the time of injury or surgery.

Chronic osteomyelitis results from inadequately treated acute osteomyelitis. Osteomyelitis is extremely resistant to antibiotic therapy. It is theorized that this is partially because of the avascular nature of cortical bone. Appropriate quantities of antibodies may never reach the infected tissue. Bone infections are extremely difficult to eradicate, and even treatment by surgical drainage and débridement with appropriate antibiotic therapy are often insufficient to eliminate the disease.

QUESTIONS

▼ *Circle the letter preceding each item that correctly answers the question or completes the statement. More than one answer may be correct.*

1. Which of the following fractures is illustrated in the accompanying diagram (see **A**)?
   a. Segmental
   b. Compression
   c. Greenstick
   d. Transverse
2. Which type of fracture is illustrated in the accompanying diagram (see **B**)?
   a. Oblique
   b. Greenstick
   c. Stress (fatigue)
   d. Avulsion
3. Which of the following best describes a complete fracture?
   a. The fracture crosses or involves the entire width or thickness of the bone.
   b. The fracture contains more than two fragments of bone.
   c. There is a structural discontinuity or break in a bone in which the surface opposite the break is intact.
   d. A fragment of the bone at the involved area is separated at a tendon site.
4. The initial stage in the repair of a fracture is the:
   a. Division of osteogenic cells, which causes a callus to form around the fracture site
   b. Proliferation of osteoblasts, which form trabeculae
   c. Remodeling of the fracture site
   d. Formation of a blood clot in the area
5. Opposition refers to the:
   a. Degree of severity
   b. Degrees of deviation from the normal longitudinal axis and the direction of the apex of the angle
   c. Extent of displacement of the fracture surfaces
   d. Percentage of the fractured portion of one fragment that touches its mate

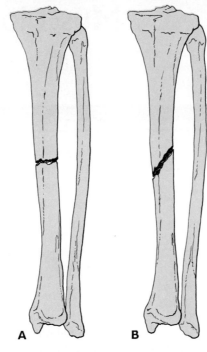

A   B

6. All the following are signs and symptoms indicative of a shoulder dislocation *except:*
   a. The patient supports the injured limb in a flexed position away from the chest or the side.
   b. The humeral head can be palpated in the anterior axilla.
   c. There is localized pain in the area of the injury.

d. Aseptic necrosis will likely occur if the dislocated shoulder is not reduced within 12 hours.
7. Before attempting to reduce a dislocated shoulder, which of the following should be observed and recorded:
   a. The amount and duration of pain the victim is experiencing
   b. The presence of tactile sensation within a small designated area over the deltoid muscle
   c. Blood pressure and pulse rate
   d. Ability of the patient to elevate minimally the injured limb away from the body
8. The important structure necessary for shoulder abduction and is most frequently injured as a complication of a shoulder dislocation is the:
   a. Radial nerve
   b. Brachial artery
   c. Axillary nerve
   d. Radial artery

▼ *Answer the following on a separate sheet of paper.*
9. Explain the changes that occur in the process of fracture healing.
10. Why is it important to diagnose osteomyelitis early, especially in children?
11. Explain why children's fractures usually heal rapidly and well.
12. Why is bayonet apposition often preferable in reduction of children's fractures?

▼ *Match the type of fracture in column A with its characteristic in column B. Each letter may be used more than once.*

Column A	Column B
13. _____ Spiral	a. Heals rapidly; occurs in children
14. _____ Oblique	b. Results from torsion of a limb
15. _____ Greenstick	c. Occurs in people who have recently increased their activity level
16. _____ Pathologic	d. Is typical in ski injuries
17. _____ Stress (fatigue)	e. Is usually caused by primary or metastatic tumors
18. _____ Comminuted	f. Proceeds at an angle across the bone
	g. Contains more than two fragments of bone

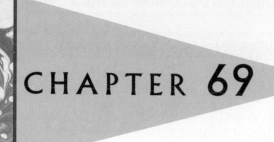

CHAPTER 69

Tumors of the Musculoskeletal System

MICHAEL A. CARTER

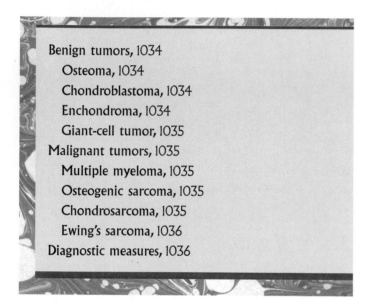

A number of types of neoplasms can occur in bone tissue. These neoplasms may originate in the bone tissue itself or may spread to the bone from other primary sites.

Bone tumor cells produce factors that stimulate osteoclast function, leading to bone resorption that can be seen radiographically. Some tumors cause increased osteoblast activity with an increased density that also can be seen radiographically. Generally, bone tumors are recognized because of a mass in the soft tissues around the bone, deformity of the bone, pain and tenderness, or pathologic fractures.

Primary bone tumors can be benign or malignant. Benign tumors are much more common, and malignant tumors are often fatal. Malignant tumors tend to grow rapidly, spread, and invade irregularly. These tumors are seen most often in adolescents and young adults.

A number of neoplasms that originate in other tissues can spread to bone by way of the bloodstream. The most common primary sites of these neoplasms are prostate, breast, lung, thyroid, kidney, and bladder. The most common bones affected are the vertebrae, proximal femur, pelvis, ribs, sternum, and proximal humerus.

BENIGN TUMORS

Osteoma

Osteomas are benign bone lesions characterized by an abnormal outgrowth of bone. The classic osteoma presents as a slowly growing, painless, hard bump. Radiographically, peripheral osteomas present as radiopaque lesions that extend from the surface of bone; central osteomas are seen as well-delineated sclerotic masses inside the bone. Surgical excision of the osteoma is the preferred treatment when the lesion is symptomatic, enlarging, or causing disability. Removal is also done for diagnostic purposes for large lesions. Excision usually produces curative results.

Chondroblastoma

Chondroblastoma is a rare, usually benign tumor. It occurs most frequently in adolescent males. This tumor is uniquely found in the epiphysis. The most common site of occurrence is the humerus. The most frequent symptom is joint pain arising from cartilaginous tissue. Treatment consists of surgical excision. Recurrence is treated with surgical excision, cryosurgery, or radiotherapy.

Enchondroma

Enchondroma, or *central chondroma,* is a benign tumor of dysplastic cartilage cells occurring in the metaphysis of tubular bones, particularly of the hands and feet. Radiographically, spotty calcification in the circumscribed, enlarged, rarefied lesion is characteristic of this tumor. It is believed to develop during the growth period in children and adolescents. This condition increases the likelihood of pathologic fractures. Surgical curettage and bone grafting are usually the treatments of choice for this lesion.

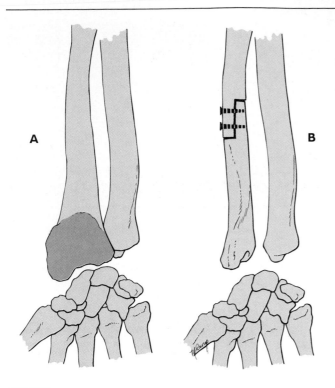

FIG. 69-1   **A,** Giant-cell tumor of the distal radius. **B,** Use of a bone transplant to reconstruct the limb after total excision of a giant-cell tumor.

Giant-Cell Tumor

A characteristic feature of a giant-cell tumor is the vascular and cellular stroma make up of oval-shaped cells containing small, elongated, darkly staining nuclei. The giant cell is large and has pink-staining cytoplasm; it contains numerous nuclei, which are vesicular and appear similar to stromal cells. Although this tumor is usually considered benign, there are varying degrees of malignancy, depending on the sarcomatous nature of the stroma. In the malignant types the tumor becomes anaplastic and has areas of necrosis and hemorrhage.

Giant-cell tumors occur chiefly in young adults. They occur more frequently in women. The common sites are the ends of the long bones, especially at the knee and the lower end of the radius. The most common symptom is pain. Joint motion limitation and weakness may also be seen. After biopsy identification this type of tumor usually requires a definitive gross local excision, including removal of a safe border of normal tissue. This tumor tends to be locally recurrent (probably 60% or greater) and of increasingly malignant character after incomplete excision. With prior biopsy, diagnosis, and gross local removal, an immediate reconstruction of the area may be possible. In the case of a large giant-cell tumor of the distal radius (Fig. 69-1, *A*) the patient's proximal fibula can be substituted to reconstruct the forearm (Fig. 69-1, *B*).

MALIGNANT TUMORS

Multiple Myeloma

The most common malignant bone tumor is multiple myeloma, which is caused by a malignant proliferation of plasma cells. Multiple myeloma is rarely seen in individuals younger than 40 years. Men are more often affected, and African Americans have twice the incidence of whites.

Bone pain is the most common symptom, and the back and rib areas are the most common sites of this pain. Palpable bone lesions may occur, especially in the skull and clavicles. Lesions in the back can lead to vertebral collapse and occasionally spinal cord compression. Treatment involves a number of activities, since multiple myeloma affects many organs. Long-term survival depends on the stage of the illness at diagnosis but is generally not more than 5 years (see Chapter 18).

Osteogenic Sarcoma

Osteogenic sarcoma, or *osteosarcoma,* is a malignant primary neoplasm of bone. The tumor arises in the metaphysis of the bone. The most common sites are at the ends of the long bones, especially at the knee. The incidence of osteogenic sarcoma is greatest in adolescents and young adults, but it may also affect people with Paget's disease who are over 50 years of age. Severe pain associated with bone destruction and erosion is a usual symptom of this condition.

The gross appearance of osteogenic sarcoma is variable. It may be (1) osteolytic, in which the bone is destroyed and the soft tissue is invaded by the lesion, or (2) osteoblastic as a result of the formation of new sclerotic bone. Periosteal new bone may be deposited adjacent to the lesion itself, appearing as a triangle on radiographs (Fig. 69-2). Although this is seen with many malignancies of bone, it is characteristic of osteogenic sarcoma; the tumor itself may produce a somewhat abortive form of bone. The radiographic appearance of such a lesion is referred to as a "sunburst," as depicted in Fig. 69-3.

Some primary tumors such as osteogenic sarcoma may be best treated by amputation or radical ablative surgery. Although chemotherapy and immunotherapy appear to have some potential benefits, complete surgical removal of the tumor and all surrounding tissue is usually necessary.

Chondrosarcoma

Chondrosarcoma is a malignant tumor composed of anaplastic chondrocytes and may occur as a central or peripheral bone tumor. It occurs most often in men over 35 years of age. A painless mass of long duration is the most frequent presenting symptom. For example, peripheral

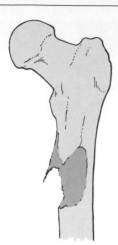

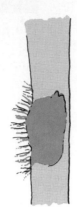

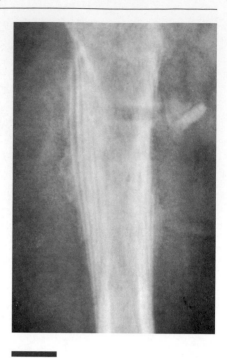

FIG. 69-2 Osteogenic sarcoma with Codman's triangle.

FIG. 69-3 Radiographic "sunburst" appearance seen in osteogenic sarcoma.

FIG. 69-4 Radiographic "onion skin" appearance seen in Ewing's sarcoma. (Courtesy of William Martel, MD.)

lesions are often asymptomatic for long periods, presenting with only minor discomfort and palpable enlargement. However, rapid aggressive growth may occur. The pelvis, femur, ribs, shoulder girdle, and craniofacial bones are the most frequent sites of the lesion.

Chondrosarcomas appear as radiolucent areas with stippled and blotchy calcification of radiographs. Radical surgical excision is the treatment preferred; however, cryosurgery, radiotherapy, and chemotherapy may also be used. For large, aggressive, or recurrent lesions, amputation may be an appropriate treatment.

Ewing's Sarcoma

Ewing's sarcoma is most often seen in teenage children, and the most common site is the shaft of long bones. The gross appearance is a soft, gray tumor arising into the bone marrow reticulum that erodes bone cortex from within. Under the periosteum, layers of new bone are deposited parallel to the shaft, producing an onion skin effect (Fig. 69-4). The typical signs and symptoms are pain, tender swelling, fever (38° to 40° C), and leukocytosis (20,000 to 40,000 leukocytes/mm³). Treatment consists of radiation therapy, cytotoxic drugs, and surgical removal of the tumor. A poor prognosis is associated with this tumor.

DIAGNOSTIC MEASURES

As a general rule the radiographic appearance of a lesion may help determine its relative malignancy. For example, a lesion with discrete rounded margins tends to be benign. Such a lesion frequently has a sclerotic margin, indicating that the bone has had the time and ability to re-

spond to the mass. The lack of a definable margin indicates invasion of the tumor into adjacent bone (Fig. 69-5, A). This lesion is growing rapidly, and the bone has not had sufficient time or a defense response to react against it. Extension of the lesion through the cortex of the bone is typical of a malignancy. When the tumor penetrates the cortex, the periosteum may be lifted off. The bone may respond by depositing a thin layer of reactive bone, which is then lifted off, and the periosteal reaction begins again. As mentioned previously, this produces an onion skin effect typical of Ewing's sarcoma (Fig. 69-5, B).

Although the previous signs indicate the degree of malignancy of a lesion, other specific radiologic signs lead to a more definitive diagnosis. For example, a radiolucent lesion located within the epiphysis of a growing bone is apt to be a chondroblastoma (Fig. 69-6). A sclerotic marginated cystic lesion in the metaphysis of a long bone near an active growth plate is likely to be a benign unicameral bone cyst (Fig. 69-7). A radiolucent lesion in an adult in the metaphysis near the old growth plate is likely to be a giant-cell tumor (Fig. 69-8).

A large, destructive lesion penetrating the cortex of the metaphysis of a long bone of an adolescent or young adult is indicative of osteogenic sarcoma. A reticulated, spotty, and extensive radiolucent cortical lesion in a child is likely to be Ewing's sarcoma. A "target" or "bull's-eye" lesion, sclerotic bone around a radiolucent area surrounding a central dense nucleus, in an individual with night pain that responds to salicylates is nearly always an osteoid osteoma.

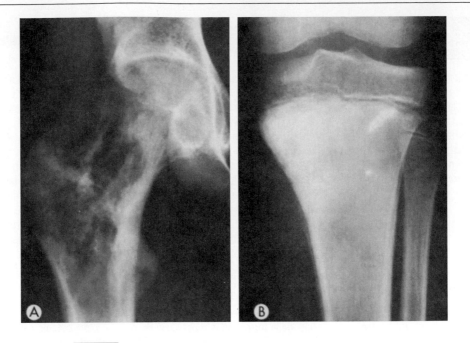

FIG. 69-5   Radiographic appearance of a malignant tumor. **A,** Femur. **B,** Tibia. (Courtesy of William Martel, MD.)

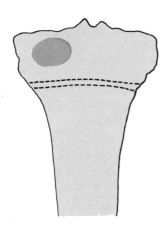

FIG. 69-6   Chondroblastoma.

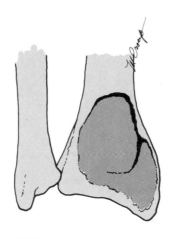

FIG. 69-7   Unicameral bone cyst.

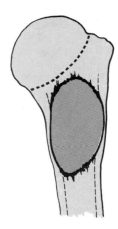

FIG. 69-8   Giant-cell tumor.

? QUESTIONS

▼ *Answer the following on a separate sheet of paper.*

1. What is the rationale for treatment of a lesion that is benign as opposed to a lesion that is less certainly benign?
2. What is the relationship of osteoclast activity to the formation of bone tumors?
3. Differentiate between benign and malignant tumors as to incidence, growth, and invasiveness.
4. What are the most common primary sites of bone neoplasms?
5. List the bones most frequently affected by neoplasms.

▼ *Circle T if the statement is true and F if it is false. Correct any false statements.*

6. T F Osteochondroma occurs often near joints and has a potential for malignant change.
7. T F Pathologic fractures usually do not result from metastasis of malignant tumor to bone.
8. T F Benign giant-cell bone tumors have a tendency to become aggressive and spread locally if there is incomplete surgical removal and/or unsuccessful radiation therapy.
9. T F The major type of bone tumor found in children results from metastasis from the primary tumor site to bone.
10. T F Chondrosarcoma occurs most often in men over 35 years of age.

▼ *Circle the letter preceding each item below that correctly answers the question or completes the statement. More than one answer may be correct.*

11. Which of the following is(are) characteristic of an osteoma?
    a. Usual presentation as a slowly growing, painless, hard bump
    b. Typically affects older men
    c. Increased likelihood of pathologic fractures
    d. Benign bone lesion occurring near the joints in children and adolescents
12. The onion skin pattern of subperiosteal new bone formation is most likely seen in which of the following tumors involving long bones?
    a. Ewing's sarcoma
    b. Osteosarcoma
    c. Chondroblastoma
    d. Reticulum cell sarcoma
13. The bone most frequently involved in chondroblastoma is the:
    a. Femur
    b. Humerus
    c. Tibia
    d. Ulna
14. Concerning chondroblastoma, which of the following is *false?*
    a. The tumor is found in the epiphysis.
    b. Severe pain associated with bone destruction is frequently encountered.
    c. It occurs most frequently in male adolescents.
    d. It is a rare, usually benign tumor.
15. James B., age 16, was admitted to the hospital with an enlarging primary mass in the right distal femur at the knee. Microscopic studies revealed numerous abnormal bone-forming cells with great variation in size and shape. Radiologic studies revealed extension of the tumor into adjacent soft tissue—cortical breakthrough. Which one of the following diagnoses would you suspect?
    a. Ewing's sarcoma
    b. Osteogenic sarcoma
    c. Osteoid osteoma
    d. Giant-cell tumor
16. A radiolucent lesion located within the epiphysis of a growing bone is likely to be:
    a. Ewing's sarcoma
    b. Chondroblastoma
    c. Osteoma
    d. Giant-cell tumor
17. The most common type of malignant bone tumor is:
    a. Multiple myeloma
    b. Osteoma
    c. Chondrosarcoma
    d. Ewing's sarcoma

CHAPTER 70 ▶ Osteoarthritis

MICHAEL A. CARTER

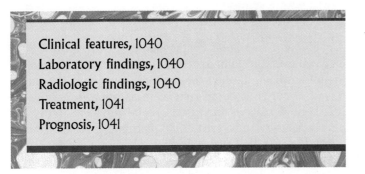

Osteoarthritis is a disorder of movable joints. The disease is chronic, slowly progressive, noninflammatory, and characterized by the deterioration and abrasion of articular cartilage and the formation of new bone at the articular surface.

Osteoarthritis, the most common form of arthritis, constitutes slightly more than half of all cases of arthritis. The disorder is more common in women than in men and is found primarily in persons over age 45. This disorder was once thought to be a normal consequence of the aging process, since the incidence increases with age. Osteoarthritis was given the name of "wear and tear" arthritis, based on the idea that the joint wore out with age. However, newer findings of the biochemistry and biomechanics of the joint have disproved this theory.

Chondrocytes are the cells responsible for the formation of the proteoglycans and collagen in the articular cartilage. For unknown reasons, the synthesis of proteoglycans and collagen is greatly increased in osteoarthritis. However, these substances are degraded at an even more rapid rate, resulting in a net loss over time. As small amounts of type I cartilage replace the normal type II, changes in the collagen fiber diameters and orientation occur that alter the biomechanics of the cartilage. The articular cartilage then loses its unique compressibility. Although the actual cause of osteoarthritis remains unknown, it appears that the aging process is related to changes in chrondrocyte functioning, causing the composition of the articular cartilage to alter and leading to the development of osteoarthritis.

Genetic factors play a role in some forms of osteoarthritis. The development of osteoarthritis of the distal interphalangeal joints of the hands (Heberden's nodes) is gender influenced and dominant in females. Women develop Heberden's nodes 10 times more often than men.

Sex hormones and other hormonal factors seem to be related to the development of osteoarthritis. The relationship between estrogens and bone formation and the prevalence of osteoarthritis in women both strongly suggest that hormones play an active part in the disease's development and progression.

The joints most often affected in osteoarthritis are the weight-bearing joints, including the knees, hips, lumbar and cervical spine, and the phalangeal joints. A distinguishing feature of osteoarthritis is that the proximal and distal phalangeal joints are often affected, whereas the metacarpophalangeal joints are usually unaffected. In rheumatoid arthritis, however, the proximal phalangeal joints and the metacarpal joints are affected, and the distal interphalangeal joints are spared.

Osteoarthritis primarily involves biochemical and biomechanical changes within the joint; it is not an inflammatory disorder. Synovitis frequently accompanies the changes seen in the joint, however, and causes pain and discomfort.

In addition to the common form of osteoarthritis, there are several variants. *Primary generalized osteoarthritis* is different in that there is an increase in the number and severity of the joints involved. *Erosive inflammatory osteoarthritis* primarily affects the finger joints and is associated with acute inflammatory episodes that lead to deformities and ankylosis. *Ankylosis hyperostosis* involves ossification of the vertebrae. *Secondary osteoarthritis* develops as a consequence of some other illness, such as rheumatoid arthritis or gout.

CLINICAL FEATURES

The most common feature of osteoarthritis is pain in the joint, especially with movement or weight bearing. This dull, aching pain is relieved by rest and exacerbated by motion or weight bearing. The patient may have stiffness after resting, but this goes away with motion. Morning stiffness, if present, usually lasts only a few minutes, as compared with the much longer period of morning stiffness characteristic of rheumatoid arthritis. Muscle spasm or pressure on the nerves in the region of the joint is likely to be the source of pain. Other features include restriction of range of motion (especially full extension), local tenderness, bony enlargements around the joint, small effusions, and crepitation.

Characteristic changes occur in the hands. Heberden's nodes, or bony enlargements of the distal interphalangeal joints, are frequently seen. Less common are Bouchard's nodes (Fig. 70-1), which are bony enlargements of the proximal interphalangeal joints.

Characteristic changes are also seen in the spine, which becomes painful, stiff, and limited in range of motion (ROM). Bony overgrowths or spurs may irritate the nerve roots as they pass through the vertebrae. This re-sults in neuromuscular changes, such as pain, stiffness, and limited ROM. Some people complain of headaches that are a direct result of osteoarthritis of the cervical spine.

LABORATORY FINDINGS

Osteoarthritis is a local arthritic disorder, so no specific blood tests are used in the diagnosis. Laboratory tests are sometimes used to exclude other forms of arthritis. Rheumatoid factor may be present in the serum, since it normally increases in frequency with aging. The erythrocyte sedimentation rate may be slightly elevated if there is extensive synovitis.

RADIOLOGIC FINDINGS

A common radiographic characteristic of osteoarthritis is narrowing of the joint space. This happens because of loss of cartilage. In the knee the joint space may be narrowed in only one compartment. In addition to narrowing, bone density is increased around the joint. *Osteophytes* (spurs) can be seen at the marginal aspects of the joint (Fig. 70-2). Cystic changes of various sizes are sometimes seen.

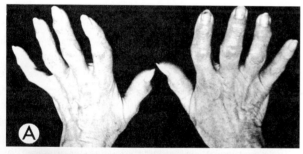

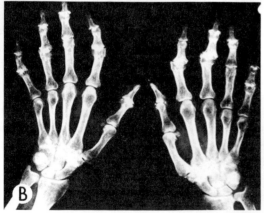

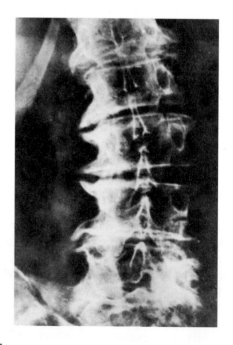

FIG. 70-1   Osteoarthritis. **A,** Primary osteoarthritis of the hands with marked proximal interphalangeal involvement (Bouchard's nodes) along with distal interphalangeal joint involvement. **B,** Radiograph of the same hands. (From Hollander JL, editor: *Arthritis and allied conditions: a textbook of rheumatology,* ed 8, Philadelphia, 1972, Lea & Febiger.)

FIG. 70-2   Spine radiograph of osteoarthritis. This anteroposterior projection of the lumbar spine shows scoliosis and narrowing of the intervertebral spaces on the concave side, where extensive osteophyte formation is present. The osteophytes are not continuous, as is seen in ankylosing spondylitis. Adjacent bony margins are sclerosed. (Reproduced from the Arthritis Foundation, New York, 1972.)

The extent of the change in the joints noted radiographically may not be related to the presence of symptoms. Radiologic evidence of osteoarthritis can be demonstrated in as many as 85% of persons over age 75, although a much lower percentage actually complain of pain and stiffness.

Specialized radiographs may help evaluate osteoarthritis. Weight-bearing radiographs of the knees may give a better picture of the effects of the illness than non-weight-bearing views. Osteoarthritis is not a symmetric disorder, so views of the contralateral joint can be helpful.

TREATMENT

The treatment of osteoarthritis is multifocal and consists of an individualized plan. The goals of treatment are to prevent or retard further damage to the joint, to manage pain and stiffness, and to maintain mobility.

Protecting the joints from additional trauma is important in slowing the progression of the disorder. Evaluating work patterns and activities of daily living assists in eliminating those activities that increase the load-bearing strain to an affected joint. Canes and walkers can significantly decrease the weight load on knees and hips. Reducing weight, if the person is overweight, can greatly decrease the load placed on knees and hips.

Physical therapy measures are important for relieving pain and preserving muscle strength and ROM. The use of ice or heat on the involved joints may provide temporary relief of pain. ROM exercises may help maintain full ROM of involved joints. Isometric exercises help build the muscles that support the joints. Isotonic exercises should not be used with resistance, since this can further stress the joint.

Drug therapy is designed to control the pain in the joint and any synovitis. Over-the-counter analgesic drugs such as acetaminophen, aspirin, and ibuprofen are usually adequate for pain relief. Aspirin and ibuprofen have the added advantage of controlling the synovitis. Other nonsteroidal antiinflammatory drugs are frequently used for pain and synovitis control. Adverse effects of these drugs are generally more common in older persons; drug therapy should be considered carefully in this age-group, since so many have osteoarthritis.

Disease-modifying antirheumatic drugs are not used in the treatment of osteoarthritis because this is not a systemic disorder. Oral corticosteroids are usually contraindicated. These agents are generally ineffective in improving symptoms, and their toxic potential makes their use risky. Intraarticular injections can provide relief of synovitis. If used too frequently, the agents deplete the normal ground substance of the cartilage and can accelerate the arthritic progression.

Surgical treatment of osteoarthritis is designed to remove loose bodies, repair damaged supporting tissues, or replace the entire joint. Arthroscopic surgery allows a variety of surgical procedures to be performed with much less morbidity than that associated with open surgeries. Particles of cartilage can be removed as efficiently as in other surgical procedures.

Another form of surgery used in osteoarthritis is angulation osteotomy. This is used to treat osteoarthritis of the knee that affects only one compartment. Pain is relieved in the joint by correcting the varus or valgus deformity and bringing healthy articular cartilage into contact with other healthy articular cartilage.

Total joint replacements for hips and knees have been successful in maintaining near-normal function for many people with osteoarthritis. Osteoarthritis is a hypertrophic form of arthritis, which means that the bone adjacent to the artificial joint is strong, forming an excellent base for attachment. Various complications can occur with joint replacement, and these are weighed against the acquired benefits. Long-term evaluation studies of total prostheses for finger and other joints are still underway.

Joint fusions may be necessary for the relief of pain in advanced cases of osteoarthritis. The cervical spine is an area in which joint fusion can provide dramatic pain relief.

PROGNOSIS

Osteoarthritis generally progresses slowly. The major problems encountered are pain on the use of a joint and increasing instability with weight bearing, particularly in the knee. These problems mean that the person usually must develop a new life-style. This new life-style often includes altering lifelong patterns of eating and exercise, manipulating complex drug regimens, and using adaptive and assisting devices.

QUESTIONS

▼ *Answer the following on a separate sheet of paper.*

1. Define osteoarthritis.
2. Describe the synthesis of proteoglycans and collagen in osteoarthritis.
3. Explain why the aging process seems to be related to the development of osteoarthritis.
4. Explain the rationale for total joint replacements for hips and knees in osteoarthritis.
5. Explain the radiologic findings for osteoarthritis.
6. Identify the goals of treatment of osteoarthritis.

▼ *Circle the letter preceding each item below that correctly answers the question or completes the statement. More than one answer may be correct.*

7. The pathogenesis of osteoarthritis develops with changes in the:
   a. Articular cartilage
   b. Articular joints

   c. Collagen of the cartilage, where a small amount of type I cartilage replaces normal type II
   d. Diameters and orientation of collagen fibers
8. The highest incidence of osteoarthritis is found in persons in which age group?
   a. 15 to 20 years old
   b. 25 to 34 years old
   c. 35 to 44 years old
   d. 45+ years old
9. In osteoarthritis the development of Heberden's nodes in the distal interphalangeal joints of the hands occurs how many times more frequently in which sex?
   a. 5 times more in men
   b. 10 times more in men
   c. 5 times more in women
   d. 10 times more in women
10. The joints most often affected in osteoarthritis include the:
    a. Lumbar and cervical spine
    b. Knees

    c. Distal phalangeal joints
    d. Metacarpophalangeal joints
11. Common clinical features of osteoarthritis include:
    a. Morning stiffness of less than 30-minute duration
    b. Aching pain in the joint with working
    c. Restriction of range of motion
    d. Muscle spasm or pressure on nerves in the region of the joint

▼ *Circle T if the statement is true and F if it is false. Correct any false statements.*

12. T F Osteoarthritis is considered an inflammatory disease.
13. T F Erosive inflammatory osteoarthritis is a variant of osteoarthritis that involves ossification of the vertebrae.
14. T F Oral corticosteroids are used in the treatment of osteoarthritis.
15. T F Evidence of positive rheumatoid factor is indicative of osteoarthritis.

CHAPTER 71 ▶ Rheumatoid Arthritis

MICHAEL A. CARTER

Rheumatoid arthritis is a chronic disorder that affects multiple organ systems. This disorder is one of a group of diffuse connective tissue diseases that are immune mediated and of unknown cause. Patients usually have progressive joint destruction, although the episodes of joint inflammation may have periods of remission (Fig. 71-1).

Rheumatoid arthritis affects women about $2\frac{1}{2}$ times more frequently than men. The incidence increases with age, especially in women. The peak incidence is between 40 and 60 years of age. The disease is seen worldwide in all racial groups. About 1% of all adults have definite rheumatoid arthritis, and about 750 new cases per million population are reported each year in the United States.

The causes of rheumatoid arthritis are still unknown, even though much is known about the pathogenesis. The disorder cannot be shown to have a definite genetic link. There is an association with the genetic markers of HLA-Dw4 and HLA-DR5 in whites. Only an association with HLA-Dw4 has been shown in African Americans, Japanese, and Chippewa Indians.

Destruction of the tissues in the joint occurs in two ways. First, a digestive destruction is brought about by the production of proteases, collagenases, and other hydrolytic enzymes. These enzymes break down the cartilage, ligaments, tendons, and bones in the joints and are released along with oxygen radicals and arachidonic acid metabolites by polymorphonuclear leukocytes in the

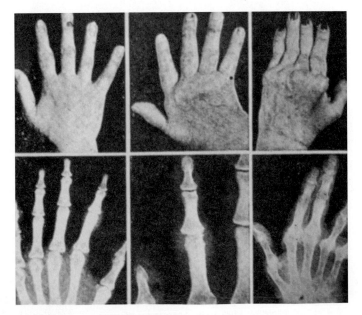

FIG. 71-1 Early, moderate, and advanced rheumatoid arthritis in the hands. Note the swelling of the second proximal interphalangeal (PIP) joint as part of the early changes. In the moderate stage, swelling of the metacarpophalangeal (MCP) joints occurs. The advanced stage shows subluxation of the MCP joints. (From Ensign DC: *Mod Med,* March 1, 1955, p 128, copyright 1955 by Harcourt Brace Jovanovich.)

synovial fluid. The process is thought to be part of an autoimmune response to locally produced antigens.

Tissue destruction also occurs through the action of rheumatoid pannus. This is a vascular granulation tissue that forms from the inflamed synovium and later extends into the joint. Along the edge of the pannus, destruction of collagen and proteoglycans occurs through the production of enzymes by cells in the pannus.

CLINICAL FEATURES

Several common clinical features are seen in persons with rheumatoid arthritis and are listed next. These may not all be present at one time in any particular individual, since the disorder is so variable.

1. *Constitutional symptoms:* these include fatigue, anorexia, weight loss, and fever. At times the fatigue can be disabling.
2. *Symmetric polyarthritis,* primarily of peripheral joints: this includes the joints of the hands, usually sparing the distal interphalangeal joints. Almost any diarthrodial joint can be affected.
3. *Morning stiffness* greater than 1 hour: this may be generalized stiffness but primarily involves the joints. This stiffness is different from the stiffness seen in osteoarthritis, which usually lasts only a few minutes and always less than an hour.
4. *Erosive arthritis:* radiologic characteristic of this disorder. The chronic inflammatory response results in loss of the marginal aspects of the bones (Fig. 71-2).
5. *Deformity:* destruction of the supportive structures of the joints occurs as the disease progresses. Ulnar drift

EXTRAARTICULAR MANIFESTATIONS OF RHEUMATOID ARTHRITIS

Skin	Subcutaneous nodules
	Vasculitis, causing brown spots
	Ecchymotic lesions
Heart	Pericarditis
	Pericardial tamponade (rare)
	Inflammatory lesions in myocardium and valves
Lungs	Pleurisy, with or without effusion
	Pulmonary inflammatory lesions
Eyes	Scleritis
Nervous system	Peripheral neuropathy
	Peripheral compression syndromes, including carpal tunnel syndrome, ulnar nerve neuropathy, peroneal palsy, and cervical spine abnormalities
Systemic	Anemia (common)
	Generalized osteoporosis
	Felty's syndrome
	Sjögren's syndrome (keratoconjunctivitis sicca)
	Amyloidosis (rare)

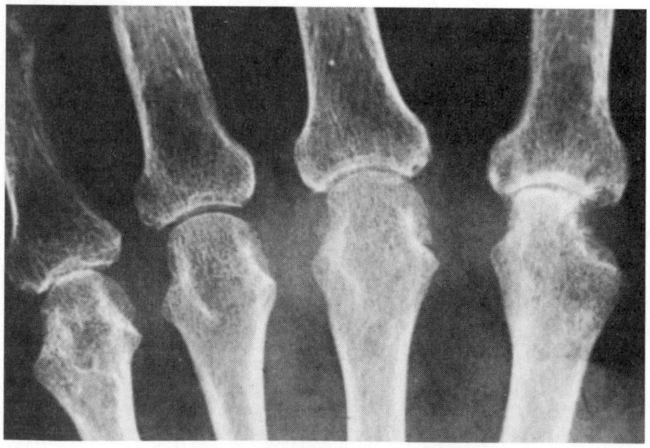

or deviation of the fingers, subluxation of the metacarpophalangeal joints, and boutonniere and swan neck deformities (Fig. 71-3) are some of the common deformities of the hands. There is a protrusion of the metatarsal heads secondary to metatarsal subluxation

FIG. 71-2   Radiograph of a rheumatoid hand. Note the erosion of the second metacarpal head and early erosion of the third metacarpal head. The cortex of the fourth metacarpal head remains indistinct. Compare this with the well-defined cortex of the fifth metacarpal head. (From the Canadian Arthritis and Rheumatism Society, JB Houpt, editor.)

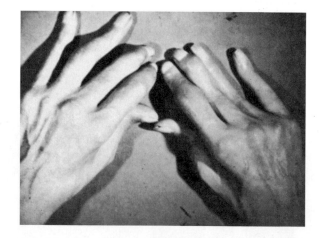

FIG. 71-3   Rheumatoid hand with boutonniere and swan neck deformities. Polyarthritis of the joints of the hands is seen. Among the advanced deforming changes is the muscle wasting in the anatomic snuffbox (between thumb and forefinger). Boutonniere deformity affects the left fourth digit, and swan neck deformity involves the right third and fourth digits. (From the Arthritis Division, University Hospital, University of Michigan.)

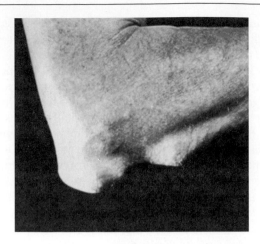

FIG. 71-4   Rheumatoid nodules in the elbow. Two large subcutaneous nodules are located about the elbow. One is in the olecranon bursa, and the other is on the extensor surface of the forearm. Nodules may be fixed or movable and are usually tender. They occur most frequently at the elbow but may also be found elsewhere, as on the feet, fingers, occiput, heels, and buttocks. Nodules occur in about 20% of patients with rheumatoid arthritis, may fluctuate in size, and are usually associated with high titers of rheumatoid factor. (From the Arthritis Foundation, New York, 1972.)

in the feet. Large joints may also be involved and have decreased range of motion, primarily in extension.

6. *Rheumatoid nodules:* subcutaneous masses occurring in about one third of adults with rheumatoid arthritis. The most common site for these is in the olecranon bursa (elbow) or along the extensor surface of the forearm; however, they can occur elsewhere. The presence of these nodules is usually indicative of an active or more severe disease (Fig. 71-4).

7. *Extraarticular manifestations:* rheumatoid arthritis may involve organs other than the joints. The heart (pericarditis), lungs (pleuritis), eyes, and blood vessels can be damaged. The box on p. 1044 outlines extraarticular manifestations of this disorder.

LABORATORY FINDINGS

Several laboratory tests are used to diagnose rheumatoid arthritis. *Rheumatoid factor* is found in the serum of about 85% of the individuals who have rheumatoid arthritis. This autoantibody is an anti–gamma globulin factor, immunoglobulin M (IgM), that reacts against altered IgG. Higher titers, greater than 1:160, are usually associated with rheumatoid nodules, severe disease, vasculitis, and a poor prognosis. Rheumatoid factor is a helpful diagnostic indicator, but it is not an exclusive test for rheumatoid arthritis. A positive test can indicate other connective tissue disorders, such as systemic lupus erythematosus, progressive systemic sclerosis, and dermato-

myositis. Furthermore, about 5% of normal people have a positive test. The incidence of positive rheumatoid factor in the normal population increases with age. As many as 20% of people over 60 years of age may have positive factors with low titers.

The erythrocyte sedimentation rate (ESR) is a nonspecific index of inflammation. Patients with rheumatoid arthritis may have high values (100 mm/hour or higher). This means that the ESR may be useful for monitoring disease activity.

Rheumatoid arthritis can cause a normocytic normochromic anemia by acting on the bone marrow. This anemia does not respond to the usual forms of therapy and can make the person feel fatigued. Iron deficiency anemia often occurs as a consequence of drug therapy for the illness. This form of anemia may respond to iron replacement.

Normal synovial fluid is a clear, light-yellow fluid with a white blood cell (WBC) count of less than 200/mm^3. In rheumatoid arthritis the synovial fluid loses its viscosity, and the WBC count is increased to 15,000 to 20,000/mm^3. This makes the fluid turbid. The fluid may clot, but the clot is usually poor and friable.

RADIOLOGIC FEATURES

In the early stages of the illness, no radiologic findings other than soft tissue swelling may be seen. As the joint damage progresses, narrowing of the joint space may occur because of the loss of articular cartilage. Bone erosions at the margin of the joint and decreased bone density occur. These changes are not usually reversible.

DIAGNOSTIC CRITERIA

The diagnosis of rheumatoid arthritis can be a complex process. In the early stages, there may be only a few or no positive laboratory tests; the joint changes can be minor; and the symptoms can be transitory. The diagnosis does not rest on any single characteristic but is based on the evaluation of a number of signs and symptoms. The diagnostic criteria are as follows:

1. Morning stiffness (lasting at least 1 hour)
2. Arthritis of three or more joint areas
3. Arthritis of hand joints
4. Symmetric arthritis
5. Rheumatoid nodules
6. Serum rheumatoid factor
7. Radiographic changes (erosions or bony decalcification)

Rheumatoid arthritis is said to be present if at least four of the seven criteria are met. The first four criteria must be present for at least 6 weeks.

TREATMENT

The treatment of rheumatoid arthritis is based on an understanding of the pathophysiology of the disorder. In addition, attention needs to be directed toward the psychophysiologic manifestations and the attendant psychosocial disruptions caused by the chronic, fluctuating course of the problem. Making an accurate diagnosis may take years, but treatment is initiated early.

The overall goals of the therapeutic program are as follows:
1. To relieve pain and inflammation
2. To maintain joint function and maximum functional capacity of the person
3. To prevent and/or correct joint deformities

There are a number of therapeutic prescriptions designed to achieve these goals: education, rest, exercise and thermotherapy, nutrition, and medication.

The first step of the therapeutic program is to provide an adequate *education* about the illness to the patient, the family, and those with whom the patient comes into contact. This education includes an understanding of the pathophysiology, causes, and prognosis of the illness and all the components of the management program, including the complex drug regimen, sources of assistance for coping with the illness, and effective methods of management offered by the health care team. The educational process is a constant one. Assistance is provided by patient clubs, community agencies, and other people with rheumatoid arthritis and their families.

Rest is important because rheumatoid arthritis usually is accompanied by profound fatigue. Although the person may have some fatigue each day, at times the person will be better or worse. Stiffness and discomfort may worsen with rest. This means that the person can frequently awaken at night with pain. Methods of decreasing nighttime pain should be advised, such as long-acting antiinflammatory drugs and analgesia. In addition, the treatment plan should cover activity pacing. The person should break each day into periods of activity followed by rest. If a particularly heavy activity is planned, such as a party, the rest period should be before that activity.

Specific *exercises* are useful in maintenance of joint function. These include active and passive range of motion to all affected joints at least twice a day. Pain medications may be necessary before beginning these exercises. *Heat* applications to painful and swollen joints may decrease pain. Special temperature-regulated paraffin baths and contrast baths of heat and cold can be used at home. The exercise and thermotherapy program is best prescribed by a health care provider who has special training, such as a physical therapist or an occupational therapist. Overuse of exercise can tear supporting structures of the joint that are already weakened by the illness.

Adaptive and assistive equipment may be necessary for the person to perform activities of daily living. The Arthritis Foundation or one of its many local chapters can provide materials that show how to use these devices and where to purchase them.

No specific nutritional prescription exists for rheumatoid arthritis. There are many unproven claims about various types of dietary interventions. The general principle is that a well-balanced diet is important. The illness may affect the temporomandibular joint, making chewing difficult at times. A number of the medications used to treat the illness can cause stomach discomfort and decrease adequate nutrition. Keeping the body weight in the proper limits is important. Weight can be easily gained, since activity levels usually are low. This increased weight can place additional stress on hip, knee, and foot joints. Referral to a registered dietitian may be of assistance.

Medication therapy is an important part of the overall treatment program. Medications are prescribed to reduce pain, decrease the inflammation of the illness, and attempt to modify the course of the illness. Different drugs may be used for each of these goals.

Pain is a constant part of rheumatoid arthritis. This means that the use of dependency-causing drugs should be kept to a minimum. Therapeutic measures such as heat and exercise can do much to diminish pain.

The mainstay of drug therapy in rheumatoid arthritis is the use of *nonsteroidal antiinflammatory drugs* (NSAIDs). This class of drugs reduces inflammation by interrupting the cascade of production of inflammatory mediators. Specifically, they inhibit either cyclooxygenase or prostaglandin synthetase. These enzymes convert the endogenous systemic fatty acid arachidonic acid to prostaglandins, prostacyclins, thromboxanes, and oxygen radicals. The historical standard drug in this class is aspirin, and all other NSAIDs are considered equally effective as aspirin at appropriate doses of each drug.

Additional drug therapy is indicated when the NSAIDs do not control the rheumatoid arthritis. These include a group of diverse, slow-acting drugs such as gold compounds, antimalarials, penicillamine, azathioprine, and methotrexate. Several of these do not have U.S. Food and Drug Administration approval for the treatment of rheumatoid arthritis. The goals of treatment with slow-acting drugs are to control the clinical manifestations and to arrest or slow the progression of the illness. The onset of response to these drugs is often gradual and can take as long as 3 to 6 months. Maximum response usually occurs after 1 year of therapy.

At least four indications exist for the use of corticosteroid therapy. Chronic oral therapy is used in those persons with rheumatoid arthritis who do not respond to NSAIDs and slow-acting drugs. The second indication is for the control of symptoms during the waiting period before the onset of action of slow-acting drugs. Third, intraarticular injections are indicated for acute exacerbations of synovitis in single joints in which mobility is significantly impaired. The fourth indication is high-dose oral therapy for short periods for severe attacks. The mechanism of action of these agents is twofold through antiinflammatory and immunosuppressive properties. Inflammation is reduced by blockage of prostaglandin formation, inhibition of leukocyte and monocyte chemotaxis and phagocytosis, stabilization of lysosomal enzymes, and prevention of changes in capillary membranes. Immunosuppression is caused by decreased reticuloendothelial, or monocyte-macrophage, procession of antigens and altered functions of lymphocytes. Many adverse effects occur from the use of these drugs, particularly with chronic use. Almost all organ systems are disturbed by their effects.

JUVENILE RHEUMATOID ARTHRITIS

Children can develop rheumatoid arthritis similar to the disease in adults. In the United States, 13.9 per 100,000 children will develop this illness. There are three subtypes of juvenile rheumatoid arthritis based on the onset of the symptoms.

Systemic onset (Still's disease) accounts for about 20% of all cases. Boys and girls are equally affected, and this form can occur at any age. As the name implies, there is systemic involvement of multiple organ systems in addition to a chronic polyarthritis. This subtype has the poorest prognosis of the three types and can lead to growth retardation.

Polyarticular onset accounts for about 40% of all cases. Girls are affected at a 2:1 ratio over boys, and this form can occur at any age as well. Five or more joints are involved at one time, but generally with only moderate extraarticular involvement. This form has a better prognosis than systemic onset but can also cause growth retardation.

Pauciarticular onset accounts for about 40% of all cases. Girls are affected 6:1 over boys. This form usually occurs before age 6. No more than four joints are involved, generally with few, if any, extraarticular involvements. This form has the best prognosis of the three forms.

Treatment of juvenile rheumatoid arthritis is similar to the treatment in adults, but with some important differences. Several of the drugs used in adults are not approved for use in children. Systemic corticosteroids can lead to growth retardation, osteoporosis, and cataracts. Some of the immunosuppressive agents can cause bone marrow suppression, sterility, and malignancy in children.

QUESTIONS

▼ *Answer the following on a separate sheet of paper.*

1. Define rheumatoid arthritis.
2. What is the association between the genetic markers HLA-Dw4 and HLA-DR5 and the development of rheumatoid arthritis?
3. Describe the two ways in which destruction of tissues in the joint occurs in rheumatoid arthritis.
4. List the seven diagnostic criteria for rheumatoid arthritis.
5. What are the overall goals of the therapeutic program for rheumatoid arthritis?
6. Describe the mechanism by which nonsteroidal antiinflammatory drugs (NSAIDs) reduce inflammation.
7. Cite the four indications for the use of corticosteroid therapy in persons with rheumatoid arthritis.
8. What is the mechanism of action of these corticosteroid drugs?
9. Discuss two of the systemic organ involvements that may be seen in rheumatoid arthritis.

▼ *Circle the letter preceding each item below that correctly answers the question or completes the statement. More than one answer may be correct.*

10. Rheumatoid arthritis typically affects which of the following segments of the population?
    a. Both sexes equally
    b. Females more than males (2.5:1)
    c. Males more than females (2.5:1)
11. The peak incidence of rheumatoid arthritis is between which years of age?
    a. 10 to 20
    b. 40 to 60
    c. 20 to 40
    d. 60 to 80
12. The joints most frequently affected by symmetric polyarthritis are the:
    a. Joints of the hands, including distal interphalangeal joints
    b. Peripheral joints
    c. Symphysis pubis
    d. Intervertebral disks
13. Common clinical features seen in rheumatoid arthritis are:
    a. Skin rash, psoriasis

b. Sun sensitivity
    c. Fatigue, anorexia, weight loss
    d. Morning stiffness lasting less than 1 hour
    e. Joint swelling of the hands, including distal interphalangeal joints
14. Which of the following laboratory findings is (are) indicative of rheumatoid arthritis?
    a. Rheumatoid factor in the serum
    b. An erythrocyte sedimentation rate of less than 100 mm/hour
    c. Urate crystals in the synovial fluid
    d. A positive mucin clot test
15. Typical radiologic findings found in rheumatoid arthritis are:
    a. Asymmetric soft tissue tophi
    b. Narrowing of the joint space
    c. Irregular loss of joint space
    d. Bony cystic erosion
16. The therapeutic program for rheumatoid arthritis usually includes:
    a. Rest periods and decreased activity during the day
    b. An educational program covering the pathophysiology, etiology, manage-

Continued.

QUESTIONS—cont'd

ment (drugs, sources of assistance), and prognosis

c. A vigorous exercise program to strengthen structures of the joint

d. Specific dietary prescriptions recommending either high-dose B or C vitamins

e. Initial prescription of slow-acting drugs

17. Which of the following subsets of juvenile rheumatoid arthritis has the best prognosis?
   a. Polyarticular onset
   b. Systemic onset (Still's disease)
   c. Pauciarticular onset

18. Rheumatoid factor is detected in the serum of what percentage of patients with rheumatoid arthritis?
   a. 50%
   b. 60%
   c. 85%
   d. 90%

▼ *Circle T if the statement is true and F if it is false. Correct any false statements.*

19. T F In the United States, 20 per 100,000 children will develop juvenile rheumatoid arthritis.

20. T F Systemic onset (Still's disease) occurs in approximately 20% of all patients with juvenile rheumatoid arthritis.

21. T F An association with the genetic marker HLA-DR5 has been shown in African Americans and Japanese.

22. T F The most common site for rheumatoid nodules is the olecranon bursa.

23. T F Rheumatoid factor is a measure of the IgM antibody, which reacts against the altered IgG and is detected in about 99% of patients with rheumatoid arthritis.

CHAPTER 72

Systemic Lupus Erythematosus

MICHAEL A. CARTER

Systemic lupus erythematosus (SLE) is a multisystem, chronic autoimmune disease. The signs and symptoms of this disorder can be diverse, transitory, and difficult to diagnose. Therefore the exact number of people with the disorder is difficult to obtain. SLE affects women about eight times as often as men. The disorder frequently begins in late adolescence or early adulthood. In the United States, African-American women are affected about three times more often than white women. The disorder is usually milder and more easily controlled if SLE develops after age 60.

SLE was originally described as a skin disorder in the 1800s and given the name lupus because of the characteristic "butterfly rash" across the bridge of the nose and the cheeks that resembles the bite of a wolf (*lupus* is the Latin word for wolf). *Discoid lupus* is the name now given to the disorder when it is limited to cutaneous involvement.

SLE is one of a group of diffuse connective tissue disorders of unknown etiology. These include SLE, scleroderma, polymyositis, rheumatoid arthritis, and Sjögren's syndrome. These disorders frequently have overlapping symptoms and may be present at the same time, making an accurate diagnosis difficult. SLE can vary from a mild disorder to one that is rapidly fulminating and fatal. The most common situation, however, is one of exacerbations and near remissions that can last for long periods. Early identification and treatment of SLE usually lead to a more favorable prognosis.

CLINICAL FEATURES

The clinical picture of SLE can be confusing, particularly in the early stages of the disorder. The most common symptom is a symmetric arthritis or arthralgia that is present 90% of the time, often as an initial manifestation. The most frequently affected joints are the proximal joints of the hands, wrists, elbows, shoulders, knees, and ankles. The polyarthritis of SLE differs from that of rheumatoid arthritis in that it is rarely erosive or deforming. Also, subcutaneous nodules are rarely seen in SLE.

Constitutional symptoms of fever, fatigue, weakness, and weight loss generally occur early and may recur throughout the course of the disorder. Fatigue and weakness may be secondary to a mild anemia that is caused by SLE.

Skin manifestations include an erythematous rash that may appear on the face (Fig. 72-1), neck, extremities, or trunk. About 40% of individuals with SLE have the characteristic butterfly rash. Exposure to sunlight may aggravate this rash. Alopecia (hair loss) can develop and can sometimes be severe. Hair growth usually returns without major problems. Small ulcerations of the oral or nasopharyngeal mucous membranes can occur.

Pleurisy (chest pain) may occur as a result of the chronic inflammatory process of SLE. SLE can also cause carditis involving the myocardium, endocardium, or pericardium.

Raynaud's phenomenon occurs in about 40% of those with SLE. Some cases may be so severe that gangrene of the digits occurs. Vasculitis may affect all sizes of arteries and veins.

Lupus nephritis occurs as the antinuclear antibody (anti-DNA) attaches to its antigen (deoxyribonucleic acid, or DNA) and is deposited in the renal glomerulus. DNA is not normally antigenic in humans but becomes so

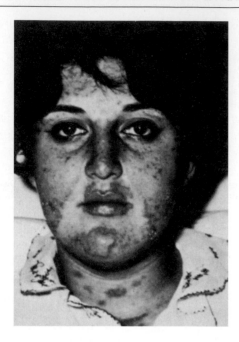

FIG. 72-1 Systemic lupus erythematous (SLE). Widespread discrete and confluent erythematous lesions are present on the face and neck. Typical peeling is noted on the chin and cheeks. (From the Arthritis Foundation, New York, 1972.)

in SLE. Complement is fixed to this immune complex, and the inflammatory process begins. Renal inflammation, tissue damage, and scarring may result.

About 65% of persons with SLE develop some renal involvement. Only 25%, however, develop severe problems. Lupus nephritis is detected by examining the urine for protein, red blood cells (RBCs), or casts. A kidney biopsy may be necessary for an accurate diagnosis.

SLE may affect the central or peripheral nervous system. Symptoms include behavioral changes (depression, psychosis), convulsions, cranial nerve disorders, and peripheral neuropathies. Central nervous system (CNS) changes are often associated with severe forms of the disorder and are frequently fatal.

DIAGNOSIS

The American Rheumatism Association has developed revised criteria for the classification of SLE. The presence of four or more of the following 11 criteria either serially or simultaneously is considered diagnostic:

1. Malar rash
2. Discoid rash
3. Photosensitivity
4. Oral ulcers
5. Arthritis: nonerosive, of two or more peripheral joints
6. Serositis: pleuritis or pericarditis

7. Renal disorder: persistent proteinuria with greater than 0.5 g/day, or cellular casts
8. Neurologic disorder: seizures or psychosis
9. Hematologic disorder: hemolytic anemia, leukopenia, lymphopenia, or thrombocytopenia
10. Immunologic disorder: positive lupus erythematosus (LE) cells, anti-DNA, anti-Sm, or a false-positive serologic test for syphilis
11. Antinuclear antibody (ANA)

DRUG-INDUCED SLE

A number of drugs can induce in susceptible individuals a syndrome that is similar to SLE. This syndrome includes most of the symptoms of SLE, including positive tests for ANA, but renal and CNS effects rarely occur. The SLE symptoms begin to disappear within a few weeks after the discontinuation of these drugs. The positive ANA test reverts to negative after several months. Hydralazine and procainamide are two of the more common drugs that can cause this reaction. A number of other drugs are capable of producing a positive ANA, including penicillamine, isoniazid, chlorpromazine, and anticonvulsants such as barbiturates, phenytoin, ethosuximide, methsuximide, and primidone. Some drugs can cause an exacerbation of SLE in patients who are in a remission. These include sulfonamides, penicillin, and oral contraceptives.

LABORATORY TESTS

Antinuclear antibodies are positive in more than 95% of those with SLE. This test indicates whether there are antibodies capable of destroying the nucleus of one's own body cells. In addition to the presence of ANA, the ANA pattern and the specific antibodies are evaluated. The pattern refers to the appearance of the slide when viewed under ultraviolet light. A differential evaluation of the specific types of ANA is now available and is useful in differentiating SLE from other types of disorders. Antibodies to double-stranded DNA (dsDNA) is a specific test for SLE. Other rheumatologic disorders can cause a positive ANA, but anti-DNA antibodies are rarely found except in SLE.

The erythrocyte sedimentation rate is usually elevated in SLE. This is a nonspecific test measuring inflammation and does not relate to the level of disease involvement in SLE.

A laboratory test that was previously used and may occasionally be used today is the LE factor. The LE cell is formed by damaging some of the person's white blood cells (WBCs) so that they will release their nucleoprotein. This protein reacts with immunoglobulin G (IgG),

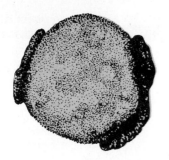

FIG. 72-2   SLE:LE cell; a neutrophil containing homogeneous material, the LE body. The nucleus is pushed to one side and flattened around the mass.

and the complex is phagocytosed by the remaining WBCs. The resulting cell is easily identified (Fig. 72-2). This factor can usually be demonstrated at some time in the course of the disorder if enough tests are done. LE cells can be demonstrated in other immune-mediated systemic forms of rheumatic disorders.

Urine is examined for the presence of protein, WBCs, RBCs, and casts. These tests are used both to determine the presence of renal complications of SLE and to monitor the progression of the illness.

TREATMENT

The treatment of the person with SLE is multifaceted and includes counseling, complex drug therapy, and preventive measures. The most frequent onset period of SLE is during late adolescence, and early adulthood for women. Because these are the prime reproductive years, much counseling is needed to assist in making the decision concerning having children. Pregnancy may cause a flare of SLE, which can be dangerous for women with renal damage. Cytotoxic drugs may be necessary to control the illness, and these can potentially affect the fetus. Contraceptive methods cannot usually include oral contraceptives, since these may aggravate SLE. The intrauterine device can be a problem for women taking systemic corticosteroids because of the potential for infection.

Drug therapy for SLE includes nonsteroidal antiinflammatory drugs (NSAIDs), corticosteroids, antimalarials, and immunosuppressive agents. The selection of appropriate drug therapy depends on the specific organs affected by the illness. NSAIDs are used to control the arthritis and arthralgia. Aspirin is used less frequently now because it produces the highest incidence of hepatotoxicity and some patients with SLE have hepatic involvement. Persons with SLE are at a higher risk of the cutaneous, hepatic, and renal adverse effects of NSAIDs and should be monitored closely.

Antimalarial therapy is sometimes effective if the NSAIDs cannot control the symptoms of SLE. Antimalarials are usually given at an initially high dosage to achieve a remission. The clearance of skin lesions offers a monitoring parameter to use in dosage adjustment. Immunosuppressive therapy (cyclophosphamide or azathioprine) can be used to suppress the autoimmune activity of SLE. These drugs are usually prescribed when there is (1) a well-established diagnosis, (2) the presence of severe, life-threatening symptoms, (3) failure of other therapeutic measures, such as a failure to respond to steroids or the need for reduction of steroids because of the adverse effects, and (4) the absence of infection, pregnancy, and neoplasm.

Acute flares of SLE, especially in those with interstitial nephritis, are treated with high-dose oral corticosteroids for short periods. These drugs are then gradually reduced in dosage over the next several weeks. Both SLE and systemic corticosteroids can produce behavioral changes, and the cause can be difficult to distinguish.

An important aspect of the prevention of flares of SLE is avoidance of exposure to ultraviolet (UV) light. Just how the sun causes SLE to flare is not fully understood. One explanation is that DNA exposed to UV light normally becomes antigenic, which leads to the flares seen after sun exposure. Patients with SLE should be encouraged to use umbrellas, hats, and long-sleeved shirts when outdoors. There may be problems getting teenagers to follow these suggestions. A sunscreen with a protection factor of 15 should be used to block the UV light exposure. The sunscreen should be reapplied after swimming or heavy exercise. The person should receive a list of drugs that can cause exacerbations so that this type of flare can be avoided.

PROGNOSIS

The prognosis for SLE varies and depends on the severity of the symptoms, the organs involved, and the length of time remissions may be maintained. No cure exists for SLE, and treatment is focused on the management of the symptoms. The prognosis is related to how well the symptoms are managed.

QUESTIONS

▼ *Answer the following on a separate sheet of paper.*

1. Formulate a definition of systemic lupus erythematosus (SLE).
2. Contrast the antinuclear antibody (ANA) test with the LE factor test.
3. Discuss the importance of counseling females of childbearing age regarding SLE.
4. Explain the rationale in SLE for avoidance of exposure to the sun.
5. What is the rationale for the selection of drugs used in the treatment of SLE?

▼ *Circle the letter preceding each item below that correctly answers the question or completes the statement. More than one answer may be correct.*

6. In SLE, women are affected approximately how many times more than men?
   a. 5
   b. 7
   c. 8
   d. 10
7. The most common initial manifestation of SLE is:
   a. Symmetric arthritis or arthralgia
   b. Subcutaneous nodules
   c. Fatigue and weakness
   d. Weight loss
8. Which of the following laboratory tests will be positive in greater than 95% of those with SLE?
   a. ANA
   b. Increased serum complement levels
   c. Decreased erythrocyte sedimentation rate
   d. Positive rheumatoid factor
9. Which of the following drugs are able to induce a syndrome (symptoms of SLE) that is similar to SLE?
   a. Isoniazid
   b. Procainamide
   c. Hydralazine
   d. Chlorpromazine
10. The serial or simultaneous presence of which of the criteria listed below is considered diagnostic of SLE?
    a. Photosensitivity, positive ANA test, symmetric joint swelling, subcutaneous nodules
    b. Malar rash, pain on motion, morning stiffness less than 30 minutes, ulcers
    c. Photosensitivity, malar rash, positive ANA test, hemolytic anemia
    d. Photosensitivity, positive rheumatoid factor, oral ulcers, pleuritis
11. The formation of antibodies against which of the following antigens is considered diagnostic of SLE?
    a. Membrane protein
    b. IgM
    c. Double-stranded DNA
    d. RNA
12. Drug therapy for SLE generally includes:
    a. Corticosteroids
    b. NSAIDs
    c. Immunosuppressive agents
    d. Cytotoxic drugs

▼ *Circle T if the statement is true and F if it is false. Correct any false statements.*

13. T F The onset of SLE is most frequently seen in late adolescence or early adulthood.
14. T F Cyclophosphamide or azathioprine is prescribed for SLE to control the symptoms and achieve a remission.
15. T F Lupus nephritis is a serious disorder that occurs in more than 80% of the individuals with SLE.
16. T F DNA is not usually antigenic to humans with SLE.

CHAPTER 73 ► Scleroderma

MICHAEL A. CARTER

Scleroderma, or *systemic sclerosis,* is an uncommon connective tissue disorder characterized by fibrosis of the skin and other organs. Scleroderma can be classified into one of three groups based on the extent of the skin disease. *Generalized scleroderma* (systemic sclerosis) can be one of two types: (1) diffuse cutaneous systemic sclerosis with truncal skin involvement, widespread visceral disease, and rapid progression or (2) limited cutaneous systemic sclerosis, including the CREST variant (see Clinical features). *Localized scleroderma* usually affects only limited skin areas and does not affect visceral organs. *Occupational and environmental scleroderma-like syndromes* can be seen after exposure to agents such as vinyl chloride, bleomycin, and rapeseed oil.

Systemic sclerosis leads to fibrosis and degenerative changes in the synovium, digital arteries, and parenchyma and small arteries of the esophagus, intestine, lungs, heart, kidney, and thyroid gland. The cause of progressive systemic sclerosis is not known, although a number of serologic and cellular immune reaction abnormalities exist, indicating that an immunologic mechanism is involved.

The disorder is seen worldwide in all races. Women are affected three times more often than men. The disease onset is usually in the third to fifth decades of life; only rarely does the disorder affect children. The disease occurs with particularly high frequency in coal miners, leading to the suggestion that silicosis is a predisposing factor.

Scleroderma is similar to other connective tissue disorders in that remissions and exacerbations may occur, with a generally slow progression that allows for a reasonably long life. The disorder may be rapidly progressive, however, and lead to an early death when vital organs are affected and damaged. Renal failure is the leading cause of death for persons with systemic sclerosis.

The changes seen in the skin and other organs are the result of the overproduction of collagen. Why this is so is not known. The changes in the blood vessels are similar. The lesions that develop in the small arteries and arterioles begin as proliferations on the intimal side of the internal elastic membrane. A medial thinning then occurs, and finally the deposit of a connective tissue cuff rich in collagen proceeds. All these changes are thought to be brought on by alterations in B cell and T cell activity.

CLINICAL FEATURES

Raynaud's phenomenon (Fig. 73-1) is the most common manifestation seen in persons with systemic sclerosis. *Raynaud's phenomenon* is a paroxysmal vasospastic disorder in which an abnormal spasm of the arteries of the hand occurs in response to cold temperatures or extreme emotions. This causes the digits to become white (vasospasm), then blue (cyanosis), and then red (reactive hyperemia). Other common symptoms are swelling and puffiness of the hands and gradual thickening and tightening of the skin of the fingers and other body parts. The fingers develop a sausagelike appearance. The skin slowly thickens and becomes taut, shiny, and tightly bound to the underlying subcutaneous tissue. This process progresses proximally, involving the arms, chest, and face. The face becomes taut (Fig. 73-2), the oral orifice becomes wrinkled, and the opening of the orifice is restricted. The forehead loses its normal wrinkles. Polyarthralgia, joint stiffness, and polyarthritis are also seen.

One form of systemic sclerosis is the *CREST* variant. This mnemonic stands for the first letter in calcinosis, Raynaud's phenomenon, esophageal dysmotility, sclerodactyly, and telangiectasia (Fig. 73-3).

The colon may be affected, which results in diarrhea or constipation, cramping, malabsorption, and in a few patients, perforation.

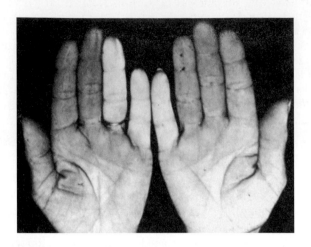

FIG. 73-1   Scleroderma: Raynaud's phenomenon. The marked pallor of the fourth and fifth digits of the left hand and the fifth digit of the right hand is characteristic of Raynaud's phenomenon. Vasospastic changes are common in systemic sclerosis. (From the Arthritis Foundation, New York, 1972.)

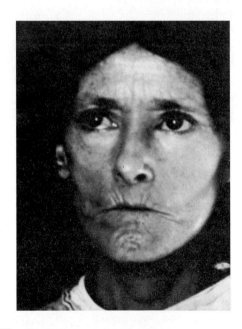

FIG. 73-2   Scleroderma: skin changes. This young woman demonstrates many features of systemic sclerosis: drawn, pursed lips, shiny skin over the cheeks and forehead, and atrophy of muscles of the temple, face, and neck. Such facial changes are known as *Mauskopf* ("mouse head"). (From the Arthritis Foundation, New York, 1972.)

Exertional dyspnea is usually the first sign of pulmonary involvement. Pulmonary function studies may show alteration in the gas exchange, that is, a decrease in breathing capacity and an increase in residual air. Pericarditis, dysrhythmias, and electrocardiogram changes may occur with cardiac involvement.

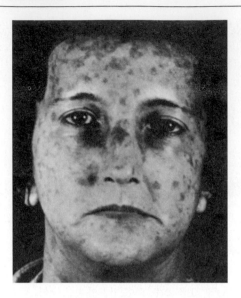

FIG. 73-3   Scleroderma: telangiectasia. Multiple telangiectases are present on the face and blanch with pressure. Telangiectasia occurs frequently in scleroderma, at times leading to confusion in differentiation from hereditary hemorrhagic telangiectasia. (From the Arthritis Foundation, New York, 1972.)

Renal involvement, manifested as proteinuria, microscopic hematuria, and hypertension, may rapidly deteriorate to renal failure. Any vital organ involvement, especially when rapidly deteriorating, indicates a poor prognosis.

LABORATORY AND RADIOLOGIC FINDINGS

The erythrocyte sedimentation rate may be elevated in patients with scleroderma. A small group of patients may demonstrate rheumatoid factor in their serum. A positive reaction to antinuclear antibody and hypergammaglobulinemia may be demonstrated. Skin biopsies are the most specific way of making the diagnosis but are usually not necessary because of the striking clinical picture.

Radiologic examination may demonstrate subcutaneous calcifications of the digits of the hand (Fig. 73-4). Esophageal and intestinal abnormalities may also be detected.

TREATMENT

Currently, no effective therapy will reverse the fibrosis of scleroderma. A variety of drugs are used to help manage symptoms. Penicillamine, dimethyl sulfoxide (DMSO), immunosuppressive drugs, and alkylating agents are sometimes used.

Protection of the hands to help avoid Raynaud's phenomenonon is an important part of the management plan.

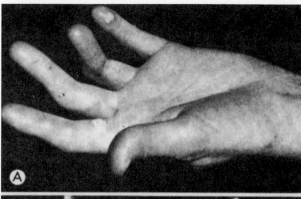
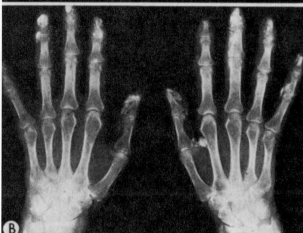

FIG. 73-4   Scleroderma: subcutaneous calcification. **A,** Hand of an adolescent girl with systemic sclerosis. Note the circumscribed lesions of calcinosis in the skin of the volar surface of the proximal portion of the second digit and the distal portion of the fifth digit. **B,** Radiograph of the hands of a woman with systemic sclerosis, as depicted by the extensive subcutaneous calcinosis in the fingers and near the joint of the right hand. (From Hollander JR, editor: *Arthritis and allied conditions: a textbook of rheumatology,* ed 8, Philadelphia, 1972, Lea & Febiger.)

Grasping a cold glass can initiate an attack. Gloves may be necessary most of the time. The person should stop the use of all tobacco products because of the adverse effects of nicotine on the blood vessels. Vasodilators are sometimes of benefit in treatment of Raynaud's phenomenon. Low dosages of corticosteroids may relieve joint complaints but are usually not of great benefit for treatment of systemic sclerosis. Nonsteroidal antiinflammatory agents can be used to decrease discomfort.

Antibiotics have been used with some success in the treatment of small-bowel involvement. The hypomotility of the bowel allows for an overgrowth of microorganisms, and these interfere with absorption. Treatment with antibiotics reduces the overgrowth.

Physical therapy is an important component of therapy. The characteristic restriction of the opening of the mouth can interfere with the person's ability to eat. Mouth function can be greatly improved through stretching and muscle strengthening.

QUESTIONS

▼ *Answer the following on a separate sheet of paper.*

1. Differentiate among generalized scleroderma, localized scleroderma, and occupational and environmental scleroderma-like syndromes as to the extent of the skin disease.
2. Describe the changes in skin and other organs in scleroderma.
3. Describe the CREST variant of scleroderma.
4. Identify the therapeutic measures used for patients with scleroderma.

▼ *Circle the letter preceding each item below that correctly answers the question or completes the statement. More than one answer may be correct.*

5. In scleroderma, women are affected how many times more often than men?
   a. 2   c. 4
   b. 3   d. 6
6. Dysfunction of which of the following organs is the leading cause of death in scleroderma?
   a. Heart   c. Brain
   b. Spleen   d. Kidney
7. The initial organ system affected by scleroderma is the:
   a. Skin and appendages
   b. Respiratory system
   c. Renal system
   d. Cardiovascular system
8. The most common manifestation associated with scleroderma is:
   a. Perforation of the colon

   b. Raynaud's phenomenon
   c. Pericarditis
   d. Exertional dyspnea

▼ *Circle T if the statement is true and F if it is false. Correct any false statements.*

9. T F   Raynaud's phenomenon is a paroxysmal vasospastic disorder in which an abnormal spasm of the arteries of the hand occurs in response to cold temperature or extreme emotions.

10. T F   Radiographic studies of systemic sclerosis may demonstrate subcutaneous calcifications of the great toe.

11. T F   Currently an experimental drug is available that will reverse the fibrosis of scleroderma.

CHAPTER 74 ▶ Gout

MICHAEL A. CARTER

Gout is a metabolic disorder that was described by Hippocrates in ancient Greece. Early theories indicated that gout was a problem only of the elite social class and was caused by overindulgence in food, wine, and sex. Many etiologic and therapeutic theories have been proposed over the ages, but today much is known about gout, and treatment has a high success rate.

Gout is a term used for a group of at least nine metabolic disorders characterized by an elevation in the serum uric acid concentration *(hyperuricemia)*. Gout may be primary or secondary. *Primary gout* is the direct result of the body's overproduction of or decreased excretion of uric acid. *Secondary gout* occurs when the overproduction or decreased excretion of uric acid is secondary to another disease process or medication.

The problem develops when crystals of monosodium urate monohydrate form in the joints and surrounding tissues. These needlelike crystals are responsible for the acute inflammatory reaction that develops, resulting in the severe pain typically associated with an acute gouty attack. These crystal deposits can lead to extensive joint and soft tissue damage if left untreated.

CLINICAL FEATURES

The serum urate level in men normally begins to increase after puberty. The urate level does not increase in women until after menopause, since estrogens increase the renal excretion of uric acid. After menopause the serum urate levels of women begin to rise to those of men.

Gout is seldom seen in women. Men account for almost 95% of the cases. Gout is seen worldwide in all racial groups. A familial prevalence suggests a genetic basis. A number of factors likely influence the expression of the illness, however, including diet, body weight, and life-style.

There are four stages in the clinical progression of untreated gout. The first stage is *asymptomatic hyperuricemia*. The normal value of serum uric acid in men is 5.1 ± 1.0 mg/dl, and in women the value is 4.0 ± 1.0 mg/dl. These levels rise to an average of 9 to 10 mg/dl in persons with gout. At this stage the person has no symptoms other than an elevated serum uric acid. Only 20% of the people with asymptomatic hyperuricemia go on to develop an acute gouty attack.

The second stage is *acute gouty arthritis*. At this stage the person has a sudden onset of exquisitely painful swelling and tenderness, usually of the great toe and metatarsophalangeal joint (Fig. 74-1). The arthritis is monarticular and shows signs of local inflammation. The person may have fever and an elevated white blood cell count. The attack may be precipitated by surgery, trauma, drugs, alcohol, or emotional stress. This stage usually leads the person to seek prompt medical attention. Other joints can be affected, including the finger joints, knees, ankles, wrists, and elbows. Acute gouty attacks usually resolve if untreated but may take 10 to 14 days to do so.

The development of the acute attack of gout generally follows a set sequence of events. First, a supersaturation of urate occurs in the plasma and body fluids, followed by a deposition into and around the joints. The mechanism of the crystallization of urates out of the serum is not clearly understood. Gouty attacks frequently follow local trauma or the rupture of *tophi* (deposits of sodium urate), which accounts for a rapid increase in local concentrations of uric acid. The body may not be able to handle this increase appropriately, resulting in the precipitation of uric acid out of the serum. Crystallization and deposition of the uric acid then trigger the gouty attack.

These uric acid crystals initiate a phagocytic response by leukocytes, and as the leukocytes ingest the urate crystals, the responses of other inflammatory mechanisms are triggered. The inflammatory response may be influenced by the site and magnitude of uric acid crystal deposition. The inflammatory reaction may become self-propagating and self-enhancing because of the deposition of additional crystals from the serum.

The third stage, which follows the acute gouty attack, is the *intercritical stage*. There are no symptoms during this period, which may last for months to years. Most people have a repeat gouty attack in less than 1 year if they are untreated.

The fourth stage is the *chronic gout stage,* in which the urate pool continues to expand over years if treatment is not begun. Chronic inflammation from the presence of urate crystals results in the development of pain, aching, and stiffness as well as large and nodular joint swelling.

Acute attacks of gouty arthritis may occur during this stage. Tophi develop in chronic gout because of the relative insolubility of urates (Fig. 74-2). The onset and the size of tophi may be proportionally related to the level of serum urate. The olecranon bursa, Achilles tendon, extensor surface of the forearm, infrapatellar bursa, and helix of the ear (Fig. 74-3) are the most common sites for tophi. These tophi may be difficult to distinguish clinically from rheumatoid nodules. Tophi are rarely seen today and will resolve with appropriate therapy.

Gout can damage the kidneys, leading to even poorer excretion of uric acid. Uric acid crystals can form in the

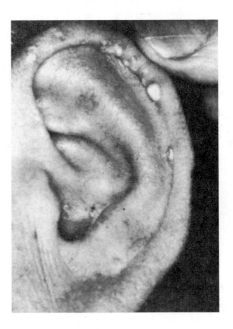

FIG. 74-3 In this patient with gout, small tophi can be seen on the helix of the ear, having a typical whitish appearance as a result of urate deposition. Small cartilaginous nodules are usually present in the ears of normal individuals and can be mistaken for tophi. A tophus characteristically stands out as a discrete white nodule when pressed by the examiner's fingers; in contrast, the cartilaginous nodule blanches out and blends with the rest of the ear. Transillumination reveals an opaque center in the tophus but not in the cartilaginous nodule. (From the Arthritis Foundation, New York, 1972.)

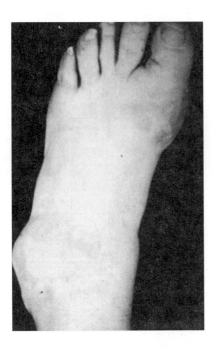

FIG. 74-1 Typical inflammatory response of gout involving the great toe. This is the most common site of acute gout. (From the Arthritis Division, University Hospital, University of Michigan.)

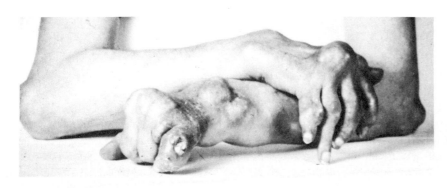

FIG. 74-2 Many tophi are present on the hands of this patient with gout. One asymmetrically shaped tophus on the little finger has ulcerated. Tophi are also present in both olecranon bursae; these are common sites for tophi. Swelling of some joints as a result of synovitis is also present. (From the Arthritis Foundation, New York, 1972.)

medullary interstitium, papillae, and pyramids, leading to proteinuria and mild hypertension. Uric acid kidney stones can also occur secondary to gout. These stones are usually small and round and do not show up on radiographs.

DIAGNOSTIC CRITERIA

Gout should be considered in men who develop monarticular arthritis, particularly of the great toe, that is acute in onset. An elevated serum uric acid is helpful in making the diagnosis but not specific, since a number of drugs can elevate the serum uric acid level. Also, a fairly large number of people have asymptomatic hyperuricemia.

Another test used to diagnose gout is the response of the joint symptoms to colchicine. *Colchicine* is a drug that inhibits phagocytic leukocytes and thereby produces a dramatic and rapid relief of symptoms. Radiologic changes other than soft tissue swelling are usually not present in the early stages of gout. The demonstration of urate crystals in the synovial fluid of an involved joint is considered diagnostic (Fig. 74-4).

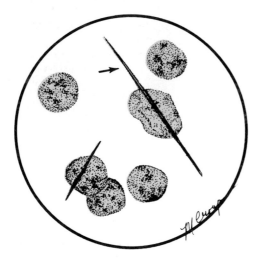

FIG. 74-4   Gout: one uric acid crystal in a white blood cell in synovial fluid.

CONTRIBUTING FACTORS

The factors that contribute to the development of gout depend on the cause of the hyperuricemia. A diet high in purines can trigger a gouty attack in a person with one of the inborn errors of purine metabolism that cause an overproduction of uric acid. A low-purine diet, however, will not usually lower the serum urate level to any great extent.

The ingestion of alcohol can bring on a gouty attack because alcohol increases urate production. Blood lactate levels increase as a by-product of the normal metabolism of alcohol. Lactic acid blocks the renal excretion of uric acid with a concomitant rise in serum levels.

A number of drugs can block the renal excretion of uric acid and lead to a gouty attack. These include aspirin in low doses (less than 1 to 2 g/day), most diuretics, levodopa, diazoxide, nicotinic acid, acetazolamide, and ethambutol.

TREATMENT

The treatment of gout depends on the stage. Asymptomatic hyperuricemia usually requires no treatment. The acute attack of gouty arthritis is treated by the use of nonsteroidal antiinflammatory drugs or colchicine. These are

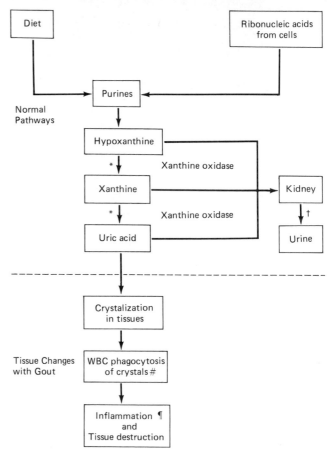

Sites for the drugs' mechanisms of action.

* Allopurinol
† Probenecid and sulfinpyrazone
# Colchicine
¶ NSAIDS

FIG. 74-5   Gout pathophysiology and drug actions. [From Weiner MB, Pepper GA: *Clinical pharmacology and therapeutics in nursing,* ed 2, New York, 1985, McGraw-Hill.]

given in high doses or in loading doses to reduce the acute inflammation of the joint. The dosage is then decreased gradually over the next few days.

The treatment of chronic gout is based on decreasing the production of uric acid or on increasing the renal excretion of uric acid. The drug allopurinol blocks the formation of uric acid from its precursors (xanthine and hypoxanthine) by inhibiting the enzyme xanthine oxidase. This drug can be given in a convenient once-a-day dose.

Uricosuric agents enhance the excretion of uric acid by blocking renal tubular reabsorption. Adequate kidney function is necessary for uricosuric agents to be effective. The creatinine clearance is evaluated to determine kidney function (normal is 115 to 120 ml/minute). Probenecid

and sulfinpyrazone are two widely used uricosuric agents. Fluid intake of at least 1500 ml/day is needed to promote the excretion of uric acid while a patient is taking a uricosuric agent. All aspirin products should be avoided because they block the uricosuric action of these drugs. Fig. 74-5 depicts gout pathophysiology and drug actions.

Strict dietary modifications are not usually necessary in the treatment of gout. The person can be helped to avoid those factors that precipitate an attack, but this is usually determined by trial and error for each person. Obviously, products high in purines may be problematic. These include organ meats such as liver, kidneys, sweetbreads, and brains as well as a number of luncheon meats. Excessive use of alcohol can also precipitate an attack.

QUESTIONS

▼ *Answer the following on a separate sheet of paper.*

1. Formulate a definition for gout.
2. Differentiate between the causes of primary and secondary gout.
3. Explain the rapid response to colchicine in gout.
4. Discuss the contributing factors that result in development of gout.
5. State the rationale for the treatment of chronic gout.
6. Explain why gout can damage the kidneys.

▼ *Circle the letter preceding each item below that correctly answers the question or completes the statement. More than one answer may be correct.*

7. The pathogenesis of gout is characterized by:
   a. Changes in the composition of articular cartilage, which results in loss of compressibility
   b. Formation of crystals of monosodium urate monohydrate in joints and tissue
   c. Formation of an antinuclear antibody (anti-DNA) that attaches to its antigen (DNA), whereby complement is fixed to this immune complex and an inflammatory process results

   d. Changes in the collagen of the cartilage where type II replaces type I cartilage, resulting in an alteration of the biomechanics of the cartilage

8. In asymptomatic hyperuricemia the serum uric acid levels usually average how many mg/dl?
   a. 4 to 5   c. 8 to 9
   b. 5 to 6   d. 9 to 10

9. In the first stage of gout the individual usually experiences:
   a. Painful swelling and tenderness
   b. Fever and an elevated white blood cell count
   c. No symptoms
   d. Elevated serum uric acid

10. In acute gouty arthritis, which of the following joints is usually involved?
    a. Wrist
    b. Bursae
    c. Metatarsophalangeal
    d. Metacarpophalangeal

11. The most common sites for tophi in chronic gout are the:
    a. Helix of the ear
    b. Olecranon bursa
    c. Cervical vertebrae
    d. Achilles tendon

12. A classic sign of gout that is acute in onset in a 50-year-old man is:

    a. Fusion of the dorsal spine into kyphosis
    b. Monarticular arthritis of the great toe
    c. Inflammation of the distal joints of the hands and feet
    d. Severe heel pain

13. Tophi develop in chronic gout because of:
    a. Relative insolubility of urates
    b. Chronic inflammation from the presence of calcium crystals
    c. Biochemical changes that occur within a joint
    d. Recent viral illness such as infection by Epstein-Barr virus

14. Which of the following depict(s) the third stage of gout?
    a. Development of tophi
    b. Asymptomatic hyperuricemia, which may last for months or years
    c. Pain, stiffness, large nodular swelling
    d. A repeat gouty attack in an untreated person

15. Treatment of an acute attack of gouty arthritis consists of initially administering high doses or loading loses of:
    a. Allopurinol
    b. Nonsteroidal antiinflammatory drugs
    c. Aspirin
    d. Colchicine

CHAPTER 75

Seronegative Spondyloarthropathies

MICHAEL A. CARTER

Seronegative spondyloarthropathies are a group of related disorders that include ankylosing spondylitis, psoriatic arthritis, and Reiter's syndrome. These disorders are called *seronegative* because rheumatoid factor is lacking in the serum. In addition, these disorders are associated with the HLA-B27 (HLA, human leukocyte antigen). These arthropathies are distinct in that they involve the sacroiliac and peripheral joints and usually have a higher incidence in men.

ANKYLOSING SPONDYLITIS

Ankylosing spondylitis is a chronic inflammatory disease that can be progressive. The illness usually involves the sacroiliac joints and the spinal articulations. The hips and costovertebral articulations can be affected as the disease progresses. Ankylosing spondylitis was once thought to be a variant of rheumatoid arthritis. This is no longer the case, based on the criteria of negative rheumatoid factor, the absence of rheumatoid nodules, and the differences in the bone changes in the spine. The 9:1 male/female ratio of the illness is no longer believed accurate now that better criteria for diagnosis have been established. Men tend to have a more progressive spinal disease and are more likely to be diagnosed as having ankylosing spondylitis. This gives a clinical ratio of about three men for each woman with spinal involvement. Ankylosing spondylitis occurs less frequently in Japanese and African Americans but more frequently in Pima Indians.

Ankylosing spondylitis affects the cartilaginous and fibrocartilaginous joints of the spine and paravertebral ligaments. Calcification of the joints and articular structures occurs when intervertebral disks become invaded by vascular and fibrous tissue and later become calcified. Calcified soft tissue bridges one vertebra to another. The synovial tissue around the joints involved becomes inflamed. Heart disease can also occur with ankylosing spondylitis.

The causes of ankylosing spondylitis are still unknown. A genetic factor appears to be involved. Approximately 90% of persons diagnosed as having ankylosing spondylitis have a positive HLA-B27 antigen.

Clinical Features

Ankylosing spondylitis has an insidious onset, beginning with feelings of fatigue and intermittent lower back or hip pain. Morning stiffness relieved by mild activity may occur. The symptoms can be so mild and unprogressive that many people are never diagnosed. In addition, the symptoms of ankylosing spondylitis can be confused with those of mechanical back problems.

The evaluation indicates a basically healthy person who gives a history of persistent back pain with insidious onset. The person is usually under 40 years of age. The back pain improves with exercise and worsens with rest

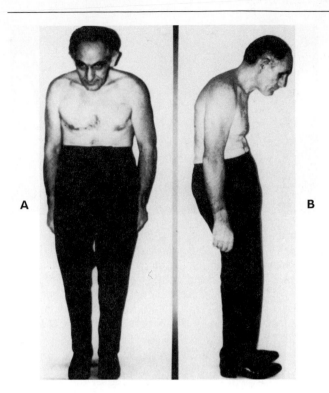

FIG. 75-1   Ankylosing spondylitis. **A,** Frontal view demonstrates the characteristic upward gaze of the eyes when they look straight ahead, necessitated by the flexion deformity of the neck. **B,** Lateral view demonstrates forward protrusion of the head, flattening of the anterior chest wall, thoracic kyphosis, protrusion of the abdomen, and flattening of the lumbar lordotic curvature. Slight flexion of the hip is also present because of hip involvement. (From the *Revised clinical slide collection on the rheumatic diseases,* 1981, Arthritis Foundation, New York.)

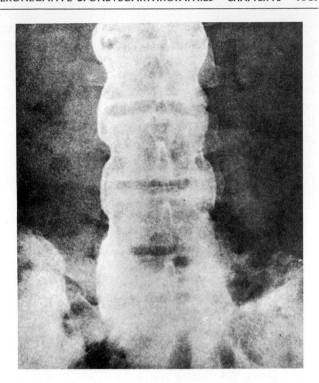

FIG. 75-2   Radiograph depicting advanced ankylosing spondylitis of the lumbar spine. There is generalized symmetric osseous bridging between the vertebrae (syndesmophytes). The apophyseal and sacroiliac joints are fused. (From Hollander JL, editor: *Arthritis and allied conditions: a textbook of rheumatology,* ed 8, Philadelphia, 1972, Lea & Febiger.)

and has diffuse radiation throughout the lower back and buttock. The physical examination shows no scoliosis, a symmetric decrease in range of motion, diffuse tenderness, and a negative straight-leg-raising test. The peripheral neurologic system is usually unchanged. As the illness progresses, there is a loss of normal lumbar lordosis, fusion of the dorsal spine into kyphosis, and restriction of thoracic excursion. In the late stages of the illness, fusion of the spine can result in hip flexion contractures, and the patient uses flexed knees to maintain an erect position (Fig. 75-1). Pain is usually diminished after ankylosis is complete, and synovitis is markedly decreased.

Laboratory Findings

No specific laboratory tests are used in diagnosing ankylosing spondylitis. The erythrocyte sedimentation rate (ESR) is usually elevated during active phases of the illness. The rheumatoid factor is usually negative. The antigen HLA-B27 is likely to be positive, but this is not specific to ankylosing spondylitis.

Radiologic Findings

Characteristic radiologic changes occur in ankylosing spondylitis. In the early stages of the illness, there may be only blurring of the sacroiliac joint and diffuse osteoporosis of the spine. As the illness progresses, joint erosion, squaring of the vertebrae, and narrowing of the disk spaces are seen. In the last stages of the illness, calcification of the disks and paravertebral ligaments occurs. Vertical bony growths, called *syndesmophytes,* can be demonstrated bridging the gaps between the vertebrae (Fig. 75-2). About 25% of patients with ankylosing spondylitis have complete fusing of the spine, including the cervical spine.

Treatment

Treatment of ankylosing spondylitis is multifocal and related to the stage of the illness. A focused intervention is aimed at increasing the patient's and family's understanding of the illness. Changes in work patterns may be necessary, since bending, lifting, and prolonged static positions are difficult. Medication therapy is aimed at decreasing the synovitis and resulting pain. Nonsteroidal antiinflammatory drugs (NSAIDs) are used for this purpose, particularly those with high prostaglandin-blocking ability and a long half-life. Indomethacin is frequently the drug of choice. Corticosteroids, slow-acting drugs, and muscle relaxants are of limited value. An active program of physical therapy is often helpful, focusing on breathing exercises, muscle strengthening, maintaining or improving posture, and range of motion exercises. Braces and splints may be used for limited times to decrease muscle spasm and pain.

Prognosis

About 20% of people with ankylosing spondylitis develop the disabling stages of the illness. About half have a slow, extended course that can last for decades. A number of the remaining persons can be successfully treated with a focused program of education, drug therapy, and physical therapy. These individuals can develop a fulfilling life-style within the confines of their illness. Less than 5% develop fatal manifestations of their illness.

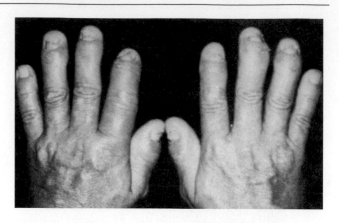

FIG. 75-3 Psoriatic arthritis. Swelling and deformity of distal interphalangeal joints are present, together with typical psoriatic involvement of the skin and nails. Several digits, including the left thumb and index finger, are diffusely swollen, suggesting a sausagelike appearance. (From the *Revised clinical slide collection on the rheumatic diseases,* 1981, Arthritis Foundation, New York.)

PSORIATIC ARTHRITIS

About 7% of persons with psoriasis (see Chapter 79) develop inflammatory joint disease. Usually the arthritis occurs after the appearance of the skin lesions, but it can occur before or at the same time as the skin lesions. The male/female ratio of this illness is nearly equal.

Clinical Features

Psoriatic arthritis most often occurs as an asymmetric inflammation involving only a few peripheral joints at a certain time. The distal joints of the hands and feet are the ones usually affected (Fig. 75-3), but other joints that can become affected include all joints of the hands, feet, knees, and hips. The activity of the arthritis tends to vary with the psoriasis, particularly the nail involvement of psoriasis. Psoriatic arthritis can present as a symmetric arthritis resembling rheumatoid arthritis; as arthritis mutilans, in which the entire joint is completely resorbed; or as spondylitis similar to that of ankylosing spondylitis. Psoriatic arthritis generally tends to be much less debilitating than rheumatoid arthritis.

Laboratory and Radiologic Findings

No specific laboratory tests exist for psoriatic arthritis. The ESR can be elevated during acute phases of the illness. The antigen HLA-B27 is positive about 20% of the time. This increases to a 50% positive rate if the person has sacroiliac inflammation with the illness.

Radiographs in the early stages of the illness are usually normal. A characteristic finding in later stages is the "pencil-in-cup" sign. The distal end of the proximal phalanx erodes to a rather sharp point, with a concomitant

bony overgrowth of the proximal end of the distal phalanx where the tendons insert.

Treatment

The treatment for psoriatic arthritis is appropriate doses of aspirin or other NSAIDs. These measures are combined with treatment of the skin lesions. Corticosteroids are not generally used because such large doses are required and the adverse effects are beyond acceptable levels. Other drug therapies include gold and immunosuppressive agents. These drugs are usually reserved for patients with severe illness who do not respond to other forms of therapy.

The long-term treatment involves a multifocal approach that includes physical therapy, alterations in activities of daily living, and occasionally hospitalization and surgery. Most people with psoriatic arthritis, however, do not require extensive medical intervention. They have frequent periods of remission that last for several months.

REITER'S SYNDROME

Reiter's syndrome is one of the leading causes of arthritis in young men. The syndrome is named for Hans Reiter, who described the clinical picture of nongonococcal urethritis, arthritis, and conjunctivitis in 1916. This syndrome rarely occurs in women, children, or older persons. In the United States the syndrome begins suddenly, usually following venereal exposure. In other parts of the world the syndrome follows an infection with *Shigella flexneri.*

Reiter's syndrome is accompanied by a triad of symp-

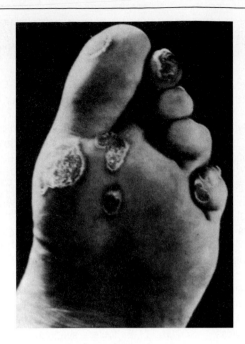

FIG. 75-4   Discrete, circinate, scaly, and plaquelike lesions on the foot (keratoderma blennorrhagicum) are caused by Reiter's syndrome and resemble secondary syphilis and psoriasis. Note two small lesions in an early phase of keratoderma. (From the Arthritis Foundation, New York, 1972.)

toms: urethritis, arthritis, and conjunctivitis. Oral mucocutaneous lesions, keratoderma blennorrhagicum (a characteristic dermatitis; Fig. 75-4), and balanitis circinata are also seen.

The causes are unknown. An association exists between HLA-B27 and the development of Reiter's syndrome. Psoriatic arthritis and Reiter's syndrome may be nearly the same disease, since the dermatitis and nail changes are very similar in the two. A history of sexual exposure or dysentery leads to the suspicion that these illnesses are immune responses to some infectious agent.

Clinical Features

Constitutional symptoms, weight loss, and fever may occur at the onset of Reiter's syndrome. A purulent or watery urethritis that the person may think is a venereal disease is often the factor that prompts a visit to seek health care.

Articular manifestations most often involve the joints of the feet and ankles, the knees, and the sacroiliac joints. Heel pain is fairly common. Conjunctivitis can occur with a purulent discharge and photophobia. The oral and penile lesions are usually painless. A few patients have electrocardiographic changes and aortic valve involvement.

The course of the illness is unpredictable. Reiter's syndrome can be acute, subacute, or chronic. Most people recover from the first attack in several months, but most have one or two more attacks within 2 years. Thirty percent develop long-term disability or permanent sequelae, including residual joint damage after severe joint involvement and long-term back pain after sacroiliac involvement.

Laboratory and Radiologic Findings

No specific laboratory tests exist for Reiter's syndrome. Ninety percent of patients with Reiter's syndrome have a positive antigen HLA-B27, but the frequency of positive rheumatoid factor is equal to that in the general population. Synovial fluid is inflammatory, with 15,000 to 20,000 white blood cells/mm³.

There are radiographic changes specific for Reiter's syndrome, including a tendency for joints of the lower extremities to be involved, isolated osteoporosis, articular erosive changes, periostitis at the insertion of the Achilles tendon, calcaneal spurs, sacroiliac inflammations, and nonmarginal spurs along the vertebral column.

Treatment

The treatment of Reiter's syndrome is primarily symptomatic. Therapeutic doses of NSAIDs are used to relieve the inflammation and pain. The use of corticosteroids systemically or locally is controversial. Antibiotics are not of proven value.

ENTEROPATHIC ARTHRITIS

Arthritis occurs in about 20% of persons who have ulcerative colitis and Crohn's disease. This arthritis is similar to the other spondyloarthropathies in that the peripheral joints are affected. The arthritis activity reflects the activity of the inflammatory bowel disease. Effective treatment of the bowel disease usually causes the arthritis to resolve.

? QUESTIONS

▼ *Answer the following on a separate sheet of paper.*

1. Explain the goals of the treatment measures and the prognosis for ankylosing spondylitis.
2. What is the relationship between psoriasis and psoriatic arthritis?
3. What are the components of the treatment program for Reiter's syndrome?

▼ *Circle the letter preceding each item below that correctly answers the question or completes the statement. More than one answer may be correct.*

4. The group of related disorders known as seronegative spondyloarthropathies includes:
   a. Psoriatic arthritis
   b. Reiter's syndrome
   c. Polyarthritis
   d. Ankylosing spondylitis
5. Which of the following statements is *false* concerning seronegative disorders?
   a. There is a high titer of rheumatoid factor in the serum in 95% of the patients.
   b. Rheumatoid factor in serum is usually negative.
   c. The antigen HLA-B27 is likely to be positive.
   d. No specific laboratory tests are used in diagnosing these conditions.
6. The joints most often involved in Reiter's syndrome are the:
   a. Weight-bearing joints (feet and ankles, knee)
   b. Sacroiliac joints

c. Hips and costovertebal articulations
d. Cartilaginous and fibrocartilaginous joints of the spine

7. Ankylosing spondylitis usually involves the:
   a. Distal joints of the hands and feet
   b. Joints of the ankles
   c. Sacroiliac joints
   d. Spinal articulations
8. Which of the following clinical features is (are) seen in the late stages of ankylosing spondylitis?
   a. Erosion of the distal and proximal phalanx
   b. Increase in pain over sacroiliac joints
   c. Hip flexion contractions and flexed knees
   d. Evidence of increased synovitis
9. Radiologic findings that occur in the early stages of ankylosing spondylitis are:
   a. Blurring of the sacroiliac joint
   b. Joint erosion and squaring of the vertebrae
   c. Diffuse osteoporosis of the spine
   d. Calcification of the disks and paravertebral ligaments
10. The drugs of choice prescribed for ankylosing spondylitis are:
    a. Nonsteroidal antiinflammatory drugs
    b. Corticosteroids
    c. Slow-acting drugs
    d. Muscle relaxants
11. In patients with severe psoriatic arthritis who are unresponsive to antiinflammatory drug therapy, the drugs used are:
    a. Corticosteroids

b. Gold
c. Immunosuppressive agents
d. Muscle relaxants

12. The male/female ratio is nearly equal in which of the following conditions?
    a. Psoriatic arthritis
    b. Reiter's syndrome
    c. Enteropathic arthritis
    d. Ankylosing spondylitis

▼ *Circle T if the statement is true and F if it is false. Correct any false statements.*

13. T F The psoriasis usually precedes the arthritis in psoriatic arthritis.
14. T F Psoriatic arthritis is usually much more destructive to the joints than rheumatoid arthritis.
15. T F Reiter's syndrome is characterized by a triad of symptoms: urethritis, arthritis, and conjunctivitis.
16. T F The male/female ratio for the occurrence of ankylosing spondylitis is 9:1.
17. T F About 35% of individuals with ankylosing spondylitis develop disabling stages of the illness.
18. T F Enteropathic arthritis activity reflects the severity of the associated ulcerative colitis, in that effective treatment of the inflammatory bowel disease usually causes the arthritis to resolve.

BIBLIOGRAPHY ▼ PART XII

Carter MA et al: Immune and inflammatory disorders. In Weiner MB, Pepper GA: *Clinical pharmacology and therapeutics in nursing,* New York, 1985, McGraw-Hill.

Crenshaw AH, editor: *Campbell's operative orthopaedics,* ed 8, St Louis, 1992, Mosby.

Guyton AC: *Textbook of medical physiology,* ed 8, Philadelphia, 1992, Saunders.

Kelley WN et al, editors: *Textbook of rheumatology,* ed 4, Philadelphia, 1993, Saunders.

McCarty DJ, editor: *Arthritis and allied conditions: a textbook of rheumatology,* ed 12, Philadelphia, 1992, Lea & Febiger.

Schumacher HR, editor: *Primer on the rheumatic diseases,* ed 10, Atlanta, 1993, Arthritis Foundation.

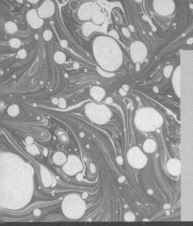

PART THIRTEEN

DERMATOLOGIC SYSTEM DISORDERS

Dermatology is concerned with the structure, function, and diseases of the skin. The skin forms a protective barrier around the entire body and has a role in body thermoregulation, glandular secretion, and sensory communication with the external environment. Any structure of the skin has a potential for disease. A skin disorder may be restricted to cutaneous involvement or be indicative of a systemic disease.

This section includes a review of skin anatomy and physiology. Selected cutaneous diseases and their etiology, pathogenesis, and treatment are also discussed. ▼

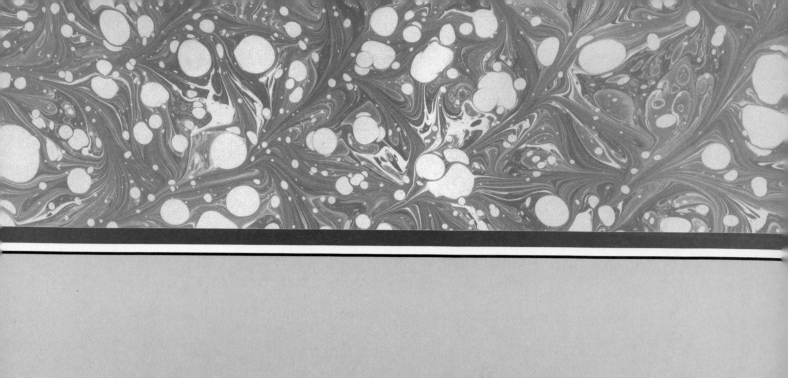

CHAPTER 76

Anatomy and Physiology of the Skin

MAREK A. STAWISKI

DERMATOLOGIC VOCABULARY

annular lesion   A ring-shaped lesion with an active margin and often a clear center; *example:* ringworm (see Fig. 80-12).

atrophy   A loss of epidermal and dermal substance; *example:* atrophy after treatment with topical steroids (see Fig. 78-3).

burrow   A linear trail produced by a parasite; *example:* scabies (see Fig. 82-2).

circinate lesion   An arcuate lesion; *example:* urticaria (Color plate 36).

comedo   A plugged pilosebaceous opening; *example:* acne vulgaris (see Fig. 77-3).

confluent   Blending into adjacent lesions; *example:* tinea versicolor (Color plate 43).

crust   An excessive accumulation of serum and cellular, bacterial, and squamous debris; *example:* impetigo (Color plate 45).

eczematoid lesion   An eczema-like inflammatory lesion with scale, vesiculation, crust, and weeping; *example:* poison ivy (Color plate 34).

erosion   A loss of epidermis only; *example:* impetigo (Color plate 45).

excoriations   A linear erosion; frequently, self-inducement is implied; *example:* neurotic excoriation (see Fig. 78-2).

fissure   A crack in the skin extending to the dermis; *example:* hand eczema (Color plate 35).

guttate   Drop sized; *example:* guttate psoriasis (see Fig. 79-2).

herpetiform   Having groups of vesicles; *example:* herpes simplex (see Fig. 80-5).

hyperkeratosis   A lesion with excessive scales; *example:* psoriasis (Color plate 38).

iris, or target, lesion   Two or three concentric circles that form an irislike lesion; *example:* erythema multiforme (see Fig. 78-9).

Koebner's phenomenon   Lesions that form in areas of previous trauma of the skin; *example:* psoriasis.

lichenification   An area of accentuated skin markings associated with a thickening of the skin caused by scratching and rubbing; *example:* neurodermatitis (see Fig. 78-1).

macule   A nonpalpable circumscribed area usually demarcated by a change of color; *example:* tinea versicolor (Color plate 43).

morbilliform lesions   A small confluent maculopapular lesion; *example:* a viral exanthem.

nodule, tumor   A palpable lesion usually larger than 5 mm; *example:* basal cell carcinoma (Color plate 47).

nummular lesion   A coin-shaped lesion; *example:* nummular eczema.

papule   An elevated palpable lesion usually smaller than 5 mm; *example:* a blue nevus (Color plate 52).

photodistribution   Distribution in areas exposed to sunlight; *example:* sunburn.

plaque   A palpable lesion that has a greater dimension in area than in thickness; *example:* psoriasis (Color plate 38).

pustule   A lesion that contains pus; *example:* acne vulgaris (see Fig. 77-4).

scale   An excessive accumulation of keratin; *example:* psoriasis (Color plate 38).

telangiectasis   A dilation of superficial vessels; *example:* dilated vessels in a basal cell carcinoma (Color plate 47).

ulcer   A loss of epidermis and dermis; *example:* early squamous cell carcinoma (Color plate 48).

verrucous   Wartlike; *example:* verruca vulgaris (see Fig. 80-1).

vesicle, bulla   A fluid-filled, elevated lesion; *example:* a vesicle of herpes simplex (see Fig. 80-5).

wheal   A transitory palpable lesion; *example:* urticaria (hives) (Color plate 36).

zosteriform   Having a linear dermatomal distribution; *example:* herpes zoster (shingles) (Color plate 41).

The skin, which is the largest organ of the human body, envelops the muscles and internal organs. It is an endless network of blood vessels, nerves, and glands, all of which have a potential for disease. Because the number of cutaneous diseases is extensive, only the most frequently encountered are discussed in this section. The most common dermatologic condition, acne, and new advances in its treatment are described. Another frequently seen disease is eczema, which can be inherited or caused by allergens. Psoriasis is thought to be the most economically ravaging skin disease. Most dermatologic hospital admissions are caused by severe exacerbations of psoriasis.

Cutaneous infections with viruses causing warts and herpes simplex have captured the attention of not only the health care community but also the press and public. Fungal infections are responsible for ringworm, athlete's foot, and jock itch. Presentation and treatment of these fungal infections and bacterial skin infections are included.

Neoplasms of the skin are the most common of the cancers encountered in humans. They range from nonmetastatic basal cell carcinomas to aggressive and frequently fatal melanomas. Description of diagnostic features and etiology of these tumors should help the reader to diagnose and prevent these malignancies. Diagnosis, prevention, and treatment of Lyme disease and infestation with scabies and lice are discussed. These conditions can be a considerable challenge to nurses, especially public health, community health, or school nurses. However, before the various skin diseases are considered, this chapter summarizes the basic structure and functions of the skin.

FUNCTIONS OF SKIN

The skin protects the body from trauma and shields it from bacterial, viral, and fungal infections. Heat loss and conservation are regulated by cutaneous vasodilation or secretion by the sweat glands. After complete loss of skin, essential body fluids evaporate and electrolytes are lost within hours; an example of this is seen in burn patients. The pleasant or unpleasant odors of the skin serve as social and sexual signs of acceptability or rejection. Epidermal appendages of the skin, such as nails and hair, have their well-established cosmetic values unique to specific cultures. The skin also provides the sensations of touch, pressure, temperature, pain, and pleasure by an intricate network of nerve endings.

SKIN STRUCTURE

Microscopically the skin consists of three layers: epidermis, dermis, and subcutaneous fat (Fig. 76-1). The *epidermis,* the outermost portion of the skin, is divided into two main layers: a stratum of anucleate cornified cells (the *stratum corneum,* or horny layer) and the inner, malpighian layer, from which the surface cornified cells arise by differentiation. The *malpighian layer* is subdivided into the (1) basal cell layer (or stratum germinativum), (2) stratum spinosum, and (3) stratum granulosum.

The *basal layer* consists largely of undifferentiated epidermal cells that undergo constant mitosis, renewing the epidermis. When such a cell undergoes mitosis, one of the daughter cells remains in the basal layer to divide again while the other cell migrates outward toward the stratum spinosum.

The major differentiating cell of the *stratum spinosum* is the *keratinocyte,* which produces keratin, a fibrous protein. As keratinocytes leave the stratum spinosum and move upward, they undergo changes in shape, orientation, cytoplasmic structure, and composition. This leads to the transformation of viable, actively synthesizing cells into the dead, cornified cells of the stratum corneum, a process termed *keratinization.* The *stratum granulosum* lies just below the stratum corneum and has an important function in the production of stratum corneum proteins and chemical bonds. Keratinocytes of the basal layer are cylindric in shape. They become polyhedral in the stratum spinosum, flatter in the granular layer, and lamellar in the stratum corneum. Important changes also occur in their cytoplasmic constituents, the nucleus, and the cell membranes. The keratinocytes synthesize tonofilaments, or filamentous proteins. In the stratum germinativum the tonofilaments are arranged in bundles that surround the nucleus of the cell. In the stratum spinosum, synthesis continues and these tonofilament bundles become more compact, forming an interlacing network extending through the cytoplasm. As they move through the stratum granulosum, keratohyalin granules appear within these cells, deposited within and around the tonofilament bundles. In the stratum corneum the granules appear tightly packed. *Keratohyalin* is not sufficiently defined chemically, and its final role in the keratinization process is not clear. It does appear to contribute to the amorphous, electron-dense matrix of the cornified cells.

It appears that during differentiation, keratinocytes pass through a synthetic phase in which tonofilaments, keratohyalin, lamellar bodies, and other cell constituents are formed. Finally they enter a transition phase, in which the cytoplasmic components are dissociated and degraded. The remaining cell constituents form a fibrous, amorphous complex surrounded by a reinforced impermeable membrane, the horny cell. This programmed process of epidermal cell migration normally takes about 28 days.

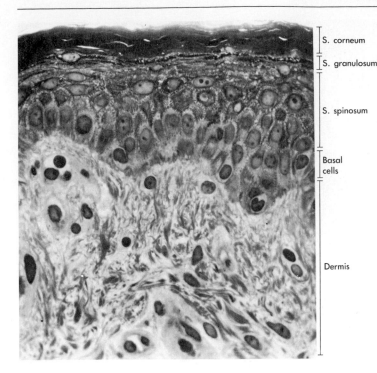

S. corneum

S. granulosum

S. spinosum

Basal cells

Dermis

FIG. 76-1   Epidermis and upper layer of the dermis. Superficial capillaries are seen in the upper dermis. Subcutaneous layer is below the dermal layer. (From Fitzpatrick TB et al, editors: *Dermatology in general medicine,* ed 2, New York, 1979, McGraw-Hill.)

The second (after keratinocytes) major cell of the epidermis is the *melanocyte,* found in the basal layer. The ratio of basal cells to melanocytes is 10:1. Within the melanocyte, pigment granules called *melanosomes* are synthesized. Melanosomes contain brown biochrome called *melanin.* The melanosomes are transferred to keratinocytes through long dendritic processes. Each melanocyte is connected through these projections, and about 36 keratinocytes form what is referred to as the *epidermal melanin unit* (Fig. 76-2). Melanosomes are hydrolyzed at varying rates by enzymes. The amount of melanin within the keratinocyte determines the color of the skin. Melanin protects the skin from harmful effects of the sun. Paradoxically it is the sun's rays that increase the production of melanosomes and melanin. African Americans and whites each have the same number of melanocytes. African Americans have large melanosomes that resist destruction by the hydrolyzing enzymes, whereas whites have smaller melanosomes that are more readily destroyed.

The *dermis* is located immediately below the epidermis and is composed of collagen fibers, elastin, and reticulin embedded in a ground substance. The dermal matrix contains blood vessels and nerves, which provide support and nourishment to the growing epidermis. Surrounding the small blood vessels are lymphocytes, histiocytes, mast cells, and polymorphonuclear neutrophils (PMNs), which protect the body from infections and foreign body invasion. Specialized collagen fibers anchor the epidermal basal cells into the dermis.

Underlying the dermis is the third layer of skin, the *subcutaneous fat.* This layer provides a cushion for the

skin, insulation to maintain body heat, and a store of energy. Cosmetically, subcutaneous fat influences the attractiveness of either gender.

Sweat (eccrine) glands are present almost everywhere on the skin except in the ears and on the lips. These glands produce a hypotonic solution that is clear and watery and has a high content of urea and lactate. Sweat glands aid in maintaining the appropriate body temperature.

Sebaceous glands are lobulated structures that consist of lipid-filled cells. The lipid oily substance referred to as *sebum* is passed to the central duct and drained to the pilosebaceous ducts of the hair follicles (Fig. 76-3). Sebaceous glands are concentrated over the face, chest, back, and proximal arms. Their activity is hormonally regulated primarily by androgenic hormones.

The *apocrine glands* are found primarily in the axilla, in the genital skin, around the nipples, and in the perianal area. The apocrine duct empties into the hair follicle above the entrance of the sebaceous duct (Fig. 76-4). The apocrine secretions do not serve any useful function in humans but contribute to the axillary odor when apocrine secretions are decomposed by bacteria. Apocrine glands produce a milky, viscous substance that results from a high content of organic components. They begin their secretory activity at puberty.

Hair is formed from keratin. By a predetermined differentiating process, certain epidermal cells form the hair follicle. The hair follicle is supported by dermal matrix and differentiates into the hair (Fig. 76-5). An epithelial canal is formed, through which the hair passes to the surface. Hair is dead keratin just as is a scale, and it is formed at a predetermined rate. Cystine and methionine,

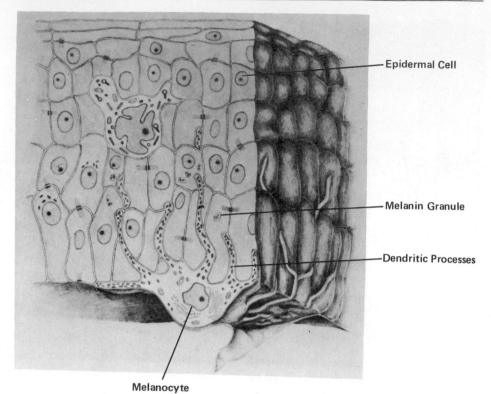

FIG. 76-2 The epidermal melanin unit. Relationship of a single melanocyte to multiple epidermal cells is well illustrated. (From Fitzpatrick TB et al, editors: *Dermatology in general medicine*, ed 2, New York, 1979, McGraw-Hill.)

Epidermal Cell

Melanin Granule

Dendritic Processes

Melanocyte

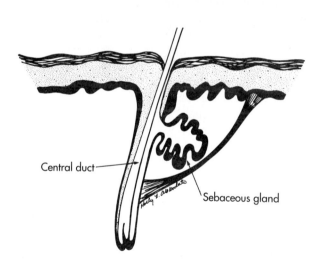

Central duct

Sebaceous gland

FIG. 76-3 Sebaceous gland opens into the central duct. (From the Biomedical Media Production Unit, University of Michigan Medical Center.)

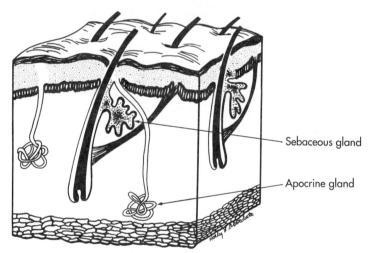

Sebaceous gland

Apocrine gland

FIG. 76-4 Apocrine gland empties above the entrance of the sebaceous duct. (From the Biomedical Media Production Unit, University of Michigan Medical Center.)

sulfur-containing amino acids, contribute strong covalent bonds, giving strength to hair. On the scalp the rate of the growth of hair is usually 3 mm/day. Each hair follicle goes through a cycle of growth *(anagen hair)*, intermediate stage *(catagen hair)*, and involution *(telogen hair)*. The anagen stage on the scalp lasts about 3 years, and the telogen stage lasts only about 3 months. Once the hair follicle reaches the telogen stage, the hair falls out. Eventually, the hair follicle regenerates into the anagen stage

and a new hair is produced. This cycle of activity for hair follicles is independent for each hair follicle. The mosaic pattern prevents the occurrence of temporary baldness of the scalp. When the process stops, the person becomes permanently bald. Various commercial preparations advertised to strengthen hair are of questionable value. Protein shampoos affect only the dead keratin and not the hair follicle and therefore cannot prevent hair loss. Recent developments have shown that male and female pat-

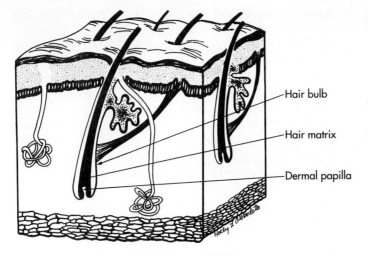

FIG. 76-5   Hair matrix is supported by a dermal papilla and differentiates into hair. (From the Biomedical Media Production Unit, University of Michigan Medical Center.)

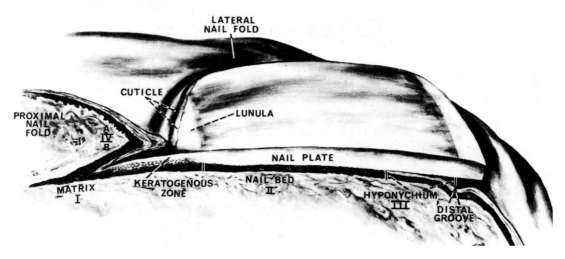

FIG. 76-6   Diagrammatic drawing of normal adult fingernails. (From Fitzpatrick TB et al, editors: *Dermatology in general medicine,* ed 2, New York, 1979, McGraw-Hill.)

terns of baldness can sometimes be treated with topical 2% minoxidil (Rogaine).

The *nail* is a dead keratin plate produced by epidermal cells of nail matrix (Fig. 76-6). The nail matrix is located beneath the proximal portion of the nail plate in the dermis. It is visible as a white area, called the *lumula,* which is covered by the proximal nail fold and cuticle. Because both nail and hair are dead keratin structures, they have no nerve endings and no blood supply.

SKIN EXAMINATION

Skin should be examined in a well-illuminated room, preferably in natural daylight. A dimly illuminated hospital room is the least desirable place to inspect the skin, and examination there may lead to serious errors in diagnosis. The color of the skin should be recorded. Purplish,

cyanotic discoloration of the toes or fingers can provide a useful clue to the presence of internal diseases. Pallor can be a sign of anemia (see Chapter 17). Skin has turgor and elasticity on palpation. Excessive dryness causes this organ to be scaly and wrinkled. This may indicate dehydration or thyroid disease. Skin ridges are visible over the palms and feet and are also present over the entire body surface. They are called *dermatoglyphics* and form the pattern unique for every individual and species (Fig. 76-7). The dermatoglyphics over the volar aspects of the fingers are used for fingerprinting. They are useful in criminology; however, health care professionals are also interested in the presence of these whorls. Their disappearance over fingertips can be a first sign of vascular insufficiency, as in systemic sclerosis (scleroderma; see Chapter 73).

There is an expected pattern of hair distribution in males and females. In many men, and some women, temporal and occipital scalp hair thinning becomes evi-

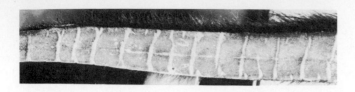

FIG. 76-7   Underside of the spider monkey with characteristic dermatoglyphics. (From Fitzpatrick TB et al, editors: *Dermatology in general medicine,* ed 4, New York, 1994, McGraw-Hill.)

dent with advancing age. However, a sudden hair loss over the scalp or even the entire body may indicate possible thyroid abnormalities (see Chapter 60). The lack of hair over distal extremities can be the first sign of vascular insufficiency, whereas abnormal hair growth over the face, especially in females, should be investigated for a hormone-producing tumor.

Nails can be damaged and thinned in many diseases, such as psoriasis, fungal infections, and thyroid abnormalities. Excessive sweat production can be a sign of anxiety or an underlying internal illness.

? QUESTIONS

▼ *Circle the letter preceding each item below that correctly answers the question or completes the statement. More than one answer may be correct.*

1. Which of the following are functions of the skin?
   a. Regulating heat loss and conservation
   b. Protecting against trauma and infection
   c. Replacing utilized corticosteroids
   d. Providing tactile sensations
2. The epidermis contains the:
   a. Stratum corneum
   b. Basal cell layer
   c. Hair roots
   d. Collagen fibers
3. The dermis is composed of:
   a. Stratum germinativum
   b. Melanocytes
   c. Blood vessels and nerves
   d. Elastin and reticulin
4. Which of the following skin conditions is most likely to have greatest economic impact?
   a. Herpes simplex
   b. Psoriasis
   c. Basal cell carcinoma
   d. Scabies
5. Which of the following is the major differentiating cell of the epidermis?
   a. Mast cell
   b. Keratinocyte
   c. Histocyte
   d. Melanocyte
6. Male and female patterns of baldness may be treated with:
   a. Topical 2% minoxidil solution
   b. Topical steroids
   c. Topical biotin
   d. Oral multivitamins

▼ *Answer the following on a separate sheet of paper.*

7. Explain the skin proliferation process by identifying the layer of the skin that produces new cells and the direction of movement of the new cells.
8. List the function of the two adnexal structures of the skin: eccrine (sweat) glands and sebaceous glands.
9. Describe the essential elements of a skin examination.
10. What is the function of the subcutaneous fat layer of the skin?

▼ *Circle T if the statement is true and F if it is false. Correct any false statements.*

11. T F   The patient with abnormal hair loss from the scalp should be investigated for possible thyroid abnormalities.
12. T F   The absence of whorls over the fingertips may indicate vascular insufficiency, as in scleroderma.
13. T F   The stratum granulosum layer contains the partially keratinized epidermal cells.
14. T F   Hair is composed of particular living keratinocytes bonded together with sulfur bonds into longitudinal strands.
15. T F   Nails are composed of keratin produced by epidermal cells.
16. T F   Melanocytes are hydrolyzed by enzymes.
17. T F   Racial differences in pigmentation are caused by differences in the number of melanocytes.
18. On the following diagram, label the three layers of the skin: epidermis, dermis, and subcutaneous fat.

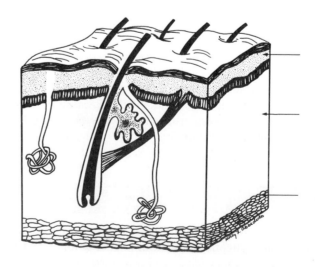

CHAPTER 77

Acne and Related Conditions

MAREK A. STAWISKI

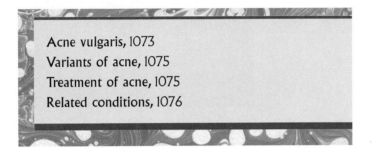

ACNE VULGARIS

Acne is a chronic inflammatory process of sebaceous glands. It generally occurs among most adolescents and young adults and usually spontaneously resolves about 20 to 30 years of age. However, many middle-age adults experience acne eruptions. Acne is usually associated with a high rate of sebum secretion. Androgens are known stimulants of sebum secretion, and estrogen reduces sebum production. Without androgens, sebaceous glands remain small. Acne is not observed in males castrated before puberty or in oophorectomized women.

A sudden onset of severe acne associated with hirsutism or menstrual abnormalities may indicate an endocrine disorder in a female patient. Acne in women in their 20s, 30s, and 40s is frequently caused by comedo-producing oil-based cosmetics and moisturizers. Mechanical factors, such as rubbing, friction pressure, and stretching of the skin rich in sebaceous glands, can make the existing acne worse. The more common mechanical causes include football helmets, surgical tape, and shirt collars. Acne can also be exacerbated by such comedogenic agents as petrolatum and greasy cosmetics.

Medications can also precipitate the onset of acne. Chronic oral corticosteroids used for treatment of other conditions (e.g., systemic lupus erythematosus, renal transplants) can trigger superficial pustules over the face, chest, and back. Oral contraceptives usually are helpful in acne treatment because of their estrogen content. In some women, however, oral contraceptives can exacerbate the

condition. Other drugs known to aggravate or precipitate acne are bromides, iodides, diphenytoin, lithium, or iso-nicotinic acid hydrazide. Industrial workers may be exposed to chlorinated hydrocarbons, which are acnegenic.

Management of acne patients requires a careful history to rule out acnegenic factors and more serious endocrine abnormalities. Most acne patients have a family history of acne.

The distribution of acne corresponds to the areas of sebaceous glands and occurs over the face, neck, chest, back, and shoulders (Fig. 77-1). The earliest lesion to appear in the skin is the *comedo. White comedones,* or closed comedones, are more likely to progress to inflammatory papules and pustules of acne. *Black comedones,* or open comedones, have a dark, horny material plugging up dilated pilosebaceous ducts. These comedones obstruct the flow of sebum to the surface. The sebum, bacteria *(Propionibacterium acnes),* and fatty acids are thought to be responsible for the development of inflammation around the pilosebaceous ducts and sebaceous glands.

Once the flow of sebum to the surface is obstructed by comedones, *P. acnes* produces lipases that break down sebum triglycerides into free fatty acids. These acids, in combination with bacteria, produce an inflammatory response in the dermis. This inflammation leads to formation of erythematous papules, inflammatory pustules, and inflammatory cysts (Fig. 77-2). The pustules and cysts drain and heal over time. Deeper papules and cysts can leave permanent scars, whereas mild acne resolves without scarring. The tendency to scar varies among individuals and is greater when the person attempts to empty the lesions. All scarring except the keloidal type improves with time.

Acne is classified as comedonal (black and white comedones) (Fig. 77-3), papulopustular (papules and pustules) (Fig. 77-4), or cystic (Color plate 31). Comedonal and papulopustular acne are given numeric grades. Grade I acne has less than 10 comedones, papules, or pustules on one side of the face (Fig. 77-3), grade II, 10 to 20 comedones, papules, or pustules; grade III, 25 to 50; and grade IV, more than 50 (Color plate 31).

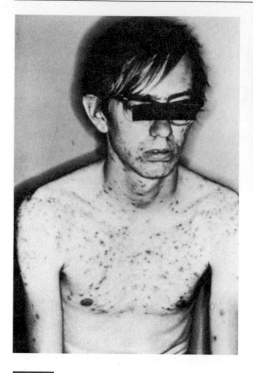

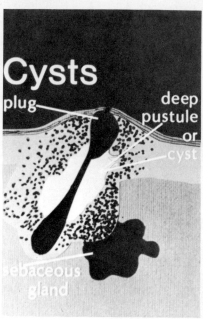

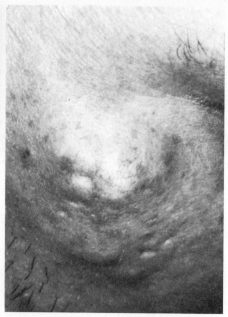

FIG. 77-1   Characteristic distribution of acne pustules over the face, chest, and shoulders.

FIG. 77-2   Inflammation around the pilosebaceous glands that leads to formation of papules, pustules, and cysts.

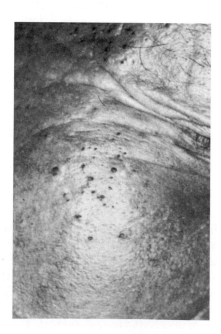

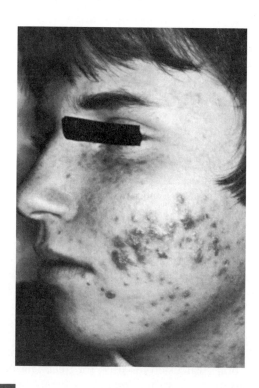

FIG. 77-3   Multiple comedones in a superficial comedonal acne.

FIG. 77-4   Severe scarring can follow obsessive manipulation of acne papules and pustules.

VARIANTS OF ACNE

Several variants of acne should be recognized. *Excoriated acne* occurs in individuals who obsessively manipulate the acne lesions; doing this can cause extreme scarring. *Conglobate acne,* or *acne conglobata,* is the most severe cystic acne, with deep cysts, multiple comedones, and marked scarring. It can be associated with malaise and fever and may even require hospitalization (Fig. 77-4 and Color plate 31). Individuals with *acne keloidalis* have multiple scars and keloids in the areas where acne lesions were present (Fig. 77-5).

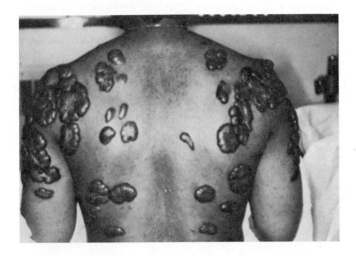

FIG. 77-5 Keloids can complicate a course of acne vulgaris.

TREATMENT OF ACNE

The goal of acne therapy is to decrease the inflammatory process of pilosebaceous glands until spontaneous remission occurs. Treatment of acne and related conditions improves the patient's cosmetic appearance and self-image and prevents scars related to acne.

Acne treatment includes halting the use of all exacerbating factors such as oil-based makeup and moisturizing creams. Dietary restrictions are usually not required or effective. However, it is reasonable to omit certain foods such as colas, chocolate, milk products, and iodides if the patient reports flare-ups of acne after ingesting these.

Cleaning and scrubbing the face with soap remove the surface oil and dislodge some comedones. The affected areas should be washed twice daily. Soaps such as Lava, Dial, Pernox, Fostex, Neutrogena, and Desquam-X Wash are recommended. An abrasive sponge such as a Buf-Puf is useful in dislodging superficial comedones. A keratolytic agent such as benzoyl peroxide at a concentration of 5% to 10% is used daily. Benzoyl peroxide is now available over the counter. Many patients have tried this

on their own, developing excessive dryness and irritation. Precipitated sulfur (1% to 2%) is useful in drying pustules, especially acne rosacea. Vitamin A acid (Retin-A) cream (0.025%, 0.05%, or 0.1%) and gel (0.01% or 0.025%) are useful because of their keratolytic effect on superficial comedones. However, Retin-A derivatives can enhance skin irritability from exposure to the wind, sun, or cold weather. Recently, topical tretinoin (Retin-A, 0.025% to 0.1% cream) has received much attention for its antiwrinkle properties. Although the drug is not indicated for this use, it is widely prescribed by many physicians. Tretinoin should be used with caution because it can cause irritant dermatitis. Other popular compounds used for their antiacne and antiwrinkle effects are glycolic acids; no reliable studies support their popularity. Topical antibiotics used to treat superficial acne papules and pustules include clindamycin (1% Cleocin T gel or solution), erythromycin (2% Erygel, 2% Eryderm, A/T/S), and meclocycline (Meclan). Meclan and Akne-Mycin cream (topical erythromycin) achieve the therapeutic effect without causing excessive dryness. This is especially useful for women with sensitive skin, as well as for older patients. Topical antibiotics are frequently used in the morning and benzoyl peroxides or Retin-A compounds at bedtime.

Systemic antibiotics remain the principal mode of therapy of deep pustular, deep papular, and cystic acne. Patients are usually treated with tetracycline, erythromycin, or minocycline. For superficial pustular acne the dose of tetracycline is 250 to 500 mg daily. For severe, deep papulopustular or cystic acne, 1000 mg of tetracycline is administered daily. Long-term tetracycline therapy has been shown to be safe. Children under 12 are not treated with tetracycline because permanent staining of the teeth can occur. Tetracycline is not given to pregnant women, since enamel hypoplasia and permanent discoloration of the teeth may occur in newborns. Some patients may develop photosensitivity, nausea, and candidiasis while receiving tetracycline. Oral tetracycline can make oral contraceptives less effective, and women can become pregnant. This is especially true if a patient has breakthrough bleeding while taking tetracycline and oral contraceptives together. Erythromycin is less effective in treatment of acne. This antibiotic is used at a dose of 250 to 500 mg daily. Patients can develop gastrointestinal irritation while taking erythromycin. A derivative of tetracycline, minocycline, at a dose of 50 to 100 mg daily, is the most effective antibiotic for acne. Minocycline is a more expensive antibiotic than tetracycline and can also cause dizziness and a reversible bluish discoloration of the skin at higher doses. The pharmacologic action of tetracycline and minocycline on acne is not completely understood. The antibiotics decrease the population of *P. acnes* in the pilosebaceous gland. This bacterium produces lipases that hydrolyze sebum to fatty acids. Fatty acids may be responsible for inflammation of the pilosebaceous duct. Tetracycline also inhibits these lipases.

Outpatient therapy for acne includes acne surgery, which consists of removal of comedones and opening and drainage of pustules. Self-manipulation of acne lesions usually results in more scar formation and should be discouraged. The benefit of ultraviolet light is minimal, and home sunlamps are not recommended. Cryotherapy has been very effective in the treatment of superficial pustules and cysts.

An oral drug, *isotretinoin* (Accutane), was approved by the U.S. Food and Drug Administration for treatment of severe antibiotic-resistant cystic-conglobate acne. A single (4 month) course of 1 mg/kg/day results in remission of the disease in about 80% to 90% of patients. In many of these patients, remission appears to be permanent, even after a 3-year follow-up. Truncal acne and acne in young teenagers relapse more frequently. Some patients require a second course of Accutane therapy. Accutane, if used in the early course of acne, can prevent most of the scarring caused by deep papules and pustules.

The exact mechanism of isotretinoin is unknown. Chemically it is related to vitamin A. In contrast to vitamin A, however, isotretinoin is not stored in the liver but is rapidly excreted; the half-life of oral isotretinoin is approximately 10 to 20 hours. Consequently, the drug has fewer side effects than vitamin A. Isotretinoin inhibits sebaceous gland function, and this presumably is its mechanism of action in acne.

Because isotretinoin is a known teratogen, *it must not be used in women who are pregnant or who intend to become pregnant* while undergoing therapy or soon after completion of therapy. Before isotretinoin is administered to women of childbearing age, a pregnancy test should be performed, and an effective method of contraception should be used for 2 weeks before therapy, throughout the therapy, and for 2 months after therapy is discontinued.

Cheilitis, xerosis, conjunctivitis, and drying of nasal mucosa with nosebleeds are the most common side effects, which are reversible after isotretinoin is discontinued. Other side effects include myalgias, transient arthralgias, and thinning of scalp hair. Rare but serious side effects include increased intracranial pressure with papilledema, nausea, vomiting, headaches, and visual disturbances. Since ingestion has been associated with inflammatory bowel diseases, isotretinoin should not be used in patients with inflammatory bowel diseases. If signs of increased intracranial pressure or severe diarrhea develop, isotretinoin must be stopped immediately. Transient elevation of triglycerides has been observed in 25% of patients. Furthermore, elevation of uric acid and liver enzyme levels and minor depression of red blood cell and white blood cell counts have been reported. Patients receiving isotretinoin should have blood lipid determinations, white blood cell counts, red blood cell counts, and levels of platelets, alkaline phosphatase, serum aspartate and alanine aminotransferases (AST, ALT; formerly SGOT, SGPT), and lactate dehydrogenase (LDH) obtained before and at intervals throughout therapy.

Much optimism surrounds the potential role of isotretinoin in the treatment of severe acne. Its use should be restricted to short-term, low-dosage therapy of patients with antibiotic-resistant cystic acne. Patients who are obese, diabetic, or alcoholic or who have high triglyceride levels and women planning families in the near future should not be treated with this medication. Furthermore, isotretinoin should be prescribed only by physicians who are experienced or trained in its use.

Dermabrasion is used to smooth and plane the scars and pits that develop as a result of acne. However, as a procedure that usually requires long surgery, it is reserved for more severe cases of scarring. Patients with broad-based scars obtain a better cosmetic result than those with deep, pitted lesions. The procedure involves the use of a high-speed metal brush to plane the skin to various levels. Improvement occurs in about 50% of patients. Scarring, hyperpigmentation, and hypopigmentation are the main complications. Only a dermatologist well trained in this procedure or a plastic surgeon should perform this technique on carefully screened patients.

Bovine collagen (Zyderm) has been used to improve superficial acne scars. After skin testing with bovine collagen, the preparation is injected into the dermis beneath the pitted scar, filling in the defect and making the skin surface more even. Despite enthusiastic reports by many dermatologists, many others remain skeptical about the long-term efficacy of this product.

RELATED CONDITIONS

Acne rosacea is a separate disease entity that usually occurs in persons between ages 40 and 60. It presents with pronounced erythema and superficial pustules and papules over the central portion of the face. A large, multilobulated rhinophyma is rare but can result from this acne as the sebaceous glands become larger (Fig. 77-6 and Color plate 32).

Blepharitis can complicate acne rosacea. The predisposing factors of acne rosacea are not known, but there is frequently a family history of acne rosacea and of ruddy complexion. Acne rosacea patients have an increased number of sebaceous glands over the face associated with erythema and multiple, small telangiectases. The acne rosacea patient should avoid foods and liquids that are hot in temperature. Alcohol ingestion can contribute to facial erythema. The main therapeutic modality is oral tetracycline. It is usually started at doses of 500 to 1000 mg daily. As the pustules and papules decrease in number, tetracycline is gradually tapered. Minocycline, 50 to 100 mg daily, can also be used. The topical antibiotic metronidazole (MetroGel) is helpful in the management of this type of acne. A 1% hydrocortisone cream with or

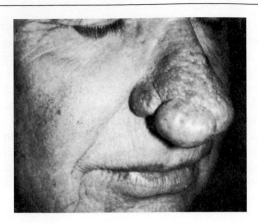

FIG. 77-6   Large rhinophyma of the nose in a patient with acne rosacea. The skin is erythematous, and multiple pustules are present.

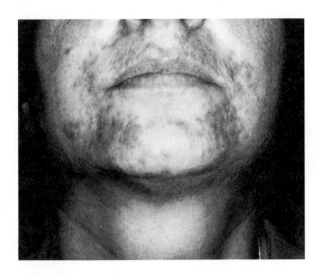

FIG. 77-7   Erythema, papules, and scaliness in perioral distribution are characteristic of perioral dermatitis.

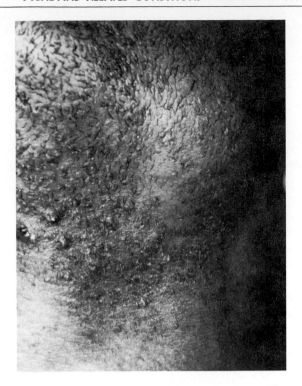

FIG. 77-8   Multiple papules and pustules in perifollicular distribution over the neck of a patient with pseudofolliculitis barbae.

without 1% or 2% precipitated sulfur can help treat the erythema and superficial pustules. Acne rosacea is a chronic disease that may have to be treated for a prolonged period. Telangiectases can be treated with a pulse dye laser, copper vapor laser, or electrodesiccation. Rhinophyma can be removed with a carbon dioxide laser.

Women in their 20s and 30s can develop superficial pustules, papules, and erythematous, greasy, scaly patches in perioral distribution (Fig. 77-7). This disorder is called *perioral dermatitis,* or *perioral acne,* and is the acne most frequently seen in adult women. Perioral acne spares the skin immediately adjacent to the lips. These patients frequently report a previous use of strong fluorinated steroid creams on the face. However, the cause of this condition is unknown. In treating this condition, all strong topical steroid creams should be stopped. A 1% hydrocortisone cream helps treat erythema and prevents

exacerbation of this acne when stronger topical steroids are stopped. Oral tetracycline, 250 to 500 mg daily, is usually effective. The antibiotic is gradually tapered over a few months. Frequently, resolution of perioral acne occurs within 4 months.

Pseudofolliculitis barbae occurs predominantly in bearded areas of African-American men. Curved, stiff beard hairs, when shaved close to the skin surface, reenter the skin and cause foreign body granulomas. The patients develop perifollicular inflammatory papules and pustules (Fig. 77-8). Scars and keloids frequently form secondary to these foreign body granulomas. The condition starts at the time when individuals begin shaving, and the most practical way to treat it is to grow a beard. Because this is not always acceptable, as in the armed forces and some places of employment, other remedies are used. Depilatories (e.g., Magic Shave) are helpful but can cause severe irritation of the skin. Using a toothbrush to comb and remove the ingrown hairs from the skin is helpful. Topical Retin-A cream (0.05%) has been helpful in some patients.

A chronic inflammation of the apocrine glands results in *hidradenitis suppurativa.* Painful nodules, cysts, scars, and sinus tracts form in the axillae, groin, perianal area, and breasts where the apocrine glands are present (Fig. 77-9). Frequently, there is a history of cystic acne in the family, and patients have cystic acne over the face, chest, and back. However, the etiology of hidradenitis suppura-

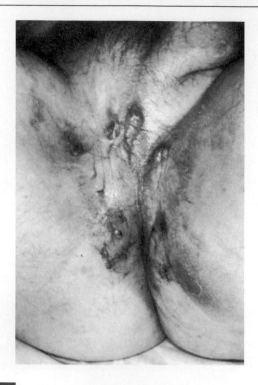

tiva is unknown. Cysts are frequently sterile or grow a common epidermal contaminant, *Staphylococcus epidermidis*. The inflammatory process of the apocrine glands may be secondary to bacteria or their breakdown products. In treating this condition, drainage of the cysts is helpful. Systemic tetracycline, minocycline, or erythromycin is useful in conservative management of inflamed, painful cysts. Patients are instructed to lose weight and clean the area of involvement with antibacterial soaps (e.g., PhisoHex). In chronic, refractory cases of hidradenitis suppurativa, surgical resection of the affected area is sometimes indicated.

FIG. 77-9 Painful nodules, cysts, and sinus tracts in hidradenitis suppurativa of the groin.

? QUESTIONS

▼ *Answer the following on a separate sheet of paper.*

1. Define acne.
2. Which age groups have the highest incidence rates of acne?
3. Describe the formation of acne lesions.
4. Explain the purpose of each of the following treatments for acne:
   a. Proper cleansing of the skin with a good soap
   b. Antibiotic therapy (identify two examples of frequently used antibiotics)
   c. Dermabrasion
5. Discuss at least two comedogenic factors contributing to the development of acne.

▼ *Circle the letter preceding the item below that correctly answers the question or completes the statement. More than one answer may be correct.*

6. Which of the following is likely to be prescribed for its antiwrinkle properties?
   a. Benzoyl peroxide
   b. Topical tretinoin, or vitamin A acid (Retin-A)
   c. Meclan
   d. 1% Cleocin T gel
7. Isotretinoin can be administered to which of the following patients?
   a. Women with severe cystic acne who stopped oral contraceptives 3 months before the flare-up of acne
   b. Patients with grade II acne that is inflammatory and scarring but that has not been treated with systemic antibiotics
   c. Women with severe cystic acne who are allergic to tetracycline and minocycline and use adequate contraception
   d. Patients with severe cystic acne who have normal triglyceride levels and borderline serum chloride levels who did not respond to oral antibiotics
8. Ms. M., 25 years old, has a sudden onset of deep, pustular acne. She is not taking oral contraceptives. Which of the following drugs would likely be contraindicated?
   a. Oral tetracycline
   b. Erythromycin
   c. Minocycline
   d. Isotretinoin
9. All of the following statements are true about hidradenitis suppurativa *except:*
   a. It involves apocrine glands.
   b. It responds well to isotretinoin (Accutane).
   c. It is usually present in the groin, breast, and axillary areas.
   d. It sometimes can be cured only by excision of the apocrine glands.
10. Acne rosacea occurs most frequently in which of the following groups?
    a. Infants
    b. Children under age 15 years
    c. Young adults (20 to 30 years)
    d. Middle-age adults (40 to 60 years)
    e. Older adults (70 to 80 years)
11. The most severe cystic acne, consisting of deep cysts, multiple comedones, and scarring, is which of the following variants?
    a. Acne rosacea
    b. Acne conglobata
    c. Excoriated acne
    d. Acne keloid

CHAPTER 78

Eczema and Vascular Disorders

MAREK A. STAWISKI

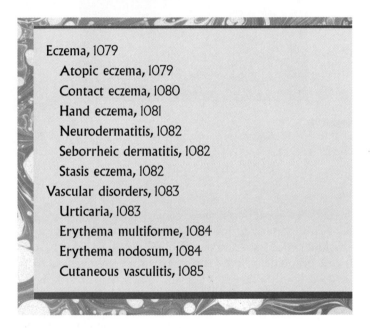

ECZEMA

Eczema encompasses all types of red, blistering, weeping, scaly, thickened, itchy skin lesions. *Acute eczema* presents with vesicles, bullae, erythema, weeping, and crusting. *Chronic eczema* has thickened, scaly, pruritic patches and plaques. Examples of eczema include the following:

1. Atopic eczema, characterized by weeping, crusted, dry, scaly, pruritic patches on the faces of infants and in the larger folds of skin found in the antecubital and popliteal fossae in adolescents and adults
2. Allergic contact eczema, characterized by pruritic vesicles, erythema, and patches in areas where patients have touched allergens such as poison ivy, poison sumac, cosmetics, rubber, and cement, among many others
3. Hand eczema characterized by erythematous, scaly, fissured patches over the hands
4. Neurodermatitis, characterized by excoriated patches and lines secondary to compulsive scratching of the skin
5. Seborrheic dermatitis, characterized by yellow-red-brown, greasy, scaly patches over the scalp and face
6. Stasis eczema, characterized by stasis edema, hyperpigmentation, and scaliness of the lower legs

Atopic Eczema

Atopic eczema, or *atopic dermatitis,* is a hereditary chronic skin disease that can appear at any age (see Chapter 9). There is often a family history of this eczema and associated allergic rhinitis or extrinsic asthma. Some children outgrow the cutaneous eczema only to develop hay fever or extrinsic asthma in later years. Infantile atopic eczema frequently presents with weeping, eroded, erythematous patches in the diaper area and on the cheeks and scalp (Color plate 33). Because the eruptions are pruritic, the infant is irritable. Secondary infections with bacteria are common. In most infants the eczema disappears spontaneously. In some infants it can progress into childhood or adult forms. Pruritus is the universal complaint of all these patients.

In children or adults the areas of involvement include the popliteal spaces, the antecubital fossae, the neck areas, and other flexural surfaces (Fig. 78-1). In adults, eczematous skin changes can become generalized over the entire body. Spontaneous remission of adulthood eczema occurs infrequently. Patients have erythematous, excoriated, thickened skin over the face, trunk, and extremities (Fig. 78-2). Changes in the weather and irritation from wool clothing, soap, and water frequently exacerbate the disease. Upper respiratory infections and bacterial skin infections can also aggravate the skin condition. Atopic eczema patients should not be vaccinated against smallpox because disseminated vaccinia can develop. Exposure to herpesvirus can result in disseminated herpetic infection of the skin.

The causes of atopic eczema are unknown. Hereditary factors definitely play a role. When two parents have atopic cczema, the child has about an 80% chance of de-

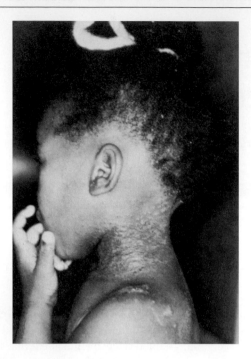

FIG. 78-1   Lichenified, thickened, scaly skin over the neck area in childhood atopic eczema.

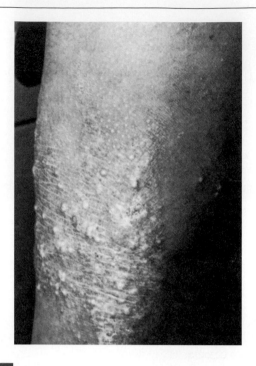

FIG. 78-2   Thickened skin with multiple excoriated papules of chronic eczema.

veloping the same skin condition. Irritation of the skin with wool, water, harsh soaps, climate changes, stress, and infection frequently result in clinical exacerbations. Many of the patients have abnormal levels of serum immunoglobulin E (IgE). Some investigators have demonstrated IgE on the surface of epidermal Langerhans cells in atopic eczema patients. Blood eosinophils are also elevated in this disease. The number of thymus-derived lymphocytes is decreased in some patients. Some investigators have postulated an abnormality in the receptors responsible for production of cyclic adenosine monophosphate (cAMP) nucleotides. How these abnormalities produce an extremely pruritic, eczematous skin is not understood.

Therapy of atopic eczema focuses on prevention and treatment. All possible exacerbating factors must be avoided or eliminated. Superfatted soaps, mineral oil, and lubricating creams are recommended. In infants, dietary restrictions may be helpful (orange juice and cow's milk), but they are not useful with older children and adults. Moisturizers such as Eucerin®, Moisturel®, and Aquaphor® are applied to dry skin. A humidifier may be installed in the house. Antibiotics are used to treat secondary bacterial infections. Pruritus is controlled with antihistaminics such as diphenhydramine (Benadryl), hydroxyzine (Atarax), or cyproheptadine (Periactin). The dosages of these medications are increased to levels that relieve pruritus or produce drowsiness, whichever comes first. Topical corticosteroids in the weakest possible strength are used for children. Topical 1% hydrocortisone is usually prescribed for infants, whereas 0.025% triamcinolone in a lubricating cream is given to adults. A 0.05% desonide or 2.5% hydrocortisone cream is used to treat eczema of the face, groin, and axillae in adults. Medium- or high-strength topical steroids used for a prolonged time can cause skin atrophy (Fig. 78-3), depigmentation, and acne formation. Ultraviolet light B (UVB) and oral psoralens combined with ultraviolet light A (PUVA) can be useful in treatment of recalcitrant, chronic atopic eczema.

Hyposensitization immunotherapy may exacerbate, benefit, or have no effect on atopic eczema. It is therefore not indicated in this form of eczema.

Contact Eczema

Contact eczema is common and occurs in localized areas where an allergen comes into contact with the skin. The skin reaction to the oil of poison ivy, *Rhus* dermatitis, is best known. Linear areas of vesiculation, weeping, and erythema occur in the places where the skin has touched the poison ivy, poison sumac, or poison oak plant (Fig. 78-4 and Color plate 34). The oil can be carried in many ways: on a pet's fur, on clothing, on shoes, or on fingernails. Once the oil is washed off, the dermatitis does not spread. *Rhus* dermatitis is not transmitted from person to person through the blister fluid.

A frequent cause of contact eczema is nickel. This

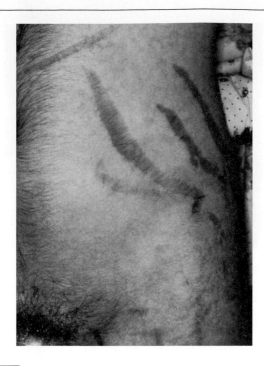

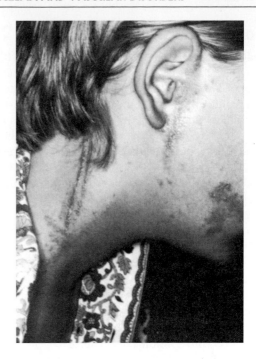

FIG. 78-3   Atrophy of skin causing striae after prolonged use of high-strength steroids.

FIG. 78-4   Grouped and linear vesicular eruptions are characteristic of poison ivy dermatitis.

metal is found in virtually all jewelry, metal eyeglass frames, and coins. A patient sensitive to nickel has crusted, well-defined patches of eczema at the site of exposure (e.g., neck, ears, wrists, abdomen). Patients allergic to potassium dichromate develop eczema when exposed to it in cement or leather shoes. Shoes can also contain rubber, which is a frequent cause of shoe contact eczema. The medications neomycin and benzocaine and the preservative ethylenediamine are common causes of allergic eczema. In *photodermatitis,* topical agents (e.g., halogenated salicylamides in soaps) or an oral medication (e.g., tetracycline) in combination with sunlight can cause erythema, edema, and occasionally vesiculation. Photodermatitis usually occurs on sun-exposed areas of the face, neck, and forearms.

Contact eczema is mediated through a cellular type IV delayed hypersensitivity (see Chapter 12). After primary exposure, a second contact with the allergen is required to produce eczema. This type of eczema can be reproduced by patch-testing the patient in whom the allergy is suspected. A careful history is required for selection of appropriate allergens to be tested. Patch testing is usually performed on the patient's back after the eczema is under control.

Therapy necessitates the removal of offending allergens. Patients must learn how to identify *Rhus* plants. Cosmetics, jewelry, and other objects that contain the allergen responsible for eczema should be avoided. Topical care of acute allergic eczema includes soaks and cor-

ticosteroid creams and gels. Frequently, severe allergic eczema, such as poison ivy, is treated with systemic steroids. A short treatment with systemic prednisone at the initial dosage of 40 to 60 mg/day is tapered over 7 to 14 days.

Hand Eczema

Hand eczema most often occurs in persons who must wash their hands frequently or who are under stress. Small vesicles appear on the lateral aspects of fingers, toes, and feet. Pruritus accompanies the appearance of vesicles. The small blisters develop into scaly, eczematous patches over the palms and soles (Color plate 35). Hand eczema is exacerbated by water, detergents, and stress. It can be a chronic problem that is extremely difficult to control. When hand eczema is exacerbated by exposure to an industrial chemical, patch testing is required to rule out allergic eczema. Heredity plays an important role in hand eczema.

Hand eczema is sometimes prevented through avoiding harsh soaps and wearing protective gloves. Oral antihistamines and strong, fluorinated topical corticosteroids (Lidex, Halog) are used to suppress this form of eczema. Occasionally a short course of a systemic corticosteroid is required, such as prednisone at a dosage of 30 to 40 mg/day initially, tapered daily over 6 to 8 days. Secondary bacterial infections are treated with appropriate systemic antibiotics.

Neurodermatitis

Neurodermatitis is caused by compulsive scratching of pruritic skin. It can be localized to the neck, scrotum, or anywhere on the body. Linear, thickened, dry patches of eczema result from persistent scratching (Fig. 78-5).

Generalized neurodermatitis frequently occurs during the cold, dry winter months in older patients who have dry, pruritic skin. Compulsive scratching can result in factitious ulcers (Fig. 78-6). These self-induced ulcers have odd angles and square borders, which should alert the examiner to this diagnosis. However, diffuse pruritus and scratching can also be caused by scabies, atopic eczema, systemic lymphoma, hypothyroidism, diabetes mellitus, cirrhosis, and severe uremia. These conditions must be carefully ruled out before the diagnosis of neurodermatitis is made.

Treatment of this condition consists of lubrication and application of topical corticosteroids to the skin. Older patients with generalized neurodermatitis should be treated only with emollients (Eucerin) or low-potency topical corticosteroids (1% hydrocortisone). The skin of older persons is thin from aging, and stronger topical steroids can lead to further atrophy and excessive bruising. Systemic antihistaminic agents (Benadryl, Atarax, Sinequan) may be useful in controlling pruritus. Topical doxepin cream (Zonalon) can be used for a limited time of about 8 days to the areas of neurodermatitis. Older patients must use systemic antihistamines with caution because excessive drowsiness or even paradoxical restlessness may occur. Localized neurodermatitis in younger patients may require stronger topical corticosteroids. Psychotherapy may be required in treating severe neurodermatitis, especially if the face is affected.

Seborrheic Dermatitis

Seborrheic dermatitis typically involves the scalp, eyebrows, nasolabial folds, ears, and anterior chest. Erythematous, scaly patches appear intermittently. The condition may begin any time from infancy to old age. It may be slightly pruritic. The cause is unknown, but genetic factors seem to play an important part. Recently, *Pityrosporum ovale* has been implicated as playing a role in the pathogenesis of seborrheic dermatitis.

Therapy of scalp seborrheic dermatitis includes shampoos that contain selenium sulfide (Selsun), ketoconazole (Nizoral), tar (Tegrin, Sebutone), and salicylic acid (Sebulex). Topical corticosteroid sprays or solutions are useful. Weak topical corticosteroids (1% hydrocortisone) combined with precipitated sulfur (0.5% to 1%) are used to treat seborrheic dermatitis of the face and the chest. Topical antifungal agents (ketoconazole) are helpful additions to the therapy. Fluocinolone acetonide in peanut oil base (Derma-smoothe/FS) can be applied under a shower cap to resistant seborrheic dermatitis of the scalp.

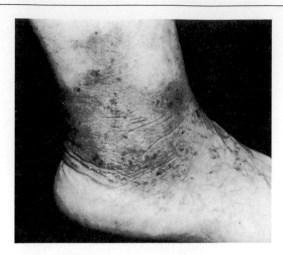

FIG. 78-5   Neurodermatitis. Persistent scratching causes a localized patch of thickened, excoriated skin. (From Fitzpatrick TB et al, editors: *Dermatology in general medicine,* ed 3, New York, 1987, McGraw-Hill.)

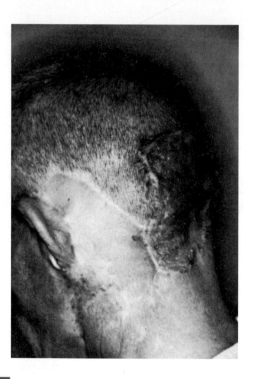

FIG. 78-6   Neurodermatitis. Compulsive scratching can result in factitious ulcers associated with hair loss.

Stasis Eczema

Stasis eczema is localized to the areas of venous stasis and edema on the lower legs. Crusted, scaly, weeping erythematous patches appear (Fig. 78-7). The eruptions are pruritic and can lead to secondary excoriations, erosions, and ulcers.

Therapy requires removal of edema fluid and improvement of circulation. The legs are elevated; wraps and

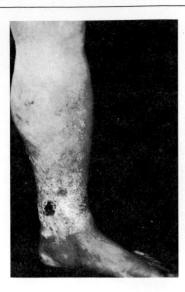

FIG. 78-7 Stasis dermatitis localized to the area of chronic venous insufficiency. Secondary ulceration is seen over the region of the malleolus medialis. (From Fitzpatrick TB et al, editors: *Dermatology in general medicine,* ed 3, New York, 1987, McGraw-Hill.)

Jobst stockings are frequently recommended. Eczema is treated with weak- or intermediate-strength topical corticosteroids (1% hydrocortisone, 0.025% triamcinolone). Ulcers are soaked, cleansed, and débrided. An occlusive dressing (Duoderm) can be used to treat venous stasis ulcers. Patients apply the occlusive dressing every 3 days.

VASCULAR DISORDERS

Urticaria

Urticaria *(hives)* is the most common cutaneous reaction in which edema and erythema result (Fig. 78-8 and Color plate 36) (see Chapter 11). Within a few hours after onset, lesions disappear. These transient skin eruptions appear as lightly erythematous wheals and papules with vasodilation of dermal and subcutaneous blood vessels accompanied by edema of surrounding tissue. Pruritus frequently occurs with urticaria. *Angioedema,* resulting in swelling of the lips, tongue, eyelids, and larynx, may accompany cutaneous urticaria. Laryngeal angioedema is a medical emergency. Angioedema may be associated with nausea, respiratory distress, vomiting, abdominal pain, and shock. Acute urticaria is frequently caused by the ingestion of a food (e.g., shellfish, nuts, food additives, food preservatives, food dyes). Virtually every drug can cause urticaria, the most common being aspirin, laxatives, and antibiotics. Connective tissue diseases, lymphomas, and carcinomas are among the internal diseases causing urticaria. Insect bites can cause papules of urticaria. Pregnant women can develop pruritic urticarial papules and plaques.

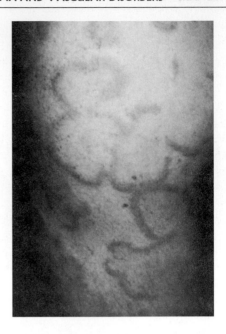

FIG. 78-8 Edema, erythema, and pruritus are the clinical features of urticarial welts.

Chronic urticaria is idiopathic in 75% to 90% of all patients but may be caused by food preservatives, collagen vascular diseases, medications, or infections. Occasionally, cold temperatures, sun, exercise, stress, or alcohol can trigger urticaria. Urticaria results from release of histamines, serotonins, bradykinins, and other mediators. These mediators result in vasodilation and edema in the dermis and subcutaneous layers. Because so many mediators of inflammation are involved in formation of urticarial lesions, treatment can be difficult. The search for an underlying cause can also be extremely difficult. Patients with chronic urticaria are evaluated by a complete history, physical examination, and blood tests, including tests for differential leukocyte count, sedimentation rate, and antinuclear factor. Blood tests should also include liver tests such as those for serum aspartate and alanine aminotransferases (AST, ALT; formerly SGOT, SGPT), lactate dehydrogenase (LDH), alkaline phosphatase, and bilirubin. Search for the infectious agent includes examination of the stool for ova and parasites, chest radiographs, sinus radiographs, and a dental checkup. Skin testing with antigens is of little merit in evaluation of urticaria. Hereditary angioedema is associated with a deficiency of the inhibitor of the first complement component. Stroking of the skin, application of ice cubes, exercising, light testing, and water testing can sometimes trigger the skin lesions.

In therapy, all precipitating factors (medications, dyes, food) should be eliminated. Elimination diets avoiding chocolate, azo dyes, cheeses, shellfish, nuts, eggs, milk, tomatoes, and fresh berries can be tried. Urticaria is treated symptomatically. Acute urticaria with angioedema is treated with subcutaneous epinephrine. Less se-

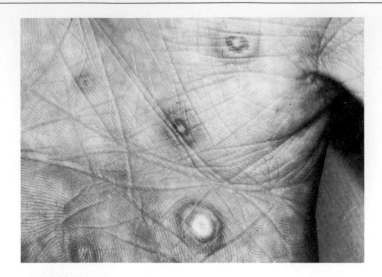

FIG. 78-9   Targetlike lesions are seen in erythema multiforme.

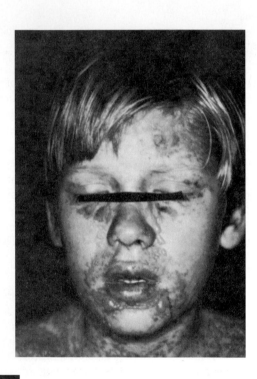

FIG. 78-10   Erosions of the lips and conjunctiva associated with fever in this boy with Stevens-Johnson syndrome.

vere urticaria is treated with oral H_1-receptor antihistamines, such as diphenhydramine, hydroxyzine, and cyproheptadine. These medications can cause severe drowsiness and sleepiness; patients should be advised about these potentially dangerous side effects. Nonsedating H_1-receptor antihistamines include terfenadine, astemizole, and loratidine and are slightly less effective. A tricyclic antidepressant such as doxepin can be used in patients resistant to therapy. H_2-receptor antihistamines such as cimetidine are also useful. Prophylaxis of hereditary angioedema can be achieved with antifibrinolytic agents (E-aminocaproic acid) and androgens (danazol).

Erythema Multiforme

Patients with erythema multiforme present with macules, papules, and vesicles. The characteristic lesion has the central "target" discoloration or necrosis (Fig. 78-9). The lesions are symmetric and frequently involve the palms of the hands. Erythema multiforme is usually asymptomatic but can be painful and pruritic.

When the mucous membranes of the lips, mouth, genitalia, and conjunctiva are involved, erythema multiforme is called *Stevens-Johnson syndrome* (Fig. 78-10). These patients are toxic and febrile. Corneal scarring can result. Maculopapular lesions can become confluent, forming large areas of bullae and necrosis. This is called *toxic epidermal necrolysis;* death occurs in about 50% of these patients. Complications of erythema multiforme include postinflammatory hyperpigmentation, keratitis with visual impairment, and pneumonia. The causes of erythema multiform include drugs (sulfa, penicillin, barbiturates, diphenylhydantoin) and infections (herpes simplex, *Mycoplasma*). However, in more than 50% of patients the cause is idiopathic. Severe erythema multiforme, or Stevens-Johnson syndrome, is treated with systemic corticosteroids.

Erythema Nodosum

Patients with erythema nodosum present with painful, erythematous nodules usually localized to the anterior aspect of the lower legs. This condition is more common in women. Fever, arthritis, and arthralgia accompany the eruptions. Specific causes can be determined in only about 20% to 30% of patients. These include streptococcal infections, sarcoidosis, drug ingestion, and inflammatory bowel disease. Resolution of the disease occurs in 3 to 6 weeks. Chest radiography, complete blood count, throat culture, and antistreptolysin O titer are obtained to elucidate underlying causes of erythema nodosum. Patients are usually treated with bedrest and aspirin and occasionally with oral corticosteroids.

Cutaneous Vasculitis

In cutaneous vasculitis, persistent palpable urticarial lesions, hemorrhagic macules, papules, ulcers, and purpura are observed (Color plate 37). The lesions are usually found over the distal extremities. Cutaneous vasculitis can be associated with systemic vasculitis of the kidney, gastrointestinal tract, and other organs. Therefore a pa-

tient may have fever, arthralgia, gastrointestinal bleeding, or hematuria. The causes of vasculitis include drugs, infections (particularly streptococcal), collagen vascular diseases (rheumatoid arthritis, systemic lupus erythematosus), and hepatitis type B virus. In most patients the cause is idiopathic. Patients with clinical lesions of cutaneous vasculitis require skin biopsy to confirm this diagnosis. The biopsy reveals infiltrates of polymorphonuclear leukocytes, which are associated with necrosis of the blood vessel walls. Once the diagnosis is established, patients are evaluated for systemic involvement through urinalysis, creatinine clearance, and tests for the presence of cryoglobulins, antinuclear factor, rheumatoid factor, and hepatitis B antigen. Therapy is based on the severity of cutaneous involvement and on systemic involvement. Systemic corticosteroids usually help in resolution of the process. Cyclophosphamide and colchicine may also be used.

QUESTIONS

▼ *Answer the following on a separate sheet of paper.*

1. Describe the characteristic lesions of acute and chronic eczema.
2. List five of the causes of allergic contact eczema.
3. What are the most frequent causes and treatments of hand eczema?
4. List the drugs most often used in the treatment of acute urticaria.

▼ *Circle the letter preceding each item below that correctly answers the question or completes the statement. More than one answer may be correct.*

5. Bill, 15 years old, presents with erythematous, excoriated, scaly, thickened skin over antecubital and popliteal fossa. He has a history of erythematous pruritic eruptions during childhood, but no known allergies. The condition is most likely:
   a. Contact eczema

   b. Atopic eczema
   c. Neurodermatitis
   d. Stasis eczema
   e. Urticaria
6. Which of the following are typical of the skin lesions of stasis eczema?
   a. Localization to the area of the lower legs
   b. Involvement of the scalp, eyebrows, and ears
   c. Crusted, scaling, weeping patches over the arms
   d. Lesions that are frequently erythematous, scaly patches
7. Mrs. A., 70 years old, has a history of dry, pruritic skin, particularly in the cold, dry months. Persistent scratching of her arms and legs has resulted in factitious ulcers with odd angles and square bodies. Her diagnosis is generalized neurodermatitis. The treatment of choice would be:
   a. Low-potency topical corticosteroids

   b. Atarax
   c. Benadryl
   d. Eucerin

▼ *Circle T if the statement is true and F if it is false. Correct any false statements.*

8. T F Urticaria is a common cutaneous reaction in which edema, erythema, and pruritus are usually present.
9. T F Application of ice cubes and light testing are useful in establishing the causative agent(s) in urticaria.
10. T F A skin biopsy is frequently necessary to confirm the diagnosis in cutaneous vasculitis.
11. T F *Pityrosporum ovale* has been implicated as playing a role in the pathogenesis of seborrheic dermatitis.

CHAPTER 79

Psoriasis and Pityriasis Rosea

MAREK A. STAWISKI

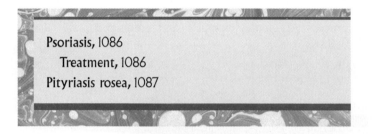
Disorders of the skin characterized by the presence of plaques, patches, and scales are called *papulosquamous diseases.* These include psoriasis and pityriasis rosea.

PSORIASIS

Psoriasis is reported in 2 to 5 million Americans. It appears as thick, erythematous plaques and papules covered by a silvery white scale. The plaques are usually located over the knees, elbows, and scalp (Fig. 79-1 and Color plate 38). However, the skin eruptions can affect any part of the body, with the exception of the mucous membranes. The nails frequently appear thickened, with yellowish discoloration, multiple pits, and separation from the nailbed. Arthritis can also accompany this skin disease and classically involves the distal interphalangeal joints. In these patients the rheumatoid factor is not present. Arthritis does not always correlate with severity of the psoriasis. Psoriasis is usually not pruritic; however, some patients report severe pruritus, especially associated with the development of new papules.

Psoriasis is a chronic disease that can occur at any age. Fluctuations mark the natural course of this condition. For example, sunlight, relaxation, and the summer season are usually beneficial to psoriasis patients. An upper respiratory tract infection can trigger an acute exacerbation of psoriasis, as evidenced by eruptions of multiple small papules over the trunk (Fig. 79-2). Psoriasis can also be

exacerbated by medications (lithium, beta-blockers, corticosteroids, antimalarials) and sunburn. Generalized psoriasis, as characterized by multiple pustules with inflammatory plaques, is called *pustular psoriasis.* This condition can be accompanied by chills, high fever, and electrolyte imbalances. Pustular psoriasis is a medical emergency that can be fatal and frequently requires hospitalization.

Psoriasis is an inherited disease, although the mode of inheritance is not well understood. A family history of psoriasis is found in 66% of psoriasis patients. Histocompatibility antigens HLA-B13, HLA-B17, and HLA-Cw6 are increased fourfold in persons with psoriasis. Environmental factors also play a significant role in the disease. Trauma to the skin can produce new lesions of psoriasis, especially in the area where the skin is punctured, scraped, or cut.

Histopathologic examination of a psoriatic skin biopsy reveals thickened epidermis and stratum corneum and dilated upper dermal blood vessels. The number of basal cells undergoing mitosis is markedly increased. These fast-dividing cells move rapidly to the surface of the thickened epidermis. This rapid proliferation and migration of epidermal cells result in thick epidermis covered by a thick keratin (silvery scale). Abnormal levels of cyclic nucleotides, especially cyclic adenosine monophosphate (cAMP) and cyclic guanosine monophosphate (cGMP), may be partially responsible for this rapid mitosis rate of epidermal cells. Prostaglandins and polyamines are also abnormal in the disease. The exact role of these abnormalities in influencing the formation of a psoriatic plaque is not clearly understood. Numerous neutrophils are attracted to the epidermis. Promoters of this neutrophil chemotaxis (complements, peptides, leukotrienes) may be abnormal in psoriasis. Epidermal proteinases that activate complement and attract neutrophils are also elevated.

Treatment

Therapy of chronic psoriasis requires knowledge of various treatment modalities, patience, and an experienced physician. The treatment must be flexible, and alternative therapy must be administered if the patient fails to respond to the original program of treatment. Localized disease is treated with topical corticosteroids over the face and intertriginous areas, and in children, weak steroids such as 1% hydrocortisone are used. Over the trunk, extremities, and scalp, intermediate-strength steroids such as triamcinolone or fluocinolone are recommended. The strong steroids—fluocinonide, halcinonide, and betamethasone—are reserved for resistant plaques.

A tar preparation of cream or shampoo is frequently used. A bath oil with tar (Balnetar) is also helpful. All these medications result in decreased cell proliferation, which makes the epidermis thinner and causes the plaques and scales of psoriasis to disappear. A new vitamin D derivative, 1,25-dihydroxy vitamin D_3 (Dovonex) ointment, can be used with great efficacy in about 30% of patients who have plaque psoriasis.

Severe generalized psoriasis requires hospitalization for intensive topical steroid, tar, and ultraviolet light therapy. Unfortunately, relapses of psoriasis often occur 3 to

6 months after hospitalization. The newest outpatient modality of treatment combines the use of psoralen, an oral photosensitizing medication, with long ultraviolet light (PUVA). This treatment is not indicated in patients with a previous history of x-ray irradiation, skin cancer, or cataracts. This therapy can result in squamous cell carcinoma, especially over the scrotum. Shorter ultraviolet light (UVB) is used successfully in the treatment of psoriasis in psoriasis treatment centers. Long ultraviolet light (UVA) is not effective unless it is used in combination with psoralen. Commercial tanning booths produce mainly UVA light and are not effective in treating psoriasis. An oral antineoplastic medication, methotrexate, may be useful in treating patients with severe plaque-type psoriasis, pustular psoriasis, or debilitating arthritis. However, this oral agent may cause irreversible cirrhosis of the liver or bone marrow suppression. The newest treatment modality for psoriasis is oral etretinate (Tegison). This new oral aromatic retinoid is excellent for treating pustular and erythrodermic psoriasis and useful for recalcitrant plaque psoriasis. The drug should not be given to women who are of childbearing age because it is a powerful teratogen. It also elevates liver enzyme, cholesterol, and triglyceride levels. Side effects include dryness of skin and mucous membranes, hair loss, headaches, diarrhea, myalgia, and arthralgias. If used for longer than 12 months, radiographic studies of the bones should be obtained to check for calcium deposits in the joints.

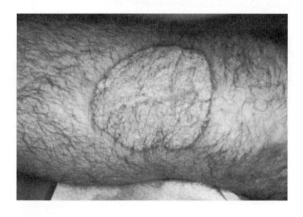

FIG. 79-1   Thick psoriatic plaques with a white silvery scale as seen in the psoriatic patient.

PITYRIASIS ROSEA

In contrast to psoriasis, pityriasis rosea is an acute, self-limited eruption seen in young adults and adolescents. Pityriasis rosea begins with an oval, scaly lesion called

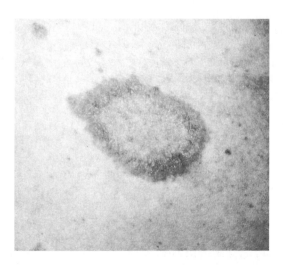

FIG. 79-3   Oval-shaped, scaly lesion of pityriasis rosea; a so-called "herald patch" with typical peripheral scale.

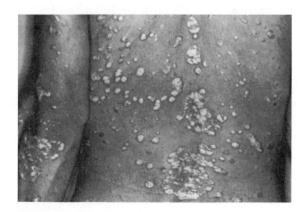

FIG. 79-2   Multiple small psoriatic papules can erupt after an upper respiratory infection. This form of psoriasis is termed *guttate psoriasis.*

the "herald patch." Within a week, multiple, pale-red, oval patches with a fine scale around the periphery appear over the neck, trunk, and proximal extremities (Figs. 79-3 and 79-4 and Color plate 39). Pruritus is usually not severe. Lesions of pityriasis rosea usually do not occur on the face, palms, and soles, in contrast to secondary syphilis. The cutaneous eruptions, which can be accompanied by malaise and fever, persist for 4 to 8 weeks and rarely recur. The cause of this common disease is unknown; however, viral agents have been suspected.

Obtaining an adequate history is necessary to rule out drug eruptions and viral exanthems. Syphilis can mimic pityriasis rosea, so serology is required (see Chapter 66). Treatment for pruritus consists of oral antihistamines and topical corticosteroids. Exposure to sunlight usually results in faster disappearance of the lesions.

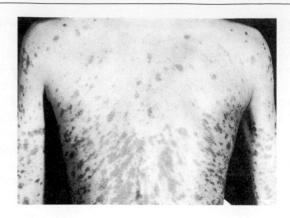

FIG. 79-4   Oval-shaped papules and patches in pityriasis rosea showing the dermatome-type pattern. (From Fitzpatrick TB et al, editors: *Dermatology in general medicine*, ed 2, New York, 1979, McGraw-Hill.)

QUESTIONS

▼ *Answer the following on a separate sheet of paper.*

1. What is the latest treatment modality for psoriasis? What are contraindications for its use?
2. What is the latest topical treatment modality for psoriasis?
3. Describe the histopathologic examination of a psoriatic skin biopsy and the clinical appearance and distribution of psoriasis.

▼ *Circle the letter preceding each item below that correctly answers the question or completes the statement. More than one answer may be correct.*

4. An oval, scaly lesion termed the "herald patch" is characteristic of:
   a. Psoriasis
   b. Pityriasis rosea
   c. Neurodermatitis
   d. Atopic eczema

5. Psoriasis can be treated with the use of psoralen and long ultraviolet light (PUVA) therapy. The treatment is contraindicated in patients who:
   a. Are heavy cigarette smokers (more than two packs/day)
   b. Have a previous history of x-ray irradiation
   c. Have been treated with topical steroids
   d. Have a history of skin cancer

6. Treatment of pruritus associated with pityriasis rosea is:
   a. Benzoyl peroxide
   b. Topical corticosteroids
   c. Tar preparation in cream
   d. Oral antihistamines

7. The incidence of psoriasis is reported in how many million Americans?
   a. More than 1
   b. 2 to 3
   c. 2 to 5
   d. 8 to 10

8. Psoriasis is a genetic disease associated with elevated:
   a. HLA-B13 antigen
   b. HLA-B17 antigen
   c. HLA-Cw6 antigen
   d. All the above

9. The most common complication of strong topical steroids used on the groin area or face or in children is:
   a. Hypertrichosis
   b. Obesity
   c. Diabetes mellitus
   d. Atrophy and striae of the skin

10. Methotrexate is a useful oral drug for treatment of psoriasis. Its usefulness is limited by:
   a. Hepatotoxicity
   b. Bone marrow suppression
   c. Elevation of cholesterol and triglyceride levels
   d. Dryness and hair loss

CHAPTER 80 ▷ Cutaneous Infections

MAREK A. STAWISKI
SYLVIA A. PRICE

WARTS

Verrucae vulgaris, or warts, are caused by the human papillomavirus (HPV). The virus replicates in the epidermal cells and is transmitted from person to person. Warts also disseminate to the patient's self by autoinoculation. The virus is contagious to those individuals who lack the virus-specific immunity in the skin. The immunity to warts is not well understood. Verrucae appear as rough, warty nodules over the trunk, legs, hands, arms, feet, genitalia, and even mucous membranes of the mouth (Fig. 80-1). Flat warts are more prevalent on the face. Plantar warts grow into the thick stratum corneum of the foot and have small black dots within, which represent infarcted capillaries. In the genitalia and the mucous membranes of the vagina, rectum, and urethra, the verrucae are called *condylomata acuminata.* They appear as verrucous, moist nodules that may occur in large numbers (Fig. 80-2). Condyloma acuminata has been associated with cervical squamous cell cancer in women and premalignant bowenoid papulosis in men. Eighty-five percent of cervical squamous cell cancers are associated

with HPV types 16 and 18. The warts usually resolve spontaneously within 2 years when immunity against the virus develops. However, the development of this immune response can be delayed for many years.

Verrucae are usually removed by cryosurgery or curettage combined with electrodesiccation. Large numbers of those that occur in children are removed with preparations of salicylic acid (Occlusal-HP) or Duofilm. Salicylic acid preparations are preferred in treatment of plantar warts (Sal-Acid Plaster). A podophyllin derivative (Condylox) is usually applied to condylomata acuminata. Treatment of warts is often difficult, prolonged, and frustrating and can be painful. Recalcitrant warts of the feet, groin, and periungual areas are frequently treated with a carbon dioxide laser. If genital warts are present, sexual partners should be examined and treated. Abstinence or condoms should be used until the warts are eradicated from both partners. Perianal warts in children can be a sign of sexual abuse.

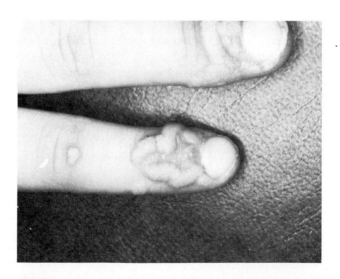

FIG. 80-1   Rough nodules of verrucae vulgaris (warts) over the fingers.

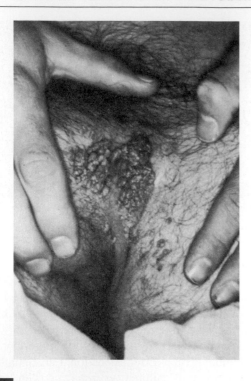

FIG. 80-2   Moist verrucous nodules of condyloma accuminatum in the groin area.

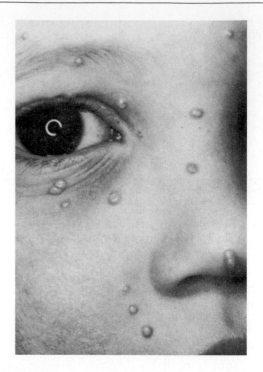

FIG. 80-3   Smooth, umbilicated, dome-shaped nodules of molluscum contagiosum over the face of a child.

MOLLUSCUM CONTAGIOSUM

Molluscum contagiosum is a dome-shaped, smooth, umbilicated nodule (Fig. 80-3). It is caused by a deoxyribonucleic acid (DNA) virus of the pox family. It is transmitted from person to person. The virus is contagious to people who lack immunity to this specific virus. Most often the lesions occur in children, frequently on the head and trunk. In young adults they usually appear in the groin area. The preferred modes of treatment are cantharidin solution in children and gentle curettage or liquid nitrogen cryosurgery in adults. In both adults and children, spontaneous resolution occurs in about 2 years. Widespread molluscum lesions in children are usually followed without therapy. They disappear spontaneously without leaving any scarring.

HERPES SIMPLEX

Herpes simplex infection is caused by a DNA virus. An infectious DNA particle enters the nucleus of the cell and uses the reproductive machinery of the cell for its own replication. The number of patients with genital herpes increased from 29,000 in 1966 to 261,000 in 1979. It is estimated that more than 25 million persons have or have had the infection today. Herpes labialis of the lip is even more common. There are two types of herpes: type I and type II. *Type I* usually affects the lips, mouth, nose, and cheeks. This form of herpes is acquired from close contact with an infected family member or friend in a nonsexual manner. It is transmitted by kissing, touching, and the use of common towels. *Type II* herpes simplex virus usually infects the genital areas. It frequently follows a sexual encounter, but not necessarily. It is estimated that as many as 20% of sexually active persons in the United States have or have had herpes type II.

Multiple, grouped, painful vesicles appear after primary exposure of the patient to the virus. Primary infections occur anywhere on a person's skin, although they usually occur around the mouth and nose, causing gingivostomatitis; around the eyes, causing conjunctivitis; the fingers, causing herpetic whitlow; and the buttocks and genitals, causing vulvovaginitis. Primary infections cause intense skin edema, extensive vesiculation, and exquisite pain (Fig. 80-4). Nurses frequently develop extremely painful edematous vesicles on their fingers. This herpetic whitlow follows exposure to a patient with herpetic infection. This primary infection lasts for as long as 6 weeks, and the nurse should not have contact with surgical, debilitated, or immunosuppressed patients during this time. During the primary infection the virus ascends via peripheral nerves to dorsal root ganglia, where it is present in the dormant stage. Some patients are subject to recurrent activations of the latent virus. Most patients do not experience recurrent infections. Recurrent infections are usually less painful and frequently localized to the lips and genitals. Recurrences can be triggered by fever,

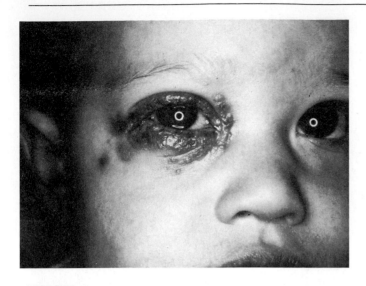

FIG. 80-4 Multiple vesicles, edema, and erythema in a primary herpetic infection causing conjunctivitis.

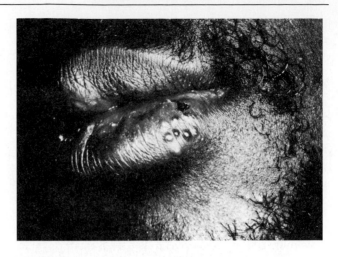

FIG. 80-5 Grouped, localized, painful vesicles of recurrent herpes simplex of the lips.

sunlight, or trauma. Grouped vesicles (Fig. 80-5) become pustules within a few days and usually resolve spontaneously within 2 weeks.

Herpes progenitalis has been the most prominent sexually transmitted disease in the United States during the past 10 years. Recurrent herpes progenitalis causes painful vesicles and ulcers. The recurrent herpetic infection can follow primary infection within weeks, months, or years. Because the initial herpetic infection can be mild, a patient may not realize that she or he has had the primary infection. Years later, when a recurrent infection appears, mistaken accusations of infidelity by a partner can arise. In humans, only 14% of patients with type I herpes acquire recurrent herpes, whereas 60% of herpes type II infections become recurrent. Ninety-eight percent of recurrent genital herpes are caused by type II virus. Many factors affect recurrence. It can be triggered by fever, emotional stress, fatigue, ovulation, and physical trauma.

Herpes infection has serious implications if the infection occurs in the eye, around the cervix, in newborns, or in immunosuppressed individuals. The herpes infection of the eye may lead to herpetic keratitis. Scarring of the cornea, and even corneal perforation, can result. A pregnant woman with active genital herpes at the time of delivery can transmit the virus to the baby as it passes through the birth canal. Severe encephalitis in a newborn can result in death or mental retardation. Cesarean section is indicated in women who have genital herpes at the time of delivery. Similarly, if the mother or a person working in the nursery has active vesicles of herpes on the lips or the hands, the baby can become infected. Infection with herpes type I can result in the same severe condition as type II herpes infection. Herpes infection in seriously ill or immunosuppressed patients can result in

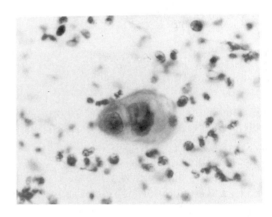

FIG. 80-6 Giant cells seen in vesicles of a patient with herpes simplex. The cells are surrounded by neutrophils. Slide is stained with 1% toluidine blue.

chronic, nonhealing ulcers (Color plate 40), dissemination, and encephalitis.

The diagnosis of herpes is usually made on the basis of history and clinical appearance. The diagnosis can be confirmed by a herpetic culture, which is positive in about 80% of the patients with herpes. The *Tzanck test* is positive in 50% to 80% of patients with herpes. In this test the material from the vesicle is placed on a glass slide and stained with 1% toluidine blue. Large multinucleated giant cells can be seen in smears taken from a patient with herpes simplex (Fig. 80-6). The Tzanck test takes only a few minutes to perform and is much less expensive than a herpes culture, but it is less accurate.

No adequate treatment exists for cutaneous herpes infections. No vaccine has been developed to prevent these infections from recurring. Recurrent episodes of herpes of the lips can sometimes be prevented by use of opaque sunscreens or avoidance of excessive sun exposure. Sexual spread of genital herpes is frequently avoided by use of rubber condoms when vesicles are present and for 7 days afterward. Sexual abstinence when vesicles are present is an alternative method of prevention. Furthermore, towels, underclothing, and swimming suits should not be shared. Acyclovir is the treatment of choice in herpes simplex infections. This drug administered in tablets or intravenous fluids is effective in treating cutaneous herpes infections. The drug is an inhibitor of herpes simplex virus DNA synthesis. Acyclovir ointment does not prevent recurrence or shorten the duration of the herpetic eruption in otherwise healthy individuals. Usually, patients with primary herpes are treated symptomatically, using soaks, topical antibiotics, pain medication, and oral acyclovir, 200 mg five times a day for 5 to 10 days. Recurrent herpetic infections are treated with acyclovir, 200 mg orally five times a day for 5 days. Acyclovir, 400 mg orally three times a day, helps suppress frequent attacks of recurrent herpes simplex. Long-term suppression appears safe and free of side effects.

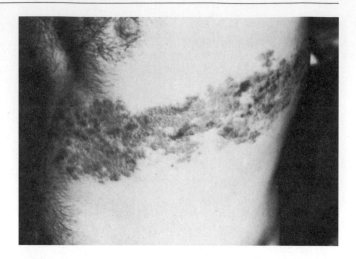

FIG. 80-7   Inflammatory vesicles appear along a single dermatome on edematous and hemorrhagic skin of herpes zoster.

CHICKENPOX (VARICELLA) AND HERPES ZOSTER

The virus that causes varicella is a DNA virus. When the disease is active, it is highly contagious. The incubation period is 14 to 21 days. The infection usually occurs in school-age children but occasionally affects young adults. Varicella is characterized by malaise and fever, followed by the eruption of multiple small erythematous macules, papules, and vesicles.

The vesicles become purulent and crusted and heal spontaneously, usually within 1 week. Characteristically, multiple stages of the lesions are present. The lesions initially appear on the trunk and face and spread peripherally to the extremities. Adults can develop varicella pneumonitis or encephalitis. In immunosuppressed children, complications from varicella infection include pneumonitis and encephalitis, both of which can be fatal. Acyclovir, 800 mg five times daily for 7 days, helps to shorten the severity and duration of the infection.

Herpes zoster is caused by the same herpes virus as varicella, or chickenpox. After the primary varicella infection, the virus apparently persists in the dorsal root ganglia. Herpes zoster, or *shingles,* usually occurs in older individuals. The dormant varicella virus is activated, and inflammatory vesicles appear unilaterally along a single dermatome. The adjacent skin is edematous and hemorrhagic (Fig. 80-7 and Color plate 41). This condition is usually preceded or accompanied by intense pain and/or burning. Even though any nerve can be involved, the thoracic, lumbar, and cranial nerves are most often affected. Herpes zoster persists for about 3 weeks. The pain that may follow an attack of herpes zoster is referred to as *postherpetic neuralgia* and fre-

quently may persist for several months or, rarely, many years. Postherpetic neuralgia is more common in older individuals. Dissemination of herpes zoster to the entire body surface, lungs, and brain can be fatal. This dissemination is usually seen in patients with lymphoma or leukemia. Thus any patient who develops disseminated herpes zoster should be evaluated for a possible underlying malignancy.

Treatment of localized herpes zoster is symptomatic with soaks and pain medication. If the ophthalmic branch of the trigeminal nerve is affected, an ophthalmologist should also be consulted because corneal perforations may result from the infection. Early administration of systemic corticosteroids may be helpful in the prevention of postherpetic neuralgia. Oral acyclovir, 800 mg five times daily for 10 days, can shorten the duration of herpes zoster infection. This drug decreases pain, reduces new lesion formation, and shortens time of healing. Topical capsaicin (Zostrix) seems to be occasionally effective for postherpetic neuralgia.

VIRAL EXANTHEMS

Rubeola, or measles, is caused by a ribonucleic acid (RNA) myxovirus. About 2 weeks after exposure, the patient develops fever, cough, headache, and conjunctivitis. The exanthem appears on the face, trunk, and proximal extremities. It consists of brightly erythematous, confluent macules. Over the buccal mucosa or the upper palate, mottled bright spots called *Koplik's spots* appear. Pneumonia and otitis media are present in many patients. Atypical measles occurs in individuals immunized with a killed-virus vaccine. Atypical measles usually presents without the Koplik's spots. In this type of measles a poly-

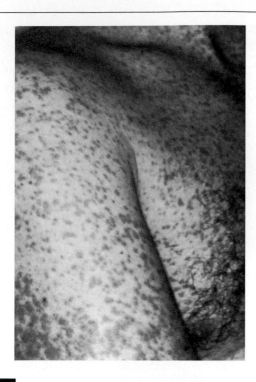

FIG. 80-8   Confluent, bright, erythematous macules after administration of ampicillin to a patient with infectious mononucleosis.

morphous rash appears on the distal extremities, and the incidence of pneumonia is very high. Typical measles eruptions last 5 to 10 days. Treatment of this infection is symptomatic. Administration of the rubeola vaccine has substantially decreased the incidence of the disease.

Rubella, or German measles, is also caused by an RNA myxovirus. The disease occurs 2 to 3 weeks after exposure and is associated with malaise and a mild fever. Pale-red macules appear over the face and within a day spread to the trunk. The exanthem fades within a few days. Painful postauricular and suboccipital enlarged lymph nodes are usually present. The diagnosis is confirmed by rising antibody titers of rubella-specific immunoglobulin M (IgM) molecules. If the infection occurs in the first trimester of pregnancy, congenital defects (cataracts, mental retardation, heart defects, deafness) are common. Therapy is symptomatic; vaccination of school-age children and women of childbearing age with low rubella titers is advisable.

Erythema infectiosum, also called fifth disease, is a viral disease usually seen in children. It is caused by a parvovirus. Pale, reticulated macules appear over the cheeks and extremities, sometimes accompanied by a low-grade fever, malaise, and pruritus of skin eruptions. The infection persists for 1 to 2 weeks, and no treatment is necessary.

Infectious mononucleosis is caused by the Epstein-Barr virus. The infection presents with malaise, fever, exudative pharyngitis, postauricular adenopathy, and hep-

atosplenomegaly. The cutaneous eruptions occur over the trunk as erythematous macules and papulovesicles. Patients with mononucleosis who receive ampicillin invariably develop erythematous, confluent, hemorrhagic macules, and therefore this therapy is contraindicated (Fig. 80-8).

An interesting infection caused by coxsackievirus A16 or enterovirus 71 is *hand-foot-and-mouth disease.* Multiple oval-shaped vesicles surrounded by erythema appear on the palms, fingers, soles, and mucous membranes of the mouth. The infection subsides within a week. It can be associated with low-grade fever, sore mouth and throat, and malaise. The infection resolves in 10 to 14 days. Only symptomatic therapy with oral acetaminophen-diphenhydramine elixir and topical lidocaine (Xylocaine Viscous) is given to patients.

FUNGAL SKIN INFECTIONS

Superficial fungal infections can involve the skin, hair, and nails. Fungal infections of the scalp and the skin are known as *ringworm infections.*

Most fungal infections in humans are caused by three genera of fungi: *Microsporum, Trichophyton,* and *Epidermophyton.* The fungi are transmitted from human to human (anthropophilic), from animal to human (zoophilic), or from soil to human (geophilic). A suspected fungal infection can be confirmed by microscopic examination of skin scrapings in a solution of potassium hydroxide (Fig. 80-9). Multiple hyphae can be found on microscopic examination of the skin scrapings of a patient with a fungus infection.

A fungal culture is done to identify the fungus responsible for the infection, to confirm a diagnosis, and to suggest a mode of transmission (Fig. 80-10).

Tinea capitis, or fungal infection of the scalp, is usually caused by *Trichophyton tonsurans* or *Microsporum canis. T. tonsurans* is transmitted by child-to-child contact and results in oval patches of hair loss. Individual hairs are broken at various lengths, and the scalp surface is scaly and crusted with discrete papules (Fig. 80-11). *M. canis* is usually transmitted from young kittens to children and causes inflammatory, purulent patches of hair loss. The patch is frequently crusted with multiple pustules and can result in permanent alopecia. Every patch of hair loss associated with scaly, crusted scalp should be suspected for a possible fungal infection. Inflammatory lesions can form large, tender, boggy masses called *kerions.* To confirm the diagnosis of tinea capitis, hairs are plucked, examined under a microscope after potassium hydroxide treatment, and cultured.

Tinea corporis is a fungal infection of the skin over the face, trunk, and extremities. Frequently a peripheral scale associated with erythema and pustules appears with a ringlike shape (Fig. 80-12). This infection can be con-

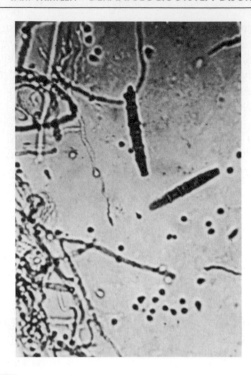

FIG. 80-9   Multiple hyphae and spores can be seen on microscopic examination of skin scrapings from a patient with superficial fungal infection of the skin.

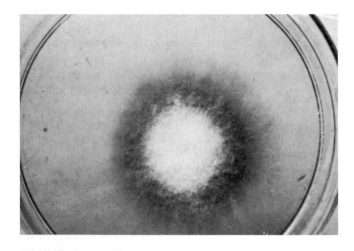

FIG. 80-10   *Trichophyton rubrum,* the most common cause of superficial fungal skin infection, as seen on fungal culture grown at room temperature.

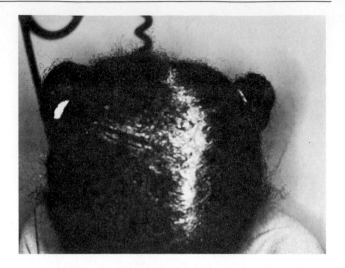

FIG. 80-11   Scaly patches of hair loss in a young child with tinea capitis.

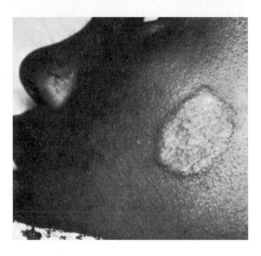

FIG. 80-12   Tinea corporis of the face, with peripheral scale and ringlike shape.

tracted from animals with *M. canis* or *Trichophyton mentagrophytes* and from humans with *Trichophyton rubrum.* The diagnosis is confirmed by potassium hydroxide examination and fungal culture.

Tinea cruris is a fungal infection of the groin. The infection is more frequent in males and is associated with severe pruritus and annular or arclike lesions with peripheral erythema and scale that frequently extends to the thighs. The scrotum is usually not involved. A common term for this infection is jock itch (Color plate 42).

Tinea pedis and *tinea manuum,* fungal infections of the feet and hands, are probably the most common fungal infections. *T. rubrum* causes scaly, erythematous patches on the soles and palms. Both feet and only one hand are frequently involved. *T. mentagrophytes* causes inflammatory, crusty, pustular eruptions on the feet. Tinea pedis, manuum, and cruris are confirmed by microscopic examination of potassium hydroxide–treated skin scrapings and fungal cultures.

Tinea barbae presents with scaly, crusted patches associated with pustules over the beard area. Large, verrucous nodules can appear, resembling kerion infection of the scalp. The infection usually results from exposure to cattle and is caused by *T. mentagrophytes.*

Fungal infection of the nails, *onychomycosis,* presents with dystrophic nails. The patient has subungual hyperkeratosis and separation of the nail plate from the nailbed (Fig. 80-13). The diagnosis is confirmed by fungal cul-

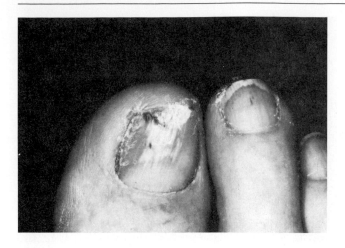

FIG. 80-13   Subungual hyperkeratosis and discoloration of the nail plate seen in onychomycosis.

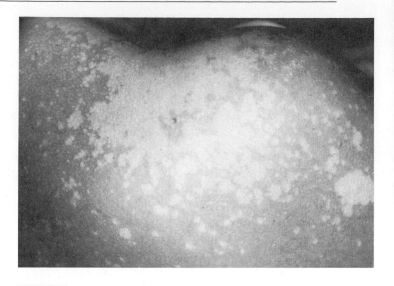

FIG. 80-14   Sharply marginated, scaly, hypopigmented patches of tinea versicolor are usually seen over the back.

tures and potassium hydroxide examination. This common fungal infection is extremely resistant to therapy and frequently recurs when treatment is discontinued.

Tinea versicolor is caused by *pityrosporum orbiculare.* Sharply marginated, scaly, white or brownish patches appear over the trunk, neck, and extremities (Fig. 80-14 and Color plate 43). The infection is more apparent in the summer. Microscopic examination of potassium hydroxide–treated scales confirms the diagnosis. Multiple short hyphae and spores are present.

Treatment

The usual treatment of tinea pedis, tinea cruris, and tinea corpuris is with topical antifungal agents, which include miconazole (Micatin), clotrimazole (Mycelex), ciclopirox olamine (Loprox), terbinaphine (Lamisil), oxiconazole (Oxistat), haloprogin (Halotex), and ketoconazole (Nizoral). These agents are used twice daily, generally for 1 month. Patients are also instructed in proper foot hygiene and told to wear loose-fitting cotton underwear and nonocclusive shoes. For prevention of infections, the useful agents available include undecylenic acid (Desenex) and tolnaftate (Tinactin).

Resistant infections of the feet and pruritic infections of the groin can also be treated with oral griseofulvin, an effective antifungal agent. Oral griseofulvin is also used for infections of the scalp and severe infections of the nails. The treatment is continued until the organisms are eradicated. Tinea capitis usually requires 4 to 6 weeks of 250 to 500 mg of griseofulvin daily; tinea corporis, 2 to 4 weeks; tinea pedis, 4 to 8 weeks; and tinea unguium, 6 to 12 months. It is important to note that this drug is phototoxic and interferes with the activity of such medications as warfarin and barbiturates. Bone marrow and liver toxicity occur extremely infrequently in patients who have no preexisting liver disease. The most common side effects from griseofulvin are headaches and gastrointestinal symptoms.

Ketoconazole is an oral agent approved for the treatment of serious systemic and skin fungal infections resistant to griseofulvin or for patients who develop side effects from griseofulvin. Serious liver disorders can complicate therapy with ketoconazole. Tinea versicolor is treated with selenium sulfide (Selsun shampoo) or ketoconazole (Nizoral shampoo), which is applied twice weekly to the affected areas for at least 60 minutes. Pigmentary changes secondary to tinea versicolor may persist for several months. Localized patches of tinea versicolor can be treated with topical Loprox, Mycelex, or Nizoral creams.

CANDIDIASIS

Candidiasis, a type of yeast infection, is caused by *Candida albicans.* The organism is normally present in the gastrointestinal tract, but it can cause an opportunistic infection (see Chapter 6). Persons who are obese, have diabetes mellitus, or are taking broad-spectrum antibiotics (tetracycline) or corticosteroids can develop the cutaneous infection. In the groin and intertriginous areas, candidiasis presents with erythema, whitish pseudomembrane, and peripheral papules and pustules (Fig. 80-15 and Color plate 44). The infection frequently occurs in infants and obese patients. *Candida* infection of the paronychial area causes swelling, erythema, and pus formation. *Candida* of the mouth, or *thrush,* presents with a white coating of the tongue and occasional macerated, fissured patches in the corner of the mouth. Disseminated candidiasis can be a life-threatening infection in immunocompromised patients with leukemia, cancer, or acquired immunodeficiency syndrome (AIDS). This systemic candidiasis can cause candidal meningitis, endo-

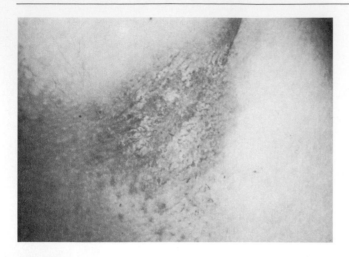

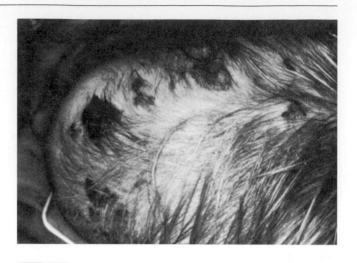

FIG. 80-15   Plaque of candidiasis in the axilla with a whitish pseudomembrane and peripheral papules.

FIG. 80-16   Crusted, eroded patches of impetigo on the scalp.

carditis, or septicemia. Diagnosis of *Candida* infection is confirmed by a microscopic examination of a potassium hydroxide–treated skin scraping and culture.

Treatment consists of removing predisposing factors. Cutaneous *Candida* infections are treated with oral or topical nystatin, topical miconazole, topical clotrimazole, or amphotericin cream. These medications are also used for vaginal candidiasis. Systemic infection is treated by intravenous amphotericin B. An oral medication, ketoconazole (Nizoral), is also effective in treatment of systemic candidiasis.

CUTANEOUS BACTERIAL INFECTIONS

Impetigo is the most common bacterial infection of the skin. It is caused by streptococci and staphylococci. The infection is frequently transferred by human-to-human contact, usually among children. Hot, humid temperatures and poor hygiene predispose one to this infection. Cuts, insect bites, and abrasions are sometimes complicated by impetigo. Patients with eczema occasionally develop impetigo secondary to excoriations of pruritic skin lesions. Impetigo begins as a purulent vesicle. As the lesion spreads, it becomes eroded and a golden crust develops on the surface (Fig. 80-16 and Color plate 45). The infection usually starts on the face and extremities but can spread to any surface of the body. In fewer than 1% of cases, poststreptococcal glomerulonephritis can develop.

Treatment should include instructions in proper hygienic techniques to control spread of the infection. Topical antibiotics (polymixin, neomycin, bacitracin) and antiseptics (Betadine) are used. Mupirocin (Bactroban) ointment used topically three times a day is the most ef-

fective topical agent for impetigo now available. Oral penicillin or erythromycin therapy is indicated when large or multiple lesions are present. This can prevent the incidence of poststreptococcal glomerular nephritis, especially in children. Impetigo usually heals without scar formation.

Cellulitis is a streptococcal infection that presents with spreading areas of erythema, fever, and lymphangitis. Oral penicillin is the treatment of choice.

Erysipelas is a serious, toxic, streptococcal infection of the skin. The lesions are brightly erythematous, sharply marginated, and tender. Bullae are hemorrhaged and may be seen within the inflamed skin (Color plate 46). They frequently occur over the face or extremities. The patient has high fever and malaise and is toxic. Regional lymph nodes are enlarged. Complications such as endocarditis and septicemia may result. Patients with erysipelas are usually hospitalized and treated with intravenous penicillin. Occasionally, prolonged treatment is required to eradicate the infection. Repeated episodes of erysipelas may produce lymphedema and predispose to further infections.

Erythrasma causes erythematous, dry, scaly patches in the intertriginous areas. It is caused by *Corynebacterium minutissimum.* The infection is most often seen in obese individuals and can be confirmed by a characteristic coral-red fluorescence under a Wood's light examination. Erythrasma is usually treated with topical antibiotics (clindamycin), but systemic erythromycin is also effective.

Trichomycosis axillaris is an infection of the axillary hair and rarely the pubic hair. Yellow, red, or black concretions form on the hair (Fig. 80-17). The infection is asymptomatic and not contagious. Patients report an abnormal coloring of sweat and possibly an axillary odor. *Corynebacterium* species isolated from these infections can be treated by topical applications of antibiotics (e.g.,

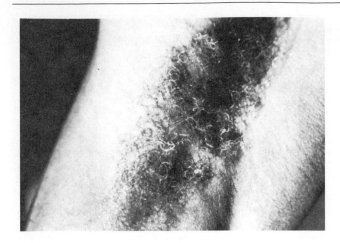

FIG. 80-17   Trichomycosis axillaris with yellow concretions on the hair.

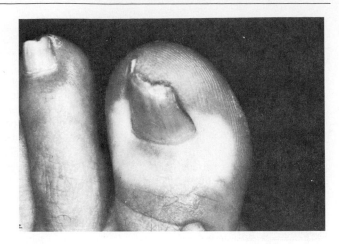

FIG. 80-18   Swollen, painful toe secondary to bacterial paronychia. The whitish area contains purulent material.

erythromycin) or by shaving the hair from the affected areas.

Superficial folliculitis, caused by staphylococci, presents with small pustules surrounded by erythema found at the opening of hair follicles. The scalp and extremities are the usual sites. Poor hygiene practices, maceration, and excoriations are the predisposing factors of this infection. Treatment is with antibacterial soaps (e.g., pHisoHex) and, occasionally, systemic antibiotics. *Recurrent chronic folliculitis* can be difficult to eradicate and may require systemic antibiotics after specimens for appropriate bacterial cultures and sensitivity studies are obtained.

Hot tub folliculitis is seen in patients exposed to inadequately disinfected whirlpools and hot tubs. These eruptions are usually localized to bathing trunk areas and are caused by *Pseudomonas aeruginosa.* Ciprofloxacin (Cipro) is effective treatment of this infection. Deep staphylococcal infections are responsible for furuncles (boils) and carbuncles (multiple confluent furuncles). Deep-seated, erythematous, tender nodules frequently occur over the buttocks, neck, and axillae. The nodules become fluctuant in a few days and discharge a purulent, necrotic material. Furuncles can be painful when located in the nasal area, axillae, or ears. They are treated with surgical draining, hot, wet dressings, and appropriate systemic antibiotics. The antibiotics are selected after aerobic and anaerobic cultures and sensitivity studies are performed.

Infection of the nail fold with staphylococci and streptococci can lead to a painful infection called *paronychia.* The infection can follow a hangnail and is common among individuals whose hands are frequently immersed in water. The nail folds are erythematous, swollen, and painful in this infection (Fig. 80-18). Because paronychia can also be caused by *Candida,* fungal cultures are required to confirm the disease. Acute bacterial paronychia is treated with systemic antibiotics, and localized pus is drained. Chronic paronychia is treated by avoidance of prolonged exposure to water. Broad-spectrum topical antibacterial and antifungal solutions such as clotrimazole (Mycelex) or mupirocin (Bactroban) can be used.

QUESTIONS

▼ *Circle the letter preceding each item below that correctly answers the question or completes the statement. More than one answer may be correct.*

1. The etiology of verrucae (warts) and herpes simplex is similar. The causative agent is:
   a. *Candida albicans*
   b. DNA virus
   c. RNA virus
   d. Bacteria

2. Untreated warts over the finger area:
   a. Persist indefinitely
   b. Invade the dermis
   c. Usually disappear spontaneously in 2 to 5 years
   d. Are not infectious

3. Ms. P., 55 years of age, presented with a series of many small, painful vesicles appearing on an edematous, hemorrhagic area of the skin on her trunk. These inflammatory vesicles appeared unilaterally along a single dermatome, starting at its origin on the back and continuing to her midline. Her history revealed chickenpox as a child. You would suspect which of the following?
   a. Herpes simplex
   b. Herpes zoster
   c. Molluscum contagiosum
   d. Rubeola

Continued.

QUESTIONS—cont'd

4. Herpes zoster is usually self-limiting and lasts:
   a. 3 to 4 days
   b. 3 to 4 weeks
   c. 1 to 2 months
   d. 3 to 4 months

5. A highly effective vaccine is used to control which of the following?
   a. Herpes simplex
   b. Rubella
   c. Verrucae
   d. Infectious mononucleosis

6. The usual mode of transmission of type II herpes simplex is by:
   a. Use of common towels
   b. Kissing and touching
   c. Sexual encounters
   d. Contaminated drinking water

7. The recurrence rate of herpes type I infections is approximately what percent?
   a. 10
   b. 14
   c. 50
   d. 80

8. The percentage (or number) of sexually active individuals who have had type II herpes simplex is estimated to be:
   a. 5 (5 million)
   b. 10 (10 million)
   c. 20 (20 million)
   d. 50 (50 million)

▼ Circle T if the statement is true and F if it is false. Correct any false statements.

9. T F Tinea versicolor is characterized by white scaly patches over the trunk, neck, and extremities.

10. T F Candidiasis can be treated with nystatin.

11. T F Candida albicans is a type of yeast that causes skin infections.

12. T F Erysipelas is a serious, toxic, streptococcal infection of the skin.

13. T F Impetigo is a viral infection.

14. T F Human papillomavirus is associated with 85% of cervical squamous cell cancers in women.

▼ Answer the following on a separate sheet of paper.

15. Describe the two tests used to attempt to confirm the diagnosis of herpes simplex.

16. What are the therapeutic measures that can be used in an attempt to prevent recurrent infections of cutaneous herpes infections?

17. Describe the serious complications associated with herpes simplex infection of the eye.

18. Describe the lesion characteristic of impetigo.

19. Contrast impetigo and erysipelas as to etiologic agent and pathogenesis.

20. State the predisposing factors associated with superficial folliculitis.

21. Describe the treatment for herpes zoster.

CHAPTER 81

Tumors of the Skin

MAREK A. STAWISKI
SYLVIA A. PRICE

Cutaneous tumors can derive from various cell types in the skin, such as epidermal cells and melanocytes. These tumors can be benign or malignant and either localized in the epidermis or invasive to the dermis and subcutaneous tissue.

MALIGNANT SKIN TUMORS

Basal Cell Carcinoma

Basal cell carcinoma is the most common malignant tumor of the skin. Approximately 500,000 new cases are diagnosed in the United States each year. It arises from epidermal cells along the basal layer of the epidermis. The incidence of basal cell carcinoma is directly proportional to the age of the patient and inversely proportional to the amount of melanin pigment in the epidermis. A direct correlation also exists between this condition and the total lifetime exposure to sunlight. About 80% of basal cell cancers occur on the sun-exposed areas of the face, head, and neck. Fortunately, the tumor rarely metastasizes.

However, a patient with a single basal cell cancer is likely to develop future skin cancers and must be followed indefinitely on an annual basis.

The carcinogenic range in the solar spectrum lies primarily between 280 and 320 nm. This spectrum is primarily responsible for burning of the skin exposed to the sun. Sunscreens, sun blocks, and avoidance of excessive sunlight exposure are recommended for patients with a family history of skin cancer and for fair-skinned individuals who have a tendency to sunburn easily. Also, patients with a history of basal cell carcinoma should use sunscreens or protective clothing to avoid carcinogenic sun rays. Most sunscreens contain *para*-aminobenzoic acid, which absorbs the carcinogenic rays.

Other causes of basal cell carcinoma include previous radiologic therapy of other skin disorders, contact with arsenic, and rare genetic disorders (xeroderma pigmentosum, nevoid basal cell carcinoma syndrome). The long ultraviolet light (UVA) in suntanning booths also damages the epidermis and is considered to be carcinogenic.

The tumor is characterized by an erythematous, smooth, pearly nodule (Fig. 81-1). The borders are frequently elevated and have telangiectatic vessels on the surface. Central ulceration and bleeding are frequently observed (Fig. 81-2 and Color plate 47). The tumor bleeds frequently, invades the dermis, and destroys normal tissue.

Basal cell carcinoma should be treated promptly. Treatments include curettage with electrodesiccation, scalpel surgery, irradiation, chemosurgery, and cryosurgery. A small basal cell cancer less than 2 cm in diameter is usually treated with scalpel excision or electrodessication and curettage after biopsy is obtained to confirm the diagnosis. The cure rate is about 95%. Roentgen therapy may be used in patients over age 60 to 70 years who have very large tumors around the eyelids, earlobes, or lips. Chemosurgery is useful in the treatment of large, infiltrating, and recurrent cancers, especially around the ears, nasolabial folds, and eyes. In chemosurgery, the microscopic excision of the tumor is accomplished by removing layer by layer with a scalpel; frozen sections are prepared, and a map of the tumor is constructed; then the un-

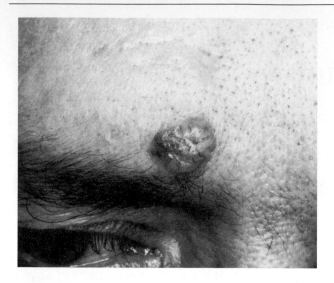

FIG. 81-1   A smooth, pearly nodule of early basal cell carcinoma.

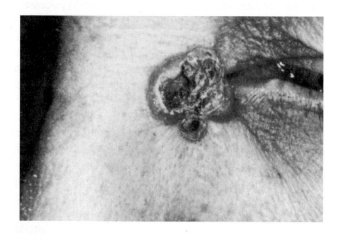

FIG. 81-2   Ulcerated tumor with elevated smooth borders in a patient with advanced basal cell carcinoma.

dersurface of each removed frozen section is examined for evidence of basal cell cancer. This is the most tedious, effective, and expensive technique, but it has a cure rate of more than 97%. Cryosurgery uses liquid nitrogen, and the cure rate is similar to that for electrodesiccation and curettage.

Squamous Cell Carcinoma

Squamous cell carcinoma is a malignant neoplasm of keratinocytes. It arises from more differentiated cells of epidermis (keratinocytes). Frequently the tumor is seen in older, fair-skinned individuals. Typically it arises on sun-damaged skin with multiple actinic keratoses present. Sunlight is the main etiologic factor causing squamous cell carcinoma of the skin. As in basal cell carcinoma,

sunlight in the ultraviolet light (UV) spectrum between 280 and 320 nm (UVB spectrum) is responsible. However, recent cooperative studies on the use of long ultraviolet light, between 320 and 400 nm (UVA spectrum), combined with oral psoralen in treatment of psoriasis have demonstrated that prolonged, chronic exposure to UVA with psoralen can also produce squamous cell carcinoma.

Fair-skinned persons of Celtic origin who are chronically exposed to the sunlight (e.g., farmers, sailors) have a high incidence of squamous cell carcinomas. Both basal cell carcinomas and squamous cell carcinomas are much more common in sunbelt areas of the United States than in midwest or northeast areas. The incidence of skin squamous cell carcinoma and basal cell carcinoma in African Americans is extremely low.

Other causes of squamous cell carcinoma include ingestion of arsenic, x-ray irradiation, burns, scars, and genetic susceptibility. Patients who were treated for acne or hemangiomas with radiologic therapy many years ago can develop basal cell cancers and squamous cell cancers. Those individuals who 50 years ago were treated with arsenic for psoriasis or asthma, ingested arsenic in their drinking water, or inhaled it in smelting plants have a tendency to develop squamous cell carcinomas. A few rare genetic diseases (albinism, xeroderma pigmentosum) also predispose individuals to these cancers. Excessive use of suntanning booths will likely lead to an increased incidence of squamous cell carcinoma in future years.

Squamous cell carcinomas that arise in sun-damaged skin usually do not metastasize and rarely cause death. Squamous cell cancers arising on areas not exposed to the sun (lips, buttocks, groin), after ingestion of arsenic, or on an old scar have the greatest risk of metastasis. Squamous cell carcinoma that occurs on areas not exposed to the sun can be a cutaneous marker of internal malignancy. Once it is diagnosed, a thorough history and physical examination are required.

A variant of squamous cell carcinoma is localized to the epidermis and is called *Bowen's disease.* Bowen's disease is usually caused by chronic sun exposure. It can also be caused by ingestion of arsenic. Some sources believe that there is an increased incidence of internal malignancies with this tumor. Patients with Bowen's disease should undergo a workup, including a complete history and physical examination, if this cancer occurs on areas not exposed to the sun.

Squamous cell carcinoma presents with an ulcerated, scaly, thickened nodule or tumor that bleeds occasionally (Fig. 81-3 and Color plate 48). The nodules usually arise on sun-damaged skin of the face, scalp, ears, neck, hands, or forearms. Frequently they are surrounded by multiple actinic keratoses, many of which, if left untreated, would degenerate into squamous cell cancers. Bowen's disease presents as an erythematous plaque with undulating borders, scaliness, and frequently central erosion. It can be

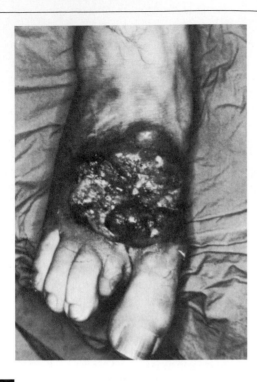

FIG. 81-3   Verrucous, ulcerated tumor of squamous cell carcinoma after radiographic therapy to the foot.

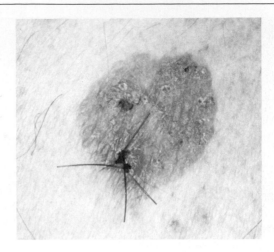

FIG. 81-4   Undulating borders and central erosion of a plaque in Bowen's disease.

indistinguishable from eczema or psoriasis (Fig. 81-4 and Color plate 49). A longstanding lesion of psoriasis or eczema unresponsive to appropriate therapy should therefore be biopsied.

The treatment of squamous cell carcinoma and its variant, Bowen's disease, is primarily surgical excision. Radiation therapy, cryosurgery, and chemosurgery have cure rates of 95% to 98%. The lymph nodes are not removed if they are clinically negative, but they should be carefully palpated during the surgical procedure. Metastatic lesions of squamous cell carcinoma do not respond well to chemotherapy. As with basal cell carcinoma patients, those with squamous cell carcinomas must be followed indefinitely, since there is a high risk for development of new squamous cell carcinomas. The lymph nodes are palpated during these follow-up visits. Of these patients, 20% to 50% with one squamous cell carcinoma eventually develop another squamous cell carcinoma or basal cell carcinoma.

Melanoma

Malignant melanoma makes up only 3% of all primary cutaneous malignancies but is responsible for almost all the deaths secondary to skin cancers. Furthermore, the incidence of melanoma is increasing. Early diagnosis and surgical treatment are the only ways to ensure long-term survival and even cure. Unless recognized and treated early, melanomas invade deeper layers of the dermis and the subcutaneous tissues and metastasize to distant sites.

Most melanomas occur in the 40- to 70-year age-group, but the number of cases has increased among the 20- to 40-year age-group. One of the explanations for this increased incidence is a greater sun exposure secondary to recreation and attire changes. Further evidence for the role of UV light in causing melanomas is the increased frequency of this tumor in sunbelt states. The mode of inheritance of melanomas is undetermined, and only a small percentage of melanoma patients (about 2%) have a family history of melanoma. However, all family members should be examined by an experienced dermatologist for atypical nevi. Atypical nevi in individuals with a family history of melanomas should be removed, since they can degenerate to malignant melanomas. Large congenital nevi give rise to malignant melanomas in 2% to 13% of patients, and these should be surgically excised.

Diagnosis is based on the change in shape, color, size, and configuration of a pigmented lesion. Irregular pigmentation with shades of blue, purple, red, and brown should alert the examiner. The borders of this tumor are irregular, and the surface is frequently ulcerated (Fig. 81-5). The lesion is asymmetric and is frequently greater than 6 mm in diameter. Satellite lesions and diffusion of pigment into the surrounding skin are also observed (Fig. 81-6 and Color plate 50). Clinical manifestations of early melanoma can be remembered by four rules of appearance of this tumor: A, asymmetry of lesion; B, border irregularity; C, color variegation; and D, diameter greater than 6 mm.

The superficial spreading melanoma is the most common type (60% to 80%) and has the best prognosis. It presents as a flat growth with bizarre colors and configuration (Fig. 81-6). The nodular melanoma is less common (20%) and presents as a tumor (Fig. 81-7). This variant has the worst prognosis. The lentigo maligna melanoma arises on a preexisting, irregularly pigmented, brown

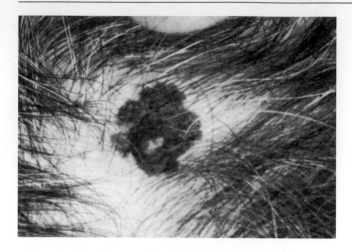

FIG. 81-5 Irregular borders, uneven pigmentation, and ulceration in a superficial, spreading malignant melanoma.

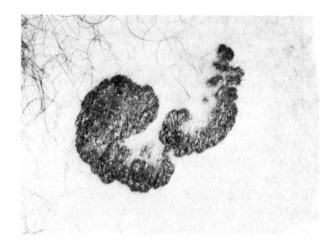

FIG. 81-6 Irregular borders in a superficial, spreading malignant melanoma.

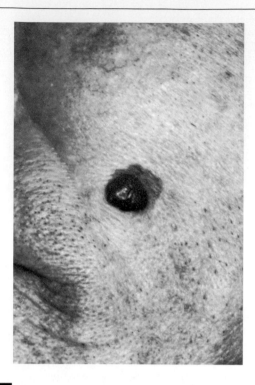

FIG. 81-7 Nodule with diffusion of pigment in nodular malignant melanoma.

patch (lentigo maligna) (Color plate 51). This tumor is even less common (5% to 10%) and, if detected early, has a good prognosis.

The prognosis for patients with malignant melanoma is not as poor as once thought. The great majority of patients survive for 5 years or more, and many are cured. Early diagnosis and surgical treatment are responsible for these improved statistics. Several factors determine the survival of melanoma patients. Patients with superficial spreading melanoma have the best prognosis, followed by lentigo maligna melanoma; nodular melanoma has the worst prognosis. Lesions located over the head, neck, trunk, hands, and feet in patients over age 50 and in males have a worse prognosis. Clinical ulceration of the tumor carries a poor prognosis. Histologic levels of primary ma-

lignant melanoma invasion of the dermis, as defined by Clark, determine prognosis: the best survival rates are seen with levels I and II melanomas, confined to the epidermis and upper dermis; intermediate survival rates are seen with levels III and IV, extending to the lower dermis; and the worst rates are seen with level V, invading the subcutaneous tissue. Breslow was able to correlate vertical tumor thickness with prognosis of malignant melanomas; melanomas less than 1 mm in thickness do not usually metastasize if removed locally, melanomas between 1 and 2 mm in thickness can develop metastasis, and tumors greater than 2 mm are likely to metastasize.

The treatment of malignant melanoma is primarily surgical. Controversy exists over whether levels I, II, and III melanomas should be widely excised. Many authorities believe that a narrow excision with 1 to 2 cm margins is adequate. Levels IV and V melanomas should receive a wide excision and possible elective regional lymph node dissection, if feasible. Patients with disseminated melanomas receive chemotherapy using dacarbazine (DTIC) with alpha-interferons. Intensive melphalan or carmustine therapy combined with autologous bone marrow transplantation can sometimes result in remission. Immunotherapy using interleukin-2 to expand T cells with antitumor reactivity may induce response of the tumor. Unfortunately, disseminated melanoma has a 1-year mortality as high as 83%. The most effective treatments of melanoma remain early detection and aggressive surgical removal.

BENIGN SKIN TUMORS

Acquired nevi, or *moles,* are the most common tumors derived from the melanocyte. The melanin pigment produces a uniform brown, dark-brown, light-brown, or blue color in flat or elevated nevi (Fig. 81-8 and Color plate 52). Flat nevi do not infiltrate the dermis and can occur anywhere on the body. Nevi are rarely excised unless they become irritated, bleed, grow rapidly, or change in appearance. Acquired nevi appear between the ages of childhood and 25 years. The lesions become flatter with age and disappear in older age (80 to 90 years).

The *compound nevus* is an elevated nodule, usually brown in color. It is elevated because melanocytes are found in the dermis. It is also composed of melanocytes in the epidermis and can occur anywhere on the body. Surgical excision is not necessary unless it is irritated by clothing or is cosmetically unattractive (Fig. 81-9).

Large nevi present at birth are called *giant congenital nevi* (Fig. 81-10). Because melanomas can arise in giant congenital nevi, they should be excised by surgical removal down to the layer of subcutaneous fat. Regrowth of the nevus will occur if this is not done. The skin should be replaced with grafts if necessary.

Large nevi greater than 6 mm in diameter with irregular color, borders, configuration, and atypical histologic appearance are called *dysplastic nevi* (Fig. 81-11). An individual who has such nevi and a family history of melanoma is at high risk for developing melanoma. He or she should be examined by a physician every 3 to 6 months, avoid sun exposure, use sunscreens when playing or working outside, and self-examine the skin every few weeks. At least some of these nevi should be biopsied. Nevi in patients with dysplastic nevi and a family

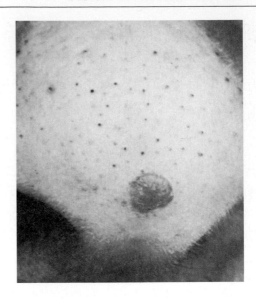

FIG. 81-9   Brownish, elevated papule with uniform color and no history of recent change is typical of a benign compound nevus.

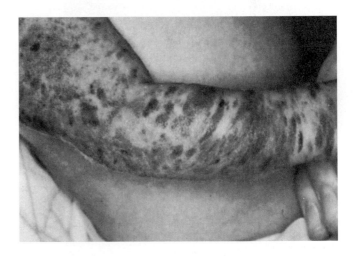

FIG. 81-10   Giant pigmented nevus present at birth has an increased incidence of progression to a melanoma.

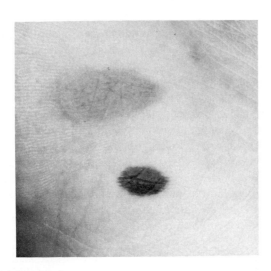

FIG. 81- 8   Dark-brown, flat macules with uniform pigment; no skin ulceration; and no history of recent change are typical of benign junctional nevi.

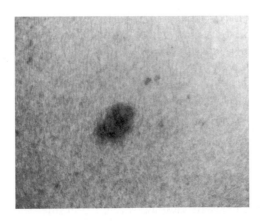

FIG. 81-11   A large nevus with irregular surface, color, and configuration typical of dysplastic nevus.

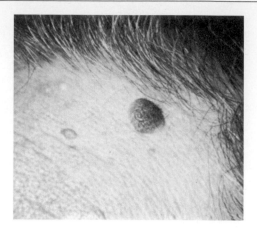

FIG. 81-12   Verrucous, superficial nodule of seborrheic kerato-sis, which appears to be glued to the surface.

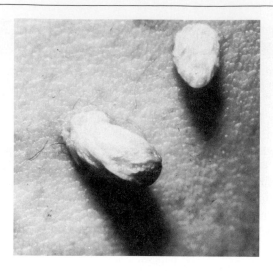

FIG. 81-14   Pedunculated, filiform lesions of acrochordons over the neck.

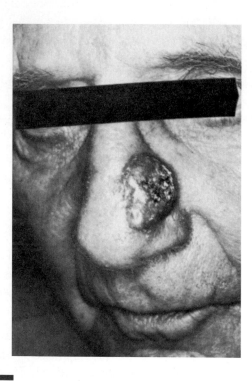

FIG. 81-13   Rapidly growing, dome-shaped tumor with central keratotic crater is a benign keratoacanthoma.

history of melanoma should be biopsied if a change in color, shape, or size is noted.

Seborrheic Keratosis

Seborrheic keratosis manifests as a verrucous, brown growth that appears to be glued to the surface of the epidermis (Fig. 81-12). The cause of this benign tumor is unknown. The tumor cells are derived from small basal cells localized in the epidermis. Older patients develop multiple seborrheic keratoses over the trunk, face, and upper

extremities. Treatment is not necessary except for cosmetic or diagnostic reasons.

Actinic Keratosis

Actinic keratosis usually occurs on the sun-exposed areas of the face, neck, scalp, and extremities. It appears as an erythematous, scaly, rough surface lesion (Color plate 53). The lesion is caused by chronic exposure to sun, particularly in older patients. This premalignant growth can develop into squamous cell carcinoma and should be treated. Treatment measures include electrodesiccation with curettage or cryosurgery. Patients are warned about future exposure to the sun and instructed in the use of sunscreens. Sunscreens that block UV_1B and UVA light with a protection factor of 15 or 30 are recommended (UVA-Guard, Neutrogena, Solbar). Also effective in the treatment of actinic keratosis is 1% to 5% topical 5-fluorouracil applied daily for 30 days.

Keratoacanthoma

Keratoacanthoma is a dome-shaped tumor with a central keratotic crater or ulceration (Fig. 81-13). The tumor grows rapidly over a few months and usually occurs in fair-skinned, older persons. The tumor is benign and may undergo spontaneous involution. Because the tumor can resemble squamous cell carcinoma, it should be excised and examined by a histopathologist.

Dermatofibroma, Acrochordon, and Keloid

Three common benign tumors are dermatofibromas, acrochordons (skin tags), and keloids. *Dermatofibroma* is a brown nodule usually found on the legs, the trunk, or

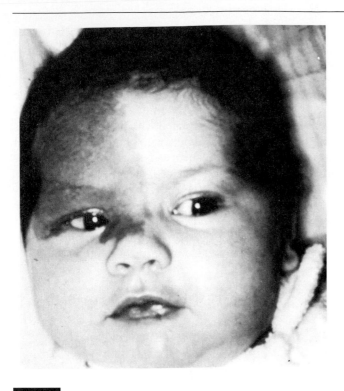

FIG. 81-15   Proliferation of capillaries causes a pink skin discoloration known as *nevus flammeus* or *capillary hemangioma*.

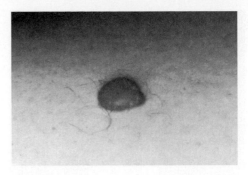

FIG. 81-17   Elevated, erythematous papule of cherry angioma.

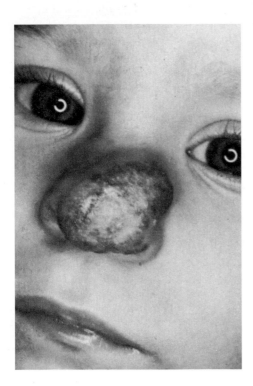

FIG. 81-16   Strawberry angioma presents with an elevated, erythematous tumor, shown here over the nose.

the arms. On palpation it has a hard buttonlike consistency. The tumor is excised only for cosmetic or diagnostic reasons, since it is benign. *Skin tags (acrochordons)* are common over the neck, axilla, and groin of middle-age and older persons (Fig. 81-14). Acrochordons are more common in obese patients and in pregnant women. They are excised if associated with pain and for cosmetic reasons. *Keloids* are caused by an abnormal scar formation after even a minor injury (see Fig. 77-5). They are more common in African Americans, and the tendency to form them is genetic. Surgical excision of keloids may be attempted for cosmetic reasons. Excision of keloids in combination with injection of corticosteroids into the lesions is frequently an effective treatment.

Benign Tumors of Blood Vessels

Among the numerous tumors of blood vessels of the skin, the most frequently encountered are nevus flammeus, strawberry angioma, cherry angioma, spider angioma, and pyogenic granuloma.

Proliferation of mature capillaries producing a pink discoloration of the skin on newborns is called *nevus flammeus* (Fig. 81-15). When the capillaries follow a branch of the trigeminal nerve, the condition has been associated with angioma of the ipsilateral eye and the central nervous system *(Sturge-Weber syndrome)*. This can lead to glaucoma and contralateral seizures. Nevus flammeus can fade or persist indefinitely. If the lesion persists, a cover-up makeup (e.g., Covermark) is recommended. The pulsed, tunable dye laser has been useful in treatment of these hemangiomas.

Strawberry angioma arises after birth and involutes spontaneously by age 7 in 70% to 95% of cases. Proliferating capillaries in the dermis cause an elevated bluish red nodule (Fig. 81-16 and Color plate 54), usually on the head or upper trunk, but it can occur anywhere on the body's surface. Because most of these tumors involute spontaneously, no treatment is usually required.

Cherry angiomas are red, slightly elevated papules

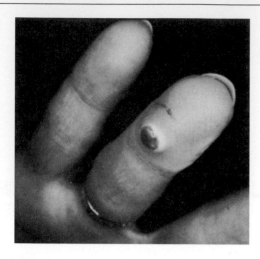

over the trunk and extremities of middle-age and older persons (Fig. 81-17). They are asymptomatic and benign, and treatment is not necessary.

Spider angiomas appear in women during pregnancy, in alcoholics, and also in children. A central arteriole feeds multiple small branches of this tumor. Multiple spider angiomas can be associated with liver disease such as cirrhosis. Most spider angiomas in children and pregnant women resolve spontaneously. Persistent spider angiomas can be electrodesiccated.

Pyogenic granuloma is caused by an abnormal proliferation of granulation tissue. The tumor occurs after trauma to the site. A red or purple, pedunculated, moist nodule appears (Fig. 81-18). This benign tumor bleeds occasionally and is treated by surgical removal.

FIG. 81-18   Pedunculated, red, moist nodule of pyogenic granuloma of the finger.

QUESTIONS

▼ *Answer the following on a separate sheet of paper.*

1. Describe the characteristic appearance of malignant melanoma.
2. What are the predisposing factors and common sites of occurrence of basal cell carcinoma?
3. Discuss the preventive measures recommended for patients with a family history of melanoma or dysplastic nevi and for fair-skinned individuals.
4. What is the usual treatment of basal cell carcinoma?
5. Describe the causes, pathogenesis, type of lesion, and treatment of squamous cell carcinoma.

▼ *Circle the letter preceding each item below that correctly answers the question or completes the statement. More than one answer may be correct.*

6. Carcinogenic sun rays in the solar spectrum occur primarily in what nm range (UVB spectrum)?
   a. 50 to 100
   b. 100 to 150
   c. 175 to 200
   d. 280 to 320
7. Cutaneous tumors are derived from which of the following skin cell types?
   a. Fibroblasts
   b. Melanocytes
   c. Epidermal cells

8. The classic presentation of squamous cell carcinoma of the skin is:
   a. Irregular pigmentation with shades of blue and purple
   b. Ulcerated, hyperkeratotic nodules with evidence of dermal invasion on palpation
   c. A smooth, pearly appearance with multiple telangiectases
9. The natural history of untreated basal cell carcinoma is characterized by:
   a. Involvement of regional lymphatics
   b. An ulcerated tumor
   c. Gradual local enlargement
   d. Metastasis
10. A benign, verrucous, flat lesion frequently found in older persons that appears to be glued to the skin surface is called:

    a. Melanoma
    b. Urticaria
    c. Seborrheic keratosis
    d. Psoriasis
11. Mr. M., 47 years old, a construction worker, presents with several lesions many months in duration on his forearm. Examination reveals erythematous, ulcerated plaques with undulating borders. A biopsy is negative for psoriasis and eczema. The most likely condition is:
    a. Melanoma
    b. Basal cell carcinoma
    c. Seborrheic keratosis
    d. Bowen's disease

▼ *Match the type of tumor in column A with the appropriate letter in column B.*

Column A	Column B
12. _____ Flat nevi	a. Elevated, nodular, usually brown in color, composed of melanocytes in the epidermis and dermis
13. _____ Compound nevi	b. Caused by abnormal scar formation after injury
14. _____ Giant congenital nevi	c. Sharply marginated, caused by proliferation of melanocytes, characterized by uniform pigment, flat in appearance
15. _____ Keloids	d. Arising after birth, involuting spontaneously in 70% to 95% of all patients
16. _____ Strawberry angiomas	e. Treated by surgical removal of nevi to the subcutaneous layer
	f. Do not infiltrate the dermis

CHAPTER 82

Lyme Disease and Infestations

MAREK A. STAWISKI
SYLVIA A. PRICE

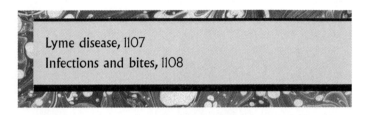

LYME DISEASE

Lyme disease is the most common anthropod-borne infection in the United States. More than 15,000 cases in 39 states have been reported to the Centers for Disease Control and Prevention since its initial description in 1975. The disease is caused by the spirochete *Borrelia burgdorferi*. The spirochetes are found in the guts of the tick *Ixodes dammini*. It appears that white-tailed deer and white-footed mice are the main reservoirs of this disease-causing spirochete. The spirochete is injected into the bloodstream through saliva and regurgitated contents from the gut of infected ticks. Lyme disease seems to be endemic and occurs chiefly in the United States along the northeastern coast (Connecticut, Massachusetts, Rhode Island, New York), in the middle west (Minnesota, Wisconsin), and in the west (California, Oregon, Utah, Nevada).

The disease has three clinical stages. *Stage I* usually occurs in the summer and early fall with single or multiple lesions of *erythema chronicum migrans* (ECM) and is frequently accompanied by flu-like symptoms (fatigue, headache, chills, fever, sore throat, stiff neck, nausea, myalgias, arthralgias). ECM begins as an erythematous papule where the tick bite occurred. The papule expands with central clearing, measuring up to 25 to 50 mm in diameter (Fig. 82-1). It usually disappears spontaneously without therapy within 1 month. The lesion may itch, sting, or burn. The thighs, groin, and axillae are particularly common sites of involvement.

ECM is the most characteristic early sign of the disease and occurs in 80% of patients. A history of a tick bite is obtained in only 60% of patients.

Patients who are not treated can enter stage II of the disease. *Stage II* Lyme disease occurs weeks to months later. It is characterized by the triad of meningitis, cranial nerve palsies, and peripheral neuropathy. Fewer than 10% of patients experience cardiac manifestations.

In *stage III, oligoarticular arthritis* occurs from 6 weeks to several years after the tick bite. Fifty percent of patients who were not treated in stages I and II will evolve to this stage. Recurrences are common, and patients may develop a chronic erosive arthritis.

Laboratory diagnosis is not completely accurate in diagnosis of Lyme disease. *B. burgdorferi* cannot be readily isolated from blood or skin biopsies. The diagnosis can be confirmed by two serologic tests: indirect immunofluorescence assay (IFA) or enzyme-linked immunosorbent assay (ELISA). Both tests are poorly stan-

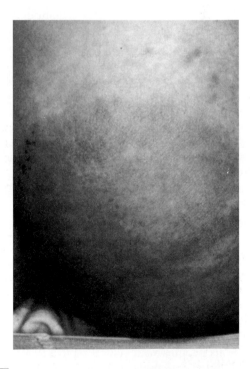

FIG. 82-1 An enlarging erythematous patch with central clearing, typical of erythema chronicum migrans.

dardized, and false-negative and false-positive results can occur.

Early Lyme disease is treated with doxycycline or amoxicillin or erythromycin for 10 to 21 days. Neurologic disease, arthritis, or cardiac disease is treated with doxycycline or amoxicillin for 1 month or intravenous penicillin for 10 to 14 days.

Lyme disease caused by the spirochete *B. burgdorferi* causes a multisystem disease affecting the skin, nervous system, heart, and musculoskeletal system. Early recognition of the symptoms and characteristic lesions of ECM should lead to early treatment and cure.

INFECTIONS AND BITES

Scabies is a common infestation caused by the mite *Sarcoptes scabiei*. It is transmitted by close human contact. The infection is especially common among children and sexually active adults. The incubation period may vary from 3 days to 3 weeks. Pruritus is the chief complaint of these patients. Excoriated linear papules and vesicles are classically found between the fingers and over the elbows, wrists, breasts, and genitalia (Fig. 82-2). Scabies must be suspected if one or more family members develop nocturnal pruritus. The diagnosis is confirmed by microscopic demonstration of the female mite or hatching larvae from a skin scraping (Fig. 82-3). Occasionally the microscopic examination is negative for scabies. Treatment consists of application of gamma benzene hexachloride (Kwell) or 5% permethrin cream (Elimite) for two 12-hour periods. Secondary irritant eczema can complicate the treatment and result in persistence of pruritus. All family members must be treated prophylactically overnight with gamma benzene hexachloride or permethrin, even if they present no evidence of scabietic lesions or pruritus.

Pediculosis pubis (pubic crabs) is a frequent infection of the pubic hair and skin. The infection is transmitted by human contact. Lice and nits, which attach to the pubic hair and can be seen with the naked eye, cause intense pruritus (Fig. 82-4). *Pediculosis capitis* (head lice) is caused by lice transmitted from person to person and can often cause epidemics, particularly in schools. Pruritus usually is the only complaint. Kwell shampoo or pyrethrins (RID) shampoo is the treatment of choice for both types of louse infestations. Patients are instructed to apply the shampoo two times. Nits may also be removed with a fine-toothed comb soaked in vinegar.

Flea bites are caused by animal fleas that live on pets and furniture, carpeting, and so forth. A flea bites a person and then leaves the skin; the usual result is a group of erythematous papules with central puncta that are localized to the lower extremities (Fig. 82-5). Only some family members may react with pruritus and clinical lesions, even though all members are bitten. Household furniture

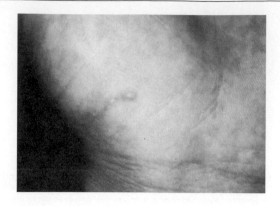

FIG. 82-2   Linear, pruritic papules of scabies on the wrist with a typical linear burrow.

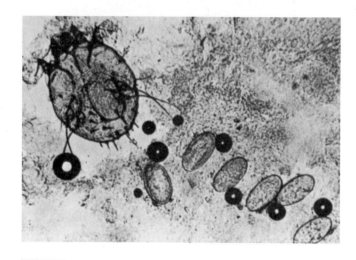

FIG. 82-3   Microscopic examination of scraped scabies reveals a mite and multiple eggs.

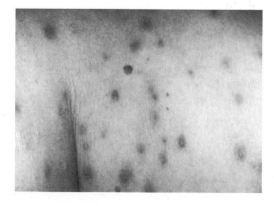

FIG. 82-4   Multiple pubic lice located in the suprapubic area.

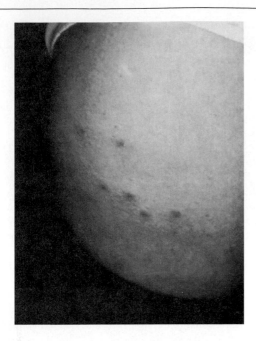

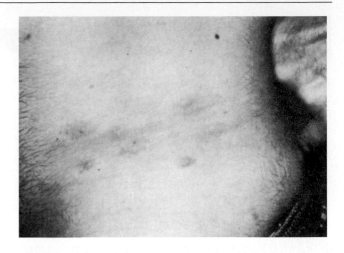

FIG. 82-6   Erythematous, urticarial papules secondary to chigger bites over the trunk.

FIG. 82-5   Grouped erythematous papules secondary to flea bites over the knee area.

(e.g., carpeting) must be treated with an appropriate insecticide to eliminate the fleas. Bites are treated symptomatically with topical steroids and oral antihistamine agents.

Chigger bites are caused by a venomous harvest mite. The bites are usually seen in warm months of July through September. The bites usually occur in lines under tight-fitting clothing. Multiple pruritic, erythematous papules or vesicles with central puncta are observed (Fig. 82-6). Symptomatic relief from these bites with antipru-

ritics and topical corticosteroids is usually helpful. Repellents containing permethrin can also be used.

Bedbugs live in wood surfaces near beds or in bedding. Bites occur during the night and characteristically appear as grouped vesicles and erythematous papules. Extermination of the bedbugs is required, and clinical lesions are treated symptomatically.

Ticks live in forests, in grass, and on animals. Once attached to the skin, the tick will engorge itself with blood and remain attached. It can be removed with a forceps. Ticks can transmit viral encephalitis, Rocky Mountain spotted fever, and Lyme disease. When visiting certain areas, people should be warned about the possibility of developing Rocky Mountain spotted fever.

QUESTIONS

▼ *Answer the following on a separate sheet of paper.*

1. Describe the appearance of erythema chronicum migrans (ECM) and other early symptoms of Lyme disease.
2. Describe the etiology, signs and symptoms, and treatment for scabies and pediculosis pubis.

▼ *Circle the letter preceding each item below that correctly completes the statement. More than one answer may be correct.*

3. Mr. M., a 35-year-old man who likes to go hunting in Rhode Island, developed a

lesion of ECM over his buttock. The way to confirm the diagnosis is:
   a. Flulike symptoms are present during the first 2 months after the bite.
   b. History of a tick bite is found in 100% of patients.
   c. Serologic tests are positive but can sometimes be negative.
   d. If not treated, he has 50% chance of developing arthritis 6 weeks to several years later.

▼ *Circle T if the statement is true and F if it is false. Correct any false statements.*

4. T F A common cause of nocturnal pruritus around the pubic area is scabies.
5. T F Treatment with gamma benzene hexachloride destroys pubic lice.
6. T F Pediculosis capitis is transmitted from person to person and may result in epidemics, particularly in schools.

BIBLIOGRAPHY ▼ PART XIII

Akers WA, Naverson DN: Diagnosis of chronic urticaria, *Int J Dermatol* 17:616-627, 1978.

Akers WA, Allen AN, Botkus D: Isotretinoin versus placebo in the treatment of cystic acne, *J Am Acad Dermatol* 6:735-745, 1982.

Anderson TF: Psoriasis, *Med Clin North Am* 66(4):769-794, 1982.

Arndt KA: *A manual of dermatological therapeutics,* ed 5, Boston, 1995, Little, Brown.

Breathnach AS, Wolff K: Structure and development of skin. In Fitzpatrick TB et al, editors: *Dermatology in general medicine,* ed 2, New York, 1979, McGraw-Hill.

Callen JP: Squamous cell carcinoma of the skin, *Prim Care* 5(2):299-311, 1978.

Callen JP: *Cutaneous aspects of internal disease,* Chicago, 1981, Year Book.

Callen JP, Stawiski MA, Vorhees JJ: *Manual of dermatology,* Chicago, 1980, Year Book.

Chanda JJ: Primary cutaneous malignant melanoma, *Prim Care* 5(2):325-337, 1978.

Chanda JJ, Callen JP: Erythema multiforme and the Stevens-Johnson syndrome, *South Med J* 71(1):566-570, 1978.

Demis DJ, Dobson RL, McGuire JI: *Clinical dermatology,* Philadelphia, 1988, Lippincott.

Ellis CN, Stawiski MA: The treatment of perioral dermatitis, acne rosacea, and seborrheic dermatitis, *Med Clin North Am* 66(4):819-830, 1982.

Fisher AA: *Contact dermatitis,* ed 3, Philadelphia, 1986, Lea & Febiger.

Fitzpatrick TB et al, editors: *Dermatology in general medicine,* ed 4, New York, 1994, McGraw-Hill.

Hurwitz S: Erythema chronicum migrans and Lyme disease, *Pediatr Dermatol* 2(4):266-274, 1985.

Kligman AM, Plewig G: Classification of acne, *Cutis* 17(3):520-522, 1976.

Kraemer KH, Greene MH: Dysplastic nevus syndrome: familial and sporadic precursors of cutaneous melanoma, *Dermatol Clin* 3(2):225-237, 1985.

Maize JC: Atopic dermatitis, *Int J Dermatol* 15(8):555-556, 1976.

Melanby K: *Scabies,* ed 2, Oxfordshire, England, 1943, Classey.

Metcalf JS, Maize JC: Melanocytic nevi and malignant melanoma, *Dermatol Clin* 3(2):217-224, 1985.

Monroe EW, Jones HE: Urticaria, *Arch Dermatol* 113(1):80-90, 1977.

Moschella SL, Pillsburg DM, Hurley HI, editors: *Dermatology,* ed 3, Philadelphia, 1992, Saunders.

Nahmias HJ: Herpes simplex virus infection: present status of diagnosis and management, *South Med J* 68(10):1191-1194, 1975.

Olsen TG: Therapy of acne, *Med Clin North Am* 66(4):851-872, 1982.

Provost TT, Farmer ER: *Current therapy in dermatology,* Philadelphia, 1985, Decker.

Rassner GR: *Atlas of dermatology,* Baltimore, 1978, Urban and Schwartzgenberg.

Rook A, Wilkinson DS, Ebling FJ: *Textbook of dermatology,* ed 4, Oxford, 1986, Blackwell.

Sams WM, Lynch PJ, editors: *Principles and practice of dermatology,* New York, 1990, Churchill Livingstone.

Shelley WB: *Consultations in dermatology with Walter B. Shelley,* vols 1 and 2, Philadelphia, 1973, Saunders.

Soter NA: Clinical presentations and mechanisms of necrotizing angitis of the skin, *J Invest Dermatol* 67(1):354-359, 1977.

Soter NA, Wilkinson DS, Fitzpatrick TB: Clinical dermatology, part 1, *N Engl J Med* 289(5):189-195, 1973.

Soter NA, Wilkinson DS, Fitzpatrick TB: Clinical dermatology, part 2, *N Engl J Med* 289(5):242-249, 1973.

Soter NA, Wilkinson DS, Fitzpatrick TB: Clinical dermatology, part 3, *N Engl J Med* 289(6):296-302, 1973.

Stawiski MA: Basal cell carcinoma, *Prim Care* 5(2):283-297, 1978.

Stechenberg BW: Lyme disease: the latest great great imitator, *Pediatr Infect Dis J* 7:402-409, 1988.

ANSWERS

CHAPTER 1

1. *Pathology* is the science or study of disease. It includes study of the pathogenesis of disease and structural and functional alterations that result from disease. Pathology is literally abnormal biology, the study of biologic processes gone awry and of individuals who are ill or disordered. *Pathophysiology* deals with dynamic aspects of disease processes. It is concerned with the disruption of normal physiology: with the alterations, derangements, and mechanisms involved in disruption and how they are manifested as signs, symptoms, and as physical and laboratory findings. Pathophysiology provides the basic link between the sciences of anatomy, physiology, and chemistry and their application to clinical practice.

2. *Anatomic pathology* is the study of the morphology of cells, organs, and tissues in disease. *Clinical pathology* refers to the application of laboratory techniques to the study of disease. Examples of anatomic pathology include surgical pathology, exfoliative cytology, and autopsy pathology. Examples of clinical pathology include clinical chemistry, microbiology, hematology, immunology, and immunochematology.

3. *Pathogenesis* is the way disease unfolds, the mechanism of development.

4. The concept of *normalcy* is complex and difficult to define succinctly. Selecting any parameter that might be applied to an individual or group, the concept of *normal* involves some average value for that parameter. For example, average values for height and weight are derived from observations of many individuals. Implicitly a certain amount of variation from the aver-

age is accepted as being permissible or normal. The usual concept of normalcy involves an average value and some range of variation either above or below that value.

5. A given disease is a dynamic phenomenon with a rhythm and pattern of its own. Each disease has a natural history, typical pattern of evolution, impact, and duration unless the disease is successfully modified by some intervention.

6. b
7. a
8. a
9. a
10. c
11. b

CHAPTER 2

1. *Mitosis* is the process by which a somatic cell splits into two new daughter cells. Once each chromosome has been replicated to form the two chromatids, mitosis follows. All 46 pairs of chromatids are separated, forming two separate sets of 46 daughter chromosomes, which are identical to the mother cell. No genetic information is lost in this process. *Meiosis* is a type of cell division of germ cells (sperm or ova) in which two successive divisions of the nucleus produce cells that contain half the number of chromosomes present in somatic cells. When fertilization occurs, the nuclei of the sperm and ovum fuse and produce a zygote with the full chromosome complement.

2. Because almost all DNA is located in the nucleus of the cell yet most of the functions of the cell are carried out in the cytoplasm, the genes must have a means of controlling the chemical reactions in the cytoplasm. This is achieved through an intermediary, RNA, which

is controlled by the DNA in the cell nucleus. This is accomplished through a process called *transcription* in which DNA transfers its code to RNA. The RNA then diffuses from the nucleus into the cytoplasm, where it controls protein synthesis. During the synthesis of RNA, the two strands of DNA separate temporarily; one of the strands is then used as a template for constructing the RNA molecule. The code triplets in the DNA cause the formation of complementary code triplets called *codons* in the RNA; these codons in turn control the sequence of amino acids in a protein to be synthesized later in the cytoplasm, a process called *translation.* The transcription process is under the influence of an enzyme called *RNA polymerase,* which interacts with promoter and terminator sites on the DNA to initiate and stop the process.

3. A trait is *dominant* if it is observable in the heterozygote and may be expressed by all individuals with that allele. A *recessive* trait is only observable in the *homozygote;* an individual who is *heterozygous* for the allele would be a carrier but not express the trait.

4.

	B	b
B	BB	Bb
b	Bb	bb

25% of the offspring will be normal (BB); 50% will be carriers (Bb); and 25% will have the disease (bb).

5. Since females are homozygous for the sex chromosomes and 50% of their X chromosomes are inactivated at random, if a female inherits an X-linked

disorder, only part of the cells express the disorder, while other cells are totally unaffected *(mosaics)*. Thus the clinical symptoms depend on the percentage of cells inactivating the normal allele for each tissue. Because of mosaicism, an X-linked disorder is likely to be milder in the female than in the hemizygous male.

6. Translocations are often associated with hematologic malignancies, since many genes expressed by cells of the immune system normally require structural changes to become functional. During this normal process, pathologic translocations may occur, resulting in a malignancy.

7. The advantages of chorionic villus sampling compared with amniocentesis are that it can be performed earlier in the pregnancy and is faster; the disadvantage is that a nonrepresentative sample may result, since the sample is obtained from the placenta and not the fetus.

8. Dominant genetic disorders are associated with the overproduction of a protein or the production of an abnormal protein. Overproduction of the gene can be controlled by using an antisense gene to cause down-regulation. When the antisense gene is expressed, it makes the complement (antisense) of the mRNA for the defective gene, blocking the ability of the ribosome from binding to the mRNA. Consequently, the protein coded by the defective gene cannot be made. Thus antisense genes limit the expression of the defective gene by controlling its translation.

9. a, d
10. a, b, c
11. c
12. d
13. a
14. b
15. d
16. a
17. d
18. a, b
19. a, b, c
20. False; unlike DNA, RNA is usually a short-lived, single-stranded molecule.
21. True
22. True
23. True
24. False; autosomal chromosomes are all the chromosomes except the X and Y chromosomes.
25. True
26. True
27. True

28. False; X-linked disorders are more common in males.
29. False; mitochondrial disorders are equally probable in both sexes.
30. True
31. False; RFLP analysis is usually an indirect measure of mutation.
32. False; recessive disorders are more likely to be good candidates for replacement therapy than dominant disorders.
33. False; PCR has strongly influenced molecular diagnosis of genetic disorders for the amplification of small samples of the patient's DNA.
34. b
35. d
36. a
37. d
38. b
39. c
40. c
41. d
42. c
43. c
44. b
45. a

CHAPTER 3
1. d
2. b
3. c
4. d
5. e
6. b
7. a
8. c
9. b
10. a
11. d
12. a
13. b
14. c
15. b, d
16. Biochemical; functional; anatomic
17. Central nervous; brain
18. Dystrophic; metastatic
19. Rigor mortis
20. d
21. f
22. b
23. e
24. a
25. c

CHAPTER 4
1. d
2. c
3. a, b, c
4. a, c, e
5. b, d
6. a, c

7. a, b, c
8. a, c
9. b
10. a, c, d
11. b
12. b, c
13. c, d
14. c
15. d
16. e
17. c
18. a
19. a, b, d
20. a, c
21. All are correct.
22. b, c
23. a, c, d
24. All are correct.
25. b, d, e
26. a, c
27. a, b, c
28. b, d, e
29. All are correct.
30. a, b, c
31. a, d
32. a, b, c
33. a, c
34. True
35. True
36. True
37. False; the host is capable of forming and liberating endogenous substances with a chemotactic effect.
38. True
39. True
40. True
41. True
42. False; it is called a macrophage.
43. True
44. True
45. True
46. True
47. False; they are formed by fusion of macrophages.
48. False; this is characteristic of chronic inflammation; subacute inflammation involves only early repair.
49. False; it is caused by abnormal production or remolding of collagen in the healing wound.
50. True
51. True
52. b
53. e
54. a
55. d
56. c
57. Abscess
58. Ulcer
59. Empyema
60. Fistula
61. -itis

62. Margination
63. Emigration
64. Resolution
65. Repair
66. Lymphadenitis
67. a, b, e, d, c

CHAPTER 5

1. b
2. b
3. d
4. b
5. d
6. c; the thymus and bone marrow are primary lymphoid organs; the remaining lymphoid organs are secondary, such as the spleen, lymph nodes, and nonencapsulated tissue (e.g., MALT, GALT).
7. a
8. b
9. b
10. c; cytokines are chemicals that are low-molecular-weight proteins released from cells participating in the immune response. Cytokines act as potent messengers between the cells involved in the immune response by promoting cell growth and activation, directing cellular traffic, stimulating macrophage function, and destroying antigens.
11. a; when an antigen presenting cell raises the epitope–major histocompatibility complex (MHC) to the cell surface, CD4 cells are activated, gamma interferon is produced, and the immune response is amplified. The other answers illustrate effector functions.
12. a
13. d; natural killer cells are not true T cells, but rather perform a nonspecific effector function by recognizing "nonself" cells by nonspecific means, such as unusual electrical charges on the cell surface.
14. b; class I MHC antigens are found on the surface of almost all nucleated cells. When cells become infected with viruses, the viral epitope is presented on the surface of the cell by the MHC class I antigen.
15. a
16. b; B cells mature in two phases. The first phase is in the bone marrow, when stem cells mature first to pre-B cells, then to B cells that express immunoglobulins. The second phase is antigen dependent, when the B cell interacts with an immunogen, becomes activated (plasma cell), and produces immunoglobulins.
17. d

18. b
19. a; the variable portion of the CD4 protein is composed of varying amino acid sequences that form the epitope-binding sites. This portion has variability because of the immune system's specificity. A host of epitope-specific immunoglobulins are needed by the body to combine with a host of different epitopes.
20. c
21. b
22. d; the functions of complement include lysis (building of the MAC, which inserts pore-forming molecules into the cell membrane of bacteria to cause cell death), production of immune mediators that lead to vasodilation at the site of inflammation, and opsonization.
23. a
24. b
25. b
26. c
27. c
28. a; type II hypersensitivity reactions are cytotoxic and occur when circulating immunoglobulins interact with epitopes to cause cell death.
29. d
30. d
31. e
32. c
33. d
34. a
35. b
36. e
37. c
38. b
39. d
40. a

CHAPTER 6

1. *Infection* can be said to be present if some microbial agent has been able to adhere to the body surface or to colonize and invade the tissues of the host and then grow and multiply. The presence of infection, however, only indicates the relation of the parasite to the host and does not necessarily indicate disease. Infectious disease is usually manifested by clinical illness. Infection may be totally asymptomatic.
2. *Skin* (especially if traumatized): ordinarily the multilayered epithelium, dry keratin layer, and shedding of cells provide a mechanical barrier to infection. The chemical properties of sweat and sebaceous secretions have a mild bactericidal effect, and the normal flora provides a biologic barrier.

Mouth, pharynx, gastrointestinal tract: the entire alimentary canal is lined with mucous membrane, which, along with the protective layer of mucus, provides a mechanical barrier to invasion by microbes. The flow of saliva washes away many microbes mechanically. Rapid peristalsis in the stomach and especially in the small intestine provides another mechanical barrier. The high acidity of the stomach provides an excellent chemical barrier. Finally, the normal flora of the mouth, throat, and especially the large intestine provides a biologic barrier to microbial proliferation and invasion. The gastrointestinal mucus contains antibodies that provide immunologic defense.

Respiratory tract: a mechanical barrier is provided by a layer of mucus covering the surface and the constant action of the cilia, which move the secretions toward the exterior of the body. Antibody is present in respiratory secretions, and motile macrophages in the alveoli engulf and destroy microbes.

Urinary tract: defense is provided by the multilayered epithelium and the flushing action of urine flow.

Eyes: the flow of tears is a defense; antibody also is present in tears.

The defenses of the body surfaces against microbial invasion are mechanical, chemical, biologic (normal flora of each surface area), and immunologic.

3. The microorganisms may spread locally along fascial planes or tubular structures, such as a bronchus or ureter. The organisms may be passively carried by the fluid currents of the body. They may spread via lymphatics, ultimately to infect lymph nodes, or may be transferred to another location by a phagocyte if it does not kill the ingested organism. The next step is systemic spread of the microorganisms via the circulating blood. Organisms may even enter blood vessels directly in the local area of initial invasion.

4. If an infectious agent is not contained locally by the inflammatory response or the regional lymph nodes, the microorganisms may enter the systemic blood (bacteremia) and possibly disseminate throughout the body. The phagocytic cells of the monocyte-macrophage system, chiefly in the liver and spleen, cleanse the blood of the microorganisms.

5. An infectious disease is produced in a debilitated host by an organism ordi-

narily harmless to a healthy individual with intact defenses.

6. (a) Antimicrobial therapy, which would suppress part of the normal flora and allow a normal resident organism to overgrow or might cause the treated person to become susceptible to an exogenous invader. (b) Adrenocorticosteroids, which would be affecting inflammatory and immunologic mechanisms, might allow overgrowth of bacteria that would ordinarily be held in check. (c) Radiation therapy and cancer chemotherapy, which might depress the bone marrow and lymphoid tissue, possibly resulting in severe infection. (d) Immunosuppressive therapy (used to prevent rejection of a transplanted organ) causes a depression of immune defenses against microbes. (e) Unavoidable situations in hospitalized patients: anesthesia, shock, and burns, which lower many defenses. (f) Primary disease conditions: for example, virus infection of upper respiratory tract, which may be followed by bacterial pneumonia. (g) Environmental factors: overcrowding, famine, weather, etc.

7. Bacterial flora modifies the surface on which it grows and, by competitive or direct inhibition, prevents others potentially more pathogenic microorganisms from establishing residence.

8. Some pathogenic organisms may damage tissue by immunologic means, producing cellular hypersensitivity (tuberculosis), or may produce circulating antigen-antibody complexes (poststreptococcal glomerulonephritis). Others may produce exotoxins or endotoxins. Viruses act as intracellular parasites, altering cellular metabolism and synthetic activity.

9. d
10. c
11. b, d
12. c
13. b
14. c
15. b
16. a
17. d
18. b
19. a
20. c

CHAPTER 7

1. In *active congestion,* more blood than usual is actively flowing into the area. This increase in local blood flow is accomplished by dilation of arterioles,

which behave as valves governing the flow into the local microcirculation. In *passive congestion,* some impairment of drainage of blood from the area occurs. Anything that compresses the venules and veins draining a tissue or otherwise hinders flow may produce passive congestion.

2. When the heart fails in its pumping action, impaired venous drainage results. For example, if the left side of the heart fails in its pumping action, the flow of blood returning to the heart from the lung will be impaired. The blood will be dammed back into the lung, producing passive congestion of the pulmonary vasculature.

3. If the passive congestion is short-lived, there are no effects on the involved tissue. In chronic passive congestion, however, there may be permanent effects on the tissue, because in a passively congested area, if the change in blood flow is severe enough, an element of tissue hypoxia may lead to shrinkage or loss of cells of the involved tissue. Also, in many areas there is evidence of local breakdown of red blood cells, which results in the deposition of certain pigments within the tissues. Fibrosis may also ensue.

4. Edema is an accumulation of excess fluid between the cells of the body or within the various body cavities or, according to some, within cells.

5. c, d
6. c
7. a, d
8. c
9. a, c
10. a, b, c
11. c
12. a, c
13. b
14. c

15. The most common cause of hemorrhage is loss of integrity of vascular walls, permitting the escape of blood. This is most often the result of external trauma, as with injuries accompanied by bruising.

16. (a) Blood platelet system. With a small hole in the blood vessel, the blood platelets may aggregate over the hole and simply plug it up. (b) Blood-clotting system. A fibrin clot is formed by the activation of a series of clotting factors in the blood.

17. The local effects of hemorrhage are related to the presence of extravasated blood in the tissues and can range from trivial to lethal. The most trivial local

effect is perhaps a bruise, which may be of only cosmetic importance, whereas a small volume of hemorrhage in a vital area of the brain can produce death. Systemic effects depend on two factors: (a) rate of loss and (b) volume of blood extravasated. If blood loss is rapid, the patient may actually die or may go into hemorrhagic shock. With survival and the passage of time, the patient may develop blood-loss anemia.

18. (a) Thrombosis may result in obstruction of an artery or vein, with possible ischemia or congestion, respectively. (b) It provides a source of possible emboli.

19. (a) Thrombus in an artery, (b) narrowing of an atherosclerotic artery, (c) embolus in an artery, (d) tumor pressing on a vessel.

20. (a) Functional disturbance (pain, such as angina), (b) atrophy of ischemic tissue, (c) infarction of ischemic tissue.

21. All are correct.
22. a
23. a
24. c
25. a, c
26. a, b
27. d
28. b
29. a, c
30. a
31. b
32. False; Mönckeberg's sclerosis is not clinically significant; the lining of the involved vessel is not roughened, and the lumen is not narrowed.
33. True
34. True
35. False; atherosclerosis is a multifactoral disease.
36. True
37. True
38. False; infarct is used to denote tissue necrosis caused by a circulatory abnormality.

CHAPTER 8

1. c
2. d
3. f
4. e
5. a
6. g
7. b
8. b, c
9. b
10. a
11. b
12. b
13. a, c

14. c
15. d
16. c
17. d
18. b, d
19. a
20. b
21. True
22. True
23. False; the tumor is sometimes referred to as *scirrhous.*
24. True
25. True
26. False; this neoplasm is classified as a leiomyosarcoma.
27. True
28. Ischemia; advancing age related to decreasing hormone production (e.g., breast tissue); disuse (e.g., a cast).
29. The ability to invade normal tissue; the ability to form metastases.
30. Via lymphatic channels; via direct "transplantation," such as across serosal cavities (or, in fact, into incisions via surgical instruments); via the bloodstream.
31. Neoplasms can produce a variety of local-mechanical symptoms by impinging on normal structures, producing obstruction of passages, destroying vital functions, etc. They may ulcerate, may become secondarily infected, or may give rise to hemorrhages. Neoplasms may have endocrine function and produce signs and symptoms on that basis. Advanced malignant growths may produce cachexia.
32. The most important criterion is the distinction between benign and malignant biologic behavior. That is, if a neoplasm has invaded neighboring non-neoplastic tissue or has produced metastases, it is malignant. When neither invasion nor metastasis is evident, a neoplasm can still be classified as malignant if its potential for malignant behavior can be predicted by its microscopic appearance alone; untreated neoplasms of certain types will invade and metastasize. Also included is the cell type of origin of the neoplasm and the organ of origin of the neoplasm.
33. CIN III is severe dysplasia and is tantamount to preinvasive cancer. Destruction of foci of cervical dysplasia can prevent frankly invasive cancer.
34. It is likely related to the effects of cytokines generated within the tumor or part of the response to the tumor.
35. This concept is not completely understood at present. It is thought that the behavior of cancer cells is "antisocial"

with regard to normal cells of the body. Malignant cells disobey the usual territorial rules and grow in inappropriate locations. Evidence is beginning to accumulate indicating that the important abnormalities of cancer cells seem to lie within the cell membrane. On the cell membrane, homeostatic signals are received from other cells and from other points in the body and are transmitted to the interior of the cell. Abnormalities in this membrane may result in abnormal reception of control signals or abnormal responses to them. Evidence also indicates that events at the cell membrane are important in controlling cellular proliferation. The antigenic structure of cell membranes is important with regard to the immunologic interactions of the cell with its surroundings.
36. Ultraviolet radiation (as in sunlight); ionizing radiation (gamma rays, x-rays, atomic particles); many chemicals, most of which are mutagenic; aromatic hydrocarbons and amines, nitrosamines, azo dyes; certain viruses.
37. (a) A classic notion is that of somatic mutation, which suggests that the basic carcinogenic event involves a chemical change in the DNA of a cell, that is, a mutation. This type of mutation would involve a nongerm cell, or somatic cell. This theory of mutation would explain why once a cell is transformed into a neoplastic cell, its characteristics breed true, giving rise to an expanding clone of cells with similar properties, determined by the mutated DNA. (b) Another explanation for the expression of malignant behavior is the "addition" of genetic information to the cell by viral infection, with the "new" genetic information expressed as abnormal cellular behavior. (c) Finally, some evidence indicates that malignancy may be a matter of abnormal differentiation, that is, abnormal and inappropriate expression of genetic information always present in each cell of the body but usually kept repressed except, for instance, in embryonic life.
38. *T* refers to the primary tumor (T1 is smaller than T4); *N* is the status of regional lymph nodes (N0 designates absence of nodal metastases, and N1, N2, and N3 indicate increasing metastatic involvement); *M* refers to distant metastasis, with appropriate adscripts.
39. It is becoming evident that some genetic abnormalities may be inherited, yielding a predisposition for the devel-

opment of a tumor in a given family. Molecular methods of analysis identify specific genes and gene products involved in familial cancer syndromes. Persons at higher than normal risk of developing tumors can be identified, and preventive or intervention strategies can be designed and implemented.
40. The means used include the confirmation of the neoplasm's presence by physical examination and by radiographic, ultrasonographic, and/or endoscopic means. A final step in determining the diagnosis of neoplasm involves morphologic examination based on microscopic features of the tissue. Decisions about treatment are related to the clinical stage of the cancer. The concept of staging is based on a given type of cancer being likely to manifest a certain progression. Several different modalities of cancer treatment exist, including extirpation of the cancerous tissue surgically, radiotherapy, application of ionizing radiation to the neoplasm, chemotherapy (based on the differential sensitivity of proliferating cancer cells and normal cells to a variety of cytotoxic chemical agents), and immunotherapy. The approach is not limited to the use of a single treatment modality but is based on the needs of the individual patient with a particular neoplasm at a given clinical stage.

CHAPTER 9

1. *Hypersensitivity* denotes the immunologic capacity, acquired through contact with a specific, chemically characterizable agent, to hyperreact to that agent. The cellular events that follow exposure and establish a capacity for responses of hypersensitivity are termed *sensitization.*
2. *Angioedema* reflects a localized inflammatory increase in vascular permeability without frank injury to small veins and capillaries, usually reversible within a short period, whereas *lymphedema* results from abnormal pressures (caused by an obstruction to flow upstream) that promote passage to fluid out into tissues.
3. Evidence suggests that clinical anaphylaxis in both animals and humans involves a sudden multifocal reaction of allergen with mast cell–bound, specific IgE followed by widespread tissue response to the mediator substances (e.g., histamine, SRS-A, leukotrienes) released.
4. This seems to reflect differences among

species in both the distribution of mast cells and the relative responsiveness of tissues to mediator substances.

5. This generally requires the injection of potent allergens, although certain gastrointestinal and respiratory parasites also elicit prominent IgE responses. Many persons also make specific IgE responses to mucosal contact with innocuous materials, including foods, pollens, and animal emanations (danders). In addition, individual capacities to overproduce IgE and to respond immunologically to specific antigens also seem to be involved.

6. Efforts to reduce allergen (and irritant) exposure; suppressive medications to mitigate symptom severity nonspecifically; and specific hyposensitization to reduce responsiveness to unavoidable challenge.

7. Measures taken to reduce the risk of an anaphylactic reaction include (a) avoidance of known offenders (allergens), which is critical in reducing the risk of anaphylaxis, and (b) susceptible persons are urged to carry commercially prepared, preloaded syringes of epinephrine whenever possible.

8. c
9. d
10. b
11. a, c
12. d
13. a, b, d
14. c
15. c
16. b
17. c
18. a, b, c, f
19. d
20. b
21. b, c, d
22. b
23. b
24. d
25. d
26. a
27. a
28. c
29. b
30. a, b, d
31. True
32. True
33. False; strongly positive reactions indicate only the immunologic "apparatus" for response and provide no assurance that symptoms arise from exposure to the allergens in question.
34. False; aqueous extracts are used, and testing by pricking through the skin is usually done first; negative reactors

are considered for intracutaneous (IC) tests; however, where IC tests are done exclusively, dilute materials must be used.

35. True
36. False; neither the sensitivity nor the specificity of in vitro procedures exceeds that of conventional skin tests.
37. True

CHAPTER 10

1. A clinically defined condition marked by recurrent, discrete episodes of reversible bronchial narrowing, separated by periods in which ventilation approaches normal. These events occur in asthma-prone subjects by a variety of stimuli; this denotes a state of bronchial hyperactivity. Asthma is an abnormal pattern of response rather than a discrete disease.

2. Bronchial narrowing produces an increased resistance to airflow, which underlies an inability to achieve normal rates of flow during respiration, especially expiration. This results in uneven lung aeration and a loss of the normal spatial matching of ventilation and pulmonary blood flow. These defects may produce no symptoms or merely a sense of tracheal irritation; alternatively, respiratory distress may be intolerable.

3. Although atopy is implicated in many instances of bronchial asthma, in a substantial number of asthmatic persons, no allergic factors are demonstrated even after exhaustive study. These persons are often said to have "intrinsic" asthma, although their problem is more properly idiopathic. In addition, many allergic (atopic) asthmatic persons also respond adversely to nonallergic factors.

4. Asthmatic airways behave as if their beta-adrenergic innervation were incompetent, and, at least functionally, partial beta blockage seems to exist. Without adequate bronchodilator tone, bronchoconstrictor influences, known to be mediated normally by parasympathetic (cholinergic) and alpha-adrenergic pathways, would tend to predominate. In clinical practice the bronchial lability of asthmatic patients may be confirmed by demonstrating their brisk airway obstructive responses to extremely low concentrations of inhaled histamine and methacholine.

5. Since invading organisms frequently destroy ciliated epithelium and localize agents of inflammation in labile bronchi, their adverse effect on asthma

is predictable. In addition, animal studies have suggested that microbial substances may further weaken beta-adrenergic activity.

6. (a) The overall severity of impairment from asthma differs widely among individuals and typically varies with time in any affected person; (b) treatment programs of increasing potency (and complexity) are appropriate to control asthma of mounting severity; (c) antiinflammatory drugs are fundamental treatment for all but the most minimal asthma; and (d) increasing symptom intensity should prompt a *preplanned* set of remedial behaviors designed to improve the individual's functional status.

7. The effectiveness of these agents is thought to reflect direct stimulation of an enzyme, adenyl cyclase, which promotes the synthesis of cyclic AMP. Cyclic AMP–induced effects (e.g., relaxation of bronchial smooth muscle and inhibition of mediator release from mast cells and basophils) are promoted both by beta-adrenergic agents and by theophylline, and additive effects of these two groups of drugs often result.

8. Failure to synchronize inhalation and nebulizer discharge; inadequate time before passive exhalation occurs to permit aerosol mixing and deposition in the airways; interception and effective loss of rapidly moving particles by oropharyngeal baffles (e.g., teeth, tongue). Many of these deficiencies are reduced when metered-dose inhalers (MDIs) are used with spacers. Such devices are essential for children and many adult users to increase substantially lung deposition of drug.

9. Steroid-dependent asthmatic persons require regular oral corticosteroid treatment to maintain acceptable function. Symptoms are controlled with the lowest possible daily dose of a rapidly metabolized agent such as prednisone. Administration of moderate doses on alternate days may also be effective while reducing systemic side effects and suppressing hypothalamic-pituitary-adrenal function. The latter treatment benefits must reflect brief periods (longer than 36 hours after dosing) when no drug effect remains, since the required alternate-day doses are often more than twice those necessary in daily administration.

10. d, e
11. b
12. b, d, e

13. a, c
14. e
15. b
16. a, b, c, d
17. a, b, c
18. b, c, d
19. b
20. a
21. a
22. False; EIA is most often evident in children and characteristically appears in subjects who are symptom free before beginning exertion.
23. False; other conditions, such as the impaction of a foreign body or growth of a localized tumor in the bronchi, as well as pulmonary emphysema, may lead to diffuse wheezing, simulating asthma.
24. True
25. True
26. True
27. b, d
28. a, c
29. e

CHAPTER 11

1. Anaphylactic reaction and urticaria can result from IgE-mediated responses to protein allergens. In both situations the implicated agents usually are: (a) ingestants such as egg, fish, shellfish, and nuts, including peanuts; (b) drugs and drug metabolites that are capable of stable bonding to proteins (e.g., penicillins) or that are themselves complete antigens; (c) many drugs also appear to cause urticaria, although not typical anaphylaxis, by mechanisms exclusive of IgE (e.g., aspirin).
2. Since bouts of hives generally are self-limited and vary in duration as well as severity, the value of treatment measures for affected individuals often is difficult to discern. Epinephrine has demonstrated effectiveness in speeding resolution. Agents such as diphenhydramine and hydroxyzine also are acknowledged to have value in this condition. Adrenal corticosteroids have been beneficial in severe acute hives. Hydroxyzine often is the most valuable agent in chronic urticaria.
3. Hives (urticaria) probably affect at least 25% of the population at some time.
4. Treatment modalities for urticaria are difficult to evaluate, since bouts of hives tend to be self-limiting and vary in duration as well as severity.
5. a
6. b
7. a, b, d
8. a, c, d

9. a, b, c
10. b
11. c
12. a, b, c
13. c
14. d
15. a
16. b, d
17. b, d
18. a
19. c, d
20. b, d
21. False; these factors probably act by direct contact with an abraded epidermis but are rarely implicated.
22. True
23. False; these drugs should be reserved for their antiinflammatory properties, with bland lubricants used to soften and moisten the skin.
24. True
25. False; tars are rarely used today to reduce lichenification and cracking; urea-containing ointments are more cosmetically acceptable agents to promote healing and restoration of skin texture, and topical corticosteroids are also quite helpful for this purpose.
26. False; organic solvents that defat normal skin must be avoided.
27. True
28. False; the resemblance of urticarial wheal to IgE-mediated skin reactions has promoted this false inference.
29. True
30. True

CHAPTER 12

1. The appearance of *autoantibodies* (antibodies that react with autologous tissue components) provides valuable diagnostic markers. However, these serum factors seldom inflict direct tissue injury. Their appearance implies either an acquired mutation among immunocompetent cells or the reactivation of cells that had been suppressed but not eliminated. Several mechanisms may result in autoimmunity.
2. In certain instances the inciting antigens are normally sequestered and may remain "foreign" even to mature tissue. These responses could arise after subtle injury incident to microbial invasion. The possibility that infecting bacteria and viruses may produce limited changes in host tissue components, rendering them "foreign" to immune surveillance, has been proposed. Antibodies (or sensitized lymphocytes) resulting from this process might have specificities broad enough to permit re-

action with native as well as modified tissue determinants. Autoimmune phenomena could arise if an invading organism and host tissues shared an antigen or closely similar antigenic groups as a result of parallel evolution. Mutant ("forbidden") clones of lymphoid cells programmed to recognize normal host components as "foreign" could be involved, as well. Such cells might be antigen-specific or nonspecific T_H (helper/promoter lymphocytes) that foster the immune responses of both T and B lymphocytes. Alternatively, a decline of suppressor (T_S) lymphocytes that normally inhibit these responses might be implicated.
3. Circulating antibodies, reactive with glomerular and alveolar basement membrane glycoproteins, are usually present and, along with complement components, form linear deposits at these sites in vivo. The associated tissue damage is thought to reflect, in part, complement-mediated cytotoxicity and local effects of recruited neutrophils.
4. Chills, fever, and low back pain occasionally preceded by urticaria or flushing, uneasiness, and mild air hunger. When cell lysis is massive, the resulting debris may trigger wide-spread intravascular clotting with depletion of coagulation factors and bleeding from wounds and venipuncture sites.
5. All the following measures must be used to prevent or mitigate hemolytic transfusion reactions:
   a. The source and proper recipient of blood products must be identified.
   b. There must be continual surveillance of persons receiving blood, especially those whose mobility or awareness is impaired.
   c. Any serious evidence suggestive of an incipient reaction should prompt discontinuance of the questioned unit, maintenance of IV access, and careful clinical observation.
   d. A carefully drawn venous sample from the recipient should be checked for serum hemoglobin, a sign of intravascular red cell breakdown, and the compatibility of donor and recipient reconfirmed.
   e. All materials used for transfusion should be saved to facilitate serologic and microbiologic testing.
   f. Special precautions to monitor urine output are essential, and examination of serial centrifuged urine specimens for hemoglobin is

useful, since clearance of serum hemoglobin is rapid.

g. Maintenance of adequate hydration and urine flow are important considerations in all survivors, and osmotic diuresis with cautiously administered IV mannitol may help in achieving this goal.

h. Safe fluid therapy demands precise and regular evaluation of cardiopulmonary and renal function. Measures to combat shock, pulmonary edema, acute renal failure, and/or defibrination with bleeding may be required.

6. Recipients of leukoagglutinins have developed fever, cough, shortness of breath, and lung shadows on chest radiographs; several days have been required for full resolution.

7. False; platelets and red blood cells are attacked predominantly.

8. True

9. True

10. True

11. False; viral invasion may damage T_s suppressor cells that normally repress T and B cell responses to "self" components.

12. a, d

13. c

14. d

15. c

16. b

17. c

18. a, c

19. e

20. a, c

21. b, c

22. b

23. a

24. d

25. c

CHAPTER 13

1. a, c, d

2. a, c

3. c

4. a, b, d

5. b

6. c, d

7. a, b

8. All are correct.

9. False; since this response to injected antigens is to be expected in most persons, it is not confined to the atopic population.

10. True

11. True

12. True

13. e

14. a, c

15. b, c, d

16. f

17. b, d

18. c

19. Initially, complexes of host IgG or IgM and drug (or drug protein conjugate) become attached to one or more blood cell types. Complement components are localized to the cell surface, and their interaction results in discrete membrane lesions, the formed elements being injured as "innocent bystanders" rather than direct participants. After fixation of complement factors, the immune complexes often dissociate from affected membranes.

20. (a) Syncope, hypotension, cardiac rhythm disturbances, and at times, convulsions. (b) These reactions are probably a direct toxic effect of the large doses required for local infiltration.

21. a. An effective approach to the prevention of adverse drug reactions requires knowledge of the potential complications of medication and a willingness to consider adverse drug reactions as a possible cause of any unexpected clinical event.

b. Since adverse responses usually are repetitive, no drug should be given without first assessing the individual's past experience with that agent. The clinical data base requires no less than a comprehensive assessment of past drug reactivity. Health care personnel must also be prepared to accept, at face value, reports of past problems arising from medication until these have been disproved conclusively.

c. Close surveillance can reveal the earliest stigmata of drug reactions, facilitating prompt withdrawal of the offender and often abbreviating morbidity. Once recognized, adverse reactivity must be clearly indicated in the clinical record and, if possible, the sensitivity identified for the patient or responsible family members. Documentation is aided if the patient carries a card, bracelet, or medallion indicating medication(s) to be avoided. Exhaustive instruction is necessary when a risk of reaction from related agents exists or when the offender has many readily available, poorly identified sources.

CHAPTER 14

1. d

2. c, d

3. c

4. a, b, c

5. a

6. True

7. True

8. True

9. False; T cell defects are generally more evident.

10. False; relatively complete absence of T cell function occurs selectively when the thymus fails to develop.

11. True

12. False; T helper cells bearing the CD4 membrane marker are the principal lymphocyte subset promoting B cell proliferation and development into Ig-secreting plasma cells.

13. (a) Determination of naturally occurring (IgM) antibodies to ABO blood group substances absent from the subject's red cells. Normal persons consistently demonstrate such isohemagglutins by age 1 year. (b) Schick testing of persons previously immunized with diphtheria toxoid. If adequate levels of (IgG) specific antibody have been produced, tissue breakdown at the site of toxin injection is prevented. (c) Determination of antibody titers before and after nonviable immunizing materials such as tetanus toxoid and typhoid vaccine.

14. Intradermal injections are performed with 0.1 ml portions of substances that elicit DTH and to which a previous sensitizing exposure may be assumed; commonly used materials include PPD (of the tubercle bacillus) and streptokinase and streptodornase (enzymes of beta-hemolytic streptococci). Test sites are observed and palpated after 48 hours, and an indurated area with a diameter of 10 mm or larger generally is regarded as a positive reaction. Using a battery of such materials, at least one positive test should be evident in the vast majority of nomal persons (excluding infants). For nonreactors, the next step is the determination of B and T cell categories using monoclonal antibodies to tag their cell membrane components. Automated approaches to such assays (by flow cytometry) can estimate levels of helper/inducer, suppress/cytotoxic, and null cells as well as functional subcomponents within these groups.

15. (a) Response of lymphocytes in short-term tissue culture to antigens and nonspecific agents that stimulate cell division and associated nucleic acid synthesis. An increase in the incorporation of thymidine tagged with tritium is ob-

served normally in response to these agents. (b) Peripheral aggregation of sheep red blood cells around human peripheral cells (T lymphocytes) when the two are mixed and incubated. Normally, more than 60% of lymphocytes demonstrated rosetting, although a teleologic basis for the sheep cell receptor is unknown. (c) Assays of lymphokines produced in response to appropriate antigens added to lymphocyte preparations. Currently available monoclonal antibodies provide an expanding variety of specific reagents.

16. The numbers and functional state of T lymphocytes also affect antibody secretion, since antigen recognition by T cells must precede most antibody (humoral) responses.

CHAPTER 15

1. c
2. d
3. b, c
4. d
5. c
6. a
7. a
8. c; no, it is not stable, which will make the development of a vaccine more difficult.
9. a
10. d
11. c
12. d
13. b
14. c
15. d
16. d
17. b
18. e
19. e
20. c
21. b
22. b
23. c
24. d
25. b
26. a
27. e
28. a
29. c
30. a
31. e
32. b
33. d
34. f
35. True
36. True
37. False; the molecules are single-stranded RNA with positive polarity.
38. False; many other cells have CD4+

molecules on their surface and can be infected (e.g., monocytes, macrophages).
39. True
40. True
41. True
42. False; heterosexual contact is the most common mode.

CHAPTER 16

1. A science that deals with blood and the blood-forming tissues. It is the study of blood, its nature, function, and disease.
2. The hematologic system includes blood and blood-forming tissues and monocyte-macrophage system located throughout the body (spleen, liver, lymph nodes, bone marrow). It phagocytizes foreign materials (microorganisms to dying red blood cells). Disorders arising from these systems are called *blood dyscrasias*.
3. Red blood cells (erythrocytes, red corpuscles, or RBCs); white blood cells (leukocytes, white corpuscles, or WBCs); platelets (or thrombocytes).
4. Since RBCs, WBCs, and platelets have a finite life span, a constant optimum production is necessary to maintain levels required to meet tissue needs. In adults, this production, called *hematopoiesis* (formation and maturation of blood cells), takes place in the bone marrow of the skull, vertebrae, pelvis, sternum, ribs, and proximal epiphyses of the long bones. However, during periods of increased demand (e.g., hemorrhage or cell destruction), production may resume in all the bones, as is normal in children. All normal cells are thought to derive from a single pluripotential stem cell. The stem cell can differentiate into lymphoid and hematopoietic stem cells that become progenitor cells. Progenitor cells differentiate along a single pathway. Through a series of divisions and maturational changes, these cells become specific mature cells in the circulating blood.
5. A complete history or profile (including past and current illnesses, drug exposure, bleeding tendencies, nutritional habits, family history), physical assessment, and selective diagnostic studies. These studies attempt to quantitate the various constituents of blood and bone marrow.
6. c
7. c
8. c
9. b
10. b

11. a, b, c, d
12. c
13. d
14. a
15. g
16. b
17. e
18. i
19. c
20. j
21. h
22. f
23. False; men, 4.7 to 6.1; women 4.2 to 5.2.
24. True
25. True
26. False; 4000 to 10,000
27. False; 150,000 to 400,000
28. True
29. Poikilocytosis
30. Hypochromic
31. Protein hemoglobin (Hb)

CHAPTER 17

1. The major component of the red blood cell (RBC) is the protein hemoglobin (Hb), which transports O_2 and CO_2 and maintains the normal pH through a series of intercellular buffers. The Hb molecule consists of two pairs of polypeptide chains (globin) and four heme groups, each one containing an atom of ferrous iron. This configuration allows the most expedient exchange of gases.
2. It is postulated that RBC production is stimulated by a glycoprotein, *erythropoietin*, believed to originate in the kidney. It is theorized that erythropoietin production is influenced by tissue hypoxia caused by such factors as changes in atmospheric O_2, decreased O_2 content of arterial blood, and decreased Hb concentration. The stem cells committed to erythrocyte production appear to be the targets of erythropoietin and initiate proliferation and maturation of RBCs.
3. *Anemia* is a reduction below the normal level in the number of RBCs, the quantity of Hb, and the volume of packed RBCs (hematocrit) per deciliter of blood.
4. Pallor (nailbeds, palms, mucous membranes of the mouth and conjunctivae), tachycardia, shortness of breath, dyspnea, headache, dizziness, faintness, tinnitus.
5. (a) Increased RBC loss: direct loss from the circulation through bleeding. Bleeding from trauma or ulcers, polyps in the colon, malignant growth,

hemorrhoids, menstruation. (b) Destruction of RBCs in the circulation (hemolysis). Hemoglobinopathies (inherited abnormal Hb): sickle cell disease, impaired globin synthesis, thalassemia; RBC membrane defects: hereditary spherocytosis; enzyme deficiencies: glucose-6-phosphate dehydrogenase (G6PD) deficiency.

6. (a) Normocytic, normochromic anemia: RBCs are of normal size and shape, contain the normal amount of Hb (MCV and MCHC are normal or low-normal). Examples are acute blood loss, hemolysis, renal disease, and metastatic infiltrative diseases of the bone marrow. (b) Macrocytic, normochromic anemia: RBCs are larger than normal but are normochromic because the Hb concentration is normal (MCV is increased, MCHC is normal). Examples are deficiency states of vitamin B_{12} and/or folic acid; cancer chemotherapy. (c) Microcytic, hypochromic anemia: microcytic means small, hypochromic means containing less than the normal amount of Hb (MCV and MCHC are decreased). Examples are iron deficiency anemia, chronic blood loss, and thalassemia.

7. (a) Treatment necessitates identification of the cause of the anemia. (b) If possible, resolve the underlying cause. (c) Start specific treatment only if indicated.

8. Excess (poly-) of all the cell lines (-cythemia), but generally used for conditions in which the RBC mass exceeds normal.

9. It may be classified as primary or secondary. (a) *Primary polycythemia:* in polycythemia the pluripotential stem cell is abnormal. There is marked erythrocytosis, leukocytosis, and thrombocytosis. (b) *Secondary polycythemia:* secondary to underlying medical problems (e.g., cardiopulmonary diseases) that decrease arterial O_2 saturation, stimulating erythropoiesis, and renal tumors, which increase erythropoietin production.

10. Compare your drawing with Fig. 17-1.

11. Erythrocytes containing Hb S traverse the microcirculation more slowly than normal erythrocytes, resulting in deoxygenation. Hb S erythrocytes adhere to endothelium, retarding blood flow. Increased deoxygenation may take the abnormal RBCs below a critical point, causing sickling within the microvasculature.

12. Life-threatening disorder of the stem cell in the bone marrow in which an insufficient number of blood cells are produced. May be congenital, idiopathic, or secondary. Deficient in all types of blood cells (pancytopenic).

13. Antineoplastic or cytotoxic agents; radiation therapy; certain antibiotics; miscellaneous drugs (e.g., anticonvulsants, thyroid medications); chemicals (e.g., benzene, organic solvents, insecticides).

14. Transplantation with compatible donors (e.g., siblings with matching HLA antigens). Success rate is about 60% to 70% long-term survival.

15. c
16. a
17. c
18. b, c
19. b, c, e
20. a, c
21. b
22. a
23. b
24. c, d, e, f
25. c
26. a, d
27. True
28. True
29. False; 1:600
30. False; this treatment is in investigative stages.
31. Normocytic, normochromic
32. Visceral sequestration crisis with sickling and pooling of blood, especially in the chest.

CHAPTER 18

1. d, e
2. g, i
3. h
4. a, e
5. c
6. b
7. f
8. CSFs are glycoproteins that are part of a group of white blood cell (WBC) regulators known as cytokines. These are continuously synthesized by cells (e.g., lymphocyte/macrophage system, fibroblasts, endothelial cells in the bone marrow). CSFs are believed to circulate fully and attach themselves to specific receptors on the cell surface of hematopietic precursors, committing them to differentiation, which in the case of the WBCs, to the neutrophil and monocyte cell lines.
9. Morphologic classification based on differentiation and maturation of the predominant leukemic cells in the

bone marrow, as well as cytochemical studies.

10. Familial leukemia is rare, but there appears to be a higher incidence of leukemia in siblings of affected children, with the incidence increasing to 20% in monozygotic (identical) twins. Persons with chromosomal abnormalities seem to have a 20-fold increase in the incidence of acute leukemia.

Chemicals are being implicated with increased frequency, especially the alkylating agents. There is a likelihood of increased incidence of leukemia in patients treated with both radiation and chemotherapy.

11. Neoplastic plasma dyscrasias arising from a single clone (monoclonal) of plasma cells, manifested by the uncontrolled proliferation of immature and mature plasma cells in the bone marrow.

12. Younger patients: nontender, "rubbery" enlarged lymph node in the low cervical or supraclavicular area or a nonproductive cough secondary to hilar adenopathy. Older patients: unexplained fever and/or night sweats. Constitutional symptoms such as anorexia, cachexia, weight loss, and fatigue are seen in disseminated disease.

13. Multiple myeloma: treatment is aimed at reducing the number of malignant cells and preventing and controlling the complications.

Waldenström's macroglobulinemia: treatment is aimed at decreasing the IgM plasma load and bone marrow infiltration and lymphoid tissues.

14. False; T cell lymphomas have higher relapse rates with shorter relapse-free intervals.
15. True
16. False; plasma cells do not normally circulate and are found in small numbers in the bone marrow.
17. False; *neutropenia* refers to a decrease in the absolute neutrophil count.
18. True
19. False; 70% of the non-Hodgkin's lymphomas are of B cell origin.
20. False; these cells are called basophils.
21. c, d
22. a
23. a, b, c
24. b, d
25. a, b, d
26. d
27. a, b
28. c
29. All are correct.
30. b
31. a, c

32. b
33. All are correct.
34. a
35. Leukemia
36. Reed-Sternberg cells
37. Leukopenia
38. Chronic granulocytic leukemia
39. a. Neutrophils (neutrophilia)
    b. Eosinophils (eosinophilia)
    c. Basophils (basophilia)
40. i
41. b, g
42. a, d, g, j
43. g, h, j
44. f
45. c, g
46. e

CHAPTER 19

1. Platelets are derived from a noncommitted pluriopotential stem cell, which on demand and in the presence of thrombopoietin, differentiates into the committed stem cell pool to form the *megakaryoblast*. This cell, through a maturation sequence, becomes a megakaryocyte. The cell cytoplasm eventually breaks up into individual platelets.

2. Vasoconstriction is an immediate response to the injury, followed by adhesion of platelets to collagen in the vessel wall exposed by the injury. ADP is released by the platelets, causing them to aggregate. Minute amounts of thrombin stimulate platelet aggregation. Platelet factor III also accelerates plasma clotting. In this way a platelet plug forms. Platelets also play a role in the formation of fibrin and in clot retraction.

3. Factors V and X

4. It is thought that once the platelet level reaches a certain peak level, spontaneous aggregates of platelets occur. In the large vessels this has little effect, but the platelets plug the tiny capillaries. In the process the capillary wall is damaged and bleeding occurs into the tissues. Examples of primary thrombocytosis are polycythemia vera and chronic granulocytic leukemia. Examples of secondary thrombocytosis are those occurring temporarily after stress or exercise with storage pool release from the spleen or accompanying increased bone marrow demand states (hemorrhage or hemolytic anemia).

5. von Willebrand's disease is the most common inherited coagulation disorder. Most common subtype is type I. Except for types II and III, which are autosomal recessive, all are inherited as an autosomal dominant trait. von Willebrand's factor facilitates platelet adhesion to components in the vascular subendothelium under conditions of high flow and shear stress. It is also the intravascular carrier for factor VIII to sites of active hemorrhage.

6. Treatment options: cryoprecipitate, factor VIII concentrates, desmopressin (DDAVP), fresh-frozen plasma, and estrogens. Goal is to increase availability of von Willebrand's factor.

7. Treatment is aimed at replacement of the deficient plasma coagulation factors. Teaching patients and their families safety measures and home infusion of factor concentrates at the earliest signs of bleeding has improved the quality of life.

8. DIC refers to a multifaceted complex syndrome in which a normally homeostatic and physiologic system of maintaining fluidity of blood becomes a pathologic system, leading to diffuse fibrin thrombi occluding the microvasculature of the body. DIC is initiated by the introduction of a procoagulant material or activity into the circulating blood.

9. Heparin's role is to neutralize thrombin activity inhibiting the consumption of the coagulation factors and fibrin deposition. Increasing the concentration of clotting factors and platelets with infusions of plasma and platelets should then inhibit the bleeding diathesis.

10. Improved donor screening, HIV testing of blood, development of virucidal methods, and recombinant (genetically engineered) factor preparations (factors VIII and IX)

11. False; platelets function to maintain capillary integrity and to initiate and retract clots.

12. False; administration of factor VIII

13. False; factor III (tissue thromboplastin) and factor IV (calcium ion) are the exceptions.

14. True

15. True

16. False; factor VIII is not synthesized by the liver.

17. True

18. False; the partial thromboplastin time (PTT) measures the intrinsic and common pathway.

19. False; the son of a carrier female has a 50% chance of being a hemophiliac.

20. b
21. a
22. c
23. b
24. d

25. b, d
26. a
27. d
28. b
29. a
30. d
31. b, d
32. e
33. a
34. d
35. b

CHAPTER 20

1. Intracellular, intravascular, and interstitial
2. See the box on p. 249 for a review.
3. Blood buffers, kidneys, and lungs
4. a
5. b
6. d; she has 60 lb of fluid (0.5 × 120), and $^2/_3$ of this is in the ICF, or 40 lb; 1 L = about 2 lb, so ICF = 20 L.
7. d
8. a, c
9. b
10. e
11. b
12. b, d
13. d
14. a
15. d
16. a
17. c; (=600 mOsm/400 mOsm/L)
18. b
19. a, b, d, e
20. c
21. a
22. b, c, d
23. b, c, d
24. b
25. False; active transport
26. True
27. True
28. True
29. False; causes sodium reabsorption
30. True
31. True
32. False; 2 L
33. False; requires data from history and clinical observations
34. False; only when the ion valence is one
35. True

CHAPTER 21

1. a
2. d
3. b
4. b, c, d
5. a
6. b, c, d
7. All are correct.
8. a; b and c are nonspecific; d is less sen-

sitive and specific; serum sodium reflects osmotic concentration, not volume changes.

9. a, c, e

10. b; since the patient is hypovolemic and hypokalemic

11. d; BSA of 70 kg man = 1.76 m²; fluid loss moderate; 1.76 × 2400 ml = about 4200 ml, or according to 4 kg weight loss, fluid loss = 4 L

12. a, b, c

13. c

14. b

15. b

16. a

17. (a) The effective circulating blood volume would decrease; (b) and (c) plasma osmolality and Na⁺ concentration would not change, since the fluid loss is isotonic with equal amounts of sodium and water lost; (d) ADH secretion would increase because of ECF volume depletion; (e) and (f) urine osmolality and thirst would increase because of the increased ADH secretion; (g) blood pressure would decrease because of hypovolemia.

18. Hyponatremia and hypoosmolality would occur.

19. (a) $2/3$ of pure water losses would come from the ICF, whereas $1/3$ would come from the ECF because these compartments make up 40% and 20% of the fluid, respectively, of the 60% of the body weight that is fluid. Isotonic fluid loss, on the other hand, comes from the ECF entirely. Therefore there is a greater decrease in the ECF volume and in the blood pressure with isotonic fluid losses; (b) the plasma osmolality will increase as a result of the loss of pure water but will not change with isotonic losses; (c) the brain cells will shrink and become dehydrated with pure water losses, but the volume does not change with isotonic losses.

20. Normal (isotonic) saline remains in the ECF and is effective in restoring the effective circulating blood volume and tissue perfusion. The 5% dextrose in water (D₅W) is metabolized to pure water; only $1/3$ remains in the ECF, whereas $2/3$ enters the ICF. Therefore D₅W has less effect on restoring the ECF volume and tissue perfusion. In addition, the D₅W would cause a dilutional hyponatremia.

21. a

22. a; (2 × [Na⁺] = 280 or 2 × [Na] + glucose/18 = 285); Na and Cl provide

most of the osmotically active solute particles; glucose particles contribute little to the osmolality under normal circumstances because glucose can enter cells.

23. b

24. All are correct.

25. c, d; since the patient has both a fluid volume deficit and hyponatremia as well as hypokalemia

26. c

27. d

28. d

29. a

30. b, c, d, e

31. c

32. a

33. a, b, d

34. All are correct.

35. a, b, d

36. d

37. d

38. b

39. c

40. b

41. All are correct.

42. All are correct.

43. a, b

44. e

45. a

46. e

47. d

48. c

49. c

50. a

51. c

52. c

53. a

54. b

55. c

56. a

57. b, c

58. a

59. d

60. a, b, c

61. b

62. d

63. a

64. c

65. a, b

66. a

67. b

68. a

69. d

70. a, c, e

CHAPTER 22

1. Cellular enzymes that maintain the life processes can only function within a narrow pH range. Cardiac function, in particular, is adversely affected by a pH less than 7.25 or greater than 7.55. Con-

tractility is depressed, and dysrhythmias may occur.

2. *pH* is the negative log of the hydrogen ion concentration [H⁺]. It has an inverse relationship to the actual [H⁺]. An *acid* is a compound that releases a H⁺ when in a solution with water (proton donor). A *base* is a H⁺ acceptor; that is, it incorporates H⁺ into its molecular structure by removing it from solution. The *pK* of a buffer system is the pH at which the buffer is 50% dissociated and has its maximum buffering capacity. The carbonic acid/bicarbonate buffer system would be more effective as a blood buffer if its pK were 7.4 rather than 6.1. A *buffer* system consists of a weak acid and its salt (or a weak base and its salt) and is only partially dissociated in solution. It acts as a chemical sponge. It can soak up extra H⁺ or release them to prevent fluctuations in the pH.

3. A volatile acid (carbonic acid) is one that can change from a liquid to a gas ($CO_2 + H_2O$) and is excreted by the lungs. Nonvolatile acids or fixed acids (e.g., phosphoric acid, sulfuric acid, lactic acid, ketoacids) cannot be excreted by the lungs but must be excreted by the kidneys.

4. The bicarbonate/carbonic acid system is the major buffer system of the ECF. The phosphate, hemoglobin, and protein buffer systems are primarily intracellular.

5. The kidney tubules excrete excess H⁺ in combination with phosphate and ammonia buffers. The H⁺ is excreted in exchange for Na⁺. The kidneys restore the bicarbonate level in the blood by absorbing HCO_3^- and Na⁺.

6. The lungs excrete CO_2, which is the anhydride of carbonic acid (minus a water molecule), and thus help to regulate [H⁺] in the blood. Hyperventilation means that CO_2 is being excreted by the lungs (blown off) faster than it is produced in the body, as indicated by a low Paco₂. Hyperventilation cannot be identified accurately by observing an increased rate and depth of breathing. The rate could be normal. Hypoventilation means that the lungs are deficient in eliminating CO_2 so that the Paco₂ is increased.

7. The anion gap is actually a calculation of anions in the body that are unmeasured, such as organic acids. It is calculated by subtracting the sum of the concentration of the major ECF anions from the cations. The

normal value is 8 to 16, with a mean of 12. $Na^+ - (Cl^- + HCO_3^-)$. The anion gap helps to identify the type of metabolic acidosis.

8. *The isohydric principle* states that all buffer systems in a solution are in equilibrium with the same H^+. Thus one only needs to measure and analyze one buffer system. Clinically, we need only measure the $PaCO_2$ and HCO_3^- to assess the acid-base status in the body.

9. The CO_2 content measures the alkali reserve of the body, which is primarily bicarbonate but also contains the carbonic acid component (which is small). It is measured using venous blood. The CO_2 content should not be confused with the $PaCO_2$, which is a measure of the pressure (tension) of dissolved CO_2 gas in arterial blood and is influenced by the lungs. The standard bicarbonate is measured after the blood specimen is equilibrated with CO_2 at a $PaCO_2$ of 40 mm Hg, thus "eliminating" the effect of respiration on the bicarbonate concentration, and is therefore said, to represent only metabolic changes in acid-base balance. In reality, it is no more accurate in estimating the bicarbonate concentration than the CO_2 content measure. The base excess (BE) is a method of identifying and assessing the severity of acid-base disorders. A positive value ($>+2$) means there is an excess of alkali (metabolic alkalosis), and a negative value (<-2) means there is a deficit of alkali (metabolic acidosis). Some authorities have criticized the BE, in particular, as misleading. Normal values: CO_2 content = 21 to 29 mEq/L; $PaCO_2$ = 40 mm Hg; standard HCO_3^- = 22 to 26 mEq/L.

10. a. Examine the clinical history for potential causes.
   b. Note clinical signs and symptoms, which might indicate an acid-base imbalance.
   c. Examine laboratory data of electrolytes and other data for disease processes associated with acid-base disorders.
   d. Examine pH.
   e. Examine the $PaCO_2$ and HCO_3^- in relationship to the pH and make a tentative decision about the primary disorder.
   f. Estimate the expected compensatory response to the primary acid-base disturbance.
   g. Calculate the anion gap and compare its change to the change in the bicarbonate concentration.
   h. Make the final interpretation

11. A value greater than or less than expected suggests a mixed acid-base disturbance.

12. (a) It can shut off the respiratory drive, since the pH of the CSF may be increased; (b) it may cause postacidosis respiratory alkalosis as a result of persistent hyperventilation; (c) a complicating respiratory alkalosis may cause tissue hypoxia, since the oxyhemoglobin dissociation curve is shifted to the left; (d) metabolic alkalosis may result if $NaHCO_3$ is given to a patient with DKA; (e) a serious metabolic alkalosis may result in the treatment of cardiopulmonary arrest; (f) tetany and convulsions may occur in a patient with renal failure; (g) it may cause hypervolemia and pulmonary edema.

13. b
14. c
15. c
16. a
17. c
18. All are correct.
19. a
20. b
21. b
22. a
23. a, b, c
24. H^+; HCO_3^-
25. H^+; HCO_3^-
26. Hyperventilation or blowing off CO_2
27. Hypoventilation or CO_2 retention
28. a
29. c, f, g, k
30. b, e, h
31. d
32. i
33. j, l
34. c
35. b, d
36. e
37. a
38. f
39. b
40. a
41. c
42. e
43. b
44. b
45. b
46. c
47. a
48. c, d
49. d
50. a, b, d
51. a. The diarrhea suggests possible metabolic acidosis.
   b. Physical assessment data (orthostatic hypotension, weakness, poor skin turgor, dry mucus membranes) suggest an ECF volume deficit and is supported by the low urinary sodium. She may even have a K^+ deficit, since it is normal and not elevated in the presence of an acidosis.
   c. The pH shows an acidemia. The HCO_3 and $PaCO_2$ are both decreased (change in the same direction) suggesting a compensated metabolic acidosis.
   d. For every 1 mEq decrease in HCO_3, expect 1.2 mm Hg drop in the $PaCO_2$: change in HCO_3 = 12 (24 − 12); expected change in $PaCO_2$ = 25.6 [40 − (12 × 1.2)]; actual $PaCO_2$ = 28 mm Hg. Thus it represents a simple compensated metabolic acidosis.
   e. AG = 142 − (118 + 12) = 12 mEq/L = normal anion gap
   f. Conclusion: normal anion gap, compensated metabolic acidosis

52. a. History suggests probable metabolic acidosis, an expected chronic disturbance with this condition.
   b. The creatinine and BUN indicate severe renal insufficiency.
   c. pH reveals acidemia. The HCO_3 and $PaCO_2$ change in the same direction, showing that there is respiratory compensation. The HCO_3 of 8 mEq/L indicates a moderately severe metabolic acidosis.
   d. The acid-base values fall within the metabolic acidosis confidence band on the acid-base nomogram, so it is probably not a mixed disorder. Change in HCO_3 = 16 (24 − 8). Expected drop in $PaCO_2$ = 20.8 [40 − (16 × 1.2)]. Actual $PaCO_2$ = 24 mm Hg. Might be a small amount of respiratory acidosis from fluid overload and wet lungs (data unavailable).
   e. AG = 137 − (102 + 8) = 27 mEq/L; increased anion gap common in renal failure because of the retention of fixed acids: sulphates, phosphates
   f. Conclusion: high anion gap, partly compensated metabolic acidosis

53. a. History suggests possible metabolic acidosis.
   b. Physical assessment and chest radiograph suggest acute respiratory acidosis.
   c. pH shows acidemia; the $PaCO_2$ and HCO_3 have changed in opposite directions, suggesting a mixed disorder. Increase in the $PaCO_2$ is much greater than the decrease in the

HCO$_3$, so perhaps the respiratory acidosis is primary.

d. Expected rise in HCO$_3$ = 1 mEq/L for every 10 mm Hg rise in the Paco$_2$; change in Paco$_2$ = +20 (60 − 40) = 2 × 10. Expected HCO$_3$ = 24 + (2 × 1) = 26 mEq/L; actual = 15 mEq/L; rise less than expected suggests mixed disorder.

e. No data available

f. Conclusion: acute respiratory acidosis superimposed on chronic metabolic acidosis

54. Acute respiratory acidosis secondary to probable pulmonary infection; no data are available to state whether man also has COPD in addition to probable pulmonary edema from CHF.

55. Chronic respiratory acidosis; kidneys are retaining HCO$_3$.

56. The patient has developed metabolic alkalosis secondary to diuretic therapy.

57. Posthypercapneic metabolic alkalosis; this is related to chloride deficiency, which occurred during the development of chronic respiratory acidosis and was worsened by the administration of diuretics.

58. See answers 54 to 57 for probable causes.

59. True

60. False; they have an inverse relationship; when bicarbonate increases, chlorides decrease, and vice versa.

61. False; hypoventilation

62. False; need history, signs and symptoms, and laboratory values, which must be interpreted together so that a complete clinical picture emerges.

63. True

CHAPTER 23

1. Transportation of ingested material from the pharynx to the stomach.

2. Lower esophageal closure strength has not developed fully in the infant. In adults, regurgitation reflects both LES incompetence and failure of the UES to serve as a regurgitation barrier.

3. Varicose veins of the esophagus (enlarged, tortuous veins). Esophageal varices develop in cases of hepatic cirrhosis and portal hypertension because of the communication between the portal and esophageal veins, providing a bypass of the liver to the vena cava. Esophageal varices may rupture, causing a fatal hemorrhage, because they are unable to withstand the high-pressure flow.

4. An *esophagomyotomy* is a surgical procedure on the lower esophagus to enlarge the opening into the stomach. A *pyloroplasty* is a procedure to repair the pylorus, especially to enlarge the gastric outlet. These procedures are often used to treat achalasia and are often combined, since incompetence of the LES and reflux esophagitis may follow the myotomy. Enlarging the gastric outlet helps to prevent gastric reflux into the esophagus.

5. Avoid hot, cold, or spicy foods; eat bland foods.
Eat slowly and chew food well before swallowing.
Sleep with head of bed elevated.
Take antacids.
Avoid eating just before going to bed.
Avoid tight clothes.
Lose weight, if overweight.
Avoid stooping, bending.
Avoid straining to have a bowel movement (stool softeners may be necessary).
Eat in a quiet, relaxed environment.
Avoid alcohol and tobacco.

6. Check your drawing with Fig. 23-5. The most important mechanism preventing reflux is the zone of high pressure between the esophagus and stomach (physiologic LES). The acute gastroesophageal angle produces a flap-valve effect. The phrenoesophageal ligament produces a pinchcock-valve effect.

7. Chronic reflux esophagitis causes esophageal inflammation, ulcer formation, bleeding, and eventually scarring and stricture.

8. Because these patients often aspirate esophageal or gastric contents into the lungs, especially during sleep

9. The symptom of pyrosis, or heartburn, is poorly correlated with the presence or absence of esophagitis. Some patients with heartburn do not have evidence of esophagitis, and some patients with esophagitis caused by reflux may not have symptoms until the condition is advanced. The acid perfusion test is the best method of identifying esophagitis.

10. d
11. c
12. b
13. c
14. a
15. b
16. a
17. a, c
18. a
19. a

20. a
21. a, c, d
22. b
23. b
24. d
25. c
26. a, c
27. a
28. b
29. c
30. b, c
31. True
32. True
33. False; it is possible to swallow liquid while standing on one's head or in a spaceship under conditions of zero gravity.
34. True
35. False; the throat may be sprayed with a local anesthetic.
36. True
37. True
38. c
39. e
40. d
41. a
42. b
43. b
44. c, e
45. a, d

CHAPTER 24

1. Refer to Fig. 24-1.

2. The outer layer of the stomach consists of peritoneum, which is reflected off the lesser curvature as the lesser omentum and off the greater curvature as the greater omentum.

3. Mucosal folds that allow for expansion of the stomach.

4. Pepsinogen is converted to pepsin in the presence of a low pH. Pepsin and HCl begin the process of protein digestion.

5. The extrinsic nerve supply of the stomach is entirely from the autonomic nervous system. Parasympathetic fibers travel via the vagus nerve and control gastric motor and secretory activity. Sympathetic fibers travel via the greater splanchnic nerves. Sympathetic stimulation inhibits gastric secretion and motility, which is opposite to the effect of vagal stimulation. Auerbach's and Meissner's nerve plexuses are involved in local reflexes and help to coordinate peristalsis. These plexuses constitute the intrinsic gastric innervation.

6. Celiac artery comes off the aorta; right and left gastric and gastroepiploic arteries supply most of the stomach.

7. Because posterior wall duodenal ulcers frequently erode into the gastroduode-

nal and pancreaticoduodenal arteries located just behind the duodenum.

8. Reservoir function, mixing function, and emptying function.

9. Approximately 1 to 2 L; there is a receptive relaxation of the smooth muscle as food and liquids are ingested.

10. Intrinsic factor combines with vitamin B_{12} and is necessary for its absorption in the ileum. Vitamin B_{12} is necessary for the normal maturation of red blood cells.

11. There is a basic intrinsic rhythm to the peristaltic activity of the stomach that is modified by nervous and hormonal factors. Gastrin stimulates gastric motility, as does parasympathetic stimulation, whereas sympathetic stimulation inhibits motility. Gastric emptying is also controlled by nervous and hormonal factors elicited by distention of the duodenum and the physical and chemical state of the chyme as it enters the duodenum.

12. The gastric mucus forms a protective coat for the gastric mucosa against mechanical and chemical injury (Hollander). The mucus in the columnar epithelial cells and the tight junctions between the epithelial cells prevent back diffusion of hydrogen ion (Davenport). Aspirin, alcohol, and bile salts are the most common substances causing disruption of the gastric mucosal barrier. The result is increased back diffusion of H^+, mucosal injury, and ulceration caused by the action of gastric acid and pepsin.

The duodenum is protected by secretion of a highly alkaline, viscid mucus that neutralizes the acid chyme from the stomach. It is produced by Brunner's glands in the duodenum.

13. Increases closure strength of the LES, thus preventing gastric reflux into the esophagus during gastric mixing; increases pyloric sphincter tone, thus preventing gastric emptying until mixing is completed; stimulates the secretion of acid and pepsin in the stomach so that protein digestion may begin; promotes receptive relaxation of the stomach so that filling can occur without an increase in intragastric pressure; stimulates gastric and intestinal motility so that mixing and propulsion of chyme is promoted; stimulates secretion of insulin, bile, and pancreatic juice.

14. Superficial inflammation of the gastric mucosa. If you have ever had "food poisoning" or "intestinal flu" with nausea, vomiting, or diarrhea,

you no doubt have had acute superficial gastritis.

15. *Cephalic phase:* sight, smell, or thought of food is mediated through parasympathetic fibers of the vagus nerve, which stimulates gastric acid secretion.

Gastric phase: antral distention is the prime stimulus to release of the hormone gastrin, which stimulates gastric acid secretion.

Intestinal phase: of little importance in stimulating gastric acid secretion; influence is mainly inhibitory.

16. d
17. a, b, c, d
18. a, c, d
19. a, b, e
20. b
21. a, c, d
22. c
23. a
24. c, d
25. c
26. d
27. a, c, d
28. c
29. a, c
30. d
31. b
32. a, b, d, c
33. e
34. e
35. a, b, c
36. False; pepsinogen
37. True
38. True
39. True
40. True
41. True
42. a
43. b
44. a, b, d
45. a, b, e, f

CHAPTER 25

1. Cytotoxic drugs interfere with the metabolism of all rapidly proliferating cells (cancer and leukemic cells). Since hair cells and the epithelial cells of the gastrointestinal mucosa are the most rapidly proliferating cells in the body, they are especially vulnerable to the effects of these drugs. Cell division is inhibited, resulting in atrophy of both the villi and the crypts of Lieberkühn, and sometimes there is ulceration and bleeding of the mucosa.

2. The secretion of bile from the liver aids the digestive process by emulsifying fats so that a greater surface area is presented for pancreatic action. Bile

salts act as detergents solubilizing fatty acids, glycerides, and fat-soluble vitamins by the formation of micelles. These substances are thus held in solution until absorption takes place.

3. *Maldigestion* means that digestion of a particular nutrient failed to take place somewhere in the stepwise process of food breakdown into the simplest products that can be absorbed. Maldigestion could be caused by general lack of a secretion containing enzymes (pancreatic insufficiency) or lack of a specific enzyme (lactase insufficiency). Other causes of maldigestion are lack of mechanical breakdown of food particles, so that digestive enzymes cannot reach all the food substances, or a transit time through the intestine that is too rapid to allow time for hydrolysis by enzymes. Maldigestion always results in malabsorption, since nutrients cannot be absorbed until they have been hydrolized into the simplest substances.

Malabsorption refers to lack of transport of a substance across the intestinal mucosa.

4. The stool is pale, large in volume, greasy, frothy, and tends to float. It tends to stick to the side of the toilet and is difficult to flush away.

5. The lesion is granulomatous and similar to the lesion of tuberculosis. Since the tubercular lesion represents a hypersensitivity reaction (cellular immune mechanism), medical scientists have looked for an infectious agent and autoantibodies but have not been successful in identifying either.

6. Valvulae conniventes, villi, and microvilli

7. (a) Inadequate digestion as a result of rapid emptying of stomach and poor mixing; (b) insufficient stimulation of CCK release (which stimulates pancreatic secretion) caused by bypass of duodenum in Billroth II gastrectomy; (c) deconjugation of bile salts by abnormal bacterial proliferation in blind loop after Billroth II; (d) loss of reservoir function, resulting in dumping of stomach contents into small bowel, with rapid transit time.

8. When the small bowel is obstructed either mechanically or functionally, it loses its absorptive and forward propulsive capacity, so gastrointestinal secretions pool within the lumen. The resulting ischemia of the intestinal wall from the distention further compromises the absorptive and motile

function of the bowel, so a vicious cycle of degeneration develops. The pooling of fluids in the gut depletes the ECF volume, resulting in hypovolemic shock. Bacterial proliferation occurs in the pooled fluids, and increased permeability of the ischemic mucosa allows absorption of bacteria and their toxins into the circulation, causing septicemia and toxemia.

9. Superior mesenteric
10. Pyloric; ileocecal
11. Mesentery
12. Greater omentum; infection
13. Ligament of Treitz
14. Valvulae conniventes
15. Villi
16. Crypts of Lieberkühn
17. Lacteal
18. Umbilicus; iliac; appendix
19. d
20. b
21. a, b, d
22. b
23. c
24. c
25. d
26. a, b, c, d
27. c
28. a, b, c, d, e
29. c
30. c, d, e
31. a, b, d
32. a, b, c, d
33. d, f
34. c, g
35. a, h
36. b, e
37. c
38. e
39. c
40. c
41. c
42. e
43. a
44. c
45. b
46. d, e
47. f
48. g
49. c, h
50. a, f
51. b
52. d
53. g, e
54. b
55. c
56. a
57. c
58. True
59. False; sympathetic fibers
60. True
61. True
62. True

CHAPTER 26

1. Check your drawing with Fig. 26-1.
2. The absorption of water and the elimination of the wastes of digestion
3. The large intestine is half as long as the small intestine. It has a diameter more than twice that of the small intestine. The external anal sphincter is under voluntary control, whereas the sphincters at each end of the small intestine are under autonomic control. The large intestine has no villi, its longitudinal muscle layer is incomplete throughout most of its length, and the mucosa contains more goblet cells than that of the small intestine. These structural differences between the small and large intestine are in keeping with their primary functions. The villi, large volume of secretions, and active motility pattern of the small intestine serve well its primary function of digestion and absorption. In contrast, the large intestine is much less motile, and although one of its main functions is absorption of water, it only absorbs about $1/13$ the amount absorbed by the small intestine. The decreased motility allows more time for absorption, since its ability to absorb is lessened by its lack of villi. One of the functions of the large intestine is to act as a reservoir until elimination can take place. The increased number of goblet cells and increased mucus secretion are important since the feces are semisolid in the large intestine and lubrication is more necessary for propulsion of the fecal mass.
4. *Haustral churning* refers to back-and-forth pendular movements especially prominent in the transverse colon, caused by annular contractions of short segments of the bowel, especially the circular muscles. These movements allow time for the absorption of water. *Mass peristalsis* is a contraction involving a long segment of the large intestine that propels a large amount of fecal material forward. Feces are frequently moved into the rectum by mass peristalsis and the defecation reflex is initiated.
5. Hemorrhoids, constipation, cancer of the rectum, anorectal abscesses, fissures, and fistulas.
6. *Palpation of abdomen:* presence of mass, tenderness.
   Rectal digital examination: palpation of tumors, hemorrhoids.

Proctosigmoidoscopic examination: direct visualization of tumors, internal hemorrhoids, ulcerated or hyperemic mucosa; biopsy or cell washings may also be obtained for histologic study (lower 25 cm of bowel observed).
Colonoscopy: direct visualization of entire large bowel with same information obtained as above.
Barium enema radiography: neoplasms, strictures, diverticula, and polyps may all be visualized.
Stool examination: blood, parasites, shape, size, etc. may give clues to many disorders of the GI tract.

7. Only a small percentage of the patients with diverticulitis require surgery. Surgery is indicated when there is severe and extensive disease or complications such as perforation. During an attack of acute diverticulitis, the medical treatment usually consists of bedrest, liquid diet, stool softeners, and antibiotics.
8. Ulcerative colitis of more than 10 years' duration; certain types of colonic polyps; eating a diet low in fiber and high in refined carbohydrates.
9. Burkitt proposed that slow transit with low-fiber diets permits bacterial action on bile acids or other normal bowel constituents to produce carcinogens, which then act on the colonic mucosa.
10. Since the superior hemorrhoidal vein is connected to the portal system, increased portal pressure may cause backflow into these veins and hemorrhoids.
11. A *fissure in ano* is a persistent crack in the perianal skin. A *fistula in ano* is an abnormal granulation-lined tract connecting two epithelial sufaces—in this region running between the anal canal and the skin of the perianal area. It is the consequence of anorectal abscess that has been inadequately treated. Any of these conditions may be a complication of hemorrhoids. Crohn's disease of the colon is especially likely to be associated with anorectal fistulas.
12. a
13. a
14. e
15. a
16. a, b, c, d
17. a, b, c
18. e
19. e
20. c
21. b
22. a, c, d, e
23. e
24. a

25. b, c, d
26. c
27. e
28. a, c, e
29. d
30. a, b, c, e
31. b
32. All are correct.
33. b, d, e
34. b
35. c
36. a
37. d
38. b
39. a, c, d
40. a, b, d, e
41. a, b, c
42. a
43. Diverticulosis; diverticulitis
44. Pedunculated; juvenile; villous; familial polyposis
45. Annular; polypoid
46. Direct extension to adjacent structure; metastasis via lymph nodes; metastasis via bloodstream
47. Superior; middle; inside; inferior
48. Bleeding; thrombosis; strangulation
49. d
50. a
51. c
52. a
53. a
54. b
55. b
56. b
57. b
58. a
59. c
60. a
61. a-2; b-1; c-3
62. True
63. False; it is under voluntary control.
64. False; only a few severe or complicated cases
65. False; vitamin K and some of the B group
66. True
67. True
68. False; they are inside both sphincters.
69. True
70. False; 35%
71. True
72. True
73. True
74. True

CHAPTER 27

1. Blood circulation through the liver is unusual because a mixture of portal venous blood and arterial blood flows through the liver sinusoids. The portal blood contains many nutrients absorbed from the intestines that are metabolized in the liver.

2. The *gallbladder* is a pear-shaped hollow muscular bag that has a capacity of about 45 ml. Its primary function is to concentrate hepatic bile transported to the gallbladder via the cystic duct. Bile is stored in the gallbladder and released as needed for digestion of fats in the intestine. Cholecystokinin-pancreozymin stimulates the gallbladder to contract and release bile.

   The *pancreas* is about 6 inches long and $1\frac{1}{2}$ inches wide and resembles a bunch of grapes. The main pancreatic duct runs through the entire length of the organ and opens into the duodenum. An accessory pancreatic duct (duct of Santorini) may also open into the duodenum at a different point. The pancreas has an exocrine secretion, pancreatic juice from the acini, and endocrine secretions, glucagon and insulin, produced by the alpha and beta cells in the islands of Langerhans. The release of pancreatic juice is controlled by CCK and secretin.

3. Formation and excretion of bile; carbohydrate metabolism, including synthesis, storage, and release of glucose to maintain proper blood level; protein metabolism, including synthesis of most proteins, urea formation, and storage of amino acids; fat metabolism, including cholesterol synthesis and fat storage; storage of many vitamins and minerals; metabolism of steroid hormones; detoxification of both endogenous and exogenous substances potentially harmful; acts as flood chamber and filter.

   The liver is called an organ of defense because of its large concentration of phagocytic Kupffer cells lining the sinusoids. These cells are actually part of the monocyte-macrophage (reticuloendothelial) defense system.

   The liver detoxifies drugs and other potentially harmful chemicals by oxidation, reduction, hydrolysis, or conjugation so that they become physiologically inactive. Conjugation with glucuronic acid, for example, makes the substance water soluble so that it may be excreted in the urine.

   The liver is capable of holding a liter or more of blood and holds a strategic position between the intestinal and general circulation. It can serve as a reservoir (flood chamber) when blood backs up, as in right ventricular failure. Sudden release of the blood from the reservoir could cause circulatory overload and pulmonary congestion.

   The liver is the central chemical laboratory for the metabolism of carbohydrates, fats, and proteins, and this role alone makes the liver essential for life. It plays a major role in the regulation of blood glucose, serum lipids, serum proteins, and coagulation factors.

4. Excess production of bilirubin exceeding the processing ability of the liver; impaired uptake of unconjugated bilirubin; impaired conjugation; and impaired excretion of bilirubin.

5. *Kernicterus* is the deposition of bilirubin in lipid-rich brain, especially the basal ganglia, causing damage to the cells by its toxic action. Kernicterus occurs when there are high lvels of unconjugated bilirubin (lipid-soluble) in the blood.

6. The jaundice is physiologic because the immaturity of the liver leads to relative deficiency of the glucuronyl transferase, which conjugates free bilirubin with glucuronic acid. The acceptor proteins may also be inadequate, so uptake by the hepatocyte is also deficient.

7. No, it is useful only in helping to prevent hepatitis in exposed individuals, especially hepatitis A.

8. *Community:* safe and inspected water supply and sewage disposal; inspection of all wells and septic tanks; restaurant inspection; inspection of public swimming pools and beaches for safety of water.
   Home: good general sanitary habits—handwashing, separate drinking glasses and eating utensils, adequate dish washing and sterilization.
   Clinical unit: use of disposable syringes, needles, and catheters; screening of blood for hepatitis B antigen; careful disposal of urine and feces from infected patients; handwashing; avoidance of needle puncture; isolation of infected patients in a private room with separate bathroom facilities, disposable dishes, and gowns and gloves worn by those attending patient.

9. About 90% removal or destruction of the liver is still compatible with life. Complete removal results in death in about 10 hours.

10. (a) Triangular, 1500, right upper; (b) kidney, gallbladder; (c) stomach,

pancreas; (d) falciform; (e) capsule of Glisson

11. (a) Bile, hepatic, hepatic; (b) cystic, bile; (c) pancreatic, Vater; (d) Oddi

12. (a) Hepatic portal, hepatic, vena cava; (b) portal; (c) hepatic; (d) spleen, esophageal, rectal

13. (a) Lobule; (b) sinusoids, Kupffer; (c) canaliculi

14. b

15. d

16. a, b, c, d

17. d; bile is catabolized in the intestine.

18. All are correct.

19. c

20. c

21. c

22. a

23. c

24. c

25. d

26. a

27. a, b, d

28. d

29. b

30. d

31. d

32. d

33. d

34. a, c, d, e

35. e

36. f

37. a

38. b

39. h

40. c

41. d

42. g

43. *Alcoholic hepatitis* is a lesion characterized by hepatocellular necrosis and infiltration with inflammatory cells. It is associated with alcohol ingestion and is believed to be the critical lesion in the development of Laennec's cirrhosis.

44. Because cirrhosis is generally silent until far advanced, when major signs and symptoms appear. Early symptoms are vague and nonspecific, so patients do not seek medical help.

45. *Portal hypertension* is a sustained elevation of the portal venous pressure above the normal 6 to 12 cm H_2O. The primary mechanism causing portal hypertension is increased resistance to blood flow through the liver. This could occur in cirrhosis, congestive heart failure (backup of blood from right atrium), and hepatic vein thrombosis. Increased inflow through the splanchnic arteries in cirrhosis also contributes to portal hypertension.

46. Compression of varices by esophageal and gastric balloons (Sengstaken-Blakemore tube); vasopressin infusion. It is important to remove the blood from the gastrointestinal tract, since large amounts of ammonia may be produced from the action of gut bacteria on the blood protein. The ammonia may reach the systemic circulation, causing hepatic encephalopathy by interfering with cerebral metabolism. Recurrent bleeding from esophageal varices may be prevented by reducing the pressure and blood flow through the varices by creating a surgical shunt between the portal and systemic circulation. Flow through the esophageal veins is reduced, but ammonia and other protein metabolites may pass directly into the systemic circulation, causing hepatic encephalopathy.

47. *Hepatic encephalopathy* is a form of cerebral intoxication caused by ammonia and/or other protein metabolites. It is manifested clinically by a neuropsychiatric syndrome characterized by mental clouding and neuromuscular dysfunction progressing to coma.

    It occurs when more ammonia is presented to the liver than the failing cells can synthesize into urea or when the ammonia bypasses the liver through shunts and enters the systemic circulation.

    It is important to detect hepatic encephalopathy during the early stages, since prompt treatment may be successful in reversing the process. The mortality is high if it progresses to an advanced stage.

48. *Asterixis* is a peripheral manifestation of impaired cerebral metabolism characterized by a peculiar flapping tremor of the wrists and metacarpophalangeal joints. It is tested by having the patient extend both arms out with fingers spread.

49. *Constructional apraxia* is the inability to construct simple diagrams or to write legibly in the absence of paralysis or motor weakness. Deterioration in the ability to perform purposeful, skilled construction or to write reflects the progress of the encephalopathy, and a serial record can be kept in the patient's records.

50. *Stage I:* slowness of mentation and affect, untidiness, slurred speech, personality change, inappropriate behavior, disordered sleep rhythm

Stage II: accentuation of stage I, inappropriate behavior, lethargy, asterixis, muscle tremor

Stage III: sleeps most of time but can be aroused; marked confusion, may be abusive and violent; abnormal EEG pattern

Stage IV: comatose, positive Babinski's sign, hyperactive reflexes, abnormal EEG, hepatic fetor sometimes detected

51. In *acute cholecystitis* the patient has a sudden onset of severe pain in the right upper quadrant that may last for several hours. It is often associated with the passage of a gallstone through the cystic or common bile duct. There may be tenderness over the gallbladder. *Chronic cholecystitis* is characterized by symptoms that are much milder. There may be episodes of mild pain in the right upper quadrant and a long history of dyspepsia, flatulence, heartburn, and fat intolerance.

52. Because the liver acts as a filter, with about one third of the cardiac output traversing it each minute. Malignant cells transported from the intestines, stomach, or pancreas through the portal vein are readily trapped in the liver capillary bed.

53. a, b, c, d

54. c

55. d

56. a

57. d

58. a, c, d

59. a, c

60. b

61. a, b, d

62. c

63. d

64. e

65. d

66. c

67. b

68. c, d

69. d

70. b

71. c

72. a, b, c, d, e

73. a

74. d

75. a, b, d

76. a, b, c

77. False; it is within the peritoneal cavity.

78. True

79. True

80. False; more common in females; history of alcoholism more common in males

81. True
82. True
83. False; pure bilirubin stones
84. False; a pseudocyst forms outside the pancreas, often within lesser omental sac.
85. False; they are uncommon in the United States and are usually diagnosed late, when they are beyond hope; early symptoms are insidious.
86. True
87. True
88. True
89. False; it is a cholecystectomy.
90. d
91. b
92. c
93. i
94. a
95. g
96. e
97. f
98. h
99. f
100. c
101. a
102. b
103. e
104. d
105. The primary mechanism causing *ascites* is resistance to blood flow through the liver resulting in portal hypertension. Portal hypertension raises the hydrostatic pressure in the intestinal vascular bed, which favors the transudation of fluid from the intravascular space to the interstitial space, resulting in ascites. Other mechanisms contributing to the development of ascites include hypoalbuminemia (decreased liver synthesis), which causes decreased colloid osmotic pressure (COP), favoring transudation; increased production and flow of hepatic lymph (caused by the portal hypertension), which "weeps" a high-protein fluid into the ascitic fluid in the peritoneal cavity and raises the COP in ascitic fluid, which favors more transudation; and retention of Na^+ and water because of increased aldosterone (because less is inactivated by the failing liver cells).

    Signs and symptoms of ascites include increased abdominal girth, bulging flanks, and shortness of breath when the volume is large.

    Treatment consists of a low-sodium diet and the judicious use of diuretics. Paracentesis should only be used if the volume of fluid is great enough to cause respiratory distress and for diagnostic purposes.

CHAPTER 28

1. Venae cavae → right atrium → pulmonary artery → lung capillaries → pulmonary veins → left atrium → left ventricle → aorta → systemic arteries → arterioles → capillaries → venules → systemic veins.
2. The AV node delays the wave of electrical excitation to allow time for ventricular filling during atrial contraction before ventricular contraction. It also prevents an excessive number of electrical impulses from reaching the ventricles.
3. The thickness of the right ventricle is only one third that of the left ventricle. These differences in muscular size reflect their respective pumping functions in the circulatory system. The right ventricle pumps blood through the low-pressure, low-resistance pulmonary circuit. The workload of the left ventricle is much greater than that of the right, since it must generate pressure about five times as high to overcome the high resistance of the systemic circulation.
4. To support the AV valves during ventricular contraction and prevent leaflet eversion into the atria.
5. Three; aortic valves; sinuses of Valsalva; to protect the coronary orifices from occlusion by the aortic valve cusps during ventricular ejection.
6. The visceral and parietal pericardium. This small space contains a small amount of lubricating fluid that functions as protection against friction.
7. Lymph is propelled by muscle compression of the lymph vessels. Flow is aided by lymphatic peristalsis.
8. Sympathetic stimulation of the alpha receptors causes vasoconstriction, while stimulation of beta receptors causes vasodilation. This vasodilatory effect is produced by beta$_2$-receptors. In contrast, the beta$_1$-receptors produce cardiac effects of increased heart rate, force of contraction, and velocity of AV conduction. The beta$_2$-receptors produce vasodilation.
9. d
10. c
11. c
12. b
13. b
14. c
15. d
16. c
17. d
18. b
19. a, b, c
20. a, c, d
21. e
22. c, e, f, a d, b
23. c, d
24. a, b
25. c
26. a
27. e
28. d
29. b
30. f
31. Automaticity; excitability; conductivity; rhythmicity
32. Valves
33. Collateral
34. Right coronary; left anterior descending
35. 60 to 100; 40 to 60; 20 to 30

CHAPTER 29

1. Systole and diastole represent the mechanical activity of the heart. *Systole* is the period when the heart muscle contracts; *diastole* indicates the resting period of the heart when the muscles relax. The terms *systole* and *diastole* are typically used in referring to ventricular activity. The *electrocardiogram* (ECG) represents a body surface recording of the summated electrical activity of all the myocardial cells. An action potential is an intracellular recording of the electrical activity of a single cell. Electrical activity stimulates mechanical activity.
2. *Starling's law of the heart* states that, within limits, the force of contraction is a function of the length of muscle fibers, that is, their end-diastolic length. Thus the horizontal axis of the ventricular function curve represents the stretching of the myocardium. It can be seen that as the degree of stretch and end-diastolic volume (EDV) increases, the stroke volume (SV), or ventricular performance, increases (vertical axis). However, where the curve flattens, there is no increase in performance as EDV increases. Then, with further EDV increases, dyspnea and finally pulmonary edema develop. The position of the ventricular function curve represents the degree of contractility. When the curve is shifted to the left (increased contractility caused by influence of norepinephrine or Ca^{++}), there is greater increase in ventricular performance or SV at a given EDV or degree of muscle fiber length (the

curve is steeper). A shift of the curve to the right represents myocardial depression and decreased contractility, so there is a smaller increase in SV for increments in stretch or EDV. The ejection fraction (EF), SV/EDV, is a good index of contractility. Thus the steeper the curve, the greater the contractility. It can be seen from these relationships that contractility has a greater influence on ventricular performance than the Starling mechanism (increasing EDV to increase performance).

3. *Poiseuille's law,* stated in terms of the circulation, says that the volume of blood circulated per minute is directly related to the systemic blood pressure gradient and inversely related to the resistance ($F = \Delta P/R$). The systemic blood pressure gradient is calculated by subtracting pressures at the arterial and venous end of the circulation (i.e., mean arterial pressure − central venous pressure).

4. SV = EDV − ESV = 100 ml − 30 ml = 70 ml (this is in the normal range). CI = CO ÷ body surface area = 4.5 L/minute ÷ 1.5 m^2 = 3.0 (this is also in the normal range). EF = SV/EDV = 70/100 = 0.70 (the EF should be $^2/_3$, or 0.67, so it is normal).

5. a
6. c
7. All are correct.
8. c
9. a, c
10. a
11. a
12. All are correct.
13. a, c
14. b
15. b
16. d
17. b
18. a
19. All are correct.
20. a, h, d, f, g, c, i, b, e
21. d
22. c
23. a
24. e
25. b
26. f
27. Absolute refractory; relative refractory
28. Negatively; potassium; sodium
29. Open; closed
30. Closed; open
31. AV node
32. c
33. b
34. d
35. b

36. c
37. a, d
38. f
39. e

CHAPTER 30

1. Class III
2. The left carotid may be partially occluded, possibly because of an atherosclerotic plaque. Her mean arterial pressure (MAP) is about 126 mm Hg. MAP = diastolic blood pressure + pulse pressure/3 = 100 + 78/3 = 126.
3. The *hepatojugular test* is performed by manually applying pressure over the right upper quadrant of the abdomen for 30 to 60 seconds and simultaneously observing the jugular veins. A rise in the level of the venous pressure head in the neck veins indicates a positive test. A positive test signifies that the right side of the heart was not able to accept the increased venous return (main source, venous reservoir in the liver, which is being compressed), which could result from right ventricular failure.
4. The *hexaxial reference system* is a representation of all the limb leads of the electrocardiogram (ECG). It is formed by moving the bipolar limb leads centrally so that these lines intersect. The position of the heart may be pictured at the center of this electrical reference system. When the unipolar limb leads are added to the reference system, the hexaxial reference system is produced. Using this reference system, the summation vector, or electrical axis, for the P, QRS, and T waves can be derived. An analysis of deviations of the electrical axis from the various leads assists in diagnosing conditions such as conduction abnormalities and chamber enlargement.
5. Pressures in the various cardiac chambers and great vessels may be recorded and the waveforms of the pressure tracings analyzed to detect valvular stenosis and regurgitation. The injection of radiopaque material into the various cardiac chambers allows visualization of chamber size and wall movement so that deviations from normal may be detected. Cardiac output may also be determined. Sampling of oxygen content in the right and left sides of the heart allows detection of right-to-left shunts, as from a ruptured septum. Selective coronary artery angiography allows detection of lesions in these vessels.

6. Indications for coronary angiography: (a) to determine the feasibility of coronary bypass surgery; (b) to evaluate atypical angina; and (c) to evaluate the results of coronary revascularization surgery.
7. d
8. c
9. a, c
10. b
11. d
12. d
13. b
14. b
15. d
16. All are correct.
17. d
18. a
19. b, c
20. c
21. c
22. c
23. c
24. b
25. b
26. a
27. b
28. d
29. b
30. c
31. a
32. d
33. a
34. c
35. d
36. c
37. b
38. c
39. False; it is on top of the foot.
40. True
41. False; the CVP increases during inspiration.
42. True
43. False; it is normal.
44. True
45. False; they are caused by turbulent blood flow through the partially occluded artery during the recording of blood pressure in an extremity.
46. True
47. c
48. d
49. b
50. f
51. a
52. e
53. c
54. b
55. a
56. a
57. d
58. c

59. c
60. c
61. d
62. b
63. a
64. b
65. c
66. ' a
67. b
68. c
69. a
70. b
71. d
72. e
73. b
74. c
75. a
76. f
77. f
78. a
79. b
80. e
81. c
82. g
83. h
84. d
85. Regurgitation
86. 5 mm Hg; aortic stenosis
87. Turbulent

CHAPTER 31

1. Oxygen demand is greater for the left ventricle than for the right because of its greater workload and larger muscle mass. Oxygen supply is more restricted because little coronary perfusion of the left ventricle occurs during systole. The firm compression of blood vessels by the thick muscular wall limits perfusion during systole. On the other hand, the thinner-walled right ventricle continues to have some perfusion during systole.

2. Atherosclerotic lesions tend to occur in the epicardial proximal segments of the right and left coronary arteries and at points of abrupt curvature, as where the left coronary artery branches into the left anterior descending.

3. Size and location of the infarct; function of the uninvolved myocardium; collateral circulation; cardiovascular compensatory mechanisms.

4. It is a reflex parasympathetic response resulting from pain or stimulation of parasympathetic ganglia in the myocardium. The effect is to slow the heart rate and reduce the blood pressure and cardiac output. Thus the response has an adverse effect in myocardial infarction, since sympathetic support of the compromised circulation is needed.

5. Severe, prolonged chest pain; elevated serum cardiac enzymes; ECG changes in leads overlying the area of necrosis (deep Q waves, ST segment elevation, inverted T waves).

6. Since cardiac output is a function of heart rate and stroke volume, a slow heart rate can reduce the total volume ejected in a given time by lowering the frequency of ejection. A rapid rate reduces ventricular filling time, so less blood is ejected per beat. Tachycardia also reduces the length of diastole, so perfusion time of the myocardium is limited. Thus oxygen supply is reduced at the same time that demand is increased because of the increased cardiac work.

7. Heart rate, force of contraction, and arterial pressure (a determinant of wall tension).

8. Because the diseased coronary blood vessels have a limited ability to dilate and thus increase perfusion and oxygen delivery to the myocardium. Total coronary perfusion is not increased by nitroglycerin, although there is some improvement of flow to ischemic areas by dilation of collaterals.

9. To allow healing of the infarcted tissue, decrease the incidence of complications, and salvage the ischemic zone surrounding the infarct.

10. In *congestive heart failure,* digitalis, diuretics, and restriction of fluid and salt intake are used to improve cardiac function and prevent the development of pulmonary edema.

    The first priority in the treatment of severe *pulmonary edema* is to reduce the increased intravascular volume and pressure in the pulmonary vessels and thus reduce transudation of fluid. This may be achieved quickly by elevation of the trunk with the legs dependent. Additional treatment includes the use of morphine, which causes peripheral dilation and helps pool blood in the extremities. Aminophylline relieves bronchospasm and increases the contractility of the heart. Oxygen therapy helps to correct the hypoxemia, and positive-pressure breathing may reduce transudation by opposing the increased pulmonary hydrostatic pressure.

    Cardiogenic shock is treated with vasopressor drugs (and sometimes vasodilators) and sometimes circulatory assistance devices to reduce the cardiac workload. Sodium bicarbonate is used to correct acidosis.

11. The patient needs individualized guidance and teaching to achieve maximum functional ability. Both psychologic and physical variables are involved.
12. b
13. b
14. c
15. All are correct.
16. c
17. c
18. b
19. b
20. a
21. a
22. b
23. c
24. d
25. c
26. All are correct.
27. a, b, d, e
28. c
29. c
30. b
31. d
32. e
33. All are correct.
34. d
35. c
36. d
37. a, d, e
38. d
39. All are correct.
40. b
41. c
42. a
43. b
44. a
45. b
46. True
47. True
48. False; this is a complication of saphenous vein bypass graft.
49. False; it increases muscle mass and oxygen demand.
50. False; they are a protective response to sinus node failure.
51. Ischemia
52. Increases
53. b, d, a, c
54. a
55. b
56. b
57. a
58. b
59. a
60. a
61. a
62. b
63. b
64. c
65. d
66. a

67. d
68. a
69. c
70. b
71. c
72. a
73. b
74. e
75. d
76. b
77. c
78. b, c, d
79. c
80. b
81. d
82. d
83. c
84. b
85. d

CHAPTER 32

1. Recurrent attacks of rheumatic fever: most common cause
   Subacute bacterial endocarditis: most infections in patients with rheumatic or congenital heart deformities
   Papillary muscle dysfunction or rupture: may be a complication of myocardial infarction
   Congenital malformations
   Inborn defects of connective tissue
2. It is regurgitation secondary to chamber enlargement. As a result of ventricular chamber enlargement, the papillary muscles and chordae tendineae are unable to anchor the valve leaflets securely. The valvular annulus may also enlarge.
3. Prophylactic antibiotics are necessary to reduce the risk of bacterial endocarditis in susceptible patients, including those with a history of rheumatic carditis and those with cardiac deformities. Even minor procedures such as dental work and catheterization may cause a transient bacteremia and the implantation of organisms on the endocardial surface.
4. Pulmonary congestion: diuretics to decrease blood volume; digitalis to increase heart contractility
   Atrial fibrillation: antidysrhythmic drugs
   Systemic emboli: anticoagulant drugs
5. Splitting of fused valvular commissures by the surgical introduction of an instrument to dilate them by blunt pressure or by inflating a balloon
6. The *Jones criteria* consist of a list of major and minor manifestations used to help establish a diagnosis of

rheumatic fever. If evidence indicates that the subject has had a preceding streptococcal infection (positive throat culture, ASO titer) and also has two major manifestations or one major and two minor manifestations, a diagnosis of rheumatic fever is made. Major manifestations include carditis, polyarthritis, erythema marginatum, and subcutaneous nodules. Minor manifestations are fever, arthralgia, elevated ESR or CRP, and prolonged PR.

7. a
8. c, b, d, a
9. a
10. c
11. d
12. b
13. c
14. c
15. b
16. b
17. c
18. c
19. All are correct.
20. b
21. c
22. d
23. c
24. a
25. b
26. c
27. e
28. c
29. a
30. All are correct.
31. c
32. b
33. b
34. c or d
35. c
36. c
37. b, d
38. c
39. c
40. c
41. a, c, e, f
42. b, d, f
43. b
44. All are correct.
45. a, c, e

CHAPTER 33

1. c
2. a
3. b
4. d
5. b, d
6. a
7. b
8. b, g

9. b
10. a, c, d, f
11. c
12. b
13. b
14. a
15. d
16. b, c, e
17. f
18. c
19. b
20. b
21. d
22. a, c
23. d
24. b
25. a, d
26. c
27. Circulatory; pump
28. Left atrial pressure; pulmonary venous; pulmonary edema
29. Heart failure
30. 40
31. Patient; reservoir
32. Venae cavae; oxygenator; aorta; femoral artery
33. 3, 5, 1, 7, 2, 4, 6
34. Concentric; eccentric; dilation
35. b, e, f
36. a, c, d
37. b
38. e
39. f
40. a
41. c
42. d
43. c
44. a
45. b
46. a
47. c
48. b
49. a
50. a, d
51. a
52. c
53. a
54. e
55. d

CHAPTER 34

1. a-4, b-3, c-6, d-2, e-5, f-8, g-1, h-7
2. *Varicose veins* are dilated, tortuous veins generally seen in the lower extremities. Pathogenic factors include inflammatory destruction of valves, weak vein walls and increased venous pressure (as in pregnancy), all causing varying degrees of valvular incompetence and regurgitation. The two major complications of varicosities are thrombosis

and venous ulcer, both resulting from venous stasis. A *varicosity* differs from an aneurysm in that the vessel is affected throughout a significant segment of its length, whereas an aneurysm generally involves a short segment of a blood vessel.

3. Deep venous thrombosis is more serious because of the potential complication of pulmonary embolus. The superficial veins may become distended as a result of impaired deep venous drainage.

4. Early ambulation, leg exercises, oral anticoagulants, external intermittent compression, elastic stockings, and elevation of the lower extremities to promote deep venous drainage are all methods of preventing deep venous thrombosis.

5. An *aneurysm* is a localized dilation of the arterial wall, resulting from degeneration and weakening of the medial layer of the artery. Aneurysms are frequently asymptomatic. The first sign of disease may be a serious, potentially life-threatening complication such as rupture, acute thrombosis, or embolization.

6. The deposition of the products of red blood cell destruction such as hemosiderin, caused by venous stasis with subsequent capillary destruction, results in the brownish skin discoloration seen in patients with chronic venous insufficiency.

7. Stasis of blood flow, endothelial injury, and hypercoagulability.

8. a
9. b
10. c
11. d
12. d
13. c
14. b, c
15. d
16. b, c, d; generally temperature not elevated to this extent; Homans' sign unreliable
17. a, d, e
18. b
19. b
20. Thrombophlebitis; phlebothrombosis
21. Thromboangiitis obliterans
22. d
23. a
24. b
25. c
26. b
27. a
28. c

29. d
30. c
31. a
32. b
33. d
34. c
35. b
36. a
37. False; it is called embolectomy.
38. False; they should be slightly dependent.
39. True
40. False; it is called an embolus.

CHAPTER 35

1. Infections, malignant diseases, and chronic bronchitis and emphysema

2. *Respiration* is the combined activity of the various mechanisms that supply oxygen (O_2) to the body cells and remove carbon dioxide (CO_2).

3. The blanket of mucus serves to trap dust and bacteria, which are then moved by ciliary action to the pharynx, where they are swallowed or expectorated. Inspired air is also humidified and warmed by the mucus blanket and underlying vascular network.

4. The right mainstem bronchus is larger and runs a more vertical course from the trachea than the left.

5. The lung would collapse (atelectasis).

6. The lung has a dual blood supply: the bronchial and the pulmonary circulation. (Did you remember to include the bronchial circulation?) The pulmonary circulation is a low-pressure, low-resistance system (the mean pulmonary artery pressure, at 15 mm Hg, is only about one-sixth that of the systemic circulation, at about 90 mm Hg).

7. Yes, there is a net pressure of 10 mm Hg in the direction of the alveolus.

8. Larynx or glottis
9. Surfactant; surface tension
10. Ventilation; respiratory bellows; diaphragm
11. Hering-Breuer
12. Pons and medulla
13. c
14. c
15. c
16. e
17. a
18. b
19. e
20. d
21. c
22. c
23. a-6, b-3, c-1, d-5, e-7, f-8, g-9, h-4,

i-10, j-2, k-12, l-11
24. a-4, b-5, c-2, d-1, e-7, f-6, g-3
25. c
26. b
27. a
28. c
29. c
30. b
31. Because of dilution with water vapor and other gases in the anatomic dead space

32. The volume of anatomic dead space is equal to 1 ml/pound of body weight; if you weigh 120 pounds, your anatomic dead space is about 120 ml.

33. Diffusion; the driving force is the pressure gradient between the partial pressure of the gas in the alveolus and in the pulmonary capillary.

34. No; perfusion increases going from the apex to the base of the lungs because of the effect of gravity in the low-pressure, low-resistance pulmonary circulation. The overall ventilation/perfusion ratio ($\dot{V}/\dot{Q}$) is 0.8, which is less than unity.

35. $\dot{V}/\dot{Q} = 3$ L/minute $\div 6$ L/minute $= 0.5$. This value would represent wasted perfusion and would be present in a shunt-producing disease.

36. More O_2 could be transported to the tissues in physical solution, which might make the critical difference in cases where there is very little hemoglobin (Hb) available to transport O_2 to the tissue cells.

37. No; an increased concentration of O_2 in the inspired air will be wasted, since the blood is already 97% to 98% saturated when it leaves the lungs and the O_2 content is normal. An examination of the oxyhemoglobin dissociation curve (flat upper portion) shows that little if any advantage could be gained.

38. The S shape of the oxyhemoglobin dissociation curve indicates that under normal environmental conditions, large changes of the oxygen tension (Po_2) of the inspired air cause only small changes in oxyhemoglobin saturation. Even at a Po_2 of 50 mm Hg in the alveoli, Hb is 80% to 85% saturated with O_2, which is sufficient to meet tissue demands for O_2 under most conditions.

39. The Bohr effect is the slight shift to the right of the oxyhemoglobin dissociation curve caused by the increase in acidity as a result of the effect of CO_2 being released from the tissues. The rightward shift in the curve causes O_2 to be more easily released from its as-

sociation with Hb and thus facilitates tissue uptake of O_2.

40. Although alveolar Po_2 may be increased slightly by hyperventilation, this does not significantly increase the O_2 content of the arterial blood, because of the sigmoid shape of the O_2 dissociation curve and because blood leaving normally ventilated alveoli is already almost fully saturated with O_2. The CO_2 dissociation curve, however, is linear in shape, indicating that the CO_2 content of the blood is directly related to the alveolar Pco_2. When CO_2 is "washed out" of the lungs during hyperventilation, the CO_2 content of the blood is likewise reduced.

41. If diffusion were impaired enough to affect CO_2 transport, the patient would be dead. CO_2 diffuses more readily than O_2 at the same pressure gradient. Even a minute pressure gradient (less than 1 mm Hg) is enough to ensure elimination of all the CO_2 produced at rest.

42. No; knowledge of the blood gases does not give information about how well the tissues are being perfused, how much O_2 is being delivered to the tissues, and the Po_2 in the tissue cells. One must have data on Hb concentration and adequacy of cardiac function and make other clinical observations to assess the adequacy of respiratory function. All data must be correlated, and the final judgment is a clinical one.

43. All the following are examples of altered mechanisms or conditions that may interfere with normal respiration: (1) low Po_2 of inspired air: high altitudes; (2) depression of respiratory center: barbiturate overdose; (3) alveolar hypoventilation from inadequate bellows function: obesity, deformed chest cage, weak respiratory muscles; (4) impaired diffusion of gases at the alveolocapillary membrane: pulmonary edema or fibrosis; (5) $\dot{V}/\dot{Q}$ imbalance: pneumonia or pulmonary embolism; (6) impaired transport of blood gases by systemic circulation: anemia, carbon monoxide poisoning, inadequate cardiac output or shunting by tissues as in shock; (7) impairment of gas diffusion at tissue level: edema.

44. Stage 1 is *ventilation:* flow of air into and out of the lungs effected by the respiratory bellows.
Stage 2 is *transportation:* includes the diffusion of gases between the alveo-lus and the pulmonary blood and between the tissue cells and the systemic blood. Transportation also includes the distribution of the pulmonary and systemic blood and the distribution of air in the lungs.
Stage 3 is *cell respiration:* oxidation of cell metabolites with the production of energy, water, and CO_2.

45. Normal inspiration is principally caused by contraction of the diaphragm and the muscles elevating the rib cage (sternocleidomastoids, serrati, scalene, scapular elevators). There is increased activity in these muscles during forceful inspiration. Expiration involves the relaxation of these muscles and is largely passive. The internal intercostal and abdominal muscles are more active during forced expiration.

46. 201 ml/minute (12 g/dl $\times$ 1.34 ml/g $\times$ 5000 ml/minute $\times$ 0.25)

47. Mixed venous blood containing reduced Hb from the bronchial circulation is mixed with oxygenated pulmonary blood leaving the lungs, thus accounting for the slight reduction in Hb saturation.

48. Decreases; increases (alkalosis); shifts to the left so that Hb is reluctant to release O_2 to the tissues

49. 42 mm Hg [(247 − 47) $\times$ 0.21]; no, a Po_2 of 42 would barely be able to supply tissue O_2 requirements at rest. The climber might be expected to pass out unless he uses cylinder O_2 supply.

50. a

51. a, b, c

52. b

53. Increase; decrease; less; into

54. Ascends; decreasing

55. Increase; more; out of

56. Normal; low; low

57. Decrease; increase; alkalosis

58. Right; decreased

CHAPTER 36

1. Routine chest radiography, fluoroscopy, bronchography, angiography, lung scans, and tomography, including CT scan

2. (a) Status of the thoracic cage, including the ribs, pleura, and contour of the diaphragm and of the upper airway as it enters the chest; (b) the size, contour, and position of the mediastinum and hilus of the lung, including the heart, aorta, lymph nodes, and root of the bronchial tree; (c) the texture and degree of aeration of the lung parenchyma; (d) the size, shape, number, and location of pulmonary lesions, including cavitation, fibrous markings, and zones of consolidation.

3. c

4. c

5. a

6. b

7. h

8. d

9. e

10. i

11. f

12. g

13. d

14. e

15. a, f, g

16. c

17. b

18. f

19. The chief value of ventilatory function tests is that quantitative data are provided to assess the degree of pulmonary disability, follow the progress of the disability, and assess response to treatment. Ventilatory function test data are not in general specifically diagnostic, although patterns of disordered pulmonary function may be discerned. Blood gas measurements, as well as ventilatory function tests, provide quantitative data to assess the degree of respiratory insufficiency and are particularly helpful in guiding oxygen therapy, but these data do not provide all the information necessary to assess total respiratory function.

20. Alveolar ventilation takes into account the amount of air wasted in ventilating the dead space.

21. Measurements of the change in volume at different degrees of lung inflation and the change in alveolar or intrapleural pressure measured by means of an esophageal balloon are made simultaneously. Compliance is then calculated by the following formula:

$$\text{Compliance} = \frac{\Delta \text{ volume}}{\Delta \text{ pressure}}$$

22. Causes of decreased lung compliance include pulmonary fibrosis, pulmonary edema, pneumonia, and deficiency of surfactant. Causes of decreased thoracic cage compliance include obesity, abdominal distention, and skeletal deformities of the chest cage.

23. The emphysema patient whose main problem is increased airways resistance caused by premature collapse of the airways during expiration adopts a slow, deep pattern of respiration to mini-

mize the work of breathing. Airflow is less turbulent with slow, deep respirations.

24. The chief problem for a patient with stiff lungs is an increase in the elastic resistance. The work of breathing is minimized by a rapid, shallow pattern of respiration.

25. The radial artery is usually chosen for the arterial puncture because of its easy access. The wrist is extended (positioned over a rolled towel) and the artery is stabilized with two fingers of one hand while the arterial puncture is made with the other hand, using a heparinized syringe. Air is displaced from the blood specimen. Finally, the specimen is placed on ice and taken to the blood gas laboratory.

26. *Hyperventilation* can occur as a result of anxiety, brain injury, and pneumonia. It may also be secondary to metabolic acidosis occurring as a compensation. Causes of *hypoventilation* include narcotic or barbiturate overdose and increased physiologic dead space. It may also occur as a compensation for metabolic alkalosis.

27. *Hypoxemia* is caused by ventilation-perfusion imbalance, alveolar hypoventilation, impaired diffusion, and intrapulmonary anatomic shunts. Hypoxemia caused by intrapulmonary anatomic shunting is not corrected by oxygen administration because the blood bypasses the pulmonary unit.

28. False; the reason is incorrect. In this case, less effective ventilation results because the total amount of air wasted as dead space ventilation is greater.

29. True
30. False; $\dot{V}_A = (200 - 120) \times 30 = 2.4$ L/minute
31. True
32. True
33. True
34. True
35. a
36. b
37. c
38. c
39. b
40. d
41. a, b
42. a, c
43. d
44. e
45. f
46. c
47. d
48. e

49. b
50. a
51. h
52. g
53. Check your answer by referring to Table 36-5 and text.

CHAPTER 37

1. c
2. f
3. g
4. b
5. a
6. e
7. d
8. True
9. False; a PaO_2 less than 85 mm Hg may or may not be associated with hypoxia. One can be fairly certain, however, that there is associated hypoxia if the PaO_2 is persistently below 50 mm Hg.
10. False; the detection of cyanosis is difficult, the cause is highly variable, and it may be absent in the presence of severe hypoxia or present when there is no hypoxia.
11. True
12. False; anemic persons (e.g., hemoglobin [Hb] = 7 g/dl) may never develop cyanosis even though they have severe hypoxia, since it would be difficult to have 5 g out of 7 g/dl reduced Hb at any one time. Even in patients with normal Hb concentration, cyanosis generally is an advanced sign of respiratory insufficiency.
13. True
14. True
15. False; alveolar hyperventilation is the cause of hypocapnia.
16. True
17. *Digital clubbing* refers to a loss of the base angle of the nail so that this angle is greater than the normal 160 degrees; bulbous changes in the digital tips are also indicative of clubbing. Loss of the base angle is the earliest sign of digital clubbing, whereas the bulbous change is a late sign. Digital clubbing is important to detect because it is frequently associated with pulmonary disease (especially bronchogenic carcinoma), cardiovascular disease, and gastrointestinal disease.
18. Inspection of the buccal mucosa, especially under the tongue, is the most reliable method of detecting central cyanosis in African-American and white patients. The lighting must be good, preferably daylight.

CHAPTER 38

1. An increased resistance to airflow
2. All three diseases may exist in the pure form, although it is more common for patients to manifest aspects of all these diseases. It is especially common for patients to have features of chronic bronchitis and emphysema at the same time. This overlap and difficulty in separating the diseases are the reason for the label COPD.
3. An asthmatic attack is characterized by orthopnea (having to sit up to breathe), dyspnea, fear of suffocation, prolonged wheezing expirations, and later, cough and sputum production. Treatment consists of bronchodilator drugs and oxygen if the blood gases are abnormal. Corticosteroid drugs are used occasionally for severe attacks. Long-term therapy consists in desensitization and avoidance of known allergens. Status asthmaticus is a prolonged, severe attack of asthma that may cause ventilatory insufficiency so severe that death results.

4.

Feature	CLE	PLE
Sex prevalence	More common in males	Equal sex distribution
Etiology	Associated with smoking	Possible genetic factor
Pathologic anatomy	Respiratory bronchioles primarily affected	Entire acinus affected
Part of lung affected	Uneven distribution; upper lobes may be more severely affected	Uniform in distribution; basal lung more severely affected
Type of associated COPD	Chronic bronchitis	Primary emphysema; chronic bronchitis; aging

5. Measures to relieve obstruction of the small airways; cessation of smoking; avoidance of air pollutants; prompt treatment of infection; cautious oxygen administration
6. Excessive production of mucus, chronic cough; 3 months per year and 2 consecutive years

7. Abnormal enlargement of the alveoli and alveolar ducts and destruction of the alveolar walls
8. Blebs; ruptured alveoli
9. Bullae; check valve obstruction of the bronchiole
10. In asthma there is hypersensitivity of the tracheobronchial tree to various stimuli, manifested by periodic, reversible airway narrowing caused by bronchospasm.
11. Chronic inflammation causes weakening of the bronchial walls so that they become dilated. The dilated areas may be cylindric or saccular in shape. The dilated areas serve as a reservoir for the collection of sputum. The stagnant sputum collection, in turn, may lead to chronic reinfection, so progressive destruction and persistence of the process occur. Precipitating factors include whooping cough, measles, pneumonia, aspiration of a foreign body, and bronchial obstruction from a tumor.
12. Chronic loose cough, expectoration of a large amount (up to 200 ml/day) of foul-smelling sputum, malnutrition, digital clubbing, cor pulmonale, and right ventricular failure
13. Daily bronchial hygiene with postural drainage, antibiotics
14. Removal of the obstructing bronchial secretions
15. b
16. a
17. c
18. a, c, d
19. b, d
20. c
21. b
22. a, b, c
23. d
24. True
25. True
26. False; cystic fibrosis is more common in whites.
27. True
28. True
29. True
30. False; the prognosis is poor; average survival time is 26 years.
31. a
32. b
33. a
34. b
35. a
36. b
37. b
38. b
39. a
40. b
41. b, e

42. a, c
43. d, e
44. d
45. c
46. b
47. d
48. b
49. b
50. b

CHAPTER 39

1. f
2. e
3. a
4. b
5. d
6. c
7. True
8. False; *pectus excavatum* is a congenital deformity in which the lower end of the sternum is attached to the thoracic spine by fibromuscular bands, giving the lower end of the anterior chest a "caved-in" appearance.
9. True
10. False; the deformity is symmetric.
11. c
12. a
13. d
14. b
15. Alveolar hypoventilation and an inability to maintain normal blood gas tensions
16. *Traumatic:* penetrating wound to the chest (knife or gunshot wound)
Spontaneous: rupture of blebs and bullae in emphysema, pneumonia, neoplasm
17. Airtight seal is placed over the wound immediately.
18. Air gains access to the pleural cavity through the defect.
19. A large pneumothorax (more than 20% lung collapse) is treated by closed (water-sealed) chest tube drainage. A large pleural effusion may be removed by thoracentesis. If a pleural effusion is an exudate, it is treated by closed chest tube drainage to prevent fibrothorax.
20. Pleural effusion
21. Pulmonary venous pressure
22. An exudate
23. A transudate
24. (a) Invasion by bacteria, viruses, fungi, malignant cells: infection and destruction of lung tissue; (b) inhalation of irritating dusts: inflammation and pulmonary fibrosis; (c) inhalation of irritating gases: inflammation and pulmonary fibrosis; (d) damage to the alveolocapillary endothelium: edema; (e) deficiency of pulmonary surfactant: atelectasis.

25.

	Absorption atelectasis	Compression atelectasis
Common cause	Intrinsic obstruction of airway by mucus plug	Extrinsic pressure on lung from pleural effusion, hemothorax, pyothorax, or pneumothorax
Mechanism	Obstruction prevents air from entering alveoli distal to obstruction; air in alveoli is gradually absorbed into bloodstream; alveoli collapse	External pressure from fluid or air causes compression collapse of alveoli

26. These small pores (between the alveoli) provide a path for collateral ventilation between alveoli and whole segments of the lung in case the normal airway is obstructed. Deep inspiration is effective in opening up the pores and providing ventilation to adjacent obstructed alveoli. Collapse caused by absorption of gases into the bloodstream is thus prevented. (Once collapse occurs, reexpansion is much more difficult.) During expiration the pores close and pressure builds up, aiding in the expulsion of the mucus plug.
27. *Engorgement* (4 to 12 hours): serous exudate from leaking blood vessels pours into alveoli.
Red hepatization (next 48 hours): lung is red and granular in appearance (RBCs, PMNs, and fibrin fill alveoli).
Gray hepatization (3 to 8 days): lung has grayish appearance (leukocytes and fibrin consolidate in alveoli).
Resolution (7 to 11 days): lysis and resorption of exudate by macrophages and restoration of tissue to normal.
28. Administration of antibiotic effective against the specific infecting organism, oxygen therapy for hypoxemia, and treatment of complications

29. *Size of dust particles:* those 1 to 5 μm can easily reach alveoli.
   Concentration and length of exposure: high concentration and long exposure generally are needed to produce adverse affects.
   Nature of the dusts: some organic dusts produce an allergic alveolitis; the chemical nature of inorganic dusts is important; some are harmless and inert, whereas others harm macrophages, by which they are phagocytized and form fibrotic nodules.
30. Histoplasmosis, coccidioidomycosis, and blastomycosis
31. Decreased lung compliance; interference with the gas diffusion pathway
32. Restrictive lung disease
33. Interstitial
34. Parenchyma; lung abscess, empyema; poor
35. True
36. True
37. False; the prognosis is generally good.
38. False; erythromycin is effective against mycoplasmal pneumonia; antibiotics are not effective against viral infections.
39. True
40. False; this statement describes hypostatic pneumonia.
41. True
42. True
43. c
44. a
45. b
46. c, g, j
47. d, h, i
48. a, f
49. b, e
50. c, f, h, i
51. a, b, g
52. d, e
53. c, h
54. c
55. f, g
56. d
57. a, e
58. b
59. h
60. b, c, d, e
61. b, e, f
62. a
63. a, c, e, g
64. d
65. a
66. b
67. e
68. c
69. d
70. b
71. c
72. a

73. a, b
74. a
75. a
76. c
77. d
78. d
79. b, d
80. b
81. b
82. e
83. a, c, d
84. a, b

CHAPTER 40

1. Local injury to the vascular wall; stasis of blood flow; hypercoaguability
2. Chronic obstructive pulmonary disease
3. Increased hydrostatic pressure within the pulmonary capillaries, decrease in the colloid osmotic pressure (as in nephritis), damage to the capillary wall (as when noxious gases are inhaled), left ventricular heart failure
4. It is the name given to attacks of dyspnea caused by pulmonary edema at night. The increased hydrostatic pressure in the lungs is caused by the horizontal position in patients with chronic passive congestion of the lungs resulting from left ventricular failure.
5. It is the condition in which hypertrophy and dilation of the right ventricle develop from disease affecting the structure and function of the lung. (Congenital and left heart disease are not included.)
6. When the left ventricle fails while the right ventricle continues to pump blood, the pulmonary hydrostatic pressure rises until pulmonary edema results. Yes.
7. Prevent the recurrence of pulmonary embolism; relieve symptoms resulting from the embolism; surgically remove a massive embolus
8. To improve the underlying pulmonary disorder and correct the hypoxemia
9. Two mechanisms leading to increased pulmonary vascular resistance are (a) anatomic alterations in the pulmonary blood vessels leading to a reduction of the pulmonary vascular bed and (b) hypoxic vasoconstriction.
10. a, b, c; d is associated with a massive pulmonary embolism; e is associated with infarction, an uncommon event with pulmonary embolism.
11. c
12. a, b, d
13. c
14. b, c, d, e
15. c

16. a, c
17. c
18. a
19. a, b, c, d
20. a
21. d
22. b, d
23. True
24. True
25. True
26. False; appearance similar
27. Embolism
28. Pulmonary hypertension

CHAPTER 41

1. *Respiratory insufficiency* refers to an impairment of the normal ability to oxygenate arterial blood and eliminate CO_2, so there is an inability to maintain normal arterial blood gas levels under conditions of increased demand such as increased activity or exercise.
2. Chronic obstructive pulmonary disease (COPD)
3. Hypoxemia without hypercapnia (hypoxemic respiratory failure, or oxygenation failure); hypoxemia with hypercapnia (hypercapnic respiratory failure, or ventilatory failure)
4. High concentrations of O_2 will reduce the hypoxic drive for breathing (which patients with this condition depend on) and may aggravate hypoventilation and CO_2 retention.
5. Pao_2 about 40 mm Hg; $Paco_2$ 60 to 70 mm Hg
6. Liquefy and remove secretions by adequate hydration and administration of expectorants and aerosols; supervise patient's coughing; use suctioning, percussion, vibration, and postural drainage; treat respiratory infection with the appropriate antibiotic.
7. Ensure that hypoxemia, acidosis, and hypercapnia do not reach hazardous levels.
8. Retained respiratory tract secretions, infection, and bronchospasm, which are all related. For example, bronchospasm can be a response to inflammation and infection or to the inhalation of irritants such as smoke or allergens. Injudicious administration of sedatives or narcotics or inhalation of high O_2 concentration are important iatrogenic factors. Refer to the box on p. 623 for a list of other common factors.
9. A $\dot{V}/\dot{Q}$ mismatch means that some regions of the lung have high $\dot{V}/\dot{Q}$ ratios, whereas others have low $\dot{V}/\dot{Q}$ ratios. The high $\dot{V}/\dot{Q}$ gas-exchanging units compensate for the units with a low

$\dot{V}/\dot{Q}$ in the case of CO_2 because of the linear relationship between CO_2 content and $Paco_2$; consequently the $Paco_2$ does not rise. The $Paco_2$ is a function of overall alveolar ventilation and CO_2 production. In the case of the Pao_2, the high $\dot{V}/\dot{Q}$ units cannot compensate for the low $\dot{V}/\dot{Q}$ units, since O_2 content increases little even when there is a large increase in ventilation (flat part of oxyhemoglobin dissociation curve). Thus the Pao_2 is greatly affected by regional $\dot{V}/\dot{Q}$ imbalance, but the $Paco_2$ is not.

10. $Pao_2 = Pio_2 - (Paco_2/R)$
    $Pio_2 = Fio_2 \times (PB - PH_2O)$
    $Pio_2 = 0.21 (760 - 47) = 149.7$ mm Hg (breathing air)
    $Pio_2 = 0.50 (760 - 47) = 356.5$ mm Hg (breathing 50% O_2)
    $Pao_2 = 149.7 - (80/0.8) = 49.7$ mm Hg (predicted breathing air)
    $Pao_2 = 356.5 - (80/0.8) = 256.5$ mm Hg (predicted breathing 50% O_2)
    $P(A - a)o_2 = 49.7 - 50 =$ essentially 0 (breathing air)
    $P(A - a)o_2 = 256.5 - 246 = 10.2$ mm Hg (breathing 50% O_2)
    The hypoxemia is caused by pure hypoventilation, since his A − a gradient breathing air is essentially zero (normal, less than 20, allowing for some measurement error). The depression of the Pao_2 is accounted for by the increase in $Paco_2$ in the situation when he is breathing air and when he is breathing 50% O_2. Note that his hypoxemia was corrected by O_2 therapy but that his $Paco_2$ was not. This is because overall alveolar ventilation is reduced because of depression of the respiratory center by the narcotic. He may eventually need to be mechanically ventilated.

11. $Pao_2 = 0.21 (747 - 47) - (55/0.8) = 78.25$ mm Hg (predicted on admission)
    $P(A - a)o_2 = 78.25 - 35 = 43.25$ mm Hg (on admission)
    $Pao_2 = 0.24 (747 - 47) - (40/0.8) = 111.75$ (predicted 2 days later)
    $P(A - a)o_2 = 111.75 - 50 = 61.75$ mm Hg (2 days later)
    Since A − a gradient breathing air on admission is greater than 20, he probably has $\dot{V}/\dot{Q}$ imbalance in addition to hypoventilation. Two days later, on 24% O_2, his condition appears to be deteriorating (even though his Pao_2 has increased) because the A − a gradient has increased. He is not hypoventilating because $Paco_2$ is now normal, but his $\dot{V}/\dot{Q}$ imbalance has probably become worse.

12. False; the point when respiratory insufficiency has progressed to failure is difficult to detect in these patients, since they have adapted somewhat to the abnormal blood gas tensions.

13. False; it is highly unreliable. (If you missed this question, go back and read the section on cyanosis in Chapter 37.)

14. True

15. True

16. False; hyperventilation causes this.

17. True

18. True

19. True

20. False; the Pao_2 should fall about 12 mm Hg for every 10 mm Hg rise in the Pco_2. Since the Pco_2 rose by 30 mm Hg above the value $(70 - 40 = 30)$, the Pao_2 should be expected to fall by 36 mm Hg to a value of 59 mm Hg $(95 - 36 = 59)$. Since the Pao_2 is 45 mm Hg, the patient probably has some $\dot{V}/\dot{Q}$ imbalance or shunting. (You could have used the alveolar gas equation to solve this problem if you had been given data on the barometric pressure, patient's temperature, and Fio_2. The rule-of-thumb approach has been used here on the assumption that the patient is breathing air.)

21. False; hypoventilation and hyperventilation refer to CO_2 homeostasis and can be assessed only by the measurement of the $Paco_2$. CO_2 homeostasis is related to both CO_2 production and alveolar ventilation. One can infer that CO_2 production is increased when the work of breathing is increased (because of airway obstruction or thoracic wall or lung restriction) or when the patient's temperature is increased. On the other hand, CO_2 elimination depends on alveolar ventilation, which in turn is determined by tidal volume, dead space, and breathing frequency. The balance between the CO_2 production and elimination processes cannot be determined accurately by clinical observation.

22. True; an FVC less than 15 ml/kg of ideal body weight indicates a serious reduction of ventilatory reserve. A normal FVC for a 70 kg man is about 4550 to 5250 ml (70×65 to 75). See Table 41-1.

23. True; predicted $Pao_2 = 1.0 (747 - 47) - (24/0.8) = 670$ mm Hg $P(A - a)o_2 = 670 - 80 = 590$ mm Hg

24. False; life cannot be sustained with a 50% shunt except by breathing 100% O_2, which in itself is toxic to the lung when given for prolonged periods.

25. True; this occurs with breathing more than 50% O_2 for longer than 48 hours.

26. False; it causes increased cerebral blood flow (CBF) and increased intracranial pressure (ICP).

27. True

28. True; increased $Paco_2 \rightarrow$ increased CBF $\rightarrow$ increased ICP $\rightarrow$ papilledema and headache

29. False; directly related to CO_2 production and inversely related to alveolar ventilation. See formula.

30. True; both hypoxemia and hypercapnia are generally present in terminal respiratory failure.

31. d
32. b, c
33. a
34. b, c
35. a, b, c, d
36. c, d
37. a, b
38. e
39. d
40. b, d
41. All are correct.
42. d
43. b, d
44. b, c
45. b, c
46. All are correct; cardiac output is increased at first but decreases later as myocardial tissue hypoxia becomes severe.
47. $c \rightarrow d \rightarrow a \rightarrow e \rightarrow b \rightarrow g \rightarrow f$. Actually, d could occur during sleep, but here it is considered as indicating an exacerbation of the chronic bronchitis. Both a and d cause a further rise in the $Paco_2$ beyond the patient's chronic level.
48. d
49. c
50. a, b, c
51. a, b, d, e
52. All are correct.
53. All are correct.
54. a, c, d
55. a, b, c
56. All are correct.
57. d
58. c, d, e, g
59. a, b, f
60. f
61. a
62. c
63. e
64. b
65. d
66. Hypoxemia
67. Hypoventilation
68. 5.73 mm Hg; yes

$PAO_2 = FiO_2$ $(P_B - 47$ mm Hg$) -$
$PaCO_2/0.8$
$= 0.21 (760 - 47) - 84/0.8$
$= 149.73 - 105$
$= 44.73$ mm Hg
$P(A - a)O_2 = PAO_2 - PaO_2$
$= 44.73 - 39$
$= 5.73$ mm Hg

69. 10.08 ml O_2/dl; NO (normal, 18 to 20 ml/dl blood)
$CaO_2 = SaO_2 \times$ Hb (g/dl) $\times$
1.34 (ml O_2/g Hb)
$+ (PaO_2 \times 0.0031)$
$= 0.62 \times 12$ g/dl $\times 1.34$
$= 0.12$
$= 9.96$ ml O_2/dl $+ 0.12$
$= 10.08$ ml O_2/dl

70. b
71. b
72. b
73. a

CHAPTER 42

1. The *carcinoid syndrome* is a symptom complex characterized by attacks of anxiety, tremulousness, hypotension, flushing, dyspnea, and cyanosis resulting from bronchoconstriction. It is caused by the elaboration of serotonin and other biologically active substances secreted by a carcinoid type of bronchial adenoma.

2. Cough, chest pain, sputum expectoration, mild dyspnea, digital clubbing, and hemoptysis are common, but symptoms may be minimal. Diagnosis on the basis of symptoms is difficult, since the onset may be insidious and the symptoms are not specific. Lung cancer may imitate a number of other lung disorders.

3. *Radiology:* "coin lesion" seen on radiograph
Bronchoscopy: direct visualization of tumor and biopsy identification of malignant cells
Cytology: examination of sputum, bronchial washings, or pleural fluid for malignant cells

4. a, f, i
5. a, e, h, j
6. b, c, g, i
7. b, d, i
8. True
9. False; there is a positive relationship; the greater the number of cigarettes smoked, the greater the risk.
10. False; it is asbestos.
11. False; secondary metastases are more common.
12. True
13. True

14. a, c
15. c
16. a, c, d
17. c
18. e

CHAPTER 43

1. In the United States, about 10% of those infected with tuberculosis (TB) will develop clinical TB during their lifetime, but the risk is higher for immunosuppressed individuals, especially those with human immunodeficiency virus (HIV) infection. It is estimated that during 1990-1999 worldwide, 88 million persons will develop TB, and 8 million of these cases will be attributed to HIV infection.

2. (a) Risk of acquiring the infection and (b) risk of developing clinically active disease after infection has occurred. The risk of acquiring the infection and developing disease depend on the existence of infection in the population, especially among persons infected with HIV, immigration of persons from areas of high prevalence of TB, high-risk racial and ethnic minority groups (e.g., African Americans, Native Americans, Alaskan natives, Asians, Pacific Islanders, Hispanics), and transmission of TB within high-risk environments (e.g., correctional facilities, homeless shelters, hospitals, nursing homes).

3. At least two drugs are used in treatment of TB because of the possibility of drug resistance. For example, a 6-month drug regimen consisting of isoniazid (INH), rifampin, and pyrazinamide given for 2 months followed by INH and rifampin for 4 months is recommended for the initial therapy of TB for patients with fully susceptible organisms who adhere to treatment. A 4-month regimen of isoniazid and rifampin, preferably with pyrazinamide for the first 2 months, is recommended for adults who have active TB and who are smear and culture negative, if minimal possibility of drug resistance exists.

4. Principles on which treatment for TB is based include (a) regimens must include multiple drugs to which the organisms are susceptible; (b) the drugs must be taken regularly; and (c) drug therapy must continue for a sufficient period to provide the safest and most effective therapy in the shortest time.

5. Isoniazid, 300 mg/day for adults for 12 months, is the recommended preven-

tive therapy regimen for HIV-infected persons with a positive tuberculin skin test reaction.

6. BCG vaccination is not generally recommended against TB in the United States because of the low risk of infection and the variable effectiveness of the vaccine. The CDC recommends that the vaccine should be given only to infants and children with negative skin test results who cannot be given preventive isoniazid therapy but who are continuously exposed to a person with infectious TB; who will be continuously exposed to a person with infectious TB that is resistant to isoniazid or rifampin; or who belong to groups for whom the rate of new infection exceeds 1% per year and for whom the usual surveillance and treatment programs have not been successful.

7. The purpose of DOT therapy is to foster adherence and ensure that patients take the TB drugs as prescribed.

8. Risk factors for MDR-TB in patients with no previous history of TB treatment include exposure to a patient who has drug-resistant TB, being from a country with a high prevalence of drug resistance, and greater than 4% primary resistance to isoniazid in the community.

9. TB eradication involves a combination of effective chemotherapy, prompt case and contact identification and follow-up, management of persons exposed to patients with infectious MDR-TB, and chemoprophylatic therapy of high-risk population groups.

10. b, c
11. b
12. a
13. c
14. c
15. d
16. b
17. b
18. c
19. d
20. d
21. a, b, c, d
22. c
23. c, d, g, l
24. k, m
25. d, g, j
26. a
27. f, l
28. b, g
29. False; a four-drug regimen is recommended, consisting of INH, rifampin, pyrazinamide, and ethambutol.

30. False; 10% to 25% of patients with TB disease have negative reactions when tested with the tuberculin skin test.
31. False; PCR technique is in the experimental phase and is currently not available for routine diagnosis of TB.
32. True
33. False; short-course therapy involves at least two and preferably three drugs; for example, a 4-month regimen of INH and rifampin, preferably with pyrazinamide for the first 2 months, for adults who have active TB and who are smear and culture negative, if there is little possibility of drug resistance.
34. False; it is estimated that 10% of infected persons will likely develop clinical TB during their lifetime.

CHAPTER 44

1. 1, Left kidney; 2, right kidney; 3, ureter; 4, bladder; 5, urethra; 6, urinary meatus
2. 1, Eleventh rib; 2, twelfth rib; 3, transversus abdominus muscle; 4, psoas major muscle
3. 1, Fibrous capsule; 2, cortex; 3 medulla; 4, column of Bertin; 5, papilla; 6, pyramid; 7, minor calyx; 8, major calyx; 9, renal pelvis; 10, ureter
4. 1, Proximal convoluted tubule; 2, glomerular capillary tuft; 3, Bowman's capsule; 4, efferent arteriole; 5, juxtaglomerular cells; 6, afferent arteriole; 7, macula densa; 8, loop of Henle; 9, distal convoluted tubule; 10, collecting duct
5. Check your drawing with Fig. 44-1. The hilus of each kidney should be at about the level of the second lumbar vertebra. The superior pole of the left kidney is at about the level of the lower border of the eleventh rib, while the right is at about the level of the twelfth rib.
6. (a) Bowman's capsule; (b) proximal convoluted tubule; (c) distal convoluted tubule; (d) collecting ducts; (e) papillary ducts of Bellini; (f) minor calyces; (g) major calyces; (h) renal pelvis; (i) ureter; (j) bladder
7. (a) Abdominal aorta; (b) renal artery; (c) interlobar arteries; (d) arcuate arteries; (e) interlobular arterioles; (f) afferent arterioles; (g) glomerular capillaries; (h) efferent arterioles; (i) peritubular capillaries; (j) interlobular veins; (k) arcuate veins; (l) interlobar veins; (m) renal vein; (n) inferior vena cava
8. More than 25% of the population has more than one renal artery supplying a kidney, which may cause technical difficulties for the surgeon. Some difficulties presented by aberrant blood vessels may be insurmountable.
9. A decrease in the hydrostatic pressure of the blood flowing through the afferent arteriole sensed by the JG cells or a decrease in sodium concentration in the distal tubule filtrate sensed by the macula densa cells causes the release of renin from the JG cells. This results in the conversion of angiotensinogen to angiotensin I and finally to the active form, angiotensin II. Angiotensin II increases arterial blood pressure by causing peripheral vasoconstriction and stimulates the secretion of aldosterone. Increased aldosterone levels cause increased sodium reabsorption in the distal tubule. More water is then reabsorbed, resulting in an increase in plasma volume. Both vasoconstriction and increased plasma volume help to elevate blood pressure. An increase in the blood pressure in the afferent arteriole has the opposite effect. An increase in the Na^+ concentration of the distal tubule, however, does not affect renin output.
10. A severe blunt impact over the back, flank, or even the abdomen can cause trauma to the kidney. This situation is common in motor vehicle accidents. The most common trauma in such cases results from the kidney being pushed against a transverse process or being punctured by a fractured twelfth rib. The resulting injury can vary from a simple bruise to a shattering of the renal parenchyma. Complete transection of a kidney by the twelfth rib may occur in severe cases.
11. d
12. f
13. b
14. e
15. c
16. a
17. d
18. d
19. c
20. b
21. d
22. c
23. c
24. a
25. It is called *ultrafiltration* because the glomerular filtrate has the same composition as plasma with the absence of proteins—almost everything is filtered through and at a high flow rate.
26. The differences in pressure between the glomerulus and Bowman's capsule tend to force fluid into the capsule. Net filtration pressure = intracapillary hydrostatic pressure − oncotic pressure of the blood − intracapsular hydrostatic pressure.
27. The GFR is the rate of appearance of glomerular filtrate from filtration of the blood at the glomerulus. The average GFR in men is 125 ml/minute and in women, 110 ml/minute.
28. To measure the GFR, a substance must be used that is freely filtered by the glomerulus but is neither secreted nor reabsorbed along the tubules. A substance that was cleared by both filtration and secretion along the tubule would cause the apparent GFR to be higher than the true GFR. A substance that was both filtered and reabsorbed would cause the apparent GFR to be lower than the true GFR.
29.

$$GFR = \frac{UV}{P}$$

$$= \frac{(500 \text{ mg/dl})(2 \text{ ml/minute})}{25 \text{ mg/dl}}$$

$$= 40 \text{ ml/minute}$$

A GFR of 40 ml/minute indicates that this patient has moderately severe impairment of renal function. The calculated value is normally corrected for body surface area (BSA) by means of a nomogram. The standard BSA is 1.73 m^2 (BSA of an average man). The final result is then reported in milliliters per minute per 1.73 m^2.

30. Regulation of water and acid-base balance. Water is reabsorbed in the presence of ADH. Acid-base balance is regulated by regeneration of bicarbonate and hydrogen ion excretion in combination with phosphates and ammonia.
31. The lungs control the excretion of carbon dioxide, and the kidneys control the reabsorption of bicarbonate, both important components of the bicarbonate–carbonic acid buffer system in the blood. The ratio of these two components is important in maintaining a normal blood pH.
32. H^+ is excreted in the urine by combining with $HPO_4^=$ to form $H_2PO_4^-$ and by combining with NH_3 to form NH_4^+.
33. (a) Maintains plasma osmolality at 285 mOsm by varying water excre-

tion; (b) maintains ECF volume and tissue perfusion by varying Na^+ excretion; (c) maintains plasma pH near 7.4 by regulating acid-base balance; (d) maintains concentration of each individual electrolyte within the normal range; (e) excretory route for most drugs; (f) excretes nitrogenous end products; (g) secretes/activates certain hormones: erythropoietin, prostaglandins, 1,25-dihydroxyvitamin D_3; (h) degradation of polypeptide hormones, especially insulin.

34. (a) Vapor pressure is lowered, (b) boiling point is elevated, (c) freezing point is lowered, (d) osmotic pressure is increased. Osmotic pressure refers to the external pressure that would have to be applied to a solution with a greater number of particles to prevent water from diffusing across a semipermeable membrane from a solution with a lesser number of particles. It is a measure of water concentration, and there are no real physical pressures present in the solutions—the pressure is that used to characterize the system. Adding particles to water lowers its chemical potential (molar free energy), and water always flows from an area of higher potential (more dilute) to an area of lower potential (more concentrated). The attainment of equilibrium by the application of pressure to the more concentrated solution is because its chemical potential is raised so that it is equal to the water in the more dilute solution on the other side of the membrane. The application of pressure prevents an increase in volume in the more concentrated solution because of water diffusion.

35. The osmometer is an apparatus for measuring the freezing point of a solution. The freezing point depression below that of pure water can then be used to calculate accurately the osmotic concentration of the solution, since it depends only on the number of particles in solution. The urinometer actually measures the density or specific gravity of a solution and does not measure true concentration, which depends on the number of particles in solution. Therefore the osmometer is more accurate in estimating the concentration of a solution.

36.

$$\text{Osmolality} = \frac{\Delta T}{K_f} = \frac{-0.53}{-1.86}$$

$$\times 1000 = 285 \text{ mOsm}$$

The result is multiplied by 1000 to convert to milliosmols.

37. Check your drawing with Fig. 44-15. Cortical glomeruli should be located high in the cortex, with relatively short loops of Henle, which extend slightly into the medullary area. Juxtamedullary glomeruli should be located deep in the cortex next to the medulla, and the loops of Henle should be relatively long, extending deep into the medulla.

38. The vasa recta are medullary blood vessels that form hairpin loops beside the juxtaglomerular loop of Henle. They help maintain the concentration gradient of the medullary interstitial fluid.

39. The purpose of the countercurrent mechanism is the conservation of water (or the concentration of urine) by the kidney. The two basic processes involved are the loop of Henle acting as a countercurrent multiplier of concentration to build up the concentration gradient in the medulla and the vasa recta acting as a countercurrent exchanger to prevent washing out the hyperosmolality built up by the loop of Henle.

40. d
41. a
42. b
43. c
44. c
45. d, e
46. a, b
47. a
48. e
49. e
50. d, e
51. c
52. e
53. c, d
54. b, c
55. a, d
56. b
57. a
58. c
59. c
60. d
61. b
62. c
63. a
64. c
65. a
66. e
67. c; increase in medullary blood flow washes out medullary hypertonicity.
68. a
69. b
70. c
71. d
72. b; it is hyperosmotic even during diuresis.
73. b; maximum urine concentration $\approx$ 1400 mOsm; plasma concentration is 285 mOsm.
74. a
75. d
76. c
77. b, c
78. a, c, d; reabsorption in the proximal tubule is obligatory; increases permeability of the collecting ducts to water.
79. a; b is a function of the renin-angiotensin-aldosterone system.
80. b
81. d; under conditions of volume expansion, NaCl delivery to the distal tubule macula densa cells is increased, resulting in a signal to suppress renin release; under conditions of volume contraction, NaCl delivery is decreased and renin secretion is increased.
82. b, d
83. c
84. e
85. a
86. a
87. b
88. a
89. a
90. a
91. b
92. a
93. c
94. b
95. d; hypoosmotic during diuresis because of Na^+ reabsorption, and water cannot passively follow; isosmotic when water is reabsorbed with Na^+ during antidiuresis.
96. a, b, or c
97. c
98. b
99. a
100. b
101. c
102. c

CHAPTER 45

1. A normal healthy adult may excrete up to 150 mg of protein in the urine per day. The amounts in excess of 150 mg/day are considered pathologic and occur most frequently in renal disease, particularly glomerulonephritis. Patients with the nephrotic syndrome excrete more than 3.5 g of protein/day and may excrete as much as 20 to 30 g.

2. The direct cause of proteinuria is always an increase in glomerular permeability.

3. When urine stands for a period of time, urea breaks down to ammonia and the urine becomes more alkaline.

4. Uric acid is derived principally from the catabolism of nucleoproteins in the cells. Cytotoxic drugs cause increased degradation of the rapidly proliferating cells, and thus uric acid production is increased. Two thirds of the uric acid is normally excreted by the kidneys. The uric acid may crystallize and obstruct the tubules under conditions of acid urine.

5. (a) Infection with urea-splitting organisms producing alkaline urine; (b) hypercalciuria caused by prolonged immobilization; (c) urinary stasis as a result of low fluid intake. All three of these conditions are often present in patients with chronic illness who are confined to bed, thus favoring the formation of urinary calculi, which form in alkaline urine. Calcium salts are mobilized from bone, and precipitation is favored by highly concentrated, alkaline urine.

6. High fluid intake

7. (a) Check the accuracy of the urinometer using distilled water; (b) gently mix urine to ensure a uniform solution; (c) avoid errors of surface tensions; (d) read the calibrated units from top to bottom at eye level; and (e) correct for temperature.

8. Creatinine is a nitrogenous end product of muscle metabolism. The normal plasma level is 0.7 to 1.5 mg/dl. The plasma level is constant in the healthy person and depends on muscle mass.

9. A substance that is filtered by the glomerulus is neither secreted nor reabsorbed by the tubules is required for a true measurement of GFR. Creatinine is secreted by the tubules, and there is an error inherent in the laboratory method of measuring the plasma level. These two large errors nearly cancel each other out so that creatinine clearance approximately equals GFR.

10. GFR decreases with increasing age. After age 30 it decreases at the rate of about 1 ml/minute each year.

11. The PAH excretion test is the most accurate test of effective renal plasma flow.

12. The plasma creatinine level, because its production rate in the body is constant. It depends on muscle mass, which changes very little. Urea production varies with dietary protein intake and catabolism of body protein. Azotemia means that there is an increase in nitrogenous substances in the blood. This occurs when the kidneys are not able to excrete these substances as rapidly as they are produced.

13. (a) The correct interpretation of a "trace" reading must take into account the concentration of the urine specimen and the time of day it is collected. A trace reading in an early-morning concentrated specimen is probably within normal limits. If the urine is collected later in the day and is dilute, a trace response might indicate excessive proteinuria. (b) Contamination by vaginal secretions in the female (contain protein).

14. Albumin; Tamm-Horsfall

15. 6

16. a; alkaline

17. b, c; nocturnal acid

18. 285

19. 1.001, 1.040; to maintain the osmolality of the ECF at a constant value.

20. 28%; this is the minimum for normal renal function; average excretion is 35%.

21. 1.025, 1.003

22. Urine acidification or ammonium chloride; 5.3

23. Sodium conservation; a

24. c

25. c

26. a, c

27. c:

$$C_{cr} = \frac{U_{cr}V}{P_{cr}}$$

$$= \frac{50 \text{ mg/dl} \times 1 \text{ ml/min}}{2 \text{ mg/dl}}$$

$$= 25 \text{ ml/min}$$

It is necessary to convert the 24-hour urine volume to milliliters per minute to calculate the problem: 1400 ml/24 hours × 24 hours/1440 minutes = 1 ml/minute.

28. b; decrease is at the rate of 1 ml/minute a year after the age of 30. A decrease of 60 ml/minute is expected in this 90-year-old man, which is about a 50% decrease from the normal GFR in a young, healthy man.

29. Red blood cells, white blood cells, casts, bacteria

30. A bacterial count of 10^5 (100,000) CFUs/ml of urine is considered significant and is an indication of urinary tract infection (more than three or four WBCs per high-power field during microscopic examination of the urine sediment suggests significant bacteriuria and indicates that a bacterial count should be done). However, the urine must not have been contaminated by bacteria from other sources, as from the container or from the genitalia. Therefore the genitalia must be cleansed with soap and water before voiding into the sterile specimen bottle, and care must be taken to avoid contamination of the urine by the labia or vaginal secretions in the female ("sterile-voided"). Catheterization gives greater insurance that the specimen is "sterile." The urine must be examined immediately or a preservative should be added and the specimen refrigerated to avoid bacterial growth.

31. An IVP is accomplished by injecting into a vein radiologic contrast medium, which is then excreted by the kidneys, while in the retrograde pyelogram a catheter is passed up a ureter and contrast medium is injected directly into the renal pelvis.

   The purpose of an IVP is to visualize the cortex, calyces, renal pelvis, ureters, and bladder. The adequacy of filling of the calyces and renal pelvis may also be determined. The purpose of the retrograde pyelogram is to obtain better visualization when the IVP is not clear and to investigate a nonfunctioning kidney.

32. (a) Hypertension: may be caused by renal artery stenosis or other obstruction; (b) possible neoplasm: blood vessels of tumor can be visualized; (c) transplant: to visualize the precise vascular supply before surgery; (d) to visualize the blood supply to the cortex: may have patchy appearance indicating ischemia.

33. The GFR is probably low and the dye will not be excreted well; the pyelogram will be difficult to visualize.

34. The entry site should be checked periodically for signs of hematoma or inflammation. Vital signs are checked every 15 minutes until stable and then every 4 hours for 24 hours. Peripheral pulses (in the leg when the femoral artery is used as the entry site) should be checked for diminished strength at the same time intervals as above to detect occlusion of blood flow as a result of thrombus or embolus formation. Color and skin temperature are other signs that should be observed to detect occlusion.

35. The patient should lie prone with a sandbag under the abdomen for 30 minutes after a renal biopsy. Firm pressure with 4×4 sponges is applied over the biopsy site for 10 minutes, followed by application of a pressure dressing. The patient should be kept in bed and as quiet as possible for 24 hours. Vital signs are checked and the abdomen observed for swelling during this period. The urine should also be observed for gross and occult blood.

36. (a) Microscopic; (b) bacteriologic; (c) radiology; (d) biopsy

37. Tamm-Horsfall; distal

38. Cylindruria, protein

39. Culture and sensitivity

40. Clubbing (also may be seen in some other forms of chronic renal disease)

41. b

42. a

43. c

44. a; death occurs in only 0.17% of the cases.

45. c

46. d

47. a

48. b

49. b

50. c

51. d

52. a

CHAPTER 46

1. The period of development of the disease condition; chronic renal failure is a progressive, slow process over a period of years, whereas acute renal failure develops over a few days to weeks. In both cases the kidneys lose their ability to keep the internal environment of the body normal.

2. Stage I, decreased renal reserve: up to 75% of nephron mass destroyed. Stage II, renal insufficiency: 75% to 90% nephron mass destroyed. Stage III, uremia or end-stage renal failure: 90% or more of the nephron mass destroyed.

3. First stage: BUN and plasma creatinine levels both normal; second stage: BUN and plasma creatinine levels rising just above normal, unstable; third stage: BUN and plasma creatinine levels both rising sharply with each decrement of GFR.

4. The creatinine clearance progresses toward zero as nephrons are progressively destroyed by the renal disease process (creatinine clearance rate gives a fairly good estimate of the true GFR in the middle range but is much less accurate at either high or low filtration rates).

5. Polyuria means an increase in the volume of urine, whereas oliguria is just the opposite—urine output is decreased below the normal range. (Do not confuse polyuria and frequency, a common mistake made by students. Frequency means an increase in the number of voidings, but there is not necessarily an increase in the volume. With moderate polyuria, there is not necessarily an increase in frequency.) Nocturia means that a person has to get up more than once to void during normal sleeping hours or output is 700 ml or more during the night.

6. Polyuria and nocturia occur because of the solute diuresis and inability to concentrate the urine. Both symptoms occur early in the course of progressive renal failure and are compensatory. When most of the nephrons are destroyed, the patient becomes oliguric because the total net filtration rate is low (because there are few nephrons), even though the GFR for each individual intact nephron may be high (decompensation stage). Primary lesions of the medulla may interfere with the chloride pump, the countercurrent mechanism, and tubular secretion and reabsorption, whereas lesions of the glomerulus may prevent glomerular filtration from occurring or cause the loss of protein and formed elements into the urine.

7. An increased solute load may be induced in a normal person by ingestion of a high-protein diet or by giving mannitol intravenously. The usual solute load of the kidneys is thus extended many times. Each normal nephron is undergoing an osmotic diuresis, which results in an obligatory loss of water. The kidney loses its flexibility to either concentrate or dilute the urine from the plasma osmolality of 285 mOsm under the stress of water deprivation or overload. Identical principles are involved in progressive renal failure, and both conditions are explained by the intact nephron hypothesis.

8. The remaining intact nephrons compensate by hypertrophying. Filtration rate, solute load, and tubular reabsorption per nephron are all increased, and glomerular-tubular balance is maintained until most of the renal nephrons are destroyed.

9. The renal disease may not be diag-nosed until it is far advanced, when functional and morphologic characteristics may be similar for a number of chronic renal diseases.

10. a. Obstruction of urinary outflow of any cause, such as urethral valves or stricture, calculi, or tumors, usually results in UTI if the obstruction is partial or acute renal failure if the obstruction is complete.

    b. Females are at greater risk for UTI presumably because of their short urethra and proximity of the urinary meatus to the anus; males have the greater risk for UTI during infancy because of congenital structural defects of the urinary tract and during old age because of obstruction from prostatic hypertrophy.

    c. The regurgitation of infected urine into the renal pelvis and interstitium in severe VUR predisposes to UTI and the development of chronic PN.

    d. Instrumentation of the urinary tract, especially the use of indwelling catheter, is associated with a high incidence of UTI.

    e. UTI and ESRD is common in patients with neurogenic bladder (e.g., diabetes, paraplegics) since urinary drainage is impaired.

    f. UTI is typically associated with analgesic nephropathy.

    g. UTI is a common complication in ESRD probably because of defective immunity and damaged kidneys are more susceptible to infection.

    h. Metabolic disturbances such as gout, diabetes, and hypercalcemia are frequently associated with UTI.

11. School-aged girls with significant bacteriuria (whether symptomatic or asymptomatic) are more likely to have recurrent UTI during their childbearing years. All children with significant bacteriuria should be screened for VUR (especially boys), since they may have a correctable structural defect of the urinary tract that, if treated, could prevent the development of progressive renal disease.

12. a, VUR; b, intrarenal reflux; c, infection

13. According to this theory, progressive renal failure continues when a critical mass of nephrons has been destroyed, even in the absence of the original destructive factor (e.g., reflux or infection), because of compensatory intrarenal hypertension in

the remaining healthy nephrons. If this theory is correct, lowering intraglomerular pressure by restricting dietary protein and administering antihypertensive drugs (especially ACE inhibitors) would slow down the progression to renal failure.

14. Acute, rapidly progressive, and chronic glomerulonephritis (GN) are the three clinical types of renal disease that initially and primarily cause diffuse inflammation of the glomeruli. The classic case of acute GN follows a beta-hemolytic streptococcal infection of the throat, typically in a child, causing hematuria, albuminuria, hypertension, and edema. More than 90% have a complete recovery, death occurs in a few, and the remainder may develop rapidly progressive GN or chronic GN. Rapidly progressive GN refers to a type of GN with a fulminant course and progression to end-stage renal disease (ESRD) within a few months. Goodpasture's syndrome is a good example of this type, and the prognosis is poor. Chronic GN is characterized by slow destruction of nephrons from longstanding GN until ESRD is reached (2 to 30 years). A number of systemic diseases can cause chronic GN, and often the cause is unknown. In most cases, chronic GN has no known relationship to acute or rapidly progressive GN. However, an acute nephritic syndrome may occur during the course of chronic GN.

15. b
16. c
17. b
18. c; $\dfrac{900 \text{ mOsm}}{285 \text{ mOsm/L}} \approx 3 \text{ L}$
19. c
20. c
21. a
22. e; see Fig. 46-4.
23. b-1, c-2, d-3, a-4 (polycystic kidney disease and chronic glomerulonephritis are tied for third place.)
24. d
25. d
26. d
27. b
28. b
29. All are correct.
30. e
31. b
32. d
33. a
34. d
35. b
36. d

37. d
38. a
39. b
40. a
41. d
42. a
43. b
44. b
45. e
46. a
47. d
48. d
49. a
50. d
51. e
52. c
53. a
54. b
55. a
56. b
57. e
58. c
59. c
60. d
61. e
62. a
63. d
64. a
65. e
66. d
67. d
68. e
69. d; answer a is a screening test.
70. c
71. c
72. e
73. a
74. e
75. b
76. b
77. e
78. All are correct.
79. c
80. a
81. a
82. a, b
83. b
84. c
85. d
86. b
87. e
88. c
89. a
90. d
91. c
92. b
93. a
94. b, c, g
95. a, d, e, f, h
96. c, d
97. b, e
98. a, e

99. b, f
100. b, g
101. b, c, d, i, j
102. b, c, i
103. a, b
104. b, h
105. d
106. e
107. False; not if the contralateral kidney has developed nephrosclerosis. The ischemic kidney may have better function than the contralateral kidney, so the latter should be removed.
108. False; about two thirds or more
109. True
110. True
111. False; the loss of protein is usually not sufficient to cause hypoproteinemia.
112. False; it is often small with a granular surface resulting from ischemia.
113. True
114. True
115. False; it signifies a highly advanced state of destruction; prognosis is poor.
116. True
117. True
118. True
119. True
120. True
121. PMNs; tubules; lymphocytes; plasma
122. a, Atrophied tubule with cast; b, normal tubule; c, area of interstitial fibrosis; d, hypertrophied tubule with atrophy of epithelial cells; e, PMNs

CHAPTER 47

1. The uremic syndrome refers to a symptom complex that results from or is associated with retention of nitrogenous metabolites related to renal failure.

2. The first group of symptoms relates to deranged regulatory and excretory functions (such as fluid and electrolyte disturbances, acid-base imbalances). The second group of symptoms refers to cardiovascular, neuromuscular, gastrointestinal, and other system abnormalities. The middle molecular hypothesis postulates that molecules of intermediate size present in uremia (guanidines, indican, phenols, amines, etc.) may act as toxins and may be responsible, in part for the multifarious systemic manifestations of the uremic syndrome. The theory also implies that a treatment method allowing effective removal of middle molecules will reduce the symptoms of the uremic syndrome.

3. Because the total number of nephrons is decreased, not because of a tubular transport problem.

4. H^+ is probably being buffered by calcium carbonate from the bones. No doubt this process contributes to the dissolution of bone, although it is not as important as the increased parathormone levels.

5. Because of the increased solute load of each intact nephron. The osmotic diuresis results in obligatory salt losses.

6. Milk of magnesia and magnesium citrate

7. A fixed urine specific gravity of 1.010 means that the patient has severe renal failure with no ability to either concentrate or dilute the urine. Consequently there is little ability to regulate the fluid balance in the body, and fluid intake must be carefully prescribed.

8. When the GFR falls to about 5 ml/minute in terminal renal failure, both men and women lose their libido and are generally sterile. Men are generally impotent, and women cease to menstruate.

9. Poor nutrition, overhydration, indwelling catheters and cannulas, immunosuppressive drugs.

10. White-skinned person—waxy yellow (bronze) cast to the skin; brown-skinned person—yellowish brown coloration; black-skinned person—ashen gray with yellow tones. All these skin color changes are caused by the anemia and retention of urochrome pigments in the uremic patient. Skin color changes in dark-skinned persons are caused by a loss of the red undertones that give the dark skin a "look-alive" appearance. Yellow tones are more evident in the conjunctiva and on the palms and soles.

11. • GI bleeding → hypotension →
    ↓ renal perfusion → ↓ GFR
    • GI bleeding → digestion of blood
    protein → ↓ BUN
    • Vomiting → dehydration →
    hypovolemia → ↓ renal perfusion→
    ↓ GFR
    • Diarrhea → loss of HCO_3^- →
    aggravation of acidosis

12. You might expect the patient to complain of tiring easily, of not being able to work long without resting, and of being unable to sleep at night or being lethargic during the day. You might observe that the patient's affect seemed flat and the patient had difficulty following a complex train of thought. Muscular weakness and muscular twitching might be complaints.

The untreated patient in terminal renal failure will eventually become confused and comatose and may have convulsions, especially if severely hypertensive.

13. *Stage I:* nerve conduction test reveals decreased velocity of nerve conduction. Patient may complain of needing to walk or move the legs (restless leg syndrome). *Stage II:* sensory nerve changes. Patient complains of burning sensation on the soles of the feet and numbness or prickling sensation moving up legs in stockinglike fashion; may have parethesias of the hands. *Stage III:* motor nerve involvement. Loss of motor function usually is first observed as footdrop and may progress to paraplegia.

14. Check your illustration with the radiograph of the hand in Fig. 47-2. The radial aspect of the bone is eroded and has a jagged appearance.

15. See Fig. 47-3 if you have forgotten this sequence of events. Bone disorders associated with secondary hyperparathyroidism might include "honeycombing" demineralization of the bone, especially notable on skull radiograph, and subperiosteal bone resorption, giving the phalanges a ragged border. Pathologic fractures of the long bones and ribs may result. Calcium salts may be deposited in the soft tissues of the body, around joints, in the arteries, and in the eyes.

16. This patient has a calcium-phosphate cross-product of $8 \times 10 = 80$, which exceeds the solubility product of calcium and phosphate by a large margin. Soft tissue deposition of calcium phosphate would certainly be expected.

17. Check your illustration with Fig. 47-4. Irritation from the calcium salts deposited in the eye may cause conjunctivitis, called "uremic red eye" from its appearance.

18. b
19. c
20. a
21. c
22. b
23. a
24. c
25. b, c, d
26. c
27. a, b, c, d
28. a, b, c, e
29. a, c
30. d

31. c
32. d
33. a
34. c
35. c
36. True
37. False; if you missed this question, review the description in this chapter.
38. True
39. True
40. True
41. False; certain amino acids are elevated, whereas others are depressed.
42. False; uremic patients are often hyperglycemic.
43. True
44. True
45. Urea; ammonia; infection
46. (a) Osteitis fibrosa; (b) osteomalacia (rickets); (c) osteosclerosis
47. c
48. a, d
49. b, e
50. b
51. f
52. d
53. e
54. c
55. a

CHAPTER 48

1. When the patient becomes azotemic. Four causes of sudden deterioration of renal function include (a) ECF volume depletion; (b) urinary tract obstruction; (c) infection, especially of urinary tract; and (d) severe or malignant hypertension. The principles of conservative measures are based on regulating individual solute and fluids to achieve as normal an internal milieu as possible in view of the kidney's decreased ability to adapt to a variable intake. Phosphate-binding medications should be given early in the course of chronic renal failure.

2. Dialysis, renal transplantation, or death in terminal renal failure

3. About 500 ml + 500 ml = 1000 ml

4. Chronic intermittent dialysis and renal transplantation. Dialysis may be used for long-term maintenance of the end-stage renal failure patient. Even if the patient chooses renal transplantation as the mode of therapy, dialysis will undoubtedly play a role in treatment. Dialysis can be used to restore and maintain an optimal physical state in the uremic patient before the transplanted kidney is available and as a backup treatment

modality should the transplanted kidney fail. The patient who has chosen maintenance home or satellite-center dialysis may also opt for a transplant at a later date.

5. *Dialysis* is the process by which water and small-molecular-weight solutes pass through a semipermeable membrane from one fluid compartment to another and achieve equilibrium.

6. An artificial shunt is a device for diverting arterial blood to a vein so that the pressure and flow are great enough to allow hemodialysis and provide for easy blood access. With an *external shunt* or cannula system, an external silicone rubber tubing directs or shunts blood from artery to vein. An *internal shunt* can be created by anastomosing an artery to a nearby vein (AV fistula) or using a graft of bovine carotid artery.

7. d

8. a, c, d

9. a

10. b

11. b, c, d; a BUN of 60 mg/dl is not in itself an indication for dialysis.

12. c

13. c

14. c

15. a; not entirely true—some albumin does pass through the pores in the semipermeable membrane. The amount of albumin lost from the blood is generally insignificant during hemodialysis but is quite substantial during peritoneal dialysis.

16. b

17. d

18. b; the purpose is to provide a blood-flow rate high enough for hemodialysis. The enlarged vein allows large-bore needles to be easily inserted.

19. b

20. a, b

21. c, d

22. b

23. a, b

24. b

25. c

26. a, d, e

27. d

28. c

29. d

30. a

31. a, b, d, i

32. g

33. e, k

34. h

35. f

36. j

37. c

38. b

39. a

40. d

41. c

42. True

43. True

44. False; most recipients go through an acute rejection episode during the first few weeks after transplantation, requiring dialysis because of renal insufficiency. This occurs even when the kidney eventually functions well.

45. False; the only exception might be an identical twin donor who is genetically identical with the recipient. There are undoubtedly other minor and major antigens yet undiscovered that are not matched and that play a role in the immunologic response.

46. True

47. True

48. (a) Rapid serologic testing for HLA-DR antigens is highly predictive of success rate. Thus, when a cadaver becomes available, there is sufficient time to find the best match with the aid of a national computer bank of potential recipients. If the cadaver graft success rate improves sufficiently, it may be possible to solicit nonrelated living donors. (b) Pretransplant blood transfusions greatly improve kidney graft success rate. Patients who become sensitized to certain antigens in the donor population are not given a transplant from donors with those antigens. (c) Cyclosporin A has greatly increased cadaver graft survival.

49. Hemofiltration; CAPD; oral sorbents. All are supposedly more successful in removing middle molecules.

50. e

51. d

52. a

53. a

CHAPTER 49

1. Because the fumes of CCl_4 (and other organic solvents) inhaled and the ingested ethyl alcohol react chemically in the body to produce a potent nephrotoxin, which may produce acute tubular necrosis

2. Nephrotoxic injury and renal ischemia

3. Acute renal failure is superimposed on chronic renal insufficiency because of intrinsic renal disease. Precipitating causes include nausea, vomiting, and infections.

4. Two basic types of lesion are involved in ATN, though in some cases they may be mixed. The less serious lesion results in necrosis of the tubular epithelium only. This lesion commonly results from mild doses of CCl_4 or $HgCl_2$. When only epithelial damage takes place, complete healing of the lesion commonly occurs in 3 to 4 weeks. In the second type of lesion there is necrosis of the epithelium and also the basement membrane. This is commonly associated with severe renal ischemia. The prognosis of this type of lesion depends on the extent of the damage. When the basement membrane is disrupted, epithelial regeneration occurs in a haphazard manner, frequently leading to obstruction of the nephron at the site of necrosis.

5. Acute cortical necrosis means that the entire nephron is infarcted. It is commonly associated with pregnancy complications such as postpartum hemorrhage, premature separation of the placenta, eclampsia, and septic abortion. The prognosis is generally poor. If the patient survives the acute phase of illness, calcification and permanent renal damage often occur in the area of cortical necrosis. Glycol (antifreeze) poisoning may also cause this lesion.

6. Infection

7. This classification stresses the identification of extrarenal causes (prerenal, postrenal) and the prevention of progression to intrinsic acute renal failure. The categories provide a systematic diagnostic approach, since the diagnosis of ARF is made on the basis of exclusion of extrarenal (immediately reversible) causes.

8. Bladder outlet obstruction: benign or malignant prostatic hypertrophy; cancer of cervix or rectum. Bilateral ureteral obstruction: cellular debris from necrotizing papillitis in a person with diabetes mellitus; obstruction of the ureter by a calculus in a patient with one functioning kidney; trauma or accidental ligation during extensive pelvic surgery. Intrarenal obstruction: uric acid crystallization in the renal collecting ducts in a leukemic patient receiving chemotherapy; obstruction of the renal tubules with Bence-Jones protein in a patient with multiple myeloma (see also Chapter 18). Inadequate hydration and hypovolemia are important predisposing factors in both cited examples of renal tubule obstruction.

9. Penicillin: methicillin; aminoglycosides: neomycin, gentamicin, kana-

mycin, tobramycin. Chronic renal insufficiency and advanced age (>60 years) are characteristics of patients at high risk for drug-induced ARF.

10. All the theories concerning the pathogenesis of ARF attempt to explain the severe reduction in the GFR. Suggested mechanisms include the following.

(a) Mechanical obstruction of the renal tubule lumina by necrotic tubular cells that have sloughed off; cellular swelling may also collapse the tubules, blocking them off.

(b) Backleak of filtrate into the peritubular circulation through damaged tubular cells.

(c) Impermeability or reduction in surface area of the glomerular filtration membrane.

(d) Intrarenal vascular dysfunction, with redistribution of blood from cortex to medulla maintained by the release of renin from the juxtaglomerular cells, activation of angiotensin II, and consequent vasoconstriction of the afferent arterioles. Inhibition of prostaglandin synthesis may also play a role in the intrarenal vascular dysfunction.

(e) Stimulation of renin-angiotensin, with consequent vasoconstriction of the afferent arterioles through the tubuloglomerular feedback mechanism.

11. Fractional excretion of sodium (FE$_{Na}$). It is actually the ratio of the renal clearance of sodium to that of creatinine (C$_{Na}$/C$_{cr}$ × 100%). Formula for calculation:

$$FE_{Na} = \frac{U_{Na} \times P_{cr}}{P_{Na} \times U_{cr}} \times 100\%$$

The measurement should be done before a diuretic is given, and only fresh urine should be used. Intermittent urinary tract obstruction and preexisting chronic renal insufficiency cause problems in interpretation. These factors are hazards in the use of renal indices to differentiate prerenal azotemia from ATN. Since the laboratory tests are simple, they should be repeated several times.

12. Mannitol and furosemide
13. c
14. b
15. a, b, d, f
16. e
17. b, c, d
18. All are correct.
19. d (associated with severe renal infection)

20. d
21. c
22. b
23. a
24. True; azotemia characterizes both oliguric and nonoliguric ARF.
25. False; the opposite happens, causing cortical ischemia and shunting renal blood to normally relatively ischemic medulla.
26. True; a nephrotoxic chemical is produced by reaction with ethyl alcohol.
27. False; myoglobin is released from the muscle and excreted in the urine and may induce ARF.
28. False; obstructive uropathy is suggested.
29. True; urea, being a small molecule, back-diffuses because the sluggish movement of filtrate through the tubules gives it more exposure time for this to occur, whereas creatinine is not reabsorbed because it is a larger molecule. The fever, bleeding, and trauma often associated with prerenal azotemia also produce a catabolic state, further increasing the BUN.
30. b
31. c
32. a
33. a
34. a
35. a
36. b

CHAPTER 50

1. True
2. True
3. False; toward the cell body
4. False; nerves do not exist in the CNS; cranial nerves are part of the PNS, although their nuclei are located in the CNS.
5. False; most of them are, but they also exist in ganglia outside the CNS.
6. True
7. False; oligodendroglia perform this function in the CNS; Schwann cells do not exist in the CNS.
8. True
9. True
10. False; it forms the craniosacral outflow.
11. True
12. True
13. True
14. True
15. True
16. False; they are bipolar.
17. False; this is the definition of a Golgi type I neuron.
18. False; transmission of impulses between neurons can occur only at synapses, and the transmission is unidirectional from presynaptic terminal to postsynaptic membrane (called the law of Bell-Magendie).
19. True; proteins are transported from the cell body down the axon by axoplasmic flow.
20. True
21. True
22. False; it covers nerve fibers only in the PNS.
23. True
24. False; they are properly called fiber tracts or nerve fiber tracts to distinguish them from nerves that exist in the PNS.
25. False; lower level of L1
26. False; they are CNS tracts.
27. True
28. e
29. a, c
30. a
31. c, d
32. d
33. b
34. c
35. d
36. c
37. d
38. d
39. c
40. a
41. b, c
42. e
43. d
44. b
45. a
46. b
47. a, b, c, d
48. a, b, e
49. c, d
50. d
51. c
52. a, b, d
53. a, c, d
54. b
55. a, b, c, d
56. a, b, c, e
57. a, b, c, d
58. c
59. a, b, c
60. b
61. a, b
62. c
63. c
64. c
65. a
66. d
67. a, c, d
68. b
69. c, d, e

70. a, b, d
71. b
72. b
73. b
74. All are correct.
75. a, b, c, d
76. a, c, d
77. a, b, c
78. b, c
79. b, c
80. a
81. b, c, d
82. a, c, d
83. c
84. b
85. d
86. a, b, c
87. b
88. c
89. a, b
90. a, b, c, d
91. b
92. c, d
93. d
94. e
95. a
96. c
97. b
98. c, d, e
99. a, b, f
100. Anatomic components of the extrapyramidal system (although difficult to define anatomically) probably include the basal ganglia and their connections to the cerebral cortex, cerebellum, reticular formation, and certain thalamic nuclei. The substantia nigra, red nucleus, and subthalamic nucleus in the brainstem are also considered part of the extrapyramidal system. The main function of this system is to provide coarse control of voluntary muscular movement.

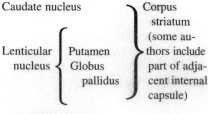

Caudate nucleus

Lenticular nucleus { Putamen / Globus pallidus } Corpus striatum (some authors include part of adjacent internal capsule)

Amygdaloid nucleus
Claustrum
Red nucleus
Substantia nigra
Subthalamic nucleus (corpus Luysii) } Structures closely associated with basal ganglia

The basal ganglia function in some way to prevent oscillation and after-discharge in motor systems, probably by direct action on the midbrain centers and in part as inhibitory feedback to the motor cortex. They are also involved in the control of stretch reflexes and in the generation of mannerisms and automatic activity.

CHAPTER 51

1. Neurologic illness is usually well defined, and a clear history will provide clues that will assist in an accurate assessment of the patient's condition.
2. Examination of the motor system (e.g., testing the gait, voluntary muscle strength, muscle tone)
   Sensory examination (e.g., pain, temperature, vibration sense, examination of the reflexes)
   Coordination of arms and legs
   Examination of mental status and speech
   Examination of cranial nerves
   Examination of reflex status
3. False; the parietal cortex
4. True
5. False; the left hemisphere is dominant.
6. True
7. e
8. h
9. d
10. g
11. a
12. f
13. b
14. c
15. b, d
16. c
17. b
18. c
19. c
20. b
21. a
22. b
23. c
24. b
25. b
26. a, c
27. a
28. True
29. False; these are signs of upper motor neuron involvement.
30. True
31. d
32. i
33. f
34. g
35. j
36. b
37. e
38. h
39. a
40. b

41. c
42. a
43. d
44. (a) Superficial tactile sense; (b) proprioceptive (motion or position) sense; (c) vibratory sense; (d) cortical sensory function
45. Romberg
46. L5 to S1
47. b
48. b
49. d

CHAPTER 52

1. b
2. c
3. a
4. b, c
5. e
6. c, d
7. c
8. a, c
9. b, c, d
10. c
11. a
12. b
13. a
14. d
15. d
16. c
17. b
18. b
19. a
20. b, c, d
21. c, d
22. c, d, e
23. a
24. d
25. d
26. e
27. e
28. a, b, c
29. b
30. e
31. a, c, e
32. d
33. a
34. b
35. c
36. c
37. c
38. c, d
39. b
40. b
41. a
42. a
43. a
44. b
45. b
46. c
47. b
48. a

49. b
50. c
51. a
52. a, c
53. c
54. e
55. d
56. a
57. c
58. b
59. b
60. a
61. a
62. c
63. d
64. True
65. True
66. False; ipsilateral neck or shoulder
67. True
68. Location; onset; pattern (timing, frequency, duration); aggravating/relieving factors; quality; intensity; associated symptoms; effects on life-style; methods of relief
69. Observation of patient's verbal and nonverbal behavior that may indicate pain (e.g., abnormal posture or gait, muscle guarding, moaning, expressions of anger); autonomic hyperactivity such as increased blood pressure or heart rate; tenderness or muscle guarding on palpation
70. The major function of the pain sensory system is to prevent injury. Individuals who have a congenital insensitivity to pain (very rare) do not react to or avoid noxious stimuli and are not particularly disturbed by them. These persons repeatedly injure themselves by failing to avoid high temperatures, intense pressure, extreme twisting, or corrosive substances. They may be totally unaware of internal diseases that would be painful to a normal person. These individuals typically have pressure sores, missing digits, and damaged joints. Although lack of pain sensitivity might seem to be an advantage on superficial examination, the multiple injuries present in persons with this "advantage" attest to its disadvantage.
71. c
72. e
73. a, b, c, e
74. b, c, e
75. a, b, e
76. a, d, e
77. All of these
78. False; this is a description of classic migraine.
79. True; presumably because it is caused by persistent leakage of CSF through the needle site
80. True
81. True
82. True
83. True
84. Questions need to be asked concerning the onset, frequency, duration, location, precipitating/relieving factors; whether there are prodromal symptoms or associated symptoms such as dizziness, nausea, vomiting, or blurred vision; type of pain and whether it is incapacitating; whether other members of the family have a headache problem; and whether there has been head injury in the past. Medical conditions must be considered in relation to the headache pattern.
85. Anterior; trigeminal
86. Posterior; upper cervical
87. b, c, e, i, j
88. a, c, h, j
89. d, f, a, k
90. b
91. e
92. d
93. b
94. Nucleus pulposus
95. Annulus fibrosus
96. Annulus; posterior longitudinal

CHAPTER 53

1. b
2. b, c
3. c
4. b, d
5. The internal carotid enters the skull through the carotid canal, where it gives rise to the ophthalmic artery. It then divides into the anterior and middle cerebral arteries. The anterior cerebral artery supplies the medial surface of the cerebrum and anastomoses with the anterior communicating artery. The middle cerebral artery supplies the lateral surfaces of the cerebral cortex. This branch joins, via the posterior communicating artery, the posterior cerebral branch of the basilar artery. The cerebral arteries and their communicating branches to the basilar artery form the circle of Willis. The basilar artery supplies the cerebellum and the brainstem. It terminates in two posterior cerebral arteries, which supply the inferior surfaces of the temporal and occipital lobes. They communicate with the middle cerebral artery via the posterior communicating artery to complete the circle of Willis.
6. *Extrinsic factors:* (a) Systemic blood pressure: if the BP drops below 60 mm Hg, the autoregulatory mechanism of the brain becomes less effective. If the BP continues to drop until cerebral blood flow (CBF) is decreased to 30 ml/100 g of tissue per minute, signs of cerebral ischemia will appear. (b) Cardiovascular function: if cardiac output is decreased by more than one-third, CBF is likely to fall. (c) Blood viscosity: CBF may increase by as much as 30% with anemia; in polycythemia it may decrease by 50%.
Intrinsic factors: (a) Cerebral autoregulatory mechanism is related to cerebral perfusion pressure (difference between the cerebral artery and veins). When systemic BP decreases, there is a compensatory increase in cerebral vascular pressure, whereas when BP increases, the opposite occurs. (b) Cerebral blood vessels: these vessels are considered the most important factor relating to crebrovascular resistance. A myogenic response suggests that parenchymal tissue of arterioles releases a vasodilatory metabolite in response to their oxygen needs and thereby exerts control on arterial smooth-muscle tone. (c) Intracranial pressure (ICP): an increase in the ICP will increase cerebrovascular resistance. However, CBF does not decrease until ICP has increased to 450 mm H_2O.
7. 200,000; 2 million
8. (a) Transient ischemic attacks (TIAs): focal neurologic deficits that develop suddenly and disappear within a few minutes to hours. (b) Progressive (CVA [stroke] in evolution): evolution of stroke is gradual although acute. (c) Completed CVA: deficits are maximal at onset, with little improvement.
9. c, d, b, a
10. All are correct.
11. e
12. True
13. True
14. False; cerebral tissue necrosis is not associated with TIA.
15. True
16. a
17. d
18. a
19. b
20. d
21. c
22. c
23. c
24. a, b, c
25. c
26. b
27. b
28. All are correct.

29. These factors are (a) stabilization of vital signs—maintaining a patent airway and BP control on an individualized basis, (b) detection and correction of cardiac dysrhythmias, (c) bladder care, (d) proper positioning stressed immediately (frequent turning, range of motion).

30. (a) Vasodilators have increased CBF experimentally but have not proved beneficial in human stroke (CVA) victims. It should be noted that the use of vasodilators may exert an adverse effect on CBF by lowering systemic BP and thereby decreasing intracerebral anastomotic flow. (b) Platelet antiaggregants such as aspirin may be given for prophylaxis against platelet aggregation and subsequent clotting in persons at risk of a CVA. The long-term effectiveness of the therapy needs further evaluation.

31. The primary goal of surgical intervention is improvement of the CBF.

32. (a) A revascularization technique by which a superficial temporal artery is anastomosed to a superficial cortical artery or a segment of the saphenous vein is anastomosed to the subclavian artery and the proximal end of the internal carotid. (b) A carotid endarterectomy in which the neck of the carotid artery is exposed. The vessel is incised at the site of stenosis, and the clot and plaque material are removed.

33. To prevent recurrent hemorrhage

34. (a) Decrease in salt intake, especially with the elderly, and extreme care to maintain BP during surgical procedures; (b) avoidance of oversedation and prolonged bed rest; (c) increased activity; (d) weight control, especially with obese patients; (e) cessation of cigarette smoking

CHAPTER 54

1. Basal ganglia; slow degeneration of nerve cells; below the cortex (subcortical)

2. Extrapyramidal motor nerve tract; it regulates semiautomatic movements, such as coordination of hand movements and swallowing.

3. *Parkinson's syndrome* is a chronic disorder of the central nervous system characterized by a specific group of symptoms that become progressively worse until the patient is unable to perform the activities of daily living and becomes bedridden. Parkinson's syndrome may be idiopathic, posten-

cephalitic, or drug induced (the last a type of pseudoparkinsonism).

4. Parkinson's disease (PD) results from a loss of dopaminergic neurons in the substantia nigra and other pigmented nuclei. As a result, deficiency of dopamine (a neurotransmitter) within the nigrostriatal pathway running from the substantia nigra to the basal ganglia occurs. This leads to an imbalance between dopamine (inhibitory) and acetylcholine (excitatory) neurotransmitters and underlies most of the symptoms of PD. PD is best treated by a combination of L-Dopa plus carbidopa (Sinemet). Dopamine cannot be given directly, since it does not cross the blood-brain barrier.

5. (a) *Resting tremor:* fine or coarse rhythmic alternating contraction of opposing muscle groups, occurring at rest in disease of the basal ganglia and decreasing with voluntary motion; (b) *choreiform movement:* rapid, irregular, jerky, purposeless contractions of random muscle groups followed by prompt relaxation; (c) *athetoid movement:* continuous slow, writhing movements that may be tonic avoiding or grasping reactions; (d) *dystonia:* slow, powerful movements, such as bending a lead pipe; (e) *hemiballism:* flailing, intense violent movements involving one side of the body

6. Phenothiazine, *Rauwolfia* agents

7. Hyperactive glabellar reflex; resting tremor (pill-rolling); expressionless face; festinating gait; micrographia; monotone voice; plastic or cogwheel rigidity

8. Acute disseminated encephalomyelitis, in which patchy areas of demyelination occur in the brain and spinal cord. Preventive measures include regular vaccination for measles in children and avoidance of routine smallpox vaccination. The newer, killed-duck-embryo rabies vaccine should be used when it is necessary to give rabies vaccinations.

9. There are widespread patches of myelin destruction and gliosis in the central nervous system. If the patient reported a temporary blurring of vision in one eye or blindness or an episode of weakness or tingling in an extremity, this would be grounds for suspicion.

10. The major theories are (a) slow viruses, (b) autoimmune process, and (c) aluminum toxicity.

11. b, c, e

12. c

13. a

14. a, c

15. c
16. b
17. b
18. d
19. c
20. c
21. c
22. d
23. c
24. d
25. c
26. All are correct.
27. a, c, e
28. e
29. e
30. a
31. a
32. True
33. False; also have been noted in lead encephalopathy and Down's syndrome
34. True
35. True
36. False; the cause is unknown.
37. True
38. False; thiamine is the therapy of choice.
39. True
40. False; it is a very serious condition.
41. False; it does not provide complete protection against invasion by viruses.
42. True
43. True

CHAPTER 55

1. *Epilepsy* is a paroxysmal disorder of the nervous system characterized by recurrent attacks of loss or alteration of consciousness with or without motor convulsive phenomena. This is usually caused by excessive, uncontrolled local discharges of a group of cerebral neurons, usually in the cortex.

2. The incidence is estimated to be about 0.5% or slightly higher. The incidence in the offspring of epileptic persons is higher than that in the general population.

3. Head injury, hypoglycemia, vitamin B_6 deficiency, alcohol withdrawal, encephalitis, brain tumors

4. Midbrain, thalamus, cerebral cortex

5. Current theory postulates epileptic neurons that have lower thresholds for firing abnormal discharges. A deafferented neuron has been identified in some focal lesions. These neurons are hypersensitive and in a chronic state of depolarization. The cytoplasmic membranes exhibit increased permeability, making them susceptible to activation by various factors (hypoxia, hyperthermia) and circumstances (repeated sensory stimuli).

6. Metabolic needs are increased during convulsions; the electrical discharges of motor nerve cells may be increased to 1000/second. Cerebral blood flow is increased, and there is some increase in respiration and glycolysis. Acetylcholine appears in the cerebrospinal fluid during and after seizures. Glutamic acid may be depleted during seizure activity.

7. *Status epilepticus* refers to a state in which there is a succession (two or more) of generalized seizures with no recovery of consciousness between them.

8. a, b, c, d
9. a, b
10. c
11. d
12. b, d
13. a, b, c, d
14. b
15. c
16. a
17. e
18. f
19. d

CHAPTER 56

1. Normal intracranial pressure (ICP) is about 4 to 15 mm Hg. The basic cause of increased ICP is an expanding mass within the rigid, bony cranium that allows very little room for expansion (about 5 cm³) before pressure starts to increase. Normally the cranial contents consist of tissue, blood, and cerebrospinal fluid (CSF). An increase in ICP can be caused by increased tissue (as from a growing tumor), blood (hematoma secondary to rupture of a blood vessel), blockage of the flow of CSF and its accumulation, and cerebral edema (typically associated with cerebral trauma). Increased ICP is dangerous because it causes cerebral ischemia, hypoxia, compression of the cortex, and herniation of the brain stem through the foramen magnum. This compression causes cessation of function of the vital regulatory centers within the brain stem and death.

2. Compression of cortex: hemiparesis is caused by compression of motor cortex; seizures may result from local cortical disruption; mental dysfunction occurs because cortex is involved in higher thought processes.

   Displacement of brain stem down into foramen magnum, causing its compression: reticular formation in brain stem is involved in level of consciousness; systolic blood pressure increases

so that it will be higher than ICP and cerebral circulation will be maintained; this also causes decerebrate rigidity from removal of normal influence of higher centers on muscle tone.

   Compression of the oculomotor nerve by herniated uncus causes ipsilateral dilated pupil.

3. (a) Local tissue damage from direct force (penetration or compression by missiles or bone fragments or damage as a result of displacement of cranial contents in rapid acceleration or deceleration); (b) cerebral ischemia caused by lack of autoregulation secondary to increasing ICP.

4. Forceful thrusting of the brain contents against the inner surface of the skull on the side opposite the impact. The areas most likely to be damaged in a decelerating motor vehicle accident are the anterior portion of the frontal and temporal lobes and the upper section of the midbrain.

5. The most common sites are those at which a relatively mobile portion of the vertebral column meets a relatively fixed segment. These sites occur between the lower cervical and upper thoracic spine, between the lower thoracic and upper lumbar spine, and between the lower lumbar spine and the sacrum.

6. Stabilize the spinal column to prevent contusion, laceration, and further damage to the spinal cord from bony fragments and foreign bodies.

7. *Epidural hematomas* usually result from a tear in the middle meningeal artery. The bleeding occurs between the dura mater and the skull, usually in the temporal area. The development of clinical symptoms and the course are rapid and proceed to completion within a few hours, since the bleeding is arterial. On the other hand, *subdural hematomas* usually result from the tearing of veins that pass from the surface of the brain to one of the major dural sinuses. Blood escapes between the dura and the arachnoid. Since bleeding is under venous low pressure, the accumulation of blood may be much more prolonged and the clinical course much more protracted.

8. a
9. All are correct.
10. d
11. b, c
12. c; treatment b might cause herniation of the uncus.
13. b
14. a, b, c

15. b, d
16. c
17. a
18. c; loss of vibration sense because of destruction of dorsal (uncrossed ascending) columns and increased touch threshold because of destruction of ventral spinothalamic tract (crossed ascending axons)
19. c, d
20. c, e
21. a, d
22. b
23. False; it is between the dura and skull.
24. False; this causes quadriplegia.
25. True
26. True
27. True
28. False; surgical decompression is controversial; all agree that it should be done if there is progressive neurologic deficit.
29. True
30. True
31. d
32. b
33. c
34. d
35. b
36. d
37. b
38. a
39. e
40. a
41. b
42. b

CHAPTER 57

1. b
2. d
3. a
4. c
5. e
6. d
7. b
8. a
9. c
10. g
11. f
12. c
13. d
14. b
15. a
16. e
17. It is difficult because the symptoms are diverse and depend on the location and size of the growth. However, the symptoms tend to progress. The most common general symptoms are headache, vomiting, and papilledema, all a result of increased intracranial pressure from the expanding mass.

18. d
19. c
20. d
21. a
22. a, c, e
23. a
24. b
25. d
26. b
27. c
28. c
29. f
30. d
31. e
32. a
33. b
34. True
35. True
36. False; microglia function as phago-cytes
37. True
38. True
39. False; most often in thoracic region
40. False; this is amaurosis fugax; pap-illedema involves engorgement and swelling of the optic disc.
41. a
42. b
43. c
44. d
45. c
46. b

CHAPTER 58

1. One mechanism by which hormones work on cells is the adenyl cyclase system. In this case the polypeptide hormones interact with a specific membrane receptor. As a result of this interaction, adenylate cyclase is acti-vated and ATP is converted to cyclic AMP. Cyclic AMP binds to the regu-latory subunit of a protein kinase, lib-erating a catalytic subunit of the en-zyme. This in turn initiates the phos-phorylation of certain enzymes that either activate or inactivate the bio-logic potency of these enzymes.

   A second mechanism by which hormones work on target cells is ex-emplified by steroid hormones, which work directly inside the cell by en-tering the cell across the cell mem-brane and binding to cytosol receptor proteins. The steroid receptor com-plex then is translocated to the nu-cleus of the cell, where it binds specifically to its locus on the chro-matin, activating RNA polymerase with ultimate synthesis of one or sev-eral specific messenger RNAs. These products travel from the nucleus to the ribosome, where they direct the synthesis of proteins. By changing messenger RNA, steroids can modify the way protein is synthesized.

2.

Type of hormone	Location of production	Examples
Proteins (polypep-tides, glycopro-teins)	Posterior pituitary gland	Pitressin
	Beta cells of islets of Langer-hans	Insulin
	Thyroid gland	Thyroxine
	Parathyroid gland	Parathyroid hormone
	Anterior pituitary	Tropic hor-mones
Steroids (lipids)	Adrenal cortex	Cortisol
	Gonads	Estrogen Progesterone

3. A decrease in the pressure of the blood flowing through the afferent ar-teriole of the renal glomerulus is sensed by JG cells, causing release of renin. This results in the following sequence of events:

   Renin → Renin substrate
               ↓
           Angiotensin I
               ↓
           Angiotensin II
               ↓
           Adrenal cortex
               ↓
           Aldosterone

4. The hypothalamus possesses a variety of nuclei made up of neurons having a secretory function. These neurons manufacture proteins, called releasing hormones, secreted through axons into blood vessels. The hypothalamus re-ceives fibers from other areas of the brain that influence hypothalamic neu-ronal function.

5. This anatomic mechanism permits the movement of neurostimuli from the hypothalamus to the pituitary gland; this is the mechanism by which the CNS influences the pituitary gland.

6. Any neurostimuli reaching the CR cen-ter causes release of CRH into the por-tal system. CRH causes release of ACTH by cells in the anterior pituitary gland. ACTH stimulates the adrenal cortex to produce cortisol, which af-fects the rate and amount of CRH-ACTH secreted by the hypothalamic-pituitary axis.

7. ACTH production typically exhibits a cyclic pattern throughout the 24-hour period. The levels usually go up early in the day, go down later in the day, and go up again during the night, to reach a peak level by the next morning.

8. The two postulated mechanisms for en-docrine disorders are those (1) in which the hormone concentrations are primar-ily disturbed and (2) in which the re-ceptors are primarily defective. Most endocrine disorders can be understood conceptually in terms of the metabolic action of the hormone(s) involved.

9. If a disease arises from excessive pro-duction of a hormone, the problem may be treated surgically by removing the gland or part of the gland that pro-duces the hormone. This is followed by replacement with normal amounts of the hormone. If a disease is caused by hormone deficit, the treatment is re-placement of the hormones that are not being produced.

10. b, c, d
11. b
12. c
13. a
14. True
15. True
16. False; they are specific.

CHAPTER 59

1. b
2. a
3. a
4. c
5. d
6. e
7. g
8. a
9. c
10. b
11. h
12. f
13. a, b, c, d
14. c, d
15. a, c, d
16. c
17. b, c, e
18. e
19. b

20. b, c
21. All are correct.
22. a, d
23. All are correct.
24. a, b, d
25. a, c
26. c
27. True
28. False; human growth hormone is the only one effective in humans and is used in experimental study for the treatment of hypopituitary dwarfism.
29. True
30. False; radiographic examination of the pituitary gland is mandatory in patients with suspected pituitary disease, since pituitary tumors are a common cause of these disorders.
31. True
32. Medical treatment using a somatostatin analog is currently being tested. This analog can induce sustained suppression of growth hormone and somatomedin C levels, decrease in tumor size, and marked clinical improvements.
33. It is produced by recombinant DNA techniques.
34. (a) Pituitary tumor that destroys normal pituitary cells; (b) vascular thrombosis leading to necrosis of the normal pituitary gland; (c) infiltrative granulomatous diseases that destroy the pituitary; and (d) idiopathic or possible autoimmune destruction of pituitary cells
35. Their urine specific gravity fails to increase, and urine osmolality remains low. Thirst may become intense, and they may develop orthostatic hypotension and experience significant weight loss. Rationale for administration of aqueous pitressin: urine volume decreases; specific gravity increases.
36. Treatment of SIADH is based on water restriction to less than 1000 ml/day; administration of 3% to 5% sodium chloride solutions with furosemide. Diuretic induces loss of water and sodium chloride, which is restored in hypertonic form. Demeclocycline can be used effectively to reverse the hypoosmolality associated with SIADH.

CHAPTER 60
1. a
2. a
3. c
4. b, c
5. a, b, c
6. b
7. b, c
8. a, b
9. a
10. a, b
11. b
12. a, c
13. True
14. False; a lesion in thyroid gland
15. True
16. True
17. True
18. True
19. The thyroid gland located below the cricoid cartilage in the neck is made up of nodules of tiny follicles. These follicles are lined by cuboidal epithelium, and their lumen is filled with colloid. The follicular epithelial cells initiate the synthesis of thyroid hormones and activate their release into the circulation. The thyroid hormones produced by the follicles are thyroxine and triiodothyronine.
20. The process of biosynthesis of thyroid hormones is as follows: (a) Trapping of iodine by the thyroid follicular cells. The thyroid takes up and concentrates large amounts of iodine from the circulating iodide pool. (b) Oxidation of iodide to iodine. The thyroid plasma gradient is 20 to 30 : 1 at a wide range of plasma inorganic iodide concentrations. Iodide is catalyzed by an iodide peroxidase enzyme and converted to iodine. (c) Organification of iodine into monoiodotyrosine. Iodine is incorporated into a tyrosine molecule, which occurs at the cell-colloid interphase. (d) Coupling of iodinated precursors. The resulting compounds, monoiodotyrosine and diiodotyrosine, are coupled as follows: two molecules of diiodotyrosine make thyroxine (T_4), and one molecule of diiodotyrosine and one molecule of monoiodotyrosine make triiodothyronine (T_3). (e) Storage. The coupling of these compounds and the storage of the resulting hormones take place within thyroglobulin. (f) Hormone release from storage. This release occurs by incorporation of colloid droplets into the follicular cells by a process called pinocytosis. Thyroglobulin is hydrolyzed, and the hormones are released into the circulation.
21. Tests presently used in the diagnosis of thyroid disease are (a) serum thyroxine and triiodothyronine, (b) T_3 resin uptake, (c) free thyroxine, (d) serum TSH levels, and (e) radioisotope thyroid uptake.
22. The significance of elevated serum thyroglobulin in patients with metastatic disease is indicative of recurring disease.
23. This uptake test measures the ability of the thyroid gland to trap and organify iodide. The patient receives a trace dose of ^{123}I, which the thyroid traps and concentrates over 24 hours. Radioactivity present over the thyroid is calculated. Normally, uptake ranges from 10% to 35% of the administered dose. Values are high in hyperthyroidism and low when the thyroid gland has been suppressed.
24. 20 to 30
25. 5
26. 4 to 11; 80 to 160
27. Graves' disease; toxic nodular goiter

CHAPTER 61
1. a, b, c, d
2. b
3. c
4. a, b, c
5. a, c
6. b
7. b
8. b
9. a, c
10. a
11. d
12. d
13. a, c
14. a, c, d
15. All are correct.
16. All are correct.
17. c
18. c
19. All are correct.
20. c
21. a, b
22. The catabolic effect of glucocorticoid excess causes a decrease in the ability of protein-forming cells to synthesize protein from amino acids.
23. Interferes with the action of insulin in the peripheral cells, which results in the impairment of the ability of the receptor cells to metabolize glucose.
24. Stress causes the CNS to activate the corticotropin-releasing center, causing CRH and ACTH to be released. Increased ACTH leads to an increase in cortisol release. The important concept is that stress causes an increased secretion of cortisol by the adrenal gland.
25. 9Alpha-fluorocortisol has a fluorine group in the 9alpha-position of the cortisol molecule. Prednisolone has a double bond between carbons 1 and 2 of this molecule. The metabolic effects of these compounds are different from

those of the parent compound. For example, prednisolone, compared with cortisol, has less sodium-retaining activity and more antiinflammatory activity per milligram. 9Alpha-fluorocortisol has much greater sodium-retaining activity than cortisol.

26. Pituitary irradiation, removal of a pituitary tumor, and adrenalectomy. The excess cortisol is eliminated if the procedure is successful.

27. Surgical removal of the neoplasm

28. In congestive heart failure, patients are unable to pump blood normally and cardiac output decreases. The renal afferent arteriole experiences a change in perfusion pressure, causing increased production of renin, which activates synthesis of angiotensin. This stimulates aldosterone production, causing resorption of sodium and water and volume expansion.

29. True

30. True

31. True

32. False; CRF directly initiates the secretion of ACTH.

33. False; deficiency of 21-hydroxylase causes a decrease in cortisol production and increase in ACTH secretion.

CHAPTER 62

1. b
2. c
3. a, c
4. a
5. a, c
6. b
7. c
8. b, d
9. a, c
10. c

CHAPTER 63

1. a, b
2. a, b
3. c
4. a
5. c
6. a, b, c
7. d
8. b
9. a, b
10. a
11. b
12. c
13. a
14. a, b, c, d
15. a, b
16. Fasting plasma glucose is measured to check the function of the regulating

mechanisms that control carbohydrate metabolism. This measurement can help evaluate the integrity of the mechanism regulating plasma glucose. In general, these levels become abnormal only in the advanced state of a disease. Therefore it does not provide information about early abnormalities in glucose metabolism.

17. Insulin. In people without diabetes, a rise in blood glucose stimulates release of insulin, which triggers disposal of excess glucose.

18. This system assists diabetics in managing their own diets. The food exchange lists help patients identify food alternatives.

19. The newer, second-generation sulfonylureas have advantages over the first-generation compounds in that they have little or no antidiuretic effect.

20. The recognition of individuals at risk for developing insulin-dependent diabetes (IDDM) may lead to early detection of the autoimmune process causing destruction of beta cells and treatment with specific immunosuppressive agents. Once the disease has developed, pancreatic transplantation may restore insulin-secreting capacity. In non-insulin-dependent diabetes (NIDDM) patients, a better understanding of the molecular mechanism of insulin resistance may lead to the development of pharmacologic agents that could specifically enhance insulin action.

21. c
22. d
23. a
24. b
25. True
26. False; 75% of diabetic patients eventually die of vascular disease; heart attacks, kidney failure, strokes, and gangrene are the major complications.
27. False; exercise appears to facilitate the transport of glucose into cells.
28. True
29. b
30. a
31. c
32. a
33. b
34. c
35. c
36. a, b
37. a, b, c
38. c
39. c
40. b

41. All are correct.
42. a
43. b, c, e
44. d
45. c
46. a, d
47. d

CHAPTER 64

1. The development and release of ova (oogenesis) and the production of steroid hormones (estrogens, estrone [E_1], estradiol [E_2], estriol [E_3], androgens, progesterone)

2. During menopause, estradiol levels decrease and the ovary decreases in size and is virtually devoid of follicles. The decrease in circulating estradiol levels increases, by negative feedback, pituitary gonadotropin secretion.

3. Treatment of amenorrhea is often based on the underlying disorder causing the problem. For example, patients with prolactin-secreting pituitary adenomas should be treated with either transphenoidal resection of the pituitary tumor or suppression of prolactin secretion with bromocriptine. Patients with hypothalamic-pituitary or ovarian deficiency should receive replacement therapy with estrogens and progesterone administered cyclically.

4. During the years of reproductive maturity, cyclic changes occur in the ovaries and uterus that serve the purpose of preparing the ovum and endometrium each month for a pregnancy. These cyclic changes are regulated by hormones of the hypothalamic-pituitary-gonadal axis. The outline below presents a simplified summary of these changes.

A. Normal menstrual cycle: average length of cycle = 28 days

B. Ovarian cycle
   1. Follicular phase
      a. FSH levels rise on day 1 of 28-day cycle, peaks on day 7, and declines thereafter
      b. FSH initiates maturation of several ovarian follicles (ovum and surrounding cells)
      c. FSH stimulates follicles to secrete estrogens
   2. Luteal phase
      a. LH levels rises on about day 9 of 28-day cycle, peaks at day 14 (ovulation), and gradually decreases during premenstrual phase
      b. LH induces ovulation (ap-

proximately day 14 but variable) of maturing ovum and formation of corpus luteum

    c. Corpus luteum secretes increasing amounts of progesterone and small amounts of estrogen

C. Endometrial or menstrual cycle

    1. Proliferative or postmenstrual (preovulatory) phase

      a. Days 6 to 14 of 28-day cycle

      b. Rising estrogens levels stimulate proliferation and thickening of endometrium

    2. Ovulation (approximately day 14)

    3. Secretory of premenstrual phase

      a. Days 15 to 28 of 28-day cycle

      b. Increasing progesterone levels produced by corpus luteum stimulate endometrium to become vascular, edematous, and with a thicker mucosa capable of implanting a fertilized ovum

    4. Menstrual phase

      a. If ovum unfertilized, corpus luteum begins to regress on day 23 or 24 of 28-day cycle

      b. As luteal function degenerates, progesterone and estrogen levels decline, causing degeneration of uterine endometrium and initiation of menstruation

      c. Superficial endometrial lining is sloughed, accompanied with menstrual bleeding lasting about 5 days (day 1 to day 5 of 28-day cycle).

5. The anatomic structure of the female reproductive system, with access from outside the body to internal structures, allows ascent of organisms from the lower tract to the upper tract and potentially the perineal cavity, as well as descent from the upper tract, where there is hematogenous spread of the organism from a primary site of infection elsewhere in the body.

6. High-risk factors for ovarian cancer are early menarche, late menopause, nulliparous, or first pregnancy late; and if two or more first-degree relatives have ovarian cancer, a woman has a 50% chance of developing it. Some physicians recommend prophylactic oophorectomy at age 35 years for women in the latter high-risk group.

7. The breast changes are cystic formation, ductal epithelial proliferation, diffuse papillomatosis, and ductal adenosis with formation of fibrous tissue. Fibrocystic breast disease occurs during childbearing years; the cause is likely a relative excess of estrogen and a deficiency of progesterone during the luteal phase of the menstrual cycle.

8. Breast cancers develop from epithelial tissues, with most being in the duct system. Initially there is hyperplasia of the cells with development of atypical cells that progress to carcinoma in situ and then to stromal invasion. A cancer takes about 7 years to grow from a single cell to a mass large enough to palpate (about 1 cm in diameter). At that size about one fourth of breast cancers have already metastasized.

9. Detection and diagnosis begin with obtaining a thorough history of pertinent information related to the breasts and a physical examination of the breasts. Mammography is essential, since it can detect masses too small to be felt and in many instances reveal the probable nature of a palpable mass. Tissue-sampling procedures done to obtain specimens for microscopic examination include fine-needle aspiration, core needle biopsy, and open biopsy. If the specimen is malignant, further evaluation is needed.

10. a, d

11. b

12. c

13. d

14. a, d

15. b

16. c

17. a, c, d

18. d

19. c, d

20. a

21. a

22. b

23. c

24. d

25. c

26. True

27. False; primary amenorrhea is the failure to begin spontaneous menstruation by age 17.

28. True

29. True

30. True

31. False; a leiomyoma is a benign, well-circumscribed uterine tumor.

32. False; treatment is radical vulvectomy, bilateral inguinal lymphadenectomy, and removal of a portion of the distal urethra or vagina, and/or a portion of the rectum with postoperative pelvic irradiation.

33. True

CHAPTER 65

1. Primary functions are to produce mature spermatozoa and to deposit sperm in the female reproductive tract with coitus.

2. Spermatogenesis begins with puberty (about age 13) and continues throughout life. In the seminiferous tubules, spermatogonia begin to proliferate. Some of the daughter cells remain spermatogonia, and others move to the lumen of the seminiferous tubule and enlarge into primary spermatocytes. These cells undergo meiotic division to form two secondary spermatocytes. Each secondary spermatocyte undergoes a second meiotic division, resulting in two spermatids. One spermatogonium produces four sperm. Each spermatid undergoes a maturation and differentiation process to develop the head, neck, body, and tail of the mature sperm. This process takes place continuously throughout life. Sperm are stored in the epididymides and vasa deferens and retain their fertility for as long as 42 days.

3. A clomiphene or GnRH stimulation test should be done if low gonadotropins are present with low serum testosterone. In this case, clomiphene should cause a 50% increase in the interstitial cell–stimulating hormone (ICSH). If ICSH does not increase, the test indicates a hypothalamic-pituitary insufficiency. However, administering GnRH should cause a peak level three times the control of luteinizing hormone (LH) within minutes. With hypothalmaic dysfunction, a response may not occur until repeated injections are given over several days. An exaggerated response indicates a reduced feedback response secondary to low levels of testosterone and estradiol.

4. It is difficult to separate the decline of reproductive function with the decline in physical fitness that occurs with advancing age; the latter decline may be responsible for the decrease in reproductive function. The seminiferous tubules of the testes continue to produce sperm but in less numbers with advancing age. Testosterone levels gradually decrease. The number of Leydig cells may decrease as the abil-

ity of the remaining cells to produce testosterone decreases. Failure to attain or maintain erection of the penis (impotence) is more common with advanced age. Psychologic as well as physiologic factors are involved, such as veins and arteries that supply the erectile tissue of the penis being subject to sclerosis.

5. The factors responsible for infections of the genital organs in men are venereal transmission, a manifestation of systemic disease, or a result of instrumentation (catheterization, surgery).

6. As the tumor progresses, there can be direct extension to the urethra, bladder neck, and seminal vesicles. It can also spread via lymphatic or hematogenous routes. Most common site of metastasis is by the hematogenous route to the bones of the pelvis, lumbar spine, femur, thoracic spine, and ribs. Organ metastases are to the liver and lung.

7. d
8. c
9. a
10. b
11. b
12. b
13. d
14. a
15. a
16. c
17. b
18. a
19. a, b, c
20. c
21. c
22. a
23. e
24. d
25. b

CHAPTER 66

1. Venereal or sexually transmitted diseases (STDs) are infections that are primarily transmitted by heterosexual or homosexual intercourse or by intimate contact with the mouth, genitalia, or rectum.

2. These include sterility, genital tract carcinoma, and possibly death. A variety of perinatal infections may be transmitted to the fetus or neonate. The economic consequences of chlamydia illness in the United States are an estimated annual cost of more than $2.4 billion.

3. The causative organism is *Treponema pallidum.*

4. Primary, secondary, and early latent stages are treated with parenteral penicillin G.

5. Single-dose treatments are IM ceftriaxone or cefixime, ciprofloxacin, or ofloxacin orally.

6. The recurrent vesicles and ulcers are infectious to sexual partners until the ulcers heal completely. The herpesvirus has been recovered from the cervix up to 3 months after a primary infection without evidence of an active lesion. There is no treatment that will eradicate the herpes simplex virus (HSV). Acyclovir has reduced the ulcerative phase and duration of viral shedding.

7. The human papillomavirus (HPV) thrives in the moist areas of the urogenital, perineal, and perianal regions. Incubation period is several weeks to months after contact. The warts vary in color from tan, pink, or white papules. In males they occur on the frenulum and coronal sulcus, along the penile shaft, and in anal and perianal areas; in females, lesions occur on the labia majora and minora, introitus, perianal and anal regions, thighs, vagina, and cervix. Direct extension from the point of innoculation can occur, and single warts will multiply into cauliflower-like growths several centimeters in diameter. Range of symptoms from local irritation to secondary bacterial infection. High association between the virus and genital tract malignancies exists.

8. Treatment is necessary to prevent potentially serious complications of chlamydial infection; asymptomatic partners should also be treated because transmission rate is high. An oral preparation of doxycycline or Azithromycin is recommended for uncomplicated urethral, endocervical, or rectal chlamydial infections in men and nonpregnant women. Erythromycin is the drug of choice for pregnant women and neonates.

9. b
10. b
11. a, b, d
12. c
13. a, b, c
14. a, b, d
15. a
16. c
17. a, b, c
18. True
19. False; the papillomavirus that causes condylomata acuminata is different than the papovaviruses that cause common warts.
20. True

21. False; candidiasis is not a venereal disease. However, vaginitis, vulvovaginitis, balanitis, and balanoposthitis caused by this organism have been identified after sexual contact.

22. True

CHAPTER 67

1. The structures of the musculoskeletal system include bones, joints, skeletal muscles, tendons, ligaments, bursae, and the specialized tissues that connect these structures.

2. *Woven bone* is a type of bone seen with rapid growth (e.g., in fetal development or after a fracture; in adults it is found at ligament or tendon insertions). *Lamella bone* is mature bone found throughout the body of adults. The structure of lamella bone is highly organized, mineralized plates rather than a solid cystalline mass, which provides substantial strength for bone.

3. Joints are held together by joint capsules, fibrous bands, ligaments, tendons, fasciae, or muscles.

4. The joint is lubricated by synovial fluid and by hydrostatic changes in the interstitial fluid of the cartilage. Pressure on the cartilages causes fluid to move to an area of less pressure. As the joint glides forward, this weeping fluid moves ahead to the load. The fluid moves back into the portions of the cartilage from which the pressure is relieved. Articular cartilage and the bones of the joint are normally held apart during action by the film of the fluid.

5. The process of bone resorption occurs because the osteoclasts produce proteolytic enzymes that break down matrix and several acids that cause dissolution of the bone minerals. Calcium and phosphorus are released into the bloodstream during this process.

6. Osteoid is the organic matrix of bone that is about 70% type I collagen. This type of collagen is rigid, giving bone its high tensile strength.

7. The significance of joints innervated by peripheral nerves crossing the articulation is that pain from one joint may be reported as coming from another (e.g., pain arising in the hip can be felt by the person as knee pain).

8. b
9. a
10. d
11. a, d
12. a
13. a
14. a

15. c
16. b
17. b
18. c, d
19. a
20. a
21. b
22. False; it is often difficult to distinguish periarticular pain from pain arising from a joint.
23. True
24. False; the mucin clot test is less effective with the more inflammatory fluids, because the acetic acid added to the synovial fluid forms a precipitate by interaction with hyaluronic acid. The hyaluronic acid has been broken down by the lysosomal enzymes and is not available to precipitate when treated with acetic acid.
25. True
26. False; articular cartilage has few cells and a large amount of ground substance.
27. c
28. a
29. d
30. b
31. Refer to Fig. 67-1.

CHAPTER 68

1. d
2. a
3. a
4. d
5. c, d
6. d
7. b, d
8. c
9. When a fracture occurs, the periosteum is generally torn, blood vessels are damaged, and bone fragments are separated. A blood clot forms, and granulation tissue develops within which osteogenic cells differentiate into chondroblasts and osteoblasts. A band (callus) forms around a fragment at the fracture site and continues to thicken and expand, converging with the band from the opposite fragment and fusing with it. Fushion of the two fragments and fracture healing progress as osteoblasts form trabeculae, which adhere to the bone and extend across the fracture site. The bony callus remodels to assume the shape of intact bone, as osteoblasts form new bone and osteoclasts remove the damaged and temporary bone.
10. Early diagnosis of osteomyelitis, especially in children, is important so that appropriate antibiotic and surgical treatment can be administered to prevent the local spread of infection and crippling destruction of the entire bone.
11. In children the periosteal sleeve around the tubular bones is strong and active, allowing for rapid healing.
12. Children's limbs grow quickly; bayonet apposition is often used to achieve equal length by adulthood.
13. b, d
14. f
15. a
16. b
17. c
18. g

CHAPTER 69

1. When a lesion is definitely diagnosed as benign and self-limiting, no further diagnostic studies are generally needed. However, when a lesion is diagnosed as benign with a lesser degree of certainty, the patient should be reexamined at regular intervals with repeat radiographs. If over several months there is no change in the lesion or in the patient's condition, follow-up visits may be discontinued. The patient must be instructed to return for further examination if any changes occur. It is important to assess whether the patient and the family are responsible and will follow through with the repeated examination.
2. Bone tumor cells produce factors that stimulate osteoclast activity, which leads to bone resorption. Some tumors cause increased osteoblast activity and increased density.
3. Benign tumors are much more common, although malignant tumors are often fatal. Malignant tumors tend to grow rapidly and spread and invade irregularly; most often they occur in adolescents and young adults.
4. Most common primary sites of bone neoplasms are prostrate, breast, lung, thyroid, kidney, and bladder.
5. The most common bones affected by neoplasms are vertebrae, proximal femur, pelvis, ribs, sternum, and proximal humerus.
6. True
7. False; pathologic fractures are generally the result of metastasis of malignant tumor to bone.
8. True
9. False; metastasis from a primary site to bone is frequently found in adults, not in children.
10. True
11. a, d
12. a

13. b
14. a
15. b
16. b
17. a

CHAPTER 70

1. *Osteoarthritis* is a disorder of the movable joints. The disorder is chronic, slowly progressive, and noninflammatory and is characterized by the deterioration and abrasion of articular cartilage and the formation of new bone at the articular surface.
2. The synthesis of proteoglycans and collagen in the joint is greatly increased in osteoarthritis. There is a net loss of proteoglycans and collagen over time, since degradation is even more rapid.
3. The aging process seems to be related to the development and progression of osteoarthritis through changes in chondrocyte functioning. Chondrocytes are the cells responsible for the formation of the proteoglycans and collagen in the articular cartilage. The aging chondrocytes may lose their ability to function appropriately.
4. Total joint replacements for hips and knees have been successful in maintaining near-normal function for many people with osteoarthritis. Osteoarthritis is a hypertrophic form of arthritis; that is, the bone adjacent to the joint is strong, forming an excellent base for attachment of the artificial joint. A number of complications can occur with joint replacement, and these must be weighed against the benefits.
5. Narrowing of the joint space is typically seen in osteoarthritis because of loss of cartilage. Radiologic findings also reveal an increase in bone density around the joint. Cystic changes of various sizes are sometimes seen. Osteophytes (spurs) can be seen at the marginal aspects of the joint.
6. The goals of the treatment of osteoarthritis are retardation or prevention of further damage to the joint and management of pain and stiffness to maintain mobility.
7. a, c, d
8. d
9. d
10. a, b, c
11. a, b, c
12. False; osteoarthritis is a noninflammatory disease.

13. False; erosive inflammatory osteoarthritis affects primarily the finger joints.
14. False; oral corticosteroids are contraindicated in the treatment of osteoarthritis.
15. False; no specific blood tests are used in the diagnosis of osteoarthritis.

CHAPTER 71

1. *Rheumatoid arthritis* is a chronic disorder that affects multiple organ systems and is one of a group of diffuse connective tissue diseases that are immune mediated and of unknown etiology. There is usually progressive joint destruction, although the episodes of joint inflammation may alternate with periods of remission.
2. The association of the genetic markers HLA-Dw4 and HLA-DR5 in whites with the development of rheumatoid arthritis.
3. Destruction of the tissues in the joints occurs in the following ways. (a) There is a digestive destruction caused by the production of proteases, collagenases, and other hydrolytic enzymes. These enzymes break down the cartilage, ligaments, tendons, and bones in the joints and are released along with oxygen radicals and arachidonic acid metabolites by PMNs in the synovial fluid. (b) Destruction of tissue appears to take place through the action of rheumatoid pannus. Along the edge of the pannus there is destruction of collagen and proteoglycans through the production of enzymes of cells in the pannus.
4. The diagnostic criteria are (a) morning stiffness (at least 1 hour), (b) arthritis of three or more joint areas, (c) arthritis of hand joints, (d) symmetric arthritis, (e) rheumatoid nodules, (f) serum rheumatoid factor, and (g) radiographic changes (erosions of bony decalcification).
5. The overall goals of the therapeutic program for rheumatoid arthritis are to relieve pain and inflammation, maintain joint function and the patient's maximum functional capacity, and prevent and/or correct joint deformities.
6. NSAIDs reduce inflammation by interrupting the cascade of production of inflammatory mediators. They act by inhibiting either cyclooxygenase or prostaglandin synthetase. These enzymes are responsible for the conversion of the endogenous systemic fatty acid arachidonic acid to prostaglandins, prostacyclins, thromboxanes, and oxygen radicals.

7. The indications for corticosteroid therapy are as follows. (a) Chronic oral therapy is used in those persons with rheumatoid arthritis who do not respond to NSAIDs and slow-acting drugs. (b) It is used for control of symptoms while awaiting the onset of action by slow-acting drug therapy. (c) Intraarticular injections are indicated for acute exacerbations of synovitis in single joints where mobility is significantly impaired. (d) High-dose oral therapy is used for short periods for a severe attack.
8. Corticosteroid agents act through their antiinflammatory and immunosuppressive properties. Inflammation is reduced by blockage of prostaglandin formation, inhibition of leukocyte and monocyte chemotaxis and phagocytosis, stabilization of lysosomal enzymes, and prevention of changes in capillary membranes. Immunosuppression results from the decreased reticuloendothelial, or monocyte-macrophage, procession of antigens and the altered function of lymphocytes.
9. Rheumatoid arthritis may involve the heart (pericarditis), lungs (pleuritis), eyes, and blood vessels. Refer to box on p. 1044.
10. b
11. b
12. b
13. c
14. d
15. b, d
16. a, b
17. c
18. c
19. False; in the United States, 13.9 children/100,000 will develop juvenile arthritis.
20. True
21. False; only an association with HLA-Dw4 has been shown in African Americans and in Japanese.
22. True
23. False; rheumatoid factor is detected in about 85% of patients with rheumatoid arthritis.

CHAPTER 72

1. Systemic lupus erythematosus (SLE) is a multisystem, chronic, autoimmune disease. The signs and symptoms of this disorder can be diverse and transitory.
2. The antinuclear antibody (ANA) test indicates whether there are antibodies capable of destroying the nucleus of the subject's own body cells. In addition to the presence of ANA, the ANA

pattern and the specific antibodies are evaluated. The LE factor test may occasionally be used today to identify the lupus erythematosus factor. The LE cell is formed by damage to some of a person's white cells, causing release of their nucleoprotein, which reacts with IgG; this complex is phagocytosed by the remaining white cells. The resulting cell is easily identified.
3. The onset of SLE occurs most frequently during late adolescence and early adulthood in women. Counseling is needed to assist those affected regarding the decision about having children. Pregnancy may cause a flare-up of SLE, which can be dangerous for women with renal damage. Cytotoxic drugs may be necessary to control the illness, and these can affect the fetus. Contraceptives, including birth control pills, cannot be prescribed, since they may aggravate SLE.
4. Just how the sun causes SLE to flare up is not fully understood. One explanation is that DNA exposed to ultraviolet light normally becomes antigenic, and this leads to the flares seen after sun exposure.
5. The selection of appropriate drug therapy depends on the specific organs affected by the illness. NSAIDs are used to control the arthritis and arthralgia. Aspirin is used less frequently because it produces the highest incidence of hepatotoxicity, and some people with SLE have hepatic involvement.
6. c
7. a
8. a
9. b, c
10. c
11. c
12. a, b, c
13. True
14. False; cyclophosphamide or azathioprine can be used in an effort to suppress the autoimmune activity of SLE.
15. False; lupus nephritis occurs in more than 65% of those with SLE.
16. False; DNA is antigenic to humans with SLE.

CHAPTER 73

1. *Generalized* scleroderma (systemic sclerosis) can be either diffuse cutaneous systemic sclerosis with truncal involvement, widespread visceral disease, or limited cutaneous systemic sclerosis including the CREST variant; *localized* scleroderma usually only affects limited skin areas and does not af-

fect visceral organs; *occupational and environmental* scleroderma-like syndromes can be seen after exposure to substances such as chloride, bleomycin, and rapeseed oil.

2. The skin and other organ changes in scleroderma are the result of the overproduction of collagen. Lesions that develop in the small arteries and arterioles begin as proliferations on the intimal side of the internal elastic membrane. A medial thinning then occurs, and finally a connective tissue cuff rich in collagen is deposited.

3. One form of systemic sclerosis is the CREST variant. The colon may be affected, which results in diarrhea or constipation, cramping, and malabsorption. Exertional dyspnea is usually the first sign of pulmonary involvement; pulmonary function studies may show alterations in gas exchange (decrease in breathing capacity and increase in residual air); pericarditis; dysrhythmias; electrocardiogram changes with cardiac involvement; renal involvement manifested as proteinuria, microscopic hematuria, and hypertension may rapidly deteriorate to renal failure.

4. Drugs such as penicillamine, dimethyl sulfoxide (DMSO), immunosuppressive drugs, and alkylating agents are sometimes used to manage symptoms. Protection of the hands to help avoid Raynaud's phenomenon is an important part of the management plan. Nonsteroidal antiinflammatory agents can be used to decrease discomfort. Physical therapy is an important component of the treatment plan.

5. b
6. d
7. a
8. b
9. True
10. False; radiographic studies of systemic sclerosis may demonstrate calcifications of the digits of the hand.
11. False; currently no effective therapy will reverse the fibrosis of scleroderma.

CHAPTER 74

1. *Gout* is a term used for a group of at least nine metabolic disorders that are characterized by an elevation in the serum uric acid concentration (hyperuricemia).
2. Primary gout is the direct result of the body's overproduction or decreased excretion of uric acid. Secondary gout occurs when the overproduction or de-

creased excretion of uric acid is secondary to another disease process or to medication.
3. Colchicine is a drug that inhibits phagocytic leukocytes and produces a dramatic and rapid relief of the symptoms of gout.
4. The factors that contribute to the development of gout depend on the cause of the hyperuricemia. For example, a diet high in purines can trigger a gouty attack in a person with one of the inborn errors of purine metabolism. The ingestion of alcohol can produce a gouty attack because blood lactate levels increase as a byproduct of the normal metabolism of alcohol. Lactic acid blocks the renal excretion of uric acid, with a concomitant rise in serum levels.
5. The treatment of chronic gout is based on decreasing the production of uric acid or increasing the renal excretion of uric acid.
6. Gout can damage the kidneys, leading to an even poorer excretion of uric acid. These uric acid crystals can form in the medullary interstitium, papillae, and pyramids, leading to proteinurea and mild hypertension. Uric acid kidney stones can also occur secondary to gout.
7. b
8. d
9. c
10. c
11. a, b, d
12. b
13. a
14. b
15. b, d

CHAPTER 75

1. The goals of the treatment of anklosing spondylitis are multifocal and relate to the stage of the illness. There is a focused intervention aimed at increasing the understanding of the illness by the patient and the family. Changes in work patterns may be necessary, since bending, lifting, and prolonged static positions will be difficult. Medication is aimed at decreasing the synovitis and pain. An active exercise program is often focused on breathing exercises, muscle strengthening, and reducing limitations in range of motion.
2. About 7% of people with psoriasis develop inflammatory joint disease (psoriatic arthritis). Usually the arthritis occurs after the appearance of the skin le-

sions, but it can occur before or at the same time as the skin lesions.
3. The treatment of Reiter's syndrome is primarily symptomatic. Therapeutic doses of nonsteroidal antiinflammatory drugs are used to relieve the inflammation and pain. Antibiotics are not of proven value.
4. a, b, d
5. a
6. a, b
7. c, d
8. c
9. a, c
10. a
11. b, c
12. a
13. True
14. False; psoriatic arthritis generally tends to be much less debilitating than rheumatoid arthritis.
15. True
16. True
17. False; about 20% of individuals with ankylosing spondylitis develop disabling stages of the illness.
18. True

CHAPTER 76

1. a, b, d
2. a, b
3. c, d
4. b
5. b
6. a
7. The basal layer consists largely of undifferentiated cells that undergo constant mitoses, renewing the epidermis. One of the daughter cells migrates outward toward the stratum spinosum. These undifferentiated basal-layer cells are precursors of keratinocytes. Keratinocytes migrate upward through the stratum granulosum to the stratum corneum to form a fibrous-amorphous complex surrounded by a reinforced impermeable membrane, the horny cell.
8. Eccrine (sweat) glands produce a hypotonic solution and allow excess heat to be eliminated from the body, which aids in maintaining appropriate temperature. Sebaceous glands produce sebum, which lubricates the epidermis.
9. (a) Skin should be examined in a well-illuminated room, preferably in natural daylight. (b) Color should be recorded (e.g., purplish, cyanotic discoloration, pallor). (c) Skin characteristics such as turgor and elasticity on palpation should be noted. (d) Hair distribution and condition of nails should be recorded.

10. The subcutaneous layer provides a cushion for the skin; insulation to maintain body heat, and a store of energy.
11. True
12. True
13. True
14. False; hair is composed of dead keratin, not living keratinocytes.
15. True
16. True
17. False; African Americans have large melanosomes that resist destruction by the hydrolyzing enzymes; whites have smaller melanosomes that are easily destroyed.
18. Refer to figure below.

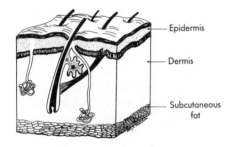

Epidermis

Dermis

Subcutaneous fat

CHAPTER 77

1. Acne is a chronic inflammatory process of the sebaceous glands.
2. Acne generally occurs among adolescents and young adults and spontaneously resolves around 20 to 30 years of age.
3. The earliest lesion is the comedo. White comedones are likely to progress to the inflammatory papules and pustules of acne. Black comedones obstruct the flow of sebum to the surface. The sebum, bacteria, and fatty acids are thought to be responsible for the development of inflammation around the pilosebaceous ducts and sebaceous glands. This inflammation leads to the formation of papules, inflammatory pustules, and cysts. The cysts open in time, drain, and heal. Deeper papules and cysts can leave permanent scars, whereas mild acne resolves without scarring.
4. (a) To remove the surface oil and to dislodge some comedones. (b) Tetracycline. This antibiotic eliminates *Propionibacterium acnes* in the sebaceous gland. Tetracycline has an inhibitory effect on the enzyme lipase, thus preventing breakdown of fat into fatty acids. (c) Dermabrasion is used to smooth and plane the scars and pits that develop as a result of acne.

5. (a) Oil-based makeup and (b) external oils can exacerbate acne.
6. b
7. c, d
8. d
9. b
10. d
11. b

CHAPTER 78

1. The characteristic lesions of eczema are pruritic, erythematous, crusty, weepy, and scaly eruptions. Acute eczema presents with many vesicles and bullae and with erythema, weeping, and crusting, whereas chronic eczema presents with thickened (lichenified), scaly, pruritic patches and plaques.
2. (a) Skin reaction to the oil of poison ivy, (b) nickel sensitivity, (c) allergic reaction to potassium and dichromate, (d) allergic reaction to shoes that contain rubber, (e) allergic reaction to medications such as neomycin or benzocaine.
3. Dyshidrotic hand eczema occurs in persons who must wash their hands frequently or are under stress. It is exacerbated by water, detergents, and stress. There is hereditary predisposition to this edema.
4. Acute urticaria with angioedema is treated with subcutaneous epinepherine. Less severe urticaria is treated with oral antihistamines, such as diphenydramine hydroxyzine and cryproheptadine.
5. b
6. a
7. All are correct.
8. True
9. True
10. True
11. True

CHAPTER 79

1. The latest treatment modality for psoriasis is oral etretrinate (Tegison). This oral aromatic retinoid is excellent for the treatment of pustular and erythrodermic psoriasis and is useful for recalcitrant plaque psoriasis. This drug should not be given to women of childbearing age because it is a powerful teratogen. It also elevates liver enzymes, cholesterol, and triglycerides. Side effects include dryness, hair loss, headaches, diarrhea, myalgia, and arthralgias. If used longer than 6 months, radiographic studies of the bones should be done to check for calcium deposits in the joints.

2. A vitamin D derivative, 1,25-dihydroxy-vitamin D_3, can be used for psoriasis.
3. A psoriatic skin biopsy reveals thickened epidermis and stratum corneum and dilated upper dermal blood vessels. The number of basal cells undergoing mitosis is increased. These fast-dividing cells move rapidly to the surface of thickened epidermis. This rapid proliferation and migration of epidermal cells result in thick epidermis covered by a thick keratin (silvery scale) over the trunk. Abnormal levels of cyclic nucleotides, especially cyclic AMP and GMP, may be partially responsible for this rapid mitosis of epidermal cells. Prostaglandins and polyamines are also possibly abnormal in the disease. The role of these abnormalities in influencing the formation of a psoriatic plaque is not clearly understood.
4. b
5. b, d
6. b, d
7. c
8. d
9. d
10. a, b

CHAPTER 80

1. b
2. c
3. b
4. b
5. b
6. c
7. b
8. c
9. True
10. True
11. True
12. True
13. False; impetigo is the most common bacterial infection of the skin.
14. True
15. The diagnosis of herpes can be confirmed by a positive herpetic culture in about 80% of patients. Another test is the Tzank test, which is positive in 50% to 80% of patients with herpes. In this test the material from the vesicle is placed on a glass slide and stained with 1% toluidine blue. Large, multinucleated giant cells can be seen in patients with herpes. This test can be performed in a few minutes; it is cheaper than a herpetic culture but less reliable.
16. At present there is no vaccine to prevent herpes infections from recurring. Recurrent episodes of herpes of the lips can sometimes be prevented by

use of opaque sunscreens or avoidance of sun exposure. Oral acyclovir (Zoviraz) at a dose of 400 mg twice daily frequently prevents recurrent eruptions of herpes simplex. Sexual spread of genital herpes is frequently aborted by use of rubber condoms when vesicles are present and for 7 days afterward. Sexual abstinence when vesicles are present is an alternative method of prevention. Towels, underclothing, and swimming suits should not be shared.

17. A primary herpes simplex infection can cause severe conjunctivitis and even blindness.

18. Impetigo first appears as a purulent lesion. As the lesion spreads, it becomes eroded, and a golden crust develops on the surface.

19. Impetigo is caused by streptococci and staphylococci. The infection is transferred by human-to-human contact, usually among children. Heat, humidity, and poor hygiene predispose to this infection. Erysipelas, on the other hand, is a serious toxic infection of the skin. The patient has a high fever and malaise and is toxic.

20. Poor hygiene and excoriations

21. Treatment of localized herpes zoster is symptomatic with soaks and pain medication. If the ophthalmic branch of the trigeminal nerve is affected, an ophthalmologist should also be consulted because corneal perforations may result from the infection. Early administration of systemic corticosteroids may be helpful in the prevention of postherpetic neuralgia. Oral acyclovir at the dose of 800 mg 5 times daily for 7 days can shorten the duration of herpes zoster infection.

CHAPTER 81

1. Characteristic of malignant melanoma is an irregular pigmented lesion with shades of blue, purple, red, and brown. The borders of the tumor are irregular, and the surface is frequently ulcerated. Satellite lesions and diffusion of pigment into the surrounding skin are also observed.

2. Basal cell carcinoma is derived from epidermal cells in the skin. This tumor rarely metastasizes. The most common sites of occurrence are on the sun-exposed areas of the face, head, and neck.

3. The preventive measures for patients with a history of melanoma and for fair-skinned individuals are sunscreens, sun blocks, and avoidance of excess sunlight. Any individual who has dysplastic nevi and a family history of melanoma is at high risk for developing melanoma. He or she should be examined by a physician every 3 to 6 months, should avoid sun exposure, should use sunscreens when outside, and should self-examine the skin every few weeks.

4. Treatment includes curettage with electrodesiccation, scalpel surgery, irradiation, or cyrosurgery.

5. Squamous cell carcinoma is a tumor that arises from keratinocytes in the epidermis. This tumor develops in older, fair-skinned persons. The tumor usually presents as an ulcerated, hyperkeratotic nodule with evidence of dermal invasion on palpation. Squamous cell carcinoma of the skin arising in sun-exposed areas rarely metastasizes. This cancer is treated with scalpel surgery, curettage with electrodesiccation, or irradiation.

6. d
7. All are correct.
8. b
9. b, c
10. c
11. d
12. c
13. a
14. e
15. b
16. d

CHAPTER 82

1. Erythema chronicum migrans (ECM) begins as an erythematous papule where the tick bite occurred. The papule expands with central clearing, measuring up to 25 to 50 mm in diameter. It usually disappears spontaneously without therapy within 2 months. The lesion may itch, sting, or burn. The thighs, groin, and axillae are common sites of involvement. Other symptoms occur weeks to months later in patients who are not treated. These symptoms are characterized by the triad of meningitis, cranial nerve palsies, and peripheral neuropathy. Fewer than 10% of patients experience cardiac manifestations.

2. *Scabies* is caused by the mite *Sacoptes scabiei*. It is transmitted by close contact, especially among children and sexually active adults. Pruritus is the chief complaint. Excoriated linear papules and vesicles are classically found between the fingers, over the elbows, wrists, breasts, and genitalia. Treatment consists of application of gamma benzene hexachloride (Kwell) for two 24-hour periods. Children under 5 years of age are treated for a limited time with 5% permethrin. Secondary irritant eczema can complicate treatment and result in persistence of pruritus. All family members must be treated prophylactically overnight with gamma benzene hexachloride or permethrin, even if they present no evidence of scabietic lesions or pruritus. *Pediculosis pubis* (pubic crabs) is a frequent infection of the pubic hair and skin and is transmitted by human contact. Lice and nits, which attach to the pubic hair, can be seen with the naked eye and cause intense pruritus. Kwell shampoo is the treatment of choice and should be applied twice. Nits may also be removed with a fine-toothed comb soaked in vinegar.

3. a, c, d
4. True
5. True
6. True

Index